Contents

labelled   over leaf →

Overview of CDC Hand Hygiene Guidelines.

The Centers for Disease Control and Prevention recently released new recommendations for hand hygiene in health care settings. Hand hygiene is a term that applies to either handwashing, use of an antiseptic hand rub, or surgical hand antisepsis. Evidence suggests that hand antisepsis, the cleansing of hands with an antiseptic hand rub is more effective in reducing nosocomial infections than plain handwashing.

Follow These Guidelines in the Care of *All Patients*.

- Continue to wash hands with either plain soap or an antimicrobial soap and water (see Skill 8-1, page 192) whenever the hands are visibly soiled.
- Use an alcohol-based hand rub to routinely decontaminate the hands in the following clinical situations (NOTE: if alcohol-based hand rubs are not available, the alternative is handwashing.):
  - Before and after client contact.
  - Before donning sterile gloves when inserting central intravascular catheters.
  - Before performing nonsurgical invasive procedures (e.g., urinary catheter insertion, nasotracheal suctioning).
  - After contact with body fluids or excretions, mucous membranes, nonintact skin, and wound dressings.
  - If moving from a contaminated body site (rectal area or mouth) to a clean body site (surgical wound, urinary meatus) during client care.
  - After contact with inanimate objects (including medical equipment) in the immediate vicinity of the client.
  - After removing gloves.
- Before eating and after using a restroom, wash hands with a nonantimicrobial or an antimicrobial soap and water.
- Antimicrobial-impregnated wipes (i.e., towelettes) are not a substitute for using an alcohol-based hand rub or antimicrobial soap.
- If exposure to *Bacillus anthracis* is suspected or proven, wash hands with a nonantimicrobial or an antimicrobial soap and water. The physical action of washing and rinsing hands is recommended because alcohols, chlorhexidine, iodophors, and other antiseptic agents have poor activity against spores.

Method for decontaminating hands
When using an alcohol-based hand rub, apply product to palm of one hand and rub hands together, covering all surfaces of hands and fingers, until hands are dry. Follow the manufacturer's recommendations regarding the volume of product to use.

Follow These Guidelines for Surgical Hand Antisepsis.

- Surgical hand antisepsis reduces the resident microbial count on the hands to a minimum. See Skill 36-1, page 1218, for the surgical hand scrub procedure.
  - The CDC recommends using an antimicrobial soap, and to scrub hands and forearms for the length of time recommended by the manufacturer, usually 2 to 6 minutes. The Association of Operating Room Nurses recommends 3 to 4 minutes. Refer to agency policy for time required.
  - When using an alcohol-based surgical hand-scrub product with persistent activity, follow the manufacturer's instructions. Before applying the alcohol solution, prewash hands and forearms with a nonantimicrobial soap and dry hands and forearms completely. After application of the alcohol-based product as recommended, allow hands and forearms to dry thoroughly before donning sterile gloves.

General Recommendations for Hand Hygiene.

- Use hand lotions or creams to minimize the occurrence of irritant contact dermatitis associated with hand antisepsis or handwashing.
- Do not wear artificial fingernails or extenders when having direct contact with clients at high risk (e.g., those in intensive-care units or operating rooms).
- Keep natural nails tips less than 1/4-inch long.
- Wear gloves when contact with blood or other potentially infectious materials, mucous membranes, and nonintact skin could occur.
- Remove gloves after caring for a client. Do not wear the same pair of gloves for the care of more than one client.
- Change gloves during client care if moving from a contaminated body site to a clean body site.

(Modified from Centers for Disease Control and Prevention: *Morbidity and Mortality Weekly Report [MMWR],* October 25, 51[RR16]:1-44, 2000. Available at www.cdc.gov/handhygiene.)

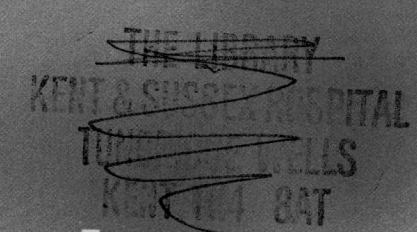
Clinical Nursing Skills & Techniques

Clinical Nursing Skills & Techniques

Anne Griffin Perry, RN, MSN, EdD, FAAN

Professor and Chair
Department of Primary Care and Health Systems Nursing
Southern Illinois University
Edwardsville, Illinois

Patricia A. Potter, RN, PhD, CMAC, FAAN

Nursing Research Scientist
Barnes-Jewish Hospital
St. Louis, Missouri

With over 1100 illustrations

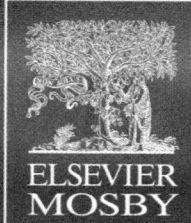
ELSEVIER
MOSBY

6th edition

**ELSEVIER
MOSBY**

11830 Westline Industrial Drive
St. Louis, Missouri 63146

Clinical Nursing Skills & Techniques
Copyright © 2006, Mosby Inc.

ISBN 0-323-02839-X

NOTICE

Nursing is an ever-changing field. Standard safety precautions must be followed, but as new research and clinical experience broaden our knowledge, changes in treatment and drug therapy may become necessary or appropriate. Readers are advised to check the most current product information provided by the manufacturer of each drug to be administered to verify the recommended dose, the method and duration of administration, and contraindications. It is the responsibility of the licensed prescriber, relying on experience and knowledge of the patient, to determine dosages and the best treatment for each individual patient. Neither the publisher nor the authors assume any liability for any injury and/or damage to persons or property arising from this publication.

Previous editions copyrighted 2004, 2002, 1998, 1994, 1990, 1986

NCLEX, NCLEX-RN, and NCLEX-PN are federally registered trademarks and service marks of the National Council of State Boards of Nursing, Inc.

International Standard Book Number 0-323-02839-X

Executive Editor: Susan R. Epstein
Senior Developmental Editor: Jean Sims Fornano
Publishing Services Manager: John Rogers
Senior Project Manager: Beth Hayes
Senior Designer: Kathi Gosche

Printed in the United States of America

Last digit is the print number: 9 8 7 6 5 4 3 2 1

As always this book is dedicated to my children. To be their mother has brought into my life great joy, honor, and a strong sense of humor. They are truly my shinning stars. As children grow, things change, and I now dedicate this text to:

My daughter: Rebecca Lacey Perry Bryan and her husband, Robert Donald Bryan, and my son: Horace Mitchell "Mitch" Perry IV

Anne Perry

To the dedicated professional nursing staff of Barnes-Jewish Hospital. You inspire me daily.

Patricia Potter

Contributors

JEANNETTE ADAMS, PhD, MSN, APRN, CRNI
Nursing Consultant
Coconut Grove, Florida

BARBARA J. BERGER, RN, MSN
Clinical Nurse Specialist for Nursing Practice and Nursing
    Informatics
Southwest General Health Center Partnering with
    University Hospitals Health Systems
Middleburg, Ohio

JANICE C. COLWELL, RN, MS, CWOCN
Clinical Nurse Specialist
University of Chicago Hospitals
Chicago, Illinois

EILEEN CONSTANTINOU, RN, MSN
Professional Practice Consultant
Barnes-Jewish Hospital
St. Louis, Missouri

WANDA CLEVELAND DUBUISSON, RN, PhD(C)
Associate Professor
Joseph and Mary Fail School of Nursing
William Carey College School of Nursing
Hattiesburg, Mississippi

SHARON EDWARDS, RN, MSN, PhD
Assistant Professor
University of South Florida
Tampa, Florida

SUSAN JANE FETZER, RN, BA, BSN, MSN, MBA, PhD
Associate Professor
College of Nursing
University of New Hampshire
Durham, New Hampshire

LEAH W. FREDERICK, RN, MSN, CIC
Consultant
Infection Control Consultants
Scottsdale, Arizona

AMY HALL, RN, BSN, MS, PhD
Associate Professor
Saint Francis Medical Center College of Nursing
Peoria, Illinois

LINDA C. HAYNES, PhD, RN
Associate Professor
University of Northern Colorado
Greeley, Colorado

DIANE HILDWEIN, RN, BC, MA
Director of Clinical Education
St. Luke's Hospital
Chesterfield, Missouri

MAUREEN B. HUHMANN, MS, RD
Clinical Instructor and Clinical Dietician
University of Medicine and Dentistry
Newark, New Jersey

JUDITH ANN KILPATRICK, RN, DNSC
Assistant Professor
Widener University School of Nursing
Chester, Pennsylvania

JILL FELDMAN MALEN, RSN, MS, NS, ANP
Clinical Nurse Specialist
Barnes-Jewish Hospital at Washington University
    Medical Center
St. Louis, Missouri

MARY K. MANTESE, RN, MSN
Director of Patient Care Services/Chief Nurse Executive
Barnes-Jewish West County Hospital
St. Louis, Missouri

NELDA K. MARTIN, RN, MSN, BC, ACC, ANP
Critical Care Clinical Nurse Specialist and Adult Nurse
    Practitioner
Barnes-Jewish Hospital
St. Louis, Missouri

MARY MERCER, RN, MSN
Coordinator
Cardiac Rehabilitation
St. John's Mercy Medical Center
Creve Coeur, Missouri

ELAINE K. NEAL, RN, BSN, MSN
Nursing Instructor
Graham Hospital School of Nursing
Canton, Illinois

MEGAN NOBLE, PhD, RN
Staff Nurse
MICU, Strong Memorial Hospital
University of Rochester Medical Center
Rochester, New York

JANE RUHLAND, MSN, BSN, RNC
Patient Safety and Quality Consultant
Barnes-Jewish Hospital
St. Louis, Missouri

JACKIE RAYBUCK SALEEBY, PhD, RN, BC
Associate Professor
Jewish Hospital College of Nursing and Allied Health
St. Louis, Missouri

KELLY M. SCHWARTZ, RN, BSN
Professional Practice Consultant
Barnes-Jewish Hospital
St. Louis, Missouri

JULIE S. SNYDER, MSN, RN, BC
Adjunct Clinical Faculty
Old Dominion University School of Nursing
Norfolk, Virginia

LAURA SOFIELD, MSN, APRN, BC
Director of Clinical Practice
Meridian Institute for Aging, Senior Health Center
Manchester, New Jersey

PATRICIA A. STOCKERT, RN, BSN, MS, PhD
Saint Francis Medical Center College of Nursing
Peoria, Illinois

NANCY TOMASELLI, RN, MSN, CS, CRNP, CWOCN, CLNC
President and CEO
Premier Health Solutions, LLC
Cherry Hill, New Jersey

RIVA TOUGER-DECKER, PhD, RD, FADA
Associate Professor/Program Director
Graduate Program in Clinical Nutrition
Division of Nutrition, Department of Diagnostic Sciences
New Jersey Dental School
Newark, New Jersey

JOAN DOMIGAN WENTZ, MSN, RN
Assistant Professor
Barnes-Jewish Hospital College of Nursing and Allied
    Health
St. Louis, Missouri

TERRI L. WOOD, RN, PhD
Assistant Professor
Barnes-Jewish Hospital College of Nursing and Allied
    Health
St. Louis, Missouri

RITA WUNDERLICH, BSN, MSN, PhD
Assistant Professor
Saint Louis University School of Nursing
St. Louis, Missouri

RHONDA YANCEY, RN, BSN
Consultant, Professional Practice
Barnes-Jewish Hospital
St. Louis, Missouri

Clinical Consultants

TINA MARRELLI, MSN, MA, RN
Health Care Consultant and Writer
President, Marrelli and Associates, Inc.
Boca Grande, Florida

DULA F. PACQUIO, EdD, RN, CTN
Professor and Director
Transcultural Nursing Institute and MSN Program
Kean University
Union, New Jersey

CYNTHIA VISHY, RN, BSN
Manager, Clinical Education
St. Louis Children's Hospital
St. Louis, Missouri

Reviewers

MARIANNE ADAM, MSN, CRNP
Assistant Professor of Nursing
Moravian College
Bethlehem, Pennsylvania

JEANNETTE ADAMS, PhD, RN, APRN, CRNI
Nursing Consultant
Coconut Grove, Florida

MARIE H. AHRENS, RN, MS
Clinical Instructor
University of Tulsa School of Nursing
Tulsa, Oklahoma

SUSAN J. APPEL, PhD, ACNP, FNP, BC
Assistant Professor
School of Nursing
University of Alabama
Birmingham, Alabama

SHARON A. ARONOVITCH, PhD, APRN, BC, CWOCN
Assistant Professor of Nursing
Florida State University
Tallahassee, Florida

SYLVIA K. BAIRD, BSN, MN
Manager, Patient Safety
Spectrum Health
Grand Rapids, Michigan

DORIS BARTLETT, RN, MS
Assistant Professor
Bethel College
Mishawaka, Indiana

JULIE BAYLOR, RN, PhD, MSN
Assistant Professor
Bradley University
Peoria, Illinois

MARGARET W. BELLAK, RN, MN
Associate Professor
Indiana University of Pennsylvania
Indiana, Pennsylvania

JANICE BOUNDY, PhD, RN
Professor, Director of Graduate Program
Saint Francis College of Nursing
Peoria, Illinois

THERESE M. BOWER, EdD, MSN, CNS, RN
Nursing Educator
Firelands Regional Medical Center School of Nursing
Sandusky, Ohio

SUSAN BURCHIEL, RN, MSN, C
Instructor of Nursing
Cuesta College
San Luis Obispo, California

JAQUELINE ROSENJACK BURCHUM, DNSc, APRN, BC
Assistant Professor
The University of Memphis, Loewenberg School of Nursing
Memphis, Tennessee

SUSAN BURKETT, RN, MSN, CPNP, CPN
Chief Administrative Officer
TC Thompson Children's Hospital
Chattanooga, Tennessee

JEANIE BURT, RN, MA, MSN
Assistant Professor
School of Nursing
Harding University
Searcy, Arkansas

DARLENE NEBEL CANTU, MSN, RNC
Director
Baptist Health System
School of Professional Nursing
San Antonio, Texas
Faculty
San Antonio College
San Antonio, Texas

KATHLYN CARLSON, BSN, MA, CPAN
Staff Nurse
Abbott Northwestern Hospital
Minneapolis, Minnesota

BARBARA M. CARRANTI, MS, RN, CNS
Instructor
Syracuse University School of Nursing
Syracuse, New York

BARBARA CATON, RN, BSN, MSN
Assistant Professor
Southwest Missouri State University–West Plains
West Plains, Missouri

D. SUE CLARREN, RNC, ND
Assistant Professor
University of Nevada, Las Vegas
Las Vegas, Nevada

LAURA CLAYTON, MSN, FNP, RN
Assistant Professor of Nursing Education
Shepherd University
Shepherdstown, West Virginia

PATRICIA CONLEY, RN, BSN, MSN
Med Specialty Nurse
Veterans Administration Medical Center
Kansas City, Missouri

JANET COURTNEY, RN, MSN
Chair, Department of Nursing
Holyoke Community College
Holyoke, Massachusetts

MARCIE L. DAVIS, RN, BC, BSN
Nursing Instructor
Ulster County BOCES Career and Technology Center
New Paltz, New York

KAREN DELRUE, RN, MSN, CEN
Clinical Nurse Specialist–Emergency Services
Spectrum Health
Grand Rapids, Michigan

GAY OYCO DIVINAGARCIA, RNC, MA
Associate Professor
Nursing Department
Indian River Community College
Fort Pierce, Florida

SUSAN ERUE, BSN, MS
Instructor
Wesleyan College
Mount Pleasant, Iowa

MARGARET B. EWING, RN, SNP, MEd
School Health, School Nurse Coordinator
Maple Newton
Newtown, Pennsylvania

SUSAN JANE FETZER, PhD, BSN, BS, MSN, MBA
Associate Professor
University of New Hampshire
Durham, New Hampshire

MARGARET S. FREEL, RN, MSN, CNRN, APN/CS
Clinical Instructor and Clinical Simulation Lab Coordinator
Neihoff School of Nursing
Loyola University Chicago
Chicago, Illinois

YVETTE GLENN, MSN, FNP, APRN, BC
Wound Care Specialist
VA Illiana Healthcare System
Danville, Illinois

LOIS C. HAMEL, PhD, RN, MSN
Adult Nurse Practitioner/Adjunct Assistant Professor
University of New England/University of Vermont Medical School
Portland, Maine

ADRIENNE HENTEMANN, RN, BSN, MS
Administrative Associate
Spectrum Health
Grand Rapids, Michigan

MONICA M. HENTEMANN, RN, BSN
Registered Nurse
Spectrum Health Downtown
Grand Rapids, Michigan

BETH HOGAN-QUIGLEY, RN, BSN, MSN, CRNP
Clinical Lecturer
University of Pennsylvania School of Nursing
Philadelphia, Pennsylvania

SARAH M. HOWELL, RN, MSN
Assistant Professor of Nursing
Mississippi University for Women
Columbus, Mississippi

MINTIE INDAR-MARAJ, RN, BC, EdD
Adjunct Professor
New York University School of Nursing
New York, New York

HELEN JACKSON-RUIZ, RN, MSN
Instructor
Nebraska Methodist College
Omaha, Nebraska

SUSAN JUNAID, MSN, ARNP, WHNP
Assistant Professor
Allen College
Waterloo, Iowa

MARY DORSEY KELLERMANN, RN, MS, CRNP
Adult Nurse Practioner/Gerontological Nurse Practioner
President, Educational Entities
Associate Professor
Coppin State University
Baltimore, Maryland

LINDA L. KERBY, RNC, BSN, MA, BA
Educational Consultant
Leawood, Kansas

KATHLEEN M. LAMAUTE, EdD, FNP
Assistant Professor and Coordinator FNP Program
Molloy College
Rockville Centre, New York

RONNETTE C. LANGHORNE, RN, MS
Nursing Instructor
Norfolk State University
Norfolk, Virginia

SHEILA LAWTON, MSN, ARNP, CCRN
Nursing Instructor
College of Saint Mary
Omaha, Nebraska

VIRGINIA D. LESTER, RN, BSN, MSN, CS
Assistant Professor of Nursing
Angelo State University
San Angelo, Texas

BERNADETTE M. LOMBARDI, RN, MSN, MS, MA
Assistant Director of Nursing
Memorial and Samaritan Schools of Nursing
Albany, New York

ROSEMARY MACY, RN, MSN
Assistant Professor
Boise State University
Boise, Idaho

JOAN SIMS MARSH, RN, MSN
Assistant Professor/Chair, Division of Nursing Education
University of Virgin Islands, St. Croix Campus
St. Croix, U.S. Virgin Islands

MARY JO MATTOCKS, PhD, RN, MN
Chief Nursing Officer
Mesa View Regional Hospital
Mequite, Nevada

MARY ANNE S. MCLAUGHLIN, MSN, RN
Manager, Disease Management
Penn Home Care & Hospice Services
University of Pennsylvania Health System
Bala Cynwyd, Pennsylvania

CLAUDIA LOUTH MITCHELL, RN, BS, MS
Professor of Nursing
Santa Barbara City College
Santa Barbara, California

TERI A. MURRAY, PhD, MSN, MEd, BSN, RN
Director, Undergraduate Nursing Program
Barnes College of Nursing
University of Missouri–St. Louis
St. Louis, Missouri

RUTH NOVITT-SCHUMACHER, BSN, MSN
Clinical Instructor
School of Nursing
University of Illinois
Chicago, Illinois

BONNIE OZAROW, RN, BSN, MSA
Manager, Corporate Safety and Regulations
Spectrum Health
Grand Rapids, Michigan

ROBIN E. PATTILLO, PhD, MSN, MEd, RN
Associate Professor
School of Nursing
Auburn University
Auburn, Alabama

ROXANNE PERUCCA, MS, CRNI
Nurse Manager/Clinical Nurse Specialist
University of Kansas Hospital
Kansas City, Kansas

ELAINE PRINCEVALLI, RN, BSN, MSN
Instructor, Practical Nurse Education Program
State of Connecticut Department of Education
Hamden, Connecticut

Contributors to Previous Editions

We would like to acknowledge the following people who participated in the fifth edition.

MAUREEN CARTY, MSN, OCN
Oncology Clinical Nurse Specialist
Genesis Medical Center
Davenport, Iowa

MARY F. CLARKE, MA, RN
Informatics Nurse Specialist
Genesis Medical Center
Davenport, Iowa

EILEEN COSTANTINOU, RN, BSN, MSN
Professional Practice Consultant
Barnes-Jewish Hospital
St. Louis, Missouri

WANDA CLEVELAND DUBUISSON, BSN, MN
Assistant Professor
University of Southern Mississippi, College of Nursing
Hattiesburg, Mississippi

MARTHA E. ELKIN, RN, MSN
Lactation Counselor
Stephens Memorial Hospital
Norway, Maine

AMY HALL, PhD, MS, BSN, RN
Assistant Professor
Saint Francis Medical Center, College of Nursing
Peoria, Illinois

MARILEE KUHRIK, RN, MSN, PhD
Associate Professor
Colorado Mountain College
Glenwood Springs, Colorado

NANCY S. KUHRIK, RN, MSN, PhD
Associate Professor
Colorado Mountain College
Glenwood Springs, Colorado

RUTH LUDWICK, PhD, MSN, BSN, RNC, CNS
Associate Professor
Kent State University
Kent, Ohio

RITA MERTIG, MS, BSN, RNC, CNS
Professor
John Tyler Community College
Richmond, Virginia

JANE RUHLAND, RN, MSN, BSN
Education Coordinator
Barnes-Jewish St. Peters Hospital
St. Peters, Missouri

JACQUELINE RAYBUCK SALEEBY, PhD, RN, CS
Associate Professor
Jewish Hospital College of Nursing and Allied Health
St. Louis, Missouri

JULIE SNYDER, MSN, RNC
Faculty
Louise Obici School of Nursing
Suffolk, Virginia

ANNE FALSONE VAUGHAN, MSN, BSN, CCRN
Clinical Instructor
Bellarmine College, Lansing School of Nursing
Louisville, Kentucky

RITA WUNDERLICH, PhD (CAND), MSN(R), CCRN
Doctoral Candidate, Saint Louis University
Instructor
Clinical Nurse
Saint Louis University Hospital
St. Louis, Missouri

Clinical Consultants to the fifth edition

ELIZABETH A. AYELLO, PhD, MS, BSN, RN, CS, CWOCN
Clinical Assistant Professor
New York University, Division of Nursing
New York, New York

MARGARET BENZ, RN, MSN, CSANP
Adjunct Assistant Professor
Saint Louis University
St. Louis, Missouri

GALE CARLI, MSN, MHED, BSN, RN
Assistant Professor
Ohlone College
Fremont, California

ELLEN CARSON, PhD, CLINICAL SPECIALIST
Associate Professor
Pittsburg State University
Pittsburg, Kansas

PATRICIA A. DETTENMEIER, MSN(R), BSN, CS, ANP
Adult Nurse Practitioner
Saint Louis University Health Sciences Center
St. Louis, Missouri

MARTHA E. ELKIN, MSN
Lactation Counselor
Stephens Memorial Hospital
Norway, Maine

SUSAN JANE FETZER, PhD, MBA, MSN, BSN, BA
Assistant Professor, Coordinator RN to BSN
University of New Hampshire
Durham, New Hampshire

LEAH FREDERICK, MS, RN, CIC
Infection Control Consultant
Infection Control Consultants
Scottsdale, Arizona

THELMA HALBERSTADT, EdD, MS, BS, RN
Professor
Northern Essex Community College
Lawrence, Massachusetts

AMY HALL, PhD, MS, BSN, RN
Assistant Professor
Saint Francis Medical Center College of Nursing
Peoria, Illinois

RUTH LUDWICK, PhD, MSN, BSN, RNC, CNS
Associate Professor
Kent State University
Kent, Ohio

MARY KAY MACHECA, MSN(R), RN, CS, ANP, CDE
Certified Adult Nurse Practitioner and Certified Diabetes
    Educator
The Bortz Diabetes Control Center
Richmond Heights, Missouri

MARY K. MANTESE, MSN, RN
Regulatory Compliance Manager
Barnes-Jewish West County Hospital
St. Louis, Missouri

NORMA METHENY, PhD, MSN, BSN, FAAN
Professor and Dorothy A. Votsmier Chair in Nursing
Saint Louis University School of Nursing
St. Louis, Missouri

SHARON M. J. MUHS, MSN, RN
Registered Nurse
Saint Luke's Hospital
Chesterfield, Missouri

ELAINE K. NEEL, MSN, BSN
Nursing Instructor
Methodist Medical Center School of Nursing
Peoria, Illinois

CATHERINE A. ROBINSON, BA, RN
Clinical Nurse Manager
Barnes-Jewish Hospital

SHARON SOUTER, MSN, BSN
Director of Nursing Program
New Mexico State University at Carlsbad
Carlsbad, New Mexico

PATRICIA A. STOCKERT, RN, BSN, MS, PhD
Associate Professor
Saint Francis Medical Center College of Nursing
Peoria, Illinois

PAMELA BECKER WEILITZ, MSN(R), RN, CS, ANP
Adult Nurse Practitioner
South City Health, LLC
St. Louis, Missouri

We would like to acknowledge the following people, who participated in editions three and four.

DELLA ARIDGE, RN, MSN
Clinical Nurse Specialist
Abdominal Organ Transplant Service
Saint Louis University Health Sciences Center
St. Louis, Missouri

ELIZABETH A. AYELLO, PhD, MS, BSN, RN, CS, CWOCN
Clinical Assistant Professor
New York University, Division of Nursing
New York, New York

LYNDAL GUENTHER BRAND, RN, BSN, MSN
Instructor, Missouri Baptist Medical Center
School of Nursing
St. Louis, Missouri

PEGGY BRECKINRIDGE, RN, BSN, MSN, FNP
Associate Professor of Nursing
College of Health Sciences
Roanoke, Virginia

VICTORIA M. BROWN, RN, BSN, MSN, PhD
Associate Professor, School of Nursing
Georgia College & State University
Milledgeville, Georgia

GINA BUFE, RN, BSN, MSN(R), PhD, CS
Psychiatric Clinical Nurse Specialist
Private Practice
Hyannis, Massachusetts

DOROTHY McDONNELL COOKE, RN, PhD
Associate Professor of Nursing
Saint Louis University Health Sciences Center
St. Louis, Missouri

SHEILA A. CUNNINGHAM, RN, BSN, MSN
Assistant Professor of Nursing
Neumann College
Aston, Pennsylvania

RICK DANIELS, RN, BSN, MSN, PhD
Associate Professor of Nursing
Oregon Health Sciences University at Southern
Ashland, Oregon

MARDELL DAVIS, RN, MSN, CETN
School of Nursing
University of Alabama
Birmingham, Alabama

CAROLYN RUPPEL D'AVIS, RN, BSN, MSN
Director, Baccalaureate Program/Adjunct Assistant
Professor
The Catholic University of America
Washington, D.C.

PATRICIA A. DETTENMEIER, RN, BSN, MSN(R), CCRN
Assistant Clinical Professor, School of Nursing
Instructor in Medicine, School of Medicine
Saint Louis University
St. Louis, Missouri

DEBORAH OLDENBURG ERICKSON, RN, BSN, MSN
Instructor, School of Nursing
Methodist Medical Center of Illinois
Peoria, Illinois

DEBRA FARRELL, BSN, CNOR
Operating Room Staff Nurse
Saint Anthony's Medical Center
St. Louis, Missouri

LINDA FASCIANI, RN, BSN, MSN
Assistant Professor of Nursing
County College of Morris
Randolph, New Jersey

SUSAN JANE FETZER, PhD, MBA, MSN, BSN, BA
Assistant Professor, Coordinator RN to BSN
University of New Hampshire
Durham, New Hampshire

MARLENE S. FOREMAN, BSN, MN, RNCS
Associate Professor of Nursing
Louisiana State University at Eunice
Eunice, Louisiana

CAROL P. FRAY, RN, MA
Associate Professor, Adult Health Nursing
College of Nursing
University of North Carolina at Charlotte
Charlotte, North Carolina

PAULA GOLDBERG, RN, MS, MSN
Oncology Clinical Coordinator
Barnes Hospital
St. Louis, Missouri

NANCY C. JACKSON, RN, BSN, MSN, CCRN
Pulmonary Clinical Nurse Specialist
St. Mary's Health Center
St. Louis, Missouri

RUTH L. JILKA, RD, CDE
Diabetes Educator
Barnes Hospital
St. Louis, Missouri

TERESA M. JOHNSON, RN, MSN, CCRN
Clinical Nurse Specialist
The Medical Center of Central Georgia
Macon, Georgia

CARL KIRTON, RN, BSN, MA, CCRN, ACRN, ANP
Clinical Assistant, Professor of Nursing
New York University
New York, New York

DIANE M. KYLE, RN, BSN, MS
Doctoral Candidate,
Supervisor of Clinical Services/Clinical Nurse Specialist
East Hartford Visiting Nurse Association, Inc.
East Hartford, Connecticut

LOUISE K. LEITAO, RN(C), BSN, MA
Director of Clinical Services
East Hartford Visiting Nurses Association, Inc.
East Hartford, Connecticut

GAIL B. LEWIS, RN, MSN
Associate Professor
Barnes College
St. Louis, Missouri

MARY KAY MACHECA, MSN(R), RN, CS, ANP, CDE
Certified Adult Nurse Practitioner and Certified Diabetes
    Educator
The Bortz Diabetes Control Center
Richmond Heights, Missouri

JILL MALEN, RN, BSN, MS
Pulmonary Clinical Nurse Specialist
Barnes-Jewish Hospital at Washington University Medical
    Center
St. Louis, Missouri

ELIZABETH MANTYCH, RN, MSN
University of Missouri at St. Louis School of Nursing
St. Louis, Missouri

MARY MERCER, RN, MSN
Coordinator, Cardiac Rehabilitation
St. John's Mercy Medical Center
Creve Coeur, Missouri

MARY DEE MILLER, RN, BSN, MS, CIC
Nurse Epidemiologist
Mercy Hamilton/Fairfield Hospitals
Hamilton, Ohio

KATHLEEN MULRYAN, RN, BSN, MSN
Professor of Nursing
LaGuardia Community College
Long Island City, New York

ELAINE K. NEEL, RN, BSN, MSN
Instructor, School of Nursing
Methodist Medical Center of Illinois
Peoria, Illinois

MARSHA EVANS ORR, RN, BS, MS, CS
Zone Clinical Manager
Apria Healthcare
Phoenix, Arizona

SHARON PHELPS, RN, BSN, MS
Nursing Practice Consultant
Barnes-Jewish Hospital
St. Louis, Missouri

JUDITH ROOS, RN, MSN
Associate Professor
Jewish Hospital College of Nursing and Allied Health
St. Louis, Missouri

JAN RUMFELT, RNC, MSN, EdD
Associate Professor, School of Nursing
Southern Illinois University at Edwardsville
Edwardsville, Illinois

LINETTE M. SARTI, RN, BSN, CNOR
OR Charge Nurse
Bayfront Medical Center
St. Petersburg, Florida

APRIL SIEH, RN, BSN, MSN
Assistant Professor
Delta College
University Center, Michigan

MARLENE SMITH, RN, BSN, MEd
Staff Development Specialist
St. Louis Regional Medical Center
St. Louis, Missouri

SHARON SOUTER, RN, BSN, MSN
Director of Nursing Program
New Mexico State University at Carlsbad
Carlsbad, New Mexico

MARTHA A. SPIES, RN, MSN
Assistant Professor
Deaconess College of Nursing
St. Louis, Missouri

SANDRA ANN SZEKELY, RN, BSN
Director, Clinical & Infusion Services
Comfort Care of Michigan
Troy, Michigan

PAMELA BECKER WEILITZ, MSN(R), RN, CS, ANP
Adult Nurse Practitioner
South City Health, LLC
St. Louis, Missouri

LAUREL WIERSEMA, RN, MSN
Surgical Clinical Nurse Specialist
Barnes Hospital
St. Louis, Missouri

Preface to the Student

Skill List highlights the skills you will focus on in each chapter.

Media Resources details the electronic resources available for each chapter.

Learning Objectives highlight key information to follow.

Key Terms are listed at the beginning of each chapter to call attention to critical terminology.

Evidence-Based Practice Trends provide an overview of recent research findings and their implications for quality nursing practice.

Cultural Considerations provide guidance for care of culturally diverse clients.

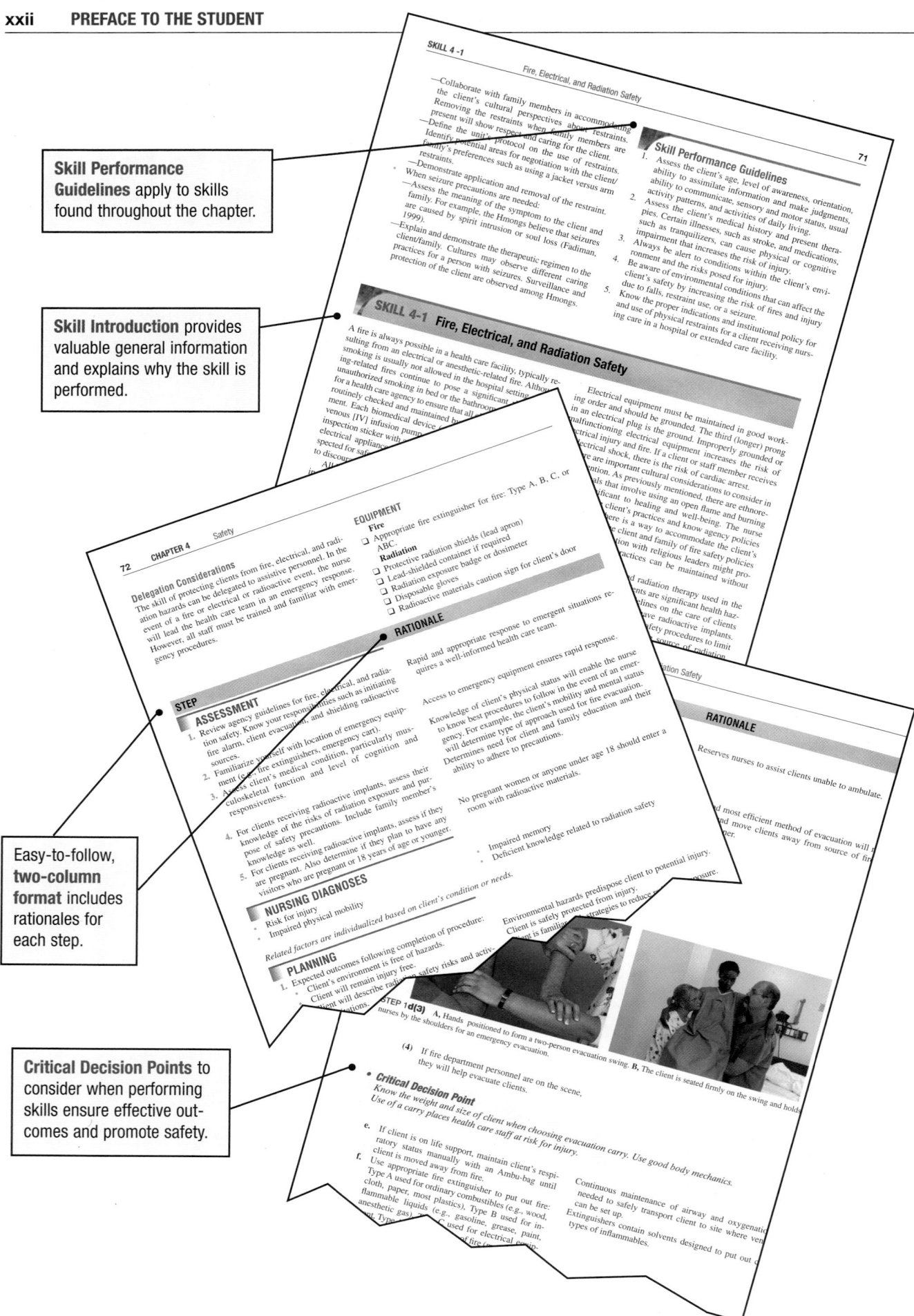

Skill Performance Guidelines apply to skills found throughout the chapter.

Skill Introduction provides valuable general information and explains why the skill is performed.

Easy-to-follow, **two-column format** includes rationales for each step.

Critical Decision Points to consider when performing skills ensure effective outcomes and promote safety.

SKILL 4-1

Fire, Electrical, and Radiation Safety

Skill Performance Guidelines   71

1. Assess the client's age, level of awareness, orientation, ability to assimilate information and make judgments, ability to communicate, sensory and motor status, usual activity patterns, and activities of daily living.
2. Assess the client's medical history and present therapies. Certain illnesses, such as stroke, and medications, such as tranquilizers, can cause physical or cognitive impairment that increases the risk of injury.
3. Always be alert to conditions within the client's environment and the risks posed for injury.
4. Be aware of environmental conditions that can affect the client's safety by increasing the risk of fires and injury due to falls, restraint use, or a seizure.
5. Know the proper indications and institutional policy for and use of physical restraints for a client receiving nursing care in a hospital or extended care facility.

—Collaborate with family members in accommodating the client's cultural perspectives about restraints. Removing the restraints when family members are present will show respect and caring for the client.
—Define the unit's protocol on the use of restraints. Identify potential areas for negotiation with the client/family's preferences such as using a jacket versus arm restraints.
—Demonstrate application and removal of the restraint.
—Assess the meaning of the symptom to the client and family. For example, the Hmongs believe that seizures are caused by spirit intrusion or soul loss (Fadiman, 1999).
—Explain and demonstrate the therapeutic regimen to the client/family. Cultures may observe different caring practices for a person with seizures. Surveillance and protection of the client are observed among Hmongs.

When seizure precautions are needed:

SKILL 4-1 Fire, Electrical, and Radiation Safety

A fire is always possible in a health care facility, typically resulting from an electrical or anesthetic-related fire. Although smoking is usually not allowed in the hospital setting, unauthorized smoking in bed or the bathroom... smoking-related fires continue to pose a significant... for a health care agency to ensure that all... routinely checked and maintained by... venous [IV] infusion pump... ment. Each biomedical device... inspection sticker with... electrical appliance... spected for saf... to discour...

Electrical equipment must be maintained in good working order and should be grounded. The third (longer) prong in an electrical plug is the ground. Improperly grounded or malfunctioning electrical equipment increases the risk of electrical injury and fire. If a client or staff member receives electrical shock, there is the risk of cardiac arrest.

As previously mentioned, there are important cultural considerations to consider in... als that involve using an open flame and burning... ificant to healing and well-being. The nurse... client's practices and know agency policies... re is a way to accommodate the client's... e client and family of fire safety policies... tion with religious leaders might pro... ractices can be maintained without...

d radiation therapy used in the... nts are significant health haz... lines on the care of clients... ave radioactive implants... afety procedures to limit... source of radiation

ation Safety

RATIONALE

Reserves nurses to assist clients unable to ambulate.

...d most efficient method of evacuation will... and move clients away from source of fir... er.

72   CHAPTER 4   Safety

Delegation Considerations

The skill of protecting clients from fire, electrical, and radiation hazards can be delegated to assistive personnel. In the event of a fire or electrical or radioactive event, the nurse will lead the health care team and familiar with emergency response. However, all staff must be trained and familiar with emergency procedures.

EQUIPMENT

Fire
☐ Appropriate fire extinguisher for fire: Type A, B, C, or ABC.
Radiation
☐ Protective radiation shields (lead apron) if required
☐ Lead-shielded container if required
☐ Radiation exposure badge or dosimeter
☐ Disposable gloves
☐ Radioactive materials caution sign for client's door

RATIONALE

STEP	RATIONALE
ASSESSMENT	
1. Review agency guidelines for fire, electrical, and radiation safety. Know your responsibilities such as initiating fire alarm, client evacuation, and shielding radioactive sources.	Rapid and appropriate response to emergent situations requires a well-informed health care team.
2. Familiarize yourself with location of emergency equipment (e.g., fire extinguishers, emergency cart).	Access to emergency equipment ensures rapid response.
3. Assess client's medical condition, particularly and musculoskeletal function and level of cognition and responsiveness.	Knowledge of client's physical status will enable the nurse to know best procedures to follow in the event of an emergency. For example, the client's mobility and mental status will determine type of approach used for fire evacuation.
4. For clients receiving radioactive implants, assess their knowledge of the risks of radiation exposure and purpose of safety precautions. Include family member's knowledge as well.	Determines need for client and family education and their ability to adhere to precautions.
5. For clients receiving radioactive implants, assess if they are pregnant. Also determine if they plan to have any visitors who are pregnant or 18 years of age or younger.	No pregnant women or anyone under age 18 should enter a room with radioactive materials.

NURSING DIAGNOSES
• Risk for injury
• Impaired physical mobility
• Impaired memory
• Deficient knowledge related to radiation safety

Related factors are individualized based on client's condition or needs.

PLANNING
1. Expected outcomes following completion of procedure:
   • Client's environment is free of hazards.
   • Client will remain injury free.
   • Client will describe radi... safety risks and activ...
   ...ions.

Environmental hazards predispose client to potential injury.
Client is safely protected from injury... strategies to reduce...
...nt is famili...

STEP 1d(3) A, Hands positioned to form a two-person evacuation swing. B, The client is seated firmly on the swing and holds nurses by the shoulders for an emergency evacuation.

(4) If fire department personnel are on the scene, they will help evacuate clients.

• **Critical Decision Point**
Know the weight and size of client when choosing evacuation carry. Use good body mechanics.
Use of a carry places health care staff at risk for injury.

e. If client is on life support, maintain client's respiratory status manually with an Ambu-bag until client is moved away from fire.
f. Use appropriate fire extinguisher to put out fire: Type A used for ordinary combustibles (e.g., wood, cloth, paper, most plastics), Type B used for inflammable liquids (e.g., gasoline, grease, paint, anesthetic gas)... Type C used for electrical equip...

Continuous maintenance of airway and oxygenation needed to safely transport client to site where ven... can be set up.
Extinguishers contain solvents designed to put out... types of inflammables.

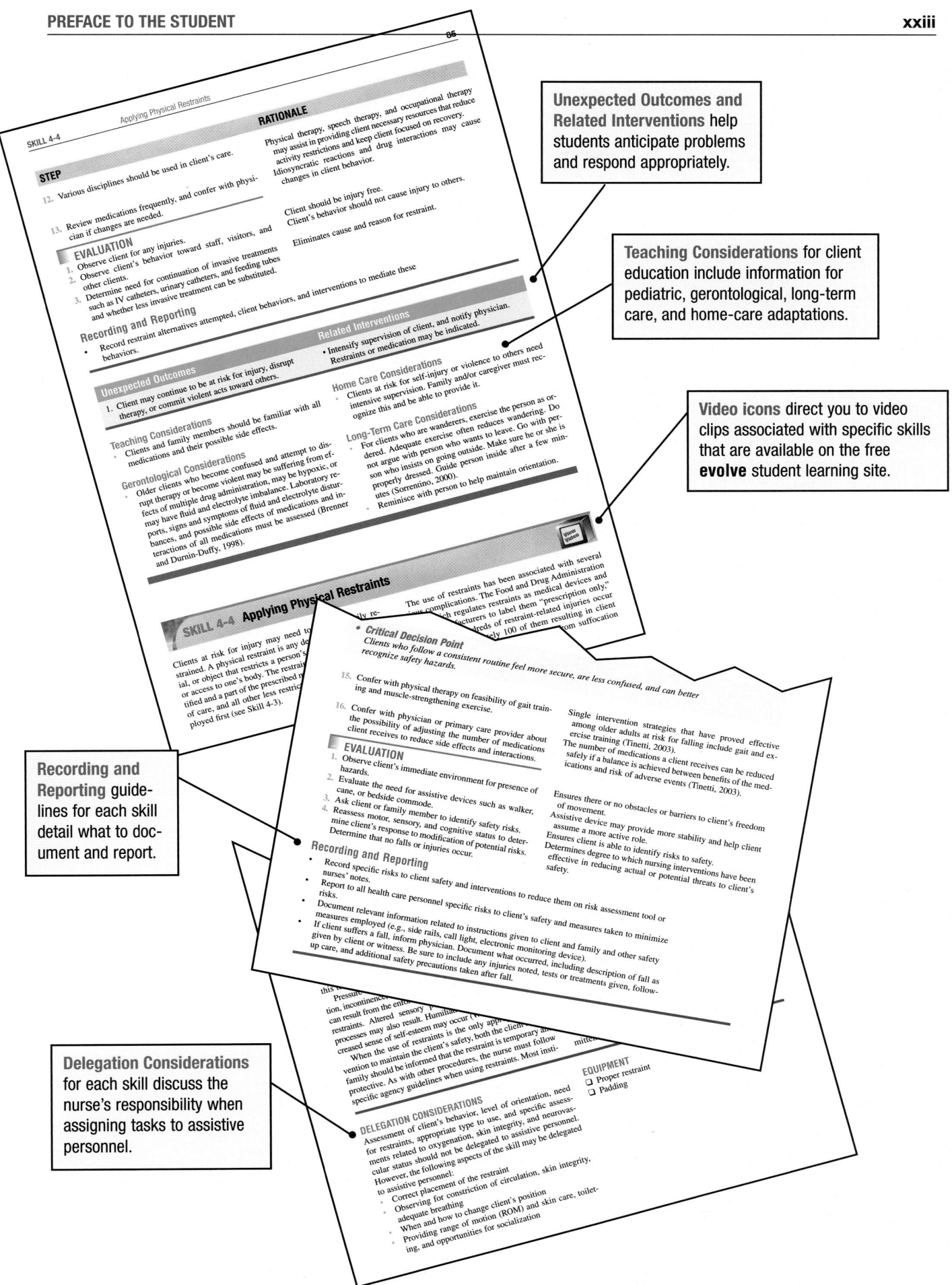

SKILL 4-4

Applying Physical Restraints

RATIONALE

STEP

12. Various disciplines should be used in client's care.

Physical therapy, speech therapy, and occupational therapy may assist in providing client necessary resources that reduce activity restrictions and keep client focused on recovery. Idiosyncratic reactions and drug interactions may cause changes in client behavior.

13. Review medications frequently, and confer with physician if changes are needed.

EVALUATION

1. Observe client for any injuries.
2. Observe client's behavior toward staff, visitors, and other clients.
3. Determine need for continuation of invasive treatments such as IV catheters, urinary catheters, and feeding tubes and whether less invasive treatment can be substituted.

Client should be injury free.

Client's behavior should not cause injury to others.

Eliminates cause and reason for restraint.

Recording and Reporting

• Record restraint alternatives attempted, client behaviors, and interventions to mediate these behaviors.

Unexpected Outcomes

1. Client may continue to be at risk for injury, disrupt therapy, or commit violent acts toward others.

Related Interventions

• Intensify supervision of client, and notify physician. Restraints or medication may be indicated.

Home Care Considerations

Clients at risk for self-injury or violence to others need intensive supervision. Family and/or caregiver must recognize this and be able to provide it.

Teaching Considerations

• Clients and family members should be familiar with all medications and their possible side effects.

Gerontological Considerations

• Older clients who become confused and attempt to disrupt therapy or become violent may be suffering from effects of multiple drug administration, may be hypoxic, or may have fluid and electrolyte imbalance. Laboratory reports, signs and symptoms of fluid and electrolyte disturbances, and possible side effects of medications and interactions of all medications must be assessed (Brenner and Durnin-Duffy, 1998).

Long-Term Care Considerations

• For clients who are wanderers, exercise the person as ordered. Adequate exercise often reduces wandering. Do not argue with person who wants to leave. Go with person who insists on going outside. Make sure he or she is properly dressed. Guide person inside after a few minutes (Sorrentino, 2000).
• Reminisce with person to help maintain orientation.

SKILL 4-4 Applying Physical Restraints

Clients at risk for injury may need to [be re]strained. A physical restraint is any de[vice, materi]al, or object that restricts a person's [movement] or access to one's body. The restraint [must be jus]tified and a part of the prescribed [course] of care, and all other less restric[tive means em]ployed first (see Skill 4-3).

The use of restraints has been associated with several [serio]us complications. The Food and Drug Administration [whi]ch regulates restraints as medical devices and [manuf]acturers to label them "prescription only," [hun]dreds of restraint-related injuries occur in client [approximat]ely 100 of them resulting in client [death from] suffocation

Critical Decision Point

Clients who follow a consistent routine feel more secure, are less confused, and can better recognize safety hazards.

15. Confer with physical therapy on feasibility of gait training and muscle-strengthening exercise.

Single intervention strategies that have proved effective among older adults at risk for falling include gait and exercise training (Tinetti, 2003).

16. Confer with physician or primary care provider about the possibility of adjusting the number of medications client receives to reduce side effects and interactions.

The number of medications a client receives can be reduced safely if a balance is achieved between benefits of the medications and risk of adverse events (Tinetti, 2003).

EVALUATION

1. Observe client's immediate environment for presence of hazards.
2. Evaluate the need for assistive devices such as walker, cane, or bedside commode.
3. Ask client or family member to identify safety risks.
4. Reassess motor, sensory, and cognitive status to determine client's response to modification of potential risks. Determine that no falls or injuries occur.

Ensures there or no obstacles or barriers to client's freedom of movement.

Assistive device may provide more stability and help client assume a more active role.

Ensures client is able to identify risks to safety.

Determines degree to which nursing interventions have been effective in reducing actual or potential threats to client's safety.

Recording and Reporting

• Record specific risks to client safety and interventions to reduce them on risk assessment tool or nurses' notes.
• Report to all health care personnel specific risks to client's safety and measures taken to minimize risks.
• Document relevant information related to instructions given to client and family and other safety measures employed (e.g., side rails, call light, electronic monitoring device).
• If client suffers a fall, inform physician. Document what occurred, including description of fall as given by client or witness. Be sure to include any injuries noted, tests or treatments given, follow-up care, and additional safety precautions taken after fall.

this c...

Pressure...
tion, incontinence...
can result from the enfo...
restraints. Altered sensory...
processes may also result. Humilia...
creased sense of self-esteem may occur (...

When the use of restraints is the only app...
vention to maintain the client's safety, both the clie...
family should be informed that the restraint is temporary an...
protective. As with other procedures, the nurse must follow ...
specific agency guidelines when using restraints. Most insti...

mitted ...

EQUIPMENT

❑ Proper restraint
❑ Padding

DELEGATION CONSIDERATIONS

Assessment of client's behavior, level of orientation, need for restraints, appropriate type to use, and specific assessments related to oxygenation, skin integrity, and neurovascular status should not be delegated to assistive personnel. However, the following aspects of the skill may be delegated to assistive personnel:

• Correct placement of the restraint
• Observing for constriction of circulation, skin integrity, adequate breathing
• When and how to change client's position
• Providing range of motion (ROM) and skin care, toileting, and opportunities for socialization

---

Unexpected Outcomes and Related Interventions help students anticipate problems and respond appropriately.

Teaching Considerations for client education include information for pediatric, gerontological, long-term care, and home-care adaptations.

Video icons direct you to video clips associated with specific skills that are available on the free **evolve** student learning site.

Recording and Reporting guidelines for each skill detail what to document and report.

Delegation Considerations for each skill discuss the nurse's responsibility when assigning tasks to assistive personnel.

Focus on Clinical Practice at the end of each chapter includes case scenarios with critical thinking questions.

NCLEX® Review Questions assess your mastery of the chapter material and help you prepare for the exam.

References direct you to the background material on which procedures and practices are based.

FOCUS on CLINICAL PRACTICE

Mrs. Gladys Dean has been admitted to the general medicine unit for workup for malignant melanoma. She is 73 years old and is currently taking Synthroid, Lasix, Catapres, low-dose aspirin, and Colace. She has the early stages of Parkinson's disease and has a characteristic mild propulsive gait. Mrs. Dean is alert and asks the nurses numerous questions about planned tests for her condition. She wears a hearing aid in her right ear.

1. List three physiological alterations that increase Mrs. Dean's risk of falling.
2. Among the medications Mrs. Dean receives, which may predispose to conditions for falling?

3. When the nurse assesses Mrs. Dean's fall risk, the "Get up and Go" test is designed to measure:
   A. Client's perceived energy level
   B. Client' ability to remain oriented
   C. Client's balance when rising from a chair
   D. Client's knowledge of environmental barriers
4. Mrs. Dean's daughter comes to visit her mother and immediately raises all four side rails. What would be your reaction to this?
5. Explain why Mrs. Dean might benefit from a physical therapy referral to minimize her risk for falling.

NCLEX REVIEW QUESTIONS

1. Which of the following statements is true about fall prevention?
   1. Falls are most successfully prevented by making the client's environment safe.
   2. The early use of restraints in a restless client will effectively reduce falls.
   3. A bed alarm when used alone will prevent falls.
   4. Falls are most often prevented by linking client characteristics to prevention strategies.
2. In the event you discover a fire, do all of the following to secure the fire except:
   1. Place wet towels along base of doors
   2. Have client place blanket over fire
   3. Close all windows and doors
   4. Turn off oxygen sources

3. Mr. Joseph weighs 200 pounds and has a cast that extends from his hip down to his ankle. A fire begins in Mr. Joseph's bathroom. The best method for evacuating Mr. Joseph is:
   1. The "seat" carry
   2. Evacuation in bed
   3. The "back strap" method of evacuation
   4. Placing Mr. Joseph on floor and dragging out on a blanket
4. A physician's order for a restraint must include all of the following except:
   1. Time limitation for application of restraint
   2. Type of restraint to apply
   3. Type of behavior that requires use of restraint
   4. Alternatives to be used before restraint is used.

References

Beare P, Myers J: *Principles and practice of adult health nursing*, ed 2, St. Louis, 1994, Mosby.
Brenner Z, Durnin-Duffy K: Toward restraint free care, *Am J Nurs* 98(12):16f, 1998.
Brians LK and others: The development of the RISK tool for fall prevention, *Rehabil Nurs* 16(2):67, 1991.
Capezuti E and others: Physical restraint use and falls in nursing home residents, *J Am Geriatr Soc* 44(6):627, 1996.
Centers for Disease Control and Prevention: Web-based Injury Statistics Query and Reporting System (WISQARS), National Center for Injury Pre...
Disease Contr...

Centers for Medicare and Medicaid Services: *Conditions of participation; interpretive guidelines*, Bethesda, Md, 2004, US Department of Health and Human Services.
Ebersole P and others: *Toward healthy aging: human needs and nursing process*, ed 6, St. Louis, 2004, Mosby.
Hockenberry MJ and others: *Whaley and Wong's nursing care of infants and children*, ed 7, St. Louis, 2003, Mosby.
Ignatavicius DD, Workman ML: *Medical-surgical nursing: critical thinking for... orative care*, Philadelphia, 2002, WB ...
...ccreditation of Healthcare Organizations:
...itation manual for hospitals, Chicago.

Joint Commission on Accreditation of Healthcare Organizations: *2005 National Patient Safety Goals*, Chicago, 2004, The Commission.
Lambert V: Patient restraints, *FDA Consum* 26(3):9, 1992.
Lannon S: Epilepsy in the elderly, *Clin Nurs Pract Epilepsy* 2(2):5, 1995.
Lueckenotte AG: *Gerontologic nursing*, St. Louis, 2000, Mosby.
McKenry L, Salerno E: *Mosby's pharmacology in nursing*, ed 20, St. Louis, 1999, Mosby.
National Institute of Neurological Disorders and Stroke: *Seizures and epilepsy: hope through research*, Bethesda, Md, 2001, National Institutes of Health.
North American Nursing Diagnosis Association International: *Nursing diagnoses: definitions and classification 2003-2004*, Philadelphia, 2003, NANDA International.
Pacquiao DF: Cultural competence in ethical decision-making. In Andres M, Boyle J: *Concepts in transcultural nursing*, Philadelphia, 2003, Lippincott, Williams, & Wilkins.
Patterson JE and others: Nursing consultation to reduce restraints in a nursing home, *Clin Nurse Spec* 9(4):231, 1995.
Phipps W and others: *Medical-surgical nursing: ...ical practice*, ed 6, St. Louis, 1999, Mosby.
Robinson G: *Essential Judaism: a complete guid... toms, and rituals*, New York, 2000, Pocket Boo...
Shantz D, Spitz M: What you need to know about... 23(11):34, 1993.
Skidmore-Roth L: *Mosby's drug guide for nurse... 2005, Mosby.
Sorrentino SA: *Assisting with patient care*, St. Lo...
Sorrentino SA: *Mosby's textbook for nursing ass... 2000, Mosby.

Sterling DA and others: Geriatric falls: injury severity is high and disproportionate to mechanism, *J Trauma* 50(1):116, 2001.
Tideiksaar R: Home safe home: practical tips for fall-proofing, *Geriatr Nurs* 11(6):280, 1989.
Weick M: Physical restraints: an FDA update, *Am J Nurs* 92(11):74, 1992.

Research References

American Geriatrics Society, British Geriatrics Society, American Academy of Orthopedic Surgeons Panel on Falls Prevention: Guideline for the prevention of falls in older persons, *J Am Geriatr Soc* 49:664, 2001.
Campbell AJ and others: Falls prevention over 2 years: a randomized controlled trial in women 80 years and older, *Age Ageing* 28:513, 1999.
Fadiman A: *The spirit catches you and you fall down*, New York, 1999, Farrar, Straus & Giroux.
Halfon P and others: Risk of falls for hospitalized patients: a predictive model based on routinely available data, *J Clin Epidemiol*

Research References highlight current research and selected evidence-based "best" practice sources in the literature.

Mosby's
NURSING SKILLS CD-ROM
POTTER • PERRY

Mosby's Nursing Skills CD-ROM student version contains video covering 126 basic, intermediate, and advanced skills.

Preface to the Instructor

Today's nursing students are preparing for careers in an environment of ongoing change. A strong foundation in all levels of nursing skills is central to their success. With that goal in mind, this sixth edition of *Clinical Nursing Skills & Techniques* incorporates comprehensive coverage of 200 basic, intermediate, and advanced nursing skills within a nursing process framework. Because successful performance is based on understanding, students are presented with both the evidence-based practice trends and rationales for techniques. Numerous features encourage the student to consider the many factors influencing their clients, including age and cultural background. New end-of-chapter exercises focus on clinical practice and NCLEX® style review. As always, *Clinical Nursing Skills & Techniques* provides your students with a comprehensive resource that will serve them for many years to come.

Classic Features

- **200 basic, intermediate, and advanced nursing skills** are presented.
- **Five-step nursing process** format provides a consistent presentation that helps students apply the process while learning each skill.
- **Two-column format** is easy to follow.
- **Skills List, Objectives,** and **Key Terms** open each chapter.
- **Over 1100 full-color photos and drawings** help students master the material covered.
- **Skill Performance Guidelines** appear early in each chapter to focus student attention on the key principles about to be presented.
- **Rationales** are given for steps within skills so students learn the *why*, as well as the how, of each skill.
- **Critical Decision Points** alert students to key steps that affect safety and help them modify care as needed to meet individual client needs.
- **Recording and Reporting** sections follow the evaluation discussion and alerts students to what information should be documented in each situation.
- **Delegation Considerations** discuss the nurse's responsibility when delegating to assistive personal and high-

lights which tasks are appropriate for delegation and which are not.
- **Teaching Considerations** remind students to incorporate this essential nursing activity while performing skills.
- **Unexpected Outcomes** and **Related Interventions** remind students to be alert for possible problems and help them determine appropriate responses.
- **Home Care Considerations** teach students how to adapt skills for the home setting.
- **Glossary** includes all key terms.

New Features

- **New Chapter on Disaster Preparedness** provides a frame of reference for nursing care in the disaster environment, highlights how various responding agencies interact, and provides specific information on biological, chemical, and radiation exposures.
- **Eleven new skills**
  Code Management
  Communicating With a Depressed Client
  Fire, Electrical, and Radiation Safety
  Local Anesthetic Infusion Pump
  Care of the Grieving Family
  Care of the Dying Patient
  Care of Clients With Immobilization Devices
  Using an Automated External Defibrillator (AED)
  Wound Vacuum Assisted Closure
  Measuring Occult Blood in Gastric Secretions
- **Evidence-Based Practice Trends** present students with the scientific foundation on which procedures and protocols are based. Recent research findings are discussed and their implications for the successful care of clients.
- **Cultural Implications** discuss various cultural beliefs and preferences that may affect the performance of the skills presented in the chapter.
- **Expanded Pediatric Considerations** detail special considerations and variations for pediatric patients.
- **Focus on Clinical Practice** sections present a case study with a set of questions. Students will develop analytical

and problem-solving skills as they resolve the issues of the case.

- **NCLEX Review Questions** may be found at the end of each chapter to help familiarize students with this testing format in preparation for their certification exams.
- **Answers to End-of-Chapter Exercises.** The complete set of answers allows students to check their proficiency as they study.
- **Research References** direct students to the documentation supporting evidence-based practice trends discussed in each chapter.

Ancillaries

- **Skills Performance Checklists** allow you and your students to evaluate skill performance. Students may purchase the checklists separately or at a special price when packaged with the text.
  Skills Performance Checklists: ISBN 0-323-03159-5
  Text/Checklist Package: ISBN 0-323-03160-9
- **Instructor's Resource Manual with updated Test Bank** includes Educational Strategies with classroom activities and clinical activities, ideas for independent learning projects, cross curriculum guide, a table of abbreviations commonly used on patient charts, and answers to end-of-chapter exercises.
  Instructor's Resource Manual (print): ISBN 0-323-03669-4
  Instructor's Resources Guide (CD-ROM): ISBN 0-323-03588-4
- **Evolve Online Courseware** includes weblinks, instructor's resource manual, computerized test bank, procedure checklists, and skills video clips.
- **Mosby's Nursing Skills CD-ROM.** Innovative, action-packed videos give students a visual model of key skills. Contemporary concepts such as delegation, client rights, standard CDC precautions, and communications techniques are integrated throughout. Includes 126 basic, intermediate, and advanced skills.
  Mosby's Nursing Skills CD-ROM (Student Version): ISBN 0-323-03333-4
- **Mosby's Nursing Skills Videos.** Three sets of videos for classroom presentation demonstrate 126 skills.
  Basic Nursing Skills: ISBN 0-323-03156-2
  Intermediate Nursing Skills: ISBN 0-323-03176-7
  Advanced Nursing Skills: ISBN 0-323-01387-2

Contents

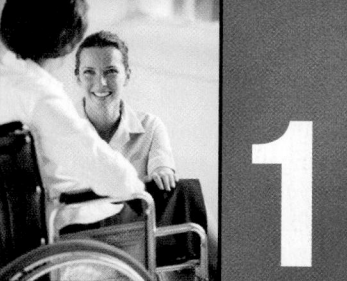

1

Admitting, Transfer, and Discharge

MEDIA RESOURCES

Evolve Site *evolve*

http://evolve.elsevier.com/Perry/skills
- Weblinks
- Video clips

OBJECTIVES

Mastery of content in this chaper will enable the nurse to:

- Describe the nurse's role in maintaining continuity of care through a client's admission, transfer, and discharge from an acute care facility.
- Explain the purpose and importance of advance directives.
- Identify clients in need of comprehensive discharge planning.
- Explain the importance of including the client's family in the admission, transfer, or discharge process.
- Perform the following skills: admit a client to an agency, admit a client to a nursing division, transfer a client to a different agency, discharge a client.

KEY TERMS

Advance directives

Centers for Medicare and Medicaid Services (CMS)

Condition of participation

Continuum of care

Discharge planning

Emergency Medical Treatment and Labor Act (EMTALA)

Health Insurance Portability and Accountability Act (HIPPA)

Joint Commission on Accreditation of Healthcare Organizations (JCAHO)

Patient's Rights

Patient Self-Determination Act

A client often has numerous needs when entering the health care system. In the acute care setting a variety of services are provided by multiple caregivers, and the nurse plays a key role in coordinating the client's care from admission to discharge. The nurse spends more time with clients than do other caregivers and thus is in the best position to understand the client's needs from a holistic perspective. The nurse coordinates the many resources required to ensure a smooth transition from the hospital to the next level of care. To separate the processes of admission and discharge is a critical error; the two are simultaneous and continuous. Discharge planning should begin at the time of admission. The nurse identifies clients' health care needs; anticipates physical, psychological, and social deficits that have implications for resuming normal activities; involves family and significant others in a plan of care; provides for health education; and assists in making health care resources available to the client. Ultimately the client and family should be prepared to understand the implications of any health problems and the responsibilities for continued care either in the home or next level of care setting.

Evidence-Based Practice Trends

Clients receive a variety of health care services in multiple settings from numerous caregivers. It is important for caregivers to view the patient care they provide as part of an integrated system of settings, services, health care practitioners, and care levels that make up a continuum of care.

The continuum of care is defined by the Joint Commission on Accreditation of Healthcare Organizations (JCAHO) as matching an individual's ongoing needs with the appropriate level and type of medical, psychological, health, or social care or services within a organization or across multiple organizations (JCAHO, 2004). This continuum flows from before admission to the admission process, throughout the acute care hospitalization, before discharge as the discharge plan is developed, and post hospitalization upon discharge to home or to another health care setting. It is imperative for all disciplines involved in the care of the client to work collaboratively in assisting the client's transition from one level of care or service to another. The client and family must be integrally involved in the planning and decision making in each step of the health care continuum.

Cultural Considerations

When admitting clients from diverse cultures and religions it is important to understand their cultural and religious practices. Some client's cultural practices include family decision making. When this is the case, it may be necessary to accommodate large groups of people who stay at the client's bedside and/or stay in the vicinity (Galanti, 2003).

- Develop trust by working with the established family and social hierarchy, recognizing those in authority and allowing them to participate in making decisions about the client's care.
- The oldest family member present may respond for the client. Observe client's behaviors and interactions with family members (Bodnar, 1995).

For client's who are Orthodox Jews, schedule the admission or transfer so the client can begin observance of the Sabbath (sundown on Friday to sundown on Saturday) undisturbed. Orthodox Jews follow the tenets of their religion closely (Robinson, 2000).

- Prepare the unit or setting for the transfer. During Sabbath, Orthodox Jews generally avoid using electrical equipment (telephone, call light, elevators).
- Have Kosher meals and snacks available
- Answer the client's telephone
- Make frequent and regular rounds to the client's bedside because he or she will not use the call light

Assess use of cultural healers and other healing modalities; for example, Hmongs may attribute health and illness to religious and supernatural forces (Fadiman, 1999).

Skill Performance Guidelines

1. Screen all clients upon admission to a health care setting for possible discharge needs.
2. Include the client, family, and relevant health care professionals early in planning for all moves through the health care system.

3. Consider the client's past experiences in health care settings.
4. Consider the client's cultural, socioeconomic, and educational background when discharge planning.

5. All appropriate health care providers who contribute to the client's care must collaborate in developing a plan of care for discharge.
6. Assist other health care personnel in assessing appropriate resources needed as clients move through the health care system.

SKILL 1-1   Admitting Clients

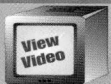

A client can access the health care system in a variety of ways (e.g., hospital, urgent care center, clinic, or physician's office). Commonalities exist for the type of procedures used to admit clients to these settings (Box 1-1). However, a client's condition determines the extent of the admitting procedure. For example, a client entering through the emergency department may not be in a condition to undergo the same registration process that takes place in a hospital admitting office. In this case family members may provide pertinent information for the hospital's records while the client is being cared for. In contrast, an older adult client who can no longer attend to daily chores but who is still independent enough to perform some self-care activities undergoes extensive screening before being accepted as a nursing home resident.

Admitting officers, secretaries, and technicians are the personnel primarily involved with the preliminary admission procedures, such as interviewing clients and reviewing information about insurance, demographic data, and general agency procedures. Technicians may collect routine specimens and perform screening procedures such as electrocardiograms (ECGs). Some hospitals have a small satellite admitting office within the emergency department.

Role of the Admitting Clerk or Secretary

The role of the admitting clerk or secretary includes specific activities such as initiating and maintaining a courteous and professional relationship with the client and providing for the client's safety, legal rights, and privacy. Privacy can be maintained by escorting the client and family to an admitting interview area where important identifying information is collected, including the client's full legal name, age, birth date, address, next of kin, physician, religious preference,

occupation, and type of insurance (Figure 1-1). If the client does not speak English or has a severe hearing impairment, an interpreter may be called to assist during the admission procedure to ensure that correct information is gathered.

At this time, an identification (ID) band legibly stating the client's full legal name, hospital or agency number, physician, and birth date should be applied securely to the client's wrist. The ID band serves to identify the client when therapies or procedures are performed. If a client is unconscious, identification may not be made until family members arrive. Also, a client who has been a victim of crime may be safer with an anonymous name under an agency's "blackout" procedure.

The admitting clerk or secretary should provide for the client's legal rights by instructing the client or legal guardian to read the general consent form for treatment. At the time of admission, all clients are to receive information regarding their rights related to the health care services they will encounter. In 1999 the Centers for Medicare and Medicaid Services (CMS) introduced a Patients' Rights Condition of Participation that all hospitals must meet to receive Medicare and Medicaid reimbursement. This new condition set forth the requirement that each client is notified of his or her rights (Box 1-2). Other regulatory agencies, such as the JCAHO, also require institutions to provide for specific patient rights (Box 1-3). Each institution will have policies and procedures describing the client's rights and the role of the nurse in ensuring those rights.

BOX 1-1   Common Procedures for Admission to a Health Care Agency

- Placement of client in appropriate receiving area
- Explanation of client's rights and elements of advance directives
- Orientation to the health care agency's policies and procedures
- Assessment of client's health care problems and needs
- Preliminary testing and screening (specific for each agency and client's condition)
- Development of an individualized plan of care
- Determination of client's payment source for health care

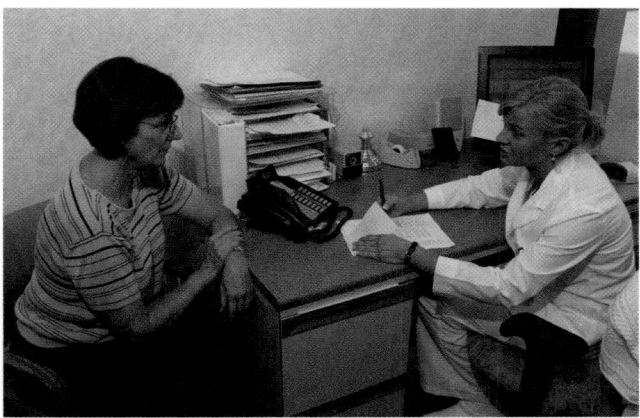

FIGURE 1-1 The admitting clerk gathers important information from the client.

BOX 1-2   Key Principles of Patients' Rights Provided for by CMS

- Patient's right to notification of his or her rights
- Patient's right to the exercise of his or her rights in regard to his or her care
- Patient's right to privacy and safety, including the freedom to be free from all forms of abuse or harassment
- Patient's right to confidentiality of his or her records and access to his or her records in a reasonable period of time
- Patient's right to freedom from restraints used in the provision of acute medical and surgical care unless clinically necessary
- Patient's right to freedom from seclusion and restraints used in behavioral management unless clinically necessary

CODE OF FEDERAL REGULATIONS TITLE 42, CHAPTER IV PART 482 SEC. 482.13 CONDITION OF PARTICIPATION: PATIENTS' RIGHTS.

- A hospital must protect and promote each patient's rights.
- A hospital must inform each patient, or when appropriate, the patient's representative of the patient's rights, in advance of furnishing or discontinuing patient care whenever possible.
- The hospital must have a process for prompt resolution of patient grievances and must inform each patient whom to contact to file a grievance.
- The patient has the right to participate in the development and implementation of his or her plan of care.
- The patient or his or her representative has the right to make informed decisions regarding his or her care.
- The patient's rights include being informed of his or her health status, being involved in care planning and treatment, and being able to request or refuse treatment. This right must not be construed as a mechanism to demand the provision of treatment or services deemed medically unnecessary or inappropriate.
- The patient has the right to formulate advance directives and to have hospital staff and practitioners who provide care in the hospital comply with these directives.
- The patient has the right to have a family member or representative of his or her choice and his or her own physician notified promptly of his or her admission to the hospital.
- The patient has the right to personal privacy.
- The patient has the right to receive care in a safe setting.

- The patient has the right to be free from all forms of abuse or harassment.
- The patient has the right to the confidentiality of his or her clinical records.
- The patient has the right to access information contained in his or her clinical records within a reasonable time frame.
- The patient has the right to be free from restraints of any form that are not medically necessary or are used as a means of coercion, discipline, convenience, or retaliation by staff. The term "restraint" includes either a physical restraint or a drug that is being used as a restraint. A physical restraint is any manual method or physical or mechanical device, material, or equipment attached or adjacent to the patient's body that he or she cannot easily remove that restricts freedom of movement or normal access to one's body. A drug used as a restraint is a medication used to control behavior or to restrict the patient's freedom of movement and is not a standard treatment for the patient's medical or psychiatric condition.
  - —A restraint can only be used if needed to improve the patient's well-being and less restrictive interventions have been determined to be ineffective.
  - —The use of a restraint must be selected only when other less restrictive measures have been found to be ineffective to protect the patient or others from harm; and in accordance with the order of a physician or other licensed independent practitioner.
  - —This order must never be written as a standing or on an as needed basis (that is, prn); and be followed by consultation with the patient's treating physician, as soon as possible, if the restraint is not ordered by the patient's treating physician.
  - —The use of a restraint must be:
    - In accordance with a written modification to the patient's plan of care;
    - Implemented in the least restrictive manner possible;
    - In accordance with safe and appropriate restraining techniques; and
    - Ended at the earliest possible time.
  - —The condition of the restrained patient must be continually assessed, monitored, and reevaluated.
  - —All staff who have direct patient contact must have ongoing education and training in the proper and safe use of restraints.

Modified from Centers for Medicare and Medicaid Services: Patient rights: conditions of participation, *Federal Register* 482.13, 2002.

During off-shifts and weekends, when the admitting department is closed, the responsibilities of the admitting clerk or secretary may become the role of the nurse who will be caring for the client.

The Patient Self-Determination Act, effective December 1, 1991, requires all Medicare- and Medicaid-recipient hospitals to provide clients with information about their right to accept or reject medical treatment. Clients must receive at the time of registration information about advance directives and be referred to appropriate resources if they want to discuss advance directives or receive help in completing an advance directive document (Box 1-4).

At the time of registration the admitting clerk must also provide the client with information about the Health Insurance Portability and Accountability Act (HIPAA). HIPAA is a federal law to protect the privacy of client health information, referred to as PHI or protected health information. The first key concept of HIPAA is that institutions must inform clients of the privacy rights they have and how the institution will handle their PHI. This requirement is typically completed by the admitting clerk by giving the client a written summary or "notice" of his or her rights under HIPAA (CMS, 2002b).

A second concept is that the institution and the health care providers are to use or disclose the client's PHI only for the purposes of treatment or payment or for health care operations. If PHI is to be used for anything else, the institution must first obtain the client's specific authorization.

A third concept is that health care providers should disclose only the minimum amount of PHI necessary to accomplish the purpose of the use. PHI should be disclosed only on a need-to-know basis. For example, if a technician is called into the room to obtain a blood specimen, it is not

BOX 1-3   JCAHO Patient Rights Standards

- The hospital respects the rights of patients.
- Patients receive information about their rights.
- Patients are involved in decisions about care, treatment, and services provided.
- Informed consent is obtained.
- Consent is obtained for recording or filming made for purposes other than the identification, diagnosis, or treatment of the patients.
- Patients receive adequate information about the person(s) responsible for the delivery of their care, treatment, and services.
- Patients have the right to refuse care, treatment, and services in accordance with law and regulation.
- The hospital addresses the wishes of the patient relating to end-of-life care decisions.
- Patients and, when appropriate, their families are informed about the outcomes of care, treatment, and services, including unanticipated outcomes.
- The hospital respects the patient's right to and need for effective communication.
- The hospital addresses the resolution of complaints from patients and their families.
- The hospital respects the needs of patients for confidentiality, privacy, and security.
- Patients have a right to an environment that preserves dignity and contributes to a positive self-image.
- Patients have the right to be free from mental, physical, sexual, and verbal abuse, neglect, and exploitation.
- Patients have the right to pain management.
- Patients have a right to access protective and advocacy services.
- The hospital protects research subjects and respects their rights during research, investigation, and clinical trials involving human subjects.

BOX 1-4   Advance Directives

- An advance directive is a document that gives a client's directions about future medical care or designates another person(s) to make medical decisions if the individual loses decision-making capacity.
- An advance directive conveys the client's choice in continuing medical care when the client is unable to speak or make decisions.
- Advance directives may include a living will, power of attorney for health care, or a notarized handwritten document.
- A copy of the document should be available in the client's medical record. If not available, the substance of the advance directive should be documented in the medical record, and a family member should be asked to bring the advance directive to the hospital.
- The attending physician is notified of the client's advance directive.
- Witnesses for an advance directive document should not be medical personnel, nor should they be related to the client or heirs to the client's estate.

necessary for the nurse to tell the technician all of the details of the client's past psychosocial issues. The technician simply needs to know what test is to be drawn and any clinically relevant patient safety issues. The HIPAA privacy regulations give clients the right to access their records, request amendments to the PHI contained in their records, request restriction of certain uses or disclosures of their PHI, request that they be sent information at an alternate address or telephone number, and request an accounting of PHI disclosures. It is important to be familiar with the institution-specific policies and procedures related to HIPAA.

Role of the Nurse

Nurses should be directly involved in assigning clients to rooms, completing a thorough nursing assessment, reviewing any advance directives, ensuring that necessary diagnostic testing is completed, and providing for continuity of care when the client is admitted through the emergency department. The nurse should also identify any known allergies and, if any exist, place an allergy band on the client and properly document the known allergies in the medical record. Admitting personnel should confer with nursing staff to ensure that a client's room is assigned based on the client's condition, health care needs, and personal preferences. For example, a client who is acutely ill and receiving multiple treatments may best be cared for in a room close to the nurses' station.

When a client is admitted through the emergency department, the emergency department nurse should notify the nursing division and give a report of the client's admission information, including the client's name, admitting physician, chief complaint, any treatments or testing completed and the outcome, diagnosis, and pertinent information related to the client's condition (e.g., initial vital signs, allergies, level of consciousness, and intravenous [IV] fluid infusing). A full report and timely review of physician orders ensures adequate preparation for the client's arrival and prompt treatment (Clark and Normile, 2002). The client and family members should be transported to the nursing division with an escort and introduced to the nurse assuming the client's care. Any pertinent observations about the client's behavior (e.g., anxiety or fear or level of knowledge regarding need for health care) can be shared with the nursing staff at this time to foster continuity of care and assist the client and family in coping with a new environment and procedures.

Clients admitted the morning of a surgical procedure or treatment are called "same day" admissions. The nurse should provide them with basic instructions regarding the purpose of the surgery or treatment, preparatory procedures, and postsurgical or posttreatment care. Admission forms, consent forms, diagnostic tests, and instructions may be completed before the actual day of surgery. Informational booklets pertaining to the client's surgery or treatment are often available to clients well in advance of their surgery date.

The nurse plays an active role in coordinating the initial admission process for all clients. A client's condition influences the extent and type of admission activities. When a critically ill client reaches a hospital's nursing division, the client must undergo extensive examination and treatment procedures almost immediately. Little time is available for the nurse to orient the client and family to the division or learn of their fears or concerns. When a client enters a hospital for elective treatment, the nurse may have more time to prepare the client psychologically for hospitalization. Early psychological preparation when the client is still at home can be very helpful in preparing clients for hospitalization.

The nurse must always be conscious of the client's level of fatigue and comfort. The admission process can be exhausting. When the client is experiencing physical or psychological symptoms, the nurse determines whether any portion of the admission process can be completed later.

DELEGATION CONSIDERATIONS

The skill of assessing clients during admission to a health care facility should not be delegated to assistive personnel. However, the following activities may be delegated: preparation of the client's room and equipment before admission, gathering and securing the client's personal care items, assisting with escorting and orienting the client and family to the nursing unit, and collecting specimens.

EQUIPMENT

- ❏ Bedpan and urinal
- ❏ Washbasin, bath towel, and washcloth
- ❏ Toiletry items (e.g., soap, toothpaste, hand lotion; optional in some hospitals)
- ❏ Facial tissues
- ❏ Water pitcher and drinking cup
- ❏ Kidney or emesis basin
- ❏ Disposable thermometer (see agency policy)
- ❏ Sphygmomanometer
- ❏ Stethoscope
- ❏ Documentation forms (see agency policy)

STEP	RATIONALE

ROOM PREPARATION

1. Perform hand hygiene, and prepare room equipment and furniture. Prepare bed by adjusting it to the lowest horizontal position. Turn down top sheet and spread. Arrange room furniture for easy access to bed.

Promotes client's comfort by preventing delays during care. Proper position of bed lessens likelihood of client falls and of back injuries to staff assisting the client into the bed.

2. Be sure equipment is in working order. Then assemble any special equipment such as suction, oxygen supplies, or IV pole in client's room.

Prevents delays in delivering immediate treatment and provides for smooth transition between caregivers.

ASSESSMENT

3. Greet client and family cordially. Introduce yourself by name and job title; explain your responsibilities in client's care. (Primary nurse may be assigned at this time.)

Reduces anxiety about admission, clarifies staff roles, and expedites client requests.

4. If client is not able to speak English or has a severe hearing impairment, arrange for a translation service so that a nursing assessment can be conducted.

Translation services are preferred over use of family members to ensure correct translation of medical terminology.

5. Assess client's general appearance, noting signs or symptoms of physical distress.

Provides baseline assessment.

- **• Critical Decision Point**
  If client is having acute physical problems, postpone routine admission procedures until client's immediate needs are met. The nurse may complete a focused assessment at this point.

6. Escort client and family to assigned room. Introduce them to roommate if semiprivate room is assigned at this time.

Orientation begins with introduction to roommate.

7. Assess client's and family's psychological status by noting nonverbal behaviors and verbal responses to greetings and explanations.

Anxiety influences how well client adapts to a health care environment and retains instruction.

8. Assess vital signs (see Chapter 17) and height and weight (see Chapter 18).

Provides baseline measurement to compare future findings. Determines alterations from normal range.

STEP	**RATIONALE**
9. Have family or friends leave room unless the client wishes to have them assist client with undressing. Close door and curtains. Help client undress, and assist client into comfortable position.	Provides for privacy and prepares client for examination.
10. Obtain nursing history organized by standards of nursing care adopted by hospital (e.g., functional health patterns). Data will include:	The JCAHO requires each client to have an admission assessment prepared by an RN (JCAHO, 2004). Each institution must set time frame for completion of admission assessment (maximum time 24 hours).
a. Client's perception of illness and health care needs **b.** Past medical history **c.** Presenting signs and symptoms	The nursing assessment should be completed as soon as possible following the client's arrival at the nursing division. This will allow the nurse to: **1.** Establish a baseline of the client's clinical status **2.** Identify signs and symptoms should the client's condition deteriorate
d. Complete review of health status based on standards such as elimination, nutrition and metabolism, activity and exercise, self-concept, values and beliefs, cultural factors, social support, and cognitive function	A comprehensive health history provides a holistic view of client's health problems and response to those problems.
e. Risk factors for illness	Allows nurse to institute preventive care measures and to educate client about health promotion behaviors.
f. History of allergies, including type of substance and a description of the reaction client has previously experienced	Client may have a sensitivity to a drug or substance rather than a true allergy; this should be clarified. Specify all allergens to prevent accidental exposure.

- *Critical Decision Point*
  Provide client with allergy arm band listing allergies to foods, drugs, latex, or other substances; document allergies according to hospital policy.

STEP	**RATIONALE**
g. Risk factors for falling (e.g., neurological disorders, history of previous falls, urinary urgency, use of sedatives and analgesics, history of unsteady gait, use of assistive devices, history of orthostatic hypotension, memory deficits such as forgetfulness)	Identification of risk factors may lead to placement of client on fall precautions (see agency policy).
h. Medication history, including prescribed, over-the-counter (OTC), and alternative therapies such as herbs and hormones	A complete medication history helps to assess potential for drug interactions and may explain client's presenting signs and symptoms.
i. Client's knowledge of health problems and expectations of care	Enables the nurse to recognize and meet client expectations when possible.
11. Conduct physical assessment of appropriate body systems (Chapter 18). If not obtained in admitting, instruct client to provide a urine specimen. Inform client as to blood specimens to be collected or tests to be performed.	Provides objective data for identifying health problems. Preparation of client can relieve anxiety that is created when unannounced procedures are performed.
12. Check physician's orders for treatment measures that should be initiated immediately.	Delay can cause deterioration of client's condition.
13. Orient client to nursing division.	
a. Introduce staff members who enter room. Always introduce client by last name unless client indicates otherwise.	Helps client to recognize caregivers. Shows respect for client.
b. Tell client and family the name of head nurse or charge nurse of the division, and explain that person's role in solving problems.	Provides means for client to communicate problems.

STEP	RATIONALE
c. Explain visiting hours and their purpose.	Provides knowledge about and increases willingness to observe visiting hours policy, which ensures client will receive adequate rest.
d. Discuss smoking policy, and identify smoking areas for client and family.	The JCAHO requires a hospital-wide smoking policy that prohibits the use of smoking materials throughout the hospital. Exceptions are authorized for a client by a physician prescription (JCAHO, 2004).
e. Demonstrate use of equipment (e.g., bed, over-bed table, lighting).	Client's safety depends on understanding correct use of equipment.
f. Show client how to use nurse call light, and position it in a convenient place. Have client demonstrate use of light.	Ensures client knows how to call for assistance.
g. Escort client to bathroom (if able to ambulate).	Client's safety depends in part on understanding how to use toilet facilities.

• *Critical Decision Point*
Ensure that client knows how to call for assistance while in bathroom. (An emergency call light is installed in bathrooms.)

h. Explain hours for mealtime and nourishments to client and family.	Family may wish to visit during evening to assist with meals.
i. Describe services available (e.g., chaplain, beauty shop, activity therapy).	Offers client options for making decisions.

NURSING DIAGNOSES
- Anxiety
- Ineffective coping
- Deficient knowledge regarding hospital procedures and planned therapies

- Fear
- Risk for injury
- Powerlessness

Related factors are individualized based on client's condition or needs.

PLANNING

1. Expected outcomes following completion of procedure:
   - Client is able to explain purpose and schedule of planned treatments and procedures.
   - Client will demonstrate how to call for nurse when assistance is needed.
   - Client will be able to ambulate (if condition permits) in room free of obstacles and safely and efficiently use equipment in the room.
   - Client is able to verbalize understanding of smoking policy, visiting hours, mealtimes, and services available.

Understanding treatment plan gives client a better sense of control and reduces anxiety about the unknown.

Falls commonly occur when clients attempt to reach toilet facilities or a chair without assistance.

Equipment used in care of client can pose hazards and can assist in reducing some anxiety.

Knowledge of hospital policies assists client in adapting to the health care environment.

IMPLEMENTATION

1. Inform client about procedures or treatments scheduled for the next shift or day (e.g., visits by physician or dietitian). These vary based on nature of client's condition.
2. Give client and family chance to ask questions about procedures or therapies. (If client is unresponsive or unable to understand, review with family.)
3. Collect valuables client chooses to keep at facility. Complete listing sheet (see agency policy), and have client or family member sign it. Place valuables in agency safe, or send home with family.

Client has right to be informed of any scheduled procedures or treatments. Being able to anticipate planned therapies minimizes anxiety.

Provides opportunity to clarify expectations and misconceptions.

Accounts for placement of valuables and prevents loss.

STEP	**RATIONALE**
4. Ensure client and family have time together alone, if desired.	Admission can be stressful and fatiguing. Allows time for decision making.
5. Be sure call light is within easy reach and bed is in low position. (Check agency policy regarding use of side rails.)	Provides for client's safety. Side rails are typically used to reduce the chance of falls but can be considered a restraint if the side rail inhibits client's ability to get out of bed when desired (JCAHO, 2004).
6. Perform hand hygiene.	Reduces spread of microorganisms.

▌ EVALUATION

1. Confirm client's understanding of hospital policies, tests, and procedures through discussion and questions.	Learning and understanding are demonstrated through client feedback.
2. Observe client for nonverbal signs (e.g., restlessness, poor eye contact, facial tension).	Such signs may indicate anxiety.
3. Monitor client's ability to ambulate independently. Assess for fall risk using scale with grading criteria as per agency policy.	Provides data to judge client's ability to ambulate without injury.
4. Check client's room setup regularly.	Determines if care area is free of obstacles.

Recording and Reporting

- Record history and assessment findings on appropriate forms.
- If client has an advance directive, place copy in the medical record. In the absence of the actual advance directive, the substance of the directive is documented in the medical record (JCAHO, 2004).
- Notify physician of client's arrival; report any unusual findings. Secure admission orders if not previously provided.
- Begin to develop nursing plan of care. Confer with client and family as needed.

Unexpected Outcomes	**Related Interventions**
1. Client denies understanding hospital policies or knowing purpose or schedule for tests and procedures.	• Schedule a follow-up session with client. • Keep information focused and specific to client's situation. Include family if helpful.
2. Client becomes restless, expresses concerns, or displays tension in body movements.	• Give client time to discuss fears and concerns. • Show caring and compassion so that client becomes willing to communicate openly.
3. Client falls or is injured.	• Nurse must attend to client's immediate physical needs, inform physician of the injury or fall, reassess the client's environment, ensure that the environment is free of safety hazards, and complete incident report (see Chapter 3).

Teaching Considerations

- Complete a learning needs assessment to identify the client's and family's educational needs and learning preferences.
- Explain to client that a different nurse provides care on each shift. Explain time frame for how assignments are made.
- Teaching can occur throughout the admission process. A nurse can provide information regarding physical assessment findings, planned diagnostic procedures, or hospital routines. A formal teaching plan should not begin until assessment is completed and a care plan is developed.
- Teaching begins early in a client's hospitalization. Nurse introduces instruction when client is able to be attentive and learn from the information. Information should be specific, focusing on topics such as the nature of client's illness, medications needed for treatment, and use of equipment in self-care (e.g., dressings, ambulatory devices).
- In an emergency situation or if the client is unable to perform aspects of his or her care, instruct family members in the rationale for any procedures and routines to be used in client's care.

Pediatric Considerations

- Allow and encourage parental involvement in the child's care. Hospitalization is a major crisis for children with stress resulting from separation, loss of control, bodily injury, and pain. Separation anxiety is most evident from middle infancy throughout the toddler years, especially ages 16 to 30 months. The child experiences protest, despair, and detachment. Preschoolers are better able to tolerate brief periods of separation, but their protest behaviors are more subtle than those in younger children (e.g., refusal to eat, difficulty sleeping, withdrawing from others). School-age children are able to cope with separation but have an increased need for parental security and guidance (Hockenberry and others, 2003). Allow parents to assist with routine care activities (e.g., bathing, eating) and when possible to remain with the child during procedures.
- The nurse can play an important role in making the hospital experience a chance for children to develop new socialization skills and to broaden their interpersonal relationships. The nurse fosters parent-child relationships, offers educational opportunities, and provides for socialization with other children (Hockenberry and others, 2003).

Gerontological Considerations

- Hospitalized older adults with some functional disabilities often rapidly regress into a helpless state during hospitalization. Interventions that may help to retain functional status during an episodic illness include daily orientation cues for client, allowing the client to be independent as tolerated, reassurance regarding probability of transient delirium, getting client up and out of room at least daily, using physical therapy (PT) and occupational therapy (OT) daily, keeping the environment pleasant and comfortable, and personalizing the environment (Ebersole and others, 2004).
- Clients who characteristically fall in the hospital are those who have been recently admitted and are unfamiliar with surroundings, have several pathological conditions, take medications with sedative or tranquilizing effects, or have had multiple recent transfers. In addition, visual changes that occur with aging can lead to falls in hospitalized older adult clients (Ebersole and others, 2004).

SKILL 1-2 Transfering Clients

Clients transfer to new patient care units and new agencies to receive different forms and levels of therapy and services and to have care continued closer to home. When clients transfer, continuity of vital aspects of nursing care must be ensured. The argument is that better continuity of care ensures better client outcomes. The client and family benefit when care is continued as smoothly as possible without interruptions in therapy that may hinder progress toward recovery.

The nurse collaborates early with physicians and members of the other health care disciplines to ensure efficient client transfer with good client outcomes. This collaboration is important when clients transfer, for example, from an intensive care unit (ICU) to a general nursing unit or transfer from a postsurgical floor to a skilled nursing facility for acute rehabilitation. It is only through open collaboration and effective communication that the ultimate goal of enhancing client care can be realized.

When a client is transferred from one division to another within an institution, the transfer process may be completed with little interruption to care activities because policies and procedures are usually similar throughout the institution. The nurse should first provide a telephone report to the receiving nurse. This will allow the receiving nurse to prepare for the client (e.g., preparing the room and securing necessary equipment). As clinically appropriate, the nurse or a technician may accompany the client during transport, provide the receiving nurse with the client's medical record, introduce the client to the receiving nurse, and provide an updated report including any changes in clinical status or plan of care.

In the emergency department, when a client is transferred from one institution to another, the nurse should complete the transfer in compliance with the Emergency Medical Treatment and Labor Act (EMTALA). EMTALA is a federal law intended to protect clients from being transferred against their wishes and thus defines how an appropriate facility-to-facility transfer is accomplished. An appropriate transfer includes:

- Informing the client of the risks and benefits of the transfer
- Obtaining the client's written consent for transfer
- Having the transferring hospital provide medical treatment within its capacity
- Having available space and qualified personnel for treatment of the client at the receiving institution and agreement to accept transfer of the client and to provide treatment
- Making copies of all relevant medical records, including a transfer form, sent by the transferring institution to the receiving facility

- Transporting the client using qualified personnel and transportation equipment (i.e., ambulance with advanced cardiac life support [ACLS] versus basic life support [BLS])

Although this law primarily affects the emergency department, the nurse should be familiar with the institution's EMTALA policies and transfer policies that relate to inpatient transfers because many institutions follow the same policies for all client transfers.

DELEGATION CONSIDERATIONS

Because of the related assessment and decision making, the skill of transferring clients should not be delegated to assistive personnel. However, the following activities may be delegated: dressing the client, gathering and securing the client's personal belongings and any equipment that may accompany the client, and assisting with escorting the client to the nursing unit or transport area.

EQUIPMENT

- ❑ Transfer forms
- ❑ Copies of medical records, radiology films, laboratory test results, etc. (as appropriate)
- ❑ Special equipment as needed: wheelchair or stretcher, emesis basin, bedpan and urinal, oxygen tank and tubing, IV pole, cardiac monitor, and emergency medications.

STEP	RATIONALE

ASSESSMENT

1. Obtain transfer order from sending physician. Order should include name of receiving agency (when applicable), receiving physician's name, and statement of client's stability for transfer.

Physician is legally responsible for releasing client from medical care and arranging for receiving physician. Client has legal right to refuse transfer against medical advice.

2. In collaboration with the physician and members of other health care disciplines, assess reason for client's transfer (e.g., change in condition, services available at agency, client or family preferences regarding client's location).

Client should have access to agency with best resources to meet health care needs. Physician determines client's physical stability for transfer.

3. Explain purpose of transfer thoroughly, and provide time to discuss client's and family's feelings about the change in care setting. As necessary, obtain client's written consent to transfer.

Transfers are sometimes planned quickly. Client requires adequate psychological preparation. The client must consent to transfer to a different facility. If the client is unable to consent, the client's family must provide this consent. In the event of a clinical emergency in which the client and the client's family are unable to consent, this consent may be waived and the client may be transferred to a higher level of care based on the clinical judgment of the physician requesting the transfer.

4. Assess client's current physical condition, and determine method for transport. When transferring to new agency, assess method of transport to transferring vehicle (e.g., wheelchair or stretcher) (consult agency policy).

Client's condition can change quickly and may influence stability for transfer and type of support needed during transport.

- *Critical Decision Point*

  Determine if client's status and safety require life support equipment. Staff assisting with transfer should be trained in life support measures. When transporting to new agency, a vehicle equipped with life support equipment is necessary.

5. Assess if client requires pain relief or other medications for symptom management before transfer.

Ensures client's comfort.

6. Ensure that client's family or significant others have been notified of transfer as desired by client.

Provides adequate communication with family or significant others to assist with client's emotional and psychological adjustment to the transfer.

STEP	RATIONALE

NURSING DIAGNOSES

- Anxiety
- Fear
- Deficient knowledge regarding transfer procedure

- Pain, acute and chronic
- Powerlessness
- Risk for relocation stress syndrome

Related factors are individualized based on client's condition or needs.

PLANNING

1. Expected outcomes following completion of procedure:
   - Client's vital signs and physiological status are unchanged following transfer.
   - Client incurs no injury during transport procedures.

   - Client or family is able to explain purpose of transfer and procedure for transport.
   - Receiving nursing staff acquires and confirms written plan of care.
2. Arrange for client's transport to an agency by chosen vehicle (may require support from social worker).
3. When transfer is to a new agency, contact the agency and arrange for bed in appropriate setting. Confirm willingness of agency to accept client (may be completed by social worker or discharge coordinator).

Treatments planned so as not to interrupt physical support of client during transfer.
Safety measures are successful in transferring client from wheelchair or stretcher to transport vehicle.
Understanding provides client with sense of control.

Ensures continuity of care.

Transfer should occur without delays so that client has access to all needed resources at all times.
Prevents delays when client arrives at destination. Receiving hospital must ensure that there is available space and qualified personnel to treat clients. Hospital must also agree in advance to transfer.

IMPLEMENTATION

1. Make sure documentation in client's record is complete. Nursing care measures should be individualized based on client need.
2. Complete nursing care transfer form according to agency policy. (When transfer is to a different nursing unit, entire medical record accompanies client.)
3. Gather client's personal care items, clothing, and valuables. Secure in suitcase or container.
4. Anticipate problems client may develop just before or during transfer. Perform necessary nursing therapies such as suctioning or changing a dressing.
5. Assist in transferring client to stretcher or wheelchair using proper body mechanics (see Chapter 10).
6. Perform and document final assessment of client's physical stability.

Accurate information is necessary for receiving agency to assume client's care.

Form provides summary of client's pertinent nursing care needs to ensure continuity of care and prevents unnecessary duplication of services.
Articles can be easily lost in transfer.

Ensures client's comfort and safety during transport.

Client transported to outside agency is more easily moved by stretcher into transport vehicle.
Minimizes risk of client developing complications during transfer.

- *Critical Decision Point*
  Be sure to check vital signs, check for clear airway, inspect patency of intravenous lines and accuracy of infusion rate, and note client's level of consciousness.

7. When transfer is to an outside agency, accompany client to transport vehicle.
8. Call receiving agency/unit and notify of impending transfer and client's status (check agency policy).

Ensures medically qualified personnel are in attendance until client leaves agency/unit.
Notification of nurse in charge or nurse assuming care of client will ensure better continuity of care at time of client's arrival.

STEP	RATIONALE

EVALUATION

1. During the final assessment compare data with previous findings.

   Determines if client's condition is changing.

2. Inspect client's alignment and positioning on stretcher/wheelchair.

   Proper alignment and positioning reduces risk of an injury occurring during transport.

3. Confirm client's understanding of transfer and procedures through discussion and questions.

   Learning is demonstrated through client feedback.

4. Determine if receiving agency/nurse has questions about client's care.

   Provides for clear communication and continuity of care.

Recording and Reporting

- Sending nurse documents client's status, including vital signs and other assessment findings, nursing plan of care, time of transfer, and method of transport.
- Receiving nurse documents client's arrival at agency by recording date and time of arrival, reason for transfer, method of transport, client's condition, and care provided at time of arrival.

Unexpected Outcomes	Related Interventions
1. Client's physical status deteriorates during preparation.	• Call physician immediately. • Initiate necessary interventions to stabilize client's condition.
2. Client sustains injury during transfer to wheelchair or stretcher.	• Stabilize client and call physician. • Complete incident report.
3. Client is confused or uncertain about transfer.	• Provide clarification or additional explanation.
4. Receiving staff misinterprets directions for client's care.	• Sending agency should have representative nurse or physician call to confirm that there are no questions regarding client's care.

Teaching Considerations

- A transfer can create anxiety for client and family members. It may become necessary for the nurse to carefully repeat instructions regarding transfer at a time when client and family can better attend to nurse's explanation.

Pediatric Considerations

- Information sharing is critical whenever a child is transferred either within a hospital or between facilities. Children need their parents' comfort and security; thus parents need to be well informed. Older children need to be involved in any discussion regarding transfers.
- If possible, a parent should be allowed to accompany a child in the transfer.

Gerontological Considerations

- When an older adult client is transferred to a new facility, relocation is stressful. The nurse should ensure that

significant support persons are still accessible and that client is thoroughly oriented to new surroundings, is allowed to take important memorabilia, and has opportunity to make decisions about care.

Long-Term Care Considerations

- It is important that clients receive the level of services appropriate to their physical and mental health needs. Participation of social worker or discharge planner in transfer process will ensure that transfer to a long-term care facility is appropriate.
- Upon client's arrival at long-term care agency, nurse will complete resident assessment instrument (RAI). The RAI consists of the minimum data set (MDS), resident assessment protocols, and utilization guidelines specified in state operations guidelines (Lueckenotte, 2000).

SKILL 1-3 Discharging Clients

Discharge planning is a process that facilitates the transition of the client from a health care agency to the most independent level of care, whether that is home or another agency. The overall goal of discharge planning is to provide the most appropriate level and quality of care throughout all stages of the client's illness. Every hospitalized client requires discharge planning. The trend toward a shortened length of stay in the acute care setting can make discharge planning increasingly difficult, but all the more essential (Wells and others, 2002). Federal regulations identify the elements of a comprehensive discharge planning model (Box 1-5).

The discharge planning process must be comprehensive and multidisciplinary, including all caregivers who are involved in the care of the client. Successful discharge planning ensures that the client has a safe and realistic plan for continuing care after leaving the hospital (Hou and others, 2001). This process should facilitate a prompt and well-coordinated discharge from acute care to ensure that adequate care is continued either in a client's home or in a restorative care setting.

Development of a plan with outcomes mutually accepted by the client and caregivers and ongoing communication about its progress are essential (Cleary and others, 2003). The discharge process may be described as occurring in three phases: acute, transitional, and continuing care (Figure 1-2). In the acute phase, medical attention dominates discharge planning efforts. During the transitional phase the need for acute care is still present, but its urgency declines and clients begin to address and plan for their future health care needs. In the continuing care phase the clients are able to participate in planning and implementing continuing care activities needed after discharge.

Probably the greatest challenge in effective discharge planning is communication. The communication problem can be minimized when an organization has a discharge coordinator or case manager responsible for discharge planning (Zander, 2002). Staff in these roles are responsible for thoroughly assessing a client's health care needs at discharge, identifying available and needed resources, linking the client and family to the proper resources, coordinating services (as appropriate), and following up on the client's progress following discharge.

Discharge from an agency can be stressful for the client and family members. Before a client is discharged, the client

BOX 1-5 Federal Requirements for Discharge Planning Process

- Hospitals must identify at an early stage of hospitalization clients who are likely to suffer adverse health consequences upon discharge if there is no planning.
- The hospital must provide a discharge planning evaluation.
- A registered nurse, social worker, or other qualified person must develop or supervise development of the evaluation.
- Discharge planning must include an evaluation of the likelihood of the client needing posthospital services and of the availability of the services.
- Discharge planning must include an evaluation of the likelihood of a client's capacity for self-care.
- Upon request of the client's physician, the hospital must arrange for development and implementation of the client's discharge plan.
- The evaluation must be completed on a timely basis so that appropriate arrangements for posthospital care are made before discharge and to avoid unnecessary delays in discharge.
- The discharge planning evaluation must be in the client's medical record, and the results must be discussed with the client and/or significant others.
- The client and family members must be counseled to prepare them for posthospital care.

Modified from Centers for Medicare and Medicaid Services: Discharge planning: conditions of participation, *Federal Register* 482.43, 2002.

and family must know how to manage care in the home and what to expect in regard to any continuing physical problems. Without the necessary equipment and professional resources, the client risks loss of rehabilitation gains made before discharge. Failure to understand restrictions or implications of health problems may cause a client to develop complications. For example, to control blood glucose levels, an adolescent newly diagnosed with diabetes mellitus must receive education on diabetes self-management, supplies (such as insulin, syringes, and a blood glucose monitor), and information regarding community resources. Without any one of these components, the adolescent is at risk for developing hyperglycemia, hypoglycemia, or long-term vascular complications associated with the disease. Poor discharge planning ignores the client's needs within the home and increases the chance of the client needing to reenter the health care system prematurely.

DELEGATION CONSIDERATIONS

The skill of discharging clients should not be delegated to assistive personnel. However, the following activities may be delegated: gathering and securing the client's personal items and any supplies that may accompany the client, and assisting with transporting the client to the discharge transport vehicle.

EQUIPMENT

- ❑ Wheelchair or stretcher
- ❑ Discharge instruction forms

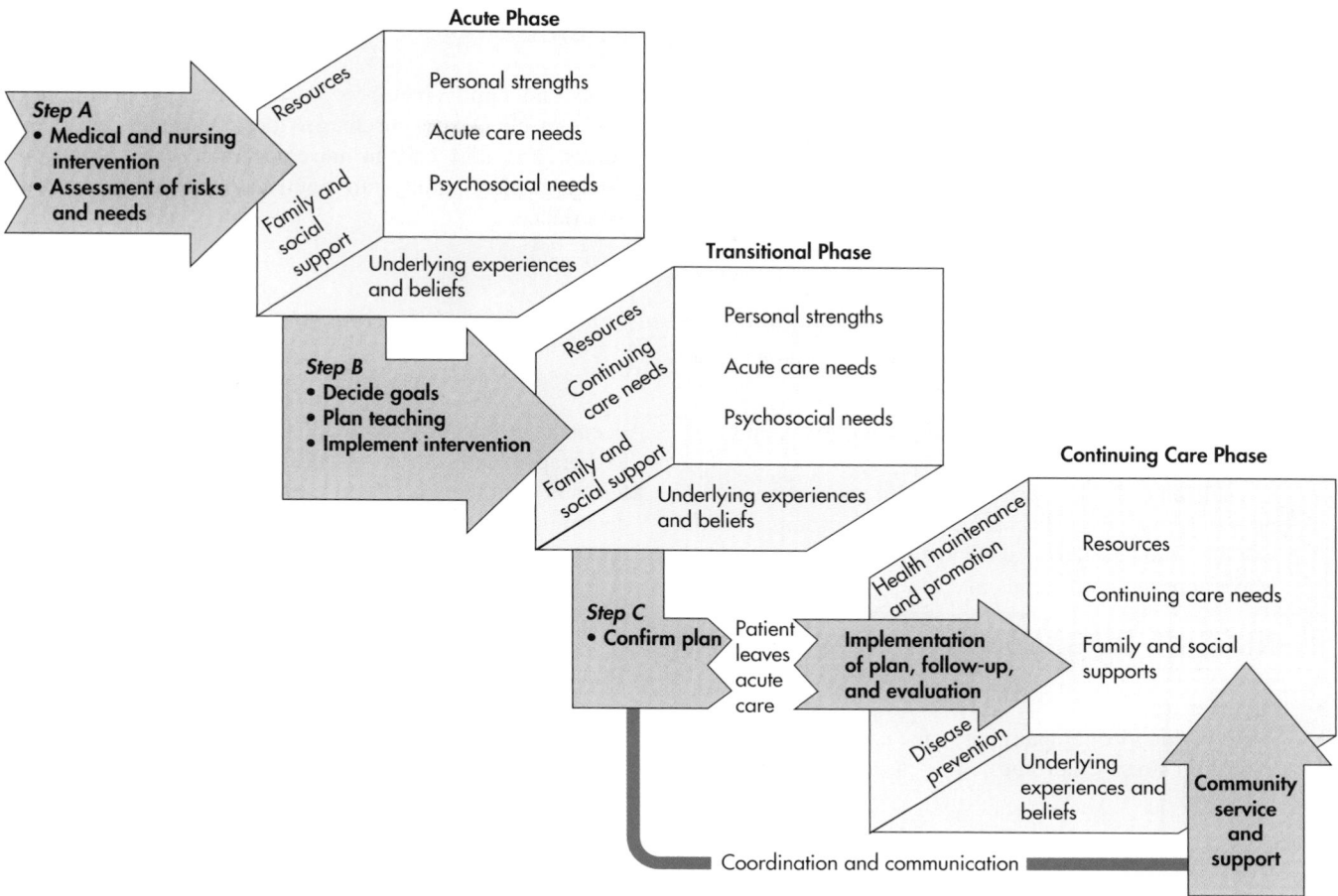

FIGURE **1-2** Phases of discharge planning process. (Redrawn from Rorden JW, Taft E: *Discharge planning guide for nurses,* Philadelphia, 1990, W.B. Saunders.)

STEP	RATIONALE

ASSESSMENT

1. From time of admission, assess client's discharge needs using nursing history, discussions with client, and care plan; focus on ongoing assessments of client's physical health, functional status, psychosocial support system, financial resources, health values, cultural and ethnic background, level of education, and barriers to care.

Plan for discharge begins at admission and continues throughout client's stay in agency. Discharge planning interventions will focus on assisting clients in achieving maximal functioning.

2. Assess client's and family's need for health teaching related to how to perform home therapies, use of home medical equipment, restrictions resulting from health alterations, and possible complications.

Improves understanding of health care needs and ability to achieve self-care at home. Inclusion of family member in teaching sessions provides client with available resource.

3. Assess with client and family for any environmental factors within home that might interfere with self-care (e.g., size of rooms, doorway clearances, steps, bathroom facilities, availability of utilities). (A home care nurse may be available on referral to assist with assessment.)

Environmental factors within the client's home may pose safety risks. For example, throw rugs may be a fall hazard for a client discharged with crutches or a walker (see Chapter 41).

4. Collaborate with physician and staff in other disciplines (e.g., physical therapy) in assessing need for referral for skilled home care services or extended care facility.

Clients eligible for home care are confined to home as result of illness, are under physician's care, and require skilled nursing care on an intermittent basis. A multidisciplinary assessment ensures a comprehensive discharge plan.

STEP	RATIONALE
5. Assess client's and family's perceptions of continued health care needs outside the hospital. Include an assessment of family caregiver's perceived ability to provide care to client.	Clients and family members may disagree on health care needs of client after discharge. Identifying these discrepancies early may help in more accurately developing the discharge plan. Family caregiving can be a highly stressful experience.

• *Critical Decision Point*
It may be necessary to talk with client and family separately to learn about true concerns or doubts.

6. Assess client's acceptance of health problems and related restrictions.	Acceptance of health status can affect willingness to adhere to therapies and restrictions after discharge.
7. Consult other health care team members about anticipated needs after discharge (e.g., dietitian, social worker, clinical nurse specialist, home care nurse). Make appropriate referrals in a timely manner.	Members of all health care disciplines should collaborate to determine client's needs and functional abilities.

NURSING DIAGNOSES

- Anxiety
- Caregiver role strain
- Deficient knowledge regarding home care restrictions
- Relocation stress syndrome

- Interrupted family processes
- Fear
- Self-care deficit: feeding, toileting, dressing/grooming, bathing/hygiene
- Impaired home maintenance

Related factors are individualized based on client's condition or needs.

PLANNING

1. Expected outcomes following completion of procedure:	
• Client or family caregiver is able to explain how health care is to continue in home (or other facility), what treatments or medications are needed, and when to seek medical attention for problems.	Increases likelihood of care not being interrupted in home (or other facility).
• Client is able to demonstrate self-care activities (or family member is able to administer care measures).	Feedback ensures learning.
• Obstacles to client's mobility and ambulation are removed in home setting. Items that are hazards because of client's health restrictions are removed.	Client may be physically weakened or have physical changes resulting from illness that predispose client to injury.

IMPLEMENTATION

PREPARATION BEFORE DAY OF DISCHARGE

1. Suggest ways to change physical arrangement of home to meet client's needs (see Chapter 41).	Client's level of independence and ability to retain function can be maintained within safe environment.
2. Provide client and family with information about community health care resources (e.g., medical equipment companies, Meals on Wheels, adult day care). Referrals can be made while client is in hospital.	Community resources may offer services client or family cannot provide.

STEP	**RATIONALE**

3. After determining any barriers to learning and client's readiness to learn, conduct teaching sessions with client and family as soon as possible during hospitalization (e.g., signs and symptoms of complications, information regarding medications, use of medical equipment, follow-up care, diet, exercise, restrictions imposed by illness or surgery). Pamphlets, books, or videotapes may be given to client. Client may also be referred to resources on the Internet.

Gives client opportunities to practice new skills, ask questions, and obtain necessary feedback to ensure learning.

• *Critical Decision Point*
Different types of educational materials may be effective with different individual learning styles. Assess how client prefers to learn (e.g., read, watch video, listen to instructions). If printed material is to be used, be sure material at proper reading level is available.

4. Communicate client's and family's response to teaching and proposed discharge plan to other health care team members involved in client's care.

Facilitates development of individualized discharge plan.

DAY OF DISCHARGE

• *Critical Decision Point*
If any of the following activities can be completed before day of discharge, planning will be more effective.

5. Let client and family ask questions or discuss issues related to home care. A final opportunity to demonstrate learned skills may also be helpful.

Allows for final clarification of information previously discussed. Helps relieve anxiety.

6. Check physician's discharge orders for prescriptions, change in treatments, or need for special medical equipment. (Orders should be written as early as possible.) Arrangements should be made for delivery and setup of equipment before the client arrives home (e.g., hospital bed, oxygen, feeding pump).

Discharge is authorized only by physician. Early check of orders permits nurse to attend to any last-minute treatments or procedures well before discharge.

7. Determine whether client or family has arranged for transportation home.

Client's condition at discharge determines method of transport.

8. Offer assistance as client dresses and packs all personal belongings. Provide privacy as needed.

9. Check all closets and drawers for belongings. Obtain copy of valuables list signed by client, and have security or appropriate administrator deliver valuables to client.

Prevents loss of personal items. Client's signature verifies receipt of items and relieves nursing department of liability for losses.

10. Provide client with prescriptions or pharmacy-dispensed medications ordered by physician. Offer a final review of any information needed to facilitate safe medication self-administration.

Review of drug information provides feedback to determine client's success in learning about medications.

11. Provide information on any follow-up appointments to the physician's office.

Ensure continuity of care to prevent rehospitalization.
Source of concern for many clients is whether agency has accepted insurance or other payment forms.

STEP	RATIONALE

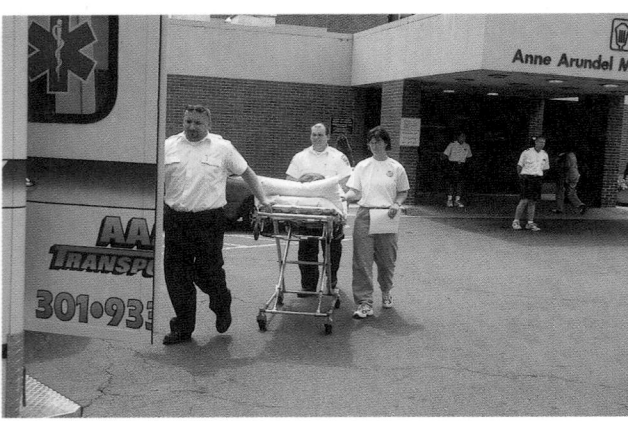

A

B

STEP **14 A,** Nurse escorts the client to the transport vehicle at the time of discharge via a wheelchair. **B,** Many clients are discharged via stretcher.

12. Contact agency's business office to determine whether client needs to finalize arrangements for payment of bill. Arrange for client or family to visit office.

Provides for safe transport.

13. Acquire utility cart to move client's belongings. Obtain wheelchair for clients unable to ambulate. Clients leaving by ambulance are transported on ambulance stretchers.

14. Assist client to wheelchair or stretcher using proper body mechanics and transfer techniques. Escort client to entrance of agency where source of transportation is waiting (see agency policy) (see illustrations). Lock wheelchair wheels. Assist client in transferring into automobile or transport vehicle. Help family place personal belongings in vehicle.

Prevents injury to nurse and client. Agency policy requires escort to ensure client's safe exit. Agency's liability ends once client is safely in vehicle.

15. Return to division, and notify admitting or appropriate department of time of discharge. Notify housekeeping of need to clean client's room.

Allows agency to prepare for admission of next client.

EVALUATION

1. Ask client or family member to describe nature of illness, treatment regimens, and physical signs or symptoms to be reported to a physician.

Measures client's or family's learning.

2. Have client or family member perform any treatments to be continued in the home.

Return demonstrations allow nurse to evaluate level of learning.

3. Home care nurse inspects home, identifies obstacles that pose risks for client, and recommends revisions.

Continuity of care is achieved.

Recording and Reporting

- Complete documentation of client's discharge on discharge summary form (Box 1-6). Client should receive signed copy of form.
- Document any unresolved problems and description of arrangements made for resolution in nurses' notes.
- Complete documentation in nurses' notes of client's vital signs and status of client's health problems at time of discharge.

BOX 1-6   Elements of a Written Discharge Summary Form

- Mode of discharge: ambulatory, wheelchair, stretcher
- Instructions for self-care activities: activity, diet, medications, special treatments such as wound care, self-catheterization, tracheostomy care
- List of discharge medications with dose, frequency, and route
- Signs and symptoms of complications or drug reactions to be observant for

- Signs and symptoms that are to be normally expected by the client
- Correct settings for any equipment required
- Planned follow-up appointment at physician's office, clinic
- Explanation of pertinent emergency procedures
- Client's signature, showing understanding of instructions

Unexpected Outcomes	Related Interventions
1. Client or family is unable to explain self-care measures.	• Provide immediate clarification or offer reinstruction.
2. Client or family demonstrates treatment measures incorrectly.	• Plan additional time to demonstrate treatment measures to client and family. • Ask client to explain what aspect of procedure is difficult to perform and why.
3. Risks continue to be present in home.	• Family or client may discount risk or may not have resources to make needed changes. • Home care nurse should attempt to problem solve and seek appropriate solution.
4. Client or family resists discharge plans and refuses assimilation of new roles needed for home care.	• Contact additional resources (e.g., social work, home care, pastoral care) to assist client and family with home care needs.
5. Client refuses continued treatment and requests to leave the hospital before planned discharge.	• Talk with client to determine why they are requesting to leave the hospital. As possible, attempt to resolve the pressing issue for the client; involve family and social work as appropriate. • Notify physician to allow physician to talk with client and explain the risks of leaving the hospital with unresolved health care needs and the benefits of continued treatment. • Request that client sign discharge against medical advice (AMA) form documenting that he or she understands the risk of leaving. • Complete incident report, and document thoroughly all communications/action taken in attempt to have client continue treatment.

Teaching Considerations

- Assess client's fatigue and pain levels before undertaking any teaching activity. Keep focused on the important teaching topics to cover. Include family or significant other as appropriate.
- Consider client's cultural, social, and educational background when developing a discharge teaching plan.

Pediatric Considerations

- Once family members have learned how to perform any necessary caregiver skills, have them assume care before child returns home. Many hospitals incorporate a trial period requiring family to manage care before child's discharge home (Hockenberry and others, 2003).
- The goal for home care program for infants, children, or adolescents with chronic conditions is provision of comprehensive, cost-effective health care within a nurturing home environment (American Academy of Pediatrics, 1995).

Gerontological Considerations

- Research has demonstrated that older adults are vulnerable to poor outcomes during the first few weeks after discharge. This reinforces the importance of either telephone or home care follow-up for older adults after discharge to address needs associated with functional decline and, in doing so, to prevent costly readmissions (Naylor and others, 1994).

- Older adults and their families may overestimate their ability to manage care after discharge. They may also disagree about what postdischarge care includes.

Home Care Considerations

- Assess availability and skill of primary caregiver (e.g., spouse or neighbor): assess time availability, ability and willingness to give care, emotional and physical stamina, and knowledge of caregiving. Assess additional resources, including friends or neighbors who are available to help.
- Assess attitude of immediate family members: ability to adjust to demands of client care, impact of care demands on their lives (e.g., reducing noise levels in home, preparing special diets), and potential ongoing nature of client's needs. Family members who are not properly prepared for their role as caregivers may be overwhelmed by client's needs, which can lead to neglect or unnecessary hospital readmissions.

- Assess referral for appropriateness of client admission to home care agency based on the following admission criteria:
  - Client is confined to place of residence (homebound).
  - Client is under care of a physician.
  - Client needs part-time or intermittent skilled nursing services.
  - Reasonable expectation exists that client's medical, nursing, and social needs can be adequately met by home care agency in client's place of residence.
  - Home care services are necessary and reasonable for treatment of client's illness or injury.
- Document client intake information on home care admission referral form. Ensure that information is complete. Discrepancies have been noted between information home care nurses deem essential and information that they actually receive from agency discharging client (Anderson and Helms, 1995).
- Inform client or family member and client's physician as to decision to accept or not accept client for admission to home care agency.

FOCUS *on* CLINICAL PRACTICE

Mr. Johnston, a 78-year-old retired accountant, presented to the emergency department (ED) with acute confusion. He has a history of congestive heart failure, type 1 diabetes, and falls. He is being admitted to your nursing division. The emergency department nurse calls you to give report on the assessment she has made and the care provided in the ED. She notes the admitting diagnosis, vital signs (temperature, pulse, respiration, blood pressure, and pain level), and ED physician orders, and she lists which of those orders have been implemented.

1. What other information would you like to have about this client?
2. The admitting clerk calls you to determine the appropriate room location for Mr. Johnston. What can you do to reduce the risk of falls for Mr. Johnston?

3. The technician arrives with Mr. Johnston in a wheelchair; he is accompanied by his wife. You introduce yourself to Mr. and Mrs. Johnston, explain that you are the nurse that will be caring for Mr. Johnston during the day shift, and accompany them to the assigned room. During your interactions it is clear that Mr. Johnston is very anxious and only comforted by the presence and reorientation of his wife. What interventions would you select to reduce the client's anxiety and increase his level of orientation?
4. Mrs. Johnston states her husband has an advance directive. What is the role of the nurse in understanding a client's advance directive?

NCLEX REVIEW QUESTIONS

1. During the registration process, the admission clerk should not provide the client with:
    1. Information about client rights
    2. Information about advance directives
    3. Identification band
    4. Allergy band

2. The client discharge plan should be developed by:
    1. Team members of each discipline involved in the care of the client
    2. The discharge planner
    3. The primary nurse
    4. The nurse manager

3. The clinical status of the client should be assessed and documented immediately before transfer or discharge to:
    1. Increase reimbursement to the hospital
    2. Identify any potential changes in clinical needs of the client that may prevent transfer/discharge or may require nursing intervention to provide for client safety during transport
    3. Fulfill hospital documentation requirements
    4. Provide the necessary information to reflect a discharge plan for accrediting agencies

References

Centers for Medicare and Medicaid Services: Discharge planning: conditions of participation, *Federal Register* 482.43, 2002.

Centers for Medicare and Medicaid Services: Emergency Medical Treatment and Labor Act, *Federal Register* 413.65, 2002a.

Centers for Medicare and Medicaid Services: Health Insurance Portability and Accountability Act, *Federal Register* 164, 2002b.

Centers for Medicare and Medicaid Services: Patient rights: condition of participation, *Federal Register* 482.13, 2002.

Galanti GA: *Caring for patients with different cultures,* Philadelphia, 2003, University of Pennsylvania Press.

Joint Commission on Accreditation of Healthcare Organizations: *Comprehensive accreditation manual for hospitals: the official handbook,* Chicago, 2004, The Commission.

Lueckenotte AG: *Gerontologic nursing,* St. Louis, 2000, Mosby.

Robinson G: *Essential Judaism: a complete guide to beliefs, customs and rituals,* New York, 2000, Pocket Books.

Zander K: Nursing case management in the 21st century: intervening where margin meets mission, *Nurs Adm Q* 26(5):58, 2002.

Research References

American Academy of Pediatrics, Committee on Children With Disabilities: Guidelines for home care of infants, children, and adolescents with chronic disease, *Pediatrics* 96(1):161, 1995.

Anderson M, Helms L: Communication between continuing care organizations, *Res Nurs Health* 18(1):49, 1995.

Bodnar A, Leinenger M: Transcultural nursing care of American Gypsies: In Leininger, editor: *Transcultural nursing, concepts, theories, research, and practice,* New York, 1995, McGraw-Hill.

Cleary M and others: Consumer feedback on nursing care and discharge planning, *J Adv Nurs* 42(3): 269, 2003.

Clark K, Normile B: Delays in implementing admission orders for critical care patients associated with length of stay in emergency departments in six mid-Atlantic states, *J Emerg Nurs* 28(6):489, 2002.

Ebersole P and others: *Toward healthy aging: human needs and nursing response,* ed 6, St. Louis, 2004, Mosby.

Fadiman A: *The spirit catches you and you fall down,* New York, 1999, Farrar, Straus & Giroux.

Hockenberry MJ and others: W*ong's nursing care of infants and children,* ed 7, St. Louis, 2003, Mosby.

Hou JW and others: Can physicians' admission evaluation of patients' status help to identify patients requiring social work interventions? *Soc Work Health Care* 33(2):17, 2001.

Naylor M and others: Comprehensive discharge planning for the hospitalized elderly: a randomized clinical trial, *Ann Intern Med* 120(12):999, 1994.

Wells DL and others: Evaluation of an integrated model of discharge planning: achieving quality discharges in an efficient and ethical way, *Can J Nurs Res* 34(3):103, 2002.

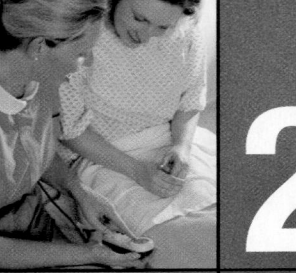

2

Communication

MEDIA RESOURCES

Evolve Site *evolve*

http://evolve.elsevier.com/Perry/skills

- Weblinks
- Video clips
- Mosby's Nursing Skills Video Exercises

Mosby's Nursing Skills Videos/CD-ROM

- *Basic Principles Video:* Communication, including oral, written, nonverbal reporting, charting end-of-shift report, guidelines for effective communication; roles and responsibilities of nursing team members

OBJECTIVES

Mastery of content in this chaper will enable the nurse to:

- Identify guidelines to use in therapeutic communication.
- Explain the communication process.
- Identify the purpose of therapeutic communication, communication in various phases of the nurse-client relationship, and special issues related to communication.
- Develop skills for therapeutic communication in various phases of the nurse-client relationship and special situations related to communication.

KEY TERMS

Active listening
Cadence
Clarifying
Comforting
De-escalation
Empathy
Interviewing
Orientation phase

Paraphrasing
Reflecting
Restating
Summarizing
Termination phase
Therapeutic silence
Working phase

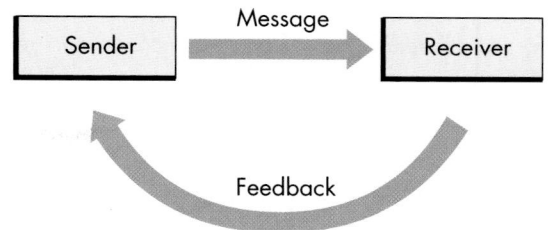

FIGURE **2-1** Communication is a two-way process.

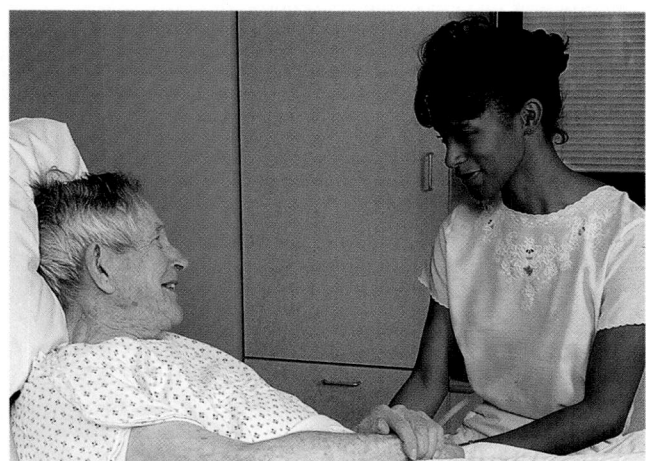

FIGURE **2-2** An open, relaxed posture conveys interest.

A nurse's responsibility to effectively communicate extends beyond the client to include family members/significant others and members of the health care team. Therefore nurses must possess effective communication skills as a part of their fundamental nursing knowledge base. This chapter does not intend to give a complete introduction to the complicated process of communication. Rather, the purpose of this chapter is to provide a framework by which nurses can develop therapeutic skills that are essential to the communication process.

Communication is an interaction between two or more persons that involves the exchange of information between a sender and a receiver (Figure 2-1). It is an essential component of the human experience, involving the expression of emotions, ideas, and thoughts through verbal (words or written language) and nonverbal (behaviors) exchanges. Therapeutic communication is an application of the process of communication to promote the well-being of the client.

Verbal communication includes both spoken word and written word. The sender of verbal communication must be aware of the tone, volume, and cadence (pace or rate) of voice to send an accurate message. In addition, the sender of verbal communication must be aware of cultural differences between sender and receiver, such as the use of jargon or slang. Other issues the sender must consider with written communication include barriers such as cognitive and visual impairments of the receiver. In addition, the developmental perspectives of the client should be taken into consideration, because these may influence the method of communication used.

Nonverbal communication describes all behaviors that convey messages without the use of words. This type of communication includes body movement, physical appearance, personal space, and touch. The sender of nonverbal communication must be aware of body language, which includes the sender's posture, body position, gestures, eye contact, facial expression, and movement (Figure 2-2). For clarity, nonverbal communication should be consistent with the spoken word. When assessing a client's needs, one should assess the nonverbal messages received from the client and validate them. For example, if the client is observed to be wringing his or her hands and sighing often, the nurse may ask, "You seem anxious today. Is there anything on your mind?" Problems in language behavior can be avoided through the consistent use of clear, mutually understood verbal terminology and nonverbal gestures. A nurse must be aware of any cultural norms or values (e.g., eye contact) to which the client may adhere to avoid misinterpretation of nonverbal cues (see Skill 2-4).

Communication is essential to excellent nursing practice. Nurses use communication skills in caring for clients by providing information, providing comfort, promoting understanding, clarifying misinformation, assisting in developing plans of care, and facilitating wellness through client teaching. The nurse-client relationship promotes a connection, which is an essential component of the healing process.

There are several key components of effective communication: self-awareness, empathy, genuineness, and respect for the client as a unique person. Self-awareness enables both the nurse and the client to be aware of the feelings they have about themselves and others, as well as the feelings about the content of the messages sent and received. Genuineness, empathy, and respect also are key elements for the nurse to possess. Each helps to convey a sense of caring. Other components that may affect therapeutic nurse-client communication include nonverbal cues, culture, and previous experience. When initially interviewing the client, the nurse assesses personal, family, and community strengths and resources. Special situations with clients that may hinder the communication process include the noncommunicative client, the hostile/aggressive client, and the noncompliant client.

Evidence-Based Practice Trends

Effective communication with clients across the life span is essential for effective nursing practice. Nurses have developed creative modes of communicating with clients in a variety of settings. For example, when interacting with clients with severe communication impairments, nurses have employed alternative modes of communication. These include use of augmentative communicative devices, including picture books and communication software, and collaboration with speech pathologists (Hemsley and others, 2001).

Managing clients with behavioral and/or cognitive impairments is challenging and requires communication skills to assess and redirect the client and to modify any negative behaviors. Research has shown that specific behavior management strategies learned during formal staff training was effective in reducing agitation and improving interactions with behaviorally disturbed clients who reside in nursing homes (see Skills 2-2 and 2-3) (Burgio and others, 2002). In addition, nurses employed in geriatric settings who participated in video training programs on the use of effective communication skills reported having increased knowledge and competence when interacting with clients who have communication difficulties. For example, the nurses used more open-ended questions with clients. Also, the nurses who took part in the training were perceived more positively by the clients (Bryan and others, 2002; Caris-Verhallen and others, 2000).

Physiological factors such as pain may hinder communication between the nurse and the client. Initial research on nurses' assessment of discomfort and pain in clients with dementia, who were unable to adequately report their physical condition, showed that the assessment protocol helped the nurses to identify pain in these clients and to provide pharmacological and nonpharmacological pain relief (Kovach and others, 2001). Regarding pain management in the pediatric setting, study findings concluded that poor communication between the nurses and the parents, as well as the nurses' knowledge deficits regarding the assessment of pain in children, contributed to ineffective pain management in postoperative pediatric clients. Two key nursing implications that arose from this research were the need to increase the nurses' knowledge about pain and the need for nurses to have realistic expectations of the parents. Both of these implications improved communication (see Skill 2-3) (Simons and Roberson, 2002).

Communicating With Culturally Diverse Clients

Nurses face challenges when communicating with culturally and linguistically diverse clients. Effective communication between the client and the nurse is essential to improve health outcomes. Research has demonstrated that providing both general and disease-specific information to clients in a culturally sensitive manner may improve chronic illness self-management (Piette and others, 2003). A survey conducted among nurses who work with culturally and linguistically diverse clients found the following factors essential to effectively care for these clients: (1) use of appropriate linguistic services (e.g., interpreter or bilingual health care workers) and/or other communication strategies and (2) a display of empathy and respect for culturally and linguistically diverse clients (Cioffi, 2003).

When nurses are communicating with clients of diverse cultures, an interpreter may be necessary. When using an interpreter, address the client and family directly; do not direct questions or comments to the interpreter. Take care to determine if understanding was achieved. Speak slowly in normal tones, and avoid overly technical jargon or terms unique to a culture (Box 2-1). Adopting a flexible, respectful attitude that also communicates interest in the client helps to bridge any communication barriers that exist due to cultural differences between client and caregiver.

Anxiety, anger, and depression are not conceptualized in some cultures in the same way as in Western culture, and they may be presented as somatic complaints because some cultures view illness as holistic and combine physical, psychological, and spiritual symptoms together (Park and others, 2002). For example, a client may speak of lack of sleep and appetite but deny sensation of anxiety. East Asian cultures, Cambodians, and Laotians may describe communicat-

---

BOX 2-1 Special Approaches to Clients Who Speak Different Languages

- Use a caring tone of voice and facial expressions to help alleviate clients' fears and anxieties.
- Speak slowly and distinctly, but not loudly.
- Use gestures, pictures, and playacting to help the client understand.
- Repeat the message in different ways if necessary.
- Be alert to and use words the client seems to understand.
- Keep messages simple.
- Avoid jargon.
- Use an appropriate language dictionary.

From Giger J, Davidhizar R: *Transcultural nursing: assessment and interventions*, ed 3, St. Louis, 1999, Mosby.

ing with dead ancestors as a coping mechanism for anxiety, and this is normal within their culture (Yick and Gupta, 2002). In addition, anger may be internalized and expressed in somatic complaints of heat, indigestion, or tachycardia.

Skill Performance Guidelines

1. Listen to what and how the client communicates, including content and verbal and nonverbal messages. Some clients express themselves clearly without difficulty. Often, however, indirect and nonverbal cues communicate a client's needs.

2. Nonverbal communication involves transmission of messages without the use of words. Personal appearance, tone of voice, facial expression, posture, gait, gestures, and touch are ways to convey nonverbal messages.

3. Know your own attitudes toward the client or situation. Being unaware of personal feelings can lead to negative consequences in communication. To control what and how issues are communicated, nurses must first be aware of their personal feelings.

4. Control external factors in both the environmental setting (temperature of room, privacy issues) and the psy-chological setting (emotional state of the nurse and client) that influence or hinder communication. If the nurse is talking with the client about the client's personal concerns, privacy is important. When teaching, the nurse may want to have a family member/significant other present with whom to reinforce the content of the instruction. If the client is experiencing subjective distress in the form of pain or anxiety, measures should be taken to minimize these subjective experiences. Controlling noise level and interruptions may also be important.

5. Establish and understand the purpose of interaction. This is an essential quality of effective communication. Without this quality, communication is casual and superficial.

6. Guide the interaction depending on the client's condition and response. Client needs remain the focus of the interaction. For example, a nurse establishes that the purpose of the interaction is client teaching; however, the client just learned about of the death of a loved one and expresses the need to talk about the death. The nurse assists the client with grieving and thus remains flexible and creative in the interaction.

SKILL 2-1   Establishing the Nurse-Client Relationship

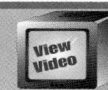

A therapeutic nurse-client relationship is considered the foundation of nursing care and involves client-centered goal-directed interactions using therapeutic communication skills (Hagerty and Patusky, 2003). The primary goal of effective therapeutic communication for the nurse is to promote wellness and personal growth in clients. Therapeutic communication empowers clients to make decisions but differs from social communication in that it is client centered and goal directed with limited disclosure from the professional. Social communication involves equal opportunity for personal disclosure, and both participants seek to have personal needs met (Keltner and others, 2003). Nurses do not share intimate details of their personal lives with clients. However, the use of personal self-disclosure is used with caution and only in selected situations. Personal self-disclosure by the nurse may be used for the following goals: (1) to educate the client, (2) to build the therapeutic alliance with the client, and (3) to foster the client's autonomy (Fortinash and Holoday-Worret, 2004). For example, nurses may share selected personal thoughts and life experiences with clients to demonstrate that they understand what the client is going through.

Skills that are essential to therapeutic communication include active listening, clarifying, comforting, focusing, genuineness, informing, interviewing, paraphrasing, reflecting, restating, summarizing, suggesting, use of therapeutic si-lence, and use of open-ended statements/questions. Some of these skills are defined with case illustrations identifying therapeutic and nontherapeutic examples of their use (Box 2-2). Paraphrasing involves restating the client's original message by transforming the message into the nurse's own words without losing the meaning. Empathy in communication is achieved through the use of the aforementioned skills. Empathy is being sensitive and understanding of the client's feelings and communicating this understanding to the client. It differs from sympathy in that sympathy is nonobjective and noncritical.

Barriers to therapeutic communication include giving an opinion, offering false reassurance, being defensive, showing approval or disapproval, stereotyping, and asking "why?" The therapeutic nurse-client relationship is goal directed, with the client moving toward productive modes of interpersonal functioning. The nurse-client relationship is characterized by three overlapping phases: orientation, working, and termination (Hagerty and Patusky, 2003). The orientation phase involves learning about the client and any initial concerns and needs. In the orientation phase, roles of the nurse or other health care providers are clarified, information is collected, goals are established, misunderstandings are clarified, and rapport is established between the nurse and the client. When the strategies of the orientation

BOX 2-2   Therapeutic Communication Techniques

TECHNIQUE: LISTENING

Definition: An active process of receiving information and examining one's reaction to messages received

Example: Within the cultural practice of your client, maintain eye contact and be receptive to nonverbal communications.

Therapeutic Value: Nonverbally communicates nurse's interest and acceptance to client

Nontherapeutic Threat: Failure to listen, interrupting client

TECHNIQUE: BROAD OPENINGS

Definition: Encouraging client to select topics for discussion

Example: "What are you thinking about?"

Therapeutic Value: Indicates acceptance by nurse and value of client's initiative

Nontherapeutic Threat: Domination of interaction by nurse; rejecting responses

TECHNIQUE: RESTATING

Definition: Repeating main thought client has expressed

Example: "You say that your mother left you when you were 5 years old."

Therapeutic Value: Indicates nurse is listening and validates, reinforces, or calls attention to something important that has been said

Nontherapeutic Threat: Lack of validation of nurse's interpretation of message; being judgmental; reassuring; defending

TECHNIQUE: CLARIFICATION

Definition: Attempting to put into words vague ideas or unclear thoughts of client to enhance the nurse's understanding or asking client to explain what he or she means

Example: "I'm not sure what you mean. Could you tell me again?"

Therapeutic Value: Helps to clarify client's feelings, ideas, and perceptions and to provide an explicit correlation between them and the client's actions

Nontherapeutic Threat: Failure to probe; assumed understanding

TECHNIQUE: REFLECTION

Definition: Directing back to client ideas, feelings, questions, or content

Example: "You're feeling tense and anxious, and it's related to a conversation you had with your sister last night?"

Therapeutic Value: Validates nurse's understanding of what client is saying and signifies empathy, interest, and respect for client

Nontherapeutic Threat: Stereotyping client's responses, inappropriate timing of reflections; inappropriate depth of feeling of reflections; inappropriate to the cultural experience and educational level of the client

TECHNIQUE: HUMOR

Definition: Discharge of energy through comic enjoyment of the imperfect

Example: "This gives a whole new meaning to 'Just relax.'"

Therapeutic Value: Can promote insight by making conscious repressed material, resolving paradoxes, tempering aggression, revealing new options, and is a socially acceptable form of sublimation

Nontherapeutic Threat: Indiscriminate use; belittling client; screen to avoid therapeutic intimacy

TECHNIQUE: INFORMING

Definition: Skill or informing giving

Example: "I think it would be helpful for you to know more about how your medication works."

Therapeutic Value: Helpful in client education about relevant aspects of client's well-being and self-care

Nontherapeutic Threat: Giving advice

TECHNIQUE: FOCUSING

Definition: Questions or statements that help client expand on a topic of importance

Example: "I think it would be helpful if we talk more about your relationship with your father."

Therapeutic Value: Allows client to discuss central issues related to problem and keeps communication process goal directed

Nontherapeutic Threat: Allowing abstractions and generalizations; changing topics

TECHNIQUE: SHARING PERCEPTIONS

Definition: Asking client to verify nurse's understanding of what client is thinking or feeling

Example: "You're smiling, but I sense that you are really very angry with me."

Therapeutic Value: Conveys nurse's understanding to client and has potential for clearing up confusing communication

Nontherapeutic Threat: Challenging client; accepting literal responses; reassuring; testing; defending

TECHNIQUE: THEME IDENTIFICATION

Definition: Underlying issues or problems experienced by client that emerge repeatedly during nurse-client relationship

Example: "I've noticed that in all the relationships that you have described, you've been hurt or rejected by the man. Do you think this is an underlying issue?"

Therapeutic Value: Allows nurse to best promote client's exploration and understanding of important problems

Nontherapeutic Threat: Giving advice; reassuring; disapproving

TECHNIQUE: SILENCE

Definition: Lack of verbal communication for a therapeutic reason

Example: Sitting with client and nonverbally communicating interest and involvement

Therapeutic Value: Allows client time to think and gain insights, slows the pace of the interaction, and encourages client to initiate conversation, while conveying nurse's support, understanding, and acceptance

Nontherapeutic Threat: Questioning client: asking for "why" responses; failure to break a nontherapeutic silence

TECHNIQUE: SUGGESTING

Definition: Presentation of alternative ideas for client's consideration relative to problem solving

Example: "Have you thought about responding to your boss in a different way when he raises that issue with you? For example, you could ask him whether a specific problem has occurred."

Therapeutic Value: Increases client's perceived options or choices

Nontherapeutic Threat: Giving advice, inappropriate timing; being judgmental

Modified from Stuart GW, Laraia M: *Principles and practice of psychiatric nursing*, ed 7, St. Louis, 2001, Mosby.

phase are successful and the client is ready, the work toward effective goal attainment can begin with the working phase of the nurse-client relationship. The termination phase consists of evaluation and summary of progress toward pre-scribed goals. A nurse prepares for termination generally at the beginning of the relationship. The nurse must communicate effectively with clients throughout all three phases of the nurse-client relationship.

DELEGATION CONSIDERATIONS

Therapeutic communication is a goal of all client interactions, delegated or not. Establishing therapeutic communication is a skill that can be delegated to assistive personnel following appropriate instruction. However, before delegation of this skill, assistive personnel must be informed of the proper way to interact verbally and nonverbally with the client and of environmental considerations, such as privacy and confidentiality. The following skills should be reviewed: communicating with the cognitively or sensorially impaired client, the older client, the pediatric client, the anxious client, and the potentially violent client if warranted according to the nursing assessment.

STEP	RATIONALE

ASSESSMENT

1. First contact nurse has with client occurs during the orientation phase when nurse assesses the following behaviors: client's needs, coping strategies, defenses, and adaptation styles.

   Recurrent themes in client's response help to identify problem areas related to health status (e.g., avoidance of questions, request for information, expression of a loss).

2. Determine client's need to communicate (e.g., client who constantly uses call light, client who is crying, client who does not understand an illness, client who has just been admitted to the hospital or nursing home).

   Clients in need of support, comfort, knowledge, or encouragement can benefit from meaningful communication.

3. Assess reason client needs health care.

   Nature of illness can affect client's coping ability and effectiveness in communicating needs and concerns.

4. Assess factors about self and client that normally influence communication: perceptions, values, and beliefs; emotions; sociocultural background; severity of illness; knowledge; age; verbal ability; roles and relationships; environmental setting; physical comfort or discomfort (Figure 2-3).

   Communication is a dynamic process influenced by interpersonal and intrapersonal processes. By assessing factors that influence communication, nurse can more accurately assess experiences of client (Parsons, 2002).

5. Nurse assesses own barriers to communication with client (e.g., bias toward client's condition, anxiety from inexperience).

   Barriers prevent nurse from conveying empathy and caring and obtaining relevant assessment information (Leonard and Plotnikoff, 2000).

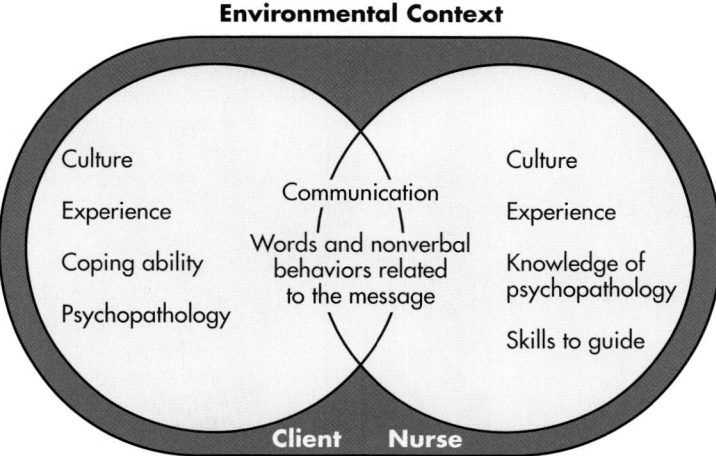

FIGURE 2-3 Essential and influencing variables of the therapeutic communication environment. (Modified from Keltner NL and others: *Psychiatric nursing,* ed 4, St. Louis, 2003, Mosby.)

STEP	RATIONALE

6. Assess client's language and ability to speak. Does client have difficulty finding words or associating ideas with accurate word symbols? Does client have difficulty with expression of language and/or reception of messages? What is client's primary language?

Assessment determines need for special communication techniques (e.g., picture boards; aids, such as an interpreter) (Figure 2-4) (Happ, 2001).

7. Assess client's ability to hear. Be sure hearing aid is functional if worn. Be sure client hears and understands words.

Clients with hearing deficits require techniques to enhance hearing reception (e.g., speaking in normal tone, speaking so client can see face).

8. Observe client's pattern of communication and verbal or nonverbal behavior (e.g., gestures, tone of voice, eye contact).

Client's patterns of communication may determine type of and manner of communication used by nurse.

9. Assess resources available in selecting communication methods:
    a. Review information available through chart, care plan, past experience, nursing assessment, client interview.
    b. Consult with family, physician, and other health care team members concerning client's condition, problems, impressions.

Relying totally on information from client can restrict the quality of interaction. Additional resources provide insight into best methods of communicating. The greater amount or quality of information nurse has, the greater the ability to understand and communicate with client. Collaboration with other health care team members facilitates nurse's response to client based on integration of knowledge (Dube and others, 2000).

10. Before initiating the working phase of nurse-client relationship, nurse assesses client's readiness to work toward goal attainment.

Client's goals are identified and agreed upon by effective communication skills such as restating and clarifying.

11. Consider when client is due to be discharged or transferred from health care agency.

Allows nurse to anticipate the amount of time available to work with client and when termination of relationship is to occur.

NURSING DIAGNOSES

- Anxiety
- Impaired verbal communication
- Ineffective coping (specify)
- Decisional conflict (specify)

- Fear
- Deficient knowledge (specify)
- Noncompliance (specify)
- Impaired social interaction

Related factors are individualized based on client's condition or needs.

PLANNING

1. Expected outcomes following completion of procedure:
    - A therapeutic relationship is established between nurse and client.

An effective connection is based on the client and the nurse getting to know each other. Trustworthiness is built when the nurse is honest regarding intentions (Keltner, and others, 2003).

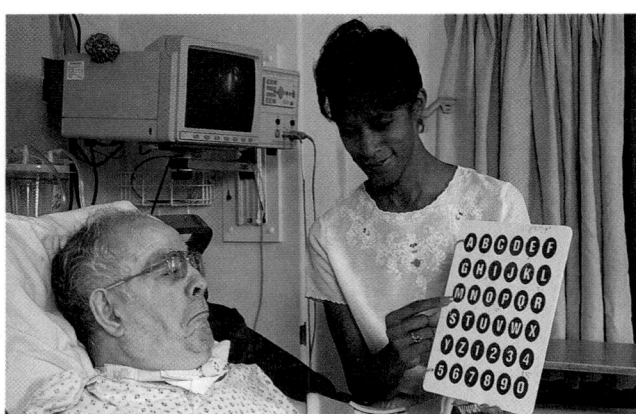

FIGURE **2-4** Tracheostomy interferes with speech.

STEP	RATIONALE
• Client is able to express ideas, fears, and concerns clearly and openly with relief of anxiety.	Once clients are able to talk directly about emotions, the focus can be on coping more effectively with them (Keltner and others, 2003).
• Client goals are identified and achieved.	Interaction remains client focused.
• Client understands information communicated by nurse.	This provides a means to build trust and develop a knowledge base for client to make decisions.
2. Prepare for communication during orientation phase by providing a warm and accepting environment, establishing trust, formulating individualized client goals, considering time allocation, formulating initial questions, and mentally preparing to keep one's mind clear of other concerns or distractions.	Preparation is part of planned process that facilitates communication and interaction. Planning for orientation phase assists in identifying actual or potential problems, current health status, and experience. Without understanding purpose of interaction, allowing adequate time, or preparing for communication, a greater risk exists of casual non–goal oriented communication that may fail to assist client in reaching a greater potential toward physical, psychological, social, and spiritual health.
3. Prepare client and environment physically by providing a quiet environment conducive to interaction, maintaining privacy, reducing distractions or interruptions, and taking care of client's physical needs before beginning discussion (e.g., attending to immediate comfort or hygiene needs).	Certain environments are more conducive to therapeutic interactions than others. Privacy is less threatening to client and promotes freer expression of feelings. Distractions and interruptions hinder adequate reception of the message. Taking care of basic needs decreases client distractions.
4. Prepare for communication during working phase by identifying strategies to achieve established goals, which includes development of a realistic plan to meet identified health goals of clients.	Preparation promotes goal attainment and avoids risk of misinterpretation.
5. Prepare for communication during termination phase by identifying methods of summarizing and synthesizing information pertinent for aftercare.	Effective communication by summarizing and synthesizing information reinforces behavior change.

IMPLEMENTATION

ORIENTATION PHASE

1. Create a climate of warmth and acceptance, considering both environmental factors (temperature of room, noise level) and emotional and physical state of client (presence of pain or anxiety). Be aware of nonverbal cues that are both sent and received. Provide comfort and support to client.	This facilitates open exchange without fear or anxiety.
2. Address client by name and introduce self and role on health care team ("Hello, my name is Sally, and I am the registered nurse assigned to take care of you today . . ."). Use clear, specific communication (verbal and nonverbal) to provide information and clarify concerns.	Congruent verbal and nonverbal communication conveys warmth and respect and helps to establish rapport. Clear, specific communication decreases confusion and anxiety.
3. Use appropriate nonverbal behaviors (e.g., good eye contact, open relaxed position, sitting eye level with client [see Figure 2-2]).	This facilitates communication by providing a nonverbal message that conveys nurse is interested in what client has to say.
4. Observe client's nonverbal behaviors, including body language. If client's verbal behaviors do not match nonverbal behaviors, nurse should seek clarification.	Congruence between client's verbal and nonverbal behaviors ensures correct message is received by nurse.
5. Explain purpose of interaction when information is to be shared.	Information and explanation can decrease anxiety about the unknown.

STEP	RATIONALE

- *Critical Decision Point*
  Establish a therapeutic environment in which client feels at ease, as well as conveying empathy to client while gathering data and helping client to identify the problem.

6. Use active listening.	Conveys interest in the client's needs, concerns, and problems; conveys empathy.
7. Identify client's expectations in seeking health care.	This conveys a level of interest in client's needs.
8. Interview the client to obtain information about the client's health state, lifestyle, support systems, patterns of health and illness, and strengths and limitations.	The interview process facilitates a positive nurse-client relationship and facilitates the development of trust, putting the client at ease.
9. Encourage client to ask for clarification at any time during the communication.	This gives client a sense of control and keeps channels of communication open.
10. Use therapeutic communication techniques when interacting with client (refer to Box 2-2).	Techniques serve to establish a greater understanding of messages sent and received.

WORKING PHASE

1. Use effective communication skills such as restating, reflecting, and paraphrasing to identify and clarify strategies for attainment of mutually agreed-upon goals.	Effective communication ensures clear understanding on part of client and improves ability of client to participate in care.
2. Problem areas are discussed and prioritized.	Client's anxiety is minimized through the nurse's nonjudgmental, supportive approach.
3. Provide information to client, and help client express needs and feelings.	Client is able to respond to help and fully participates in realistic plan to attain health-related goals. This helps client develop workable solutions based on goals that have meaning to client and that are supportive of client well-being (Fortin, 2002).
4. Use questions carefully and appropriately. Ask one question at a time, and allow sufficient time to answer. Use direct questions. Use open-ended statements as much as possible.	Assist clients in expressing self and allows nurse to obtain thorough information about client's needs and concerns.

- *Critical Decision Point*
  Avoid asking questions about information that may not have yet been disclosed to the client (e.g., human immunodeficiency virus [HIV] status). Avoid asking "why" questions; this may cause increased defensiveness in the client and may hinder communication.

5. Avoid communication barriers as discussed earlier in this chapter.	Communication breakdown occurs when a message is not received, is distorted, or is not understood. Communication may be hindered by nontherapeutic responses.

TERMINATION PHASE

1. Use effective communication skills to discuss discharge/termination issues and to guide discussion related to specific client changes in thoughts and behaviors.	Effective communication skills reinforce behaviors/skills learned during working phase of relationship.
2. Summarize with client what was discussed during interaction, including goal achievement.	Summary signals close of interaction, allows nurse and client to depart with same idea, and provides a sense of closure at completion of discussion. It mutually confirms understanding.

STEP	RATIONALE

EVALUATION

1. Observe client's verbal and nonverbal responses to your communication, noting client's willingness to share information and concerns during orientation phase.

2. Note your response to client and client's response to you. Evaluate effectiveness of therapeutic techniques used in establishing rapport with client. Consider use of alternative techniques if previous skills were ineffective.

3. During working phase, evaluate client's ability to work toward identified goals. Elicit feedback (verbal and nonverbal) to determine success of goal attainment. Evaluate client's health status in relation to identified goals. Reevaluate and identify barriers if client goals are not met.

4. During termination phase, use communication skills such as summarizing and restating. Client's strengths are reinforced, issues still requiring work are outlined, and an action plan is developed.

Both verbal and nonverbal feedback reveal client's interest and willingness to communicate and reflect client's ability to form a therapeutic relationship with nurse.
Sensitivity to one's own ability at using therapeutic communication skills can improve ability to adjust techniques when necessary.

Feedback is an essential step in evaluating new behaviors. Modifications must be made if goals cannot be met.

Client progress is evaluated, and recommendations are communicated. Health status of client is evaluated in terms of attainment of mutually agreed-upon goals.

Recording and Reporting

- Record in nurses' notes communication pertinent to client's health, response to illness or therapies, and responses that demonstrate understanding or lack of understanding (include verbal and nonverbal cues).
- Report any pertinent information obtained through client's verbal and nonverbal behaviors to members of health care team.

Unexpected Outcomes	Related Interventions
1. Client continues to verbally and nonverbally express feelings of anxiety, fear, anger, confusion, distrust, and helplessness. Client may be responding to internal and external factors and cues. Client may speak a different language.	• Assess client's level of anxiety, fear, and distrust. • Repeat message to client at a later time. • Use a caring tone of voice and facial expression to help alleviate fears of client who may speak a different language. • Assess for barriers to communication.
2. Feedback between nurse and client reveals a lack of understanding. Barriers to communication exist. ■ Nurse may have let own personal issues interfere with establishment of a therapeutic nurse-client relationship. ■ Nonverbal cues (e.g., poor eye contact, facial expressions, gestures) indicate ineffective communication, which may be due to misunderstanding, cultural issues, pain, or other health-related issues. ■ Client may speak a different language.	• Make appropriate adjustments to communication style. Use special approaches for clients who speak a different language, for example, use of gestures, pictures, and playacting to help client understand. • Consider cultural norms associated with eye contact, use of touch, personal space, and nonverbal behaviors. • Repeat message in different ways if necessary. • Avoid using medical terms that client may not understand. • Be alert to words client seems to understand, and use them frequently.
3. Nurse is unable to acquire information about client's ideas, fears, and concerns. Techniques used by nurse fail to promote client's willingness to communicate openly. Trust is not established. Goals are not identified and therefore cannot be achieved.	• Use alternative communication techniques to promote client's willingness to communicate openly. • Offer another professional for client to talk with to obtain necessary information.

Teaching Considerations

- Be aware of cultural and gender differences when interacting with clients. Plan for identified communication difficulties associated with culture, language, age, and gender. Use gestures, pictures, and playacting to help client understand. Be alert to literacy status. Be alert to words client seems to understand, and use them frequently.
- Client teaching should be individually tailored to meet needs of client. Teaching should always be conducted toward meeting client's learning needs with consideration for client's preferred methods for learning. This may include, but is not limited to, communicating through return demonstrations, computer-assisted learning tools, written information, audiovisual media, and checklists.

Pediatric Considerations

- Communicating with children requires an understanding of feelings and thought process from the child's perspective (Hockenberry and others, 2003).
- Use vocabulary that is familiar to child, based on child's level of understanding (age and development appropriate). Nurse must evaluate child's usual patterns of communication (Rutishauser, 2003).
- Nurse needs to understand child's cognitive, developmental, and functional level to select most appropriate communication techniques. Some age-appropriate communication techniques include storytelling and drawing (Hockenberry and others, 2003).

Gerontological Considerations

- Be aware of any cognitive or sensory impairment. Each client must be assessed individually, and nurse must avoid stereotyping older adults as having cognitive or sensory impairments (Moore and Miller, 2003).
- It is important to understand the value of good communication skills and importance of history and personality within older adult population in terms of providing both human and therapeutic responses. Regression to earlier defenses is normal and adaptive with this population, particularly when facing illness.
- Nurse should make sure older client with visual impairments uses assistive devices such as eyeglasses and large-print reading material to aid in communication.

Home Care Considerations

- Identify primary caregiver for client. This individual may be family member, friend, or neighbor.
- Assess level of understanding of client and primary caregiver regarding client's condition.
- Avoid making unnecessary changes in client's lifestyle, and incorporate client's daily habits into communication event (e.g., bathing and dressing client).

SKILL 2-2 Communicating With the Anxious Client

Clients in the health care setting may experience anxiety for a variety of reasons. A newly diagnosed illness, separation from loved ones, threat associated with diagnostic tests or surgical procedures, and expectations of life changes are just a few factors that can cause anxiety. How successfully a client copes with anxiety depends in part on previous experiences, the presence of other stressors, the significance of the event causing anxiety, and the availability of supportive resources. The nurse can be a support to the client. The nurse can help to decrease anxiety through effective communication. Communication methods reviewed in this skill assist the nurse in helping the anxious client clarify factors causing anxiety and to cope more effectively. There are four stages of anxiety with corresponding behavioral manifestations: mild, moderate, severe, and panic (Box 2-3).

BOX 2-3 Behavioral Manifestations of Anxiety: Stages of Anxiety

MILD ANXIETY

Increased auditory and visual perception
Increased awareness of relationships
Increased alertness
Able to problem solve

MODERATE ANXIETY

Selective inattention
Decreased perceptual field
Focus only on relevant information
Muscle tension; diaphoresis

SEVERE ANXIETY

Focus on fragmented details
Headache, nausea, dizziness
Unable to see connections between details
Poor recall

PANIC STATE OF ANXIETY

Does not notice surroundings
Feeling of terror
Unable to cope with any problem

DELEGATION CONSIDERATIONS

Communication with an anxious client is best managed by a professional nurse. However, therapeutic communication is important in all client interactions. Communicating effectively with the anxious client is a skill that assistive personnel must be able to perform. However, before delegation of this skill, assistive personnel must be informed of the proper way to interact verbally and nonverbally with the client, and the staff member must understand why the client is anxious. The skills necessary for communicating with the anxious client should be reviewed with assistive personnel.

STEP	RATIONALE

ASSESSMENT

1. Assess for physical, behavioral, and verbal cues that indicate client is anxious, such as dry mouth, sweaty palms, tone of voice, frequent use of call light, difficulty concentrating, wringing of hands, and statements such as "I am scared."

   Anxiety can interfere with usual manner of communication and thus interfere with client's care and treatment. Extreme anxiety can interfere with comprehension, attention, and problem-solving abilities.

2. Assess for possible factors causing client anxiety (e.g., hospitalization, unknown diagnosis, fatigue).

   Client's feeling of anxiety may be unknown to nurse. Understanding the source of anxiety can assist nurse in client support and communication.

3. Assess factors influencing communication with client (e.g., environment, timing, presence of others, values, experiences, need for personal space because of heightened anxiety).

   Understanding factors that influence communication helps nurse identify effective communication strategies.

4. Assess own level of anxiety, and make a conscious effort to remain calm.

   Anxiety is highly contagious, and one's own anxiety can heighten client's anxiety.

5. Nurse may need to confer with family members about possible causes of client's anxiety.

   Gathering information about client from a family perspective is useful because family may shed new light on situation (Keltner and others, 2003).

STEP	RATIONALE

NURSING DIAGNOSES

- Anxiety
- Impaired verbal communication
- Decisional conflict (specify)
- Ineffective coping

- Fear
- Deficient knowledge
- Impaired social interaction

Related factors are individualized based on client's condition or needs.

PLANNING

1. Expected outcomes following completion of procedure:
   - Client's anxiety is reduced through use of effective communication techniques.

Client is given resource to cope with stressor(s).

- *Critical Decision Point*
  First acknowledge and take care of anxious client's physical and emotional discomfort, but avoid dwelling on physical complaints. Focus on understanding client, providing feedback and assisting in problem solving, and providing atmosphere of warmth and acceptance.

   - Client is able to discuss area of concern.

   Communication techniques dispel anxiety and allow client to focus on problem.

2. Prepare for communication by considering the following: client goals, time allocation, and resources.

   Effective communication allows client to establish rapport, to achieve a sense of calm, and to begin to analyze source of anxiety.

3. Recognize and control own anxiety (breathe slowly and deeply). Be aware of nonverbal cues that indicate own anxiety (e.g., body language, posture, cadence of speech).

   Nurse's own anxiety can increase client's anxiety.

4. Prepare environment physically by providing a quiet, calm area, allowing ample personal space.

   Decreasing stimuli can have a calming effect. Invasion of personal space is known to increase anxiety.

IMPLEMENTATION

1. Provide brief, simple introduction; introduce yourself, and explain purpose of interaction.

   Anxiety may limit amount of information client can understand.

2. Use appropriate nonverbal behaviors and active listening skills, such as staying with client at bedside.

   Nonverbal messages to client convey nurse's interest and help to alleviate anxiety.

3. Use appropriate verbal techniques that are clear and concise to respond to anxious client. Use brief statements that both acknowledge current feeling state and provide direction to client.

   Appropriate techniques and statements provide reassurance and prevent further escalation of anxiety.

4. Help client acquire alternate coping strategies, such as progressive relaxation, slow deep-breathing exercises, and visual imagery (see Chapter 6).

   Coping mechanisms provide foundation for effective communication so that client can explore causes of anxiety and steps to alleviate anxious feelings.

5. Minimize noise in physical setting.

   A less stimulating environment can create a calming, stress-free atmosphere that reduces anxiety.

6. Provide necessary comfort measures.

   Pain can heighten client's anxiety (Kovach and others, 2001).

EVALUATION

1. Observe for continuing presence of physical signs and symptoms or behaviors reflecting anxiety.

   Observation determines extent to which planned interaction relieved client's anxiety.

2. Have client discuss ways to cope with anxiety in the future and make decisions about own care.

   This measures client's ability to assume more health-promoting behavior.

3. Evaluate client's ability to discuss factors causing anxiety.

   Evaluation measures client's ability to attend or focus on area of concern.

Recording and Reporting

*   Record in nurses' notes cause of client's anxiety and any exhibited signs and symptoms of behaviors.
*   Report methods used to relieve anxiety and client's response to ensure continuity of care between nurses.

Unexpected Outcomes	Related Interventions
1. Physical signs and symptoms of anxiety continue. Nurse's interaction may have increased client's anxiety, or source of anxiety is not resolved.	• Utilize refocusing or distraction skills, such as relaxation or guided imagery, to reduce anxiety (Fortinash and Holoday-Worret, 2004).
2. Client displays difficulty in decision making, and preparation of facts may be altered. Client avoids nurse's efforts at focusing discussion or is unable to discuss real concerns. Anxiety continues to prevent client from problem solving.	• Be clear and direct when communicating with client to avoid misunderstanding. • Touch, when used appropriately, may help control feelings of panic. Clients respond positively to touch as a warm, caring nursing approach.
3. Anxiety continues to escalate.	• Continue to use previous steps. • Be very direct and clear when making requests. If client needs to deal with stimulus causing anxiety, reintroduce when client is less anxious. • Touch, while therapeutic, requires individualized assessment of client's anxiety level and need for personal space and may be perceived as threatening. When used appropriately, reassurance through human touch may help control feelings of panic. As a last resort, administer an antianxiety medication (per orders).

Teaching Considerations

*   Teaching client to identify possible sources of anxiety, such as illness, hospitalization, knowledge deficits, or other known stressors, gives client knowledge of anxiety and increases client's sense of control over anxiety.

Pediatric Considerations

*   Children often demonstrate anxiety through physical and behavioral signs but are unable to express anxiety verbally. Children may express anxiety through restless behavior, physical complaints, or behavioral regression. It is important to note any changes in child's behavior that occur during illness or hospitalization (Hockenberry and others, 2001; Tommet, 2003).

Gerontological Considerations

*   Anxiety is one of the most common symptoms seen in older adults. Clients often become ritualistic and intent on performing activities a certain way. Anxiety can develop as a result of a specific event or a general pattern of change (e.g., decline in health) (Lueckenotte, 2000).
*   Anxiety may be seen in long-term care settings, such as residential care facilities and assisted living facilities, and should be managed based on client's presenting behaviors with consideration of any cognitive/physical impairments.
*   Psychosocial factors such as anxiety and confusion, lack of mobility, and spacial organization of long-term care institution are factors that decrease social contacts, thus hindering communication with both peers and health care providers. This leads to further feelings of isolation, boredom, and increased anxiety.

Home Care Considerations

*   Anxiety may be seen in home care settings and should be managed based on client's presenting behaviors with a consideration of any cognitive/physical impairments.
*   Older adults who are socially isolated, have multiple medical problems, including physical impairments, may be more likely to have anxious and/or depressive symptoms. In addition, they may be less likely to seek care for these symptoms.
*   Anticipation of a home care visit may increase a client's anxiety and may lead to exacerbation of symptoms. Therefore some clients may avoid home care visits (Fortinash and Holoday-Worret, 2004).

SKILL 2-3   Communicating With the Angry Client

Anger is the common underlying factor associated with potential for violence. A client can become angry for a variety of reasons. The anger may be directly related to a client's experience with illness, or it can be associated with problems that existed before the client entered the health care setting. In the health care setting, the nurse has frequent contact with a client and thus often becomes the target of the client's anger. It is important for the nurse to understand that in many cases the client's ability to express anger is important to recovery. For example, when a client has experienced a significant loss, anger becomes a means to help cope with grief. A client may express anger toward the nurse, but the anger often hides a specific problem or concern. For example, a client diagnosed as having cancer may voice displeasure with the nurse's care instead of expressing a fear of dying.

It can be very stressful for a nurse to deal with an angry client. Anger can represent rejection or disapproval of the nurse's care. A nurse's efforts at satisfying the needs of one angry client can result in a failure to meet the priorities of other clients.

The nurse must allow the client to express anger openly, and the nurse must not feel threatened by the client's words. However, the client's anger should not be allowed to threaten or compromise care. Skills for communicating with an angry client or a potentially violent client allow a nurse to assist the client in dealing with anger constructively and in refocusing emotional energy toward effective problem solving. De-escalation skills are useful techniques that can be used to manage the potentially violent client; these skills range from using nonthreatening verbal and nonverbal messages to safely disengaging and controlling the aggressor physically (Fortinash and Holoday-Worret, 2004).

DELEGATION CONSIDERATIONS

De-escalation is a skill best performed by a professional nurse. However, assistive personnel must be able to communicate effectively with the potentially violent client, provided that communication with this type of client is not beyond the skill level of assistive personnel. Before delegation of this skill, assistive personnel must be informed of the proper way to interact verbally and nonverbally with the client. The skills for communicating with the potentially violent client and methods of de-escalation should be reviewed with assistive personnel, as well as approaches that have previously been successful and unsuccessful.

STEP	RATIONALE
ASSESSMENT	
1. Observe for behaviors that indicate client is angry (e.g., pacing, clenched fist, loud voice, throwing objects) and/or expressions that indicate anger (e.g., repeat questioning of nurse, nonadherence to requests, belligerent outbursts, threats).	Anger is a normal expression of frustration or response to feeling threatened. However, its expression can interfere with or block communication and interactions.
2. Assess factors that influence communication of angry client, such as refusal to comply with treatment goals, use of sarcasm or hostile behavior, having a low frustration level, or being emotionally immature.	Allows nurse to accurately assess situation or experiences of client that can hinder or facilitate communication (Burgio and others, 2002).
3. Consider resources available to assist in communicating with potentially violent client, such as members of health care team or family members.	May assist in clarifying cause and intervention required to deal with client's anger.

- **Critical Decision Point**
  With some violent behaviors (e.g., physical aggression) nurse may be unable to de-escalate the situation. When this potential exists, nurse must know whom to call for assistance (e.g., trained psychology technicians, security staff).

STEP	RATIONALE

NURSING DIAGNOSES

- Anxiety
- Impaired verbal communication
- Decisional conflict
- Ineffective coping

- Fear
- Impaired social interaction
- Risk for self-directed or other-directed violence

Related factors are individualized based on client's condition or needs.

PLANNING

1. Expected outcomes following completion of procedure:
   - Client no longer exhibits verbal and nonverbal expressions of anger.
2. Prepare for interaction with angry client:
   a. Pause to collect own thoughts, feelings, and reactions.
   b. Determine what client is saying.
   c. Attempt a calm, firm, assertive approach. Attempt to talk in comfortable, reassuring voice.
3. Prepare environment to de-escalate potentially violent client.

   a. Encourage other people, particularly those who provoke anger, to leave room or area.
   b. Maintain adequate distance.

   c. Maintain open exit. Position self closest to the door to facilitate escape from a potentially violent situation. Do not block exit so client feels escape is unattainable; this may potentiate a violent outburst.
   d. Make sure gestures are slow and deliberate rather than sudden and abrupt.
   e. When anger begins to disturb others, close door. This is particularly important if client is becoming agitated.

De-escalation techniques successfully allow client to express anger in a constructive way.

Awareness and control of your own reaction and responses can facilitate more constructive interaction.

Potentially violent client needs to be in an environment with decreased stimuli and to have protection from injury to self or against others.
Encourages client's expression of anger rather than provokes it.
Avoids pressuring client; the nurse maintains safe distance if anger becomes out of control.
Prevents feeling of being trapped for both nurse and client.

Less chance of misinterpretation of message and less threatening.
Agitation and anxiety can spread to others. Some hospital rooms may be equipped with security windows or cameras to allow for observation of client.

- *Critical Decision Point*
  Clients may be disruptive to each other, especially those who are hyperactive, intrusive, threatening, or exhibiting bizarre behaviors. For these clients, nurses should first try least-restrictive measures before using more-restrictive measures, such as seclusion.

   f. Reduce disturbing factors in room (e.g., noise, drafts, inadequate lighting).
   g. Take care of client's physical and emotional needs and discomforts (e.g., offer analgesic for pain).

Reduces irritating factors.

Physical and emotional needs may be factors in client's anger; sometimes client is not aware of these needs (Feldt, 2000).

IMPLEMENTATION

1. Create climate of acceptance for client. Maintain non-threatening verbal and nonverbal communication skills when interacting with angry or potentially violent client.
2. Respond to the potentially violent client.
   a. Use therapeutic silence, and allow client to ventilate feelings.

A relaxed atmosphere may prevent further escalation.

Often de-escalates anger because anger expends emotional and physical energy; client runs out of momentum and energy to maintain anger at high level.

STEP	RATIONALE
b. Answer questions as appropriate; if client asks power struggle type of question (challenging or confrontational type), redirect and set limits by giving clear, concise expectations. Inform client of potential consequences without sounding threatening, and follow through with consequences if behaviors are not altered.	By setting limits on power-struggle questions, structure is provided, and anger is diffused.
c. If client is making verbal threats to harm others, remain calm yet professional, and continue to set limits on inappropriate behavior.	Angry client loses ability to process information rationally and therefore may impulsively express anger through intimidation.

- *Critical Decision Point*
  If strong likelihood of imminent harm to other is present upon discharge, nurse should notify proper authorities (e.g., nurse manager).

d. Maintain personal space and safety with client who is making verbal threats of violence directed at others. Maintain nonthreatening position, nonverbal including body language, position, and cadence.	Avoiding sudden movements and loud tones prevents nurse from giving the appearance of an attack.

- *Critical Decision Point*
  The potentially violent client can be impulsive and explosive, and therefore nurse must keep personal safety skills in mind. In this case touch should be avoided.

e. If client appears to be calm and anger is defused, explore alternatives to situation or feelings of anger.	Processing with client may prevent future explosive outbursts and teach client effective ways of dealing with anger.

EVALUATION

1. Observe for continuing behaviors of verbal expressions of anger.	Indicates success of communication efforts.
2. Note client's ability to answer questions and problem solve.	Determines whether anger has lessened so that client can focus on alternative coping skills.

Recording and Reporting

- Record in nurses' notes cause of client's anger (if determined) and behaviors client exhibits.
- Record and report technique used to de-escalate and client's response.

Unexpected Outcomes	Related Interventions
1. Client continues to demonstrate behaviors or verbal expression of anger or violence. Nurse is unable to assist client in relieving source of anger or in expressing anger openly without violent acts.	• Reassess factors contributing to anger. Also remove or alter factors contributing to anger. • Take charge with calm, firm directions. Give as-needed (prn) medications as ordered for agitation/escalating behaviors. Direct client to a quiet area for a "time out." • Fellow staff should be available to assist if necessary.

Teaching Considerations

- Clients experiencing emotionally charged situations may not comprehend instruction. Focus on understanding client, providing feedback and assisting in problem solving, and providing an atmosphere of safety, warmth, and acceptance.
- Teaching client to identify possible factors that contribute to angry outbursts, such as inadequate coping skills, low frustration levels, illness, hospitalization, knowledge deficits, or other known stressors, may give client a sense of control.
- Once anger has been de-escalated, teach client new adaptive methods of coping with anger.

Pediatric Considerations

- Set limits for inappropriate behaviors exhibited by child.
- Apply such limits immediately because children tend to have less internal control over their own behaviors (Hockenberry and others, 2001).

Gerontological Considerations

- Clients who have cognitive impairments may exhibit tantrumlike behaviors in response to real or perceived frustration. Nurse can use distraction techniques to remove cognitively impaired older adult client from disturbing stimuli, or nurse can use redirection to activity that is pleasurable to client (Lueckenotte, 2000).

Home Care Considerations

- Personal safety for nurse against potentially violent client or family member extends to all health care settings, including client's home. Nurse may be in potentially dangerous situation while giving care to client at home; nurse may give care to client without support from other staff members.
- Be aware of physical surroundings of home, including possible exits.
- If de-escalation does not occur and nurse feels safety may be threatened, nurse should call for assistance or remove self from situation.

SKILL 2-4   Communicating With the Depressed Client

Depression is a feeling state that is more than just sadness. It is a common psychiatric condition that affects a person's ability to function in day-to-day activities. There are many symptoms of depression, the most common being apathy, feelings of sadness, fatigue, guilt, poor concentration, sleep disturbances, and suicidal thoughts. Depression results in both subjective and objective behaviors (Box 2-4). Subjective behaviors include report of feelings of sadness, tearful, report of no energy, and increase in physical complaints. Some clients report feeling anxious when depressed. Objective signs include decrease in performance of activities of daily living (ADLs), and decreased time spent in social activities (altered social interaction).

Many clients in acute care settings suffering from either acute or chronic health conditions have symptoms of depression. Some clients may have been formally diagnosed and treated with medications and/or psychotherapy, and yet others may not have been diagnosed and therefore have not been treated. The nurse uses the nursing process to develop nursing interventions, expected outcomes, and evaluation of those outcomes for clients with depression. The intervention strategies emphasize use of therapeutic communication strategies within the context of the nurse-client relationship.

BOX 2-4 Symptoms of Depression	
COMMON SYMPTOMS	**OTHER SYMPTOMS**
Apathy	Fatigue
Sadness	Thoughts of death
Sleep disturbances	Decreased libido
Hopelessness	Ruminations of inadequacy
Helplessness	Psychomotor agitation
Worthlessness	Verbal beratings of self
Guilt	Spontaneous crying
Anger	Dependency, passiveness

From Keltner NL and others: *Psychiatric nursing*, ed 4, St. Louis, 2003, Mosby.

Delegation Considerations

Communication with a depressed client is best managed by a professional nurse. However, therapeutic communication is important in all client interactions. Communicating effectively with the depressed client is a skill that assistive personnel must be able to perform. However, before delegation of this skill, assistive personnel must be informed of the proper way to interact verbally and nonverbally with the client, and the staff member must understand possible causes and signs and symptoms of depression. The skills necessary for communicating with the depressed client should be reviewed with assistive personnel.

STEP	RATIONALE
ASSESSMENT	
1. Assess for physical, behavioral, and verbal cues that indicate client is depressed, such as feelings of sadness, tearfulness, difficulty concentrating, increase in reports of physical complaints, and statements such as "I am sad/depressed."	Depression can interfere with usual manner of communication and thus interfere with client's care and treatment. If depression is severe, it can interfere with comprehension, attention, and problem-solving abilities.
2. Assess for possible factors causing client's depression (e.g., acute or chronic illness, personal vulnerability, past history).	Client's depressive state may be unknown to nurse. Understanding the possible cause of depression may assist nurse in client support and communication.
3. Assess factors influencing communication with client (e.g., environment, timing, presence of others, values, experiences, poor concentration).	Understanding factors that influence communication helps nurse identify effective communication strategies.
4. Nurse may need to confer with family members about possible causes of client's depression, including past history of the illness.	Gathering information about client from a family perspective is useful because family may shed new light on situation (Keltner and others, 2003).

NURSING DIAGNOSES

- Impaired verbal communication
- Decisional conflict
- Ineffective coping
- Hopelessness

- Self-care deficit
- Impaired social interaction
- Risk for self-directed violence

Related factors are individualized based on client's condition or needs.

STEP	RATIONALE
PLANNING	
1. Expected outcomes following completion of procedure: • Client's depression is reduced through use of effective communication techniques.	Client is given resources to cope with feelings of depression.
2. Prepare for communication by considering the following: client goals, time allocation, and resources.	Effective communication allows client to establish rapport, to achieve a sense of calm, and to begin to analyze source(s) of depression.
3. Be aware of your own nonverbal cues that affect communication with depressed client (e.g., body language, posture, cadence of speech). Remain nonjudgmental.	Nurse's personal feelings regarding depression may negatively affect interaction with client.
4. Prepare environment physically by providing a quiet, calm area, allowing ample personal space.	Decreasing stimuli can have a calming effect. Invasion of personal space is known to increase anxiety, thereby hindering communication with the depressed client.

- *Critical Decision Point*
  First acknowledge and take care of depressed client's physical and emotional discomfort, but avoid dwelling on physical complaints. Focus on understanding client, providing feedback and assisting in problem solving, and providing atmosphere of warmth and acceptance.

STEP	RATIONALE
IMPLEMENTATION	
1. Provide brief, simple introduction; introduce yourself, and explain purpose of interaction.	Symptoms associated with of depression may limit amount of information client can understand.
2. Accept client as he or she is and focus on positive aspects of client. Provide positive feedback.	Depressed clients often have low self-esteem, and this approach helps to focus on their strengths.
3. Be honest and empathic.	Facilitates the development of trust.

STEP	RATIONALE
4. Use appropriate nonverbal behaviors and active listening skills, such as staying with client at bedside.	Nonverbal messages to client convey nurse's interest and help to alleviate depressive symptoms.
5. Use appropriate verbal techniques that are clear and concise to respond to depressed client. Use brief statements that both acknowledge current feeling state and provide direction to client.	Appropriate techniques and statements provide reassurance to depressed client. Conveys empathy.
6. Use open-ended questions, such as "Tell me about how you are feeling" or "You seem sad, tell me about your sadness."	Encourages the client to continue talking, facilitating an in-depth discussion of symptoms.
7. Reward small decisions and independent actions. Or when necessary, make decisions that clients are not ready to make. Present situations that require no decision making.	Depressed clients may be overly dependent and indecisive.
8. Respond to anger therapeutically, and encourage verbal expression of anger.	Depressed clients may be angry; the nurse can understand that anger is a symptom of their depression. Tension may be reduced with verbal expression.
9. Provide necessary comfort measures.	Depressed clients often have multiple somatic complaints; the nurse needs to address and adequately treat the physical complaints (e.g., pain, nausea) (Solnek and Seiter, 2002).
10. Spend time with client who is withdrawn.	By spending time with client, the nurse is communicating the client's worth.
11. Ask client about suicidal ideation and presence of a plan.	Depressed clients are at increased risk for suicide. Other risk factors include general medical conditions, hopelessness, male gender, increased age. The more developed the plan, the greater the risk of suicide (Keltner and others, 2003).

EVALUATION

1. Observe for continuing presence of physical signs and symptoms or behaviors reflecting depression.	Observation determines extent to which planned interaction relieved client's depressive symptoms.
2. Have client discuss ways to cope with depression in the future and make decisions about own care.	This measures client's ability to assume more health-promoting behavior.
3. Evaluate client's ability to discuss factors causing depression.	Evaluation measures client's ability to attend or focus on area of concern.

Recording and Reporting

- Record in nurses' notes both objective and subjective behaviors (associated with depression) the client is displaying and objective behaviors (associated with depression) observed by the nurse.
- Report methods used to improve these behaviors and client's response to ensure continuity of care between nurses.

Unexpected Outcomes	Related Interventions
1. Depressive behaviors continue. Nurse's interaction has been ineffective at relieving depressive symptoms.	• Continue to use therapeutic communication skills when interacting with depressed client. • Refer client to mental health professional for consultation regarding use of pharmacological agents and/or formal psychotherapy to treat depression.
2. Client reports suicidal ideation with/without plan.	• Refer client to mental health professional for evaluation and possible admission to an inpatient psychiatric treatment facility.

Teaching Considerations

- Teaching client to identify possible sources of depression, such as acute/chronic illness, personal vulnerability, ineffective coping, or other known stressors, gives client knowledge of depression and increases client's sense of control over depression.
- Teaching modifications should be made with a consideration of impaired concentration and memory related to the client's depressed status (e.g., present a small amount of material at a time).

Pediatric Considerations

- Children often demonstrate symptoms of depression that differ from adults with depression. They manifest depression through physical (increased somatic complaints) and behavioral signs (poor school performance, social isolation) and may be unable to express depression verbally. Children may express depression through restless behavior or behavioral regression. It is important to note any changes in child's behavior that occur during illness or hospitalization (Hockenberry and others, 2001; Son and Kirchner, 2000).

Gerontological Considerations

- Depression among older adults is a major health concern. It is important to differentiate between depression and any underlying medical illness in this population because the symptoms may overlap. In addition, suicide risk is increased in older adults (Keltner and others, 2003).

Home Care Considerations

- Depression may been seen in home care settings and should be managed based on client's presenting behaviors with a consideration of any cognitive/physical impairments.

FOCUS on CLINICAL PRACTICE

You are assigned to care for Mrs. Garcia, an 82-year-old woman who was admitted to the hospital 5 days ago after falling at home. She had emergency surgery to repair a fractured right hip. During shift report, the nurse tells you that Mrs. Garcia is a problematic client. She is demanding and never seems satisfied with anything. When you approach her to perform an initial assessment, she is babbling incoherently and seems disoriented. She appears disheveled, and her lunch tray is untouched. She is wincing and grimacing. You ask the client if she is complaining of pain, but you get a response that you cannot understand. After repeating the question, "Are you in pain? Please rate your pain on a scale from 0 to 10," the client yells at you and throws the water pitcher across the room.

1. What other information would you like to have about this client?
2. How will you best manage pain control with this client?
   A. Use interpreter or daughter to assist in communicating with client about nature of pain.
   B. Use a visual analog scale to have client rate her pain.
   C. Medicate client as ordered by physician.
   D. Use comfort measures (e.g., back massage, repositioning pillows, decreasing stimulation such as light and noise).
   Explain your choice(s).

3. How will you manage the client's negative behaviors?
   A. Use interpreter or daughter when communicating with client.
   B. Use therapeutic communication techniques to set limits with inappropriate/negative behaviors, such as throwing objects or yelling
   C. Maintain a calm demeanor.
   D. Tell client you will not care for her if she is mean/angry.
   Explain your choice(s).
4. How can you help the client manage her ADLs? Because she is 5 days after surgery, nursing protocol dictates her pain should be subsiding and she should be ambulating with assistance and attending physical therapy.
   A. Use interpreter or daughter when communicating with client.
   B. Assist the client in performing ADLs while encouraging the client to do as much for herself as possible.
   C. Provide privacy for client.
   D. Convey empathy by remaining calm and nonjudgmental; give positive feedback for her accomplishments.
   Explain your choice(s).

NCLEX REVIEW QUESTIONS

1. Which of the following reflects an obstacle to nurse-client communication?
   1. Discussing fears about client with members of the health care team
   2. Validating client information with the family
   3. Admitting and apologizing to clients for a mistake
   4. Avoiding issues that are uncomfortable for clients

2. Which of the following statements by the nurse best reflects therapeutic communication?
   1. "I think your doctor needs to know that you are still in pain."
   2. "What do you want me to do about all of your problems?"
   3. "When it comes to pain, your doctor tends to undermedicate all of his clients."
   4. "Just get a good night's sleep, and your pain will be better in the morning."

3. A client recovering from a bilateral mastectomy for breast cancer tearfully tells you she is feeling depressed and worthless as a woman. Which of the following is an ineffective communication technique?
   1. "Often women have body image issues after undergoing surgery such as you have."
   2. "Tell me more about how you feel."
   3. "Why do you feel depressed and worthless?"
   4. "How long have you been feeling depressed and worthless?"

References

Dube CE and others: Communication skills for preventive interventions, *Acad Med* 75(suppl 7): S45, 2000.

Feldt KS: The checklist of nonverbal pain indicators (CPNI), *Pain Manag Nurs* 1(1):3, 2000.

Fortin AH: Communication skills to improve patient satisfaction and quality of care, *Ethn Dis* 12(4): S3, 2002.

Fortinash K, Holoday-Worret P: *Psychiatric mental health nursing*, ed 3, St. Louis, 2004, Mosby.

Giger J, Davidhizar R: *Transcultural nursing: assessment and interventions,* ed 3, St. Louis, 1999, Mosby.

Happ MB: Communicating with the mechanically ventilated patients: state of the science, *AACN Clin Issues* 12(2):247, 2001.

Hockenberry MJ and others: *Wong's care of infants and children,* ed 7, St. Louis, 2003, Mosby.

Keltner N, Schwecke L, Bostrom C: *Psychiatric nursing*, ed 4, St. Louis, 2003, Mosby.

Leonard, BJ, Plotnikoff GA: Awareness: the heart of cultural competence, *AACN Clin Issues,* 11(1):51, 2000.

Lueckenotte A: *Gerontologic nursing*, ed 2, St. Louis, 2000, Mosby.

Moore LW, Miller M: Older men's experience of living with severe visual impairment, *J Adv Nurs* 43(1):10, 2003.

Parsons LC: Transcultural communication: the cornerstone of culturally competent care, *SCI Nurs* 19(4):160, 2002.

Rutishauser C: Communicating with young people, *Paediatr Resp Rev* 4(4):319, 2003.

Solnek BL, Seiter T: How to diagnose and treat depression, *Nurse Pract* 27(10):12, 2002.

Son SE, Kirchner JT: Depression in children and adolescents, *Am Fam Physician* 62(10):2297, 2000.

Stuart G, Laraia M: *Stuart and Sundeen's principles and practice of psychiatric nursing*, ed 7, St. Louis, 2001, Mosby.

Tommet PA: Nurse parent dialogue: illuminating the evolving patterns of families with children who are medically fragile, *Nurs Sci Q,* 16(3):239, 2003.

Research References

Bryan K and others: Working with older people with communication difficulties: an evaluation of care worker training, *Aging Ment Health* 6(3):248, 2002.

Burgio LD and others: Teaching and maintaining behavior management skills in the nursing home, *Gerontologist* 42(4):487, 2002.

Caris-Verhallen WM and others: Effects of video interaction analysis training on nurse-patient communication in the care of the elderly, *Patient Educ Couns* 39(1):91, 2000.

Cioffi J: Communicating with culturally and linguistically diverse patients in an acute care setting: nurses' experiences, *Int J Nurs Stud* 40(3):299, 2003.

Hagerty BM, Patusky KL: Reconceptualizing the nurse-patient relationship, *J Nurs Scholarsh* 35(2):145, 2003.

Hemsley B and others: Nursing the patient with severe communication impairment, *J Adv Nurs* 35(6): 827, 2001.

Kovach CR and others: Use of the assessment of discomfort in dementia protocol, *Appl Nurs Res* 14(4):193, 2001.

Park Y-J and others: The conceptual structure of Hwa-Byuun in middle-aged Korean women, *Health Care Women Int* 23:389, 2002.

Piette JD and others: Dimensions of patient-provider communications and diabetes self-care in an ethnically diverse population, *J Gen Intern Med* 18(8):624, 2003.

Simons J, Roberson E: Poor communication and knowledge deficits: obstacles of effective pain management of children's postoperative pain, *J Adv Nurs* 40(1):78, 2002.

Yick AG, Gupta R: Chinese cultural dimensions of death, dying, and bereavement: focus group findings, *J Cult Divers* 9(2):32, 2002.

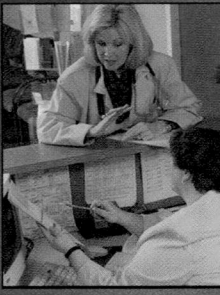

3

Recording and Reporting

3-1   Giving a Change-of-Shift Report

3-2   Documenting Nurses' Progress Notes

3-3   Incident Reporting

MEDIA RESOURCES

Evolve Site *evolve*

http://evolve.elsevier.com/Perry/skills
- Weblinks
- Video clips
- Mosby's Nursing Skills Video Exercises

Mosby's Nursing Skills Videos/CD-ROM
- *Basic Principles Video:* Communication, oral, written, nonverbal reporting, charting end-of-shift report
- *Safe Medication Administration Video:* Documenting medications, elements of documentation, if patient refuses medication, and when patient asks for medication when medication cannot be given

OBJECTIVES

Mastery of content in this chaper will enable the nurse to:

- Describe guidelines for effective documentation and reporting.
- Describe elements of a change-of-shift report given to a nursing team.
- Complete an incident report accurately.
- Write a nurse's progress note using SOAP, SOAPIE, PIE, and focus charting formats.
- Describe information found in a patient care profile and nursing Kardex.
- Complete a nursing flow sheet.
- Explain guidelines used in documentation of home care and long-term care.
- Describe the role of critical pathways in multidisciplinary documentation.
- Discuss the role of computerization in documentation.

KEY TERMS

Acuity records	Incident report
Case management	Kardex
Change-of-shift report	Objective data
Charting by exception (CBE)	PIE
Computer-based patient care record (CPCR)	Problem-oriented medical record (POMR)
Consultation	Resident
Critical pathway	SOAP
DAR	SOAPIE
Documentation	Standardized care plan
Evidence-based practice	Subjective data
Flow sheet	Transfer reports
Focus charting	Variance
Graphical user interface	

Nursing documentation continues to be an essential and challenging component of health care delivery. Documentation is anything written or printed that is relied on as a record or proof for authorized persons. Documentation is a vital aspect of nursing practice and a vital link between the provision and evaluation of health care (Iyer and Camp, 1999). One of the most challenging nursing issues is how to document quality client care within the constraints imposed by regulations, limited resources, and finances. Information in the client record provides a detailed account of the level of quality of care delivered to clients. Effective documentation ensures continuity of care, saves time, and minimizes the risk of errors (Yocum, 2002). Quality documentation depends on members of the health care team being able to communicate effectively with one another in both written and spoken word. Furthermore, technology has increased the variety and methods of documen-

tation, which potentially heightens the productivity and scope of nursing practice (Mathews and Zadak, 1993). Nurses are accountable for their actions, and, as a result, written information must be clear and logical, exactly describing all client care delivered. Information that is documented and reported to others is confidential and must be protected.

Accreditation agencies such as the Joint Commission on Accreditation of Healthcare Organizations (JCAHO) specify guidelines for documentation. Under the prospective payment system, hospitals are reimbursed a set dollar amount by Medicare for each diagnosis-related group (DRG). Everything that is done for the client must be documented in the medical record for the health care institution to recover its costs. If information regarding client care is not recorded, organizations may not be adequately reimbursed.

Confidentiality

Like all members of the health care team, nurses are legally and ethically obligated to keep client information confidential. Nurses may not discuss client's examinations, observations, conversations, or treatments with other clients or staff not involved in the client's care. Only staff directly involved with specific aspects of a client's care have legitimate access to the client's health care records. Clients may request copies of their records, and they have a right to read their records. Agencies have specific policies for controlling the manner in which records are shared. Most commonly clients are required to provide a written permission for the release of medical information.

In 2003 legislation to protect client privacy for health information in the form of the Health Insurance Portability and Accountability Act (HIPAA) was finalized. This legislation governs all areas of health information management, which includes, for example, reimbursement, coding, security, and client records. Previously the rule required written consent for disclosure of all client information. Under new regulations, in order to eliminate barriers that could delay access to care, providers are required only to notify clients of their privacy policy and make a reasonable effort to get written acknowledgment of this notification. As a result, clients have more control over their personal health care information and who has access to this information.

When students are in a clinical setting, confidentiality and compliance with HIPAA legislation are part of professional practice. Only information needed to provide safe, efficient care is obtained from the medical record. For example, when assigned to provide complete care for a client, the student needs to review the current medical record and plan of care. However, this information is not shared with other classmates, nor can students access the medical records of other clients on the specific clinical area. To further maintain confidentiality and protect client privacy, written materials used in student clinical practice should not have client identifiers, such as room number, date of birth, medical record number, or other identifiable demographic information.

HIPAA requires that disclosure or requests for health information be limited to the minimum, which would include only the specific information required for a particular purpose. For example, if a client's home telephone number is needed to reschedule an appointment, access to the medical record would be limited solely to the telephone information. Clients will have new rights to understand and control how their health information is used (U.S. Department of Health and Human Services [USDHHS], 2003).

Standards

Current JCAHO standards require that all clients who are admitted to a health care institution have an assessment of physical, psychosocial, environmental, self-care, client education, and discharge planning needs (JCAHO, 2004b). Documentation of nursing care is within the context of the nursing process, as well as evidence of client and family teaching and discharge planning. Documentation of care should include the evaluation of client outcomes, including the client's response to treatments, education, and preventive care. If more that one discipline regularly cares for a client, the JCAHO also expects a multidisciplinary care plan.

The documentation of care and client information is vital in ensuring client safety in health care organizations. Electronic records and information create complexities in information management. The goal of information management is to support decision making and to improve client outcomes, improve health care documentation, ensure client safety, and improve performance in client care, treatment, and services; governance; management; and support processes (JCAHO, 2004b).

Multidisciplinary Communication Within the Health Care Team

An optimum level of client care requires proficient communication among the members of the health care team. Records and reports communicate specific information about a client's health status and the interventions that all health care team members contribute toward improving the client's health. When information is communicated clearly and accurately in a timely way, health care is more efficient and the client benefits.

A client's record is a confidential, permanent legal document containing information relevant to a client's health care. Information about the client's health care is recorded after each client contact. The record is a continuing account of the client's health status and needs, the treatments delivered, results of diagnostic tests, and the client's response to therapy.

Reports are oral, written, or audiotaped exchanges of information between caregivers (Figure 3-1). Reports can include information about a client's clinical status, observations made about the client's behavior, data pertaining to diagnostic tests, and directions for changes in therapy. Common reports given by nurses include change-of-shift re-

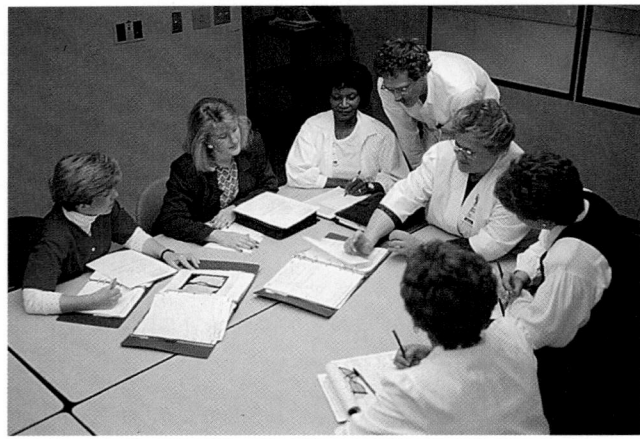

FIGURE **3-1** Communication among members of the health care team.

ports (see Skill 3-1), telephone reports, transfer reports, and incident reports (see Skill 3-3). In addition, a physician may call a nursing unit to receive a verbal report on a client's condition and progress. The laboratory submits written reports about the results of diagnostic tests.

Information is also communicated through discussions among health care team members. For example, a discharge planning conference often involves members of all disciplines (e.g., nursing, medicine, social work, physical therapy, and dietary), who meet to discuss the client's progress toward established discharge goals.

Consultations are another form of discussion whereby one professional caregiver provides formal advice about the care of a client. For example, a dietitian may consult with the nurse on the best foods to meet a client's dietary restrictions. Consultations and conferences should be documented in a client's record so that all caregivers benefit from the information and plan the client's care accordingly.

Guidelines for Quality Documentation and Reporting

Quality documentation and reporting enhance efficient, individualized client care and is achieved through the use of standard guidelines. Accurate documentation is one of the best defenses of legal claims associated with nursing care (Martin, 2001; Sullivan, 2004). To limit liability, nursing documentation must clearly indicate that individualized, goal-directed nursing care was provided to a client based on the nursing assessment. The recorded information in the client's record must describe exactly what happened to a client. This is best achieved when the nurse charts immediately after care is provided (Sullivan, 2000). Nurses must include all assessment findings, interventions (including client education), client responses, and consultations/referrals in the medical record.

Five common issues in malpractice caused by inadequate documentation include (1) not charting the correct time

TABLE 3-1   LEGAL GUIDELINES FOR RECORDING

GUIDELINES	RATIONALE	CORRECT ACTION
Do not erase, apply correction fluid, or scratch out errors made while recording.	Charting becomes illegible: it may appear as if you were attempting to hide information or deface record.	Draw single line through error, write word "error" above it, and sign your name or initials. Then record note correctly. Check agency policy.
Do not write retaliatory or critical comments about client or care by other health care professionals.	Statements can be used as evidence for nonprofessional behavior or poor quality of care.	Enter only objective descriptions of client's behavior; client comments should be quoted.
Need to add additional client information.	New information is acquired.	If additional information is to be added to an existing entry, write the date and time of the new entry on the next available space, and include "Addendum to note of (date and time of prior note)" (Sullivan, 2000).
	Forgot to chart during a shift.	Write the current date and time in the next available space, and write "Late entry for (date and time/shift missed)" (Sullivan, 2000).
Correct all errors promptly.	Errors in recording can lead to errors in treatment.	Avoid rushing to complete charting; be sure information is accurate.
Record all facts.	Record must be accurate and reliable.	Be certain entry is factual; do not speculate or guess.
Do not leave blank spaces in nurses' notes.	Another person can add incorrect information in space.	Chart consecutively, line by line; if space is left, draw line horizontally through it, and sign your name at end.
Record all entries legibly and in black ink.	Illegible entries can be misinterpreted, causing errors and lawsuits; ink cannot be erased; black ink is more legible when records are photocopied or transferred to microfilm.	Never erase entries or use correction fluid, and never use pencil.
If order is questioned, record that clarification was sought.	If you perform order known to be incorrect, you are just as liable for prosecution as the physician is.	Do not record "physician made error." Instead, chart that "Dr. Smith was called to clarify order for analgesic."
Chart only for yourself.	You are accountable for information you enter into chart.	Never chart for someone else. **Exception:** if caregiver has left unit for day and calls with information that needs to be documented, include the name of the source of information in the entry, and include that the information was provided via telephone.
Avoid using generalized, empty phrases such as "status unchanged" or "had good day."	Specific information about client's condition or case can be accidentally deleted if information is too generalized.	Use complete, concise descriptions of care.
Begin each entry with time, and end with your signature and title.	This guideline ensures that correct sequence of events is recorded; signature documents who is accountable for care delivered.	Do not wait until end of shift to record important changes that occurred several hours earlier; be sure to sign each entry.
For computer documentation, keep your password to yourself.	Maintains security and confidentiality.	Once logged into the computer, do not leave the computer screen unattended.

when events occurred, (2) failing to record verbal orders or failing to have them signed, (3) charting actions in advance to save time, (4) documenting incorrect data, and (5) failing to give a report, or giving an incomplete report, to an oncoming shift (Table 3-1).

Factual

A record or report must contain descriptive, objective information about what a nurse sees, hears, feels, and smells. An objective description is the result of direct observation and measurement.

The use of vague terms, such as *appears, seems,* or *apparently,* is not acceptable because these words suggest that the nurse is stating an opinion. For example, the description "the client seems anxious" does not accurately communicate the facts and does not inform other caregivers of the details regarding the anxious behavior. The phrase "seems anxious" infers a conclusion without any supporting facts. To correct for this inaccurate statement the nurse may include subjective descriptions and objective assessment findings.

A subjective description includes the recording of subjective data using the client's exact words. Using the previous example, the nurse may record "Clients states, 'I feel nervous.'" The nurse also includes objective assessment findings such as increased pulse rate, increased respirations, and increased restlessness.

Accurate

The use of exact measurements establishes accuracy. For example, a description such as "Intake, 360 ml of water" is more accurate than "Client drank an adequate amount of fluid." These measurements can later be used as a means of determining whether a client's condition has changed. Charting that an abdominal wound is "5 cm in length without redness, drainage, or edema" is more descriptive than "large wound healing well."

Documentation of concise data is clear and easy to understand. It is essential to avoid the use of unnecessary words and irrelevant detail. For example, the fact that the client is watching TV is only necessary when this activity is significant to the client's status and plan of care.

Use of an institution's accepted abbreviations, symbols, and system of measures (e.g., metric) ensures that all staff members document accurately. The nurse should use abbreviations carefully to avoid misinterpretation. To minimize errors, abbreviations are spelled in their entirety when abbreviations can be confusing. The JCAHO has an established list of abbreviations that should never be used because these increase errors (JCAHO, 2004a). For example, the abbreviation for every day (qd) **should no longer be used** (Chapter 19). If a treatment or medication is needed daily, the written order or care plan should write out the word *daily* or *every day*. The abbreviation od (every day) can be misinterpreted to mean O.D. (right eye).

Correct spelling demonstrates a level of competency and attention to detail. Many terms can easily be misinterpreted (e.g., dysphagia or dysphasia and dram or gram). Some spelling errors can also result in serious treatment errors; for example, the names of certain medications such as digitoxin and digoxin or morphine and Numorphan are similar and must be transcribed carefully to ensure that the client receives the correct medication.

JCAHO standards (JCAHO, 2004c) require that "all entries in medical records are dated and a method is established to identify the authors of entries." Therefore each entry in a client's record ends with the caregiver's full name or initials and status, such as "Julie Smith, RN." Each time initials are used, the full name and status must previously appear on the same page so the individual entering initials can be readily identified. A nursing student enters full name, student nurse abbreviation (e.g., SN, NS), and educational institution, such as "David Jones, SN (student nurse), CMTC (Central Maine Technical College)."

Records need to reflect accountability during the time frame of the entry, which is best accomplished when nurses only chart their own observations and actions. The signature holds that nurse accountable for information recorded. If information was inadvertently omitted from the record, it is acceptable for nurses to ask colleagues to chart information after they leave work. The entry needs to clearly show what was done and by whom (e.g., "At 11 AM Sam Turner, RN, called and reported that at 8 AM Demerol 100 mg IM was administered to client for abdominal pain").

Complete

The information within a recorded entry or a report needs to be complete, containing appropriate and essential information. Criteria for thorough communication exist for certain health problems or nursing activities (Table 3-2). The nurse makes written entries in the client's medical record, describing nursing care that is administered and the client's response. An example of a thorough nurses' note follows:

> 1915 Client verbalizes sharp, throbbing pain localized along lateral side of right ankle, beginning approximately 15 minutes ago after twisting his foot on the stairs. Client rates pain as 8 on a scale of 0 to 10. Pain increased with movement, slightly relieved with elevation. Pedal pulses equal bilaterally. Right ankle circumference 1 cm larger than left. Ice applied. Percocet 2 tabs given for pain.

> 1945 Client states pain somewhat relieved following application of ice and rates pain as 6 on a scale of 0 to 10. Physician notified for new analgesic order. Lee Turno, RN.

Current

Timely entries are essential in the client's ongoing care (JCAHO, 2004c). To increase accuracy and decrease unnecessary duplication, many health care agencies use records kept near the client's bedside, which facilitate immediate documentation of information as it is collected from a client. Activities or findings to communicate at the time of occurrence include the following:

- Vital signs
- Administration of medications and treatments
- Preparation for diagnostic tests or surgery
- Change in client's status and who was notified, (e.g., physician, manager, client's family)
- Admission, transfer, discharge, or death of a client
- Treatment for a sudden change in client's status

This information is often included in flow sheets kept at the bedside. Nurses often keep notes on a worksheet when caring for several clients, making notes as the care occurs to ensure that entries recorded later in the record are accurate.

Most health care agencies use military time, a 24-hour system that avoids misinterpretation of AM and PM times (Figure 3-2). Instead of two 12-hour cycles in standard time, the military clock is one 24-hour time cycle. For example, 1:00 PM is 1300 military time; 10:22 AM is 1022 military time.

Organized

The nurse communicates information in a logical order. For example, an organized note describes the client's pain, nurse's assessment and interventions, and the client's response. To write notes about complex situations in an organized fashion the nurse thinks about the situation and often make notes of what is to be included before beginning to write in the permanent legal record.

TABLE 3-2   EXAMPLES OF CRITERIA FOR REPORTING AND RECORDING

TOPIC	CRITERIA TO REPORT OR RECORD
ASSESSMENT	
Subjective data	Describe episode/event in client's words in quotation marks.
	When possible, clarify onset, location, description of condition (severity, duration, frequency, precipitating, aggravating and relieving factors)
Client behavior (e.g., anxiety, confusion, hostility)	Onset, behaviors exhibited, precipitating factors
Objective data (e.g., rash, tenderness, breath sounds)	Onset, location, description of condition (severity; duration; frequency; precipitating, aggravating, and relieving factors)
NURSING INTERVENTIONS AND EVALUATION	
Treatments (e.g., enema, bath, dressing change)	Time administered, equipment used (if appropriate), client's response (objective and subjective changes) compared to previous treatment; for example, "client denied pain during dressing change" or "client reported severe abdominal cramping during enema"
Medication administration	Immediately after administration document time medication given, preliminary assessment (e.g., pain level, vital signs), client response or effect of medication; for example, "1500 Pain reported at 6 (scale 0-10). Tylenol 500 mg given PO 1530: Client reports pain level 2 (scale 0-10)" or "Pruritus and hives developed over lower abdomen 1 hour after penicillin was given"
Client teaching	Information presented, method of instruction (e.g., discussion, demonstration, videotape, booklet), client response, including questions and evidence of understanding such as return demonstration or change in behavior
Discharge planning	Measurable client goals or expected outcomes, progress toward goals, need for referrals

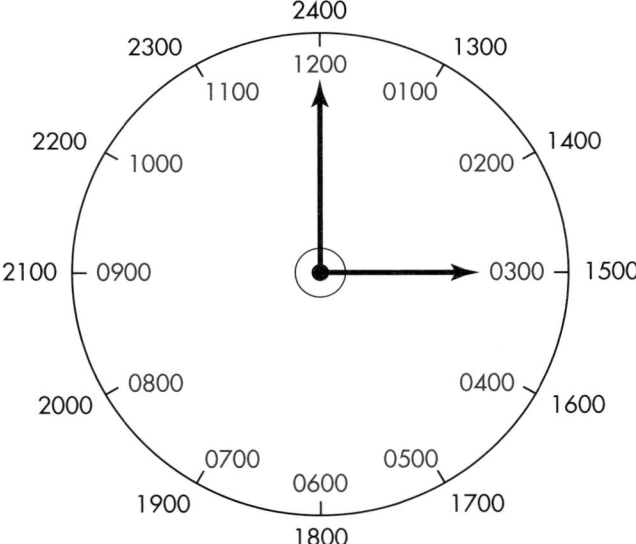

FIGURE 3-2   Military time clock. Instead of two 12-hour cycles, the military clock in one 24-hour time cycle (e.g., 3 PM is 1500 military time).

Common Record-Keeping Forms and Formats

A variety of forms are available that are designed for the type of information nurses routinely document. The categories within a form are usually derived from institutional standards of practice or guidelines established by accrediting agencies.

Admission Nursing History Forms

A nursing history form is completed when a client is admitted to a nursing care unit. The history form guides the nurse through a complete assessment to identify relevant nursing diagnoses or problems. Data on history forms provide baseline data that can be compared with changes in the client's condition. Each institution designs a nursing history form differently, based on the standards of practice and philosophy of nursing care.

Flow Sheets and Graphic Records

Flow sheets are forms that allow nurses to quickly and easily enter assessment data about the client, including vital signs, intake and output, and routine repetitive care, such as hygiene measures, ambulation, meals, weights, and safety and restraint checks. Flow sheets use a coding system for data entry (Figure 3-3). If an occurrence on the flow sheet is unusual or changes significantly, a focus note is needed. For example, if a client's blood pressure becomes dangerously high, the nurse completes a focus assessment and records this, as well as action taken, in the progress notes. Flow sheets provide a quick, easy reference for the health care team members in assessing a client's status. Critical care and acute care units commonly use flow sheets for all types of physiological data.

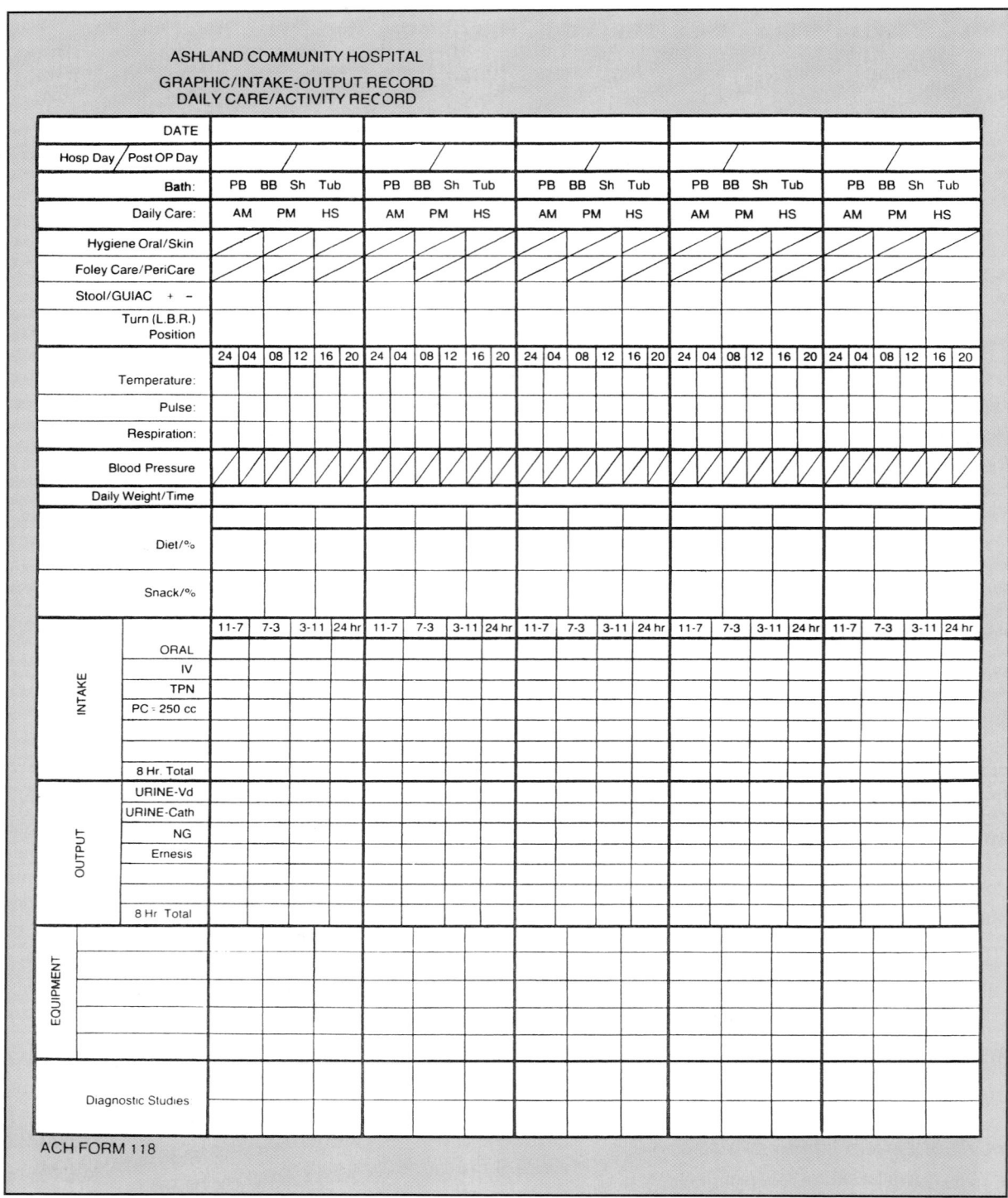

FIGURE **3-3** Graphic and intake-output record. (Courtesy Ashland Community Hospital, Ashland, Ore.)

Client Care Summary or Kardex

Many hospitals now have computerized systems that provide basic, summative information in the form of a client care summary. This is printed out for each client during each shift. This summary is continually updated and provides the nurse with a current detailed list of orders, treatment, and diagnostic testing. In some settings, a Kardex, a portable "flip-over" file or notebook, is kept at the nurses' station. Most Kardex forms have an activity and treatment section and a nursing care plan section, which organize information for quick reference as nurses give change-of-shift reports or make walking rounds. An updated Kardex eliminates the need for repeated referral to the chart for routine information throughout the day. In many institutions Kardex entries are done in pencil because of the need for frequent revisions as the client's needs change. In settings in which the Kardex is a permanent part of the client's record, entries are made in ink.

Information commonly found on the client care summary or Kardex includes the following:

- Basic demographic data (e.g., age, religion)
- Physician's name
- Primary medical diagnosis
- Current physician's treatment orders to be carried out by the nurse (e.g., dressing changes, ambulation, glucose monitoring)
- Nursing care plan
- Nursing orders (e.g., education sessions, symptom relief measures, counseling)
- Scheduled tests and procedures
- Safety precautions to be used in the client's care
- Factors related to activities of daily living
- Nearest relative/guardian or person to contact in an emergency
- Emergency code status
- Allergies

Acuity Records

Acuity records provide a method of determining the hours of care and staff required for a given group of clients. A client's acuity level is based on client need, including the type and number of nursing interventions required for providing care in a 24-hour period. Typically nurses enter acuity data the same time each day. The acuity level determined by the nursing care allows clients to be rated in comparison with one another. For example, an acuity system might rate bathing clients from 1 to 5 (1 is totally dependent, 5 is independent). A client returning from surgery requiring frequent monitoring and extensive care may be listed with an acuity level of 1. On the same continuum another client awaiting discharge after a successful recovery from surgery has an acuity level of 5. Accurate acuity ratings may also be used to justify overtime and the number and qualifications of staff needed to safely care for clients. The client-to-staff ratios established for a unit depend on a composite gathering of data for the 24-hour interventions that are necessary for each client receiving care.

Standardized Care Plans

Many institutions have attempted to make documentation easier for nurses with standardized care plans. The plans, based on the institution's standards of nursing practice, are preprinted, established guidelines that are used to care for clients who have similar health problems. After a nursing assessment is completed, the staff nurse identifies the standard care plans that are appropriate for the client. The care plans

are placed in the client's medical record. Modifications can be made in ink to the standardized plans to individualize the therapies. Most standardized care plans also allow the nurse to write in specific goals or desired outcomes of care and the dates by which these outcomes should be achieved.

One advantage of standardized care plans is establishment of clinically sound standards of care for similar groups of clients. These standards can be useful when quality improvement audits are conducted. Another advantage is education. Nurses learn to recognize the accepted requirements of care for clients. The standardized care plans can also improve continuity of care among professional nurses.

The use of standardized care plans is controversial. The major disadvantage is the risk that the standardized plans inhibit nurses' identification of unique, individualized therapies for clients. When standardized care plans are used in a health care facility, the nurse remains responsible for an individualized approach to care. Standardized care plans cannot replace the nurse's professional judgment and decision making. In addition, care plans need to be updated on a regular basis to ensure that content is current and appropriate. There is the trend among many hospitals to computerize care plans. With such a system, daily computer-generated care plans are printed and incorporate several nursing diagnoses or problems in a single care plan. Such a system facilitates the process of revision and individualization of plans.

Discharge Summary Forms

Much emphasis is placed on preparing a client for an effective, timely discharge from a health care institution. A prospective payment system based on DRGs encourages health care institutions to be more efficient and to discharge the client as soon as possible. The earlier a client is discharged, the more likely it is that a hospital will be fully reimbursed. However, it is important to ensure that a client's discharge results in desirable outcomes. Multidisciplinary involvement in discharge planning helps to ensure that a client leaves the hospital in a timely manner with the necessary resources (Box 3-1).

Ideally discharge planning begins at admission. Nurses revise the plan of care as the client's condition changes. There needs to be evidence of the involvement of the client and family members in the discharge planning process so that the client and family have the necessary information and resources to return home. The JCAHO (2004c) has established standards for client education necessary for effective discharge planning. In addition to the JCAHO standards, a common standard in nursing practice is to educate clients about the nature of their disease process, its likely progress, and the signs and symptoms of complications. When a client is discharged from inpatient care, the various members of the health care team prepare a discharge summary. The summary is given to the client or family, or home care, rehabilitation, or long-term care agency (JCAHO, 2004c). Discharge summary forms make the summary con-

- Use clear, concise descriptions in client's own language.
- Provide step-by-step description of how to perform a procedure (e.g., home medication administration). Reinforce explanation with printed instructions.
- Identify precautions to follow when performing self-care or administering medications.
- Review signs and symptoms of complications that should be reported to a physician.
- List names and phone numbers of health care providers and community resources that the client can contact.
- Identify any unresolved problem, including plans for follow-up and continuous treatment.
- List actual time of discharge, mode of transportation, and who accompanied the client.

cise and instructive. A summary form emphasizes previous learning by the client and family and care that should be continued in any restorative care setting. When given directly to clients the form may be attached to pamphlets or teaching brochures.

Methods of Recording

As there are multiple documentation forms, there are also multiple documentation systems for recording client information and progress. The nursing service within each agency selects a documentation system to be used; this system may be used hospital-wide or throughout a specific health care system. The type of documentation system selected reflects the philosophy of the nursing service.

Problem-Oriented Medical Records (POMR)

The POMR is a method of documentation that places emphasis on the client's problems. Data are organized by problem or diagnosis. Ideally each member of the health care team contributes to a single list of identified client problems. This approach assists in coordinating a common plan of care (see Skill 3-2).

Source Records

In a source record the client's chart is organized so that each discipline (e.g., nursing, medicine, social work, and respiratory therapy) has a separate section in which to record data. One advantage of a source record is that caregivers can easily locate the proper section of the record in which to make entries.

A disadvantage of the source record is that details about a specific problem may be distributed throughout the record. For example, the nurse describes the character of abdominal pain and use of relaxation therapy and analgesic medication in the nurses' notes. The physician's notes describe the progress of the client's bowel obstruction and the plan for surgery in a separate section of the

record. The results of x-ray examinations that show the location of the bowel obstruction are in the test results section of the record. The method by which source records are organized does not show how information from all disciplines is related or how care is coordinated to meet all of the client's needs.

Charting by Exception

Charting by exception (CBE) is an approach that is used to eliminate redundancy, ensure concise documentation of routine care, emphasize abnormal findings, and identify trends in clinical care. While making documentation more effective it can significantly reduce time spent in charting (Cummins, 1999). It is a shorthand method for documenting normal findings and routine care based on clearly defined standards of practice and predetermined criteria for nursing assessments and interventions. Clearly defined standards of practice that specify nurses' responsibilities to clients provide the framework for routine care of all clients. With standards integrated into documentation forms, such as predefined normal assessment findings or predetermined interventions, a nurse need document only significant findings or exceptions to the predefined norms. In other words, the nurse writes a progress note only when the standardized statement on the form is not met. Assessments are standardized on forms so that all caregivers evaluate and document findings consistently (Figure 3-4).

Because the standard assessments are located in the chart, client data are already present on the permanent record, so nurses do not have to keep temporary notes for later transcription and caregivers have easy access to current data. The assumption with charting by exception is that all standards are met unless otherwise documented. When nurses see entries in the chart, they know that something out of the ordinary has been observed or has occurred. For that reason, when changes in a client's condition develop, it is easy to track them. Any exceptions should be thoroughly described so that staff can monitor and intervene appropriately. The exception is recorded consistently until it is resolved.

Documenting Standards Of Care

Documentation of care should reflect the standards of care established by a specific agency within the guidelines established by the JCAHO. Nurses in specific agencies define their practice and most often base their care standards on evidence-based practice, which may include client assessment and monitoring practices, recommended nursing interventions, and outcome criteria that were shown to be effective when tested in clinical research. For example, clinical research on enteral nutrition identified safe practice for the assessment and management of enteral feeding tubes (chapter 30). This research changed the way nurses verified the location of feeding tubes (Metheny and Stewart, 2002). As a result, the risk of aspiration of tube feedings was reduced and client safety improved.

```
┌─────────────────────────────────────┐   ┌──────────────────────────────────┐
│                                     │   │  789651458 X                     │
│     BARNES-JEWISH HOSPITAL          │   │  Collins, Phil                   │
│                                     │   │                                  │
│   Nursing Shift Assessment  C-6     │   │                  S.S.            │
│                                     │   │  Dr.                             │
│                                     │   │  Unit:      Bed:                 │
│  Requested by: CAROL                │   │                                  │
└─────────────────────────────────────┘   └──────────────────────────────────┘
```

Search Interval   From: 05-Dec-1999 at 07:00
                    To: 06-Dec-1999 at 14:51

Patient Assessment

		Monday 12/06 07:00
N/S	**NEUROSENSORY STANDARD** Alert and awake. If asleep awakens to name. Verbal appropriate, clear, and understandable. Swallows without coughing. Oriented to time, place, person and situation. Behavior is appropriate to situation. Moves all extremities well, ambulates with steady gait.	Within Normal Limits
RESP	**RESPIRATORY STANDARD** Respirations are even and unlabored. Nailbeds and mucous membranes are pink. Patent airway. Lung sounds clear to auscultation. No cough noted	Within Normal Limits
CARD	**CARDIOVASCULAR STANDARD** Regular palpable pulses. Skin pallor within patient's norm. Skin warm and dry. No edema.	Within Normal Limits
SKIN	**SKIN INTEGRITY STANDARD** Skin and mucous membranes intact without notable lesions or impaired integrity. Mucous membranes moist and pink. Braden Score greater than 17.	* Exception as noted below
	Braden Risk Assessment	Mobility: Slightly Limited (3) Sensory: Slightly Limited (3) Moisture: Occasionally Moist (3) Activity: Walks Occasionally (3) Nutrition: Adequate (3) Friction/Shear: Potential Problem (2) Total Score 17
	Casts, Splints, Braces Type: Fiberglass Cast Site: Right Lower Leg	Maintains correct anatomical position No pressure areas noted Distal extremity pink warm to touch Palpable distal pulse Capillary Refill <3 seconds Sensation normal Able to move distal phalanges.
	VASCULAR ACCESS STANDARD IV SITE: Site free of redness, swelling, pain, bleeding, drainage, IV patent, dressing occlusive and intact.	
NUTR	**NUTRITION STANDARD** Tolerating prescribed diet without nausea and vomiting. Eating at least 75% of each meal without difficulty. Feeds self.	Within normal limits
	Diet Type	Regular
GI	**GASTROINTESTINAL STANDARD** Abdomen soft. Bowel sounds active all 4 quadrants. No pain with palpation. Having bowel movements within patient's normal pattern, consistency, and color.	Within Normal Limits
GU	**GENITOURINARY STANDARD** Continent of urine. Urine clear and yellow to amber color.	Within Normal Limits
PSYCH	**PSYCHOSOCIAL STANDARD** Accepts situation and facial expressions are appropriate. family support available and patient receives visitors. Able to communicate without assistance.	Within Normal Limits
EDU	Health Status Teaching	
	Tests/Procedures/Therapies	
	Medication Teaching	
	Nutrition Teaching	
	Medical Equipment Teaching	
HMGT	Equipment	
Charted By		cl

Signatures:
cl   C. Logan, RN

Printed: 06-Dec-1999 at 14:51

FIGURE 3-4 Charting by exception—assessment form. When standards in far left column are not met, a detailed note explaining findings must be entered. (Courtesy Barnes-Jewish Hospital, BJC Health System, St. Louis, Mo.)

Standardized Language

Standardized language is becoming recognized as the means by which nurses can communicate consistent information to describe a clinical situation (Micek and others, 1996). When nurses use the same language to identify client problems and plan client outcomes, nursing care becomes more effective and appropriate to client needs. There are classification systems that provide standardized language. The North American Nursing Diagnosis Association (NANDA International) (2002) has developed standardized nursing diagnoses to describe clients' responses to health problems. The Nursing Interventions Classification (NIC) provides a label name, a definition, and a list of activities that a nurse might do to carry out the intervention (Dochterman and Bulechek, 2004). Use of this standardized language in documentation may prove useful to communicate client care needs more clearly.

Another standard form of language being used throughout health care is client outcomes. The Nursing Outcomes Classification (NOC) provides an outcome label, a definition, and a list of interventions that might result in the outcome (Moorhead and others, 2004). The use of outcomes is essential when evaluating the achievement of the quality and appropriateness of client care. "An outcome is defined as a desired health state, condition, or behavior" (Micek and others, 1996).

Outcome statements require a target date for completion, which can vary greatly depending on the outcome desired. Once the date is established, nurses evaluate the client's progress toward achievement at the prescribed intervals. Each evaluation of progress determines if the client's problem or diagnosis is resolved or if the plan must be revised or extended. In some cases a different plan needs to be implemented. Each outcome is individualized for the particular client using specific measurement criteria. Such a process promotes continuity of care across the continuum of a client's care and centers on the client's and family's ability to restore, maintain, or improve the client's health.

Case Management and Critical Pathways

Case management is a care management approach that coordinates and links health care services to clients and their families while streamlining costs and maintaining quality (Dadich, 2003). It is a "collaborative process which assesses, plans, implements, coordinates, monitors, and evaluates the options and services required to meet an individual's health needs, using communications and available resources to promote quality, cost effective outcomes" (Case Management Society of America, 2003). The uniqueness of case management is that clinicians, either as individuals or as part of a collaborative group, oversee the management of clients with specific case types (e.g., specific diagnoses with complex nursing and medical problems) and are usually held accountable for some standard of cost management and quality.

Case management programs use a multidisciplinary plan of care that is often summarized into critical pathways. The critical pathways are multidisciplinary care plans that include key interventions and expected outcomes within an established time frame (Figure 3-5). Critical pathways are evidence based and the assessment/monitoring, interventions, and expected outcomes are based on research and/or clinical evidence within the literature.

A computerized charting system may be used to allow for integration of the chart by many disciplines. The nurse and other team members such as physicians, dietitians, social workers, physical therapists, and respiratory therapists use the same critical pathway to monitor the client's progress during each shift or in the case of home care, every visit. With the computerized record available at every computer terminal, each care provider can access it at any time.

Critical pathways promote integration of information so that each discipline has access to notes written by others. It also reduces duplication and the amount of charting (Brugh, 1998). Unexpected occurrences, unmet goals, and interventions not specified within the critical pathway time frame are called variances. A variance occurs when the activities on the critical pathway are not completed as predicted or the client does not meet the expected outcomes. An example of a variance is when a postoperative client develops pulmonary complications requiring oxygen therapy and monitoring with pulse oximetry. A positive variance occurs when a client progresses more rapidly than expected (e.g., use of a Foley catheter may be discontinued a day early). A variance analysis is necessary to review the data for trends and for developing and implementing an action plan to respond to the identified client problems. In addition, variances may result from changes in the client's health or may occur as a result of other health complications not associated with the primary reason for which the client requires care. The nurse's responsibility is to address the variance and to justify the actions taken to manage the critical pathway deviation (Iyer and Camp, 1999). Over time the reoccurrence of similar variances may lead the health care team to revise a critical pathway.

Home Care Documentation

The home care business continues to grow with shorter hospitalizations and larger numbers of older adults requiring home care services. Medicare has specific guidelines for establishing eligibility for home care reimbursement. Documentation in the home care system has different implications than in other areas of nursing. One primary difference is that the majority of care is witnessed by the client and family rather than the nurse. Nurses must have precise and accurate assessment skills to gather the needed information about changes in the client's health care status. In addition, documentation systems need to provide the entire health care team with the necessary information to work together effectively (Box 3-2). The documentation is both the quality control and the justification for reimbursement from Medicare, Medicaid, or private insurance companies. Nurses need to document all their services for payment (e.g.,

Norman Regional Hospital CareMap®						Page 1
Community Acquired Pneumonia		Check (✓) Precautions				
		☐ Falls	☐ Skin	☐ DNR		

Admitting Physician:	Primary Care Physician:	Consulting Physician(s):	Expected LOS	M&R LOS
Allergy/Reaction			Secondary Diagnosis	

Prob	Patient Problem	Expected Outcome (Responsible Discipline)	Outcome	Date	Signature
#1 ★	Infection	Blood cultures obtained prior to start of antibiotics? (RN)	☐ YES ☐ <u>NO</u>		
#2	Activity Tolerance	Patient is at or above baseline activity (endurance) level? (RN)	☐ YES ☐ <u>NO</u>		
#3	Knowledge Deficit	Patient able to verbalize understanding of pneumonia signs and symptoms? (RN)	☐ YES ☐ <u>NO</u>		
#4 ★	Timeliness of Antibiotic Administration	First dose of antibiotic administered within 2 hours of order? (RN, RPh)	☐ YES ☐ <u>NO</u>		
#5 ★	Discharge Preparation	Patient switched from IV to oral antibiotic within 48hrs after delivery of 1st dose? (RN, RPh)	☐ YES ☐ <u>NO</u>		
★ = Key Exception — = Documentaion Required		Copyright©2000 Norman Regional Hospital			Patient Sticker

Statement of Intent:
The CareMap® serves as an optional guideline for patient care and is subject to alteration based on the individual needs of the patient.
(CareMap® used with permission of the Center for Case Management.)

Authors: **Rosalie Lavon, M.D., Jerry Leu, M.D., John McCarter, M.D., Tom Merrill, M.D., Bruce Naylor, M.D., J. Kin Pirtle, M.D., Joe Riddle, M.D., Christian Sieck, M.D., Jackie Evans, Linda Fielder, Vicki Johnson, Wanda Maddox, Yvette Morrison, Wanda Morrow, Joyce Nolen, Barbara Poe, Michelle Rausch, Darin Smith, Brenda Wilson**
Date: 7/00   Form# CMAP 114   Revised:

FIGURE **3-5** Example of a critical pathway for pneumonia. (From Norman Regional Hospital CareMap, Community Acquired Pneumonia. Copyright 2000, Norman Regional Hospital. Used with permission of Normal Regional Hospital, Norman, Okla.)

Continued

Norman Regional Hospital CareMap®
Community Acquired Pneumonia
CareMap® Summary

PATIENT STICKER

Time Admitted: _____

	Day #1 (ER/Floor) Date _____	Day #2 Date _____
Assessments/Monitoring	VS qshift (and Temp q4h if T>99.5) Nursing Assessment qshift Weight I&O Pain Assessment	VS qshift (and Temp q4h if T>99.5) Nursing Assessment qshift I&O Pain Assessment
Consults	Respiratory Therapy Assess need for Social Work Consult	
Procedures/Tests	CBC with diff, Basic Metabolic Panel, UA, Sputum gram stain + C&S Stat (induce if necessary), Blood cultures x2 (15 minutes apart), CXR (PA & Lateral)	CBC with diff
Treatments	Oxygen Therapy per protocol C&DB q2hr Suction prm Albuterol AN treatments/MDI per RT/RN if ordered Incentive Spirometry q2hr WA @ bedside if ordered	Continue oxygen therapy per protocol, evaluate for discontinuation of O2 RT to convert to MDI prm Incentive Spirometry q2hr WA @ bedside if ordered
Medications/IV	Initial Antibiotic STAT (to be administered within one hour of order) IV Fluids	Cont Abx–consider oral switch Evaluate and change to HL or DC IV if applicable
Nutrition	Diet as tolerated Encourage oral fluids if appropriate	Diet as tolerated Encourage oral fluids if appropriate Goal: 3-4 glasses H_2O if not fluid restricted
Activity/Safety	Activity as tolerated (Encourage up in chair for meals) Fall prevention program initiated if appropriate	Activity as tolerated (Encourage up in chair for meals) Goal: Ambulate 25-50ft x 2
Patient/Family Education	Assess knowledge level concerning disease process and medication Teach use of MDI if applicable	Reasses patient's ability to use MDI Reinforce med education, activity and follow-up
Discharge Planning	RN/SW initiates discharge planning	Interview patient/family re: discharge planning
Psychosocial/Emotional/ Spiritual	Explain procedures Encourage verbalization of feelings	Notify Chaplain to visit if requested
CMAP # 114		

Page 2

Additional Daily Treatments/Other

Isolation Precautions

Special Procedures/Surgeries:

Additional Daily Lab:
Order for CareMap entered into computer: initial (RN/US) _____

Other Pertinent Information:

Family Spokesperson:

Emergency Phone #: _____

FIGURE **3-5, cont'd** Example of a critical pathway for pneumonia. (From Norman Regional Hospital CareMap, Community Acquired Pneumonia. Copyright 2000, Norman Regional Hospital. Used with permission of Normal Regional Hospital, Norman, Okla.)

direct skilled care, client instructions, skilled observation, and evaluation visits) (JCAHO, 2004c).

Some parts of the record are needed in the home with the client; other information is needed in an office setting. Thus duplication of documentation is necessary, or agency policies are needed regarding what forms nurses need to leave at their office versus what forms need to be taken into the homes. Computerized client records are evolving as one means of addressing these different needs. With the use of modems and laptop computers it is becoming possible for the records to be available in multiple locations, which allows greater access to the multidisciplinary needs that are often present in home care.

Long-Term Health Care Documentation

An increasing number of older adults require care in long-term health care facilities. Because many individuals will live in this setting for the rest of their lives, they are referred to as residents rather than clients. In the long-term care setting, nursing personnel face challenges much different from those in the acute care setting (Iyer and Camp, 1999).

In long-term care, governmental agencies are instrumental in determining the standards and policies for documentation. For example, the Omnibus Budget Reconciliation Act of 1987 included extremely significant Medicare and Medicaid legislation for long-term care documentation. Each resident is viewed holistically by using the Resident Assessment Instrument. This assessment requires a registered nurse who has clinical competence, observational skills, and assessment expertise. The overall goal is a system of clinical documentation that provides improved care for residents and increased reimbursement for that care (Boroughs, 1999).

In addition, the department of health in each state governs the frequency of written nursing records of the residents in long-term care facilities. Since residents are often stable, daily documentation is done using flow sheets. Assessments done several times a day in the acute care setting may be required only weekly or monthly in the long-term care setting.

Long-term care agencies also may have skilled care units where clients require increased levels of care in response to mandates for shorter hospital stays. Multidisciplinary communication among such health care providers as nurses, social workers, recreational therapists, and dietitians is essential in these settings as well. The fiscal support for long-term care residents hinges on the justification of nursing care as demonstrated in documentation of the services rendered.

Computerized Documentation

Nurses have been using computerized systems for supplies, equipment, stock medications, and diagnostic testing for some time. However, most larger hospitals have also been using computerized documentation systems. There is now a rapidly growing trend for computerized documentation even in smaller community hospitals. Computerized documentation systems are drastically changing. Many computerized systems are developed in standardized formats with the ability to easily gain access to data across the continuum (regardless of setting) and the ability to capture useful information from both individual clients and population groups.

Software programs increasingly allow nurses to quickly enter specific assessment data, fill in forms with typical entry choices, allow narrative for unique situations, have adequate computer memory for large amounts of data, and automatically transfer information to different reports. Computers also help generate nursing care plans and document all facets of client care.

Typical user interfaces (e.g., keyboard and monitor) require typing skills and can result in data entry errors. Graphic user interfaces (e.g., touch pads, mouse, and icons) are not well suited for nursing. Pen-based or automated speech-recognition (ASR) or voice-recognition technology may eventually become extremely effective for nursing documentation. A notebook-sized computer is available, allowing nurses to document with ease and flexibility not possible in the current systems.

A complete computer-based patient care record (CPCR) is a comprehensive system that uses many components of data collection (Box 3-3). The CPCR permits the nurse to have an instrumental role in development of this form of documentation. In addition, this type of record system is an effective way to influence nursing practice and to record the care planned and/or given to an individual client (Currell and Urquhart, 2004).

The transition to computerized documentation presents both opportunities and challenges to nurses and nurse managers (Figure 3-6). The successful implementation of a computerized documentation system requires preparation, involvement, and commitment of the entire nursing staff. The transition from paper to computer presents challenges for nursing staff. Tools for transforming existing documents into interactive interdisciplinary computerized forms have been developed. Some studies, however, have shown that during the transition when charting must be

BOX 3-3 Objectives of Computer-Based Patient Care Recording (CPCR)

Improved uniformity, accuracy, and retrievability of data about client care

Confidentiality of health care information ensured in the system

Access for authorized health care providers from any department

Ability to retrieve information selectively and choose various formats for examining it

Assistance with clinical application, including analysis tools, risk assessment, and clinical reminders

Support for data collection in a manner that adequately supports health care providers' direct entry and stores information according to a defined vocabulary

Easy access to client data, fast retrieval, and versatile data display that facilitates improved health care delivery

Availability of a lifelong record of health-related events incorporating records from various settings and time periods

Modified from National Coordination Office for Computing, Information, and Communications: *High performance computing and communications FY 1997 implementation plan,* Washington, DC, 1996, US Government Printing Office, http://www.ccic.gov/pubs/imp97/136.html, accessed July 2004.

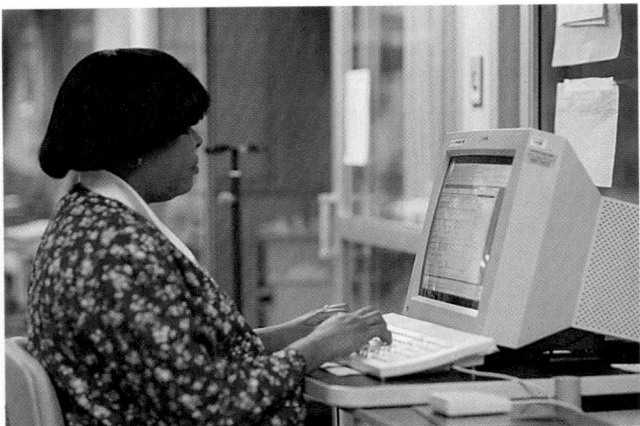

FIGURE **3-6** Computerized documentation provides many benefits.

done on both paper and the computer, the amount of time spent on documentation was not excessive (Korst and others, 2003).

Evidenced-Based Practice Trends

Computer-based health care records, informatics, and implementation of the electronic patient record all have major implications for the practice of nursing and the documentation of nursing care. Computer-based documentation systems are integral to improving and documenting quality nursing care (Helleso and Ruland, 2001). Such a system maintains a continual record of care planned and/or provided to a client by nurses and other members of the health care team and shows improvement in meeting selected agency's documentation standards (Currell and Urquhart, 2004). Studies have shown that the inclusion of the nursing process within the computerized record is a positive and important factor in influencing acceptance of the new system (Ammenwerth and others, 2001, 2003). There are important preconditions for the success of computer-based nursing process documentation, including a high acceptance of the nursing process, careful preparation of predefined care plans, and organizational preparation and inclusion of future users in the development process. It is also essential to have sufficient technical equipment with integration into the hospital information system (Ammenwerth and others, 2003).

SKILL 3-1 Giving a Change-of-Shift Report

In addition to written documentation, nurses report information about their assigned clients to the nurses working the next shift. The purpose of the report is to provide continuity of care for the client. A change-of-shift report may be given orally in person, by audiotape recording, or during "walking-planning" rounds at each client's bedside. Oral reports are given in conference rooms, with staff members from both shifts participating. An advantage of oral reports is that it allows staff members to ask questions or clarify explanations. When nurses make rounds, the client and family members also have the opportunity to participate in any decisions. The nurses can see the client together to perform needed assessments, evaluate progress, and discuss the interventions best suited to the client's needs. An audiotape report is given by the nurse who completed the client's care, and it is left for the nurse on the next shift to review. Taped reports can improve efficiency by taping report before the end of the shift when time is available and by avoiding social conversations between peers. It is essential to schedule an opportunity for the oncoming nurses to ask questions for clarification after listening to the taped report. Regardless of the form of the change-of-shift report, confidentiality must be maintained.

DELEGATION CONSIDERATIONS

The skill of giving a change-of-shift report may not be delegated to assistive personnel. However, nurses should instruct assistive personnel what to report back to them so that any pertinent information can be reassessed by the nurse, validated, and later included in the change-of-shift report.

EQUIPMENT

❑ Worksheets, nursing Kardex (or patient care profile [PCP]), nursing care plan or multidisciplinary treatment plan or critical pathway
❑ Tape recorder (according to agency policy)

STEP	RATIONALE

ASSESSMENT

1. Gather information from worksheets, assistive personnel report, or other relevant documents.

Nurse will not read forms during report that the next nurse can easily read independently. However, data used in reports must be current and reflect an overview of client's progress during shift.

PLANNING

1. Prioritize information based on client's needs and problems; for example, report on immediate treatment planned for newly admitted client, report on educational progress of client about to be discharged home.

Data reported need to reflect client changes during the shift and be pertinent, specific, and accurate.

● *Critical Decision Point*
Report only relevant information to next shift to ensure staff's timely responsiveness.

IMPLEMENTATION

1. Develop an organized format for delivering report that includes a description of client's needs and concerns. For each client the following information may be included:

   a. *Background information:* Include client's name, sex, age, current primary reason for hospitalization, and brief history. Also include any known allergies, code status (i.e., do not resuscitate), and special needs as related to any physical challenges (e.g., blind, hearing deficit, amputee).

   Data are organized based on priorities and individualized by reporting nurse.

   b. *Assessment data:* Provide objective observations and measurements made during shift. Describe client's condition, and emphasize any recent changes. Include any *relevant* information reported by client, family, or health care team members, such as laboratory data and diagnostic test results.

   Oncoming nurse will use data as baseline for comparison during next shift.

   c. *Nursing diagnoses:* Include nursing diagnoses appropriate for client.

   This clarifies client's current responses to health problems.

   d. *Interventions, outcomes, and evaluation:* (steps can be combined in a report).

   (1) Describe therapies or treatments administered during shift and expected outcomes (e.g., relief of pain, improved airway patency). Specify how interventions are uniquely implemented for this client. Explain client's response and whether outcomes are met.

   Staff learn the effect interventions are having on client's recovery and progress.

   (2) Format for evaluation could be a mechanism for reporting on client progress and variance documentation.

STEP	**RATIONALE**
(3) Describe instructions given in teaching plan and client's ability to demonstrate learning.	Continuity of teaching is ensured, minimizing repetition but communicating any needs for reinforcement.
e. *Family information:* Report on family visitation or involvement, specifically as it influenced client. Explain if family members were included in care procedures or instruction.	Report informs staff as to level of involvement family members have assumed in client's care.
f. *Discharge plan:* Client's progress toward discharge is reviewed during each change-of-shift report. Discharge plan identifies interventions and outcomes needed to allow client to have a smooth transition from hospital or health care facility to home. This plan also identifies health care referrals, roles and responsibilities of multidisciplinary team, and their follow-up visits.	All team members collaborate to follow plan of care that promotes discharge.
g. *Current priorities:* Explain clearly the priorities to which oncoming nurse must attend.	Provides for continuity of care.
2. *Clarify:* Ask staff from oncoming shift if they have any questions regarding information reported.	This allows for clarification of misinterpretation and discussion of additional areas of interest.

• *Critical Decision Point*
Find specific nurses from next shift who will be directly providing care to clients for whom report was given.

SKILL 3-2 Documenting Nurses' Progress Notes

A medical record is a comprehensive descriptive document of a client's health status and needs and the services provided for a client's care. Accurate documentation reflects the quality of care and provides evidence of each health care team member's accountability in giving care. The purpose of the client's record is to provide information for communication, education, assessment, research, financial billing, auditing, and legal documentation (Table 3-3).

Nurses involved in the direct care of clients are responsible for recording assessments of a client's condition, changes in a client's condition, a detailed accounting of nursing interventions, and an evaluation of the client's progress toward established outcomes. The nursing department of each health care agency selects the method used for documentation of client care. The method should reflect the philosophy of the nursing service and incorporate the standards of care and practice for the department. For example, if a nursing department's standards of practice use nursing diagnosis or a framework such as Gordon's functional health patterns (1994), the documentation system uses diagnoses or health patterns in care plans and other forms.

The problem-oriented medical record (POMR) is a format for documentation that places emphasis on the client's problems. Data are organized by problem or diagnosis, and narrative notes include assessment, planning, intervention, and evaluative information specific to the client's health status. In a true POMR system, all caregivers contribute to a single list of identified client problems. Most institutions use a modified POMR system whereby nursing staff contribute to a single list of nursing diagnoses or problems. Clients benefit from a POMR charting method because all health care team members can contribute to a common plan of care. A POMR has a database, problem list, care plan, and progress notes.

Database

The database section contains all available assessment information pertaining to the client (e.g., history and physical examination, the nurse's admission history and ongoing assessment, the dietitian's assessment, laboratory reports, and radiological test results). The database is the foundation for identifying client problems and planning care. As new data

TABLE 3-3	PURPOSES OF RECORDS
PURPOSE	**DESCRIPTION**
Communication	The record is a means for health care team members to communicate processes in the client's *care* (e.g., individual therapies, client education, use of referrals) and the client's *progress* (e.g., response to therapies). Anyone reading the record should have a clear understanding of the plan of care.
Education	The record contains a variety of information, including medical and nursing diagnoses, successful and unsuccessful therapies, and diagnostic findings. Students of nursing, medicine, and other health-related disciplines use records as educational resources.
Assessment	Records provide data that nurses use to identify and support nursing diagnoses and plan proper interventions for care. Information from records adds to the nurse's own observations and assessment. Information in medical progress notes allows the nurse to anticipate the status of the client and to conduct an assessment that augments, validates, or confirms physician findings.
Research	Statistical data relating to the frequency of clinical disorders, complications, use of specific medical and nursing therapies, deaths, and recovery from illness can be gathered from client records. Records describe characteristics of the client populations in a health care agency.
Financial billing	The medical record is a document that shows the extent to which hospitals should be reimbursed for services. For the facility to obtain full reimbursement, the record must show that all physicians' orders were completed adequately and correctly, and it must reflect results of those orders.
Auditing	A regular review of information in client records gives a basis for evaluation of the quality and appropriateness of care provided in an institution. The JCAHO requires health care institutions to establish quality assessment and improvement programs to conduct objective, ongoing reviews of client care. Review of records can reveal information about the processes and outcomes of care.
Legal documentation	A medical record must be accurate because it is a legal document. In case of a lawsuit, the medical record, not the nursing care, is on trial. Nursing care may have been excellent; however, care not documented is care not done as far as a court of law is concerned.

become available, the database is revised. It accompanies clients through successive hospitalizations or clinic visits.

Problem List

After data are analyzed, problems are identified and a single list is made. The problem list includes the client's physiological, psychological, social, cultural, spiritual, developmental, and environmental needs. The problems are listed in chronological order and filed in the front of the client's record to serve as an organizing guide for the client's care. New problems are added as they are identified. When a problem has been resolved, the date is recorded and it is highlighted or a line is drawn through the problem and its number.

Nursing Care Plan

A care plan is developed for each problem by the disciplines involved in the client's care. Nurses document the plan of care in a variety of formats. Generally these plans of care include nursing diagnoses, expected outcomes, and interventions.

Progress Notes

Health care team members monitor and record the progress of a client's problems (Box 3-4). The information can be expressed in various formats of structured notes. One method is the SOAP charting. SOAP is a mneomonic for S—subjective data (verbalizations of the client), O—objective data (that which is measured and observed), A—assessment (diagnosis based on the data), P—plan (what the care-giver plans to do). An I and E are sometimes added (i.e., SOAPIE) in some institutions. The I stands for intervention, and the E represents evaluation. The logic for SOAP notes is similar to that of the nursing process. Collect data about the client's problems, draw conclusions, and develop a plan of care. The nurse numbers each SOAP note and titles it according to the problem on the list.

A second progress note method is the PIE format. It is similar to SOAP charting in its problem-oriented nature. However, it differs form the SOAP method in that PIE charting has a nursing origin, whereas SOAP originated from medical records. The format simplifies documentation by unifying the care plan and progress notes. PIE differs from SOAP notes because the narrative does not include assessment information. A nurse's daily assessment data appear on flow sheets, preventing duplication of data. The narrative note includes P—problem, I—intervention, and E—evaluation. The PIE notes are numbered or labeled according to the client's problems. Resolved problems are dropped from daily documentation after the nurse's review. Continuing problems are documented daily.

A third narrative format is focus charting. It involves use of DAR notes, which include D—data (both subjective and objective), A—action or nursing intervention, and R—response of the client (i.e., evaluation of effectiveness). One distinction of focus charting is its movement away from charting only problems, which has a negative connotation. Instead the notes are structured according to client concerns: a sign or symptom, a condition, a nursing diagnosis, a be-

---

BOX 3-4   Formats for Recording Progress Notes

SOAP (ACRONYM FOR SUBJECTIVE DATA, OBJECTIVE DATA, ASSESSMENT, AND PLAN)

Usually based on a numbered list of problems or nursing diagnoses.

Example:

S (Subjective data—the client's statements regarding the problem): Client states, "I am dreading this surgery because last time I had a terrible reaction to the anesthesia and had such terrible pain when they made me get out of bed."

O (Objective data—observations that support or are related to subjective data): Noted muscle tension and loud, agitated voice.

A (Assessment/analysis—conclusions reached based on data): Fear related to pain/anesthesia.

P (Plan—the plan for dealing with the situation): Notified anesthesiologist, Dr. M, of client's prior experience. Discussed alternatives for anesthesia/pain control options. Stressed importance of activity for circulation/healing. Encouraged to keep nurses informed of pain level/need for medication and that pain may be present, but manageable.

PIE (ACRONYM FOR PROBLEM, INTERVENTION, AND EVALUATION)

Problem-oriented system in which progress notes are written based on a list of identified problems, and detailed data may be entered by any member of the health care team.

Example:

P (Problem): Client states, "I am dreading this surgery because last time I had a terrible reaction to the anesthesia and had such terrible pain when they made me get out of bed." Noted muscle tension and loud, agitated voice.

I (Intervention): Notified anesthesiologist, Dr. M, of client's prior experience. Discussed alternatives for anesthesia and pain-control options. Stressed importance of activity for circulation/healing. Encouraged to keep nurses informed of pain level/need for medication and that pain may be present, but manageable.

E (Evaluation): Client stated she was "very relieved." Stated she would tell the nurses about pain.

FOCUS OR DAR CHARTING

A way to organize progress notes to make them more clear and organized.

Example:

D (Data): Client states, "I am dreading this surgery because last time I had a terrible reaction to the anesthesia and had such terrible pain when they made me get out of bed." Noted muscle tension and loud, agitated voice.

A (Nursing Action): Notified anesthesiologist, Dr. M, of client's prior experience. Discussed alternatives for anesthesia and pain-control options. Stressed importance of activity for circulation/healing. Encouraged to keep nurses informed of pain level/need for medication and that pain may be present, but manageable.

R (Client Response): Client stated she was "very relieved." Stated understanding of the importance of informing the nurses about pain.

NOTE: Some agencies add P (Plan) and refer to this as DARP charting.

Example:

P (Plan): Assess pain level at least every 4 hours postoperatively. Provide nonpharmacological pain management techniques, and administer medication as needed.

NARRATIVE NOTE

Describes client data in a narrative paragraph.

Example:

Client states, "I am dreading this surgery because last time I had a terrible reaction to the anesthesia and had such terrible pain when they made me get out of bed." Noted muscle tension and loud, agitated voice. Notified anesthesiologist, Dr. M, of client's prior experience. Discussed alternatives for anesthesia and pain-control options. Stressed importance of activity for circulation/healing. Encouraged to keep nurses informed of pain level/need for medication and that pain may be present, but manageable.

---

havior, a significant event, or a change in a client's condition. Documentation is written in accordance with the nursing process. Nurses are encouraged to broaden their thinking to include any client concerns, not just problem areas, and to apply critical thinking. Focus charting is easily understood by caregivers and adaptable to most health care settings. Focus charting helps track the client's condition and progress (Smith, 2000).

DELEGATION CONSIDERATIONS

The skill of writing a progress note should not be delegated to assistive personnel. The documentation of repetitive care activities on flow sheets (e.g., intake and output [I&O], height, and weight) may be delegated to assistive personnel.

The nurse should instruct assistive personnel what to report so that any pertinent information can be reassessed by the nurse, validated, and included in the report.

The RN is responsible for any follow-up to validate client outcomes.

EQUIPMENT

❑ Progress note forms (manual or computer)
❑ Pen

STEP	RATIONALE

ASSESSMENT

1. Review all necessary assessments and nursing interventions required by client. Evaluate client's response and status of each diagnosis.

Nursing process organizes nursing care and directs care toward appropriate client problems.

IMPLEMENTATION

1. Identify forms to be maintained and their location.

   a. Forms at bedside or on chart holder just outside door may include graphic chart for vital signs, intake and output record, checklist or flow sheet for routine care or a critical pathway, medication administration record, and nurses' progress notes.

   b. Other nursing forms may be included: intravenous (IV) flow sheets; diabetic record; pain management flow sheet; admission, transfer, and discharge forms; and teaching forms. Follow guidelines for charting (see Table 3-1) to ensure quality documentation.

2. After each client contact, identify information that needs to be documented. Consider the following:

   a. Abnormal findings
   b. Changes in status
   c. New problems identified

3. Document in a timely fashion without leaving open spaces between notes, and include date and time.

4. Using agency format, determine the most effective way to include significant client changes, including the following:

   a. Pertinent factual objective data
   b. Selected subjective data that validates or clarifies
   c. Nursing actions taken
   d. Client responses to actions taken
   e. Additional plans needing to be implemented
   f. To whom information has been reported, including name and status

5. Sign progress note with full name or first initial and last name and status according to agency policy. Do not leave an open space between this note and the previously written note. Students may be required to indicate their level of education and school affiliation.

Comprehensive documentation requires that proper information be entered on all necessary forms.
Accurate clinical decisions are often based on information completed in correct format.

Prompt documentation increases accuracy and promotes effective communication to other members of health care team.

Prompt documentation provides accurate record of client status and avoids omissions resulting from unexpected events.
Consistent use of agency format assists communication of client care in a logical, organized, and complete format.

When additional follow-up is needed, documenting to whom this has been reported shares responsibility with that individual.
Signatures identify persons accountable for client care.

SKILL 3-3 Incident Reporting

An incident is any event not consistent with the routine operation of a health care unit or routine care of a client. The client, visitor, or employee may be at risk when anything unusual occurs in a health care area. Examples of incidents include a client fall, accidental needle-stick injury, medication administration error, a visitor experiencing symptoms of illness, or carelessness in performance of a procedure that leads to actual or potential client injury. When an incident occurs, the nurse involved or the nurse who witnessed the incident completes an incident report. Reporting of incidents helps in the identification of high-risk trends in nursing care or daily unit operations that warrant correction. The report is completed even if an injury does not occur or is not apparent. The information from incident reports helps nursing staff find solutions to prevent repeated incidents. The reports are an important part of a unit's quality improvement program (Table 3-4). Incident reports are not a part of the permanent medical record, but they are kept by the facility to track reoccurring or high-risk problems so as to develop appropriate policies.

TABLE 3-4 EXAMPLES OF INCIDENT REPORT ENTRIES

PROPER ENTRY	INCORRECT ENTRY
6 PM Client found on floor at foot of bed; able to respond to name when called. 2-cm abrasion noted across left forehead. Vital signs stable. Dr. Smith notified and arrived on floor at 6:15 PM. Placed client on fall-prevention protocol.	Client found on floor at foot of bed, probably fell on way to bathroom. Small abrasion over left forehead. Dr. Smith notified. Client instructed to use call light when needing to go to bathroom.
Administered morphine sulfate 10 mg at 4 PM; 6 mg morphine sulfate ordered. Monitored vital signs q 15 minutes; called Dr. Jones; vital signs remain stable.	Administered 10 mg morphine sulfate at 4 PM without checking order before administering. 6 mg morphine sulfate ordered.
Needle stick to right index finger, caused minimal bleeding. Notified employee health department.	Needle stick to right index finger, likely due to needle left in bed linen after blood drawing. Notified employee health.

DELEGATION CONSIDERATIONS

The skill of incident reporting should not be delegated to assistive personnel. Incident reporting often involves assistive personnel who actually find the client in the situation that must be reported. Caregivers need to know their responsibility in actions to take, in reporting what they have found, and in explaining their actions to resolve the situation.

* The nurse should instruct assistive personnel to report an event such as a fall, incorrect treatment, an adverse reaction, etc.
* The nurse is responsible for assessing the client, obtaining all information about the incident, and completing the incident report.

EQUIPMENT
❑ Incident report form
❑ Pen

STEP	RATIONALE

ASSESSMENT

1. Use critical thinking skills to systematically and carefully determine what was involved in the incident. Either report the incident as witnessed or determine from AP what specifically occurred. Record the exact sequence of events involved in incident, including time and type of incident; injury to client, nurse, or other staff; and observation of factors that may have contributed to incident (e.g., wet floor discovered in area of client fall, loose needle in client's bed linen).

Report must include objective, chronological information in the event incident leads to a lawsuit or investigation into institutional policy and procedure. Nurse who witnessed incident or who found client at time of incident files report.

STEP	RATIONALE

- **Critical Decision Point**

  Prepare an incident report on any questionable event. Do not avoid incident reporting based on the notion that punitive actions are taken whenever incident reports are filed.

2. Assess extent of any injury to client or others, including client's subjective report and objective physical examination findings.

   Indicates type of treatment or action needed.

IMPLEMENTATION

1. If incident involves an injury, take steps to restore individual's safety, such as stabilizing client's position after a fall and assessing for further injuries.

   A priority is to stabilize any injury to prevent worsening of individual's condition.

2. When client sustains an injury, call a physician immediately.

   Ensures prompt medical attention.

3. When visitor or staff member sustains an injury, refer to emergency department or appropriate treatment setting.

4. Complete incident report form.

   Prompt recording ensures accurate data.

- **Critical Decision Point**

  Document on incident report form as quickly as possible. The closer to the event, the more accurate the recording. (NOTE: This also necessitates that staff readily know where incident forms are kept and which forms to use for clients, visitors, and staff.)

   a. Record time of incident, and describe exactly what occurred or was observed, using objective findings and observations (see Table 3-4).

   Prevents inferences and misinterpretation.

- **Critical Decision Point**

  It is extremely important to use words that are objective in nature and to use language that does not allow for subjective interpretation. Do not include personal opinions or feelings. Direct quotes by victim can be documented as victim's interpretation of incident.

   b. Describe objectively client's or staff member's condition when incident was discovered or observed.

   Establishes baseline for comparison with any later changes.

   c. Describe measures taken by any caregivers at time of incident.

   Provides standard in determining appropriateness of therapies.

   d. Send completed report to designated department.

   Data are used for facility's risk management and quality improvement programs.

5. When client is involved, document events of incident in client's chart.

   a. Do not duplicate all information from incident report.

   Incident report can include factors nurse observed that may be contrary to policy and procedure. Client's chart should include only objective description of incident.

   b. Do not record that incident report was completed.

   Client's chart is legally recoverable and can be used in court. Incident reports are property of institution but are recoverable through subpoena.

STEP	RATIONALE
c. Simply enter objective description of what happened.	Medical record is for purpose of documenting client's health status and medical care, not to blame or justify events of incident.
d. Record any assessment and intervention activities initiated as a result of incident.	Nurse is responsible for documenting the actions taken following a client injury or mishap.
6. If client was injured, implement any ordered therapies and begin routine assessment of body systems influenced by injury.	Ensures continuity of client care and ongoing assessment of client needs.

FOCUS on CLINICAL PRACTICE

You and your nurse assistant have been caring for Mr. Klein, a 45-year-old man with a degenerative neurological condition, who was admitted for a colon resection. This is his second postoperative day. Elements of his care concern monitoring vital signs every 4 hours, ambulating every 6 hours, and wound assessment.

1. Noting the three elements of care listed above, list those elements for which documentation may be delegated to the nurse assistant.
2. As you correctly noted, wound assessment cannot be delegated. Because the nurse assistant will be providing other aspects of Mr. Klein's care, what information would the nurse need to include in a report to the nurse assistant about the wound?
3. When you assess the wound, it is important that you record your findings. Select the method of recording used in your agency, and do a sample recording of the wound assessment.
4. The nurse assistant walks Mr. Klein and reports to you that he "feels funny" after walking. List your actions in order of priority.
5. The nurse assistant notifies you that Mr. Klein fell out of his chair. What are your actions in order of priority?

NCLEX REVIEW QUESTIONS

1. Recorded or reported information must be recorded timely and correctly. Identify an incorrect guideline for documentation information.
    1. Data are recorded immediately after care or treatment.
    2. Record information provided by another nurse.
    3. Begin each new entry with the time.
    4. Draw a single line through an error entry.
2. Military time is frequently used to document care. You provided oral hygiene at 4:00 PM. The correct military time is:
    1. 0400
    2. 1400
    3. 1600
    4. 2400
3. There are multiple types of charting. Focus charting includes:
    1. Data-Action-Response
    2. Problem-Intervention-Evaluation
    3. Subjective-Objective-Assessment-Plan
    4. Subjective-Evaluation-Assessment-Plan-Implementation-Evaluation
4. There are four purposes for charting by exception. Three of these purposes are to eliminate redundancy, to ensure concise documentation for routine care, and to emphasize abnormal findings. The fourth purpose is to:
    1. Identify a change in the client's condition
    2. Identify a change in the client's medical orders
    3. Identify trends in clinical care
    4. Identify trends in resource utilization
5. The major purpose of the change-of-shift report is to:
    1. Ensure notification of new physician orders
    2. Identify any new trends in care
    3. Provide continuity of care
    4. Determine any client risks
6. An incident report is completed to:
    1. Document poor care
    2. Document an injury
    3. Identify high-risk trends
    4. Identify poor nursing management

References

Boroughs DA: Documentation in the long-term care setting, *J Nurs Adm* 29(12):46, 1999.

Brugh LA: Automated clinical pathways in the patient record: legal implications, *Nurse Case Manag* 3(3):131, 1998.

Case Management Society of America: Membership information, http://www.cmsa.org/membership, 2003.

Cummins KM: Charting by exception, a timely format for you? *Am J Nurs* 99(3):24G, 1999.

Dadich KA: Care delivery strategies. In Yoder-Wise PS, editor: *Leading and managing in nursing,* ed 3, St. Louis, 2003, Mosby.

Dochterman J, Bulechek GM: *Nursing Interventions Classification (NIC),* ed 4, St. Louis, 2004, Mosby.

Gordon M: *Nursing diagnosis: process and application,* ed 3, St. Louis, 1994, Mosby.

Iyer PW, Camp NH: *Nursing documentation: a nursing process approach,* ed 3, St. Louis, 1999, Mosby.

Joint Commission on Accreditation of Healthcare Organizations: *FAQs about the 2004 National Patient Safety Goals,* http://www.jcaho.org/accredited+organizations/patient+safety, accessed July 2004a.

Joint Commission on Accreditation of Healthcare Organizations: *Management of information,* http://www.jcaho.org/, accessed July 2004b.

Joint Commission on Accreditation of Healthcare Organizations: *The medical records guide to the 2004 JCAHO standards,* Chicago, 2004c, The Commission.

Martin BA: Torts-r-us, *Vermont Nurse Connection* 4(1):4, 2001.

Mathews J, Zadak K: Managerial decisions for computerized patient care planning, *Nurs Manage* 24:7, 1993.

Moorhead S and others: *Nursing Outcomes Classification (NOC),* ed 3, St. Louis, 2004, Mosby.

National Coordination Office for Information Technology Research and Development: *High performance computing and communications FY 1997 implementation plan,* Washington, DC, 1996, U.S. Government Printing Office.

National Institutes of Health: *Standards for privacy of individually identifiable health information*: the privacy rule—final modification, http://www.cms. hhs.gov/hipaa.

North American Nursing Diagnosis Association: *Nursing diagnoses: definitions and classification 2002-2004,* Philadelphia, 2002, The Association.

Smith LS: How to use focus charting, *Nursing* 30(6):76, 2000.

Sullivan GH: Keep your charting on course, *RN* 63(5):74, 2000.

Sullivan GH: Legally speaking, does your charting measure up? *RN* 67(3):61, 2004.

Yocum RF: Documenting for quality patient care, *Nursing* 32(8):58, 2002.

Research References

Ammenwerth E and others: Nursing process documentation systems in clinical routine: prerequisites and experiences, *Int J Med Inf* 64(2-3):187, 2001.

Ammenwerth E and others: Factors affecting and affected by user acceptance of computer-based nursing documentation: results of a two-year study, *J Am Med Inform Assoc* 10(1):69, 2003.

Currell R, Urquhart C: Nursing record systems: effect on nursing practice and health care outcomes: The Cochrane Library (Oxford) 1:(2004) (ID#CD002099).

Helleso R, Ruland CM: Developing a module for nursing documentation integrated in the electronic patient record, *J Clin Nurs* 10(6):799, 2001.

Korst L and others: Nursing documentation time during implementation of an electronic medical record, *J Nurs Adm* 33(1):24, 2003.

Metheny NA, Stewart BJ: Testing feeding tube placement during continuous tube feedings, *Appl Nurs Res* 15:254, 2002.

Micek WT and others: Patient outcomes: the link between nursing diagnoses and interventions, *J Nurs Adm* 26(11):29, 1996.

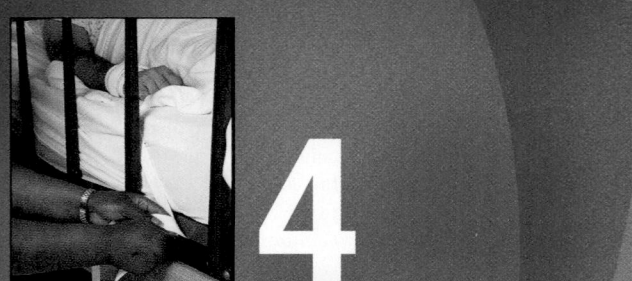

4

Safety

MEDIA RESOURCES

Evolve Site *evolve*

http://evolve.elsevier.com/Perry/skills

- Weblinks
- Video clips
- Mosby's Nursing Skills Video Exercises

Mosby's Nursing Skills Videos/CD-ROM

- *Safety and Restraints Video:* Preventing accidents and falls; using restraint alternatives, side rails, bed and wheelchair locks; safe use of restraints, physician's orders, delegation guidelines; applying restraints—vest restraint, extremity restraints, finger-control mittens; monitoring restraint use

OBJECTIVES

Mastery of content in this chaper will enable the nurse to:

- Discuss methods to reduce physical and environmental hazards in all health care settings.
- Discuss specific risks to safety as they pertain to the older adult client.
- Describe nursing interventions taken in the event of a fire.
- Describe nursing interventions specific for reducing the risk of falls.
- Describe steps in the design of a restraint-free environment.
- Describe nursing interventions for a client who experiences generalized seizures.
- Describe methods to evaluate interventions designed to maintain or promote a client's safety.

KEY TERMS

Aspiration	Mummy restraints
Belt restraints	Physical restraint
Extremity restraints	Seizure
Mitten restraints	Seizure precautions

BOX 4-1   2005 JCAHO Patient Safety Goals for Fall Prevention

GOAL: REDUCE THE RISK OF PATIENT HARM RESULTING FROM FALLS

- Assess and periodically reassess each patient's risk for falling, including the potential risk associated with the patient's medication regimen.
- Implement a fall reduction program, including a transfer protocol, and evaluate the effectiveness of the program.
- Evaluate and as appropriate, modify the environment of care to minimize harm to patients if they fall.
- Install bed alarms for use with patients at high risk for falling.
- Use "low beds" for patients at high risk for falling.
- Do not use full length bed rails.

Modified from Joint Commission on Accreditation of Healthcare Organizations: *2005 National Patient Safety Goals,* Chicago, 2004, The Commission.

Health promotion and illness prevention involve maintaining the client's safety. Maintenance of a client's safety in the home, community, and health care environment is essential. Promoting client safety prevents the frequency of treatment-related accidents and reduces the length and cost of treatment when hospitalization occurs, the potential for lawsuits, and the number of work-related injuries to personnel. In addition, a safe environment encourages clients to assume a more active role in their health care practices.

The impetus to maintain client safety within health care organizations is well supported by accrediting and governmental agencies. For example, the Joint Commission on Accreditation of Healthcare Organizations (JCAHO) established in July of 2002 its first set of national patient safety goals for improving the safety of patient care in health care organizations. All JCAHO-accredited health care organizations are surveyed for implementation of the goals. Each year the goals are revised, and new goals applicable to the safety conditions within health care organizations are adopted. Each patient safety goal has a set of requirements that must be met by a health care organization, unless the goal does not pertain to the agency. Nurses are accountable within their institutions for adhering to the safety goal requirements. Chapter 19 discusses the patient safety goals pertaining to medication administration. Box 4-1 lists the new 2005 patient safety goals pertaining to fall prevention.

In the home, community, and health care setting accidents are a primary threat to the safety of older adults. Beginning at about age 70, the death rate from falls increases dramatically, and the rate continues to increase with age. In 2001 more than 11,600 people ages 65 and older died from fall-related injuries (Centers for Disease Control and Prevention [CDC], 2003). Falls are a leading cause of injury in hospitalized older adult clients as well. Injuries to older adults can be related to psychogenic factors, physiological changes occurring because of the aging process, pathological conditions, medications, and/or environmental hazards. Ebersole and others, (2004) identify the following areas for nurses to consider when attempting to provide a safe environment for the older adult: housing, relocation stress, institutionalization, migration patterns, transportation and mobility, community and neighborhood supports, adaptational capacity of older adults, and environmental safety and convenience.

Safety can be maintained for clients of any age by preventing self-injury. Accidents classified as client-inherent accidents include self-inflicted cuts, injuries, and burns; ingestion or injection of foreign substances; self-mutilation or setting fires; and pinching fingers in drawers or doors. Client-inherent accidents can occur in both oriented and disoriented clients of all ages.

Measures designed to promote client safety are the result of individualized assessment findings. Often it is the conclusion of the nurse that a client's safety is at risk, and subsequent nursing interventions are implemented. A safe environment is one in which clients' basic needs are met, physical hazards are reduced or eliminated, transmission of microorganisms is reduced, and sanitary measures are carried out. Physical hazards, especially those implicated in falls, can be minimized within the home after a thorough home risk assessment (see Chapter 41). In addition, in the hospital or long-term care setting, safety is enhanced by staff remaining alert to clients' risks for injury and implementing use of safety devices such as call lights, signaling devices, and electronic devices that trigger an audio alarm to alert staff to clients who may need assistance. These safety devices are especially useful for older adult clients who are at greater risk for injury during the evening and nighttime due to unfamiliarity with the environment, decreased lighting, and the frequent need to use bathroom facilities.

Clients at risk for injury from falling or other injuries may need restraints temporarily. Restraints are not a solution for a client problem; they are a temporary means to control behavior. Restraints do not necessarily prevent falls. In fact, it has been shown that clients may suffer fewer injuries if left unrestrained (Capezuti and others, 1996; Patterson, Strumpf, and Evans, 1995). Many complications are associated with the use of restraints, the most severe resulting in client death. *There are many alternatives to the use of restraints, and all should be employed before using restraints.* Ideally nurses should collaborate to design fall prevention programs and a restraint-free environment for clients. When restraints are necessary for client safety, the nurse must follow agency-specific policies. A physician's time-limited order is needed, and the appropriate restraint must be used and applied correctly. The client or family member's informed consent is necessary in the long-term care setting. In addition, measures to prevent the hazards of immobility and other complications must be instituted.

A client with a unique risk for injury is one who suffers a seizure disorder (see Skill 4-5). Certain forms of seizures involve sudden, violent, involuntary muscle contractions along with loss of consciousness. During a seizure clients can injure themselves from falls or when their bodies convulsively strike hard surfaces. Nurses caring for clients who have a seizure disorder must be familiar with seizure precautions to provide adequate protection to the client. Nursing interventions are designed to protect a client from traumatic injury, maintain a patent airway, and maintain a positive sense of self-esteem.

Another source of environmental hazard in health care settings is the use of radioactive materials in the diagnosis and treatment of clients, such as during x-ray procedures or radioactive implants. The Nuclear Regulatory Commission strictly regulates safe handling, use, and disposal of radioactive materials. Care providers need to be familiar with agency policies governing use of these materials. Safety measures relating to time, distance, and shielding must be instituted with the goal of reducing exposure of clients, visitors, and staff to radiation.

Evidence-Based Practice Trends

Most research on falls has been conducted in samples from the community and in nursing homes, concentrating on the older adult population (Halfon and others, 2001). Less is known about falls among hospital inpatients, and only a few studies conducted used strong methodological design. The research does show evidence that regardless of clinical setting, fall prevention consists of identifying a client's risk factors and implementing targeted strategies or interventions aimed at reducing risk. Fall prevention strategies should be linked to the client characteristics that lead to a fall and implementation of a comprehensive program that targets interventions that are appropriate and effective (Morse, 2002). Assessment of fall risk should include fall history, medication review, acute or chronic medical problems, mobility level, examination of vision, gait and balance, and basic neurological and cardiovascular function (American Geriatrics Society, British Geriatrics Society, American Academy of Orthopedic Surgeons Panel on Falls Prevention [AGS, BGS], 2001). Successful interventions, based upon the client's assessment, include such things as balance and gait training, exercise programs, medication modification, frequent toileting, postural hypotension treatment, environmental hazard modification, and behavioral and educational programs (AGS, BGS, 2001; Tinetti, 2003). Although some interventions, such as assistive devices (bed alarms, canes, walkers) and behavioral and educational programs, do not prevent falls when used in isolation, they do demonstrate benefit as a part of a multifaceted intervention program. It is clear that the combined effect of multiple interventions produces the best outcomes.

Nurses play a key role in fall prevention in any setting. In addition to promoting a safe environment for clients, educating clients about why falls occur and how they can be prevented promote increased awareness and most importantly behavioral changes regarding fall prevention.

Cultural Considerations

- Become aware of ethnoreligious rituals such as use of open flame and burning that are significant to healing and well-being in some cultural groups. Buddhists (Fadiman, 1999) and Hindus (Pacquiao, 2003) burn incense at the bedside to promote healing. Hindus light an eternal flame at the bedside at the time of the client's death. Orthodox Jews light candles throughout Sabbath (Robinson, 2000).
  —Be prepared to negotiate with the client to find an alternative because open flame is prohibited at the bedside.
    • Battery-operated candles are appropriate for observant Jews who avoid use of electrical appliances during Sabbath. An area may be specially designated for burning incense, herbs, and candles in close proximity to the client's bedside.
- Assess the client's routine and care needs in collaboration with family caregivers. Cultures emphasizing privacy will prevent a client from asking a nonrelated caregiver of the opposite sex for assistance.
- When restraints are needed:
  —Assess the meaning of restraints to the client and the family. Asian families may view the retraining of elders as disrespectful. Holocaust survivors may view restraints as imprisonment or persecution.

—Collaborate with family members in accommodating the client's cultural perspectives about restraints. Removing the restraints when family members are present will show respect and caring for the client.

—Define the unit's protocol on the use of restraints. Identify potential areas for negotiation with the client/family's preferences such as using a jacket versus arm restraints.

—Demonstrate application and removal of the restraint.

- When seizure precautions are needed:

  —Assess the meaning of the symptom to the client and family. For example, the Hmongs believe that seizures are caused by spirit intrusion or soul loss (Fadiman, 1999).

  —Explain and demonstrate the therapeutic regimen to the client/family. Cultures may observe different caring practices for a person with seizures. Surveillance and protection of the client are observed among Hmongs.

Skill Performance Guidelines

1. Assess the client's age, level of awareness, orientation, ability to assimilate information and make judgments, ability to communicate, sensory and motor status, usual activity patterns, and activities of daily living.
2. Assess the client's medical history and present therapies. Certain illnesses, such as stroke, and medications, such as tranquilizers, can cause physical or cognitive impairment that increases the risk of injury.
3. Always be alert to conditions within the client's environment and the risks posed for injury.
4. Be aware of environmental conditions that can affect the client's safety by increasing the risk of fires and injury due to falls, restraint use, or a seizure.
5. Know the proper indications and institutional policy for and use of physical restraints for a client receiving nursing care in a hospital or extended care facility.

SKILL 4-1 Fire, Electrical, and Radiation Safety

A fire is always possible in a health care facility, typically resulting from an electrical or anesthetic-related fire. Although smoking is usually not allowed in the hospital setting, smoking-related fires continue to pose a significant risk due to unauthorized smoking in bed or the bathroom. It is important for a health care agency to ensure that all electrical devices are routinely checked and maintained by the engineering department. Each biomedical device (e.g., suction machine, intravenous [IV] infusion pump, ventilator) should have a safety inspection sticker with an expiration date. If a client brings an electrical appliance to the hospital, the device must be inspected for safe wiring and function before use. It is preferred to discourage clients from bringing nonhospital equipment.

All health care agencies routinely have employees participate in fire safety training, including the use of fire extinguishers and methods for client evacuation. If a fire occurs in a health care agency, the obvious first priority is to protect the client from immediate injury. Health care personnel report the exact location of the fire, contain it, and extinguish it if possible. All personnel are then mobilized to evacuate clients. The best intervention is to prevent fires. Nursing measures include complying with the agency's smoking policies and keeping combustible materials away from heat sources. Some agencies have fire doors that are held open by magnets and close automatically when a fire alarm sounds. It is important to keep equipment away from these doors.

Electrical equipment must be maintained in good working order and should be grounded. The third (longer) prong in an electrical plug is the ground. Improperly grounded or malfunctioning electrical equipment increases the risk of electrical injury and fire. If a client or staff member receives an electrical shock, there is the risk of cardiac arrest.

There are important cultural considerations to consider in fire prevention. As previously mentioned, there are ethnoreligious rituals that involve using an open flame and burning that are significant to healing and well-being. The nurse must assess the client's practices and know agency policies to determine if there is a way to accommodate the client's needs. Informing the client and family of fire safety policies is essential. Consultation with religious leaders might provide insight on how practices can be maintained without creating a fire risk.

Radioactive materials and radiation therapy used in the diagnosis and treatment of clients are significant health hazards. Hospitals have strict guidelines on the care of clients who receive radiation and who have radioactive implants. Staff must strictly follow radiation safety procedures to limit time of exposure and distance to the source of radiation. Oftentimes clients are restricted to specific floors of a hospital where radioactive materials are used (e.g., oncology units). The nurse must be familiar with established agency protocols and policies.

Delegation Considerations

The skill of protecting clients from fire, electrical, and radiation hazards can be delegated to assistive personnel. In the event of a fire or electrical or radioactive event, the nurse will lead the health care team in an emergency response. However, all staff must be trained and familiar with emergency procedures.

EQUIPMENT

Fire

❏ Appropriate fire extinguisher for fire: Type A, B, C, or ABC.

Radiation

❏ Protective radiation shields (lead apron)
❏ Lead-shielded container if required
❏ Radiation exposure badge or dosimeter
❏ Disposable gloves
❏ Radioactive materials caution sign for client's door

STEP	RATIONALE

ASSESSMENT

1. Review agency guidelines for fire, electrical, and radiation safety. Know your responsibilities such as initiating fire alarm, client evacuation, and shielding radioactive sources.

2. Familiarize yourself with location of emergency equipment (e.g., fire extinguishers, emergency cart).

3. Assess client's medical condition, particularly musculoskeletal function and level of cognition and responsiveness.

4. For clients receiving radioactive implants, assess their knowledge of the risks of radiation exposure and purpose of safety precautions. Include family member's knowledge as well.

5. For clients receiving radioactive implants, assess if they are pregnant. Also determine if they plan to have any visitors who are pregnant or 18 years of age or younger.

Rapid and appropriate response to emergent situations requires a well-informed health care team.

Access to emergency equipment ensures rapid response.

Knowledge of client's physical status will enable the nurse to know best procedures to follow in the event of an emergency. For example, the client's mobility and mental status will determine type of approach used for fire evacuation.

Determines need for client and family education and their ability to adhere to precautions.

No pregnant women or anyone under age 18 should enter a room with radioactive materials.

NURSING DIAGNOSES

- Risk for injury
- Impaired physical mobility

- Impaired memory
- Deficient knowledge related to radiation safety

Related factors are individualized based on client's condition or needs.

PLANNING

1. Expected outcomes following completion of procedure:
   - Client's environment is free of hazards.
   - Client will remain injury free.
   - Client will describe radiation safety risks and activity limitations.

Environmental hazards predispose client to potential injury.
Client is safely protected from injury.
Client is familiar with strategies to reduce radiation exposure.

IMPLEMENTATION

1. **Fire Safety**
   a. When a fire is located, sound the fire alarm immediately. Follow agency policy for alerting staff to respond.

   b. Protect client from immediate injury.

   c. Secure the fire.
      (1) Close all doors and windows.
      (2) Turn off oxygen and electrical equipment.
      (3) Place wet towels along base of doors.

Summons emergency assistance and initiates evacuation plan.

Clients close to fire must be removed from area or shielded to avoid burns.
Strategies prevent spread of fire and close off source of oxygen to fire.

STEP	**RATIONALE**

d. Evacuate clients.

   (1) Direct ambulatory clients to walk by themselves to a safe area. Know the fire exits and emergency evacuation route. — Reserves nurses to assist clients unable to ambulate.

   (2) Move bedridden clients by stretcher, bed, or wheelchair.

   (3) Use appropriate carrying method when needed: (a) Place blanket, and drag client out of area of danger. (b) Use two-person swing: Place client in sitting position, and have two staff members form a seat by clasping forearms together. Lift client into "seat," and carry out of area of danger (see illustrations). (c) Use a "back-strap" method: stand in front of client and place client's arms around your neck. Grasp client's wrists firmly against your chest. Pull client onto your back, and carry out of danger. — Safest and most efficient method of evacuation will reduce injuries and move clients away from source of fire in a timely manner.

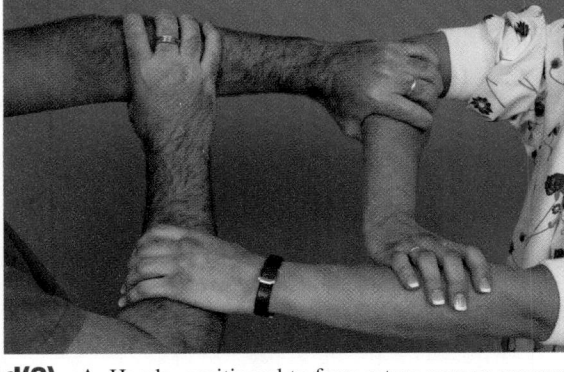
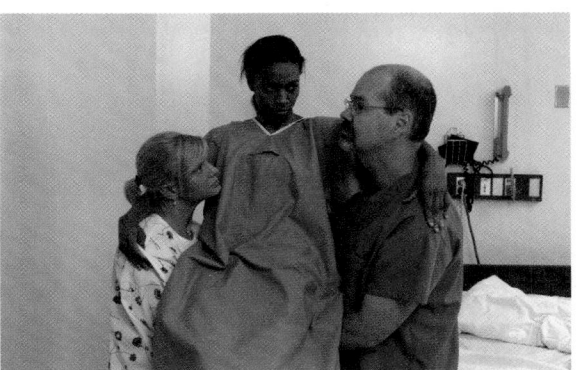

STEP 1d(3)   **A,** Hands positioned to form a two-person evacuation swing. **B,** The client is seated firmly on the swing and holds the nurses by the shoulders for an emergency evacuation.

   (4) If fire department personnel are on the scene, they will help evacuate clients.

• *Critical Decision Point*

Know the weight and size of client when choosing evacuation carry. Use good body mechanics. Use of a carry places health care staff at risk for injury.

e. If client is on life support, maintain client's respiratory status manually with an Ambu-bag until client is moved away from fire. — Continuous maintenance of airway and oxygenation are needed to safely transport client to site where ventilator can be set up.

f. Use appropriate fire extinguisher to put out fire: Type A used for ordinary combustibles (e.g., wood, cloth, paper, most plastics), Type B used for inflammable liquids (e.g., gasoline, grease, paint, anesthetic gas), Type C used for electrical equipment, Type ABC for any type of fire (most common extinguisher in use). — Extinguishers contain solvents designed to put out certain types of inflammables.

STEP	RATIONALE

(1) To use an extinguisher pull the pin (see illustration), aim the nozzle at the base of the fire (see illustration), squeeze the extinguisher handles (see illustration), and sweep from side to side to coat the area evenly.

Proper technique extinguishes fire quickly and safely.

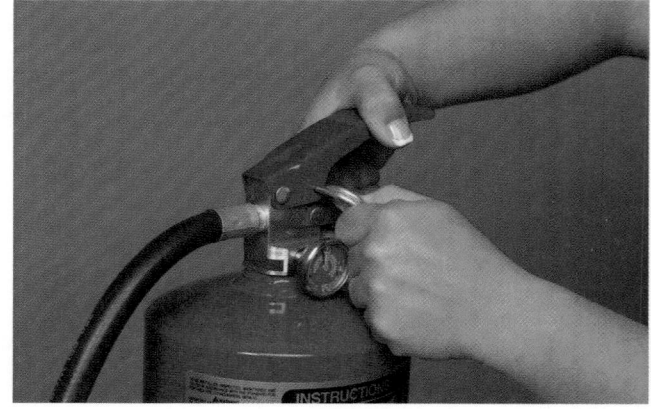

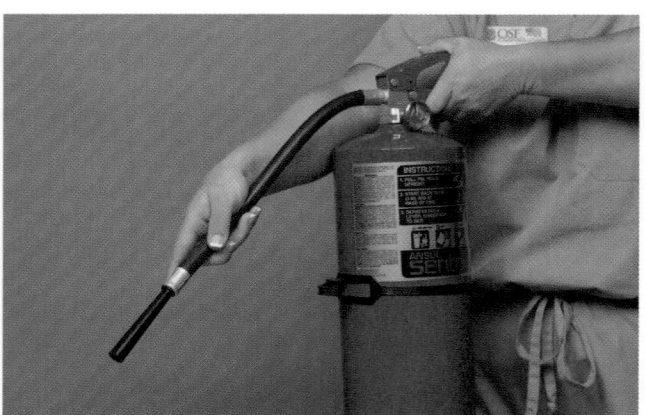

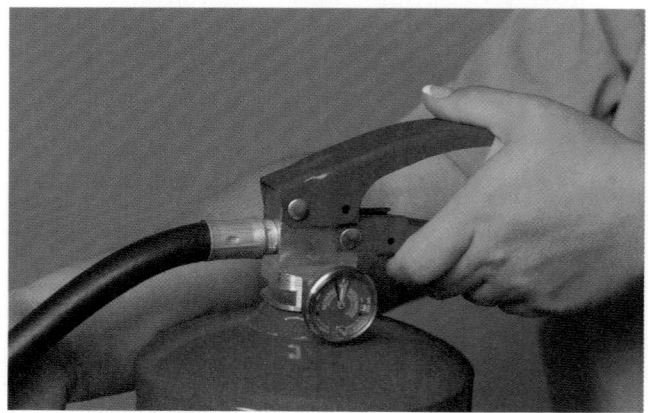

STEP 1f(1)   Using a fire extinguisher. **A,** Remove the safety pin. **B,** Direct the hose at the base of the fire. **C,** Push the top handle down. (From Sorrentino SA: *Assisting with patient care,* St. Louis, 1999, Mosby.)

2. **Electrical Safety**
   a. If client receives an electrical shock, immediately assess the presence of a pulse.
   b. If client is pulseless, institute cardiopulmonary resuscitation (see Chapter 26).
   c. Notify emergency personnel and client's physician.
   d. If client has a pulse and remains alert and oriented, obtain vital signs and assess the skin for signs of thermal injury.

3. **Radiation Safety**
   a. When caring for clients receiving radiation therapy or who have radioactive implants, wear a radiation exposure dosimeter (see illustration).

Electrical shock can cause cardiac arrest, asystole.

Necessary in order to attempt to restore client's circulation.

Emergency medical procedures will be initiated.
Electrical current will cause burn at point of entry and exit from the body.

Dosimeters track the cumulative exposure to radiation.

STEP	RATIONALE

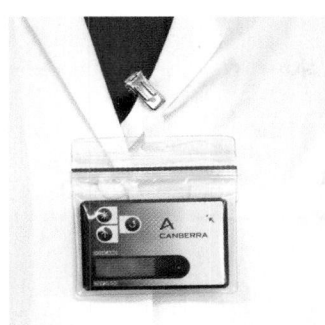

STEP **3a**   Radiation dosimeter.

b. Explain treatment plan to client and family, including activity limitations, safety regulations, and time and distance limits. (For example, visitors are usually limited to 30 minutes a day and must stay 6 feet away from radiation source.)

Improves likelihood of client's adherence to safety guidelines.

c. Place client in a private room with private bath, and place sign ("Caution: Radioactive Material") on door, indicating radioactive materials are in room.

Prevents unnecessary exposure of other clients to radiation.

d. Provide activities and distractions for client undergoing radiation therapy (music, reading materials, planned calls from family members).

Client undergoing radiation is often on bed rest and limited in activities that can be initiated. Social isolation can cause anxiety, loneliness, and depression.

e. Rotate care providers during client's length of stay on unit.

Minimizes time any one staff member is in the presence of a radioactive source.

f. When entering client's room, wear a protective lead apron and gloves. Have family members wear protective gear as well.

Prevents exposure to radiation.

g. Follow agency policy for removal of laboratory specimens, dietary tray, dressings, linens, trash, and body fluids.

Body excretions and secretions and items in contact with client will carry radiation and must be disposed of in a manner to prevent transmission to others.

h. After caring for client, wash gloves before removing, and dispose of them in designated waste container. Perform thorough hand hygiene.

Minimizes contact of hands with radiation source.

i. When client is discharged from facility, request a radiation safety officer to conduct a survey of sources of radiation.

Ensures all sources of radiation have been removed following client's treatment.

EVALUATION

1. Regularly inspect client's room for fire or electrical hazards.

Maintains safe environment for client.

2. Have client describe steps used to minimize radiation exposure and associated risks of exposure.

Demonstrates client's learning and ability to adhere to restrictions.

Recording and Reporting

- Follow agency policy for the report of a fire or electrical accident.
- Document in nurses' notes any education provided to client.
- Complete an incident report for any client receiving a thermal or electrical burn.
- Follow agency policy for the report of any radiation exposure or leak.

Unexpected Outcomes	Related Interventions
1. Hazards are found in client's hospital room.	• Report to appropriate safety or maintenance staff. • Inform fellow health care workers of any risk until hazard is removed.
2. Client unable to describe precautions to avoid radiation exposure and associated risks.	• Reinstruct client and use age-appropriate instructional material. • Include family members in discussion as appropriate.

Teaching Considerations

• Explain to clients who receive brachytherapy (radiation source that is in direct, continuous contact with tumor tissues) that they emit radiation for a period of time and thus can pose a hazard to others unless proper precautions are followed.

• In the event a radioactive implant becomes dislodged, explain to clients and visitors to never touch the radioactive source. Have them call the nurse immediately.

SKILL 4-2   Fall Prevention in a Health Care Facility

In 2001 more than 1.6 million older adults were treated in emergency departments for fall-related injuries, and nearly 388,000 were hospitalized (CDC, 2003). Of those who fall, 20% to 30% suffer moderate to severe injuries such as hip fractures or head trauma that reduce mobility and independence and increase the risk of premature death (Sterling and others, 2001). Frail older adults are especially at risk. Frail older adults with impaired strength, mobility, balance, and endurance are twice as likely to fall as healthier persons of the same age (CDC, 2003). It is therefore essential for nurses to accurately assess clients and their environment for fall risk factors. In this way measures may be instituted to reduce and/or eliminate hazards before client injury occurs. In the home older clients are more likely to fall in the bedroom, bathroom, and kitchen. These falls most often occur while transferring from beds, chairs, and toilets; getting into or out of bathtubs; tripping over carpet edges or doorway thresholds; slipping on wet surfaces; and descending stairs (Tideiksaar, 1989). Therefore it is important to carefully assess the environment and to inform the client of potential hazards. Chapter 41 covers home safety assessment in depth and recommends strategies for making the home safer.

In the hospital setting a tool, such as the RISK for falls assessment tool, may be used to identify a client at risk for falling (Box 4-2). The client's physical status, mental status, medications, and devices used to ambulate are assessed to determine the degree of risk. Based on an individual client's condition and environment, nursing measures are instituted to ensure safety. The call light/intercom system (Figure 4-1) should be explained to the client and family.

Be sure side rails are used appropriately. A full set of raised side rails (two to a bed or four to a bed) may be considered a physical restraint. Raising only one of two or three of four side rails gives clients room to exit a bed safely and to maneuver within the bed. Beds and wheelchairs are locked, and beds are kept in the low position after care is provided (Figure 4-2). Clients may be placed in a Geri chair, or a wedge cushion (Figure 4-3) may be used on the chair or wheelchair to hinder unassisted ambulation. Seating in lounges or dayrooms should be arranged to encourage client interaction. Various types of seating should be available, such as lounge chairs and recliners. Wheelchairs should be used only to transport clients. Visual cues, such as color-coded arm bands or signs on the door or at the bedside, are found to be effective in easily identifying risk-prone clients within an institution, so that staff know which clients may need special assistance.

For clients who continue to attempt to ambulate without necessary assistance, electronic bed and chair alarm devices may be used. These devices are designed to warn nursing staff that a client is attempting to leave the bed or a chair unassisted. A device known as the Ambularm is worn on the leg and signals when the leg is in a dependent position, such as over a side rail or on the floor (Figure 4-4). The device is used for clients who climb out of bed unassisted and are in danger of falling. Additional devices include pressure-sensitive strips placed beneath the client and under the buttocks on either a bed or chair (Figure 4-5), and a tether alarm that is clipped to the client's garment. These devices alert staff that a fall situation is occurring. In this way staff can respond to the client in a timely fashion and provide needed assistance. An alternative

BOX 4-2   Risk for Falls Assessment Tools

TOOL 1: RISK ASSESSMENT TOOL FOR FALLS

Directions: Place a check mark in front of elements that apply to your client. The decision of whether a client is at risk for falls is based on your nursing judgment. Guideline: A client who has a check mark in front of an element with an asterisk (*) or four or more of the other elements would be identified as at risk for falls.

General Data

___Age over 60
___History of falls before admission*
___Postoperative/admitted for surgery
___Smoker

Physical Condition

___Dizziness/imbalance
___Unsteady gait
___Diseases/other problems affecting weight-bearing joints
___Weakness
___Paresis
___Seizure disorder
___Impairment of vision
___Impairment of hearing
___Diarrhea
___Urinary frequency

Mental Status

___Confusion/disorientation*
___Impaired memory or judgment
___Inability to understand or follow directions

Medications

___Diuretics or diuretic effects
___Hypotensive or central nervous system suppressants (e.g., narcotic, sedative, psychotropic, hypnotic, tranquilizer, antihypertensive, antidepressant)
___Medication that increases gastrointestinal motility (e.g., laxative, enema)

Ambulatory Devices Used

___Cane
___Crutches
___Walker
___Wheelchair
___Geriatric (Geri) chair
___Braces

TOOL 2: REASSESSMENT IS SAFE "KARE" (RISK) TOOL

Directions: Place a check in front of any element that applies to your client. A client who has a check mark in front of any of the first four elements would be identified as at risk for falls. In addition, when a high-risk client has a check mark in front of the element "Use of a wheelchair," the client is considered to be at greater risk for falls.

___Unsteady gait/dizziness/imbalance
___Impaired memory or judgment
___Weakness
___History of falls
___Use of a wheelchair

Modified from Brians LK and others: The development of the RISK tool for fall prevention, *Rehabil Nurs* 16(2):67, 1991.

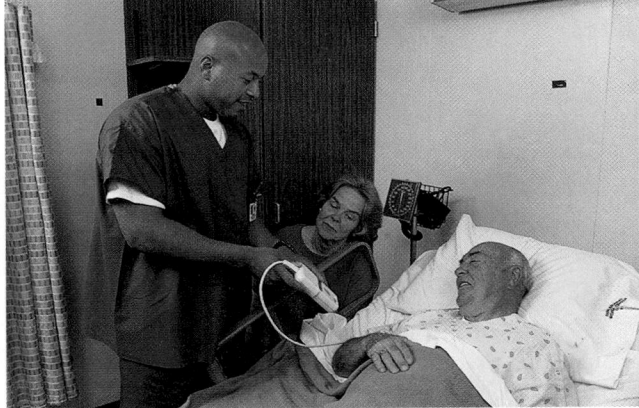

FIGURE **4-1**   The nurse demonstrates the use of the call light to the client and secures it in an accessible position.

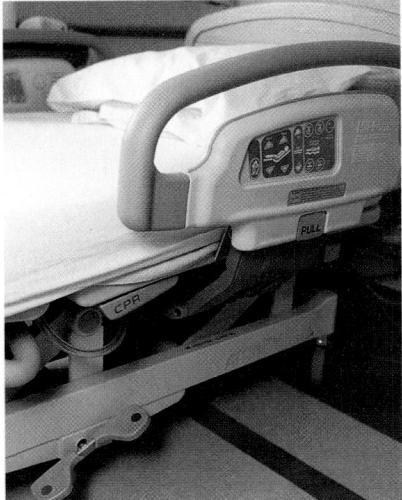

FIGURE **4-2**   The hospital bed should have the wheels locked, be kept in the low position, and have the side rails up (when appropriate).

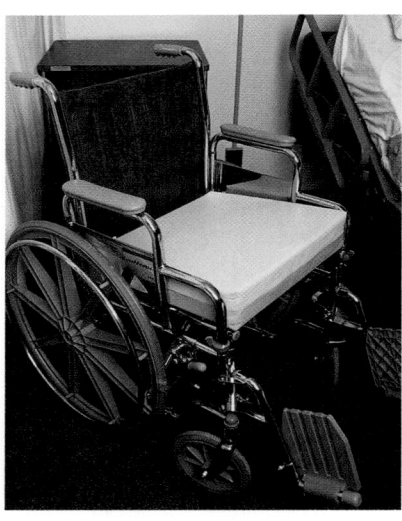

FIGURE **4-3**   A wedge pillow on the seat is thicker at the front, deterring the client from getting up without assistance.

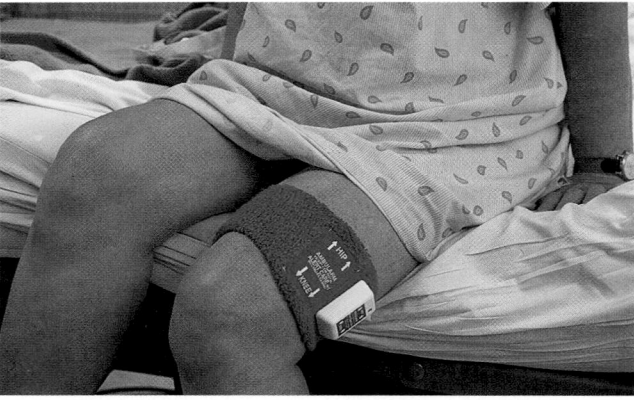

FIGURE **4-4**   Position-sensitive switch triggers an audio alarm when client approaches a near vertical position when getting out of bed. (Courtesy Alert Care, Mill Valley, Calif.)

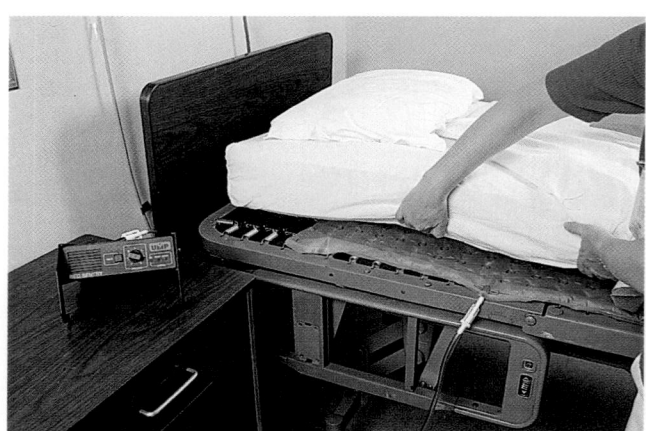

FIGURE **4-5**   Pressure-sensitive pad triggers an audio alarm when client's weight is removed from the bed. (From Sorrentino SA: *Assisting with patient care,* St. Louis, 1999, Mosby.)

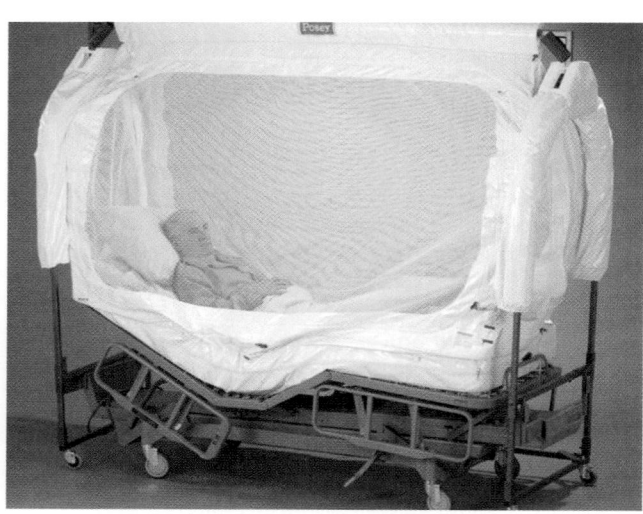

FIGURE **4-6**   The Vail Enclosed Bed.

to a physical restraint is the Posey® Bed Enclosure (see Figure 4-6). Less restrictive than a chemical or vest restraint, the Bed Enclosure allows the client freedom of movement, within a protected environment. This freedom of movement reduces the side effects caused by physical restraints. The Bed Enclosure attaches to most beds and is designed to reduce the risk of entrapment that has been associated with other bed enclosure systems. The bed works particularly well with the cognitively impaired.

At home or in the health care setting it is very important that clients have adequate footwear when ambulating. Clients need well-fitting, sturdy shoes with nonskid rubber soles. A walking shoe or sneaker is recommended. In addition, clients should wear cotton socks, which absorb moisture and prevent friction. Finally, whenever a client attempts to ambulate it is important that a clear path for walking is available. The nurse should remove any barriers or clutter that may create a risk for tripping or misstepping.

DELEGATION CONSIDERATIONS

Assessment of a client's risk for falling should not be delegated to assistive personnel. However, the skills necessary to prevent falls can be delegated. When delegating safety measures, stress the importance of the following:

- Client's mobility limitations and any specific measures to minimize risks
- Specific environmental safety precautions (e.g., bed locked and in low position, call bell and personal items within reach, clear pathway, nonskid footwear)
- What to do when a client starts to fall while being assisted with ambulation (i.e., ease client into a sitting position in a chair or on the floor, and alert the nurse)

EQUIPMENT

- ❑ A risk assessment tool for falls
- ❑ Hospital bed with side rails
- ❑ Call light

STEP	RATIONALE

ASSESSMENT

1. Assess older adult directly, and review medical history for physiological alterations that increase risk of falling: impaired memory and cognition, osteoporosis, osteoarthritis, decreased hearing, decreased night vision, cataracts or glaucoma, orthostatic hypotension, decreased balance, slowed nervous system response, history of stroke or parkinsonisms, incontinence, and decreased energy or fatigue.

Physiological alterations predispose client to falls (e.g., postmenopausal woman is prone to osteoporosis and therefore at risk of breaking hip or ankle when walking: fall results from stress fracture; fracture is not caused by fall).

2. Review client's medication history (including over-the-counter medications) for use of: diuretics, antihypertensives, psychotropics, and polypharmacy (use of multiple medications).

Select medications may cause physical or cognitive impairment that leads to falls. Antihypertensive medications and diuretics may cause hypotension. Diuretics increase the need to make trips to a bathroom. Multiple use of medications has been associated with falls. Narcotics and tranquilizers may cause drowsiness.

3. Assess risk factors in health care facility that pose a threat to older adult's safety (e.g., improperly lighted room, obstructed walkway, clutter of supplies and equipment).

Provides opportunity to decrease risk of accidents.

4. Perform the timed "Get Up and Go" test, which involves looking for unsteadiness as a client gets up from a chair without using his or her arms, walks a few feet, and returns.

Examination easily incorporated into clinical encounters with client is useful in screening for altered balance and gait (Tinetti, 2003).

5. Determine if client has had a history of falls or other injuries within the home. Be specific in your assessment. Follow this acronym, SPLATT:
   Symptoms at time of fall
   Previous fall
   Location of fall
   Activity at time of fall
   Time of fall
   Trauma postfall (Lueckenotte, 2000)

Key symptoms can be helpful in identifying cause for fall. Onset, location, and activity associated with fall provide further details on causative factors and how future falls might be prevented.

6. Determine what client knows about risks for falling and steps he or she takes to prevent falls.

Client's own knowledge of risks influences ability to take necessary precautions in reducing falls.

NURSING DIAGNOSES

- Deficient knowledge related to safety precautions
- Risk for injury
- Impaired physical mobility
- Risk for falls

- Disturbed sensory perception
- Impaired memory

Related factors are individualized based on client's condition or needs.

STEP	RATIONALE

PLANNING

1. Expected outcomes following completion of procedure:
   - Client's environment is free of hazards.
   - Client or family member is able to identify safety risks.
   - Client does not suffer a fall or injury.

Environmental hazards predispose client to potential injury.
Client awareness of risks promotes cooperation and an understanding of treatment plan.
An injury due to a fall can be life threatening, causing dependency or immobilization.

IMPLEMENTATION

1. Introduce self to client, including both name and title or role.
2. Identify client by checking arm band and having client state name, if possible.
3. Explain the plan of care.
4. Gather equipment and perform hand hygiene.

5. Provide privacy. Position and drape client as needed.
6. Adjust bed to proper height, and lower side rail on side of client contact.

7. Call light/intercom system (see Figure 4-1):
   a. Explain and demonstrate how to turn call light/ intercom system on and off at bedside and in bathroom.

Reduces client uncertainty.

Prevents client care errors.

Promotes client cooperation.
Promotes organization and reduces transmission of microorganisms.
Prevents lowering of client's self-esteem.
Allows for proper body mechanics and prevents injury. Height of bed allows ambulatory client to easily get in and out of bed safely.

Knowledge of location and use of call light is essential to client safety.

- *Critical Decision Point*
  Observe client in a return demonstration to ensure learning has taken place.

   b. Consistently secure call light/intercom system to an accessible location.
8. Side rails (see Figure 4-2):
   a. Explain to client and family the two main reasons for using side rails: preventing falls and turning self in bed.
   b. Check agency policies regarding side rail use.

   c. Keep top two side rails up and bed in low position with bed wheels locked when client care is not being administered and client is an older adult, weak, confused, sedated, or sleeping.
   d. Leave one side rail up and one down on side where oriented and ambulatory client gets out of bed.

Ensures client can reach immediately when needed.

Promotes client and family cooperation.

Side rails may be considered a restraint device when used to prevent ambulatory client from getting out of bed (Centers for Medicaid and Medicare Services [CMS], 2004).
Prevents client from falling out of bed. With bed in low position, if client climbs out of bed and falls, trauma may be reduced.

Getting into bed is easier; client can use side rail to position self once in bed.

- *Critical Decision Point*
  Side rails have the potential to cause entrapment of the head and body, especially in clients who are confused or restless. Assess for excessive gaps and openings between bed frame and mattress. Use side rail netting or protective padding to prevent mattress from being pushed to one side.

STEP	**RATIONALE**
9. Provide clear instructions to client and family regarding any mobility restrictions, ambulation and transfer techniques.	Promotes client independence and understanding of treatment plan.
10. Explain to client specific safety measures to prevent falls (e.g., wear well-fitting, flat footwear with nonskid soles; dangle feet for a few minutes before standing; walk slowly; ask for help if dizzy or weak).	Promotes client understanding and cooperation. Dangling provides adjustment to orthostatic hypotension, allowing blood pressure to stabilize before ambulating (see Chapter 11).
11. Make sure ambulatory client's pathway to bathroom facilities is clear.	Eliminates potential hazards and promotes client independence.
12. Provide adequate, nonglare lighting throughout room.	Reduces likelihood of falling over objects or bumping into them. Glare is a major problem for older adults.
13. Remove unnecessary objects from rooms (e.g., suction machines, extra IV poles).	Eliminates potential hazards when client gets out of bed or ambulates.
14. Arrange necessary objects in a logical way, placing them consistently in easy-to-reach locations.	Placing items such as eyeglasses, dentures, hearing aid, and telephone within client's reach allows client to carry out self-care activities safely.

- *Critical Decision Point*
  Clients who follow a consistent routine feel more secure, are less confused, and can better recognize safety hazards.

15. Confer with physical therapy on feasibility of gait training and muscle-strengthening exercise.	Single intervention strategies that have proved effective among older adults at risk for falling include gait and exercise training (Tinetti, 2003).
16. Confer with physician or primary care provider about the possibility of adjusting the number of medications client receives to reduce side effects and interactions.	The number of medications a client receives can be reduced safely if a balance is achieved between benefits of the medications and risk of adverse events (Tinetti, 2003).

EVALUATION

1. Observe client's immediate environment for presence of hazards.	Ensures there or no obstacles or barriers to client's freedom of movement.
2. Evaluate the need for assistive devices such as walker, cane, or bedside commode.	Assistive device may provide more stability and help client assume a more active role.
3. Ask client or family member to identify safety risks.	Ensures client is able to identify risks to safety.
4. Reassess motor, sensory, and cognitive status to determine client's response to modification of potential risks. Determine that no falls or injuries occur.	Determines degree to which nursing interventions have been effective in reducing actual or potential threats to client's safety.

Recording and Reporting

- Record specific risks to client safety and interventions to reduce them on risk assessment tool or nurses' notes.
- Report to all health care personnel specific risks to client's safety and measures taken to minimize risks.
- Document relevant information related to instructions given to client and family and other safety measures employed (e.g., side rails, call light, electronic monitoring device).
- If client suffers a fall, inform physician. Document what occurred, including description of fall as given by client or witness. Be sure to include any injuries noted, tests or treatments given, follow-up care, and additional safety precautions taken after fall.

Unexpected Outcomes	Related Interventions
1. Client is unable to identify safety risks.	• Reinforce identified risks with client, or involve family member/friend and review safety measures needed to prevent a fall.
2. Client suffers a fall despite all measures taken. Safety measures were unsuccessful.	• Nurse must attend to client's immediate physical needs, inform physician of fall and any apparent injury, re-assess client's environment to ensure that environment is free of safety hazards, complete incident report, and communicate to other care providers that client is at risk for falls.

Teaching Considerations

- Make available to clients and families the Centers for Disease Control and Prevention's (CDC's) *Tool Kit to Prevent Senior Falls.* It contains fact sheets, health education materials, and a home assessment checklist. Materials are based on research conducted and sponsored by the CDC. Information is available at http://www.cdc.gov/ncipc/fact_book.
- Client should be instructed to have yearly vision and hearing examinations. Adaptive devices, such as a hearing aid or glasses, may be needed or modified.
- In a health care facility, client and family should be thoroughly oriented to surroundings, with special emphasis given to call lights and/or intercom devices.
- Emphasize to client the need to always look ahead when ambulating and to use good posture.

Pediatric Considerations

- Injuries from falls are more often related to the child's activity level and curious nature. Eliminating places for the child to climb will help limit injuries. Assessing the client for the proper bed and safety restrictions such as crib hoods will also eliminate many falls.
- Toddlers and preschoolers in hospital beds should have side rails kept down or only half raised to allow for easy exit without feeling the need to crawl over the rails.
- When caring for infants, caregivers must always keep a hand on the child when turned away from the bedside, even for a second.

Gerontological Considerations

- Older adults, especially postmenopausal women, are at risk for fractured hips. Fractures can cause independent clients to become more dependent or immobilized (Lueckenotte, 2000).
- Older adult clients with short-term memory loss or cognitive dysfunction may be unable to follow directions and may attempt to climb out of bed or get up from chair unassisted.
- Increasing lower body strength and improving balance through regular physical activity may reduce risk of falling (Campbell and others, 1999). Tai chi is one type of exercise program shown to be effective (Wolf and others, 1996).

Home Care Considerations

- When establishing a safe home environment, a thorough home safety assessment is needed (Chapter 41).
- Night-lights, grip bars, handrails, raised toilet seats, and skidproof strips or surfaces for tub or shower should be used. Remove obstacles from the home such as clutter and throw rugs.
- Client may need hospital bed, with side rails, and bell to signal caregiver or family, especially at night.

Long-Term Care Considerations

- Clients who wander from a facility are at risk for injury. Specific interventions such as electronic wandering devices can be used to reduce this risk (see Chapter 41).

SKILL 4-3 Designing a Restraint-Free Environment

There are clients at risk for falling or wandering who present special challenges in maintaining their safety. Wandering, a common problem in clients with dementia, is defined as meandering, aimless, or repetitive locomotion that exposes a client to harm and is frequently incongruent with boundaries, limits, or obstacles (North American Nursing Diagnosis Association International [NANDA], 2003). The use of restraints is one safety strategy that can protect clients from injury, but they must be used with extreme caution. Physical restraints should be the last resort and used only when reasonable alternatives have failed.

Restraints may become necessary to prevent serious injury to clients due to falling and wandering, to protect from self-injury (e.g., pulling out tubes, removing dressings), and to prevent violence toward others. Some medications, such as those given to calm an agitated client, can be considered a chemical restraint when they are not a standard part of the client's treatment plan.

Recently the public, the media, and the government have grown increasingly concerned about the need to ensure basic protections for client health and safety in health care facilities, especially with regard to the use of restraints and seclusion. Regulatory agencies such as the Joint Commission on Accreditation of Healthcare Organizations (2004) and the Centers for Medicaid and Medicare Services (2004) outline standards regarding the safe use of restraints. The agencies define clients' rights and choices regarding restraints and clearly state the reasons for using physical restraints. The use of mechanical or physical restraints must be part of the prescribed medical treatment, all less restrictive interventions must be tried first, other disciplines must be used, and supporting documentation must be provided. For example, a nurse caring for a client who is attempting to dislodge a tube must try less restrictive measures first, such as camouflage or diversional activity. If the alternatives fail, the nurse may consider use of a restraint to prevent injury.

A restraint-free environment should be the goal for all clients, whether in a health care facility or home. Measures can be taken to ensure safety for those clients who are at risk for self-injury by interrupting therapy and those who may inflict injury on others.

DELEGATION CONSIDERATIONS

The skills necessary to assess client behaviors and make decisions about less restrictive interventions should not be delegated to assistive personnel. Promoting a safe environment (e.g., client positioning) and monitoring client behavior for risk of injury may be delegated to assistive personnel. The nurse must instruct assistive personnel to report to the nurse specific behaviors and actions, such as client confusion, getting out of bed unassisted, pulling at tubes, combativeness, and so on.

EQUIPMENT

- ❑ Visual or auditory stimuli (e.g., calendar, clock, radio, television, pictures)
- ❑ Diversional activities (e.g., puzzle, game, music, stuffed animal, dummy tube)

STEP	RATIONALE
ASSESSMENT	
1. Assess client's physical and mental status, such as orientation; level of consciousness; ability to understand, remember, and follow directions; balance; gait; vision; hearing; bowel/bladder routine; level of pain; laboratory values; and presence of orthostatic hypotension.	Accurate assessment helps to identify safety risks and physiological causes for behavior and ensures proper interventions.
● *Critical Decision Point* *Inability to understand or follow directions indicates client needs constant supervision.*	
2. Review prescribed medications (e.g., sedatives, hypnotics, analgesics, diuretics).	Medication interactions or side effects often contribute to falling or altered mental status.
3. Assess client's knowledge of condition and treatment.	Knowledge of treatment protocols and rationales may increase client's cooperation.

STEP	RATIONALE

NURSING DIAGNOSES

- Risk for injury
- Deficient knowledge regarding need for restricted activity

- Risk for trauma

Related factors are individualized based on client's condition or needs.

PLANNING

1. Expected outcomes following completion of procedure.
   - Client will be injury free and/or will not inflict injury on others while in a restraint-free environment.

Restraints and/or alternatives are successful in preventing injury.

IMPLEMENTATION

1. Orient client and family to surroundings, introduce to staff, and explain all treatments and procedures.

   Promotes client understanding and cooperation.

2. Encourage family and friends to stay with client. Sitters or companions may be used. In some institutions, volunteers can be effective companions.

   Reduces client anxiety and increases safety when one person provides care and supervision is constant.

3. Place client in a room that is easily accessible to caregivers.

   Allows for frequent observation.

4. Provide appropriate visual and auditory stimuli. Choose a stimulus meaningful to the specific client (e.g., clock, calendar, radio [with client's choice of music], television, and family pictures may be indicated).

   Orients client to day, time, and physical surroundings. Strategy must be individualized to be effective.

5. Meet client's basic needs (e.g., toileting, relief of pain, relief of hunger) as quickly as possible.

   Basic needs provided in a timely fashion decreases client discomfort and anxiety.

- *Critical Decision Point*

   Getting out of bed for toileting purposes is one of the most common events leading to a client's fall, especially during evening or night hours, when rooms may be darkened.

6. Approach client in a calm, nonthreatening, professional manner.

   Reduces tension in the environment.

7. Provide the same caregivers to the extent possible.

   Provides stability of routine care and consistency in approach.

- *Critical Decision Point*

   A sufficient number of staff should be readily available quickly for emergency situations.

8. Provide scheduled ambulation, chair activity, and toileting. Organize treatments so client has long uninterrupted periods throughout the day.

   Provides for sleep and rest periods. Constant activity may irritate client.

9. Position IV catheters, urinary catheters, tubes/drains out of client view, or use camouflage by wrapping IV site with bandage or stockinet, placing undergarments on client with urinary catheter, or covering abdominal feeding tubes/drains with loose abdominal binder.

   Facilitates medical treatment and reduces client access to tubes/lines.

10. Stress reduction techniques, such as back rub, massage, and imagery, may be employed (see Chapter 6).

    Reduced stress allows client energy to be channeled more appropriately.

11. Use diversional activities such as puzzles, games, books, folding towels, drawing/coloring, or an object to hold. Be sure it is an activity client consents to.

    Meaningful diversional activities provide distraction, help to reduce boredom, and provide tactile stimulation. Minimize occurrences of wandering.

STEP	RATIONALE
12. Various disciplines should be used in client's care.	Physical therapy, speech therapy, and occupational therapy may assist in providing client necessary resources that reduce activity restrictions and keep client focused on recovery.
13. Review medications frequently, and confer with physician if changes are needed.	Idiosyncratic reactions and drug interactions may cause changes in client behavior.

EVALUATION

1. Observe client for any injuries.	Client should be injury free.
2. Observe client's behavior toward staff, visitors, and other clients.	Client's behavior should not cause injury to others.
3. Determine need for continuation of invasive treatments such as IV catheters, urinary catheters, and feeding tubes and whether less invasive treatment can be substituted.	Eliminates cause and reason for restraint.

Recording and Reporting

• Record restraint alternatives attempted, client behaviors, and interventions to mediate these behaviors.

Unexpected Outcomes	Related Interventions
1. Client may continue to be at risk for injury, disrupt therapy, or commit violent acts toward others.	• Intensify supervision of client, and notify physician. Restraints or medication may be indicated.

Teaching Considerations
• Clients and family members should be familiar with all medications and their possible side effects.

Gerontological Considerations
• Older clients who become confused and attempt to disrupt therapy or become violent may be suffering from effects of multiple drug administration, may be hypoxic, or may have fluid and electrolyte imbalance. Laboratory reports, signs and symptoms of fluid and electrolyte disturbances, and possible side effects of medications and interactions of all medications must be assessed (Brenner and Durnin-Duffy, 1998).

Home Care Considerations
• Clients at risk for self-injury or violence to others need intensive supervision. Family and/or caregiver must recognize this and be able to provide it.

Long-Term Care Considerations
• For clients who are wanderers, exercise the person as ordered. Adequate exercise often reduces wandering. Do not argue with person who wants to leave. Go with person who insists on going outside. Make sure he or she is properly dressed. Guide person inside after a few minutes (Sorrentino, 2000).
• Reminisce with person to help maintain orientation.

SKILL 4-4 Applying Physical Restraints

Clients at risk for injury may need to be temporarily restrained. A physical restraint is any device, garment, material, or object that restricts a person's freedom of movement or access to one's body. The restraint must be clinically justified and a part of the prescribed medical treatment and plan of care, and all other less restrictive measures must be employed first (see Skill 4-3).

The use of restraints has been associated with several serious complications. The Food and Drug Administration (FDA), which regulates restraints as medical devices and requires manufacturers to label them "prescription only," estimates that hundreds of restraint-related injuries occur each year, approximately 100 of them resulting in client death. Most client deaths have resulted from suffocation

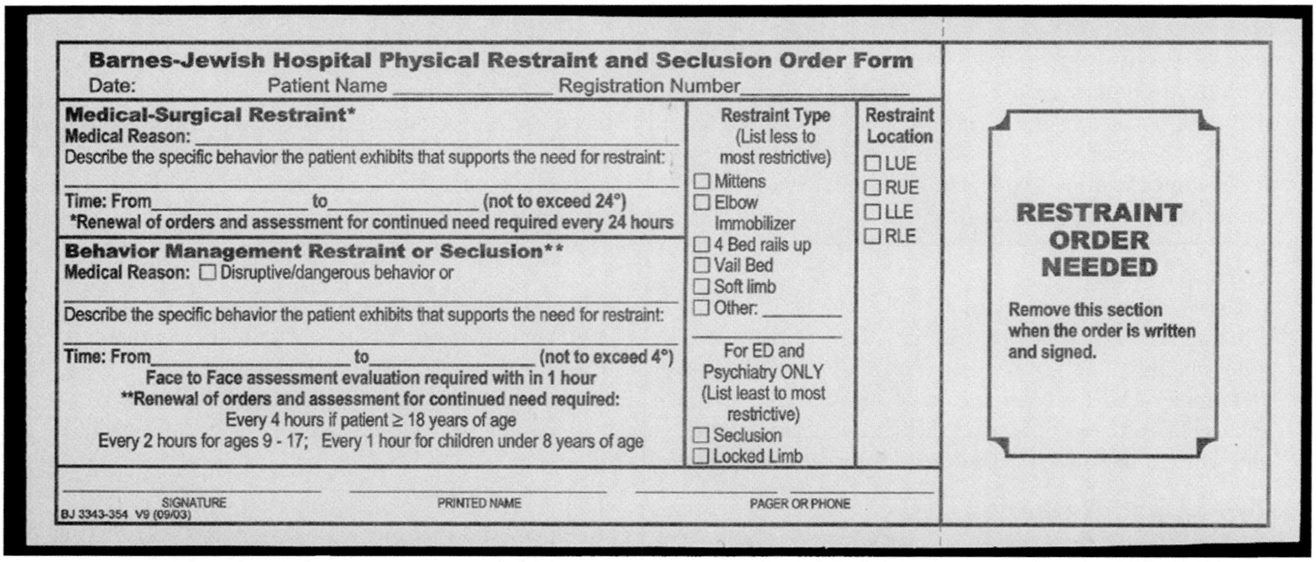

Barnes-Jewish Hospital Physical Restraint and Seclusion Order Form

Date: Patient Name ______________ Registration Number______________

Medical-Surgical Restraint*
Medical Reason: ______________
Describe the specific behavior the patient exhibits that supports the need for restraint:
____
Time: From______________ to______________ (not to exceed 24°)
*Renewal of orders and assessment for continued need required every 24 hours

Behavior Management Restraint or Seclusion**
Medical Reason: ☐ Disruptive/dangerous behavior or
____
Describe the specific behavior the patient exhibits that supports the need for restraint:
____
Time: From______________ to______________ (not to exceed 4°)
Face to Face assessment evaluation required with in 1 hour
**Renewal of orders and assessment for continued need required:
Every 4 hours if patient ≥ 18 years of age
Every 2 hours for ages 9 - 17; Every 1 hour for children under 8 years of age

Restraint Type (List less to most restrictive)
☐ Mittens
☐ Elbow Immobilizer
☐ 4 Bed rails up
☐ Vail Bed
☐ Soft limb
☐ Other: ________

For ED and Psychiatry ONLY (List least to most restrictive)
☐ Seclusion
☐ Locked Limb

Restraint Location
☐ LUE
☐ RUE
☐ LLE
☐ RLE

SIGNATURE PRINTED NAME PAGER OR PHONE
BJ 3343-354 V9 (09/03)

RESTRAINT ORDER NEEDED

Remove this section when the order is written and signed.

FIGURE 4-7 Restraint order form. (Courtesy Barnes-Jewish Hospital, BJC Health Care, St. Louis, Mo.)

from a vest or jacket restraint (Lambert, 1992). Numerous institutions have stopped using vest restraints. For these reasons the use of vest restraints will not be described in this text.

Pressure ulcer formation, hypostatic pneumonia, constipation, incontinence, contractures, and neurovascular impairment can result from the enforced immobility that results from using restraints. Altered sensory perception and altered thought processes may also result. Humiliation, fear, anger, and a decreased sense of self-esteem may occur (Weick, 1992).

When the use of restraints is the only appropriate intervention to maintain the client's safety, both the client and the family should be informed that the restraint is temporary and protective. As with other procedures, the nurse must follow specific agency guidelines when using restraints. Most institutions require a physician's order (Figure 4-7), which should specify the type of behavior or condition requiring restraint, the type of restraint, and time limitations for restraint application. A face-to-face assessment by the physician is required. Orders should be renewed according to agency policy and based upon reassessment and reevaluation of the restrained client.

Not all clients will be able to easily accept the use of restraints. Cultural values affect how clients and family members perceive use of restraints. The nurse assesses the meaning of restraints to both the client and family. If the nurse collaborates closely with family members, culturally sensitive care can be provided, such as removing restraints when family members are present or choosing the use of mitten restraints over that of belt restraints.

DELEGATION CONSIDERATIONS

Assessment of client's behavior, level of orientation, need for restraints, appropriate type to use, and specific assessments related to oxygenation, skin integrity, and neurovascular status should not be delegated to assistive personnel. However, the following aspects of the skill may be delegated to assistive personnel:

- Correct placement of the restraint
- Observing for constriction of circulation, skin integrity, adequate breathing
- When and how to change client's position
- Providing range of motion (ROM) and skin care, toileting, and opportunities for socialization

EQUIPMENT

- ❑ Proper restraint
- ❑ Padding

STEP	RATIONALE

ASSESSMENT

1. Determine client's need for restraint if other less restrictive measures fail to prevent interruption of therapy or injury to self or others. Confer with physician or primary health care provider.

Restraints may be needed when other less restrictive measures fail to prevent interruption of therapy such as traction, IV infusions, or nasogastric tube feedings; to prevent the confused or combative client from removing Foley catheters, surgical drains, or life support equipment; to reduce risk of injury to others by client; and at times to reduce risk of client falling out of bed or wheelchair.

2. Assess client's behavior, such as confusion, disorientation, agitation, restlessness, combativeness, or inability to follow directions.

If client's behavior continues despite attempts to eliminate cause of behavior, use of physical restraint may be needed.

3. Review agency policies regarding restraints. Check physician's order for purpose of restraint and type, location, and time or duration of restraint. Determine if signed consent for use of restraint is needed.

Physician's order is necessary to apply restraints. The least restrictive type of restraint should be ordered. Because restraints limit client's ability to move freely, nurse must make clinical judgments appropriate to client's condition and agency policy. If nurse restrains client in emergency situation because of violent or aggressive behavior that presents an immediate danger, a face-to-face physician assessment within 1 hour is needed (CMS, 2004).

4. Review manufacturer's instructions for restraint application before entering client's room. Determine the most appropriate size restraint.

Nurse should be familiar with all devices used for client care and protection. Incorrect application of restraint device may result in client injury or death.

5. Inspect area where restraint is to be placed. Note if there is any nearby tubing or devices. Assess condition of skin, sensation, and range of motion of joint (if applicable) of underlying area on which restraint is to be applied.

Restraints may compress and interfere with functioning of devices or tubes. Assessment provides baseline to monitor client's skin integrity and neuromuscular status.

- *Critical Decision Point*
  Restraints should not interfere with equipment such as IV tubes. They should not be placed over access devices, such as an arteriovenous (AV) dialysis shunt.

NURSING DIAGNOSES

- Impaired physical mobility
- Risk for impaired skin integrity
- Risk for peripheral neurovascular dysfunction
- Anxiety

- Risk for situational low self-esteem
- Risk for self-directed or other-directed violence
- Risk for injury
- Self-care deficit

Related factors are individualized based on a client's condition or needs.

PLANNING

1. Expected outcomes following completion of procedure:
   - Client remains free from injury.

   Injury can be life threatening, cause dependency or immobilization, and increase length of stay.

   - Client's therapy (e.g., IV tube, catheters) is uninterrupted.

   Disruption of therapy can cause client injury, pain, or discomfort and increase risk of infection.

   - Client's self-esteem and dignity are maintained.

   Physical restraints can have a detrimental effect on psychosocial well-being of client.

IMPLEMENTATION

1. Identify client by checking arm band and having client state name, if possible.

Prevents client care errors.

2. Approach client in a calm, confident manner. Explain what you plan to do.

Reduces client anxiety and promotes cooperation.

STEP	RATIONALE

3. Gather equipment, and perform hand hygiene.

Promotes organization and reduces transmission of microorganisms.

4. Provide privacy. Position and drape client as needed.

Prevents lowering of client's self-esteem.

5. Adjust bed to proper height, and lower side rail on side of client contact.

Allows nurse to use proper body mechanics and prevent injury.

6. Be sure client is comfortable and in correct anatomical position.

Prevents contractures and neurovascular impairment.

7. Pad skin and bony prominences (as necessary) that will be under the restraint.

Reduces friction and pressure from restraint to skin and underlying tissue.

8. Apply appropriate size restraint: **Always refer to manufacturer's directions.**

   a. **Belt restraint:** Have client in a sitting position. Apply over clothes, gown, or pajamas. Remove wrinkles or creases from front and back of restraint while placing it around client's waist. Bring ties through slots in belt. Help client lie down if in bed. Avoid placing belt too tightly across client's chest or abdomen (see illustrations).

Restrains center of gravity and prevents client from rolling off stretcher or sitting up while on stretcher or from falling out of bed. Tight application may interfere with ventilation.

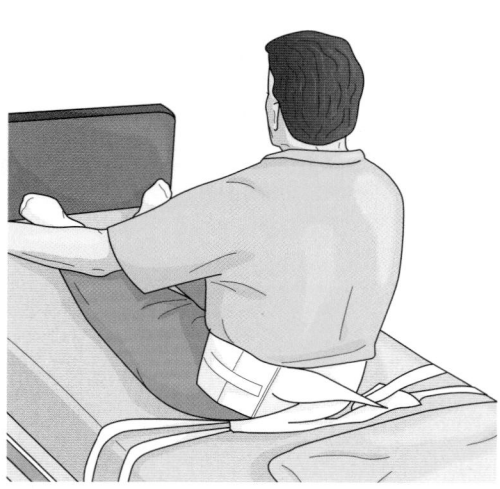
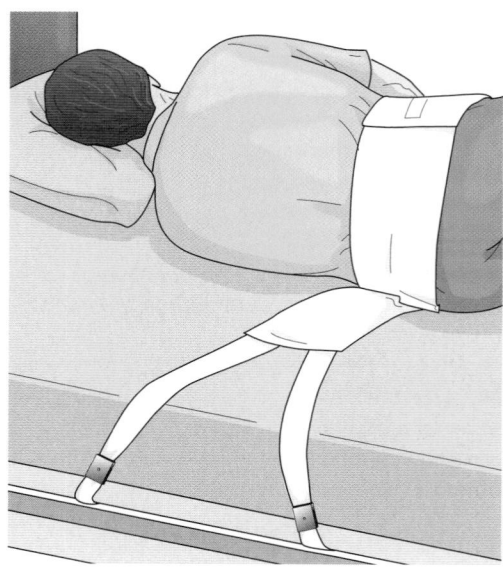
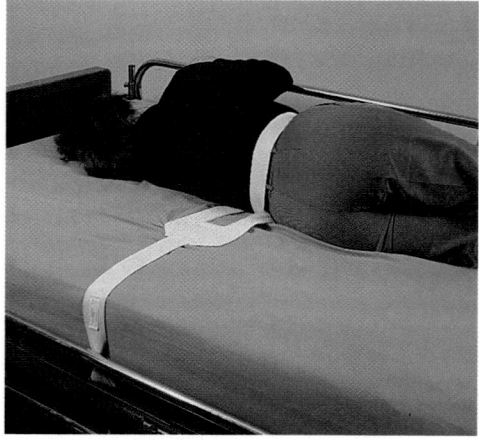

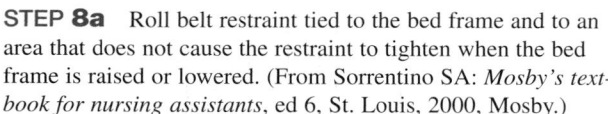

STEP **8a**   Roll belt restraint tied to the bed frame and to an area that does not cause the restraint to tighten when the bed frame is raised or lowered. (From Sorrentino SA: *Mosby's textbook for nursing assistants*, ed 6, St. Louis, 2000, Mosby.)

STEP	RATIONALE

b. Extremity (ankle or wrist) restraint: Restraint designed to immobilize one or all extremities. Commercially available limb restraints are composed of sheepskin or foam padding (see illustration). Limb restraint is wrapped around wrist or ankle with soft part toward skin and secured snugly in place by Velcro straps.

Maintains immobilization of extremity to protect client from injury from fall or accidental removal of therapeutic device (e.g., IV tube, Foley catheter). Tight application may interfere with circulation.

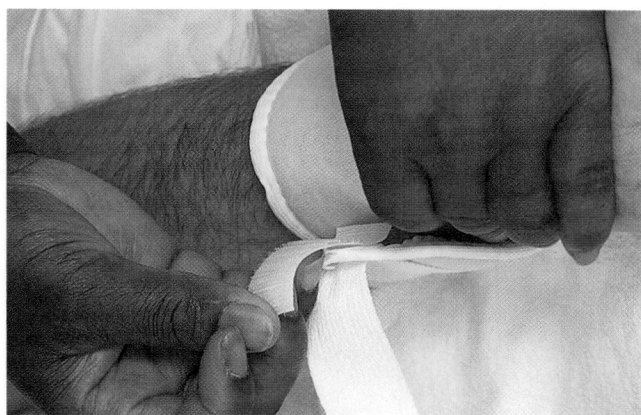

STEP 8b   Securing an extremity restraint. (Courtesy J.T. Posey Co., Arcadia, Calif.)

• **Critical Decision Point**
Client with wrist and ankle restraints is at risk for aspiration if placed in supine position. Place client in lateral position rather than supine.

c. Mitten restraint: Thumbless mitten device to restrain client's hands. Place hand in mitten, being sure Velcro strap(s) is around the wrist and not the forearm (see illustration).

Prevents clients from dislodging invasive equipment, removing dressings, or scratching.

d. Elbow restraint (freedom splint): Restraint consists of piece of fabric with slots in which tongue blades are placed. Insert client's arm so that elbow joint rests against padded area with tongue blades, keeping joint rigid (see illustration).

Commonly used with infants and children to prevent elbow flexion (e.g., when IV placed in antecubital fossa).

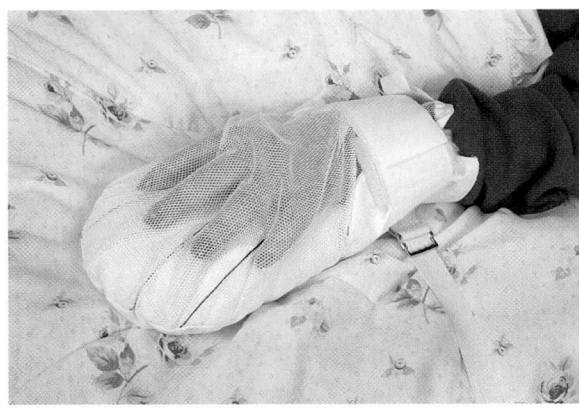

STEP 8c   Mitten restraint. (From Sorrentino SA: *Assisting with patient care,* St. Louis, 1999, Mosby.)

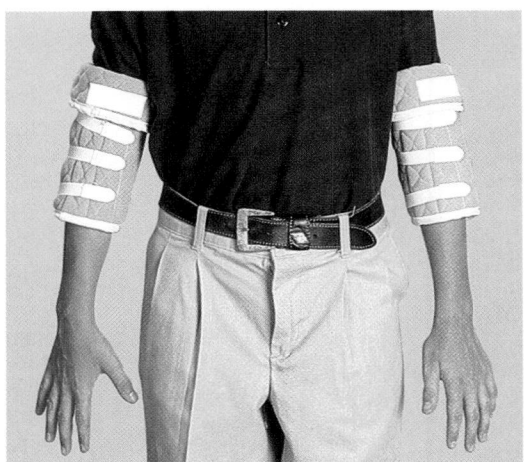

STEP 8d   Elbow restraints. (Courtesy J.T. Posey Co., Arcadia, Calif.)

STEP	RATIONALE

9. Attach restraint straps to bed frame when head of bed is raised or lowered (see illustration). **Do not attach to side rails.** Restraint may also be attached with client in chair or wheelchair to chair frame.

Client may be injured if restraint is secured to side rail and it is lowered.

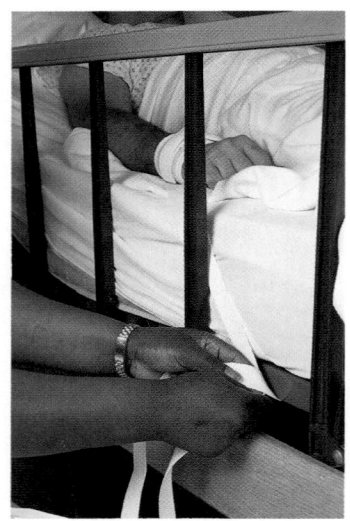

STEP **9**   Restraints should be tied to the bed frame and to an area that does not cause the restraint to tighten when the bed frame is raised or lowered.

10. Secure restraints with a quick-release tie (see illustrations).

Allows for quick release in an emergency.

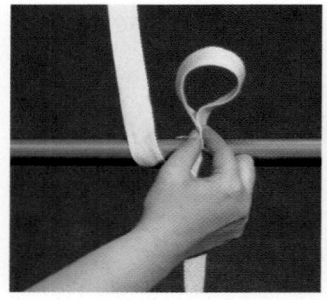 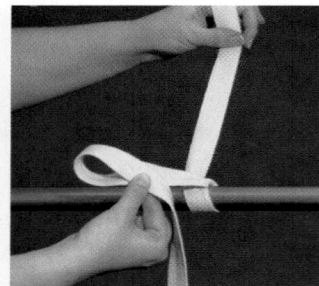 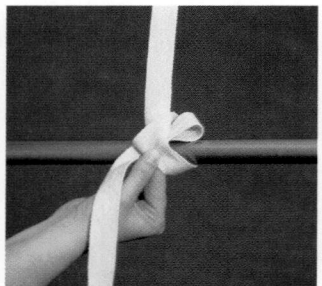 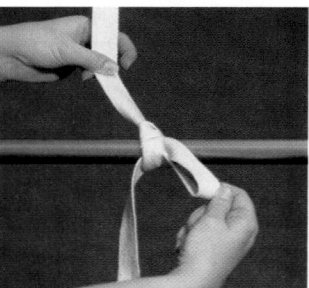

STEP **10**   The Posey quick-release tie. (Courtesy J.T. Posey Co., Arcadia, Calif.)

11. Insert two fingers under secured restraint (see illustration).

Checking for constriction prevents neurovascular injury. A tight restraint may cause constriction and impede circulation.

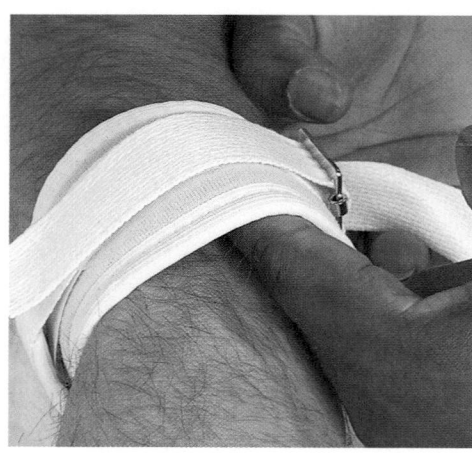

STEP **11**   The nurse checks restraints for constriction by inserting two fingers under the restraint.

STEP	RATIONALE
12. Restraints should be removed at least every 2 hours (JCAHO, 2004). If client is violent or noncompliant, remove one restraint at a time and/or have staff assistance while removing restraints.	Provides opportunity to change client's position, perform full ROM, toileting, and exercise and to provide food or fluids.

• **Critical Decision Point**
Violent or aggressive client should not be left unattended while restraints are off.

13. Secure call light or intercom system within reach.	Allows client, family, or caregiver to obtain assistance quickly.

• **Critical Decision Point**
Restraints restrict movement, making clients unable to perform their activities of daily living without assistance. Providing food/fluids and assisting with toileting and other activities is essential.

14. Leave bed or chair with wheels locked. Bed should be in the lowest position.	Locked wheels prevent bed or chair from moving if client attempts to get out. If client falls when bed is in lowest position, chances of injury are reduced.
15. Perform hand hygiene.	Reduces transmission of microorganisms.

EVALUATION

1. Evaluate proper placement of restraint, skin integrity, pulses, temperature, color, and sensation of the restrained body part **at least every 2 hours or sooner** according to client need and according to agency policy (JCAHO, 2004).	Frequent assessments prevent complications, such as suffocation, skin breakdown, and impaired circulation.
2. Inspect client for any injury, including all hazards of immobility, while restraints are in use. Also inspect during routine removal of restraint.	Client should be free of injury and not exhibit any signs of complications from immobility.
3. Observe IV catheters, urinary catheters, and drainage tubes to determine that they are positioned correctly and that therapy remains uninterrupted.	Reinsertion can be uncomfortable and can increase risk of infection or interrupt therapy.
4. Reassess client's need for continued use of restraint at least every 24 hours or more often depending on purpose of restraint (e.g., behavioral use requires review every 2 to 4 hours). Face-to-face reassessment by physician is required and new order obtained if restraint is to be continued (see agency specific policy).	The intent is to discontinue restraint at the earliest possible time (JCAHO, 2004).

Recording and Reporting

• Record nursing interventions employed to ensure client's safety before use of restraints.
• Record client's behavior before restraints were applied, level of orientation, and client's or family member's understanding of purpose of restraint and consent for application.
• Record in nurses' notes or restraint flow sheet type and location of restraint applied, time restraint was applied, and specific assessments related to oxygenation, skin integrity, musculoskeletal system, and peripheral vascular integrity.
• Record client's behavior after restraints were applied, times client was assessed while restraints were on and findings, attempts to use alternatives to restraint and client's response, times restraint is released (temporarily and permanently), and client's response when restraints were removed.

Unexpected Outcomes	Related Interventions
1. Client experiences impaired skin integrity related to improper or prolonged use of restraint.	• Reassess need for continued use of restraint and if other alternative measures can be employed. If restraint is needed to protect client or others from injury, ensure restraint is applied correctly and provide adequate padding. • Check skin under restraint for abrasions, and remove restraints more frequently. • Institute appropriate skin/wound care. • Change wet or soiled restraints to prevent skin maceration.
2. Client has altered neurovascular status of an extremity, such as cyanosis, pallor and coldness of skin, or complaints of tingling, pain, or numbness.	• Remove restraint immediately, and notify physician.
3. Client exhibits increased confusion and disorientation.	• Evaluate cause for altered behavior, and attempt to eliminate cause. • Provide appropriate sensory stimulation, reorient as needed, and attempt restraint alternatives.
4. Client releases restraint and suffers a fall or other traumatic injury.	• Attend to client's immediate physical needs, inform physician of fall or injury, and reassess type of restraint and its correct application.

Teaching Considerations
- Explain thoroughly the use of restraints. Caution family against removing, repositioning, or retying restraint.

Pediatric Considerations
- The use of restraints should be limited to clinically appropriate and adequately justified situations after all appropriate alternatives have been used. Restraints of children are only used to restrict movement when clients are at risk of injuring themselves or others.
- When a child needs to be restrained for a procedure, it is best that the person applying the restraint not be child's parent or guardian.
- A mummy restraint is a safe, efficient, short-term method to restrain small child or infant for examination or treatment. Open a blanket and fold one corner toward the center. Place child on blanket with shoulders at fold and feet toward opposite corner (Figure 4-8, *A*). With child's right arm straight down against body, right side of blanket is pulled firmly across right shoulder and chest and secured beneath left side of body (Figure 4-8, *B*). Left arm is placed straight against body, and left side of blanket is brought across shoulder and chest and locked beneath child's body on right side (Figure 4-8, *C*). Lower corner is folded and brought over body and tucked or fastened securely with safety pins (Figure 4-8, *D*) (Hockenberry and others, 2003).

Gerontological Considerations
- Advanced age is not in itself an indication for use of restraints. Promoting functional restoration by performing individual assessment of risk factors, orienting client as needed, modifying the environment, teaching muscle strengthening exercises, and meeting older client's needs in activities of daily living will help prevent falls and other traumatic injuries (Ebersole and others, 2004).

Home Care Considerations
- A physical restraint is a device that requires a physician's order. It should not be sent home with family unless device is needed to protect client from injury. If client's family wishes to use restraint at home, a physician's order is required and clear instructions should be given regarding proper application, care needed while in restraints, and complications to look for. Family should be carefully assessed for competency and understanding of intent for using restraint.

Long-Term Care Considerations
- Unnecessary restraint is false imprisonment. The person must understand reason for restraint. The person is told how restraint will help planned medical treatment and risk of restraint use.
- Restraints are not used to discipline a person or for staff convenience (Sorrentino, 2000).

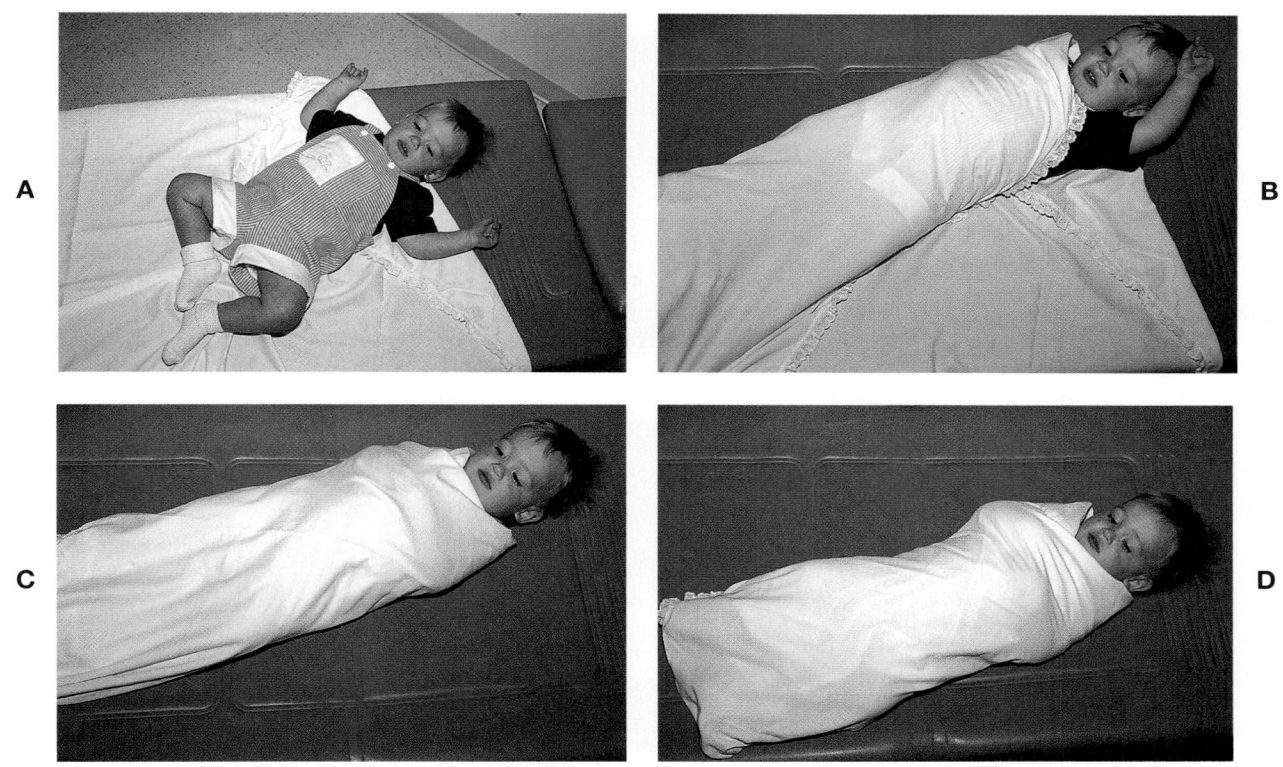

FIGURE **4-8**   Mummy restraint.

SKILL 4-5   Seizure Precautions

A seizure is a hyperexcitation of neurons in the brain leading to a sudden, violent, involuntary series of muscle contractions that may be paroxysmal and episodic, as in a seizure disorder, or transient and acute, as after a head injury. A generalized tonic-clonic or grand mal seizure lasts from 1 to 2 minutes (no longer than 5 minutes) and is characterized by a cry, loss of consciousness, tonicity (muscle rigidity), clonicity (rhythmic muscle jerking), and incontinence. Before a convulsive episode a few clients may report an aura, which serves as a warning or sense that a seizure is about to occur. An aura may be a bright light, smell, or taste (Shantz and Spitz, 1993). Following the seizure there is a postictal phase, lasting for up to an hour, during which the client may be fatigued, confused, and lethargic (Ignatavicius and Workman, 2002).

Status epilepticus is characterized by prolonged seizures lasting more than 10 minutes or a series of seizures that occur in rapid succession over 30 minutes (Ignatavicius and Workman, 2002). It is a potential complication of all types of seizures and constitutes a medical emergency requiring intensive monitoring and treatment.

Seizure precautions include all nursing interventions to protect the client from traumatic injury: side-lying position for adequate ventilation and drainage of secretions, providing privacy, and providing support following the seizure. Traditionally oral airways have been used with the purpose of maintaining the client's airway during a seizure. However, forcing something in the client's mouth could result in injury to the jaw, tongue, or teeth and cause stimulation of the gag reflex causing vomiting, aspiration, and respiratory distress (National Institute of Neurological Disorders and Stroke, 2001). Forcing an airway into a client's mouth is no longer recommended. An airway is inserted only when there is clear access for insertion. Padded tongue blades do not belong at the bedside and should never be inserted into the client's mouth after a seizure begins (Ignatavicius and Workman, 2002).

Observation during a seizure is critical because it may assist in determining the type of seizure. It is important that the nurse observe the client carefully before, during, and after the seizure so that the episode can be documented accurately.

DELEGATION CONSIDERATIONS

Assessment of a client's need to be placed on seizure precautions cannot be delegated to assistive personnel. Setting up seizure precautions and protecting clients at risk for seizures may be delegated to assistive personnel. Measures to emphasize if a client is at risk for a seizure include the following:

* The importance of protecting the client from a fall
* Avoiding attempts to restrain client
* Not placing anything in the client's mouth

Equipment

❑ Padding for side rails and headboard
❑ Suction machine
❑ Oral airway
❑ Oral suction equipment
❑ Oxygen via nasal cannula or face mask
❑ Equipment for intravenous access
❑ Clean disposable gloves

STEP	RATIONALE

ASSESSMENT

1. Assess client's seizure history and knowledge of precipitating factors, noting frequency of seizures, presence of aura, and sequence of events, if known. Use family as resource if necessary.

Knowledge about seizure history enables nurse to anticipate onset of seizure activity.

2. Assess for medical and surgical conditions that may lead to seizures or exacerbate existing seizure condition (e.g., electrolyte disturbances such as hypoglycemia, hyperkalemia; heart disease, excess fatigue; alcohol or caffeine consumption).

Common conditions that may precipitate seizures.

3. Assess medication history and client's adherence. Also assess therapeutic drug levels of anticonvulsants if test results available.

Seizure medications must be taken as prescribed and not stopped suddenly. This may precipitate seizure activity.

4. Inspect client's environment for potential safety hazards if seizure occurs. Prepare bed with padded side rails and headboard, bed in low position, and client in side-lying position when possible.

Prevents client from injury sustained by striking head or body on furniture or equipment.

5. For clients with a history of seizures, oxygen setup, suction apparatus, clean gloves, and pillows should be visible for immediate use in a hospital setting.

This ensures prompt, organized intervention.

6. Assess a client's cultural perspective about the meaning of seizures and their treatment. For example, the Hmongs believe that seizures are caused by spirit intrusion or soul loss (Fadiman, 1999). Performing a ritual led by a shaman will appease the spirits and restore the client's well-being.

Cultures may observe different caring practices for a person with seizures.

NURSING DIAGNOSES

* Risk for aspiration
* Ineffective airway clearance
* Situational low self-esteem

* Deficient knowledge regarding safety precautions during seizure activity
* Noncompliance with medications

Related factors are individualized based on a client's condition or needs.

PLANNING

1. Expected outcomes following completion of procedure:
   * Client remains free of traumatic injury while experiencing seizure.

   Injury from a fall or from jerking may occur as a result of onset of seizure activity.

   * Client's airway remains patent during seizure activity.

   Airway occlusion and aspiration are potential complications of seizure activity.

   * Client does not experience a lowered sense of self-esteem following seizure episode.

   Loss of bowel or bladder control is common in tonic-clonic seizures, causing client to feel embarrassment or shame.

STEP	RATIONALE

IMPLEMENTATION

1. When seizure begins, position client safely. If standing or sitting, guide client to floor and protect head by cradling in nurse's lap or placing pillow under head. Clear surrounding area of furniture. If client is in bed, raise side rails, pad, and put bed in low position.

Position protects client from traumatic injury, especially head injury.

2. If possible, provide privacy. Have staff control flow of visitors in area.

Embarrassment is common after a seizure, especially if others witnessed the seizure.

3. If possible, turn the client on side, with head flexed slightly forward.

Position prevents tongue from blocking airway and promotes drainage of secretions, thus reducing risk of aspiration.

4. Do not restrain client. Loosen clothing.

Prevents musculoskeletal injury and airway obstruction.

5. Do not force any objects into client's mouth such as fingers, medicine, tongue depressor, or airway when teeth are clenched.

Prevents injury to mouth and possible aspiration.

- ### *Critical Decision Point*
  Injury may result from forcible insertion of hard object. Soft objects may break or come apart and be aspirated.

6. Maintain the client's airway, and suction as needed. Provide oxygen by nasal cannula or mask if ordered. *Use oral airway only if easy access to oral cavity is possible.*

Prevents episode of hypoxia during seizure activity.

7. Stay with client, observing sequence and timing of seizure activity.

Continued observation ensures adequate ventilation during and following seizure and will assist in documentation, diagnosis, and treatment of seizure disorder.

8. After seizure is over, explain what happened, and answer client's questions.

Informing clients of type of seizure activity experienced will assist them in participating knowledgeably in their care.

9. For clients experiencing status epilepticus:
   a. Put on clean gloves.

Clean gloves prevent nurse from coming in contact with client's saliva.

   b. Insert an oral airway (see illustration) when jaw is relaxed between seizure activity. Hold airway with curved side up, insert downward until airway reaches back of throat, then rotate and follow natural curve of tongue (see Chapter 26).

Airway occlusion and aspiration are potential complications.

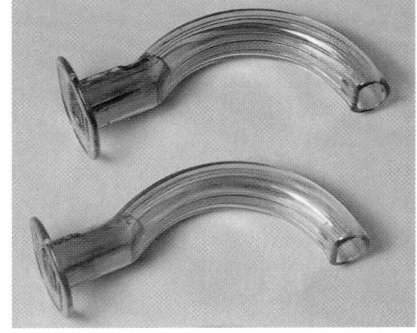

STEP **9b** Oral airways.

   c. Access oxygen and suction equipment, and prepare for IV insertion.

Intensive monitoring and treatment are required for this medical emergency.

- ### *Critical Decision Point*
  Do not place fingers near or in client's mouth. Client may inadvertently bite nurse's fingers during a seizure. Do not forcibly insert airway if client's teeth are still clenched.

STEP	RATIONALE
10. Pad side rails and headboard (see illustration).	Traumatic injury may be reduced. Avoid use of pillows to pad side rails because suffocation could occur.

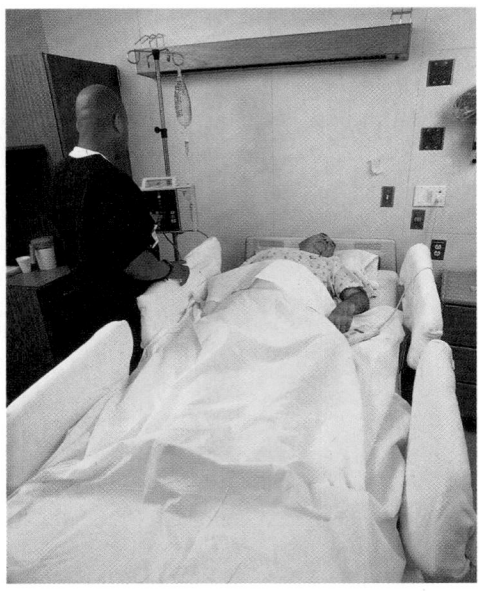

STEP **10**   Padded side rails and headboard.

11. Following seizure, assist client to position of comfort in bed with padded side rails up and bed in lowest position. Place call light or intercom system within reach, and provide a quiet nonstimulating environment.	Provides for continued safety. Clients are often confused and sleepy following a seizure.
12. Offer psychosocial support; stay with client to explain what has occurred. Foster an atmosphere of acceptance and respect, and provide time for client to express feelings and concerns.	Clients who accept the reality of a disease and integrate this reality into their own self-concept experience higher levels of self-esteem.
13. Perform hand hygiene.	Reduces transmission of microorganisms.

▌EVALUATION

1. Observe progression of seizure, noting type of body movement, duration.	Data assists in identification of type of seizure and source.
2. Conduct a head-to-toe assessment to determine presence of any traumatic injuries resulting from seizure activity.	Injury may occur during seizure activity.
3. Assess client's mental status after seizure (level of consciousness, confusion, hallucinations).	Temporary mental status changes are common following a seizure.
4. Assess for bowel or bladder incontinence.	Loss of bowel or bladder control can increase client anxiety and risk of skin breakdown.

• *Critical Decision Point*
Inspect oral cavity for breaks in mucous membrane due to bites and broken teeth.

5. Observe client's color and respiratory rate and pattern during and after seizure.	Client may experience shallow irregular breathing during seizure, but normal color and respirations should be apparent following the episode.
6. If possible, ask client to verbalize feelings after seizure.	Therapeutic interaction may enable client to recognize feelings associated with having a seizure disorder. Client self-esteem is maintained.

Recording and Reporting

- Record timing of seizure activity and sequence of events.
- Record presence of aura (if any), level of consciousness, posture, color, movements of extremities, incontinence, and client's status immediately following seizure.
- Report to physician immediately as seizure begins. Status epilepticus is an emergency situation requiring immediate medical therapy.

Unexpected Outcomes	Related Interventions
1. Client suffers traumatic injury.	• Attend to client's immediate physical needs, inform physician of injury, reassess client's environment to ensure that environment is free of safety hazards, complete incident report, and communicate to other care providers measures taken to reduce risk for further injury.
2. Client's airway becomes occluded, and materials are aspirated.	• Turn onto side, insert oral airway (if possible), and apply suction to remove materials and maintain patent airway. • Maintain nasal oxygen.
3. Client verbalizes negative feelings following a seizure.	• Offer support to client, and allow for verbalization of feelings.

Teaching Considerations

- Clients should be thoroughly familiar with prescribed medications. Medication should never be stopped suddenly because this may precipitate seizures.
- Alcohol should be avoided because it may be incompatible with anticonvulsive medications. It may intensify central nervous system depression.
- Proper oral hygiene and frequent dental care are necessary when client takes phenytoin (Dilantin) long term, because gingival hyperplasia is a side effect (Skidmore-Roth, 2005).
- Client should wear a medical alert bracelet or carry identification card noting presence of seizure disorder and listing medications taken.
- Hypoglycemia, fatigue, stress, and illness have potential to initiate seizure activity (Beare and Myers, 1994). Therefore clients should eat a balanced diet at regular intervals, get enough sleep, and consult their doctor promptly when ill.
- A seizure condition usually imposes driving limitations. It is recommended that a waiting period of 1 seizure-free year elapse before client attempts to drive or operate dangerous equipment (Phipps and others, 1999).
- Some antiepileptic medications (AEDs) may interfere with effectiveness of oral contraceptives, making pregnancy a possibility. In addition, taking a single AED causes a threefold increase in risk of birth defects. Although pregnancy is rarely contraindicated, client should be counseled about potential effects (Rolak, 1998).

Pediatric Considerations

- Parents should be taught what to observe for in seizures because many times they are present at the onset.

- Children with severe atonic seizures may be encouraged to wear a helmet to protect them when they fall. A child with tonic-clonic seizures should have side rails padded and suction and oxygen available to manage respiratory secretions for airway maintenance.

Gerontological Considerations

- Older adults may have various symptoms that can impede the recognition of a seizure disorder. Confusion lasting several days, receptive and expressive language problems, and unusual behaviors may be the result of a seizure (Lannon, 1995).
- Older adults tend to metabolize anticonvulsants more slowly; therefore drugs may accumulate, resulting in toxicity. Many anticonvulsants have known blood levels for therapeutic ranges, so blood levels should be monitored carefully in clients of all ages (McKenry and Salerno, 1999).
- If client has dentures, do not try to remove them during a seizure. If they loosen, tilt head slightly forward and remove after seizure (Lannon, 1995).

Home Care Considerations

- Family members need to be familiar with care of client experiencing a seizure.
- Client's home should be assessed for environmental hazards in light of seizure condition.
- Until seizure condition is well controlled (usually for at least 1 year), client should not take a tub bath or engage in activities such as swimming unless knowledgeable family member is present.
- Referral to the Epilepsy Foundation or a similar group may help to improve client's self-esteem and coping ability.

FOCUS on CLINICAL PRACTICE

Mrs. Gladys Dean has been admitted to the general medicine unit for workup for malignant melanoma. She is 73 years old and is currently taking Synthroid, Lasix, Catapres, low-dose aspirin, and Colace. She has the early stages of Parkinson's disease and has a characteristic mild propulsive gait. Mrs. Dean is alert and asks the nurses numerous questions about planned tests for her condition. She wears a hearing aid in her right ear.

1. List three physiological alterations that increase Mrs. Dean's risk of falling.
2. Among the medications Mrs. Dean receives, which may predispose to conditions for falling?

3. When the nurse assesses Mrs. Dean's fall risk, the "Get up and Go" test is designed to measure:
   A. Client's perceived energy level
   B. Client' ability to remain oriented
   C. Client's balance when rising from a chair
   D. Client's knowledge of environmental barriers
4. Mrs. Dean's daughter comes to visit her mother and immediately raises all four side rails. What would be your reaction to this?
5. Explain why Mrs. Dean might benefit from a physical therapy referral to minimize her risk for falling.

NCLEX REVIEW QUESTIONS

1. Which of the following statements is true about fall prevention?
   1. Falls are most successfully prevented by making the client's environment safe.
   2. The early use of restraints in a restless client will effectively reduce falls.
   3. A bed alarm when used alone will prevent falls.
   4. Falls are most often prevented by linking client characteristics to prevention strategies.
2. In the event you discover a fire, do all of the following to secure the fire except:
   1. Place wet towels along base of doors
   2. Have client place blanket over fire
   3. Close all windows and doors
   4. Turn off oxygen sources

3. Mr. Joseph weighs 200 pounds and has a cast that extends from his hip down to his ankle. A fire begins in Mr. Joseph's bathroom. The best method for evacuating Mr. Joseph is:
   1. The "seat" carry
   2. Evacuation in bed
   3. The "back strap" method of evacuation
   4. Placing Mr. Joseph on floor and dragging out on a blanket
4. A physician's order for a restraint must include all of the following except:
   1. Time limitation for application of restraint
   2. Type of restraint to apply
   3. Type of behavior that requires use of restraint
   4. Alternatives to be used before restraint is used.

References

Beare P, Myers J: *Principles and practice of adult health nursing,* ed 2, St. Louis, 1994, Mosby.

Brenner Z, Durnin-Duffy K: Toward restraint free care, *Am J Nurs* 98(12):16f, 1998.

Brians LK and others: The development of the RISK tool for fall prevention, *Rehabil Nurs* 16(2):67, 1991.

Capezuti E and others: Physical restraint use and falls in nursing home residents, *J Am Geriatr Soc* 44(6):627, 1996.

Centers for Disease Control and Prevention: Web-based Injury Statistics Query and Reporting System (WISQARS) [online], National Center for Injury Prevention and Control, Centers for Disease Control and Prevention (producer), www.cdc.gov/ncipc/wisqars, cited Nov. 24, 2003.

Centers for Medicare and Medicaid Services: *Conditions of participation: interpretive guidelines,* Bethesda, Md, 2004, US Department of Health and Human Services.

Ebersole P and others: *Toward healthy aging: human needs and nursing process,* ed 6, St. Louis, 2004, Mosby.

Hockenberry MJ and others: *Wong's nursing care of infants and children,* ed 7, St. Louis, 2003, Mosby.

Ignatavicius DD, Workman ML: *Medical-surgical nursing: critical thinking for collaborative care,* Philadelphia, 2002, WB Saunders.

Joint Commission on Accreditation of Healthcare Organizations: *Comprehensive accreditation manual for hospitals,* Chicago, 2004, The Commission.

Joint Commission on Accreditation of Healthcare Organizations: *2005 National Patient Safety Goals,* Chicago, 2004, The Commission.

Lambert V: Patient restraints, *FDA Consum* 26(8):9, 1992.

Lannon S: Epilepsy in the elderly, *Clin Nurs Pract Epilepsy* 2(2):5, 1995.

Lueckenotte AG: *Gerontologic nursing,* St. Louis, 2000, Mosby.

McKenry L, Salerno E: *Mosby's pharmacology in nursing,* ed 20, St. Louis, 1999, Mosby.

National Institute of Neurological Disorders and Stroke: *Seizures and epilepsy: hope through research,* Bethesda, Md, 2001, National Institutes of Health.

North American Nursing Diagnosis Association International: *Nursing diagnoses: definitions and classification 2003-2004,* Philadelphia, 2003, NANDA International.

Pacquiao DF: Cultural competence in ethical decision-making. In Andres M, Boyle J: *Concepts in transcultural nursing,* Philadelphia, 2003, Lippincott, Williams, & Wilkins.

Patterson JE and others: Nursing consultation to reduce restraints in a nursing home, *Clin Nurse Spec* 9(4):231, 1995.

Phipps W and others: *Medical-surgical nursing: concepts and clinical practice,* ed 6, St. Louis, 1999, Mosby.

Robinson G: *Essential Judaism: a complete guide to beliefs, customs, and rituals,* New York, 2000, Pocket Books.

Shantz D, Spitz M: What you need to know about seizures, *Nursing* 23(11):34, 1993.

Skidmore-Roth L: *Mosby's drug guide for nurses,* ed 6, St. Louis, 2005, Mosby.

Sorrentino SA: *Assisting with patient care,* St. Louis, 1999, Mosby.

Sorrentino SA: *Mosby's textbook for nursing assistants,* St. Louis, 2000, Mosby.

Sterling DA and others: Geriatric falls: injury severity is high and disproportionate to mechanism, *J Trauma* 50(1):116, 2001.

Tideiksaar R: Home safe home: practical tips for fall-proofing, *Geriatr Nurs* 11(6):280, 1989.

Weick M: Physical restraints: an FDA update, *Am J Nurs* 92(11):74, 1992.

Research References

American Geriatrics Society, British Geriatrics Society, American Academy of Orthopedic Surgeons Panel on Falls Prevention: Guideline for the prevention of falls in older persons, *J Am Geriatr Soc* 49:664, 2001.

Campbell AJ and others: Falls prevention over 2 years: a randomized controlled trial in women 80 years and older, *Age Ageing* 28:513, 1999.

Fadiman A: *The spirit catches you and you fall down,* New York, 1999, Farrar, Straus & Giroux.

Halfon P and others: Risk of falls for hospitalized patients: a predictive model based on routinely available data, *J Clin Epidemiol* 54:1258, 2001.

Morse JM: Enhancing the safety of hospitalization by reducing patient falls, *Am J Infect Control* 30:376, 2002.

Tinetti ME: Preventing falls in elderly persons, *N Engl J Med* 348(1):42, 2003.

Wolf SL and others: Reducing frailty and falls in older persons: an investigation of tai chi and computerized balance training—Atlanta FICSIT Group, Frailty and Injuries: Cooperative Studies of Intervention Techniques, *J Am Geriatr Soc* 44(5):489, 1996.

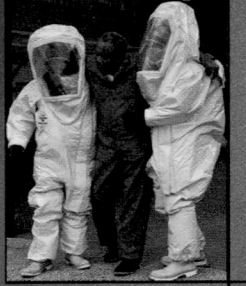

5

Disaster Preparedness

MEDIA RESOURCES

Evolve Site *evolve*

http://evolve.elsevier.com/Perry/skills

• Weblinks

OBJECTIVES

Mastery of content in this chaper will enable the nurse to:

- Discuss the characteristics of different types of disasters.
- Identify actions to take in the event of biological, chemical, and radiation exposure.
- Describe the type of personal protective equipment used when dealing with biological, chemical, and radiological exposures.
- Explain the Centers for Disease Control and Protection's five focus areas for emergency and disaster planning.
- Apply triage concepts to selected disaster scenarios.
- Evaluate the role of the nurse as a member of the multidisciplinary disaster team.
- Discuss guidelines for client care in the event of mass care casualty.
- Discuss methods used for decontamination.
- Describe precautions used when caring for contaminated clients.
- Describe psychosocial effects of disasters on clients.
- Discuss common interventions used in treatment of biological, chemical, and radiological exposure.

KEY TERMS

All-hazards event
All-hazards preparedness
Biological agent
Biological disaster
Bioterrorism/bioterrorist attack
Casualty
Chemical decontamination
Chemical warfare agents
Contamination
Decontamination
Department of Homeland Security (DHS)
Detection and surveillance
Disaster
Disaster management
Disaster planning
Disaster response
Disaster triage
Emergency responders
Exposure
Field triage tag
First responders

Hazard/hazard identification
Hazardous material
Incident Command System (ICS)
Incubation period
International Nursing Coalition for Mass Casualty Education (INCMCE)
Manmade disaster
Mass casualty incident (MCI) or event
Mass casualty triage
Medical disaster
Mutual aid agreement
Natural/environmental disaster
Nuclear event
Postdisaster evaluation
Shelter-in-place
Technological disaster
Triage
Weapons of mass destruction (WMD)

Although disaster preparedness and the possibility of terrorist attacks have been a subject of discussion and research for over 20 years, the attacks on the World Trade Center and Pentagon on September 11, 2001, forever changed the reality and sense of security felt by citizens of the United States. These attacks demonstrated the vulnerabilities, including the very serious lack of preparedness of the health care community, in the event of a mass casualty incident (MCI). The attacks increased public awareness of not only possible or probable future terrorist attacks but also increased public awareness of the more common natural or environmental disasters affecting individuals on a more regular basis.

Throughout history nurses have played a role in the multidisciplinary team approach in preparing for and responding to disasters. Nurses have heeded the call for help when the nation has been at war or when natural disasters have occurred. Now nurses recognize the need to prepare for a different type of disaster, terrorist attack, which may lead to mass casualties. Information gathered from postdisaster evaluations have provided critical data to aid health care workers and communities to recover from disasters, diminish the human toll caused by the events, and to update and improve disaster response. As a result, a considerable body of knowledge and experience has been compiled to improve the response of the entire health care team and the many agencies/individuals involved in disaster response (e.g., police, firefighters, administrators, and paramedics). The newly formed Department of Homeland Security has identified preparedness and education of the nation as an essential component to national security against domestic and foreign threat.

HOMELAND SECURITY

The National Strategy for Homeland Security and the Homeland Security Act of 2002 were enacted to secure the homeland from terrorist attack. The Department of Homeland Security (DHS) was established to provide a unifying core as the basis for efforts to prevent and deter terrorist attacks. This governmental agency was designed to coordinate the efforts of the extensive network of organizations that were in place to secure and maintain the safety of our nation. In performing its function the DHS established five strategic goals (DHS, 2004):

Increase awareness: To identify and understand threats, assess vulnerability, and disseminate timely information

Prevention: To detect, deter, and mitigate threats to homeland security, including the safeguarding of people's freedom and the infrastructure of the nation

National leadership: To lead national, state, local, and private efforts to restore service and rebuild communities in the event of terrorist act, natural disaster, or other emergency

Service to the public: To effectively facilitate lawful trade, travel, and immigration

Organizational excellence: To value individuals and create a culture of mutual respect, accountability, and teamwork

TERRORISM PREPAREDNESS

In addition to the activities of the DHS, the Centers for Disease Control and Prevention (CDC) is recognized as the leading federal agency designed to protect the health and safety of people at home and abroad. The CDC's mission (2003) is to ensure that the nation is well prepared to respond to an act of terrorism. The agency provides a national focus for the development and application of disease prevention and control, environmental health, and health promotion and education. The core competencies of public health provide the foundation for the CDC's effort (2003) to protect the public's health from terrorist attacks. The CDC has developed a strategic plan in the event of a disaster. Preparedness, the first focus of the CDC strategic plan, is key to the impact any disaster has on the individuals or communities involved. Preparedness requires that nurses, as the largest sector of the health care workforce, have a basic understanding of the science of a disaster and an understanding of the key components of any plan to deal with an MCI (CDC, 2003).

In the event of a biological, chemical, or radiation attack the CDC's strategic plan includes the following:

- *Preparedness and prevention*—The comprehensive preparedness required to manage self, family, and/or the community when an event occurs that is likely to result from a catastrophic and or destructive event that disrupts normal functioning.
- *Detection and surveillance*—Awareness of the environment, recognizing what might be unusual or different, and knowing what these differences may mean.
- *Diagnosis and characterization of biological, chemical, and radiological agents*—The ability of an individual to recognize or identify clusters of data indicating a biological, chemical, or radiological MCI event has occurred.
- *Response*—The systematic, coordinated, and effective delivery of services when disaster strikes.
- *Communication*—The establishment of protocols and standing orders in the event of a disaster to successfully manage health care and to use the media for communicating information to the public (e.g., directions to treatment facilities, evacuation routes). Traditional modes of communication may be interrupted in the event of an MCI (e.g., the telephone system, the Internet); therefore part of disaster preparedness involves backup plans for maintaining public and intraagency/interagency communication (e.g., use of two-way radios and satellite phones).

Although the CDC's plan is designed for mass casualty disaster events or community-wide incidents, the plan clearly applies to any disaster event.

The CDC and the American Red Cross are advocates of preparedness and coordination of prompt, effective emergency efforts. This preparedness coordination goes far beyond these individual agencies and includes outreach to other agencies or groups through mutual aid agreements. These agreements might include the willingness of one agency to provide shelter (e.g., a church, school, or recreation center), while other agencies provide clothing (e.g., department stores, the Salvation Army, or Goodwill), and still other agencies agree to provide vehicular support in the time of a disaster. Referring to this short list of just a few of the needs required at the time of a disaster, the nurse quickly becomes aware that disaster planning is not only a multidisciplinary task but also a multiagency task. Although the average citizen, government agency, and other health care workers play a vital role in disaster preparedness, nurses will always have a unique responsibility within this multidisciplinary and multiagency coalition.

Disaster Defined

A disaster is any unexpected event whose effect leads to significant destruction and/or adverse consequences. More specifically, a disaster is any event in which needs exceed available resources. Box 5-1 provides common disaster terminology definitions. Although these definitions serve to standardize the events of an MCI, it is important to understand that each disaster is unique in the way it affects individuals, families, and communities.

When most Americans hear the term *disaster,* they immediately think terrorist attack. In reality the most common forms of disaster are natural and manmade (e.g., major fires, hurricanes, tornadoes, and floods). Individuals often recognize their vulnerability with regard to natural disasters; they recognize the possibility of mass casualties, significant destruction, and adverse consequences. However, neither public nor professional attention has been historically given to the threats posed by an MCI resulting from a biological, chemical, or nuclear attack. Because of September 11, 2001, Americans now realize the inevitability of an MCI.

This chapter will begin to prepare nursing students and keep nurses aware of the possibility for disasters, along with the action to take in the event of an MCI. To further support the need for health care providers to increase their preparedness, new laws are being enacted in some states that require disaster training as part of the continuing education requirement for licensure. However, only disaster planning, education, training, and drills on a local, national, and global level will effectively prepare health care providers, volunteers, and other individuals needed in the event of an MCI. Nurses can and should help influence, develop, practice, and carry out policies that will improve the safety and quality of health care of individuals and communities at the time of a mass casualty disaster.

Alerting the Public

At the current time there is no specific warning system for an MCI, nor is there a specific set of responses for health care providers, volunteers, and other individuals who wish to respond to community threats. However, the Department of Homeland Security established a color-coded national framework to provide officials and citizens with information regarding the nature and degree of terrorist threat (Figure 5-1).

BOX 5-1 Disaster Definitions and Types

- **Disaster**—A catastrophic and/or destructive event that disrupts normal functioning; it may include any anticipated or unexpected event whose effects lead to significant destruction and/or adverse consequences
- **Mass casualty incident or event (MCI)**—Any event or situation that results in multiple casualties and/or deaths; an MCI exists when health care needs exceed health care resources
- **All-hazards event**—Multiple manmade or natural events with destructive capacity to cause multiple casualties
- **All-hazards preparedness**—The comprehensive preparedness necessary to manage casualties resulting from a disaster regardless of etiology
- **Casualty**—Any individual who is ill, injured, missing, or killed as a result of an MCI
- **Medical disasters**—Catastrophic events that result in human casualties that overwhelm the available health care resources
- **Natural/environmental disasters**—Catastrophic events that result from an ecologic event that exceeds the capacity of the community (e.g., the impact of hurricanes or tornados on a community)
- **Manmade disasters**—Catastrophic events whose principal direct cause is attributable to human action
- **Technological disasters**—Catastrophic events in which people, property, community infrastructure, and economic welfare are adversely affected by the disruption of technology (e.g., industrial accidents, unplanned release of nuclear waste)

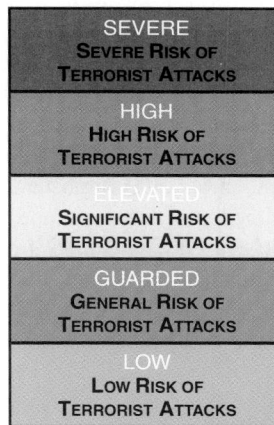

HOMELAND SECURITY
ADVISORY SYSTEM

SEVERE
SEVERE RISK OF
TERRORIST ATTACKS

HIGH
HIGH RISK OF
TERRORIST ATTACKS

ELEVATED
SIGNIFICANT RISK OF
TERRORIST ATTACKS

GUARDED
GENERAL RISK OF
TERRORIST ATTACKS

LOW
LOW RISK OF
TERRORIST ATTACKS

FIGURE 5-1 The Homeland Security Advisory System indicates the potential risk level for serious, terrorist activity.

To determine the current advisory level for the nation, individuals can visit the Department of Homeland Security website at http://white-house.gov/homeland.

Green designates that there is a low risk level for terrorist attacks. At the green level, government agencies are charged with refining and exercising appropriate preplanned protective measures, ensuring personnel receive proper training. At this level of threat government agencies also have the charge to ensure facilities are regularly assessed for vulnerability to terrorist attack. At the same time citizens are encouraged to develop and share family emergency plans, create emergency supply kits, get informed, and know how to "shelter-in-place." Shelter-in-place is a precaution designed to keep individuals safe while remaining indoors. Sheltering-in-place does not mean seeking a shelter, but rather taking refuge in a small interior room with no or few windows. It does not require an entire home or office be sealed. When the security alert is at the green level, individuals are encouraged to learn how to turn off utilities, examine volunteer opportunities, provide community service, and consider completing emergency preparation courses (e.g., cardiopulmonary resuscitation [CPR] and first aid).

Condition blue (guarded) is declared when there is a general risk for terrorist attack. In addition to the green level activities, government agencies communicate with designated emergency response or command locations, review and update emergency response procedures, and provide the public with information to strengthen the ability to act appropri-

ately. Citizens are encouraged to complete the steps recommended at the green level, review stored disaster supplies, replace outdated items, and be alert to suspicious activity.

Condition yellow is declared when there is significant risk of terrorist attacks. Government agencies continue activities listed with the less severe levels of threat and also increase surveillance of critical locations, coordinate emergency plans, assess the characteristics of the threat, refine preplanned protective measures, and implement appropriate contingency and emergency response plans. Citizens continue to complete the steps recommended at the lower levels of alert, ensure their disaster supply kit is stocked and ready, and check important telephone numbers. Citizens should also develop a family emergency plan to identify and practice alternative routes to and from school and work and should continue to be alert to suspicious activity, which should be reported to authorities (e.g., 911).

Condition orange indicates there is a high risk of terrorist attack. Government agencies continue with the above activities and begin coordinating necessary security, take additional precautions at public events, prepare to execute contingency procedures, and restrict access to a threatened facility to essential personnel only. Citizens continue to complete recommendations at the lower levels of alert, exercise caution when traveling, review the family emergency plan with all family members, be patient and expect delays, and check on neighbors or others who may need assistance in an emergency.

Red is the highest level of alert, which suggests a severe risk of terrorist attacks. Generally it is not expected that this level of alert will be maintained for extended periods. Increased numbers of emergency personnel will be redirected to respond to critical emergency needs; to assign emergency personnel to monitor, redirect, and constrain transportations systems; and to close public and government facilities, as needed. At the same time citizens are encouraged to continue to complete emergency preparedness recommendations at the lower levels of alert, listen to local emergency management officials, stay tuned to TV or radio for current information, prepare to shelter-in-place or evacuate, expect delays and restrictions, provide volunteer services only as requested, and contact schools and/or businesses to determine the status of the school or workplace.

When alerting the public, it is important that all messages are consistent, immediate, accurate, and open. Therefore close collaboration with the media is important, because members of the media can play a key role in providing accurate information and possibly reducing the number of concerned individuals who unnecessarily come to hospitals. Key message topics include (CDC, 2003):

If you think you are exposed, take these steps . . .

If you are injured . . .

Likely effects of biological or chemical exposure/radiation contamination include . . .

To avoid contamination . . .

Available resources, experts/contacts for medical information include . . .

THE D-I-S-A-S-T-E-R PARADIGM

The American Medical Association (AMA) developed a series of National Disaster Life Support (NDLS) courses "designed to provide a uniform, coordinated approach to All-Hazards disaster management" (AMA, 2002). This unified all-hazards training program is designed to prepare the health care community to recognize and manage health care needs of victims of a disaster. The D-I-S-A-S-T-E-R model put forth in the training program is designed to standardized methods for recognizing a disaster, managing the scene, and providing care to disaster victims.

Detection

Detection is the first goal in an MCI and includes (a) determining the presence of an MCI or public health emergency (PHE), (b) recognizing the cause of the incident, and (c) becoming aware of the environment or more specifically changes in the environment (e.g., an unusual pattern of client presentation, unusual smells, or suspicious individuals). Although many events may have a clear cause, others may have an insidious onset. For example, if a large number of otherwise healthy young adults start showing up in an emergency department with similar but unexplained symptoms, the nurse and other health care providers should begin to suspect something is not right. Detection may simply be the awareness of an unusual health care situation.

It is important to remember that to be able to provide care the nurse must first ensure personal safety. It is essential that rescue workers avoid becoming victims. When the scene of a disaster is in a clearly designated area outside the health care agency, security of the scene must be deter-

---

BOX 5-2 Potential Organisms for Bioterrorism by CDC Category

CATEGORY A—GREATEST THREAT

Anthrax (Bacillus anthracis)
Botulism (Clostridium botulinum toxin)
Plague (Yersinia pestis)
Smallpox (Variola major)
Viral hemorrhagic fevers (Ebola, Marburg, Lassa, Machupo)

CATEGORY B—HIGH RISK

Brucellosis (Brucella species)
Epsilon toxin of Clostridium perfringens
Food safety threats (e.g., Salmonella, Escherichia coli, Shigella)
Ricin toxin from Ricinus communis (castor beans)
Staphylococcal enterotoxin B
Water safety threats (e.g., Vibrio cholerae, Cryptosporidium parvum)

CATEGORY C—EMERGING BIOLOGICAL WEAPONS FOR TERRORIST USE

Nipah virus
Hantavirus

---

mined. Nurses should always consider external scenes of disasters, such as sites of explosions or severe storm damage, unsafe until trained professionals arrive and determine the scene is safe.

The thought of nuclear and radiological incidents creates considerable apprehension and fear for many individuals. In the case of these events the cause for disseminating radioactive material is generally known. A fire or an explosion is often associated with nuclear attacks; however, devices designed to disseminate radioactive material may not always be obvious. In the event of a terrorist attack, a nuclear blast is the least likely scenario, whereas a "dirty bomb" is the more likely cause for dispersal of radioactive material. The effects of nuclear and radiological events are dependent on the amount of radiation exposure. Most victims will have delayed onset of symptoms (including nausea, vomiting, and diarrhea), whereas some will have obvious burns. Generally the sooner symptoms appear, the greater the exposure to radioactive material.

Dispersal of biological agents is a real and psychological terrorist threat. Incubation periods and initially common clinical symptoms make detection of a biological attack difficult. Box 5-2 presents common biological agents recognized as potentials for terrorist use.

Another form of MCI is the dissemination of a toxic chemical agent. The agent may be disseminated via a number of methods (e.g., fire or explosion). Health care providers are often at risk for becoming secondary victims when chemical agents are used to create an MCI. Chemical agents are categorized based on their mechanism of injury. These include pulmonary agents, blistering agents, blood agents, and nerve agents.

HOSPITAL EMERGENCY INCIDENT COMMAND SYSTEM

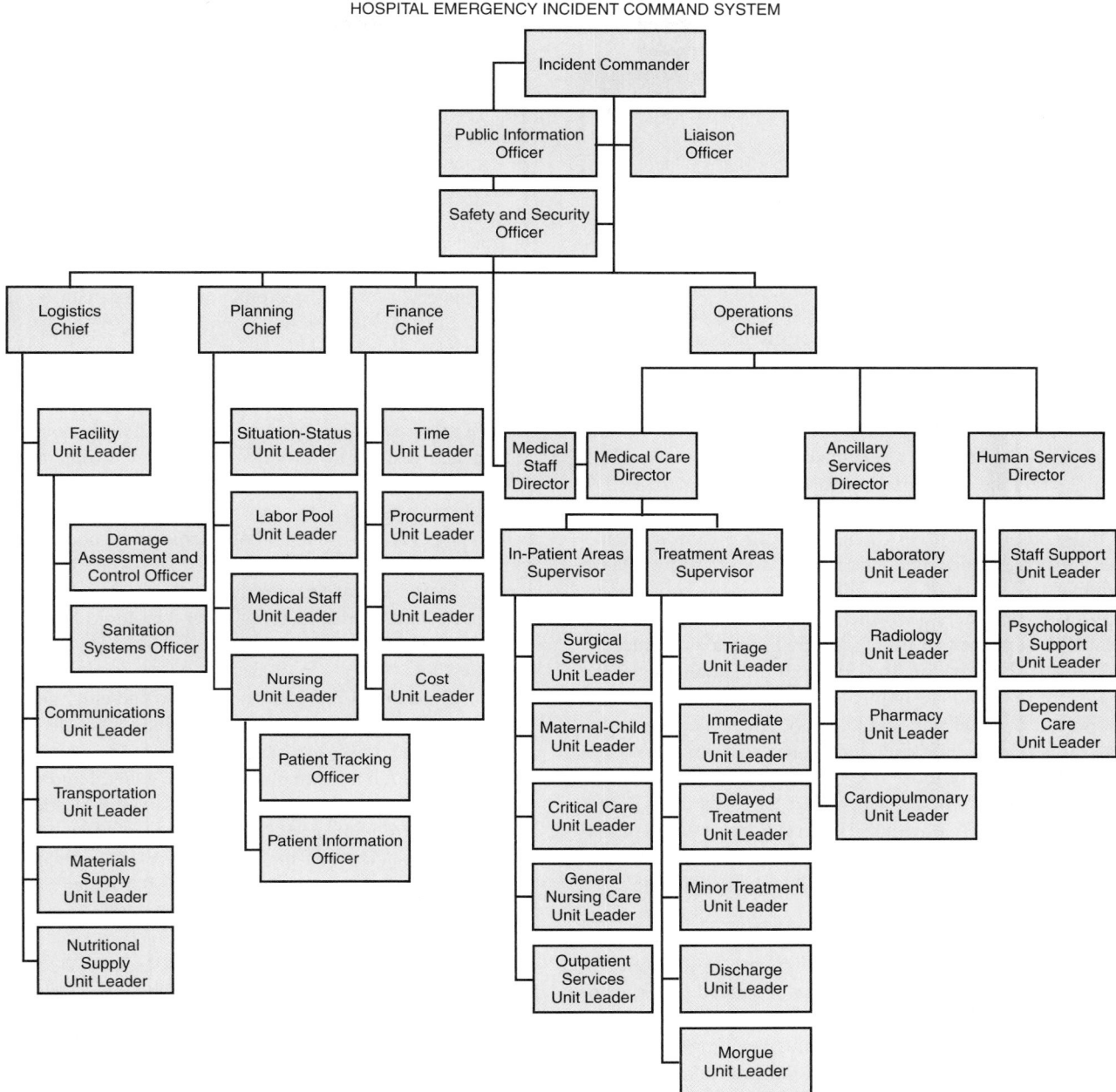

FIGURE **5-2** The Hospital Emergency Incident Command System prepares all response teams to work smoothly in a disaster situation.

Incident Command

Incident command refers to the need for the emergency system to be activated when a threat or hazard is suspected. For most individuals this means activating the 911 system, so that emergency responders can be brought in to assume command. Emergency responders initially remain outside the possible contaminated area. Therefore their arrival can be impeded by the impact of the disaster on roads, traffic, and availability of resources. An incident command system represents a unified command structure where a single indi-

vidual coordinates the organization, planning, logistics, financial, and operation systems. Figure 5-2 offers an example of a general chain of command in an MCI.

Scene Security and Safety

Nurses should never be responsible for determining the security and safety of a disaster scene. This task is the responsibility of trained emergency personnel (e.g., firefighters and police). When a health care agency is the scene of the disaster or a secondary site for a disaster, trained personnel are re-

TABLE 5-1 THE DO'S AND DON'TS OF SCENE SAFETY AND SECURITY	
DO	**DON'T**
Stay out of a disaster scene unless well trained and invited. Call 911.	Don't enter the scene unless invited. Don't needlessly disturb the scene; important evidence could be lost or contaminated by an eager but untrained helper. Don't interfere with the services of other emergency personnel when uninvited or untrained. Don't open suspicious packages.

sponsible for determining scene security and safety. A health care agency can become a secondary disaster site when contaminated by the agent from the original disaster scene. For example, a client has been exposed to mustard gas. This is an oily chemical that is difficult to remove from a client's body. If not properly decontaminated, the victim contaminated by the mustard gas will inadvertently contaminate health care providers and others in the immediate environment. The same can be true for many biological agents.

When caring for clients at or from a disaster scene, the rescuer must avoid becoming a victim. Recognizing who can declare a scene safe and knowing when it is safe to enter a disaster area is designed to protect disaster workers. It is also important for those trained to recognize the extent of a disaster to alert workers when the scene is actually larger than is immediately obvious. The first priority at any disaster scene is to protect yourself and other team members. The second priority is to protect the public, clients, and the environment (Table 5-1).

In order to be properly protected, the nurse must understand which personal protection equipment (PPE) is used to minimize the risk of contact with contaminated materials or individuals. Proper use of many advanced forms of PPE requires training and fitting and an understanding that not all PPE will protect against all potential hazards and that, when used inappropriately, PPE can become a source of hazard (e.g., dehydration, decreased vision, decreased mobility, and decreased ability to communicate). Some of these hazards result because while using advanced forms of PPE the user cannot eat, drink, or go to the bathroom.

Personal protection equipment is graded by the level of safety provided. Level A protection provides maximum protection because it offers a self-contained breathing apparatus, fully encapsulates the individual, and includes chemical-resistant boots and gloves (Figure 5-3). Highly trained personnel use the level of protection in heavily contaminated areas. If not wearing this type of protection and others are or if you are near an area where level A PPE is being used, the general rule is to get out or do not enter. Level B protection provides respiratory protection but less skin protection. Used

by trained responders, this PPE includes a self-contained breathing apparatus, hooded chemical-resistant suit, and face, boot, and glove protection. Level B protection also requires training and fitting. Level C protection also requires that the user be trained and properly fitted. First responders (those emergency personnel first on the scene) and hospital personnel are trained and fitted to use this type of protection. As with level A and B protection, level C protection presents danger to the user, primarily dehydration and hyperthermia. Standard work uniform or work clothes offer level D protection. There is no respiratory protection. Standard precautions are an integral part of the protection afforded with level D protection. Depending on the circumstances, the health care provider may also choose to use a fluid-impermeable gown, cap, eye protection, mask, gloves, and shoe covers.

The most recently labeled level of protection is BioPPE. BioPPE requires the use of standard work clothes along with contact and respiratory protection. Double gloving and an N95 mask or better respirator is recommended. Hand hygiene that includes washing with soap and water followed by use of an alcohol gel is important not only at this level but at all other levels. BioPPE protection is not adequate when caring for clients exposed to toxic chemicals; however, it provides adequate protection against radiological and biological agents.

Assessment

Assessing hazards is more important than knowing the exact cause of a disaster. By allowing trained individuals to assess a disaster scene, the nurse can avoid becoming a victim. In a disaster situation it is important to have general knowledge of potential threats to health and well-being. In addition, health care providers and volunteers must learn to shift thinking and realize that the MCI can result in secondary hazards that come in many forms. Box 5-3 provides a partial list of potential hazards in the event of an MCI.

Support

In terms of a disaster, *support* means, "Give me what I need to get the job done." The earlier support is summoned, the better. Support varies with the situation and task at hand. Support resources necessary during a disaster include human resources, agencies, facilities, supplies, and vehicles. For example, although there may not be enough hospitals to accommodate all victims, a school or recreation center could easily be turned into a makeshift hospital if there had been preparation for unforeseen disasters. There may not be adequate ambulances to transport victims of a disaster, but a mutual aid agreement with a school district laid out before an unforeseen disaster could turn school buses into vehicles to transport less injured victims.

Chaos is common in every disaster. Chaos can be managed, but it is difficult to control. In the event of a disaster many "walking well" (injured individuals who are able to transport themselves to a health care facility or even frightened individuals who fear contamination) will leave a disaster scene. Within 30 minutes the hospital nearest the disas-

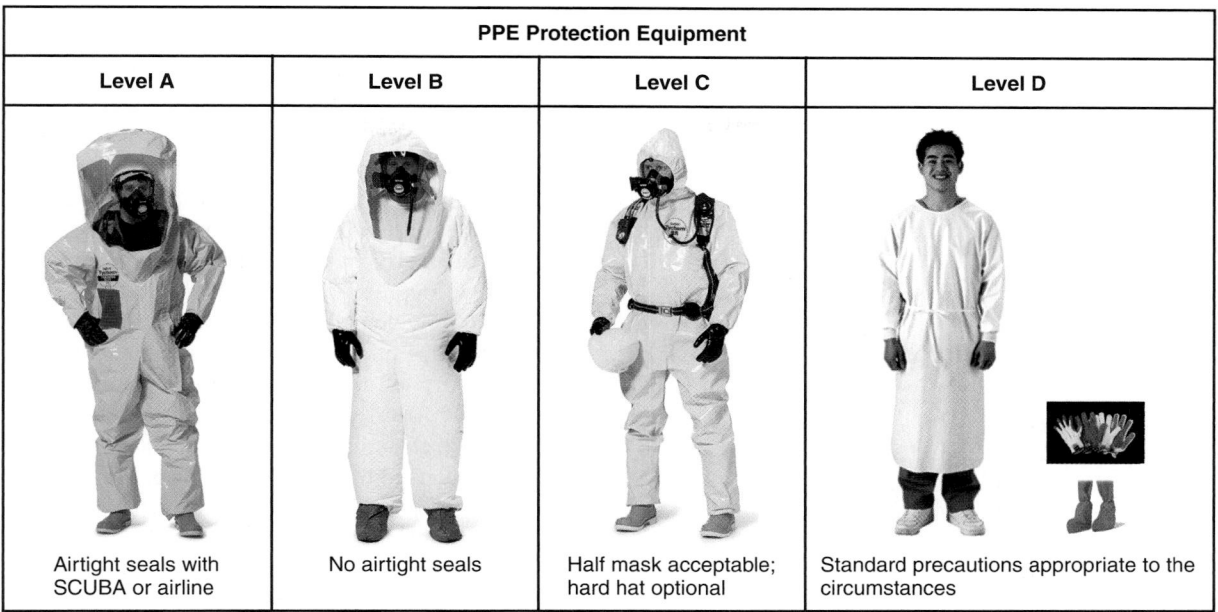

PPE Protection Equipment			
Level A	**Level B**	**Level C**	**Level D**
Airtight seals with SCUBA or airline	No airtight seals	Half mask acceptable; hard hat optional	Standard precautions appropriate to the circumstances

FIGURE 5-3 The Occupational Safety and Health Administration (OSHA) defined personal protective equipment for the four levels of hazardous exposure. (**A, B, C,** courtesy DuPont Personal Protection, Wilmington, Del. **D,** courtesy Kappler, Guntersville, Ariz.)

BOX 5-3   Potential Hazards at the Scene of a Disaster

- Downed power lines
- Smoke/toxic gases
- Debris that can result in trauma
- Fractured/leaking gas lines
- Fire resulting in burns
- Structural collapse
- Blood and other body fluids
- Inclement weather
- Hazardous materials
- Nuclear, biological, or chemical exposure
- Flooding and the threat of drowning
- Radiation exposure
- Explosion, particularly secondary explosions
- Snipers
- Darkness
- Infection
- High-velocity projectiles and the pressure wave after an explosion
- Becoming incapacitated and unable to protect yourself or your client

---

ter scene will be overrun by these individuals, leaving the most highly injured individuals at the site of the disaster. Added to the chaos at the health care facility is the responsibility to care for sick and injured individuals already admitted to the hospital or emergency department.

First health care responders must be able to quickly distinguish between actual victims with exposure to the weapon (chemical, biological, or nuclear) of mass destruction that has led to the MCI. Regardless of the lethality of any biological, nuclear, or chemical terrorist attack, the "shock" to the community and society may well serve the intended purpose of the terrorist. The "worried well" must also be recognized as victims because they are obviously suffering fear and anx-

iety. However, they cannot detract the nurse from the job of rescuing as many potential survivors as possible. Quickly differentiating "worried well" from actual injured clients will prevent wasting valuable time. Furthermore, it will help alleviate community-wide hysteria and unnecessary, costly, and potentially humiliating decontamination procedures (Drody and Ackerman, 2003).

The security of a health care facility must also be considered in disaster planning. Health care providers offer a valuable resource that cannot be wasted on maintaining the security of the health care facility. The local police in collaboration with agency administration and security force personnel have the responsibility to maximize the protection of lives and assets of the health care agency. Ensuring security officers are kept informed as to the incident history, current status, and potential problems is one step in managing chaos following an MCI. As part of this protection, roadblocks, checkpoints, and facility lockdown procedures may be put in place.

Triage, Treat, and Evacuate

Triage refers to the sorting of individuals by the seriousness of their condition and the likelihood of their survival (AMA, 2004). Unfortunately, there are many different modern triage systems used to classify, tag, and treat victims of MCI. These various systems use a variety of symbols, colors, and other devices to classify individuals as to the need for treatment. The disaster triage model described here is the "MASS" triage system adopted by the NDLS Family of Courses (AMA, 2002). Mass casualty triage is an initial sorting of victims into groups. Victims are then individually assessed, sorted into "ID-me" victim categories, and evacuated for

TRIAGE OVERVIEW
D-I-S-A-S-"T"-E-R

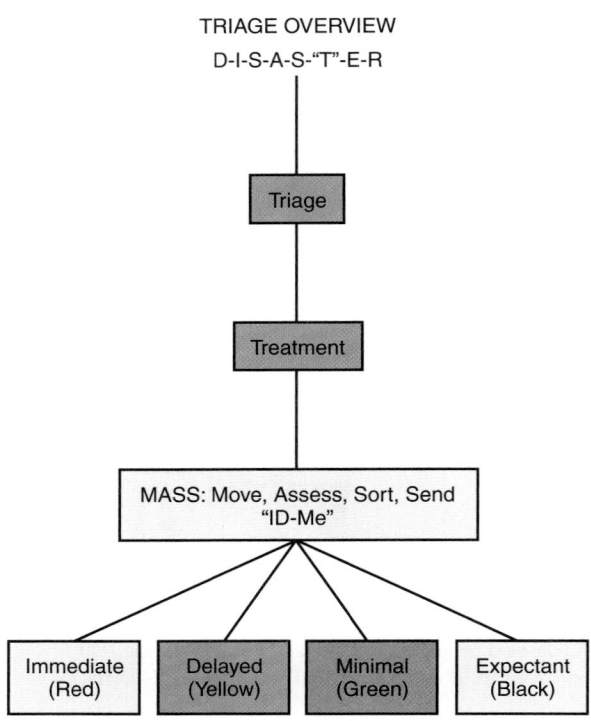

FIGURE **5-4** "Mass" triage system.

treatment. Figure 5-4 provides an overview of this triage system. The ultimate goal is to move, assess, sort, and send victims for treatment. The initial assessment is a very crude form of assessment, yet health care providers remain constantly vigilant because victims can quickly deteriorate and require immediate health care.

At the scene of a disaster, step one of this triage system, "move," requires victims who can walk to move to a specified collection area. These clients are identified as the minimally injured individuals requiring the least amount of care. A brief screening of these individuals will reveal that their airway, breathing, and circulation are intact; their mental status is intact to the extent that they can follow directions; and they are not likely to have low blood pressure or have difficulty breathing. Although this group is constantly monitored, the individuals in the green or minimal group have been identified as those who will undergo formal individualized medical assessment last. By managing this group first, (a) it is less likely individuals will transport themselves to the nearest hospital, thus immediately overwhelming that hospital, which should be designated for the most injured victims, and therefore (b) limited hospital resources can be reserved for the more injured individuals.

The "move" phase also allows rescue workers to identify those individuals who can follow commands but may not be able to walk. This group becomes the yellow or delayed group. The ability to follow commands suggests individuals in this group have the mental ability to follow commands; however, the injuries may prevent them from moving to a designated location. These injuries can vary from low blood

pressure to broken bones or lost limbs. Rescue workers recognize this group is at greater risk than the green group; further they recognize the classification is not based on individual assessment. There is the recognition that the injuries of these individuals may quickly deteriorate and require them to be triaged to a more critical group.

The second step of the triage process, "assess," allows rescue workers to focus on the remaining victims, who are presumed more critically injured. This group is now the red, immediate, group. Rescuers immediately assess these individuals and provide potentially life-saving interventions focusing priorities on airway, breathing, circulation, mental status, and level of consciousness (LOC). As individuals in this group are assessed they may be resorted into either the delayed or expectant group. For example, an individual may not have responded to early commands because of a hearing loss, and thus on individual assessment it is determined the individual fits in a less critically injured group. Within this group the goal is to obtain an accurate count of the most severely injured victims who still have a chance of survival if proper treatment can be delivered quickly (AMA, 2004). Similarly the dead and individuals with serious injuries that cannot be treated quickly may necessitate a "black tag." An enormous emotional toll is placed on triage personnel when a black tag is placed on a living human, even though this action is imperative to identify the greatest number of individuals likely to survive a mass casualty disaster.

During the "assess" triage process, personnel actually begin the "sort" task. Using the "ID-me" system, mnemonic tags are placed on individuals to identify priority need for care (e.g., red—immediate, yellow—delayed, green—minimal, and black—expectant). Table 5-2 provides examples of how victims might be sorted based on injury.

During the third step of the triage process, an individual is sorted or triaged into a group, a tag is securely tied to the person's body, not the clothing because clothing is removed for decontamination, evaluation, or treatment. At this point workers obtain an accurate count of victims in the red group. This information is sent to the incident commander, who can alert receiving hospitals of the expected number of casualties they will receive. These victims are then transported to receiving hospitals. Victims remaining from the other triage groups can now be reassessed and retriaged.

The final step in the MASS triage system is "send." Rescue workers evacuate, transport, or release all living clients as soon as possible. Immediate (red) clients are sent first, then delayed (yellow), followed by minimal (green), and then expectant (black). The dead are not initially moved. Movement of these individuals is the responsibility of law enforcement officials.

EVIDENCE-BASED PRACTICE

Research in disaster situations offers many challenges from a scientific, legal, and ethical standpoint. Consequently, much information gained has historically been gathered through retrospective study. These studies have been essen-

TABLE 5-2   ID-ME — ASSESS, TREAT, AND SEND

IMMEDIATE RED	DELAYED YELLOW	MINIMAL GREEN	EXPECTANT BLACK
Unconscious or unresponsive Altered mental status Severe breathing difficulty Uncontrollable bleeding Amputations above elbow or knee Cyanosis Rapid or weak pulse Open abdominal wounds	Deep lacerations Open fractures with controlled bleeding and strong pulses Finger amputations Abdominal injuries with stable vital signs Closed head injuries without altered level of consciousness	Abrasions Contusions Minor lacerations No apparent injuries Other injuries of similar severity	Victims still alive but so severely injured as to have little chance of survival Victims who have died

tial to improving preparedness and preventing past mistakes in the event of future mass casualty events. However, studies that focus on preparedness, planning efforts, and education designed also to improve outcomes do not necessarily have to be retrospective. As with any other research agenda, a study of disaster science begins with an assessment of current strengths and areas of weakness. Furthermore, disaster science research should be structured with a focus on individuals, families, communities, health care workers, and the health care system (Walker and others, 2003).

Nursing research that focuses on MCI and disasters is of paramount importance because nurses play a key role as members of the interdisciplinary team that responds to a disaster. Through research, nurses can identify strategies for educating the profession and influencing the health care delivery system. These studies should be outcomes driven or designed to improve the outcomes of care in a disaster situation. Nurses have conducted/published very few studies related to bioterrorism outside the arena of military nursing, which has focused on care of injured individuals in wartime or in deployed environments. Since the terrorist attacks on September 11, these studies have become more relevant to nurses caring for the civilian population living in the United States (Walker and others, 2003).

Future evidence-based studies need to be conducted to measure quality of care from the time a disaster is detected through recovery from the event. Ideally, nurses will collaborate with individuals from other disciplines to plan ahead and seek opportunities for research in all areas of disaster care: preparedness, response, and recovery (Walker and others, 2003).

Skill Performance Guidelines

When considering all forms of disaster, there are basic guidelines for a nurse or other health care provider to follow:

1. Rapid response is crucial. Health care providers must be familiar with their agency's policies for disaster response and the specific role each must follow.
2. Health care providers are responsible for ensuring that the contaminated, injured, and those concerned about potential exposure to a hazardous agent are medically treated in an efficient manner.
3. The potential for public alarm and major disruption of everyday life is enormous because of widespread fear of the unknown. Health care providers must be familiar with crisis intervention and stress management techniques.
4. A health care agency such as a hospital is part of a community. Hospitals and other agencies must work with their communities in developing and instituting plans for notification and communication.
5. In an MCI a large majority of people will self-triage and go directly to a local hospital, bypassing triage and treatment whether contaminated, exposed, or not. Plans are needed to transfer clients to other medical facilities.

SKILL 5-1   Care of the Client After Biological Exposure

Bioterrorism or a biological attack is the result of the release of a biological agent into a specified environment. Early recognition of a biological event offers several challenges. Although other types of weapons of mass destruction (WMD) typically present with an overt, sudden, onset in a localized area, biological events tend to present in a more insidious fashion. The biological attack may be unannounced or covert and the onset of symptoms delayed by an incubation period, the time between exposure and onset of symptoms. Differing biological agents intended to cause mass casualties may have incubation periods from 1 or 2 days to several weeks. During this period of incubation, some of these biological agents may be transmitted as the infected client exposes others. The mode of transmission of the biological agent will determine the severity of the biological disaster. In order to understand how to protect oneself from becoming a victim of bioterrorism, the nurse must understand the mode of transmission and precautions to take to maintain biosafety. Table 5-3 offers a summary that includes mode of transmission, precautions, and treatment options for biological agents.

DELEGATION CONSIDERATIONS

The assessment of a client exposed to a biological agent cannot be delegated to assistive personnel. However, assistive personnel may provide supportive care to survivors and administer care after death to those clients who do not survive. The nurse provides assistive personnel with information, assistance, and direction, including:

- Appropriate use of PPE to prevent exposure
- Techniques for handling a body after death to prevent contamination

EQUIPMENT

Choice of equipment depends on the route of transmission of the infecting agent. The following is a general list of supplies needed in the event of release of the most contagious biological agents. Not all of the following equipment will be needed in all situations.

- ❑ Biohazard bags with label
- ❑ Soap and water
- ❑ 0.5% diluted bleach or Environmental Protection Agency (EPA)-approved germicidal agent
- ❑ Negative-pressure room (high-efficiency particle air filtration may be required) with anteroom
- ❑ Gloves
- ❑ Gown
- ❑ Shoe covers
- ❑ Head covers
- ❑ Mask
    —Standard face mask
    —N95 mask
- ❑ Face shield

STEP	RATIONALE

▮ ASSESSMENT

1. Conduct a focused health history and physical examination (e.g., pulmonary assessment—O_2 saturation, lung sounds, sputum character; cardiac—heart sounds; neurological—Glascow Coma Scale, reflexes). Review history of client's presenting symptoms, and determine pattern.

Symptom identification and clustering of data is the first step to accurately determine exposure to type of biological agent and client's response.

2. Measure client's vital signs.

Provides baseline to later evaluate client's response to therapy.

3. Review results of diagnostic tests, and consult with physician or primary care provider.

Initial signs and symptoms of exposure to biological agent may suggest common disorders (e.g., flu). Further review of diagnostic findings may help to rule out other common disorders.

4. Assess the client for other health risks (e.g., history of heart disease, pulmonary disease, cancer) that would complicate the effects of contamination with exposure to a biological agent.

Clients with preexisting medical conditions may require additional treatment or may be at greater risk for death.

5. Assess client's immediate psychological response following exposure. Individual responses to biological weapons will vary. Clients may present with dissociative symptoms (e.g., feeling as though "not there" or sensing everything is outside of the person), disorientation, depression, anxiety, psychosis, and an inability to care for self. Even without direct exposure to a biological agent many individuals, spurred by feelings of fear and doom, will present for emergency services.

Aids the nurse to be able to provide appropriate crisis intervention and stress management. Remaining calm and projecting confidence while assessing individuals for clinical symptoms versus feelings of panic will go a long way in reducing the anxiety of the ill and worried well as they experience the general sense of panic associated with a biological event.

6. Identify resources available (e.g., critical incident stress debriefing teams, counselors, psychiatric/mental health nurse practitioners).

Expert resources can assess extent of psychological impact of disaster.

TABLE 5-3   SUMMARY OF SELECTED CLASS A BIOLOGICAL WARFARE AGENTS

DISEASE/ INFECTIOUS AGENT	FORM AND INCUBATION/ ONSET OF SYMPTOMS	UNTREATED COURSE OF DISEASE		PROBABLE ROUTE OF CONTAMINATION FOR USE AS A BIOLOGICAL WARFARE AGENT	TREATMENT OF MASS CASUALTIES	PROPHYLAXIS/ VACCINE
		EARLY-ONSET SYMPTOMS	LATE-ONSET SYMPTOMS			
BACTERIAL BIOLOGICAL AGENTS						
Anthrax *Bacillus anthracis*, a spore-forming gram-positive bacillus	Inhalation or pulmonary (usually within 48 hours but may incubate for up to 60 days)	Febrile flulike symptoms (malaise, low-grade fever, dry cough, and headache)	Severe respiratory distress, hemodynamic failure, and death	Aerosol; no person-to-person transmission	Ciprofloxacin or doxycycline	Ciprofloxacin or, if susceptible, doxycycline; vaccine available, but in short supply
	Cutaneous (1-12 days)	Local urticaria; painless papular lesions usually located on head, forearms, or hands	Papular lesions become vesicular; later developing black eschar and edema	Person-to-person transmission with direct contact with skin lesions		
	Gastrointestinal (1-7 days)	Abdominal pain, nausea, vomiting, and diarrhea	Gastrointestinal bleeding, fever; usually followed by toxic sepsis and death	Contaminated food and/or water		
Plague Acute, severe bacterial infection secondary to a gram-negative bacillus *Yersinia pestis*	Bubonic Onset of symptoms dependent upon route of transmission (1-6 days)	Swollen tender lymph nodes (most notable femoral and inguinal), high fever, rapid pulse	Hypotension, extreme exhaustion, death	Aerosol and then human-to-human by droplet inhalation	Ciprofloxacin or doxycycline	Ciprofloxacin or doxycycline; no vaccine available at the present time
	Pneumonic (1-6 days)	High fever, chills, tachycardia, headache	Fulminate pneumonia (foamy hemoptysis, tachypnea, and dyspnea), sepsis, and death			
Botulism Anaerobic gram-positive bacillus that produces a potent muscle-paralyzing neurotoxin	Foodborne (12-36 hours)	Nausea, vomiting, diarrhea	Symmetrical cranial nerve paralysis, descending flaccid paralysis (progressive paralysis of arms, respiratory muscles, and legs), and death	Contaminated food	Passive immunization (antitoxin); supportive care	Passive immunization (antitoxin); antitoxin available in short supply
	Inhalational (2 hours-8 days)	No fever, no changes in mental status	Symmetrical cranial nerve paralysis, descending flaccid paralysis (progressive paralysis of arms, respiratory muscles, and legs), and death	Inhalation of aerosolized toxin		
Typhoidal tularemia *Francisella tularensis*, an extremely infectious bacteria	Contaminated water, food or via aerosol distribution (1-14 days)	Flulike symptoms (headache, cough, fever and chills, malaise)	Pharyngeal ulcers, pleuritic chest pain, pneumonia, pericarditis, respiratory failure, sepsis, and death	Inhalation of aerosolized bacteria	Ciprofloxacin or doxycycline	Ciprofloxacin or doxycycline; vaccine available, only limited supply; vaccine offers incomplete protection
MAJOR VIRAL BIOLOGICAL AGENT OF CONCERN—SMALLPOX						
Smallpox *Variola* virus	Distribution via airborne droplets, aerosols, and fomites (7-17 days; weaponized smallpox when delivered aerosolized has an incubation period of only 3-5 days)	Acute viral symptoms (high fever, myalgia, headache, and backache)	Continued viral symptoms, high fever, prostration, and synchronous onset of rash progressing from macules to papules to vesicles, and eschar formation	Transmitted by large droplets; therefore spread may be by inhalation of aerosolized virus, oral secretions, by infected human vector exposure, or by exposure to contaminated objects	Supportive therapy only	None; vaccine available in short supply

STEP	RATIONALE

- ***Critical Decision Point***
A biological event should be considered when large numbers of ill persons present who have unexplained yet similar symptoms; when there are unexplained deaths, particularly among young and healthy populations; when there is an unusual pattern associated with the symptoms (e.g., geographical, season, client population); when the client fails to respond to traditional therapy; when a single client presents with symptoms suggestive of an uncommon agent (e.g., anthrax or smallpox). Once a biological event is suspected, incident command must be notified immediately.

NURSING DIAGNOSES

- Decreased cardiac output
- Altered tissue perfusion
- Diarrhea
- Risk for imbalanced fluid volume
- Nausea
- Impaired oral mucous membrane
- Impaired swallowing
- Disturbed thought processes
- Acute pain
- Ineffective airway clearance
- Risk for aspiration
- Impaired gas exchange
- Acute confusion
- Risk for peripheral neurovascular dysfunction
- Disturbed sensory perception
- Risk for imbalanced body temperature
- Impaired skin integrity
- Risk for suffocation
- Anxiety
- Compromised family coping
- Post-trauma syndrome
- Fear
- Disturbed body image

Related factors are individualized based on client's condition or needs.

PLANNING

1. Expected outcomes following completion of procedure:
   - Client will be comforted.

     In some cases the only care that is available is palliative, with comfort as the focus. The nurse and other health care providers must not underestimate the value of COMFORT as CARE.
   - Client's vital signs will return to baseline.

     When there are no underlying medical conditions and *if* the client's disease process is responsive to treatment (when treatment is available), vital signs will return to normal. Returning to normal may take days or weeks.
   - Client's work of breathing will decrease.

     Treatment aimed at improving gas exchange and cardiac output.
   - Client's skin integrity will return to baseline.

     Antibiotic and antitoxin therapy will aid in resolution/healing of lesions over time.
   - Client's LOC will return to baseline.

     Treatment measures restore neurological function and oxygenation status.
   - Client's mental health status will return to a pre-trauma level of functioning.

     With early identification of individuals at risk for psychiatric complications, appropriate interventions can be implemented to alleviate long-term emotional distress. Clients with unrelieved symptoms of stress and ongoing symptoms of despair and hopelessness may warrant long-term mental health services.

2. Dispense timely and accurate information, including an accurate description of the agent client is exposed to and implications, to the client and family.

   Information helps to allay anxiety and fear.

STEP	RATIONALE
IMPLEMENTATION	
1. Perform hand hygiene.	Reduces transmission of microorganisms.
2. Institute transmission-based isolation precautions. (Refer to Table 5-3 for mode of transmission of the category A biological agents.)	Reduces transmission of microorganisms and the likelihood of additional secondary sites of contamination.
3. Administer appropriate antibiotics and/or antitoxins.	Various biological agents are commonly treated with ciprofloxacin and/or doxycycline (e.g., anthrax, plague, typhoidal tularemia), and botulism requires supportive care and use of an antitoxin. For smallpox and other viral pathogens, treatment is only supportive. Postvaccination for 3 to 7 days post exposure along with administration of appropriate immune globulin preparations may prove effective.
4. Administer immunizations (e.g., smallpox).	In the event smallpox is used as a biological weapon, the best treatment is prevention by immunization with vaccinia vaccine before the onset of symptoms. There is no specific treatment of smallpox after the onset of illness other than palliative/supportive care.
5. Administer fluid and nutrition therapy.	Various biological agents commonly cause gastrointestinal (GI) disturbances that may result in dehydration.
6. Administer oxygen therapy.	Various biological agents commonly cause respiratory symptoms that may result in an altered gas exchange.
7. Provide supportive care (e.g., comfort measures, including pain management).	Some victims of a biological attack will not survive; supportive palliative care is essential (see Chapter 7).
8. Counsel client and family on both acute and potential long-term psychological effects of exposure. Offer access to trained counselors.	Reaction of clients to exposure will include shock, immobilization, and fear. Long-term psychological effects could arise without proper counseling (CDC, 2004).

• *Critical Decision Point*
Collaborate with the physician and other rescue workers for an ongoing plan for managing the client exposed to a biological agent while also caring for other clients who may already be present in the health care agency seeking care for illness unrelated to the current MCI.

EVALUATION	
1. Observe for improved airway maintenance, breathing, circulation, level of consciousness, and neurological functioning.	Evaluates the client's response to available treatment and/or supportive care.
2. Inspect the condition of client's skin; note character of remaining lesions.	Evaluates client's response to antibiotic therapy.
3. Evaluate the client for changes that suggest either improvement or deterioration of psychological status; ask client, "How do you feel right now?" Check level of orientation and ability to conduct conversation.	Evaluates client's response to emotional trauma.

Recording and Reporting

- Report suspected cases of a biological incident to physician or emergency officer.
- Record in nurses' notes client status and response to treatment and/or comfort measures.
- Report any unexpected outcome to physician or nurse in charge.

Unexpected Outcomes	Related Interventions
1. Client's physical symptoms progress despite appropriate treatment.	• Notify physician or nurse in charge. • Continue to provide comfort care.
2. Client becomes more anxious or delusional or develops suicidal ideations.	• Notify mental health treatment team. • Remain calm, offer reassurance, and protect self and others from physical harm. • Continue to provide comfort measures.
3. Client death.	• Handling of bodies should take into account continued risk for contamination; therefore those handling bodies should be fully informed regarding proper procedure.
4. Secondary contamination of rescue workers.	• Rescue workers immediately report symptoms to a physician or nursing supervisor.

Teaching Considerations

- Preparation for a mass casualty disaster will go a long way in preventing casualties and chaos. Public education of the likelihood of a mass casualty biological event is needed. This education should include information regarding types of biological agents, mode of transmission, symptoms, and appropriate treatment.
- Education of the public should include locations of shelters and disaster treatment sites.
- Families should be encouraged to prepare for the unexpected.
  - Create an emergency communication plan.
  - Establish a meeting place.
  - Assemble a disaster supply kit.
  - Know the disaster emergency plan for school-age children (American Red Cross, 2001).
- Disaster teams should routinely implement disaster drills.

Pediatric Considerations

- "Children are vulnerable to the stresses of evacuation, which include living in shelters and losing their homes, schools, parents, pets, and loved ones" (Bernardo, 2001).
- Children are particularly vulnerable to environmental toxins because (a) they are closer to the ground and thus more likely to inhale the toxin, (b) they breathe more air per kilogram of body weight, (c) their organ systems tend to be more sensitive than those of adults, and (d) they have more years of life expectancy over which to develop complications from the toxic exposure (Claudio and others, 2003).
- Asthma is a special concern in children. Asthma symptoms (e.g., wheezing, shortness of breath, chest discomfort) can be triggered by exposure to a biological agent (Claudio and others, 2003).
- Children entrapped during a disaster are more likely to develop infections following the disaster due to exposure to pollutants, waterborne and airborne infectious agents, and contact with their own vomit and feces (Goodman and Hogan, 2002).

- Children are triaged by nurses and physicians using the same criteria as triage for other disaster victims; the more severely injured are treated first regardless of age.
- Parents and family members should be allowed to be with injured children as soon as possible.
- The death of a child as a result of a disaster is always traumatic; should a parent express the desire to be present during pediatric resuscitation, ideally this should be allowed; a nurse should be available to explain to the parent what is happening (Plum and Veenema, 2003).

Gerontological Considerations

- Under disaster conditions, older adults should be triaged according to injuries, not age.
- Because the older adult may have a myriad of concurrent illnesses, possible exposure to a biological agent may exacerbate that condition and result in the need for more immediate care than an initial triage may have suggested.

Home Care Considerations

- Preparing for a biological disaster
  - A disaster kit should be assembled before disaster strikes. The Federal Emergency Management Agency and the American Red Cross offer free literature establishing home care preparedness.
  - Individuals with special needs (e.g., hearing impairment, impaired mobility, individuals without vehicles, individuals with special diets) will all require additional planning to be prepared in the event of a disaster.
  - One of the most important steps to prepare for a disaster is to have a household disaster plan.
  - In case of a disaster many schools and employers have disaster plans; individuals should familiarize themselves with these plans along with their own home disaster plan.
  - Post emergency telephone numbers by the telephone, and teach children how and when to call 911.
  - Family members should have a mechanism in place to ensure they are able to stay in contact in case they are

separated (e.g., a designated meeting place, a family member or friend to call to notify when separated from the family).

- An individual of the family should know how to turn off water, gas, and electricity in case of a disaster because emergency management personnel may make this request of civilians in the event of a disaster.

- To reduce the risk of complications from a biological infectious agent during a disaster, as many members of the family as possible should take a first aid class. A first aid kit should be maintained in an accessible location in the home. Family members should also know what type of PPE is needed to protect the family from secondary exposure.

- When biological disaster becomes a reality
  - Listen to the radio or television for special instructions.
  - Remain isolated, and advise friends and relatives not to visit if family members are symptomatic.
  - Use the appropriate PPE needed to protect the family; this may include sheltering-in-place.

- Maintain strict hand hygiene for both well and symptomatic family members after using the bathroom, before eating and drinking, and after contact with pets.
- Wear gloves (vinyl or latex) when in contact with a sick individual's blood or body fluids.
- When a sick individual's symptoms worsen, transportation should be to the nearest designated hospital.
- Monitor the temperature of the symptomatic individual, and provide him or her with plenty of food and fluids.

- Change the sick person's clothing and bed linens frequently; wash them separately from those of other family members, using any commercial detergent.
- Disinfect any surfaces the symptomatic person comes in contact with, using an appropriate disinfectant (e.g., Lysol), especially when soiled by blood or other body fluids.
- The caregiver's highest priority is to avoid becoming a victim. Therefore this individual should get plenty of rest, drink fluids frequently, and eat a healthy diet. Should the caregiver develop symptoms, appropriate medical care should immediately be obtained.

SKILL 5-2 Care of the Client After Chemical Exposure

A chemical disaster is defined as the dispersal of a toxic chemical agent into the environment. The mechanism of dispersal may or may not be known. In fact, the dispersal mechanism such as an explosion or fire may be a secondary terrorist attack designed to create greater fatalities. Explosions spread toxic chemical in uncontrolled directions, creating more victims. Symptoms resulting from chemical exposure are usually apparent within minutes but may be delayed up to 24 hours. Early recognition of a chemical event is a priority because many chemical antidotes must be administered quickly. Biological events are often unannounced or covert; the same can be said of toxic chemical incidents. Use of chemical agents by terrorists is intended to cause mass casualties and induce fear and/or mass hysteria.

Chemical events are generally confined to small areas, though larger dispersal of these agents may occur (e.g., via a crop duster). The nature and scale of contamination is also dependent on the state of the agent used (e.g., gas versus liquid), the particular characteristics of the chemical used (e.g., heavy or lighter than air), and where the event occurs (e.g., indoors, where ventilation systems affect dispersal, or outdoors, where wind and velocity affect speed and direction of dispersal). Safety of rescue workers requires they be located upwind and uphill from a toxic chemical disaster scene in order to avoid exposure. There is one unique exception to this rule and that is in the event that cyanide gas is the chemical agent that has been released. Cyanide is lighter than air and will thus travel uphill. It has the unique smell of bitter almonds. If the smell is detected, a rescue worker must evacuate the area immediately, though exposure may have already occurred.

Because symptoms are almost immediate, it is important to evacuate victims as quickly as possible from the contaminated zone to a decontamination zone. Special respiratory and skin PPE is required to prevent contamination of rescue workers. In addition, before decontamination, victims are a potential source of contamination for rescue workers. It is imperative that the nurse protect against toxic chemical contamination when in contact with the contaminated client. Secondary contamination is high with toxic chemical incidents. A summary of common chemical warfare agents, presenting symptoms, and untreated course of exposure is presented in Table 5-4.

The rapid chemical decontamination of victims of a toxic chemical incident is more important than determining the exact toxic chemical. When decontamination is required, trained personnel are required. Decontamination is categorized as either gross or technical, which generally occurs at the scene. Decontamination also is provided at the hospital when a contaminated individual presents for treatment. The nurse and all other health care personnel should use appropriate precautions to avoid becoming a victim.

TABLE 5-4 SUMMARY OF SELECTED CHEMICAL WARFARE AGENTS

CHEMICAL AGENT	ONSET OF SYMPTOMS	UNTREATED COURSE OF CHEMICAL EXPOSURE
"Lethal" agents—nerve agents (tabun, sarin, soman, and VX)	Symptoms are generally immediate.	Pinpoint pupils and shortly thereafter salivation, runny nose, dyspnea, chest tightness, nausea, muscle twitching, coma, seizures, and death
"Blood" agents—hydrogen cyanide	Rapid onset of symptoms though cyanide poisoning is often associated with the smell of bitter almonds.	Death due to asphyxiation
"Blister" agents—mustard and lewisite	Symptoms may be immediate or delayed.	Skin irritation and blistering
"Choking" agents—phosgene and chlorine	Symptoms can be immediate or may be delayed up to 24 hours.	Coughing, choking, and disruption in pulmonary function that can lead to death

Delegation Considerations

The assessment of a client exposed to a chemical agent cannot be delegated to assistive personnel. However, assistive personnel may provide supportive care to survivors and administer care after death to those clients who do not survive. The nurse provides assistive personnel with information, assistance, and direction, including:

- Appropriate use of PPE to prevent exposure
- Techniques for handling a body after death to prevent contamination

Equipment

The following is a general list of supplies needed in the event of release of the most toxic chemical agents.

- ❏ Decontamination room or area (adult decontamination rooms may not meet the needs of children requiring decontamination; decontamination areas for ambulatory victims will not meet the needs of those who are not ambulatory)
- ❏ Scissors or some other tool to cut off clothing rather than further contaminating the individual by pulling the clothing over the victim's head
- ❏ Biohazard bags with labels
- ❏ Large volumes of water
- ❏ Appropriate PPE for use by trained personnel

STEP	RATIONALE

▌ ASSESSMENT

1. Assess the client's symptoms. Perform appropriate focused physical examination (pulmonary, skin, gastrointestinal, neurological).

2. Observe for presence of liquid on client's skin or clothing and odor (e.g., chlorine).

3. Assess the client for preexisting medical conditions that would complicate the effects of the toxic chemical exposure.

Symptom identification and clustering of data is the first step to accurate identification of client's problem and response.

Common conditions present when chemical exposure has occurred.

Clients with preexisting medical conditions may require additional treatment or may be at greater risk for death.

• *Critical Decision Point*

A toxic chemical event should be considered when large numbers of ill persons present who have unexplained yet similar symptoms; the primary objective for initial care is decontamination. Decontamination is the process used to remove harmful contaminants from the surface of the skin. It is achieved by removing clothing, scrubbing the skin, and by hydrolysis, a process of chemical dilution using large volumes of water.

STEP	RATIONALE
4. Assess client's immediate psychological response following exposure. Individual responses to chemical exposure will vary. Clients may present with dissociative symptoms, disorientation, depression, anxiety, psychosis, and inability to care for self. Even without direct exposure to a chemical agent many individuals, spurred by feelings of fear and doom, will present for emergency services. These worried well can quickly overwhelm available emergency services.	Aids the nurse in being able to provide appropriate crisis intervention and stress management. Remaining calm and projecting confidence while assessing individuals for clinical symptoms versus feelings of panic will go a long way in reducing the anxiety of the ill and worried well as they experience the general sense of panic associated with chemical exposure.
5. Identify resources available (e.g., critical incident stress debriefing teams, counselors, psychiatric/mental health nurse practitioners).	Expert resources can assess extent of psychological impact of disorders.

NURSING DIAGNOSES

- Decreased cardiac output
- Ineffective tissue perfusion
- Diarrhea
- Risk for imbalanced fluid volume
- Nausea
- Impaired oral mucous membrane
- Impaired swallowing
- Disturbed thought processes
- Acute pain
- Ineffective airway clearance
- Impaired gas exchange

- Risk for aspiration
- Acute confusion
- Risk for peripheral neurovascular dysfunction
- Disturbed sensory perception
- Impaired skin integrity
- Risk for suffocation
- Impaired verbal communication
- Compromised family coping
- Anxiety
- Post-trauma syndrome
- Fear

Related factors are individualized based on client's condition or needs.

PLANNING

1. Expected outcomes following completion of procedure:
   - Client will be comforted.

   - Client's vital signs will return to baseline.

   - Client's work of breathing will decrease.
   - Client's skin integrity will return to baseline.

   - Client's LOC will return to baseline.

   - Client's mental health status will return to a pretrauma level of functioning.
2. Explain care to the client and family, including decontamination and treatment. Explain your role, orient to location and activities to perform, explain what client has experienced, and ask, "How are you feeling right now?" Assure them they will be seen by medical personnel.

Because of the fatal nature of many chemical agents, the only care available is palliative. Comfort is a focus in managing clients.

When there are no underlying medical conditions and *if* the client's condition is responsive to treatment (when treatment is available), vital signs will return to normal as a result of hemodynamic stability. Returning to normal may take days or weeks.

Indicates improvement in gas exchange and cardiac output.

Minimizing exposure of skin to chemical agent will reduce severity and extent of skin lesions.

Neurological stability achieved when exposure to chemical is minimized or when appropriate antitoxin is given quickly.

Crisis intervention is successful in reducing client's anxiety, fear, and dissociative symptoms.

Information helps to allay anxiety and fear.

STEP	RATIONALE

IMPLEMENTATION

1. Perform hand hygiene.
2. Only trained personnel using required PPE decontaminate clients with toxic chemical contamination.

Reduces transmission of and damage from toxic chemicals.
Reduces likelihood of secondary toxic chemical contamination to untrained personnel attempting decontamination.

● *Critical Decision Point*
Hold victim outside decontamination area until preparations are completed for decontamination procedure. If client is grossly contaminated, consider decontamination before entry into building.

3. Provide for client privacy by closing room curtains or closing door.
4. Decontaminate the client:
   a. Act quickly; avoid touching contaminated parts of clothing as much as possible.
   b. Remove all of client's clothing. CAUTION: Do not pull over the client's head; instead, cut garments off.
   c. Use copious amounts of soap and water to wash the client thoroughly.

   d. If eyes are burning or vision is blurred, rinse eyes with plain water for 10 to 15 minutes. If the client wears contacts, remove and place with contaminated clothing; do not reinsert in eyes. Wash eyeglasses with soap and water; reapply when completed (CDC, 2004).
5. Dispose of client's contaminated clothing in an appropriate biohazard bag and seal. Then place bag in another plastic bag and seal (see agency policy).
6. Initiate treatment for chemical agent using appropriate chemical agent protocol.

7. Control bleeding.
8. Administer fluid and nutrition therapy.

Prevents discomfort and embarrassment when clothing is removed.

Cutting off clothing prevents contamination of head and hair.

Copious amounts of soap and water will lead to chemical dilution (CDC, 2004) and in some cases will prevent client death.
Flushes toxins from the eye.

Reduces the likelihood of secondary chemical contamination.

Appropriate chemical agent protocol will vary with client exposure (e.g., linesterase, nerve agent, chlorine, lewisite) (Box 5-4).
Various chemical agents cause extensive bleeding.
Various chemical agents commonly cause GI disturbances that may result in dehydration.

BOX 5-4   Examples of Chemical Exposure Protocols

CHLORINE PROTOCOL

1. Dyspnea?
   Try bronchodilators
   Admit to hospital
   Oxygen by mask
   Chest x-ray
2. Treat other problems and reevaluate (consider phosgene)
3. Respiratory system OK?
   Yes—go to 5
4. Is phosgene poisoning possible?
   Yes—go to Phosgene Protocol
5. Give supportive therapy: treat other problems or discharge.

MUSTARD PROTOCOL

1. Airway obstruction?
   Yes—tracheostomy
2. If there are large burns:
   Establish IV line—do not push fluids as for thermal burns
   Drain vesicles—unroof large blisters and irrigate area with topical antibiotics
3. Treat other symptoms appropriately:
   Antibiotic eye ointment
   Sterile precautions prn
   Morphine prn

Modified from Centers for Disease Control and Prevention: *Emergency room procedures in chemical hazard emergencies: a job aid,* www.cdc.gov/nech/demil/articles, accessed April 28, 2004.

STEP	RATIONALE
9. Establish airway if needed; administer oxygen therapy.	Various chemical agents commonly cause respiratory symptoms that may result in altered gas exchange.
10. Provide supportive care (e.g., comfort measures, including pain management).	Some victims of a chemical attack will not survive; it is essential for the nurse to provide palliative symptom control.
11. Counsel client and family on both acute and potential long-term psychological effects of exposure. Offer access to trained counselors.	Reaction of clients to exposure will include shock, immobilization, and fear. Long-term psychological effects could arise without proper counseling (CDC, 2004).

• *Critical Decision Point*
Collaborate with the physician and other rescue workers for an ongoing plan to manage clients exposed to a toxic chemical agent while also caring for other clients who may already be present in the health care agency seeking care for illness unrelated to the current MCI.

EVALUATION

1. Observe for improved airway maintenance, breathing, circulation, level of consciousness, and neurological functioning.	Evaluates the client's response to available treatment and/or supportive care.
2. Inspect condition of skin; note extent of blistering.	Determines extent of healing.
3. Evaluate client's level of orientation, ability to problem solve, and perception of condition.	Evaluates the client's psychological status and ability to make decisions.

Recording and Reporting

• Report suspected cases of a toxic chemical event to physician or emergency officer.
• Record in nurses' notes client's status and response to treatment and/or comfort measures.
• Report any unexpected outcome to physician or nurse in charge.

Unexpected Outcomes	Related Interventions
1. Secondary contamination of rescue workers.	• Rescue workers immediately remove their clothing, scrub their bodies, and use copious amounts of soap and water. • Clothes are contained in appropriate biohazard bags. • Clean clothes are provided.
2. Client's physical symptoms progress despite appropriate treatment.	• Notify physician or nurse in charge. • Continue to provide comfort care.
3. Client's psychological symptoms progress despite appropriate treatment. Client exhibits anxiety, disorientation, and suicidal ideation.	• Notify mental health treatment team. • Remain calm, offer reassurance, and protect self and others from physical harm. • Continue to provide comfort measures.
4. Client death.	• Handling of bodies should take into account continued risk for contamination; therefore those handling bodies should be fully informed regarding proper procedure. Delegation of preparation of the deceased should always take into account the level of training of those managing the body.

Teaching Considerations

- Preparation for a mass casualty disaster will go a long way in preventing casualties and chaos. Public education of the likelihood of a mass casualty chemical event is needed. This education should include information regarding types of chemical agents, mode of dissemination, symptoms, and treatment.
- Education of the public should include locations of shelters and disaster treatment sites.
- See Skill 5-1 for family disaster plan and preparation.

Pediatric Considerations

- Adult decontamination facilities may not be appropriate to meet the needs of children. The special protective equipment worn by rescue workers may frighten young children. Considerable stress and anxiety can be anticipated by the cleaning process and possible separation from uncontaminated parents. Additional health care workers may be needed to ensure adequate decontamination has taken place. Verbal encouragement and praise can be effective in facilitating the process (Bernardo, 2001).
- Children are vulnerable to the stresses of evacuation; living in shelters; and losing their homes, schools, parents, pets, and loved ones. (Bernardo, 2001).
- Disasters may result in relocation of children and their families to new homes. When this new home is located in an area of differing culture, customs, or other life patterns, the child is further exposed to stress (Bernardo, 2001).
- Children are particularly vulnerable to environmental toxins because (a) they are closer to the ground and thus more likely to inhale the toxin, (b) they breathe more air per kilogram of body weight, (c) their organ systems tend to be more sensitive than those of adults, and (d) they have more years of life expectancy over which to develop complications from the toxic exposure (Claudio and others, 2003).
- Asthma is a special concern in children. Asthma symptoms (e.g., wheezing, shortness of breath, chest discomfort) can be triggered by exposure to a chemical agent (Claudio and others, 2003).

- Children trapped during a disaster are more likely to develop infections following the disaster due to exposure to pollutants, waterborne and airborne infectious agents, and contact with their own vomit and feces (Goodman and Hogan, 2002).
- Parents and family members should be allowed to be with injured children as soon as possible.
- The death of a child as a result of a disaster is always traumatic; should a parent express the desire to be present during pediatric resuscitation, ideally this should be allowed; a nurse should be available to explain to the parent what is happening (Plum and Veenema, 2003).

Gerontological Considerations

- Under disaster conditions, older adults should be triaged according to injuries, not age.
- Because the older adult may have a myriad of concurrent illnesses, it is possible chemical exposure may exacerbate that condition and result in more immediate care than an initial triage may have suggested.

Home Care Considerations

- See Skill 5-1.
- Keep upwind and uphill from the release of the toxic chemical unless it has been identified to be cyanide.
- Use appropriate PPE needed to protect the family; this may include sheltering-in-place.
- When a family member becomes contaminated, have him or her cut his or her clothes off, scrub his or her body, and use copious amounts of soap and water; avoid direct contact with the family member until there is reasonable certainty that decontamination has been achieved.
- When possible, have the contaminated individual place all contaminated clothing and other items in a plastic bag that can be sealed.
- When an individual exposed to toxic chemicals develops symptoms following decontamination, transportation to the nearest designated hospital becomes a priority.
- Decontaminate any surfaces the contaminated individual may have contacted by donning gloves, scrubbing the area, and using copious amounts of soap and water.

SKILL 5-3 Care of the Client After Radiation Exposure

Radiological events differ from nuclear events. A radiological event is the dispersal of radioactive material via a "dirty bomb" or by deliberate contamination of food supplies, water supplies, or over the terrain. A nuclear event involves a device that releases nuclear energy in an explosive manner as a result of a nuclear chain reaction. Early symptoms of radiation exposure are similar to those experienced by anxious individuals. Thus once radiation release becomes publicly recognized, an enormous number of "worried well" will compromise incident management, scene security, and triage (Veenema, 2003).

Radiation comes in a variety of forms. Alpha particles are the least dangerous, traveling only a few centimeters. They do not penetrate materials easily. An individual's clothing will block alpha particles from reaching the skin. Alpha particles are only harmful if ingested. Beta particles do penetrate a short distance into the skin. Protective clothing is required for protection from beta particles. Gamma rays pose the greatest health risk because the waves penetrate deeply, causing severe burns and internal injury. Lead shielding is required for protection. Blasts caused by a nuclear explosion not only cause injury resulting from radiation exposure but also traumatic injuries and burns. Any victim may present with many combined forms of injury requiring treatment. Although the most feared terrorist threat is a nuclear explosion, this is the least likely threat posed by terrorists. Nuclear devices and their delivery systems are not readily available and are complicated to use (AMA, 2002).

The sooner symptoms begin to appear, the greater the client's exposure to the radiation. Early symptoms, within a few hours, suggest the individual has received a lethal dose of radiation. Early symptoms include nausea, vomiting, di-

TABLE 5-5 CHARACTERISTICS OF A NUCLEAR EVENT AND A RADIOLOGICAL EVENT		
CHARACTERISTICS	NUCLEAR EVENT	RADIOLOGICAL EVENT
Event recognition	Obvious	Not obvious
Thermonuclear explosion	Yes	No
Casualties	Large	Small
Amount of radiation release and contamination	Large	Small
Likelihood of terrorism	No	Yes

From American Medical Association: *Core disaster life support: provider manual* (version 1.01), Chicago, 2002, American Medical Association. Used with permission of the AMA.

arrhea, and a possible burn. Hair may begin to fall out, and the victim quickly becomes immunocompromised.

Nuclear incidents will usually result in wide destruction requiring specialized equipment and resources at the scene to assess structural damage and levels of radioactivity. Radiological events usually cover much smaller areas but may be difficult to define. Table 5-5 presents characteristic differences between a nuclear event and a radiological event. Specialized equipment and training are required to assess the source of radioactivity and determine the scope of contamination. Decontamination is important with radiation exposure; however, it must be provided in an area where there is not continued radiological release. Radiological decontamination requires specialized training and equipment. The principles to follow to protect individuals from exposure involve distance, time, and shielding.

Delegation Considerations

The assessment of a client exposed to radiation cannot be delegated to assistive personnel. However, assistive personnel may provide supportive care to survivors and administer care after death to those who do not survive. The nurse provides assistive personnel with information, assistance, and direction, including:

* Appropriate use of PPE to prevent exposure
* Technique for handling a body after death to prevent contamination

Equipment

The following is a general list of supplies needed in the event of release of the most radiological exposure.

❏ Decontamination room or area (Adult decontamination rooms may not meet the needs of children requiring decontamination; decontamination of ambulatory victims will not meet the needs of those who are not ambulatory.)
❏ Scissors or some other tool to cut off clothing
❏ Depending on the type of radiological exposure, containers for clothing will be needed
❏ Appropriate PPE for use by trained personnel
❏ Equipment for select specimen collection (see Chapter 43)

STEP	RATIONALE

ASSESSMENT

1. Assess the client's symptoms by performing a focused physical examination (e.g., pulmonary, cardiac, skin, neurological, gastrointestinal).

Symptom identification and clustering of data is the first step to determine client's condition and response.

• *Critical Decision Point*

Before assessment a specially trained technician will conduct a radiation survey of the client, initially conducting a scan of the face, hands, and feet using a radiation survey instrument. If meter results are positive, a thorough survey (5 to 8 minutes per person) is conducted (CDC, 2003).

2. Assess the client for secondary traumatic wounds: location, drainage, size, appearance.

Radioactive fragments may be imbedded in a wound. Can be indicated by very high, localized levels of internal contamination (CDC, 2003).

• *Critical Decision Point*

Do not touch the wound if it is suspected that radioactive fragments are present.

3. Assess the client for preexisting medical conditions that would complicate the effects of the radiological exposure.

Clients with preexisting medical conditions may require additional treatment or may be at greater risk for death.

4. Determine client's allergies, specifically allergy for iodine sensitivity.

Clients with iodine sensitivity should avoid taking potassium iodide, the treatment of choice for radioactive iodine exposure.

5. Assess individual psychological response to radiological event. Clients may present with dissociative symptoms (e.g., feeling as though "not there," sensing that experiences are outside the person), disorientation, depression, anxiety, psychosis, and an inability to care for self. Ask the client, "How do you feel now?" Determine level of orientation, ability to follow conversation.

Aids the nurse in being able to provide appropriate crisis intervention and stress management. Remaining calm and projecting confidence while assessing individuals for clinical symptoms versus feelings of panic will go a long way in reducing the anxiety of the ill and worried well as they experience the general sense of panic associated with a radiological event.

6. Identify resources available (e.g., critical incident stress debriefing teams, counselors, psychiatric/mental health nurse practitioners).

Expert resources can assess extent of psychological impact of disaster.

• *Critical Decision Point*

A radiological event is the most feared event by most individuals. Many are uneducated regarding the dangers of and differences between radiation materials. The health care agency can expect to be overrun by anxious, frightened individuals who can potentially create a danger to the environment.

NURSING DIAGNOSES

- Nausea
- Deficient fluid volume
- Diarrhea
- Risk for infection
- Impaired tissue integrity

- Acute pain
- Compromised family coping
- Anxiety
- Post-trauma syndrome
- Fear

Related factors are individualized based on client's condition or needs.

STEP	RATIONALE

PLANNING

1. Expected outcomes following completion of procedure:
   - Client will be comforted.

   - Client will be successfully decontaminated.

   - Client's vital signs will return to baseline.

   - Client will be free of nausea and diarrhea.

   - Client's skin integrity will return to baseline.

   - Client's immune system will return to baseline.
   - Client's work of breathing will decrease.

2. Explain care to the client and family. Explain your role, orient to location and activities to perform, explain what client has experienced, and ask, "How are you feeling right now?" Assure them they will be seen by medical personnel.

In some cases the only care that is available is palliative and focused on client's comfort.
Decontamination procedures remove radioactive materials from client's skin.
When there are no underlying medical conditions and *if* the client's disease process is responsive to treatment (when treatment is available), vital signs will return to normal. Returning to normal may take days or weeks.
GI alterations are common following radiation exposure and typically respond to antidiarrheal and antiemetic medications.
Radiological burns will be minimized through successful decontamination.
Exposure to radiation successfully minimized.
Supportive treatment aimed at improving gas exchange and cardiac output.
Crisis intervention is aimed at reestablishing client's orientation and sense of reality.

IMPLEMENTATION

1. Perform hand hygiene.
2. Only trained personnel use required PPE to decontaminate clients with radiological contamination.
3. Provide for client privacy by closing room curtains or door.
3. Decontaminate the client:
   a. Remove client's clothing.

   b. Wash client's skin thoroughly with water and soap, taking care not to abrade or irritate the skin. Do not allow radioactive material to be incorporated into any wounds.
   c. Have radiation technician resurvey the client after washing. Rewash as necessary.
   d. Isolate and cover any area of the skin that is still positive for radiation by using a plastic bag or wrap (CDC, 2003).
4. Client's contaminated clothing is bagged and tagged for further evaluation and placed in an appropriate biohazard container (CDC, 2003).

Reduces transmission of microorganisms.
Reduces likelihood of secondary radiological contamination to untrained personnel attempting decontamination.
Prevents anxiety or embarrassment when clothes are removed.

Removal of clothing should eliminate 70% to 90% of contamination (CDC, 2003).
Use of copious amounts of water is critical in decontamination.

Reduces the likelihood of secondary chemical contamination when containers designed to contain the radiological particle are used.

- *Critical Decision Point*
  Collaborate with the physician and other rescue workers for an ongoing plan to manage clients exposed to radiological materials while also caring for other clients who may already be present in the health care agency seeking care for illness unrelated to the current nuclear or radiological event.

5. Prepare for possibly obtaining a complete blood count (CBC), urinalysis, fecal specimen, and swabs of body orifices.

CBC establishes baseline to determine client's immunological status over time. When internal contamination is suspected, collection of urine, feces, and body orifice swabs will be ordered to analyze for radionuclides (CDC, 2003).

STEP	RATIONALE
6. Treat symptoms according to ordinary treatment practices: provide intravenous (IV) fluid support, antidiarrheal therapies, antiemetic medications, and potassium iodide tablets (CDC, 2004).	Client exposed to radiation is at risk for GI alterations and fluid imbalance. Potassium iodide reduces risk of thyroid cancer from radioactive iodine exposure.

▌EVALUATION

1. Observe for improved fluid balance, GI status, level of consciousness and neurological functioning, and further improvement of other radiological agent–specific symptoms.	Evaluates the client's response to available treatment and or supportive care.
2. Monitor CBC and other appropriate laboratory tests.	Determines client's immune response.
3. Evaluate client's level of consciousness, orientation, and ability to relate events. Ask if client remembers what has occurred; observe affect.	Determines if psychological status has improved.

Recording and Reporting

- Record in nurses' notes client's status and response to treatment and/or comfort measures.
- Report presence of open wound and any suspected radioactive fragment to physician or nurse in charge.
- Report any unexpected outcomes to physician.

Unexpected Outcomes	Related Interventions
1. Secondary contamination of rescue workers.	• Institute appropriate decontamination of the rescue worker.
2. Client's symptoms progress despite appropriate treatment.	• Notify physician or nurse in charge. • Continue to provide comfort care.
3. Client's psychological state deteriorates with development of disorientation, suicidal ideation, violence toward others.	• Notify mental health treatment team. • Remain calm, offer reassurance, and protect self and others from physical harm. • Continue to provide comfort care.
4. Client death.	• Handling of bodies should take into account continued risk for contamination; therefore those handling bodies should be fully informed regarding proper procedure. Delegation of preparation of the deceased should always take into account the level of training of those managing the body.

Teaching Considerations

- See Skill 5-1 for family disaster plan and preparation.

Pediatric Considerations

- Adult decontamination facilities may not be appropriate to meet the needs of children. The special protective equipment worn by rescue workers may frighten young children. Considerable stress and anxiety can be anticipated by the cleaning process and possible separation from uncontaminated parents. Additional health care workers may be needed to ensure adequate decontamination has taken place. Verbal encouragement and praise can be effective in facilitating the process (Bernardo, 2001).
- Children are particularly vulnerable to radiation because (a) their organ systems tend to be more sensitive than those of adults and (b) they have more years of life expectancy over which to develop complications from the radiological exposure (Claudio and others, 2003).
- Children trapped during a disaster are more likely to develop infections following the disaster due to exposure to

pollutants, waterborne and airborne infectious agents, and contact with their own vomit and feces (Goodman and Hogan, 2002).

- Parents and family members should be allowed to be with injured children as soon as possible.
- The death of a child as a result of a disaster is always traumatic; should a parent express the desire to be present during pediatric resuscitation, ideally this should be allowed; a nurse should be available to explain to the parent what is happening (Plum and Veenema, 2003).

Gerontological Considerations

- Under disaster conditions, older adults should be triaged according to injuries, not age.
- Because the older adult may have a myriad of concurrent illnesses, it is possible radiological agents may exacerbate these conditions and result in the older adult needing more immediate care than an initial triage may have indicated.

Home Care Considerations

- See Skill 5-1.
- When a radiological or nuclear event becomes reality, listen to the radio or television for special instructions, including appropriate means for maintaining a safe shelter.
- Keep upwind and uphill from the release of the radioactive materials (AMA, 2002).
- The caregiver's highest priority is always to avoid becoming a victim. Therefore this individual should avoid becoming contaminated, get plenty of rest, drink fluids frequently, and eat a healthy diet. Should the caregiver develop symptoms, appropriate medical care should immediately be obtained (AMA, 2002).

FOCUS on CLINICAL PRACTICE

You are working in the emergency department (ED) in a large metropolitan area. You note that an unusually large number of clients are being admitted to the ED with fever, cough, chills, and in some cases confusion, given that these symptoms are relatively rare during the summer months in your geographical location. You and other health care providers in the ED begin to cluster data obtained from this large group of individuals who are presenting to the ED. You find that many of the clients work in the same high-rise office building and the vast majority of the clients are relatively young, 25 to 45 years of age. Generally, most of the affected clients report a sudden onset of symptoms within the last 72 hours. Some of these same clients have presented to the ED with family members who are presenting with the same symptoms. Among the clients you are caring for are Mr. Slone, a 45-year-old-executive, and Mrs. Jason, a 35-year-old administrative assistant to Mr. Slone. Each of the clients has presented to the ED with their symptomatic spouses. Mrs. Jason has also brought in her symptomatic 7-year-old son.

1. In all of your clients you notice fever, cough, and chills. The clients generally appear very uncomfortable. You decided to do a focused assessment. What systems will you assess, and what information will you obtain?

2. Mr. Slone begins to rapidly deteriorate as he experiences greater shortness of breath. You start him on oxygen therapy via nasal cannula at 2 L/min. You and the other health care workers in the ED begin to recognize that the ED has received a large number of ill individuals (a) with symptoms that are inconsistent with the season, (b) who are generally healthy, and (c) who have a common geographical relationship because all of the clients are either employed in the specified high-rise structure or are relatives of employees from this building. In addition to providing appropriate treatment for these clients, what are other priority actions that health care personnel should take?

3. As the number of clients arriving to the ED increases, the health care needs quickly begin to exceed the health care resources. An MCI is declared. What action should be taken to ensure adequate supplies are available to treat not only the incoming clients but also those clients already present in the ED and those coming in for symptoms other than those similar to the incoming biologically exposed individuals?

4. Because many of the ED health care staff did not initially recognize the potential threat admitted clients posed, the ED has become a secondary site of contamination, because it appears the primary site of exposure

Continued

FOCUS *on* CLINICAL PRACTICE

was the high-rise building. Mr. Slone and his administrative assistant report his having received a letter that contained some unusual white powder. Mr. Slone stated that he disregarded the potential threat because the metropolitan area in which they live was not a likely terrorist site; furthermore, the terrorist threat level was yellow. Several staff members begin to express anxiety as it becomes apparent that they may have been exposed to a potentially lethal biological agent. Many of the staff express a desire to go home. Obviously their reasons for wishing to go home are not valid. Your rationale for this decision includes the following:

5. As the day progresses, it becomes apparent many of the clients admitted to the ED will require hospital admission. A terrorist attack has been determined, and the clients have been diagnosed with inhalation anthrax. What preparations should be made for the transport and admission of these clients to the assigned unit?

NCLEX REVIEW QUESTIONS

1. Why is a clearly defined, executable, and practiced emergency response plan the best indicator that an institution is more likely to be successful in a disaster situation?
   1. Practice makes staff more familiar with disaster protocols in the event of a true disaster.
   2. Practice of protocols meets regulatory agency guidelines.
   3. Practice prevents the likelihood of acute traumatic stress disorder.
   4. Practice is cost-effective in the long term because less staff will be required to handle the disaster because more staff are better prepared.
2. Which nurse is most likely to demonstrate signs of acute traumatic stress disorder?
   1. An experienced nurse who has been delegated to care for the community patients currently admitted to the emergency department.
   2. An experienced nurse assigned to triage disaster victims transported to the emergency department but able to walk in to the triage area.
   3. An experienced nurse who is assigned to care for clients on an as-needed basis.
   4. An experienced nurse who must inform a mother that her three children ages 2, 3, and 4 years of age did not survive the plane crash.

3. Which disaster victim should receive the highest level of priority for care?
   1. A disaster victim who arrives at the ED without a pulse
   2. A disaster victim who arrives at the ED with labored respirations, cool skin, a pulse of 120, and a blood pressure of 90/60
   3. A disaster victim who is a noted politician with an open fracture of his left arm
   4. All disaster victims under the age of 6 years
4. What type of precautions should be used when a client is admitted with cutaneous anthrax?
   1. Standard
   2. Contact
   3. Respiratory
   4. Airborne

References

American Medical Association: *Core disaster life support: provider manual* (version 1.01), 2002, Chicago, The Association.

American Red Cross: *Terrorism: preparing for the unexpected*: Washington, DC, 2001, American Red Cross.

Bernardo L: Pediatric implication in bioterrorism. I. Physiologic and psychosocial differences, *Int J Trauma Nurs* 7(1):14, 2001.

Centers for Disease Control and Prevention: *Interim guidelines for hospital response to mass casualties from a radiological incident,* Atlanta, 2003, CDC.

Centers for Disease Control and Prevention: *Emergency room procedures in chemical hazard emergencies: a job aid,* www.cdc.gov/nech/demil/default.htm, accessed May 6, 2004.

Claudio L and others: Addressing environmental health issues. In Levy BS, Sidel VW, editors: *Terrorism and public health: a balanced approach to strengthening systems and protecting people,* New York, 2003, Oxford Press.

Department of Homeland Security: Securing our homeland: U. S. Department of Homeland Security strategic plan, Washington, DC, 2004, Department of Homeland Security.

Doyle, CJ: Mass casualty incident: integration with prehospital care, *Emerg Med Clin North Am* 8(1):163, 1990.

Drody E, Ackerman G: Biological and chemical terrorism: a unique threat. In Veenema TG, editor: *Disaster nursing and emergency preparedness for chemical, biological, and radiological terrorism and other hazards,* New York, 2003, Springer Publishing.

Goodman C, Hogan D: Urban search and rescue. In Hogan D, Burstein J, editors: *Disaster Medicine*, Philadelphia, 2002, Lippincott, Williams & Wilkins.

Guha-Sapir, D: Rapid needs assessment in mass emergencies: review of current concepts and methods, *World Health Stat Q* 44:171, 1991.

HEICS III: Hospital emergency incident command system update project: a project of the San Mateo County Emergency Medical Services Agency with support and funding from the California Emergency Medical Services Authority, http://www.emsa.ca.gov/Dms2/heics3.htm.

Levy BS, Sidel VW, editor: *Terrorism and public health: a balanced approach to strengthening systems and protecting people,* New York, 2003, Oxford Press.

Plum KC, Veenema TG: Management of psychosocial effects. In Veenema TG, editor: *Disaster nursing and emergency preparedness for chemical, biological, and radiological terrorism and other hazards,* New York, 2003, Springer Publishing.

Veenema TG, editor: *Disaster nursing and emergency preparedness for chemical, biological, and radiological terrorism and other hazards,* New York, 2003, Springer Publishing.

Walker JH and others: Directions for nursing research and development. In Veenema TG, editor: *Disaster nursing and emergency preparedness for chemical, biological, and radiological terrorism and other hazards,* New York, 2003, Springer Publishing.

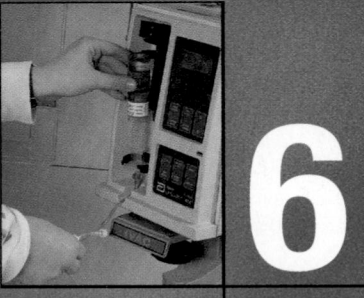

6

Comfort

MEDIA RESOURCES

Evolve Site *evolve*
http://evolve.elsevier.com/Perry/skills
- Weblinks
- Video clips
- Mosby's Nursing Skills Video Exercises

Mosby's Nursing Skills Videos/CD-ROM
- *Post-operative Nursing Care Video:* Pain management, including the use of PCA

OBJECTIVES

Mastery of content in this chaper will enable the nurse to:

- Assess a client's level of comfort.
- Identify skills appropriate for relieving a client's specific pain report.
- Plan care based on a client's history and physical assessment.
- Assist a client in positioning and splinting to achieve pain relief.
- Describe delivery of medication through a patient-controlled analgesia (PCA) device.
- Teach a client to use a PCA device.
- Monitor and manage the client receiving epidural analgesia.
- Monitor and manage the client receiving a local anesthetic infusion pump for pain management.
- Identify various nonpharmacological pain-relief measures.
- Discuss mechanisms by which nonpharmacological measures relieve pain.
- Assist a client in the use of nonpharmacological measures to relieve pain.
- Evaluate the effectiveness of pain management techniques.

KEY TERMS

Acute pain	Nonopioids
Addiction	Nonpharmacological
Bioavailability	Opioids
Chronic pain	Pain intensity
Cutaneous stimulation	Pain rating scales
Distraction	Patient-controlled analgesia
Drug tolerance	(PCA)
Effleurage	Pétrissage
Epidural	Pharmacological agents
Friction	Physical dependence
Guided imagery	Preemptive analgesia
Intraspinal	Pseudoaddiction
Intrathecal	Relaxation
Massage	Splinting

Pain is a complex phenomenon that is much more than a single sensation caused by a specific stimulus. The stimulus for pain can be physical and/or mental in nature. Pain is subjective and highly individualized. It involves the individual's behavioral and emotional responses to the pain experience. Pain is tiring and demands a person's physical, emotional, and mental energy. It can interfere with personal relationships and influence the meaning of life. Certain types of pain create predictable signs and symptoms, but the nurse can only assess pain by relying on the client's report and behavior. The client is the only one who knows whether pain is present and what the experience is like. In McCaffery and Pasero (1999), McCaffery states, "Pain is whatever the experiencing person says it is, existing when she/he says it

does." It is not the responsibility of clients to convince the nurse that they have pain; it is the nurse's responsibility to believe them. Pain has been defined as "an unpleasant sensory and emotional experience associated with actual or potential tissue damage, or an experience described in terms of such damage" (American Pain Society, 2003).

The physiology of acute pain involves four stages: transduction, transmission, perception, and modulation. Transduction is the conversion of mechanical, chemical, or thermal noxious energy to electrical energy in sensory nerves that then initiates an action potential. Transmission is the movement of impulses along sensory nerves via the spinal cord and to the brain. Perception is the process whereby the brain interprets the stimuli to be noxious and thus begins to respond to the stimuli. Modulation involves brain activation of descending pathways that attempt to block pain transmission. Knowledge of these four processes assists in pain management.

Pain is difficult to categorize on duration or pathology alone. However, the literature commonly identifies three types of pain: acute, chronic/persistent, and cancer pain (American Pain Society, 2003). Because cancer pain differs from chronic noncancer pain in significant ways (time frame, pathology, treatment strategies), currently it merits a discrete category (Berry and others, 2001).

Acute pain or transient pain is pain that:

- Has an identifiable cause
- Has a rapid onset
- Varies in intensity
- Is of short duration
- Generally disappears with healing

Chronic pain or persistent pain is pain that:

- Extends beyond the period of healing
- Often lacks identified pathology
- Rarely is accompanied by autonomic signs
- Does not provide a protective function
- Disrupts sleep and activities of daily living
- Degrades health and function of individual
- May be cancer or noncancer/nonmalignant in origin

Cancer pain is pain that:

- May be acute, chronic, or intermittent
- Is usually related to tumor recurrence or treatment

Because an individual's experiences are quite personal, pain management requires an individualized approach. The most effective pain management involves a combined approach of nonpharmacological strategies with the administration of pharmacological agents: nonopioids and opioids (Table 6-1).

Timely administration before a client's pain becomes severe is crucial to ensure that the client gains optimal relief. Pain is easier to prevent than to treat. In most circumstances, administration of pharmacological agents at regular intervals "around-the-clock" rather than on an "as-needed" (prn) basis

TABLE 6-1 TWO ANALGESIC GROUPS: EXAMPLES WITHIN EACH GROUP

Nonopioids	Opioids
a. *Acetaminophen* (Tylenol)	a. *Mu agonists** (full agonists)—Examples:
b. *NSAIDs*—Short acting—Examples:	Codeine
Aspirin	Fentanyl (Duragesic patch)
Trisalicylate (Trilisate)	Hydrocodone
Ibuprofen (Motrin, Advil)	Hydromorphone (Dilaudid)
Ketorolac (Toradol)	Levorphanol (Levo-Dromoran)
Ketoprofen (Orudis)	Meperidine (Demerol)
Naproxen (Naprosyn)	Methadone
Piroxicam (Feldene)	Morphine
c. *NSAIDS*—Long acting—Examples:	Oxycodone
Bextra	Propoxyphene (Darvon)
Celebrex	Tramadol hydrochloride (Ultram)
Vioxx	b. *Agonist-antagonists*—Examples:
d. Topicals—Examples:	Buprenorphine (Buprenex)
Lidocaine (Lidoderm)	Nalbuphine (Nubain)
Eutectic mixture of lidocaine and prilocaine (EMLA)	Pentazocine (Talwin)
ELA-MAX (OTC)	
Capsaicin	

Modified from McCaffery M, Pasero C: *Pain: clinical manual,* ed 2, St. Louis, 1999, Mosby.
*Many of the pure opioids are also found in combination with nonopioids. Several are also available in long-acting formulations.

is preferable. This approach alleviates pain before it becomes severe and can facilitate an earlier recovery (Acute Pain Management Guideline Panel, 1992; Jacox and others, 1994).

Often a combination of nonopioids and opioids is effective in managing pain. Although clients, family members, and caregivers may fear that frequent administration of pain medications will result in the client's psychological dependence (addiction) on the opioid, such dependence is actually rare (American Pain Society, 2003). Clients may exhibit drug-seeking behaviors when in fact they are seeking pain relief. This is termed pseudoaddiction. Occasionally a physician may order a placebo to discredit a client's report of pain. This is unethical and should be avoided (American Pain Society, 2003). Clients are also concerned about drug tolerance. Therefore it is important for the nurse to understand the differences between addiction, physical dependence, and drug tolerance (Box 6-1) in order to educate the client, family members, and other health care providers (McCaffery and Ferrell, 1999).

Complementary strategies for pain relief include nonpharmacological interventions. These interventions provide an opportunity for the client to assume an active role in achieving a higher level of comfort and, in some instances, freedom from pain. It is recommended that an integrated approach that considers both pharmacological and nonpharmacological therapies in managing pain be used (Berry and others, 2001).

Promoting comfort with nonpharmacological interventions, as with pharmacological agents, requires careful attention to assessment and planning. The experience of pain is influenced by a client's age; level of cognition; personality; culture and ethnicity; coping style; emotional, physical,

BOX 6-1 Terminology Related to the Use of Opioids in Pain Treatment

PHYSICAL DEPENDENCE

"Physical dependence is a state of adaptation that often includes tolerance and is manifested by a drug class specific withdrawal syndrome that can be produced by abrupt cessation, rapid dose reduction, decreasing blood level of the drug, and/or administration of an antagonist."

ADDICTION

"Is a primary, chronic, neurobiologic disease, with genetic, psychosocial, and environmental factors influencing its development and manifestations. It is characterized by behaviors that include one or more of the following: impaired control over drug use, compulsive use, continued use despite harm, and craving."

DRUG TOLERANCE

"A state of adaptation in which exposure to a drug induces changes that result in a diminution of one or more of the drug's effect over time."

American Society of Addiction Medicine: *Consensus document,* retrieved April 9, 2004, http://www.asam.org/ppol/paindef.html, 2001.

and spiritual needs; state of health; and past pain experiences. The effectiveness of any therapy will be minimal if clients do not perceive as helpful what they receive. It is important for clients to actively participate in any attempts to alleviate discomfort, because they are the best authority on their pain (Jacox and others, 1994; McCaffery and Pasero, 1999).

TABLE 6-2 MISCONCEPTIONS: BARRIERS TO THE ASSESSMENT AND TREATMENT OF PAIN	
Misconception	**Correction**
1. The best judge of the existence and severity of a client's pain is the physician or nurse caring for the client.	The client's self-report is the most reliable indicator of the existence and intensity of pain.
2. Clinicians should use their personal opinions and beliefs about the truthfulness of the client to determine the client's true pain status.	Allowing each clinician to act on personal beliefs presents the potential for different pain assessments by different clinicians, leading to different interventions from each clinician. This results in inconsistent and often inadequate pain management. It is essential to establish the client's self-report of pain as the standard for pain assessment.
3. Visible signs, either physiological or behavioral, always accompany pain and can be used to verify its existence and severity.	Even with severe pain, periods of physiological and behavioral adaptation occur, leading to periods of minimal or no observable signs of pain. Lack of pain expression does not necessarily mean lack of pain.
4. The pain rating scale preferred for use in daily clinical practice is the visual analog scale (VAS).	The preferred pain rating scale depends on the client's cognitive and physical ability, culture, developmental level, and tool availability.
5. Cognitively impaired older adult clients are unable to use pain rating scales.	When an appropriate pain rating scale (e.g., 0-10) is used and the client is given sufficient time to process information and respond, many cognitively impaired older adults can use a pain rating scale.
6. If clients hurt enough they will tell you.	Clients are often hesitant to report pain for fear of being labeled as complainers, hypochondriacs, or addicts.
7. Psychosocial interventions alone will reduce or alleviate pain.	Nonpharmacological interventions are synergistic with medications, but are not a substitute for pharmacological management of pain.

Modified form McCaffery M, Pasero C: *Pain: clinical manual*, ed 2, St.Louis, 1999, Mosby.

Evidence-Based Practice Trends

Because pain is now considered a comorbid medical condition and not simply a symptom of a pathological state, the trend, if possible, is to prevent pain. Preemptive analgesia and balanced anesthesia are two methods of preventing pain while reducing opioid use. Consumption of opioids and the implication of addiction are of major concern to clients in pain, health care providers, and the judicial system. Understanding the influence of genes (Fagerlund and Braaten, 2001; Flores and Mogil, 2001; Pohl and Braz, 2001; Pohl and others, 2003) and gender (Chang and Heitkemper, 2002; Robinson and others, 2003; Weisse and others, 2003) in pain management has just begun. Furthermore, the use of herbals, homeopathy (Soeken, 2004), and dietary therapies (Tall and Raja, 2004) to treat pain is evolving. The goal is to develop an individualized pain management plan that provides optimum pain relief with minimal adverse effects.

The concept of clients as authoritative participants makes pain control an ethical and legal issue. Pain can dehumanize, destroy autonomy, and create a sense of hopelessness and powerlessness in the client, yet the treatment of pain is regularly and systematically inadequate. Although pain experience is strictly subjective and qualitative, it is often treated objectively and quantitatively by health care providers who inadequately assess and often undermedicate clients (McCaffery and Ferrell, 1999). Pain that is caused or persists as a result of nurses' or physicians' attitudes and outdated practices therefore becomes a matter of ethics. For example, a nurse who does not believe that clients have pain because they are watching TV or visiting with friends or a physician who orders only Demerol for a dying client with intractable pain. McCaffery and Pasero (1999) have identified common misconceptions about pain that health care professionals need to consider when planning client care (Table 6-2).

Barriers to effective pain management occur in clients and health care providers and within the health care system (Glajchen, 2001). Managing a client's pain can be challenging and rewarding, especially in clients with chronic pain. Freedom from pain is not always a realistic goal. In these clients pain management may have to be directed toward pain control rather than complete pain relief.

In the early 1990s the Agency for Health Care Policy and Research (AHCPR) issued guidelines for effective pain management for clients with acute and cancer pain (Acute Pain Management Guideline Panel, 1992; Jacox and others, 1994). These guidelines are designed to help caregivers, clients, and clients' families understand the nature and treatment of pain. In 1999 the Joint Commission on Accreditation of Healthcare Organizations (JCAHO, 2003), which accredits 80% of the nation's hospitals encompassing 98% of hospital beds, set standards for the assessment and treatment of clients in pain. Organizations are being called on to confront and overcome institutional barriers that may prevent adequate pain management for clients (Box 6-2).

The following are skills for improving the effectiveness of pain management that the nurse may use alone or in combination, depending on client needs. Many of the measures discussed can be taught to the client and family for use in the home.

BOX 6-2　**JCAHO Pain Standards**

The 2003 JCAHO standards call upon health care organizations to:
- Recognize the right of patients to appropriate assessment and management of pain
- Assess pain in all patients
- Record the assessment in a way that facilitates regular reassessment and follow-up
- Educate providers/patients and families
- Establish policies that support appropriate prescription or ordering of pain medicines
- Include patient needs for symptom control in discharge planning
- Collect data to monitor effectiveness and appropriateness of pain management

From Joint Commission on Accreditation of Healthcare Organizations: *Comprehensive accreditation manual for hospitals: the official handbook,* Oak Brook Terrace, Ill, 2003, The Commission.

Cultural Considerations

- Understand cultural differences in pain expression.
  - Cultures vary in when to recognize pain, what words to use in expressing pain, when to seek treatment, and what treatments are desired. Russians, Asians, and Native Americans tend to be stoic, whereas Italians, Puerto Ricans, and Jews tend to be more expressive (Garwick, 2000; Nayak and others, 2000).
- Explore generic beliefs about pain/discomfort with the client. Cultures with a holistic worldview of health and illness mix religious/spiritual, natural (hot and cold), and the supernatural in their beliefs system.
- Assess the meaning of pain to the client.
  - Pain associated with terminal illness may be borne by a Hindu client who believes that his or her suffering is a consequence of actions in previous life. For example, a belief in the concept of Karma motivates the client to bear the pain, refuse pain medications, and suffer in silence (Pacquiao, 2003). Jews view pain as a communal suffering that should be shared with others to affirm one's life experience (Bonura and others, 2001).
- Assess multiple modalities used by the client/family for relief of pain.
  - Individuals and cultural groups use complementary and alternative modalities of pain relief such as aromatherapy, imagery, and acupressure along with biomedical interventions (Ludwig-Beymer, 2003).
- Assess meanings of cultural artifacts that clients bring with them. Do not remove these objects without the client's consent (Purnell and Paulanka, 2003).
- Collaborate with the client's identified religious or cultural healers in planning holistic interventions for the client. Hispanics often consult a curandero who empowers people to look at their emotional, physical, and spiritual life so that their bodies might heal (Vanderbilt, 2001); Southeast Asians may consult a shaman or faith healers (Andrews and Boyle, 2003).
- Recognize cultural variations in tolerance and metabolism of analgesics and central nervous system (CNS) depressants. Asians require much smaller doses of analgesics (Campinha-Bacote, 1998; Purnell and Paulanka, 2003).
- Assess cultural variables influencing the operation of patient-controlled analgesia (PCA).
  - Orthodox or Observant Jews may not use electrical equipment during the Sabbath and Holy Days; therefore the staff should program the PCA to achieve optimum pain relief.
  - Some groups may refuse these invasive pain-relief measures because of their cultural and religious beliefs.
  - Southeast Asians may not want any intravenous lines inserted into the child's scalp because the head is considered the seat of the life force. Invasive procedures to the head are believed to allow life to escape from the puncture wound (Orque, 1983).

Skill Performance Guidelines

1. Know the client's past and current medical history, type of therapy, and current medications, including over-the-counter products. Clients with prior pain conditions can alert the nurse to pain-relieving measures that were successful. Clients currently receiving opioids for chronic pain may require higher doses of analgesics to alleviate new pain. Drug-drug interactions, including enhanced or reduced effects or side effects, may occur with polypharmacy.
2. Determine the client's perception of the pain experience. A thorough assessment of factors contributing to the client's pain will enable the nurse to select appropriate therapies. In addition, assess the effects of pain on self-care abilities, quality of life, and sleep.
3. Demonstrate respect for the client's evaluation of the quality and quantity of pain experienced and the response to methods of pain management. It is important to assess the client's acceptable level of comfort so that both client and nurse are striving for the same outcome.
4. Control environment factors that may influence the client's response to discomfort, such as too much stimuli or fatigue, as well as the effectiveness of comfort measures used.
5. Decide the frequency for assessing a client's comfort. It is the nurse's responsibility to assess the client's response to comfort measures and expression of discomfort. The collection of data leading to establishment of pain trends and a comparison of changes in pain patterns is useful in making therapeutic decisions.
6. Communicate to the physician significant changes in the client's comfort level and possible need for changes in pain management regimen. There is no firm guide for the best time to report changes in comfort. However, the nurse who knows the client well and evaluates a client's response to the pain management interventions can identify along with the client when pain-relieving measures are no longer effective or no longer necessary and when the type and quality of pain have changed.

SKILL 6-1 Providing Pain Relief

Alleviating suffering is a major nursing responsibility. Because pain is often an element of suffering, promoting optimal pain relief is a primary goal. Through a comprehensive pain assessment the nurse can begin to understand the impact of pain on a client's life. Effectively managing a client's pain does not necessarily mean eliminating pain. Pain management requires the nurse, working with the client and family, to identify an acceptable intensity of pain that allows maximum client function. Further, collaboration with other health care providers is essential for the best possible pain relief.

The nursing process offers a systematic method of pain management that results in improved pain relief for a majority of clients. This process recognizes distinct differences in client perceptions and responses to pain and thus the importance of individualized pain-relieving interventions. Acknowledging the client as a unique person is essential to optimal pain management. The nurse uses the nursing process to come to know the client and develop an individualized pain management plan.

Management of pain is such a priority that the American Society for Pain Management Nursing (ASPMN), in cooperation with the American Nurses Association (ANA), is rewriting its *Scope and Standards* of pain management for the nurse generalist and nurse specialist. From these standards a certification examination in pain management will be offered in October 2005 (ASPMN, 2004).

DELEGATION CONSIDERATIONS

The nurse cannot delegate pain assessment; however, assistive personnel may screen clients for pain and provide selected nonpharmacological pain-reducing strategies (back rubs, heat, cold, massage, elevation, etc.) as instructed by the nurse. When delegating skills to assistive personnel, instruct them to:

- Eliminate environmental conditions that might enhance pain
- Provide maximum rest periods
- Turn and place client in a position of comfort
- Ask client to report pain using pain intensity tool chosen by client with nurse
- Report to the nurse client reports of pain intensity above predetermined goal
- Report to the nurse nonverbal behaviors suggestive of pain
- Screen for pain during client transfer or activity

EQUIPMENT
❏ Pain intensity tool

STEP	RATIONALE

ASSESSMENT

1. Assess client's risk for pain (e.g., those undergoing invasive procedures, anxious clients, clients unable to communicate).

2. Ask clients if they are in pain. However, clients from various cultures may not admit to having pain; thus additional pain assessment techniques may be necessary.

3. Assess client's response to pharmacological interventions.

4. Examine site of client's pain or discomfort. Include inspection (discoloration, swelling, drainage), palpation (change in temperature, area of altered sensation, painful area, areas that trigger pain, areas that reduce pain), and range of motion of involved joints (if applicable). Percussion and auscultation also helps to identify abnormalities (e.g., lung consolidation or crackles) and determine cause of pain.

Allows nurse to anticipate client's needs and to intervene in a timely manner, possibly preventing pain.

There is no objective test that can measure pain. The clinician must accept the client's report of pain (American Pain Society, 2003). In clients of differing cultures, watch for nonverbal indicators of pain, and ask significant others if they believe the client is in pain (Andrews and Boyle, 1999).

Determines extent to which therapies have been successful.

Clinical observations clarify information from client. Site of discomfort may direct nurse to specific types of pain-relief measures.

STEP	**RATIONALE**
5. Assess for physical, behavioral, and emotional signs and symptoms of pain.	Combination of signs and symptoms may help reveal source and nature of pain.
a. Moaning, crying, whimpering, vocalizations ("Stop, stop!")	
b. Decreased activity	
c. Facial expressions (e.g., grimace, clenched teeth)	
d. Change in usual behavior	
e. Abnormal gait	
f. Irritability	
g. Guarding of body part	
h. Increased blood glucose level	The stress of unrelieved pain causes the endocrine system to release excessive amounts of hormones and decreased insulin levels. The metabolic responses can include hyperglycemia.
i. Diaphoresis	
j. Change in mental status (e.g., confusion)	Confusion may be a sign of unrelieved pain and not opioids, as is commonly assumed (McCaffery and Pasero, 1999).
k. Decreased gastrointestinal (GI) motility, nausea, and vomiting	Signs and symptoms typically occur with pain originating from involvement of visceral organs and result from stimulation of the parasympathetic nervous system.
l. Muscle tension, restlessness, exhaustion	Continued stimulation of sympathetic nervous system depletes energy stores.
m. Insomnia, anorexia, fatigue	These physical manifestations may in turn increase the perception of pain.
n. Depression, hopelessness, anger, fear, social withdrawal, powerlessness, stoicism	Depression frequently occurs in clients with chronic pain and can increase perception and intensity of pain (Bair and others, 2003).
o. Concomitant symptoms: symptoms that often occur with pain (e.g., headache, constipation, restlessness)	Signs and symptoms of sympathetic nervous system stimulation caused by stress and unrelieved pain (McCaffery and Pasero, 1999).

- **Critical Decision Point**
  Physiological responses (e.g., tachycardia, hypertension) to acute pain are of short duration and return to normal within minutes. Be aware that if pain has been prolonged, a client will not usually exhibit physical signs and symptoms.

STEP	**RATIONALE**
6. Assess characteristics of pain: The PQRSTU of pain assessment.	Guides clinician in collecting information about client's pain experience.
a. **P**rovocative/**P**alliative factors (For example, "What makes your pain better or worse?")	Certain types of pain may be precipitated or aggravated by select factors. Allows nurse to identify the nature and source of discomfort. No single approach is right for every client. A combination of interventions is often the most effective approach to pain relief (Acute Pain Management Guideline Panel, 1992).
b. **Q**uality (For example, use open-ended questions such as "Tell me what your pain feels like.")	Assists in identifying the underlying pain mechanism (e.g., somatic or neuropathic pain) necessary for determining appropriate treatment (McCaffery and Pasero, 1999).
c. **R**egion/**R**adiation (For example, "Show me where your pain is.")	Allows nurse to identify possible causative factors.

STEP	RATIONALE

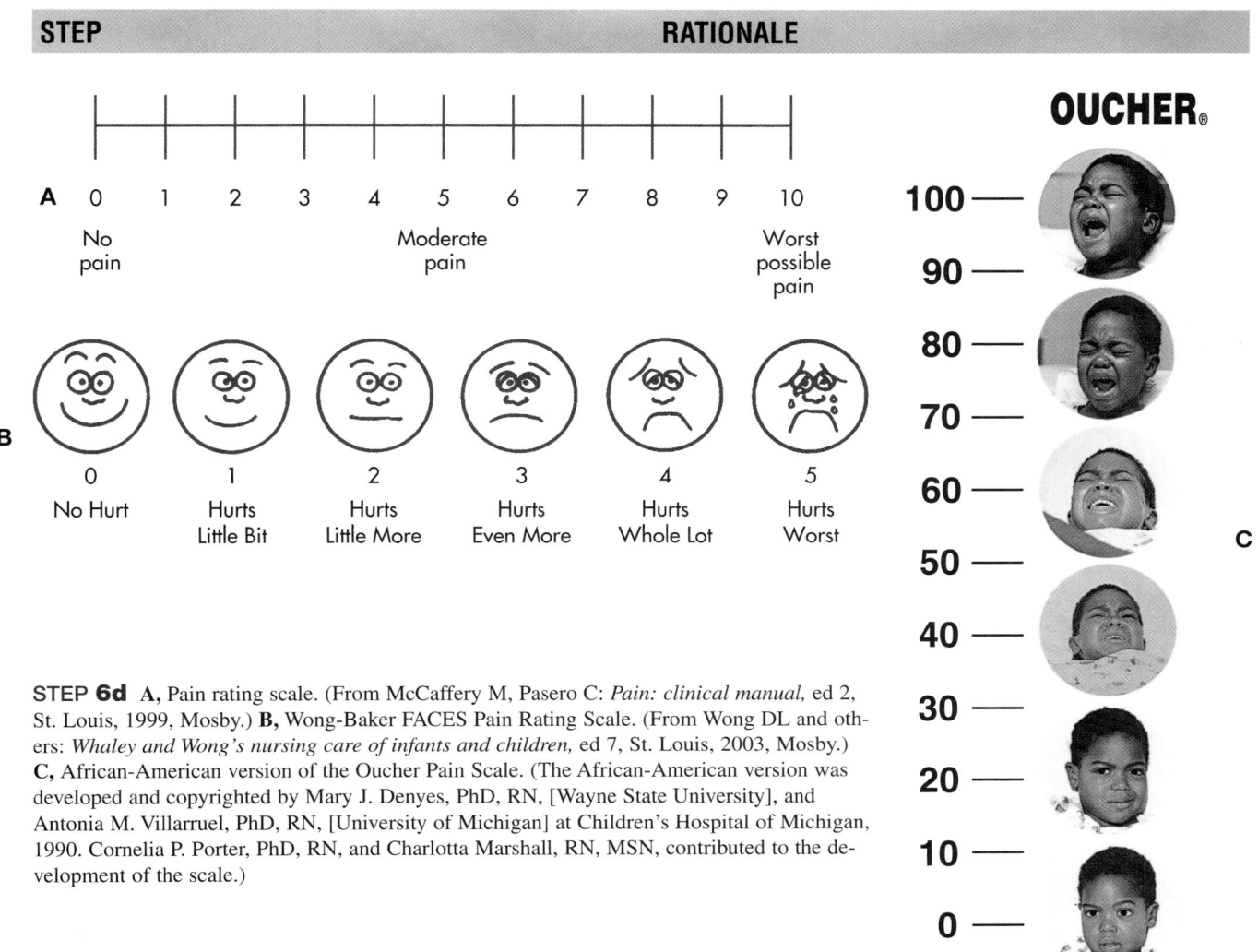

STEP 6d A, Pain rating scale. (From McCaffery M, Pasero C: *Pain: clinical manual,* ed 2, St. Louis, 1999, Mosby.) **B,** Wong-Baker FACES Pain Rating Scale. (From Wong DL and others: *Whaley and Wong's nursing care of infants and children,* ed 7, St. Louis, 2003, Mosby.) **C,** African-American version of the Oucher Pain Scale. (The African-American version was developed and copyrighted by Mary J. Denyes, PhD, RN, [Wayne State University], and Antonia M. Villarruel, PhD, RN, [University of Michigan] at Children's Hospital of Michigan, 1990. Cornelia P. Porter, PhD, RN, and Charlotta Marshall, RN, MSN, contributed to the development of the scale.)

d. Severity: Using a pain intensity scale appropriate to client's age, developmental level, and comprehension, ask the client to rate pain (see illustrations).

Pain is a subjective experience; therefore client's evaluation should be accepted. An appropriate pain rating scale should be reliable, easily understood, and easy to use and should reflect changes in pain intensity (McCaffery and Pasero, 1999). Assists in identify causes of pain.

e. Timing: Ask client if pain is constant, intermittent, continuous, or a combination. Also ask if pain increases during specific times of the day, with particular activities, or in specific locations.

Environmental stimuli, such as loud noises, bright lights, strong odors, or temperature extremes, can alter client's response to pain.

f. How is the pain affecting you (**U**) in regard to activities of daily living (ADLs), work, relationships, enjoyment of life?

Mild to moderate pain significantly interferes with function (McCaffery and Pasero, 1999).

• *Critical Decision Point*
Occasionally a client will be unable to report the pain intensity. In this situation it is prudent for the nurse to ask if the pain is "a lot, a little, or in between?" This provides the nurse with some idea of the level of pain intensity.

STEP	**RATIONALE**

- **Critical Decision Point**

  It is important to consistently use the same pain intensity tool with the same client. Different tools (VAS, NRS, colors, FACES, etc.) may be used with different clients depending on their preference, age, developmental level, and/or comprehension ability.

NURSING DIAGNOSES

- Activity intolerance
- Deficient knowledge
- Anxiety
- Pain (acute, chronic)
- Fear
- Powerlessness
- Ineffective coping
- Interrupted family processes

- Fatigue
- Hopelessness
- Ineffective role performance
- Self-care deficit
- Disturbed sleep pattern
- Situational low self-esteem
- Impaired home maintenance
- Impaired physical mobility

Related factors are individualized based on client's condition or needs.

PLANNING

1. Expected outcomes following completion of interventions:

   - Client verbalizes full or partial relief from pain.

     The client's self-report of pain is the single most reliable indicator of pain.

   - Nonverbal behaviors, such as relaxed face and absence of squinting, reflect a reduction in pain.

     Nonverbal behaviors are valid and reliable indicators of pain, especially in the cognitively impaired client (Feldt, 2000).

   - Client's function improves. There is improvement in sleep, nutrition, physical activity, and personal relationships.

     Adequate pain relief permits client to participate in usual ADLs.

2. Prepare client's environment:
   - **a.** Temperature suited to client — Temperature extremes can alter client's response to pain.
   - **b.** Lighting — Bright or very dim lighting can aggravate pain sensation.
   - **c.** Sound — Loud or irritating sounds can aggravate pain.
   - **d.** Activity. Prevent unnecessary interruptions, coordinate activities, and plan for rest periods. — Fatigue accentuates perception of pain.
   - **e.** Close room door or curtain. — Provides privacy and reduces stimuli that may increase pain.
3. Explain steps to be taken to minimize pain stimuli. — Reduces fear and anxiety.

IMPLEMENTATION

1. Perform hand hygiene, and apply disposable gloves if indicated. — Reduces transmission of infection.
2. Administer pain-relieving medications as ordered. — Analgesics are the cornerstone of pain management.
3. Remove painful stimulus:
   - **a.** Assist client with attaining comfortable position within normal body alignment. — Turning and repositioning reduce stimulation of pain and pressure receptors. Also maximizes response to pain-relieving interventions.
   - **b.** Smooth wrinkles in bed linens. — Reduces pressure and irritation to skin.
   - **c.** Loosen any constrictive bandage or device: blood pressure cuff, elastic wrap bandages, band of elastic hose, intravenous (IV) dressings, identification bands. — Bandage or device encircling extremity may restrict circulation.

- **Critical Decision Point**

  Be sure to assess clients' pain when they are moving, not just lying in bed or sitting in a chair.

   - **d.** Reposition underlying tubes, wires, or equipment.

STEP	RATIONALE
4. Applying splinting (e.g., pillow or folded blanket)	
a. Explain purpose of splinting to client.	Promotes client's cooperation.
b. Assist client to place hands firmly over area of discomfort (see illustration).	Splinting immobilizes painful area.
c. Assist client to splint during coughing, deep breathing, and turning.	Splinting decreases movement and subsequent pain during activity.
d. Assist client to attain comfortable position within normal body alighment.	Turning and repositioning reduce stimulation of pain and pressure receptors.
e. Use pillow to support body position.	
5. Provide psychosocial interventions that assist the client with relaxing, such as reducing environmental stimuli, alleviating anxiety by giving information, praying with client, or providing distraction through watching TV or listening to music.	Thoughts influence feelings, which can change perception and behaviors. Thus feelings can reduce the perception of pain (McCaffery and Pasero, 1999).
6. If used, remove and dispose of gloves. Perform hand hygiene.	Reduces transmission of infection.

EVALUATION

1. Within 1 hour of an intervention, ask client to verbalize how well the pain has been relieved and what his or her pain intensity is now (0 to10).	Evaluates effectiveness of pain-relieving interventions in a timely manner after each intervention.
2. Compare client's current pain intensity with personally set pain intensity goal.	Assists in determining appropriate changes to the pain management plan.
3. Compare the client's ability to function and perform ADLs before and after pain interventions.	Contributes to determining effectiveness of pain-relieving interventions, especially in nonverbal clients.
4. Evaluate for presence of analgesic side effects.	Side effects of analgesics may be controlled by reducing the dose, increasing time intervals, or administering other medications (e.g., stimulant laxative for opioid-induced constipation) (Plaisance and Ellis, 2002).

Recording and Reporting

- Report inadequate pain relief (not reaching goal), a reduction in client function, and/or adverse effects from pain interventions (pharmacological and nonpharmacological).
- Record findings of ongoing assessment, interventions completed (including notification of physician, if done), and client's response to interventions. Documents client's response, provides improved continuity of care for future pain experiences, and communicates to all health care providers.

Unexpected Outcomes	Related Interventions
1. Client verbalizes continued pain that exceeds pain intensity goal, describes worsening of pain, displays nonverbal behavior reflecting pain, or identifies pain in a different location.	• Perform a complete pain assessment. • Implement nonpharmacological pain-relief measures. • Ask family members what might be helpful. • Notify physician.
2. Client experiences adverse reaction to medication.	• Assess adverse reaction effects on client. • Notify physician. • Be prepared to administer antidote (e.g., antiemetic, antihistamine, opioid-reversing agent). • Monitor for effectiveness of antidote. • Complete adverse reaction documentation, and record in client's medical record according to agency policy.

Teaching Considerations

- Review client and family's understanding of the pain intensity tool used to rate the pain.
- Explain to client and family about behavioral changes that can be caused by pain.
- Fear of addition is a primary concern of clients and family members; thus the nurse asks them about this potential fear.

Pediatric Considerations

- Although validity and reliability scores of pain rating scales generally increase with age, some rating tools can be used with a child as young as 3 years of age (Hockenberry and others, 2003).
- Children may be reluctant to report pain because they may have misconceptions about the cause of their pain or they may fear the consequences (e.g., another painful procedure or an injection).
- Infants and children experience pain but may respond to pain differently than adults do because of their different developmental levels. For example, they may cry and thrash about, have sleep disturbances, have a shortened attention span, suck or rock, refuse to eat or play, or be quiet and withdrawn. Still others become active when they are in pain; variations in activity levels are related to the child's personality, developmental level, and previous pain experiences (Hockenberry and others, 2003).
- Parents can be a helpful source of information when assessing a child's pain and when planning pain-relief therapies. Most parents know how their child exhibits pain and which pain-relief interventions have been successful or unsuccessful.
- Children with verbal skills can rate their level of pain on the Wong-Baker FACES Pain Rating Scale or the Oucher Pain Scale.

- Additional pain assessment scales for neonates, newborns, and nonverbal children are available.

Gerontological Considerations

- Older clients tend to have inadequately managed pain because of concerns regarding adverse effect of pharmacological treatments (Herr, 2002a).
- Older adults may require more time to explain the pain management tool selected.
- Pain is not a natural occurrence of aging, although older adult clients are at risk for experiencing more pain-causing conditions (American Geriatrics Society Guidelines, 2002).
- Older adult clients with pain may underreport pain (Herr, 2002a). As the nurse, explain the importance of honesty in reporting their pain.
- Older adult clients with conditions that are painful, but who are nonverbal, receive fewer analgesics than similar clients who are able to report their pain (Herr, 2002b).
- A final strategy for assessing pain in older adult, nonverbal clients with painful conditions is an around-the-clock analgesia trial and observing their behaviors (Herr, 2002b).

Home Care Considerations

- Home living conditions, such as type of bed, stairs, and environmental stimuli, should be considered. Supportive bed and quiet environment will enhance sleep and promote pain management.
- Pain management attitudes of the primary care provider (significant other) requires investigation, because without their participation successful pain management in the client experiencing pain will not be realized.
- Administration (around-the-clock versus prn) and storing of analgesics requires planning.
- Assess situation for others in environment who might take the medications.

SKILL 6-2 Patient-Controlled Analgesia

Patient-controlled analgesia (PCA) is an interactive method of pain management that permits client control over pain through self-administration of analgesics (Pasero, 2003b). A client simply depresses the button on a PCA device and a regulated dose of analgesic is delivered. Thus it is crucial that candidates for PCA be able to understand how, why, and when to self-administer the medication (American Pain Society, 2003). It is used extensively in clients with acute (e.g., postoperative) and chronic (e.g., cancer) pain. Available routes of PCA administration include subcutaneous (Sub-Q), IV, and epidural. Occasionally, nurse-con-

trolled analgesia (NCA) may be ordered, whereby the nurse depresses the button after first assessing the client. In addition, family-controlled analgesia (FCA) has been used in children with cognitive or physical disabilities (Lehr and BeVier, 2003). PCA is not recommended in situations in which oral analgesics could easily manage pain (American Pain Society, 2003).

A PCA may be electronic (Figure 6-1) or nonelectronic, consisting of an infusion device, a prefilled drug reservoir, and tubing that delivers the medication from the infuser through the patient-control module to tubing connected to IV

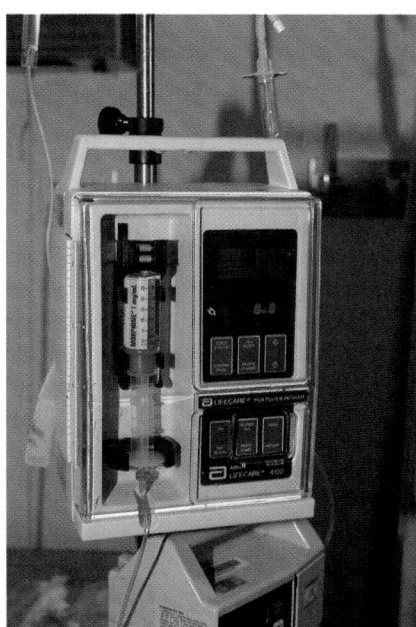

FIGURE **6-1** Patient-controlled analgesia (PCA) device.

fluid, which runs at a continuous rate. PCAs are individually programmed to automatically deliver a specific physician-prescribed continuous infusion (basal rate) of medication, a bolus dose (patient initiated), or both. Overdosing is prevented by interposing a preprogrammed delay time or "lock-out" (usually 6 to 16 minutes) between client-initiated doses. In addition, the total amount of opioid that the client may receive in 1 or 4 hours can be limited (Pasero, 1999). The use

of basal (continuous) infusions should be used cautiously because studies have not shown analgesic benefit. Continuous infusion could increase the risk of opioid overdose (American Pain Society, 2003).

The PCA has several advantages. It allows more constant serum levels of the opioid and, as a result, avoids the peaks and troughs of a large bolus. Because the blood level is maintained within a narrow range of the minimum effective analgesia concentration for the individual, pain relief is enhanced and the incidence of side effects, such as sedation and respiratory depression, is decreased (Pasero, 2003b). A second advantage is that when used postoperatively, fewer complications may arise because earlier and easier ambulation occurs as a result of effective pain relief. Increased client control and independence are other advantages of PCA. Because the device provides medication on demand as soon as the client feels the need, the total amount of opioid use can be reduced. PCA allows the client to manage pain with minimal nursing intervention and therefore also saves nursing time. Clients are not as dependent on the nursing staff for pain medication administration.

Potential concerns involving PCA use are client-related, pump failure, or operator errors. Clients may misunderstand how PCA therapy works, mistake the PCA button for the nurse call button, or have family members who operate the demand button. The pump may fail to deliver drug on demand, have a faulty alarm or low battery, or lack free-flow protection. Operators may incorrectly program the dose, concentration, or rate. They may fail to clamp or unclamp tubing, improperly load syringe or cartridge, fail to monitor for side effects/overdose, or not respond to alarms (Leavitt, 2003). Thus PCA requires careful monitoring.

DELEGATION CONSIDERATIONS
The administration of PCA should not be delegated to assistive personnel. However, certain aspects of the client's care, such as hygiene and vital signs, might be delegated. The nurse must instruct assistive personnel:
- In signs of unrelieved pain and sedation and to report them when they occur
- To immediately report any new symptom or change in client status to the nurse
- To never administer a PCA dose for the client

EQUIPMENT
- ❏ PCA system
- ❏ Identification label and time tape (may already be attached and completed by pharmacy)
- ❏ 18- or 20-gauge needle (if not using a needless system)
- ❏ Alcohol swab
- ❏ Adhesive tape
- ❏ Disposable gloves, if applicable

STEP	RATIONALE

ASSESSMENT

1. Assess client's cognitive ability.	Determines appropriateness of client to be able to use PCA for pain management.
2. Assess for physical, behavioral, and emotional signs and symptoms of pain or discomfort (see Skill 6-1).	Combination of signs and symptoms may reveal source and nature of pain.
3. Assess characteristics of pain (see Skill 6-1).	Guides clinician in collecting information about client's pain experience.
4. Assess environment for factors that contribute to pain.	

STEP	RATIONALE
5. If client has had surgery, apply disposable gloves and inspect incision. Palpate gently for tenderness.	Can reveal evidence of tissue trauma or damage, which stimulates peripheral pain receptors to transmit impulses to cortex to create conscious awareness of pain (McCaffery and Pasero, 1999).
6. Assess patency of existing IV infusion line (see Chapter 21).	IV line must be patent with fluid infusing for medication to reach venous circulation.
7. Assess venipuncture site for infiltration or inflammation (see Chapter 21).	Confirmation of placement of IV needle or catheter and integrity of surrounding tissues ensures medication is administered safely.
8. Assess knowledge and effectiveness of previous pain management strategies.	Response to pain-control strategies assists in identifying learning needs and affects client's willingness to try therapy.
9. Check physician's order for name of medication, dose, frequency of medication (continuous or demand or both), and lockout period.	Opioid medication administration is a dependent nursing function and requires physician's prescription. Commonly prescribed medications delivered via PCA include morphine sulfate, fentanyl, and hydromorphone (American Pain Society, 2003).
10. Check client's history of drug allergies.	Avoids placing client at risk for allergic reaction.

NURSING DIAGNOSES

- Activity intolerance
- Deficient knowledge regarding patient-controlled analgesia.
- Anxiety
- Pain (acute, chronic)

- Fear
- Powerlessness
- Ineffective coping
- Risk for infection

Related factors are individualized based on client's condition or needs.

PLANNING

1. Expected outcomes following completion of procedure:	
• Client verbalizes pain relief.	Drug is given safely and is effective in providing pain control.
• Client exhibits relaxed facial expression and body position.	Points to successful pain relief.
• Client remains alert and oriented.	Indicates freedom from sedating effects of opioids.
• Client increasingly participates in self-care activities.	Suggests successful pain relief.
• Client correctly operates PCA device.	Demonstrates learning and appropriate operation of PCA device.
2. Explain purpose and demonstrate function of PCA to client and family:	Effective explanations allow client participation in care and independence in pain control. Preoperative education about PCA therapy has been shown to improve postoperative pain relief (Knoerl and others, 1999).
a. Device is programmed to deliver ordered type and dose of pain medication, lockout interval, and 1- or 4-hour maximum dose limit (see Figure 6-1).	Ensures safety by implementing parts of the six rights of drug administration.

• *Critical Decision Point*
Be sure the family is taught not to push the button for the client unless directed to do so by the nurse or physician.

b. Device allows client to push medication demand button on timing unit instead of calling nurse.	Gives client control of pain. Client does not have to call and wait for nurse to prepare and deliver medication.
c. Provides lockout time between demand doses to prevent overdose.	Relieves client's fear of possibe overdose. System has built-in safeguards to help prevent accidental administration of doses or overdosing.

STEP	**RATIONALE**
d. Infuser will be on IV pole or attached to bed clothing or wrist.	
e. Device administers small but frequent amounts of medication as needed to provide comfort and minimize side effects.	Small dosing with client-controlled administration produces constant serum drug levels rather than peaks and troughs associated with prn nurse-administered therapy (Pasero, 2003b).

• *Critical Decision Point*
Instruct client to check with nurse or physician with questions and concerns or if medication is not controlling pain. Drug may need to be changed, or dosage may need to be adjusted.

3. Check infuser and patient-control module for accurate labeling or evidence of leaking.	Avoids medication error. Damage to system can occur in shipping and handling; inspect to avoid injury or harm to client, self, or others.
4. Program computerized PCA pump to deliver prescribed medication dose and lockout interval.	Ensures safe, therapeutic drug administration.
5. Draw curtains around client's bed, or close door to room.	Maintains client's privacy.
6. Position client comfortably for procedure. Maintain any position restrictions. Venipuncture or central line site needs to be accessible.	Comfortable position enhances effectiveness of analgesia.

IMPLEMENTATION

1. Perform hand hygiene.	Reduces transmission of microorganisms.
2. Follow the "six rights" to be sure of correct medication (see Chapter 19). Check client's identification band, and call client by name.	Minimizes risk of medication error and harm to client.
3. Attach drug reservoir to infusion device and prime tubing.	Locks system and prevents air from infusing into IV tubing.
4. Apply gloves.	Reduces potential contact with blood when working with IV line.
5. Attach 18- or 19-gauge needle to exit tubing adapter of patient-control module or attach needleless system adapter.	Needed to connect with IV line.
6. Wipe injection port of maintenance IV line with alcohol if closed port is being used.	Alcohol is a topical antiseptic that minimizes entry of surface microorganisms during needle insertion.
7. Insert needleless adapter or needle into injection port nearest client.	Establishes route for medication to enter main IV line. Prevents delay of medication delivery to client.
8. Secure connection with tape and immobilize PCA tubing.	Prevents dislodging of needle from port. Facilitates ambulation.
9. Administer loading dose of analgesia as prescribed.	A one-time dose may be given manually by nurse or programmed into PCA pump.
10. Discard gloves and supplies in appropriate containers. Perform hand hygiene.	Reduces transmission of infection.
11. If client is experiencing pain, demonstrate use of PCA system; if not, have client repeat instructions given earlier.	Repeating instructions reinforces learning. Checking client's understanding through return demonstration helps nurse determine client's level of understanding and ability to manipulate device.
12. Monitor and record PCA use according to agency policy.	Complies with documentation of Schedule II drugs.
13. Dispose of empty cassette or syringe in compliance with institutional policy.	Control and dispensation of opioids are regulated by the Controlled Substances Act.
14. If PCA is discontinued before device is completely empty, record drug wastage on PCA medication record per institutional policy. Note date, time, amount of drug wasted, and reason for wastage. Wastage must be witnessed and record signed by two registered nurses.	

STEP	**RATIONALE**

EVALUATION

1. Use pain rating scale to evaluate client's pain intensity.

Determines response to PCA dosing. Documenting "PCA in use" or "PCA effective" is not an adequate record of the client's pain level.

2. Observe for signs of adverse reactions, especially excessive sedation (Box 6-3).

Intravenous medications produce rapid effects.

BOX 6-3 **Sedation Scale**

S = Sleep, easy to arouse
1 = Awake and alert
2 = Slightly drowsy, easily aroused
3 = Frequently drowsy, arousable, drifts off to sleep during conversation
4 = Somnolent, minimal or no response to physical stimulation

From McCaffery M, Pasero C: *Pain: clinical manual,* St. Louis, 1999, Mosby.
Box 6-3 illustrates a scale that can be used to assess sedation levels in clients receiving opioid analgesia.

---

3. Have client demonstrate dose delivery.
4. Evaluate number of attempts (number of times client pushed the button) and delivery of demand doses (number of times drug actually given) as well as basal dose, if ordered, according to agency policy (usually every 4 to 8 hours).

Evaluates skill in use of PCA.
Assists in evaluating effectiveness of PCA dose and frequency in relieving pain.

Recording and Reporting

- Record drug, dose, and time begun on appropriate medication form. Specify concentration and diluent. Note lockout time, demand and/or basal dose.
- Record regular periodic assessments of client status on PCA medication form if required, in the narrative notes, pain assessment flow sheet, or other documentation tool used in the institution. Forms may vary from institution to institution, but information required is similar. Indicate vital signs, if appropriate; sedation status; pain rating; status of vascular access site; amount of solution infused; amount of solution remaining; amount of drug received.

Unexpected Outcomes	**Related Interventions**
1. Client verbalizes continued or worsening discomfort, or displays nonverbal behaviors indicative of pain.	• Underlying medical or surgical condition may have changed, or client may be undermedicated. • Perform complete pain assessment. • Assess for possible complications. • Inspect IV site for possible catheter occlusion or infiltration. • Evaluate number of attempts and deliveries initiated by client. • Check that maintenance IV fluid is continuously running. • Evaluate pump for operational problems. • Consult with physician.

Unexpected Outcomes	Related Interventions
2. Client is sedated and not readily arousable.	• Stop PCA. • Elevate head of bed 30 degrees, unless contraindicated. • Instruct client to take deep breaths. • Apply oxygen at 2 L/min per nasal cannula. • Assess vital signs. • Evaluate amount of opioid delivered within past 4 to 8 hours. • Ask family members if they depressed the button without client knowledge. • Review medication administration record for other possible sedating drugs. • Notify physician. • Prepare to administer an opioid reversing agent. • Observe client frequently.
3. Client unable to manipulate PCA device to maintain pain control.	• Consult with physician regarding alternative medication route. • Discuss with physician possible basal (continuous) dose. • Assess client support system for significant other who can manipulate PCA device.

Teaching Considerations

- Instructions are best given during pain-free or pain-reduced states and before initiating therapy. If preoperative client, instruct before surgery.
- Encourage client to push button on timing unit whenever pain is felt. Tell client not to delay interval if he or she is experiencing pain. Pain is easier to prevent than to treat.
- Explain regimen to family so that they can support and assist client.
- Instruct family not to push timing device for the client unless client is unable to push the button himself or herself and the nurse has instructed family.
- Inform client of nonpharmacological pain management strategies that may supplement or enhance pharmacological intervention.
- Inform client and family that client cannot overdose with PCA if only the client pushes the button.

Pediatric Considerations

- Patient-controlled analgesia can be an effective means of pain control in children who can understand the concept. When selecting pediatric candidates for PCA use, consideration must be given to developmental level, cognitive level, and motor skills. Ordinarily PCA use is safe and effective for clients as young as 8 to 9 years old (Lehr and BeVier, 2003). From a developmental perspective, use of PCA is particularly effective with adolescents, because it leads to feeling of control.
- Patient-controlled analgesia can be used by clients as young as 5 to 6 years of age depending on their ability to understand the concept and physically push the button. Family members must be instructed and reminded not to push the button for the child. Some facilities have allowed parents with specific guidelines and training to push the button for children too young or unable to control device on their own. This practice remains controversial (Hockenberry and others, 2003).
- Pharmacological pain support is safe and effective in pediatric clients when dose is calibrated according to child's weight (Lehr and BeVier, 2003). As with adults, doses may need adjusting after initiation of medication to obtain optimal analgesia with minimal side effects (Acute Pain Management Guideline Panel, 1992).
- Delivery of the PCA dose on the upstroke of the button (review device insert) prevents accidental depression of the button when the child falls asleep (Lehr and BeVier, 2003).
- It is important that family members be reminded not to push the button for the pediatric client unless they have been designated as the primary pain manager. FCA is an acceptable alternative to PCA, but it may increase the risk of overdosing (Lehr and BeVier, 2003).
- There are no reports of addiction secondary to the use of PCA in pediatric clients.

Gerontological Considerations

- Older clients appear more sensitive to analgesic properties and side effects of opioids (American Geriatrics Society Guidelines, 2002). Older adults' reduced renal and liver function slows opioid metabolism and excretion. This causes a faster peak effect and a longer duration of action of the opioid (American Pain Society, 2003). In addition, their decrease in water concentrates hydrophilic opioids, possibly resulting in increased side effects. Thus start with a low dose, and titrate upward slowly.

- If confusion occurs while using a PCA, the dose should be lowered, the lockout lengthened, or a nonopioid analgesic added to reduce the opioid dose (Pasero, 1999). Nurse-activated around-the-clock dosing is another alternative (McCaffery and Pasero, 1999).

SKILL 6-3 Epidural Analgesia

The term intraspinal refers to both the epidural or intrathecal (subarachnoid) space that surrounds the spinal cord, where analgesics can be administered. The epidural space is a potential space that contains a network of vessels, nerves, and fat. The intrathecal/subarachnoid space contains cerebral spinal fluid (CSF) that bathes the spinal cord. The brain and spinal cord are covered by three meninges or membranes. The dura mater is the outermost protective membrane. The epidural space is a potential space that lies between the vertebral column and the dura, thus above the dura mater. It extends from the foramen magnum to the sacral hiatus. The intrathecal/subarachnoid space lies between the arachnoid and the pia mater and contains cerebrospinal fluid. Intrathecal (spinal) drugs are administered only by physicians and/or nurse anesthetists. Registered nurses, as regulated by their State Boards of Nursing, are not allowed to administer analgesics into the subarachnoid space, thus discussion will be limited to epidural analgesia only.

Drugs administered in the epidural space can be distributed (1) by diffusion through the dura mater into the CSF, where it acts directly on receptors in the dorsal horn of the spinal cord; (2) via blood vessels in the epidural space and delivered systemically; and/or (3) by means of absorption by fat in the epidural space, creating a depot where the drug is slowly released into the systemic circulation (Pasero, 2003a).

Opioids and local anesthetics, separately or in combination, are often used in epidural analgesia, although adjuvants may also be given (Guay, 2001). Because opioids are delivered close to their site of action (CNS) they have greater bioavailability and thus require much smaller doses to achieve adequate pain relief. Common opioids administered via the epidural route are morphine, hydromorphone (Dilaudid), fentanyl, and sufentanil. These opioids vary in their lipophilic (fat loving) and hydrophilic (water loving) properties, which alter absorption rate and duration of action. Fentanyl and sufentanil are lipophilic, causing them to have a quicker onset and shorter duration of action (2 hours). Morphine and hydromorphone are hydrophilic, resulting in a longer onset and duration of action (up to 24 hours with a single bolus dose) (Pasero, 1999). In addition, hypdrophilic opioids adminis-

tered via the epidural route readily circulate toward the brain (rostrally), resulting in analgesia at many levels along the spinal cord. However, lipophilic opioids do not circulate readily, resulting in "segmental" analgesia (Pasero, 2003a).

Epidural local anesthetics, bupivacaine (Marcaine) and ropivacaine (Naropin) (Pasero, 2003a) block generation and conduction of pain nerve impulses in the CNS. These local anesthetics significantly block sensory nerves while having a minimal effect on motor nerves. Thus, the client is able to ambulate (Pasero, 1999). Combining opioids with local anesthetics improves pain control and reduces complications (CNS and cardiotoxicity) while lowering opioid doses (Pasero, 2003a).

For epidural catheter placement the client is placed in the lateral decubitus or sitting position with shoulders and hips squared and hips and head flexed (McCaffery and Pasero, 1999). Usually an anesthesiologist or nurse anesthetist places a catheter into the epidural space (Figure 6-2) below the second lumbar vertebra, where the spinal cord ends; however, thoracic epidurals may also be inserted. When the catheter is intended for temporary or short-term use, it may not be sutured in place and exits from the insertion site on the back (Figure 6-3). By contrast, a catheter intended for permanent or long-term use is "tunneled" subcutaneously and exits on the side of the body or on the abdomen. Tunneling decreases the chance of infection or dislodging of the catheter. In both cases the catheter is covered with a sterile occlusive dressing and secured to the client. The only way to ensure proper placement of an epidural catheter is radiologically.

Epidural medication can be administered either intermittently via bolus injection by the clinician, demand injection by the client (patient-controlled epidural analgesia [PCEA]), or continuously via a controlled delivery system such as an infusion pump (see Chapter 20). If PCEA is used, there is a continuous infusion of medication and the PCEA bolus dose is used to treat breakthrough pain (Pasero, 2003a).

Although the use of epidural opioids for pain control has many advantages for the client, it requires astute nursing ob-

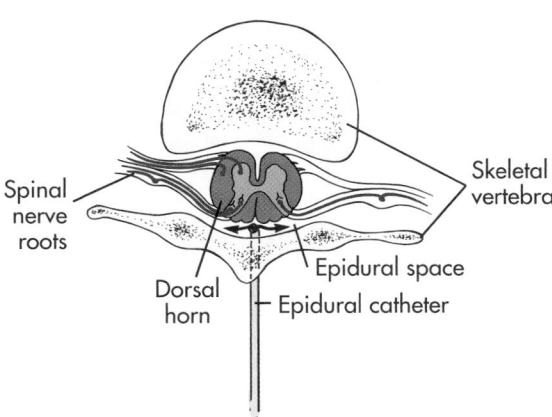

FIGURE 6-2 Anatomical drawing of epidural space. (From Sinatra S: *Spinal opioid analgesia: an overview.* In Sinatra RS and others, editors: *Acute pain management,* St. Louis, 1992, Mosby.)

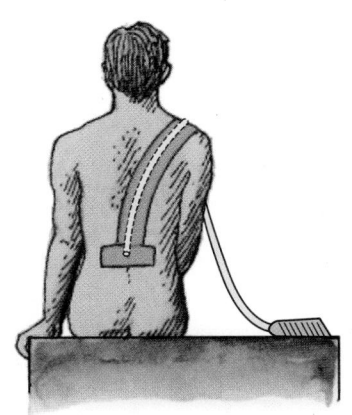

FIGURE 6-3 Epidural catheter taped in place. (Courtesy Astra Zeneca Pharmaceuticals, Wilmington, Del.)

servation and care. The catheter poses a threat to client safety because of its anatomical location, its potential for migration through the dura, and its proximity to spinal nerves and vessels. An epidural catheter migration into the subarachnoid space can produce medication levels too high for intrathecal use. Epidural and intrathecal doses are not equivalent. Intrathecal doses are much smaller than epidural doses. As an example, the epidural dose of morphine is 10 to 20 times greater than that required for an intrathecal dose (Rawal, 1999).

Assisting the client in obtaining pain control or relief, evaluating the analgesic effect, and intervening appropriately in the event of a complication or occurrence of side effects are the responsibilities of the nurse caring for these clients. In addition, the nurse should question administering concurrent oral medications that are known to cause sedation and/or respiratory depression (e.g., muscle relaxants or anxiolytics). The nurse should obtain approval for their use from the health care professional managing the epidural analgesia (Pasero and others, 1999).

DELEGATION CONSIDERATIONS

Administration of epidural anesthesia should not be delegated to assistive personnel. The nurse is responsible for pain assessment and management. However, other aspects of care such as hygiene and position may be delegated. The nurse must instruct assistive personnel to:

- Pay particular attention to the insertion site when repositioning or ambulating clients to prevent disruption of the catheter
- Report any catheter disconnection immediately
- Immediately report to the nurse any change in client status or comfort level

EQUIPMENT

- ❑ Disposable gloves
- ❑ Prediluted preservative-free opioid or local anesthetic as prescribed by physician and prepared for use in IV infusion pump (usually prepared by pharmacy)
- ❑ Infusion pump
- ❑ Infusion pump and compatible tubing without Y-ports. Some infusion pumps have tubing color coded for intraspinal use.
- ❑ Tape
- ❑ Label (for tubing)

STEP	RATIONALE

ASSESSMENT

1. Assess client's comfort level, presenting medical/surgical condition, and appropriateness for epidural analgesia.

Certain conditions may make epidural analgesia the method of choice for pain control: postoperative states, clients with trauma or advanced cancer that is not responsive to other pain management modalities, and those predisposed to cardiopulmonary complications because of preexisting medical condition or surgery.

2. Check to see if client recently received anticoagulants.

Recent anticoagulants may contraindicate the placement of epidural catheter because of the inability to apply pressure at the epidural insertion site (Regional anesthesia, 2003).

STEP	RATIONALE

3. Check to see if client routinely takes herbals and if so which ones.

Some herbals interfere with the clotting mechanism and could predispose to bleeding at the epidural insertion site. Currently there is no contraindication to their use (Regional anesthesia, 2003). It is prudent to recognize herbs a client uses.

• *Critical Decision Point*
Contraindications to epidural analgesia include coagulopathies, abnormal clotting studies, history of multiple abscesses, sepsis (McCaffery and Pasero, 1999). Additional contraindications may include skeletal or spinal abnormalities.

4. Check client's history of drug allergies.

Avoids placing client at risk for allergic reaction.

5. Assess for physical, behavior, and emotional signs and symptoms of pain (see Skill 6-1).

Combination of signs and symptoms provides baseline to later determine efficacy of analgesia.

6. Assess characteristics and intensity of pain (see Skill 6-1).

Serves as a baseline to later determine efficacy of analgesia.

7. Assess environment for factors that may be contributing to pain.

Nurses can eliminate environmental stimuli that aggravate client's response to pain.

8. Assess sedation level of client by assessing level of wakefulness or alertness, ability to follow commands, and drowsiness.

Establishes a baseline before first dose. Sedation always precedes respiratory depression from opioids (Young-McCaughan and Miaskowski, 2001).

9. Assess rate, pattern, and depth of respirations (see Chapter 17).

Establishes baseline.

10. Assess blood pressure (see Chapter 17).

Establishes a baseline. Vasodilation can occur, and hypotension, including orthostatic hypotension, is common.

11. Assess initial motor and sensory function (see Chapter 18) of lower extremities.

Establishes a basline. Excess analgesia can cause adverse neurological effects.

12. Check to see if catheter is secured to client's skin from the back or front (see illustration).

Aids in preventing dislodging or migration of catheter.

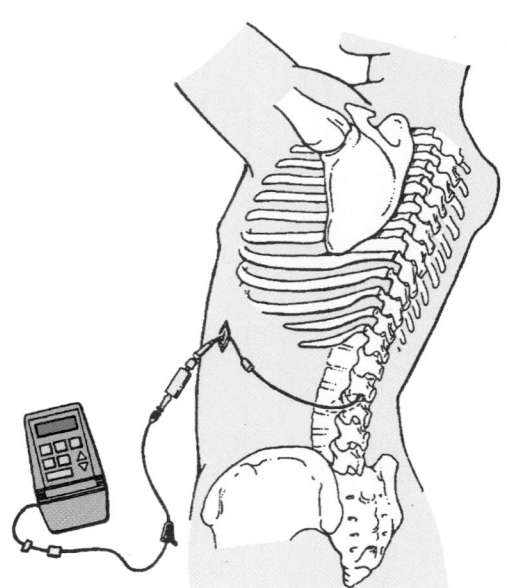

STEP **12** External catheter and ambulatory infusion pump. (Courtesy SIMS Deltec, Inc., St. Paul, Minn.)

STEP	RATIONALE
13. Assess catheter insertion site every 2 to 4 hours for:	
a. Redness, warmth, tenderness, swelling	Local inflammation and superficial skin infection at insertion site can occur.
b. Drainage	Purulent drainage is sign of infection. Clear drainage may indicate puncture of dura, causing medication to be delivered into subarachnoid space or causing cerebrospinal fluid leakage. Bloody drainage may indicate catheter entered blood vessel.
14. Check physician's order for medication, dosage, and infusion method.	Medication administration is dependent nursing function and requires physician's prescription.
15. If continuous infusion, check infusion pump for proper calibration and operation.	Ensures client will obtain prescribed analgesic dose. Be mindful of catheter placement, either epidural or intrathecal, because there is a substantial difference in dosage according to the route.
16. If continuous infusion, check patency of tubing.	Kinked tubing will interrupt analgesic infusion.
17. Keep a patent IV in place until 24 hours after epidural analgesia has ended.	Allows for IV access in case IV medications have to be given to counteract adverse reactions.

NURSING DIAGNOSES

- Pain (acute, chronic)
- Deficient knowledge regarding epidural analgesia
- Activity intolerance
- Disturbed sensory perception

- Anxiety
- Risk for injury
- Impaired physical mobility
- Risk for infection

Related factors are individualized based on client's condition or needs.

PLANNING

1. Expected outcomes following completion of procedure:

• Client verbalizes pain relief.	Indicates drug and dose are effective in relieving pain, catheter is intact, and equipment is functioning properly in compliance with physician order.
• Catheter and injection cap or infusion pump tubing are securely taped and labeled.	Closed, intact system prevents entry of pathogens and disruption of flow of medication.
• Client remains normotensive, and heart rate stays in normal range.	Indicates absence of potential side effects of epidural opioids.
• Client is alert and oriented.	Indicates absence of excessive sedation.
• Respirations are regular, of adequate depth, and equal to or greater than 8 breaths per minute.	Indicates adequate ventilation and reduced risk for respiratory depression from opioids (Pasero, 1999).
• Client does not experience headache.	Indicates catheter in epidural space.
• Epidural dressing is dry and intact.	No cerebrospinal fluid leakage.
• Catheter and infusion tubing are free of knots and kinks.	Helps to ensure that system is patent.
• No redness, warmth, exudates, tenderness, or swelling is evident at catheter insertion site. Client is afebrile.	Indicates absence of inflammation or infection.
• Client voids without difficulty, in adequate amounts, and absence of distended bladder.	Indicates absence of urinary retention (a potential side effect).

STEP	RATIONALE
• Client has no or minimal pruritus and no paresthesias of lower extremities.	Indicates absence of potential side effect of epidural medications.
2. Identify client by checking arm band and asking client's name, hospital number, and/or date of birth.	Ensures correct client receives ordered drug.
3. Explain purpose and function of epidural analgesia and expectations of client during procedure. For example, ask client to call for assistance before getting out of bed.	Proper explanation enhances client cooperation and effective results.
4. Attach "epidural line" label to tubing.	Labeling helps to ensure medication analgesic is administered into correct line and into epidural space.
5. Use tubing *without* Y-ports for continuous infusions.	Use of tubing without Y-ports prevents accidental injection or infusion of other medication meant for vascular space into epidural space.
6. Draw curtains around client's bed or close door to room.	Maintains client's privacy.

IMPLEMENTATION

STEP	RATIONALE
1. Perform hand hygiene and apply gloves.	Reduces transmission of microorganisms.
2. Administer continuous infusion:	
a. Attach container of diluted preservative-free medication to infusion pump tubing and prime tubing (see Chapter 27).	Tubing should be filled with solution and free of air bubbles to avoid air embolus.
b. Attach proximal end of tubing to pump and distal end to epidural catheter. Tape all connections. Give ordered bolus or start infusion. (See Chapter 27 for use of infusion pump.)	Infusion pumps propel fluid through tubing. Taping maintains a secure, closed system to help prevent infection. A filter may be needed on tubing depending on institutional policy.
c. Check infusion pump for proper calibration and operation. Many institutions have two nurses check settings.	Maintains patency and ensures client is receiving proper dose and pain relief.
3. Administer bolus dose of medication:	
a. Draw up prediluted, preservative-free opioid solution through filter needle.	Preservative may be toxic to nerve tissue (Cosentino, 2000).
b. Change from filter needle to regular 20-gauge needle or needleless adapter.	Prevents infusion of microscopic glass particles and allows medication to be injected.
c. Clean injection cap with povidone-iodine. (Do not use alcohol.)	Sterilizing injection port prevents inadvertent introduction of microorganisms into CNS. Alcohol causes pain and is toxic to neural tissue (Pasero, 2003a).
d. Dry injection cap with sterile gauze.	Reduces possible injection of povidone-iodine.
e. Insert needle attached to syringe into injection cap. Or if using a needleless system, attach syringe directly to injection cap. Aspirate.	Aspiration of more than 1 ml of clear fluid or bloody return means catheter may have migrated into subarachnoid space or into a vessel (Pasero, 1999). Do not inject drug. Notify physician.
f. Inject opioid at a rate of 1 ml over 30 seconds.	Slow injection prevents discomfort by lowering the pressure exerted by fluid as it enters the epidural space (Cox, 2001).
g. Remove needle or syringe from injection cap. There is no need to flush with saline.	The catheter is in a space, not a blood vessel, thus flushing with saline is not required (McCaffery and Pasero, 1999).
h. Dispose of needle and syringe in sharps container.	Prevents accidental needle sticks and exposure to blood.
4. Remove and dispose of gloves. Perform hand hygiene.	Reduces transmission of microorganisms.
5. Before removal of epidural catheter, check for presence of therapeutic anticoagulation.	Removal of epidural catheter while a client is anticoagulated increases the risk of spinal hematoma because of anticoagulation and inability to compress vessels (Regional anesthesia, 2003).

STEP	RATIONALE

EVALUATION

1. Evaluate comfort level, and compare with original assessment data.

2. Observe for signs of adverse reactions to epidurally administered opioid or local analgesic.

3. Observe respiratory rate, rhythm, depth, and pattern; sedation level; and skin color. Monitor respiratory rate and depth at least every 1 to 2 hours depending on institutional policy.

4. Observe respiratory rate, rhythm, and pattern every 2 hours for 12 to 24 hours after epidural bolus of opioid to an opioid-naive client (someone who has not received opioids on an around-the-clock basis for more than 5 to 7 days) (Passero, 1999).

Determines if response to analgesia has been effective and if catheter is securely in place.

Although pain is relieved with smaller doses and side effects are less severe with epidural opioid analgesia, side effects can still occur.

Respiratory depression may result from epidural opioid use as long as 24 hours after initiation.

• *Critical Decision Point*

Be prepared to deliver an ampule of naloxone (Narcan), a strong opioid antagonist, 0.4 mg diluted in 9 ml of saline at 1 to 2 ml/min, if respirations fall below 8 breaths per minute and are shallow. Desired effect is to increase respirations, not reverse analgesia. Rapid reversal of opioids by Narcan could result in profound withdrawal, seizures, dysrhythmias, pulmonary edema, and severe pain (American Pain Society, 2003). Continue to assess respiratory status after Narcan administration because renarcotization with resulting respiratory depression could occur (American Pain Society, 2003).

5. Monitor blood pressure and pulse. Assist client when changing positions.

6. Monitor intake and output. Assess for bladder distention. Observe for frequency or urgency.

7. Observe for pruritus, especially of face, head, neck, and torso.

8. Observe for nausea and vomiting.

9. Check insertion site for clear or bloody drainage. Assess for reports of headache.

10. Monitor temperature. Observe insertion site for signs of inflammation.

11. Evaluate for motor weakness or numbness and tingling of lower extremities (paresthesias).

12. After removal of epidural catheter, evaluate for signs and symptoms of hematoma formation: motor or sensory changes below level of catheter.

Postural hypotension, vasodilation, and heart rate changes may occur.

Urinary retention may occur as a result of effects of medication on spinal nerves innervating the bladder.

Itching is the most common side effect when opioids are delivered via the intraspinal route (McCaffery and Pasero, 1999).

Nausea and vomiting can begin 4 to 6 hours after a bolus because of time needed for drug to reach chemoreceptor trigger zone. Nausea from epidural analgesia is exacerbated by movement.

Headache and cerebrospinal fluid leakage can occur from a dural puncture. Bloody drainage may occur if catheter has migrated into a vessel.

Infection can occur from poor sterile technique or systemic bacteremia.

Excessive analgesia, infusion of drugs toxic to central nervous system, or contact of catheter with neural tissue may cause adverse sensory deficits (Acute Pain Management Guideline Panel, 1992). Indicates need to notify physician immediately. Unwanted motor and sensory deficits may be eliminated by reducing epidural dose.

Although rare, unrecognized spinal hematoma formation could result in permanent neurological damage.

Recording and Reporting

- Record drug, dose, and time begun and ended on appropriate medication record. Specify concentration and diluent.
- Record any supplemental analgesic requirements.
- Review pump settings and usage with the next shift.
- Record regular, periodic assessment of client's status in nurses' notes or on appropriate flow sheets or in narrative notes. Indicate vital signs, intake and output, sedation level, pain status, neurological status, status of epidural site, presence or absence of adverse reactions to medication, and presence or absence of complications resulting from placement and maintenance of epidural catheter.
- Report any adverse reactions or complications to physician.

Unexpected Outcomes	Related Interventions
1. Client states pain is still present. Primary causes are insufficient drug dose or catheter blockage, breakage, or improper position.	• Check all tubing, connections, medication doses, and pump settings.
2. Client is sedated or not easily arousable.	• Stop epidural infusion. • Administer opioid reversing agent per physician order. • Monitor continuously until client is easily arousable.
3. Client experiences periods of apnea or respirations are less than 8 breaths per minute, shallow, or irregular.	• Instruct client to take deep breaths. • Stop or reduce rate of epidural infusion. • Notify physician. • Prepare to administer opioid reversing agent per physician order. • Monitor every 30 minutes until respirations are 8 or above and of adequate depth.
4. Client reports sudden headache. Clear drainage is present on epidural dressing or more than 1 ml of fluid can be aspirated from catheter. Possible indication that catheter has migrated into the subarachnoid space.	• Stop infusion. • If receiving bolus doses, do not administer. • Notify physician.
5. Blood is present on epidural dressing or can be aspirated from the catheter. Probable indication that catheter has punctured a blood vessel.	• Stop infusion. • Notify physician.
6. Redness, warmth, tenderness, swelling or exudates is noted at catheter insertion site. Client is febrile. Signs and symptoms of infection.	• Notify physician.
7. Client experiences minimal urinary output, urinary frequency or urgency, bladder distention, pruritus, or nausea and vomiting.	• Consult with physician about reducing the dose of opioid. • Discuss treatment for side effects.

Teaching Considerations

- Describe catheter placement and use to client as appropriate. Drawing or showing pictures helps.
- Teach client the purpose, action, and signs and symptoms of adverse reactions to opioid or local anesthetic to be administered.
- Teach client to report pain level using mutually acceptable pain scale.
- Inform client of other pain management strategies that may supplement or enhance pharmacological intervention (e.g., imagery, distraction, relaxation).
- Tell client of pain management strategies that may interfere with pharmacological interventions such as over-the-counter medications and herbals.
- Explain that pain relief begins within 30 to 60 minutes of initiation of epidural infusion.
- Explain therapy to family or significant others so that they can support and assist client.
- Some clients may feel so much better after obtaining pain relief that they attempt to ambulate without assistance or to overdo their activities. Caution them to begin slowly to avoid injury and to call for nurse to assist.

Pediatric Considerations

- The use of epidural analgesia has increased in children.
- EMLA cream can be applied to the site 2 hours before catheter insertion. Because the same analgesics are administered to children as are given to adults, children are at risk for the same side effects and adverse reactions (McCaffery and Pasero, 1999).

Gerontological Considerations

- Older adults are at the same risk for complications and medication adverse effects as other adult clients. Careful assessment remains key.

Home Care Considerations

- Clients needing long-term or permanent therapy are discharged with a tunneled catheter. Before consideration of catheter placement in preparation for discharge and care in the home, several variables need to be assessed, including fine motor skills, cognitive ability, stage of disease and prognosis, and degree of involvement of family or significant others.
- Teach client and caregiver proper dosage and administration of medication. Evaluating client's technique for catheter care and administering medication, as well as reinforcing instructions, are priorities.
- Explain pain assessment based on pain scale and available drug and dosage for breakthrough pain. Inform client how to contact clinician for increase in dosage if highest level prescribed is ineffective.
- Teach client and caregiver aseptic technique for medication administration as needed and for all catheter care procedures, including dressing changes. Instruct client to change dressing every week (policy will vary with home care agency). Teach signs and symptoms of infection, and instruct client to report to nurse or physician immediately should signs and symptoms appear.
- Teach client and caregiver about signs and symptoms of adverse reactions to medication being used and interventions to alleviate side effects.
- Urinary retention: Teach how to perform straight catheterization.
- Pruritus: Advise client to wear clean, lightweight, cotton clothing; keep room cool; use cool moist compresses; lubricate skin; apply cornstarch.
- Teach client and caregivers about medications to control side effects.
- Give phone numbers of clinicians to contact in emergency.
- Teach client about resources in the community.

SKILL 6-4 Local Infusion Pump Analgesia

During surgery for joint replacement, surgeons may insert an infusion pump (Figure 6-4) to deliver a local anesthetic (Marcaine) to the surgical site through a one-way catheter. Thus pain relief is provided directly to the surgical site. Oral analgesics may also be needed by the client, but the total dose is often reduced (Pasero, 2000). The pump has both a demand (4 to 6 ml per bolus) and a continuous rate (2 to 4 ml/hour) feature. Continuous reservoirs hold 100 ml, whereas the client-controlled units have a 60-ml reservoir. The device remains in place for about 48 hours. The client is taught to remove the catheter at home. This device is meant for one-time use only. Nursing care is directed toward assessment of catheter connections, evaluation of local anesthetic side effects, and client teaching.

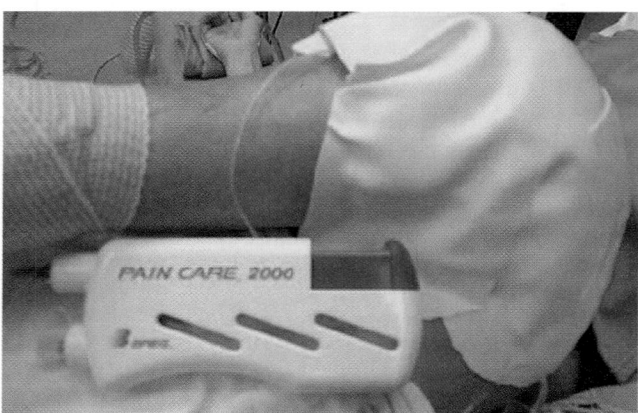

FIGURE **6-4** Local anesthetic infusion pump. (Courtesy Breg, Inc., Vista, Calif.)

Delegation Considerations

Administration of a local anesthetic infusion should not be delegated to assistive personnel. The nurse is responsible for pain assessment and management of the anesthetic infusion. These are aspects of care such as hygiene and ambulation that can be delegated. The nurse must instruct assistive personnel to:

* Pay particular attention to the insertion site when providing care, to avoid dislocation.

* Report any catheter disconnection immediately.
* Notify nurse immediately of a change in client's status or level or comfort.

Equipment
❏ Pump in place from surgery (see Figure 6-4)

STEP	RATIONALE

ASSESSMENT

1. Assess surgical dressing and site of catheter insertion.

2. Assess catheter connections.

3. Assess for blood backing up in tubing.

4. Read label on device.

5. Determine extremity activity level from physician orders.
6. Assess for signs of Marcaine toxicity: hypotension, dizziness, tremor, severe itching, swelling of the skin or throat, irregular heartbeat, palpitations, confusion, ringing in the ears, muscle twitching, numbness around the mouth, metallic taste, seizures.

Dressing should be dry and intact. If not, stop infusion and notify physician. Catheter may not be properly placed.
Should be firmly attached. If connections become detached, do NOT reattach because infection could occur. Notify physician.
Stop infusion, and notify physician. Indicates possible displacement of catheter into blood vessel.
Provides information regarding type of anesthetic, concentration, volume, flow rate, date and time prepared, and name of person who prepared it.
Excessive activity may cause displacement of catheter.

Early identification of Marcaine toxicity prevents possible complications.

STEP	RATIONALE

NURSING DIAGNOSES

- Activity intolerance
- Deficient knowledge
- Anxiety
- Pain (acute, chronic)

- Fatigue
- Self-care deficit
- Ineffective role performance
- Disturbed sensory perception

Related factors are individualized based on client's condition or needs.

PLANNING

1. Expected outcomes following completion of interventions:

   - Client verbalizes full or partial relief from pain.

   - Reduction of nonverbal pain behaviors indicative of pain, such as grimacing, clenching teeth, rocking.
   - Client sleeps and eats better; is more active, and communicates easily with family and friends.

   The client's self-report of pain is the single most reliable indicator of pain.

   Nonverbal behaviors are valid and reliable indicators of pain, especially in the cognitively impaired client (Feldt, 2000).
   Adequate pain relief allows client to participate in usual ADLs.

IMPLEMENTATION

1. For catheter removal:
   a. Perform hand hygiene.
   b. Remove surgical dressing using clean gloves.
   c. Have client in relaxed position.

   d. Grasp catheter firmly, and pull outward from skin with steady motion.

   e. Look for mark on end of catheter tip.
   f. Once catheter is removed, place a sterile dressing over the area and apply pressure for at least 2 minutes.
   g. Discard soiled dressing and gloves. Perform hand hygiene.
   h. Document findings.

   Decreases number of microorganisms on skin.
   Prevents exposure to body fluids.
   Relaxes joint muscles, reducing traction from muscle tension, and provides distraction.
   If resistance felt, stop pulling. Reposition extremity, and try again. If tubing continues to stretch and demonstrates resistance, stop pulling, cover area with sterile dressing, and notify physician.
   Indicates complete removal of catheter.
   Prevents hematoma formation.

   Reduces transmission of microorganisms.

EVALUATION

1. Ask client to rate pain intensity using appropriate scale.
2. Observe for signs of adverse drug reaction.

3. Observe client's position, mobility, relaxation, and participation in ADLs.
4. Inspect condition of surgical dressing.

   Determines client response to local injection of medication.
   Local analgesics can result in systemic adverse effects if absorbed by veins.
   Indicates successful pain management.

   A wet dressing indicates possible catheter migration out of wound.

Recording and Reporting

- Record drug, concentration, date inserted, and if continuous or demand feature.
- Record pain assessment.
- Document additional analgesics necessary to control pain.
- Record any adverse reactions to local anesthetic.

Unexpected Outcomes	Related Interventions
1. Client verbalizes pain intensity greater than previously determined goal or demonstrates nonverbal behaviors indicative of pain. Catheter may be displaced, clogged, or surgical site may be developing complications.	• Check reservoir for presence of medication. • Notify physician.
2. Client reports symptoms of local anesthetic adverse reaction. Possible hypersensitivity to local anesthetic, displacement of catheter into vein, pump failure (releasing too much drug into site).	• Notify physician.

Teaching Considerations

- Client instruction is best given preoperatively because client emerges from operating room with device in place.
- If device is on demand (not continuous), instruct client to depress button every 6 hours.
- Instruct client to inform nurse if pain meets or exceeds pain intensity goal because oral and/or IV analgesics are also available for breakthrough pain.
- Instruct client to notify physician if excessive fluid or bleeding on the dressing occurs.
- Provide written instructions regarding the possible adverse reactions to Marcaine that should be reported to the physician immediately.
- Provide verbal and written instructions as to how and when to discontinue device when at home. Catheter should be placed in a plastic bag and brought with client to first follow-up visit with physician.
- Provide instructions regarding extremity movement.

Pediatric Considerations

- As of this date, local infusion pumps have not been used in the pediatric population.

Gerontological Considerations

- No special considerations except if the client is mentally compromised. Continuous dosing may be administered, but demand doses require a mentally competent adult. In addition, special precautions must be taken to protect the catheter.

Home Care Considerations

- Provide instructions as described under Teaching Considerations.

SKILL 6-5   Nonpharmacological Aids to Promote Comfort

There are a variety of nonpharmacological interventions to assist in lessening a client's pain that can be used in acute care, in the home, and in restorative care settings. These pain-relief measures should be used in combination with pharmacological interventions, not in place of medications. Nondrug techniques may diminish the physical effects of pain, alter the client's perception of pain, and provide the client with a greater sense of control. Distraction, relaxation, guided imagery, and cutaneous stimulation such as massage and acupressure are examples of effective nonpharmacological pain-relief measures. Austin (2004) reviews the evidence for several mind-body therapies. The AHCPR guidelines for acute pain management cite nonpharmacological interventions to be appropriate for clients who find such interventions appealing, express anxiety or fear, may benefit from avoiding or reducing drug therapy, and have incomplete pain relief with pharmacological interventions alone (Acute Pain Management Guideline Panel, 1992).

Clients often must undergo a number of painful diagnostic and therapeutic procedures. The degree of discomfort depends in large part on a client's knowledge and perceptions of the experience. Because perception is greatly influenced by higher centers in the brain, the pain experience is a product of a person's past pain experiences, values, cultural expectations, and emotions. The nurse has a variety of nonpharmacological interventions to relieve pain (e.g., biofeedback, therapeutic touch, physical therapy, and transcutaneous electrical nerve stimulation) that can augment medications (Slucka, 2001). The nurse also has an excellent opportunity to assist clients in controlling their pain by teaching them a variety of nonpharmacological techniques (Box 6-4) that may modify their view of and reaction to pain. By participating in the pain management plan the client takes an important step in achieving pain relief. Because everyone responds differently to these techniques, finding those that work best for the client will take time. A

BOX 6-4 **Nonpharmacological Strategies for Pain Management**	
RELAXATION AND POWER OF THE MIND	**SPIRITUALITY AND REFLECTION**
Self-comfort Muscle relaxation Autogenics training Breathing exercises Music relaxation Visual imagery	Thoughts and stress Enhancing spirituality Humor medicine Set aside time to focus on what is Share your stress Journaling
PUT YOUR BODY TO WORK	**WHAT TO DO WHEN YOUR PAIN FLARES**
Exercise Pacing Energy conservation Body mechanics	Cultivating endorphins Cold and hot packs Ball therapy Contrast baths Hand massage

Modified from *When your pain flares up*, Pain Management Center, Fairview Health Services, Minneapolis, 2002, Fairview Press.

combination of nonpharmacological techniques may be beneficial.

Cutaneous Stimulation

Massage

A gentle massage, a form of cutaneous stimulation, is the application of touch and movement to muscles, tendons, and ligaments without manipulation of the joints (Haldeman and Hooper, 1999). A proper massage not only blocks perception of pain impulses but also helps relax muscle tension and spasm that otherwise might increase pain (Piotrowski and others, 2003). Massage hastens the elimination of wastes stored in muscles, improves oxygenation of tissues, and stimulates the relaxation response in the nervous system (Weavers, 1999). A superficial massage of the back, shoulders, and lower part of the neck is sometimes referred to as a back rub. A nurse should offer a back rub after a bath or before a client prepares for sleep to promote relaxation and comfort, to relieve muscle tension, and to stimulate circulation. An effective back rub takes 3 to 6 minutes and is an important intervention for decreasing pain and improving sense of well-being. Massage may also involve the feet and hands. Massage should not be performed over bruised, swollen, or inflamed areas or bones of spine. The use of therapeutic touch for the treatment of pain has also been shown to be effective in a number of studies (O'Mathuna, 2000).

Heat/Cold

Heat and cold applications (see Chapter 40) relieve pain and promote healing. The selection of heat versus cold varies with client preference and the client's condition. Heat produces vasodilation, reduced blood viscosity, reduced muscle tension, and increased tissue metabolism. Heat helps relieve muscle spasms and joint stiffness. Cold produces vasoconstriction, reduced cell metabolism, and increased blood viscosity. Cold is effective for inflamed joints and muscles (Sauls, 1999; Smith and others, 2002). Although the physiological responses to heat and cold may differ, superficial heat or cold applications may provide comfort in similar conditions such as muscle spasms, strains, and localized joint pain. Caution should be exercised in using heat or cold applications with clients who are unconscious or have impaired sensation. Frequent skin assessment should be performed.

Relaxation

Relaxation is a cognitive and/or physical strategy that provides pain relief or reduces pain to an acceptable level. The client's full participation and cooperation are necessary for relaxation techniques to be effective. The techniques are particularly useful for chronic pain, labor pain, and relief of procedure-related pain. Relaxation interventions involve progressive muscle relaxation, massage, quiet breathing, deep breathing, guided imagery, or a combination.

Guided Imagery

Guided imagery is a creative sensory experience that can effectively reduce pain perception and minimize reaction to pain. It draws on internal experience of memories, dreams, fantasies, and visions; explores the inner world of experience; protects the privacy of the client; and fosters the imagination. The goal of imagery is to have the client use one or several of the senses to create an image of the desired result. This image creates a positive psychophysiological response. Thus focus of the imagination helps clients change their perceptions about their disease, treatment, and healing ability, which may help relieve pain, tension, or stress. Choosing images that clients find pleasant requires a careful assessment by the nurse (Kwekkeboom and others, 2003). Otherwise, the nurse may mistakenly describe images of objects or things that the client fears or dislikes. For example, a scene of rolling waves at the seashore may be restful to one client but desolate or frightening to another.

Distraction

Distraction is a technique that diverts an individual's attention away from the pain sensation. By introducing meaningful stimuli, the nurse helps the client refocus attention. It is believed that a person can consciously attend to only one stimulus, thus diverting the attention away from pain (McCaffery and Pasero, 1999). Distraction strategies the nurse can offer the client include changing activity, listening to music (Burns and others, 2003; Good and others, 2000), reading, focusing on another person, walking, napping, writing, concentrating on a simultaneously mental and physical activity (playing a musical instrument), learning something new (completing a crossword puzzle), and listening to or watching a comedy program (Weavers, 1999). When the distraction is removed, the client may have a heightened awareness of pain.

DELEGATION CONSIDERATIONS

Selected nonpharmacological pain-relieving strategies may be delegated to assistive personnel. In hospitalized clients, many may require a physician order. When delegating to assistive personnel, the nurse must:

- Identify and explain which nonpharmacological measures work best for the client
- Make clear the expected client response
- Instruct to report a worsening of client's pain

EQUIPMENT

- ❏ *Massage:* lotion or oil, folded sheet, bath towel
- ❏ *Relaxation:* relaxation tape and tape player
- ❏ *Distraction:* based on type of distraction (e.g., tape player, assorted music tapes, puzzles, video games, other games).

STEP	RATIONALE

ASSESSMENT

1. Have client identify intensity of pain or discomfort.

There is no objective test that can measure pain. "The clinician must accept the patient's report of pain" (American Pain Society, 2003).

2. Assess physiological, behavioral, and emotional responses to pain or discomfort (see Skill 6-1, step 4).

Physiological responses of individuals vary with severity and duration of pain. Responses serve as means to evaluate effectiveness of pain-relief measures. Overt signs and symptoms may not be present with chronic pain. Physical signs and symptoms may indicate change in comfort level.

3. Assess characteristics of pain and underlying probable cause (see Skill 6-1).

Determines if nonpharmacological approaches are appropriate. Massage is contraindicated in cases of muscle, bone, or joint injury.

- **Critical Decision Point**
  It may be helpful the first time to administer an analgesic before implementing a nonpharmacological strategy so that client can gain a level of comfort needed to practice noninvasive approaches.

4. Examine site of client's pain or discomfort. Include inspection (discoloration, swelling, drainage), palpation (change in temperature, area of altered sensation, painful area, areas that trigger pain, areas that reduce pain), and range of motion of involved joints (if applicable).

Clinical observations clarify information from client. Site of discomfort may direct nurse to specific types of pain-relief measures.

5. Review physician's orders.

In some acute care settings, a medical order will be needed to perform nonpharmacological therapies.

6. Assess client's willingness to receive nonpharmacological pain-relief measures.

Clients have the right to decide about their own care. Participation increases effectiveness. If client is reluctant to try activity, accept this uncertainty and provide information about suggested therapy so that client can make decision.

7. Assess activities client participates in at home that may serve as distraction (e.g., jigsaw puzzles, crocheting or knitting, board games, music, imagery, and relaxation tapes).

Doing these activities in health care setting increases likelihood that client will participate.

STEP	**RATIONALE**
8. Assess client's language level, and identify descriptive terms that will be used when employing nonpharmacological pain-relieving strategies.	Provides clarification of information.

NURSING DIAGNOSES

- Activity intolerance
- Deficient knowledge regarding nonpharmacological methods of pain control
- Anxiety

- Pain (acute, chronic)
- Ineffective coping
- Powerlessness

Related factors are individualized based on client's condition or needs.

PLANNING

1. Expected outcomes following implementation of non-pharmacological technique:	
• Client demonstrates and describes pain-relief measures.	Demonstrates client learning.
• Client is relaxed and comfortable after technique as evidenced by slow, deep respirations; calm facial expressions; calm tone of voice; relaxed muscles; relaxed posture.	Nonpharmacological strategies assist client with relaxing and experiencing less discomfort. Physiological response to relaxation procedures and massage is deep relaxation. Distraction promotes comfort by diverting attention from one situation to another.
• Client verbalizes pain relief.	The client's subjective expression is the most reliable indicator of the presence of pain (American Pain Society, 2003).
2. Explain purpose of technique and what will be expected of client during activity.	Proper explanation of activity results in enhanced client participation.
3. Plan time to perform technique when client is able to concentrate.	Increases opportunity for success.
4. Prepare environment by:	
a. Controlling lighting in room	Darkened room can be relaxing.
b. Controlling distractions by visitors or staff	Distractions prevent client from attending to pain-reduction or pain-control techniques.
c. Maintaining comfortable room temperature (sheet or light blanket prevents chilling)	Temperature extremes can alter client's response to pain.
d. Closing curtains around client's bed or closing door	Maintains client's privacy, helps control lighting, and reduces anxiety.
5. Assist client to comfortable position for technique chosen, such as semi-Fowler's or Sims' position.	Client comfort enhances relaxation and participation in skills.

IMPLEMENTATION

Massage

1. Perform hand hygiene.	Reduces transmission of microorganisms.
2. Adjust bed to high, comfortable position, and lower upper side rails on side nurse is standing.	Ensures proper body mechanics and prevents strain on nurse's back muscles.
3. Place client in comfortable position such as prone or side-lying position. Clients with respiratory difficulties may lie on side with head of bed elevated.	Enhances relaxation and exposes area to be massaged.
4. Drape client to expose only area to be massaged.	Maintains client's privacy and warmth.
5. Ensure client is not allergic to lotion. Then warm lotion in hands or in basin of warm water.	Warm lotion is soothing, and warmth helps to produce local muscle relaxation.

STEP	**RATIONALE**

6. Choose stroke technique based on desired effect:
   a. Effleurage (Massaging upward and outward from vertebral column, and back again) (see illustration)

   Gliding stroke, used without manipulating deep muscles, smoothes and extends muscles, increases nutrient absorption, improves lymphatic and venous circulation.

   b. Pétrissage (see illustration)

   Use on tense muscle groups to "knead" muscles, promote relaxation, and stimulate local circulation.

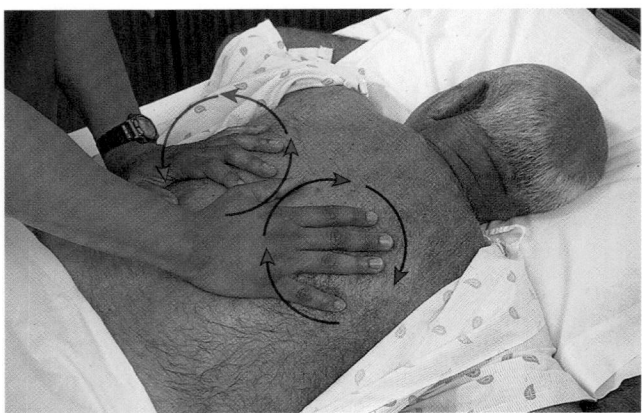

STEP **6a** Effleurage.

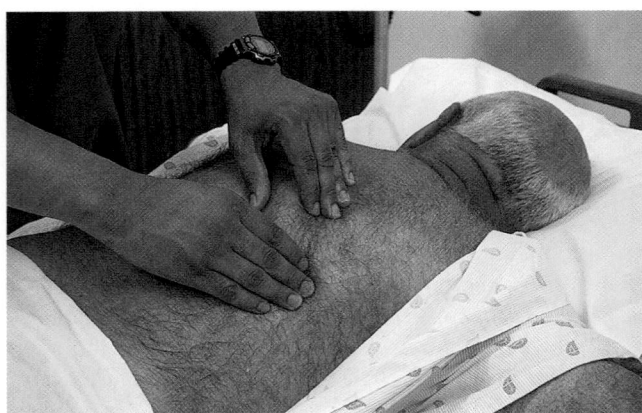

STEP **6b** Pétrissage.

   c. Friction

   Strong circular strokes bring blood to surface of skin, thereby increasing local circulation and loosening tight muscle groups.

7. Encourage client to breathe deeply and relax during massage.

   Potentiates effects of massage.

8. Standing behind client, stimulate scalp and temples.
9. Supporting client's head, rub muscles at base of head.

   Strong circular strokes (friction) stimulate local circulation and relaxation.

10. With client supine, massage hands and arms, as appropriate:

    Releases tension in hands and arms. Studies indicate that anxious behaviors may be significantly reduced with hand massage (Mok and Woo, 2004).

    a. Support hand, and apply friction to palm using both thumbs.
    b. Support base of finger, and work each finger in corkscrewlike motion.
    c. Complete hand massage using effleurage strokes from fingertips to wrist.
    d. Knead muscles of forearm and upper arm between thumb and forefinger, as appropriate.

    Encourages relaxation; enhances circulation and venous return.

11. After determining client has no neck injury or condition that contraindicates neck manipulation, massage neck as appropriate:
    a. Place client in prone position unless contraindicated.

    Provides access to neck muscles.

    b. Knead each neck muscle between thumb and forefinger.

    Reduces tension that often localizes in neck muscles.

    c. Gently stretch neck by placing one hand on top of shoulders and other at base of head and gently move hands away from each other.

    Helps relax muscle body.

STEP	**RATIONALE**

12. Massage back, as appropriate:

    a. Keep client in prone position unless contraindicated; side-lying position is an option.

    b. Do not allow hands to leave client's skin.

Continuous contact with skin's surface is soothing and stimulates circulation to tissues. Breaking contact with skin can startle client.

    c. Apply hands first to sacral area; massage in circular motion. Stroke upward from buttocks to shoulders. Massage over scapulas with smooth, firm stroke. Continue in one smooth stroke to upper arms and laterally along sides of back down to iliac crests (see illustration). Continue massage pattern for 3 minutes.

General firm pressure applied to all muscle groups promotes relaxation.

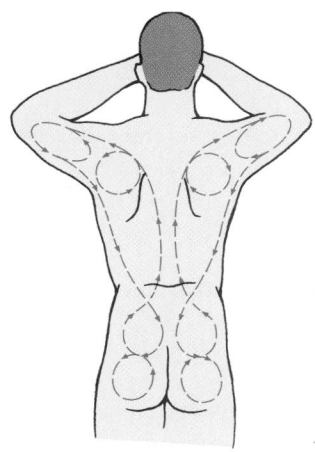

STEP **12c** Circular massage.

    d. Use effleurage along muscles of spine in upward and outward motion.

Massage follows distribution of major muscle groups.

    e. Use pétrissage on muscles of each shoulder toward front of client.

Area often tightens because of tension.

    f. Use palms in upward and outward circular motion from lower buttocks to neck.

Brings blood to surface of skin.

    g. Knead muscles of upper back and shoulder between thumb and forefinger.

These muscles are thick and can be vigorously massaged.

    h. Use both hands to knead muscles up one side of back, then other.

    i. End massage with long stroking effleurage movements.

Most soothing of massage movements.

13. Massage feet, as appropriate:

    a. Place client in supine position.

Returns client to comfortable anatomical position.

    b. Hold foot firmly. Support ankle with one hand or support sides of foot with each hand while performing massage.

Maintains joint stability during massage.

    c. Make circular motions with thumb and fingers around bones of ankle and top of foot.

Relaxes muscles.

    d. Trace space between tendons with firm finger pressure, moving from toe to ankle.

    e. Massage sides and top of each toe.

    f. Use top of fist to make circular motions on bottom of foot.

    g. Knead sides of foot between index finger and thumb.

    h. Conclude with firm, sweeping motions over top and bottom of foot.

Light strokes may tickle.

STEP	RATIONALE
14. Tell client you are ending massage.	Informs and prepares client for inhalation and exhalation (next step).
15. When procedure is complete, instruct client to inhale deeply, exhale, and then initially move about slowly after resting a few minutes.	Returns client to more awake and alert state. When deeply relaxed, client may experience dizziness on arising too rapidly.
16. Wipe excess lotion or oil from client's body, where applied, with bath towel.	Excess lotion or oil can irritate skin and lead to breakdown.
17. Return bed to low position, and raise side rails as appropriate when massage is finished. Perform hand hygiene.	Reduces spread of microorganisms.

Progressive Relaxation

STEP	RATIONALE
1. Instruct client to take several slow, deep breaths.	Increased oxygen can lessen anxiety and prevent shortness of breath with relaxation. Breaths should be diaphragmatic and deep to avoid hyperventilation.
2. Have client close eyes, if desired.	Client may be less easily distracted.
3. Instruct client to:	
a. Alternate tightening and relaxing all muscle groups for 6 to 7 seconds, beginning at feet and working upwards toward head.	Alternating tension and relaxation in muscle groups allows client to feel difference.
b. Instruct client to tighten muscles during inhalation and relax muscles during exhalation.	Relaxation is integrated response associated with diminished sympathetic nervous system arousal; decreased muscle tension is desired outcome. Relaxation decreases pulse and respiration rates and blood pressure and reduces anxiety.
c. As each muscle group is completed, ask client to enjoy relaxed feeling and allow mind to drift and think how nice it is to be relaxed; ask client to breathe deeply.	Distracts client from perceiving pain. Enhances the relaxation response. Breathing deeply prevents Valsalva response, which can increase intrathoracic pressure and compromise cardiac function.
d. Calmly explain during exercise that client may feel sensations of tingling, heaviness, floating, or warmth as relaxation occurs.	Prevents anxiety should sensation occur without warning.
e. Ask client to continue slow, deep breaths.	Allows opportunity to enjoy feelings of relaxation.
4. When exercise is complete, instruct client to inhale deeply, exhale, and then initially move about slowly after resting a few minutes.	Returns client to more awake and alert state. When deeply relaxed, client may experience dizziness on arising too rapidly.

Deep Breathing

STEP	RATIONALE
1. Instruct client to sit comfortably with feet uncrossed. If client unable to sit, move to a supine position with small pillow under head.	Encourages relaxation.
2. Place one hand on the chest and the other on the abdomen.	Allows client to focus on chest and then abdomen.
3. Inhale deeply through the nose, allowing the abdomen to rise and the hand to move outward.	Provides steady timing of inhalation and focuses the client on stretching abdominal muscles.
4. When the abdomen is partially expanded, continue to breathe and allow chest to expand, moving the upper hand outward.	Affords maximal inhalation.
5. Pause for a few seconds.	
6. Exhale slowly through pursed lips.	Permits optimal exchange of oxygen and carbon dioxide.
7. Repeat for 4 to 6 minutes.	Provides slow, controlled release of air.

STEP	**RATIONALE**

Guided Imagery

1. Direct client through guided imagery exercise:
   a. Instruct client to imagine that inhaled air is ball of healing energy.

   Development of specific images assists in removal of pain perception.

   b. Imagine inhaled air travels to area of pain.

   Client's ability to concentrate decreases pain perception.

2. Alternatively nurse may direct imagery:
   a. Suggest client think about going to pleasant place such as beach or mountains.

   Directs imagery after selection of restful place by nurse and client.

   b. Direct client to experience all sensory aspects of restful place (e.g., for beach: warm breeze, warm sand between toes, warmth of sunshine, rhythmic sound of waves, smell of salt air, gulls gliding and swooping in air).

   Helps client concentrate and relax through stimulation of numerous senses.

   c. Direct client to continue deep, slow, rhythmic breathing.

   Promotes relaxation through muscle relaxation.

   d. Direct client to count to three, inhale, and open eyes. Suggest client move about slowly initially.

3. Provide client time to practice exercise without interruption.

   Guided imagery requires an intense level of concentration that may take time to achieve.

Distraction

1. Direct client's attention away from pain with distraction techniques.

   Redirection of attention alters emotional or cognitive aspects of pain.

2. Ask client to close eyes or to focus on single object in room.

   Directs attention inward and protects client from external distraction.

3. Instruct client to concentrate on slow, rhythmic breathing. Guide breathing, or instruct client to control and concentrate on breathing by thinking: "in, one, two; out, one, two."

   Promotes relaxation by concentrating on kinesthetic action, thus reducing ability to concentrate on pain.

4. Continue distraction using chosen activity.
   a. Use music of client's choosing. Emphasize listening to rhythm and adjust volume as pain increases or decreases.

   Focusing on an activity diverts attention from painful sensation.

   b. Direct client to give detailed account of an event or story.

   Stress details of event to enhance distraction from pain stimulus.

   c. Engage client in conversation; encourage participation of family members and visitors.

   Visitors can help direct attention away from mild to moderate pain.

EVALUATION

1. Evaluate client's physiological and behavioral response to technique. Observe character of respirations, body position, facial expression, tone of voice, mood, mannerisms, verbalization of discomfort.

   Determines effectiveness of procedure, level of relaxation, degree of pain relief achieved, and which procedures were most effective.

2. Use pain rating scale to evaluate comfort level.

   Objectively measures change in pain intensity.

3. Observe client perform pain-control measures.

   Confirms learning.

Recording and Reporting

- Record in nurses' notes client's assessment findings, procedure and technique, preparation given to client, client's response to procedure or technique, and further comfort needs related to event. Incorporate pain-relief technique into nursing care plan.
- Record alterations in client's condition (e.g., changes in blood pressure, pulse, respiration, condition of client's skin, complaints of dizziness).
- Report client's response to nonpharmacological interventions to the staff at change of shift.
- Report any unusual responses to techniques (e.g., uncontrolled or aggravated pain) to nurse in charge or physician. Unexpected findings or occurrences during procedure should be reported because additional assistance or time with client may be needed.

Unexpected Outcomes	Related Interventions
1. Client may not be able to concentrate on technique because of intense pain.	• Administer analgesics before nonpharmacological strategy. • Ensure environment conducive to technique.
2. Client states pain intensity unchanged or escalating, or client is demonstrating nonverbal behaviors indicative of pain.	• Fully assess pain. • Consider administering analgesics before technique. • Consider a different technique or a combination (e.g., elevation and cold) of nonpharmacological strategies. • Focus on helping client to relax. • Answer any questions or concerns.

Teaching Considerations

- Clients need information about nonpharmacological pain therapies because pain is an "experience," with both physical and psychosocial components. Nondrug therapies affect both components to varying degrees.
- Techniques may require more practice before results are achieved. Pharmacological intervention may be required to lessen pain so that client can achieve relaxation and to augment other methods of pain control.
- Teach client to rest between periods of activity because fatigue increases pain perception.
- Discuss and practice with client possible techniques to use at home. Upon discharge, include written instructions.
- If appropriate, teach family member how to perform massage (if not contraindicated) as part of home care.

Pediatric Considerations

- A number of nonpharmacological pain management therapies can be used successfully with children. Distraction and relaxation strategies work for all ages and should be suited to the developmental level of the child (e.g., a pacifier can be used for the infant, reading or playing a recording of a favorite story is appropriate for the preschooler, listening to music on a portable cassette or CD player with headphones may work for a teenager).
- Because children have an active imagination, relaxation can be a powerful adjuvant in pain control.
- Parents can be very helpful in providing pain relief. They often provide comfort, for example, by their presence, by their conversation, and by holding and cuddling their child (Acute Pain Management Guideline Panel, 1992; Hockenberry and others, 2003; Jacox and others, 1994).

Gerontological Considerations

- Visual, hearing, cognitive, and motor impairments may make it difficult for older adults to be able to effectively use procedures such as distraction, relaxation, or guided imagery (Acute Pain Management Guideline Panel, 1992). However, do not assume these techniques will not work.
- Ask the client what other interventions have helped relieve pain in the past.

Home Care Considerations

- Family members may need to collaborate planning time to reduce noise and other stimuli in the home to promote client's relaxation.
- Discuss nonpharmacological interventions with client's family and friends.

FOCUS *on* CLINICAL PRACTICE

You are caring for Mr. Johnson, a 78-year-old man who has had a stroke. He has global aphasia (unable to understand words and unable to speak) and seems confused. At the time of his stroke he fell and fractured his left hip. It has been 2 days since his surgery for hip repair, and he is drinking small amounts of liquids without difficulty. He had been receiving morphine via a PCA at 1 mg every hour on a continuous/basal basis, but the physician has ordered that the PCA be discontinued. There is now an order for Percocet: one tablet for mild to moderate pain and two tablets for severe pain by mouth every 6 hours, prn. There are no other medications ordered. He has not had a bowel movement since admission. He has hypoactive bowel sounds, and his abdomen is slightly distended.

1. How and when will you assess this client's pain?
   A. Use the 0 to 10 pain scale, and assess with each vital sign.
   B. Use the FACES pain scale, and assess every 8 hours.
   C. Observe for nonverbal pain behaviors during activity.
   Explain your choice.
2. When you discontinue the PCA, what procedural steps are required in order to be in compliance with the Controlled Substances Act and your agency policy?

3. When you are turning Mr. Johnson to change the linen, you notice that he groans. It has been 4 hours since his PCA was discontinued, and he has not had any analgesics. What nursing action should you take?
   A. Administer 1 Percocet tablet now.
   B. Administer 2 Percocet tablets now.
   C. Notify the physician.
   Explain your choice.
4. Because of his aphasia, you are concerned that Mr. Johnson will not be able to tell his future nurses if he is in pain or not. What pain management regimen should you discuss with the physician?
   A. Placing him back on a continuous/basal dose of morphine
   B. Ordering the Percocet around-the-clock
   C. Switching to acetaminophen (Tylenol) prn
   Explain your choice.
5. You are concerned about Mr. Johnson's bowels because of the morphine he had been receiving and his reduced mobility. What intervention should you request from the physician?
   A. Metamucil (stool softener)
   B. Senokot (laxative)
   C. Fleet's enema
   Explain your choice.

NCLEX REVIEW QUESTIONS

1. A client with chronic/persistent pain who was on opioids around-the-clock for the past month suddenly stopped taking them because of the cost. About 24 hours later he experiences shaking chills, sweating, and abdominal pain. The nurse recognizes these as symptoms of:
   1. Addiction
   2. Drug tolerance
   3. Physical dependence
   4. Pseudoaddiction
2. When assessing pain in a client who is nonverbal it is important for the nurse to observe for painful behaviors during:
   1. Family visits
   2. Meals
   3. Movement
   4. Sleep

3. When assessing a client receiving continuous and demand doses of an opioid via a PCA, the nurse becomes concerned when the client:
   1. Drifts off to sleep while talking
   2. Is drowsy but arousable
   3. Rates the pain a 3 out of 10
   4. Sleeps through the night
4. The nurse teaches the family of a client receiving a PCA the importance of:
   1. Alerting the nurse when the client appears to be sleeping
   2. Encouraging the client to depress the button every hour
   3. Not pushing the button for the client
   4. Reporting to the nurse if the client's pain intensity falls below 3 out of 10

Continued

NCLEX REVIEW QUESTIONS

5. Before assisting in the insertion of an epidural catheter for pain management, the nurse evaluates the client for a history of the following conditions that could contraindicate this invasive procedure:
   1. Allergy to iodine
   2. History of migraine headaches
   3. Recent lumbar puncture
   4. Sepsis

6. Before injecting preservative-free epidural medication, the nurse cleans the port with:
   1. Alcohol
   2. Dakin's solution
   3. Glutaraldehyde
   4. Povidone-iodine

7. The nurse suspects Marcaine toxicity in a client connected to a local infusion pump when observing the following symptoms:
   1. Heart rate of 60
   2. Hypotension
   3. Numbness at incision
   4. Severe itching

8. When teaching a client being discharged home with a local infusion pump attached to the left elbow, the nurse instructs the client to:
   1. Bring removed catheter to the first postoperative physician visit
   2. Depress the button every 2 hours during the day
   3. Elevate the left elbow on three pillows
   4. Reinforce the dressing if it becomes saturated

9. It is important for the nurse to understand that nonpharmacological strategies to promote comfort should be used:
   1. With analgesics
   2. In place of analgesics
   3. On an intermittent basis
   4. With severe pain

10. When teaching clients about nonpharmacological strategies to manage pain, the nurse stresses the importance of:
    1. Ingesting an opioid before each nondrug strategy
    2. Taking rest periods between strategies
    3. Trying only one nonpharmacological strategy at a time.
    4. Using a nondrug strategy that has been effective in family members

References

Acute Pain Management Guideline Panel: *Acute pain management: operative or medical procedures and trauma.* Clinical practice guideline, AHCPR Pub No. 92-0032, Rockville, Md, 1992, Agency for Health Care Policy and Research, Public Health Service, US Department of Health and Human Services.

American Geriatrics Society Guidelines, *J Am Geriatr Soc* 60:S204, 2002.

American Pain Society: *Analgesic use in the treatment of acute pain and cancer pain,* ed 6, Glenview, Ill, 2003, American Pain Society.

American Society of Addiction Medicine: *Consensus document,* retrieved April 9, 2004, http://www.asam.org/ppol/paindef.htm, 2001.

American Society for Pain Management Nursing, personal communication, 2004.

Andrews A, Boyle J: *Transcultural concepts in nursing care,* ed 2, Philadelphia, 1999, Lippincott.

Austin J: Mind-body therapies for the management of pain, *Clin J Pain* 20(1):27, 2004.

Bair M and others: Depression and pain comorbidity: a literature review, *Arch Intern Med* 163(20): 2433, 2003.

Berry PH and others: *Pain: current understanding of assessment, management, and treatments,* Chicago, 2001, National Pharmaceutical Council, Inc and Joint Commission on Accreditation of Healthcare Organizations.

Campinha-Bacote J: *The process of cultural competence.* Cincinnati, 1998, Transcultural C.A.R.E. Associates.

Cosentino B: Epidural pain management, *Nurs Spectr* 12A(4):NJ1, 2000.

Cox F: Clinical care of patients with epidural infusions, *Prof Nurse* 16(10):1429, 2001.

Guay D: Adjunctive agents in the management of chronic pain, *Pharmacotherapy* 21(9):1070, 2001.

Haldeman S, Hooper PD: Mobilization, manipulation, massage and exercise for the relief of musculoskeletal pain. In Wall PD, Melzack R: *Textbook of pain,* ed 4, London, 1999, Churchill Livingstone.

Herr K: Chronic pain in the older patient: management strategies, *J Gerontol Nurs* 28(2):28, 2002a.

Herr K: Pain assessment in cognitively impaired older adults, *AJN* 102(12):65, 2002b.

Hockenberry MJ and others: *Wong's nursing care of infants and children,* ed 7, St. Louis, 2003, Mosby.

Jacox A and others: *Management of cancer pain.* Clinical practice guideline No. 9, Rockville, Md, 1994, Agency for Health Care Policy and Research, Public Health Service, US Department of Health and Human Services.

Joint Commission on Accreditation of Healthcare Organizations: *Comprehensive accreditation manual for hospitals: the official handbook,* Oak Brook Terrace, Ill, 2003, The Commission.

Knoerl D and others: Preoperative PCA teaching program to manage postoperative pain, *Medsurg Nurs* 8(1):26, 1999.

Leavitt S: Using patient-controlled analgesia (PCA) for acute pain management, *http://www.baxter.com/services/professional-education/*, retrieved December 3, 2003.

Lehr V, BeVier P: Patient-controlled analgesia for the pediatric patient, *Orthop Nurs* 22(4):298, 2003.

Ludwig-Beymer P: Transcultural aspects of pain. In Andrews M, Boyle J: *Transcultural nursing concepts,* Philadelphia, 2003, Lippincott, Williams and Wilkins.

McCaffery M, Ferrell BR: Opioids and pain management, what do nurses know? *Nursing* 29(3):48, 1999.

McCaffery M, Pasero C: *Pain: clinical manual,* ed 2, St. Louis, 1999, Mosby.

Mok E, Woo P: The effects of slow-stroke back massage on anxiety and shoulder pain in elderly stroke patients, *Complement Ther Nurs Midwifery,* 10(4):209, 2004.

Orque MS: Nursing care of the South Vietnamese patients. In Orque MS, Bloch R, Monrroy LSA, editors: *Ethnic nursing care: a multicultural approach,* St. Louis, 1983, Mosby.

Pacquiao D: Cultural competence in ethical decision making. In Andrews M, Boyle J: *Transcultural nursing concepts,* Philadelphia, 2003, Lippincott, Williams and Wilkins.

Pasero C: *Epidural analgesia for acute pain management,* Self-directed learning module, Pensacola, Fla, 1999, American Society for Pain Management Nursing.

Pasero C: Continuous local anesthetics, *Am J Nurs* 100(8):22, 2000.

Pasero C: Epidural analgesia for postoperative pain, *Am J Nurs* 103(10):62, 2003a.

Pasero C: Intravenous patient-controlled analgesia for acute pain management, Self-directed learning module, Pensacola, Fla, 2003b, American Society for Pain Management Nursing.

Pasero C, Portenoy R, McCaffery M: Using continuous infusion with PCA, *Am J Nurs* 99(2):22, 1999.

Plaisance L, Ellis J: Opioid-induced constipation, *Am J Nurs* 102(3):72, 2002.

Purnell L, Paulanka B: *Transcultural health care,* Philadelphia, 2003, FA Davis.

Rawal N: Epidural and spinal agents for postoperative analgesic, *Surg Clin North Am* 79(2): 313, 1999.

Regional anesthesia in the anticoagulated patient: defining the risks, retrieved December 20, 2003, http://www.asra.com/Concensus_Conferences/Consensus_Statements.shtml, 2003.

Sauls J: Efficacy of cold for pain: fact of fallacy? *Online J Knowl Synth Nurs* 6(8):1, 1999.

Slucka K: The basic science mechanisms of TENS and clinical applications, *APS Bull* 11(2):10, 2001.

Weavers S: Pain management patient education manual, Gaithersburg, Md, 1999, Aspen.

When your pain flares up, Pain Management Center, Fairview Health Services, Minneapolis, 2002, Fairview Press.

Young-McCaughan A, Miaskowski C: Measurement of opioid-induced sedation, *Pain Manage Nurs* 2(4):132, 2001.

Research References

Beyer J, Denyes M, Villarruel A: The creation, validation, and continuing development of pain intensity measures in children, *J Pediatr Nurs* 5(5):333, 1992.

Bonura D and others: Culturally congruent end-of-life care for Jewish patients and families, *J Transcult Nurs* 12(3), 211, 2001.

Burns V and others: A pilot study into the therapeutic effects of music therapy at a cancer help center, *Altern Ther Health Med* 7(1):48, 2003.

Chang L, Heitkemper M: Gender differences in irritable bowel syndrome, *Gastroenterology* 123(5):1686, 2002.

Fagerlund T, Braaten O: No pain relief from codeine. . . ? An introduction to pharmacogenomics, *Acta Anaesthesiol Scan* 45(2):140, 2001.

Feldt K: The checklist of nonverbal pain indicators (CNPI), *Pain Manag Nurs* 1(1):13, 2000.

Flores C, Mogil S: The pharmacogenetics of analgesia: toward a genetically-based approach to pain management, *Pharmacogenomics* 2(3):177, 2001.

Garwick A: What do providers need to know about American Indian culture? Recommendations from urban Indian family caregivers, *Fam Syst Health* 18(2):177, 2000.

Glajchen M: Chronic pain: treatment barriers and strategies for clinical practice, *J Am Board Fam Pract* 14(3):178, 2001.

Good M and others: Cultural differences in music chosen for pain relief, *J Holist Nurs* 18(3):246, 2000.

Kwekkeboom K and others: A pilot study to predict success with guided imagery for cancer pain, *Pain Manag Nurs* 4(3):112, 2003.

O'Mathuna D: Evidenced-based practice and reviews of therapeutic touch, *J Nurs Scholarsh* 32(3):279, 2000.

Nayak S and others: Culture and gender effects in pain beliefs and the prediction of pain tolerance, *Cross-Cultural Research* 34(2):135, 2000.

Piotrowski M and others: Massage as adjuvant therapy in the management of acute postoperative pain: a preliminary study, *J Am Coll Surg* 197(6):1037, 2003.

Pohl M, Braz J: Gene therapy of pain: emerging strategies and future directions, *Eur J Pharmacol* 429(1-3):39, 2001.

Pohl M and others: Gene therapy of chronic pain, *Curr Gene Ther* 3(3):223, 2003.

Robinson M and others: Altering gender role expectations: effects on pain tolerance, pain threshold, and pain ratings, *J Pain* 4(6): 284, 2003.

Smith J and others: A randomized, controlled trial comparing compression bandaging and cold therapy in postoperative total knee replacement surgery, *Orthop Nurs* 21(2):61, 2002.

Soeken K: Selected CAM therapies for arthritis-related pain: the evidence from systematic reviews, *Clin J Pain* 20(1):13, 2004.

Tall J, Raja S: Dietary constituents as novel therapies for pain, *Clin J Pain* 20(1):19, 2004.

Weisse C and others: The influence of gender and race on physician's pain management decisions, *J Pain* 4(9):505, 2003.

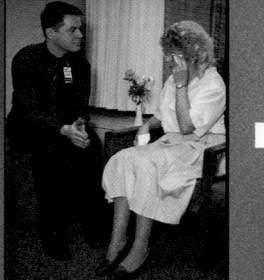

7

Palliative Care

7-1 Supporting Clients and Families in Grief

7-2 Symptom Management in Palliative Care

7-3 Care of the Body After Death

MEDIA RESOURCES

Evolve Site *evolve*

http://evolve.elsevier.com/Perry/skills
• Weblinks

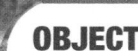

OBJECTIVES

Mastery of content in this chaper will enable the nurse to:

- Identify the nurse's role in assisting clients and families with problems related to grief and dying.
- Discuss principles of palliative care.
- Describe approaches for symptom management in the dying client.
- Discuss the needs clients present when asked about assistance in dying (AID).
- Discuss important considerations when working with families and significant others in regard to organ and/or tissue donation.
- Describe the physiological changes after death.
- Describe postmortem care techniques.
- Describe how to correctly prepare a client's body after death.

KEY TERMS

Actual loss	Organ procurement agency (OPA)
Advance directives	Organ/tissue donation
Autopsy	Palliative care
End-of-life care	Perceived loss
Hospice	Postmortem care
Loss	Rigor mortis
Maturational loss	Situational loss
Morgue	System distress

People who face life-threatening illnesses have many medical and technological advances available to either reverse the course of their disease or to prolong their lives. For clients with serious life-limiting illness, it becomes important for health care providers to find ways to help clients approach their end of life. Such is the goal of palliative care, the prevention, relief, reduction, or soothing of symptoms of disease or disorders without effecting a cure (Field and Cassel, 1997). Palliative care is not just for clients during the last days of life. Although this chapter focuses on end-of-life care for the terminally ill, it is important to understand that palliative care is for any age, any diagnosis, at any time, and not just during the last few months of life. Palliative care allows clients to make more informed choices, achieve better relief of symptoms, and have more opportunity to work on issues of life closure. A palliative care approach is a philosophy of total care that ensures that a client experiences a "good death," free of avoidable pain and suffering, in accord with the client's and family's wishes, and reasonably consistent with clinical, cultural and ethical standards (Tolle and others, 2000).

Gaining competence in providing palliative care is essential for nurses to be able to prepare clients and families for difficult and stressful life experiences. There is an impetus to provide more palliative care in the home setting. Many older adults die at home, cared for only by their family or sometimes visiting nurses or home health aides. Accordingly, it is important to offer clients and their families a more therapeutic environment in which dying and death can occur (Stajduhar, 2003).

Frequently clients who are experiencing a terminal illness are under hospice care. Hospice is a multidisciplinary, family-centered program of care designed to assist the terminally ill person with being more comfortable and maintaining a satisfactory lifestyle through the phases of dying. The focus of hospice care is palliative care. A client enters a hospice program during the terminal phase of an illness (usually 6 months or less). Hospice care is provided in the home or in health care settings as well. It is important for nurses to understand the option of hospice care, because too often clients are not admitted to hospice until they have only a few weeks to live. Hospice staff are committed to the philosophy of providing care and support for the client and family during the terminal phase of illness and at the time of death. Hospice programs offer respite care services to give family members much needed time temporarily away from caregiving activities.

Providing end-of-life care to a terminally ill client has a profound effect on the dying person, significant others, friends, and caregivers. End-of-life care is the humane provision of physical, psychological, social, and spiritual support to a client and client's family at the end of life. The fears associated with dying are often related more to the client's sense of loss, loneliness, and isolation and family members' sense of powerlessness. Loss and grief affect dying clients and survivors physically, psychologically, socially, and spiritually. The nurse's role in facilitating the grief process includes assisting clients and survivors with feeling the loss, expressing the loss, and completing the tasks of the grief process (End-of-Life Nursing Education Consortium [ELNEC], 2000). To be effective, a nurse must have a thorough understanding of a client's loss, its significance and meaning to the client and family, and how it affects the client's and family's ability to carry on.

Comfort for a dying client requires management of symptoms of disease and therapies. For many clients, symptom distress is characteristic of the dying experience (Chochinov, 2002). Symptom distress is the experience of discomfort or anguish related to the progression of a disease. Clients can experience anguish from not knowing or being unaware of aspects of their health status or planned treatment. Worry or fear is common in many dying clients and may heighten their perception of discomfort. A nurse must assess the character of the client's symptoms and the client's wishes for symptom management and then carefully select appropriate therapies (Figure 7-1).

At the time of death it is important that the nurse provide understanding and compassionate care to the client's family. Family members must often face difficult end-of-life decisions. For example, families experience considerable stress when deciding whether to withdraw life-sustaining treatments (Tilden and others, 2001). When a client dies in a hospital setting, the nurse provides postmortem care. It is important for the nurse to care for the client's body with

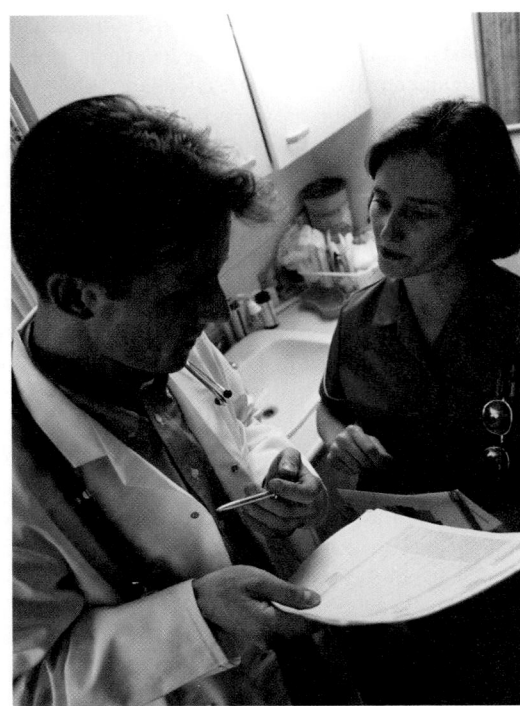

FIGURE 7-1 New staff members consult on best course of symptom management for client.

dignity, sensitivity, and in a way consistent with the client's religious and cultural beliefs. After death the body undergoes many physical changes (e.g., stiffening of the body [rigor mortis], loss of skin elasticity [algor mortis], and purple discoloration of the skin [livor mortis]). For that reason, care must be provided as soon as possible to prevent tissue damage or disfigurement of body parts.

Evidence-Based Practice Trends

There has been considerable research recently on palliative and end-of-life care. Specifically, research topics have focused on symptom management and on understanding the continuum of palliative care for clients and their family caregivers. Researchers have attempted to understand the decision-making needs of both clients and families and the barriers to optimal care of the dying (Murray and others, 2003; Tolle and others, 2000). Barriers to achieving desirable qualities of the dying experience include a mismatch of expectations between providers, patients, and families, absence of advance directives when needed, and ineffective communication style of clinicians (Hanson and others, 1997; Schneiderman and others, 1992; Tilden and others, 1995). Tolle and others studied 475 family members' perspectives about the final month of life for decedents. Their research found that control of pain for dying clients is a major issue and concern. A high percentage of family members indicated moderate to severe decedent pain in the final week of life. Despite reports of moderate and severe pain for a significant proportion of decedents, families maintained a high level of satisfaction with clinicians' efforts to manage pain (Tolle and others, 2000).

Murray and others (2003) examined terminally ill women's decisions regarding place of end-of-life care. All of the women lived in Canada and had access to a palliative care unit. The women indicated that home was the preferred location under ideal conditions, whereas the palliative care unit was considered the best location given their current circumstances. The women reported having decisional conflict that potentially delayed decision making about their care. Decisional delay could result in options being constrained or lost. The researchers suggest it is important for nurses to understand early on the decisions faced by clients and which decisions have been made and which decisions remain unresolved. Relationship building and the effect of the decision on place of care on family were important to participants of the study. Avoiding burden for family or friends was a recurrent issue. Participants also desired to achieve adequate pain and symptom management and to maintain a sense of control (Murray and others, 2003).

Cultural Considerations

It is important for the nurse to understand cultural meanings and beliefs about death and dying. For example, among Chinese, death is taboo and discussion of the topic is associated with bad luck and evil (Yick and Gupta, 2002). Some Muslims may view illness as penance for their sins and death as part of life destined by God (McKennis, 1999; Rassoul, 2000).

As with the care of any client, it is important to collaborate with family members and religious leaders to understand culture-specific practices and to address issues about prognosis, Advanced Directives, Do Not Resuscitate (DNR), and organ donation. Orthodox Jews may not leave a dying client alone and have groups of community members (minyan) praying at the bedside with the client (Schwartz, 2003). A Hindu elder's refusal of nourishment and pain medication is supported by the family to improve the person's chance for a better life in the next cycle. The belief is congruent with their religious tenet of transmigration of the soul. Such support may be upsetting to staff who do not understand the cultural meaning of their behaviors.

Among Hindus, the client's head faces east and a lamp is placed near the head to light the way. Large numbers of family members are present to chant, pray, and spread incense. They also apply ash to the forehead and put milk or water from the Ganges into the mouth of the dying client. The client will chant his or her "mantra"; if the client is unable to do so, a family member can chant it into the right ear (Kemp and Bhungalia, 2002). Other groups such as Catholics may arrange for a priest to anoint the client and give Holy Communion if possible.

Arrange for interdisciplinary conferences to increase awareness and sensitivity of staff to cultural differences. Clients from divergent cultures often have values different from those of caregivers who value biomedical approaches to care. Whereas professional care personnel value quality of life, other groups such as Orthodix Jews value the sanctity of life. Cultures that believe in the transmigration of life such as Buddhists and Hindus may view dying as an opporunity for atonement and to be reborn into a higher life form. Buddhist clients may wish to maintain consciousness throughout the process of dying and may refuse medication that may alter the level of consciousness and alleviate pain (Yick and Gupta, 2002).

Skill Performance Guidelines

1. As it becomes obvious that a person is facing a life-threatening illness, determine the status of the person's advance directives.
2. Always respect client-family choices and preferences. Be an advocate in their decision making about treatment.
3. Dignity-conserving care helps a client to feel valued and should be a standard of care for all clients nearing death. This includes vigilant symptom control, psychological and spiritual well-being, and support of the family. What defines dignity for each client and family is unique.
4. As a client's death approaches, consider if the dying person is a candidate for organ/tissue donation, and learn the client's and family's preferences.
5. Know a client's and family's culturally preferred practices for the days preceding death, the time of death, and the bereavement period afterward.
6. Following a client's death, consult agency policy regarding who is to pronounce death (e.g., attending physician or resident) and what departments (e.g., nursing supervisor, medical records) are to be notified at the time of death. Notify as directed.
7. Care for the body needs to be performed in a timely manner. If organ or tissue donation has been made, notify the organ procurement agency (OPA) as soon as death is imminent.

SKILL 7-1 Supporting Clients and Families in Grief

Throughout our lives we suffer losses. We experience necessary losses as a natural part of our lives and expect those losses to be recovered and replaced by something different or better. However, there are other losses that cause us to suffer unbearable changes in our safety and security (Hasler, 1996). For example, a terminal illness and death of a loved one can have long-term effects on a person's physical and psychological health.

Loss comes in many forms based on the values and priorities learned within a person's sphere of influence, including family, friends, society, and culture. An actual loss is any loss of a person or object that can no longer be felt, heard, known, or experienced. Examples include the loss of a body part or role at work. A perceived loss is any loss that is tangible and uniquely defined by the grieving client. It may be less obvious to others. An example is the loss of confidence or prestige. A maturational loss includes any change in a person's developmental process that is normally expected during a lifetime. One example would be a mother's feeling of loss as a child goes to school for the first time. Finally, a situational loss includes any sudden, unpredictable external event such as an automobile accident that leaves a driver paralyzed.

The type of loss and the perception of the loss influence the depth and duration of grief a person experiences. Each individual responds to loss differently and therefore grieves differently. A nurse must assess the special meaning that a loss has for a client and its effect on the client's health and well-being.

Hospitalization, chronic illness, and disability are special circumstances that have multiple associated losses. When persons enter a hospital, they lose their privacy, control over body functions and their daily routines, their modesty, and any illusions that they may have about their personal indestructibility. A chronic illness or disability also adds concern over financial security and the threat to the stability of relationships at home and work.

Death is the ultimate loss. Although death is part of the continuum of life and a universal and inevitable part of being human, it is also an event that generates anxiety and fear. Death ends relationships that bind and unite families and individuals together, and it separates people from the physical presence of persons who influence their lives. A person with an advanced, progressive, ultimately fatal illness faces many levels of suffering. So too, do family members. It is difficult to be sick, and many people dislike seeking help from others, yet nearly all want companionship in the face of death (Finucane, 2002).

Grief

Grief is the emotional response to a loss. It is manifested in a variety of ways that are unique to the type of loss and an individual's personal experiences, cultural expectations, and spiritual beliefs. Coping with grief after a loss involves the process of mourning, the outward, social expression of a loss (ELNEC, 2000). Mourning involves working through the grief until an individual accepts and adapts to the loss and adjusts his or her expectations to go on in life.

Bereavement includes grief and mourning—the inner feelings and outward reactions of the survivor (ELNEC, 2000). Survivors go through a bereavement period that is not linear. It does not proceed in sequential stages that can be precisely predicted, which may imply passivity on the part of the bereaved. Rather, an individual will move back and forth through a series of stages and/or tasks many times, possibly extending over a period of several years, before the process is completed. No one really "gets over" a loss, but the individual can heal and learn to live with a loss (ELNEC, 2000).

There are numerous theories on grief and mourning, all aimed at describing the stages of grief or mourning a person

TABLE 7-1	A COMPARISON OF THEORIES OF GRIEF AND MOURNING
THEORY	**STAGES**
Kübler-Ross's Stages of Dying	A behavioral-oriented theory that includes five stages: **Denial**—Individual acts as though nothing has happened and may refuse to believe or understand loss have occurred. **Anger**—Individual resists the loss and may strike out at everyone and everything. **Bargaining**—Individual postpones awareness of reality of the loss and may try to deal in a subtle or overt way as though the loss can be prevented. **Depression**—Individual feels overwhelmingly lonely and withdraws from interpersonal interaction. **Acceptance**—Individual accepts the loss and looks to the future.
Bowlby's Phases of Mourning	A behavior theory that includes four phases: **Numbing**—Individual describe phase as feeling "stunned" or "unreal." A period of intense emotion. Serves to protect the body from consequences of loss. Lasts from a few hours to a week or more. **Yearning and searching**—Arouses acute distress in most persons. A painful phase characterized by physical symptoms such as tightness in the chest and throat, shortness of breath, a feeling of weakness and lethargy, insomnia, and anorexia. Phase may last for months or years. **Disorganization and despair**—Individual endlessly examines how and why the loss occurred. Common time for person to express anger. Gradually phase gives way to an acceptance that loss is permanent. **Reorganization**—Individual begins to accept unaccustomed roles, acquires new skills, builds new relationships. Phase may last a year or more. Individual needs support to untie self from the lost relationships.
Worden's Tasks of Mourning	A behavioral theory that includes four tasks: **Accept reality of loss**—There is always some period of disbelief and surprise over a loss. This task involves processes required to accept that the person or object is gone and will not return. **Work through pain and grief**—Emotional pain comes as a natural part of loss. Individuals who deny or shut off the pain prolong their grief. **Adjust to environment in which the deceased is missing**—Individual does not realize full impact of loss for at least 3 months. At this point friends and associates stop calling, and the person is left to ponder the impact of loneliness. Often individual must take on roles formerly filled by the deceased. **Emotionally relocate the deceased and move on with Life**—Individual does not forget the deceased or give up the relationship with the deceased. Deceased, however, must take a new, less prominent place in a person's emotional life. People in this task fear they will forget their loved one.

experiences during a loss. The theories provide useful frameworks for understanding the behaviors a client experiences during a loss, anticipating the type of support a client requires and the progress a client makes in dealing with a loss, and in selecting grief support interventions. Table 7-1 summarizes the major theories of grief and mourning. It is important to again emphasize that there is no set time frame for a person to experience grief. An individual tends to move back and forth through the various stages of grief and mourning, depending on the type of support he or she receives, the meaning of the loss, and the person's coping strategies.

A nurse can be most helpful to clients by knowing the types of grief. Normal or uncomplicated grief consists of the normal feelings, behaviors, and reactions to a loss, such as resentment, sorrow, anger, crying, and loneliness. The normal grief response can be positive by helping a person to mature and develop as an individual. Anticipatory grief is the process of disengaging or "letting go" that occurs before an actual loss or death. For example, once a person or family receives a terminal diagnosis, they begin the process of saying good-bye and completing life affairs. The process is more stressful when a client is unable to make decisions due to deteriorating health. Unless guided by the client's explicit deci-

sions regarding end-of-life care, the family assumes responsibility for all decisions. If the process of death is extended over time, persons in the client's family may have few symptoms of grief once the death occurs.

Complicated grief occurs when a person has difficulty progressing through the normal phases or stages of grief and mourning. Bereavement becomes complicated and extended over time. A person never resolves his or her loss. The grief can be chronic (lasting over long periods of time), delayed (suppressing or postponing normal grief until unexpected time), exaggerated (overwhelming grief that may be reflected in self-destructive behaviors), and masked (person unaware that behaviors interfering with normal function are a result of his or her loss).

The following skill provides the nurse with basic knowledge needed to support clients and families in grief. The nurse should not assume how or if the client or family experiences grief. The nurse should also avoid assuming that a particular behavior indicates grief; rather, the nurse should allow clients to share what is happening in their own way. An effective nurse encourages clients to tell their stories. The skill of supporting clients and families in grief prepares a nurse for being an advocate for clients and families.

Delegation Considerations

The skill of supporting clients and families in grief should not be delegated to assistive personnel. A professional nurse has the responsibility for recognizing a client's grief and knowing the appropriate communication and counseling strategies to use. The nurse provides assistive personnel with information, assistance, and direction, including:

- Informing the nurse when the client expresses behaviors of grief (e.g., crying, anger, loss of appetite)
- Encouraging assistive personnel to conduct conversations with clients but to inform the RN when clients express needs or concerns
- Informing the nurse when family members arrive so he or she can meet with them and assess how they are coping

STEP	RATIONALE

ASSESSMENT

1. Find a private location, or close the privacy curtains in hospital room.

2. Establish a quiet presence: bring chair over to client's bedside. Establish one-to-one eye contact.

3. Begin interviewing client/family using honest and open communication. Listen carefully, and observe the client's responses and behaviors.

4. When a client exhibits a behavior or expresses what appears to be a concern, use communication techniques to confirm your observation (e.g., summarizing, paraphrasing, clarifying, sharing observations).

5. As client shares information, consider the following factors:
   Client's age, gender, race
   Client' culture
   Client's socioeconomic status

6. Determine the quality and meaning of the relationship severed by the client's grief experience.
   "Tell me what your mom means to you . . ."
   "Your illness will affect your family; who are you most concerned about?"

7. Determine how much time has passed since the loss occurred. Also assess if the loss was sudden and unexpected or if it was anticipated as a result of the client's chronic illness.

8. As you identify behaviors that suggest the stage of grief a client is experiencing, allow this information to guide the assessment.
   "I can tell you are very sad. Can you share with me your thoughts?"
   "You know your anger is a normal part of grieving; tell me your concerns."
   "You have not been eating well the last few days. Is something bothering you?"

9. Have client describe his or her loss and how it has affected him or her:
   "Tell me how knowing you have cancer makes you feel."
   "How has your illness changed your life? Tell me more."
   "What are you doing differently now that you know your diagnosis?"

Privacy promotes a sense of comfort for client to reveal inner thoughts and feelings.

Presence is a behavior that is valued by clients and that expresses caring.

In a caring relationship a nurse establishes trust, opens lines of communication, and listens to what a client has to say.

Techniques offer feedback that client's message was understood. Confirms accurate message was received. Sharing observations helps prompt client to communicate.

Age, gender, status, race, spirituality, religious beliefs, intellect, self-expression, and cultural opportunity are the basis for an individual to define and qualify the definition of life or death (Cressy, 1997). Culture affects how clients respond to loss.

The quality and meaning of the relationship severed influences the client's grief experience and ability to cope.

The suddenness of a loss can slow resolution of grief.

Identification of the type and stage of grief should be used to guide discussion and not to judge the outcomes of the grief process.

The aim of assessment is to gather a detailed database. This avoids formation of premature assumptions about the stage or phase of grief.

STEP	RATIONALE
10. Ask client to describe the coping strategies used in the past during difficult times. "When your dad died, what helped you get to a point in time to accept the loss?" "Tell me how you usually handle difficult experiences."	Client's existing coping strategies can provide potential resources in managing grief.
11. Determine how client's illness has affected family members' daily routines. Is the family providing personal care to the client?	Family is an important resource that can be significantly affected by family member's illness. Often family choose to become personal caregivers. Living with the decision to provide care at home can be life enriching as well as emotionally and physically draining (Stajduhar, 2003).
12. Assess the client's spiritual health. Focus on aspects of spirituality most likely to be affected (e.g., life satisfaction, faith/belief, hope).	Spiritual well-being seems to be tied to a person's satisfaction with life. Each person has some source of authority and guidance in life; faith in an authority provides confidence.

NURSING DIAGNOSES

- Impaired adjustment
- Anticipatory grieving
- Caregiver role strain
- Compromised family coping
- Risk for caregiver role strain
- Defensive coping
- Ineffective coping

- Readiness for enhanced coping
- Readiness for enhanced family coping
- Death anxiety
- Dysfunctional grieving
- Ineffective denial
- Fear

Related factors are individualized based on client's condition or needs.

PLANNING

1. Expected outcomes following completion of procedure: • Client will maintain relationships with significant others. • Client will express grief in own culturally accepted way. • Client will use coping strategies offered by nurse. • Client will achieve short-term goals for maintaining normal life routines.	Indicates client able to retain connections with social network during grief resolution. Client receives support necessary to retain autonomy and value as a person. Strategies will offer useful alternatives for client in managing emotional stress of grief. Client able to accommodate changing life circumstances and maintains sense of control.

IMPLEMENTATION

1. Show an empathic understanding of the client's strengths. Reinforce expressions of positive thinking and realistic goal setting.	Strategy promotes client's hope.
2. Offer information about the client's illness, and correct any misunderstanding or misinformation.	Minimizes misunderstanding that can add to client's anguish and discomfort.
3. Discuss with client ways to best use resources of family members to help him or her remain independent but still obtain necessary assistance. Focus on ways to carry on usual routines and schedules in spite of changing circumstances. Include family in discussion as appropriate	Supports a client's behavioral dimension of hope. Also enforces maintenance of normalcy, critical for dignity conservation (Chochinov, 2002).
4. Encourage client to engage in supportive relationships with family and friends.	Affiliation with significant others offers hope and energizes client by remaining active in daily life.
5. Work with client in focusing on ways to achieve short-term goals. This may include, for example, symptom relief, completion of relational tasks, resolution of relational problems.	Enforces sense of control and autonomy over life circumstances (Chochinov, 2002).

STEP	RATIONALE
6. When interacting with family, allow time for them to express grief. Use a problem-solving approach to help them identify their problems pertaining to caregiving. Lead through a step-by-step discussion of how to approach each problem. Encourage family to use available community resources (e.g., hospice, respite care).	Facilitates family mourning. Helps to reduce caregiving stress.
7. Offer frequent sessions that allow client opportunity to further express grief and discuss fears or concerns.	Continuing grief support takes time.
8. Offer to instruct client on relaxation strategies: guided imagery, relaxation, meditation.	Complementary alternative therapies can be effective in reducing level of stress, thereby providing useful coping strategy.
9. For clients in terminal stage of illness, support frequent visits with loved ones, review lifetime stories or photographs, help client engage in meaning-engendering projects such as organizing photo albums, writing journals.	Activities provide the client with a sense that he or she continues to serve a vital function and that life maintains purpose and dignity (Chochinov, 2002).

EVALUATION

1. Have client describe activities engaged in with family/friends.	Determines extent relational ties are maintained.
2. Observe client's behaviors during ongoing interactions.	Demonstrates client's ability to express grief
3. Discuss with client perceptions of benefit gained from strategies for relieving stress.	Evaluates efficacy of coping strategies.
4. Discuss with client progress toward meeting defined short-term goals.	Evaluates client's achievement of goals and need for revision.

Recording and Reporting

- Record in nurses' notes approaches used in grief support and client's response, both verbal and nonverbal.
- Keep nursing team members informed of client's grief expressions and reactions. Emphasize any changes that might affect physical health further such as change in appetite, refusal of a treatment.

Unexpected Outcomes	Related Interventions
1. Client is unable to express grief openly with care provider yet shows symptoms of extreme sorrow, anger, denial.	• Consider referral to health care professional with grief counseling experience (e.g., social worker, psychologist, pastoral care professional).
2. Family and client relationships deteriorate, little social support available to client.	• Discuss with client the difficulties encountered when family or friends are with client. • Determine if client feels he or she is a burden to family. • Consider a joint client and family discussion with nurse or health care professional.

Teaching Considerations

- When providing support to clients and their grieving family members, consider if instruction might be useful to the family. Often family members find it life enriching to be able to help clients (Stajduhar, 2003). Use contact with family members to instruct on topics such as client's signs and symptoms to observe for, ways to offer comfort or support, how to deliver personal care (e.g., bathing, oral hygiene), managing medication administration.

Pediatric Considerations

- It is important for a nurse to learn a child's understanding and experience of death. There are developmental theories for a child's concepts of death based on cognitive stage of development.
- Respect family's wishes in how and what to tell children about serious illness, dying, and death. It is important to be honest with children and to provide straightforward, yet caring explanations.

- Use of play therapy or drawing may help a child express his or her emotions, fears, and realizations about death.

Gerontological Considerations

- Freedom from loneliness and maintenance of self-esteem are major needs of the older adult. It is important not to care for these clients in a detached manner (e.g., slow to respond to physical discomforts, failing to keep room odor free, keeping the room dimly lit, speaking in hushed tones of voice). The dying person perceives such detached behaviors as abandonment (Ebersole, Hess, and Luggen, 2004).
- Older adults may not feel they have a choice in health care treatment and thus need to be involved in decisions about their care.

SKILL 7-2　Symptom Management in Palliative Care

Vigilant symptom management is a cornerstone of quality palliative care (Chochinov, 2002). Managing the dying client's symptoms begins with understanding that the symptoms are very real. The client's fears and anxieties often compound the effect and magnitude of symptoms, particularly that of pain and fear of suffocation (air hunger). Therefore symptom management includes physical care and psychological care as well.

Steinhauser and others (2000) report that clients, families, and physicians agree that pain and symptom management are important at the end of life and integral to the success of improving care for the dying. Frequently terminally ill clients ask nurses for assistance in dying (Schwarz, 1999), but it is often an expression of the need for better pain management (Ersek and others, 1995), emotional support (Quill and others, 1997), or for someone to actively listen and be present (Dixon, 1997).

The literature reports that pain is prevalent among cancer patients, especially as the disease progresses. Thirty percent of clients with cancer have pain at the time of diagnosis, and 65% to 85% have pain when their disease becomes advanced (Manfredi and others, 2003). Pain management is very complex. Pain such as neural pain that often becomes refractory to opioids (unresponsive to opioid medications) requires complex therapies that may include antidepressants, anticonvulsants, steroids, intraspinal medications, and antitumor therapy. Chapter 6 offers details on pain management approaches.

Delegation Considerations

A professional nurse is responsible for assessment of clients' symptoms and a determination of what symptoms can be independently managed and what symptoms require medical intervention. Certain symptom therapies can be delegated to assistive personnel such as positioning and environmental controls, hygiene approaches, and hydration. Therapies involving administration of opioids, anxiolytics, antidepressants, etc. require a nurse's intervention. The nurse provides assistive personnel with instruction and assistance regarding:

- When to notify nurse if client's symptoms worsen or change in nature
- Potential adverse effects of pharmacological agents and what to report to the nurse
- The need to maintain communication with dying clients, who still retain the sense of hearing

STEP	RATIONALE
ASSESSMENT	
1. Begin by asking clients to describe the symptoms they are experiencing. Use open-ended questions (e.g., "Tell me what physical changes, sources of distress, or sources of discomfort you are feeling as a result of your disease." "Tell me if any physical function has changed since your disease."	Allows client to describe illness-related concerns that are important to the client's dignity and ability to maintain normalcy as much as possible (Chochinov, 2002).
2. Give client time to describe physical symptoms; be exhaustive: "Is there anything else bothering you?" "You've told me you have pain in your _____; are you having any other pain?"	Ensures a more complete database. Prevents nurse from assuming what client's symptoms might be and prematurely halting assessment before all data is revealed.
3. If client reports pain, use the PQRST criteria for assessing the character of pain (see Chapter 6).	A detailed pain assessment is necessary for selection of appropriate therapies.

STEP	**RATIONALE**
4. Assess the condition of the skin, including upper and lower extremities (see Chapter 18).	As dying approaches, peripheral circulation is often diminished to facilitate increased circulation to vital organs.
5. Assess character of client's respirations and breathing pattern. Ask client if he or she feels a sense of suffocation or difficulty getting enough air during breathing. Does the client have copious secretions requiring suctioning?	Dyspnea or air hunger is a response to metabolic and oxygen changes of the respiratory system near the time of death. Increased respiratory secretions are common near the time of death.
6. Assess client's oral cavity; inspect condition of mucosa, tongue, and teeth (see Chapter 18).	Dehydration is commonly associated with progression of many terminal diseases. Dryness of the mucosa and development of *Candida* colonization of the oral cavity increases with aging, reduced salivary flow, radiation therapy, and immunosuppression (Butticaz and others, 2003).

7. If client reports changes in bowel function (see Chapter 33), assess the following:
  a. Client preferences for bowel management at home and success of approaches
  b. Usual bowel elimination pattern (frequency, character, time of day defecation occurs)
  c. Typical 7-day diet intake
  d. Current activity level
  e. Typical fluid intake for 24 hours (including type of fluids)
  f. Medication history (prescription and over-the-counter)
  g. Check for impaction if experiencing constipation
	Constipation is one of the most prevalent symptoms in palliative care clients. Decreased intestinal motility and increased anal sphincter tone resulting from use of opioids for pain management are common causative factors. Constipation may also be a consequence of the disease process or result of general debility (Cadd and others, 2000).
	Diarrhea often results from disease processes (e.g., colon cancer) and response to chemotherapy medications.
	Client may require suppository or enema secondary to pain medications and diet change.

8. Assess client's urinary elimination pattern (see Chapter 32), including ability to control urination. Determine need for catheterization versus use of diapers.	Urinary incontinence results from progressive disease (e.g., spinal cord involvement and reduced level of consciousness). Not all incontinent clients require catheterization.
9. Ask if client is experiencing nausea, vomiting, or decreased appetite.	Common side effect of medications and nausea may also result as concomitant symptom to severe pain.
10. Assess daily food and oral intake. Weigh client.	Findings will indicate percentage of daily recommended nutrient requirements consumed by client. Reveals risk for dehydration.

11. If client exhibits terminal restlessness, assess the following:
 	
  a. Confirm if client has pain, nausea, dyspnea, full bladder or full rectum, and joint pain as a result of inability to move.
  b. Determine if client has any unresolved concerns about death and meaning or purpose in life.
  c. Review client's medical record for dehydration, hypercalcemia, hyponatremia, and hypoglycemia.
	Terminal restlessness, also called agitated delirium, is a common condition in the terminally ill (Travis and others, 2001).
	Determines presence of common physical problems that should be treated or ruled out as causative factors.
	
	Existential causes for restlessness can be relieved with grief support and counseling.
	All factors are potential causes for delirium.

12. Review current medications taken by client, and consider common side effects or idiosyncratic effects. If client is on multiple medications, consult with pharmacist.	Untoward responses to medications and idiosyncratic effects may result in hypoactive and hyperactive states of activity.
13. Using a visual analog scale with a rating from 0 to 10, with 10 being the worst level of fatigue and 0 representing no fatigue, determine client's subjective perception (see Chapter 6). Ask if fatigue prevents client from doing what he or she wants to do.	Metabolic demands of a debilitating disease cause weakness and fatigue. Exhaustion phase of the general adaptation syndrome causes energy depletion. Side effects of medications may contribute to fatigue.

STEP	RATIONALE

NURSING DIAGNOSES

- Bowel incontinence
- Ineffective breathing pattern
- Constipation
- Risk for constipation
- Diarrhea
- Fatigue
- Deficient fluid volume
- Nausea

- Imbalanced nutrition: less than body requirements
- Impaired oral mucous membrane
- Acute pain
- Chronic pain
- Impaired swallowing
- Ineffective tissue perfusion
- Total urinary incontinence

Related factors are individualized, based on client's condition or needs.

PLANNING

1. Expected outcomes following completion of procedure:
   - Client will report reduction in severity of pain.
   - Client will report feeling warm and comfortable.

   - Client will report pleasure in drinking and eating.

   - Client will pass a soft, formed stool.

   - Skin will remain clear without irritation or breakdown.

   - Client is able to rest without becoming restless and irritable.
   - Client reports a reduction in level of fatigue.
   - Client experiences less effort to breathe.

2. Position client comfortably. Close room door or curtain.
3. Explain procedures to be performed, and have client assist in choosing the best schedule for care measures.

Indicates pain relief.
Therapies designed to improve warmth help to reverse effects of reduced peripheral circulation.
Hydration of oral mucosa improves integrity of oral tissues and client's tolerance to eating and drinking.
Indicates restoration of stool character and promotion of peristaltic activity.
Conditions of bowel or urinary incontinence may be irreversible. Goal is to protect skin from injury.
Therapies effect calming.

Indicates energy conservation accomplished.
Client less apprehensive and able to breathe at even, normal rate.
Promotes comfort and privacy.
Minimizes client's anxiety. Maintains client's autonomy.

IMPLEMENTATION

1. Refer to Chapter 6 for implementation of pharmacological and nonpharmacological pain therapies. Be sure client understands nature of pain and pattern of pain to expect from illness.
2. Provide general comfort measures:
   a. Provide daily bath with lubrication of the skin.
   b. Provide eye care to remove crusts from eyelids.
   c. Use artificial tears.

   d. Keep lips lubricated with petroleum jelly.
   e. Reposition frequently.
   f. Reposition to avoid lying over drainage or intravenous (IV) tubes and other care devices.
3. Provide oral hygiene every 2 to 4 hours while awake (see Chapter 14). Also make available sodium bicarbonate rinses 4 to 6 times a day (order required). For clients with fungal infections consult with physician regarding use of antifungal mouth rinses.

4. Treat nausea by administering ordered antiemetics (rectal route recommended). As nausea subsides, offer clear liquids and ice chips. Avoid liquids such as coffee, milk, and fruit juices.

Timely and round-the-clock management of pain is essential in the terminally ill. Aggressive pain management is more likely to relieve severity of discomfort. Client's knowledge of pain will help to reduce anxiety, which can aggravate pain.

Any source of physical irritation can worsen pain. Blink reflex diminishes near death, causing drying of cornea.

Dehydration develops as client experiences metabolic changes and fluid intake declines. As client approaches death, mouth breathing is common. Clients have reported reduction in discomfort due to oral dryness and removal of debris on tooth surfaces and mucosa following a rigorous oral hygiene regimen (Butticaz and others, 2003).
Clear liquids are more readily tolerated by gastrointestinal (GI) mucosa. Certain liquids tend to increase stomach acidity.

STEP	RATIONALE

- **Critical Decision Point**

  Do not force a terminally ill client to eat or drink if he or she does not want nourishment.

5. Provide a bowel management program including:
   a. Diet high in high-fiber foods such as prunes, fruit juices, bran, and vegetables

   Promotes peristalsis and keeps fecal matter soft.

   b. Increased fluid intake if medically appropriate and tolerated by client
   c. Regular daily exercise such as walking
   d. Daily suppository (if ordered)
6. If client has diarrhea:
   a. Provide low-residue diet.

   Slows peristalsis.

   b. Assess for fecal impaction.

   Leakage of liquid stool in the form of diarrhea can be a warning sign of impaction.

   c. Confer with physician to change medications that might be contributing to symptom.
7. Confer with physician regarding use of condom catheter, indwelling Foley, or diapers for treatment of total urinary incontinence.

   Promotes comfort of dying client and reduces exposure of skin to moisture.

8. Have client identify those tasks he or she wishes to perform; then help client conserve energy to perform those tasks:

   Strategies conserve energy and reduce sense of fatigue after activities are performed. Provides client sense of overall improved well-being.

   a. Introduce frequent rest periods during day.
   b. Determine when client typically feels more energetic.
   c. If clients are able to ambulate, allow them to be free to leave the confines of their room and associate with other clients or staff.
   d. Devise ways to reduce steps in any activity (e.g., dressing, bathing [having all supplies readily accessible], cooking [plan Meals on Wheels to be delivered or help client devise menu with pre-prepared foods].
9. Provide vigilant skin care (see Chapter 15).

   Reduces exposure of skin to external irritants and minimizes pressure over skin surfaces.

10. Provide adequate ventilation and oxygenation:
    a. Position client in semi-Fowler's or Fowler's position.

    Positioning promotes maximal ventilation and drainage of secretions.

    b. Suction when excessive pulmonary secretions accumulate.

    Suctioning may temporarily relieve severity of death rattle (Watts and Jenkins, 1999).

    c. Reposition client to relieve death rattle.
    d. Administer oxygen as ordered.
    e. Keep room cool with low humidity (not completely dry).

    Cool room aids in relief of dyspnea (Lueckenotte, 2000).

11. Establish presence with client to allay anxiety and panic felt with air hunger. Share control with client (e.g., offer choice to switch oxygen devices, type of positioning, choices of respiratory therapies). Administer morphine, Thorazine, and anxiolytics as ordered.

    Sharing control with clients helps to reduce pain and anxiety, relieving sense of breathlessness (Tarzian, 2000). Thorazine can cause a marked reduction in breathlessness as death approaches (Travis and others, 2001). Morphine and anxiolytics relieve respiratory distress.

12. Control terminal restlessness through environmental manipulation and supervised pharmacological intervention:
    a. *Environmental manipulation*—Keep client's room quiet, adequately lit, and at a comfortable temperature. Offer family members opportunities to maintain close contact. Encourage use of soft music, prayer, or reading aloud of personal passages from a favorite book.

    Reduces unnecessary external stimulation and provides a comforting space.

    Privacy allows family members chance to provide verbal assurances and touch the dying client (Travis and others, 2001). The presence of a family member to hold a hand or speak gently may provide a calming effect (Lichter and Hunt, 1990).

STEP	RATIONALE
b. *Pharmacological intervention*—Use least-sedating means possible to control restless behavior, confer with physician or pharmacy for titration of medication doses (e.g., haloperidol, Thorazine, Elavil, ABH compound [Ativan, Benadryl, Haldol]). Discontinue all nonessential medication. Administer subcutaneous, sublingual, rectal, or transdermal delivery routes.	Aim is to control delirium without rendering dying client unconscious. Control of restlessness relieves family's concern that client is in pain or distress (Fainsinger and others, 1993). Discontinuation of unnecessary medications makes it less likely that there will be interference with the medications providing comfort and relief (Travis and others, 2001). Routes are least invasive.

EVALUATION

1. Ask client to rate pain on scale of 0 to 10 and to describe level of comfort.	Client will report a reduced severity in pain and express a level of improved comfort or pain control.
2. Ask client to describe comfort of oral cavity, and inspect oral cavity.	Mucosa is hydrated. Client denies difficulty swallowing and voices pleasure in eating/drinking.
3. Inspect character of fecal mass.	Stool will be soft and formed with bowel movement (BM) every 3 days.
4. Inspect condition of skin.	Skin is without lesions or signs of pressure.
5. Observe client's behavior and/or ask family to report on status of client's agitation.	Client will be able to rest calmly without restlessness or anxiety.
6. Ask client to rate level of fatigue on scale from 0 to 10. Observe client as he or she performs routine daily activities.	If energy conservation is effective, client will have less fatigue and be able to remain active for longer periods of time.
7. Assess character of client's respirations, and ask client if he or she continues to feel out of breath.	Determines if breathlessness is relieved. Client should be able to breathe without sternal retraction, at normal respiratory rate.

Recording and Reporting

- Clearly record all client symptoms in detail in nurses' notes or appropriate flow sheets. Use consistent descriptors for comparison over time.
- Record type of interventions administered and client's response in nurses' notes.
- Record those interventions that are repeatedly successful in care plan.
- Report development of symptom or worsening of symptom to primary care provider.

Unexpected Outcomes	Related Interventions
1. Any one or a combination of symptoms may continue unresolved, with client reporting little or no relief.	• Increase the frequency of an intervention. • Provide more combination therapies (pharmacological and nonpharmacological) after consulting with primary care provider. • Attend to client, and use therapies he or she finds most effective.
2. Client becomes anxious, fearful, or exhausted as a result of continued symptoms.	• Provide information to client and family about nature of symptoms and aims of therapies. • Have client make choices as to options for therapy. • Answer call lights quickly, and explain when care is planned throughout the day.

Teaching Considerations

- Teach family how to become involved in client's care (Figure 7-2). Family caregivers can learn to perform most of the skills used in symptom management. Family will administer medications in the home setting. Offer supervised instruction and opportunities for questions. Reinforce family member when they have found an approach that is successful (as well as safe).
- Help family members learn to interact with the dying person (e.g., using attentive listening, avoiding false reassurances, conducting conversations about normal family activities or problems).
- Teach family members the signs and symptoms of death (Table 7-2).

Pediatric Considerations

- Allow young children to visit a dying parent or grandparent if all parties consent. (Some dying clients have strong feelings about possibly traumatizing children during this transition.)

Home Care Considerations

- Teach family to recognize signs and symptoms to expect as the client's condition worsens (see above) and information on whom to call in an emergency.
- When the family becomes fatigued with care activities, relieve them from their duties so that they can acquire needed rest and support. Refer them to resources for meals and lodging.

TABLE 7-2   PHYSICAL SIGNS AND SYMPTOMS ASSOCIATED WITH THE FINAL STAGES OF DYING

Physical Signs and Symptoms	Rationale	Intervention
Coolness, color, and temperature change in hands, arms, feet, and legs; perspiration may be present	Peripheral circulation diminished to shunt blood to vital organs	Place socks on feet. Cover with light cotton blanket. Keep warm blankets on client but do not use electric blanket.
Increased sleeping	Conservation of energy	Spend time with client; hold the client's hand and speak normally.
Disorientation, confusion of time, place, person	Metabolic changes	Identify self by name before speaking to client; speak softly, clearly, and truthfully.
Incontinence of urine, bowel, or both	Increased muscle relaxation and decreased consciousness	Change bedding as appropriate. Be vigilant. Use bed pads, and try to avoid use of indwelling catheter.
Congestion	Poor circulation of body fluids, immobilization, inability to expectorate secretions causes rattles and bubbling	Elevate head with pillow or raise head of bed; gently turn head to side to drain secretions.
Restlessness	Metabolic changes and decrease in oxygen to the brain	Calm client by speech and action; reduce light; gently rub back, stroke arms, or read aloud. Do not use restraints.
Decreased intake of food and fluids	Body conservation of energy for function	Do not force client to eat or drink; give ice chips, soft drinks, juice, popsicles, as possible. Provide mouth care.

Modified from Ebersole P and others: *Toward healthy aging,* ed 6, St. Louis, 2004, Mosby.

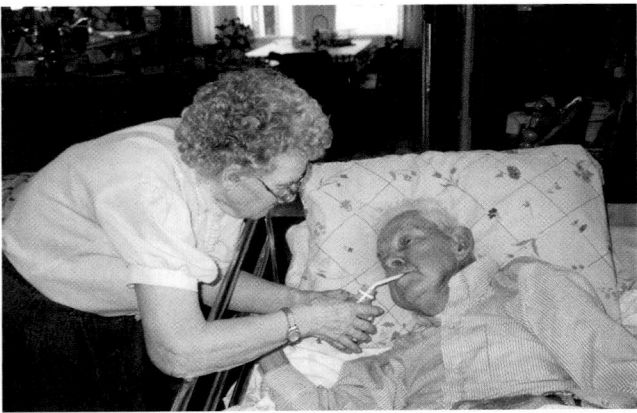

FIGURE 7-2 Involve family in client's care.

Long-Term Care Considerations

- The goal of a nursing facility is to provide a caring environment for those who are dying. However, there are many facilities that sorely lack appropriate supportive care. Compassionate care allows family members to be present whenever they choose, day or night, and involves aggressive and appropriate symptom management (Lueckenotte, 2000).
- Nighttime is a time of least attention and a time of loneliness and pain. Night is also a time of fear of dying alone and no one will know. If a friend or relative cannot stay with the client, a mature sitter is an option. A volunteer from hospice might provide the same support. For those older adults who have developed a lifestyle around aloneness, solitude might be preferred. Be sensitive to the client's preferences (Ebersole and others, 2004).

SKILL 7-3 Care of the Body After Death

When a client dies in a hospital setting, the nurse provides postmortem care. It is important for the nurse to care for the client's body with dignity and sensitivity and in a manner consistent with the client's religious or cultural beliefs. The Uniform Determination of Death Act (UDDA) definition or a similar definition of death is now accepted in all 50 of the United States as valid and legal criteria of death. The UDDA defines death as "irreversible cessation of circulatory and respiratory functions or irreversible cessation of all function of the brain, including the brainstem" (Chabalewski and Norris, 1994). After death the body undergoes many physical changes. For that reason, care must be provided as soon as possible to prevent tissue damage or disfigurement of body parts.

Federal and state legislation require hospitals to formulate policies and procedures based on current laws to consider life support and the degree of intervention the person desires at the time of death, to validate death, to identify potential organ or tissue donors, and to provide postmortem care. As part of a person's right to self-determination, every adult may accept or refuse recommended medical treatment. The Patient Self-Determination Act of 1991 requires all health care agencies serving Medicaid and Medicare clients to provide clients with information regarding advance directives options. Advance directives are legal documents that allow persons to have a say in the medical treatments they will receive if unable to make decisions. Self-determination is at the core of protecting clients from misuse of the medical system (Ebersole and others, 2004). The person can specify what types of treatments are acceptable or unacceptable and can also designate another person appointed as a proxy (durable power of attorney) to legally make treatment decisions if he or she is unable to make decisions. For example, an advance directive might address whether IV therapy, tube feedings, or use of respiratory ventilation are to be used in a client's treatment. Ideally a client has had an opportunity to discuss with family and friends his or her wishes regarding end-of-life care. For example, does the client want to be placed on a ventilator, wish to have cardiopulmonary resuscitation, wish to receive blood products? It is the nurse's responsibility to determine if the client's wishes have been assessed and if advance directives are appropriately documented in the client record. A copy of any advance directive document should be placed in the client's medical record.

Although it is legally mandated that health care agencies provide information related to advance directives, studies suggest that clients and families often have a limited understanding of advance directives and their implications. For example, once a client becomes seriously ill, what options does the family have in making decisions? If a client requires a ventilator for temporary treatment and chances of survival are good, does the advance directive supersede and require the family to withhold treatment? Many clients have not executed advance directives often because of confusion and misleading information (Rein and others, 1996). The nurse may find it beneficial to discuss advance directives with a dying person and family if the person's wishes are not clearly reflected in the record (Johns, 1996). Because agency policies and state laws differ, nurses need to be familiar with agency policies and the state laws where they are practicing.

Cardiopulmonary resuscitation (CPR) is a basic emergency procedure for life support, consisting of artificial respiration and manual external cardiac massage. It is used in cases of cardiac and/or pulmonary arrest. The procedure is performed on a client unless a "do not resuscitate" (DNR) order is written and signed by the client's physician. A DNR order may be part of a client's advance directive document. Adult clients may consent to a DNR order orally or in writing after being properly informed by a physician. Oral consents require two witnesses, one of whom must be a physician affiliated with the health care institution. A written consent requires two adult witnesses. State statutes require that physicians review DNR orders regularly (usually every 3 days) for hospitalized clients to ensure their relevance and appropriateness.

Another consideration as death approaches is one of organ/tissue donation. The 1986 Omnibus Budget Reconciliation Act (OBRA) requires a client's significant others be offered the option of organ and tissue donation (Chabalewski and Norris, 1994). Organs may be requested when the client is terminally ill but on life support. The client must be maintained on ventilatory and circulatory support until vital organs are harvested. The family must understand that the client is "brain dead," that the equipment is not keeping the client alive but keeping the physical body in a state so that organs will not be damaged before harvesting. Tissues such as eyes, bone, and skin may also be requested after death. The nurse can be very helpful in supporting families through the organ and tissue request process. It is important to provide a private area to discuss all issues with the family. The staff member designated to make organ/tissue request must offer the family clarification of what defines brain death. The family must also know who legally can give final consent, what options there are for organ or tissue donation, whether there are associated costs, and how donation will affect burial or cremation.

Most states now give citizens the option of signing the back of their motor vehicle license to designate their wish to be an organ or tissue donor. However, a family member must ultimately make the final decision. Thus it is important for persons to keep family members informed of their wishes. Nevertheless, a client's choice regarding organ and tissue donation can be included in an advance directive. Recently, more people favor organ/tissue donation and have expressed the wish to donate their own organs/tissues when they die. Following donation, most donor families report feeling positive about the donation and report that donation has helped them in working through the grieving process.

Basic principles to remember when making organ and tissue requests include:

- Find the family a private place to sit while a request is being made.
- Be sure the legal decision maker in the family is involved in the request.
- Notify the local donor registry to determine if the client qualifies. Certain disease states prohibit organ/tissue donation.
- Be sure the family is well informed about options and how the body of the deceased will be cared for.
- Be sure the family is informed about who assumes financial responsibility for harvested organs. The recipient and/or local organ retrieval agency usually assumes these costs.
- Do not place any pressure on the family to consent to donation.
- Be sensitive to the family's cultural and religious practices.

Another area that is difficult for the nurse and family concerns autopsy. An autopsy or postmortem examination is performed to confirm or determine the cause of death, gather data regarding the nature and progress of a disease, study the effects of therapies on body tissues, and provide statistical data for epidemiology and research purposes. A consent form must be signed by the most immediate family member and the physician or designated requester. Autopsies are required in circumstances of unusual death (e.g., violent trauma, unexpected death in the home), as well as for death occurring within a set time frame following hospitalization. Each state has guidelines for when autopsies are required. Autopsies normally do not delay burial, but there is a cost to families. Getting permission for an autopsy through delicate questioning is difficult at best (Dracup and Brown, 1998). Often the physician will ask for permission for an autopsy, but it is the nurse's responsibility to answer questions and support the family's choices. It may prove helpful to explain the value that an autopsy has for improving knowledge in the field of medicine. To help the living, an autopsy can lead to new therapies and new understanding of diseases.

BOX 7-1   Cultural and Religious Considerations in Care of the Body After Death

African-Americans—Prefer having member of the health care team clean and prepare the loved one's body. Some consider organ donation a taboo but may agree to an autopsy.

Chinese-Americans—Some families will prefer to bathe the client themselves. Often believe the body should remain intact; organ donation and autopsy are uncommon.

Filipino-Americans—Some families may prefer to wash the body themselves and are likely to want time for all family members to say good-bye. May not permit organ donation or autopsy.

Hispanics or Latino-Americans—Family members may help with care of the body and are likely to want time to say goodbye. Organ donation and autopsy are uncommon.

Jewish religion—Dying person may want Deathbed Confessional, Name Changing, or other prayers. Usually oppose autopsies but may consider organ donation. Body must not be left unattended until burial. Family member may remain present while body is prepared by nursing staff for transport to morgue and then to funeral home.

Roman Catholic—Dying person should receive sacraments of Penance and Anointing of the Sick within 30 days before death. Religion does not oppose autopsies or organ donation.

Muslim religion—When a person is close to death, he or she will recite the Islamic Creed with help from others. After death the person's eyes should be closed, mouth closed, and arms and legs straightened.

Hindu religion—Dying person should be in a peaceful room if not at home. Person or someone else should recite the Gita. Family members prefer to wash the body.

Buddhist religion—An ordained monk or nun should be present to care for the dying person. When the person has died, the body should be covered with a cotton sheet. The body should not be touched or manipulated in any way. **Do Not** close the eyes or mouth. No noise, talking, or crying is allowed.

Clients' and families' cultural beliefs become very important in postmortem care. Maintaining the integrity of rituals and mourning practices gives families a sense of acceptance of the client's death and an inner peace. Although there are individual variations within cultural and religious groups, general preferences are described in Box 7-1. The ability of families to express their cultural values when a client dies becomes a tool to make predictable and controllable that which is unpredictable and inevitable (Kagawa-Singer, 1998).

DELEGATION CONSIDERATIONS

Care of the body after death can be delegated to assistive personnel. However, the nurse should recognize that often the family will expect to see the nurse more than usual to provide support. Also, care after death can actually begin before the actual death so that clients and families can preserve cultural practices. Check agency policy regarding which staff members are permitted to remove invasive tubes or lines. At the time of death it may be best for the nurse and assistive personnel to work together in preparing the body.

* Inform care providers of any preferences the family might have because of cultural, religious, or ethnic beliefs that will influence the routine procedure of caring for the client's body.
* Reinforce the importance of handling the body with respect.

EQUIPMENT

❑ Disposable gloves, gown, and other protective clothing
❑ Plastic bag for hazardous waste disposal
❑ Washbasin, washcloth, warm water, and bath towel
❑ Clean gown or disposable gown for body as indicated by agency policy
❑ Shroud kit with name tags
❑ Syringes for removing Foley catheters
❑ Scissors
❑ Small pillow or towel
❑ Paper tape, gauze dressings
❑ Paper bag, plastic bag, or other suitable receptacle for client's clothing, belongings, and other items to be returned to significant others
❑ Valuables envelope

STEP	RATIONALE

ASSESSMENT

1. Confer with physician regarding time when death is pronounced. Physician may request an autopsy, especially for unusual circumstances.

2. Assess for presence of family members or significant others and whether they have been informed of the client's death. Determine who is legally defined as next of kin.

3. Approach next of kin for tissue donation or call organ/tissue request team (check agency policy). Discuss all donor options.

4. Give family a place to privately gather. Allow time for significant others to ask questions.

5. Once family has made decision, complete necessary organ/tissue donation request form.

6. Determine if family members have special requests for the preparation or viewing of the body (position of body, a special gown, shaving). Determine if family wishes to remain present or assist.

7. Check orders for any specimens or special orders needed by the physician.

8. Make arrangements for staff, minister, or others to stay with the family while preparing the body for viewing.

9. Assess the deceased for general condition of the body and any bandages, tubes, or equipment (check agency policy).

10. Determine if an autopsy is planned.

Certifies client's death. Autopsy designed to determine cause of death and extend knowledge about disease.

It is the physician's responsibility to notify significant others of the client's death. The nurse provides emotional support and prepares the body for viewing.

Organ/tissue request should be performed by staff who have received appropriate training.

Conveys caring and concern for significant other. Questions may provide valuable information about the response of significant others to their loss and their needs.

Federal guidelines require documentation that request has been made.

Respects the individuality of the client and family and their right to having their values and beliefs enforced.

Procedures may be used in determining cause of death.

Provides support to family and conveys respect for their cultural/religious preferences.

Because of the fragility of tissues following death, tissue damage can occur easily. Most agencies have specific policies about removal of tubes, wires, and equipment.

If an autopsy is planned, some procedures such as removal of tubes and lines may be contraindicated.

NURSING DIAGNOSES

For clients:
* Risk for impaired skin integrity

For family and significant others:
* Powerlessness
* Ineffective coping
* Dysfunctional grieving

Related factors are individualized based on the client's, family's, and significant others' needs.

STEP	RATIONALE

PLANNING

1. Expected outcomes following completion of procedure:
   - Deceased's body will be free of skin damage.

     Care is delivered so as to prevent additional bruises, lacerations, or abrasions.

   - Significant others will express grief.

     Significant others feel support in being able to react to loss of loved one.

2. Gather or direct assistive personnel to gather needed equipment.

   Because this is often a time of emotional intensity for significant others, organization is particularly important.

3. Have body placed in a private room or have roommate moved to another area as body is being prepared. Be sure to explain to roommate what has occurred and be supportive.

   Provides staff with an area to make the body presentable for family to visit in private.

IMPLEMENTATION

1. Check with significant others about notifying other significant family members or friends. Call the funeral home.

   Following a death, significant others may have difficulty with remembering details about what to do and how to respond and may need assistance. Funeral home must be alerted so that personnel can pick up the body promptly.

2. Discuss procedure of preparing the body with significant others. Follow the practices of the family's culture/religion.

   Having an ability to direct what is happening can increase the significant others' sense of control. Discussing personal preferences with the significant others conveys caring and concern.

3. If tissue donation has been made, consult agency policy for specific guidelines on care of the body.

   Retrieval of tissues (e.g., eyes, bone, skin) may require special preparation measures.

4. Arrange equipment at bedside.

   Ensures organized procedure.

5. Perform hand hygiene.

   Reduces transmission of microorganisms.

6. Close room door or draw bedside curtain.

   Provides privacy for the deceased and significant others.

7. Apply disposable gloves and gown or protective barriers as applicable.

   Body excretions may harbor infectious microorganisms. For example, leaking stool or withdrawal of intravenous tubing or other tubing may cause temporary bleeding.

- *Critical Decision Point*

  If significant others are assisting in the preparation of the body, be sure they too are protected from body excretions.

8. Identify the body according to agency policy. Leave identification in place as directed in agency policy.

   Ensures proper identification of the body for delivery to morgue, autopsy room, and funeral home.

9. If in keeping with agency procedures, remove all indwelling catheters, intravenous, oxygen, and other tubes. **(If an autopsy is to be performed, policy may direct to leave these devices in place.)** Dress puncture wounds with a small dressing and paper tape.

   Creates a normal appearance. Paper tape minimizes skin trauma.

10. If the person wore dentures, reinsert them. If mouth fails to close and if it is culturally appropriate to close the mouth, place a rolled-up towel under the chin.

    It is difficult to insert dentures after rigor mortis occurs. Dentures maintain the client's natural facial expression.

11. Position client as outlined in agency procedures or family's cultural preferences. Avoid placing one hand on top of the other. Check agency policy regarding need to restrain hands and feet.

    Client appears natural and comfortable. Placing one hand on top of the other can lead to discoloration of skin. Agencies often require restraining of appendages to prevent tissue damage when body is being moved.

12. Place small pillow or folded towel under the head or elevate head of bed 10 to 15 degrees.

    Prevents pooling of blood in the face and subsequent discoloration.

STEP	RATIONALE
13. Close eyes gently by grasping the eyelashes and pulling lids over corneas of eyes (unless religious preference is to keep eyes open).	Closed eyes present a more natural appearance. Pressure on lids can lead to discoloration.
14. Determine if family wants client left in unshaven state and if it was custom of client to wear a beard. Otherwise, shave male client.	Presents client in his normal appearance before death.
15. Wash body parts soiled by blood, urine, feces, or other drainage. (A mortician will provide a complete bath.)	Prepares body for viewing and reduces odors.
16. Place an absorbent pad under the client's buttocks.	Relaxation of sphincter muscles at time of death may cause release of urine or feces.

- **Critical Decision Point**
  Turning a corpse sometimes leads to a breath exhaled from the body. This is a normal event.

STEP	RATIONALE
17. Remove soiled dressings, and replace with clean gauze dressings. Use paper tape.	Paper tape minimizes skin trauma. Changing dressings helps to control odors caused by microorganisms and to create a more acceptable appearance.
18. Place a clean gown on the client (agency policy may require removal before body is wrapped).	Prepares body for viewing.
19. Brush and comb client's hair. Remove any clips, hairpins, or rubber bands.	During viewing, the client should appear well-groomed. Hard objects such as pins can damage or discolor the face and scalp.
20. Clarify personal belongings that are to stay with the body and those items to be taken home by family.	Helps to prevent loss of valuables.
21. If significant others request viewing, place a clean sheet or light blanket over the body up to the chin with arms outside covers if possible. Remove unneeded equipment from the room. Provide soft lighting, and offer chairs for family.	Maintains dignity and respect for the client and significant others. Prevents exposure of body parts.
22. Encourage the family to say goodbye through both touch, talk, or religious rituals. Do not rush this process. Give family time to be alone with client.	Compassionate care allows family to experience the death process with dignity.
23. After the significant others have left the room, remove all linen and the client's gown (refer to agency policy). Place body in body bag, or apply the shroud as required by the agency (see illustration).	Prevents injury to skin and extremities. Avoids unnecessary exposure of body parts.

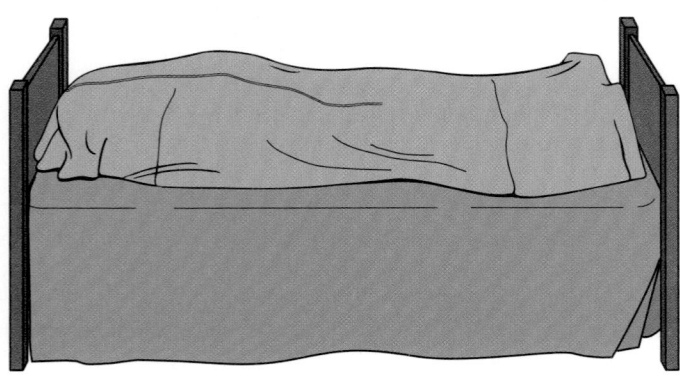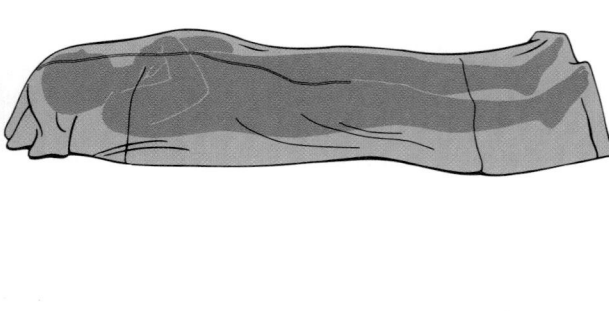

STEP 23 Body in body bag and shroud.

STEP	**RATIONALE**
24. Label the body. Be sure to note if client has an infectious disease (follow agency policy).	Ensures proper identification of the body. Reduces exposure of morgue and mortician staff to infection.
25. Arrange transportation of the body to the morgue or mortuary. If delay is anticipated before the mortician arrives, the body should be cooled in the morgue to prevent further tissue damage.	

EVALUATION

1. Observe significant others' response to the loss.	Each person's response to loss is unique, and evaluation is necessary to determine the need for referral for assistance.
2. Provide significant others with the opportunity to express feelings.	Significant others often seek chance to express feelings with someone other than an immediate family member.
3. Note appearance and condition of client's skin during preparation of the body.	Determines if damage to tissues occurs after preparation of the body.

Recording and Reporting

- Record in nurses' notes or appropriate form time of death, resuscitative measures taken to prevent death (if applicable), and who pronounced death of client.
- Record any special preparation of the body and type of organ/tissue donation. Include who was called and who came to the hospital for organ/tissue request.
- Record names of morgue, funeral home, chaplain, and relationship to the deceased of individual family members making decisions.
- Document how valuables and personal belongings were handled and who received them. Secure signatures as required by agency policy.
- Record on appropriate form personal articles left on the body (e.g., teeth or glasses) and/or jewelry taped to skin, tubes left in place.
- Record time of discharge and destination of the body. Location of identifying tags.

Unexpected Outcomes	**Related Interventions**
1. Family/significant others become immobilized by their grief and have difficulty functioning.	• Consider if a member of the family is able to act as a calming presence. Enlist his or her help in explaining what to expect in after-death care. • Call for assistance from pastoral care workers, social work staff, or a nursing staff member who has developed a close relationship with the client/family.
2. Significant others become very agitated and express their grief openly, at times by striking out against others.	• Support from security staff may be necessary. • Refer to social work or staff trained in crisis intervention.
3. Lacerations, bruises, or abrasions are noted on skin surfaces of deceased. Positioning or preparation of the body results in skin injury.	• Document according to policy.

Pediatric Considerations

- Parents should be allowed to stay with the child any time of day or night. Reassure parents that everything possible was done for the child.
- When possible, the topic of organ donation should be approached with the family before the death of the child. Many families appreciate this topic being brought to their attention because they would not think of it on their own. Many find it comforting to know they are able to help others.
- Make every effort to arrange for family members, especially parents, to be with the child at the time of death, if they wish to be present. For many, viewing the body is a sign of closure—an opportunity to finish their good-byes (Hockenberry and others, 2003).

- Parents frequently ask, "What will my child die from?" "What will happen when he dies?" Answer questions giving specific details of an impending death, while being sensitive to the family's cultural background and knowledge level (Martinson, 1995).
- Parents frequently ask to hold the child's body during viewing.

Gerontological Considerations

- Despite the family's grief and pain, the family must give the client permission to die, let the client know it is all right to let go and leave (Ebersole and others, 2004).
- Visitors should be allowed to be with the dying aged any time of day or night. Night is the most lonely and painful time.

Home Care Considerations

- As death approaches, significant others often need information about what to expect (e.g., the signs and symptoms of impending death). Encourage family to talk with client and say their last goodbyes, because the client's hearing is often still intact.
- As death approaches, the nurse needs to consider the type of support the significant others are likely to need at the time of death and make plans to put this support in place.
- Following death in the home, the nurse will need to follow agency guidelines related to body preparation and transfer of the body.
- For disposal of durable medical equipment (e.g., tubings, needles, syringes) or soiled dressings or linens, the nurse must follow the policies of the agency. The nurse may need to instruct significant others in the handling and disposal of medical waste.

FOCUS on CLINICAL PRACTICE

Mr. Weiss is a 62-year-old man who suffered a heart attack while at home. He was resuscitated and brought to the emergency department. He is now on a ventilator and vasopressor medications, which are maintaining his blood pressure and heart function. He is nonresponsive to even deep painful stimuli. Physicians are preparing to evaluate Mr. Weiss for clinical brain death. They have discussed with Mrs. Weiss the irreversibility of her husband's condition. Mr. Weiss has two adult daughters, 27 and 24 years of age. His wife has been in the waiting room as the physicians make rounds on her husband. She is seen crying and talking with her daughters at length. She is overhead telling her daughters, "This can't be happening. Your dad and I were going on a trip next weekend."

1. The loss experienced by Mrs. Weiss can best be described as a(an):
   A. Perceived loss
   B. Situational loss
   C. Actual loss
   D. Maturational loss
2. As the nurse caring for Mrs. Weiss, your assessment of her crying and statement of disbelief to her daughter suggests that you:
   A. Diagnose her grief as dysfunctional
   B. Identify her stage of grief as denial and plan interventions accordingly

   C. Gather further information regarding Mrs. Weiss's response to loss before forming a conclusion
   D. Recognize that Mrs. Weiss will progress through each stage of grief in a linear fashion
3. List three approaches you might use to assess Mrs. Weiss's loss and level of grief more fully.
4. You find in the chart a copy of Mr. Weiss's advance directives. As you sit down to talk with Mrs. Weiss, she asks, "What is an advance directive?" Your best answer would be:
   A. An advance directive is a legal document that allows your husband to have a say in the medical treatments he will receive if unable to make decisions.
   B. An advance directive is a document that defines by law which members of the family have the right to make decisions about end-of-life care.
   C. An advance directive is a document prepared by an individual before his death that outlines treatment choices that can be made by family members.
   D. An advance directive is a legal document that gives family permission to donate organs after death.
5. Mrs. Weiss's daughter approaches you and says, "The doctors want us to consider donating Dad's organs. I didn't think you could donate anything until someone dies." How might you respond? Is the daughter the best person to ask for organ donation?

NCLEX REVIEW QUESTIONS

1. Doug Brown is a 70-year-old man who comes to the neighborhood health clinic. After an eye examination, his physician explains that he has senile cataracts, which explains his progressive visual loss. Mr. Brown's situation could be described as a:
   1. Maturational loss
   2. Situational loss
   3. Perceived loss
   4. Actual loss

2. A client who exhibits terminal restlessness can best be assessed by:
   1. Reviewing laboratory values
   2. Measuring condition of respirations
   3. Assessing level of consciousness
   4. Determining level of client's fatigue

3. When preparing a body after death, you should not close the eyes of a client who practices which of the following religions:
   1. Judaism
   2. Hinduism
   3. Buddhism
   4. Catholicism

4. A priority in palliative care is symptom management. A principle to follow in symptom management is:
   1. Recognize that the dying client's symptoms are very real
   2. A client's anxiety may distract him or her from feeling pain or discomfort
   3. Symptom management focuses on physical care-giving
   4. As a terminal illness progresses, a client typically has less discomfort

References

Chabalewski F, Norris M: The gift of life: talking to families about organ and tissue donation, *Am J Nurs* 94(6):28, 1994.

Chochinov HM: Dignity-conserving care: a new model for palliative care: helping the patient feel valued, *JAMA* 287(17):2253, 2002.

Cressy D: *Birth, marriage, and death: ritual, religion and the life-cycle in Tudor and Stuart England,* New York, 1997, Oxford University Press.

Crowley LM and others: Strategies for culturally effective end-of-life care, *Ann Inter Med* 136(9), 673, 2002.

Dixon MD: The quality of mercy: reflections on provider-assisted suicide, *J Clin Ethics* 8:290,1997.

Dracup K, Brown CW: Asking difficult questions, *Am J Crit Care* 7(6):399, 1998.

Ebersole P and others: *Toward healthy aging,* ed 6, St. Louis, 2004, Mosby.

End-of-Life Nursing Education Consortium (ELNEC), American Association of Colleges of Nursing and City of Hope National Medical Center, 2000.

Ersek M and others: Priority ethical issues in oncology nursing: current approaches and future directions, *Oncol Nurs Forum* 22:803, 1995.

Fainsinger RL and others: A perspective on the management of delirium in terminally ill patients on a palliative care unit, *J Palliat Care* 9(3):4, 1993.

Field MJ, Cassel CK: *Approaching death: improving care at the end of life,* (Institute of Medicine Committee on Care at the End of Life), Washington, DC, 1997, National Academy Press.

Finucane TE: Care of patients nearing death: another view, *J Am Geriatr Soc* 50(3):551, 2002.

Hasler K: Understanding and managing bereavement, *Nurs Stand* 10(24):51, 1996.

Hockenberry MJ and others: *Wong's nursing care of infants and children,* ed 7, St. Louis, 2003, Mosby.

Johns J: Advanced directives and opportunities for nurses, *Image J Nurs Sch* 28(2):149, 1996.

Kagawa-Singer M: The cultural context of death rituals and mourning practices, *Oncol Nurs Forum* 25(10):1752, 1998.

Kemp C, Bhungalia S: Culture and the end of life: a review of major world religions, *J Hosp Palliat Nurs* 4(4):235, 2002.

Lichter I, Hunt E: The last 48 hours of life, *J Palliat Care* 6(4):7, 1990.

Lueckenotte A: *Gerontologic nursing,* ed 2, St. Louis, 2000, Mosby.

Manfredi P and others: Neuropathic pain in patients with cancer, *J Palliat Care* 19(2):115, 2003.

Martinson M: Pediatric hospice nursing, *Annu Rev Nurs Res* 13:195, 1995.

McKennis AT: Caring for the Islamic patient, *AORN J* 69(6): 1185–1189, 1191, 1194–1196, 1199–1200, 1202, 1205–1206, 1995.

Rassoul GH: The crescent and Islam: healing, nursing and the spiritual dimension, *J Adv Nurs* 32(6):1476, 2000.

Rein A and others: Advance directive decision making among medical inpatients, *J Prof Nurs* 12(1):39, 1996.

Schwartz E: Jewish Americans. In Giger JN, Davidhizer RE: *Transcultural nursing: assessment & interventions,* ed 4, St. Louis, 2003, Mosby.

Schwarz JK: Assisted dying and nursing practice, *Image J Nurs Sch* 31(4):367, 1999.

Tarzian AJ: Caring for dying patients who have air hunger, *Image J Nurs Sch* 32:137, 2000.

Travis SS and others: Terminal restlessness in the nursing facility: assessment, palliation, and symptom management, *Geriatr Nurs* 22(6):308, 2001.

Watts T, Jenkins K: Palliative care nurses' feelings about death rattle, *J Clin Nurs* 8(5):615, 1999.

Research References

Butticaz G and others: Evaluation of a nystatin-containing mouth rinse for terminally ill patients in palliative care, *J Palliat Care* 19(2):95, 2003.

Cadd A and others: Assessment and documentation of bowel management in palliative care: incorporating patient preferences into the care regimen, *J Clin Nurs* 9(2):228, 2000.

Hanson LC and others: What is wrong with end of life care? Opinions of bereaved family members, *J Am Geriatr Soc* 45:1339, 1997.

Murray MA and others: Women's decision-making needs regarding place of care at end of life, *J Palliat Care* 19(3):176, 2003.

Quill TE and others: Palliative options of last resort: a comparison of voluntarily stopping eating and drinking, terminal sedation, physician-assisted suicide, and voluntary active euthanasia, *JAMA* 278:2099, 1997.

Schneiderman LJ and others: Effect of offering advance directives on medical treatments and costs, *Ann Intern Med* 117:599, 1992.

Stajduhar KI: Examining the perspectives of family members involved in the delivery of palliative care at home, *J Palliat Care* 19(1):27, 2003.

Steinhauser KE and others: Factors considered important at the end of life by patients, family, physicians, and other care providers, *JAMA* 284:2476, 2000.

Tilden VP and others: Decisions about life sustaining treatment: impact of physicians' behaviors on the family, *Arch Intern Med* 155:633, 1995.

Tilden VP and others: Family decision-making to withdraw life-sustaining treatments from hospitalized patients, *Nurs Res* 50(2):105, 2001.

Tolle and others: Family reports of barriers to optimal care of the dying, *Nurs Res* 49(6):310, 2000.

Yick AG, Gupta R: Chinese cultural dimensions of death, dying, and bereavement: focus group findings, *J Cult Divers* 9(2):32, 2002.

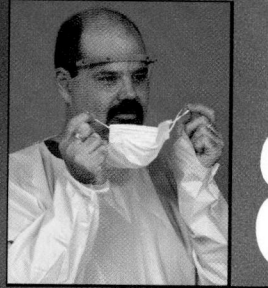

8

Medical Asepsis

8-1   Hand Hygiene

8-2   Caring for Clients Under Isolation
        Precautions

MEDIA RESOURCES

Evolve Site *evolve*
http://evolve.elsevier.com/Perry/skills
- Weblinks
- Video clips
- Mosby's Nursing Skills Video Exercises

Mosby's Nursing Skills Videos/CD-ROM
- *Basic Principles Video:* Medical asepsis, the chain of
  infection and handwashing

OBJECTIVES

Mastery of content in this chaper will enable the nurse to:

- Discuss how critical thinking applies in the prevention of the transmission of infection.
- Explain the difference between medical and surgical asepsis.
- Identify nursing care measures intended to break the chain of infection.
- Explain how each element of the infection chain contributes to infection.
- Describe factors that can influence nursing staff compliance with hand hygiene.
- Perform proper procedures for hand hygiene.
- Perform correct isolation techniques.

KEY TERMS

Asepsis	Medical asepsis
Aseptic technique	Microorganism
Colonized	Nosocomial infection
Contamination	Pathogen
Immunocompromised	Standard precautions
Infection	Surgical asepsis
Invasive procedure	Transmission-based precautions
Isolation	

Infection control practices that reduce and/or eliminate sources and transmission of infection help to protect clients and health care providers from disease. Clients in all health care settings, but particularly in acute and ambulatory care, are at risk for acquiring infections because of lower resistance to infectious microorganisms, exposure to an increased number of and more types of disease-causing organisms, and the performance of invasive procedures. Nosocomial infections are those that develop as a result of a stay or visit in a health care facility, and the infection was not present or incubating at the time of admission (Garner, 2002). A hospital is one of the most likely settings for acquiring a nosocomial infection because of staff, clients, and environmental factors that support a high population of virulent strains of microorganisms that are resistant to antibiotics. Most nosocomial infections are transmitted by health care workers and clients as a result of direct contact during the delivery of care activities.

In all settings, clients and their families must be able to recognize sources of infection and be able to institute protective measures. Nurses are in a position to influence positively others' behavior and to change their own behavior through health education. Client and family teaching should include information concerning signs and symptoms of infections, modes of transmission, and methods of prevention.

Although protection of the client is an obvious priority, nurses are at risk for contact with infectious materials or exposure to a communicable disease. Knowledge of the infectious process and disease transmission and critical thinking skills associated with use of aseptic techniques and barrier protection cannot be overemphasized. The nurse must use judgment when caring for any client who has the risk of acquiring or transmitting an infection. The nurse must know the infectious organism and how it is transmitted, the actions needed to protect the client, and the steps to take to ensure protection from exposure to the microorganism. Today's nurse plays a vital role in the prevention and control of infections.

The mere presence of a pathogen does not mean that an infection will begin. Development of an infection occurs in a cyclical process that depends on the following six elements:

1. An infectious agent or pathogen
2. A reservoir or source for pathogen growth
3. A portal of exit from the reservoir
4. A mode of transmission
5. A portal of entry to the host
6. A susceptible host

An infection develops if this chain remains intact (Figure 8-1). Nurses use infection control practices to break an element of the chain so that infection will not be transmitted (Table 8-1). The nurse's efforts to minimize the onset and spread of infection are based upon asepsis and the principles of aseptic technique. Asepsis is defined as the absence of pathogenic (disease-producing) microorganisms (DeCastro, 2002). The two types of aseptic technique the nurse practices are medical and surgical asepsis.

Medical asepsis, or clean technique, includes procedures used to reduce the number of and prevent the spread of microorganisms. Hand hygiene, barrier techniques, and routine environmental cleaning are examples of medical asepsis. Principles of medical asepsis are commonly followed in the home, as in the case of washing hands before preparing food.

Surgical asepsis, or sterile technique, includes procedures used to eliminate all microorganisms from an area. Sterilization destroys all microorganisms and their spores (Rutala, 1996). Nurses in the operating room (OR), labor and delivery, and procedural areas practice sterile technique where sterile instruments and supplies are used. The techniques used in maintaining surgical asepsis are more rigid than those performed under medical asepsis (see Chapter 9).

Evidenced-Based Practice Trends

For generations, hand washing with soap and water has been considered the best method to prevent transmission of infection from health care workers to clients. In 1846, Ignaz Semmelweis observed that cleansing contaminated hands with an antiseptic agent between client contacts apparently reduced transmission of contagious diseases. Researchers have recently shown, however, that hand washing with plain

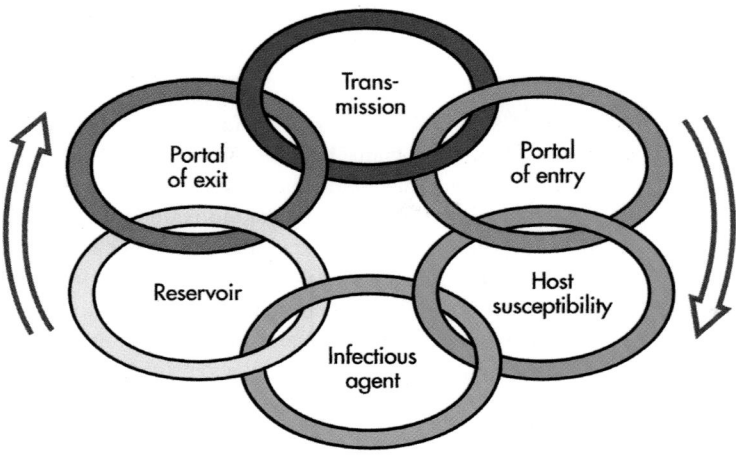

FIGURE **8-1** Chain of infection.

TABLE 8-1   BREAKING THE CHAIN OF INFECTION

Element of Infection Chain	Medical Aseptic Practices
Infectious agent (pathogenic organism capable of causing disease)	Cleanse contaminated objects. Perform cleaning, disinfection, and sterilization.
Reservoir (site or source of microorganism growth)	Control sources of body fluids and drainage. Perform hand hygiene. Bathe client with soap and water. Change soiled dressings. Dispose of soiled tissues, dressings, or linen in moisture-resistant bags. Place syringes, uncapped hypodermic needles, and intravenous needles in designated puncture-proof containers. Keep table surfaces clean and dry. Do not leave bottled solutions open for prolonged periods. Keep solutions tightly capped. Keep surgical wound drainage tubes and collection bags patent. Empty and dispose of drainage suction bottles according to agency policy.

Portal of exit (means by which microorganisms leave a site)	Respiratory
	    Avoid talking, sneezing, or coughing directly over wound or sterile dressing field.
	    Cover nose and mouth when sneezing or coughing.
	    Wear mask if suffering respiratory tract infection.
	Urine, feces, emesis, and blood
	    Wear disposable gloves when handling blood and body fluids.
	    Wear gowns and eyewear if there is a chance of splashing fluids.
	    Handle all laboratory specimens as if infectious.

Transmission (means of spread)	Reduce microorganism spread
	    Perform hand hygiene.
	    Use personal set of care items for each client.
	    Avoid shaking bed linen or clothes; dust with damp cloth.
	    Avoid contact of soiled item with uniform.
	    Discard any item that touches the floor.
	    Follow standard precautions or select transmission-based isolation precautions.

Portal of entry (site through which microorganism enters a host)	Skin and mucosa
	    Maintain skin and mucous membrane integrity, lubricate skin, offer frequent hygiene, turn and position.
	    Cover wounds as needed.
	    Clean wound sites thoroughly.
	    Dispose of used needles in puncture-proof container.
	Urinary
	    Keep all drainage systems closed and intact, maintaining downward flow.

Host (client)	Reduce susceptibility to infection.
	    Provide adequate nutrition.
	    Ensure adequate rest.
	    Promote body defenses against infection.
	    Provide immunization.

soap can result in paradoxical increases in bacterial counts on the skin (Centers for Disease Control and Prevention [CDC], 2002). Alcohol-based products have been found to be more effective for standard hand washing or hand antisepsis than soap or antiseptic soaps (CDC, 2002). Moreover, in several prospective trials, alcohol-based rinses or gels containing emollients caused substantially less skin irritation and dryness than plain or antimicrobial soaps tested. Soap and water is still necessary for hand hygiene if hands are visibly soiled (CDC, 2002). Studies have shown that health care workers with chipped nail polish or artificial nails had higher numbers of bacteria on their fingertips than those without artificial nails. For this reason, the CDC recommends artificial nails and extenders not be worn when working with high-risk clients (CDC, 2002).

Skill Performance Guidelines

1. Remember that hand hygiene using an appropriate alcohol-based instant hand antiseptic or soap and water is an essential part of client care and infection prevention.
2. Always know a client's susceptibility to infection. Age, nutritional status, stress, disease processes, and forms of medical therapy can place clients at risk.
3. Recognize the elements of the chain of infection, and initiate measures to prevent the onset and spread of infection.
4. Incorporate consistently the basic principles of asepsis into client care.
5. Protect fellow health care workers from exposure to infectious agents through proper use and disposal of equipment.
6. Be aware of body sites where nosocomial infections are most likely to develop (e.g., urinary or respiratory tract). This enables the nurse to direct preventive measures.

SKILL 8-1 Hand Hygiene

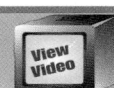

The most important and most basic technique in preventing and controlling transmission of infection is hand hygiene. Hand hygiene is a general term that applies to either hand washing, antiseptic hand wash, antiseptic hand rub, or surgical hand antisepsis. Hand washing refers to washing hands with plain soap and water. An antiseptic hand wash is defined as washing hands with water and soap or other detergents containing an antiseptic agent. An antiseptic hand rub means to apply an antiseptic hand rub product to all surfaces of the hands to reduce the number of microorganisms present. Surgical hand antisepsis is an antiseptic hand wash or antiseptic hand rub performed preoperatively by surgical personnel to eliminate transient and reduce resident hand flora. Antiseptic detergent preparations often have persistent antimicrobial activity (CDC, 2002).

Contaminated hands are a prime cause of transmission of infection. For example, a nurse caring for a client who has excessive pulmonary secretions assists the client in expectorating mucus and disposes of the tissues in a bedside container. The client's roommate asks the nurse to open containers of food on the meal tray. The nurse then leaves the client's room to pour a dose of medication due in 5 minutes. If the nurse fails to perform hand hygiene before each of these actions, organisms from the first client's mucus could easily be transmitted to the roommate's food and to the medication container. Unfortunately, health care workers function in a busy environment. Client care activities are fast paced. With an increased workload, frequent interruptions in care activity, and sometimes limited access to sinks, hand-washing compliance can be a problem. Nishimura and others (1999) have found that hand-washing compliance among intensive care unit (ICU) personnel is low. After videotaping staff as they entered the ICU, the researchers found only 71% of ICU personnel washed their hands before beginning client care. *Hand hygiene is not optional*. It is a critical responsibility for all health care workers.

When hands are visibly dirty or contaminated with proteinaceous material or visibly soiled with blood or other body fluids, hands should be washed with either a nonantimicrobial soap and water or an antimicrobial soap and water. If hands are not visibly soiled, an alcohol-based hand rub should be used for routinely decontaminating hands in the following situations:

1. Before having direct contact with clients
2. Before putting on sterile gloves and before inserting indwelling urinary catheters, peripheral vascular catheters, or other invasive devices
3. After contact with a client's intact skin (for example, when taking a pulse or blood pressure, and lifting a client)
4. After contact with body fluids or excretions, mucous membranes, nonintact skin, and wound dressings *if hands are not visibly soiled*
5. When moving from a contaminated body site to a clean body site during care
6. After contact with inanimate objects (including medical equipment) in the immediate vicinity of the client
7. After removing gloves (CDC, 2002)

Hands may also be washed with an antimicrobial soap and water in these situations.

DELEGATION CONSIDERATIONS

Hand hygiene is a basic procedure that should be performed correctly by all caregivers. When nurses observe assistive personnel, physicians or therapists, and family caregivers incorrectly perform hand hygiene, they should reinforce the importance of the technique and the correct procedural steps.

EQUIPMENT

- ❏ Alcohol-based waterless antiseptic containing emollients
- ❏ Easy-to-reach sink with warm running water
- ❏ Antimicrobial or regular soap
- ❏ Paper towels or air dryer
- ❏ Clean orangewood stick (optional)

STEP	RATIONALE

ASSESSMENT

1. Inspect surface of hands for breaks or cuts in skin or cuticles. Note condition of nails. Artificial nails and long or unkempt nails should be avoided. Report and cover any skin lesions before providing client care.
2. Inspect hands for visible soiling.
3. Inspect nails for length and presence of artificial nails or extenders.

Open cuts or wounds can harbor high concentrations of microorganisms. Agency policy may prevent nurse from caring for high-risk clients if open lesions are present on hands or if artificial or long nails are worn (CDC, 2002).

Visible soiling requires hand washing with soap and water.

Long nails and chipped or old polish increase number of bacteria residing on nails, requiring more vigorous hand hygiene. Artificial nails may increase the microbial load on hands (CDC, 2002).

NURSING DIAGNOSES

This skill is required for clients having a variety of nursing diagnoses.

PLANNING

1. Expected outcomes following completion of procedure:
   - Hands and areas under fingernails are clean and free of debris.

Transient bacteria have been removed.

IMPLEMENTATION

1. Push wristwatch and long uniform sleeves above wrists. Avoid wearing rings. If worn, remove during washing.

2. Hand antisepsis using an instant alcohol waterless antiseptic rub
   a. Dispense ample amount of product into palm of one hand (see illustration).
   b. Rub hands together, covering all surfaces of hands and fingers with antiseptic (see illustration).

Provides complete access to fingers, hands, and wrists. Wearing of rings increases number of microorganisms on hands (Garner, 1995).

Enough product is needed to thoroughly cover the hands.

Provides enough time for product to work.

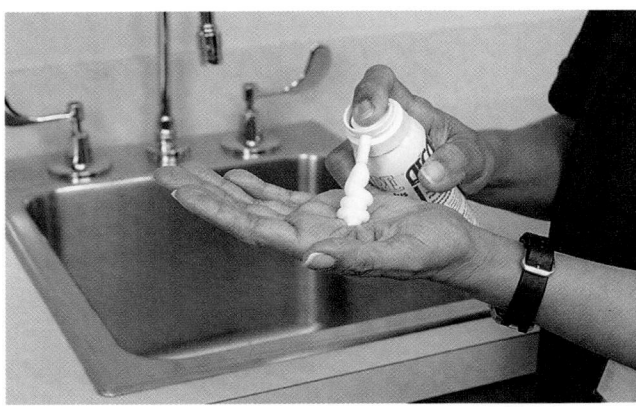

STEP **2a** Apply waterless antiseptic to hands.

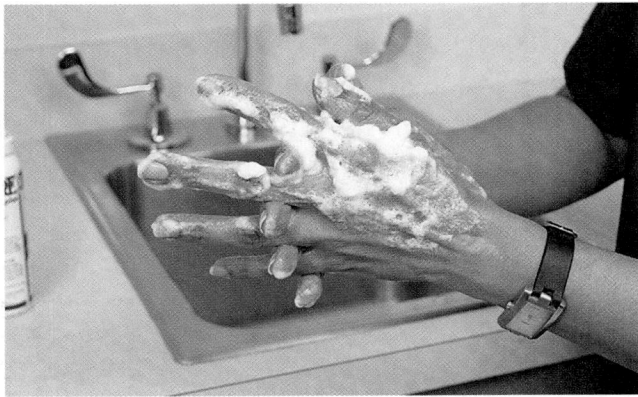

STEP **2b** Rub hands thoroughly.

STEP	RATIONALE

   c. Rub hands together until the alcohol is dry. Allow hands to completely dry before applying gloves.

Ensures complete antimicrobial action.

3. Hand washing using plain or antimicrobial soap and water

   a. Be sure fingernails are short, filed, and smooth.

Many microorganisms on hands come from the subungual region (beneath the fingernails).

   b. Stand in front of sink, keeping hands and uniform away from sink surface. (If hands touch sink during hand washing, repeat.)

Inside of sink is a contaminated area. Reaching over sink increases risk of touching edge, which is contaminated.

   c. Turn on water. Turn faucet on (see illustration), or push knee pedals laterally, or press pedals with foot to regulate flow and temperature.

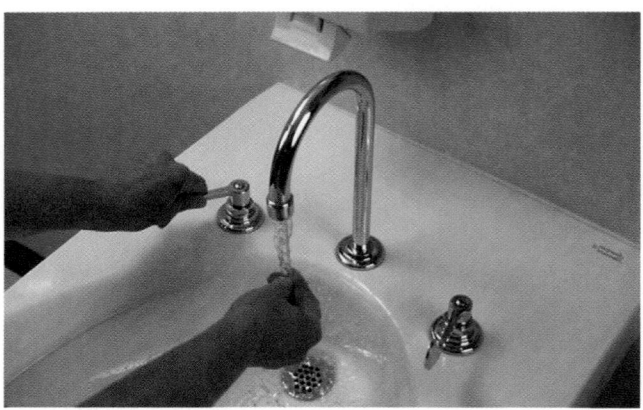

STEP **3c** Turning on water.

   d. Avoid splashing water against uniform.

Microorganisms travel and grow in moisture.

   e. Regulate flow of water so that temperature is warm.

Warm water removes less of the protective oils on hands than hot water.

   f. Wet hands and wrists thoroughly under running water. Keep hands and forearms lower than elbows during washing

Hands are the most contaminated parts to be washed. Water flows from least to most contaminated area, rinsing microorganisms into sink.

   g. Apply a small amount of soap or antiseptic, lathering thoroughly (see illustration). Soap granules and leaflet preparations may be used.

The use of antiseptic exclusively can be drying to the hands and cause skin irritations.

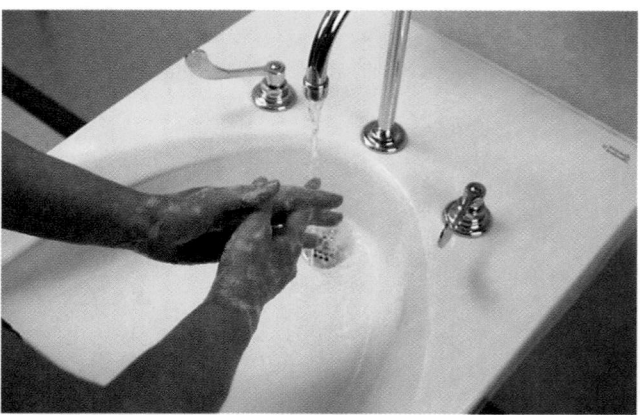

STEP **3g** Lathering hands thoroughly.

• Critical Decision Point

The decision whether to use an antiseptic or not should be dependent on the procedure to be performed and the client's immune status.

STEP	RATIONALE

h. Perform hand hygiene using plenty of lather and friction for at least 10 to 15 seconds. Interlace fingers and rub palms and back of hands with circular motion at least 5 times each. Keep fingertips down to facilitate removal of microorganisms.

Soap cleanses by emulsifying fat and oil and lowering surface tension. Friction and rubbing mechanically loosen and remove dirt and transient bacteria. Interlacing fingers and thumbs ensures that all surfaces are cleansed.

i. Areas underlying fingernails are often soiled. Clean them with the fingernails of other hand and additional soap, or clean with an orangewood stick.

Area under nails can be highly contaminated, which will increase the risk for transmission of infection from the nurse to the client.

• ***Critical Decision Point***
Do not tear or cut skin under or around nail.

j. Rinse hands and wrists thoroughly, keeping hands down and elbows up (see illustration).

Rinsing mechanically washes away dirt and microorganisms.

k. Dry hands thoroughly from fingers to wrists and forearms with paper towel, single-use cloth, or warm air dryer.

Drying from cleanest (fingertips) to least clean (forearms) area avoids contamination. Drying hands prevents chapping and roughened skin.

l. If used, discard paper towel in proper receptacle.

Prevents transfer of microorganisms.

m. To turn off hand faucet, use clean, dry paper towel, avoiding touching handles with hands (see illustration). Turn off water with foot or knee pedals (if applicable).

Wet towel and hands allow transfer of pathogens from the faucet by capillary action.

n. Apply lotion to hands. Use the facility-provided lotion if one is provided.

Helps to minimize skin dryness. The provided lotion will be compatible with antimicrobial soaps and latex.

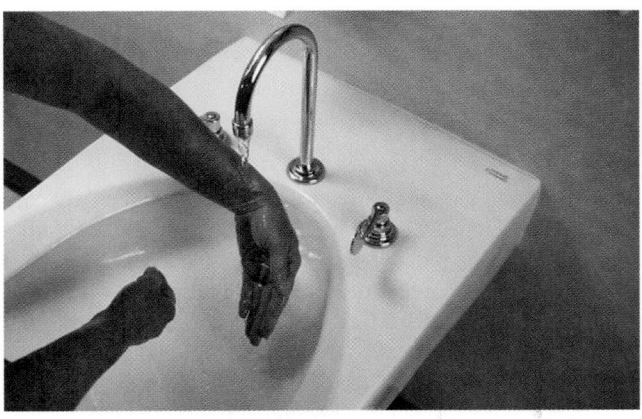

STEP 3j Rinsing hands.

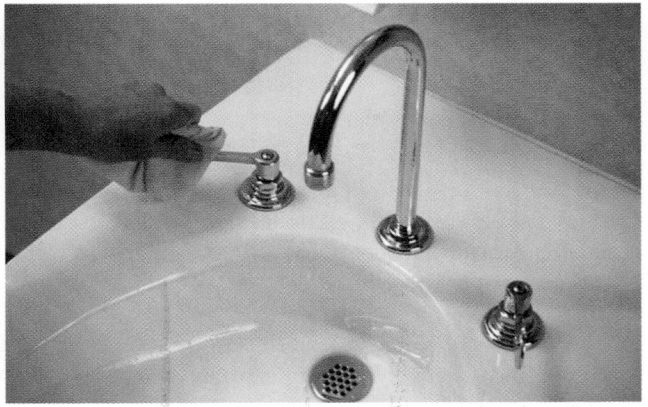

STEP 3m Turning off faucet.

▌EVALUATION

1. Inspect surface of hands for obvious signs of dirt or other contaminants.

Determines if hand washing is adequate.

Recording and Reporting

• It is not necessary to record or report this procedure.
• Report any dermatitis to employee health and/or infection control per your agency's policy.

Unexpected Outcomes	Related Interventions
1. Hands or areas under fingernails remain soiled.	• Nurse must repeat hand washing with soap and water.
2. Repeated use of soaps or antiseptic may cause dermatitis or cracked skin.	• Requires methods to alleviate complications of hand hygiene: Use the alcohol-based hand antiseptic rub whenever hands are not visibly soiled. Rinse and dry hands thoroughly after using soap and water, avoid excessive amounts of soap or antiseptic; try various products. Use hand lotions or barrier creams (small individual-use containers are preferred because large containers have been found to harbor pathogens).

Teaching Considerations

* Instruct the client and family caregiver in proper techniques and situations for hand hygiene.
* Clients are aware of the importance of hand hygiene (McGuckin and others, 1999). It has been shown that when clients are educated about the risks of infection in hospitals, they can play an important role in improving hand hygiene compliance by reminding health care workers to perform hand hygiene.

Gerontological Considerations

* The impact of infections is much greater in older adults. This is especially true in older adult day care centers, where incidence of acute respiratory infection is high.

Hand hygiene by staff attending older adults is of utmost importance and should be an ongoing continuing education requirement (Falsey, 1999).

Home Care Considerations

* Evaluate client and primary caregiver to determine their understanding of the transmission of microorganisms and their ability and motivation to perform hand hygiene according to medical asepsis.
* Evaluate the hand hygiene facilities in the home to determine the possibility of contamination, proximity of the facilities to the client, and the ability to maintain supplies and equipment.

SKILL 8-2 Caring for Clients Under Isolation Precautions

There is a risk of transmitting nosocomial infection or infectious disease among clients or health care workers. When a client has a known source of infection, health care workers follow specific infection control practices and take preventive actions.

The majority of organisms causing nosocomial infections are found in the colonized body substances of clients, regardless of whether or not a culture has confirmed infection and a diagnosis has been made (Jackson and Lynch, 1992). Body substances such as feces, urine, mucus, and wound drainage can contain potentially infectious organisms.

Isolation or barrier precautions include the appropriate use of gowns, masks, eyewear, and other protective devices or clothing. Nurses should assess the need for barrier precautions for each task they plan and for all clients regardless of their diagnoses (Lynch, 1995). Because of increased attention to the prevention of blood-borne pathogens and tuberculosis (TB), the Centers for Disease Control and Prevention (CDC) (1988, 1994) and the Occupational Safety and Health Administration (OSHA) (1994, 2001) have stressed the importance of barrier protection.

In 1996 the Hospital Infection Control Practice Advisory Committee (HICPAC) of the CDC published revised guidelines for isolation precautions. These recommendations were based on current epidemiological information regarding disease transmission in hospitals. Although primarily intended for care of clients in acute care, the recommendations can be applied to clients in subacute care or long-term care facilities. HICPAC recommended that hospitals modify the recommendations according to their needs and as dictated by federal, state, or local regulations (CDC, 1996; Garner, 1995).

The new guidelines contained two tiers of precautions. The first and most important tier (Box 8-1) is called standard precautions and is designed for care of all clients regardless of risk or presumed infection status. Standard precautions are the primary strategies for prevention of infection transmission. Standard precautions apply to contact with (1) blood, (2) body fluids, (3) nonintact skin, and (4) mucous membranes.

The second tier (Table 8-2) includes precautions designed for care of clients who are known or suspected to be infected, or colonized, with microorganisms transmitted by droplets, by airborne route, or by contact with contaminated

BOX 8-1   Standard Precautions (Tier One)* for Use With All Clients

- Standard precautions apply to blood, all body fluids, secretions, excretions, nonintact skin, and mucous membranes.
- Hand hygiene is performed if contaminated with blood or body fluid, immediately after gloves are removed, between client contact, and when indicated to prevent transfer of microorganisms between clients or between clients and environment.
- Gloves are worn when touching blood, body fluid, secretions, excretions, nonintact skin, mucous membranes, or contaminated items. Gloves should be removed and hand hygiene performed between client care encounters.
- Masks, eye protection, or face shields are worn if client care activities may generate splashes or sprays of blood or body fluid.
- Gowns are worn if soiling of clothing is likely from blood or body fluid. Perform hand hygiene after removing gown.

- Client care equipment is properly cleaned and reprocessed, and single-use items are discarded.
- Contaminated linen is placed in leakproof bag and is handled to prevent skin and mucous membrane exposure.
- All sharp instruments and needles are discarded in a puncture-resistant container. OSHA recommends that needles be disposed of uncapped or a mechanical device be used for recapping. Sharps with built-in safety features must be used when available, and these safety features must be activated after use.
- A private room is unnecessary unless the client's hygiene is unacceptable. Check with infection control professional.

Modified from Centers for Disease Control and Prevention, Hospital Infection Control Practice Advisory Committee: Guidelines for isolation precautions in hospitals, *Am J Infect Control* 24:24, 1996.
*Formerly universal precautions and body substance isolation.

TABLE 8-2   TRANSMISSION CATEGORIES (TIER TWO) (FOR USE WITH CLIENTS INFECTED OR COLONIZED WITH SPECIFIC ORGANISMS)

Category	Disease	Barrier Protection
Airborne precautions	For diseases transmitted by small droplet nuclei (smaller than 5 μm), such as measles, chickenpox, disseminated varicella zoster, pulmonary or laryngeal TB.*	Private room, negative airflow of at least six air exchanges per hour; respirator or mask.*
Droplet precautions	For diseases transmitted by large droplets (larger than 5 μm), such as streptococcal pharyngitis, pneumonia, and scarlet fever in infants or small children, pertussis, mumps, meningococcal pneumonia or sepsis, pneumonic plague.	Private room or cohort client; mask when closer than 3 ft from client.
Contact precautions	For diseases transmitted by direct client or environmental contact, such as colonization or infection with multidrug-resistant organisms, respiratory syncytial virus, major wound infections, herpes simplex, scabies.	Private room or cohort client; gloves, gowns.

Modified from Centers for Disease Control and Prevention, Hospital Infection Control Practice Advisory Committee: Guidelines for isolation precautions in hospitals, *Am J Infect Control* 24:24, 1996.
*See CDC TB guidelines.

surfaces or dry skin. The three types of transmission-based precautions—airborne, droplet, and contact—may be combined for diseases that have multiple routes of transmission, for example, chickenpox. When used either singly or in combination, they are to be used in addition to standard precautions when required by the specific infection or colonization with a specific organism. Box 8-2 summarizes the tiers of precautions and the types of clients requiring their use.

When a client requires isolation in a private room, the nurse must remember that loneliness can easily develop. Isolation disrupts normal social relationships with visitors

and caregivers. A client who suffers from an infectious disease may also experience self-concept or body image changes. When a client from another culture requires isolation, extra caution must be used to be sure the client and family understand the therapeutic purpose of isolation. For example, the isolation of a loved one is considered disrespectful and uncaring behavior in many collectivistic cultures (Hispanics, Africans, and Asians) (Mashaba, 2002).Unless the nurse acts to minimize feelings of psychological and physical isolation, the client's emotional state can interfere with recovery.

BOX 8-2   Synopsis of Types of Precautions of Clients Requiring the Precautions*

STANDARD PRECAUTIONS

Use Standard Precautions for the care of all clients

AIRBORNE PRECAUTIONS

In addition to Standard Precautions, use Airborne Precautions for clients known or suspected to have serious illnesses transmitted by airborne droplet nuclei. Examples of such illnesses include:
(1) Measles
(2) Varicella (including disseminated zoster)*
(3) Tuberculosis†

DROPLET PRECAUTIONS

In addition to Standard Precautions, use Droplet Precautions for clients known or suspected to have serious illnesses transmitted by large particle droplets. Examples of such illnesses include:
(1) Invasive *Haemophilus influenzae* type b disease, including meningitis, pneumonia, epiglottitis, and sepsis
(2) Invasive *Neisseria meningitidis* disease, including meningitis, pneumonia, and sepsis
(3) Other serious bacterial respiratory infections spread by droplet transmission, including:
  (a) Diphtheria (pharyngeal)
  (b) Mycoplasma pneumonia
  (c) Pertussis
  (d) Pneumonic plague
  (e) Streptococcal pharyngitis, pneumonia, or scarlet fever in infants and young children
(4) Serious viral infections spread by droplet transmission, including:
  (a) Adenovirus*
  (b) Influenza
  (c) Mumps
  (d) Parvovirus B 19
  (e) Rubella

CONTACT PRECAUTIONS

In addition to Standard Precautions, use Contact Precautions for clients known or suspected to have serious illnesses easily transmitted by direct client contact or by contact with items in the client's environment. Examples of such illnesses include:
(1) Gastrointestinal, respiratory, skin, or wound infections or colonization with multidrug-resistant bacteria judged by the infection control program, based on current state, regional, or national recommendations, to be of special clinical and epidemiologic significance
(2) Enteric with a low infectious dose or prolonged environmental survival, including:
  (a) *Clostridium difficile*
  (b) For diapered or incontinent clients: enterohemorrhagic *Escherichia coli* 0157:H7, *Shigella,* hepatitis A, or rotavirus
(3) Respiratory syncytial virus, parainfluenza virus, or enteroviral infections in infants and young children
(4) Skin infections that are highly contagious or that may occur on dry skin, including:
  (a) Diphtheria (cutaneous)
  (b) Herpes simplex virus (neonatal or mucocutaneous)
  (c) Impetigo
  (d) Major (noncontained) abscesses, cellulitis, or decubiti
  (e) Pediculosis
  (f) Scabies
  (g) Staphylococcal furunculosis in infants and young children
  (h) Zoster (disseminated or in the immunocompromised host)*
(5) Viral/hemorrhagic conjunctivitis
(6) Viral hemorrhagic infections (Ebola, Lassa, or Marburg)

From Centers for Disease Control and Prevention, Hospital Infection Control Practice Advisory Committee: Guidelines for isolation precautions in hospitals, *Am J Infect Control* 24:24, 1996.
*Certain infections require more than one type of precaution.
†See CDC *Guidelines for Preventing the Transmission of Tuberculosis in Health-Care Facilities.*

DELEGATION CONSIDERATIONS

The skill of caring for clients under isolation precautions can be delegated to assistive personnel.
• Review with care provider the nature and type of infection a client has.
• Warn care provider of high-risk factors for infection transmission that pertain to assigned client.

EQUIPMENT

❑ Disposable gloves, mask, eyewear or goggles, and gown
❑ Other client care equipment (as appropriate)
❑ Soiled linen and trash receptacle

STEP	RATIONALE

ASSESSMENT

1. Assess client, and review medical history for possible indications for isolation, for example, risk factors for TB, major draining wound, or purulent productive cough. Review the precautions necessary for the specific isolation system.

Mode of transmission for infectious microorganism determines type and degree of precautions followed.

2. Review laboratory test results.

Informs nurse of type of microorganism for which client is being isolated, body fluid in which it was identified, and whether client is immunosuppressed.

STEP	RATIONALE

3. Consider types of care measures to be performed while in client's room (e.g., medication administration or dressing change).

Enables nurse to organize care items for procedures and time spent in client's room.

4. Review nursing care plan notes, or confer with colleagues regarding client's emotional state and reaction/adjustment to isolation.

Determines client's need for emotional support and teaching.

5. Determine from nursing care plan, medical record, or significant other if client and family understand the purpose of isolation or procedures to anticipate.

Determines client's level of knowledge and need for instruction/reinforcement.

6. Before applying latex gloves, assess if the client has a known latex allergy (see Chapter 9).

Client with latex allergy can have a serious allergic or sensitivity reaction even after brief exposure to gloves.

NURSING DIAGNOSES

- Ineffective protection
- Deficient knowledge regarding purpose of isolation
- Impaired social interaction
- Risk for infection

Related factors are individualized based on client's condition or needs.

PLANNING

1. Expected outcomes following completion of procedure:
   - Client spontaneously engages in discussions with nurse and family.
   - Client asks for information about disease transmission.

Active interaction reveals client's willingness and/or ability to communicate and to be taught and to understand information.

   - Client explains purpose of isolation.

Instruction about precautions improves client's ability to cooperate in care.

IMPLEMENTATION

1. Perform hand hygiene (see Skill 8-1).

Reduces transmission of microorganisms.

2. Prepare all equipment needed to be taken into client's room.

Prevents nurse from making more than one trip into room.

3. Determine appropriate barriers to apply based upon isolation category and activities to be performed for client.

Ensures adequate protection to prevent transmission of infection.

4. Prepare for entrance into isolation room. Choice of barrier protection depends on type of isolation and facility policy (see Table 8-2). For example, if client is on airborne precautions, apply only a special mask and keep room door closed.

Proper preparation ensures nurse is protected from microorganism exposure.

   a. Apply either surgical mask or a fitted respirator around mouth and nose (type and fit-testing will depend on type of isolation and facility policy).

Prevents exposure to airborne microorganisms or exposure to microorganisms from splashing of fluids.

   b. Apply eyewear or goggles snugly around face and eyes (when needed).

Protects nurse from exposure to microorganisms that may occur during splashing of fluids.

   c. Apply gown, being sure it covers all outer garments. Pull sleeves down to wrist. Tie securely at neck and waist (see illustration).

Prevents transmission of infection when client has excessive drainage, discharges.

   d. Apply disposable gloves. (NOTE: A latex-free environment should be provided if the client or the health care worker has a latex allergy.) If gloves are worn with gown, bring glove cuffs over edge of gown sleeves.

Reduces transmission of microorganisms.

5. Enter client's room. Arrange supplies and equipment.

Prevents extra trips entering and leaving room.

STEP	RATIONALE

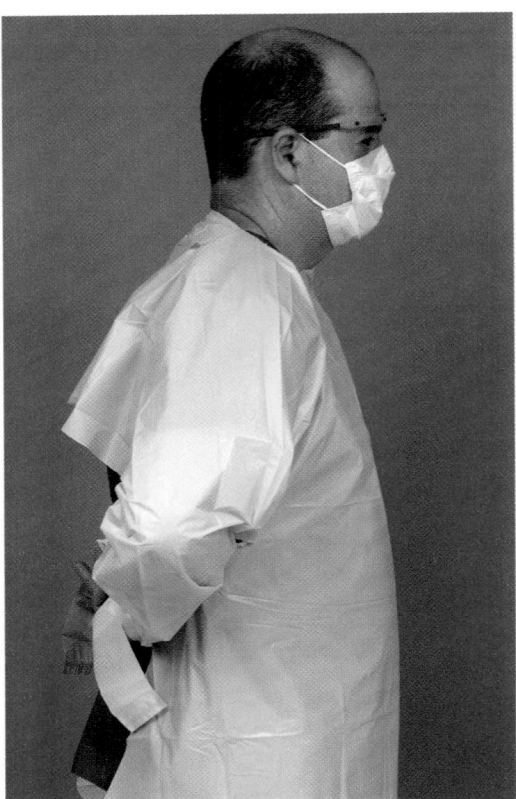

STEP **4c** Nurse with protective equipment for contact and droplet infection.

6. Explain purpose of isolation and precautions necessary to client and family. Offer opportunity to ask questions. Assess for emotions that may be related to the isolation, such as loneliness or boredom, and for signs/symptoms of depression, for example, lack of appetite or difficulty sleeping.

Improves client's and family's ability to participate in care and minimizes anxiety.

7. Assess vital signs.
  a. If the client is infected or colonized with a resistant organism (e.g., vancomycin-resistant enterococci [VRE] or methicillin-resistant *Staphylococcus aureus* [MRSA]), equipment taken into the room remains in the room or is thoroughly disinfected when removed from the room (see agency policy).

Prevents cross contamination to other clients.

  b. Avoid contact of stethoscope or blood pressure cuff with infective material. Wipe off with disinfectant as needed.

If used later on other clients, increases risk of infection being transmitted.

  c. If stethoscope is to be reused, clean diaphragm or bell with 70% alcohol or liquid soap. Set aside on clean surface.

Systematic disinfection of stethoscopes with 70% alcohol or liquid soap will minimize chance of spreading infectious agents between clients (Bernard and others, 1999).

  d. Individual or disposable thermometers should be used.

Prevents cross contamination.

8. Administer medications (see Chapters 20 and 21):
  a. Give oral medication in wrapper or cup.

Supplies are handled and discarded to minimize transfer of microorganisms.

STEP	RATIONALE

   b. Dispose of wrapper or cup in plastic-lined receptacle.

   c. Administer injection, being sure gloves are worn.

   Reduces the risk of exposure to blood.

   d. Discard disposable syringe and uncapped or sheathed needle into designated sharps container (see illustration).

   Reduces risk of needle stick injury.

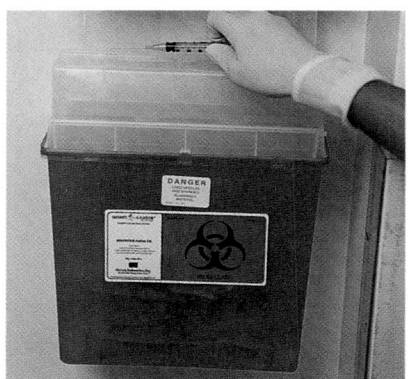

STEP **8d** Disposal of syringes and uncapped needle.

   e. Place reusable plastic syringe (e.g., Carpuject) on clean towel for eventual removal and disinfection.

   Prevents added contamination of syringe.

9. Administer hygiene, encouraging the client to verbalize any questions or concerns regarding isolation. Informal teaching may be done at this time.

   Hygiene practices further minimize transfer of microorganisms.

   a. Avoid allowing isolation gown to become wet; carry wash basin outward away from gown; avoid leaning against wet tabletop.

   Moisture allows organisms to travel through gown to uniform.

● *Critical Decision Point*

   In case of excess soiling, a gown impervious to moisture should be worn.

   b. Assist client in removing own gown; discard in impervious linen bag.

   Reduces transfer of microorganisms.

   c. Remove linen from bed; avoid contact with isolation gown. Place in impervious linen bag.

   Linen soiled by client's body fluids is handled so as to prevent contact with clean items.

   d. Provide clean bed linen and set of towels.

   e. Change gloves and perform hand hygiene if they become excessively soiled and further care is necessary.

10. Collect specimens (see Chapter 43):

   a. Place specimen containers on clean paper towel in client's bathroom.

   Container will be taken out of client's room; prevents contamination of outer surface.

   b. Follow procedure for collecting specimen of body fluids (see Chapter 43).

   c. Transfer specimen to container without soiling outside of container. Place container in a plastic bag, and label the outside of the bag or as per agency policy.

   Specimens of blood and body fluids are placed in well-constructed containers with secure lids to prevent leaks during transport.

   d. Check label on specimen for accuracy. Send to laboratory (warning labels may be used, depending on hospital policy).

STEP	**RATIONALE**

11. Dispose of linen, trash, and disposable items:
    a. Use single bags that are impervious to moisture and sturdy to contain soiled articles. Use double bag if necessary for heavily soiled linen or heavy wet trash.
    b. Tie bags securely at top in knot (see illustration).

Linen or refuse should be totally contained to prevent exposure of personnel to infective material.

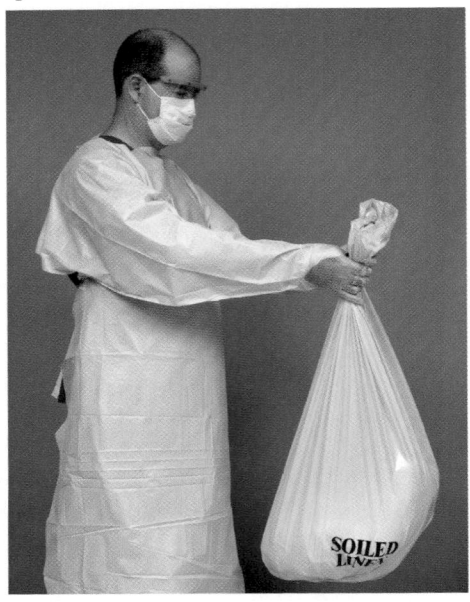

STEP **11b** Secure soiled linen in a waterproof bag.

12. Remove all reusable pieces of equipment. Clean any contaminated surfaces with hospital-approved disinfectant (Bonilla and others, 1996) (see agency policy).

All items must be properly cleaned, disinfected, or sterilized for reuse.

13. Resupply room as needed. Have staff colleague hand new supplies to you.

Limiting trips of personnel into and out of room reduces nurse's and client's exposure to microorganisms. Quality time should be spent with the client when in the room.

14. Leave isolation room. Remember, order of removal of protective barriers depends on what is worn in room. This sequence describes steps to take if all barriers were required to be worn.
    a. Remove gloves. Remove one glove by grasping cuff and pulling glove inside out over hand (see illustration). Discard glove. With ungloved hand, tuck finger inside cuff of remaining glove and pull it off, inside out (see illustration).

Technique prevents nurse from contacting contaminated glove's outer surface.

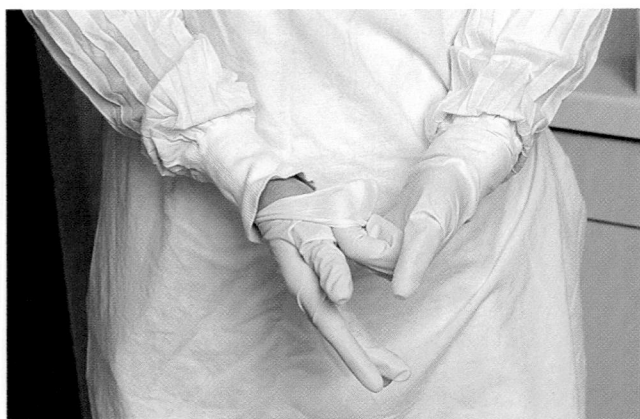
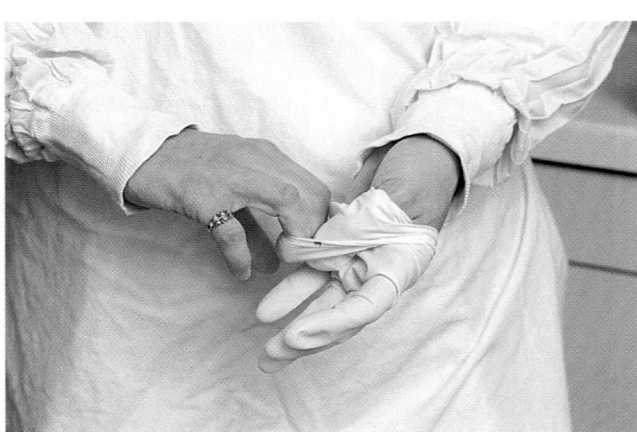

STEP **14a** Removal of gloves.

STEP	**RATIONALE**

b. Remove mask. If the mask secures over the ears, remove elastic from ears, pull mask away from face (see illustration). For a tie-on mask, untie *bottom* mask string and then top strings, pull mask away from face and drop into trash receptacle. (Do not touch outer surface of mask.)

Ungloved hands will not be contaminated by touching only elastic or mask strings. Prevents top part of mask from falling down over nurse's uniform.

c. Untie neck strings, then back strings of gown. Allow gown to fall from shoulders (see illustration). Remove hands from sleeves without touching outside of gown. Hold gown inside at shoulder seams, and fold inside out; discard in laundry bag.

Hands do not come in contact with soiled front of gown.

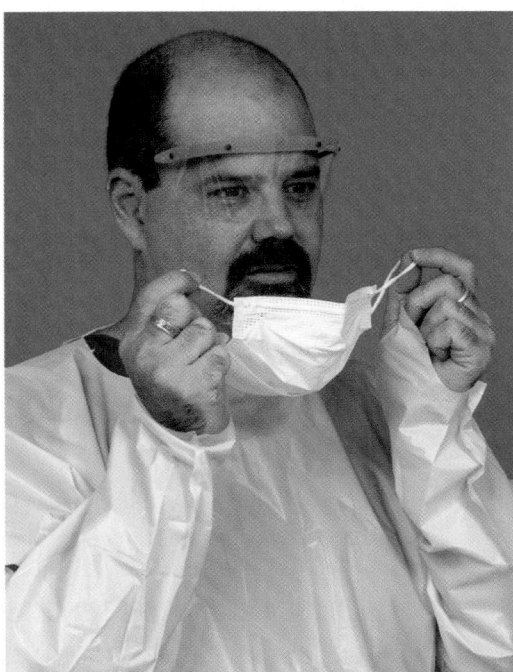

STEP **14b** Nurse removes mask.

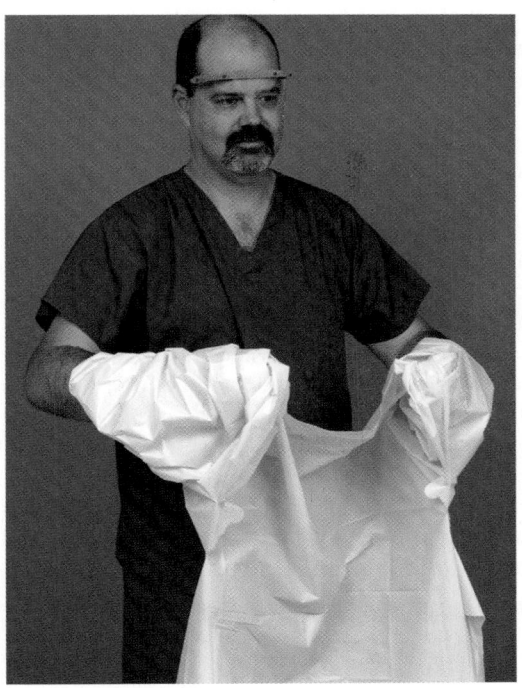

STEP **14c** Nurse removes gown.

d. Remove eyewear or goggles.

Hands have not been soiled.

e. Perform hand hygiene.

Reduces transmission of microorganisms.

f. Retrieve wristwatch and stethoscope (unless it must remain in room), and record vital sign values on notepaper.

Clean hands can contact clean items.

g. Explain to client when you plan to return to room. Ask whether client requires any personal care items. Offer books, magazines, audiotapes.

Diversions help to minimize boredom and feeling of social isolation.

h. Leave room and close door, if necessary. Door should be closed if client is in negative airflow room.

EVALUATION

1. While in room, ask if client has had sufficient opportunity to discuss health problems, course of treatment, or other topics important to client.

Measures client's perception of adequacy of discussions with caregivers.

2. Ask client to describe purpose of isolation and offer chance to ask questions.

Feedback demonstrates learning.

Recording and Reporting

* Document procedures performed and client's response to social isolation in nurses' progress notes. Also document any client education performed and reinforced.

Unexpected Outcomes	Related Interventions
1. Client avoids social and therapeutic discussions.	• Confer with family and/or significant other, and determine best approach to reduce client's sense of loneliness and depression.
2. Client or health care worker may have an allergy to latex gloves.	• Notify physician/employee health, and treat sensitivity or allergic reaction appropriately. • Use latex-free gloves for future care activities.

Teaching Considerations

* Visitors and family members are taught by the nurse how to follow the recommended isolation precautions when visiting client. They are also taught appropriate use of barrier techniques for home caregiving.

Pediatric Considerations

* Isolation creates sense of separation from family and loss of control. Strange environment adds to confusion child feels during isolation. Preschoolers are unable to understand cause-effect relationship for isolation. Older children may be able to understand cause but still fantasize.
* Children require simple explanations, for example, "You need to be in this room to help you get better." All barriers to be used must be shown to child. Parents must be actively involved in any explanations. Nurses let child see their faces before applying masks so that child does not become frightened.

Gerontological Considerations

* Isolation can be a particular concern for older adults, especially those who have signs and symptoms of confusion or depression. Many times clients become more confused when they are confronted with a nurse using barrier precautions or when they are left in a room with the door closed. Nurses must assess need for closing door (negative airflow room) along with safety of client and additional safety measures that may need to be taken.
* Older adults should be assessed for signs of depression such as loss of appetite or decrease in verbal communications. If necessary, this should be brought to attention of health care team for appropriate interventions.

Home Care Considerations

* Although isolation precautions followed in the hospital are not directly applicable to home care, caregivers should be aware of potential sources of contamination in home.

FOCUS on CLINICAL PRACTICE

Joe is assigned to Mr. Nesbitt, a 78-year-old nursing home resident. When Joe enters Mr. Nesbitt's room, he begins to conduct a physical assessment.

1. As Joe turns Mr. Nesbitt to check the condition of his skin, he notices moisture on his own hand. Joe looks more closely and realizes the moisture is from an open, oozing lesion on Mr. Nesbitt's sacral area. What should Joe do next?

2. After assessing the wound, Joe quickly checks the position and function of Mr. Nesbitt's indwelling urinary catheter and then performs hand hygiene before leaving Mr. Nesbitt's room. What method should Joe use for hand hygiene?

3. What elements of the infection chain were intact or broken as a result of Joe's care?

NCLEX REVIEW QUESTIONS

1. An alcohol-based hand rub should be used for hand hygiene:
   1. When soap and water are not available
   2. Only as an alternative to regular hand washing
   3. After contact with the environment close to the client
   4. Only if hands are visibly soiled
2. When placing a client under isolation precautions, it is important to:
   1. Consider that the client may feel lonely and provide opportunity for social interaction
   2. Keep visitors away from the client to avoid contagion
   3. Wear gloves, a gown, and face protection for each encounter
   4. Place the patient in a room with negative airflow for contact precautions
3. The use of a mask when the nurse is closer than 3 feet to a client involves which of the following:
   1. Airborne precautions
   2. Droplet precautions
   3. Contact precautions
   4. Standard precautions

References

Centers for Disease Control: Update: universal precautions for prevention of transmission of human immunodeficiency virus, hepatitis B virus, and other bloodborne pathogens in health care setting, *MMWR Morbid Mortal Wkly Rep* 37(24):377, 1988.

Centers for Disease Control and Prevention: Guidelines for preventing the transmission of *Mycobacterium tuberculosis* in health-care facilities, *Federal Register* 59(208):54242, 1994.

Centers for Disease Control and Prevention, Hospital Infection Control Practice Advisory Committee: Guidelines for isolation precautions in hospitals, *Am J Infect Control* 24:24, 1996.

Centers for Disease Control and Prevention, Hospital Infection Control Practice Advisory Committee and the HICPAC/SHEA/APIC/IDSA Hand Hygiene Task Force: Guideline for hand hygiene in health-care settings, *MMWR Morb Mortal Wkly Rep: Recommendations and Reports* 51(RR16), 2002.

DeCastro M: Aseptic technique. In *APIC text of infection control and epidemiology*, revised 2002, Washington, DC, Association for Professionals in Infection Control and Epidemiology, Inc.

Garner B: Infection control. In Meeker MH, Rothrock JC, editors: *Alexander's care of the patient in surgery*, St. Louis, 1995, Mosby.

Garner J: Isolation systems. In *APIC text of infection control and epidemiology*, revised 2002, Association for Professionals in Infection Control and Epidemiology, Inc.

Jackson M, Lynch P: Body substance isolation, *Infect Control Hosp Epidemiol* 13(14):191, 1992.

Lynch P: Barrier precautions and personal protection. In Soule B and others, editors: *Infections and nursing practices,* St. Louis, 1995, Mosby.

Occupational Safety and Health Administration: Respiratory protection, *Fed Regist* 59(219):58884, 1994.

Occupational Safety and Health Administration: Occupational exposure to bloodborne pathogens; needlesticks and other sharps injuries; final rule, 29 CFR Part 1910, *Fed Regist* 66:5318, 2001.

Rutala W: Disinfection and sterilization of patient-care items, *Infect Control Hosp Epidemiol* 17(6):377, 1996.

Research References

Bernard L and others: Bacterial contamination of hospital physicians' stethoscopes, *Infect Control Hosp Epidemiol* 20(9):626, 1999.

Bonilla HF and others: Long-term survival of vancomycin-resistant *Enterococcus faecium* on a contaminated surface, *Infect Control Hosp Epidemiol* 17(12):770, 1996.

Falsey A and others: Evaluation of a handwashing intervention to reduce respiratory illness rates in senior day-care centers, *Infect Control Hosp Epidemiol* 20(3):200, 1999.

Mashaba G: South African culturally based health-illness patterns and humanistic care practices. In Leininger M, McFarland M: *Transcultural nursing,* New York, 2002, McGraw-Hill.

McGuckin M and others: Patient education model for increasing handwashing compliance, *Am J Infect Control* 27(4):309, 1999.

Nishimura S and others: Handwashing before entering the intensive care unit: what we learned from continuous video-camera surveillance, *Am J Infect Control* 27(4):367, 1999.

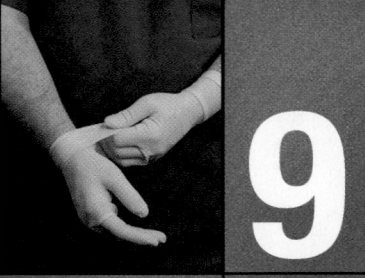

9

Sterile Technique

MEDIA RESOURCES

Evolve Site *evolve*

http://evolve.elsevier.com/Perry/skills
- Weblinks
- Video clips
- Mosby's Nursing Skills Video Exercises

Mosby's Nursing Skills Videos/CD-ROM
- *Wound Care Video:* Sterile gloving, latex precautions

OBJECTIVES

Mastery of content in this chaper will enable the nurse to:

- Discuss settings where surgical aseptic techniques may be used.
- Describe conditions when surgical asepsis should be used.
- Identify principles of surgical asepsis.
- Explain the importance of organization and caution when using surgical aseptic techniques.
- Apply and remove a cap and mask correctly.
- Identify individuals at risk for latex allergy.
- Perform the following skills: applying sterile gloves using open glove method, preparing a sterile field, applying a sterile drape correctly.

KEY TERMS

Asepsis	Sterile field
Latex allergy reaction	Strike through
Microorganisms	Surgical asepsis
Pathogenic microorganisms	Transmission-based
Standard precautions	precautions
Sterile	

BOX 9-1   Principles of Surgical Asepsis

1. All items used within a sterile field must be sterile.
2. A sterile barrier that has been permeated by punctures, tears, or moisture must be considered contaminated.
3. Once a sterile package is opened, a 2.5-cm (1-inch) border around the edges is considered unsterile.
4. Tables draped as part of a sterile field are considered sterile only at table level.
5. If there is any question or doubt of an item's sterility, the item is considered to be unsterile.
6. Sterile persons or items contact only sterile areas; unsterile persons or items contact only unsterile areas.
7. Movement around and in the sterile field must not compromise or contaminate the sterile field.
8. A sterile object or field out of the range of vision or an object held below a person's waist is contaminated.
9. A sterile object or field becomes contaminated by prolonged exposure to air; stay organized, and complete any procedure as soon as possible.

Surgical asepsis or aseptic techniques and practices are designed to render and maintain objects and areas free from pathogenic microorganisms (Decastro, 2002). As in medical asepsis, hand hygiene with an appropriate cleanser or antiseptic is essential before the initiation of an aseptic procedure. Surgical asepsis does require more precautions than medical aseptic technique (see Chapter 8). Any break in technique could result in contamination, increasing the client's risk for an infection. Although surgical asepsis is commonly practiced in operating rooms (ORs), labor and delivery areas, and major diagnostic or special procedure areas, the nurse may use surgical aseptic techniques at the client's bedside (Box 9-1) in three primary situations:

- During procedures that require intentional perforation of a client's skin (e.g., insertion of intravenous [IV] catheters [see Chapter 27])
- When the skin's integrity is broken due to a surgical incision or burns
- During procedures that involve insertion of devices or surgical instruments into normally sterile body cavities (e.g., insertion of a urinary catheter [see Chapter 32])

The skills in this chapter can be used at the client's bedside; portions of Skills 9-1 and 9-2 also can be practiced in the OR, labor and delivery, and procedure areas. Chapter 36 describes additional skills specific to the OR and labor and delivery areas. A nurse in an OR follows a series of steps toward sterile technique, such as applying a mask, protective eyewear, and a cap; performing a surgical hand scrub; ap-

plying a sterile gown; and applying sterile gloves. In contrast, a nurse performing a sterile dressing change at a client's bedside or in the home setting may only wash the hands and apply sterile gloves. Regardless of the procedures followed in different settings, the use of surgical asepsis depends on the nurse developing a surgical aseptic awareness. The nurse must always recognize the importance of strict adherence to aseptic principles (Decastro, 2002). All individuals involved in surgical asepsis have a responsibility to provide and maintain a safe environment by following aseptic principles (Association of Operating Room Nurses [AORN], 2004). The nurse can be an excellent role model and client advocate, reinforcing proper practice when another caregiver breaks technique.

In treatment areas and at the bedside, it is important to have a client's full cooperation to minimize contamination of a work area. The nurse must prepare a client before any procedure. Certain clients may fear moving or touching objects during a sterile procedure, whereas others may even try to assist. The nurse explains how a procedure is to be performed and what a client can do to avoid contaminating sterile items, including avoiding sudden body movement, refraining from touching sterile supplies, and avoiding coughing or talking over a sterile area.

The Centers for Disease Control and Prevention (CDC) (1996) has established standard precautions as the minimum standard for infection control (see Chapter 8). Standard precautions should be used for potential contact with blood and certain body fluids (peritoneal, pericardial, pleural, cerebrospinal fluid [CSF], vaginal, seminal, and amniotic). These are considered potentially infectious for human immunodeficiency virus (HIV), hepatitis B virus (HBV), hepatitis C virus (HCV), and other blood-borne pathogens. Standard precautions also apply to body fluids containing visible blood. The use of standard precautions calls for the wearing of masks in combination with eye protection devices such as goggles or glasses with solid side shields whenever splashes, spray, splatter, or droplets of blood or other potentially infectious fluids may be generated. These barriers keep the eyes, nose, and mouth free from exposure. Similarly, gowns are to be worn when there is risk of being splattered with blood or other infectious materials. All health care institutions should ensure that personal protective equipment and instructions for their use are provided to all employees (Occupational Safety and Health Administration [OSHA], 1991, 1994).

In addition to standard precautions, transmission-based precautions are a second tier of precautions used, either singularly or in combination, when required by a specific infection or colonization of an organism (see Chapter 8). For example, when a client requires airborne or droplet precautions, the nurse will wear a mask.

Evidence-Based Practice Trends

In 1860 Joseph Lister promoted the use of carbolic acid as a surgical hand scrub. Since then, using an antiseptic on the hands of surgical team members has been an accepted practice. Bacteria on the hands of health care workers can cause wound infections if they are introduced into the surgical wound. Studies have shown that antiseptics containing 60% to 95% alcohol alone, or 50% to 95% alcohol when combined with other selected antiseptics, lower bacterial counts on the skin more effectively then do other antiseptics without alcohol (CDC, 2002). In addition, bacteria appear to reproduce slowly on the hands after a surgical scrub with alcohol, and bacterial counts on hands after wearing gloves for 1 to 3 hours seldom exceed prescrub values (CDC, 2002). For this reason, an alcohol-based hand rub may be used as a preoperative hand scrub after an initial 15-second prewash with plain soap and water (CDC, 2002).

Skill Performance Guidelines

1. Always follow standard precautions with all clients.
2. Always review your agency's policies and procedures before conducting a sterile procedure.
3. Always assess the client's potential for infection before choosing the barrier to be used, such as masks or caps.
4. Use barrier techniques to decrease the transmission of microorganisms from health care personnel and the environment to the client.
5. Remember that hand hygiene is essential before initiating any sterile procedure.
6. Incorporate the principles of surgical asepsis when conducting any sterile procedure.

SKILL 9-1 Applying and Removing Cap, Mask, and Protective Eyewear

Although masks and caps are usually worn in surgical procedure areas (e.g., the operating room), there are certain surgical aseptic procedures performed at a client's bedside that also might require these barriers. For example, it may be an agency's policy for a nurse to wear a mask during the changing of a central line dressing or insertion of a peripherally inserted central catheter (PICC). Other policies might require that a nurse wear a mask and a cap to secure hair during dressing changes on a client with extensive burns. When there is a risk for the nurse to be exposed to splattering of blood or body fluid, there is also the need to apply protective eyewear.

The nurse should assess the client's potential for acquiring an infection before applying a mask (e.g., does the client have a large open wound, does the nurse have a respiratory infection, is the client immunosuppressed?). If a mask is worn, it should be changed if it becomes moist or soiled (e.g., splattered with blood). Nurses may choose to wear a surgical cap to secure loose hair that might contaminate a sterile area (Meeker and Rothrock, 1999). As in all situations that require protection from splatters from blood or body fluid, the nurse should follow standard precautions (see Chapter 8).

DELEGATION CONSIDERATIONS

The skill of applying and removing cap, mask, and protective eyewear can be delegated to assistive personnel. However, the procedures performed at a client's bedside that require cap and mask generally cannot be delegated (refer to specific skill for recommendations). Assistive personnel should learn how to be available to hand off additional sterile equipment or assist with client positioning. The RN determines if protective barriers are necessary for the other staff.

EQUIPMENT

❑ Mask (different types are available for people with different skin sensitivities)
❑ Surgical cap (NOTE: Use only if hospital policy requires, or use to secure hair if there is a possibility of contamination of a sterile field)
❑ Hairpins, rubber bands, or both
❑ Protective eyewear (e.g., goggles or glasses with appropriate side shields)

STEP	RATIONALE

ASSESSMENT

1. Consider type of sterile procedure to be performed, and consult agency's policy for use of mask/caps/eyewear.
2. If you have symptoms of a cold or respiratory infection, either avoid participating in procedure or apply a mask.
3. Assess the client's actual or potential risk for infection when choosing barriers for surgical asepsis (e.g., older adult, neonatal client, or immunocompromised client).

Not all sterile procedures require mask, cap, or eyewear.
Ensures client and nurse will be properly protected.
A greater number of pathogenic microorganisms reside within the respiratory tract when infection is present.
Some clients are at a greater risk for acquiring an infection, so nurse uses additional barriers.

NURSING DIAGNOSES

- Risk for infection

- Ineffective protection

Related factors are individualized based on client's condition or needs.

PLANNING

1. Expected outcome following completion of procedure:
   - Client will not develop signs of localized infection.

2. Prepare equipment, and inspect packaging for integrity and exposure to sterilization.

Indicates lack of microorganism transfer to client and sterile field.
Ensures availability of equipment and sterility of supplies before procedure begins.

IMPLEMENTATION

1. Applying cap
   a. If hair is long, comb back behind ears and secure.
   b. Secure hair in place with pins.

   c. Apply cap over head as you would apply hairnet. Be sure all hair fits under cap's edges (see illustration).
2. Applying mask
   a. Find top edge of mask, which usually has a thin metal strip along edge.
   b. Hold mask by top two strings or loops, keeping top edge above bridge of nose.
   c. Tie two top strings at top of back of head, over cap (if worn), with strings above ears (see illustration).

Cap must cover all hair entirely.
Long hair should not fall down or cause cap to slip and expose hair.
Loose hair hanging over sterile field or falling dander may result in contamination of objects on sterile field.

Pliable metal fits snugly against bridge of nose.

Prevents contact of hands with clean facial portion of mask. Mask will cover all of nose.
Position of ties at top of head provides tight fit. Strings over ears may cause irritation.

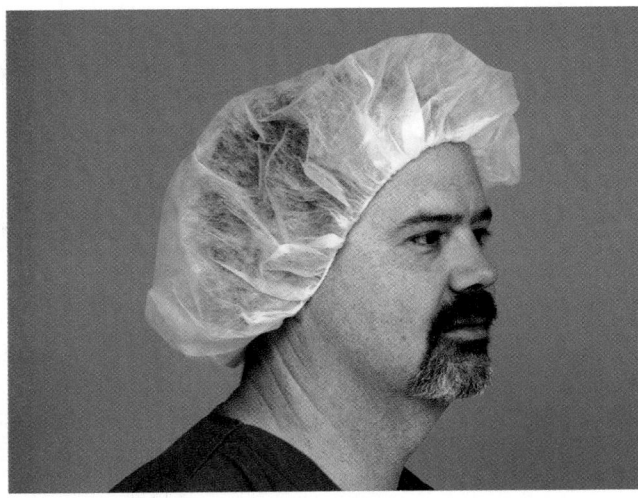

STEP **1c** Nurse applies cap over head, covering all hair.

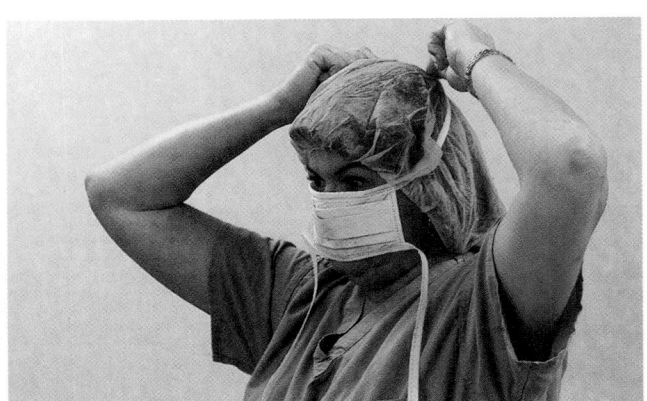

STEP **2c** Tie top strings of mask.

STEP	RATIONALE

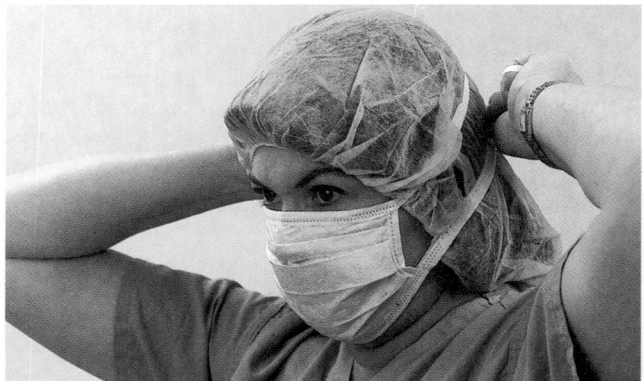

STEP **2d** Tie bottom strings of mask.

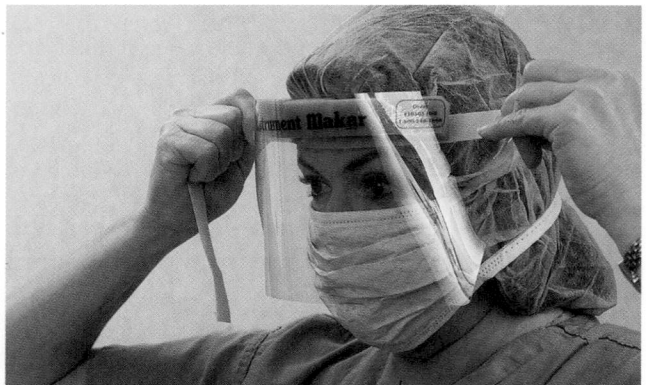

STEP **3a** Apply face shield over cap.

d. Tie two lower ties snugly around neck with mask well under chin (see illustration).	Prevents escape of microorganisms through sides of mask as nurse talks and breathes.
e. Gently pinch upper metal band around bridge of nose.	Prevents microorganisms from escaping around nose.
3. Applying protective eyewear	
a. Apply protective glasses, goggles, or face shield comfortably over eyes, and check that vision is clear (see illustration).	Positioning can affect clarity of vision.
b. Be sure eyewear fits snugly around forehead and face.	Ensures eyes are fully protected.
4. Disposing of cap and mask and removing eyewear	
a. Remove gloves first, if worn (see Skill 9-3).	Prevents contamination of hair, neck, and facial area.
b. Untie bottom strings of mask first.	Prevents top part of mask from falling down over nurse's uniform. Contaminated surface of mask could then contaminate uniform.
c. Untie top strings of mask, and remove mask from face, holding ties securely. Discard mask in proper receptacle (see illustrations).	Avoids contact of nurse's hands with contaminated mask.

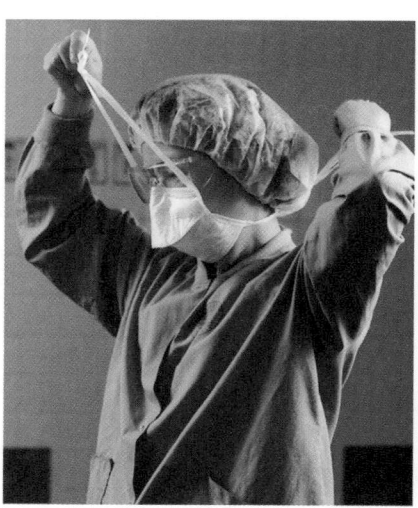

A

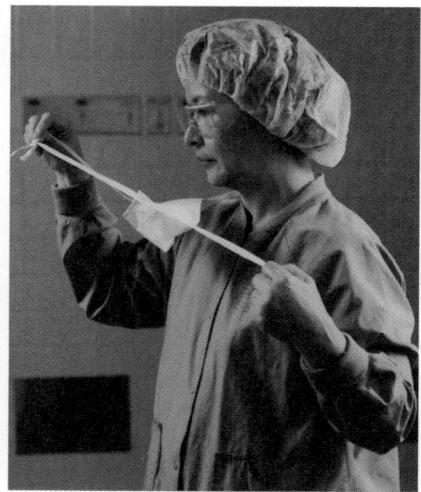

B

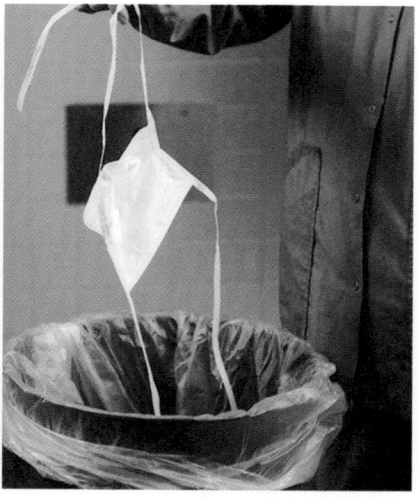

C

STEP **4c** **A,** Untying top mask strings. **B,** Removing mask from face. **C,** Discarding mask. (From Phipps W and others: *Medical-surgical nursing: concepts and clinical practice,* ed 6, St. Louis, 1999, Mosby.)

STEP	RATIONALE
d. Remove eyewear, avoiding placing hands over soiled lens.	Prevents transmission of microorganisms.
e. Grasp outer surface of cap and lift from hair.	Minimizes contact of hands with hair.
f. Discard cap in proper receptacle, and perform hand hygiene.	Reduces transmission of infection.

EVALUATION

1. Following procedure, assess area of body treated for drainage, tenderness, edema, or change in temperature or color of skin.	Rules out presence of localized infection.

Recording and Reporting

- No recording or reporting is required for this set of skills. Record specific procedure performed in nurses' progress notes, and describe client's status, for example, condition of surgical site, appearance of intravenous central catheter site.

Unexpected Outcomes	Related Interventions
1. Redness, heat, edema, pain, or purulent drainage develops at wound or treatment site, indicating possible infection.	• Notify physician of change in condition of affected area, and initiate appropriate treatments as ordered. • If there is a pattern or trend in clients developing similar infection, infection control team will investigate.

Home Care Considerations

- Instruct family caregiver as to specifics of when to apply cap, mask, and protective eyewear.

- Determine ability of family caregiver to safely implement sterile procedure.
- Instruct client and family caregiver to observe for signs of infection.

SKILL 9-2 Preparing a Sterile Field

When performing sterile aseptic procedures, the nurse must have a work area in which objects can be handled with minimal risk of contamination. A sterile field serves such a purpose. It is an area considered free of microorganisms and may consist of a sterile kit or tray, a work surface draped with a sterile towel or wrapper, or a table covered with a large sterile drape (DeCastro, 2002). Sterile drapes establish a sterile field around a treatment site, such as a surgical incision, venipuncture site, or site for introduction of an indwelling urinary catheter. Drapes also provide a work surface for placing sterile supplies and for manipulating items with sterile gloves. Drapes are available in cloth, paper, and plastic. They may be wrapped in individual sterile packages or included within sterile kits or trays. Most are fluid resistant. Many styles, shapes, and sizes are available to accommodate different areas or body parts to be covered. For example, a fenestrated drape has a slitlike opening in it to expose only the perineal area during urinary catheter insertion.

Many sterile items come prepackaged within containers that serve as both sterile fields and work areas for the nurse. For example, bladder catheterization kits and tracheal suction kits contain sterile items that can be moved within the tray and containers into which sterile solutions can be poured. Once a sterile field is created, it is the responsibility of the nurse to perform the procedure and to be sure the field is not contaminated.

The skill of preparing a sterile field incorporates skills of opening sterile packages, preparing a sterile drape, adding sterile supplies to a field, and pouring sterile solutions.

DELEGATION CONSIDERATIONS
The procedures performed at clients' bedsides that require use of a sterile field generally should not be delegated (refer to specific skill for recommendations). However, assistive personnel may assist in positioning clients and obtaining extra supplies.

EQUIPMENT
- ❑ Sterile gloves
- ❑ Sterile drape or kit that is to be used as a sterile field
- ❑ Sterile gown (see agency policy)
- ❑ Disposable cap and mask (see agency policy)
- ❑ Sterile supplies and solutions specific to the procedure
- ❑ Waist-high table/countertop surface
- ❑ Protective eyewear

STEP	RATIONALE

ASSESSMENT

1. Verify that procedure requires surgical aseptic technique.

   Some procedures require medical rather than surgical aseptic technique.

2. Assess client's comfort, oxygen requirements, and elimination needs before preparing for procedure.

   Certain procedures for which sterile field is prepared may last a long time. Nurse anticipates client's needs so that client can relax and avoid any unnecessary movement that might disrupt procedure.

- • *Critical Decision Point*
  Position client for maximum comfort and ease of breathing. Additional staff may be needed to assist with positioning so client does not contaminate sterile field.

3. Check sterile package integrity for punctures, tears, discoloration, moisture, or any other signs of contamination. If using commercially packaged supplies or those prepared by agency, check for sterilization indicator.

   The inspection of packaging ensures that only sterile items are presented to sterile field (AORN, 2004).

4. Anticipate number and variety of supplies needed for procedure.

   Not all sterile kits contain sufficient amounts or types of supplies. Failure to have necessary supplies causes nurse to leave sterile field, increasing risk of contamination.

NURSING DIAGNOSES
- • Risk for infection

- • Ineffective protection

Related factors are individualized based on client's condition or needs.

STEP	**RATIONALE**

PLANNING

1. Expected outcomes following completion of procedure:
   - The sterile field is not contaminated.
   - Client is not exposed to microorganisms.
2. Complete all other priority tasks before beginning procedure.
3. Prepare equipment at bedside.

4. Ask visitors to step out briefly during procedure. Discourage movement by staff who will assist with procedure.
5. Position client comfortably for specific procedure to be performed. If a body part is to be examined or treated, position client so part is accessible. Have assistive personnel assist with positioning as needed.
6. Explain to client purpose of procedure and importance of sterile technique.

Nurse uses correct surgical aseptic practice.

Sterile fields should be prepared as close as possible to time of use to reduce potential for contamination (AORN, 2004).
Ensures availability before the procedure and prevents break in sterile technique. (NOTE: Povidone-iodine and chlorhexidine are not considered sterile solutions unless in a sterile package and require separate work surfaces for prepping.)
Traffic or movement can increase potential for contamination through spread of microorganisms by air currents.

Client should be able to lie still in one position comfortably during procedure. Movement can cause contamination of sterile items.

Ensures client's ability to cooperate. Teaching before procedure eliminates need to talk during procedure, which can cause air-droplet contamination of sterile area.

IMPLEMENTATION

1. Apply cap, mask, protective eyewear, and/or gown as needed (consult agency policy) (see Skill 9-1).
2. Select a clean, flat, dry work surface above waist level.

3. Perform hand hygiene thoroughly using an alcohol-based hand rub or an antimicrobial soap and water (CDC, 2002).
4. Preparing sterile work surface
   a. Sterile commercial kit or tray containing sterile items
      (1) Place sterile kit or package containing sterile items on clean, dry, flat work surface above waist level.
      (2) Open outside cover, and remove kit from dust cover. Place on work surface (see illustration).

Controls spread of airborne microorganisms.

A sterile object below a person's waist is considered contaminated.
Reduces carriage of microorganisms on hands, which may be transmitted to the client.

Items placed below waist level are considered contaminated.

Inner kit remains sterile.

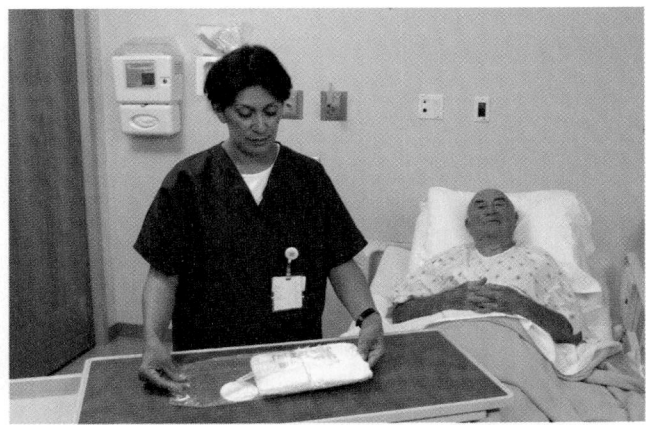

STEP **4a(2)** Open outside cover, remove kit from dust cover, place on work surface.

STEP	RATIONALE
(3) Grasp outer surface of tip of outermost flap.	Outer surface of package is considered unsterile. There is a 2.5-cm (1-inch) border around any sterile drape or wrap that is considered contaminated.
(4) Open outermost flap away from body, keeping arm outstretched and away from sterile field (see illustration).	Reaching over sterile field contaminates it.
(5) Grasp outside surface of edge of first side flap.	Outer border is considered unsterile.
(6) Open side flap, pulling to side, allowing it to lie flat on table surface. Keep your arm to side and not over sterile surface (see illustration).	Drape or wrapper should lie flat so it will not accidentally rise up and contaminate inner surface or sterile contents.
(7) Repeat step (6) for second side flap (see illustration).	
(8) Grasp outside border of last and innermost flap (see illustration).	Outer border is considered unsterile.
(9) Stand away from sterile package and pull flap back, allowing it to fall flat on table.	Never reach over a sterile field.
b. Sterile linen-wrapped package	
(1) Place package on clean, dry, flat work surface above waist level.	Items placed below waist level are considered contaminated.

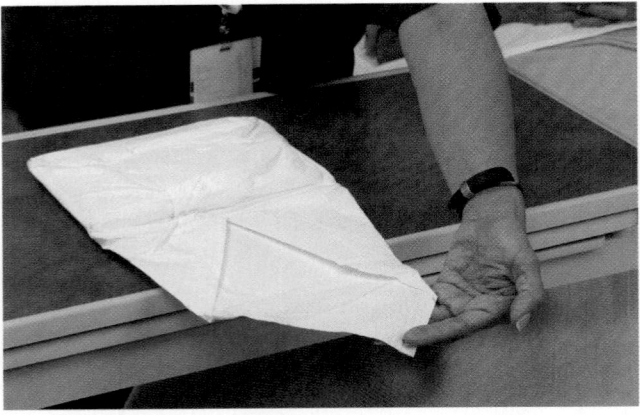

STEP 4a(4) Open outermost flap of sterile kit away from body.

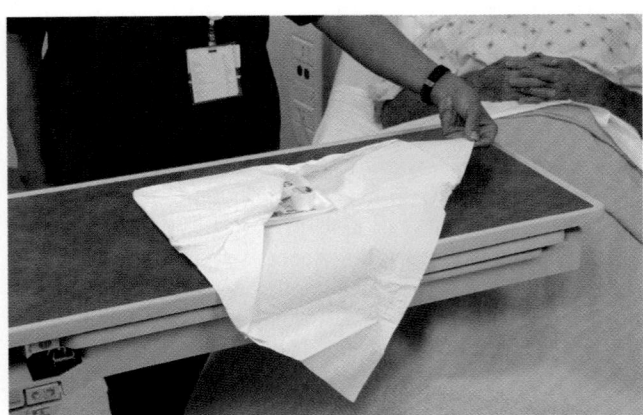

STEP 4a(6) Open first side flap, pulling to side.

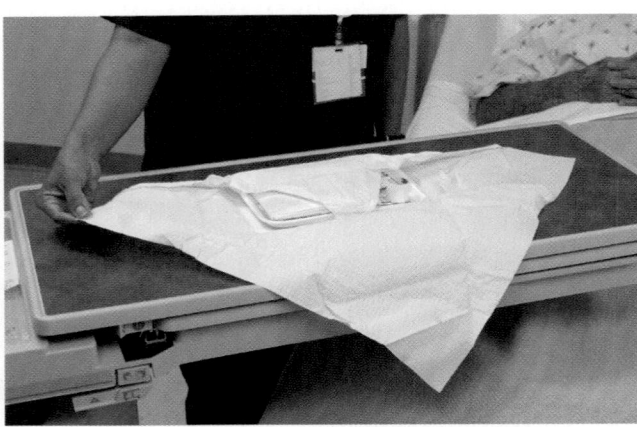

STEP 4a(7) Open second side flap, pulling to side.

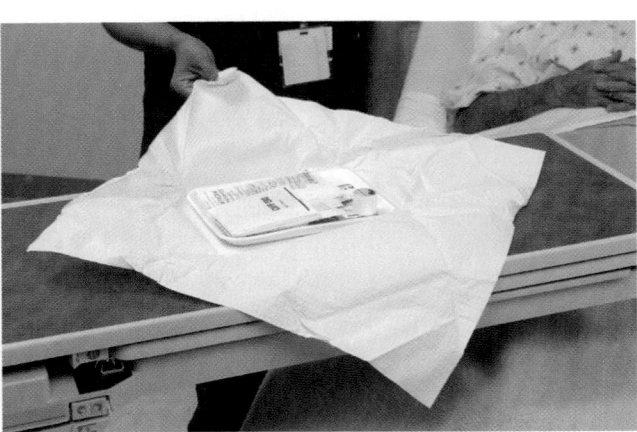

STEP 4a(8) Open last and innermost flap.

STEP	**RATIONALE**

(2) Remove tape seal, and unwrap both layers following same steps (see steps 4a(2) through 4a(9)) as with sterile kit above (see illustration).

Linen-wrapped items have two layers. The first is a dust cover. The second layer must be opened to view chemical indicator. If item is dropped on floor, it is considered contaminated.

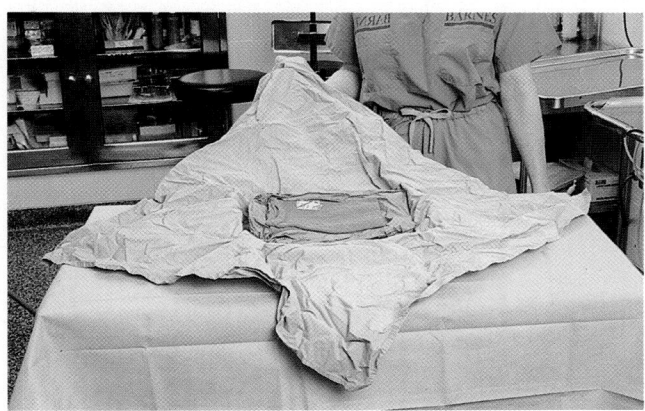

STEP 4b(2) Open sterile linen-wrapped package.

(3) Use opened package wrapper as sterile field.

Inner surface of wrapper is considered sterile.

c. Sterile drape

(1) Place pack containing sterile drape on flat, dry surface and open as described (see steps 4a(2) through 4a(9)) for sterile package.

Ensures sterility of packaged drape.

(2) Apply sterile gloves (optional, see agency policy).

A sterile object remains sterile only when touched by another sterile object. Gloves need not be worn as long as fingers grasp the one inch unsterile border of the drape.

(3) Grasp folded top edge of drape with fingertips of one hand. Gently lift drape up from its wrapper without touching any object.

If a sterile object touches any nonsterile object, it becomes contaminated.

(4) Allow drape to unfold, keeping it above waist and work surface and away from body. (Discard wrapper with other hand.)

Object held below person's waist is contaminated.

(5) With other hand, grasp adjacent corner of drape. Hold drape straight over work surface (see illustration).

Drape can now be properly placed with two hands.

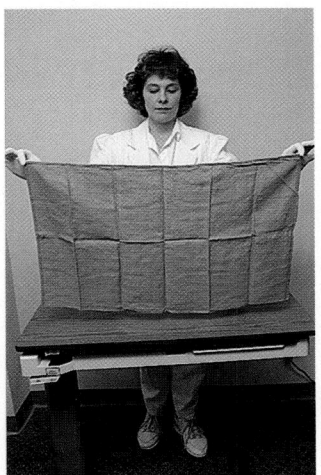

STEP 4c(5) Hold corners of sterile drape up and away from body.

STEP	RATIONALE
(6) Holding drape, first position the bottom half over top half of intended work surface (see illustration).	Prevents nurse from reaching over sterile field.
(7) Then allow top half of drape to be placed over bottom half of work surface (see illustration). A flat draped area is now available for placement of sterile supplies.	Creates flat sterile work surface.

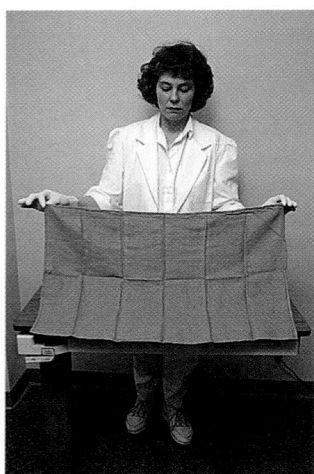

STEP **4c(6)** Position bottom half of sterile drape over top half of work surface.

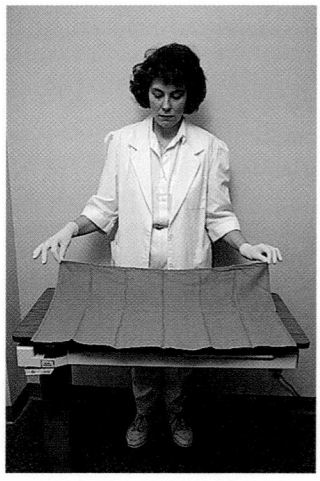

STEP **4c(7)** Allow top half of drape to be placed over bottom half of work surface.

STEP	RATIONALE
5. Adding sterile items	
a. Open sterile item (following package directions) while holding outside wrapper in nondominant hand.	Frees dominant hand for unwrapping outer wrapper.
b. Carefully peel wrapper over nondominant hand.	Item remains sterile. Inner surface of wrapper covers hand, making it sterile.
c. Being sure wrapper does not fall down on sterile field, place item onto field at an angle (see illustration). **Do not hold arm over sterile field.**	Secured wrapper edges prevent flipping wrapper and contaminating contents of sterile field (AORN, 2004).

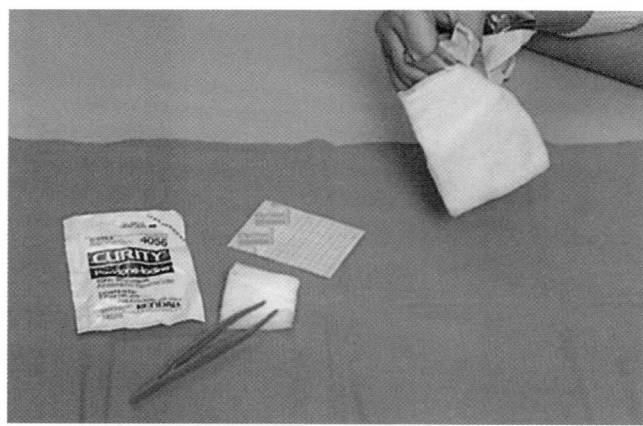

STEP **5c** Adding items to sterile field.

STEP	RATIONALE

• *Critical Decision Point*
Do not flip or throw objects onto sterile field.

<table>
<tr><td>   **d.** Dispose of outer wrapper.</td><td>Prevents accidental contamination of sterile field.</td></tr>
<tr><td>**6.** Pouring sterile solutions</td><td></td></tr>
<tr><td>   **a.** Verify contents and expiration date of solution.</td><td>Ensures proper solution and sterility of contents.</td></tr>
<tr><td>   **b.** Be sure receptacle for solution is located near table/work surface edge. Sterile kits have cups or plastic molded sections into which fluids can be poured.</td><td>Prevents reaching over sterile field during pouring of solution.</td></tr>
<tr><td>   **c.** Remove seal and cap from bottle in an upward motion.</td><td>Prevents contamination of the bottle lip.</td></tr>
<tr><td>   **d.** With solution bottle held away from field and bottle lip 1 to 2 inches above inside of sterile receiving container, slowly pour entire contents of solution container (see illustration).</td><td>Edge and outside of bottle are considered contaminated. Slow pouring prevents splashing. Sterility of contents cannot be ensured if cap is replaced.</td></tr>
</table>

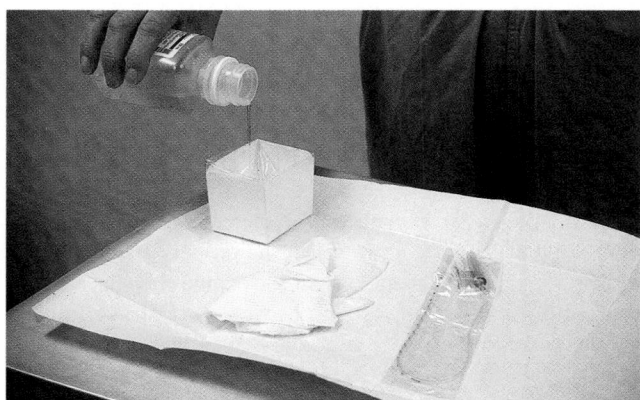

STEP **6d** Pouring solution into receiving container on sterile field.

• *Critical Decision Point*
When liquids permeate sterile field or barrier, it is called strike through, resulting in contamination.

EVALUATION

1. Observe for break in sterile technique.	Break in sterile field requires the nurse to set up new sterile field.

Recording and Reporting

• No recording or reporting is required for this set of skills. Record sterile procedure performed in nurses' progress notes, and describe client's status, for example, condition of surgical site, appearance of intravenous central catheter site.

Unexpected Outcomes	Related Interventions
1. Sterile field comes in contact with contaminated object, or liquid splatters onto drape, causing strike through.	• Discontinue field preparation, and start over with new equipment.
2. Sterile item falls off sterile field.	• Open package containing new sterile item, and add to field, unless field becomes contaminated.

Home Care Considerations

• In the home setting most care will be performed in a clean environment. In the event that a sterile environment is ordered, client and family need to be aware of the principles that apply to the sterile environment. For example, family can be taught how to correctly use package wrapper as a sterile drape/barrier when applying a sterile dressing, or family can be taught correct procedure for removing sterile item from package without contaminating item.

• Assess client's and family's understanding and ability to provide a sterile environment when needed to perform a specific procedure

---

SKILL 9-3 Sterile Gloving

Gloves help prevent the transmission of pathogens by direct and indirect contact. Nurses apply sterile gloves before performing sterile procedures such as inserting urinary catheters, changing dressings on central IV catheters, or applying sterile dressings. It is important to select the proper-size glove. The gloves should not stretch so tightly over the fingers that they can easily tear, yet they should be tight enough that objects can be picked up easily. Sterile gloves are available in sizes, such as sizes 6, 6½, and 7. However, in most clinical areas sterile gloves in "one size fits all" are available.

It is important to choose not only the right size of glove but also the correct material. Many clients and health care workers have known allergies to latex, the natural rubber used in most gloves and other medical products (DeCastro, 2002). Box 9-2 lists individuals who are at risk for latex allergy. Latex proteins enter the body in various ways—through skin or mucous membranes, intravascularly, or via inhalation. The cornstarch powder used to make latex gloves slip on easily over the hands is a carrier of the latex proteins (Burt, 1998). When gloves are applied or removed, the cornstarch particles become airborne and can remain so for hours. The latex can then be inhaled or settle on clothing, skin, or mucous membranes. Reactions to latex can be mild to severe (Box 9-3). For individuals at high risk or with suspected sensitivity to latex, it is important to choose latex-free or synthetic gloves. More health care institutions are implementing latex-safe environments for workers (Kim and others, 1998).

> **BOX 9-2 Individuals at Risk for Latex Allergy**
>
> • Spina bifida
> • Congenital or urogenital defects
> • History of indwelling catheters or repeated catheterizations
> • History of using condom catheters
> • High latex exposure (e.g., health care workers, housekeepers, food handlers, tire manufacturers, workers in industries that use gloves routinely)
> • History of multiple childhood surgeries
> • History of food allergies

Modified from Gritter M: The latex threat, *Am J Nurs* 98(9):26, 1998; and Kim KT and others: Implementation recommendations for making health care facilities latex safe, *AORN J* 67(3):615, 1998.

> **BOX 9-3 Levels of Latex Reactions**
>
> There are three types of common latex reactions which, in order of severity, include:
> 1. **Irritant dermatitis**—a nonallergic response characterized by skin redness and itching.
> 2. **Type IV hypersensitivity**—cell-mediated allergic reaction to chemicals used in latex processing. Reaction can be delayed up to 48 hours, including redness, itching, and hives. Localized swelling, red and itchy or runny eyes and nose, and coughing may develop.
> 3. **Type I allergic reaction**—a true latex allergy that can be life-threatening. Reactions vary based on type of latex protein and degree of individual sensitivity, including local and systemic. Symptoms include hives, generalized edema, itching, rash, wheezing, bronchospasm, difficulty breathing, laryngeal edema, diarrhea, nausea, hypotension, tachycardia, and respiratory or cardiac arrest.

Modified from Gritter M: The latex threat, *Am J Nurs* 98(9):26, 1998.

Once gloves are applied, the nurse should always be conscious of the position of the hands during procedures. If a sterile glove touches a clean, a contaminated, or a questionably contaminated object, it becomes unsterile and a new sterile glove must be applied. It is helpful to interlock the fingers and hold the hands together in front of the body and above waist level while waiting to handle sterile items. If a tear develops in a sterile glove, the nurse applies a new glove immediately.

DELEGATION CONSIDERATIONS

The skill of applying and removing sterile gloves can be delegated to assistive personnel. However, many procedures that require the use of sterile gloves cannot be delegated to assistive personnel. (Refer to specific skill for recommendations.)

EQUIPMENT

❑ Package of proper-size sterile gloves; latex or synthetic nonlatex (NOTE: Hypoallergenic, low-powder, and low-protein latex gloves may still contain enough latex protein to cause an allergic reaction [Burt, 1998].)

STEP	RATIONALE

◼ ASSESSMENT

1. Consider the type of procedure to be performed, and consult institutional policy on use of sterile gloves.

2. Consider client's risk for infection. For example, preexisting condition and size or extent of area being treated.

3. Examine glove package to determine if it is dry and intact.

4. Inspect condition of hands for cuts, open lesions, or abrasions. Lesions harbor microorganisms and should be covered with an impervious dressing.

5. Assess client for the following risk factors before applying latex gloves:
   a. Previous reaction to the following items within hours of exposure: adhesive tape, dental or face mask, golf club grip, ostomy bag, rubber band, balloon, bandage, elastic underwear, IV tubing, rubber gloves, condom.
   b. Personal history of asthma, contact dermatitis, eczema, urticaria, rhinitis.
   c. History of food allergies, especially avocado, banana, peach, chestnut, raw potato, kiwi, tomato, papaya.
   d. Previous history of adverse reactions during surgery, dental procedure.
   e. Previous reaction to latex product.

Ensures proper use of sterile gloves when needed.

Directs nurse to follow added precautions (e.g., use of additional protective barriers) if necessary.

Torn or wet package is considered contaminated.

When strict surgical asepsis is used, presence of such lesions may prevent nurse from participating in procedure.

Determines level of client's risk for latex allergy.

◼ NURSING DIAGNOSES

• Risk for infection
• Risk for injury

• Ineffective protection

Related factors are individualized based on client's condition or needs.

◼ PLANNING

1. Expected outcomes following completion of procedure:
   • Client will not develop signs or symptoms of infection after procedure.
   • Client will not develop latex sensitivity or latex allergy reaction.

2. Select correct size and type of gloves.

Indicates microorganisms not introduced into sterile body cavities or sites (such as skin or urinary tract).

Client at risk for latex allergy is not exposed to latex proteins.

There is less chance of contamination if correct size of gloves is worn.

• *Critical Decision Point*
   Synthetic nonlatex gloves are necessary for clients at risk or if nurse has sensitivity or allergy to latex.

STEP	RATIONALE
3. Place glove package near work area.	Ensures availability before procedure.

IMPLEMENTATION

1. Glove application

    a. Perform thorough hand hygiene.

Reduces number of bacteria on skin surfaces and reduces transmission of infection.

    b. Remove outer glove package wrapper by carefully separating and peeling apart sides (see illustration).

Prevents inner glove package from accidentally opening and touching contaminated objects.

    c. Grasp inner package, and lay it on clean, dry, flat surface at waist level. Open package, keeping gloves on wrapper's inside surface (see illustration).

Sterile object held below waist is contaminated. Inner surface of glove package is sterile.

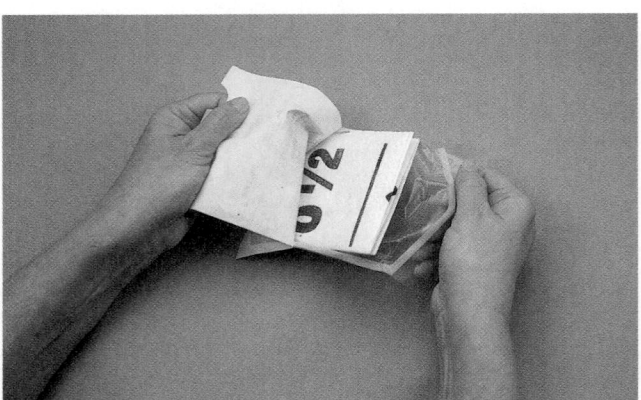

STEP 1b Open outer glove package wrapper.

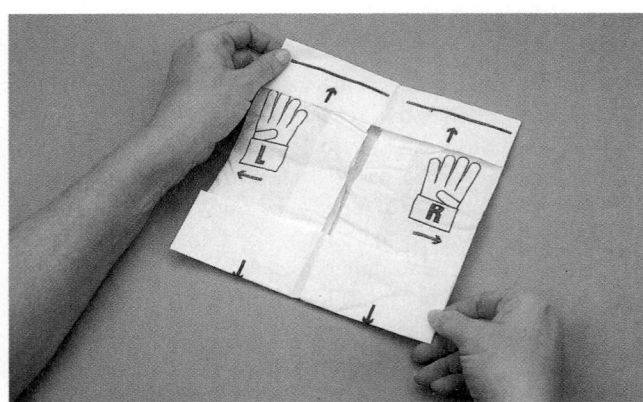

STEP 1c Open inner glove package on work surface.

    d. Identify right and left glove. Each glove has a cuff approximately 5 cm (2 inches) wide. Glove dominant hand first.

Proper identification of gloves prevents contamination by improper fit. Gloving of dominant hand first improves dexterity.

    e. With thumb and first two fingers of nondominant hand, grasp edge of cuff of glove for dominant hand. Touch only glove's inside surface (see illustration).

Inner edge of cuff will lie against skin and thus is not sterile.

    f. Carefully pull glove over dominant hand, leaving cuff and being sure cuff does not roll up wrist. Be sure thumb and fingers are in proper spaces.

If glove's outer surface touches hand or wrist, it is contaminated.

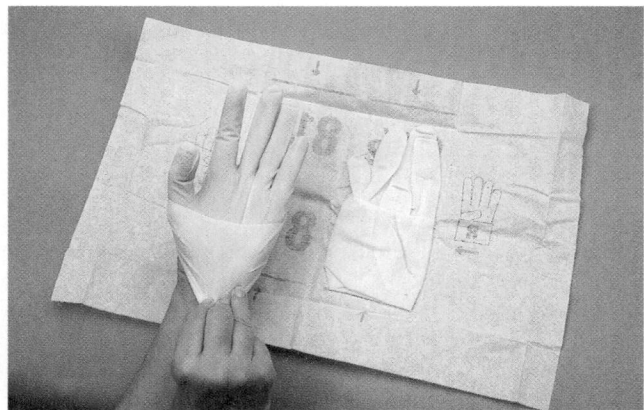

STEP 1e Pick up glove for dominant hand and insert fingers, pull glove completely over dominant hand (example is for left-handed person).

STEP	**RATIONALE**

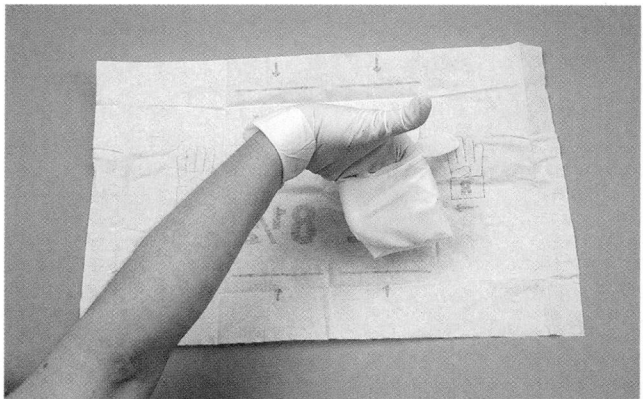

STEP **1g** Pick up glove for nondominant hand.

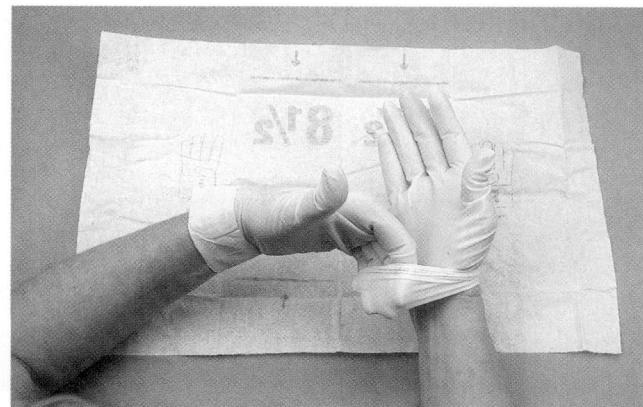

STEP **1h** Pull second glove over nondominant hand.

g. With gloved dominant hand, slip fingers underneath second glove's cuff (see illustration).

Cuff protects gloved fingers. Sterile touching sterile prevents glove contamination.

h. Carefully pull second glove over nondominant hand (see illustration).

Contact of gloved hand with exposed hand results in contamination.

• *Critical Decision Point*
Do not allow fingers and thumb of gloved dominant hand to touch any part of exposed non-dominant hand. Keep thumb of dominant hand abducted back.

i. After second glove is on, interlock hands together, above waist level. The cuffs usually fall down after application. Be sure to touch only sterile sides (see illustration).

Ensures smooth fit over fingers.

2. Glove disposal

a. Grasp outside of one cuff with other gloved hand; avoid touching wrist.

Minimizes contamination of underlying skin.

b. Pull glove off, turning it inside out. Discard in receptacle (see illustration).

Outside of glove does not touch skin surface.

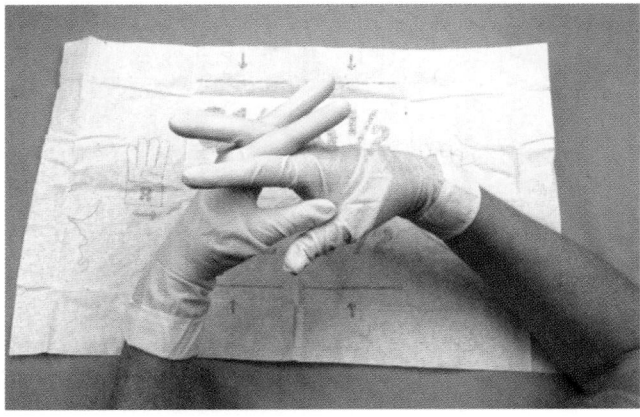

STEP **1i** Interlock gloved hands.

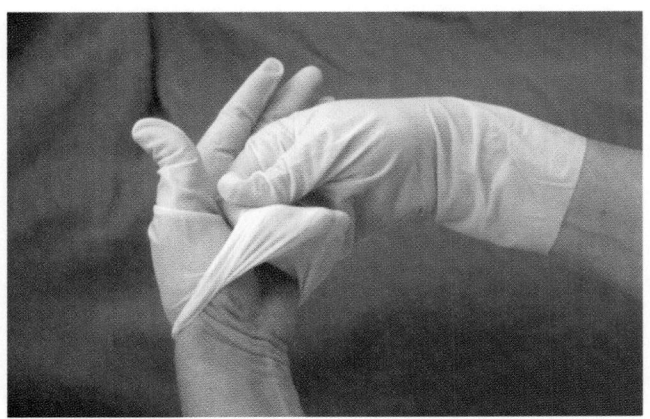

STEP **2b** Carefully remove first glove by turning it inside out.

STEP	RATIONALE
c. Take fingers of bare hand and tuck inside remaining glove cuff. Peel glove off inside out. Discard in receptacle.	Fingers do not touch contaminated glove surface.
d. Perform thorough hand hygiene.	This protects health care worker from contamination resulting from any unseen tears or pinholes in gloves, also removing powder from hands helps to prevent skin irritations.

EVALUATION

1. Assess client for signs of infection, focusing on area treated.	Improper technique may contribute to development of an infection.

Recording and Reporting

- It is not necessary to record application of gloves. Record specific procedure performed and client's response and status.
- In the event of a latex allergy reaction, record client's response in nurses' notes and vital sign flow sheet. Note type of response and client's reaction to emergency treatment.

Unexpected Outcomes	Related Interventions
1. Client develops localized signs of infection—for example, urine becomes cloudy or odorous; wound becomes painful, edematous, reddened with purulent drainage.	• Contact physician and implement appropriate treatments as ordered.
2. Client develops systemic signs of infection, for example, fever, malaise, increased white blood cell count.	• Contact physician, and implement appropriate treatments as ordered.
3. Client develops allergic reaction to latex (see Box 9-3).	• Immediately remove source of latex. • Bring emergency equipment to bedside. Have epinephrine injection ready for administration, and be prepared to initiate IV fluids and oxygen.

Teaching Considerations

- Nurse or client with a known latex allergy should wear a medical alert bracelet or tag and carry a wallet card stating "latex allergy."
- Individuals with known latex allergies should carry a quick-acting oral antihistamine and an epinephrine auto-injector at all times.

FOCUS *on* CLINICAL PRACTICE

1. You are assigned to Mrs. Smith, a 78-year-old grand-mother who is blind and is being admitted to the facility for a cholecystectomy. You enter her room to begin a series of procedures: measurement of urine for intake and output, irrigation of a nasogastric tube, insertion of a peripheral intravenous catheter, and measurement of the client's blood pressure. Which procedure requires use of sterile gloves?

2. Before performing these procedures, what explanations should be given to Mrs. Smith?

3. You prepared the peripheral site for Mrs. Smith's intravenous catheter, then attempted to insert the catheter without success, and you need to try another location. What would you do next?

4. Mrs. Smith tells you she has allergic reactions when she eats bananas or tomatoes. Based on this information, what would you ask Mrs. Smith, and what actions would you take?

5. Mrs. Smith's physician is planning to insert a central venous line. You obtained the necessary equipment, prepared a sterile drape, and opened the sterile pack. You removed the outer wrapper and placed the item on the sterile field. While doing this, you noticed the item touched the drape 2 inches from the border of the drape. What would you do next?

NCLEX REVIEW QUESTIONS

1. Sterile barriers are removed in what order?
   1. Gloves, then mask, eyewear, and cap
   2. Mask, eyewear, cap, then gloves
   3. Eyewear, cap, mask, then gloves
   4. Gloves, then eyewear, cap and mask

2. When opening a sterile pack, which of the following will compromise the sterility of the contents?
   1. Keeping the contents of the pack away from the table edge
   2. Holding or moving the object below the waist
   3. Opening the pack just before the procedure
   4. Allowing movement around the sterile field that does not touch near the sterile field

3. When putting on sterile gloves, it is important to remember to:
   1. Grab only the inside of the glove with your bare hand
   2. Grab only the cuffs of the gloves with your bare hand
   3. Wear a size that is as tight as possible
   4. Ask someone else to assist you in putting them on

References

Association of Operating Room Nurses: *Standards, recommended practices, and guidelines,* Denver, 2004, The Association.

Burt S: What you need to know about latex allergy, *Nursing* 28(10):33, 1998.

Centers for Disease Control and Prevention, Hospital Infection Control Practice Advisory Committee: Guidelines for isolation precautions in hospitals, *Am J Infect Control* 24:24, 1996.

Centers for Disease Control and Prevention, Hospital Infection Control Practice Advisory Committee and the HICPAC/SHEA/APIC/IDSA Hand Hygiene Task Force: Guideline for hand hygiene in health-care settings, *MMWR Morb Mortal Wkly Rep: Recommendations and Reports* 51(RR16), 2002.

DeCastro M: Aseptic technique. In *APIC text of infection control epidemiology*, revised 2002, Association for Professionals in Infection Control and Epidemiology, Inc.

Gritter M: The latex threat, *Am J Nurs* 98(9):26, 1998.

Kim KT and others: Implementation recommendations for making health care facilities latex safe, *AORN J* 67(3):615, 1998.

Meeker MH, Rothrock JC: *Alexander's care of the patient in surgery*, ed 11, St. Louis, 1999, Mosby.

Occupational Safety and Health Administration: Respiratory protection: proposed rule, *Fed Regist* 59(219):58884, 1994.

Occupational Safety and Health Administration: Occupational Safety and Health Act of 1991: bloodborne pathogens, www.osha.gov, 1991.

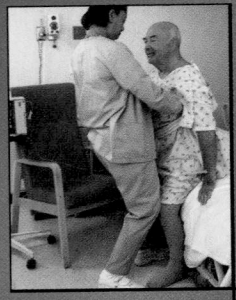

10

Body Mechanics, Transfer, and Positioning

10-1   Maintaining Body Alignment

10-2   Using Safe and Effective Transfer Techniques

10-3   Moving and Positioning Clients in Bed

MEDIA RESOURCES

Evolve Site *evolve*

http://evolve.elsevier.com/Perry/skills
- Weblinks
- Video clips
- Mosby's Nursing Skills Video Exercises

Mosby's Nursing Skills Videos/CD-ROM
- *Body Mechanics and Exercise Video:* Principles of body mechanics; moving a person up in bed with a lift/draw sheet; turning/positioning a person in side-lying position; dangling; transfer from bed to wheelchair using a transfer belt; passive range-of-motion exercises; ambulation using a gait belt; signs/symptoms of and precautions for orthostatic hypotension

OBJECTIVES

Mastery of content in this chaper will enable the nurse to:

- Describe body mechanics and its importance in caring for clients.
- Describe normal body alignment for standing, sitting, and lying down.
- Assess for alterations in body alignment.
- Describe procedures for lifting clients.
- Describe positioning techniques for the supported Fowler's, supine, prone, 30-degree lateral side-lying, and Sims' positions.
- Describe the procedures for helping a client to move up in bed, helping a client to a sitting position, logrolling a client, and transferring a client from a bed to a chair.
- Describe the procedure for a three-person carry.

KEY TERMS

Balance	Hemiplegia
Base of support	Hoyer lift (mechanical/
Body alignment	hydraulic lift)
Body mechanics	Leverage
Center of gravity	Line of gravity
Drawsheet	Logrolling
Footboard	Orthostatic hypotension
Footdrop	Paralysis
Friction	Paresis
Gravity	Posture
Hand rolls	Proprioceptive function
Hemiparesis	Weight

Health care providers are required to provide employees with safety information and training to use when transferring, positioning, and lifting clients. The Occupational Safety and Health Administration (OSHA) has identified guidelines on back safety and guidelines on the prevention of musculoskeletal injuries (OSHA, 2000; United States Department of Labor, 2003).

Before lifting, the nurse should assess the weight to be lifted and what assistance, if any, is needed (Edlich, Woodard, and Haines, 2001; United States Department of Labor, 2003). If help is needed, the nurse should assess if a second person is adequate or if mechanical assistance is needed. Once the amount of needed assistance is determined, use the following steps for proper body mechanics:

- Tighten stomach muscles and tuck pelvis; this provides balance and protects the back.
- Bend at the knees; this helps to maintain your center of gravity and lets the strong muscles of the legs do the lifting.
- Keep the weight to be lifted as close to the body as possible; this action places the weight in the same plane as the lifter and close to the center of gravity for balance.
- Maintain the trunk erect and knees bent so that multiple muscle groups work together in a synchronized manner.
- Avoid twisting. Twisting your spine can lead to serious injury.
- The best height for lifting vertically is approximately 2 feet off the ground and close to the lifter's center of gravity.

Body mechanics is the coordinated effort of the musculoskeletal and nervous systems to maintain balance, posture, and body alignment during lifting, bending, moving, and performing activities of daily living. Body mechanics also facilitates body movement so that a person can carry out a physical activity without using excessive muscle energy.

Nurses often care for clients who have conditions resulting in immobility or who require limitations in activity imposed by their treatment plan. As a result, the nurse plays an important role in positioning and moving clients safely and effectively to reduce the risks of immobilization. Positioning of clients to maintain correct body alignment is essential to prevent complications. These complications include pressure ulcers (see Chapter 15), which can develop in 24 hours and require months of time and thousands of dollars to correct (Lueckenotte, 2000); and contractures and footdrop, which can occur within a few days when muscles, tendons, and joints become less flexible because of lack of mobility and incorrect alignment. The force of gravity pulls an unsupported, weakened foot into a footdrop position, and calf muscles and heel cords shorten, complicating future attempts at walking. Pillows placed under the knees or an elevated knee gatch can produce knee and hip contractures. A sagging mattress increases the risk of hip contractures. These knee and hip contractures can cause future gait and posture problems, making mobility more difficult.

Some clients are at especially high risk for complications from improper positioning and have increased risk of injury during transfer. Examples include alterations in bone formation or joint mobility, and impaired muscle development, which results in muscle wasting and weakness. Central nervous system (CNS) damage may result in motor impairment, proprioceptive loss, or cognitive dysfunction, all of which affect mobility. The application of proper body mechanics, alignment, and the use of transfer and positioning techniques assist the client in achieving an optimal level of independence without resultant injury to the health care provider.

Evidence-Based Practice Trends

Musculoskeletal disorders are noted as the most prevalent and debilitating occupational health hazard among nurses (Trinkoff and others, 2002). Little improvement in the incidence of musculoskeletal injuries in health care workers has taken place. In 1989, 4.2 lost-workday injury cases per 100 were reported; in 2000 there were 4.1 cases per 100 (Bureau of Labor Statistics, 2003; Nelson and others, 2003). Because of the risk of injury to nurses and their clients, the American Nurses Association (ANA) put forth a position statement calling for the use of assistive equipment and devices to reposition and transfer clients to promote a safe health care environment (ANA, 2003). The use of assistive equipment and continued use of proper body mechanics can significantly reduce the risk of musculoskeletal injuries (ANA, 2003). In addition, OSHA recommends that manual lifting of clients be minimized in all cases and eliminated when feasible (United States Department of Labor, 2003). Many facilities are moving toward limited lift policies (LLP) that minimize client handling by nurses. Instead, nurses should use lift devices to reduce on-the-job injuries (Moreno, 2003). By becoming knowledgeable about safe, efficient lifting techniques and proper use of assistive equipment and devices, nurses can safely transfer clients without causing injury to the client or the nurse.

Skill Performance Guidelines

1. Know the physiological influences on body alignment and mobility that affect clients throughout the life span. The greatest impact of the physiological changes on the musculoskeletal system is observed in the early and later years of life. In the child the major consequences of decreased muscle activity are loss of muscle strength, endurance, muscle mass, and joint mobility; bone demineralization; and contracture (Hockenberry and others, 2003). Inactive older adults are at risk for muscle atrophy, loss of bony mass, contractures of joints, and pressure ulcers (Lueckenotte, 2000).

2. Know the pathological conditions that affect a client's body alignment and mobility (Edlich and others, 2001; United States Department of Labor, 2003). Postural abnormalities affect body mechanics. For example, a client with severe kyphosis may not be able to lift an object safely because the center of gravity is not aligned. Diseases affecting bone formation (e.g., osteoporosis) alter body alignment and mobility.

Degenerative joint diseases (e.g., osteoarthritis), impaired muscle development (e.g., muscular dystrophy), and central nervous system damage (e.g., paralysis) interfere with normal body alignment and mobility. Therefore the client's risk of musculoskeletal injury is increased.

3. Know history of underlying conditions such as chronic disease (e.g., diabetes, chronic obstructive pulmonary disease) or malnutrition. Clients with underlying chronic conditions are at risk for skin breakdown and other hazards of immobility and as a result require more frequent position changes.

4. Control factors that can indirectly affect body mechanics by altering the safety of the environment. Cluttered hallways and bedside areas increase the client's risk of falling (see Chapters 4 and 41).

5. Know the client's fluid balance status. Dehydration or edema may require more frequent position changes because clients with alterations in fluid balance are prone to skin breakdown. In addition, identify the client with incontinence or profuse sweating. Moisture from incontinence or sweating can decrease tensile strength and alter skin resiliency to external forces.

6. Know the client's range of joint motion (ROJM). Contractures or spasticity limit joint and muscle mobility; the nurse must take care not to position the limb in an unnatural way. This could result in injury to or dysfunction of the affected limb (see Chapter 11).

7. Determine the client's level of sensory perception. Loss of sensation increases vulnerability to the hazards of immobility. Clients with decreased sensation must have their positions evaluated and changed frequently to avoid damage to the integumentary and musculoskeletal systems.

8. Know the client's baseline vital signs. The client with low blood pressure may not be able to tolerate sudden position changes and is at risk of fainting while transferring from bed to chair.

9. Assess the client's cognitive status and stage of psychological adaptation to illness. Both factors affect the ability to learn and participate in transfer and positioning.

SKILL 10-1 Maintaining Body Alignment

The term body alignment refers to the conditions of the joints, tendons, ligaments, and muscles in various body positions. When the body is aligned, whether standing, sitting, or lying, no excessive strain is placed on these structures. Body alignment means the body is in line with the pull of gravity and contributes to body balance. Without this balance, the center of gravity is displaced, which increases the force of gravity and predisposes the person to falls and injuries. Body balance is achieved when a wide base of support exists, the center of gravity falls within the base of support, and a vertical line can be drawn from the center of gravity through the base of support. Body balance is also enhanced by posture. The better aligned the posture, the greater the balance.

DELEGATION CONSIDERATIONS

The skills of maintaining the client's body alignment can be delegated to assistive personnel. Clients who have spinal cord trauma usually require the supervision of a professional nurse during transfer and repositioning. Before delegating this skill the nurse must:

- Designate specific times throughout the shift that assistive personnel must reposition the client
- Provide assistive personnel with information regarding client's individual needs for body alignment

STEP	RATIONALE

ASSESSMENT

1. Observe alignment of client in standing, sitting, or lying position.

   Determines if client assumes normal body alignment.

2. Standing (see illustration):

   Maintains body alignment in relation to body's normal center of gravity.

   a. Head is erect and at midline.

   b. Shoulders and hips are straight and parallel.

   c. Vertebral column appears straight when viewed posteriorly.

   d. Lateral observation indicates head is erect and spinal curves are aligned in reverse-S pattern.

   In reverse-S pattern, cervical vertebrae are anteriorly convex, thoracic vertebrae are posteriorly convex, and lumbar vertebrae are anteriorly convex.

   e. Lateral observation indicates that abdomen is comfortably tucked in and knees and ankles are slightly flexed.

   Maintains abdomen and trunk directly over body's center of gravity.

   f. Arms are comfortably positioned at each side.

   g. Feet are placed slightly apart, with toes pointed forward.

   Produces broad base of support and improves balance.

   h. Center of gravity is located midline and forms vertical line from middle of forehead to midpoint between feet. **Exception:** A pregnant woman's center of gravity is more anterior. Thus she leans slightly backward, and spinal column is slightly swaybacked (see illustration).

   Laterally, the line of gravity runs vertically from middle of skull to posterior one third of foot.

   Position allows woman to adapt to normal weight gain and growing fetus

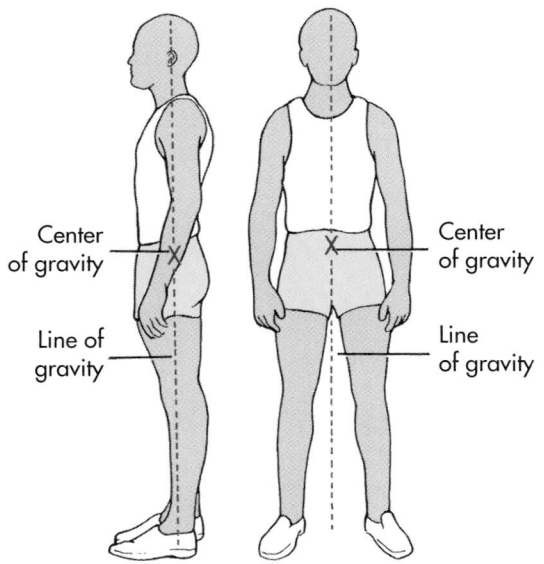

Step 2 Body alignment when standing.

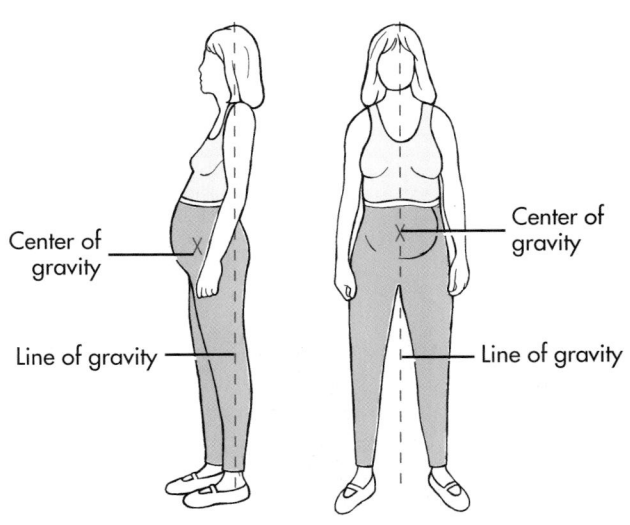

Step 2h Center of gravity in pregnant woman.

STEP	RATIONALE

3. Sitting (see illustration):
   a. Head is erect, and vertebrae are in straight alignment.
   b. Body weight is evenly distributed on buttocks and thighs.
   c. Thighs are parallel and in horizontal plane.
   d. Both feet are supported on floor, and ankles are comfortably flexed.

Prevents stress on intravertebral joints.
Prevents increased pressure over bony prominences and reduces damage to underlying musculoskeletal system.
Maintains flexion of hips and provides broad base of support.
Maintains plantar flexion and reduces risk of footdrop.

• *Critical Decision Point*
If client is unable to flex one or both knees, nurse should make sure that elevated legs are supported and ankles are flexed.

   e. A 2.5- to 5-cm (1- to 2-inch) space is maintained between edge of seat and popliteal space on posterior surface of knee.
   f. Client's forearms should be supported on armrest, in lap, or on table in front of chair.
4. Lying (see illustration):
   a. Client is in lateral position, with positioning supports removed.
   b. Client's body should be supported by adequate mattress.
   c. Vertebral column should be in alignment without observable curves.

Ensures that no excessive pressure is placed on popliteal artery or nerve, which could decrease circulation or impair nerve function.
Reduces force of gravity on shoulder joint and chance of accidental shoulder dislocation.

Allows nurse to observe spinal alignment and any pressure points.
Reduces strain on joints and ligaments.

Allows for even distribution of body weight.

• *Critical Decision Point*
Clients with lower or upper extremity weakness, decreased sensation, paralysis, or immobilization are at risk for musculoskeletal trauma because of uneven or prolonged distribution of body weight and must have their positions changed frequently.

5. Determine client's knowledge of body mechanics and positioning.

Determines if instruction is required.

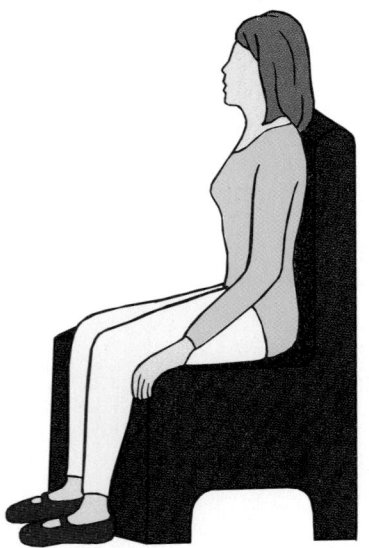

Step 3 Center of gravity when sitting.

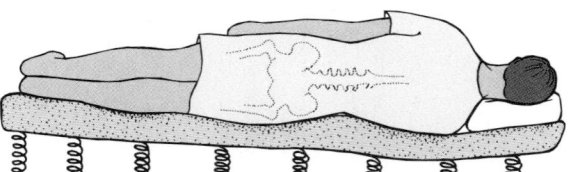

Step 4 Body alignment in lateral position.

STEP	RATIONALE

NURSING DIAGNOSES

- Impaired physical mobility
- Risk for impaired skin integrity
- Deficient knowledge concerning body mechanics and positioning

- Risk for activity intolerance
- Risk for disuse syndrome
- Risk for injury

Related factors are individualized based on client's condition or needs.

PLANNING

1. Expected outcomes following completion of procedure:
   - Body is positioned without skin surfaces being exposed to undue pressure.
   - While sitting, lying, or standing, client aligns body straight and in correct position.
   - Client is able to explain benefits of body alignment.
2. Instruct client or family caregiver regarding proper body alignment for standing, sitting, or lying.

Extremities are not crossed or aligned to cause pressure.

Avoids strain on musculoskeletal structures.

Increases likelihood of good postural habits being followed.
Provides client or family caregiver with necessary knowledge to identify potential altered body alignment.

IMPLEMENTATION

1. Demonstrate to client and family caregiver correct body alignment for standing, sitting, and lying.

2. Provide opportunity for return demonstration.
3. Discuss with client and family caregiver the hazards of prolonged immobility on body alignment and mobility (see Chapters 11 and 15).
4. Provide client and family caregiver with resources (e.g., community health agency, physician) to contact when mobility or body alignment is impaired.

Demonstration is reliable technique for teaching psychomotor skills and enables client and family caregiver to ask questions.
Allows evaluation of client or family caregiver learning.
Alerts client and family caregiver to early assessment factors associated with incorrect body alignment and impaired mobility.
Alerts resource persons to assist with minor problems of body alignment before severe, irreversible problems occur.

EVALUATION

1. Inspect skin surfaces and pressure points.
2. Have client demonstrate body alignment for standing, sitting, and lying.
3. Ask client to describe benefits of body alignment.

Reveals pressure sites.
Return demonstration reveals if learning occurred.

Evaluates cognitive learning.

Recording and Reporting

- Record in nurses' notes information presented to client and client's progress toward learning alignment and positioning.
- Report information taught to client at change of shift.
- Record time and position change of client throughout shift.

Unexpected Outcomes	Related Interventions
1. Incorrect body alignment is indicated by poor posture or decreased joint mobility.	• Indicates need for follow-up learning activities. • Instruct caregivers to step back and view the client's body alignment and look for signs of discomfort.
2. Damage to skin and musculoskeletal system (e.g., pressure sore, contracture) occurs.	• Review plan of care with client and caregiver, and modify as needed. • Post turning schedule above client's bed as a reminder. • Initiate steps to treat developing pressure ulcer (see Chapter 15).

Teaching Considerations

- Shorter clients should be taught to use a footstool when sitting so that feet rest on footstool.
- Teach family members or friends of clients who are permanently disabled proper body mechanics, alignment, transfer, and positioning techniques.
- Clients at risk for thrombophlebitis should be taught not to cross their legs and the signs and symptoms of this complication (see Chapter 11).
- If client has cognitive or sensory impairment, is a young child, is severely debilitated, or is immobilized or confined to bed, family is primary focus of instruction (see Skills 10-2 and 10-3).

Pediatric Considerations

- Teach parents that the use of play activities such as painting or drawing on a large sheet of paper placed on the bed or wall can encourage movement. Play activities to encourage ambulation include push/pull toy (toddler) and wagon (school age) (Hockenberry and others, 2003).

Gerontological Considerations

- During aging process, cervical vertebrae may become more flexed, and kyphotic posture may result (McCance and Huether, 2000).

Home Care Considerations

- Bed must be at caregiver's waist level when caregiver is assisting with alignment.
- Provide family members and caregivers a turning schedule for the client.

Long-Term Care Considerations

- Long-term care clients may have special devices or appliances such as an air mattress to increase comfort. Make sure these appliances or devices are smooth and wrinkle-free when assessing proper body alignment of the client.
- Clearly label all reusable padding or special mattresses with client's name.

SKILL 10-2 Using Safe and Effective Transfer Techniques

Transferring is a nursing skill that helps the dependent client or the client with restricted mobility attain positions to regain optimal independence as quickly as possible. Physical activity maintains and improves joint motion, increases strength, promotes circulation, relieves pressure on skin, and improves urinary and respiratory functions. It also benefits the client psychologically by increasing social activity and mental stimulation and providing a change in environment (Konradi and Anglin, 2001). Thus mobilization plays a crucial role in the client's rehabilitation.

One of the major concerns during transfer is the safety of the client and the nurse. The nurse prevents self-injury by using correct posture, minimal muscle strength, and effective body mechanics and lifting techniques. As a rule of thumb, nurses must get assistance if in doubt about their ability to transfer a client.

Many special problems must be considered during a client's transfer. A client who has been immobile for several days or longer may be weak or dizzy or may develop orthostatic hypotension (a drop in blood pressure) when transferred. A client with neurological deficits may have paresis (muscle weakness) or paralysis unilaterally or bilaterally, which complicates safe transfer. A flaccid arm may sustain injury during transfer if unsupported. As a general rule, a nurse should use a transfer belt and obtain assistance for mobilization of such clients.

DELEGATION CONSIDERATION

The skills of effective transfer techniques can be delegated to assistive personnel. Before delegating this skill the nurse must:

- Supervise assistive personnel during the transfer of clients who are transferred for the first time after prolonged bed rest, extensive surgery, critical illness, or spinal cord trauma
- Inform assistive personnel about the client's mobility restrictions, changes in blood pressure, or sensory alterations that may affect safe transfer

EQUIPMENT

- ❑ Transfer belt, sling, or lap board (as needed), nonskid shoes, bath blankets, pillows
- ❑ Slide board (friction-reducing board)
- ❑ *Wheelchair:* Position chair at 45-degree angle to bed, lock brakes, remove footrests, lock bed brakes
- ❑ *Stretcher:* Lock brakes on stretcher, lock brakes on bed
- ❑ *Option:* Mechanical/hydraulic lift: Use frame, canvas strips or chains, and hammock or canvas strips

STEP	RATIONALE

ASSESSMENT

1. Assess physiological capacity to transfer.

Determines client's ability to tolerate and assist with transfer and whether special adaptive techniques are necessary.

   a. Muscle strength (legs and upper arms)

Immobile clients have decreased muscle strength, tone, and mass. Affects ability to bear weight or raise body.

   b. Joint mobility and contracture formation

Immobility or inflammatory processes (i.e., arthritis) may lead to contracture formation and impaired joint mobility.

   c. Paralysis or paresis (spastic or flaccid)

Client with CNS damage may have bilateral paralysis (requiring transfer by swivel bar, sliding bar, Hoyer lift) or unilateral paralysis, which requires belt transfer to "best" side. Weakness (paresis) requires stabilization of knee while transferring. Flaccid arm must be supported with sling during transfer.

   d. Bone continuity (trauma, amputation)

Clients with trauma to one leg or hip may be non–weight-bearing when transferred. Amputees may use sliding board to transfer.

2. Assess presence of weakness, dizziness, or postural hypotension.

Determines risk of fainting or falling during transfer. The move from a supine to a vertical position redistributes about 500 ml of blood; immobile clients may have decreased ability for autonomic nervous system to equalize blood supply, resulting in orthostatic hypotension (Phipps and others, 2003).

3. Assess level of endurance:
   a. Assess level of fatigue during activity.

Ability to transfer may be limited by fatigue. Estimates ability to participate in transfer. Strength may be evaluated by participation in activities of daily living (ADLs). Planned rest periods before transfer may enhance function.

   b. Assess vital signs.

Vital sign changes such as increased pulse and respiration may indicate activity intolerance (see Chapter 17).

4. Assess client's proprioceptive function (awareness of posture and changes in equilibrium):

Determines stability of client's balance for transfer.

   a. Ability to maintain balance while sitting in bed or on side of bed

Determines risk of fainting or falling during transfer.

   b. Tendency to sway to or position self to one side

Clients with brain dysfunction may have proprioceptive losses. This may cause them to lean to one side or lose balance during transfer.

5. Assess client's sensory status, including adequacy of central and peripheral vision, adequacy of hearing, and presence of peripheral sensation loss.

Determines influence of sensory loss on ability to make transfer. Visual field loss decreases client's ability to see in direction of transfer. Peripheral sensation loss decreases proprioception. Clients with visual and hearing losses need transfer techniques adapted to deficits. Clients with cerebrovascular accident (CVA) may lose area of visual field, which profoundly affects vision and perception.

• *Critical Decision Point*
   Clients with hemiplegia may "neglect" one side of the body (inattention to or unawareness of one side of body or environment), which distorts perceptions of the visual field.

6. Assess client's level of comfort:
   a. Pain
   b. Muscle spasm

Pain may reduce client's motivation and ability to be mobile. Pain relief before transfer enhances client participation. A pain level reported below 4 (0 to 10 scale) has been shown to minimally affect function (Feldt, 2000).

STEP	RATIONALE
7. Assess client's cognitive status.	Determines client's ability to follow directions and learn transfer techniques.

* **Critical Decision Point**
  Clients with head trauma or CVA may have perceptual cognitive deficits that create safety risks. If client has difficulty in comprehension, simplify instructions and maintain consistency.

a. Ability to follow verbal instructions	May indicate clients at risk for injury.
b. Short-term memory	Clients with short-term memory deficits may have difficulty with transfer, initial learning, or consistent performance.
c. Recognition of physical deficits and limitations to movement	Client's knowledge of deficits can help nurse plan a safe transfer.
8. Assess client's level of motivation such as client's eagerness versus unwillingness to be mobile.	Altered psychological states reduce client's desire to engage in activity.
9. Assess previous mode of transfer (if applicable).	Determines mode of transfer and assistance required to provide continuity. Transfer (gait) belts should be used with clients who need assistance (Hignett, 2003; Zuang and others, 2000).
10. Assess client's specific risk of falling when transferred.	Certain conditions increase client's risk of falling or potential for injury. Neuromuscular deficits, motor weakness, calcium loss from long bones, cognitive and visual dysfunction, and altered balance increase risk of injury.
11. Assess special transfer equipment needed for home setting. Assess home environment for hazards.	Transfer ability at home is greatly enhanced by prior teaching of family and support persons, assessment of home for safety risks and functionality, and provision of applicable aids (see Chapter 41).

NURSING DIAGNOSES

* Activity intolerance
* Risk for injury
* Acute or chronic pain

* Impaired skin integrity
* Impaired physical mobility

Related factors are individualized based on client's condition or needs.

PLANNING

1. Expected outcomes following completion of procedure:	
• Client dangles legs or sits without dizziness, weakness, or orthostatic hypotension.	Precautions during transferring prevent vascular compromise.
• Client tolerates increased activity.	Gradual increase in number of transfers and period of time out of bed increases tolerance and endurance.
• Client can bear more weight.	Repeated transfers usually result in improved endurance and greater independence of client.
• Client transfers without injury.	Proper techniques avoid injury.
• Client is more motivated to be mobile.	
• Client transfers with minimal or no assistance.	Tolerance to activity improves.
2. Explain procedure to client. Repeat instructions simply and with continuity to client with cognitive dysfunction.	Promotes understanding and cooperation, reducing anxiety.

IMPLEMENTATION

1. Perform hand hygiene.	Reduces transfer of microorganisms.
2. **Assist client to sitting position (bed at waist level):**	
a. Place client in supine position.	Enables nurse to assess client's body alignment continually and to administer additional care, such as suctioning or hygiene needs.

STEP	RATIONALE

b. Face head of bed at a 45-degree angle, and remove pillows.

Proper positioning reduces twisting of the nurse's body when moving the client. Pillows may cause interference when the client is sitting up in bed.

c. Place feet apart with foot nearer bed behind other foot continuing at a 45-degree angle to the head of the bed.

Improves nurse's balance and allows transfer of body weight as client is moved to sitting position.

d. Place hand farther from client under shoulders, supporting client's head and cervical vertebrae.

Maintains alignment of head and cervical vertebrae and allows for even lifting of client's upper trunk.

e. Place other hand on bed surface.

Provides support and balance.

f. Raise client to sitting position by shifting weight from front to back leg.

Improves nurse's balance, overcomes inertia, and transfers weight in direction in which client is moved.

g. Push against bed using arm that is placed on bed surface.

Divides activity between nurse's arms and legs and protects back from strain. By bracing one hand against mattress and pushing against it as client is lifted, part of weight that would be lifted by nurse's back muscles is transferred through nurse's arms onto mattress.

3. **Assist client to sitting position on side of bed with bed in low position:**

a. With client in supine position, raise head of bed 30 degrees.

Decreases amount of work needed by client and nurse to raise client to sitting position.

b. Turn client onto side, facing nurse on side of bed on which client will be sitting (see illustration).

Prepares client to move to side of bed and protects from falling.

c. Stand opposite client's hips. Turn diagonally so nurse faces client and far corner of foot of bed.

Places nurse's center of gravity nearer client. Reduces twisting of nurse's body because nurse is facing direction of movement.

d. Place feet apart in a wide base of support with foot closer to head of bed in front of other foot.

Increases balance and allows nurse to transfer weight as client is brought to sitting position on side of bed.

e. Place arm nearer head of bed under client's shoulders, supporting head and neck.

Maintains alignment of head and neck as nurse brings client to sitting position.

f. Place other arm over client's thighs (see illustration).

Supports hip and prevents client from falling backward during procedure.

g. Move client's lower legs and feet over side of bed. Pivot toward rear leg, allowing client's upper legs to swing downward.

Decreases friction and resistance. Weight of client's legs when off bed allows gravity to lower legs, and weight of legs assists in pulling upper body into sitting position.

Step 3b Side-lying position.

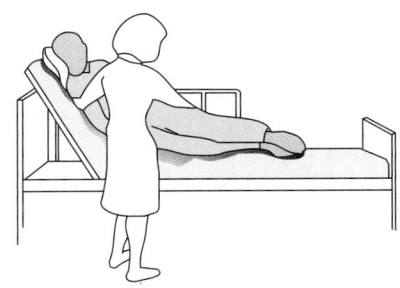

Step 3f Nurse places arm over client's thigh.

STEP	**RATIONALE**

h. At same time, shift weight to rear leg and elevate client (see illustration).

Allows nurse to transfer weight in direction of motion.

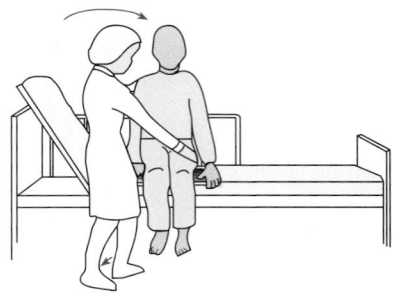

Step **3h** Nurse shifts weight to rear leg and elevates client.

• *Critical Decision Point*
Remain in front until client regains balance, and continue to provide physical support to weak or cognitively impaired client.

4. **Transferring client from bed to chair with bed in low position.**

a. Two nurses are recommended for this task.

Two nurses are recommended to transfer a client to reduce risk of musculoskeletal injury (Pan and Freivalos, 2000; Zhuang and others, 2000)

b. Assist client to sitting position on side of bed (see steps 3 a to h). Have chair in position at 45-degree angle to bed. Allow client to sit on side of the bed (dangling) for a few minutes before transferring to chair. Ask if client feels dizzy. Do not leave client unattended during dangling.

Positions chair within easy access for transfer. Dangling or allowing a client to sit on the side of the bed before transfer helps equilibrate blood pressure, reducing the risk of dizziness or fainting when standing.

c. Apply transfer belt or other transfer aids.

Transfer belt allows nurse to maintain stability of client during transfer and reduces risk of falling (Hignett, 2003; Owens and others 1999). Client's arm should be in sling if flaccid paralysis is present.

• *Critical Decision Point*
A battery-operated mechanical lift can assist the client to a standing position comfortably without undue physical stress on the nurse (Hignett, 2003).

d. Assist client with applying stable nonskid shoes. Weight-bearing or strong leg is placed forward, with weak foot back.

Nonskid soles decrease risk of slipping during transfer. Always have client wear shoes during transfer; bare feet increase risk of falls. Client will stand on stronger, or weight-bearing, leg.

e. Spread feet apart.

Ensures balance with wide base of support.

STEP	RATIONALE
a. Determine number of staff required to horizontally transfer client safely (three nurses recommended).	To prevent injury to client and/or nurses more than one nurse is recommended (United States Department of Labor, 2003).
b. Lower the head of the bed as much as client can tolerate.	Maintains alignment of spinal column.
c. Cross client's arms on chest.	Prevents injury to arms during transfer.
d. To place slide board under client, position two nurses on side of bed to which the client will be turned. Position third nurse on the other side of bed.	Distributes weight equally between nurses.
e. Fanfold the drawsheet on both sides.	Provides strong handles in order to grip the drawsheet without slipping.
f. Using the count of three, turn client onto side as one unit with a smooth, continuous motion.	Maintains body in alignment, preventing stress on any part of the body.
g. Place slide board under drawsheet (see illustration).	Prevents friction from contact of skin with board.
h. Gently roll the client back onto the slide board.	
i. Line up the stretcher with the bed. Lock brakes on stretcher and bed.	Ensure the stretcher or bed does not inadvertently move during transfer.
j. Two nurses position themselves on the side of the stretcher, while the third nurse positions self on the side of the bed without the stretcher (see illustration).	

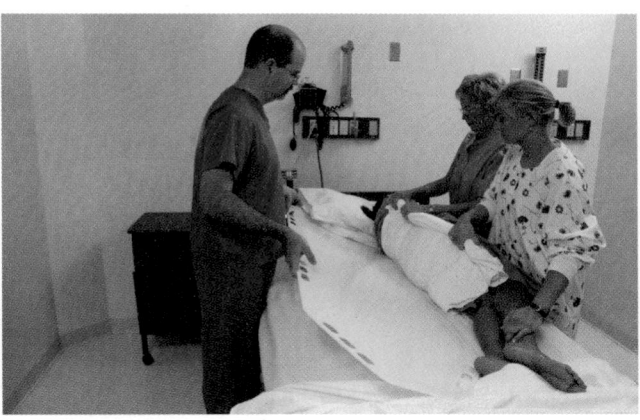

Step **5g** Placing slide board under drawsheet.

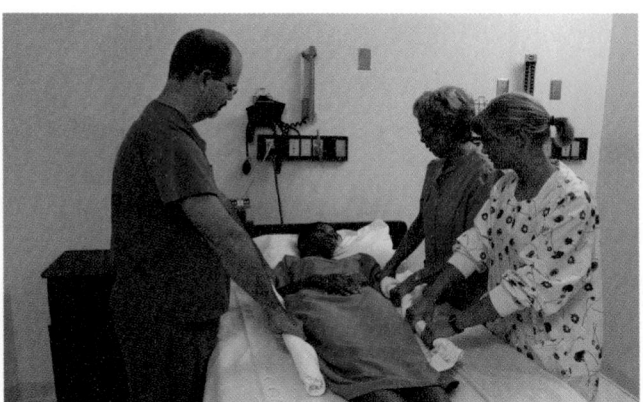

Step **5j** Positioning of nurses before transfer.

- *Critical Decision Point*
  A nurse may also be positioned at the head of the client's bed to protect and support the client's head and neck if client is weak or unable to assist.

STEP	RATIONALE
k. Fanfold drawsheet; using the count of three, the two nurses pull drawsheet with client onto stretcher while the third nurse holds the slide board in place (see illustration).	The slide board remains stationary and provides a slippery surface to reduce friction and allows the client to transfer easily to the stretcher.

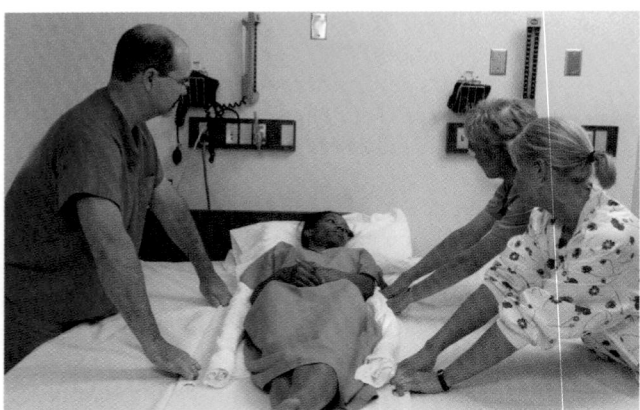

Step **5k** Transfer of client to stretcher using slide board.

STEP	RATIONALE
l. Position client in center of stretcher. Raise head of stretcher if not contraindicated.	Provides for client comfort.
6. Use mechanical/hydraulic lift to transfer client from bed to chair:	Research supports the use of mechanical lifts to prevent musculoskeletal injuries (Hignett, 2003).
a. Bring lift to bedside.	Ensures safe elevation of client off bed. (Before using lift, be thoroughly familiar with its operation.)
b. Position chair near bed, and allow adequate space to maneuver lift.	Prepares environment for safe use of lift and subsequent transfer.
c. Raise bed to high position with mattress flat. Lower side rail.	Allows nurse to use proper body mechanics.
d. Keep bed side rail up on side opposite nurse unless a second nurse is assisting.	Maintains client safety.
e. Roll client on side away from nurse.	Positions client for use of lift sling.

STEP	RATIONALE

f. Place hammock or canvas strips under client to form sling. With two canvas pieces, lower edge fits under client's knees (wide piece), and upper edge fits under client's shoulders (narrow piece).

Two types of seats are supplied with mechanical/hydraulic lift: hammock style is better for clients who are flaccid, weak, and need support; canvas strips can be used for clients with normal muscle tone. Hooks should face away from client's skin. Place sling under client's center of gravity and greatest portion of body weight.

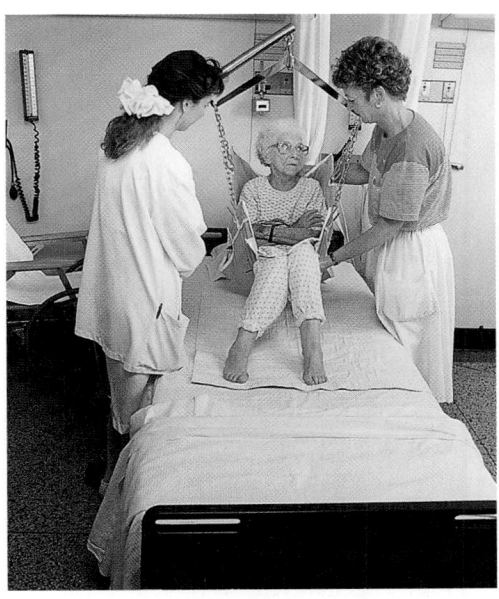

Step **6n** Sling under client and attached to lift.

g. Raise bed rail.

h. Go to opposite side of bed, and lower side rail.

i. Roll client to opposite side, and pull hammock (strips) through.

j. Roll client supine onto canvas seat.

k. Remove client's glasses, if appropriate.

l. Place lift's horseshoe bar under side of bed (on side with chair).

m. Lower horizontal bar to sling level by releasing hydraulic valve. Lock valve.

n. Attach hooks on strap (chain) to holes in sling. Short chains or straps hook to top holes of sling; longer chains hook to bottom of sling (see illustration).

o. Elevate head of bed.

p. Fold client's arms over chest.

q. Pump hydraulic handle using long, slow, even strokes until client is raised off bed.

r. Use steering handle to pull lift from bed and maneuver to chair.

s. Roll base around chair.

Maintains client safety.

Completes positioning of client on mechanical/hydraulic sling.

Sling should extend from shoulders to knees (hammock) to support client's body weight equally.

Swivel bar is close to client's head and could break eyeglasses.

Positions lift efficiently and promotes smooth transfer.

Positions hydraulic lift close to client. Locking valve prevents injury to client.

Secures hydraulic lift to sling.

Positions client in sitting position.

Prevents injury to client's arms.

Ensures safe support of client during elevation.

Moves client from bed to chair.

Positions lift in front of the chair in which client is to be transferred.

STEP	RATIONALE
t. Release check valve slowly (turn to left), and lower client into chair (see illustration).	Safely guides client into back of chair as seat descends.
u. Close check valve as soon as client is down and straps can be released.	If valve is left open, boom may continue to lower and injure client.
v. Remove straps and mechanical/hydraulic lift (see illustration).	Prevents damage to skin and underlying tissues from canvas or hooks.
w. Check client's sitting alignment, and correct if necessary.	Prevents injury from poor posture.
7. Perform hand hygiene.	Reduces transmission of microorganisms.

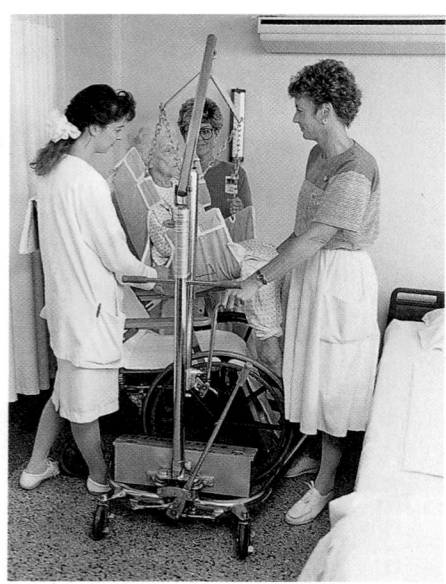

Step 6t Use of hydraulic lift to lower client into chair.

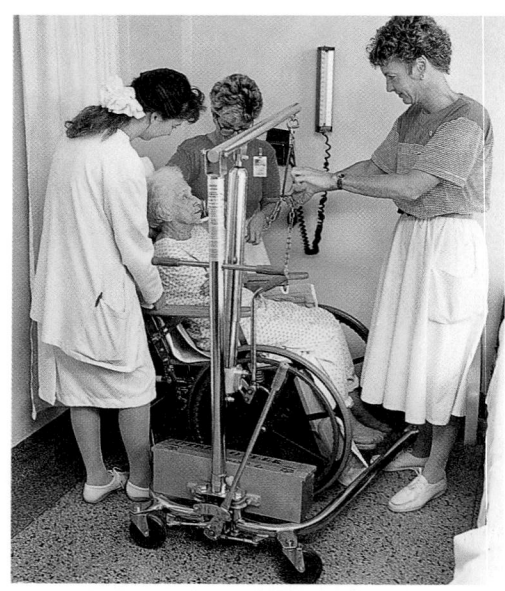

Step 6v Removal of hydraulic lift.

EVALUATION

1. Monitor vital signs. Ask if client feels dizzy or fatigued.
2. Note client's behavioral response to transfer.
3. Ask if client experienced pain during transfer.

4. Have client who transfers to chair attempt to bear weight with nurse at side.

Evaluates client's response to postural changes and activity.
Reveals level of motivation and self-care potential.
Determines need for additional pain control or alteration in technique of transferring (e.g., additional assistance).
Determines tolerance to weight bearing.

Recording and Reporting

- Record procedure, including pertinent observations: weakness, ability to follow directions, weight-bearing ability, balance, ability to pivot, number of personnel needed to assist, and amount of assistance (muscle strength) required.
- Report transfer ability and assistance needed to next shift or other caregivers. Report progress or remission to rehabilitation staff (physical therapist, occupational therapist).

Unexpected Outcomes	Related Interventions
1. Client is unable to comprehend and follow directions for transfer.	Cognitive impairment affects learning and retention. • Reassess continuity and simplicity of instruction. • Transfers may be difficult when client is fatigued or in pain; assess before transfer (allow for a rest period before transferring, or medicate for pain if indicated).
2. Client sustains injury on transfer.	Indicates improper transfer technique was used. • Evaluate incident that caused injury (e.g., assessment inadequate, change in client status, improper use of equipment). • Complete incident report according to institution policy.
3. Client's level of weakness does not permit active transfer.	• Physical impairments require increased assistance from nursing personnel. • Increase bed activity and exercise to heighten tolerance.
4. Client continues to bear weight on non–weight-bearing limb.	• Certain conditions (e.g., hip fractures) need to be non–weight bearing through healing process. • Reassess client's understanding of weight-bearing status.
5. Client is unable to stand for time required to transfer.	• Results from increased fatigue, orthostatic hypotension, or pain. • Provide for adequate assistance during transfer.

Teaching Considerations

- For many clients the return to home is coupled with enhanced psychological well-being and increased levels of motivation and ability for self-care function. Appropriate teaching of self-care skills and use of aids to maximize ability enhance outcome.
- Teach family and client transfer skills. Information should include principles of body mechanics and hazards of immobility. Incorporate return demonstration in discharge planning.

Pediatric Considerations

- Whenever possible, transporting child by stretcher, stroller, or wheelchair outside confines of room will increase environmental stimuli and provide social contact with others (Hockenberry and others, 2003).

Gerontological Considerations

- A major health concern that threatens the function of the older adult is the risk of falls (Wallman, 2001). Concern increases when the older adult is admitted to the hospital. Assess the client for the risk for falls upon admission, and a protocol to prevent falls should then be implemented (Phipps and others, 2003) (see Chapter 4).
- Use a drawsheet to avoid shearing force on the older adult client who has fragile skin.

Home Care Considerations

- Family or support person should practice transfer in hospital to achieve success before taking client home. Alternatively, client (if living alone) should practice transfer skills in bed that will be used at home. Client should be taught to transfer to chair with arms for ease of rising and sitting.
- Home should be free of hazards (e.g., throw rugs, electric cords, slippery floors). If wheelchair is used, access must be possible through all doors, and space for transfer must be available in bedroom and bathroom (see Chapter 41).
- Aids that enhance transfer ability are shower stools, commode elevators, handrails on tub, and nonskid shower surface. Many self-care devices are available for wheelchair-bound clients or clients with weak or poor muscle function. Many medical supply stores can provide excellent information and catalogs of such supplies.

SKILL 10-3 Moving and Positioning Clients in Bed

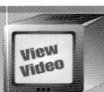

Correct positioning of clients is crucial for maintaining body alignment and comfort, preventing injury to the musculoskeletal and integumentary systems, and providing sensory, motor, and cognitive stimulation. A client with impaired mobility, decreased sensation, impaired circulation, or lack of voluntary muscle control can develop damage to the musculoskeletal and integumentary systems while lying down. The nurse must minimize this risk by maintaining unrestricted circulation and correct body alignment while moving, turning, or positioning the client.

DELEGATION CONSIDERATIONS

The skills of moving and positioning clients in bed can be delegated to assistive personnel. Before delegating this skill the nurse must:

- Report to assistive personnel any moving and positioning restrictions (e.g., avoid prone position, client has one-sided weakness).
- Designate specific times throughout the shift that assistive personnel must reposition the client.

EQUIPMENT

- ❏ Pillows
- ❏ Footboard (optional)
- ❏ Trochanter roll
- ❏ Sandbag
- ❏ Hand rolls
- ❏ Side rails

STEP	RATIONALE

ASSESSMENT

1. Assess client's body alignment and comfort level while client is lying down.

2. Assess for risk factors that may contribute to complications of immobility:

   a. *Paralysis:* hemiparesis resulting from CVA; decreased sensation

   b. *Impaired mobility:* traction, arthritis, or other contributing disease processes

   c. *Impaired circulation:* arterial insufficiency

   d. *Age:* very young, older adult

3. Assess client's level of consciousness.

4. Assess client's physical ability to help with moving and positioning, which may be affected by age, level of consciousness, disease process, strength, ROJM, and coordination.

5. Assess for presence of tubes, incisions, and equipment (e.g., traction).

6. Assess motivation of client and ability of family members to participate in moving and positioning client in bed in anticipation of discharge to home.

7. Check physician's orders before positioning client.

Provides baseline data for later comparisons. Determines ways to improve position and alignment.

Increased risk factors require client to be repositioned more frequently.

Paralysis impairs movement; muscle tone changes; sensation is affected. Because of difficulty in moving and poor awareness of involved body part, client is unable to protect and position body part for self.

Traction or arthritic changes of affected extremity result in decreased ROJM.

Decreased circulation predisposes client to pressure ulcers.

Premature and young infants require frequent turning because their skin is fragile. Normal physiological changes associated with aging predispose older adults to greater risks for developing complications of immobility.

Determines need for special aids or devices. Clients with altered levels of consciousness may not understand instructions and may be unable to help.

Enables nurse to use client's mobility, strength, and coordination. Determines need for additional help. Ensures client and nurse safety.

Will alter positioning procedure and type of positions to use. Determines approach needed for instruction.

Indicates whether instruction is necessary.

Some positions may be contraindicated in certain situations (e.g., spinal cord injury; respiratory difficulties; certain neurological conditions; presence of incisions, drains, or tubing).

STEP	**RATIONALE**

▮ NURSING DIAGNOSES

- Activity intolerance
- Impaired skin integrity

- Risk for impaired skin integrity
- Impaired physical mobility

Related factors are individualized based on client's condition or needs.

▮ PLANNING

1. Expected outcomes following completion of procedure:
   - Client retains ROJM.

   - Client's skin shows no evidence of breakdown.
   - Client's comfort is increased.
   - Client's level of independence in completing ADLs is increased.

2. Raise level of bed to comfortable working height.
3. Remove all pillows and devices used in previous position.

4. Get extra help as needed.
5. Explain procedure to client.

Correct positioning allows client to achieve optimal joint mobility and alignment.

Frequent position changes decrease risk of skin breakdown.
Proper positioning reduces stress on joints.
Maintaining good body alignment and joint mobility increases client's level of independence and overall mobility. Client with inadequate joint mobility may need assistance to carry out ADLs.

Raises level of work toward nurse's center of gravity.
Reduces interference from bedding during positioning procedure.
Provides for client and nurse safety.
Helps to decrease anxiety and increase cooperation.

▮ IMPLEMENTATION

1. Perform hand hygiene.
2. Close door to room or close bedside curtains.
3. Put bed in flat position.

Reduces transmission of infection.
Provides for client privacy.
Provides easy access to client and allows nurses to reposition client to any position without working against gravity.

• *Critical Decision Point*

Before flattening bed, account for all tubing drains and equipment to prevent dislodgment or spillage if caught in mattress or bed frame as bed is lowered.

4. **Assist client in moving up in bed (two nurses):**

This task is not a one-person task unless client can fully assist (United States Department of Labor, 2003). The use of a drawsheet is recommended to move a client up in bed (see step 5).

   a. Place client on back with head of bed flat.

   Enables nurse to assess body alignment. Reduces gravity's pull on client's upper body.

   b. Remove pillow from under head and shoulders, and place pillow at head of bed.

   Prevents striking client's head against head of bed.

   c. Face head of bed.

   Facing direction of movement prevents twisting of nurse's body while moving client.

   (1) Each nurse should have one arm under client's head and shoulders and one arm under client's thighs.

   Provides support across length of client's body.

   (2) *Alternative position if client can assist:* Position one nurse at client's upper body. Nurse's arm nearest head of bed should be under client's head and opposite shoulder; other arm should be under client's closest arm and shoulder. Position other nurse at client's lower torso. The nurse's arms should be under client's lower back and torso.

   Prevents trauma to client's musculoskeletal system by supporting shoulder and hip joints and evenly distributing weight.

STEP	RATIONALE

    d. Place feet apart, with foot nearest head of bed behind other foot (forward-backward stance).

Wide base of support increases nurse's balance. Stance enables nurse to shift body weight as client is moved up in bed, thereby reducing force needed to move load.

    e. When possible, ask client to flex knees with feet flat on bed.

Decreases friction and enables client to use leg muscles during movement.

    f. Instruct client to flex neck, tilting chin toward chest.

Prevents hyperextension of neck when moving client up in bed.

    g. Instruct client to assist moving by pushing down with feet on bed surface.

Reduces friction. Increases client mobility. Decreases nurse's workload.

    h. Flex knees and hips, bringing forearms closer to level of bed.

Increases balance and strength by bringing nurse's center of gravity closer to client. Uses thighs instead of back muscles.

    i. Warn client to push with heels and elevate trunk while breathing out, thus moving toward head of bed on count of three.

Prepares client for move. Reinforces assistance in moving up in bed. Increases client cooperation. Breathing out avoids Valsalva maneuver.

    j. On count of three, rock and shift weight from front to back leg. At the same time client pushes with heels and elevates trunk.

Rocking enables nurse to improve balance and overcome inertia. Shifting nurse's weight counteracts client's weight and reduces force needed to move load. Client's assistance reduces friction and nurse's workload.

5. **Move immobile client up in bed with drawsheet (two nurses):**

Depending upon the client's weight, it may take more than two nurses to move client.

    a. Place drawsheet under client, extending from shoulders to thighs.

Supports client's body weight and reduces friction during movement.

    b. Place client on back with head of bed flat.

Even distribution of weight makes lift easier.

    c. Position one nurse at each side of client.

Distributes weight equally between nurses.

    d. Fanfold the drawsheet on both sides, and grasp firmly near client.

Provides strong handles in order to grip drawsheet without slipping.

    e. Place feet apart with forward-backward stance. Flex knees and hips. Shift weight from front to back leg, and move client and drawsheet to desired position in bed (see illustration).

Facing direction of movement ensures proper balance. Shifting weight reduces force needed to move load. Flexing knees lowers nurses' center of gravity and uses thighs instead of back muscles.

6. Realign client in correct body alignment.

Prevents injury to musculoskeletal system. Nurses may assist client to one of the positions listed below.

    a. **Position client in supported Fowler's position (see illustration):**

        (1) Elevate head of bed 45 to 60 degrees.

Increases comfort, improves ventilation, and increases client's opportunity to socialize or relax.

        (2) Rest head against mattress or on small pillow.

Prevents flexion contractures of cervical vertebrae.

Step **5e** Moving immobile client up in bed with drawsheet.

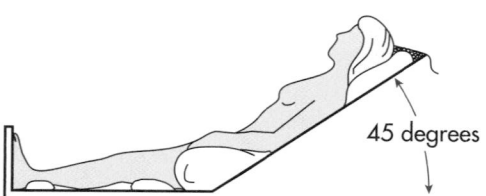

Step **6a** Footboard in place (Fowler's position).

STEP	RATIONALE
(3) Use pillows to support arms and hands if client does not have voluntary control or use of hands and arms.	Prevents shoulder dislocation from effect of downward pull of unsupported arms, promotes circulation by preventing venous pooling, and prevents flexion contractures of arms and wrists.
(4) Position pillow at lower back.	Supports lumbar vertebrae and decreases flexion of vertebrae.
(5) Place small pillow or roll under thigh.	Prevents hyperextension of knee and occlusion of popliteal artery from pressure from body weight.
(6) Place small pillow or roll under ankles.	Prevents prolonged pressure of mattress on heels.

- **Critical Decision Point**

  To keep feet in proper alignment, place footboard at bottom of client's feet, apply high-top sneakers on client's feet, or use other devices to maintain dorsiflexion.

STEP	RATIONALE
b. **Position hemiplegic client in supported Fowler's position:**	
(1) Elevate head of bed 45 to 60 degrees.	Increases comfort, improves ventilation, and increases client's opportunity to relax.
(2) Position client in sitting position as straight as possible.	Counteracts tendency to slump toward affected side. Improves ventilation and cardiac output; decreases intracranial pressure. Improves client's ability to swallow and helps to prevent aspiration of food, liquids, and gastric secretions.
(3) Position head on small pillow with chin slightly forward. If client is totally unable to control head movement, hyperextension of the neck must be avoided.	Prevents hyperextension of neck. Too many pillows under head may cause or worsen neck flexion contracture.
(4) Provide support for involved arm and hand by placing arm away from client's side and supporting elbow with pillow.	Paralyzed muscles do not automatically resist pull of gravity as they do normally. As a result, shoulder subluxation, pain, and edema may occur.

- **Critical Decision Point**

  Position flaccid hand in normal resting position with wrist slightly extended, arches of hand maintained, and fingers partially flexed; may use section of rubber ball cut in half; clasp client's hands together.

- **Critical Decision Point**

  Position spastic hand with wrist in neutral position or slightly extended; fingers should be extended with palm down or may be left in relaxed position with palm up.

STEP	RATIONALE
(5) Flex knees and hips by using pillow or folded blanket under knees.	Ensures proper alignment. Flexion prevents prolonged hyperextension, which could impair joint mobility.
(6) Support feet in dorsiflexion with firm pillow, footboard, or high-top sneakers.	Prevents footdrop. Stimulation of ball of foot by hard surface has tendency to increase muscle tone in client with extensor spasticity of lower extremity.
c. **Position client in supine position:**	
(1) Place client on back with head of bed flat.	Necessary for placing client in supine position.
(2) Place small rolled towel under lumbar area of back.	Provides support for lumbar spine.
(3) Place pillow under upper shoulders, neck, or head.	Maintains correct alignment and prevents flexion contractures of cervical vertebrae.
(4) Place trochanter rolls or sandbags parallel to lateral surface of client's thighs.	Reduces external rotation of hip.

STEP	**RATIONALE**

(5) Place small pillow or roll under ankle to elevate heels (see illustration in step 6a).

Reduces pressure on heels, helping to prevent pressure sores.

(6) Place footboard or firm pillows against bottom of client's feet, or place high-top sneakers on client's feet.

Maintains feet in dorsiflexion. Prevents footdrop.

(7) Place pillows under pronated forearms, keeping upper arms parallel to client's body (see illustrations).

Reduces internal rotation of shoulder and prevents extension of elbows. Maintains correct body alignment.

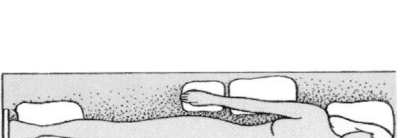

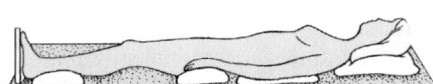

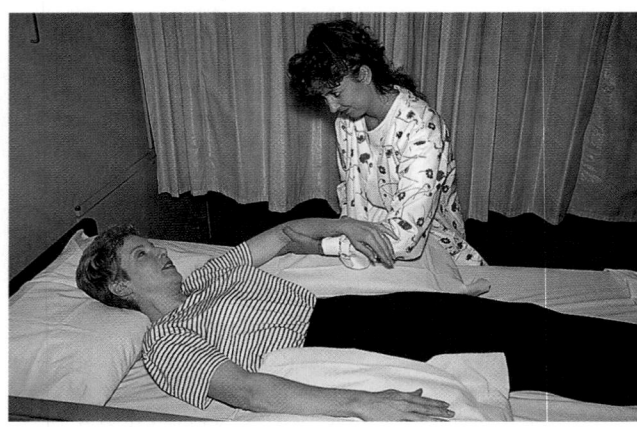

Step **6c(7)** Supine position with pillows in place.

(8) Place hand rolls in client's hands. Consider physical therapy referral for use of hand splints.

Reduces extension of fingers and abduction of thumb. Maintains thumb slightly adducted and in opposition to fingers.

d. Position hemiplegic client in supine position:

(1) Place head of bed flat.

Necessary for positioning in supine position.

(2) Place folded towel or small pillow under shoulder or affected side.

Decreases possibility of pain, joint contracture, and subluxation. Maintains mobility in muscles around shoulder to permit normal movement patterns.

(3) Keep affected arm away from body with elbow extended and palm up. Position affected hand in one of recommended positions for flaccid or spastic hand. (Alternative is to place arm out to side, with elbow bent and hand toward head of bed.)

Maintains mobility in arm, joints, and shoulder to permit normal movement patterns. (Alternative position counteracts limitation of ability of arm to rotate outward at shoulder [external rotation]. External rotation must be present to raise arm over head without pain.)

(4) Place folded towel under hip of involved side.

Diminishes effect of spasticity in entire leg by controlling hip position.

(5) Flex affected knee 30 degrees by supporting it on pillow or folded blanket.

Slight flexion breaks up abnormal extension pattern of leg. Extensor spasticity is most severe when client is supine.

(6) Support feet with soft pillows at right angle to leg.

Maintains foot in dorsiflexion and prevents footdrop. Pillows prevent stimulation to ball of foot by hard surface, which has tendency to increase muscle tone in client with extensor spasticity of lower extremity.

e. Position client in prone position:

In certain clients with pulmonary conditions, such as acute respiratory distress syndrome (ARDS), the use of the prone position can help improve oxygenation (Marion, 2001).

(1) Roll client to one side while placing arm on side to be turned, alongside of the body.

Prepares client for positioning.

(2) Roll client over arm positioned close to body, with elbow straight and hand under hip. Position on abdomen in center of bed.

Positions client correctly so alignment can be maintained.

STEP	RATIONALE
(3) Turn client's head to one side, and support head with small pillow (see illustration).	Reduces flexion or hyperextension of cervical vertebrae.
(4) Place small pillow under client's abdomen below level of diaphragm (see illustration).	Reduces pressure on breasts of some female clients and decreases hyperextension of lumbar vertebrae and strain on lower back. Improves breathing by reducing mattress pressure on diaphragm.
(5) Support arms in flexed position level at shoulders.	Maintains proper body alignment. Support reduces risk of joint dislocation.
(6) Support lower legs with pillow to elevate toes (see illustration).	Prevents footdrop. Reduces external rotation of legs. Reduces mattress pressure on toes.

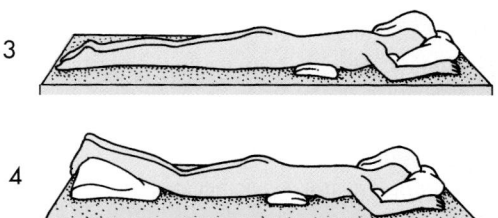

Step **6e(3-4)** Prone position with pillows in place.

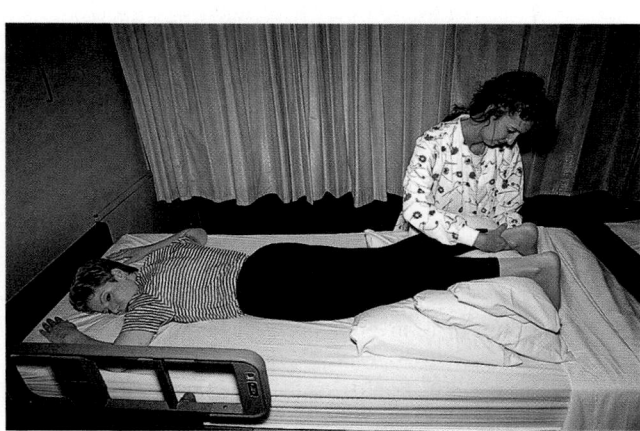

Step **6e(6)** Prone position with pillows supporting lower legs.

f. Position hemiplegic client in prone position:

- *Critical Decision Point*

  Increase frequency of positioning if pressure areas begin to appear, joint mobility becomes impaired or worsened, or client complains of discomfort. Consult with physical and occupational therapists as needed.

(1) Move client toward unaffected side.	Ensures proper alignment in center of bed when client is rolled onto abdomen.
(2) While rolling client onto side, place pillow on client's abdomen.	Prevents sagging of abdomen when client is rolled over; decreases hyperextension of lumbar vertebrae and strain on lower back.
(3) Roll client onto abdomen by positioning involved arm close to client's body, with elbow straight and hand under hip. Roll client carefully over arm.	Prevents injury to affected side.
(4) Turn head toward involved side.	Promotes development of neck and trunk extension, which is necessary for standing and walking.
(5) Position involved arm out to side, with elbow bent, hand toward head of bed, and fingers extended (if possible).	Counteracts limitation of arm's ability to rotate outward at shoulder (external rotation). External rotation must be present to raise arm over head without pain.
(6) Flex knees slightly by placing pillow under legs from knees to ankles.	Flexion prevents prolonged hyperextension, which could impair joint mobility.
(7) Keep feet at right angle to legs by using pillow high enough to keep toes off mattress and by applying high-top sneakers.	Maintains feet in dorsiflexion.

STEP	**RATIONALE**

g. **Position client in 30-degree lateral (side-lying) position:**

(1) Lower head of bed completely or as low as client can tolerate.

Provides position of comfort for client and removes pressure from bony prominences on back.

(2) Position client to side of bed opposite direction client is to be turned.

Provides room for client to turn to side.

(3) Prepare to turn client onto side. Flex client's knee that will not be next to mattress. Place one hand on client's hip and one hand on client's shoulder.

Use of leverage makes turning to side easy.

- **Critical Decision Point**

Client at risk for pressure ulcer development requires the 30-degree lateral position (see Chapter 15).

(4) Roll client onto side toward nurse.

Rolling decreases trauma to tissues. In addition, client is positioned so leverage on hip makes turning easy.

(5) Place pillow under client's head and neck.

Maintains alignment. Reduces lateral neck flexion. Decreases strain on sternocleidomastoid muscle.

(6) Bring dependent shoulder blade forward.

Prevents client's weight from resting directly on shoulder joint.

(7) Position both arms in slightly flexed position. Upper arm is supported by pillow level with shoulder; other arm, by mattress.

Decreases internal rotation and adduction of shoulder. Supporting both arms in slightly flexed position protects joint. Ventilation is improved because chest is able to expand more easily.

(8) Bring dependent hip slightly forward so that angle from hip to mattress is approximately 30 degrees.

The thirty-degree lateral position reduces pressure on trochanter.

(9) Place small tuck-back pillow behind client's back. (Make by folding pillow lengthwise. Smooth area is slightly tucked under client's back.)

Provides support to maintain client on side.

(10) Place pillow under semiflexed upper leg level at hip from groin to foot (see illustration).

Flexion prevents hyperextension of leg. Maintains leg in correct alignment. Prevents pressure on bony prominences.

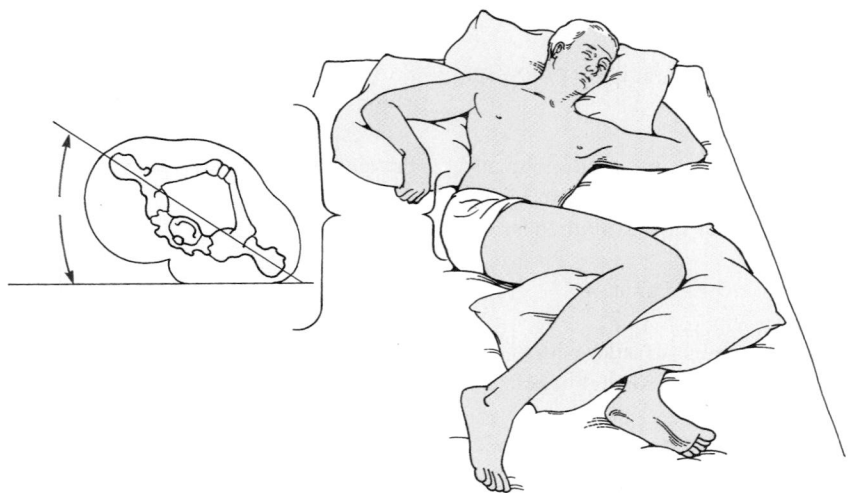

Step **6g(10)** Lateral position with pillows in place.

STEP	RATIONALE
(11) Place sandbag parallel to plantar surface of dependent foot. Place high-top sneakers on client's feet.	Maintains dorsiflexion of foot. Prevents footdrop.
h. Position client in Sims' (semiprone) position:	
(1) Lower head of bed completely.	Provides for proper body alignment while client is lying down.
(2) Place client in supine position.	Prepares client for position.
(3) Roll client on side, and position in lateral position, lying partially on abdomen, with dependent shoulder lifted out and arm placed at client's side.	Client is rolled only partially on abdomen.
(4) Place small pillow under client's head.	Maintains proper alignment and prevents lateral neck flexion.
(5) Place pillow under flexed upper arm, supporting arm level with shoulder.	Prevents internal rotation of shoulder. Maintains alignment.
(6) Place pillow under flexed upper legs, supporting leg level with hip.	Prevents internal rotation of hip and adduction of leg. Flexion prevents hyperextension of leg. Reduces mattress pressure on knees and ankles.
(7) Place sandbags parallel to plantar surface of foot (see illustration) or apply high-top sneakers.	Maintains foot in dorsiflexion. Prevents footdrop.

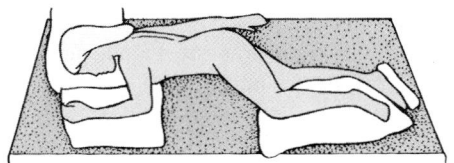

Step 6h(7) Sandbag supporting right foot in dorsiflexion.

i. Logrolling the client: (three nurses)

● *Critical Decision Point*

A nurse should supervise and aid assistive personnel when there is a physician's order to logroll a client. Clients who have suffered from a spinal cord injury or are recovering from neck, back, or spinal surgery often need to keep the spinal column in straight alignment to prevent further injury (Groeneveld and others, 2001).

(1) Place small pillow between client's knees.	Prevents tension on the spinal column and adduction of the hip.
(2) Cross client's arms on chest.	Prevents injury to arms.

STEP	**RATIONALE**

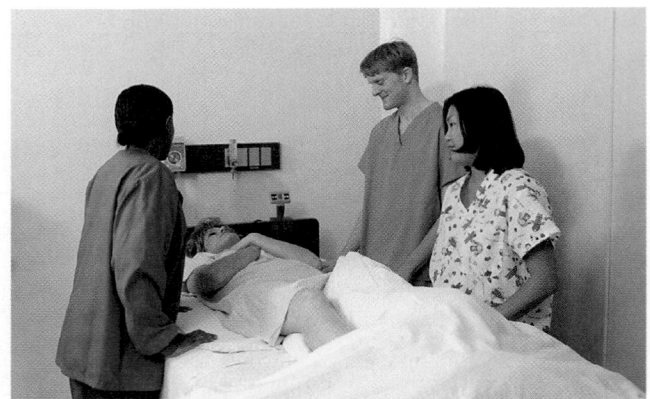 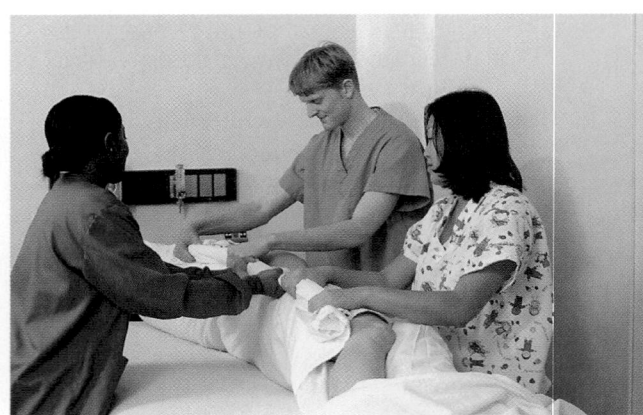

Step **6i(3-5)** Logrolling a client.

(3) Position two nurses on the side the client is to be turned toward; and one nurse on the side where pillows are to be placed (see illustration).	Distributes weight equally between nurses during turning.
(4) Fanfold the drawsheet along side of client that will be turning.	Provides strong handles to grip the drawsheet without slipping.
(5) With one nurse grasping drawsheet at lower hips and thighs, and the other nurse grasping drawsheet at client's shoulders and lower back; roll the client as one unit in a smooth, continuous motion on the count of three (see illustration).	This maintains proper alignment by moving all body parts at the same time, preventing tension or twisting of the spinal column (Groeneveld and others, 2001).
(6) Nurse on the opposite side of the bed places pillows along the length of the client for support (see illustration).	Maintains client in side-lying position.
(7) Gently lean the client as a unit back toward the pillows for support.	Ensures continued straight alignment of spinal column, preventing injury.
7. Perform hand hygiene.	Reduces transmission of infection.

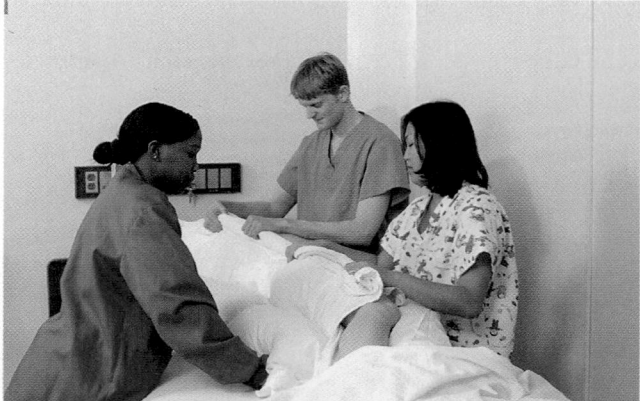

Step **6i(6)** Place pillows along client's back for support.

STEP	RATIONALE

▌EVALUATION

1. Assess client's body alignment, position, and level of comfort.

   Determines effectiveness of positioning. Additional supports (e.g., pillows, bath blankets) may be added or removed to promote comfort and correct body alignment.

2. Measure ROJM (see Chapter 11).

   Determines if joint contracture is developing.

3. Observe for areas of erythema or breakdown involving skin.

   Provides ongoing observation regarding client's skin and musculoskeletal systems. Indicates complications of immobility or improper positioning of body part.

Recording and Reporting

* Record procedure and observations (e.g., condition of skin, joint movement, client's ability to assist with positioning).
* Report observations at change of shift, and document in nurses' notes.

Unexpected Outcomes	Related Interventions
1. Joint contractures develop or worsen.	• Improper positioning results in shortening of muscles. • Increase frequency of range-of-motion exercises to affected and immobilized areas (see Chapter 11).
2. Skin shows localized areas of erythema and breakdown.	• Increase frequency of repositioning. • Place turning schedule above client's bed.
3. Client avoids moving.	• Medicate with analgesia as ordered by physician to ensure client's comfort before moving. • Allow pain medication to take effect before proceeding.

Teaching Considerations

* Include family in explanations, especially when caring for infant, young child, or confused or unconscious client.
* Teach client ways to assist with positioning, and provide opportunity for return demonstration.
* Teach client and family signs and symptoms of pressure ulcers and contractures.

Pediatric Considerations

* Children should be encouraged to be as active as their condition and restrictive devices allow. Materials or objects to stimulate activity and encouragement and participation of others must be available (Hockenberry and others, 2003).
* Children who are unable to move will need passive exercise and movement (see Chapter 11).

Gerontological Considerations

* Older adult clients must be repositioned at least every 1 to 2 hours, and a regular program of ROJM exercises must be maintained (Lueckenotte, 2000; Maas and others, 2001).

Home Care Considerations

* Assess ability and motivation of client, family members, and primary caregiver to participate in moving and positioning client in bed.
* Assess home to determine compatibility of environment with assistive devices (e.g., over-bed trapeze, Hoyer lift, hospital bed).

Long-Term Care Considerations

* Clients who have maintained bed rest for a long period of time may revert back to a favorite position. Frequently assess these clients, and turn more often as needed.
* Use drawsheet to prevent shearing force on fragile skin (Hignett, 2003; Owens, 2000; United States Department of Labor, 2003).
* Allow client to assist with moving and positioning whenever possible to promote independence.

FOCUS on CLINICAL PRACTICE

Mr. Clark is a 37-year-old man who suffered a spinal cord injury in a motor vehicle accident. He is admitted on your shift. He has sustained multiple deep lacerations on his face and trunk and facial fractures of maxillary and zygomatic bones. He rates his pain at 9 on a scale of 0 to 10.

1. The emergency department nurse was extremely busy and was unable to provide a complete report. What other information would you obtain about this client?
2. Mr. Clark is scheduled STAT for a computed tomography (CT) scan of the head and spine. He refuses to allow you to move him onto the stretcher. What interventions would you select to elicit his cooperation?
   A. Administer pain medication as ordered by the physician.
   B. Explain the purpose and importance of the CT scan.

C. Describe the method by which you will move him onto the stretcher.
D. Tell him it is a physician's order and must be carried out.
Explain your choice(s).

3. Mr. Clark has returned from CT scan. The physician has ordered Mr. Clark to be turned and positioned every 1 to 2 hours until he is taken to surgery to stabilize his spinal fracture. What do you think would be the safest technique to move Mr. Clark from side to side? Explain your answer.
4. You are very busy, and the assistive personnel state that they will turn Mr. Clark. What is the appropriate, safe action in response to assistive personnel turning Mr. Clark?
Explain your answer.

NCLEX REVIEW QUESTIONS

1. Mrs. Green is an 86-year-old woman admitted for pneumonia. She is weak and frail and has an unsteady gait. A priority nursing diagnosis related to the safety of this client would be:
   1. Pain
   2. Impaired skin integrity
   3. Altered tissue perfusion
   4. Risk for injury
2. Mr. Smith has suffered a stroke. His daughter will be caring for him in his home. You have been instructing her on proper body mechanics. Which of the following statements indicates that learning has occurred?
   1. "I'm glad I have a strong back."
   2. "As I twist to place my father in his chair, I'll make sure he doesn't fall."
   3. "I will keep my knees bent and trunk erect so my muscles work together."
   4. "I will tighten my back muscles and push my pelvis forward to provide balance when lifting my father."
3. You are transferring Mrs. Jones from the bed to the chair for the first time. Which of the following actions poses the safest method of transfer for Mrs. Jones and you?
   1. Apply a transfer belt around Mrs. Jones' waist.
   2. Use the under-axilla technique.
   3. Use the one-person transfer technique.
   4. Observe this client while she transfers to increase her independence.
4. Two assistive personnel ask for your assistance to transfer a client from the bed to a stretcher using the three-person lift technique. What is the appropriate response?
   1. "As long as we use proper body mechanics, no one will get hurt."

2. "The client only weighs 100 pounds; you should be able to handle the transfer without my assistance."
   3. "I'll go get the slide board; it is more comfortable for the client, and it will protect us from injury."
   4. "The three-person lift technique is recommended to ensure the safety of the client and nursing personnel."
5. Mr. Williams has arrived on your unit after undergoing extensive abdominal surgery. He is awake and alert. He is refusing to be repositioned in bed. What would you assess first to determine the reason for Mr. Williams's refusal? Assess level of:
   1. Consciousness
   2. Pain
   3. Motivation
   4. Knowledge related to complications of immobility
6. Mrs. Sweeney is admitted with an unstable spinal cord injury. The safest and most appropriate method of moving this client from side to side is to:
   1. Use a slide-board to move her from side to side
   2. Logroll the client with the assistance of three nurses
   3. Allow the client to move herself to promote independence
   4. Use a step-by-step method: move the trunk, then hips, and finally the leg.

References

American Nurses Association: *Position statement on elimination of manual patient handling to prevent work-related musculoskeletal disorders,* www.nursingworld.org.readroom/position/workplac/pathand.htm, June 2003.

Bureau of Labor Statistics: *Occupational industries and illnesses: industry data,* http://stats.bls.gov/bls/occupation.htm, 2004.

Ebersole P, Hess P: *Geriatric nursing and healthy aging,* St. Louis, 2001, Mosby.

Edlich R and others: Disabling back injuries in nursing personnel, *J Emerg Nurs* 27(2):150, 2001.

Feldt K: The checklist of nonverbal pain indicators (CNPI), *Pain Manag Nurs* 1(1):35, 2000.

Groeneveld A and others: Logrolling: establishing consistent practices, *Orthop Nurs* 20(2):45, 2001.

Hockenberry MJ and others: *Wong's nursing care of infants and children,* ed 7, St. Louis, 2003, Mosby.

Lueckenotte A: *Gerontologic nursing,* ed 2, St. Louis, 2000, Mosby.

Maas M and others: *Nursing care of older adults: diagnoses, outcomes, and interventions,* St. Louis, 2001, Mosby.

Marion B: A turn for the better: prone positioning of patients with ARDS, *Am J Nurs* 101(5):26, 2001.

McCance K, Huether S: *Understanding pathophysiology,* ed 2, St. Louis, 2000, Mosby.

Moreno J: Limit liability with lift programs, *Provider* 29(1):43, 2003.

Nelson A and others: Myths and facts about back injuries in nursing: the incidence rate of back injuries among is more than double that among construction workers, perhaps because misconceptions persist about causes and solutions, *Am J Nurs* 103(2):32, 2003.

Occupational Health and Safety Administration: Ergonomics standard proposal, *Fed Regist* 29 CFR Part 1910, January 24, 2000, www.osha-slc.gov/SLTC/ergonomics/index.html.

Phipps W and others: *Medical-surgical nursing: health and illness perspectives,* ed 7, St. Louis, 2003, Mosby.

Trinkoff A and others: Musculoskeletal problems of the neck, shoulder, and back and functional consequences in nurses, *Am J Ind Med* 41(3):170, 2002.

United States Department of Labor, Occupational Safety and Health Administration: *Guidelines for nursing homes: Ergonomics for the prevention of musculoskeletal disorders,* Washington, DC, 2003.

Wong DL and others: *Wong's essentials of pediatric nursing,* ed 6, St. Louis, 2001, Mosby.

Research References

Hignett S: Systematic review of patient handling activities starting in lying, sitting and standing positions, *J Adv Nurs* 41(6):545, 2003.

Konradi D, Anglin D: Moderate-intensity exercise: for our patients, for ourselves, *Orthop Nurs* 20(1):47, 2001.

Lavender S and others: Postural analysis of paramedics simulating frequently performed strenuous work tasks, *Appl Ergon* 31:45, 2000.

Owens B: Preventing injuries using an ergonomic approach, *AORN J* 72(6):1031, 2000.

Owens B and others: What are we teaching about lifting and transferring patients? *Res Nurs Health* 22:3, 1999.

Pan C, Freivalos A: Ergonomic evaluation of a new patient handling device, *Proceedings of the IEA2000/HFES 2000 Congress: the human factors and ergonomics society* 4:274, 2000.

Wallman H: Comparison of older nonfallers and fallers on performance measures of functional reach, sensory organization, and limits of stability, *J Gerontol A Biol Sci Med Sci* 56(9):M580, 2001.

Zuang Z and others: Psychophysical assessment of assistive devices for transferring patients/residents, *Appl Ergon* 31:35, 2000.

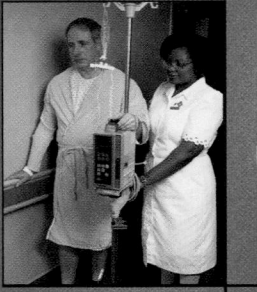

11

Exercise And Ambulation

MEDIA RESOURCES

Evolve Site *evolve*

http://evolve.elsevier.com/Perry/skills
- Weblinks
- Video clips
- Mosby's Nursing Skills Video Exercises

Mosby's Nursing Skills Videos/CD-ROM
- *Personal Hygiene Video:* Application of TED hose

OBJECTIVES

Mastery of content in this chaper will enable the nurse to:

- Discuss indications for assisting with ambulation or using devices to assist with ambulation.
- Discuss indications for performing range-of-motion and isometric exercises.
- Identify significant assessment data to be noted before and during the use of a continuous passive motion machine.
- Identify significant assessment data to be noted before assisting with ambulation and range-of-motion and isometric exercises.
- Demonstrate the following skills on selected clients: assisting with ambulation, assisting with ambulation with the use of an ambulation aid, assisting with range-of-motion exercises, assisting with isometric exercises, applying a continuous passive motion (CPM) machine, and applying elastic stockings and sequential compression device.
- Develop teaching plans for selected clients for safety precautions to use at home while using an ambulation aid, applying and monitoring effects of elastic stockings and sequential compression devices, using the CPM machine, and performing range-of-motion and isometric exercises.

KEY TERMS

Abduction	Gait belt
Active range-of-motion exercises	Hyperextension
	Immobility
Active-assisted range-of-motion exercises	Internal rotation
	Inversion
Activity tolerance	Isometric contraction
Adduction	Isometric exercise
Atrophy	Joint
Bed rest	Lateral flexion
Circumduction	Mobility
Contractures	Opposition
Crutch gait	Orthostatic hypotension
Crutch palsy	Osteoblastic
Dangling	Osteoclastic
Deep vein thrombosis (DVT)	Passive range-of-motion exercises
Dorsal	Plantar flexion
Dorsiflexion	Pronation
Eversion	Radial flexion
Exercise	Rotation
Extension	Supination
External rotation	Thrombus
Flexion	Ulnar flexion
Footboard	
Gait	

The authors acknowledge the contribution of Mary Mercer to this chapter in previous editions of this text.

Mobility refers to a person's ability to move about freely, whereas immobility refers to a person's inability to move about freely. Mobility and immobility are best understood as the end points of a continuum, with many degrees of partial mobility in between. Some clients move back and forth on the mobility-immobility continuum as a result of disease or injury. Other clients experience immobility for an indefinite period.

The level of mobility has a significant impact on an individual's physiological, psychosocial, and developmental well-being (Jitramontree, 2001). When there is an alteration in mobility, many body systems are at risk for impairment. Impaired mobility can result in altered cardiovascular functioning, disruption of normal metabolic functioning, increased risk for pulmonary complications, the development of pressure ulcers, and urinary elimination alterations (Huether and McCance 2000; Phipps and others, 2003; Quell and others, 2002; Shea and others, 2002).

The severity of a mobility impairment depends on the client's age, overall health status, nutritional status, and the degree of immobility experienced. For example, pronounced effects of immobility develop more quickly in older adult clients with chronic illnesses than in younger clients (Lueckenotte, 2000; Maas and others, 2001). Older adults are at greater risk for developing orthostatic hypotension, syncope, confusion, increased risk of fractures, and functional incontinence as a result of decreased mobility from bed rest (Ebersole and Hess, 2001; Maas and others, 2001).

Alterations in mobility also have profound psychosocial and developmental effects. Immobilization may lead to emotional, intellectual, sensory, and sociocultural alterations. For adults and older adults, immobility may alter employment, family role functions, and social interactions (Cousins and Tan, 2002). Such changes can lead to altered self-concept and lowered self-esteem. Children also are affected by immobility. Activity for them is a way of releasing energy and expressing themselves. When deprived of physical activity, children become restless and may even show signs of anger and aggression (Hockenberry and others, 2003).

Changes in a client's mobility can result from various health problems. Examples of medical conditions that can alter mobility are musculoskeletal conditions such as fractured extremities or muscle sprains, neurological conditions such as spinal cord trauma, degenerative neurological conditions such as myasthenia gravis, and head injuries. Some clients may actually be immobilized for therapeutic reasons (e.g., prescribed bed rest, reduced activity). Nursing measures attempt to maintain and/or restore optimal mobility as well as to decrease the hazards associated with immobility. Frequent repositioning, deep breathing and coughing exercises, muscle and joint exercises, increased fluid intake, and dietary intake of foods containing fiber are examples of measures that help to reduce the hazards of immobility.

Cultural Considerations

The techniques for promoting exercise and ambulation pose implications for the nurse's ability to give culturally appropriate care. Assisting with exercises and applying compression hose, for example, may place clients in positions that can be embarrassing. Follow these cultural guidelines:

- Collaborate with family members in teaching elder clients from Asian, Hispanic, and African cultures about the concept of active participation in their rehabilitation.
- Most elders expect to remain in bed until healing is completed.
- Caring and respect for elders are generally demonstrated by family members' actively doing the tasks of caring for them (Ebrahim, 1996).
- Accommodate religious practices that limit use of certain rehabilitation appliances:
  - Orthodox Jews may not be able to operate continuous passive motion machine during Sabbath and Holy Days.
  - Consult the rabbi to obtain permission for the client to use the machine.
- Nurses should be responsible for turning the machine on and off during the Sabbath and Holy Days (Galanti, 2003).
- Use gender-congruent care for women from cultures that emphasize female modesty to apply elastic stockings and sequential compression devices. Hindus, Muslims, and Orthodox women may not comply with the treatment measure for fear of being exposed to the opposite sex.
- Most elder Asian, Hispanic, and African women prefer to bare their legs and thighs only to other women.
- Provide for female privacy when assisting clients with ambulation.
- Muslim females need to be fully covered when in public because of the emphasis on *Hijab,* or female modesty (Rashidi and Rajaram, 2001).
- Southeast Asian women such as Cambodians, Vietnamese, and Laotians severely restrict exposure of their lower torso and will not likely ambulate unless properly dressed (Miller, 1995).

Evidence-Based Practice Trends

Orthostatic hypotension is a drop in blood pressure that occurs when the client changes position from a horizontal to a vertical position (Dingle, 2003; Levick, 2000). Those at higher risk are immobilized clients, those undergoing prolonged bed rest, the older adult client, and those clients with chronic illnesses such as diabetes mellitus and cardiovascular disease (Dingle, 2003; Frederiks and others, 2003; Netea and others, 2002). Signs and symptoms of orthostatic hypotension include dizziness, light-headedness, nausea, tachycardia, pallor, and even fainting.

Physiological changes associated with aging and prolonged bed rest may influence the effectiveness of the baroreceptors (Kenny, 2000). In these clients, moving to the dangling position may cause a gravity-induced drop in blood pressure; thus it is recommended to raise the head of the bed and allow a few minutes before dangling (Dingle, 2003; Kenny, 2000). This allows a less dramatic shift in blood volume and provides a gradual adjustment to the upright position. Other interventions to minimize orthostatic hypotension include movement of the legs and feet in the dangling position to promote venous return via intermittent contraction and relaxation of the skeletal leg muscles, and asking the client to take several deep breaths before and during dangling (Dingle, 2003). Dangling a client before standing is an intermediate step that allows assessment of the individual before changing positions to maintain the safety and prevent injury to the client.

Skill Performance Guidelines

1. Check the physician's orders to determine the client's activity level and type of exercises or assistive device to be used.
2. Know the client's past medical history. The nurse should know why the client needs assistance with ambulation and any contraindications or limits to exercise.
3. Know the client's normal range for vital signs. Vital signs vary. Exercise and mobility can be fatiguing and stressful, so a set of baseline vital signs is necessary.
4. Assess baseline muscle strength. The client may need muscle-strengthening exercises before ambulation.
5. Assess baseline joint function. This knowledge helps the nurse to determine whether range-of-motion exercises are needed and provides a baseline for comparison of joint function after range-of-motion exercises are performed.
6. Obtain and become familiar with the type of assistive device to be used. Nurses need to know proper preparation and use of devices to be able to teach clients to use them safely and correctly.
7. Prepare the client. Make sure client is rested and not fatigued. Obtain extra personnel to assist, safety devices, and flat, nonskid shoes for the client. Address client's fear of falling if present.
8. Determine the type and frequency of intervention. Activity that is appropriate for one day or one shift can change, resulting in an increased or decreased need for assistance with ambulation or a change in the type of intervention.
9. Know the client's home care plan. The client may need to continue the exercise regimen or use an assistive device at home.

SKILL 11-1 Performing Range-of-Motion Exercises

Regardless of whether the cause of immobility is permanent or temporary, the immobilized client must receive some type of exercise to prevent excessive muscle atrophy and joint contractures. Joint contractures can occur within 3 to 7 days; thus the nurse must be vigilant to prevent such complications (Maas and others, 2001). The total amount of activity required to prevent disuse syndrome is about 2 hours for every 24-hour period, but this activity must be scheduled throughout the day to prevent the client from remaining inactive for long periods.

Exercise prevents some of the complications of immobility and helps prepare a client for ambulation. The nurse may use range-of-motion (ROM) exercise and isometric exercises (see Skill 11-2) to help the client maintain muscle and joint function.

ROM exercises put each joint through as full a range of motion as possible without causing discomfort. ROM exercises may be *active, passive, or active-assisted*. Active range-of-motion exercises are those exercises the client is able to

perform independently, and passive range-of-motion exercises are performed for the client by someone else. Active-assisted range-of-motion exercises are performed by a client with some assistance. The type of ROM exercises are the same regardless of whether the client can do the exercises independently or some degree of assistance is required by the client. Active ROM exercises should be encouraged if the client's health status allows because these exercises involve the client in self-care and increase independence, self-control, and self-esteem. Active and active-assisted ROM exercises help to prevent muscular atrophy and joint contracture. Passive ROM exercises help to maintain joint function but do not result in sufficient muscle tension to maintain muscle tone (Maas and others, 2001). Active ROM exercises can be incorporated into activities of daily living (ADLs) (Table 11-1) as well as into children's play activities (Wong and others, 2001). Examples of exercise through play include having the child act like a butterfly or throw a bean bag or wadded piece of paper into a trash can or at a target.

TABLE 11-1   INCORPORATING ACTIVE RANGE-OF-MOTION EXERCISES INTO ACTIVITIES OF DAILY LIVING

JOINT EXERCISED	ACTIVITY OF DAILY LIVING	MOVEMENT
Neck	Nodding head yes	Flexion
	Shaking head no	Rotation
	Moving right ear to right shoulder	Lateral flexion
	Moving left ear to left shoulder	Lateral flexion
Shoulder	Reaching to turn on overhead light	Flexion, extension
	Reaching to bedside stand for book	Hyperextension
	Rotating shoulders toward chest	Abduction
	Rotating shoulders toward back	Adduction
Elbow	Eating, bathing, shaving, grooming	Flexion, extension
Wrist	Eating, bathing, shaving, grooming	Flexion, extension, hyperextension, abduction, adduction
Fingers and thumb	All activities requiring fine motor coordination (e.g., writing, eating, painting)	Flexion, extension, abduction, adduction, opposition
Hip	Walking	Flexion, extension, hyperextension
	Moving to side-lying position	Flexion, extension, abduction
	Moving from side-lying position	Extension, adduction
	Rolling feet inward	Internal rotation
	Rolling feet outward	External rotation
Knee	Walking	Flexion, extension
	Moving to and from side-lying position	Flexion, extension
Ankle	Walking	Dorsiflexion, plantar flexion
	Moving toe toward head of bed	Dorsiflexion
	Moving toe toward foot of bed	Plantar flexion
Toes	Walking	Extension, hyperextension
	Wiggling toes	Abduction, adduction

DELEGATION CONSIDERATIONS

The skill of performing range-of-motion exercises can be delegated to assistive personnel. Clients with spinal cord or orthopedic trauma usually require exercise by professional nurses or physical therapists. The nurse provides assistive personnel with information, assistance, and direction including:

- Reminding assistive personnel to perform exercises slowly and to provide adequate support to each joint being exercised.

- Cautioning assistive personnel not to exercise joints beyond the point of resistance or to the point of fatigue or pain.
- Discussing with assistive personnel the client's individual limitations or preexisting conditions such as arthritis that may affect ROM.

STEP	RATIONALE

ASSESSMENT

1. Review client's chart to determine client's medical history, and obtain physician's order if needed.

Any type of joint problem, cardiac problem, or other condition that may be aggravated by energy expenditure or joint movement indicates the need to discuss ROM exercises with client's physician. Therefore the nurse must use judgment in deciding whether to institute exercises independently or to consult the physician before beginning exercises.

2. Assess baseline joint function (see Chapter 18).

Assessment of baseline joint function is important for evaluating later ROM capabilities.

   a. Observe client's ability to perform ROM exercises during normal ADLs.

Allows nurse to observe client's functional abilities in using extremities.

3. During initial ROM exercises assess for the following:

   a. Any limitation in normal ROM or any unusual increase in mobility of joint

Decreased ROM may indicate arthritis, inflammatory process, or contracture (Phipps and others, 2003).

   b. Any signs of redness or increased heat in skin overlying joint

May indicate joint problem that contraindicates ROM exercises or may indicate inflammatory joint disease more commonly known as arthritis (Huether and McCance 2000).

   c. Tenderness on palpation in or around joint

May indicate inflammatory process.

   d. Crepitus produced by motion of joint

Crepitus, a crunching or grating sensation that is audible or palpable when the joint is moved, is an indicator of a pathological condition within the joint (Phipps and others, 2003).

   e. Deformities

Deformities suggest bony enlargement (e.g., degenerative joint disease) or contracture.

   f. Level of comfort: pain

Pain may reduce client's motivation to perform ROM exercise. Pain relief before attempting exercises may enhance client's participation.

4. Assess client's or caregiver's understanding of ROM exercises to be used.

Allows client to verbalize concerns and identifies educational needs of client or caregiver

NURSING DIAGNOSES

- Activity intolerance
- Fatigue
- Impaired physical mobility

- Pain (acute, chronic)
- Deficient knowledge regarding ROM exercise techniques

Related factors are individualized based on client's condition or needs.

PLANNING

1. Expected outcomes following completion of procedure:
   - Range of joint motion is within normal limits or client's baseline range for each joint.
   - Client denies discomfort during exercises.
   - Client demonstrates ROM during ADLs.

Indicates optimal joint mobility and decreases risk of contracture formation.
Joints are exercised safely.
Incorporation of teaching into routine care makes skill relevant to client's needs.

STEP	**RATIONALE**
2. Explain procedure and reason for performing ROM exercises.	Relieves client's anxiety and encourages cooperation and participation.
3. Assist client to comfortable position.	Positioning allows easy access to joints for complete ROM.

▌ IMPLEMENTATION

1. Perform hand hygiene.	Reduces transmission of microorganisms.
2. Fully expose only limb to be exercised.	Provides privacy and avoids embarrassing client.
3. Raise bed to comfortable position, and stand on side of bed of joints to be exercised.	Maintains proper body mechanics to prevent back strain as exercises are carried out.
4. Be sure ROM exercises are performed slowly and gently.	Prevents joint strain.

• *Critical Decision Point*

　Older adults and clients with chronic illnesses may need ROM exercises in two or more sessions to control fatigue.

5. When performing ROM exercises, support joint by holding distal and proximal areas adjacent to joint (see illustration), by cradling distal portion of extremity (see illustration), or by using cupped hand to support joint (see illustrations).	Support to joint prevents ligament and muscle strain.

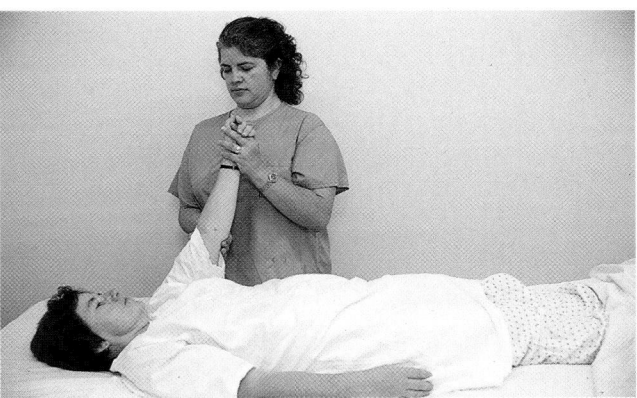

Step 5(1) Support joint by holding distal and proximal areas adjacent to joint.

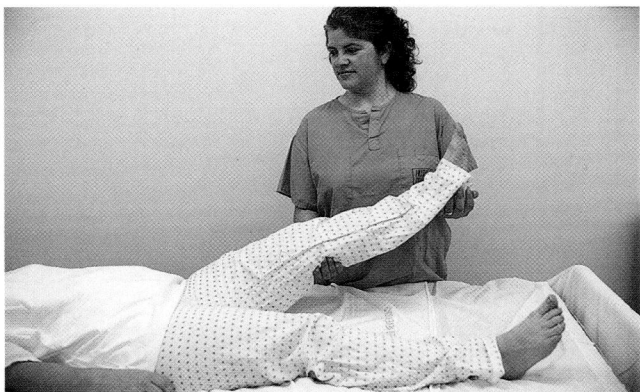

Step 5(2) Support joint by cradling distal portion of extremity.

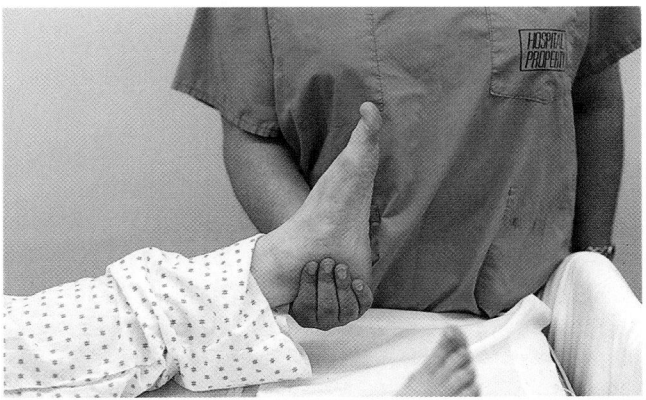

Step 5(3) Support joint by using cupped hand to support joint.

STEP	RATIONALE

6. Begin following exercises in sequence outlined. Each movement should be repeated 5 times during exercise period.

NOTE: Discontinue exercise if client complains of discomfort or if there is resistance or muscle spasm.

a. Neck
   (1) **Flexion:** Bring chin to rest on chest (ROM: 45 degrees) (see illustration).

   (2) **Extension:** Return head to erect position (ROM: 45 degrees) (see illustrations).
   (3) **Hyperextension:** Bend head as far back as possible (ROM: 10 degrees) (see illustration).
   (4) **Lateral flexion:** Tilt head as far as possible toward each shoulder (ROM: 40 to 45 degrees) (see illustration).
   (5) **Rotation:** Have client look straight ahead and rotate head in a circle (ROM: 360 degrees) (see illustrations).

It is easiest to perform exercises in head-to-toe format.

If flexion contracture of neck occurs, client's neck is permanently flexed with chin to or actually touching chest. Ultimately, client's total body alignment is altered and visual field is changed. Contractures can significantly limit the functioning of the client (Phipps and others, 2003).

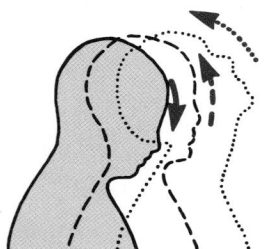

Step **6a(1-3)** Flexion, extension, and hyperextension of neck.

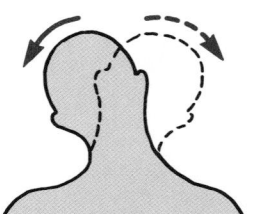

Step **6a(4)** Lateral flexion of neck.

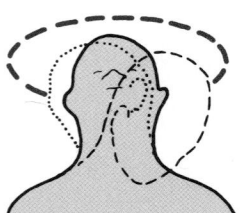

Step **6a(5a)** Rotate head in circular motion.

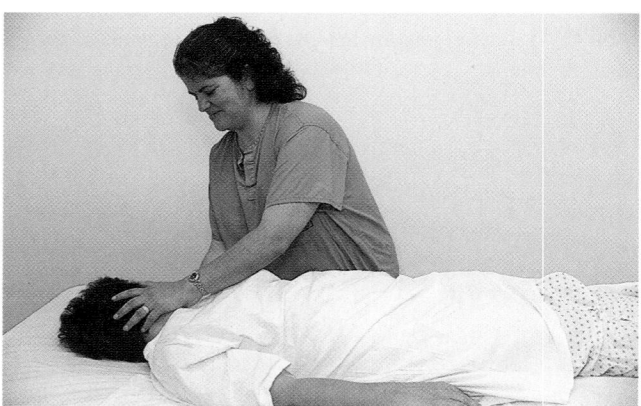

Step **6a(5b)** Rotate head in circular motion while client in supine position.

STEP	**RATIONALE**

b. Shoulder

   (1) Flexion: Raise arm from side position forward to above head (ROM: 180 degrees) (see illustration).

   (2) Extension: Return arm to position at side of body (ROM: 180 degrees).

   (3) Hyperextension: Move arm behind body, keeping elbow straight (ROM: 45 to 60 degrees) (see illustration).

   (4) Abduction: Raise arm to side to position above head with palm turned away from head (ROM: 180 degrees) (see illustration).

   (5) Adduction: Lower arm sideways and across body as far as possible (see illustrations).

   (6) Internal rotation: Move arm to side at shoulder level with elbow bent at 45 degrees. Lower arm so palm faces back (see illustration).

   (7) External rotation: With elbow flexed, move arm until thumb is upward and lateral to head (ROM: 90 degrees) (see illustration).

   (8) Circumduction: Move arm in full circle. Circumduction is a combination of all movements of ball-and-socket joint (ROM: 360 degrees) (see illustration).

Exercising shoulder effectively increases power of deltoid and triceps muscles. This strength will help if client needs to use an ambulation device, such as crutches, later.

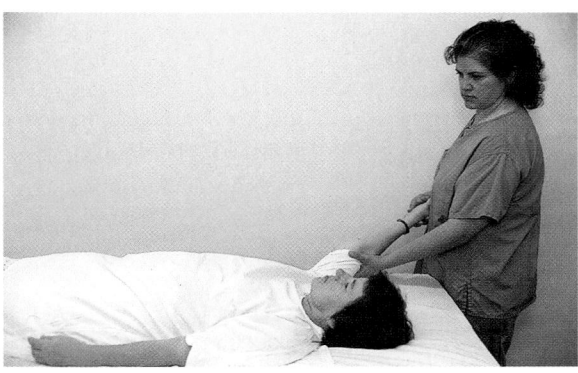

Step **6b(1)** Flexion of shoulder.

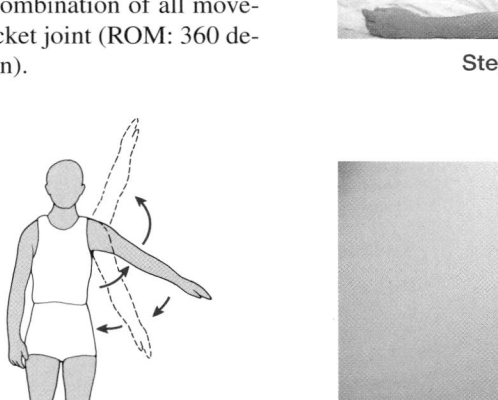

Step **6b(3)** Hyper-
extension of shoulder.

Step **6b(4-5)** Abduction and adduction of shoulder.

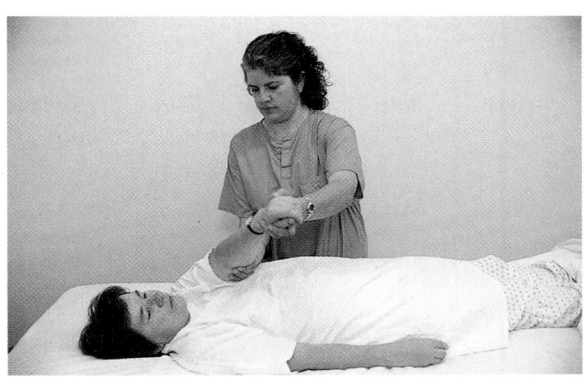

Step **6b(5)** Adduction of shoulder.

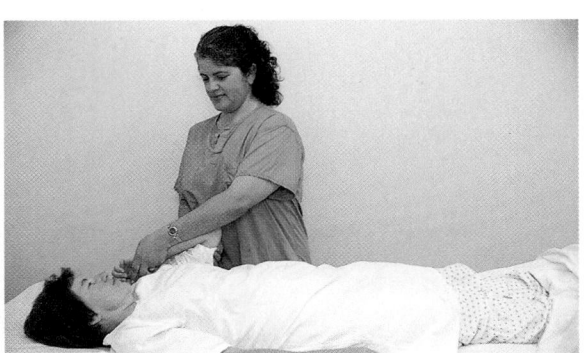

Step **6b(6)** Internal rotation of shoulder.

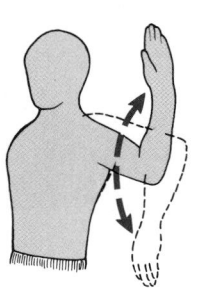

Step **6b(7)** External rotation of shoulder.

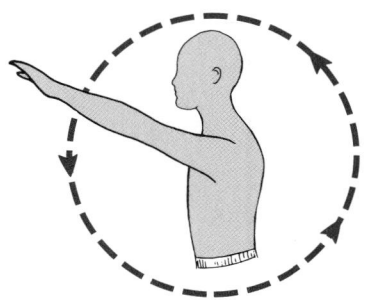

Step **6b(8)** Circumduction of shoulder.

STEP	RATIONALE

   c.   Elbow

      (1)   **Flexion:** Extend the arm then bend elbow so that lower arm moves toward the shoulder joint and hand touches shoulder (ROM: 150 degrees) (see illustration).

      (2)   **Extension:** Straighten elbow by lowering hand (ROM: 150 degrees) (see illustration).

      (3)   **Hyperextension:** Bend lower arm back as far as possible beyond normal extension (ROM: 10 to 20 degrees).

For optimal functioning, elbow must be able to fully extend and flex.

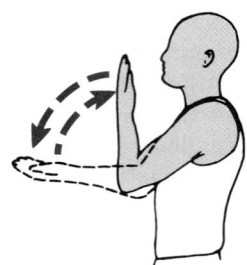

Step **6c(1-2)** Flexion and extension of elbow.

   d.   Forearm

      (1)   **Supination:** Turn lower arm and hand so that palm is up (ROM: 70 to 90 degrees) (see illustration).

      (2)   **Pronation:** Turn lower arm so that palm is down (ROM: 70 to 90 degrees) (see illustration).

For optimal functioning, forearm must be able to rotate from supination to **pronation.**

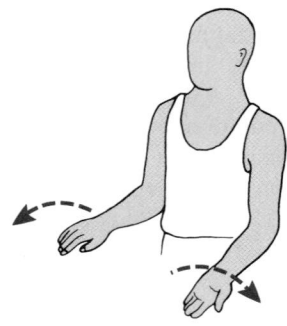

Step **6d(1-2)** Supination and pronation of forearm.

   e.   Wrist

      (1)   **Flexion:** Move palm toward inner aspect of forearm (ROM: 80 to 90 degrees) (see illustration).

      (2)   **Extension:** Move fingers so fingers, hands, and forearm are in same plane (ROM: 80 to 90 degrees).

      (3)   **Hyperextension:** Bring **dorsal** surface of hand back as far as possible (see illustration).

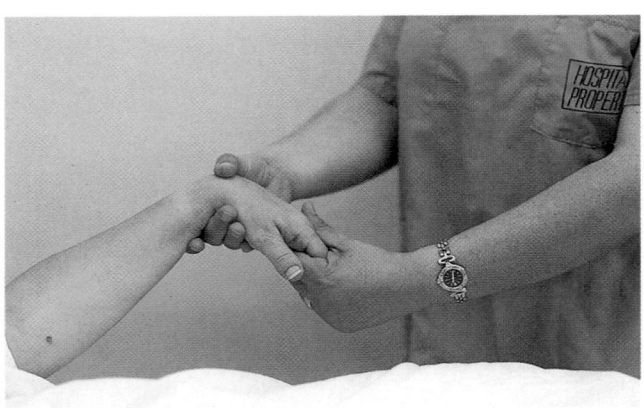

Step **6e(1)** Flexion of wrist.

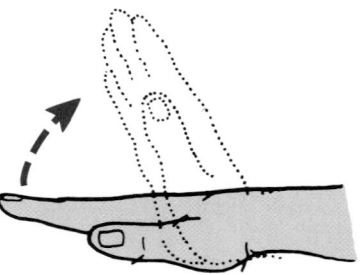

Step **6e(3)** Hyperextension of wrist.

STEP	**RATIONALE**

(4) Abduction (radial flexion): Bend wrist medially toward thumb (ROM: up to 30 degrees) (see illustration).

(5) Adduction (ulnar flexion): Bend wrist laterally toward fifth finger (ROM: 30 to 50 degrees) (see illustration).

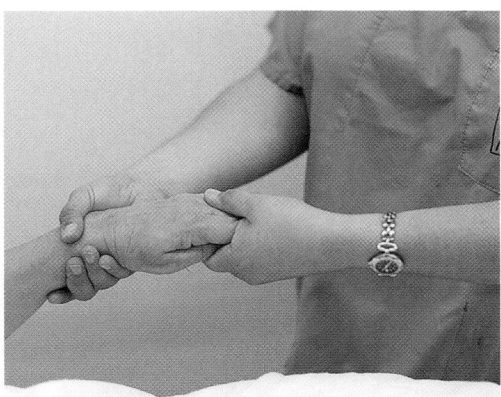

Step **6e(4)** Abduction (radial flexion) of wrist.

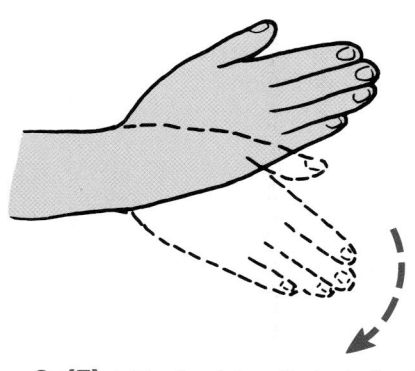

Step **6e(5)** Adduction (ulnar flexion) of wrist.

f. Fingers

(1) Flexion: Make fist (ROM: 90 degrees) (see illustration).

(2) Extension: Straighten fingers (ROM: 90 degrees).

(3) Hyperextension: Bend fingers back as far as possible (ROM: 30 to 60 degrees) (see illustration).

(4) Abduction: Spread fingers apart (see illustration).

(5) Adduction: Bring fingers together (see illustration).

Flexibility of fingers and thumb is necessary to grasp items (e.g., holding onto crutch).

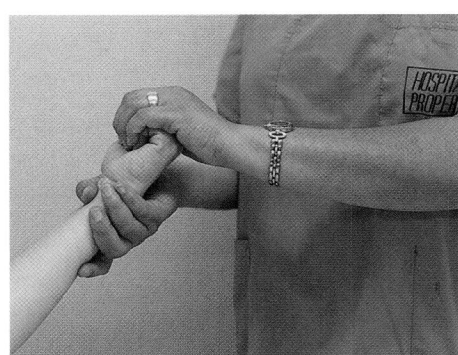

Step **6f(1)** Flexion of fingers.

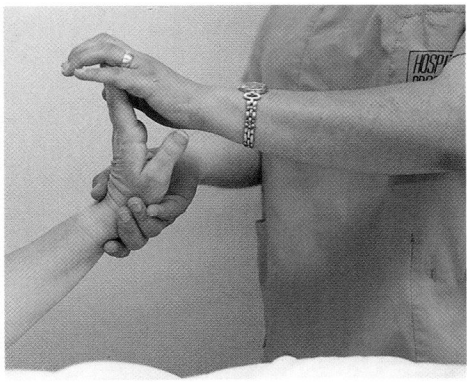

Step **6f(3)** Hyperextension of fingers.

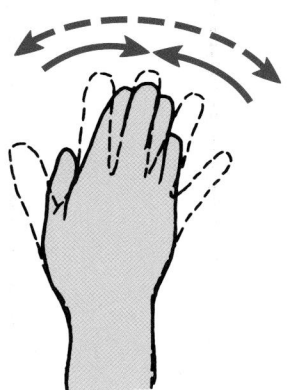

Step **6f(4-5)** Abduction and adduction of fingers.

STEP	RATIONALE

g. Thumb

   (1) Flexion: Move thumb across palmar surface of hand (ROM: 90 degrees) (see illustration).

   (2) Extension: Move thumb straight away from hand (ROM: 90 degrees).

   (3) Abduction: Extend thumb laterally (usually done when placing fingers in abduction and adduction) (ROM: 30 degrees).

   (4) Adduction: Move thumb back toward hand (ROM: 30 degrees).

   (5) Opposition: Touch thumb to each finger of same hand (see illustration).

Flexibility of thumb maintains coordination for fine motor activities.

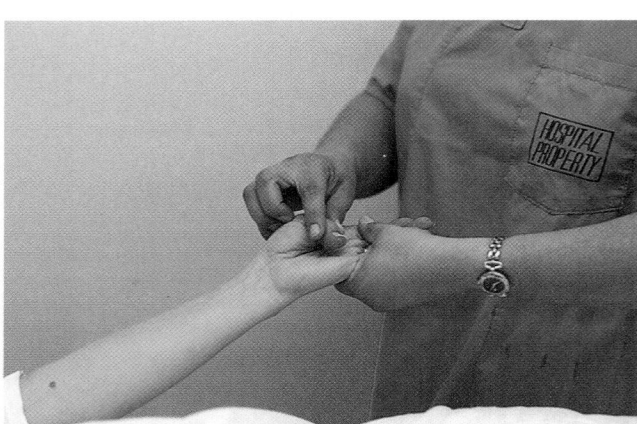

Step **6g(1)** Flexion of thumb.

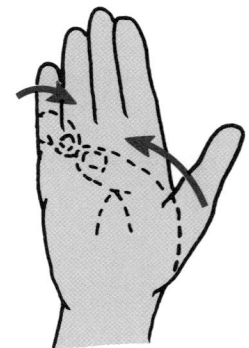

Step **6g(5)** Opposition of thumb.

h. Hip

   (1) Flexion: Move leg forward and up (ROM: 90 to 120 degrees) (see illustration).

   (2) Extension: Move leg back beside other leg (ROM: 90 to 120 degrees) (see illustration).

Contracture of hip can cause unsteady gait or difficulty ambulating.

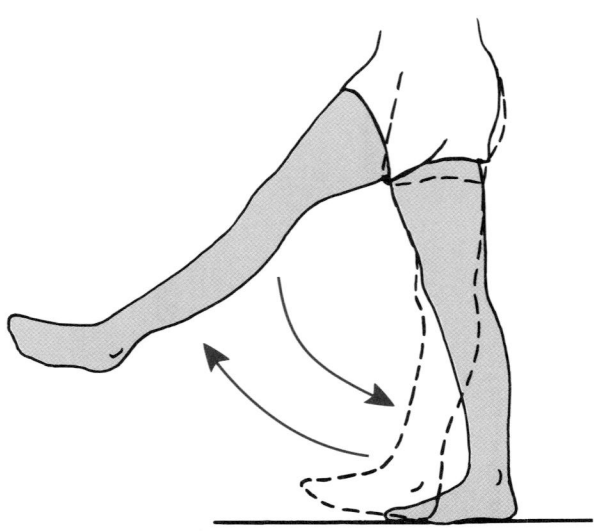

Step **6h(1-2)** Flexion and extension of hip.

STEP	RATIONALE

(3) **Hyperextension:** Move leg back beyond normal extension (ROM: 30 to 50 degrees) (see illustration).

(4) **Abduction:** Move leg laterally away from body (ROM: 30 to 50 degrees) (see illustration).

(5) **Adduction:** Move leg back toward medial position and beyond if possible (ROM: 30 to 50 degrees) (see illustration).

(6) **Internal rotation:** Turn foot and leg inward 90 degrees (see illustration).

(7) **External rotation:** Turn foot and leg outward 90 degrees (see illustration).

(8) **Circumduction:** Move leg in circle (ROM: 360 degrees) (see illustration).

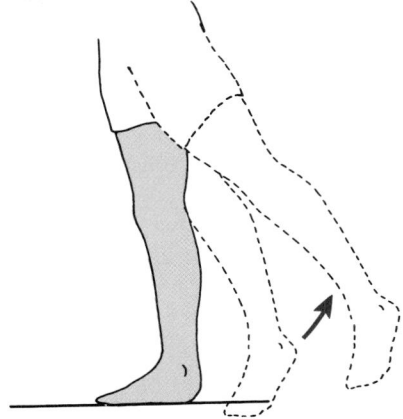

Step **6h(3)** Hyperextension of hip.

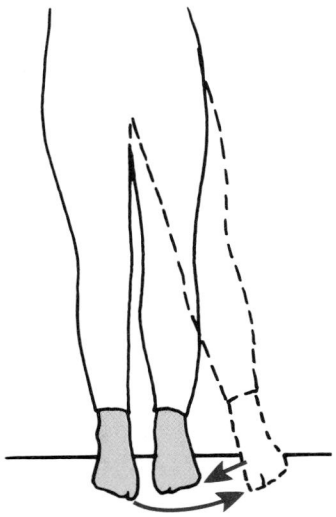

Step **6h(4-5)** Abduction and adduction of hip.

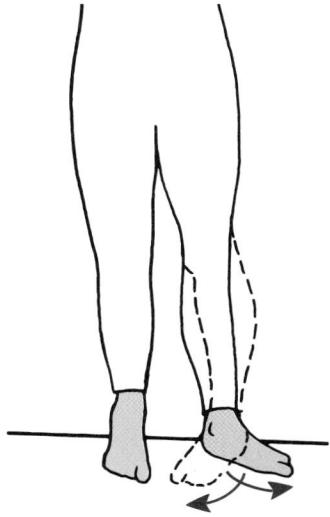

Step **6h(6-7)** Internal and external rotation of hip.

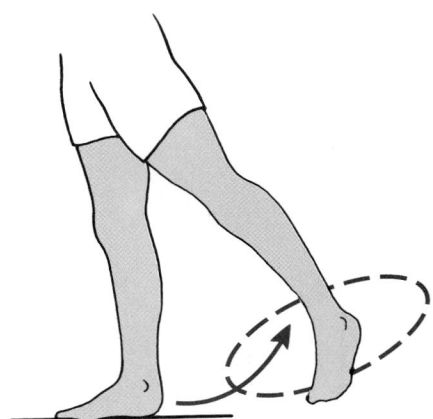

Step **6h(8)** Circumduction of hip.

STEP	RATIONALE

i. Knee

   (1) **Flexion:** Bend knee by bringing heel toward back of thigh (ROM: 120 to 130 degrees) (see illustration).

   (2) **Extension:** Return leg to floor (ROM: 120 to 130 degrees) (see illustration).

Flexibility of knee is necessary to lift objects and to ambulate.

j. Ankle

   (1) **Dorsiflexion:** Move foot so toes are pointed upward (ROM: 20 to 30 degrees) (see illustration).

   (2) **Plantar flexion:** Move foot so toes are pointed downward (ROM: 45 to 50 degrees) (see illustration).

A common, debilitating, and at times preventable contracture is footdrop. When footdrop occurs, the foot is permanently fixed in **plantar flexion.** Apply boots or high-top tennis shoes to decrease the incidence of footdrop (Phipps and others, 2003).

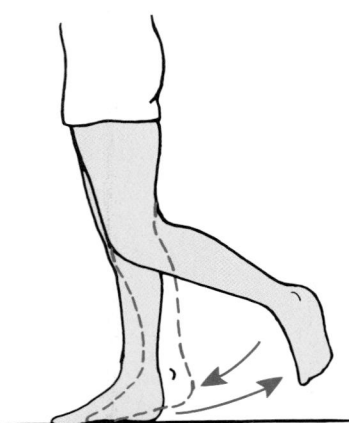

Step **6i(1-2)** Flexion and extension of knee.

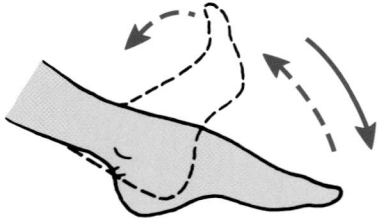

Step **6j(1-2)** Dorsiflexion and plantar flexion of ankle.

k. Foot

   (1) **Inversion:** Turn sole of foot medially (ROM: 10 degrees or less) (see illustration).

   (2) **Eversion:** Turn sole of foot laterally (ROM: 10 degrees or less) (see illustration).

Adequate ROM in feet allows client to walk.

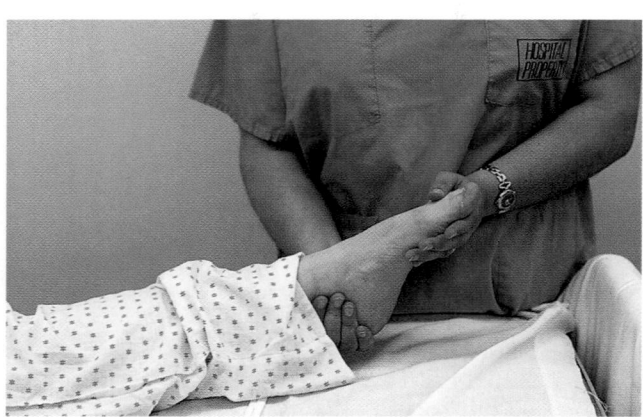

Step **6k(1)** Inversion of foot.

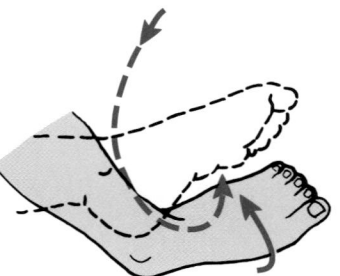

Step **6k(2)** Eversion of foot.

STEP	**RATIONALE**

(3) **Flexion:** Curl toes downward (ROM: 30 to 60 degrees) (see illustration).

(4) **Extension:** Straighten toes (ROM: 30 to 60 degrees) (see illustration).

(5) **Abduction:** Spread toes apart (ROM: 15 degrees or less) (see illustration).

(6) **Adduction:** Bring toes together (ROM: 15 degrees or less) (see illustration).

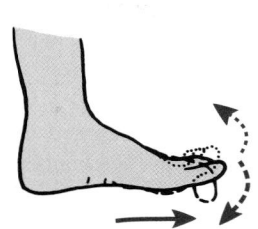
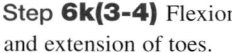
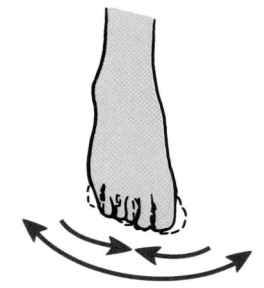

Step **6k(3-4)** Flexion and extension of toes.

Step **6k(5-6)** Abduction and adduction of toes.

7. If exercise performed in bed, lower bed to safe position.

Provides safe exit route if client is ambulatory.

8. Reposition client to position of comfort, and perform hand hygiene.

Evaluation

1. Measure range of motion of various joints as compared to baseline range of those joints.

   Determines whether exercises have had desired effect of increasing or maintaining joint mobility.

2. Ask for client's subjective statements regarding experience (e.g., complaints of discomfort, level of fatigue).

   Evaluates client's tolerance of exercise. Develop schedule for implementing the performance of ROM exercises based on client's tolerance and fatigue level.

3. Determine degree of assistance required to perform exercises.

   Establishes guidelines to maximize self-care ability.

4. Ask client to independently perform exercises.

   Determines that client performs exercises correctly.

Recording and Reporting

- Record in nurses' notes the joints exercised, type of exercise, extent to which joints can be moved, any joint abnormalities, client's subjective statements regarding tolerance of activity, and nurse's objective observation of tolerance.

- Report immediately to nurse in charge or physician if there is resistance during performance of ROM exercises, if client complains of pain on movement of joint, or if there are signs of swelling, redness, or heat in joint.

Unexpected Outcomes	**Related Interventions**
1. Client experiences discomfort on ROM exercise.	• Stop ROM exercises. • Notify physician if you suspect inflammation or infection.
2. Resistance is encountered when performing ROM exercise.	• Do not force movement of joint.
3. Spastic muscle contraction develops during ROM exercises.	• Stop movement of affected part. • Place continuous gentle pressure on muscle group until it relaxes. • Resume exercises using a slower, steady movement.

Teaching Considerations

- Instruct client to exercise only to point of resistance and to stop if pain is experienced.
- Provide opportunity for return demonstration.
- Encourage active ROM as soon as client's condition warrants independent activity.

Pediatric Considerations

- Children should have ROM exercises incorporated into play activities to encourage participation (Hockenberry and others, 2003).

Gerontological Considerations

- Inform client that studies have demonstrated that regular activity may reduce the risks of falls (Gregg and others, 2000).
- Be aware of chronic conditions (i.e., congestive heart failure, chronic obstructive pulmonary disease, hypertension) that may limit client's ability to participate in ROM exercises. Monitor fatigue, pain, and respiratory functioning frequently.

Home Care Considerations

- Assess family or primary caregiver's ability, availability, and motivation to assist client with exercises that client is unable to perform independently.
- Assist family or primary caregiver with arranging home environment to promote exercise program (e.g., space allocation, lighting, temperature, safety precautions).

Long-Term Care Considerations

- Develop a schedule for implementing the performance of ROM, preferably the same time each day.
- Consult with physical therapist for additional assistance or exercises and client's response to ROM exercises.

SKILL 11-2 Performing Isometric Exercises

In addition to ROM exercises, some immobilized clients may be able to perform muscle-strengthening exercises. Isotonic muscle contractions cause a change in muscle length. Examples of exercises that cause isotonic muscle contractions are walking, performing aerobics, and moving arms and legs against light resistance. Performing these types of exercises regularly can positively affect heart and lung function, improve muscle tone, and have beneficial effects on the entire body if performed properly (Maas and others, 2001; Oka and others, 2000). Some individuals, however, are unable to tolerate such increases in activity. For these individuals, isometric exercises are more appropriate and are easily accomplished by an immobilized client in bed. Isometric or static exercises involve tightening or tensing of muscles without moving body parts (isometric contractions). They increase muscle tension but do not change the length of muscle fibers.

Isometric exercises involve the contraction of a muscle while pushing against a stationary object or resisting the movement of an object. Examples of isometric exercises are performing push-ups and hip lifting. In hip lifting, the individual, who is in a sitting position, pushes with the hands against a sitting surface such as a chair to raise the hips. Isometric exercises help to promote muscular strength and provide the necessary stress for bone maintenance and growth. Without sufficient stress against bone, osteoclastic activity (activity by cells responsible for bone tissue absorption) increases over osteoblastic activity (activity by bone-forming cells) (Huether and McCance, 2000). The result is demineralization of the bone and eventual osteoporosis.

DELEGATION CONSIDERATIONS

The skill of performing isometric exercises can be delegated to assistive personnel. However, clients with cardiovascular disease require assessment by a nurse when initially performing these exercises. The nurse provides assistive personnel with information, assistance, and direction, including:

- Discussing with assistive personnel the amount of time and frequency of the prescribed isometric exercises
- Reminding assistive personnel to perform exercises slowly at client's pace
- Discussing with assistive personnel the client's individual limitations or preexisting conditions such as arthritis that may affect ROM needed for isometric exercises.

STEP	RATIONALE

ASSESSMENT

1. Review client's chart for contraindications to isometric exercises such as cardiovascular disease.

Isometric exercises raise blood pressure and pulse. The presence of a preexisting medical condition, such as a history of cardiac problems, may be a contraindication (Maas and others, 2001).

2. Assess client's baseline vital signs.

Isometric exercises may raise blood pressure. Documentation of baseline vital signs is necessary to determine whether exercises cause a deterioration in vital signs (Huether and McCance, 2000).

3. Assess client's baseline muscle strength:
   a. Ask client to perform task against resistance (e.g., push one foot against palm of hand).
   b. Assess grasp strength by having client grasp nurse's hands. Note whether hand grasps are equal.
   c. Have client grasp two fingers of nurse's right hand with client's left hand and two fingers of nurse's left hand with client's right hand.
   d. Observe client's ability to do daily activities (e.g., whether client has adequate strength to bathe self, pull self up in bed, move from bed to chair).
   e. Obtain client's subjective statements related to muscle strength. Does client feel weaker?

Enables nurse to compare muscle strength before and after exercise.

4. Assess client's nutritional status.

Proper nutrition is essential if client is to be able to perform exercises. Promotion of protein anabolism involves conservation and replenishment of energy stores (Lueckenotte, 2000).

5. Level of comfort: pain

Pain may reduce client's motivation to perform isometric exercises. Pain relief before attempting exercises may enhance client's participation.

6. Assess client's or caregiver's understanding of isometric exercises to be used.

Allows client to verbalize concerns and identifies educational needs of client or caregiver.

NURSING DIAGNOSES

- Activity intolerance
- Deficient knowledge regarding exercises
- Pain (acute, chronic)

- Impaired physical mobility
- Fatigue

Related factors are individualized based on client's condition or needs.

PLANNING

1. Expected outcomes following completion of procedure:
   - Client will gradually increase number of exercise repetitions.

Client will gradually become stronger and be able to increase number of repetitions. However, results can be obtained by doing even one set of exercises (Hass and others, 2000).

   - Vital signs will remain stable.

Documents client's activity tolerance.

2. Explain procedure, and demonstrate exercises.

Relieves anxiety and encourages client cooperation.

3. Assist client to comfortable position.

Reduces stress and promotes client participation.

STEP	RATIONALE

IMPLEMENTATION

1. Provide privacy.
2. Instruct client to perform the following isometric exercises as prescribed. Each exercise prescription is individualized according to the client's needs and limitations. Exercises are as follows:

Prevents client embarrassment.

Gradual build-up of exercise repetitions improves both muscle strength and endurance (Huddleston, 2002). The muscle should exert as much effort as possible for a period of 5 to 15 seconds (Maas and others, 2001).

- *Critical Decision Point*
  Clients doing isometric exercises should be taught to exhale while exerting effort. Many persons hold their breath (Valsalva maneuver), which increases intrathoracic pressure, causing a decrease in venous return to heart (Maas and others, 2001).

    a. Quadriceps isometric exercises:
        (1) Assist client to supine recumbent position.

Quadriceps enable person to ambulate and get out of chair; large muscles of thigh (quadriceps) must be strong enough for client to extend knees and stabilize them.

        (2) Instruct client to press back of the knee against mattress while trying to lift heel from bed (see illustration).

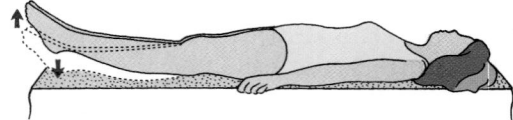

Step 2a(2) Lift heels while pressing back of knees against mattress.

        (3) Hold muscles tightly contracted for 5 to 15 seconds, and then relax completely for several seconds (Maas and others, 2001).

Nurse can assist client in learning this exercise by placing hand between the back of client's knee and mattress and asking client to press hand against mattress with the back of the knee.

        (4) Repeat exercise.
    b. Gluteal muscle isometric exercises:
        (1) Assist client to supine position.
        (2) Instruct client to pinch buttocks muscles together and hold for 5 to 15 seconds and then relax completely for several seconds (see illustration).
        (3) Repeat exercise.

Improves client's balance when sitting.

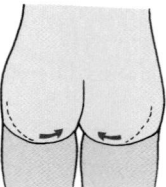

Step 2b(2) Pinch gluteal muscles together.

    c. Abdominal muscle isometric exercises:
        (1) Have client pull abdominal muscles in as tightly as possible (see illustration).
        (2) Hold for 5 to 15 seconds. Release muscles gradually.
        (3) Repeat exercise.

Improves trunk stability.

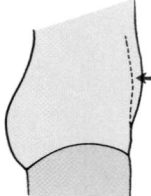

Step 2c(1) Pull abdominal muscles in tightly.

STEP	RATIONALE

d. Foot muscle isometric exercises:
   (1) Instruct client to flex foot toward and away from knee holding each position for 5 to 15 seconds.
   (2) Repeat exercise.

Increases muscle activity in leg and thereby promotes venous return to heart.

e. Hand muscle isometric exercises:
   (1) Obtain sponge rubber ball. (Size of ball depends on size of client's hand.)
   (2) Have client grip ball with entire hand 5 to 10 times.
   (3) Dig each fingertip, one at a time, into ball 5 to 10 times each.
   (4) Gradually increase frequency of exercise until client can grip ball and exercise once or twice a day.

Strengthens grip to hold onto crutch or walker more effectively.

f. Biceps isometric exercises:
   (1) Have client raise arms to shoulder height and interlock fingertips of both hands.
   (2) Try to pull hands apart using arm muscles.
   (3) Hold for 5 to 15 seconds.
   (4) Relax muscles.
   (5) Repeat exercise.

Strengthens biceps and thereby helps with ambulation if ambulatory assistive device is used.

g. Triceps muscle isometric exercises (see illustration):
   (1) Have client raise arms to shoulder height.
   (2) Make fist with one hand and place against palm of other hand.
   (3) Push hands together as hard as possible for 5 to 15 seconds.
   (4) Relax and repeat exercise.

Strengthens triceps to assist with transfer techniques and use of crutches or walker.

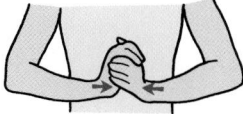

Step **2g** Triceps muscle isometric exercises.

3. Instruct client to perform the following isometric exercises:
  a. Triceps muscle isometric exercises (see illustration):
   (1) Assist client to sitting position on edge of bed or in chair. If mattress is soft, blocks or books are placed on bed under client's hands.
   (2) Instruct client to try to lift buttocks off bed or seat of chair by pressing down on mattress or chair seat with hands.
   (3) Hold muscles tight for 5 to 15 seconds, then relax.
   (4) Repeat exercise.

To use crutches or walker effectively, client must have enough strength in the triceps to extend and stabilize the elbows while lifting or shifting body weight.

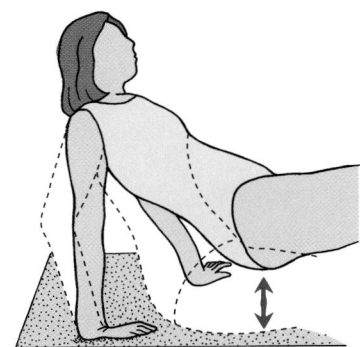

Step **3a** Triceps muscle resistive isometric exercises.

STEP	RATIONALE
b. Quadriceps muscle isometric exercises: **(1)** Have client push feet against footboard. **(2)** Hold muscles tight for 5 to 15 seconds, then relax. **(3)** Repeat exercise.	Builds strength, size, and shape of leg muscles.

EVALUATION

1. Observe client's ability to perform exercises.
2. Evaluate client's level of energy, muscular strength, and comfort following exercises.
3. Obtain vital signs.

Demonstrates client's learning.
Determines whether client is performing exercises accurately and whether the exercises are increasing muscle strength.
Determines client's tolerance to activity.

Recording and Reporting

• Record in nurses' notes type of isometric exercises used, length of time contractions held, number of repetitions of each exercise, assessment of client's muscular strength and comfort after exercises, client's subjective statements regarding muscular strength, and client's ability to perform exercises.

Unexpected Outcomes	Related Interventions
1. Client is unable to perform exercises. Client may be too weak.	• Continue ROM exercises, and reposition client to try to increase strength. • Make sure nutrition and rest are adequate.
2. Client is unwilling to perform exercises.	• Lack of understanding of significance of exercises may be the problem. • Stress importance of the exercises. • Be sure client is not experiencing distracting symptoms such as nausea or pain.
3. Muscular strength is not increasing.	• Client may not be performing exercises as described or as often as instructed. • Stress importance of following routine.
4. Client's blood pressure and heart rate increase significantly during exercises.	• Client may not be able to tolerate procedure. • Discontinue exercises, and consult physician.

TEACHING CONSIDERATIONS

• Instruct client to perform exercises before regular activities, such as breakfast or work. Building exercises into routine activities increases likelihood of adherence to exercise program.
• Instruct client to gradually increase exercise activity each day.

PEDIATRIC CONSIDERATIONS

• Exercises can be incorporated into a child's activity plan.
• Children are more likely to exercise as part of a game or in groups as opposed to exercising alone (Hockenberry and others, 2003).

GERONTOLOGICAL CONSIDERATIONS

• Physical exercise is important for older adults to maintain health, preserve functional status, and improve general quality of life (Cousins and Tan, 2002; Huddleston, 2002; Lueckenotte, 2000).
• For the older adult who has not previously participated in exercise, it is important to start with only 5 minutes of exercise and gradually work up to a 20- to 30-minute daily routine (Lueckenotte, 2000).
• Encourage older adults to drink water before and after exercising (Huddleston, 2002).

SKILL 11-3 Continuous Passive Motion Machine

The continuous passive motion (CPM) machine is designed to exercise varying joints such as the hip, ankle, knee, shoulder, and wrist. The CPM machine is most commonly used after knee surgery. The CPM machine is usually prescribed on the day of surgery or the first postoperative day, depending on the surgeon's preference and client's condition. The purpose of the CPM machine is to mobilize the joint to prevent contractures, muscle atrophy, venous stasis, and thromboembolism. The CPM machine can aid in alleviating pain, edema, stiffness, and dislocation and potentially can shorten a client's hospital stay (Babis and others, 2001; Hammesfahr and Serafino, 2002).

The electronically controlled CPM machine flexes and extends the joint to a prescribed degree and at a set speed as ordered by the physician. Velcro straps secure the extremity. When the device is turned on, the frame slides slowly back and forth, gently moving the joint through a preset ROM. The CPM machine can weigh up to 25 pounds. Using two hospital personnel to lift the machine reduces the risk of back strain and prevents risk of damage to the client's extremity.

DELEGATION CONSIDERATIONS

The skill of using the CPM machine should not be delegated to assistive personnel. The nurse may delegate aspects of care such as hygiene and instruct the assistive personnel to immediately report increased pain, skin breakdown, or joint inflammation.

EQUIPMENT

❑ CPM machine
❑ Nonsterile gloves

STEP	RATIONALE

ASSESSMENT

1. Assess the CPM machine for electrical safety.

   All electrical equipment in health care settings is routinely checked for safety. Routine observation of electrical cord and functioning of equipment each time it is used further monitors safety.

2. Assess the setup of the machine before placing on bed: check the stability of the frame, the flexion/extension controls, padding of exposed metal parts or hard surfaces, and the on/off switch.

   Ensures that all pieces of the equipment are operational and will prevent damage to the client's joint. Ensures metal parts are padded to prevent skin breakdown or chafing of skin rubbing against metal or hard surfaces.

3. Assess the client's comfort on a scale of 0 to 10 (10 being the worst pain) before and during use.

   Establishes comfort baseline. Determines how the client tolerates the CPM machine and the need for analgesia.

4. Assess client's baseline vital signs.

   Provides baseline to measure exercise tolerance.

5. Assess the client's ability and willingness to learn about the CPM machine.

   Determines readiness to learn, reduces anxiety, and promotes client participation.

NURSING DIAGNOSES

- Pain (acute)
- Activity intolerance
- Knowledge deficit regarding CPM machine
- Fatigue

Related factors are individualized based on client's condition or needs.

PLANNING

1. Expected outcomes following completion of the procedure:
   - Client will increase length of time and flexion of joint as prescribed by physician.

     CPM machine facilitates joint range of motion, prevents formation of adhesions, edema, stiffness, deformity (Babis and others, 2001; Hammesfahr and Serafino, 2002).

   - Client's vital signs will remain stable.

     Documents client's activity tolerance.

   - Client denies discomfort during or after CPM exercise.

     Providing analgesia for client assists in tolerating exercise.

2. Explain procedure and demonstrate CPM machine.

   Relieves anxiety and encourages client cooperation.

3. Assist client to comfortable position.

   Reduces stress and promotes client participation.

STEP	RATIONALE

IMPLEMENTATION

1. Perform hand hygiene.
2. Provide analgesia 20 to 30 minutes before CPM machine is needed.
3. Wear nonsterile gloves if wound drainage is present.

4. Place elastic hose on client if ordered (see Skill 11-4).
5. Place CPM machine on bed.
6. Set limits of flexion and extension as prescribed by physician.
7. Set speed control to slow or moderate range.
8. Put machine through one full cycle.
9. Stop CPM machine when in extension. Place sheepskin on CPM machine.
10. Place client's extremity in CPM machine (see illustration).
11. Adjust CPM machine to client's extremity. Lengthen and shorten appropriate sections of frame.
12. Center client's extremity on frame.
13. Align client's joint with CPM's mechanical joint.
14. Secure client's extremity on CPM machine with Velcro straps (see illustration). Apply loosely.
15. Start machine. When it reaches flexed position, stop machine and check degree of flexion.
16. Start CPM machine, and observe for two full cycles.

17. Make sure client is comfortable.
18. Provide client with on/off switch.
19. Instruct client to turn CPM machine off if malfunctioning or experiencing pain. Instruct client to notify nurse immediately.
20. Discard gloves, and perform hand hygiene.

Reduces transmission of microorganisms.
Assists client in tolerating exercise.

Gloves reduce nurse's risk of exposure to blood-borne viruses or bacteria.
Elastic hose promote venous return from lower extremities.

Prevents injury by setting machine at safe limits.

Ensures CPM machine is working properly.
Ensures all exposed hard surfaces are padded to prevent rubbing and chafing of client's skin.

Avoids pressure areas on extremity.

Prevents possible complications and ensures correct settings.

Ensures CPM machine is fully operational at the preset extension and flexion modes.

Allows client to turn on and off CPM machine if malfunctions.

Prevents transmission of microorganisms.

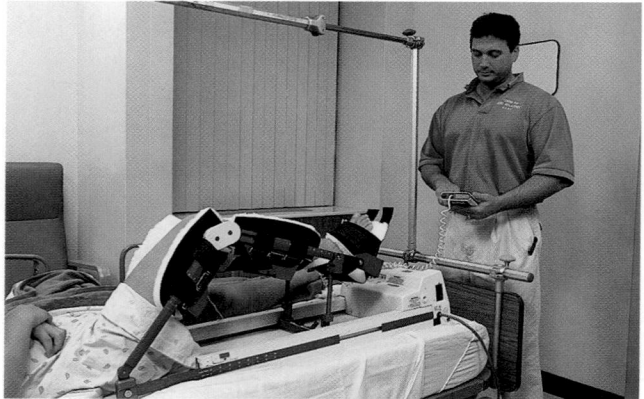

Step **10** Position leg in CPM cradle.

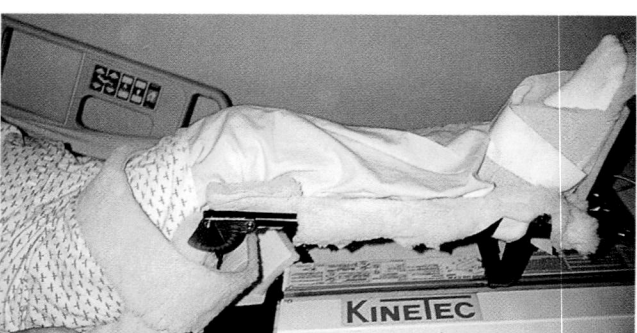

Step **14** Client's extremity properly placed and secured on CPM machine.

STEP	RATIONALE

EVALUATION

1. Inspect bony prominences and areas of skin in contact with machine at least every 2 hours.

2. Ask client to rate pain on a scale of 0 to 10.

3. Check client's alignment and positioning at least every 2 hours.

4. Observe client and CPM machine with each increase in flexion and extension.

Identifies potential skin breakdown.

Determines if analgesia is effective.

Promotes comfort and ensures proper extension and flexion of joint.

Prevents complications and ensures CPM machine is functioning properly.

Recording and Reporting

- Record in nurses' notes the client's tolerance for CPM machine, rate of cycles per minute, degree of flexion and extension used, condition of extremity and skin, condition of operative site if present, length of time CPM machine in use.
- Report immediately to nurse in charge or physician any resistance to range of motion; increased pain; swelling, heat, or redness in joint.

Unexpected Outcomes	Related Interventions
1. Client unable to tolerate increase in flexion or extension.	• Consult with physician and physical therapist to plan additional therapies to increase flexion and extension of joint. • Provide rest periods throughout day to rest the joint. • Consider need for analgesia before CPM machine is used.
2. Client experiences increased pain when using CPM machine.	• Determine efficacy of current analgesia, and obtain new orders. • Determine cause of increased pain.
3. Client develops reddened areas on bony prominences or extremity.	• Determine if hard surfaces on CPM machine are well padded. • Monitor client's alignment and positioning at least every 2 hours. • Provide skin care at least every 2 hours.

Teaching Considerations

- Instruct client in the use and importance of the CPM machine.

Pediatric Considerations

- Arrange for social or creative activities that are developmentally appropriate for the child's age (Wong and others, 2001).
- Demonstrate use of CPM machine using a large doll or stuffed animal before applying to child's extremity to relieve anxiety.

Gerontological Considerations

- Older adults have increased risk of skin breakdown because of decreased elasticity and fragility of the skin.

Pressure from the CPM machine increases the risk of pressure ulcers, especially on the heel (Lueckenotte, 2000).
- Older adults may perceive pain as a natural part of aging and may underreport its presence (Maas and others, 2001). Special attention to nonverbal cues and additional instruction in pain management may be necessary to ensure the older adult's comfort.

Home Care Considerations

- Home care physical therapist may assist client/family in continuing CPM machine in the home.
- Client/family must have specific instructions regarding the use of the CPM machine, length of time for each session, expected outcomes, and what to do if the client experiences increased pain, the client is unable to tolerate the CPM sessions, or the equipment malfunctions (Branson and Goldstein, 2001).

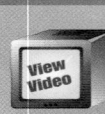

SKILL 11-4 Applying Elastic Stockings and Sequential Compression Device

Prevention is the best method to reduce the risk of deep vein thrombosis (DVT) secondary to immobility. Early ambulation remains the most effective preventive measure (Phipps and others, 2003). However, there are times when early ambulation is not an option, particularly in the critically ill client. Early application of elastic stockings and sequential compression device (SCD) along with low-molecular-weight or low-dose heparin therapy have been reported as successful in preventing the development of deep vein thrombosis (Boccalon and others, 2000; Merli, 2000; Phipps and others, 2003).

Three elements (commonly referred to as Virchow's triad) contribute to the development of DVT: hypercoagulability of the blood, venous wall damage, and stasis of blood flow (Phipps and others, 2003). Elastic stockings help reduce two of the elements: blood stasis and venous wall injury. First, they promote venous return by maintaining pressure on superficial veins to prevent venous pooling, thereby reducing the risk of clot formation in the lower extremities. Second, it has been suggested that elastic stockings prevent passive dilation of the veins, thereby decreasing the risk of endothelial tears. An increased incidence of DVT has been found in clients in whom the venous diameter had increased. In such cases the endothelial layer can tear.

Sequential compression device can be used alone or in conjunction with elastic stockings, depending upon the physician's preference. These devices consist of an air pump, connecting tubing, and extremity sleeves that sequentially inflate and deflate chambers within the sleeve. The intermittent pumping action drives superficial blood into deep veins, where it is evacuated proximally by the venous valves, thus removing pooled blood and preventing both venous stasis and the accumulation of clotting factors.

DELEGATION CONSIDERATIONS

The skill of applying elastic stockings and SCD may be delegated to assistive personnel. The nurse initially determines the size of elastic stockings and accurate application of the SCD and assesses the client's lower extremities for any signs and symptoms of impaired circulation. Before delegating this skill the nurse must:

- Remind assistive personnel to remove the SCD sleeves from the legs before allowing client to get out of bed. This ensures clients safety and avoids client becoming tangled in SCD sleeves and connectors
- Observe for signs and symptoms of allergic reactions to elastic (e.g., redness, itching, irritation) and report finding immediately

- Instruct assistive personnel to inform the nurse if one calf appears larger than the other, a calf is red and/or warm to the touch, or the calf is painful

EQUIPMENT
- ❑ Tape measure
- ❑ Powder or corn starch (optional)
- ❑ Elastic support stockings
- ❑ Disposable SDC sleeve(s)
- ❑ Tubing assembly
- ❑ Sequential compression device (motor)

STEP	RATIONALE

ASSESSMENT

1. Assess client for risk factors in Virchow's triad:

      a. *Hypercoagulability:* All clients with clotting disorders, fever, dehydration, pregnancy and/or first 6 weeks postpartum if the woman was confined to bed, or oral contraceptive use (especially if client smokes).

      b. *Venous wall abnormalities:* Local trauma, orthopedic surgeries, major abdominal surgery, varicose veins, atherosclerosis.

      c. *Blood stasis:* Immobility, obesity, pregnancy.

Potential candidates for elastic stockings and/or SCD are clients who have an alteration in one of the elements of Virchow's triad (Merli, 2000; Phipps and others, 2003). Hypercoagulability increases tendency for blood to clot.

Venous wall abnormalities can impair circulation or traumatize blood cells, both of which increase client's risk of clotting.

Stasis facilitates clotting.

STEP	RATIONALE

- ### Critical Decision Point
  Discourage clients from activities that promote venous stasis (e.g., crossing legs, wearing garters, elevating legs on pillows). When possible, have clients elevate legs to improve venous return.

2. Observe for signs, symptoms, and conditions that might contraindicate use of elastic stockings or SCD:

   a. Dermatitis or open skin lesion

   b. Recent skin graft

   c. Decreased circulation in lower extremities as evidenced by cyanotic, cool extremities and/or gangrenous conditions affecting the lower limb(s)

3. Obtain physician's order.
4. Assess client's or caregiver's understanding of application of elastic stockings and SCD sleeves.
5. Assess the condition of client's skin and circulation to the legs (i.e., presence of pedal pulses, edema, discoloration of the skin, temperature, lesions, or cuts).

Elastic stockings and SCD sleeves may aggravate a skin condition or cause it to spread. Also the physician may want medication and dressing applied to the lesion.

Recent skin grafts are delicate and should not be dislodged (Phipps and others, 2003).

Elastic stockings and SCD may further impede circulation (Phipps and others, 2003).

May be needed for reimbursement reasons.

Identifies potential educational needs of client or caregiver.

Identifies a baseline for skin integrity and the quality of peripheral pulses in lower extremities. Prevention is the best medicine to avoid the development of thrombophlebitis. Early application of elastic stockings and SCD sleeves can be instrumental in preventing this complication.

- ### Critical Decision Point
  Thrombophlebitis can develop in the lower extremities. Clinical manifestations of thrombophlebitis vary according to the size and location of the thrombus. Signs and symptoms of superficial thrombosis include palpable veins and the surrounding area being tender to touch, reddened, and warm. There may be a slight temperature elevation. Edema of the extremity may or may not occur. Signs and symptoms of DVT include a swollen extremity; pain; warm, cyanotic skin; and temperature elevation. However, up to 80% of all clients are asymptomatic (Breen, 2000). Although Homan's sign (pain in calf on dorsiflexion of foot) has been an assessment parameter in the past, it is not a reliable sign. Fewer than 20% of clients exhibit a positive Homan's sign (Phipps and others, 2003).

6. Assess client's or caregiver's understanding of proper care of elastic stockings.

Identifies potential educational needs of client or caregiver.

NURSING DIAGNOSES

- Activity intolerance
- Ineffective peripheral tissue perfusion
- Decreased cardiac output

- Deficient knowledge regarding application of elastic stockings
- Risk for impaired skin integrity
- Impaired physical mobility

Related factors are individualized based on client's condition or needs.

PLANNING

1. Expected outcomes following completion of procedure:
   - Client shows no evidence of skin irritation.

   - Client shows no evidence of thrombophlebitis.
   - Client is able to demonstrate application of elastic stockings.
   - Client has reduction of edema in lower extremities.

Proper application ensures no side effects that would impair skin integrity.

Proper application prevents trauma to venous walls.

Verifies correct psychomotor learning.

Decreases venous pooling in lower extremities.

STEP	**RATIONALE**

2. Explain procedure and reasons for applying elastic stockings and SCD.

Reduces anxiety and encourages client cooperation.

3. Use tape measure to measure client's legs to determine proper elastic stockings and SCD sleeve size.

Stockings must be measured according to manufacturer's directions. Elastic stockings and SCD sleeves come in two lengths: knee length and thigh length. The choice of length depends on the physician's order. If too large, stockings will not adequately support extremities. If too small, stockings may impede circulation.

- *Critical Decision Point*

Compare client's measurements with the manufacturer's sizing chart. The optimum elastic stocking pressure is 20 to 30 mm Hg at the ankle, decreasing to 8 mm Hg at the middle to upper thigh. This change in pressure produces the greatest increase in venous flow velocity that is both safe and practical (Collier, 1999; Phipps and others, 2003).

IMPLEMENTATION

1. Perform hand hygiene.

Reduces transmission of microorganisms.

2. Position client in supine position. Elevate head of bed to comfortable level.

Promotes good body mechanics for nurse. Client position eases application. Also the elastic stockings should be applied before the client stands to prevent stagnation of blood in the lower extremities.

3. If necessary, bathe legs and dry thoroughly. It is optional to apply a small amount of powder to legs and feet, provided client does not have sensitivity to either.

Powder reduces friction and allows for easier application of stockings. Powder should be used sparingly to prevent caking.

4. Apply elastic stockings:
   a. Turn elastic stocking inside out by placing one hand into sock, holding toe of sock with other hand, and pulling (see illustration).

Allows easier application of stocking.

   b. Place client's toes into foot of elastic stocking, making sure that sock is smooth (see illustration).

Wrinkles in elastic stocking can cause constrictions and impede circulation to lower region of extremity (Collier, 1999).

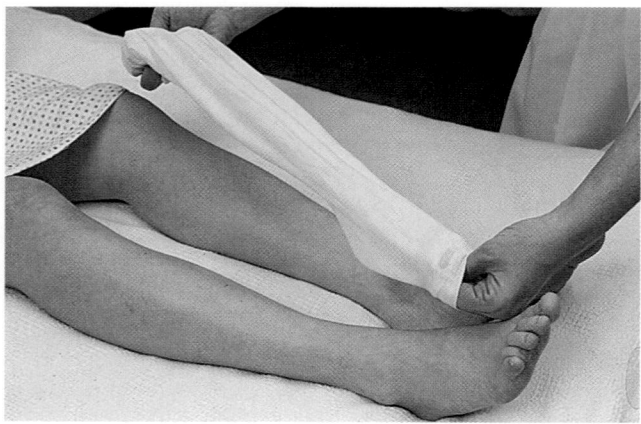

STEP **4a** Turn stocking inside out; hold toe and pull through.

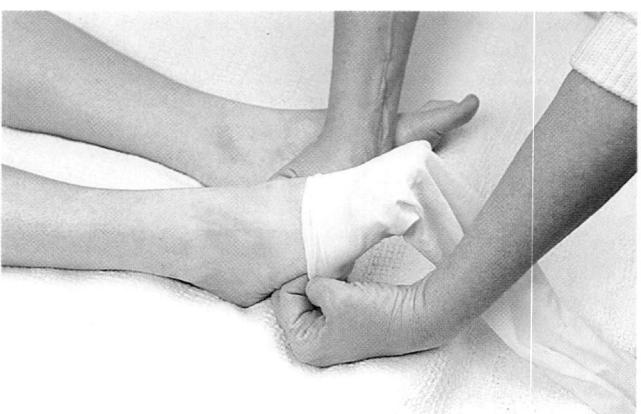

Step **4b** Place toes into foot of stocking.

STEP	**RATIONALE**
c. Slide remaining portion of sock over client's foot, being sure that the toes are covered. Make sure the foot fits into the toe and heel position of the sock. Sock will now be right side out (see illustration).	If toes remain uncovered, they will become constricted by elastic, and their circulation can be reduced.
d. Slide sock up over client's calf until sock is completely extended. Be sure sock is smooth and no ridges or wrinkles are present (see illustration).	
e. Instruct client not to roll socks partially down.	Rolling sock partially down has a constricting effect and can impede venous return.

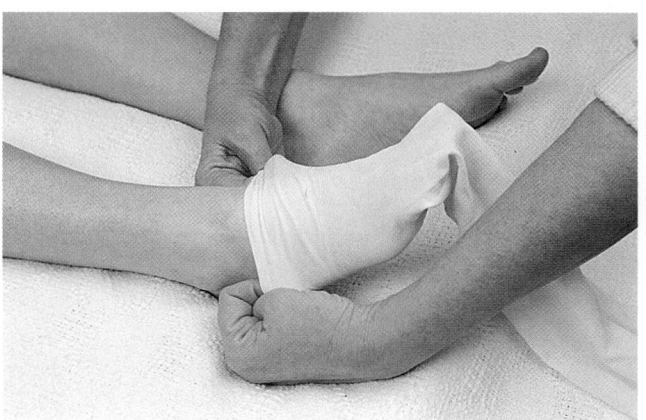

Step **4c** Slide remaining portion of sock over foot.

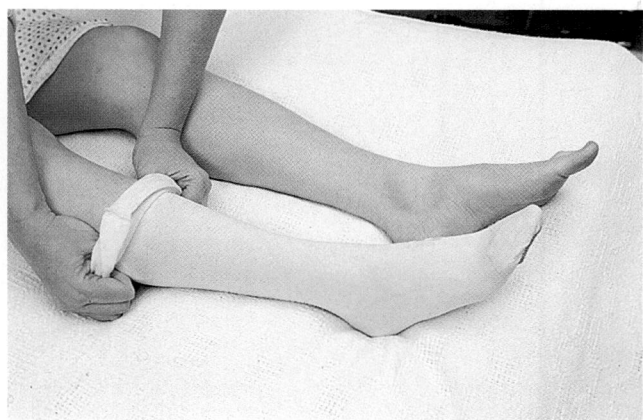

Step **4d** Slide sock up leg until completely extended.

5. Apply SCD sleeves.	
6. Remove SCD sleeves from plastic, unfold, and flatten.	
7. Arrange the SCD sleeve under the client's leg according to the leg position indicated on the inner lining of the sleeve (see illustration).	Ensures straight and even application.
a. Place client's leg on SCD sleeve.	
b. Back of ankle should line up with the ankle marking on inner lining of sleeve.	Correct application of SCD sleeve is important for proper functioning.
c. Position back of knee with the popliteal opening (see illustration).	Prevents pressure on popliteal artery.

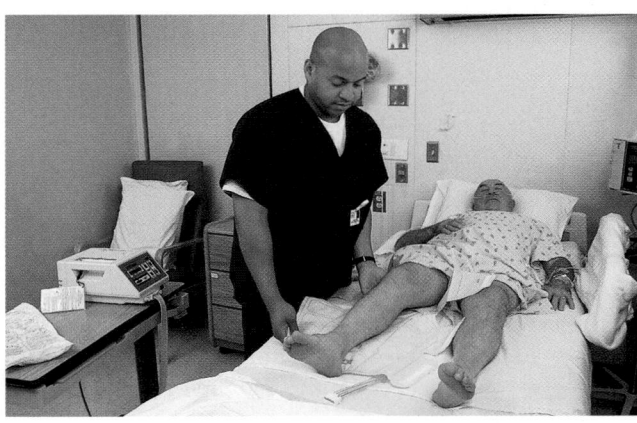

Step **7** Correct leg position on inner lining.

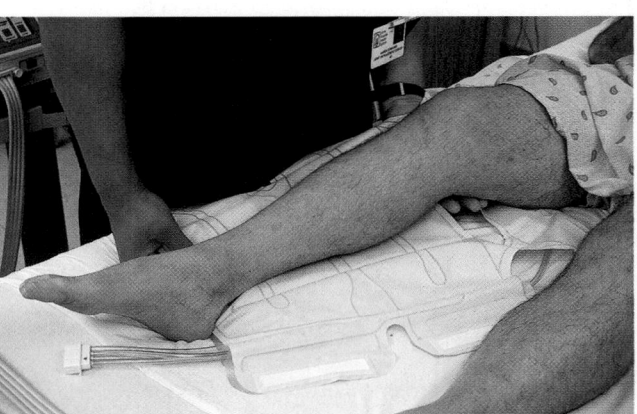

Step **7c** Position back of client's knee with the popliteal opening.

STEP	RATIONALE

- **Critical Decision Point**

  If client is wearing elastic stockings, eliminate any wrinkles and folds before applying SCD sleeves.

  d. Wrap SCD sleeves securely around client's leg.

  e. Check fit of SCD sleeves by placing two fingers between client's leg and sleeve (see illustration).

  Secure fit needed for adequate compression.

  Ensures proper fit and prevents constriction, which could impede circulation.

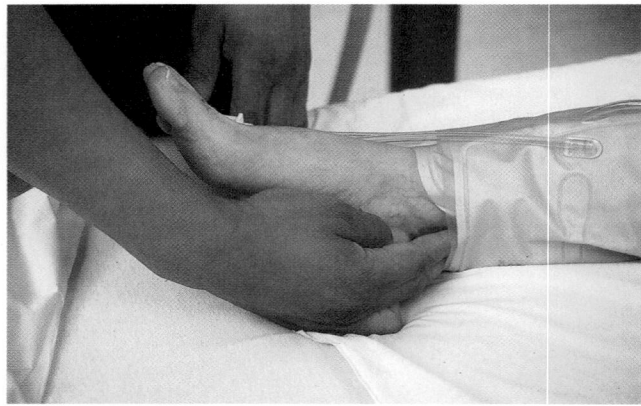

Step **7e** Check fit of SCD sleeve.

8. Attach SCD sleeve's connector to plug on mechanical unit. Arrows on connector line up with arrows on plug from mechanical unit (see illustration).

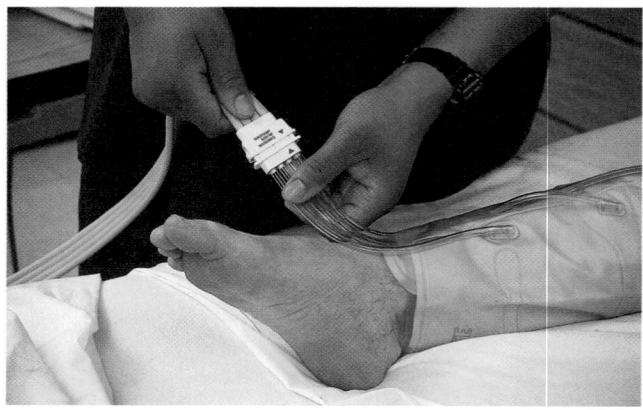

Step **8** Align arrows when connecting to mechanical unit.

- **Critical Decision Point**

  Make sure tubing and connection site are visible. Check for kinks or twisting of tubing to avoid a potential pressure ulcer.

9. Turn mechanical unit on. Green light indicates unit is functioning.

   Power source initiates sequential compression cycle.

10. Monitor functioning of SCD through one full cycle of inflation and deflation.

    Ensures proper functioning of unit and determines if SCD sleeves are too loose or constricting.

11. Reposition client to position of comfort.

    Maintains proper body alignment and promotes comfort.

STEP	RATIONALE

• **Critical Decision Point**
Remove SCD sleeves when transferring client in and out of bed to prevent injury.

12. Perform hand hygiene.	Reduces transmission of microorganisms.
13. Remove SCD sleeves at least once per shift.	

EVALUATION

1. Inspect elastic stockings to make sure there are no wrinkles or binding at top of stocking.	Wrinkles lead to increased pressure and alter circulation.
2. Observe circulatory status of lower extremities. Observe color, temperature, and condition of skin.	Ensures circulatory status in lower extremities has not been compromised.
3. Observe client's reaction to elastic stockings and/or SCD sleeves.	Ensures client is adapting to elastic stockings and/or SCD sleeves.
4. Observe client or caregiver apply elastic stockings.	Determines ability to perform skill accurately.
5. Inspect SCD for kinks or twisting in tubing.	Ensures proper functioning of unit.

Recording and Reporting

• Record in nurses' notes date and time of elastic stockings and/or SCD sleeves application, condition of skin and circulatory status of lower extremities before application, length and size of elastic stockings and SCD sleeves, time elastic stockings and SCD sleeves are removed (at least once per shift), condition of skin and circulatory status after removal.

• Immediately report signs of thrombophlebitis or impeded circulation in lower extremities to charge nurse or physician.

Unexpected Outcomes	Related Interventions
1. Skin reaction to elastic stockings develops.	• Observe for evidence of redness, skin lesions, and client's subjective report of itching or burning. • Some clients may have skin reaction to material used in elastic stockings and may indicate an allergic reaction.
2. Decrease in circulation in lower extremities develops.	• Assess for coolness in lower extremities, cyanosis, decrease in pedal pulses, decrease in blanching, and numbness or tingling sensation. • Check that elastic stockings are not too small or have wrinkles or folds that impede circulation (Breen, 2000). • Notify physician immediately; signs and symptoms may indicate obstruction of arterial blood flow.
3. Deep vein thrombosis is suspected.	• Because clinical signs may be vague, an order for more sensitive radiology tests should be obtained from a physician. Doppler compression ultrasonogram (also known as Doppler duplex) or impedance plethysmography may be carried out to rule out the presence of thrombosis (Breen, 2000; Phipps and others, 2003). • Lower extremities should not be massaged because of potential for dislodging thrombus.

Continued

Unexpected Outcomes	Related Interventions
4. Pulmonary embolism develops.	• Signs and symptoms include tachypnea, shortness of breath, anxiety, pleuritic chest pain, cough, hemoptysis, tachycardia, and signs of right ventricular failure (i.e., distended neck veins) (Phipps and others, 2003). • Notify physician immediately. • Monitor vital signs. • Administer supplemental oxygen as ordered.
5. Alarm on SCD mechanical unit is activated.	• Troubleshoot: check for kinks in tubing, air leaks, and that all connections are secure. • Get a new mechanical unit if there is failure to find reason for alarm.

Teaching Considerations

- Provide time for client to perform return demonstration of application of elastic stockings.
- Instruct client to launder elastic stockings every 2 days with mild detergent and lay flat to dry.
- Recommend client to have two pair of elastic stockings so that a clean set is available at all times.

Pediatric Considerations

- Elastic stockings are not generally used with younger children. However, they are used when their condition warrants and sizes are available for their needs. When the size is not available, ace wraps may sometimes be used. Extra caution is needed to monitor ace wrap application to ensure bandage is not constricting circulation in leg.
- SCD may be used occasionally in this client population.
- Observe younger children frequently because of the potential for an electrical hazard. Keep mechanical unit out of reach of child (Hockenberry and others, 2003).
- Keep SCD's cords and tubing away from child's reach.

Gerontological Considerations

- Perform comprehensive assessment of older adults. Normal physiological aging can mask the signs and symptoms of venous insufficiency.
- Older adults may need assistance in applying elastic stockings because of decreased strength or arthritic changes in the hands.

- Older adults may experience wasting of muscles because of the aging process; therefore, it is essential to measure these clients carefully to ensure proper fit.
- Reinforce need for the older client to call for help before transferring from bed to prevent entanglement with cord or tubing from SCD mechanical unit.

Home Care Considerations

- Assess if client is adhering to prescribed use of elastic stockings. Potential reasons for discontinuing use are expense, cosmetic concerns, discomfort, and difficulty with application.
- Elastic stockings should be removed at least twice a day, and inspection of the skin and circulation of the extremities should be carried out by the client.
- Instruct caregiver or client on troubleshooting when SCD mechanical unit alarms.
- SCD sleeves should be checked periodically for air leaks and wear and tear.

Long-Term Care Considerations

- Elastic stockings will lose elasticity over time and should be replaced at least every 6 months.
- SCD sleeves may lose their elasticity from long-term use. Check frequently for wear and tear.
- Check for proper fit. Elastic stockings and SCD sleeves may become too tight or loose if client's weight fluctuates.

SKILL 11-5 Assisting With Ambulation

Clients who have been immobile for even a short time may require assistance with ambulation. Assistance may mean walking alongside the client while providing support, or the client may require the use of an assistive device to aid in ambulation. Whenever the nurse gets a client up and out of bed or a chair, from a horizontal to a vertical position, there is a risk for orthostatic hypotension. Orthostatic hypotension or postural hypotension is a drop in blood pressure that occurs when a client changes from a horizontal to a vertical position. A drop in blood pressure of approximately 15 mm Hg in systolic pressure and 10 mm Hg in diastolic pressure with symptoms of dizziness, light-headedness, nausea, tachycardia, pallor, and fainting indicates orthostatic hypotension. The nurse uses interventions before ambulating clients that maintain muscle tone to increase venous return to the heart and to decrease stasis of blood in the lower extremities. Safety precautions are important before and during ambulation of clients to ensure they do not fall as a result of orthostatic hypotension.

An assistive device may be ordered to increase stability, to support a weak extremity, or to reduce the load on weight-bearing structures such as hips, knees, or ankles. These devices range from standard canes, which provide minimal support, to crutches and walkers, which can be used by clients who are unable to bear complete weight on the lower extremities or who bear weight on only one lower extremity. Selection of the appropriate device depends on the client's age, diagnosis, muscular coordination, and ease of maneuverability (Hoeman, 2002). Use of assistive devices may be temporary, such as during recuperation from a fractured extremity or orthopedic surgery, or permanent, as in the case of a client with paralysis or permanent weakness of the lower extremities.

Canes are lightweight, easily moveable devices that extend about waist high and are made of wood or metal. Canes help to maintain balance by widening the base of support. They are indicated for clients with hemiparesis and are used to ease the strain on weight-bearing joints. Canes are not recommended for clients with bilateral leg weakness; for such clients, crutches or a walker are more appropriate (Hoeman, 2002). There are two types of commonly used canes. The *standard crook* cane provides the least support

and is used by clients requiring only minimal assistance to walk. It has a half-circle handle, which allows it to be hooked over chairs. The *tripod cane* (pyramid cane) has three legs and the *quad cane* has four legs; the additional legs provide a wide base of support. These types of cane are useful for clients with unilateral, partial, or complete leg paralysis. They also have the advantage of standing alone, freeing the arms to help the client rise from a chair.

A crutch is a wooden or metal staff that reaches from the ground almost to the axilla. Crutches are used to remove weight from one or both legs. They are used by clients who must transfer more weight to their arms than is possible with canes. There are three types of crutches: *axillary, Lofstrand,* and *platform.* The axillary crutch is frequently used by clients of all ages on a short-term basis. The Lofstrand crutch has a hand grip and a metal band that fits around the client's forearm. Both the metal band and the hand grip are adjusted to fit the client's height. This type of crutch is useful for clients with a permanent disability, such as paraplegia. The metal arm band stabilizes and assists in guiding the crutch. The band offers other advantages as well. First, the encircling arm band allows clients to use their hands for other activities, such as opening doors, without dropping the crutches. Second, the anterior opening of the band allows clients to free themselves of the crutches if a fall occurs. The platform crutch is used by clients who are unable to bear weight on their wrists. It has a horizontal trough on which clients can rest their forearms and wrists and a vertical handle for the client to grip.

A walker is an extremely light, moveable device, about waist high, consisting of a metal frame with handgrips, four widely placed, sturdy legs, and one open side. Because it has a wide base of support, the walker provides great stability and security. A walker can be used by a client who is weak or who has problems with balance (Hoeman, 2002). In addition to the standard walker, there are several other models available: a foldable version that is easy to transport, one with a fold-down seat, and one with wheels on the front legs. Walkers with wheels are useful for clients who have difficulty lifting the walker as they walk because of limited balance or endurance. The disadvantage, however, is that the walker can roll forward when weight is applied (Hoeman, 2002).

DELEGATION CONSIDERATIONS

The skill of assisting clients with ambulation may be delegated to assistive personnel. Remind assistive personnel to safely ease a dizzy or fainting client into a sitting position in a chair or on the floor. The nurse provides assistive personnel with information, assistance, and direction, including:

- Instructing assistive personnel to immediately return the client to the bed or chair if the client is nauseated, dizzy, pale, or diaphoretic. Report these signs and symptoms immediately.

- Discussing the importance of applying safe, nonskid-soled shoes and ensuring that the environment is free of clutter and there is no moisture on the floor before ambulating client.

EQUIPMENT

- ❑ Ambulation device (crutch, walker, cane)
- ❑ Safety device (gait belt)
- ❑ Well-fitting, flat, nonskid shoes for client
- ❑ Robe

STEP	RATIONALE

ASSESSMENT

1. Review client's chart, including:
   a. Client's medical history

   b. Client's previous activity level

   c. Current activity order

2. Assess client's physical readiness:
   a. Assess client's heart rate (HR), blood pressure (BP), and orientation to time, place, and person.

   b. Assess ROM, muscle strength, and whether there is the presence of foot deformities.

   c. Assess client for any visual, perceptual, or sensory deficits.
   d. Assess environment for potential threats to client safety.
   e. Assess client for discomfort.

3. Assess client's or caregiver's understanding of technique of ambulation to be used.

4. Determine optimal time for ambulation.

5. Assess degree of assistance client needs.

Certain medications, chronic illness, and history of falling may influence the client's ability to ambulate independently.
Identifies client's previous activity level. Client may tire easily or be prone to orthostatic hypotension if bed rest has been prolonged.
Verifies if an ambulation aid is needed and specifies amount of activity permitted.

Ambulation following immobility can be fatiguing and stressful. Baseline is needed to detect orthostatic hypotension. Baseline vital signs also offer a means for comparison after exercise. The oriented client is able to understand instructions.
Determines if client has enough flexibility and muscle strength to ambulate safely and if client needs muscle-strengthening exercises. Determines if any foot deformities are present to affect ambulation.
Determines if client can use assistive device safely. Ambulation after immobility can be fatiguing and stressful.
Protects client from potential injury.

Client may be in pain or may fear pain resulting from exercise. If necessary, administer analgesic before exercise.
Allows client to verbalize concerns. Clients who have been immobile for a long time may be hesitant to ambulate. Caregiver may be hesitant to learn how to assist with ambulation.
Client's personal habits must be considered when planning activities.
For safety, another person may be needed initially to assist with client ambulation. Allow the client as much independence as possible.

NURSING DIAGNOSES

- Activity intolerance
- Ineffective peripheral tissue perfusion
- Decreased cardiac output
- Fatigue

- Risk for impaired skin integrity
- Risk for injury
- Impaired physical mobility

Related factors are individualized based on client's condition or needs.

STEP	RATIONALE

PLANNING

1. Expected outcomes following completion of procedure:
   - Client will ambulate without episode of injury.

     Precautions prevent orthostatic hypotension. Appropriate level of assistance on device ensures client's safety.

   - Client is able to ambulate without excessive fatigue or dizziness.

     Assistive device chosen requires minimal exertion.

   - Client will demonstrate correct gait.

     Demonstrates learning.

   - Client will resume social and self-care activities.

     Progressive ambulating activities increase client's endurance and independence.

2. Prepare client for procedure:
   - **a.** Explain reasons for exercise, and demonstrate specific gait technique to client or caregiver.

     Teaching and demonstration enhance learning, reduce anxiety, and encourage cooperation.

   - **b.** Decide with client how far to ambulate.

     Determines mutual goal.

   - **c.** Schedule ambulation around client's other activities.

     Scheduled rest periods between activities reduces client fatigue.

   - **d.** Place bed in low position, and slowly assist client to Fowler's upright position. If in chair, have client sit upright with feet flat on floor.

     Allows a few minutes for circulation to equilibrate. Prevents orthostatic hypotension and potential injuries (Kenny, 2000).

   - **e.** Assist client in bed to a dangling position on side of bed. Let client sit for a few minutes, taking a few deep breaths, until balance is gained. Have client move legs and feet while dangling (see illustration). Assist the sitting client to a standing position and allow to stand until balance is gained.

     Movement of legs in dangling position promotes venous return.

   - **f.** Ask if client feels dizzy or light-headed. If client appears light-headed, recheck blood pressure.

     Allows nurse to detect orthostatic hypotension before ambulation begins.

   - **g.** Care must be taken if the client has IV tubing or a Foley catheter. Obtain an intravenous (IV) pole with wheels that can be pushed as the client walks. Urinary catheter drainage bags must stay at or below the level of the bladder, so a second person may be needed to assist.

     Allows client to ambulate unencumbered.

     Urine in tubing must not reenter bladder, which would increase infection risk.

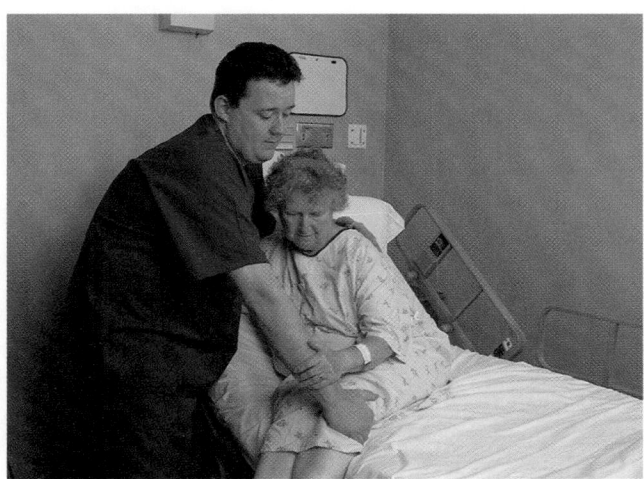

Step 2e Patient dangling.

STEP	RATIONALE

● **Critical Decision Point**
Remove obstacles from pathways, including throw rugs, and wipe up any spills immediately. Avoid crowds. Crowds increase the risk of the crutch, cane, or walker being kicked or jarred and the client losing balance.

3. If ambulation device is used, make sure it is appropriate height:

   a. *Crutch measurement:* Includes three areas: client's height, distance between crutch pad and axilla, and angle of elbow flexion. Use one of two methods:

   (1) *Standing:* Position crutches with crutch tips at 6 inches (15 cm) to side and 6 inches in front of client's feet and crutch pads 2 inches (5 cm) below axilla (Hoeman, 2002).

   (2) *Supine:* Crutch pad should be approximately 2 inches or 2 to 3 finger widths under axilla with crutch tips positioned 6 inches (15 cm) lateral to client's heel (Hoeman, 2002) (see illustration).

   (3) Instruct client to report any tingling or numbness in the upper torso.

   (4) Following correct crutch adjustment, 2 to 3 fingers should fit between top of crutch and axilla (see illustration).

Promotes optimal support and stability.

Radial nerve passes under axillary area superficially. If crutch is too long, it can cause pressure on axilla and radial nerve. Injury to radial nerve causes paralysis of elbow and wrist extensors, commonly called crutch palsy. Also, if crutch is too long, shoulders are forced upward and client cannot push body off the ground. If ambulation device is too short, client will be bent over and uncomfortable.

May mean crutches are being used incorrectly or that they are wrong size.
Adequate space prevents crutch palsy.

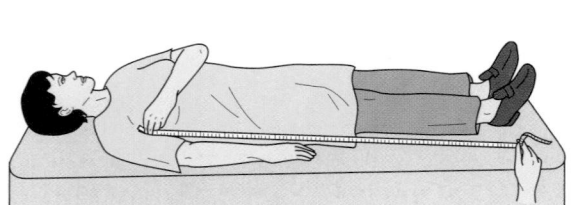

Step **3a(2)** Supine method.

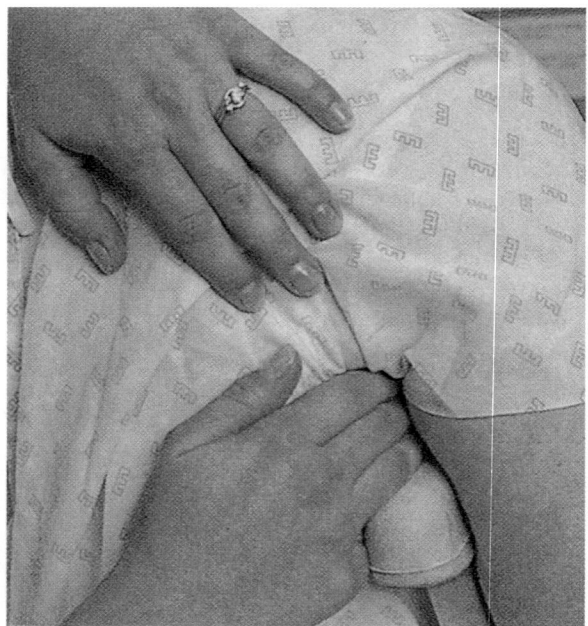

Step **3a(4)** Top of crutch.

STEP	RATIONALE

(5) With either measurement method, elbows should be flexed 15 to 30 degrees. Elbow flexion is verified with goniometer (see illustration).

Angle ensures arms can push body off ground.

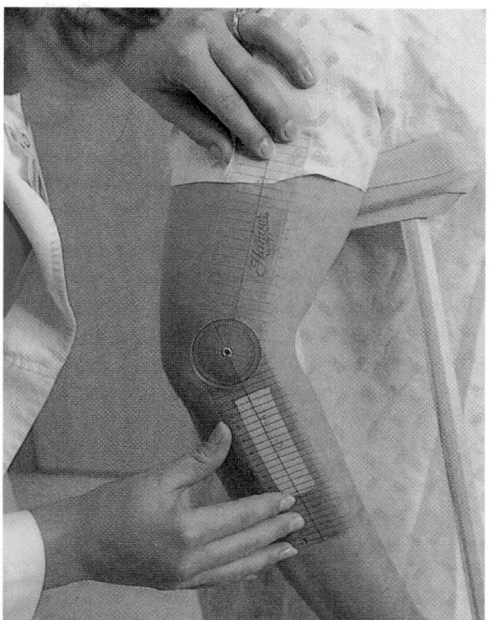

Step **3a(5)** Elbows flexed. Verification of elbow flexion.

(6) In addition to overall *length* of axillary crutch, *height* of handgrip is important. Both dimensions are adjustable on a well-made crutch, and the ability to adjust these dimensions is an important feature for a growing child. Handgrip should be adjusted so that the client's elbow is slightly flexed.

If handgrip is too low, radial nerve damage can occur even if overall crutch length is correct because the extra length between handgrip and axillary bar can force bar up into axilla as client stretches down to reach handgrip. If handgrip is too high, client's elbow is sharply flexed, and strength and stability of arms are decreased.

b. *Cane measurement:* Client should hold cane on uninvolved side 4 to 6 inches (10 to 15 cm) to side of foot. Cane should extend from greater trochanter to floor while cane is held 6 inches (15 cm) from foot (Hoeman, 2002). Allow approximately 15 to 30 degrees of elbow flexion.

Offers most support when cane is placed on stronger side of body. Cane and weaker leg work together with each step. If cane is too short, client will have difficulty supporting weight and be bent over and uncomfortable. As weight is taken on by hand and affected leg is lifted off floor, complete extension of elbow is necessary.

c. *Walker measurement:* Upper bar of walker should be slightly below client's waist. Elbows should be flexed at approximately 15 to 30 degrees when client is standing inside walker with hands on handgrips.

4. Make sure the ambulation device has rubber tips.

Rubber tips prevent the device from slipping.

5. Make sure surface client will walk on is clean and dry. Remove any objects that might obstruct the pathway.

Prevents injuries.

IMPLEMENTATION

1. Assisted ambulation with one nurse
   a. Before beginning ambulation, confirm that client does not feel light-headed.

   Helps client gain balance before attempting ambulation and ensures that client will not become faint while walking.

   b. Apply gait belt if unsure of client's stability, and assist client to standing position; observe balance.

   Prevents injury. Gait belt encircles client's waist and has space for nurse to hold while client walks. If client appears weak or unsteady, return client to bed.

STEP	RATIONALE
c. Have client take a few steps while nurse is positioned on client's stronger side. If an assistive device (e.g., cane, walker) is used, then nurse stands on client's weak side.	If client has hemiplegia (one-sided paralysis) or hemiparesis (one-sided weakness), stand next to client's unaffected side, and support client by placing arm closest to client on the walking belt.
d. Grasp walking belt in middle of client's back.	Provides support at waist so client's center of gravity remains midline.
e. Take a few steps forward with client. Then assess for strength and balance.	Ensures client has satisfactory strength and balance to continue.
f. If client becomes weak or dizzy, return client to bed or chair, whichever is closer.	Allows client to rest.
g. If client begins to fall, gently ease client to floor by holding firmly onto gait belt, stand with feet apart to provide broad base of support, extend leg, and let client gently slide to the floor. As client slides, nurse bends knees to lower body (see illustrations).	Nurse can cause more damage to self and client by trying to catch client.

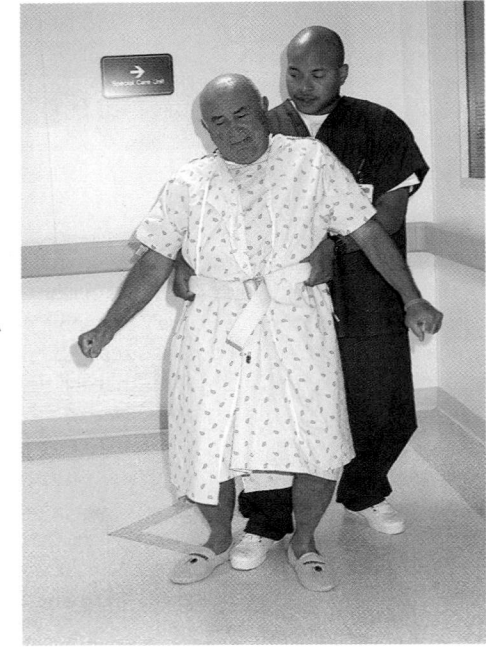

A

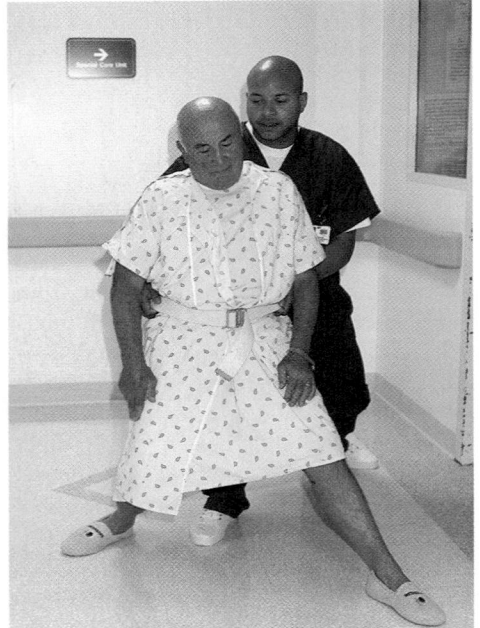

B

Step **1g A,** Stand with feet apart to provide broad base of support. **B,** Extend one leg, and let client slide against it to the floor. **C,** Bend knees to lower body as client slides to floor.

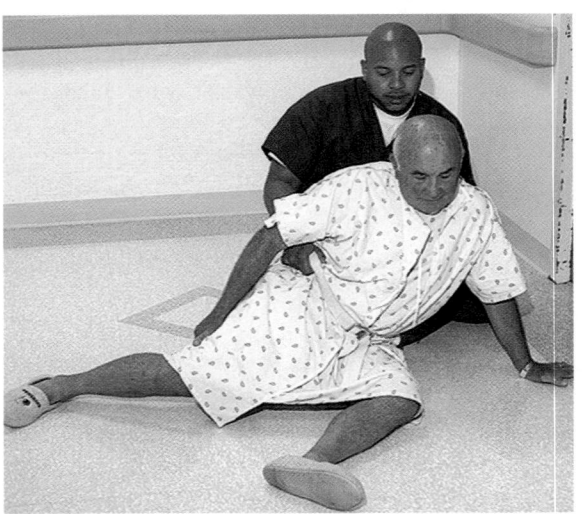

C

STEP	RATIONALE
2. Assisted ambulation with two nurses	
a. Follow steps 1a and 1b.	
b. Stand on either side of client.	
c. Both nurses grasp walking belt in middle of client's back.	Provides secure grip for each nurse.
d. Step forward in unison with client, keeping speed and step size same as client's.	Ensures stability of client.
e. Gradually increase distance walked.	Strengthens muscles, increases endurance, and prevents client from becoming too fatigued.
f. Follow steps 1f and 1g.	
3. Ambulation with assistive devices	
a. Assist client in crutch-walking by choosing appropriate crutch gait.	To use crutches, client supports self with hands and arms; therefore strength in arm and shoulder muscles, ability to balance body in upright position, and stamina are necessary. Exercises such as squeezing a rubber ball, raising and lowering both arms in a slow and rhythmic manner while holding weights, push-ups, and pull-ups will assist in strengthening the upper extremities. The type of gait the client uses in crutch-walking depends on amount of weight client is able to support with one or both legs.
(1) Four-point gait:	This is the most stable of crutch gaits because it provides at least three points of support at all times. Requires bearing weight on both legs. Each leg is moved alternately with each opposing crutch so that three points of support are on the floor all the time. Often used when client has some form of paralysis, such as for spastic children with cerebral palsy (Hockenberry and others, 2003). May also be used for arthritic clients.
(a) Begin in tripod position. Crutches are placed 6 inches (15 cm) in front and 6 inches to side of each foot. The client's weight should be placed on the handgrips, not under the arms (see illustration).	Improves client's balance by providing wide base of support. Client should have a posture of erect head and neck, straight vertebrae, and extended hips and knees.

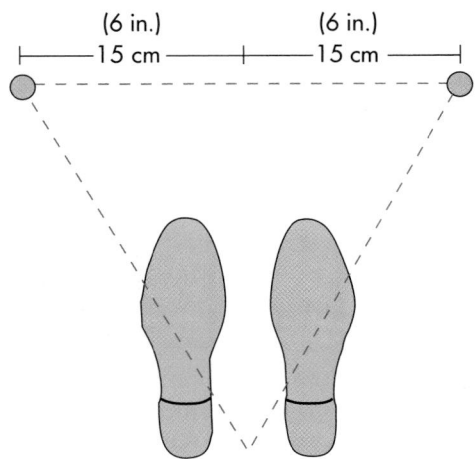

Step **3a(1)(a)** Tripod position.

STEP

RATIONALE

   (b) Move right crutch forward 4 to 6 inches (10 to 15 cm) (see illustration).

   (c) Move left foot forward to level of left crutch (see illustration).

   (d) Move left crutch forward 4 to 6 inches (10 to 15 cm) (see illustration).

   (e) Move right foot forward to level of right crutch (see illustration).

   (f) Repeat above sequence.

Crutch and foot position is similar to arm and foot position during normal walking.

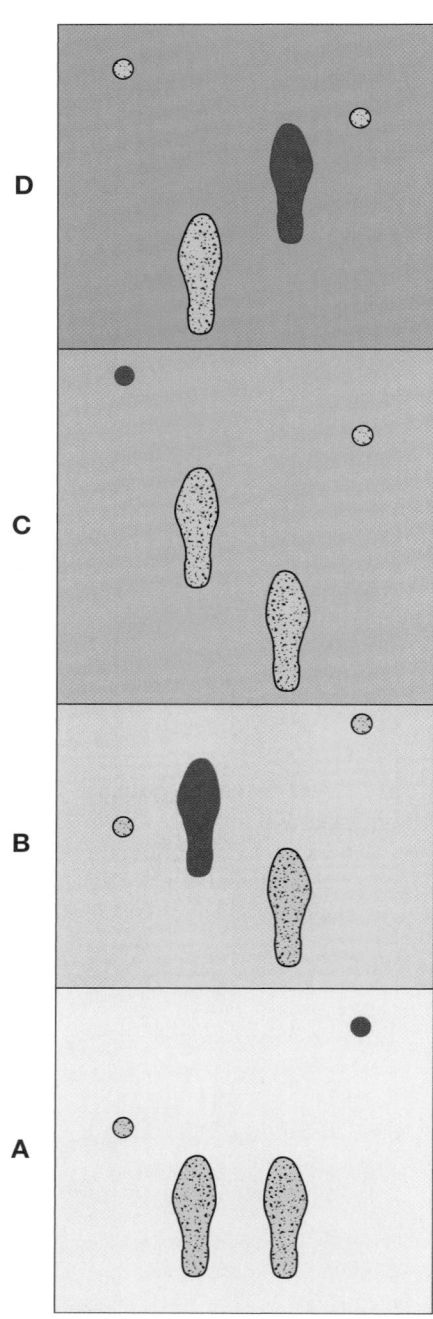

Step **3a(1)(b-e)** Four-point gait. Solid feet and crutch tips show foot and crutch tip movement in each of the four phases. (Read from bottom to top.) **A,** Right tip moves forward. **B,** Left foot moves toward left crutch. **C,** Left crutch tip moves forward. **D,** Right foot moves toward right crutch.

STEP	RATIONALE
(2) Three-point gait:	Requires client to bear all weight on one foot. Weight is borne on uninvolved leg and then on both crutches. Affected leg does not touch ground during early phase of three-point gait. May be useful for client with broken leg or sprained ankle.
(a) Begin in tripod position (see illustration A).	Improves client's balance by providing wide base of support.
(b) Advance both crutches and affected leg (see illustration B).	
(c) Move stronger leg forward, stepping on floor (see illustration C).	
(d) Repeat sequence.	

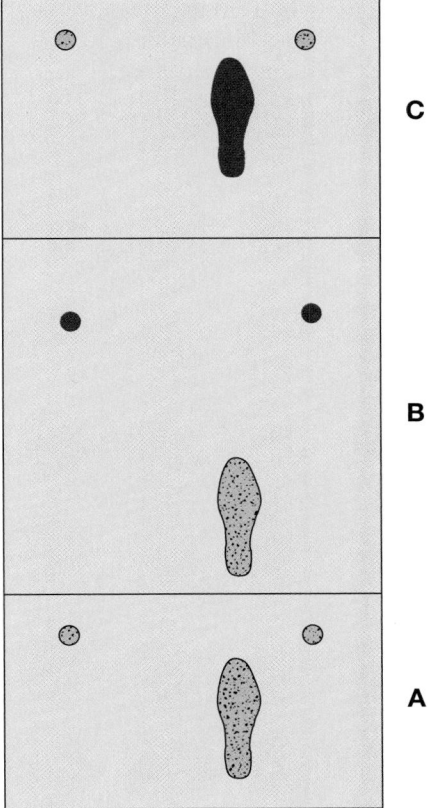

Step 3a(2)(a-c) Three-point gait with weight borne on unaffected right leg. Solid foot and crutch tips show weight bearing in each phase. (Read bottom to top.)

STEP	RATIONALE

(3) Two-point gait:

    (a) Begin in tripod position (see illustration).
    (b) Move left crutch and right foot forward (see illustration).

    (c) Move right crutch and left foot forward (see illustration).
    (d) Repeat sequence.

Requires at least partial weight-bearing on each foot. Is faster than the four-point gait. Requires more balance because only two points support body at one time (Hoeman, 2002). Improves client's balance by providing wide base of support. Crutch movements are similar to arm movement during normal walking as client moves a crutch at the same time as the opposing leg.

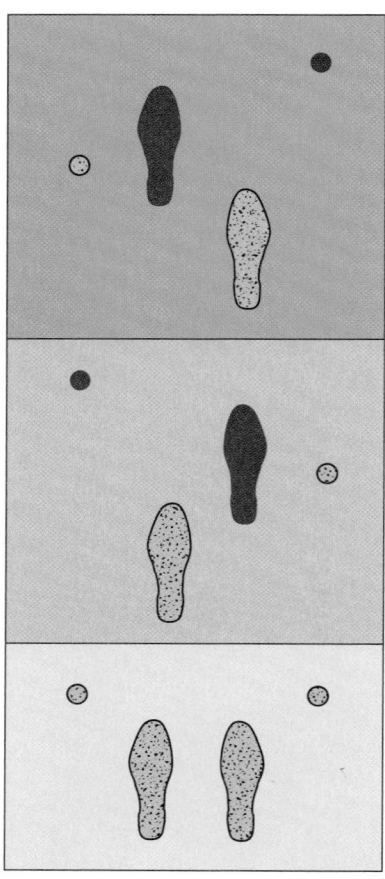

Step **3a(3)(a-c)** Two-point gait. Solid areas indicate weight-bearing leg and crutch tips. (Read from bottom to top.)

(4) Swing-to gait:

    (a) Begin in tripod position.

    (b) Move both crutches forward.

    (c) Lift and swing legs to crutches, letting crutches support body weight.
    (d) Repeat two previous steps.

Frequently used by clients whose lower extremities are paralyzed or who wear weight-supporting braces on their legs. This is the easier of the two swinging gaits. It requires the ability to partially bear body weight on both legs.

STEP	RATIONALE
(5) Swing-through gait:	Requires that client have the ability to bear partial weight on both feet.
(a) Begin in tripod position.	Improves client's balance by providing wide base of support.
(b) Move both crutches forward.	Initial placement of crutches is to increase the client's base of support so that when the body swings forward, the client is moving the center of gravity toward the additional support provided by the crutches.
(c) Lift and swing legs through and beyond crutches.	
b. Assist client in climbing stairs with crutches:	
(1) Begin in tripod position.	Improves client's balance by providing wide base of support.
(2) Client transfers body weight to crutches (see illustration).	Prepares client to transfer weight to unaffected leg when ascending first stair.
(3) Client advances unaffected leg to stair (see illustration).	Crutch adds support to affected leg. Client then shifts weight from crutches to unaffected leg.
(4) Both crutches are aligned with unaffected leg on stairs (see illustration).	Maintains balance and provides wide base of support.
(5) Repeat sequence until client reaches top of stairs.	

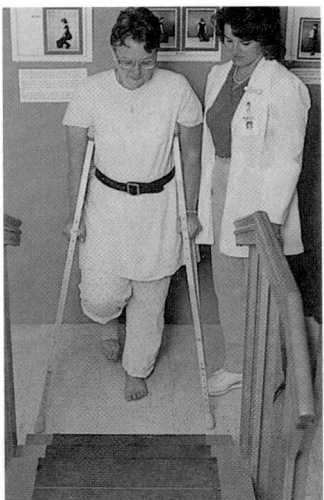

Step **3b(2)** Transfer body weight to crutches.

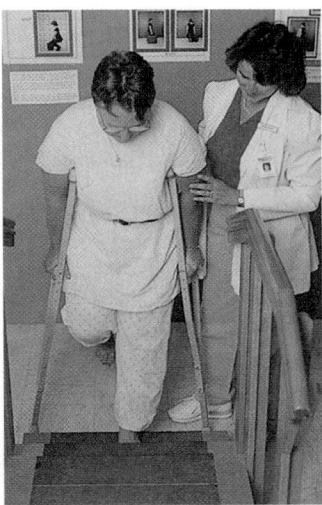

Step **3b(3)** Advance unaffected leg to stair.

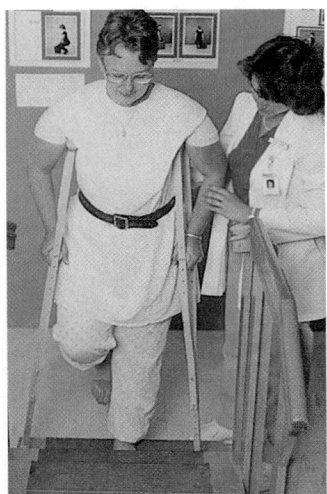

Step **3b(4)** Align crutches with unaffected leg.

STEP	RATIONALE

c. Assist client in descending stairs with crutches:

   (1) Begin in tripod position.

Improves client's balance by providing wide base of support.

   (2) Client transfers body weight to unaffected leg (see illustration).

Prepares client to release support of body weight maintained by crutches.

   (3) Move crutches to stair, and instruct client to begin to transfer body weight to crutches (see illustration) and move affected leg forward.

Maintains client's balance and base of support.

   (4) Client moves unaffected leg to stair and aligns with crutches (see illustration).

Maintains balance and provides base of support.

   (5) Repeat sequence until stairs are descended.

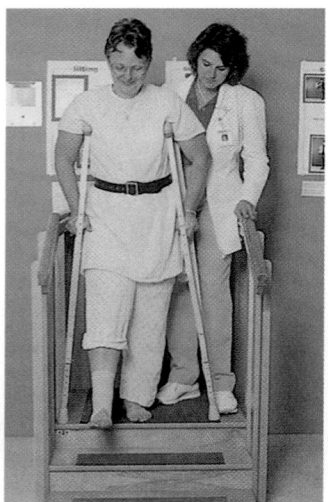

Step **3c(2)** Body weight is transferred to unaffected leg.

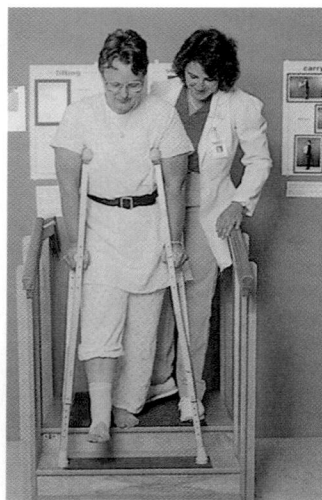

Step **3c(3)** Transfer weight to crutches.

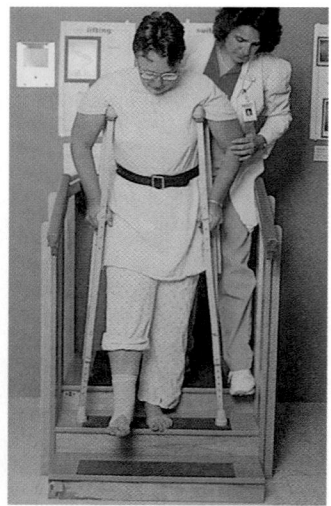

Step **3c(4)** Move unaffected leg, and align crutches.

STEP	RATIONALE

d. Assist client in ambulating with walker (see illustration):

Walker is used by clients who are able to bear partial weight. Walkers do need to be picked up, so client does need sufficient strength to be able to pick up walker. Four-wheeled model does not need to be picked up; however, it is not as stable (Hoeman, 2002).

(1) Have client stand in center of walker and grasp handgrips on upper bars.

Client balances self before attempting to walk.

(2) Lift walker, move it 6 to 8 inches (15 to 20 cm) forward, and then set it down, making sure all four feet of the walker stay on the floor. Take a step forward with either foot. Then follow through with the other leg.

Provides broad base of support between walker and client. Client then moves center of gravity toward the walker. Keeping all four feet of the walker on the floor is necessary to prevent tipping of the walker.

(3) If there is unilateral weakness, after the walker is advanced, instruct the client to step forward with the weaker leg, support self with the arms, and follow through with the uninvolved leg. If client is unable to bear weight on one leg, after advancing walker have the client swing onto it, supporting weight on hands.

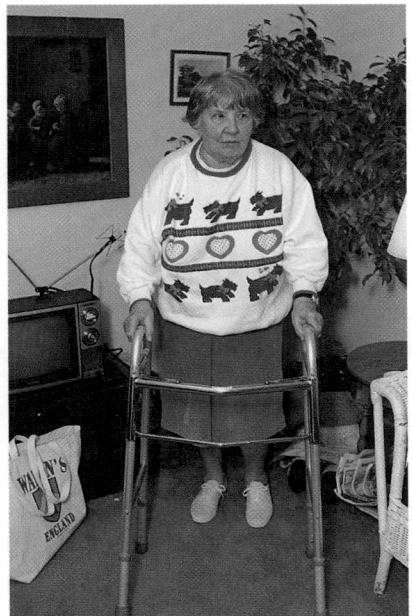

Step **3d** Walker.

STEP	RATIONALE

e. Assist client in ambulating with cane (same steps are taught whether standard or quad canes are used) (see illustration):

  (1) Begin by placing cane on the side opposite the involved leg.

  Provides added support for the weak or impaired side.

  (2) Place cane forward 6 to 10 inches (15 to 25 cm), keeping body weight on both legs.

  Distributes body weight equally.

  (3) Move involved leg forward, even with the cane.

  Body weight is supported by cane and uninvolved leg.

  (4) Advance uninvolved leg past cane.

  Body weight is supported by cane and involved leg.

  (5) Move involved leg forward, even with uninvolved leg.

  Aligns client's center of gravity. Returns client's body weight to equal distribution.

  (6) Repeat these steps.

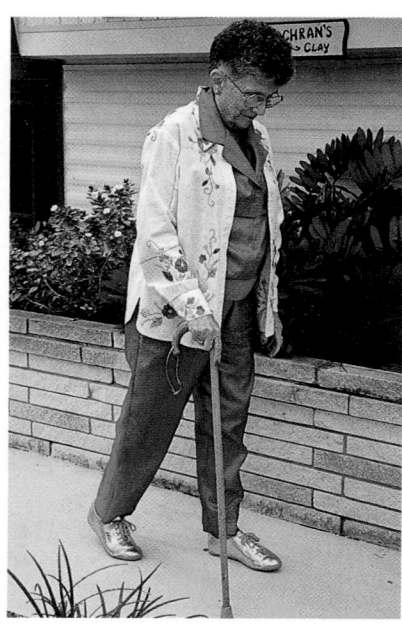
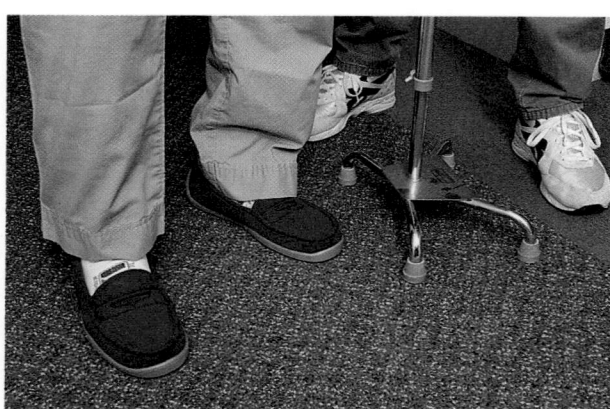

Step **3e A,** Standard cane. **B,** Quad cane.

EVALUATION

1. After ambulation, obtain client's vital signs; observe skin color, and ask about the client's energy level.

   Evaluates how client tolerated procedure and evaluates whether there was progress in ambulation. Assesses stage of client's illness and degree of convalescence when evaluating the process.

2. Evaluate client's subjective statements regarding experience.

   Evaluates activity tolerance.

3. Evaluate gait of client, observing body alignment in standing position and balance.

   Determines if client is correctly using supportive aids for ambulation. Keep in mind the client's previous manner of ambulating when assessing gait.

4. Observe client's ability to perform self-care activities.

Recording and Reporting

- Record in nurses' notes the type of gait the client used, amount of assistance required, distance walked, and activity tolerance.
- Immediately report any injury sustained during attempts to ambulate, alteration in vital signs, or inability to ambulate to nurse in charge or physician.

Unexpected Outcomes	Related Interventions
1. Client is unable to ambulate.	• Possible reasons include fear of falling, physical discomfort, upper body muscles that are too weak to use ambulation device, and lower extremities that are too weak to support body. • Initiate isometric exercise program to strengthen upper body muscles. • Provide analgesia if needed.
2. Client sustains injury.	• Obstacles in client's path, incorrect technique used, or proper safety precautions not taken. • Notify physician. Return client to bed if injury stable.

Teaching Considerations

- If a walker is used, the client is taught to examine the frame daily. When inspecting a walker, the client should observe for signs of bending or deformation of the frame, protruding screws that can scratch, and loose or missing screws that weaken the joints of the frame. Handgrips should be assessed for any cracks or signs of being loose.
- Clients should be instructed to use the arms of a chair rather than the walker to give them leverage when getting up from a chair; the walker is likely to tip if used for this purpose.
- Blistering or soreness of the hands can result from continual pressure between the hand and the handle of a crutch. Advise client to release pressure intermittently and wear gloves or pad the handle to reduce friction.

Pediatric Considerations

- For rehabilitation of a small child who has not yet learned to walk or who is unsteady, special crutches with three or four legs provide needed stability to allow the child to maintain an upright posture and learn to walk (Hockenberry and others, 2003).

- Another option for children who are just learning to walk would be front- or rear-rolling walkers.

Gerontological Considerations

- The older adult may require additional time in the morning before resuming activities.

Home Care Considerations

- Client should be instructed in how to use the ambulation aid on various terrains (e.g., carpet, stairs, rough ground, inclines). Client should also be instructed in how to maneuver around obstacles such as doors and how to use the aid when transferring to and from a chair, toilet, tub, and chair.

Long-Term Care Considerations

- Safety and maintenance checks of ambulation devices should be done on a routine basis.
- Periodic assessments should be performed to ensure that the client is using the ambulation device properly.

FOCUS on CLINICAL PRACTICE

Mr. Timber is a 78-year-old man hospitalized for a right total knee replacement. He has a past medical history of diabetes mellitus. He is now 1-day postoperative following right knee replacement. He rates his pain as 8 on a 10-point scale. Postoperative orders include ambulate with crutches today and CPM machine 4 times a day.

1. As you discuss the plan of care with Mr. Timber for the day, you include the need for ambulation with crutches. He states, "I'm not getting out of bed; I hurt and just had surgery." Discuss nursing interventions that will facilitate this client's cooperation and participation.

2. Mr. Timber has several risk factors associated with the occurrence of orthostatic hypotension. Identify these risk factors and the nursing interventions needed to minimize orthostatic hypotension (see Evidenced-Based Practice Trends).

3. You are applying the CPM machine to Mr. Timber's right leg. Discuss several measures to ensure proper and safe functioning of this intervention.

4. Mr. Timber needs crutches for approximately 4 to 6 weeks during his recovery. He is allowed no weight bearing on his right leg for the first week. What is the appropriate crutch gait for Mr. Timbers? Discuss several teaching considerations associated with the use of crutches.

NCLEX REVIEW QUESTIONS

1. A client has been on bed rest for several days. The client stands and reports dizziness and nausea. These are most likely symptoms of which of the following?
   1. Rebound hypertension
   2. Orthostatic hypotension
   3. Central venous hypotension
   4. Positional hypertension

2. Range-of-motion exercises have been ordered for your client. You note that the left elbow is resistant to extension and flexion. You should:
   1. Force the joint to full range of motion
   2. Perform range of motion to the left elbow only until resistance is met
   3. Notify the physician, and inform him or her of the client's uncooperative behavior
   4. Not perform range of motion on that joint

3. Which of the following statements best describes principles related to range-of-motion exercises?
   1. Passive range of motion sufficiently maintains muscle tone.
   2. Active range of motion is encouraged if the client's health status allows because it promotes independence and assists in maintaining muscle tone as well as joint mobility.
   3. Incorporating range-of-motion exercise into activities of daily living is not sufficient to maintain joint mobility.
   4. Monitoring the client's discomfort level during range-of-motion exercises is not necessary because it should be somewhat painful.

4. Which of the following statements is incorrect regarding isometric exercises? Instruct client to:

   1. Always inhale when exerting effort during isometric exercises.
   2. Hold muscles tight for approximately 5 to 15 seconds.
   3. Perform quadriceps isometric exercises to strengthen muscles associated with ambulation.
   4. Gradually increase frequency of isometric exercises to prevent fatigue or injury.

5. Mrs. Swain has been immobile for over 2 weeks. At this time her health status allows her to begin performing isometric exercises. Which nursing diagnosis best relates to the safety of this client?
   1. Pain
   2. Impaired skin integrity
   3. Disturbed body image
   4. Risk for activity intolerance

6. The benefits of the CPM machine include all of the following except:
   1. Provides continuous isometric muscle contractions to affected leg
   2. Promotes joint mobility of the affected joint
   3. Prevents venous stasis of the affected leg
   4. Decreases stiffness and edema in affected joint.

7. During your assessment of a client who is using a CPM machine you note a reddened area on the heel of the foot. The most likely action to prevent further skin breakdown would be:
   1. Stop use of the CPM machine
   2. Determine if hard surfaces on CPM machine are well padded
   3. Increase speed of CPM machine to improve circulation of affected leg
   4. Increase frequency of skin care to every 8 hours

NCLEX REVIEW QUESTIONS

8. The purpose of elastic stockings after surgery is to:
   1. Prevent varicose veins
   2. Prevent muscular atrophy
   3. Ensure joint mobility and prevent contractures
   4. Facilitate the return of venous blood to the heart to prevent venous stasis

9. You suspect that a client has a deep vein thrombosis in the left lower leg. The priority intervention at this time would be to:
   1. Perform Homan's sign immediately
   2. Massage the area to promote circulation
   3. Prepare the client for radiological studies such as a Doppler compression ultrasonogram
   4. Apply elastic stockings and sequential compression device

10. A client with a history of deep vein thrombosis reports shortness of breath, pleuritic chest pain, and feelings of anxiety. You note that the client has hemoptysis, tachycardia, tachypnea, and harsh cough. Because of this client's past history, you suspect this client may be experiencing:
    1. Myocardial infarction
    2. Pulmonary emboli
    3. Pneumonia
    4. Congestive heart failure

11. Which of the following activities may be delegated to assistive personnel in regard to assisting clients with ambulation?
    1. Assess client's medications to determine if any influence the ability to ambulate independently.
    2. Instruct client concerning the correct use of a walker.
    3. Inspect environment for potential threats to client safety such as spills or clutter.
    4. Evaluate client's ability to perform crutch walking.

12. You are preparing to ambulate a client with left-sided weakness. All of the following statements are true concerning safe and proper ambulation of this client except:
    1. This client is NOT using an assistive device such as a cane; therefore the nurse stands on the left side of the client.
    2. You have decided that the use of a cane would benefit this client; you need to stand on the left side of this client during ambulation when the client is using a cane.
    3. A gait belt is necessary while ambulating this client.
    4. The nurse should grasp the gait belt in the center of the client's back at waist level to ensure client's center of gravity remains at midline.

References

Branson J, Goldstein W: Sequential bilateral total knee arthroplasty, *AORN J* 73(3):608, 2001.

Breen P: DVT: What every nurse should know, *RN* 63(4):58, 2000.

Collier M: Brevet tx: anti-embolism stockings for prevention and treatment of DVT, *Brit J Nurs* 8(1):44, 1999.

Dingle M: Role of dangling when moving from supine to standing position, *Br J Nurs* 12(6):346, 2003.

Ebersole P, Hess P: *Geriatric nursing and healthy aging,* St Louis, 2001, Mosby.

Ebrahim S: Caring for older people: ethnic elders, *Br Med J* 313 (7):610, 1996.

Galanti G: *Caring for patients from different cultures,* Philadelphia, 2003, University of Pennsylvania Press.

Gregg E and others: Physical activity falls and fractures among older adults: a review of the epidemiologic evidence, *J Am Geriatr Soc* 48:883, 2000.

Hammesfahr R, Serafino M: Early motion gets the worm: continuous passive motion following total hip arthroplasty can aid in alleviating pain, edema, stiffness, deep vein thrombosis, and dislocation, and in controlling costs, *Rehab Manag* 15(2):20, 2002.

Hass D and others: Single versus multiple sets in long-term recreational weightlifters, *Med Sci Sports Exerc* 32:235, 2000.

Hockenberry MJ and others: *Wong's essentials of pediatric nursing,* ed 7, St. Louis, 2003, Mosby.

Hoeman S: *Rehabilitation nursing process, application, and outcomes,* ed 3, St Louis, 2002, Mosby.

Huddleston J: Exercise. In Edelman C, Mandle C, editors: *Health promotion throughout the lifespan,* ed 5, St Louis, 2002, Mosby.

Huether S, McCance K: *Understanding pathophysiology,* ed 2, St Louis, 2000, Mosby.

Jitramontree N: Evidence-based protocol: exercise promotion, *J Gerontol Nurs* 27(10):7, 2001.

Kenny R: Advances in the treatment of orthostatic hypotension, *Clin Geriatr* 8(7, suppl):S1, 2000.

Levick J: *An introduction to cardiovascular physiology,* ed 3, Oxford, 2000, Butterworth-Heinemann.

Lueckenotte AG: *Gerontologic nursing,* ed 2, St Louis, 2000, Mosby.

Maas M and others: *Nursing care of older adults: diagnoses, outcomes, and interventions,* St. Louis, 2001, Mosby.

Miller JA: Caring for Cambodian refugees in the emergency department, *J Emerg Nurs* 21(6): 498, 1995.

Phipps W and others: *Medical-surgical nursing: health and illness perspectives,* ed 7, St. Louis, 2003, Mosby.

Rashidi A, Rajaram S: Culture care conflicts among Asian-Islamic immigrant women in US hospitals, Holist Nurse Pract 16(1):55, 2001.

Research References

Babis G and others: Poor outcomes of isolated tibial insert exchange and arthrolysis for the management of stiffness following knee arthroplasty, *J Bone Joint Surg* 83-A(10):1534, 2001.

Boccalon and others: Clinical outcome and cost of hospital vs home treatment of proximal deep vein thrombosis with low-molecular-weight heparin, *Arch Intern Med* 160(12):1769, 2000.

Cousins S, Tan M: Sources of efficacy for walking and climbing stairs among older adults, *Phys Occup Ther Geriatr* 20(3/4):51, 2002.

Frederiks C and others: Evaluation of skills and knowledge on orthostatic blood pressure measurements in elderly patients, *Age Ageing* 31(3):211, 2003.

Merli G: Low molecular weight heparin versus unfractionated heparin in the treatment of deep vein thrombosis and pulmonary embolism, *Am J Phys Med Rehabil* 79(suppl):S9, 2000.

Netea R and others: Body position and blood pressure measurement in patients with diabetes mellitus, *J Intern Med* 251:393, 2002.

Oka R and others: Impact of a home-based walking and resistance training program on quality of life in patients with heart failure, *Am J Cardiol* 85(3):365, 2000.

Quell K and others: Is brisk walking an adequate aerobic training stimulus for cardiac patients? *Chest* 122(5):1852, 2002.

Shea R and others: Pain intensity and postoperative pulmonary complications among the elderly after abdominal surgery, *Heart Lung* 31(6):440, 2002.

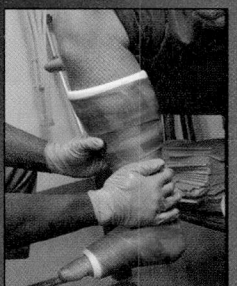

12

Orthopedic Measures

MEDIA RESOURCES

Evolve Site *evolve*

http://evolve.elsevier.com/Perry/skills

• Weblinks

OBJECTIVES

Mastery of content in this chaper will enable the nurse to:

- Explain benefits of the use of casts for clients with musculoskeletal injuries.
- Describe how to assist in application of casts.
- Describe neurovascular assessments of a client in specific casts.
- Describe techniques for drying casts.
- Describe toileting techniques for clients in casts and traction.
- Describe turning and positioning techniques for clients in casts.
- Describe elements of client education for the client with a cast and after removal of a cast.
- Explain the purposes of placing clients in skin or skeletal traction.
- Describe client conditions requiring the use of each form of skin or skeletal traction.
- Describe steps for applying each form of skin or skeletal traction.

KEY TERMS

Cast	Pearson attachment
Cast brace	Pelvic belt
Cast saw	Pelvic sling
Cast shoe	Petaling
Cast syndrome	Pulleys
Cervical halter	Reduction
Compartment syndrome	Spica cast
Countertraction	Spreader bar
Crepitation	Stockinette
External fixation	Thomas splint
Four-poster cast	Traction
Harris splint	Traction boot
Minerva jacket	Walking heel
Neurovascular assessment	

Clients in a cast, traction, or other immobilization devices are susceptible to problems that can affect all body systems. Depending on the extent of a client's injury or illness, an orthopedic device may affect a single body part or the entire body. Alterations in the client's level of mobility require extensive nursing care.

The adequacy of central and peripheral circulation to the injured area must be carefully assessed, because delivery of oxygen and removal of wastes are vital for bone healing, muscle growth and strength, and regaining mobility. Color, temperature, and capillary refill assessments provide data about the adequacy of circulation to the injured extremity. Inflammation, cellulitis, or edema may indicate venous stasis or infection.

Integumentary tissues inside and outside the cast must remain healthy and well nourished. Assessment of the tissues detects pressure, inflammation, or lesions that could lead to infection or pressure sores. Gentle and thorough cleansing of skin, careful drying, and lubrication with lotions provide moisture and stimulation to the integumentary tissues to maintain a healthy state.

Turning, positioning, and range-of-joint-motion (ROJM) exercise help to maintain the health of integumentary and musculoskeletal tissues of individuals in casts. After application of a cast, especially a spica cast or body cast (Figure 12-1) or Minerva jacket, the client must be turned from side to side and prone every 2 to 3 hours while keeping the damp cast uncovered to facilitate thorough drying of the cast. Turning also aids circulation throughout the body, decreases the development of renal calculi, and prevents the development of decubitus ulcers. Placement of pillows, rolls, or blankets helps the client to maintain the side-lying or prone position. In addition, musculoskeletal tissues maintain strength through regularly performed active ROJM exercises with or without resistance or weight. Quadriceps-, gluteus-, triceps-, biceps-, and hamstring-setting exercises, performed routinely and steadily, help to maintain muscle mass and tone (see Chapter 11).

A major challenge for nurses caring for clients in body, spica, or Minerva jacket casts is to maintain respiratory function. While turning facilitates moving air and fluids in the airways, it is also vital that clients be encouraged to breathe deeply and cough. Bed rest over time affects respiration, resulting in decreased ventilation and alveolar collapse. Clients with altered mobility who develop respiratory complications may require respiratory therapy and at times administration of antibiotics. Preventive nursing care measures should be sufficient to avoid such necessities.

Additional challenges center around intake and maintenance of functions of the gastrointestinal and genitourinary systems. Clients in casts or traction who are confined to bed frequently develop anorexia, constipation, and at times, fecal impaction. Maintaining a high (3000 ml or more) fluid intake plus a high-bulk or high-residue diet fosters proper bowel elimination. Fluid intake also facilitates renal circulation and urinary output to lessen the possibility of a urinary tract infection or development of renal calculi. Clients immobilized in casts or traction may lose weight. Diets should be high in protein, carbohydrates, vitamins, bulk, and fluids and should contain a moderate amount of fat, unless contraindicated. Because of individual metabolic and endocrine stress responses, the client will experience catabolism with muscle mass loss for a period of 10 to 20 or more days. Remodeling of bone, a process by which bone resorption and bone deposit occurs, is governed by hormones and stress placed on the bone. When serum calcium levels decrease, parathyroid hormone (PTH) is released. This stimulates osteoclast activity (bone resorption), calcium is released from the bone, and the serum calcium level rises. This can lead to poor bone replacement and the development of osteoporosis and renal calculi. With an elevated serum calcium level, calcitonin from the thyroid gland is released, bone resorption is suppressed, and calcium salts are deposited in the bone matrix.

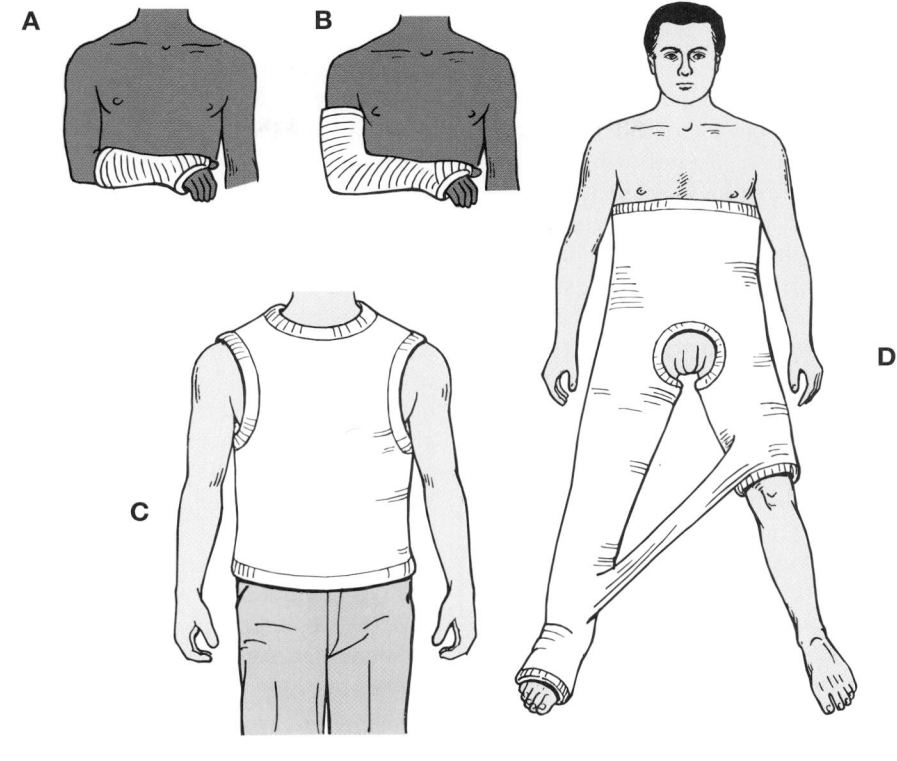

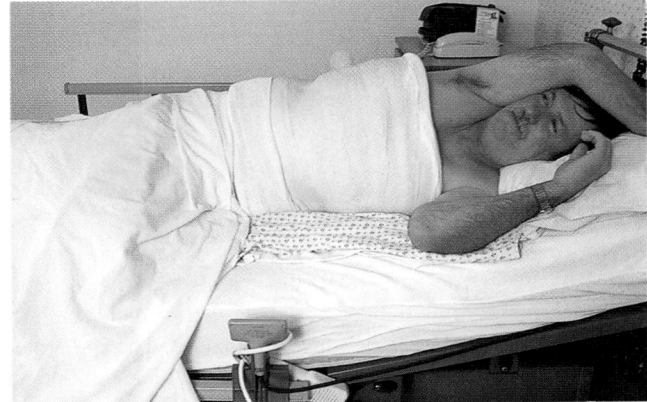

FIGURE **12-1** Types of casts. **A**, Short arm cast. **B**, Long arm cast. **C**, Plaster body jacket cast. **D**, One-and-a-half hip spica cast. **E**, Body cast.

Motor and sensory functions are greatly affected when a client is placed in a cast, sling, or splint. Motor changes may lead to muscle and joint weakness from disuse or pressure. Sensory changes, also from pressure or trauma, may lead to complaints of pain, numbness, and tingling. When such sensory signs are present, changing the client's position may relieve them. It is essential to monitor for the six P's (pain, pallor, pulselessness, paresthesia, paralysis, and pressure) of neurovascular status, because permanent damage may result if the circulation is not restored or pressure is not removed (Altizer, 2001). Bivalving, cutting the cast, or loosening the immobilizer removes the pressure or tightness and increases circulation. Motor weakness may be restored to normal ranges through ROJM exercises and physical therapy. Full

muscle function returns slowly, and consistent performance of exercises is required.

Traction is a force or pull applied to the bones directly or indirectly to overcome deformity and to help restore alignment. When bones are fractured, muscle spasms pull the distal fragments out of their normal positions, often resulting in misalignment and overriding of the bones. Sufficient pull must be applied to the injured tissues to overcome muscle spasms and thus permit the bones to realign themselves in the usual anatomical positions. In situations of severe muscle spasms, marked deformity, or displacement, traction must be applied directly to the distal fragments by means of a strong wire or pin to which traction is applied through a bar, ropes, pulleys, and weights. Such skeletal traction may be applied to one or more bones, including the bones of the skull, upper and lower extremities, and pelvic bones.

Traction to the skin, also known as "skin traction," is applied indirectly to the bones through skin around the structure. Skin traction is typically between 5 and 7 lb and is commonly used for minor trauma or immediate immobilization before surgery. Because of the lower tolerance of skin tissues to the pressure exerted, this traction is applied for shorter periods, with less weight, and at times can be interrupted. Neurovascular assessment is essential to ensure that circumferential dressings (dressings or devices that encircle an extremity) do not impede circulation or place pressure on neurological tissue. Skeletal traction, when used for severe trauma, is applied for longer periods, requires much heavier weights, and is never interrupted.

Clients in traction or those with casts who are confined to bed may become easily tired during the day and may take short, frequent naps. Thus they may be less sleepy at night and may lie awake past their usual bedtime. To offset this syndrome, clients should remain active, engage in stimulating activities, and avoid napping during the day.

Immobilized clients often experience complications of immobility such as skin breakdown and pulmonary emboli. Clients with fractures may develop complications such as fat embolism syndrome (FES), compartment syndrome, or osteomyelitis. Expert nursing care can minimize or eliminate the threat to the client from these complications.

Slings, splints, and braces are treatment devices used with musculoskeletal injury or disorder. These devices immobilize a body part, prevent deformity, protect against injury, relieve pain and muscle spasm, maintain position until healing is complete, or assist with function. Immobilization devices are applied externally to the body. They are available in many variations ranging from arm slings to back braces and finger splints. They are made from a variety of materials such as rubber, leather, metal, and plastics.

Psychologically, clients in immobilization devices may experience alterations in self-concept and body image. They may lose some independence, mobility, and work income during therapy; however, if clients perceive these changes as temporary, they usually regain full independence and mobility.

This chapter focuses on techniques designed to guide the provider in assisting with cast application and removal and care of the client with skin or skeletal traction or immobilization devices.

Evidence-Based Practice Trends

Infection leading to osteomyelitis is a serious complication of skeletal traction. With external fixators, pin tract infection is one of the most common complications. Traditionally nurses have performed pin site care to decrease the incidence of pin site infections. There has been no uniform, consistent, research-based regimen accepted as the standard of care (Gordon and others, 2000; Grossman and Bautista, 2002). The recommendations that are uniformly accepted

are that the pin sites should be inspected for infection. The frequency of pin site care, the cleansing agents, the removal of crusts, and the application of dressings are not research-based practice (Bernardo, 2001). Although some physicians and institutions recommend using hydrogen peroxide as a cleansing agent, it does not appear to be effective in preventing pin site tract infections and may in fact damage healthy tissue (Bernardo, 2001). Grossman and Bautista (2002) found in researching an evidenced-based protocol that performing pin site care every shift, with one half hydrogen peroxide and one half sterile water using sterile technique yielded improved client outcomes. Gordon and others (2000), on the other hand, found that observation of pin sites with only daily showering was as effective as complex cleaning regimens. There was no difference in infection rates between the group with no physical pin cleaning and the group with complex cleaning regimens. Pin site care is expensive because it involves not only cleaning materials but nursing time as well.

In an animal study of specially coated external fixator pins, 83.3% of the animals with antimicrobial-coated pins had no bacterial growth on day one. However, infection developed in 100% of the animals with noncoated pins (DeJong and others, 2001). More research needs to be done before this type of treatment is used in humans, but it may eventually render pin site care obsolete. For now the necessity of pin site care must be documented via research. Numerous nursing authors agree that research in pin site care should be undertaken to establish evidence-based practice for this treatment (Bernardo, 2001).

Cultural Considerations

Assess underlying cultural and religious beliefs that are affected by limited mobility. Muslim clients may not accept instructions regarding the use of the alternative hand for eating and/or personal hygiene after elimination. The right and left hands are specially designated for doing clean and dirty tasks, respectively. Muslim clients may need assistance to wash to perform their ritualized cleansing before prayers when family members are not present. Collaborate with family, religious, and community leaders to promote client's understanding.

Some cultural groups may be threatened by application of traction directly to the head. For example, Southeast Asians consider the head as the seat of life, and it should not be touched except by close kin (Miller, 1995). In addition, some Africans believe that the individual's power and soul reside in the head (Mashaba, 2002). Procedures that puncture the skin of the head are believed to allow the individual's essence or spirit to escape.

When monitoring neurovascular status for clients with casted extremities, integrate cultural differences in monitoring signs and symptoms of neurovascular status. In dark-skinned clients, poor circulation may be manifested by ashen gray appearance of the skin and nail beds instead of pallor, mottling, or bluish discoloration (see Chapter 15). In addition, monitor for associated signs and symptoms of neurovascular status such as stiffness, discomfort, coolness, and swelling.

Maintain privacy of clients with a cast or traction by closing the bedside curtains and adequately draping the client. Some cultures such as Asians, Hispanics, and Africans value female modesty (Spector, 2000). Hindus, Muslims, Amish, and Orthodox Jews emphasize female modesty especially in the presence of males.

When rehabilitative care is necessary, collaborate with family members in implementing a rehabilitative regimen for the client. For example, some cultures (Asians, Hispanics, and Africans) do not define caring as allowing the client to do things on his or her own, especially elders. It is beneficial for the client to allow family to perform direct caring tasks for the client (Andrews and Boyle, 2003). However, the care provided by the family should not impede the rehabilitation goals and return of function.

Skill Performance Guidelines

1. Identify the client's dietary preferences. Wound healing and repair of bone and tissues require additional nutritional intake. Providing foods the client can enjoy meets these additional nutritional needs.

2. Determine the limits of ROJM to the casted extremity or extremity in traction. Although it is important to maintain joint mobility, the nurse must not move the affected extremity beyond the limits imposed by the cast or traction. Excessive movement can impair wound healing, extremity alignment, and new bone growth.

3. Determine the client's level of independent functioning. Knowing what the client is capable of doing enables the nurse to properly plan for assisting the client with activities of daily living (ADLs) such as bathing, eating, dressing, and grooming.

4. Identify the client's normal elimination patterns. Restrictions on mobility imposed by the cast, traction, or use of analgesics can alter elimination patterns.

5. Determine the client's understanding of the normal bone-healing process. This knowledge assists the nurse in developing a teaching plan for the client to care for the casted extremity at home.

6. Identify the results of recent laboratory tests. Serum calcium and phosphorus are two minerals that compose callus, the precursor to bone ossification. Hemoglobin, hematocrit, and red blood cell levels will decrease in blood loss anemia.

7. Determine the frequency and type of analgesics ordered for the client by the physician. The client may experience acute, continuous pain and/or muscle spasms during the first 4 to 7 days (the acute inflammatory stage) and thus require 24-hour administration of analgesics and/or muscle relaxants during this time.

SKILL 12-1   Assisting With Cast Application

A cast is an externally applied structure used to hold musculoskeletal tissues in a specific position to permit healing of injuries or fractures or to align malpositioned tissues, such as in clubfoot or congenital hip dislocation. The rigidity of the cast overcomes the tension, tone, or rotational forces of the muscles or bones for the time required to heal or align the diseased or injured tissues. Because a cast holds tissue in the position in which it is applied, it must be applied carefully and properly to achieve the goals for its use.

Casts are made from plaster of Paris or synthetic materials (Figure 12-2). A plaster of Paris cast has multiple rolls of open-weave cotton saturated with calcium sulfate crystals. These casts are heavier than synthetic casts and can take 24 to 72 hours with no weight bearing or application of pressure while drying. Plaster of Paris is easy to mold and shape around unstable fractures. Synthetic casts are composed of polyester and cotton material, which is impregnated with a water-activated polyurethane resin. Synthetic casts are also made of fiberglass or plastic. Although the newer synthetic casts are more expensive than plaster, they can withstand contact with water without crumbling. These casts are lightweight, set in 15 minutes, and can sustain weight bearing or pressure in 15 to 30 minutes.

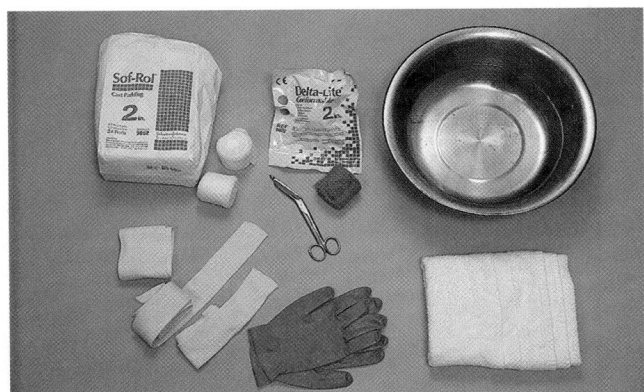

FIGURE 12-2 Plaster roll and padding material.

Client safety is important as the nurse helps apply the cast. The nurse provides optimal skin care to the client before, during, and after cast application. The nurse cleans the extremity, removing dirt, glass, or debris from areas that would be beneath the cast and would irritate the skin. After application of the cast, the nurse ensures that plaster crumbs are removed and rough edges are "petaled" to prevent skin breakdown.

DELEGATION CONSIDERATIONS

Assessment of the client's condition should not be delegated to assistive personnel. However, the skill of assisting with cast application may be delegated to assistive personnel. Before delegating the skill the nurse must:

- Inform assistive personnel to avoid client positioning that increases client discomfort
- Inform and assist assistive personnel, as needed, in the proper method of assisting with cast application

EQUIPMENT

NOTE: Equipment may be preassembled on "cast cart."

- ❑ Plaster rolls (sizes include 2-, 3-, 4-, and 6-inch rolls) or cast materials such as fiberglass, casting tape, or plastic, depending on purpose of cast or specific client condition
- ❑ Padding material (felt, stockinette, sheet wadding, Webril, or other material; available in various thicknesses and lengths)
- ❑ Plastic-lined bucket or basin filled three-fourths full with warm water
- ❑ Disposable gloves and aprons
- ❑ Scissors
- ❑ Paper or plastic sheets
- ❑ Cast saw (if old cast is to be removed)
- ❑ Cart, chair, fracture table

STEP	RATIONALE

ASSESSMENT

1. Assess client's previous health status, including conditions affecting wound healing (e.g., diabetes, peripheral vascular disease, malnutrition, age).

2. Assess client's understanding of upcoming cast application.

3. Assess condition of tissues to be in the cast, including circulation (pulse, color, temperature) to extremities, range of motion (ROM), and sensation. Note presence of skin breakdown, bruising, rash, and irritation. Skin of babies, children, and older adults may contain less subcutaneous fat.

Health status influences healing of tissues enclosed by cast.

Relieves client's anxiety and helps nurse determine whether additional information is needed.

Determines need for additional skin care before cast application. Provides baseline for close observation after cast is applied.

- *Critical Decision Point*
  Clients with skin breakdown or skin lesions may not be candidates for casting.

4. Determine client's pain status on a scale of 0 to 10.
   a. Administer analgesic per physician order.
   b. Administer muscle relaxant per physician order.

5. Determine extent to which client will be able to use casted extremity.

Fractures are painful; client responses vary, as does need for an analgesic. Administration of medications 30 minutes before procedure can lessen discomfort.

Predicts degree of assistance needed for self-care and/or ambulation.

NURSING DIAGNOSES

- Bathing/hygiene, dressing/grooming, and toileting self-care deficit
- Risk for impaired skin integrity
- Risk for peripheral neurovascular dysfunction
- Ineffective peripheral tissue perfusion

- Impaired physical mobility
- Impaired home maintenance
- Deficient knowledge regarding casting procedure
- Acute pain
- Risk for injury

Related factors are individualized based on client's condition or needs.

PLANNING

1. Expected outcomes following completion of procedure:
   - Client initially experiences only slight edema, soreness, mild pain, and some limitation of active ROJM from being in cast.

Cast limits normal function of affected tissues.

STEP	**RATIONALE**
• Skin of tissues below cast is warm and of normal color with capillary refill of 3 seconds or less. Client verbalizes no abnormal or unusual sensations and is able to move fingers or toes below casted part.	Neurovascular function to body part is maintained (McConnell, 2002).
• Skin around proximal and distal cast edges remains intact without irritation.	Skin is free of pressure and friction from cast edges (Maher and others, 2002).
• Client is able to perform limited ROJM actively.	Other joints should move without impairment.
• Client has some impaired function in mobility initially.	Cast may be heavy, or it may impair mobility because of size or area of body in cast.
• Client uses assistance with usual ADLs if head, neck, or upper extremity is in cast.	Cast can interfere with ability to dress, feed, or bathe oneself.
• Client verbalizes increase in comfort after cast in place. Rates pain less than 4 on a scale of 0 to 10.	Injured tissues and bone are stabilized.
• Client demonstrates cast-care techniques.	Demonstrates learning.
2. Instruct client, parent, and other assistants in how they can facilitate application of cast by maintaining affected part in desired position.	Cast will hold tissues in the position in which they are held during cast application. Client teaching reduces anxiety and increases cooperation.

IMPLEMENTATION

1. Administer analgesic before cast application: by mouth (PO), 30 to 40 minutes before; intramuscularly (IM), 20 to 30 minutes before; intravenously (IV), 2 to 5 minutes before. Administer muscle relaxant 30 minutes before cast application if spasms are present.	Reduces pain during cast application. Provides optimal analgesic effect. Muscle spasms may be more effectively treated with skeletal muscle relaxants than with narcotics (Lehne, 2001).
2. Perform hand hygiene, and apply gloves. Use latex-free gloves if there is risk of an allergic reaction.	Reduces transmission of microorganisms. Synthetic cast can leave gluelike resin on hands. Prevents exposure to latex allergen (Yip and Roman, 2003).
3. Position client as needed; client may be lying, sitting, or standing, depending on type of cast and tissues to be casted.	Parts to be put in cast must be supported and in optimal position for cast application.
4. Prepare skin for cast if necessary; may involve cleansing with soap and water, changing dressing, and trimming long hair. Use gentle strokes to maintain skin integrity.	Reduces complications to underlying tissues after casting. Gentle manipulation prevents pain or additional injury.
5. Explain that client may experience warmth during the cast application process.	Plaster gives off heat from a chemical reaction when drying (Maher and others, 2002).

• *Critical Decision Point*
Keep cast exposed to permit maximum dissipation of the heat. Most casts cool in about 15 minutes.

6. Depending on type of cast material being applied, do *one* of the following:	
a. With the thumb under the outer edge, submerge plaster roll under water in a casting bucket or plastic basin until bubbles stop, then squeeze slightly and give roll to person applying cast.	Dampened plaster rolls are unrolled and molded to fit part being casted. Some have resin for easy moldability.
b. Submerge synthetic cast roll in lukewarm water for 10 to 15 seconds. Squeeze to remove excess water.	Initiates chemical reaction that produces heat and hardens tape (Maher and others, 2002).

STEP	RATIONALE

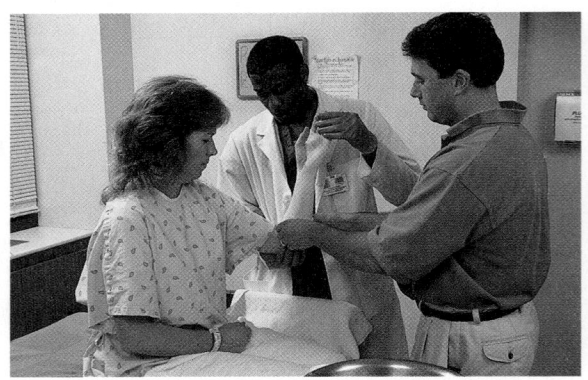 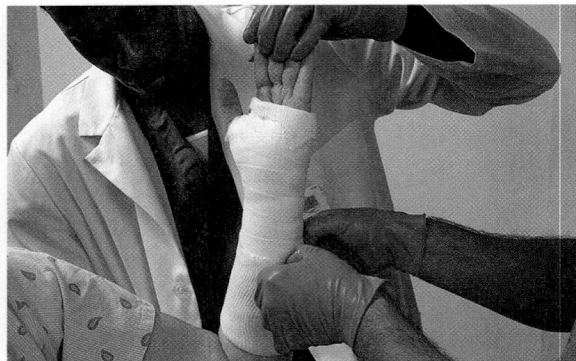

STEP 7 A and **B,** Assistant supports client's extremity as cast is applied.

7. Hold body part or parts to be put in cast in position requested by person applying cast (see illustrations).

8. Hold body part while casting tape is applied and molded. Synthetic tape is applied with slight tension. When wrapping is completed, gently compress with hands.

9. Continue to supply dampened rolls of plaster, synthetic cast roll, or cast tape or to hold parts as necessary until cast is finished. Should be able to insert two fingers between cast and limb.

10. Supply walking heel cast, cast brace, bar, or other cast stabilization material as requested by physician or practitioner.

11. Ensure that the stockinette, Webril, or other casting material is applied evenly and smoothly to prevent wadding and lumping. Damp plaster is then unrolled over padding to hold it securely outside cast. Assist with "finishing" by folding stockinette or other padding down over outer edge of cast to provide smooth edge.

12. Supply scissors to trim plaster rolls around thumb, fingers, and toes as necessary.

13. Depending on tissues casted:
    a. Place damp cast on cloth-covered pillows (two to three) to prevent deformation or pressure points as it sets. Maintain elevation at or above heart level (see Evaluation section). If ice is applied, place to the side rather than the top of the cast to prevent indentations.

Support of body part may involve applying slight manual traction, if desired, to maintain optimal position.

Casting tape is impregnated with synthetic adhesive or glass fiber materials, which dry quickly and are lightweight. Compression promotes bonding of cast layers (Maher and others, 2002).

Plaster must be of sufficient thickness to give strength to cast. More than two fingers' space in cast indicates cast is too loose and will not support limb, and less than two fingers' space indicates cast may be too tight and inhibit circulation.

Ambulation (after cast dries) may be permitted with partial weight bearing (see Chapter 11), which is facilitated by walking cast shoe, heel, or sole. Bars stabilize spica cast, or "posts" (metal poles) stabilize four-poster cast. Brace can be incorporated into cast to aid in maintaining joint motion and mobility.

Smooth edges lessen possible skin irritation. By finishing cast with stockinette, later petaling with tape is not required when cast is dry (Maher and others, 2002).

Cast should be snug but should not constrict joint movement or circulation.

Pillows prevent cast from hardening in undesirable position. Elevation enhances venous return and decreases edema. Elevation above heart level can compromise arterial blood flow if circulation is diminished (Harvey, 2001; Maher and others, 2002).

- **Critical Decision Point**
  Handle casted extremity with palms only until the cast is dry. Fingers can cause indentations that can lead to pressures areas.

STEP	**RATIONALE**
b. Place casted tissues in sling, making sure sling just holds, and does not encase, cast.	Covering (encasing) impedes air movements and delays drying.
14. Remove and dispose of gloves into appropriate receptacle. Perform hand hygiene.	Reduces transmission of microorganisms.
15. Cover client, or reclothe as needed, leaving damp, casted areas uncovered.	Covering blocks air movement, delays drying, and retains heat, which can lead to skin damage with plaster (Maher and others, 2002).
16. Assist with transfer of client to stretcher or wheelchair for return to nursing unit, to prepare client for discharge. May accompany client to room and assist with transfer to bed if necessary. Client may have cast applied in room.	Safety in transfer requires use of pillows to support cast, side rails, restraints, and sufficient personnel to support client and cast. Safety in transfer requires more than one person to accompany client in body, spica, long arm, long leg, and Minerva jacket cast to prevent falls.
17. Clean equipment (bucket, scissors, cast saw), and return to storage area; discard used materials. Perform hand hygiene.	Facilitates use of equipment and treatment area for next client. Reduces transmission of infection.
18. Explain purposes of exposure for faster drying, use of fans or lights to facilitate drying, use of elevation if pertinent, or application of ice bags if ordered.	Casts must dry from inside out for thorough drying. Fans should not be used in open areas or under cast; organisms may be blown in to cause infection. Hot blow dryers or heat lamps can burn tissues. Elevation and use of ice decrease edema formation (Maher and others, 2002).

- **Critical Decision Point**
  Synthetic casts are dry or set by time of transfer, because they set in 7 to 15 minutes. Soft tissues around affected area may swell from processes of "reducing" or manipulating before cast was applied.

19. Reposition client every 2 hours. Do not rest cast heel on pillow.	Prevents any one area of the cast from receiving continuous pressure. Avoids indentation of cast.
20. Inform client to notify personnel of any alteration in sensation, abnormal sensation, or inability to move fingers or toes in affected extremity.	Pressure within a casted extremity may increase with edema and lead to compartment syndrome. Compartment syndrome occurs when pressure within the muscle compartment increases as a result of edema, bleeding, or decreased venous return. The fascia covering the muscle group acts as a tourniquet directing the pressure to structures within the compartment: nerves, blood vessels, and muscle tissue. Neurovascular assessments are used to determine development of compartment syndrome (Harvey, 2001).
21. Cover cast with watertight plastic when bathing client. May use blow dryer on *cool* setting to dry damp areas of synthetic cast.	Plaster of Paris cast will crumble if wet. If a blow dryer is used on hot setting, it may cause the outer portion to dry while the inner section of the cast remains wet, leading to mildew development.

EVALUATION

1. Observe client for signs of pain or anxiety: ask client to rate pain on a scale of 0 to 10, observe for inability to move body parts distal to cast, pain on passive motion of distal body parts, hyperventilation, swallowing air (aerophagia), nausea and/or vomiting, tachycardia, and blood pressure elevation.	These are signs of development of compartment syndrome, cast syndrome, or severe claustrophobia from snugness of cast, common for clients in spica or body cast (Harvey, 2001; Maher and others, 2002).

STEP	RATIONALE

2. Perform neurovascular assessment every 1 to 2 hours for the first 24 hours. Assess for pain, pallor, pulselessness, paresthesia, paralysis, and pressure (Table 12-1). Compare neurovascular status with preapplication neurovascular assessment.

Neurovascular status reflects vascular supply or pressure to tissues that indicates functioning and viability of tissues (Altizer, 2001).

• *Critical Decision Point*

Deterioration in neurovascular status requires immediate action, because irreversible tissue death occurs within 4 to 12 hours of inadequate oxygenation.

3. Observe for edema distal to cast. Older adults may have concurrent dependent edema because of health state.

Edema results from trauma or venous stasis. Rarely, heat of plaster drying contributes to development of edema.

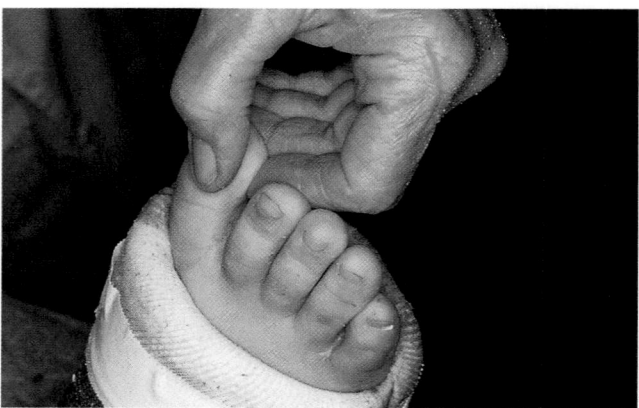

FIGURE **12-3** Assessing capillary refill. The nail bed is compressed. When released it should "pink up" in 3 seconds or less.

TABLE 12-1 6 P'S OF NEUROVASCULAR ASSESSMENT

CRITERIA	ASSESSMENT	RATIONALE
Pain	Determine amount and severity of pain if present. Ask client for descriptions; avoid coaching client with words to describe pain.	Manipulation and reduction may produce dull, aching pain as a result of pressure on nerve endings. Clients vary in perception and tolerance of pain. Pain on passive motion, unrelenting pain, or pain out of proportion is investigated further because it may signify compartment syndrome. Sudden increase in pain may signify thrombus formation (Altizer, 2001; Harvey, 2001).
Pallor	Observe color of tissues distal to cast. Older adult clients may have bluish color normally; however, no other signs of circulatory compromise should be present.	Pink indicates arterial pressure is normal, whitish color signifies decreased arterial supply, and bluish color signifies venous stasis.
Pulselessness	When possible, palpate distal pulse of casted extremity; note presence and strength of pulse. Assess capillary refill by pressing on toenail or fingernail (if cast is on extremity), releasing, and noting "pinking" of nail; nail should "pink up" in 3 seconds or less (Figure 12-3).	Weak or absent pulse may indicate decreased circulation to casted area. Blanching on pressure with subsequent capillary refill is indicative of arterial perfusion. Capillary refill is too sluggish if refill takes more than 3 seconds. It takes 2 seconds to say "capillary refill" slowly and 4 seconds to repeat it once (McConnell, 2002).
Paresthesia	Assess for numbness, tingling, or abnormal sensations.	May indicate nerve damage and/or development of compartment syndrome (Harvey, 2001).
Paralysis	Assess for motion.	May indicate nerve damage and/or development of compartment syndrome (Harvey, 2001).
Pressure	Assess skin of limb or compartment for warmth or for tight, tense, shiny appearance.	May indicate increased intra-compartmental pressure (Harvey, 2001).

STEP	**RATIONALE**
4. Evaluate temperature of tissues above and below cast. Older adult clients frequently have cooler-than-usual extremities because of decreased peripheral circulation.	Warmth of tissues distal to cast usually indicates adequate perfusion.

- **Critical Decision Point**
  Older adult clients may have slow or even poor capillary refill because of peripheral vascular conditions; use more than one neurovascular assessment to determine circulatory adequacy.

STEP	**RATIONALE**
5. Compare tissues in cast with contralateral tissues to determine current condition.	Comparison with normal tissues assists in forming judgment of neurovascular status.
6. Inspect condition of skin around edges of cast. If skin irritation is evident, "petal" the edge of the cast by overlapping strips of tape or moleskin over the edge.	This area is susceptible to pressure and friction.
7. Ask client to move parts in ROJM if possible; note if client is unable to do active ROJM of uncasted areas. Older adult clients may have stiffness of joints or edema from other health conditions.	Range of motion should be performed within limitations imposed by cast. Only tissues out of cast can, or should, be moved.
8. If client cannot do *active* ROJM to contiguous tissues, perform *passive* ROJM on these joints, noting responses or complaints of increased pain.	Passive movements decrease edema and demonstrate ability of part to be moved. However, inability to perform active ROJM and increased pain during passive movement may signify development of compartment syndrome and should be reported immediately (Harvey, 2001).
9. Ask client to describe sensations or feelings of tissues in cast. Listen for descriptions such as "pins and needles," "asleep," "numb," "burning," "tingling," or "throbbing"; do not prompt client by using those words.	May signify pressure or hypoxia to neurological tissues, affecting normal transmission of nerve impulses (Harvey, 2001).
10. Smell the cast edges; a sour smell is normal.	Detects early sign of infection (foul odor).
11. After cast is dry and set, observe client perform and verbalize knowledge of cast care.	Return demonstration objectively measures client's learning.

Recording and Reporting

- Record application of cast and condition of skin and circulation.
- Report abnormal or untoward findings from neurovascular assessments; report the following immediately: bluish color to distal parts, marked increase in edema or pain, delayed capillary refill (longer than 3 seconds), inability to palpate distal peripheral pulses if originally palpable, increased numbness or tingling, cold tissues, and inability to move tissues actively.
- Record odor and drainage from cast: Report to physician. Draw circle on cast around drainage site. Record time and date on circle.
- Document instructions given to client and family.

Unexpected Outcomes	**Related Interventions**
1. Malunion, delayed union, or nonunion of affected parts occurs because of insufficient reduction (placement) in cast or factors such as infection or foreign objects	• Ensure that cast is snug and not loose. • Report loose cast to physician; reapplication will likely be needed. • Treat infection, maintain normal blood glucose level, and provide adequate nutrition.
2. Osteomyelitis develops if open wound was present at time of casting.	• A window may be cut in cast to inspect and dress wound. *Do not* discard window cutout. Tape in place (Maher and others, 2002).

Continued

Unexpected Outcomes	Related Interventions
3. Pressure ulcer develops over bony prominence, or skin irritation occurs at cast edges.	• Cast may be split, windowed, bivalved, or removed by physician (Maher and others, 2002). • Small pieces (petals) of adhesive tape 2.5 to 5.0 cm (1 to 2 inches) are cut and taped smoothly over edge of cast.
4. Muscle weakness occurs.	• Exercise limb within limits of cast. Physician may order physical therapy.
5. Cold extremity, decreased capillary refill, swelling, pallor, diminished pulse, numbness, tingling, or altered motion of distal parts occurs as a result of decreased circulation or neurological functioning distal to cast.	• If symptoms remain, notify physician. Bivalving and cutting underlying soft dressing with spreading the cast open may be necessary to prevent permanent damage (Harvey, 2001).
6. Nausea, vomiting, feeling of abdominal fullness or pain is experienced by client in body or hip spica cast, indicating cast syndrome (superior mesenteric artery syndrome) where the duodenum is compressed between the superior mesenteric artery and the spine	• Change the client from the supine to the prone position. • Give nothing by mouth. • Notify physician, and prepare to cut abdominal window, bivalve cast, and/or insert nasogastric tube (Maher and others, 2002).
7. Client is unable to demonstrate cast care.	• Reinstruction is necessary. Adapt teaching interventions to fit client situation.

Teaching Considerations

- Clients in casts may be more comfortable than when not in cast if deformity or crepitation (the sound heard when fractured ends rub against each other) is present.
- Teach client to realign pillows to promote cast drying when client is repositioned.
- Teach client about effects of pressure from cast on underlying skin and tissue.
- Prepare client for itching sensations under cast. Client should avoid sticking objects down or in cast to scratch, because these objects can cause breaks in underlying skin and subsequent infections. May require medication to control the itching.
- If client must use crutches, instruct in crutch-walking techniques (see Skill 11-5).
- Teach client proper ROJM and isometric exercises for affected extremity.
- Caution client against drying wet cast with hair dryer; this can cause plaster to crack or skin underneath to be damaged.

Pediatric Considerations

- Synthetic casts come in a variety of colors. Allow child to choose color.
- Teach parents or other caregivers to protect cast from moisture or unnecessary wear. Plastic wrap placed around perineal area during urination or defecation prevents soiling. With a spica cast, tuck the ends of a small disposable diaper around the edges of the casted area to cover and protect the perineum in babies (Ball and Bindler, 2003).
- If child has clubfoot, parents and child should be taught that frequent cast changes are necessary. Cast changes accommodate normal bone and tissue growth and correction of abnormality (Ball and Bindler, 2003).
- Children are particularly prone to placing objects into cast to scratch. They must be monitored closely. Assess edges of cast to ensure small objects have not been inserted (Ball and Bindler, 2003). Antihistamines and a hair dryer set to cool can be used to control itching.
- Babies or children may signify pain through crying or restlessness. Gastric distention may occur in child who repeatedly screams and cries with fracture and cast application (Hockenberry and others, 2003).
- Child in body cast or spica cast may find it easier to self-feed from prone position with tray adjacent to child or on floor (Hockenberry and others, 2003).

Gerontological Considerations

- Older nonverbal clients may not verbalize pain, leading one to believe that there is no pain (Maas and others, 2001). The client may express pain through crying, agitation, or restlessness.
- Lightweight, synthetic casts are better for older adult clients. Cast is less restrictive, and light weight helps clients maintain better balance.
- Age-related decreased muscle strength in older adults is a result of loss of skeletal muscle (Maas and others, 2001) and may cause difficulty in ambulating with a cast.
- Older adult clients may have reduced sensation as a result of decreased skin receptors and may be less able to detect compression (Ebersole and Hess, 2001).

- Bone healing (remodeling cycle) takes longer to complete and rate of mineralization slows down in older adult clients (McCance and Huether, 2002).

Home Care Considerations

- Client is instructed that rest, ice, and elevation of affected extremity will help reduce swelling.
- Client must inspect cast and petal rough edges to reduce risk of trauma to underlying skin and need for cast changes.
- Client must inspect cast daily for foul odor, which indicates skin excoriation or infection under cast.

- Client must monitor neurovascular status, paying particular attention to blueness or paleness of nails, pain, feeling of tightness, numbness, or tingling sensation.
- Client must keep plaster of Paris cast dry. When bathing, casted extremity must not be submerged because cast absorbs water, loses structural integrity, and crumbles. If cast becomes wet, dry immediately.
- Synthetic casts may be cleaned with warm water and mild soap.
- Client must notify physician of any clinical manifestation of complications: fever, unrelieved pain, foul odor, or complaints that cast is too tight or rubbing skin.

SKILL 12-2   Assisting With Cast Removal

Cast removal consists of removing the cast and padding with a mechanical device such as a cast saw (Figure 12-4). The nurse must prepare for this procedure so the client remains still and cooperates during cast removal. The removal of a cast is painless but can be noisy. A child or confused client may need to be gently restrained during the procedure to prevent injury by the equipment. After the cast is removed, the nurse provides appropriate skin care.

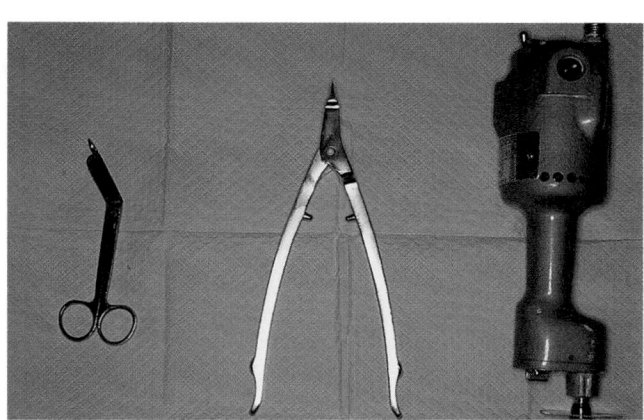

A

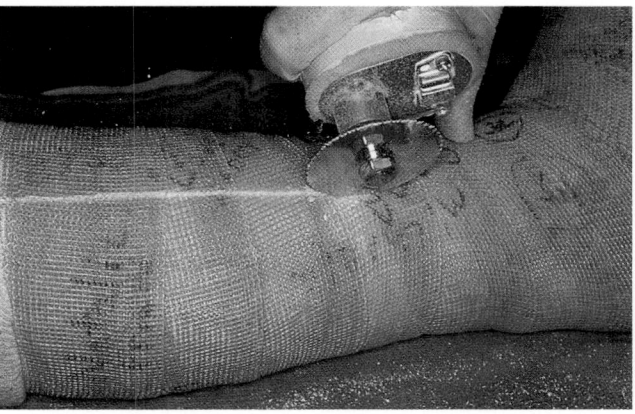

B

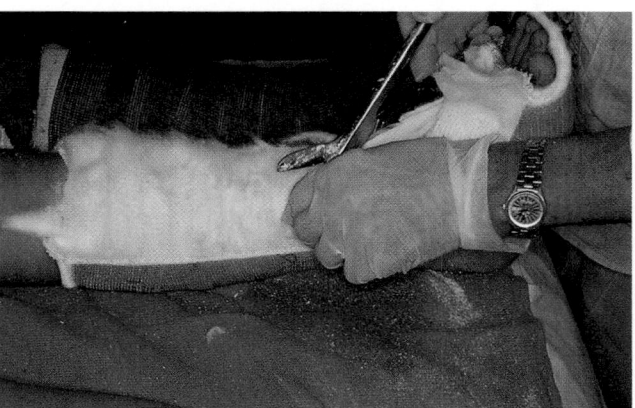

C

FIGURE **12-4** **A,** Equipment for removing a cast. *Left to right:* scissors, cast spreader, cast saw. **B,** Cast saw is used to remove cast. To bivalve a cast, it is cut longitudinally on either side and the wadding is cut with scissors. The two halves may be secured together with an elastic wrap, or the top is removed and the bottom shell of the cast becomes a posterior splint. **C,** Cutting through wadding under cast with scissors.

DELEGATION CONSIDERATIONS

Assessment of the client's condition should not be delegated to assistive personnel. However, the skill of cast removal may be delegated to assistive personnel. Before delegating this skill the nurse must:

- Instruct assistive personnel in proper method of treating skin tissues following cast removal

EQUIPMENT

- ❏ Cast saw
- ❏ Plastic sheets or papers
- ❏ Cold water enzyme wash
- ❏ Skin lotion
- ❏ Basin, water, washcloths, and towels
- ❏ Scissors
- ❏ Clean gloves
- ❏ Eye protection for client and health care professional

STEP	RATIONALE

ASSESSMENT

1. Assess client's understanding of and response to upcoming cast removal.

Helps develop a teaching plan that aids in reducing anxiety.

2. Assess client's physical readiness for cast removal (client's physical findings, physician's orders, x-ray examination results).

Determines level of healing, readiness to remove cast, and need for supportive care after removal.

3. Ask client if any itching or irritation under cast is felt.

Indicates healing and accumulation of dried skin layers.

NURSING DIAGNOSES

- Risk for impaired skin integrity
- Deficient knowledge regarding cast removal

- Anxiety
- Risk for injury

Related factors are individualized based on client's condition or needs.

PLANNING

1. Expected outcomes following completion of procedure:
   - Client incurs no underlying tissue or skin injury; there is buildup of dry, dead skin. Client's skin remains intact.

   Cast is removed safely. Layers of dead skin cells that accumulate are removed over time without scrubbing.

   - Client verbalizes understanding of normal physical sensations and procedural steps of cast removal.

   Understanding lessens anticipatory anxiety.

   - Client is able to describe and demonstrate level of activity and weight bearing allowed following cast removal.

   Allows client to safely assume activity at home.

   - Client is able to explain skin care measures.

   Allows client to assume self-care.

2. Explain physical sensations to expect during cast removal. Cast saw vibrates cast loose; client will feel heat and vibration.

   Explanation minimizes fear of possible injury.

3. Describe procedural steps for cast removal: appearance of saw, vibration sensations, removal of outer cast, appearance of padding and skin, cleansing of skin.

   Client is prepared to witness and participate in procedure. The skin will be dry and scaly, and the extremity will appear "thin" from disuse.

IMPLEMENTATION

1. Apply eye protection on client and health care professional.

2. Apply gloves if drainage is anticipated, and assist person removing cast by positioning, turning, and holding cast and tissues in cast.

   Prevents injury from saw. Use latex-free gloves if there is risk of an allergic reaction (Yip and Roman, 2003).

- ● *Critical Decision Point*

  Instruct client to remain still during cast removal.

3. After removal of cast and padding, inspect tissues for general condition, redness, warmth, and drainage.

   May signify inflammation or infection of tissues.

STEP	RATIONALE
4. If skin is intact, gently apply cold water enzyme wash to skin; let stay on skin 15 to 20 minutes.	Helps dissolve or emulsify dead cells and fatty deposits on tissues. Prevents injury to delicate tissue.

- **Critical Decision Point**

  Do not scrub skin, because this may traumatize delicate tissue and lead to skin breakdown. It may take several days before all residue is removed from skin.

STEP	RATIONALE
5. After elapsed time, gently rinse off enzyme wash; if possible, immerse tissues in basin or tub of warm water to aid in removal of tissue debris without undue rubbing or pressure using mild soap.	Removes as much debris as possible without damaging delicate tissues (James and others, 2002).
6. After patting tissues dry (avoid rubbing), apply generous coating of skin lotion, gently massaging into skin.	Rubbing could traumatize tender tissues. Lotion lubricates skin.
7. Obtain physician's order to gently put joints through active and passive ROJM. Clarify level of activity allowed.	Joints and muscles will be stiff and weak. Activity is resumed slowly to avoid reinjury.
8. Assist in transfer of client for return to room or for discharge if anticipated.	
9. Instruct client to observe for swelling and to continue to elevate the extremity to control swelling.	
10. All equipment and casts should be cleaned or discarded according to standard precautions. Remove gloves. If cast is soiled with blood, discard as biohazard waste.	Reduces transmission of microorganisms.

EVALUATION

1. Observe underlying skin.	Reveals condition of skin.
2. Assess client's verbal and nonverbal responses.	Expressions, tone of voice, and movement reveal level of anxiety or fear.
3. Ask client to explain ordered exercise plan and demonstrate exercises.	Demonstrates learning.
4. Have client explain and perform skin care.	Demonstrates learning of self-care.

Recording and Reporting

- Record cast removal, condition of tissues formerly in cast, and person removing cast in nurses' notes.
- Document instructions given to client and family and verbalization/demonstration of knowledge.
- Report changes in movement, severe swelling, and increased pain to physician.

Unexpected Outcomes	Related Interventions
1. Underlying skin may be scratched from friction of saw.	• Remind client to remain still during cast removal.
2. Client is tense, anxious, restless and withdraws from cast saw.	• Provide further explanation and support.
3. Affected tissues develop extensive edema, pain, or limited use.	• Client may have transient symptoms after cast removal. Instruct client to: • Elevate body part if edema returns. • Use nonnarcotic analgesics every 4 hours for up to 24 hours if needed. • Slowly perform ROJM exercises every 4 hours. (If marked weakness exists, physician may order client to receive physical therapy or to use sling or immobilizer for 1 to 2 days for continued rest.)

Continued

Unexpected Outcomes	Related Interventions
4. Client is unable to perform ADLs and exercises due to nonunion or pain.	• Physician will assess the fracture site by x-ray film.
5. Client is unable to explain self-care measures.	• Reinstruct or clarify as needed.

Teaching Considerations

- Inform client to expect the skin to be dry and flaky following cast removal. Inform that the amount of cellular debris under cast depends on length of time tissues are in cast and overall skin integrity (James and others, 2002).
- Instruct client to use caution with tender skin areas or joints.
- Instruct client to control swelling by elevating the extremity.
- Instruct client to call physician if unable to perform ADLs, if excessive edema occurs, if client experiences limited use of joints or muscles, or if mobility is affected. If client is treated for congenital deformity with repeated cast changes, instruct when next cast change is due; give client written appointment.
- Inform the client to expect the formerly casted limb to be stiff and smaller due to lack of muscular use. Provide client with scheduled exercises to increase mobility and muscle strength (James and others, 2002).

Pediatric Considerations

- Many young children come to regard the cast as part of themselves, which intensifies their fear of removal. Using the analogy of having fingernails or hair cut sometimes helps reduce their anxiety (Hockenberry and others, 2003).
- Babies and children may be frightened of cast saw. Demonstration of saw before removal of cast may alleviate anxiety (James and others, 2002).

- After cast removal, allowing the child to soak in a bathtub will help remove desquamated skin and sebaceous secretions. Parents must be informed that it may take several days to eliminate this completely and that they should not forcibly remove skin (Hockenberry and others, 2003).

Gerontological Considerations

- Older adult clients may experience marked stiffness or weakened muscles, depending on length of time in cast.
- Older adult client's skin is drier, thinner, and more fragile than that of a baby, child, or younger adult (Maas and others, 2001).

Home Care Considerations

- Client should have chair or bed with pillows to elevate extremity for intermittent edema.
- Suggest regular use of moisturizers for dry, scaly skin of casted extremity.
- Assess client's environment for potential safety risks.
- After cast is removed, teach client to dangle before ambulation, to proceed slowly with ambulation, and to gradually increase the time and distance ambulated.
- Client is provided instructions regarding muscle relaxants and analgesics if prescribed.

SKILL 12-3   Care of the Client in Skin Traction

Skin traction is one of the two basic types of traction used for the treatment of fractured bones and correction of orthopedic abnormalities. Skin traction applies pull to an affected body structure by straps attached to the skin around the structure. For traction to be effective, six general principles of care must be implemented (Box 12-1). Recovery is facilitated through immobilization and alignment of body parts. The nurse provides safe care through skillful application of traction. The following are the major forms of skin traction, with some variation within some of the types.

1. *Bryant's traction*—vertically held type of bilateral traction to the legs (Figure 12-5, *A*). This type of traction

can be used for children weighing less than 35 to 40 lb. Adhesive strips are applied to the lateral surfaces of each leg and wrapped with elastic bandages to secure them in place. A spreader bar is attached to the strips and then to ropes, pulleys, and weights. Bryant's traction, known as Gallow's traction in England, is used for children with fractures of the femur or to stabilize the hip joint when casting is contraindicated. After the muscle spasms are overcome and the fragments are aligned with some evidence of union, the child is removed from traction and placed in a spica cast to continue recovery and for callus formation to progress. Children may remain in Bryant's traction for only 7 to 10 days.

BOX 12-1   Six General Principles of Traction Care

1. MAINTAIN THE ESTABLISHED LINE OF PULL

This line is along the axis of the bone. Weights will hang freely, not hitting the bed or resting on the floor. The position of the weights is rechecked if the level of the bed is altered. The nurse avoids (1) bumping against the weights when walking near the bed and (2) allowing the weights to sway; both movements can cause pain for the client in traction. It is preferred that the weights not hang over the client; if this is necessary, the nurse tapes the ropes so the weights will not fall on the client.

2. MAINTAIN TRACTION EQUIPMENT

Traction rope rests in the groove of the pulley and moves easily. The rope is monitored for fraying. The nurse securely ties the knots in the traction rope and tapes the rope ends well. The rope knots are not lodged against the pulley because this will interfere with the line of pull. For the same reason the nurse ensures that the pulley, spreader bar, and foot plate do not rest against the foot of the bed.

3. MAINTAIN COUNTERTRACTION

To provide traction the nurse ensures that countertraction is maintained by the weight of the client's body, the pull of the weights in the opposite direction, or elevation of the bed. For instance, the feet of a client in Buck's traction will not touch the foot of the bed; or if the client is in cervical traction, the head will not touch the head of the bed.

4. MAINTAIN CONTINUOUS TRACTION UNLESS ORDERED OTHERWISE

The nurse will maintain continuous traction unless the physician orders intermittent traction. To change the client's position in bed, the nurse will not lift or adjust the weights if traction is continuous. The nurse will ensure correct amount of weight is used. For intermittent traction the nurse gently places and slowly removes the weights, avoiding jerking or suddenly moving the weights that could jar the client.

5. MAINTAIN CORRECT BODY ALIGNMENT

The client will have correct body alignment while lying centered in the bed. The client will be instructed regarding any restricted positions. The nurse must ensure that the client does not angle the body or lean off the side of the bed because the line of traction pull would then be changed or interrupted.

6. PREVENT FRICTION TO THE SKIN

Skin traction is removed and reapplied daily. Five to eight pounds is the usual amount of weight used for skin traction in adult clients. With any traction the nurse monitors the skin for evidence of redness, bruising, or skin breakdown. Friction or pressure from the equipment is avoided.

Modified from Maher AB and others: *Orthopaedic nursing,* ed 3, Philadelphia, 2002, Saunders.

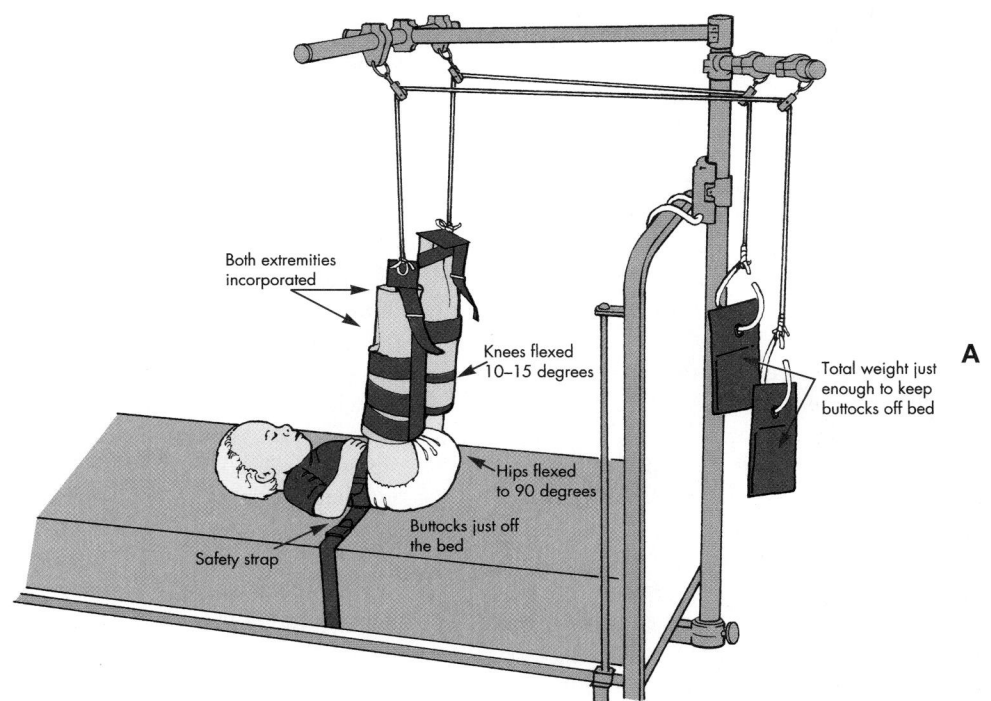

Both extremities incorporated

Knees flexed 10–15 degrees

Hips flexed to 90 degrees

Total weight just enough to keep buttocks off bed

Buttocks just off the bed

Safety strap

A

FIGURE 12-5 A, Bryant's traction. (From Folcik M and others: *Traction: assessment and management,* St. Louis, 1994, Mosby.)

Continued

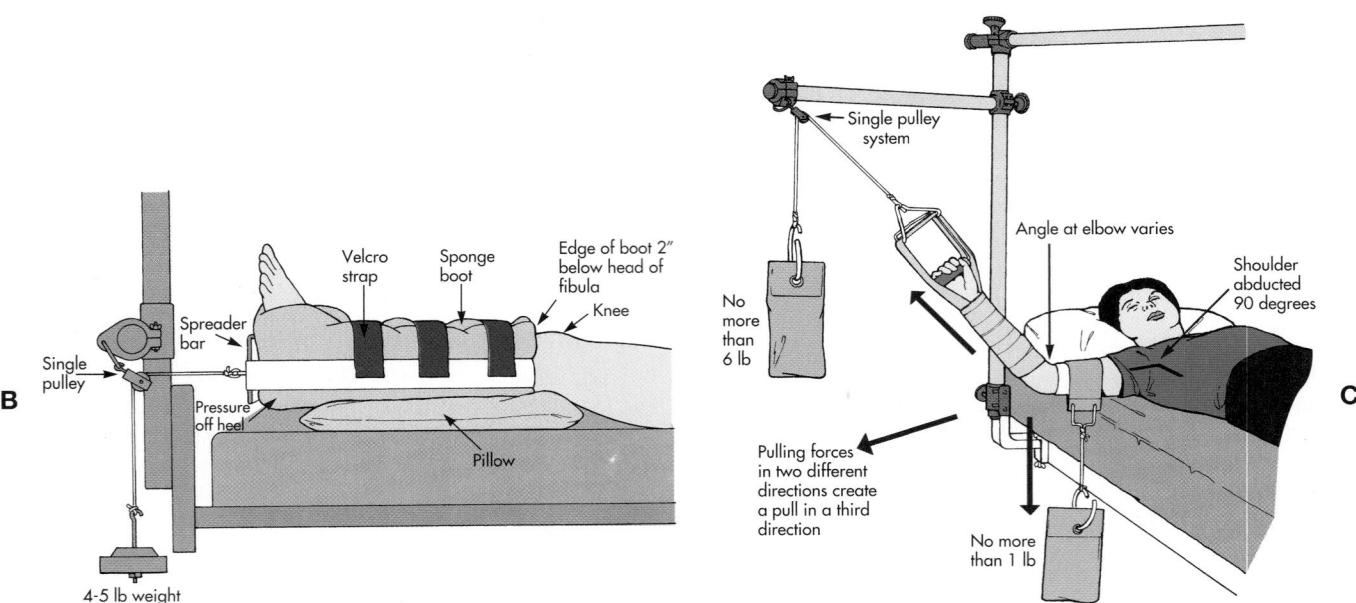

FIGURE 12-5, cont'd B, Buck's extension. **C,** Dunlop's traction. (From Folcik M and others: *Traction: assessment and management,* St. Louis, 1994, Mosby.)

2. *Buck's extension*—horizontally applied unilateral or bilateral traction (Figure 12-5, *B*). Buck's traction is applied in one of two ways: adhesive strips are applied to the lateral surfaces of the limb or limbs (usually one leg or forearm) and wrapped with elastic bandages, or a commercially prepared foam boot with Velcro straps is applied. A spreader bar is attached to the adhesive strips as in Bryant's traction or to the foam boot and then to ropes, pulleys, and weights. Buck's extension provides temporary immobilization of hip fracture until open reduction and internal fixation (ORIF) can be performed. It is also used to reduce muscle spasms, contractures, and dislocations and occasionally as an interim treatment for lumbosacral muscle spasms causing low back pain.

3. *Dunlop's traction*—simultaneous horizontal form of Buck's extension to the humerus with an accompanying vertical Buck's extension to the forearm (Figure 12-5, *C*). The horizontal Buck's extension is the "treating" traction for fractures of the humerus, whereas the vertical Buck's extension is primarily used to maintain the forearm in the desired position relative to the humerus.

4. *Cervical (head halter)*—traction involving a specially shaped halter with cutout areas for the ears, face, and top of the head (Figure 12-6, *A*). The halter cups the chin and has straps leading from the occipital skull area that attach to the chin portion and then connect to one or two spreader bars on either side of the head; the bar or bars are then attached to ropes, pulleys, and weights. Cervical traction should be used only for degenerative or arthritic conditions of the cervical vertebrae, not for fractures of the vertebrae. Because cervical traction

must be removed occasionally for client safety and care and because this traction does not result in total spinal immobilization, it is unsafe and potentially dangerous for a client with a fracture of cervical vertebrae. Release of the weights in such a situation could lead to trauma to the spinal cord and paralysis.

5. *Pelvic belt*—traction consisting of a girdlelike belt that fits around the lumbosacral and abdominal areas, fastening in the middle of the abdomen with pressure-sensitive straps or buckles (Figure 12-6, *B*). The belt has long straps that attach to a wide spreader bar beyond the feet; the bar is then connected to ropes, pulleys, and weights. The client is placed in Williams' position (supine with the head of the bed slightly elevated and the knees bent) to decrease the stress on the lumbosacral spine. This pelvic belt, or lumbosacral traction, is used for clients with low back pain, muscle spasms, and a ruptured nucleus pulposus (herniated or ruptured disk). This traction basically serves to keep the client in bed, thus relieving inflammation and irritation of the injured nerves or muscles. It does not overcome the herniation of the nucleus pulposus. Newer management principles rely on maintaining mobility rather than on promoting bed rest. Additional treatments, including diathermy, use of muscle relaxant drugs, and physical therapy, are used in conjunction with this traction.

6. *Pelvic sling (Weil sling)*—traction consisting of a hammocklike belt wherein the sling cradles the pelvis in its boundaries for treatment of one or more fractures of the pelvic bones. The sling is attached on each side to a pin threaded through a sewn tunnel; each pin is then placed

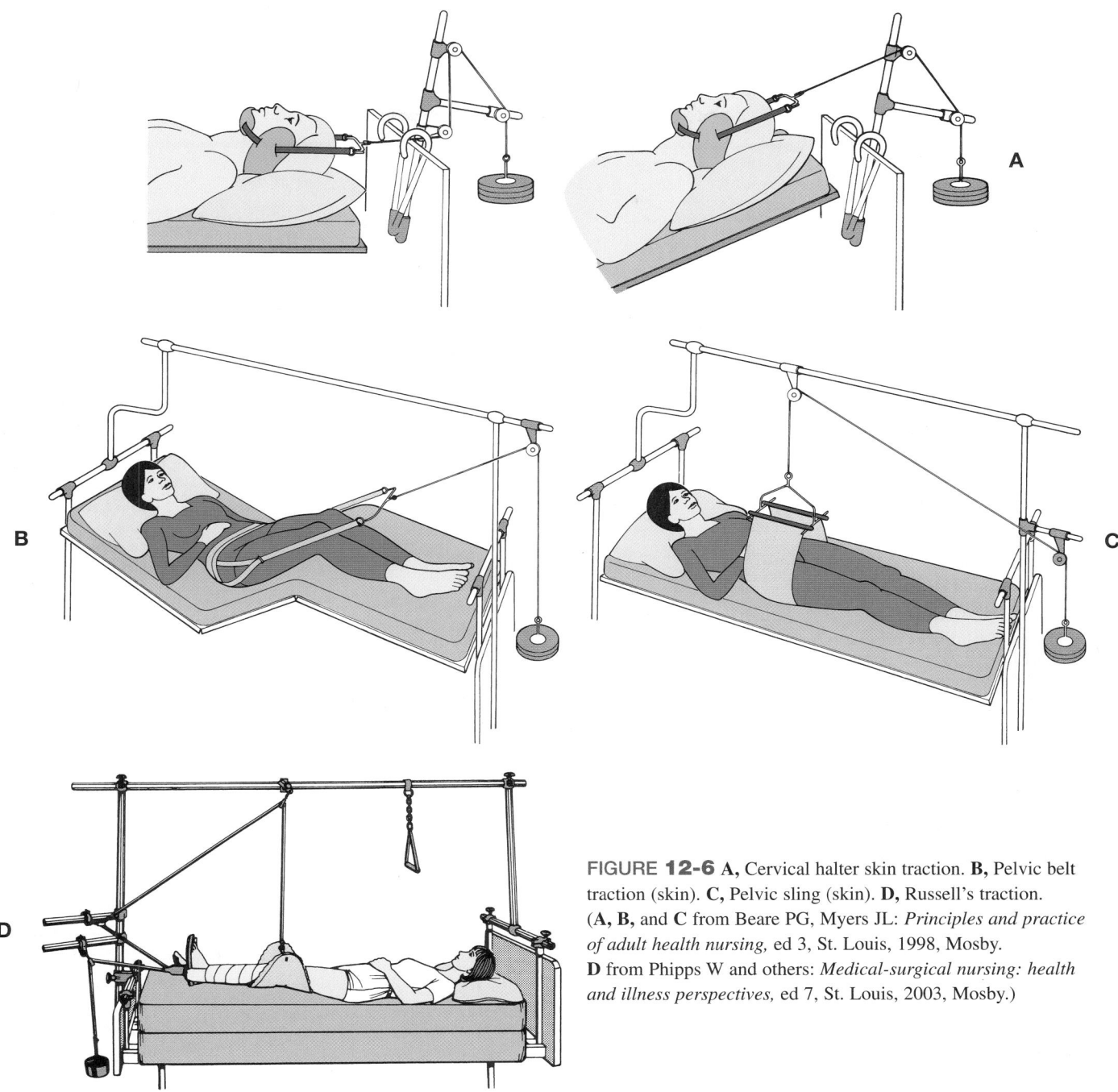

FIGURE **12-6** **A,** Cervical halter skin traction. **B,** Pelvic belt traction (skin). **C,** Pelvic sling (skin). **D,** Russell's traction. (**A, B,** and **C** from Beare PG, Myers JL: *Principles and practice of adult health nursing,* ed 3, St. Louis, 1998, Mosby. **D** from Phipps W and others: *Medical-surgical nursing: health and illness perspectives,* ed 7, St. Louis, 2003, Mosby.)

in a grooved spreader bar attached to ropes, pulleys, and weights. The sling applies gentle inward pressure to the injured tissues, thereby providing comfort and security to the client (Figure 12-6, *C*).

7. *Russell's traction*—modification of Buck's extension using Newton's third law of motion (for each force in one direction there is an equal force in the opposite direction) to double the amount of pull through the arrangement of

ropes, pulleys, and weights (Figure 12-6, *D*). Russell's traction may also be used in skeletal traction.

Because skin tissues and subcutaneous attachments cannot tolerate great amounts of weight without losing strength and continuity, skin traction uses weights varying from 1 to 2 lb for children in Bryant's traction to 7 to 10 lb for cervical skin traction. Average weights are 5 to 7 lb for Buck's extension, 7 to 10 lb for Dunlop's traction, 10 to 15 lb for pelvic belt traction (weight is distributed over the entire pelvis and lower back), and 10 to 20 lb for a pelvic sling (the sling is really a form of hammock suspension rather than traction).

Each form of skin traction mentioned above has a usual or "classic" position used for the majority of clients in that traction. Variations may be needed to treat a specific injury or condition. If pertinent, these variations are noted in the discussion of each type of traction.

DELEGATION CONSIDERATIONS

Assessment of the client and the status of traction should not be delegated to assistive personnel. However, the skill of assisting with application of skin traction may be delegated to assistive personnel. Before delegating this skill the nurse must:

- Discuss with assistive personnel any of the necessary restrictions in positioning client and in application/removal of weights
- Instruct the assistive personnel to report any change in client's skin condition or complaints of pain

EQUIPMENT

- ❑ Ropes, pulleys, weights, weight holder (Ropes are nylon for strength; weights vary from 1 to 5 lb—have several of each weight) (Babies, children, and older adults require less weight than do young adults)
- ❑ Bed frame for attachment of traction or portable frames that attach to bed
- ❑ One or more spreader bars
- ❑ Adhesive-backed moleskin
- ❑ Elastic bandages
- ❑ Heel or elbow protectors (optional)
- ❑ Knee sling for Russell's traction, traction boot for Buck's extension, cervical halter, or pelvic belt or sling
- ❑ Wastebasket with plastic bag liner

STEP	RATIONALE

ASSESSMENT

1. Assess condition of client's overall health, including degree of mobility and current medical conditions such as diabetes, peripheral vascular disease, or peripheral neuropathy.

Determines client's health state and ability to tolerate traction.

2. Assess condition of specific tissues to be placed in traction; note skin condition, excessive hair, bruises, rash, varicose veins, ulcers, dermatitis, or other lesions.

Determines ability of local tissues to tolerate traction (Maher and others, 2002).

- **• Critical Decision Point**
  Irritated or broken skin should not have skin traction placed over the damaged tissues.

a. *Cervical halter:* Assess occipital area of head, ears, chin, and neck.

Each type of traction predisposes client to area at risk for skin breakdown.

b. *Bryant's traction:* Assess both legs.
c. *Buck's extension:* Assess one or both legs.
d. *Dunlop's traction:* Assess arm and forearm.
e. *Pelvic belt:* Assess lower back and abdomen.
f. *Pelvic sling:* Assess back and abdomen.
g. *Russell's traction:* Assess lower limbs.

3. Assess client's understanding of reason for traction.
4. Assess client's level of pain on a scale of 0 to10.

Determines concerns, acceptance, and need for instruction.
Serves as baseline for later comparison and evaluation. Pain and spasms should be relieved by traction.

5. Assess client's neurovascular status.

Serves as baseline for later comparison and evaluation.

NURSING DIAGNOSES

- Bathing/hygiene, dressing/grooming, and toileting self-care deficit
- Risk for impaired skin integrity
- Risk for peripheral neurovascular dysfunction
- Impaired home maintenance

- Impaired physical mobility
- Deficient knowledge regarding the type and use of traction
- Ineffective peripheral tissue perfusion
- Acute pain

Related factors are individualized based on client's condition or needs.

STEP	RATIONALE

PLANNING

1. Expected outcomes following completion of procedure:

   • Client participates in bathing and feeding.

   • Skin around straps and moleskin, halter, boot, or sling remains intact, without irritation.

Activities are performed safely and without injury.
Skin is free of pressure and/or pulling.

   • X-ray studies confirm satisfactory alignment of fracture fragments with or without evidence of beginning callus formation (evidence of callus may not become apparent for 7 to 10 days or longer) if client is in traction for fracture.

Objective evidence is required for comparison with subjective relief of symptoms.

   • Client describes purpose of traction and follows activity restrictions.

Client learns and accepts need for restrictions.

   • Client verbalizes increase in comfort after traction application and rates pain as 4 or lower on a scale of 0 to 10.

Injured tissues and bone are stabilized.

   • As a result of being in one specific type of skin traction, one of the following occurs.

   a. *Cervical halter:* Client notes relief of spasms and pain in neck and back of neck and head (may require administration of muscle relaxant and narcotic medications while in traction).

Each type of traction is designed to relieve muscle spasms; restore alignment or lessen shortening, overriding, or rotation; relieve pain; and increase comfort (Maher and others, 2002).

   b. *Bryant's traction:* Child is able to maintain positioning with distraction by parents or caregivers.

   c. *Buck's extension:* Client is able to maintain leg in alignment. Older adult clients with severe hip pain noticeably relax.

Immobilization decreases pain. Pull of traction may decrease muscle spasms (Maher and others, 2002).

   d. *Dunlop's traction:* Same result occurs as for Buck's extension (used for upper extremity).

   e. *Pelvic belt:* Client notes lessening of spasms of lumbosacral muscles, possibly slight lessening of sensory signs of pressure on sciatic nerve (numbness, tingling, or pins and needles radiating down back of leg to toes), and possibly less pressure in vertebral area at site of injury.

Pull may lessen pressure on spinal or peripheral nerves, thereby alleviating symptoms.

   f. *Pelvic sling:* Client experiences almost immediate comfort and relief from pelvic and abdominal discomfort, pain, and feeling of "coming apart."

Sling compresses tissues together. Clients are very comfortable in sling and develop sense of security while in it.

   g. *Russell's traction:* Client notes lessening of pain in hip area (if traction is for hip trauma), relief of muscle spasms, and ease in ability to maintain more normal anatomical position of leg and thigh.

Russell's traction exerts double pull with less weight than Buck's extension because of pulley arrangement.

   • Sufficient time in traction (varying from 1 to 10 or more days) elicits symptom relief. Continuous skin traction is limited to 7 to 10 days.

Time is required for inflammation to abate and tissues to regain more normal functions. Prolonged continuous skin traction leads to skin breakdown.

   • Neurovascular status remains stable. Distal skin tissue remains warm and of a normal color with capillary refill of 3 seconds or less. Client verbalizes no abnormal sensations and is able to move fingers or toes distal to fracture site.

There is no evidence of increased pressure within the muscle compartment and no neurovascular deficit (Harvey, 2001).

   • Client verbalizes understanding of procedure, including traction setup and mobility restrictions.

Promotes cooperation and reduces anxiety.

STEP	RATIONALE

IMPLEMENTATION

1. Administer narcotic for acute pain and muscle relaxant for spasms in advance of traction application.

   Allowing drugs to reach peak effect at time of traction application will reduce pain and resultant muscle spasm.

2. Prepare client and area of body to be in traction:

   a. *Cervical halter:* Cleanse face and neck; shave man unless he has beard.

   Lessens irritation under cervical halter.

   b. *Bryant's traction:* Cleanse both legs gently if necessary (change diaper if necessary for baby).

   Prevents irritation under traction strips and bandages.

   c. *Buck's extension:* Wash affected leg (or legs) very gently and dry carefully. Do not shave legs.

   Shaving may create micro nicks that could become inflamed under traction strips.

   d. *Dunlop's traction:* Cleanse arm and forearm gently as needed.

   Prevents irritation under straps and bandages.

   e. *Pelvic belt:* Check back and iliac crests for lesions.

   Prevents skin breakdown or irritation in areas where belt is positioned.

   f. *Pelvic sling:* Ask female client to void before being placed in sling if no catheter is in place.

   Sling must be removed for placement of fracture bedpan. Male client can use urinal with no change in position of sling.

   g. *Russell's traction:* Cleanse lower extremity to knee as needed.

   Prevents irritation under bandages.

3. Position client as requested by physician:

   Position varies with part of body to be placed in traction, plus effects of weight and gravity. Body parts are kept anatomically aligned.

   a. *Cervical halter:* Client flat on back.

   b. *Bryant's traction:* Child flat on back.

   c. *Buck's extension:* Client on back; head of bed flat or elevated no more than 30 degrees.

   d. *Dunlop's traction:* Client flat on back.

   e. *Pelvic belt:* Client flat on back.

   f. *Pelvic sling:* Client flat on side or back.

   g. *Russell's traction:* Client on back; head of bed slightly elevated.

4. Assist with application of specific cervical halter, adhesive strips and elastic bandages, Buck's traction, and pelvic belt or sling as needed. Nurse may be asked to hold client in desired position or apply halter, strips, or elastic bandages while physician and other assistants hold client's tissues in desired positions.

   For lower extremity, adhesive strips are applied beginning below head of fibula on lateral surface of leg to avoid pressure over peroneal nerve. Ensures proper alignment of body parts under traction. Elastic bandages are applied from distal to proximal to prevent trapping of blood and to promote venous return (Maher and others, 2002) (see Chapter 39).

- ### *Critical Decision Point*
  Pressure on peroneal nerve as a result of bandages or traction boot can cause footdrop.

   a. Ensure that boot size is correct. Traction boot should fit snugly (not too tight or too loose).

   Too tight leads to pressure to skin, peroneal nerve, and vascular structures. Too loose leads to slipping and lack of traction force.

   b. Heel must be properly seated in traction boot. Do not pad at heel. Cut out heel section of foam boot if necessary.

   Prevents pressure over heel.

   c. Do not apply traction boot over pneumatic compression devices. Foot pumps may be used.

   Causes undue pressure on tissues and negates effects of compression device (Maher and others, 2002).

5. Assist with attachment of spreader bars, ropes, and pulleys. Ropes are tied securely in knots, passed in grooves of pulleys to weights, and are not frayed (see Box 12-1).

   Provides proper weighted traction for extremity alignment.

STEP	RATIONALE
6. When all traction materials and spreader bars are in place, weights are placed on weight holder and attached to loop in rope. The weights are then *lowered slowly and gently* until rope is taut. Physician determines exact amount of weight to be applied and position to be maintained for majority of time by client (clients should have written orders for specific traction weights, bed position, and turning regimen when pertinent).	Traction is slowly established to avoid involuntary muscle spasms or pain for client. Weight should be sufficient to create enough pull to overcome muscle spasms but not to cause distraction or marked increase in pain.
7. Before physician leaves, assess client's position and ask about additional permissible positions for client and bed.	Ensures client's safety and position for effective traction.
a. *Cervical halter:* Client stays flat on back, or head of bed may be elevated 15 to 20 degrees if ordered.	Angle of pull may allow head to be up to use body weight as countertraction.
b. *Bryant's traction:* Baby or child must stay on back at all times; buttocks are held slightly off bed if traction weight is correct amount.	Child cannot turn to side or abdomen, because traction would be ineffective and reinjury could occur (Ball and Bindler, 2003).
c. *Buck's extension:* Client is primarily on back; may be allowed to turn to unaffected side for brief periods (10 to 15 minutes).	Positioning on side permits back care and rest to tissues.
d. *Dunlop's traction:* Client must lie on back. Bed may be tilted on low shock blocks toward side opposite traction. Head of bed is kept flat.	Tilting uses body for some countertraction.
e. *Pelvic belt:* Client lies on back; knee portion of bed (Gatch) and head of bed may be raised so hips and knees are flexed at 45-degree angles (Williams' position).	Flexion of hips and knees relaxes lumbosacral muscles to lessen spasms.
f. *Pelvic sling:* Client lies on back when in sling; sling should have enough weight attached to raise buttocks slightly off bed. If weight is off, it can be used carefully as turning sheet if client's fractures permit side lying.	Hammock effect of sling is most effective with client on back. Sling must be removed for placement of bedpan.
g. *Russell's traction:* Client lies on back; head of bed may be elevated 30 to 45 degrees, depending on injury.	Low-Fowler's position creates most effective traction pull.
8. For safety, raise upper side rails as appropriate. Clients in Bryant's traction should always have someone in attendance.	Promotes client safety.
9. Gather unused materials, and return to storage areas. Perform hand hygiene.	Promotes safety and cleanliness. Reduces transmission of microorganisms.

EVALUATION

1. Observe client's participation in self-care.	Client may refrain from activity unnecessarily or may try to do too much.
2. Assess condition of skin around traction straps or bandages.	Ensures early identification of irritation or breakdown.
3. Inspect entire traction setup and functioning: observe all knots, ropes in pulleys, correct weights on weight holder; whether apparatus is hanging freely and not resting on floor; position of halter, sling, belt, and other material for specific traction; bedclothes not interfering with traction apparatus; and proper body alignment.	Reassessment is necessary to determine if traction is functioning as designed or desired or to make needed adjustments. Malfunctioning traction interferes with healing.
4. Ask if client understands mobility restrictions.	Feedback demonstrates learning.

STEP	**RATIONALE**
5. Ask client to rate pain on a scale of 0 to 10. Ask if client is also experiencing spasm, or muscle burning.	Indicates misalignment of bones or presence of muscle spasms. Initial reaction may be slight increase in soreness or pain until client is able to relax and allow traction to perform as designed.
6. Assess neurovascular status 15 minutes after application of skin traction and every 1 to 2 hours for 24 hours, then extend to every 4 hours if client is stabilizing (see Skill 12-1, Evaluation, step 2).	Provides objective data concerning peripheral perfusion to tissues. If skin traction is applied too tightly, then pressure is applied to nerves and vascular structures, resulting in a potentially irreversible deficit (Harvey, 2001).
7. Skin traction is released every 4 to 8 hours with skin condition assessed and care given. Wash, pat dry, lubricate skin, and apply a light dusting of powder before reapplication of traction.	Prevents pressure ulcers and gives early feedback regarding skin condition. Skin traction may not be removed if it is immobilizing a fracture.

Recording and Reporting

- Record assessment of skin underneath traction apparatus and nursing interventions to maintain skin integrity.
- Record neurovascular assessment of bilateral body parts (see Skill 12-1, Evaluation, step 2).
- Record length of time client is in or out of specific traction. NOTE: Clients in cervical halter and pelvic belt traction are usually in 1 to 2 hours, out 1 to 2 hours, and out to sleep.
- Document instructions given to client and family.

Unexpected Outcomes	**Related Interventions**
1. Child in Bryant's traction continues to turn to abdomen and disrupts traction	• Encourage family to stay with child and distract. Provide toys to distract child.
2. Client experiences increased pain, soreness, or stiffness from pull applied to injured tissues.	• Medicate with analgesics.
3. Client experiences muscle spasms from muscle irritation.	• Administer skeletal muscle relaxants.
4. Client experiences displaced alignment (evident on x-ray film) if fracture is present.	• Maintain proper weights, alignment, and positioning.
5. Client experiences sense of claustrophobia or being "held down" in one or another type of traction.	• Explain intervention to client, and monitor client frequently. • Administer antianxiety medication.
6. *Cervical halter:* Client experiences pain in temporomandibular joint and chin or headaches.	• Consult with physician to shorten straps between chin and occipital part of halter to direct pull from occipital area and away from chin and jaw line. • Client should describe the pull as from the back of neck, not the chin.
7. *Bryant's traction:* Client experiences edema of feet, or peripheral pulses are not palpable.	• Remove bandages and reapply.
8. *Buck's extension:* Client develops pressure area on heel or inability to dorsiflex or evert foot in traction if traction boot, adhesive straps, or elastic bandages exert pressure over head of fibula.	• Reapply traction, and reassess neurovascular status within 15 minutes.

Unexpected Outcomes	Related Interventions
9. *Dunlop's traction:* Client experiences pressure on elbow, or client is unable to approximate thumb to rest of fingers or experiences feeling of numbness of thumb or tingling along sides of thumb and index finger, or capillary refill is over 3 seconds in nail beds	• Elastic bandage is too tight over radial nerve at wrist. • Elastic bandage should be removed from forearm only and rewrapped more loosely; symptoms should then be reevaluated for alleviation or continuance.
10. *Pelvic belt:* Client experiences marked increase in pain or numbness or other sensory pressure signs when in belt.	• Remove traction to ease complaints.
11. *Pelvic sling:* Client experiences psychological dependence on sling and refuses to allow its discontinuance or becomes anxious when out of sling.	• Weaning may be required and involves releasing sling for short to longer periods of time to permit adjustment to being out of sling.
12. *Russell's traction:* Client has pain behind knee or nonpalpable popliteal pulse.	• Readjust to prevent pressure to popliteal area.
13. Client experiences burning, weeping, or drainage under adhesive strips or moleskin because of possible allergy or hypersensitivity.	• Remove traction.

Teaching Considerations
- Explain that traction may increase muscle weakness, spasms, and pain in older adult clients.
- When traction time is decreased or discontinued, client is taught to ambulate slowly within medical guidelines, gradually increasing length of time out of bed and distance walked.
- Client should be taught to notify physician of undesirable signs, such as marked increase in pain, muscle spasms, and increased numbness. Symptoms may signify reinjury or insufficient healing.

Pediatric Considerations
- Babies and children have immature musculoskeletal tissues and are almost constant "movers."
- Bryant's traction is used infrequently because of the alteration in perfusion as a result of gravitational forces and the circumferential bandages. Vasospasm and avascular necrosis may occur (Hockenberry and others, 2003).
- Always assess skin under child for small misplaced objects such as toys.
- Young children may cry when weights are initially applied but soon cease crying.

Gerontological Considerations
- Older adults may have keratoses, rashes, or other lesions that could become irritated in skin traction (Miller, 2004).
- Older adults may have long-standing conditions of musculoskeletal tissues such as arthritis or gout that could lead to inflamed tissues and skin breakdown.

- Older and chronically ill clients may have increased need for position changes resulting from limitations due to osteoporosis, osteomalacia, weakened muscles, or increased risk of skin breakdown (Miller, 2004).
- Older adults' skin heals more slowly, tears more easily, loses its elasticity, and becomes thinner than that of a younger adult (Maas and others, 2001). An alternating air pressure mattress or foam overlay on the bed may be used to decrease the risk of skin breakdown.

Home Care Considerations
- If client is to be discharged to home, relatives or caregivers should be instructed in care needs (including home traction) and mode of ambulation.
- After traction is discontinued, client is taught to dangle before ambulation, to proceed slowly with ambulation, and to gradually increase the time and distance ambulated.
- Home environment must be assessed and adapted to accommodate hospital bed and traction.
- Integrity of traction should be inspected daily—weights hang freely, traction ropes rest in groove of pulley, and client's body is not allowed to interfere with countertraction. In many cases the client's body is the countertraction.
- Client is provided instructions regarding use of muscle relaxants and analgesics if prescribed.

SKILL 12-4 Care of the Client in Skeletal Traction and Pin Site Care

Skeletal traction is the second kind of traction used for the treatment of fractures or correction of orthopedic abnormalities. As with skin traction, skeletal traction may be applied to one or several bones. Skeletal traction begins externally but continues internally directly through the bones. Weights are then attached to the skeletal pin, wire, or nail via ropes and pulleys. Amounts of weights for skeletal traction vary from 10 lb for Dunlop's skeletal traction, to 20 to 25 lb for cervical traction, to 30 to 40 lb for balanced suspension to the femur. Amounts of weights used are also dictated by age, overall condition of the client in traction, and the purpose of the traction.

The procedure can also involve external fixation, which consists of a metal frame that secures pins inserted through the bone above and below a fracture site. The external fixation stabilizes a fracture with hardware visible outside the body. It fosters the healing of complex fractured bones, usually in the lower extremities.

Skeletal traction is often used when continuous traction is desired to properly immobilize, position, and align a fractured bone during the healing process. The nurse provides safe care after skillful application of traction. Common forms of skeletal traction include the following:

1. *Balanced-suspension skeletal traction (BSST) to the femur*—traction used for displaced or overriding fractures of the femur. Balanced suspension brings about relief of muscle spasms, realignment of the fracture fragments, and callus formation (Figure 12-7). This form of traction is used less frequently because of the length of time required for hospitalization when it is used as the major form of treatment. It is now used primarily before surgical implantation of an internal fixation pin, plate, or nail until the client's condition or other injuries stabilize to permit surgery. Balanced suspension involves the use of splints under the thigh and leg to suspend them off the bed, with a Kirschner wire or Steinmann pin supplying the traction (Figure 12-8, *A* and *B*). The pin or wire is drilled through the upper tibia and attached to a spreader, which is then attached to ropes, pulleys, and weights (Figure 12-8, *C*). Sufficient weights are hung to overcome the quadriceps and hamstring muscle spasms; sometimes weights of 30 to 40 lb or more may be required initially. Suspension weights may be 7 to 8 lb, and they are balanced by 7 to 8 lb of countertraction.

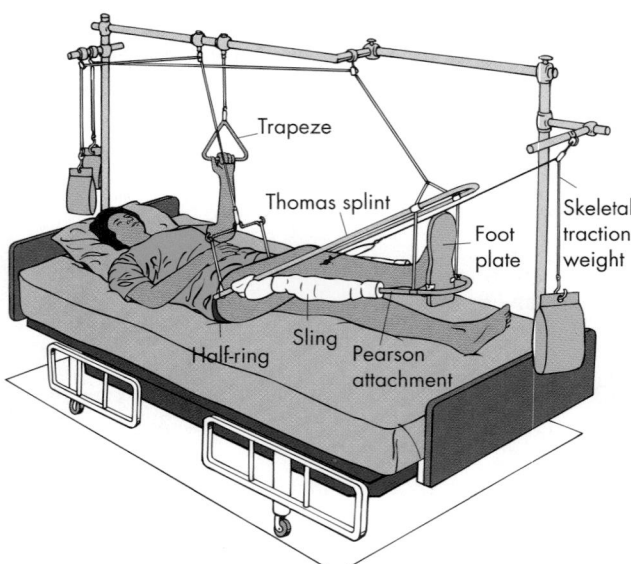

FIGURE 12-7 Balanced-suspension skeletal traction. Traction in long axis of right thigh is applied by means of Kirschner wire through proximal portion of tibia. Limb is supported by Thomas splint beneath thigh and Pearson attachment beneath leg. Foot plate attachment prevents footdrop. Weights apply countertraction to upper end of Thomas splint and suspend its lower end. By using the left arm and leg as shown, client can shift position of the hips without change in amount of traction.

2. Upper extremity traction:
   Side-arm traction—skeletal form of Dunlop's traction (Figure 12-9, *A*). The difference consists mainly of a pin drilled through the lower humerus (instead of the horizontal Buck's extension mentioned previously) and attached to a spreader, ropes, pulleys, and weights. The forearm is held in vertical Buck's extension, as it would be in Dunlop's skin traction. Side-arm skeletal traction is used for severe fractures, in which the greater pull permitted with the skeletal pin is required to overcome muscle spasms, resulting in effective alignment and union.

   Overhead 90-90 traction—humerus is placed at 90 degrees to the trunk, and elbow is flexed at 90 degrees. A sling supports the forearm. A Kirschner wire is placed through the olecranon process of the ulna (Figure 12-9, *B*).

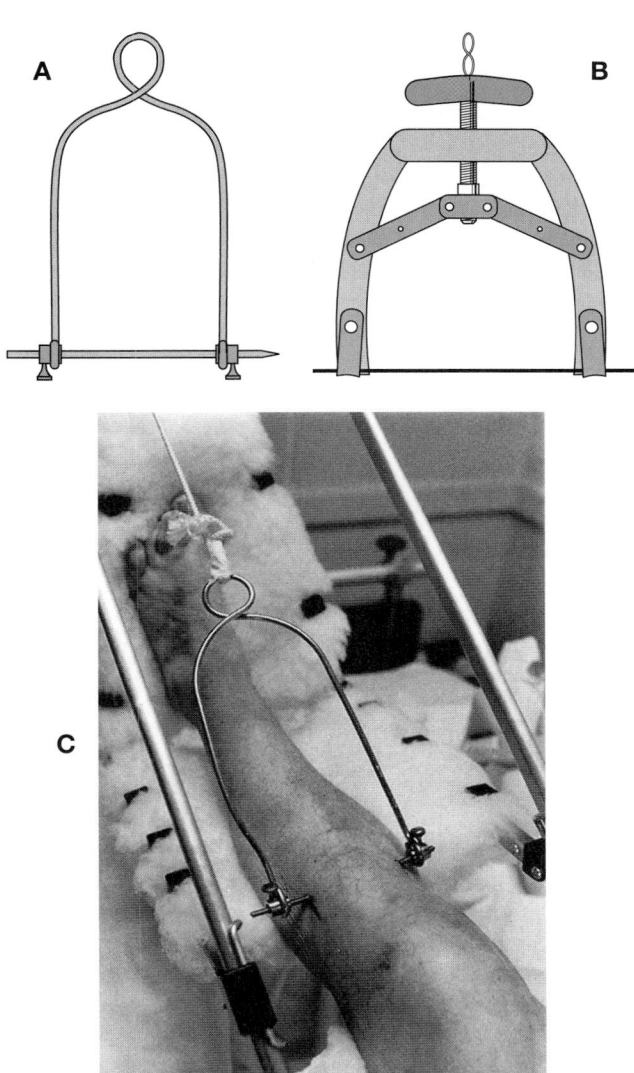

FIGURE **12-8 A,** Kirschner wire and tractor. **B,** Steinmann pin and holder. **C,** Steinmann pin placed in tibial plateau for treatment of distal femoral fracture. (**C** from Phipps W and others: *Medical-surgical nursing: concepts and clinical practice,* ed 6, St. Louis, 1995, Mosby.)

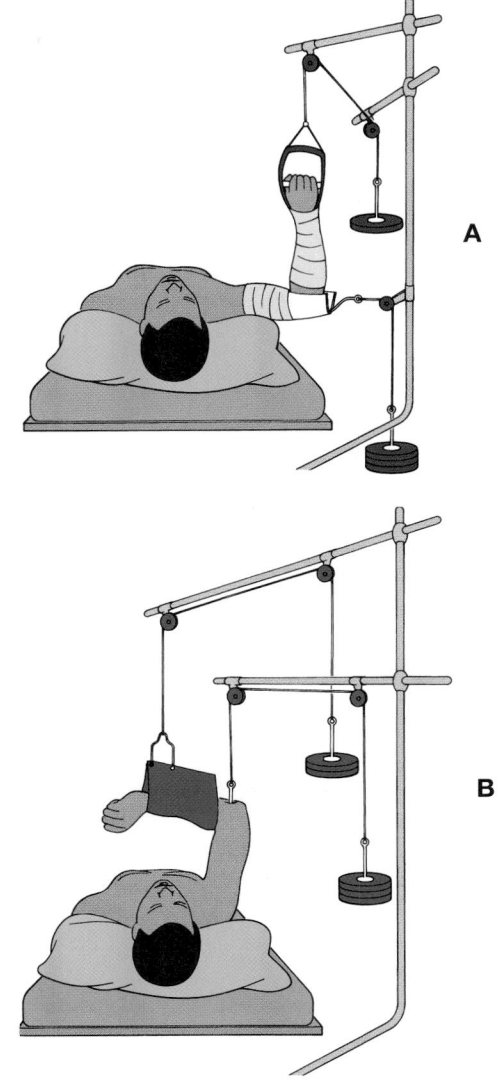

FIGURE **12-9 A,** Side-arm traction (skin/skeletal). **B,** Overhead 90-90 traction (skeletal). (From Beare PG, Myers JL: *Principles and practice of adult health nursing,* ed 3, St. Louis, 1998, Mosby.)

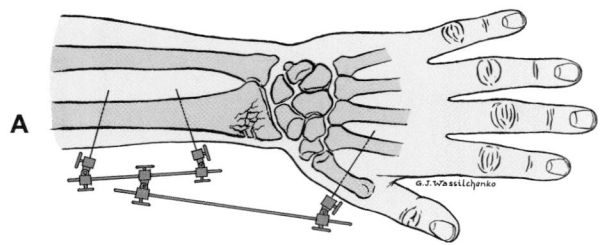

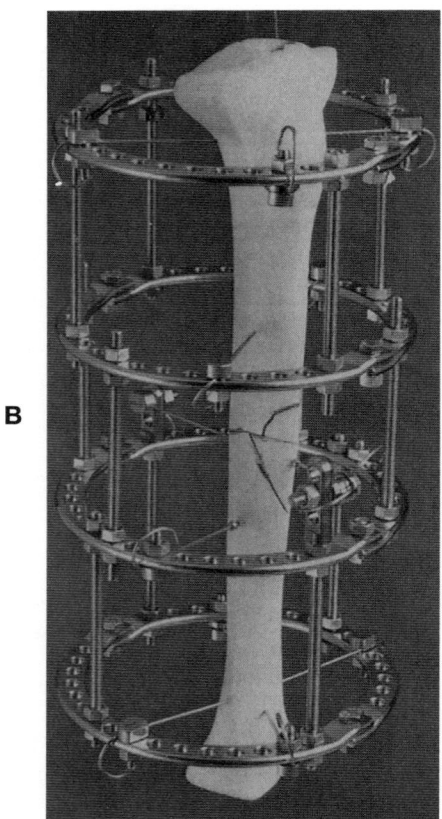

FIGURE **12-10** External fixators. **A,** Roger Anderson fixator. **B,** Ilizarhov fixator for treatment of comminuted fractures. (**B** from Phipps W and others: *Medical-surgical nursing: health and illness perspectives,* ed 7, St. Louis, 2003, Mosby).

3. *External fixation*—commonly used form of skeletal traction involving the use of one of a variety of frames to hold pins drilled into or through bones (Figures 12-10 and 12-11). External fixation is frequently used with

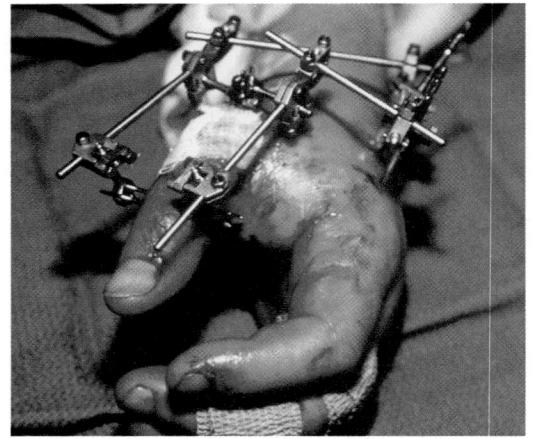

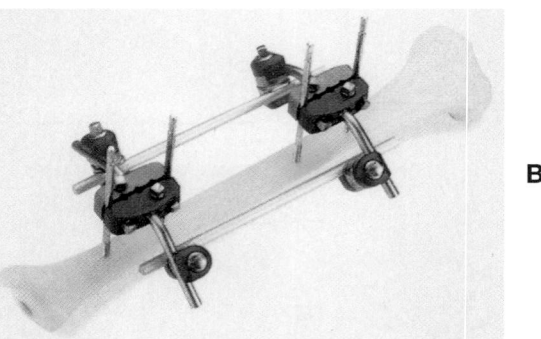

FIGURE **12-11** External fixators. **A,** Mini-Hoffman system in use on hand. **B,** Hoffman II on the tibia (standard system).

comminuted fractures having soft tissue injury. External fixation frames are used for skull and facial fractures, ribs, all bones of the upper and lower extremities, and pelvic bones. Frames may fit on one side of a bone or bones or may be attached to pins on either side of an injured limb.

4. *Skull tong traction*—traction involving the use of one of a variety of tongs (Crutchfield, Vinke, Gardner-Wells, or Barton) drilled into the skull or placed below the scalp and attached to ropes, pulleys, and weights (Figure 12-12). This type of traction is used for fractures of cervical vertebrae and involves the use of special beds or turning frames to facilitate nursing care. Halo traction is used for neurologically intact clients to prevent further spinal cord damage (Figure 12-13).

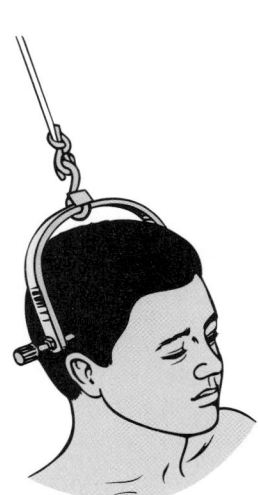

FIGURE **12-12** Gardner-Wells tongs for stabilization of cervical vertebral fractures.

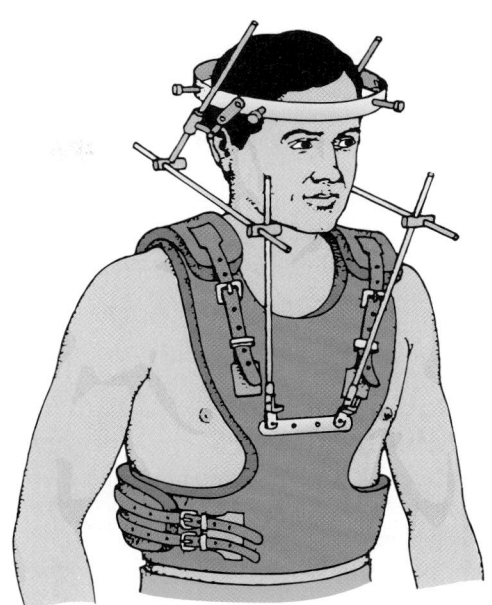

FIGURE **12-13** Halo vest. (From Beare PG, Meyers JL: *Principles and practice of adult health nursing*, ed 3, 1998, Mosby.)

DELEGATION CONSIDERATIONS

Assessment of the client's condition and status of traction should not be delegated to assistive personnel. However, the skills of assisting with insertion of skeletal pins and pin site care may be delegated to assistive personnel who are adequately trained in principles of surgical asepsis. Before delegating this skill the nurse must:

- Instruct assistive personnel to report any signs and symptoms associated with infection or inflammation at pin insertion site.

EQUIPMENT

- ❏ Sterile gloves for physician
- ❏ Wastebasket with plastic liner
- ❏ Antiseptic ointment
- ❏ Skin preparation solutions as desired

Balanced-Suspension Skeletal Traction

- ❏ Sterile tray for insertion of Kirschner wire or Steinmann pin (secure from operating suite)
- ❏ Local anesthetic of physician's choice, usually 1% to 2% lidocaine
- ❏ Thomas splint or Harris splint
- ❏ Pearson attachment
- ❏ Foot support
- ❏ Trapeze bar
- ❏ Ropes, pulleys, weights, weight holders
- ❏ Towels, felt, stockinette
- ❏ Drill and extension cord if needed
- ❏ Adhesive tape

Upper Extremity Skeletal Traction

- ❏ Sterile tray with Kirschner wire or Steinmann pin (secure from operating suite)
- ❏ Adhesive strips or moleskin
- ❏ Elastic bandages
- ❏ Handgrip bar
- ❏ Ropes, pulley, weights, and weight holders
- ❏ Low shock blocks (optional)
- ❏ Local anesthetic of physician's choice, usually 1% to 2% lidocaine

External Fixation

- ❏ External fixator, usually Hoffman or Roger Anderson apparatus, Vital fixator, AO fixator, Ilizarhov, or other fixator (see Figures 12-10 and 12-11)
- ❏ Sterile tray with pins for insertion (secure from operating room)

Skull Tong Traction

- ❏ Tongs: Crutchfield, Vinke, Gardner-Wells, Barton, or halo traction frame (see Figures 12-12 and 12-13)
- ❏ Sterile tray: Usually traction is applied in operating room
- ❏ Drill and extension cord if needed

Pin Care

- ❏ Sterile applicators
- ❏ Normal saline solution or hydrogen peroxide/normal saline solution in 1:1 solution or plain hydrogen peroxide
- ❏ Sterile containers
- ❏ Sterile gauze barrier (optional)
- ❏ Topical antibiotic ointment (optional)
- ❏ Clean gloves

STEP	RATIONALE

ASSESSMENT

1. Assess overall health condition of client, including mobility status.
2. Carefully assess specific tissues to be placed in skeletal traction. Note marked edema, rash, or other open lesions.
3. Assess client's knowledge of upcoming traction, application, and purposes.
4. Assess client's level of pain on a scale of 0 to 10.
5. Observe client's nonverbal behaviors and encourage questions.

Determines client's health state and ability to tolerate bed rest and skeletal traction.

Determines ability of tissues to tolerate traction. Skeletal pin goes through skin to bone and out through skin.

Determines willingness and ability to participate in care.

Used as baseline for later comparisons.

May reveal anxiety about impending procedure.

NURSING DIAGNOSES

- Bathing/hygiene, dressing/grooming, and toileting self-care deficit
- Risk for impaired skin integrity
- Risk for peripheral neurovascular dysfunction
- Risk for infection

- Impaired physical mobility
- Deficient knowledge regarding traction
- Acute pain
- Anxiety
- Risk for injury

Related factors are individualized based on client's condition or needs.

PLANNING

1. Expected outcomes following completion of procedure:
   - Client participates in bathing and feeding.

   - Client maintains bowel and bladder function.

   - Client's skin remains intact without redness, inflammation, or purulent drainage, especially over pressure points, proximal end of Thomas splint, and pin sites.
   - Client demonstrates adequate neurovascular functioning in extremity. Distal skin tissues remain warm and of a normal skin color with capillary refill of 3 seconds or less. Client verbalizes no abnormal sensations and is able to move fingers or toes below fracture site.
   - Client retains ROJM in unaffected extremities and verbalizes understanding of activity restrictions. Demonstrates use of trapeze.
   - Client describes purpose of skeletal traction and follows activity restrictions.
   - Client experiences reduced pain and muscle spasm and rates pain at less than or equal to 4 on a scale of 0 to 10.
   - Client does not become tense or withdrawn.
   - Client complies with restrictions imposed by traction apparatus.

Activities are performed safely, without injury. Client reduces risk of complications of immobility.

A fracture bedpan and/or urinal are used to facilitate elimination functions.

Indicates no development of pressure ulcers or infection. A small amount of clear drainage is expected from pin sites (Bernardo, 2001).

Adequate neurovascular functioning is essential to the health and well-being of the extremity (Altizer, 2001).

Routine exercise prevents contractures and muscle wasting.

Demonstrates learning and acceptance of restrictions.

Alignment of fracture reduces stress on bone fragments and adjoining muscle groups.

Demonstrates absence of anxiety.

No injury is sustained.

IMPLEMENTATION

1. Initial traction setup
   a. Position client according to physician's request. Nurse or other assistant may be asked to support tissues to be placed in traction. Client will most often be on back with head of bed slightly elevated. Client will be flat in bed for Dunlop's skeletal traction.

Ensures proper alignment during and after traction application.

STEP	RATIONALE
b. Physician performs skin preparation and discards materials in wastebasket.	Reduces possibility of wound and bone infection.
c. Physician injects local anesthetic into sites as desired. Nurse and other assistants support client, limb, or other tissues to be placed in traction. Burr holes may be drilled in the outer layer of the skull for placement of tongs.	Anesthetic acts quickly to create painless area. Client will feel pressure of pin being drilled through or into bones and will hear drill but should feel no pain.
d. Provide encouragement and praise during drilling of pin tracts.	Reduces client anxiety.
e. Assist (usually by holding spreader bar, splint, or Pearson attachment) while physician continues to use drill to insert number of pins or nails desired for traction. Support area of joints not at injury site. Do not move distal portion unnecessarily.	Movement can cause severe pain or additional trauma.
2. Prepare specific traction setups:	
a. Balanced-suspension skeletal traction (BSST)	
(1) *For lower extremity traction:* Assist with placement of Thomas or Harris splint, Pearson attachment, foot support, ropes, pulleys, and weights. Gently lower weights to establish traction. Apply antiseptic ointment to pin exit sites, and cover with sterile split dressing.	Splint and attachment are usually previously prepared for quick use. Foot plate prevents footdrop. Ointment and dressings are applied to cover open wounds to prevent infection.
(2) *For side-arm traction:* Assist with application of Buck's extension to forearm, place hand-grip, and establish skin traction by *slowly* lowering weights until rope is taut (see Figure 12-9, *A*).	Skin traction allows forearm to remain in vertical position without undue effort from client.
(3) *For 90-90 traction:* Assist with preparing sling for forearm (see Figure 12-9, *B*).	
(4) Assist with application of spreader to hold skeletal pin; tie rope to spreader and thread through pulleys to weight holder and weights. Slowly lower weights until rope is taut. Place shock blocks if requested. Apply antiseptic ointment to pin exit sites, and cover with sterile split dressing.	Amount of weight depends on severity of client's injury. Amounts vary from 5 to 10 lb or more. Shock blocks allow one side of bed to be raised to help client maintain desired position. Ointment and sterile split dressings are applied to prevent infection.
(5) Cover ends of pins (wires) with corks or tape.	Prevents injury to client or caregivers.
(6) Attach trapeze bar, and instruct in use.	Allows the client to assist in movement and to maintain upper body muscle tone.
b. External fixation	
(1) Hold affected tissues or limb while physician attaches and tightens fixator screws or clamps. Apply antiseptic ointment to pin exit sites, and cover with sterile split dressing.	Proper tension or tightness to pins is vital to prevent twist or torque, which would delay healing. Ointment and sterile split dressings are applied to prevent infection.
c. Skull tong traction	
(1) Client's cervical vertebrae are maintained in proper alignment with a Thomas cervical collar. Collar remains in place until skull tong traction is surgically placed. Traction is applied by weights ordered by physician.	Maintains proper cervical vertebrae alignment, thus reducing further injury and/or paralysis to the cervical segment of the spinal cord.
3. Assess client's initial reaction or response to traction before physician leaves.	Adjustments may be required immediately.
4. Raise side rails if appropriate.	Provides for client's safety.

STEP	RATIONALE
5. Gather equipment and supplies, and return to proper storage places. Perform hand hygiene.	Provides for safety and cleanliness and prevents transmission of infection.
6. Ensure that skeletal traction is maintained continuously	Prevents overriding of bones that could cause soft tissue damage and prevents misalignment (James and others, 2002).
7. Pin care (After traction procedure, nurse needs to discuss with physician whether pin care will be performed. Type and frequency of pin site care varies according to physician preference and institutional policy.)	Although there are commonalities in care, there are currently no accepted clinical standards for pin site care. Some institutions have policies outlining pin site care, and others permit pin site care only with a physician's orders. There is no research to support the effectiveness of pin site care in preventing infections (Bernardo, 2001).
a. Perform hand hygiene, and apply clean gloves.	Reduces transmission of infection. Use latex-free gloves if there is risk of an allergic reaction (Yip and Roman, 2003).
b. Remove old split gauze dressing around pins, and discard in receptacle. Note condition of tissues around pin site.	Evaluates ongoing condition of tissues. Can ensure early identification of infection.
c. Prepare supplies, and apply new gloves.	Aseptic technique reduces infection transmission.
d. Begin by cleaning pins on one side of extremity, then do same on other side. Never touch one pin site with material used on another.	Prevents cross contamination.
e. Dip sterile cotton-tipped applicator into sterile container of one half hydrogen peroxide and one half saline, maintaining sterile environment. Place applicator by the pin, and roll it along the skin, away from insertion site. Clean outward in a circular fashion from the pin. Dispose of applicator.	Remove crusts from pin site. Crusts can obstruct drainage, which leads to bacterial buildup. (Some institutions use only hydrogen peroxide or only saline). Although frequently used, small-sample-size studies indicate that hydrogen peroxide may not be an effective cleansing agent in preventing pin tract infection and may in fact damage healthy tissue (Bernardo, 2001).
f. Dip a new sterile applicator in normal saline; roll applicator across skin away from pin.	Removes cleansing solution to reduce skin irritation.
g. Using a sterile applicator, apply a small amount of topical antibiotic ointment to pin site, and cover with a sterile 2 × 2 split gauze dressing. (NOTE: some physicians leave site uncovered.)	Antiinfective reduces bacterial growth.
h. Repeat procedure for other pin site.	
8. Discard supplies. Remove and dispose of gloves. Perform hand hygiene.	Reduces transmission of infection.

EVALUATION

STEP	RATIONALE
1. Evaluate entire traction setup and functioning: a. Observe that knots are not caught in pulleys and that ropes are running straight through pulleys. b. Observe ropes for fraying. c. Evaluate that correct weight is hanging (do not add or remove weight without physician order) and dangling freely. d. Determine that linens are not interfering with traction apparatus. e. Observe client's body alignment.	Determines if traction is functioning as desired. Anything that inhibits the smooth movement of the traction rope in the pulley will disrupt the traction and may lead to nonunion. Poor body alignment may lead to discomfort and affect proper bone healing (Maher and others, 2002).
2. Determine client's response to traction; evaluate for presence of pain and muscle spasms on a scale of 0 to 10.	Skeletal traction takes longer for client to note relief of symptoms because of increased tissue trauma. Determines need for analgesics, muscle relaxants, and success of traction in stabilizing fracture.

STEP	RATIONALE
3. Inspect pin sites for drainage, tenderness, or inflammation.	Recognizes early signs of infection (Bernardo, 2001).
4. Assess for other indicators of infection, such as fever; elevated white blood count; continuous, dull, aching pain; redness; or warmth in extremity.	Recognizes early signs of osteomyelitis (James and others, 2002).
5. Perform neurovascular assessment (see Skill 12-1, Evaluation, step 2).	Determines peripheral perfusion to tissues, as well as client's sensation and voluntary motor activity (Altizer, 2001; Harvey 2001).
6. Assess for indicators of hypoxemia, such as restlessness or agitation.	Recognizes early signs of fat embolism syndrome (FES) (McCance and Huether, 2002).
7. Assess skin, especially around ankle, elbow, foot, or distal tibia, for fracture blisters. Do not rupture blister. Apply hydrocolloid dressing to ruptured blister.	Fracture blisters are associated with increased interstitial pressure from posttraumatic edema. Intact skin provides a barrier to prevent infection. Covering the blister with a dressing maintains a clean environment (Harvey, 2001).

Recording and Reporting

- Record in nurses' notes type of traction applied, persons applying traction, site to which traction was applied, time of application, amount of weights, and client's initial response.
- Record all findings of neurovascular assessment (see Skill 12-1, Evaluation, step 2) every 1 to 2 hours or as ordered.
- Document client teaching and verbalization of understanding.

Unexpected Outcomes	Related Interventions
1. Skeletal pin moves or slides in pin tract, leading to increased risk of infection or nonunion.	• Notify physician.
2. Client experiences delayed union, malunion, or nonunion.	• Ensure that proper amount of weight is continuously maintained. • Provide proper nutrition. • Notify physician of infection.
3. Client has severe edema, marked increase in pain, inability to actively move joints, or increased pain on passive movement, indicating compartment syndrome.	• Notify physician immediately.
4. Client develops infection at pin site or at fracture site with development of osteomyelitis.	• Maintain aseptic technique. • Notify physician. • Administer ordered antibiotics.
5. Client experiences prolonged bleeding or frank hemorrhage.	• Chronically ill or older clients may have preexistent iron deficiency anemia made worse by bleeding or hemorrhage. Replacement of blood loss may be required.

6. Client experiences nerve damage:
  ▪ Peroneal nerve: footdrop with inability to evert and dorsiflex foot
  ▪ Radial or median nerve at wrist with inability to approximate thumb and fingers (radial) and numbness and tingling of thumb, index, middle fingers (median) with wrist drop
	• Notify physician.
	
	• Notify physician.
	• Loosen elastic bandage at wrist for side-arm traction.
	• Reposition sling at wrist for overhead 90-90 traction.

Continued

Unexpected Outcomes	Related Interventions
7. Client experiences FES (more common in fractures of long bones) with symptoms of hypoxemia: restlessness, decreased level of orientation, disorientation, tachycardia, tachypnea, dyspnea, hypotension, and petechial rash over upper chest and neck.	• Maintain stability and immobilization of fracture to prevent FES. • Notify physician, and treat with oxygen.
8. Client experiences deep vein thrombosis with possible pulmonary embolus including clinical manifestations of dyspnea, chest pain, tachypnea, apprehension, tachycardia, cyanosis, and circulatory collapse.	• Teach client calf-pump exercises, maintain sequential compression devices or foot pumps, and give ordered anticoagulant as preventive measures. • Do not massage lower extremity. • Notify physician. If symptoms of pulmonary embolus are evident, elevate head of bed (if conscious), administer oxygen, and notify physician *immediately*.
9. Client experiences declining voluntary motor responses.	• Notify physician.

Teaching Considerations

- Before discharge, client is taught use of ambulatory aid (cane, walker, or crutches); written instructions are given to client and significant others.
- Client is provided written instructions for home care maintenance, especially if being discharged with external fixation (pin site care, elevate extremity when sitting or lying to prevent edema formation).
- Client is provided dietary instructions if necessary.
- Client is taught to notify physician of undesirable signs, including increase in pain, muscle spasms, increased numbness or tingling, appearance of drainage, redness, or soreness at operative or traction pin sites.

Pediatric Considerations

- External fixator devices are becoming more widely used and are eliminating some of the traction that has been used in the past. The external fixators allow earlier mobility and earlier release from the hospital. Families must be taught proper care of the devices and must be prepared for the reactions of others regarding the devices (Hockenberry and others, 2003).
- Blood loss from a fracture can become critical more quickly in the child than the adult because blood volume is 60% of total body weight in the adult and 70% to 85% in the child (Hockenberry and others, 2003).
- Bone remodeling is at its maximum rate at approximately 2½ years of age (McCance and Huether, 2002).
- Parents are taught that babies may cry when traction is established.

- Children may experience boredom, regression, and interference with schoolwork. Parents and other caregivers must look for ways to divert the child's attention and support the child. Schoolwork should be obtained from school and the child assisted when able to perform tasks. Parents are counseled regarding regression to decrease their anxiety.
- Physical activity is essential for growth and development in the child. Immobility may result in increased anxiety. Behaviors that may be demonstrated are restlessness, depression, regression, lack of concentration, dependence, acting out, and outbursts of crying or temper tantrums (Hockenberry and others, 2003).
- Children should be assured that someone will always be available to assist them while they are in traction (Miller, 2004).

Gerontological Considerations

- Older adult clients may suffer from diabetes or peripheral vascular disease, adding risks to use of traction.
- An overhead trapeze may assist the older client in maintaining upper body strength and in facilitating hygiene and repositioning.

Home Care Considerations

- After traction is discontinued, client is taught to dangle before ambulation, to proceed slowly with ambulation, and to gradually increase the time and distance ambulated.
- Client is provided instructions regarding use of muscle relaxants and analgesics if prescribed.

SKILL 12-5 Care of the Client With Immobilization Devices

Immobilization devices increase stability, support a weak extremity, or reduce the load on weight-bearing structures such as hips, knees, or ankles. A splint immobilizes and protects a body part. Temporary splints reduce pain and prevent tissue damage from further motion immediately after an injury such as a fracture or sprain. Air splints, Thomas splints, and improvised splints from material on hand are examples of temporary splints applied in emergency situations. Upper extremity fractures are sometimes managed using splints such as hand and digital splints or sugar-tong splints.

Slings are used to support splints, casts, or injured upper extremities (Figure 12-14). They are commercially available or can be made. They are available for almost any body part. Velcro or buckle closures permit these devices to be adjusted to fit a body part of almost any size and shape.

The abduction splint, used after hip replacement surgery, maintains the client's legs in an abducted position. This permits the client to be turned without changing the healing limb's position and prevents dislocation of the hip prosthesis. The device is easily removed for skin care, dressing changes, or neurovascular assessments. A posterior splint with elastic wraps is sometimes used to support an extremity.

Cloth and foam splints, known as immobilizers, provide long-term immobilization (Figure 12-15). Immobilizers treat sprains and dislocations that do not require complete and continuous immobilization in a cast or traction. Immobilizers are often used following orthopedic surgery. Other common types of immobilizers include cervical collars (soft or hard), belt-type shoulder immobilizers, and vinyl wrist forearm splints. Molded splints, made of plastic, provide support to clients with chronic injuries or diseases such as arthritis. They maintain the body part in a functional position to prevent contractures and muscle atrophy during the period of disuse. A splint goes into place and removes quickly and easily when assessing skin or a wound.

Braces support weakened structures during weight bearing or to prevent postural deformity. For this reason, they are made of sturdy materials such as leather, metal, and molded plastic. Chest and abdominal braces, such as the Milwaukee and Boston braces, immobilize the thoracic and lumbar vertebral column to treat scoliosis (curvature of the spine). The brace does not correct the curve but instead prevents its progression. Lumbar braces support lumbar and sacral tissues after spinal surgery or fusion. Leg braces hold the thigh, leg, and foot in functional positions for weight bearing and ambulation (Figure 12-16). Both short leg and long leg braces support weak leg muscles, aid in control of involuntary muscle movement, or maintain surgical correction during the postoperative healing process. They are commonly used for clients with cerebral palsy, muscular dystrophy, multiple sclerosis, and fractures and after polio (Bakker and others, 2000).

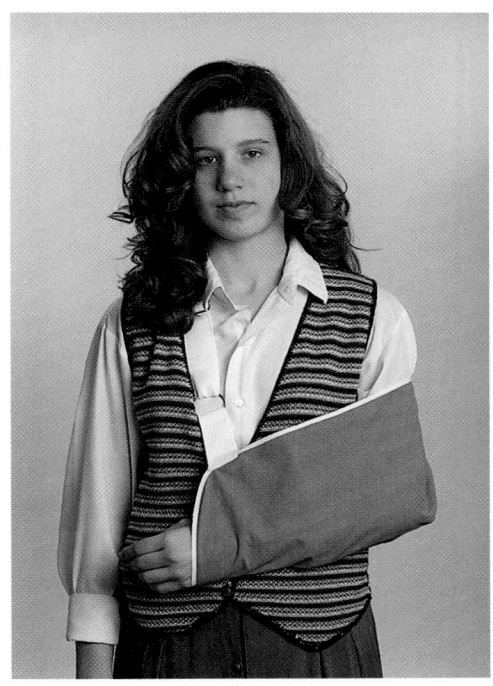

FIGURE **12-14** Sling for shoulder/arm immobilization. (From Beare PG, Meyers JL: *Principles and practice of adult health nursing*, ed 3, 1998, Mosby.)

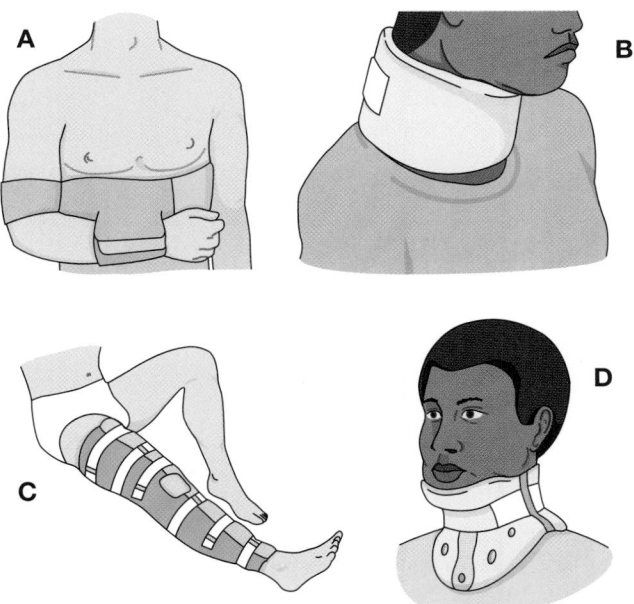

FIGURE **12-15** Examples of immobilizers. **A,** Shoulder immobilizer. **B,** Soft cervical collar. **C,** Knee immobilizer. **D,** Hard cervical collar. (From Beare PG, Meyers JL: *Principles and practice of adult health nursing,* ed 3, 1998, Mosby.)

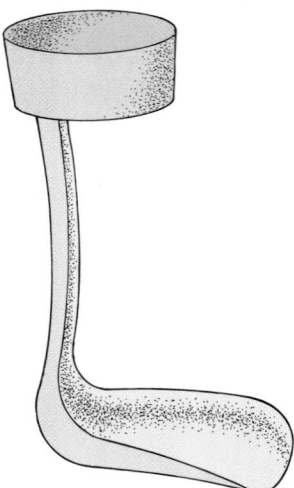

FIGURE **12-16** Ankle-foot orthosis (AFO). (From Phipps W and others: *Medical-surgical nursing: health and illness perspectives*, ed 7, St. Louis, 2003, Mosby).

DELEGATION CONSIDERATIONS

Assessment of the client's condition should not be delegated to assistive personnel. However, the skill of caring for the client wearing a brace, splint, or sling may be delegated to assistive personnel. Before delegating this skill to assistive personnel or family members the nurse must:

- Review the purpose of the brace/splint/sling as it applies to the client
- Review correct application of the brace/splint/sling and positioning of any ties or straps
- Review prescribed schedule of wear and activities permitted while in the brace/splint/sling
- Instruct assistive personnel to alert the nurse if client complains of pain, rubbing, or pressure from the brace/splint/sling or if a change occurs in client's skin condition

Equipment

❏ Brace/splint/commercially prepared sling or triangular bandage and safety pin
❏ Cotton shirt or gown

STEP	RATIONALE

ASSESSMENT

1. Review client's chart, including medical history, previous and current activity level, and description of the condition requiring immobilization.

   Reveals client's current and previous health status and purpose for the brace/splint/sling.

2. Assess client's previous experience with braces/splints/slings.

   Reveals client's baseline knowledge.

3. Assess client's understanding of reason for brace/splint/sling, care of, application of, and schedule of wear.

4. Assess client's risk for skin breakdown because of brace/splint/sling or immobilization. Look at area of skin to be in contact with support device.

   Immobile and older clients are particularly vulnerable (Miller, 2004).

5. Refer to occupational or physical therapy consult to determine type of brace to be used, desired position, and amount of activity and movement permitted.

STEP	**RATIONALE**
6. Assess client's additional need for an assistive device such as a cane, walker, or crutches.	An assistive device may be needed to provide support and promote balance during ambulation.

NURSING DIAGNOSES

- Bathing/hygiene and dressing/grooming deficit
- Risk for impaired skin integrity
- Risk for injury
- Risk for ineffective peripheral tissue perfusion
- Impaired physical mobility

- Impaired home maintenance
- Deficient knowledge regarding immobilization device
- Risk for peripheral neurovascular dysfunction
- Disturbed body image

Related factors are individualized based on client's condition or needs.

PLANNING

1. Expected outcomes following completion of procedure:	
• Client's skin remains in good condition without circulatory impairment.	Indicates no friction or pressure from device that can lead to skin breakdown or circulatory impairment.
• Client/significant other verbalizes purpose, correct application, and care of the device.	Encourages cooperation and minimizes risks and anxiety of procedure.
• Client rates pain at 2 or less (scale 0 to 10).	Indicates proper fit of device and permits safer ambulation.
• Circulation and sensation distal to brace/splint is maintained.	Reveals there are no changes in neurovascular status following application (Altizer, 2001).
• Client uses the device correctly, including schedule of wear, activity limitations, and positioning.	Demonstrates that proper immobilization promotes healing and safe ambulation without injury.
• Client demonstrates adjustment to changes in physical appearance or function	Reveals that client is confident in abilities and willing to try different strategies to enhance appearance (James and others, 2002).

IMPLEMENTATION

APPLYING SPLINT/BRACE/SLING

1. Perform hand hygiene.	Reduces transmission of microorganisms.
2. Explain reasons for the brace/splint/sling, and demonstrate how the device works.	Teaching and demonstration enhance learning, reduce anxiety, and encourage cooperation.
3. Assist the client to a comfortable position, preferably sitting or lying down.	Client's position will depend on the type of brace/splint/sling being used. Upper-extremity braces/splints/slings are applied best with the client sitting upright. Lower-extremity braces are applied best with the client lying down.
4. Prepare the skin that will be enclosed in the brace/splint/sling by cleaning the skin with soap and water; rinse, pat dry, and change any dressings (if present). If applying a back brace, put a thin cotton shirt or gown on the client. Ensure that there are no wrinkles causing pressure.	This protects the skin, absorbs moisture, and keeps the brace/splint/sling clean (Ball and Bindler, 2003).

- *Critical Decision Point*

   Instruct the client to inform the health care provider if there is a feeling of pressure, pain, numbness, rubbing, or if the skin becomes reddened.

5. Inspect the device for wear, damage, or rough edges.	Potential for skin breakdown is decreased, and correct alignment is maintained.

STEP	RATIONALE

6. Apply the brace/splint/sling as directed by physician, orthotist, physical therapist, or occupational therapist. If securing splint with elastic bandage:
  a. Apply even tension as bandage for splint is wrapped from distal to proximal.
  b. Prevent padding from gathering or bunching.
7. If applying sling using triangular bandage:
  a. Position one end of the bandage over the shoulder of the unaffected arm.
  b. Take the remaining bandage, and place the material against the chest, then under and over the affected arm, cradling the arm.
  c. Position the pointed end of the triangle toward the elbow.
  d. Tie the two ends of the triangle at the side of the neck.
  e. Fold the pointed end of the sling at the elbow in the front, and secure with a safety pin, closing the end of the sling.
  f. Adjust the length of the sling by adjusting the amount of material in the knot.
  g. Ensure the sling supports the limb comfortably without interfering with circulation.
8. Teach the client the prescribed schedule of wear and allowed activities while in the brace/splint/sling as directed by physician, physical therapist, or occupational therapist.
9. Reinforce the signs of skin breakdown, pressure, or rubbing to report.
 	
10. Assist the client with finding attractive clothes to fit over immobilizing device.
11. Teach the client how to care for the brace/splint/sling.
 	
  a. When not in use, store brace/splint in a safe but easily accessible location.
  b. Keep the brace clean, dry, and in good working order.
 	
12. Assist client with ambulating with brace/splint/sling in place.
	Proper application of the brace/splint/sling is important to avoid skin breakdown, pressure ulcers, neurovascular compromise, calluses, or worsening of the deformity.
	Prevents trapping of blood distal to immobilization device.
	
	This position cradles the arm.
	
	This prevents skin irritation to the back of the neck.
	
	This prevents pressure on the radial artery, which can impair circulation.
	Proper use of the brace/splint/sling will facilitate healing and mobility and reduce pain and stress.
	
	Brace/splint/sling may need to be adjusted. Changes may also be required because of growth or atrophy, when muscles regain or lose strength, or after reconstructive surgery. Particular attention should be given to insensitive areas of the body (Ball and Bindler, 2003).
	Improves body image and decreases feeling of alienation.
	
	Metal braces should be stored upright. Splints of molded materials should be stored away from heat. Leather materials should be treated with a leather preservative to prevent drying or cracking. Most slings can be gently washed to remove any soiling (Ball and Bindler, 2003).
	
	Plastic parts are cleaned with a damp cloth and thoroughly dried. Metal joints are cleaned with a pipe cleaner and oiled weekly. Remove rust with steel wool, and clean metal parts with a solvent.
	This will determine if client is able to ambulate safely.

- ***Critical Decision Point***
  Let the client know that although the brace/splint may seem awkward at first, after practice, the client will feel more comfortable and better able to move about. In addition, let the client know that assistance may be needed to apply and remove the brace/splint.

STEP	RATIONALE
13. Have the client apply and remove the brace/splint. Client may need assistance with application and removal of sling.	Promotes client independence; demonstration confirms level of learning skill.

EVALUATION

1. Inspect areas of the skin underneath the brace/splint/sling for signs of pressure, including redness or breakdown.	Ensures early identification of irritation or breakdown.
2. Observe the client using the brace/splint/sling.	Client may refrain from activity unnecessarily or may try to do too much.
3. Ask the client to rate level of comfort while the brace/splint/sling is in place.	Indicates proper fit of device and permits safer ambulation.
4. Palpate pulse and test sensation of extremity distal to position of brace/splint/sling.	Neurovascular status reflects vascular supply or pressure on tissues.
5. Ask the client/family the ease with which ADLs are performed while wearing the brace/splint/sling.	Determines if alternative self-care approaches necessary
6. Client states confidence in academic, physical, and social abilities related to wearing immobilizing device and is willing to try different strategies to enhance appearance.	Reveals confidence in ability and willingness to try different strategies to enhance appearance.

Recording and Reporting

- Document type of brace/splint/sling applied, schedule of wear, activity level and movement permitted, and client's tolerance of procedure in progress notes.
- Record specific assessments related to skin integrity and neurovascular status.
- Document instructions given to client and family.
- Record observations regarding client's ability to apply, ambulate with, and remove the brace/splint/sling.
- Immediately report any injury sustained while using the brace/splint/sling.

Unexpected Outcomes	Related Interventions
1. Client is unable to use the brace/splint/sling correctly	• Reassess client for correct fit. • Reassess level of comfort. • Reassess muscle strength in uninvolved extremities. • Obtain referral for physical or occupational therapy.
2. Client develops areas of pressure, redness, or skin breakdown.	• Assess device for proper fit and positioning. • Inspect brace/splint/sling for damage, wear, or rough edges. • Inform the physician. • Inform the orthotist, physical therapist, or occupational therapist so that adjustments to brace/splint can be made. • Do not allow the client to use the brace/splint until adjustments are made. • If necessary, *temporarily* pad the area of incorrect fit rather than the reddened or irritated area.
3. Circulation to the affected extremity is altered because of improper fit.	• Remove the device immediately. • Notify physician.

Teaching Considerations

- Teach parents to apply and maintain the brace/splint/sling.
- Place cotton T-shirt under upper extremity brace and long, cotton tube socks under lower extremity brace.
- Avoid lotions or powders that may irritate skin.
- Teach family exercises to perform when child is out of brace (e.g., Boston brace).
- Teach client appropriate ROM exercises within limitation of device.
- Advise client and caregiver of signs and symptoms of impaired skin integrity to report.

Pediatric Considerations

- Recognize that bracing in an adolescent often affects body image and self-esteem.
- Encourage adolescent to engage in conversation that focuses on body perception and to discuss experiences with peers (James and others, 2002).

Geriatric Considerations

- With aging there is decreased rate of epidermal proliferation, decreased skin moisture, thinner dermis, and decreased dermal blood supply (Miller, 2004).

- The older client experiences diminished muscle mass, degenerative connective tissue changes, and progressive decline in bone mass (Maas and others, 2001).
- Older clients may have limited mobility as a result of postural deviations such as increased kyphosis and decreased lordosis (Maas and others, 2001).

Home Care Considerations

- Recognize that prolonged immobility in a brace/splint may cause decreased ROM or contractures.
- Assess the ability and willingness of the client and primary caregiver regarding care required for the brace/splint.
- Remove the brace/splint when bathing or showering.
- Assess for environmental factors in the home that may interfere with safe ambulation.
- Inspect and clean braces/splints weekly.
- Assist clients with adapting clothing so that an acceptable appearance can be maintained.
- Assist client or parents with developing plan to manage ADLs while braced. If child, base plan on developmental skills and abilities.
- Enlist occupational therapy in helping client develop the highest quality of life possible.

FOCUS on CLINICAL PRACTICE

Scott, age 25, suffered multiple injuries in a motor vehicle accident (MVA) 12 hours earlier. He is admitted to the orthopedic unit, where you are assigned as his primary nurse. He sustained a simple fracture of the right tibia/fibula (tib/fib). He has a plaster of Paris cast placed on his right lower leg. In addition, he has a compound fracture of the left femur immobilized in skeletal traction with a Steinmann pin through the femur.

1. The plaster of Paris cast is still wet. The nurse must position the right leg to assist with drying of the cast. Which intervention would the nurse perform until the cast is fully dry?
   A. Cover it with plastic wrap until it is dry.
   B. Move it carefully with her fingertips.
   C. Put a foot cradle over it, and cover it with blankets.
   D. Handle it carefully with the palms of her hands.
2. As the afternoon progresses, Scott begins to complain of increasing pain in his right leg and foot. He was medicated with morphine sulfate 1 hour ago, and yet he states he has received no pain relief. You suspect he is developing compartment syndrome. What additional assessment data do you expect to collect that would support this finding?

   A. Warm skin distal to the cast
   B. Capillary refill of 2 seconds
   C. Two-point discrimination of the skin distal to the cast
   D. Numbness and tingling in the affected foot
3. The leg has been elevated above heart level and ice packs applied to the sides of the cast. The pain continues unabated with cold, pale toes evident upon inspection. After consulting with the physician, it is decided that it is necessary to bivalve the cast. The physician will:
   A. Cut in a window shape in the middle to allow visualization of the skin
   B. Cut in two lengthwise to relieve pressure
   C. Partially cut at distal and proximal ends to allow visualization of skin
   D. Partially cut at one end to relieve pressure
4. The swelling goes down, and the cast is reapplied to Scott's right leg. The nursing care plan for Scott also includes assessing for possible infection at the Steinmann pin site of the skeletal traction. Which of the following cues is least likely to indicate infection?
   A. Crusting
   B. Edema
   C. Erythema
   D. Purulent drainage

FOCUS *on* CLINICAL PRACTICE

5. To ensure that Scott's traction is working properly, which of the following principles should you follow? Check all that may apply.
   A. Ensure that the foot plate of the traction gently rests against the foot of the bed.
   B. Prevent swaying of weights when delivering care to Scott.

   C. Pulleys should be used only if Scott is allowed to move up in bed.
   D. Pulleys should not be obstructed by knots.
   E. Maintain body alignment of Scott.

NCLEX REVIEW QUESTIONS

1. How frequently would the nursing care plan call for neurovascular assessments during the first 24 hours following fracture?
   1. Every 15 to 30 minutes
   2. Every 1 to 2 hours
   3. Every 4 hours
   4. Every 12 hours
2. Nursing care for managing the client in skeletal traction includes:
   1. Explaining the purpose of the traction to the client
   2. Releasing the skeletal traction once per shift
   3. Removing the pins on the third day to prevent infection
   4. Teaching the family how to lift the weights and when changing client position.
3. When the client complains of severe itching under his cast, the nurse instructs him:
   1. "Go ahead and scratch if you are able to reach your fingers down the cast."
   2. "Itching is part of the healing process and should not be interfered with."
   3. "I'll get you a tongue blade to scratch with. Don't use your fingernails."
   4. "Scratching can cause skin breaks and infection. I'll get you some medication for the itching."
4. When caring for a client in balanced skeletal traction, the nurse will:
   1. Elevate the head of the bed 10 degrees once a day to prevent hypostatic pneumonia
   2. Eliminate the pillow under the affected part, if the client lies perfectly still

3. Teach the client how to use the trapeze bar
4. Remove some of the weights if the client complains of pain
5. While planning care of a young man's left leg with a cast, the nurse considers that the most effective way to control swelling of the fractured extremity is:
   1. Elevation and ice
   2. Heating pad and massage
   3. Massage and ice
   4. Medications and aquapad
6. When should the nurse assess a client's foot in Buck's skin traction boot?
   1. Fifteen minutes following application of the skin traction
   2. Once per shift
   3. Only when the client complains of pain
   4. Whenever the weights are adjusted
7. After removal of a cast, the client needs to be instructed to do which of the following? Check all that apply.
   1. Inspect the underlying tissues for redness or drainage
   2. Apply emollient lotion to soften the skin
   3. Begin full activities and exercise
   4. Use friction to remove dead skin by rubbing the area with a towel
8. Which of the following is the client **least likely** to complain about if there is a neurovascular deficit from too tight a splint?
   1. Pain
   2. Pressure
   3. Paraplegia
   4. Paresthesias

NCLEX REVIEW QUESTIONS

9. A 75-year-old widow is immediately placed in skin traction upon admission to the emergency department for fracture of her left hip. Which of the following are reasons the nurse should explain for the traction? Check all that apply.
   1. To decrease muscle spasms in the leg
   2. To prevent pain
   3. To improve bone healing
   4. To provide immobilization

10. The client is discharged with a large external fixator on the left leg. Your teaching plan includes which important safety guideline?
   1. Carefully clean the metal rods of the fixator daily to prevent rusting.
   2. Keep the affected leg in the dependent position.
   3. Report purulent pin site drainage to the doctor.
   4. Tighten the bolts daily.

11. The nurse suspects that the client might be developing clinical manifestations of neurovascular deficit following application of Buck's skin traction. Which of the following neurovascular assessments is the **most** significant?
   1. Capillary refill of 3 seconds in the affected foot
   2. Diminished posterior tibial pulse of the affected foot
   3. Numbness and tingling in the affected foot
   4. Pain on passive motion of the affected foot

12. Identify the appropriate interventions to teach a young girl regarding wearing a brace to prevent further progression of her scoliosis curve. Check all that apply.
   1. Wear a cotton T-shirt over the brace.
   2. Remove the brace during the day.
   3. Keep the brace clean, dry, and in good working order.
   4. Inspect the skin under the brace daily for reddened areas.

References

Altizer L: Neurovascular assessment, *Orthop Nurs* 21(4):48, 2001.

Andrews M, Boyle J: *Transcultural concepts in nursing care,* Philadelphia, 2003, Lippincott.

Ball JW, Bindler RC: *Pediatric nursing: caring for children,* ed 3, Upper Saddle River, NJ, 2003, Prentice Hall.

Ebersole P, Hess P: *Geriatric nursing and healthy aging,* St. Louis, 2001, Mosby.

Folcik M and others: *Traction: assessment and management,* St. Louis, 1994, Mosby.

Harvey C: Compartment syndrome: when it is least expected, *Orthop Nurs* 20(3):15, 2001.

Hockenberry MJ and others: *Wong's nursing care of infants and children,* ed 7, St. Louis, 2003, Mosby.

James SR and others: *Nursing care of children: principles and practice,* ed 2, Philadelphia, 2002, Saunders.

Lehne RA: *Pharmacology for nursing care,* ed 3, Philadelphia, 2001, Saunders.

Maas ML and others: *Nursing care of older adults: diagnoses, outcomes and interventions,* St. Louis, 2001, Mosby.

Maher AB and others: *Orthopaedic nursing,* ed 3, Philadelphia, 2002, Saunders.

Mashaba G: South African culturally-based health-illness patterns and humanistic care patterns. In Leininger M, McFarland M: *Transcultural nursing,* New York, 2002, McGraw Hill.

McCance KL, Huether SE: *Pathophysiology: the biologic basis for disease in adults and children,* ed 4, St. Louis, 2002, Mosby.

McConnell EA: Assessing neurovascular status in a casted limb, *Nursing* 32(9):20, 2002.

Miller CA: *Nursing for wellness in older adults: theory and practice,* ed 4, Philadelphia, 2004, Lippincott Williams & Wilkins.

Miller JA: Caring for Cambodian refugees in the emergency department, *J Emerg Nurs* 21(6):498, 1995.

Spector R: *Cultural diversity in health and illness,* Upper Saddle River, NJ, 2000, Prentice Hall.

Yip E, Roman M: Latex protein allergy and your choice of gloves: a balanced consideration, *Medsurg Nursing* 12(1):20, 2003.

Research References

Bakker JPJ and others: The effects of knee-ankle-foot orthoses in the treatment of Duchenne muscular dystrophy: review of the literature, *Clin Rehabil* 14(4):343, 2000.

Bernardo LS: Evidence-based practice for pin site care in injured children, *Orthop Nurs* 18(5):29, 2001.

DeJong ES and others: Antimicrobial efficacy of external fixator pins coated with lipid stabilized hydroxyapatite/chlorhexidine complex to prevent pin tract infection in a goat model, *J Trauma* 50(6):1008, 2001.

Gordon JE and others: Pin site care during external fixation in children: results of a nihilistic approach, *J Pediatr Orthop* 20(2):63, 2000.

Grossman S, Bautista C: Collaboration yields cost-effective, evidence-based nursing protocols, *Orthop Nurs* 21(3):30, 2002.

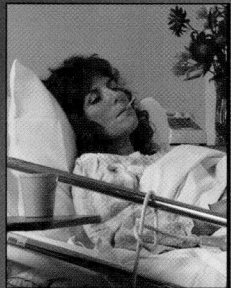

13

Support Surfaces and Special Beds

MEDIA RESOURCES

Evolve Site *evolve*

http://evolve.elsevier.com/Perry/skills

• Weblinks

OBJECTIVES

Mastery of content in this chaper will enable the nurse to:

- Identify the different types of support surfaces and specialty beds used for pressure relief.
- Explain why preventive nursing care is still essential when using support surfaces and special beds.
- Describe guidelines to follow when placing clients on support surfaces and special beds.
- Compare and contrast differences between mattress overlays and mattress replacements.
- Describe mechanisms by which skin breakdown can occur on either an air-suspension or an air-fluidized bed, a bariatric bed, a Rotokinetic bed, or a support surface mattress.
- Describe correct placement of a client on an air-fluidized bed, an air-suspension bed, a bariatric bed, a Rotokinetic bed, or a support surface mattress.

KEY TERMS

Air-fluidized bed	Kinesthetic
Air-suspension bed	Pressure ulcers
Bariatric bed	Rotokinetic bed
Flotation pad	Shearing
Friction	Weight holder
Immobility	

Despite the increasing technological advances in the world of medicine, pressure ulcers remain a major health care problem that increases client suffering, length of stay in a hospital or long-term care facility, and health care costs. Although a multidisciplinary team approach is key to reducing pressure ulcers, all agree that nurses are at the forefront of prevention and treatment of pressure ulcers in health care settings (Cullum and others, 2003; Wound Ostomy Continence Nurses Society [WOCN], 2003). Pressure ulcers are defined by the National Pressure Ulcer Advisory Panel (NPUAP) (1992) as localized areas of tissue necrosis that develop when soft tissue is compressed between a bony prominence and an external surface for a prolonged period of time. These lesions are caused by unrelieved pressure against soft tissue, usually over some bony prominence. Pressure ulcers can occur among those in any age-group or ethnic population, regardless of socioeconomic status. The occurrence of pressure ulcers is a serious and expensive health care problem in the United States, where an estimated 3% to 10% of the population in both hospital and community health care settings acquire some pressure damage. The cost to treat pressure ulcers in the United States exceeds $1 billion annually (NPUAP, 2001).

The pressure ulcer objective in *Healthy People 2010* is to reduce the prevalence of pressure ulcer diagnosis in nursing home residents from the current 0.16% to 0.08% (NPUAP, 2004). To meet this challenge, along with the challenges of health care reform to improve quality while reducing costs, it is essential for the nurse to identify clients at risk for breakdown. Factors that contribute to pressure ulcer formation are both extrinsic (e.g., moisture, friction, and shear) and intrinsic (e.g., malnutrition, loss of sensation, impaired mobility, aging skin, impaired mental status, infection, incontinence, and low arteriolar pressure).

Nurses have always been responsible for caring for persons with pressure ulcers. New knowledge and technology, including special beds and mattresses, and vigorous systematic assessment provide ways to prevent ulcers (Fulmer and Abraham, 1998). Clients at high risk of pressure ulcer development (see Chapter 15) should never be placed on ordinary foam mattresses. However, a number of support surfaces and specialty beds have been shown to reduce pressure ulcer incidence in high-risk clients (e.g., older adults, spinal cord injured, clients with burns) (Cullum and others, 2003).

The major cause of pressure ulcers is unrelieved pressure. The greater the pressure and the longer the pressure is applied, the greater the likelihood that a pressure ulcer will develop. To stay healthy, body tissues require an adequate supply of oxygen and nutrients and removal of carbon dioxide and other waste products of metabolism. This requires maintenance of adequate blood flow through the capillaries, which is normally considered to be 12 to 32 mm Hg (Pieper, 2000). When external pressure on the tissues exceeds 32 mm Hg (the capillary closing pressure), the network of capillaries collapses, and the supply of oxygen and nutrients to the cells, as well as removal of metabolic waste products, is interrupted. As a result, there is tissue ischemia and, if unrelieved, tissue death or necrosis (Monahan and Neighbors, 1998).

When a client is confined to a bed, the tissues between the skeleton and supporting bed surface become compressed, and the blood vessels within the tissues become occluded. A client lying supine on a hospital bed may exert as much as 150 mm Hg pressure (2.9 psi) on skin and soft tissue. Once pressure reaches more than 78 mm Hg for a period of time, a person usually feels discomfort and changes position. However, the client with altered sensation or one who cannot move independently is at risk for pressure ulcers of superficial and deep tissues unless pressure is significantly reduced. A classic study determined that pressures in excess of 20 to 40 mm Hg for prolonged periods cause tissue injury (Koziak, 1961). The principle behind pressure-relief strategy is dispersing the load to relieve pressure at regular intervals. At-risk clients left sitting in chairs can develop deeper and more serious pressure sores than those left in a bed because a greater pressure is being exerted on a smaller surface area, the buttocks. A client lying in bed has the pressure distributed over a greater surface area but is also at risk for developing pressure ulcers over bony prominences because they receive greater pressure than other parts of the body.

A cornerstone to the reduction of capillary tissue pressure and risk of pressure ulcers is the use of support surfaces. These products reduce this pressure over the bony prominences by maximizing contact and redistributing weight over a large area (Pieper, 2000). However, the use of support surfaces is one intervention to reduce pressure, and should be used in conjunction with other pressure ulcer risk reduction strategies (see Chapter 15).

Support surfaces have differing purposes, including pressure reduction, pressure relief, repositioning, and support of the morbidly obese client. They are used in acute, rehabilitative, long-term, and home care settings. It is important to understand the difference between a pressure-reducing and a pressure-relieving support surface. The former reduces the interface pressure between the body and support surface below 32 mm Hg. Pressure-reducing devices reduce the interface pressure, but not necessarily below capillary closing pressure (Agency for Health Care Policy and Research [AHCPR], 1994). Pressure-reducing surfaces (e.g., fiber-filled and foam overlays, gel or water support systems, air-filled mattresses, low-air-loss and air-fluidized supports) increase the area of the body in contact with the surface, thereby spreading the load and reducing

the effects of pressure. Pressure-relieving systems move under the client and reduce the amount of pressure being applied to any one area at regular intervals. Pressure-relieving devices consistently maintain external skin pressure at or below 32 mm Hg capillary closing pressure, whereas a pressure-reducing device maintains external skin pressures at a lower level than standard hospital mattresses (Fletcher, 1997). An example of a pressure-relieving system is an alternating system, in which air is pumped into an overlay or mattress by a motor.

Several support surfaces reduce friction, shear, and moisture (Table 13-1). Mattresses or beds with a slick surface help decrease friction and shear. Surfaces with porous covers allow airflow, which reduces moisture, resulting in decreased risk for skin maceration.

Frequent repositioning, which temporarily relieves pressure, is the backbone of preventive protocols. No bed or mattress totally eliminates the need for competent nursing care. Although useful, turning devices can still injure soft tissues, requiring a nurse to be especially observant for signs of pressure formation.

TABLE 13-1   SUPPORT SURFACES

CATEGORY AND MECHANISM OF ACTION	INDICATIONS FOR USE	ADVANTAGES	DISADVANTAGES
SUPPORT SURFACES AND OVERLAYS			
Foam Overlays (available as an overlay or in a full mattress)			
Reduces pressure and the cover (top) can reduce friction and shear. Base height of 3-4 inches; see manufacturer's guidelines regarding the amount of body weight supported.	Use for moderate to high-risk clients.	One-time charge. No setup fee. Cannot be punctured. Available in various sizes (e.g., bed, chair, operating room table). Little maintenance. Does not need electricity.	Hot and may trap moisture. Limited life span. Plastic protective sheet needed for incontinent clients or clients with drainage wounds.
Water Overlays (available as an overlay or in a full mattress)			
Reduces pressure and pressure points because these surfaces provide flotation with pressure reduction by evenly redistributing client's weight over the entire support surface.	Use for high-risk clients.	Readily available. Some control over motion sensations. Easily to clean.	Easily punctured. Heavy. Fluid motion may make procedures (e.g., dressing changes, CPR) difficult. Maintenance needed to prevent microorganism growth. Client transfers out of bed are difficult. Difficult to raise and lower head of bed.
Gel Overlays			
Reduces pressure and pressure points because these surfaces provide flotation with pressure reduction by evenly redistributing client's weight over the entire support surface.	Use for moderate- to high-risk clients. Useful for clients who are wheelchair dependent.	Low maintenance. Easy to clean. Multiple-client use. Impermeable to needle punctures.	Heavy. Expensive. Lacks air flow for moisture control. Variable friction control.

Data from Wound Ostomy and Continence Nurses Society: *Guideline for prevention and management of pressure ulcers*, Glenview, Ill, 2003, The Association; Bryant RA: *Acute and chronic wounds: nursing management*, ed 2, St. Louis, 2000, Mosby; Morrison MJ: *The prevention and treatment of pressure ulcers*, St. Louis, 2001, Mosby.   *Continued*

TABLE 13-1 SUPPORT SURFACES—CONT'D

CATEGORY AND MECHANISM OF ACTION	INDICATIONS FOR USE	ADVANTAGES	DISADVANTAGES
SUPPORT SURFACES AND OVERLAYS—continued			
Static Air-Filled Overlays			
Overlays are pressure reducing and can lower the mean interface pressure between the client's tissue and the mattress.	Used for moderate- to high-risk clients. Used for clients who can reposition themselves.	Easy to clean. Multiple-client use. Low maintenance. Potential repair of some air-filled products. Durable.	Damaged by punctures from needles and sharps. Requires routine monitoring to determine adequate inflation pressure. Client transfers out of bed are difficult.
Low-Air-Loss Overlay (available in a full bed or overlay)			
Maintains a constant and slight air movement against the skin to prevent moisture buildup.	Use for moderate- to high-risk clients.	Easy to clean. Maintains a constant inflation. Deflates to facilitate transfer and CPR. Moisture control. Fabric covering the overlay is air permeable, bacteria impermeable, and waterproof. Reduces shear and friction. Setup provided by the manufacturer.	Damaged by needles and sharps. Noisy. Requires electricity.
SPECIALTY BEDS			
Air-Fluidized Beds			
Bed frame contains silicone-coated beads and incorporates both air and fluid support. The silicone-coated beads become fluidized when air is pumped through the beads.	Use for high-risk clients. Use with clients with stage III or IV pressure ulcers or burns.	Less frequent turning or repositioning. Improved client comfort. Quickly becomes firm for CPR or other treatments when the device is turned "off." Reduces shear, friction, and edema to site. May facilitate management of copious wound drainage or incontinence. Setup provided by the manufacturer.	Continuous circulation of warm, dry air may increase client risk for dehydration. Bed may increase room temperature. Client may experience disorientation. Transfer of clients is difficult. Heavy. Expensive. Width of bed may preclude care to obese clients or clients with contractures.
Low-Air-Loss Beds			
Bed frame with a series of connected air-filled pillows. The amount of pressure in each pillow is controlled and can be calibrated to client need.	Indicated in clients who need pressure relief, those who cannot be frequently repositioned, or those who have skin breakdown on more than one surface. Contraindicated in clients with unstable spinal column.	Head and foot of bed can be raised and lowered. Easy transfer in and out of bed. Less frequent turning schedule. Pillows can be transferred to stretcher with client. Needs a portable motor. Setup provided by the manufacturer.	Portable motor is noisy. Bed surface material is slippery, and clients can easily slide down mattress or out of bed when being transferred.
Kinetic Therapy			
Provides continuous passive motion to promote mobilization of pulmonary secretions and also provides low air loss, which provides pressure relief.	Primarily indicated for clients needing spinal stabilization. Should not be used when the client is hemodynamically unstable.	Reduces pulmonary complications associated with restricted mobility. Reduces the risk of urinary stasis and urinary tract infections. Reduces venous stasis.	Does not reduce shear or moisture. Cannot be used with cervical or skeletal traction. Clients may have some motion sickness initially. Clients may have sensations of claustrophobia.

Data from Wound Ostomy and Continence Nurses Society: *Guideline for prevention and management of pressure ulcers,* Glenview, Ill, 2003, The Association; Bryant RA: *Acute and chronic wounds: nursing management,* ed 2, St. Louis, 2000, Mosby; Morrison MJ: *The prevention and treatment of pressure ulcers,* St. Louis, 2001, Mosby.

Evidence-Based Practice Trends

Sustained pressure on areas that support the body lead to reduced blood supply and eventually necrosis of the skin and underlying muscles. Pressure relief is a major nursing intervention for the prevention of pressure ulcers (Pieper, 2000). There are two main approaches to pressure relief. The first approach is the use of support surfaces to distribute the body weight over a large area. The second approach is to use an alternating support surface where inflatable cells alternately inflate and deflate.

Research has provided good evidence to support the effectiveness of high-specification foam over standard hospital foam. High-specification foam evenly distributes the client's body weight over the foam surface and as a result reduces pressure. In addition, clients with limited mobility have the lowest incidence of skin injury and pressure ulcers with alternating-pressure air mattresses, followed by low-pressure foam mattresses and water mattress overlays (Morrison, 2001). There is also evidence to support the use of air-fluidized and low-air-loss devices as treatments to reduce pressure ulcer risk (Cullum and others, 2003). Research offers no conclusive evidence of the effects of specialty beds. These data are inconclusive because the sample sizes are so small, but clinical data supports the use of specialty beds to reduce pressure ulcer formation in selected clients (Morrison, 2001).

Pressure ulcers can occur in any setting. Clients in the operating room are also at risk for injury to the skin and underlying tissue. This injury occurs from a combination of factors such as surgical positioning and the effects of anesthetic agents. Because the damage resulting from intraoperative pressure develops in the muscle and subcutaneous tissues and progresses outward, damage may not be visible for several days (Armstrong and Bortz, 2001). One method to reduce this risk is the use of support surfaces in the operating room. Research notes that the use of static air overlays, followed by gel pads, during surgery best reduces tissue interface pressure. Foam overlays did not reduce pressure when compared to conventional OR bed pads (Armstrong and Bortz, 2001).

Nurses caring for postoperative clients need to observe the skin for signs of injury or breakdown, even when the client is ambulatory in the postoperative setting. In addition, clients who had their surgeries in ambulatory care settings should also be instructed to observe for signs of skin breakdown.

Cultural Considerations

- Prepare the client and family members thoroughly before using any devices.
- Ethnically diverse groups may not have any experience with the type of technology used in the Western health care system.
- Some cultural groups may hesitate to ask for help or questions, especially when they have limited English communication.
- Some cultural groups such as Asians may hesitate to ask questions for fear of embarrassment.
- Use interpreters to provide explanations and demonstration for clients with limited English proficiency.
- Pace instructions slowly, and provide translated instructions.
- Give opportunities for the client and family members to manipulate the equipment/appliance under supervision.
- Anticipate precautions needed relevant to objects or articles that can damage the support surfaces.
- Accommodate cultural rituals and practices when scheduling turning of the client.
- Schedule turning to maximize contact between clients and visitors.
- Female modesty is highly valued by members of many cultures, including Amish, Muslims, Hindus, and Orthodox Jews. Cover clients when turning and positioning.

Skill Performance Guidelines

1. Perform complete assessment to determine client's risk for pressure ulcers and selection of appropriate special mattresses and beds. A complete client assessment includes use of appropriate pressure ulcer risk scales, presence of shear and friction, and the client's nutritional, fluid, mobility, and continence status (see Chapter 15).

2. Know the reason for and extent of the client's reduced mobility. The client who cannot be easily repositioned or who has pressures ulcers involving multiple surfaces benefits from pressure-relief support devices other than those used for a partially immobile client.

3. Determine if the pressure-relief support device is needed on a short-term or long-term basis. Clients in acute care settings may need the device only during the acute phase of the illness. However, clients with chronic altered mobility or decreased sensation or clients who are discharged to long-term care or home care may require long-term pressure relief. It may be more beneficial and economically sound to select one device to be used.

4. Continue to provide basic preventive care measures against the hazards of immobility, for example, regular skin assessment, turning, correct positioning, or range-of-motion exercises (when not contraindicated).

5. Use proper body mechanics when positioning or working with clients.

6. Follow all safety measures to prevent injury to clients from accidental falls or improper positioning when placing them on special beds or mattresses.

7. Encourage clients to remain as mobile as possible within the limits of their physical conditions and prescribed activity levels.

8. Educate care provider about the advantages/disadvantages and methods of operation of all support devices to ensure their proper use in all settings.

9. Collaborate with health care professionals who have expertise in this area.

10. Anticipate need to consult with social service or home care department regarding product durability, third-party reimbursement, and arrangements for delivery to and care of special beds in the home.

SKILL 13-1 Placing a Client on a Support Surface

Numerous support surfaces designed to reduce pressure on tissues overlying bony prominences are available. The wide acceptance of these devices has led many nurses to recommend their use as common preventive measures for clients with reduced mobility and risk for developing pressure ulcers. Most of the devices are easy to apply and keep clean. The extent to which the devices actually relieve pressure and prevent skin breakdown is highly variable. Few systematic studies exist that consistently find one surface is better than others (Cullum and others, 2003).

Support surfaces can be categorized as mattress (or wheelchair) overlays, mattress replacements, or specialty beds. An overlay rests on top of the hospital mattress and uses foam, air, water, gel, or combinations of these products to provide pressure relief. Mattress overlays and mattress replacements are considered to be either static (e.g., foam, gels) or dynamic (e.g., alternating-pressure surfaces).

A flotation pad is constructed of a silicone or polyvinyl chloride gel encased in a vinyl-covered square. The pad serves as an artificial layer of fat to protect bony surfaces such as the sacrum and greater trochanters. One type of flotation pad can be used for wheelchair clients.

One type of air mattress is fully integrated into the hospital bed. This bed surface may be adjusted to the client's comfort level by adding or removing air through buttons within the client's reach, or it can automatically adjust pressures to the client's position and movement when in the automatic mode. A bed sheet is always used to cover an air mattress to prevent skin from touching the plastic surface.

There are two types of foam mattresses. One is the foam mattress overlay, which may have either a flat smooth surface, foam rubber peaks ("egg-crate" variety, shown in Figure 13-1), or a cut surface. It is placed on top of the bed mattress, and usually the nurse places a sheet over the foam mattress pad overlay to prevent soiling and provide ease of cleaning. The second type is the foam specialty mattress, which completely replaces the hospital mattress and is covered by a loose-fitting cover intended to protect the mattress and minimize friction and shear. The foam mattresses are designed more for comfort rather than pressure relief.

Air mattress overlays can be static or dynamic and consist of interconnected air cells or cushions inflated by the use of a motorized blower (Figure 13-2). These mattresses use a pressure-cycling device to intermittently inflate and deflate or to maintain a constant inflation and slight air movement in the mattress.

More complex air mattresses contain several layers of tubes or support cells. A static mattress is inflated with a simple air blower after placing the mattress on a bed. An integrated air mattress connects with a pressure-cycling device

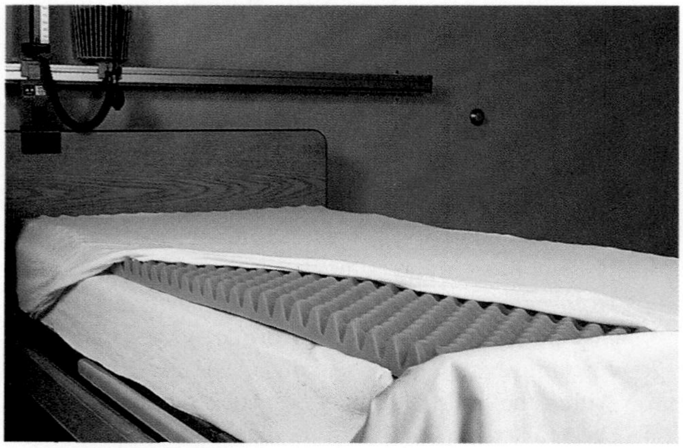

FIGURE **13-1** "Egg-crate" foam overlay is primarily for comfort.

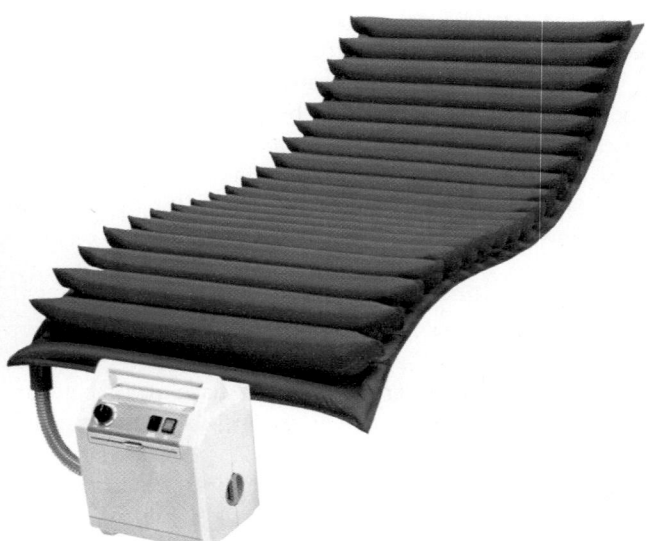

FIGURE **13-2** Dynamic air mattress overlay. (© 2002 Hill-Rom Services, Inc. Reprinted with permission. All rights reserved.)

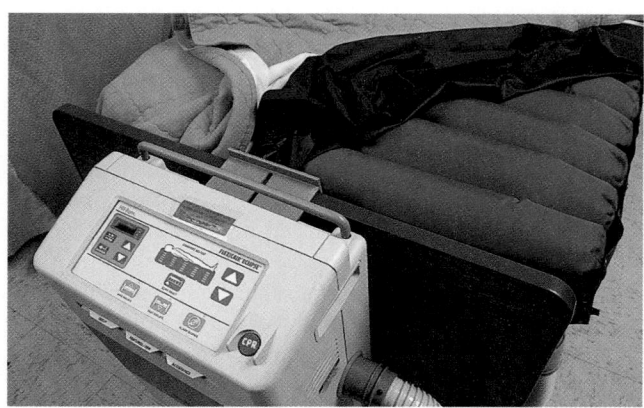

FIGURE **13-3** Motor for integrated air mattress.

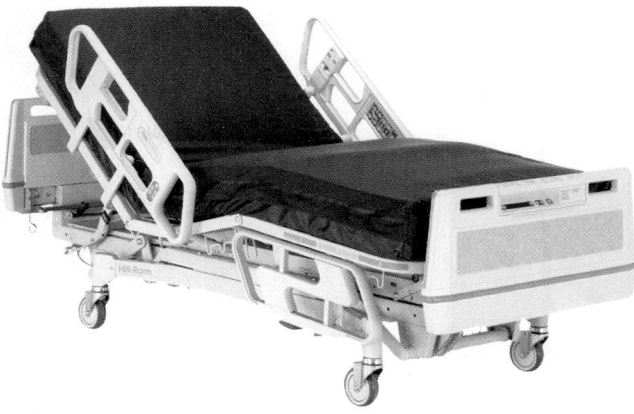

FIGURE **13-4** Air-integrated replacement mattress. (© 2002 Hill-Rom Services, Inc. Reprinted with permission. All rights reserved.)

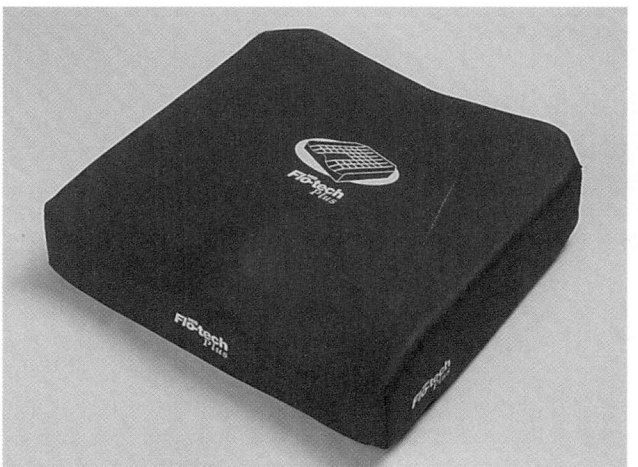

FIGURE **13-5** Low-pressure seat cushion. (Reproduced with permission from Medical Support Systems Ltd.)

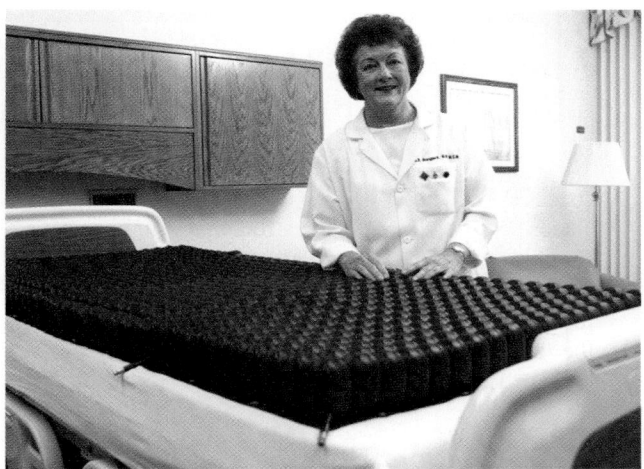

FIGURE **13-6** ROHO Dry Floatation mattress for a bed. (Courtesy the ROHO Group, Belleville, Ill.)

that intermittently inflates and deflates sections of the mattress, creating a cycling effect that minimizes pressure on bony prominences (Figure 13-3). Use a static mattress if a client can assume a variety of positions without bearing weight on a pressure ulcer. Use a dynamic support if the client cannot assume a variety of positions and if the client fully compresses a static mattress (AHCPR, 1994).

Replacement mattresses are denser, thicker, and more resilient to the client's weight and actually decrease pressure to a greater degree than some overlays (Vyhlidal and others, 1997). Replacement mattresses have foam, gel, air, or fluid sections that can be customized to the needs of a specific client with moderate to high risk for skin breakdown.

Another available option is an air-integrated replacement mattress instead of the conventional mattress (Figure 13-4). These mattresses may also be fully integrated into the bed. Air mattresses can be used for clients with moderate to high risk for skin breakdown. Air mattresses must be deflated before initiating CPR.

Another intervention is a low-pressure seat cushion (Figure 13-5) overlaid on a wheelchair or a dry static flotation mattress system (Figure 13-6) that may be overlaid on the bed or wheelchair (Figure 13-7). Through a system of controlled dynamics, low pressures are maintained by distributing pressure across the client's body surface. Thus friction and shear are minimized.

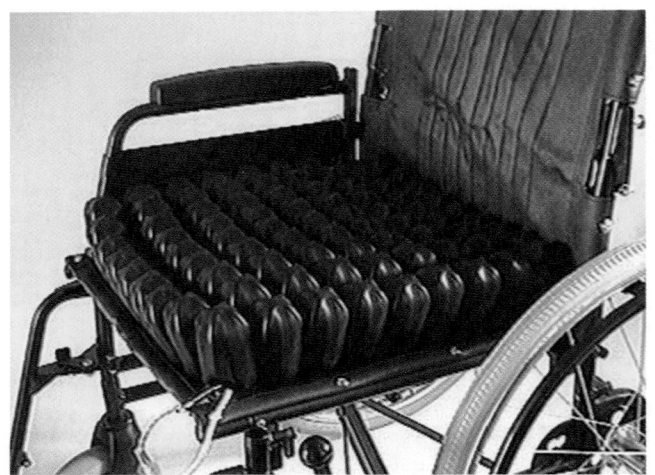

FIGURE **13-7** ROHO Dry Floatation mattress system for clients in wheelchairs. (Courtesy the ROHO Group, Belleville, Ill.)

Support surfaces aid in reducing pressure on the client's skin. They do not replace regular repositioning, meticulous skin care, or range of joint motion. The decision to place a client on a pressure-relief surface and the selection of this surface is a nursing responsibility (Box 13-1). The Support Surface Consensus Panel identified the three purposes of support: comfort, postural control, and pressure management. In addition, this panel listed nine parameters to use when evaluating and selecting a support surface: life expectancy, skin moisture control, skin temperature control, redistribution of pressure, product service requirements, fall safety, infection control, flammability, and client-product friction (Krouskop and van Rijswijk, 1995).

BOX 13-1 Procedural Guideline
Selection of pressure-reducing support surfaces

DELEGATION CONSIDERATIONS

The selection of a pressure-reducing support device should not be delegated to assistive personnel. It is the responsibility of the nurse to assess the client's skin and the risk for skin breakdown. The nurse then determines the appropriate type of pressure reduction surface (Figure 13-8).

EQUIPMENT

Agency's pressure ulcer risk assessment tool (see Chapter 15); body chart, tape measure, and/or camera to document existing areas of impaired skin integrity; documentation record; skin care products

ASSESSMENT

1. Assess client's risk for skin breakdown using a risk assessment tool.
2. Assess client's existing pressure ulcers, including areas of blistering, abnormal reactive hyperemia, and abrasion.
3. Determine need for pressure reduction surface by calculating Braden risk score.
   a. Assess risks by population: general population less than or equal to 16; intensive care unit (ICU) less than or equal to 15; older adults less than or equal to 18; and black and Latino clients less than or equal to 18 (Braden and Bergstrom, 1989; Jiricka and others, 1995; Lyder and others, 1998).

4. Identify client factors when selecting an appropriate surface. Determine (Pieper, 2000):
   a. Does the client need pressure reduction or relief? If the client cannot be repositioned or if there is a pressure ulcer, the client requires pressure relief.
   b. Is the surface needed for short- or long-term care? A short-term surface is usually needed for the acute illness and hospitalization. A long-term surface is usually needed for extended or home care.
   c. What is the potential comfort level achieved by the surface? If the client is sensitive to noise, then a device with a loud motor may increase client's discomfort.
   d. Are the client, family, and caregivers adherent to repositioning? In addition, are they aware that a support surface should never replace repositioning? In a home setting, a surface may be necessary when the family, caregiver, or client is unable to independently reposition or assist with repositioning.
   e. Does the surface have a potential to interfere with the client's independent functioning? The height of the overlay and its soft edge may affect the client's ability to transfer, and a high-air-loss bed is not appropriate for a client who needs to get in and out of bed frequently.
   f. What are the client's financial limitations?
   g. If the device is used in the home, what are the environmental limitations? Will the home and existing electrical service accommodate the surface selected?

BOX 13-1 Procedural Guideline
Selection of pressure-reducing support surfaces—cont'd

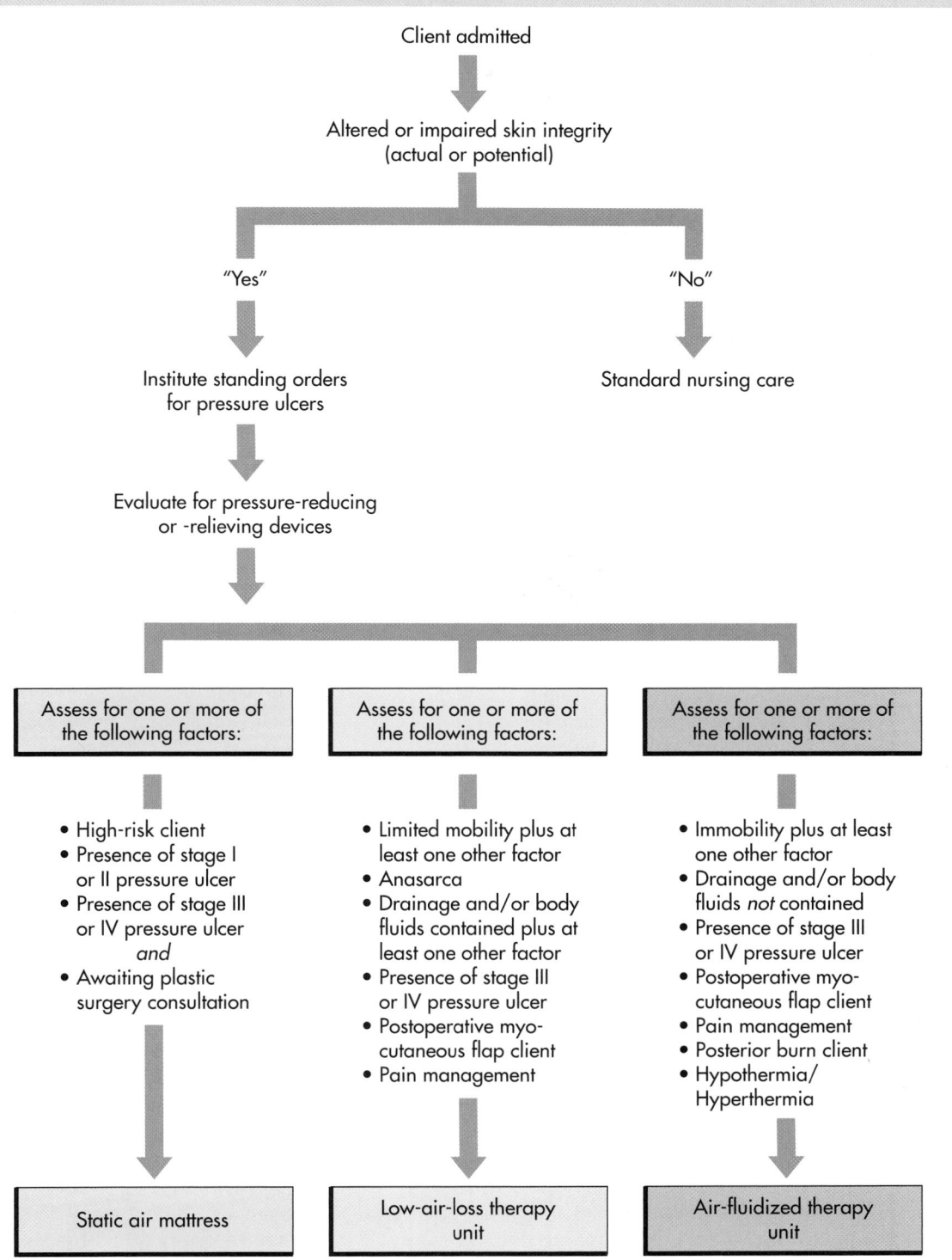

Client admitted

Altered or impaired skin integrity
(actual or potential)

"Yes"   "No"

Institute standing orders   Standard nursing care
for pressure ulcers

Evaluate for pressure-reducing
or -relieving devices

Assess for one or more of the following factors:	Assess for one or more of the following factors:	Assess for one or more of the following factors:
• High-risk client • Presence of stage I or II pressure ulcer • Presence of stage III or IV pressure ulcer *and* • Awaiting plastic surgery consultation	• Limited mobility plus at least one other factor • Anasarca • Drainage and/or body fluids contained plus at least one other factor • Presence of stage III or IV pressure ulcer • Postoperative myocutaneous flap client • Pain management	• Immobility plus at least one other factor • Drainage and/or body fluids *not* contained • Presence of stage III or IV pressure ulcer • Postoperative myocutaneous flap client • Pain management • Posterior burn client • Hypothermia/Hyperthermia
Static air mattress	Low-air-loss therapy unit	Air-fluidized therapy unit

FIGURE **13-8** Flow diagram for ordering specialty beds. (From Thomas C: Specialty beds: decision making made easy, *Ostomy Wound Manage* 23:51, 1989.)

Continued

BOX 13-1 Procedural Guideline
Selection of pressure-reducing support surfaces—cont'd

Can the caregivers and family in the home manage the surface, and does the surface have a service contract to assist the family?

h. What is the durability of the product? Is the surface easily subjected to puncture? What is the ease of cleaning the surface?

5. Determine the specific device (see Figure 13-8).

a. Pressure-reducing or pressure-relieving devices redistribute pressure over bony prominences (see Table 13-1). Surface to provide pressure reduction includes therapeutic mattress replacements, static and dynamic surfaces (i.e., moving) surfaces, low-air-loss beds and mattresses, and air-fluidized beds (WOCN, 2003). Pressure-relief surfaces would be used in the operating room for individuals assessed to be at high risk or for lengthy procedures (Cullum and others, 2000).

b. Use a static support surface if a client can assume a variety of positions without bearing weight on a pressure ulcer without bottoming out (AHCPR, 1994). Bottoming out makes the support surface ineffective. To assess for bottoming out, place a hand (palm up) under the mattress or cushion below the area of risk for pressure areas (e.g. client's pressure points with lying or sitting on surface). If there is less than 1 inch of support material felt the client has bottomed out (Bergstrom and others, 1996).

c. Select a dynamic support surface when a client can assume a variety of positions without bearing weight on a pressure ulcer, if the client fully compresses the static support surface, or if the pressure ulcer does not show evidence of healing (AHCPR, 1994). Alternating or dynamic

mattresses are associated with lower incidence of pressure ulcers when compared with standard mattresses (WOCN, 2003).

d. High-specification foam has demonstrated effectiveness in decreasing the incidence of pressure ulcers in fairly high-risk clients, including older adults and clients with fractures of the neck of the femur (Cullum and others, 2000).

e. Clients with stage III or IV pressure ulcers on multiple turning surfaces may benefit from an air-fluidized bed (AHCPR, 1994).

f. There is limited evidence that low-air-loss beds reduce the incidence of pressure ulcers in intensive care (Cullum and others, 2000; Lyder and others, 1998).

g. When excess moisture or intact skin is a potential risk, a support surface that provides airflow is important in drying the skin and reducing the incidence of pressure ulcers (AHCPR, 1994).

6. Check agency policy regarding implementing support surface.

a. Obtain a physician's order. This is usually required for the client to obtain third-party reimbursement.

b. Consult with agency's case manager or social worker to assist with the client's financial eligibility and terms and length of third-party reimbursement for the surface.

c. Consult with agency's home care or discharge planning if the device is anticipated for long-term use. Specific procedures and evaluations are needed for continuity of surface when client is transferred to extended care or discharged home.

7. Document pressure ulcer risk assessment and skin assessment in the client's record. Document the support surface selected and client response to the surface (see specific skills for recording and reporting details).

DELEGATION CONSIDERATIONS

This skill may be delegated to assistive personnel. After the nurse completes the assessment, determines the need for a support surface, and selects the specific surface, the skill of placing the device on the client's bed or wheelchair can be delegated to assistive personnel. Some types of support surfaces require that the manufacturer's representative set up and maintain the support system. When delegating aspects of care for a client on a support surface, the nurse must:

- Instruct assistive personnel to notify the nurse of any changes in the client's skin; the nurse then completes the skin assessment
- Instruct the caregiver to continue regular turning and repositioning of the client and to seek assistance for client position changes as necessary

- Instruct caregiver about the normal functioning of the support device, such as inflation and deflation cycles, and to report to the nurse any changes in inflation or deflation cycles, leakage of air, water, or gel

EQUIPMENT

- ❑ Risk assessment tool (see Chapter 15)
- ❑ Mattress support surface of choice: foam overlays (see Figure 13-1), air mattress overlay (see Figure 13-2), bed with integrated surface, air-integrated replacement mattress (see Figure 13-4).
- ❑ Sheet(s)
- ❑ Disposable gloves (if soiled linen is being handled)
- ❑ Standard bed frame (with mattress) if overlay is to be used (optional)

STEP	RATIONALE

▌ ASSESSMENT

1. Perform hand hygiene.
2. Determine client's risk for pressure ulcer formation using a validated assessment tool.

   Risk factors for pressure ulcers include nutritional deficits, shear stress, friction, alterations in mobility and perception, moisture, and abnormal serum albumin and hemoglobin levels (see Chapter 15).

Reduces transmission of microorganisms.

Risk assessment tools suggested by AHCPR and Wound Ostomy Continence Nurses Society (WOCN) (e.g., Braden scale) provide an objective measure of risk consistent between nurse assessors over time (WOCN, 2003).

- **• Critical Decision Point**

  Clients with unstable conditions may not tolerate turning or positioning required for the application of a support surface mattress.

3. Perform skin assessment. Inspect condition of skin, especially over dependent sites and bony prominences (see Chapter 15).
4. Assess client's level of comfort; ask client to rate pain on a scale of 0 to 10.

Provides baseline to measure ongoing data to determine a change in skin integrity or change in an existing pressure ulcer.

Provides baseline to determine the client's comfort needs. Nerve endings related to pressure, touch, temperature, and limb position are located in the skin. The Support Surface Consensus Panel identified client comfort as one of the main purposes of support (Krouskop and van Rijswijk, 1995).

- **• Critical Decision Point**

  Clients experiencing pain may require administration of pain medication before application of support surface of choice or transfer to another bed.

5. Assess client's understanding of purpose of support surface.
6. Verify physician's order for type of support surface.

Misconceptions can affect client's cooperation in use of mattress.

A physician's order is usually required to ensure third-party payment of support surface.

STEP	RATIONALE	

NURSING DIAGNOSES

- Anxiety
- Risk for infection
- Deficient knowledge regarding use of support surface mattress
- Impaired physical mobility

- Pain (acute, chronic)
- Risk for impaired skin integrity
- Impaired skin integrity
- Ineffective peripheral tissue perfusion

Related factors are individual based on client's condition or needs.

PLANNING

1. Expected outcomes following completion of procedure:
   - Client's skin is without erythema or mottling.

   Mottling represents hypoxia, which is an abnormal physiological response in tissues under pressure (Pieper, 2000).

   - Existing pressure ulcer shows signs of healing.

   Skin remains free of new pressure ulcers. Support surface does not interfere with circulation to dependent areas.

   - Client expresses improved level of comfort.

   Equalized pressures have eliminated localized areas of discomfort.

   - Client is removed from therapeutic surface when risk for pressure ulcers decreases.

   Provides for efficient, cost-effective care while maintaining high-quality outcomes.

2. Explain purpose of mattress and method of application to client.

   Relieves anxiety and promotes cooperation.

IMPLEMENTATION

- ### *Critical Decision Point*

  Perform application of support surface mattress or transfer to bed in an organized, efficient manner or when a client is out of bed for surgery or diagnostic testing. Clients whose medical conditions are unstable may not tolerate prolonged periods of position changes (i.e., lying flat or turning from side to side). Turning an acutely ill client to the lateral side may cause complications, such as increased oxygen demand and hypotension.

1. Close room door or bedside curtain.

   Provides client privacy and considerate care during application of mattress to bed or transfer to alternate bed.

2. Apply gloves (should be worn if linens are soiled or wet). Obtain assistance as needed.

   Gloves prevent contact with body fluids. Assistance reduces risk of friction and shear in transfer to new surface.

3. Apply support surface to bed or prepare alternate bed (bed may be occupied or unoccupied).
   a. Mattress replacement:
      (1) Apply mattress to bed frame after removing standard hospital mattress.

      Hospital mattress needs to be stored. In some instances, mattress replacements may be standard procedure.

      (2) Apply sheet over mattress. Keep linens between surfaces to a minimum.

      Sheet reduces soiling. Multiple layers decrease surface effectiveness in reducing pressure (WOCN, 2003).

   b. Air mattress/overlay:
      (1) Apply deflated mattress flat over surface of bed mattress. (There may be directions on pad indicating which side to place up.)

      Provides smooth, even surface.

      (2) Bring any plastic strips or flaps around corners of bed mattress.

      Secures air mattress in place.

      (3) Attach connector on air mattress to inflation device. Inflate mattress to proper air pressure determined by air pump or blower.

      Mattresses vary as to requiring one-time or continuous inflation cycle (Pieper, 2000). Manufacturer's directions indicate desired air pressure designed to distribute client's body weight evenly. Directions are included with each mattress.

      (4) Place sheet over air mattress, being sure to eliminate all wrinkles.

      Prevents soiling of mattress and reduces direct contact of skin with plastic surface.

STEP	RATIONALE

(5) Check air pumps to be sure pressure cycle alternates.

Alternating airflow mattress produces intermittent cycling, inflating only parts of mattress at any one time. Intermittent cycle continually alternates pressure against skin and soft tissue (Whittemore, 1998).

● **Critical Decision Point**

Keep sharp objects away from air mattress.

(6) Assist client with transferring in and out of bed.

Mattress surface is less firm and may be slippery and is difficult for some clients to assist the nurse or other personnel in transferring from bed to chair/stretcher.

c. Air-surface bed:
   (1) Obtain and place linen on bed.

In some instances bed may be available in all client rooms; if not, an ordering system exists to obtain one as needed (see agency policy).

   (2) Place switch in the "prevention" mode.

In the "prevention" mode, surface pressures change automatically with client position to equalize pressure and eliminate points of pressure.

● **Critical Decision Point**

Beds are equipped with a cardiopulmonary resuscitation (CPR) switch to instantly lower head section from an elevated position and to deflate the mattress to provide a firm surface for chest compressions (see illustration).

d. Water mattress (supplemental and self-contained):
   (1) Apply unfilled supplemental mattress flat over the surface of standard bed mattress. (Self-contained water mattress would replace bed mattress.)

Provides a smooth, even surface.

   (2) Bring any plastic strips or flaps around corners of bed mattress.

Secures water mattress in place.

   (3) Attach connector on water mattress to water source, and fill mattress to level recommended by manufacturer. Follow manufacturer's directions regarding temperature of water. Mattress should be filled in close proximity to water source. Manufacturer's directions (enclosed with mattress) indicate desired water level designed to distribute client's body weight evenly (usually determined by client weight or height and weight).

Proper water temperature prevents loss of body heat as client lies on mattress.

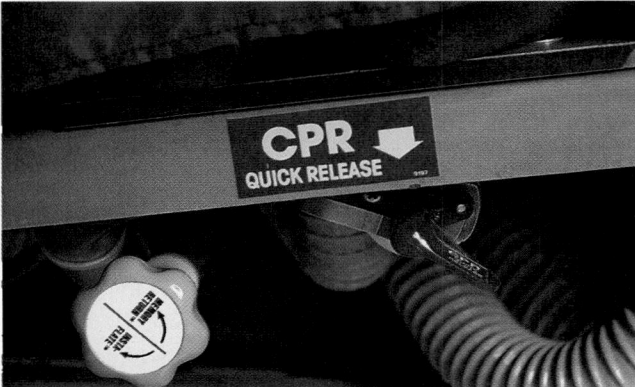

STEP **3c(2)** Cardiopulmonary resuscitation switch deflates low-air-loss bed to provide hard surface.

STEP	RATIONALE
(4) Place sheet over water mattress, being sure to eliminate all wrinkles.	Reduces soiling of mattress and prevents direct contact of skin with plastic surface.
(5) Keep sharp objects away from mattress.	Tears and punctures result in loss of water, making mattress ineffective.
4. Position client comfortably as desired over support surface. Reposition routinely.	Location of existing pressure ulcer might influence type of positioning.
5. Remove gloves, and perform hand hygiene.	Reduces transmission of microorganisms.

EVALUATION

1. Inspect and compare condition of client's skin every 8 hours or according to agency policy to determine changes in skin integrity, pressure ulcer status, and effectiveness of support surface.	Determines if pressure sores develop or if the condition of existing sores changes.
2. Reassess client's risk for pressure ulcer formation at routine intervals.	Documents change in status, which is critical for evaluating continued need for therapeutic surface.
3. Ask client to rate comfort on a scale of 0 to 10.	If pressure-relief mattress is effective, client generally experiences less discomfort.
4. Evaluate functioning of support surface periodically.	Regular inspection of mechanical components of mattress ensures proper functioning.

Recording and Reporting

- Record type of support surface applied, extent to which client tolerated procedure, and condition of client's skin in nurses' notes or skin assessment flow sheet.
- Report evidence of pressure ulcer formation to nurse in charge or to physician.

Unexpected Outcomes	Related Interventions
1. Client develops localized areas of abnormal reactive hyperemia for longer than 30 minutes (WOCN, 2003), mottling, swelling, and tenderness with evidence of breakdown.	• Modify skin care regimen. • Increase frequency of skin assessment. • Increase types of pressure-relief interventions. • Revise turning schedule. • Consult with skin care expert. • Notify physician.
2. Existing pressure areas fail to heal or increase in size or depth.	• Modify skin care regimen. • Revise turning schedule. • Consult with skin care expert. • Notify physician.
3. Client expresses discomfort while on support surface.	• Evaluate need for analgesia or mild sedation. • Evaluate need to modify support surface. • Reposition client more frequently. • Unless contraindicated, provide back massage. Do not massage reddened areas or bony prominences because massage to these areas can contribute to skin breakdown (WOCN, 2003).
4. Bed or mattress develops leak (air, water, gel).	• Take corrective action according to agency or manufacturer's policies/directions.

Teaching Considerations

- Explain risks of immobility to client and family members (see Chapter 11).
- Instruct in proper body mechanics, positioning, and pressure relief.
- Explain risks for pressure ulcers (see Chapter 15).
- Explain purpose and function of the pressure-relief surface. Include reminder that the surface augments care and does not replace the need for turning and pressure-relief maneuvers.
- Explain precautions regarding sharp objects, fire hazard, and other concerns.
- Reeducate client about need for support surface and discuss alternatives, including client's right to refuse a recommended surface.

Pediatric Considerations

- There are various pain assessment tools developed specifically for use in children (see Chapter 6).
- Parents can also be helpful in assisting the child in expressing pain and treatment preferences (Hockenberry and others, 2003).

Gerontological Considerations

- Implement preventive measures because aging skin is drier, thinner, and less pressure sensitive, increasing the risk of skin breakdown (Lueckenotte, 2000).
- Adding mattress overlays changes the bed height. Care should be taken when transferring and teaching family members to transfer from bed to chair.

Home Care Considerations

- Most of the devices covered in this section may be adapted for home use on a standard twin bed or hospital bed.
- Selection should be based on client needs and environmental audit. For example, the client on total bed rest who smokes would not be an ideal candidate for a foam mattress because of the potential for fire; the client with pets that sleep in the bed may not be suited for a water- or air-filled mattress because of the risk of puncture.
- Reimbursement varies by surface type and payer source.

SKILL 13-2   Placing a Client on an Air-Suspension Bed

Air-suspension beds are indicated for clients who are immobile or otherwise confined to the bed. The air-suspension bed supports a client's weight on air-filled cushions. The bed minimizes pressure and reduces shear in a low-air-loss system (Figure 13-9). If a client has large stage III or stage IV pressure ulcers on multiple turning surfaces, a low-air-loss bed or air-fluidized bed may be indicated (AHCPR, 1994).

For clients requiring high air loss under a given body part, for example, under the buttocks, high-air-loss cushions may be substituted. High air loss provides for selective drying while not having the effect of substantially increasing insensible fluid losses.

It is also possible to adapt the air-suspension beds to individual client needs with specialty cushions for positioning, foot support, and lateral arm supports. Clients usually require less analgesia while on the bed. Another adaptation of the air-suspension bed is the kinetic low-air-loss bed (Figure 13-10). This bed is marketed widely to intensive care areas and has the ability to provide a pressure-relief surface while rotating continuously approximately 30 to 35 degrees. This surface should not be used with a client who has an unstable spine or who is in traction.

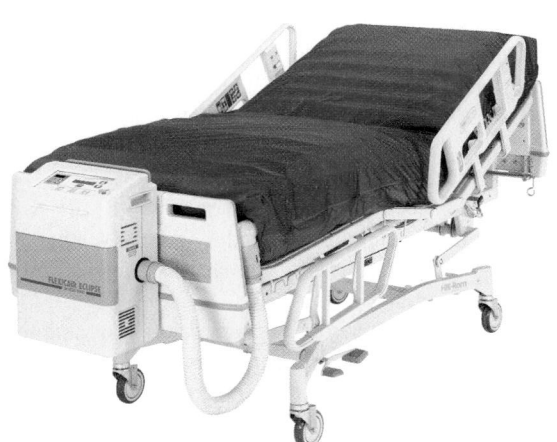

FIGURE **13-9** Low-air-loss bed. (© 2002 Hill-Rom Services, Inc. Reprinted with permission. All rights reserved.)

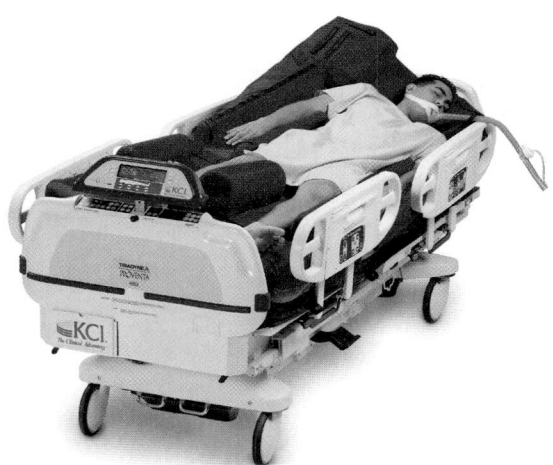

FIGURE **13-10** Lateral rotation bed. (triaDyne® Proventa™ Courtesy Kinetic Concepts, Inc, San Antonio, Tex.)

DELEGATION CONSIDERATIONS

This skill may be delegated to assistive personnel. When the nurse completes the assessment, determines the need for a specialty bed, the skill of placing the client on an air-suspension bed can be delegated to assistive personnel. Some types of specialty beds require that the manufacturer's representative set up and maintain the system. When delegating aspects of care for a client on a support surface, the nurse must:

- Instruct assistive personnel to notify the nurse of any changes in the client's skin. The nurse then completes the skin assessment.
- Instruct the caregiver to continue regular turning and repositioning of the client and to seek assistance for client position changes as necessary. This may not be necessary for clients placed on a lateral rotation air-suspension bed.

- Instruct caregiver about the normal functioning of the air-suspension bed, such as inflation and deflation cycles, and to report to the nurse any changes in inflation or deflation cycles.
- Instruct caregiver to notify the nurse if the client becomes disoriented, becomes restless, or complains of nausea.

EQUIPMENT

- ❑ Air-suspension bed
- ❑ Gore-Tex sheet (supplied by manufacturer)
- ❑ Disposable bed pads, if indicated
- ❑ Disposable gloves (optional)

STEP	RATIONALE

ASSESSMENT

1. Perform hand hygiene.
2. Determine client's risk for pressure ulcer formation using a validated assessment tool.

   Risk factors for pressure ulcers include nutritional deficits, shear stress, friction, alterations in mobility and perception, moisture, and abnormal serum albumin and hemoglobin levels (see Chapter 15).

3. Identify clients who would benefit from air-suspension therapy, such as immobilized or burn clients.

Reduces transmission of microorganisms.

Risk assessment tools as suggested by AHCPR and WOCN (e.g., Braden scale) provide an objective measure of risk consistent between nurse assessors over time (WOCN, 2003).

Beds effectively minimize pressure on fragile tissues and dependent body parts. Selected for clients who require pressure relief for treatment of or prevention of pressure ulcers.

- *Critical Decision Point*
This surface should not be used with a client who has an unstable spine or who is in traction.

4. Perform skin assessment. Inspect condition of skin, especially over dependent sites and bony prominences (see Chapter 15).
5. Assess client's level of comfort; ask client to rate pain on a scale of 0 to 10.

6. Review client's medical orders.

7. Assess client's level of consciousness.

8. Assess client's and caregiver's understanding of purpose of bed.
9. Review client's serum electrolyte levels in medical record, if available.
10. Check medical record to see if client needs to be weighed frequently.

Provides baseline to determine a change in skin integrity or change in an existing pressure ulcer over time.

Provides baseline to determine the client's comfort needs. Nerve endings related to pressure, touch, temperature, and limb position are located in the skin. The Support Surface Consensus Panel identified client comfort as one of the main purposes of support (Krouskop and van Rijswijk, 1995).

A physician's order is usually required to obtain third-party reimbursement for cost of bed.

Baseline used to detect change while client is on bed. Clients may become confused or disoriented from the flotation sensation of the bed (WOCN, 2003).

Bed inflation is maintained by one or two blowers, which make a sound that may create anxiety for the client.

The movement of air through the mattress can increase the client's risk for dehydration (WOCN, 2003).

Scales are available in some air-suspension beds and available as underbed units for clients who need to be weighed frequently or for those who cannot be moved for weighing.

STEP	RATIONALE

NURSING DIAGNOSES

- Anxiety
- Deficient fluid volume
- Risk for impaired skin integrity
- Kinesthetic sensory/perceptual alterations
- Pain (acute, chronic)

- Impaired skin integrity
- Deficient knowledge regarding use of support surface mattress
- Impaired physical mobility
- Ineffective peripheral tissue perfusion

Related factors are individualized based on client's condition or needs.

PLANNING

1. Expected outcomes following completion of procedure:
   - Client's skin remains warm, clean, and intact, or existing lesions show evidence of healing.
   - Existing pressure ulcers show evidence of healing by formulation of granulation tissue.
   - Client expresses improved sense of comfort.
   - Client remains alert and oriented or shows no change in level of orientation.
2. Explain procedure and purpose of bed to client and caregiver.
3. Prepare necessary equipment and supplies.
4. Review instructions supplied by bed manufacturer.
5. For clients with severe to moderate pain, premedicate approximately 30 minutes before transfer.
6. Obtain any additional personnel needed to transfer client to bed.

Skin is free from pressure effects of immobility.

Bed's low-pressure surface facilitates healing of existing pressure ulcers.
Bed's surface is soft, minimizing pain stimulation.
Client does not experience sensory perceptual changes from flotation.
Reduces anxiety and promotes client's cooperation.

Promotes organized transfer of client to specialty bed.
Promotes safe and correct use of bed.
Promotes client's comfort and ability to cooperate during transfer to bed. Decreases client's energy expenditure.
Ensures client's safety by having sufficient personnel to assist in transferring.

IMPLEMENTATION

1. Close client's room door or bedside curtain. Perform hand hygiene.
2. Explain steps of transfer.

3. Transfer client to bed using appropriate transfer techniques (see Chapter 10). Bed surface may be slippery, and transfers should not be attempted without assistance.
4. Once client is transferred, release Instaflate or turn bed on by depressing switch; regulate temperature.
5. Position client, and perform range-of-motion (ROM) exercises as appropriate.

6. To turn clients, position bedpans, or perform other therapies, turn on Instaflate setting. Once procedure is completed, release Instaflate.

Maintains client's privacy during transfer.

Reduces anxiety and helps client be a part of decision making during maneuvering.
Appropriate transfer techniques maintain alignment and reduce risk of injury during procedure. Company representative will adjust bed to client's height and weight.
Pressure cushions will automatically adjust to preset levels to minimize pressure, friction, and shear (Pieper, 2000).
Promotes comfort and reduces contracture formation. The bed reduces pressure on skin, but clients must still be turned and exercised to avoid joint deformity or contractures (AHCPR, 1994).
Instaflate firms the bed surface to facilitate turning and handling client. Client will not receive pressure relief while bed is in this mode.

- **Critical Decision Point**

  Client will NOT receive pressure relief when the bed is firm. Activate CPR switch to quickly deflate bed/mattress in an emergency (see Skill 13-1).

7. Know bed's special features, and use as needed.
   a. Scales
   b. Portable transport units to maintain inflation when primary power is interrupted

Facilitates ease of routine weights.
Provides for continuous pressure relief.

STEP	RATIONALE
c. Availability of specialty cushions for prone positioning, providing pressure relief, reducing moisture, preventing the client from sliding down in bed, or relieving weight from orthopedic devices	Reduces pressure, friction, and shearing forces.
d. Lateral rotation (see Figure 13-10), which allows approximately 30 degrees of turning.	Helps to reduce risk and prevent pulmonary and urinary complications of reduced mobility (Cullum and others, 2003; WOCN, 2003).
8. Remove gloves. Perform hand hygiene.	Reduces transmission of microorganisms.

▌ EVALUATION

1. Inspect condition of client's skin periodically while client is on bed.	Determines if any new pressure areas are forming.
2. Observe existing pressure ulcers for evidence of healing.	Evaluates healing progress of any existing pressure ulcers.
3. Ask client to rate level of comfort on a scale of 0 to 10.	Flotation effects of bed minimize pain stimuli.
4. Assess client's level of orientation.	Determines onset of perceptual changes.

Recording and Reporting

- Record transfer of client to bed, tolerance of procedure, and condition of skin in nurses' notes or skin assessment flow sheet.
- Report changes in condition of skin, level of orientation, and electrolyte levels to physician.
- Record teaching provided and client and/or caregiver response.
- Report restlessness or change in orientation.

Unexpected Outcomes	Related Interventions
1. Existing areas of skin breakdown or pressure areas fail to heal or increase in size or depth.	• Modify skin care regimen. • Revise turning schedule. • Consult with skin care expert. • Notify physician.
2. Client is restless, confused, or agitated.	• Notify physician. • Determine need for antianxiety medication. • Evaluate alternative pressure-relief devices.
3. Client becomes nauseated.	• Provide short-term antiemetics. • If lateral rotation is used, decrease the cycle frequency.
4. Bed malfunctions.	• Maintain client safety. • Follow agency or manufacturer's policy.

Teaching Considerations

- Explain function and purpose of air-suspension therapy.
- Explain the need to continue to change position at intervals to diminish the effects of immobility.
- Explain the need for adequate fluid intake, because bed surface may be drying and may cause dehydration.

Pediatric Considerations

- This bed is used commonly with older children. Instructions should be age appropriate and include any restrictions, such as raising the head of the bed, positioning.

- Younger children are usually easier to position, and thus the risk of pressure ulcers is easier to control

Gerontological Considerations

- When hospitalized, some older adult clients may experience misperceptions of their environment that may be intensified by the constant flotation of the air-suspension bed. Proprioception abnormalities affecting older adults are the result of nervous system and muscle changes (Lueckenotte, 2000).

Home Care Considerations

- A version of the bed is available for home use for rent or purchase; bed rental company is responsible for proper cleaning.

- Instruct family in importance of maintaining client hydration.
- Instruct family regarding the need to provide client's skin care.

SKILL 13-3 Placing a Client on an Air-Fluidized Bed

An air-fluidized bed is a dynamic device designed to distribute a client's weight evenly over its support surface (Figure 13-11). The bed minimizes pressure and reduces shearing force and friction through the principle of fluidization. Fluidization is created by forcing a gentle flow of temperature-controlled air upward through a mass of fine ceramic microspheres. The microspheres fluidize and take on the appearance of boiling milk and all the properties of a fluid. The client lies directly on a polyester filter sheet that allows air to pass through but does not allow the microspheres to escape. Clients feel as though they are floating on a surface like a warm waterbed. The contact pressure of the client's body against the filter sheet stays at 11 to 16 mm Hg.

Air-fluidized beds are useful in the care of clients who require minimal movement to prevent skin damage by shearing force and for clients who experience significant pain when being turned or positioned. Clients who can benefit from the bed include burn clients, those who have undergone extensive skin grafts or who have existing pressure ulcers, and victims of multiple trauma. Clients tend to perspire and lose body fluids while on the bed (Bryant, 2000). The surface of the filter sheet warms; as clients perspire, moisture is quickly absorbed into the circulating microspheres. Diaphoresis can go undetected, and thus insensible fluid loss may not be noticed until a client develops fluid and electrolyte imbalances. This individual is often already compromised in relation to hydration, fluids, and electrolytes; therefore the client's fluid balance status should be carefully monitored.

Conventional fluidized beds do not allow for head-of-bed position changes. Foam wedges are used to elevate the head. There are also combinations of fluidized–low-air-loss beds that allow head-of-bed elevation (Figure 13-12). These beds use air to lift the upper body, while the lower body stays on a fluidized bed surface. The weight of the bed structure makes transport extremely difficult. A pediatric version of this bed is available.

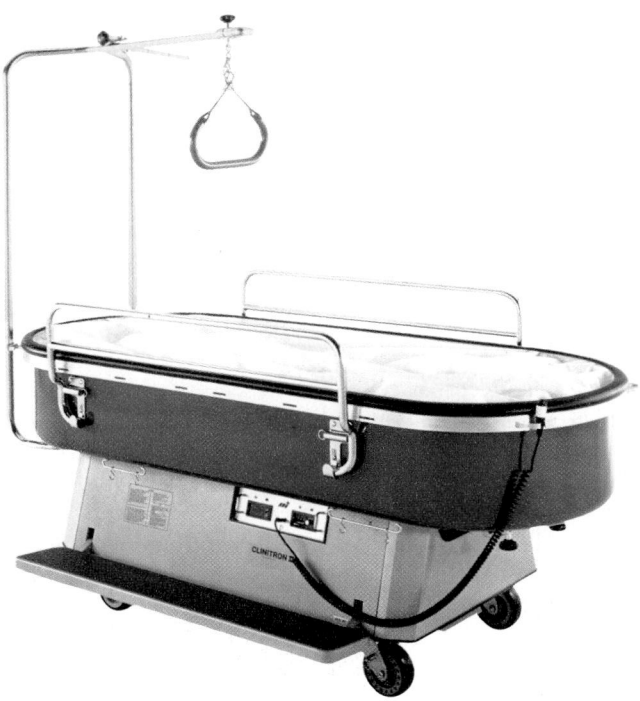

FIGURE **13-11** Air-fluidized bed. (© 2002 Hill-Rom Services, Inc. Reprinted with permission. All rights reserved.)

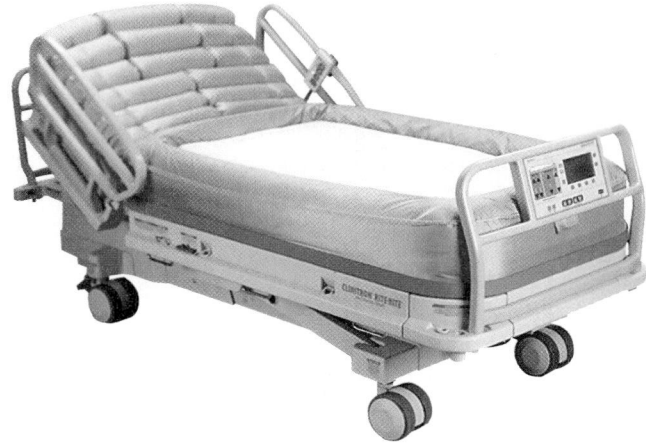

FIGURE **13-12** Combination air-fluidized therapy and low-air-loss bed. (© 2002 Hill-Rom Services, Inc. Reprinted with permission. All rights reserved.)

DELEGATION CONSIDERATIONS

This skill may be delegated to assistive personnel. When the nurse completes the assessment and determines the need for a specialty bed, the skill of placing the client on an air-fluidized bed can be delegated to assistive personnel. Some types of specialty beds require that the manufacturer's representative set up and maintain the system. When delegating aspects of care for a client on a support surface, the nurse must:

- Instruct assistive personnel to notify the nurse of any changes in the client's skin. The nurse then completes the skin assessment.
- Instruct the caregiver to continue regular turning and repositioning of the client and to seek assistance for client position changes as necessary. This may not be necessary for clients placed on a lateral rotation air-suspension bed.

- Instruct caregiver about the normal functioning of the air-suspension bed, such as inflation and deflation cycles, and to report to the nurse any changes in inflation or deflation cycles.
- Instruct caregiver to notify the nurse if the client becomes disoriented, becomes restless, or complains of nausea.

EQUIPMENT

- ❑ Air-fluidized bed
- ❑ Foam positioning wedges, if indicated
- ❑ Filter sheet (supplied by rental company)
- ❑ Disposable gloves (optional)

STEP	RATIONALE
■ ASSESSMENT	
1. Perform hand hygiene.	Reduces transmission of organisms.
2. Determine client's risk for pressure ulcer formation using a validated assessment tool. Risk factors for pressure ulcers include nutritional deficits, shear stress, friction, alterations in mobility and perception, moisture, and abnormal serum albumin and hemoglobin levels (see Chapter 15).	Risk assessment tools suggested by AHCPR and WOCN (e.g., Braden scale) provide an objective measure of risk consistent between nurse assessors over time (WOCN, 2003).

- *Critical Decision Point*
  The bed may not provide a stable surface for clients requiring skeletal traction.

STEP	RATIONALE
3. Perform skin assessment. Inspect condition of skin, especially over dependent sites and bony prominences (see Chapter 15). Pay particular attention to potential pressure sites and any existing pressure ulcers.	Data provide baseline to determine any change in client's condition while on bed.
4. Assess client's level of comfort; ask client to rate pain on a scale of 0 to 10.	Provides baseline to determine the client's comfort needs. Nerve endings related to pressure, touch, temperature, and limb position are located in the skin. The Support Surface Consensus Panel identified client comfort as one of the main purposes of support (Krouskop and van Rijswijk, 1995).
5. Assess client's level of orientation.	Baseline used to detect change while client is on bed. Flotation effect may cause altered sensory perceptions.
6. Assess client's and family members' understanding of purpose of bed.	Bed is large and makes sound when air blower is operating, which may create anxiety for client.
7. Review client's serum electrolyte levels in medical record (if available).	There is a tendency for clients to lose body fluids through diaphoresis. Baseline data are used to compare with subsequent laboratory results to determine electrolyte imbalances.
8. Identify clients at risk for complications of air-fluidized therapy: 　a. Older adult clients may become dehydrated from the airflow, which may increase insensible fluid losses. 　b. Clients receiving enteric tube feedings are at risk for aspiration due to the inability to elevate head of bed, which is limited to placing foam wedges under client's head and shoulders.	Allows nurse to anticipate need for frequent monitoring once client is placed on support surface.

STEP	RATIONALE

c. Clients who have limited ability to change positions and who are susceptible to dehydration may have tenacious pulmonary secretions that are difficult to remove.

d. Clients with specific positioning requirements such as elevating head of bed are limited to use of foam wedges.

● *Critical Decision Point*
The prone position should never be attempted.

9. Review client's medical orders.

Physician's order is usually required to obtain third-party reimbursement for cost of bed.

NURSING DIAGNOSES

- Anxiety
- Risk for imbalanced body temperature
- Risk for deficient fluid volume
- Risk for impaired skin integrity
- Impaired skin integrity
- Ineffective peripheral tissue perfusion

- Impaired physical mobility
- Pain (acute, chronic)
- Kinesthetic sensory/perceptual alterations
- Impaired home maintenance
- Risk for infection
- Deficient knowledge regarding use of support surface mattress

Related factors are individualized based on client's condition or needs.

PLANNING

1. Expected outcomes following completion of procedure:
   - Client's skin remains warm, clean, and intact, or there is evidence of healing of pressure ulcers.
   - Client expresses improved sense of comfort.
   - Skin remains well hydrated, with good turgor; mucous membranes are moist; and electrolyte levels are in normal range.
   - Client remains alert and oriented or shows no change in level of consciousness.
2. Explain procedure and purpose of bed to client and family.
3. Review manufacturer's instructions supplied by bed manufacturer.
4. For clients with severe to moderate pain, premedicate approximately 30 minutes before transfer.

5. Obtain any additional personnel needed to transfer client to bed.

Skin is free from pressure effects of immobility.

Bed's surface effective in promoting comfort.
Client's fluid and nutrient intake balance any insensible fluid loss from being on bed.

Client does not experience sensory perceptual changes from flotation.
Reduces anxiety and promotes client's cooperation.

Promotes safe and correct use of bed.

Promotes client's comfort and ability to cooperate during transfer to bed. Decreases client's energy expenditure (Krouskop and van Rijswijk, 1995).
Ensures client's safety by having sufficient personnel to assist in transferring.

IMPLEMENTATION

1. Close client's room door or bedside curtain.
2. Explain steps of transfer.

3. Perform hand hygiene, and apply gloves (if bed linens or surface is soiled).
4. Transfer client to bed using appropriate transfer techniques (see Chapter 10).

Maintains client's privacy during transfer.
Reduces anxiety and helps client be a part of decision making during maneuvering.
Reduces transmission of microorganisms.

Appropriate transfer techniques maintain alignment and reduce risk of injury during procedure.

STEP	RATIONALE

- *Critical Decision Point*

  Never attempt to place a client in a face-down position on an air-fluidized bed. Suffocation may occur.

5. Turn fluidization cycle on by depressing switch; regulate temperature.	Fluidization minimizes pressure against skin's surface and reduces friction and shear force when client moves.
6. Position client for comfort, and perform ROM exercises as appropriate.	Promotes comfort and reduces contracture formation. The bed reduces pressure on skin, but clients must still be turned and exercised to avoid joint deformity or contractures (Pieper, 2000).

- *Critical Decision Point*

  Use foam wedges on as needed (e.g., elevating the head of the client for position changes). Areas supported by the foam wedges do not benefit from the pressure relief of the bed's surface.

7. To turn clients, position bedpans, or perform other therapies, stop fluidization. Once procedure is completed, set to continuous fluidization.	Stopping fluidization provides firm, molded support that facilitates turning and handling client. Continuous fluidization provides permanent fluid support.

- *Critical Decision Point*

  In emergencies when resuscitation is required, press CPR switch and unplug unit to defluidize bed immediately (see Skill 13-1).

8. Remove gloves, and perform hand hygiene.	Reduces transmission of infection.

EVALUATION

1. Inspect condition of client's skin, including bony prominences, heels, and occipital area, according to agency policy while on bed, and monitor risk assessment.	Evaluates healing progress of any existing pressure ulcers. Determines if any new pressure areas are forming.
2. Ask client to rate level of comfort on a scale of 0 to 10.	Bed surface is soft and conforming and should assist with minimizing pain.
3. Review client's serum electrolyte levels, monitor body temperature, and note hydration status of skin and mucous membranes.	Factors may reveal fluid and electrolyte losses.
4. Measure client's level of orientation.	Determines onset of perceptual changes.

Recording and Reporting

- Record transfer of client to bed, tolerance to procedure, condition of skin, and orientation level in nurses' notes or on assessment flow sheet.
- Report changes in condition of skin and electrolyte levels to nurse in charge or to physician.
- Report teaching provided and client and/or caregiver response.
- Report changes in client's level of orientation.

Unexpected Outcomes	Related Interventions
1. Existing areas of skin breakdown or pressure areas fail to heal or increase in size or depth.	• Modify skin care regimen. • Consult with skin care expert. • Reevaluate client's risk factors affecting wound healing. • Notify physician.
2. Client's skin and mucous membranes are dehydrated.	• Provide oral fluids unless contraindicated. • If electrolyte levels are also abnormal, notify physician. • Monitor client's intake and output. • Provide intravenous fluids as ordered.
3. Client is restless or agitated or complains of nausea.	• Administer sedation or antiemetic. • Modify support surface selected. • Notify physician.
4. The filter sheet develops a tear.	• Mend tears with adhesive tape as per manufacturer's guidelines until a new bed can be provided. • Avoid use of additional sheets because they interfere with optimal bed performance.

Teaching Considerations

- Explain function and purpose of air-fluidized therapy.
- Explain that client will require assistance to change positions.
- Explain the need to maintain adequate hydration of client.

Pediatric Considerations

- This bed is used commonly with children who are burn victims. Instructions should be age appropriate and include any restrictions, such as raising the head of the bed, positioning.
- Parents need to know that the child may initially have some dizziness or nausea when first placed on the bed. This is due to the flotation sensation and will disappear as the child gets adjusted to the bed.

Gerontological Considerations

- Older adult clients are at increased risk for dehydration.
- When hospitalized, older adult client may experience significant misperceptions of their environment that may be intensified by the flotation of the air-fluidized bed.

Home Care Considerations

- Beds weigh between 1700 and 2100 lb; therefore the company leasing the bed needs to inspect the home for accessibility and structural support.
- Consult with social worker or case manager to determine third-party reimbursement.

SKILL 13-4 Placing a Client on a Bariatric Bed

A valuable resource in the care of the morbidly obese client (a person who weighs more than 100 lb above ideal weight) is the bariatric bed (Figure 13-13), a safe, adaptable surface. The bariatric bed is capable of allowing upright or sitting positions, client transport, and in-bed scales. The bed is equipped with hand controls that allow self-positioning and facilitate independence for the obese client. The full-function hand controls also allow the nurse caring for the obese client to change the bed position and thus facilitate care while reducing risk of staff injury while moving the client. The in-bed scale provides the nurse with a means of obtaining accurate weights and thus improves health care and client dignity. The bed is slightly wider than a standard hospital bed, yet it is within the guidelines for standard door width, which allows movement into and out of a room without difficulty. Because the bariatric bed is capable of supporting weights up to 850 pounds, it provides a stable balanced surface that limits hospital liability should the standard bed frame collapse or the electric motor burn out.

A full- or double-wide bariatric bed can accommodate a client up to 1000 lb. However, when a full- or double-wide bariatric bed is used, it must be assembled in the client's room and cannot be used for transfers because this bed cannot be moved through standard hospital doorways.

A limitation of this bed is the lack of pressure reduction or relief in the mattress. The at-risk obese client should have some type of pressure-relief mattress placed on the bariatric

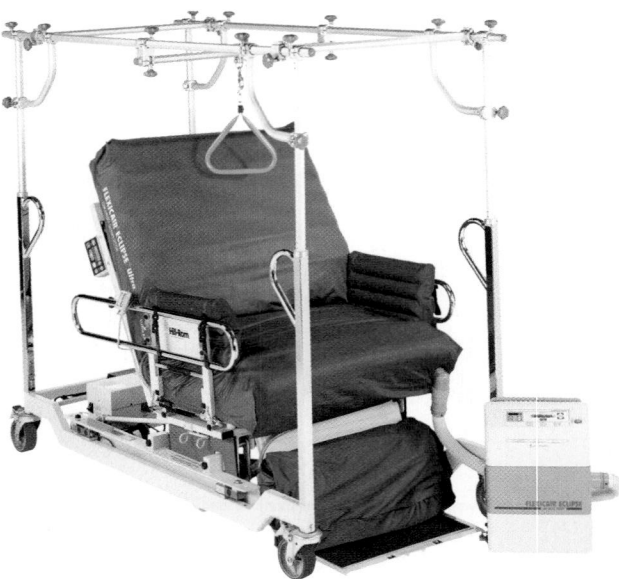

FIGURE 13-13 Bariatric bed with low-air-loss mattress replacement. (© 2002 Hill-Rom Services, Inc. Reprinted with permission. All rights reserved.)

bed. Choices for pressure relief may include static air or gel type of mattresses and low-air-loss replacement systems. These beds also have CPR switches, which permit an immediate hard surface for chest compressions.

DELEGATION CONSIDERATIONS

This skill may be delegated to assistive personnel. When the nurse completes the assessment and determines the need for a specialty bed, the skill of placing the client on a bariatric bed can be delegated to assistive personnel. The number of people needed to assist in safe client transfer from traditional to bariatric bed must be determined. Some types of specialty beds require that the manufacturer's representative set up and maintain the system. When delegating aspects of care for a client on a bariatric bed, the nurse must:

- Instruct assistive personnel to notify the nurse of any changes in the client's skin; the nurse then completes the skin assessment

- Instruct the caregiver to continue regular turning and repositioning of the client and the number of people needed to assist with client position changes
- Instruct the caregiver on specifics about applying, cleaning, and maintaining support surface

EQUIPMENT
❑ Bariatric bed
❑ Pressure-relief mattress overlay
❑ Sheets
❑ Overhead frame (optional
❑ Heavy duty lift

STEP	RATIONALE
ASSESSMENT	
1. Perform hand hygiene.	Reduces transmission of microorganisms.
2. Determine client's risk for pressure ulcer formation using a valid assessment tool (see Chapter 15).	Provides an objective measure of risk consistent between nurse assessments over time (WOCN, 2003).
3. Identify clients who would benefit from the bariatric bed system; assess their mobility status.	Selected for clients who are morbidly obese and who have the potential of being independent in positioning with assistance of a stable surface.
4. Assess condition of client's skin, paying particular attention to potential pressure sites and skinfolds. Determine the need for client to have pressure-relief mattress placed on the bariatric bed.	Data provide baseline to determine any change in client's condition while on the bed.
5. Assess client's and family members' understanding of purpose of bed.	Improves client and family compliance.
6. Review client's medical orders.	A physician's order is usually needed to obtain third-party reimbursement for cost of bed.
7. Assess need for client to be weighed.	Scales are available in many bariatric beds or as underbed scales for beds without in-bed scales.

NURSING DIAGNOSES

- Impaired physical mobility
- Impaired skin integrity
- Ineffective health maintenance
- Deficient knowledge regarding use of support surface mattress

- Ineffective peripheral tissue perfusion
- Risk for impaired skin integrity
- Pain (acute, chronic)

Related factors are individualized based on client's condition or needs.

PLANNING	
1. Expected outcomes following completion of procedure:	
• Client is independent for position changes.	Bed surface is adaptable by hand-operated controls.
• Client's skin remains intact, or existing lesions show evidence of healing.	Skin is free from pressure effects of immobility.
• Client remains free of injury.	Bed is stable to allow for positioning without tipping or bending.
2. Explain procedure and purpose of bed to client and family.	Reduces anxiety and promotes client's cooperation.
3. Review instructions supplied by bed manufacturer.	Promotes safe and correct use of bed.

- **Critical Decision Point**
  Do not exceed weight limits indicated by the manufacturer.

4. For clients with severe to moderate pain, medicate approximately 30 minutes before transfer.	Promotes client's comfort and ability to cooperate during transfer to bed. Decreases client's energy expenditure (Krouskop and van Rijswijk, 1995).
5. Obtain any additional personnel needed to transfer client to bed.	Ensures safety of client and staff by having sufficient personnel to assist in transferring.

IMPLEMENTATION

- **Critical Decision Point**
  Use of this bed is contraindicated in clients with spinal cord injuries.

1. Close client's room door or bedside curtain.	Maintains client's privacy during transfer.
2. Explain steps of transfer.	Reduces anxiety and helps client be part of decision making during maneuvering.

STEP	RATIONALE
3. Put on gloves (if needed) before assisting client to bed using appropriate transfer techniques (see Chapter 10). Depending on client's mobility status, it may be necessary to call for assistance and use a heavy duty lift.	Appropriate transfer techniques maintain alignment and reduce risk of injury to client and health care workers during procedure.
4. Place pull sheet, slide board, hydraulic lifts, or other assistive devices under the client, and transfer safely.	Reduces trauma from friction and shear to client's skin (Pieper, 2000).
5. Cover and position client, and place hand controls within reach. Be certain that the out-of-bed alarm is on, if needed. Attach overhead frame if needed.	Allows for maximal client independence. Alarm alerts caregiver that client has left the bed surface.
6. Encourage client to initiate frequent position changes and move in the bed as much as possible.	Morbidly obese clients quickly increase pressure over bony prominences. Frequent removal (e.g., every 30 to 60 minutes) of pressure from these points assists in reducing the risk for pressure ulcer formation.
7. Remove gloves, and perform hand hygiene.	Reduces transmission of microorganisms.

EVALUATION

1. Inspect condition of client's skin according to agency policy while client is on bed.	Evaluates healing of any existing pressure ulcers. Determines if any new pressure areas are forming.
2. Ask client to rate sense of comfort and safety. Encourage ROM by client	Bed frame is stable for movement and position changes.
3. Evaluate client's risk for injury.	Surface is balanced and allows maximal client independence.
4. Evaluate client's ability to move in bed.	Evaluates effectiveness of bed and education to promote independence.

Recording and Reporting

- Record transfer of client to bed, tolerance of procedure, and condition of skin in nurses' notes or skin assessment flow sheet.
- Report changes in condition of skin to nurse in charge or physician.

Unexpected Outcomes	Related Interventions
1. Existing areas of skin breakdown or pressure areas fail to heal or increase in size or depth.	• Modify skin care regimen. • Consult with skin care expert. • Notify physician.
2. Client is unable to operate bed for position changes independently.	• Reassess client's level of independence and ability to understand instructions. • Reinstruct client and family in how to operate the bed. • Provide for return demonstration regarding bed operation.

Teaching Considerations

- Explain function and purpose of bariatric bed.
- Explain function and purpose of pressure-relief mattress overlay used.
- Explain the need to continue to change position at intervals to diminish effects of immobility.

SKILL 13-5   Placing a Client on a Rotokinetic Bed

The Rotokinetic bed is used to maintain skeletal alignment while providing constant rotation (Figure 13-14). It is used in the care of spinal cord–injured and multitrauma clients. The support structure of the bed outlines the body parts and maintains proper alignment when secured properly. This bed improves skeletal alignment with constant side-to-side rotation up to 90 degrees (Tomaselli, Goldberg, and Wind, 2001). The bed rotates from side to side at a 60- to 90-degree angle every 7 minutes. Turning angles may be adjusted to meet the client's needs. Constant rotation reduces pressure ulcer development and stimulates body systems. It is recommended that the bed stay in the rotation mode for at least 20 hours a day. There is an emergency gatch that can quickly interrupt rotation when needed. To initiate CPR, the bed is returned to the horizontal position and locked in place.

The constant motion may lead to sensory distress for the client, especially older adults. This may be associated with the constant kinetic stimulation, the limited visual field, and inner ear disequilibrium. The nurse must be mindful of these complications and provide necessary emotional support. A physician's order is required for third-party payment.

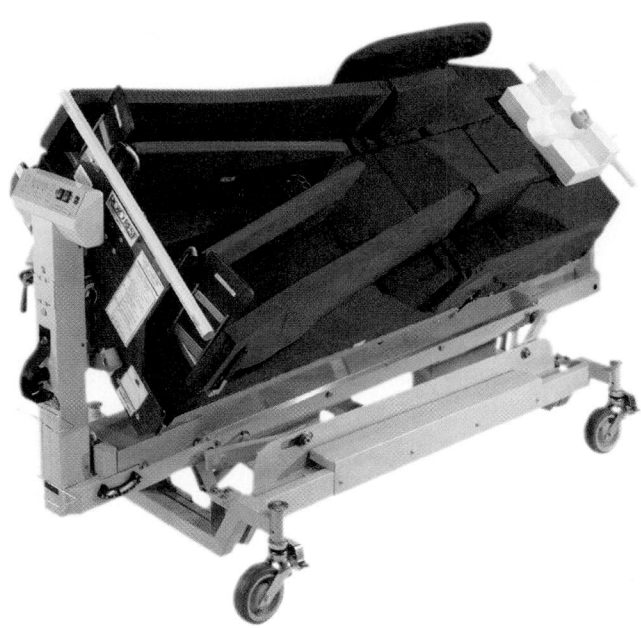

FIGURE **13-14** Rotokinetic bed. (RotoRest—Courtesy Kinetic Concepts, Inc, San Antonio, Tex.)

DELEGATION CONSIDERATIONS

The skill of placing a client on a Rotokinetic bed should not be delegated to assistive personnel. This type of bed is frequently used for clients with multiple trauma or spinal cord injuries, and the nurse must carefully determine what aspects of the client's care may be delegated to the appropriately skilled personnel. When delegating aspects of care for a client on a Rotokinetic bed, the nurse must:

- Instruct assistive personnel to notify the nurse of any changes in the client's skin; the nurse then completes the skin assessment
- Instruct the caregiver in the exact rotation frequency of the bed
- Instruct the caregiver to stop the rotation only for selected aspects of care determined by the nurse (e.g., bathing, oral hygiene, enemas)
- Instruct the caregiver to immediately notify the nurse for client confusion, nausea, and pain

EQUIPMENT
- ❑ Rotokinetic bed with support packs, bolsters, and safety straps (see Figure 13-14)
- ❑ Top sheet
- ❑ Pillowcases for bolsters

STEP	RATIONALE

ASSESSMENT

1. Perform hand hygiene.

2. Determine client's risk for pressure ulcer formation using a validated assessment tool.

    Risk factors for pressure ulcers include nutritional deficits, shear stress, friction, alterations in mobility and perception, moisture, and abnormal serum albumin and hemoglobin levels (see Chapter 15).

3. Perform skin assessment. Inspect condition of skin, especially over dependent sites and bony prominences (see Chapter 15).

Reduces transmission of microorganisms.

Risk assessment tools suggested by AHCPR and WOCN (e.g., Braden scale) provide an objective measure of risk consistent between nurse assessors over time (WOCN, 2003).

Provides baseline to measure ongoing data to determine a change in skin integrity or change in an existing pressure ulcer.

STEP	RATIONALE
4. Review client's medical orders.	Physician's order is needed to receive third-party reimbursement for cost of bed (not required in Canada).
5. Assess client's level of comfort; ask client to rate pain on a scale of 0 to 10.	Provides baseline to determine the client's comfort needs. Nerve endings related to pressure, touch, temperature, and limb position are located in the skin. The Support Surface Consensus Panel identified client comfort as one of the main purposes of support (Krouskop and van Rijswijk, 1995).
6. Assess client's level of orientation.	Baseline used to detect change while client is on bed. Constant motion may lead to sensory distress.
7. Perform pulmonary assessment, and obtain vital signs.	Provides baseline of client's pulmonary status and vital signs. Clients with severe injuries or spinal cord injuries are at risk for accumulation of pulmonary secretions. In addition, when these clients are first placed on the bed, they are at risk of changes in pulse and blood pressure (BP) due to the motion of the bed.
8. Assess client's and family members' understanding of purpose of bed.	Appearance and movement of bed may create anxiety for client and family members.

NURSING DIAGNOSES

- Pain (acute, chronic)
- Anxiety
- Ineffective health maintenance
- Risk for impaired skin integrity
- Kinesthetic sensory/perceptual alterations

- Impaired physical mobility
- Impaired skin integrity
- Risk for infection
- Deficient knowledge regarding the use of Rotokinetic bed
- Ineffective peripheral tissue perfusion

Related factors are individualized based on client's condition or needs.

PLANNING

1. Expected outcomes following completion of procedure:
   - Client's skin remains intact without evidence of abnormal reactive hyperemia or mottling.
   - Existing pressure ulcers show evidence of healing.
   - Client's musculoskeletal system is properly aligned and free of contractures.
   - Client's breath sounds improve from baseline assessment or remain clear to auscultation.
   - Client remains alert, oriented, and cooperative.

   - Client denies nausea or dizziness.
   - Client's blood pressure remains consistent with baseline vital signs.
2. Explain procedure and purpose of bed to client and family.
3. Review instructions supplied by bed manufacturer.
4. Premedicate approximately 30 minutes before transfer.

5. Obtain any additional personnel needed to transfer client to bed.

Skin is free from pressure effects of immobility.

Client is experiencing benefits of bed.
Device provides support and alignment to trunk and extremities.
Client's pulmonary congestion is improving or absent.

Client does not experience sensory perceptual changes from bed positions.
Motion of bed is not negatively affecting client.
Client not experiencing cardiovascular disturbances.

Reduces anxiety and promotes cooperation.

Promotes safe and correct use of bed.
Promotes client's comfort and ability to cooperate during transfer to bed. Decreases client's energy expenditure (Krouskop and van Rijswijk, 1995).
Ensures client's safety.

STEP	RATIONALE

IMPLEMENTATION

1. Close client's room door or bedside curtain.

2. Place Rotokinetic bed in horizontal position, and remove all bolsters, straps, and supports. Close posterior hatches.

3. Unplug electrical cord. Lock gatch.

4. Maintaining proper alignment of the client and using appropriate transfer techniques (see Chapter 10), transfer client to Rotokinetic bed.

5. Secure thoracic panels, bolsters, head and knee packs, and safety straps.

6. Cover client with top sheet.

7. Plug bed in.

8. Have company representative set optional angle as ordered by physician. May gradually increase rotation.

9. Increase degree of rotation gradually according to client's tolerance.

10. It is difficult to maintain eye contact when talking with clients during rotation. Provide adequate space for caregivers and family to move around the bed to facilitate communication.

11. The bed may be stopped for assessment and procedures. To stop the bed, permit bed to rotate to the desired position, turn the motor off, and push knob into a lock position. If necessary, the bed can be manually repositioned.

12. Inform client that there may be a sensation of lightheadedness or falling. However, reassure client that he or she will not fall because the pads are positioned to prevent this and are checked by two people to ensure proper placement.

Rationale (right column):

Maintains client's privacy during transfer.

Prevents accidental rotation during transfer.

Reduces risk of further tissue injury during transfer. May need physician available to assist in transfer.

Maintains proper alignment and prevents sliding during rotation.

Prevents unnecessary exposure.

Rotational angle is determined by physician based on the client's overall condition and tolerance to constant motion.

Gradually increasing rotation may reduce or prevent nausea, dizziness, and orthostatic hypotension (Tomaselli and others, 2001).

Allows opportunity to meet client's psychosocial needs.

Allows nurse to assess client.

Informing client of what to expect will decrease his or her anxiety.

EVALUATION

1. Inspect condition of skin (occipital region, ears, axillae, elbows, sacrum, groin, and heels) and musculoskeletal alignment every 2 hours or more often if indicated by client's condition.

2. Inspect client's pressure ulcers for evidence of healing.

3. Observe alignment and range of motion of all joints.

4. Auscultate lung sounds every shift, and compare with baseline.

5. Determine client's level of orientation once per shift while on bed.

6. Ask whether client is experiencing nausea or dizziness.

7. Monitor blood pressure.

Rationale (right column):

Evaluates healing process of any existing pressure ulcers and determines effectiveness of Rotokinetic therapy.

Evaluates healing process.

Determines if complications (e.g., atelectasis) have developed.

Provides ongoing pulmonary assessment.

Evaluates if sensory overload has developed from excess kinetic stimulation.

Determines if client experiences orthostatic hypotension from position rotation.

Recording and Reporting

- Describe condition of skin before placement on the Rotokinetic bed. A photograph may be taken to document skin condition and provide a baseline for later assessments for progress in healing.

- Record and report time of transfer to Rotokinetic bed and degree of rotation.

- Record and report subjective data indicating response to the constant rotation and presence/absence of dizziness, nausea, or blood pressure changes.

- A flow sheet may be used to document routine assessment and care, including the length of time the bed rotation stopped. The bed needs to be rotating at least 20 hours out of every 24 hours and stopped for no more than 30 minutes at a time.

Unexpected Outcomes	Related Interventions
1. Existing areas of skin breakdown or pressure areas fail to heal or increase in size or depth.	• Evaluate rotation schedule; bed should remain in rotation 20 hours a day to prevent skin breakdown. • Modify skin care regimen.
2. Client experiences hypotension.	• If severe drop in BP, stop rotation, notify physician, remain with client, and monitor vital signs every 5 minutes. • For less severe BP changes, decrease rotational angle. Gradually increase the rotation angle as client adjusts to rotation.
3. Client becomes disoriented, confused, and anxious.	• Reorient client to person, place, time. • Provide audio stimulation, via radio or tapes. • Provide television adapted to Rotokinetic bed (available from manufacturer). • Hang mirror on ceiling so client may view surroundings. • Provide symptomatic relief of motion sickness.
4. Client develops abnormal lung sounds.	• Increase frequency of pulmonary hygiene measures (e.g., cough and deep breathe, suctioning). • Have client use incentive spirometry.
5. Bed fails to rotate.	• Provide for client safety. • Position bed flat. • Follow manufacturer's/agency policies.

Teaching Considerations
- Explain function and purpose of Rotokinetic bed.
- Explain that client may feel sensation of light-headedness or falling. However, client will not fall because pads are positioned to prevent this.

Pediatric Considerations
- Provide age-appropriate education for the child. It is important that the child understand that he or she is secure in the bed and will not fall out as the bed turns.

- Distraction, such as talking books, videos, and music can help the older child adjust to the bed and the restricted mobility.

Gerontological Considerations
- Older adults are at increased risk for sensation of light-headedness or dizziness.

FOCUS *on* CLINICAL PRACTICE

You are assigned to admit Mr. Harold Kline, a 75-year-old who had a severe stroke, which resulted in bilateral sensory and motor loss. There is decreased sensation in all limbs and the trunk region, and the client is unable to change positions or transfer without assistance. He is also hard of hearing, and communicating instructions about his care is difficult. He lives with his wife of 50 years, who is in good health.

1. You anticipate that this client will need a support surface. Before selecting this surface, what assessments will you make?
2. What category of support surface will you select? What is your rationale for this selection?
3. Following consultation with physical therapy and social service, the physician orders an air-suspension bed with lateral rotation because Mr. Kline does have some blistering over bony prominences and his impaired mobility and sensation increase his risk for developing pressure ulcers. Mr. Kline begins experiencing a small amount of nausea and restlessness when initially placed on the air-suspension bed. He tells the assistive personnel, "Nurse, I am afraid that I will fall out of this bed when it tilts. Will I?" What actions should the nurse implement for Mr. Kline's nausea and anxiety?

A 72-year-old Asian-American who resides in a nursing home, Mrs. Weng, is transferred to acute care because of severe diarrhea and dehydration. Up until this illness she was independent and required minimal assistance with her activities of daily living (ADLs). She has a history of severe, painful osteoarthritis and is maintained on tube feedings for a chronic esophageal problem. She is admitted to your facility with blistering and abrasion on her coccyx. After 2 days in the hospital her tube feedings resume, and she is placed on an air-fluidized bed for ease of turning after developing a pressure ulcer on her coccyx.

4. What impact does her culture have on expression of pain, and what is the nurse's response?
5. What special considerations are necessary because of Mrs. Weng's tube-feeding requirement?
6. Ms. Long., an alert 40-year-old client, is admitted to your unit after sustaining multiple trauma from an auto accident and right lower lobe pneumonia. The physician has ordered a Rotokinetic bed. She becomes quite anxious at the appearance of the bed. The assistive personnel overheard Ms. Long. talking to family members about recent experiences with inner ear disturbances. What assessments and nursing actions should take place?

NCLEX REVIEW QUESTIONS

1. Dehydration and/or electrolyte imbalances can occur with which type of specialty bed/mattress?
   1. Egg-crate mattress
   2. Air-suspension bed
   3. Aid-fluidized bed
   4. Bariatric bed
2. Your are caring for a client on a Rotokinetic type of bed. The client complains of sudden dizziness, and you take his blood pressure and note that on lateral rotation the client develops orthostatic hypotension. Your first action is to:
   1. Have the assistive personnel notify the doctor while you assess the client further
   2. Stop the rotation of the bed and assess the client further
   3. Talk to the client and assess for factors that can make him hypotensive
   4. Increase fluids and assess the client further

3. You are caring for a client on an air-filled overlay on the mattress. As you conduct your skin assessment, you notice skin breakdown over the coccyx and left hip. You know that this client has received meticulous skin care and routine repositioning. In addition, he independently changes position when he feels pressure. What are your actions?
   1. Maintain the present mattress
   2. Increase repositioning frequency
   3. Check functioning and filling of mattress
   4. Consider changing to a pressure-relief device
4. Which factor is **not** considered when determining the need to place a client on a bariatric bed?
   1. Client's ability to assist with transfer to the bed
   2. Availability or personnel to reposition client
   3. Ability of the environment to accommodate the bed
   4. Integrity of skin on pressure areas and in skinfold regions

References

Agency for Health Care Policy and Research: *Pressure ulcers in adults: prediction and prevention,* Clinical practice guideline No. 3, Rockville, Md, 1992, U.S. Department of Health and Human Services.

Agency for Health Care Policy and Research, Panel for the Treatment of Pressure Ulcers: *Treatment of pressure ulcers,* Clinical practice guideline No. 15, AHCPR Pub No. 95-0652, Rockville, Md, 1994, U.S. Department of Health and Human Services.

Bryant RA: *Acute and chronic wounds: nursing management,* ed 2, St. Louis, 2000, Mosby.

Fletcher J: Pressure-relieving equipment: criteria and selection, *Br J Nurs* 6(6):323, 1997.

Fulmer T, Abraham I: Rethinking geriatric nursing, *Nurs Clin North Am* 33(3):387, 1998.

Hockenberry MJ and others: *Wong's nursing care of infants and children,* ed 7, St. Louis, 2003, Mosby.

Krouskop T, van Rijswijk L: Standardizing performance-based criteria for support surfaces, *Ostomy Wound Manage* 41(1):34, 1995.

Lueckenotte A: *Gerontologic nursing,* ed 2, St. Louis, 2000, Mosby.

Monahan FD, Neighbors M: *Medical-surgical nursing: foundations for clinical practice,* ed 2, Philadelphia, 1998, WB Saunders.

Morrison MJ: *The prevention and treatment of pressure ulcers,* St. Louis, 2001, Mosby.

National Pressure Ulcer Advisory Panel: *Statement on pressure ulcer prevention,* 1992, http://www.npuap.org/positn1.html, retrieved July 2004.

National Pressure Ulcer Advisory Panel: *Healthy people 2010: ulcer prevention objective,* http://www.npuap.org/HP 2010.html, retrieved July 2004.

Pieper B: Mechanical forces: pressure, shear, and friction. In Bryant RA: *Acute and chronic wounds: nursing management,* ed 2, St. Louis, 2000, Mosby.

Thomas C: Specialty beds: decision-making made easy, *Ostomy Wound Manage* 23:51, 1989.

Tomaselli N, Goldberg E, Wind S: Pressure-reducing devices: lateral rotation therapy. In Lynn-McHale DJ, Carlson KK, editors: *AACN procedural manual for critical care,* ed 4, Philadelphia, 2001, WB Saunders.

Whittemore R: Pressure-reduction support surfaces: a review of the literature, *J Wound Ostomy Continence Nurs* 25(1):6, 1998.

Wound Ostomy and Continence Nurses Society: *Guideline for prevention and management of pressure ulcers.* Glenview, Ill, 2003, The Association.

Research References

Armstrong D, Bortz P: An integrative review of pressure relief in surgical patients, *AORN Online* 73(3):645, 2001.

Bergstrom N and others: Multisite study of incidence of pressure ulcers and the relationship between risk level, demographic characteristics, diagnoses, and prescription of preventive interventions, *J Am Geriatr Soc* 44:22, 1996.

Braden B, Bergstrom BL: Clinical utility of the Braden scale for predicting pressure sore risk, *Decubitus* 2(3):44, 1989.

Cullum N and others: Beds, mattresses and cushions for pressure sore preventions and treatment, *Cochrane Review,* The Cochrane Library, Issue 3, 2000.

Cullum N and others: Beds, mattresses and cushions for pressure sore preventions and treatment, *Cochrane Database Syst Rev* 1(1), most recent update April 2003.

Jiricka MK and others: Pressure ulcer risk factors in an ICU population, *Am J Crit Care* 4(5):361, 1995.

Koziak M: Etiology of decubitus ulcers, *Arch Phys Med Rehabil* 42:19, 1961.

Lyder CH and others: Validating the Braden scale for the prediction of pressure ulcer risk in Black and Latino/Hispanic elders: a pilot study, *Ostomy Wound Manage* 44(suppl A):42s, 1998.

National Pressure Ulcer Advisory Panel Board of Directors, Cuddigan J and others: Pressure ulcers in America: prevalence, incidence, and implications for the future—an executive summary of National Pressure Ulcer Advisory Panel report monograph, *Adv Skin Wound Care* 14(4):208, 2001.

Vyhlidal S and others: Mattress replacement or foam overlay: a prospective study on the incidence of pressure ulcers, *Appl Nurs Res* 10(3):111, 1997.

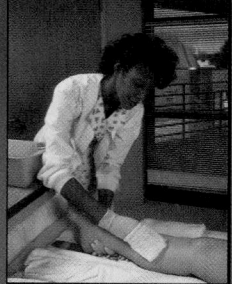

14

Personal Hygiene and Bed Making

MEDIA RESOURCES

Evolve Site *evolve*

http://evolve.elsevier.com/Perry/skills
- Weblinks
- Video clips
- Mosby's Nursing Skills Video Exercises

Mosby's Nursing Skills Videos/CD-ROM
- *Bedmaking Video:* Making the occupied bed; making a mitered corner and toe pleat
- *Personal Hygiene and Grooming Video:* Oral hygiene, oral care for the unconscious person, denture cleaning, and precautions for the person at risk of aspiration; hair care, shampooing in bed; shaving a male; nail and foot care; dressing

OBJECTIVES

Mastery of content in this chaper will enable the nurse to:

- Discuss guidelines used to provide personal hygiene to clients.
- Identify principles of aseptic technique applied while administering a bed bath.
- Administer a complete bed bath.
- Explain precautions to take when assisting clients with a tub bath or shower.
- Discuss precautions used to minimize transmission of infection during perineal care.
- Identify guidelines to follow when administering oral hygiene.
- Explain differences in providing oral hygiene to dependent versus unconscious clients.
- Administer oral hygiene correctly to a client.
- Discuss precautions used to prevent breakage of dentures.
- Identify guidelines for administering hair, nail, and foot care.
- Comb, brush, and shampoo the hair of a bedridden client.
- Shave a male or female client.
- Identify risk factors for foot and nail problems.
- Safely administer nail care.
- Change the linen on an occupied bed.

KEY TERMS

Alopecia	Mastication
Aspiration	Necrotic
Buccal	Neuropathy
Cerumen	NPO
Cheilosis	Periodontal
Cuticle	Periodontitis
Dental caries	Plaque
Dermatitis	Podiatrist
Flossing	Pruritus
Gag reflex	Sebaceous gland
Gingivae	Sebum
Gingivitis	Stomatitis
Halitosis	Tartar
Humectant	Tepid
Hygiene	Vellus
Maceration	Xerostomia

Many clients require assistance with personal hygiene or must learn or adapt new hygiene techniques. Hygiene is the science of health. Maintenance of personal hygiene is necessary for an individual's health, comfort, safety, and sense of well-being. When performing hygiene, a nurse has the opportunity to interact with clients to discuss emotional, social, and health-related concerns. In addition, administering a bath or nail care is an excellent time to conduct a physical assessment. The nurse needs to convey sensitivity and respect for the client's personal beliefs and habits and ensure a client as much privacy as possible.

The Skin

The skin is the largest organ in the body. It provides protection from the external environment and is the first line of defense against external injury and infection. The skin's functions include protection, vitamin synthesis, sensory perception, excretion, processing of antigenic substances, and temperature regulation (Sheppard and Brenner, 2000). Three primary layers make up the skin: the epidermis, dermis, and subcutaneous tissue. The skin covers the entire surface of the body and is continuous with mucous membranes of the mouth, eyes, ears, nose, vagina, and rectum. Thorough hygiene is essential for the integrity and function of each layer.

The epidermis, or outer skin layer, contains several thin layers of cells undergoing different stages of maturation. The innermost layer continually produces new cells that migrate to the outer layer, the stratum corneum, where dead cells are shed from the epidermal surface. Sebum, secreted from hair follicles from sebaceous glands, provides an acidic coating that leaves the skin with a pH between 4 and 6.8 (Sheppard and Brenner, 2000). This acid mantle protects the epidermis against penetration from chemicals and microorganisms. It also minimizes loss of water and plasma proteins.

Bacteria reside on the skin's outer surface. These resident bacteria are normal flora that do not cause disease but inhibit multiplication of disease-causing microorganisms. Transient bacteria that arise from objects coming in contact with the skin are also present. Bathing removes dead cells and bacteria and helps maintain skin integrity.

The dermis contains bundles of collagen and elastic fibers to support the epidermis. Nerve fibers, blood vessels, sweat glands, sebaceous glands, and hair follicles are found in the dermis. Sebum lubricates skin and hair. Two types of sweat glands, the eccrine and the apocrine glands, are distributed over the skin's surface. Eccrine glands secrete a watery fluid (sweat) that assists in temperature control through evaporation. The apocrine glands secrete sweat in the axillary and genital areas. Bacterial decomposition of sweat from the apocrine glands causes body odor.

The subcutaneous tissue layer contains blood vessels, nerves, lymph tissue, and loose connective tissue filled with fat cells. Fatty tissue insulates the body. Subcutaneous tissue also provides support for upper skin layers.

Because a portion of the skin is usually exposed to environmental irritants and it is an active organ sensitive to physiological changes within the body, some skin problems commonly occur (Table 14-1). The nurse assesses for the presence of such conditions while providing hygiene and suggests measures to alleviate these conditions. The client is always the best resource to explain the nature and course of skin problems as they develop. Skin problems can cause changes that affect a client's appearance and body image. The nurse should be sensitive to the client's feelings while attempting to care for a skin problem.

TABLE 14-1   COMMON SKIN PROBLEMS

Problem	Characteristics	Implications	Interventions
Dry skin	Flaky, rough, chapping skin resulting from lack of moisture in the outer stratum corneum, resulting in a less pliable epidermis (Sheppard and Brenner, 2000). Most common on anterior surfaces of lower legs, knees, elbows, and backs of hands.	Skin may crack, bleed, and become inflamed. As a result, redness, pruritus, and discomfort may develop.	Effective treatment of dry skin does not include limiting frequency of bathing, but lies in the use of moisturizers afterward (Sheppard and Brenner, 2000). Use superfatted soap (e.g., Dove) for cleansing. Rinse body of all soap well, because residue left can cause irritation and breakdown. Add moisture to air through use of humidifier. Increase fluid intake when skin is dry. Use emollient creams with vitamin E; cream forms an occlusive film that coats the skin surface to reduce evaporation (Sheppard and Brenner, 2000).
Acne Moderate acne.	Inflammatory, papulopustular skin eruption, usually involving bacterial breakdown of sebum; appears on face, neck, shoulders, and back.	Infected material within pustule can spread if area is squeezed or picked. Permanent scarring can result.	Wash hair and skin each day with warm water and soap to remove oil. Use cosmetics sparingly because oily cosmetics or creams accumulate in pores and tend to make condition worse. Dietary restrictions may need to be implemented. Foods found to aggravate condition should be eliminated from diet. Use prescribed topical antibiotics for severe acne.
Hirsutism Hirsutism.	Excessive growth of body and facial hair, especially in women.	Hirsutism may cause negative body image by giving female a male appearance.	Shaving is safest method to remove hair. Electrolysis and laser permanently remove hair. Tweezing and bleaching are temporary.
Skin rashes	Skin eruption that may result from overexposure to sun or moisture or from allergic reaction; may be flat or raised, localized or systemic, pruritic or nonpruritic.	If skin is continually scratched, inflammation and infection may occur. Rashes can also cause discomfort.	Wash area thoroughly, and apply antiseptic spray or lotion to prevent further itching and aid healing process. Warm soaks may relieve inflammation.
Contact dermatitis Contact dermatitis.	Acute or chronic eczematous rash characterized by abrupt onset with well-defined geometric margins of erythema, pruritus, pain, and appearance of scaly oozing lesions. Appears on head, neck, scalp, hands, legs, dorsum of feet, and trunk.	Dermatitis is often difficult to eliminate because person is usually in continual contact with substance causing skin reaction. Substance may be hard to identify.	Identify and avoid contributing agents (e.g., cleansers, poison ivy or oak, cosmetics, shoes/rubber). Topical, intralesional or systemic steroids are prescribed to reduce inflammation. Cool, moist compresses and tepid baths have a soothing effect (Ignatavicius and Workman, 2002).
Abrasion Abrasion of the skin.	Scraping or rubbing away of epidermis; may result in localized bleeding and later weeping of serous fluid.	Infection occurs easily as result of loss of protective skin layer.	Nurses should always be careful not to scratch clients with their jewelry or fingernails. Wash abrasions with mild soap and water. Dressing or bandage could increase risk of infection because of retained moisture.

The Mouth

The oral cavity, which is lined with a normally moist, intact mucous membrane, contains the teeth and gums. Normally the mucosa is light pink and moist. The membranous lining protects underlying organs, secretes mucus to keep the oral cavity lubricated, and absorbs water, salts, and other solutes. Saliva, a clear viscous fluid secreted by the mucous and salivary glands of the mouth, moistens the oral cavity, initiates digestion of starches, provides a means for removing cellular and bacterial debris, and aids in the chewing and swallowing of food. In a normal healthy mouth, resident florae combine with salivary proteins and glycoproteins to form plaque. Normally, the mechanical motions of chewing facilitate the production and movement of saliva around the mouth (Stiefel and others, 2000). These motions are important in suppressing bacterial and fungal colonization but are absent in unconscious clients.

The teeth are organs of chewing, or mastication. Dentin, a hard, ivory-like substance that surrounds the pulp cavity, forms the major part of a tooth (Figure 14-1). A layer of enamel, visible in the oral cavity, covers the upper portion of the tooth, or crown. The periodontal membrane, just below the gum margins, surrounds the tooth root and holds it firmly in place. A tooth receives its blood, lymph, and nerve supply from the base of the tooth socket within the jaw. Healthy teeth are smooth, shiny, and properly aligned.

The gums, or gingivae, are mucous membranes with underlying supportive fibrous tissue. They encircle the necks of erupted teeth to hold them firmly in place. The gums are normally pink, moist, firm, and relatively inelastic.

Structures of the oral cavity must receive regular hygiene to remain healthy for a person's comfort, sense of well-being, maintenance of nutrition, and protection from infection (Beighton and others, 1999). Even a minor alteration of the oral cavity, such as inflammation of the gums, can create a significant health problem. Appetite is diminished, taste may be altered, and the discomfort from inflammation can become an annoying irritant. Thorough oral hygiene maintains the integrity of oral cavity structures.

The Hair

Hair grows from follicles located within the dermis of the skin (Figure 14-2). Tiny blood vessels supply each follicle with nourishment necessary for normal hair growth. Each hair has a shaft extending from the follicle. Sebaceous glands secrete the oily substance sebum into each follicle, which lubricates the hair and scalp. The hair shaft is normally shiny and pliant and is not excessively oily, dry, or brittle.

The primary function of hair is protection. For example, hair protects the scalp from injury. Eyebrows and eyelashes protect the eyes from foreign particles. Two types of hair cover the body. Terminal hair is the long, coarse, thick hair that is easily visible on the scalp, axillae, and pubic area. Special hair care practices focus primarily on care of terminal hair. Vellus is the soft, fine hair that covers the entire body except for the palms of the hands, fingertips, soles of the feet, tips of the toes, and part of the genitalia. Hair growth, distribution, and pattern can be indicators of a person's health status. Hormonal changes, emotional and physical stress, aging, intake of toxins (e.g., arsenic, cocaine), gender, race, nutrition, infection, and certain diseases can affect hair characteristics. The hair shaft is inert; any change in its color or condition occurs as a result of hormonal activity and nutrient supply to the hair follicle. For example, a reduction in the serum protein level will result in hair becoming dry and brittle.

A person's appearance and sense of well-being often depend on the way the hair looks and feels. Illness or disability may prevent clients from maintaining daily hair care. An immobilized client's hair soon becomes tangled if not brushed or combed regularly. Dressings may leave sticky adhesive, blood, or antiseptic solutions on the hair. Diaphoresis leaves hair oily and unmanageable. Proper hair care is important to a person's body image.

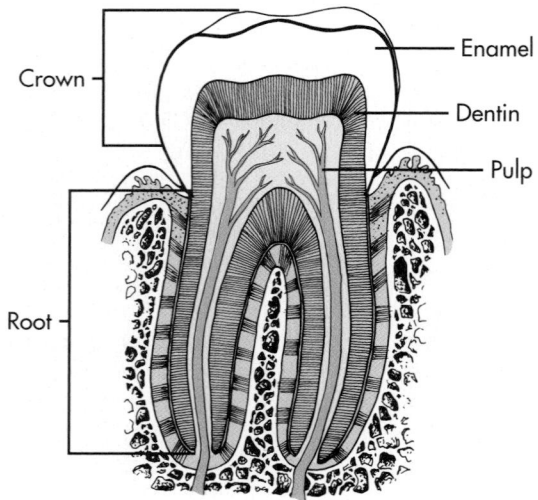

FIGURE 14-1 Normal tooth.

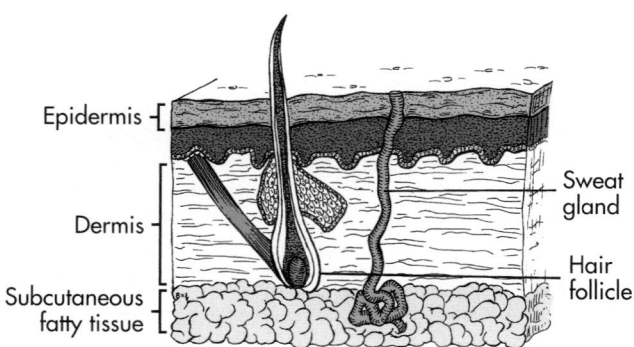

FIGURE 14-2 Cross section of hair follicle and supporting structures.

The Nails

The nails are epithelial tissues that grow from the root of the nail bed, located in the skin at the nail groove. A normal healthy nail is transparent, smooth, and convex, with a pink nail bed and translucent white tip. A normal color indicates adequate oxygenation to peripheral tissues. Pigment deposits or bands are common in nail beds of clients with dark skin. The nail bed angle should measure 160 degrees. The nail is surrounded by a cuticle, which slowly grows over the nail and must be regularly pushed back. The skin around the nail beds and cuticles should be smooth and without inflammation. Disease causes changes in the shape, thickness, and curvature of the nails.

The feet and nails require special care to prevent infection, odor, and injury. Problems typically result from abuse or poor care. The feet are important to physical and emotional health. Foot pain can often change a walking gait, causing strain on different muscle groups.

Evidence-Based Practice Trends

In a landmark study, dry skin was shown to be associated with the development of pressure ulcers (Guralnik and others, 1988). One subgroup of the population most at risk for dry skin is older adults. Research was recently conducted on interventions for reducing dry skin in older adults. Sheppard and Brenner (2000) tested the Bag Bath/Travel Bath with traditional bathing techniques for effects on skin dryness. The Bag Bath/Travel Bath, which contains a no-rinse surfactant, a humectant to trap moisture, and an emollient, significantly reduced overall skin dryness, especially skin flaking and scaling. There are now several commercial body cleansing systems available that contain the same ingredients as the Bag Bath.

Bathing can create high levels of discomfort in clients who suffer dementia. Bathing tends to increase agitation and aggression in these clients. Dunn and others (2002) measured the frequency of agitated behaviors during bathing in 15 older adult residents with dementia. The conventional tub bath was compared with the Thermal bath (no-rinse bathing with nine washcloths soaked in 300 ml of warm water and a nonrinse cleanser). For all behaviors combined, the Thermal bath caused significantly fewer agitated behaviors. Bed bath variations such as the Thermal bath may reduce agitation in the demented client.

Another area of evidence-based practice is the establishment of oral hygiene practice guidelines. Much attention has been given to the critically ill client. The colonization of bacteria within the oropharynx has been associated with several systemic diseases, including cardiovascular disease, chronic obstructive pulmonary disease, and ventilator-assisted pneumonia (Grap and others, 2003). Research has focused on the agents that best reduce bacterial growth within the oral cavity. The skill of performing mouth care for the unconscious or debilitated client (see Skill 14-3) has incorporated recommendations from three studies to improve oral hygiene in the critically ill.

Cultural Considerations

Each culture is unique in the way members perform personal hygiene. In addition, because hygiene is a personal matter, clients from different cultures will vary in their perceptions of who can assist in their care.

- Maintain privacy, especially of women from cultural groups that value female modesty.
- Uncovering the lower torso and exposing the arms should be avoided among Middle Eastern and East Asian women.
- Allow family member to participate in the care of clients by adapting the schedule of hygiene activities when they are present.
- Provide gender-congruent care for Hindu, Orthodox Jewish, Muslim, and Amish clients.
  - Male clients from these cultures prefer to be cared for by males and female clients by females.
  - Touching is taboo between unrelated males and females.
  - The client or close kin should do personal hygiene involving the lower torso if gender-congruent caregivers are not available.
- Respect cultural and religious practices relevant to hygienic practices.
  - Among Asians (Chinese, Japanese, Koreans, and Hindus) the top parts of the body are considered cleaner than the lower parts.
  - Among Hindus it is considered irreverent to show negative nonverbal communication when washing the elder's feet (Galanti, 2003).
  - Among Hindus and Muslims the left hand is used for cleaning, while the right hand is reserved for eating and praying.

Skill Performance Guidelines

1. Consider clients' cultural preferences in regard to grooming techniques.
2. Consider clients' normal grooming routines, including type of hygiene products used and the time of day when hygiene is routinely performed. Individualize your care based on clients' preferences. However, caution clients against use of products that can damage skin or teeth or injure hair and nails.
3. Wear gloves whenever there is risk of contacting body fluids.
4. Control environmental factors that may alter skin integrity, such as moisture, heat, and external sources of pressure such as wrinkled bed linen and improperly placed drainage tubing.
5. Encourage clients and family or significant other to participate in hygienic care.
6. Establish a regular oral hygiene routine that the client can easily follow at home. Ideal dental hygiene requires brushing after every meal and before bed and flossing at least once a day, the ideal being after each meal.

7. Dental hygiene can improve the client's comfort level. Persons who are mouth breathers, are using oxygen, are unable to eat or drink, have nasogastric tubes inserted, or have had trauma or surgery of the mouth will benefit from frequent oral care (e.g., every 2 hours).

8. Use the time spent providing mouth care to teach clients about factors that increase the incidence of dental or gum disease and the techniques that ensure good oral hygiene.

SKILL 14-1 Bathing and Perineal Care

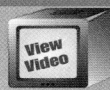

The bath has always been intended as part of the healing process (Dunn and others, 2002). Bathing removes sweat, oil, dirt, and microorganisms from the skin. It also stimulates circulation and provides a refreshed and relaxed feeling. A bath can provide a time for socialization and pleasure, especially for clients who are bedridden or seriously disabled.

The Panel for Prediction and Prevention of Pressure Ulcers (Agency for Health Care Policy and Research [AHCPR], 1992) made important recommendations for bathing. The guidelines are designed to prevent and treat pressure ulcers, but are also sound principles for good bathing techniques.

- Clean the skin at the time of soiling and at routine intervals. Frequency of cleansing should be individualized according to client need and preference. Problems such as incontinence, wound drainage, or excessive diaphoresis may require bathing several times a day.
- Avoid hot water, and use a mild cleansing agent that minimizes irritation.
- During cleansing of the skin avoid use of force and friction.
- Minimize environmental factors that lead to skin drying such as low humidity (less than 40%) and exposure to cold. Additional guidelines to apply in bathing include:
  - Protect clients from injury by assessing and controlling the bathwater temperature. This is especially important for older adults and others with reduced sensation such as diabetics with peripheral neuropathy or spinal cord–injured clients.
  - Use bathing as a time to interact with and assess a client. When giving a complete bath, a nurse can examine a variety of body systems and discuss issues of concern for the client.
  - During bathing assist clients through normal joint range-of-motion (ROM) exercises to promote circulation and joint integrity.
  - For clients who fatigue easily, consider administering a partial versus complete bed bath.

There are two categories of baths: cleansing and therapeutic. Cleansing baths include the bed bath, tub bath, sponge bath at the sink, shower, and the Bag Bath/Travel Bath (Box 14-1). The type of cleansing bath a nurse provides depends on the client's physical capabilities and the degree of hygiene required. The nurse is responsible for deciding what type of bath is most appropriate for the client. When a person is unable to perform personal care during illness or

BOX 14-1 Types of Baths

Complete bed bath—Bath administered to totally dependent client in bed.

Partial bed bath—Bed bath that consists of bathing only body parts that would cause discomfort if left unbathed, such as the hands, face, axillae, and perineal area. Partial bath also includes washing back and providing back rub. Dependent clients in need of partial hygiene or self-sufficient bedridden clients who are unable to reach all body parts receive a partial bed bath.

Sponge bath at the sink—Involves bathing from a bath basin or sink with client sitting in a chair. Client is able to perform a portion of the bath independently. Assistance is needed from the nurse for hard-to-reach areas.

Tub bath—Involves immersion in a tub of water that allows more thorough washing and rinsing than a bed bath. Client may still require the nurse's assistance. Some institutions have tubs equipped with lifting devices that facilitate positioning dependent clients in the tub.

Shower—Client sits or stands under a continuous stream of water. The shower provides more thorough cleansing than a bed bath but can be fatiguing.

Bag Bath/Travel Bath—Developed by Skewes (1994), the Bag Bath contains several soft, nonwoven cotton cloths that are premoistened in a solution of no-rinse surfactant cleanser and emollient. The Bag Bath offers an alternative because of the ease of use, reduced time bathing, and client comfort.

disability, the nurse is responsible for assisting with bathing. This also provides time for cleaning and grooming hair, shaving, and cleansing of nails. Many of the procedures can be done during or immediately after a bath.

Therapeutic baths are generally ordered by physicians for a specific effect, such as soothing the skin or promoting healing. Types of therapeutic baths include:

1. *Sitz bath*—cleanses and reduces pain and inflammation of perineal and anal areas. Used for a client who has undergone rectal or perineal surgery or childbirth or has local irritation from hemorrhoids or fissures. The client sits in a special tub or basin (see Chapter 40).

2. *Medicated bath (oatmeal, cornstarch, sodium bicarbonate, Aveeno, Burow's solution)*—aids in relief of skin irritation and creates an antibacterial and drying effect. Oatmeal has added effect of softening and lubricating the skin.

Perineal care involves thorough cleansing of the client's external genitalia and surrounding skin. A client routinely receives perineal care during a bath. However, there are clients at risk for acquiring an infection and who need more frequent perineal care. These clients include those who have fecal incontinence, an indwelling Foley catheter, or who are recovering from rectal or genital surgery or childbirth. Disposable gloves must be worn during perineal care because of the risk of contacting infectious microorganisms, such as human immunodeficiency virus (HIV), herpes virus, or *Chlamydia.*

DELEGATION CONSIDERATIONS

The skills of bathing and perineal care may be delegated to assistive personnel. The nurse provides assistive personnel with information, assistance, and direction, including:

- Importance of not massaging reddened skin areas during bathing
- Recognizing early signs of impaired skin integrity
- Proper ways to position male and female clients with musculoskeletal limitations or who have an indwelling Foley catheter or other equipment (e.g., intravenous tubing)
- When to report changes in the skin or perineal area to the nurse

EQUIPMENT

- ❑ Washcloths and bath towels
- ❑ Bath blanket
- ❑ Soap and soap dish
- ❑ Toiletry items (deodorant, powder, lotion)
- ❑ Toilet tissue or diaper wipes
- ❑ Warm water
- ❑ Clean hospital gown or client's own pajamas or gown
- ❑ Laundry bag
- ❑ Disposable gloves (when risk for contacting body fluids)
- ❑ Washbasin

Perineal Care

- ❑ Waterproof pad or bedpan
- ❑ Disposable gloves
- ❑ Additional supplies when pericare is given other than during a bath: cotton balls or swabs, a solution bottle or container filled with warm water or prescribed rinsing solution, waterproof bag

STEP	RATIONALE

ASSESSMENT

1. Assess client's tolerance for bathing: activity tolerance, comfort level during movement, cognitive ability, musculoskeletal function, presence of shortness of breath.

2. Assess client's visual status, ability to sit without support, hand grasp, ROM of extremities (see Chapter 18).

3. Assess for presence of equipment (e.g., intravenous [IV] line or oxygen tubing).

4. Assess client's bathing preferences: frequency of and time of day bathing preferred, type of hygiene products used, and other factors related to cultural diversity.

5. Ask if client has noticed any problems related to condition of skin and genitalia: excess moisture, inflammation, drainage or excretions from lesions or body cavities, rashes or other skin lesions.

6. Before or during bath, assess condition of client's skin. Note the presence of dryness, indicated by flaking, redness, scaling, and cracking. You may choose to use a tool such as the Skin Condition Data Form (SCDF) (Hardy, 1996).

7. Identify risks for skin impairment:
   a. Immobilization (e.g., clients with paralysis, immobilized extremities, traction; weakened or disabled clients)
   b. Reduced sensation (e.g., paresthesias, circulatory insufficiency, neuropathies)
   c. Nutritional and hydration alterations

Determines client's ability to perform bathing. Also determines type of bath to administer (e.g., tub bath, partial bed bath).
Determines degree of assistance needed for bathing.

Affects how nurse will plan bathing activities.

Client participates in plan of care. Promotes client's comfort and willingness to cooperate.

Provides nurse with information to direct physical assessment of skin and genitalia during bathing. Also influences selection of skin care products.

Provides a baseline for comparison over time in determining if bathing improves condition of skin.

Risk factors increase the likelihood of injury to the skin because of pressure, impaired tissue synthesis, softening of or friction on tissues, and impaired circulation (see Chapter 15).

STEP	RATIONALE

    d. Excessive moisture on skin, particularly on skin surfaces that rub against each other (e.g., under breasts, in perineal area)

    e. Vascular insufficiencies

    f. External devices applied to or around skin (e.g., casts, braces, restraints, dressings, catheters, tubes)

    g. Older adult clients

    h. Shear or friction (sliding down in bed)

    i. Incontinence (bowel or bladder)

    j. Allergies

    k. Poor score on pressure ulcer risk assessment tool (see Chapter 15)

8. Assess client's knowledge of skin hygiene in terms of its importance, preventive measures to take, and common problems encountered (see Table 14-1). — Determines client's learning needs.

9. Check physician's therapeutic bath order for type of solution, length of time for bath, body part to be attended. — Therapeutic baths are ordered for specific physical effect, which may include promotion of healing or soothing effect.

10. Review orders for specific precautions concerning client's movement or positioning. — Prevents accidental injury to client during bathing activities. Determines level of assistance required by client.

NURSING DIAGNOSES

- Activity intolerance
- Bathing/hygiene self-care deficit
- Impaired skin integrity
- Deficient knowledge regarding skin care
- Risk for impaired skin integrity

- Risk for infection
- Impaired physical mobility

Related factors are individualized based on client's condition or needs.

PLANNING

1. Expected outcomes following completion of procedure:
- Skin and genitalia are free of excretions, drainage, or odor. — Skin is clean.
- Previous skin lesions are cleaner, with less drainage. — Wound debris removed. Size of a lesion does not change after one bathing.
- Skin shows decreased redness, cracking, flaking, and scaling over subsequent baths. — Indicates reduction in skin dryness.
- Joint ROM remains same or improves from previous measurement. — Repeated ROM exercise during bathing helps prevent contractures and promotes joint movement.
- Client expresses sense of comfort and relaxation. — Bath relaxes client and removes sources of discomfort.
- Client tolerates bath without fatigue or chilling. — Fatigue during bathing can indicate worsening of chronic cardiopulmonary conditions.
- Client describes benefits and techniques of proper hygiene and skin care. — Demonstrates learning.

2. Explain procedure, and ask client for suggestions on how to prepare supplies. If partial bath, ask how much of bath client wishes to complete. — Promotes client's cooperation and participation.

3. Adjust room temperature and ventilation, close room doors and windows, and draw room divider curtain. — Warm room that is free of drafts prevents rapid loss of body heat during bathing. Privacy ensures client's mental and physical comfort.

4. Prepare equipment and supplies. — Avoids interrupting procedure or leaving client unattended to retrieve missing equipment.

5. If it is necessary to leave the room, be sure call light is within reach of client. — Provides for client's safety.

STEP	RATIONALE

IMPLEMENTATION

COMPLETE OR PARTIAL BED BATH

1. Offer client bedpan or urinal. Provide towel and wash-cloth.

    Client will feel more comfortable after voiding. Prevents interruption of bath.

2. Perform hand hygiene. Apply clean disposable gloves.

    Reduces transmission of microorganisms.

- *Critical Decision Point*

    Apply gloves if there is actual or risk for drainage or secretions on client's skin.

3. Raise bed to comfortable working height. Lower side rail closest to you, and assist client in assuming comfortable supine position, maintaining body alignment. Bring client toward side closest to you.

    Aids nurse's access to client. Maintains client's comfort throughout procedure. Nurse does not have to reach across bed, thus minimizing strain on back muscles.

4. Place bath blanket over client, and remove top sheet without exposing client. Have client hold top of bath blanket as linen is removed. Place soiled linen in laundry bag. Take care to not allow linen to contact uniform.

    Blanket provides warmth and privacy.

5. Remove client's gown or pajamas.

    Provides full exposure of body parts during bathing.

    a. If an extremity is *injured* or has reduced mobility, begin removal from *unaffected* side first.

    Undressing unaffected side first allows easier manipulation of gown over body part with reduced ROM.

    b. If client has IV line, ask for assistance from the primary nurse, charge nurse, or instructor. Steps to follow with standard IV include removing gown from arm *without* IV first (see illustrations). Then remove gown from arm with IV. Remove IV from pole, and slide IV container and tubing through arm of client's gown. Rehang IV container, and check flow rate. Regulate if necessary. Gowns with sleeves that snap may also be available for clients with IVs.

    Manipulation of IV tubing and container may disrupt flow rate.

    c. If IV pump is in use, turn pump off, clamp tubing, remove tubing from pump, and proceed as in step b. Insert tubing into pump, unclamp tubing, and turn pump on at correct rate. Observe flow rate, and regulate if necessary.

    Regulation is needed to prevent improper infusion of fluids.

6. Pull side rail up. If it is necessary to leave client's room, place bed temporarily in low position, then raise upon return. Fill washbasin two-thirds full with warm water. Check water temperature, and then have client place fingers in water to test temperature tolerance. Place plastic container of bath lotion in bathwater to warm, if desired.

    Raising side rail and lowering bed maintains client's safety as nurse leaves bedside. Warm water promotes comfort, relaxes muscles, and prevents unnecessary chilling. Testing temperature prevents accidental burns. Bathwater warms lotion for application to client's skin.

7. Place bath basin and supplies on over-bed table over bed. Then lower side rail, and remove pillow if allowed, and raise head of bed 30 to 45 degrees. Place bath towel under client's head. Place second bath towel over client's chest.

    Allows nurse to move to opposite side of bed without having to move equipment. Removal of pillow makes it easier to wash client's ears and neck. Placement of towels prevents soiling of bed linen and bath blanket.

STEP	RATIONALE

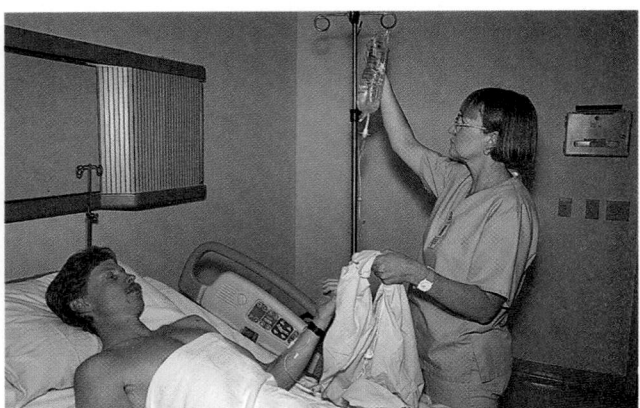

STEP **5b** **A,** Remove client's gown. **B,** Remove IV bag from pole. **C,** Slide IV tubing and bag through arm of client's gown. **D,** Rehang IV bag.

8. Wash face.
   a. Inquire if client is wearing contact lenses. If so, perform eye care as described in Chapter 16.

   b. Form mitt with washcloth (see illustration). Immerse mitt in water, and wring thoroughly.

Prevents accidental injury to eyes.

Mitt retains water and heat better than loosely held washcloth; keeps cold edges from brushing against client, and prevents splashing.

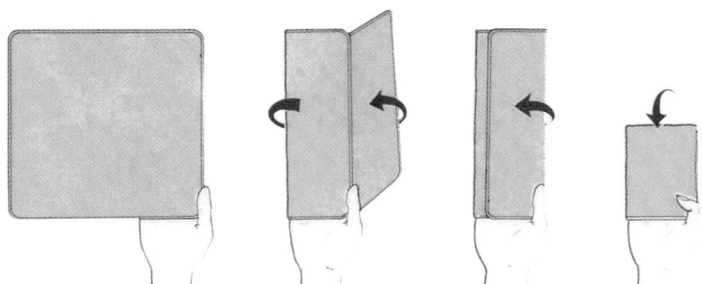

STEP **8b** Steps for folding washcloth to form a mitt.

STEP	RATIONALE

c. Wash client's eyes with plain warm water, using a clean area of cloth for each eye, bathing from inner to outer canthus (see illustration). Soak any crusts on eyelid for 2 to 3 minutes with damp cloth before attempting removal. Dry around eyes gently and thoroughly.

Soap irritates eyes. Use of separate sections of mitt reduces infection transmission. Bathing eye gently from inner to outer canthus prevents secretions from entering naso-lacrimal duct. Pressure can cause internal injury.

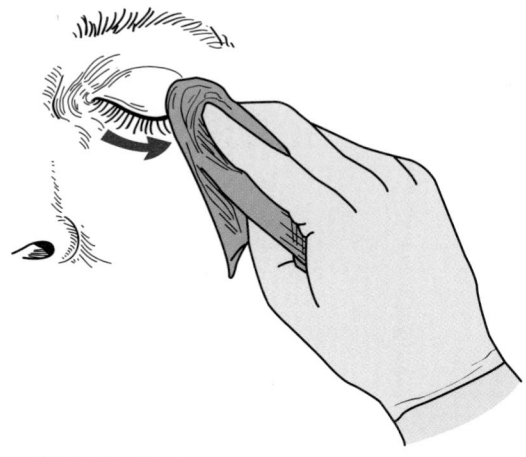

STEP **8c** Wash eye from inner to outer canthus.

d. Ask if client prefers to use soap on face. Otherwise, wash, rinse, and dry forehead, cheeks, nose, neck, and ears without using soap. Ask men if they want to be shaved (see Skill 14-4).

Soap tends to dry face, which is exposed to air more than other body parts.

9. Provide eye care for the unconscious client.
    a. Cleanse the eyelids with a washcloth from the inner to outer canthus using plain warm water.

Clients who are unconscious have lost the normal protective corneal reflex of blinking, increasing the risk for corneal drying, abrasions, and eye infection.

    b. Instill prescribed eye drops or ointment per physician's order (see Chapter 20).
    c. In the absence of a blink reflex the eyelids may be kept closed and covered with an eye patch or shield. Do not tape the eyelid.

Eyelids should be kept closed to keep eyes moist and prevent injury. Taping can injure the eyelid (American Society of Health-System Pharmacists, 2002).

10. Wash trunk and upper extremities.
    a. Remove bath blanket from client's arm. Place bath towel lengthwise under arm. Bathe with minimal soap and water using long, firm strokes from distal to proximal (fingers to axilla).

Long, firm strokes promote venous return.

STEP	RATIONALE

b. Raise and support arm above head (if possible) to wash, rinse, and dry axilla thoroughly (see illustration). Apply deodorant or powder to underarms if desired or needed.

Movement of arm exposes axilla and exercises joint's normal ROM. Respect client's preferences in use of hygienic products.

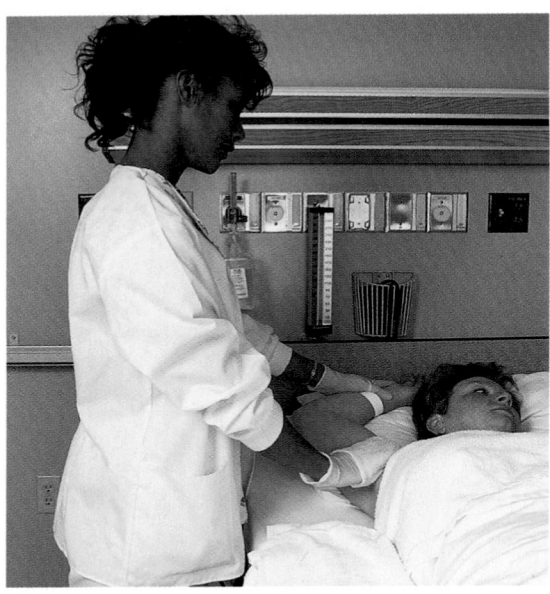

STEP 10b Positioning the arm to wash the axilla.

c. Move to other side of bed and repeat steps a and b with other arm.

d. Cover client's chest with bath towel and fold bath blanket down to umbilicus. Bathe chest using long, firm strokes. Take special care with skin under female client's breasts, lifting breast upward, if necessary, using back of the hand. Rinse and dry well.

Draping prevents unnecessary exposure of body parts. Towel maintains warmth and privacy. Secretions and dirt collect easily in areas of tight skinfolds. Skin under breasts is vulnerable to excoriation if not kept clean and dry.

11. Wash hands and nails.

a. Fold bath towel in half, and lay it on bed beside client. Place basin on towel. Immerse client's hand in water. Allow hand to soak for 3 to 5 minutes (if appropriate) before cleansing fingernails (see Skill 14-5). Remove basin, and dry hand well. Repeat for other hand.

Soaking softens cuticles and calluses of hand, loosens debris beneath nails, and enhances feeling of cleanliness. Thorough drying removes moisture from between fingers.

12. Check temperature of bathwater, and change water if necessary; otherwise continue.

Warm water maintains client's comfort.

• Critical Decision Point

If client is at risk for falling, be sure side rails are up before obtaining fresh water. Also lower bed when it is necessary to leave bedside. NOTE: All side rails raised may be considered a restraint.

STEP	**RATIONALE**

13. Wash the abdomen.

a. Place bath towel lengthwise over chest and abdomen. (Two towels may be needed.) Fold bath blanket down to just above pubic region. Bathe, rinse and dry abdomen with special attention to umbilicus and skinfolds of abdomen and groin. Keep abdomen covered between washing and rinsing. Dry well.

Keeping skinfolds clean and dry helps prevent odor and skin irritation. Moisture and sediment that collect in skinfolds predispose skin to maceration.

b. Apply clean gown or pajama top.

Maintains client's warmth and comfort. Dressing affected side first allows easier manipulation of gown over body part with reduced ROM.

● *Critical Decision Point*

If one extremity is injured or immobilized, always dress affected side first.

14. Wash the lower extremities.

a. Cover chest and abdomen with top of bath blanket. Expose near leg by folding blanket toward midline. Be sure perineum is draped.

Prevents overexposure.

b. Place bath towel under leg, supporting leg at knee and ankle. If appropriate, place client's foot in a basin to soak while washing and rinsing. (Bend client's leg at knee, and while grasping client's heel, elevate leg from mattress slightly and place bath basin on towel.) If client is unable to support leg, cleansing can simply be done by washing feet thoroughly with washcloth.

Towel prevents soiling of bed linen. Support of joint and extremity during lifting prevents strain on musculoskeletal structures. Sudden movement by client could spill bathwater. Soaking softens calluses and rough skin.

● *Critical Decision Point*

If client has diabetes or peripheral vascular disease, do not soak feet.

c. Wash leg using long, firm strokes from ankle to knee, then knee to thigh (see illustration). Do not rub or massage the back of the calf. Dry well. Wash between toes of foot. Cleanse foot, making sure to bathe between toes. Clean and clip nails as needed (see Skill 14-5). Dry toes and feet completely. Remove and discard towel.

Promotes circulation and venous return. Excess massage of calf could loosen deep vein thrombus.

Secretions and moisture may be present between toes, predisposing client to maceration and breakdown.

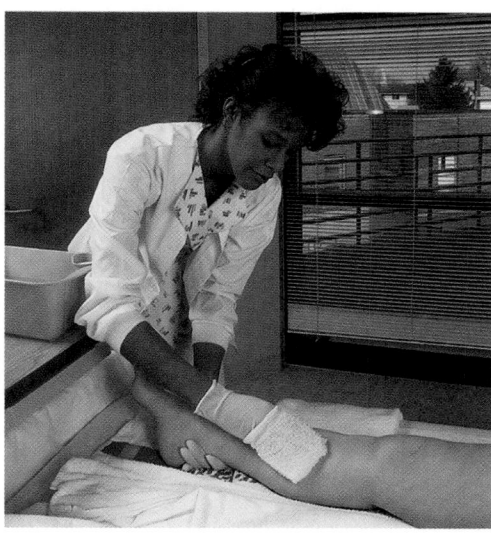

STEP **14c** Wash client's leg.

STEP	RATIONALE

- **Critical Decision Point**

  Clients with history of deep vein thromboses or blood-clotting disorders should not have their lower extremities washed with long, firm strokes. Use short, light strokes.

d. Raise side rail, move to opposite side of bed, lower side rail, and repeat steps b and c for other leg and foot. If skin is dry, apply moisturizing lotion (AHCPR, 1992). When finished, cover client with bath blanket.	Moisturizers are effective in reducing dry skin.
15. Raise side rail, and change bathwater. Remove contaminated gloves.	Decreased bathwater temperature can cause chilling. Clean water reduces microorganism transmission.
16. Wash back.	
a. Reapply clean pair of gloves. Lower side rail. Assist client in assuming prone or side-lying position (as applicable). Place towel lengthwise along client's side, and keep client covered with bath blanket.	Exposes back and buttocks for bathing. Maintains warmth and prevents unnecessary exposure.
b. If fecal material is present, enclose in a fold of underpad or toilet tissue, and remove with disposable wipes.	Skinfolds near buttocks and anus may contain fecal secretions that harbor microorganisms.
c. Keep client draped by sliding bath blanket over shoulders and thighs during bathing. Wash, rinse, and dry back from neck to buttocks using long, firm strokes. Pay special attention to folds of buttocks and anus.	Cleansing buttocks after back prevents contamination of water.
d. Cleanse buttocks and anus, washing front to back (see illustration). Cleanse, rinse, and dry area thoroughly. If needed, place a clean absorbent pad under client's buttocks.	

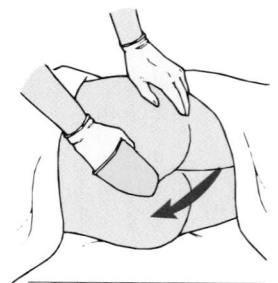

STEP 16d Cleanse buttocks from front to back.

e. Give a back rub (see Chapter 6).	Promotes client relaxation.
f. Apply body lotion to skin as needed and topical moisturizing agents to dry, flaky, reddened, or scaling areas. When finished, cover client with bath blanket.	Dry skin results in reduced pliability and cracking. Moisturizers help to prevent skin breakdown (AHCPR, 1992).

- **Critical Decision Point**

  Do not massage any reddened area on client's skin. Reddened areas may indicate tissue injury, and massaging may further injure tissue capillaries (Olson, 1989).

17. Raise side rail. Change bathwater.	Clean water should be used to provide perineal care.
18. Wash perineum.	
a. Female	
(1) If client is able to maneuver and handle washcloth, allow to cleanse perineum on own.	Maintains client's dignity and self-care ability.

STEP	**RATIONALE**

STEP **18a(2)** Drape the client for perineal care.

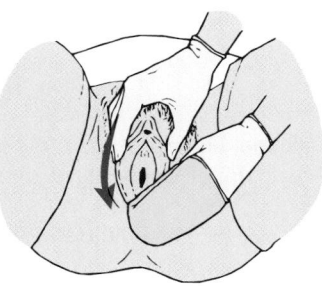

STEP **18a(5)** Cleanse from perineum to rectum (front to back).

(2) Lower side rail. Assist client in assuming dorsal recumbent position. Note restrictions or limitations in client's positioning. Be sure waterproof pad is positioned under client's buttocks. Drape client with bath blanket placed in the shape of a diamond. Lift lower edge of bath blanket to expose perineum (see illustration).

Provides full exposure of female genitalia. If client is totally dependent, provide assistance to support client in side-lying position and to raise leg as perineum is bathed. If position causes client discomfort, reduce degree of abduction in female's hips.

(3) Fold lower corner of bath blanket up between client's legs onto abdomen. Wash and dry client's upper thighs.

Keeping client draped until procedure begins minimizes anxiety. Buildup of perineal secretions can soil surrounding skin surfaces.

(4) Wash labia majora. Use nondominant hand to gently retract labia from thigh: with dominant hand, wash carefully in skinfolds. Wipe in direction from perineum to rectum. Repeat on opposite side using separate section of washcloth. Rinse and dry area thoroughly.

Perineal care involves thorough cleansing of the client's external genitalia and surrounding skin. Skinfolds may contain body secretions that harbor microorganisms. Wiping front to back reduces chance of transmitting fecal organisms to urinary meatus.

(5) Gently separate labia with nondominant hand to expose urethral meatus and vaginal orifice. With dominant hand, wash downward from pubic area toward rectum in one smooth stroke (see illustration). Use separate section of cloth for each stroke. Cleanse thoroughly around labia minora, clitoris, and vaginal orifice. Avoid tension on indwelling catheter if present, and clean area around it thoroughly.

Cleansing method reduces transfer of microorganisms to urinary meatus. (For menstruating women or clients with indwelling catheters, cleanse with cotton balls.)

Tension on catheter could cause accidental removal and pressure on bladder sphincter.

(6) Rinse area thoroughly. If client uses bedpan, pour warm water over perineal area. Dry thoroughly, using front-to-back method.

Rinsing removes soap and microorganisms more effectively than wiping. Retained moisture harbors microorganisms.

Fold lower corner of bath blanket back between client's legs and over perineum. Ask client to lower legs and assume comfortable position.

b. Male

(1) If client is able to maneuver and handle washcloth, allow to cleanse perineum on own.

Maintains client's dignity and self-care ability.

(2) Lower side rail. Assist client to supine position. Note restriction in mobility.

Provides full exposure of male genitalia. Clients unable to lie supine can be positioned on side.

STEP	RATIONALE
(3) Fold lower half of bath blanket up to expose upper thighs. Wash and dry thighs.	Buildup of perineal secretions can soil surrounding skin surfaces.
(4) Cover thighs with bath towels. Raise bath blanket up to expose genitalia. Gently raise penis, and place bath towel underneath. Gently grasp shaft of penis. If client is uncircumcised, retract foreskin. If client has an erection, defer procedure until later.	Keeps client draped to minimize anxiety. Towel prevents moisture from collecting in inguinal area. Gentle but firm handling of penis reduces chance of an erection. Secretions capable of harboring microorganisms collect underneath foreskin.
(5) Wash tip of penis at urethral meatus first. Using circular motion, cleanse from meatus outward (see illustration). Discard washcloth, and repeat with clean cloth until penis is clean. Rinse and dry gently.	Direction of cleansing moves from area of least contamination to area of most contamination, preventing microorganisms from entering urethra.

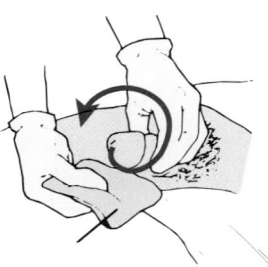

STEP 18b(5) Use circular motion to cleanse tip of penis.

STEP	RATIONALE
(6) Return foreskin to its natural position. This is extremely important in clients with decreased sensation in their lower extremities.	Tightening of foreskin around shaft of penis can cause local edema and discomfort. Clients with reduced sensation will not feel tightening of foreskin.
(7) Gently cleanse shaft of penis and scrotum by having client abduct legs. Pay special attention to underlying surface of penis. Lift scrotum carefully, and wash underlying skinfolds. Rinse and dry thoroughly.	Vigorous massage of penis can lead to an erection. Underlying surface of penis may have accumulation of secretions. Abduction of legs provides easier access to scrotal tissues. Secretions easily collect between skinfolds.
Fold bath blanket back over client's perineum, and assist client to comfortable position.	Draping promotes comfort.
19. Dispose of gloves in receptacle.	Prevents transmission of infection.
20. Assist client in grooming. Comb client's hair. Women may want to apply makeup.	Promotes client's body image.
21. Make client's bed (see Skill 14-6 and Box 14-4).	Provides clean environment.
22. Check the function and position of external devices (e.g., indwelling catheters, nasogastric tubes, IV tubes, braces)	Ensures that systems were not disrupted during bathing activities.
23. Remove soiled linen, and place in dirty-linen bag. Do not allow linen to contact uniform. Clean and replace bathing equipment. Replace call light and personal possessions. Leave room as clean and comfortable as possible.	Prevents transmission of infection. Clean environment promotes client's comfort. Keeping call light and articles of care within reach promotes client's safety.
24. Perform hand hygiene.	Reduces transmission of microorganisms.

STEP	RATIONALE

COMMERCIAL BAG BATH OR CLEANSING PACK

1. The cleansing pack contains 8 to 10 premoistened towels for cleansing (see illustration). Warm the package contents in a microwave following package directions.

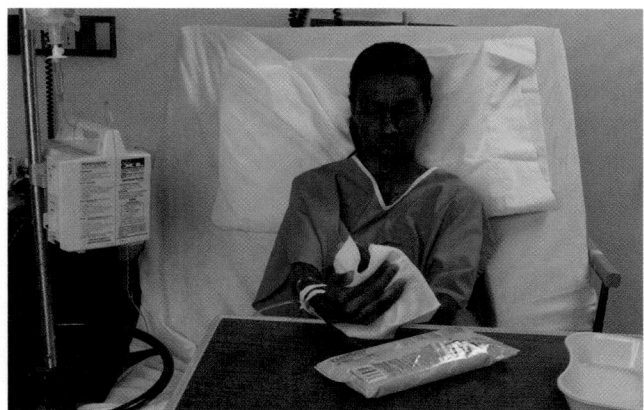
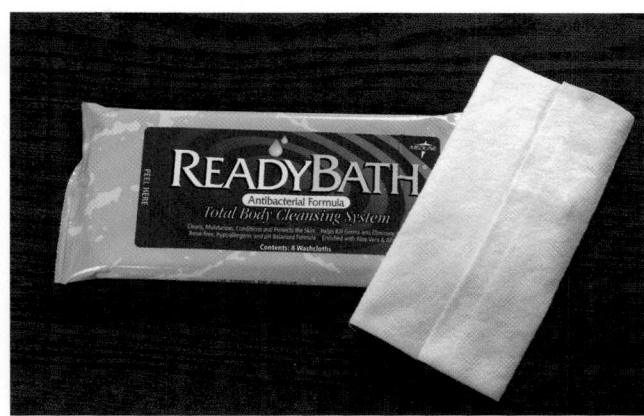

STEP **1** A bag bath.

2. Use a single towel for each general body part cleansed. Follow the same order of cleansing as the total or partial bed bath.

   Reduces transmission of microorganisms.

3. Allow the skin to air dry for 30 seconds. It is permissible to lightly cover client with a bath towel to prevent chilling.

   Drying the skin with a towel removes the emollient that's left behind after the water/cleanser solution evaporates (Skewes, 1994).

4. NOTE: If there is excessive soiling (e.g., in the perineal region), an extra bag bath may be necessary, or the nurse may use conventional washcloths, soap and water, and towels.

TUB BATH OR SHOWER

1. Consider client's condition and review orders for precautions concerning client's movement or positioning. Physician's order usually is needed for a tub bath or shower.

   Prevents accidental injury to client during bathing.

2. Schedule use of shower or tub.

   Prevents unnecessary waiting that can cause fatigue.

3. Check tub or shower for cleanliness. Use cleaning techniques outlined in agency policy. Place rubber mat on tub or shower bottom. Place disposable bath mat or towel on floor in front of tub or shower.

   Cleaning prevents transmission of microorganisms. Mats prevent slipping and falling.

4. Collect all hygienic aids, toiletry items, and linens requested by client. Place within easy reach of tub or shower.

   Placing items close at hand prevents possible falls when client reaches for equipment.

5. Assist client to bathroom if necessary. Have client wear robe and slippers to bathroom.

   Assistance prevents accidental falls. Wearing robe and slippers prevents chilling.

6. Demonstrate how to use call signal for assistance.

   Bathrooms are equipped with signaling devices in case client feels faint or weak or needs immediate assistance. Clients prefer privacy during bath if safety is not jeopardized.

7. Place "occupied" sign on bathroom door.

   Maintains client's privacy.

STEP	RATIONALE

8. Fill bathtub halfway with warm water. Check temperature of bathwater, then have client test water, and adjust temperature if water is too warm. Explain which faucet controls hot water. If client is taking shower, turn shower on and adjust water temperature before client enters shower stall. Use shower seat or tub chair and provide if needed (see illustration).

Adjusting water temperature prevents accidental burns. Older adults and clients with neurological alterations (e.g., spinal cord injury) are at high risk for burns as a result of reduced sensation. Use of assistive devices facilitates bathing and minimizes physical exertion.

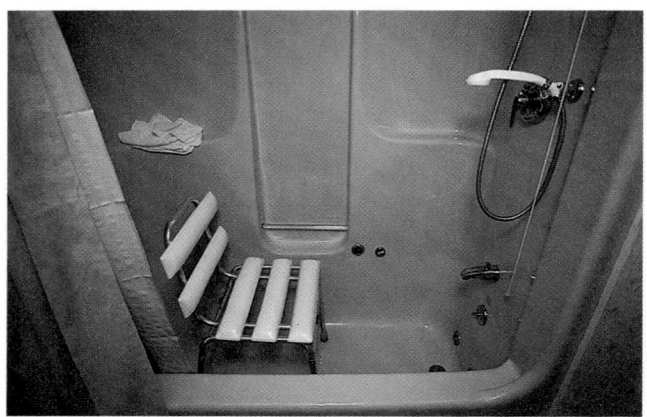

STEP **8** Shower seat for client safety.

9. Instruct client to use safety bars when getting in and out of tub or shower. Caution client against use of bath oil in tub water.

Prevents slipping and falling. Oil causes tub surfaces to become slippery.

10. Instruct client not to remain in tub longer than 10 to 15 minutes. Check on client every 5 minutes.

Prolonged exposure to warm water may cause vasodilation and pooling of blood, leading to light-headedness or dizziness.

11. Return to bathroom when client signals, and knock before entering.

Provides privacy.

12. For client who is unsteady, drain tub of water before client attempts to get out of it. Place bath towel over client's shoulders. Assist client in getting out of tub as needed, and assist with drying.

Prevents accidental falls. Client may become chilled as water drains.

- **Critical Decision Point**

  Weak or unstable clients need extra assistance in getting out of a tub. Planning for additional personnel is essential before attempting to assist the client from the tub.

13. Assist client as needed in donning clean gown or pajamas, slippers, and robe. (In home, extended care, or rehabilitation setting encourage client to wear regular clothing.)

Maintains warmth to prevent chilling.

14. Assist client to room and comfortable position in bed or chair.

Maintains relaxation gained from bathing.

15. Clean tub or shower according to agency policy. Remove soiled linen, and place in dirty-linen bag. Discard disposable equipment in proper receptacle. Place "unoccupied" sign on bathroom door. Return supplies to storage area.

Prevents transmission of infection through soiled linen and moisture.

16. Perform hand hygiene.

Reduces transfer of microorganisms.

STEP	RATIONALE

■ EVALUATION

1. Observe skin, paying particular attention to areas that were previously soiled, reddened, flaking, scaling, or cracking or showed early signs of breakdown. Use the SCDF to rate skin dryness.

   Techniques used during bathing should leave skin clean and clear. Over time dry skin should be reduced. If client shows signs of reddened areas, use a Braden scale to measure client's risk for pressure ulcer (see Chapter 15).

2. Observe ROM during bath.

   Measures joint mobility.

3. Ask client to rate level of comfort.

   Determines client's tolerance of bathing activities.

4. Ask if client feels fatigued.

   Determines client's tolerance of bathing activities.

5. Ask client to explain proper hygiene techniques.

   Evaluates client's knowledge level.

Recording and Reporting

- Record bath on flow sheet. Note level of assistance required.
- Record condition of skin and genitalia and any significant findings (e.g., reddened areas, discharge, bruises, nevi, or joint or muscle pain).
- Report evidence of alterations in skin integrity to nurse in charge or physician.

Unexpected Outcomes	Related Interventions
1. Areas of excessive dryness, rashes, or pressure ulcers appear on skin.	• Review agency skin care policy regarding moisturizing lotions. • Reassess client's history of allergies. • Increase client's hydration. • Limit frequency of complete baths or choice of soap product. • Collaborate with physician, and obtain order regarding application of ointments or creams to provide a protective barrier and help maintain moisture within skin. • Complete pressure ulcer assessment (see Chapter 15). • Obtain special bed surface if client is at risk for skin breakdown.
2. Joint ROM decreases.	• Increase ROM exercises (unless contraindicated). • Encourage more self-care by client.
3. Client becomes excessively fatigued and unable to cooperate or participate in bathing.	• Reschedule bathing to a time when client is more rested. • Clients with breathing difficulties require pillow or elevated head of bed during bath. • Notify physician if this is a change in client's fatigue level.
4. Client seems unusually restless or complains of discomfort.	• Schedule client rest periods. • Consider analgesia if client complains of pain or discomfort before the bath.
5. The rectum, perineum, or genital area is inflamed, swollen, or has foul-smelling discharge.	• Bathe area frequently enough to keep clean and dry. • Apply protective barrier or antiinflammatory cream. • Report findings to physician.

Teaching Considerations

- Clients with decreased sensation need to be cautious when entering warm bathwater. Whenever possible they need to use unaffected extremity to test water temperature to avoid accidental scalding.
- Instruct clients in how to inspect surfaces between skinfolds for signs of irritation or breakdown.
- Clients most at risk for infection of perineum are taught signs and symptoms of early infection, as well as principles and techniques for cleansing perineum correctly.

Pediatric Considerations

- Adolescents may require and/or prefer more frequent bathing as a result of more active sebaceous glands.
- Child may prefer to have parent or family help with bath. For those children who desire to be independent in some of their bathing needs, it may be necessary to assist the child in washing the ears, back, neck, and genitalia.
- Young adolescent girls should learn basic perineal hygiene measures and know why they are predisposed to urinary tract infections.
- Parents can assist their children with bathing. Helping the family to gather supplies and guiding them around special care issues (e.g., IVs, dressings) can help them feel connected to their child.

Gerontological Considerations

- Passive body heating such as a warm bath immersion for 30 minutes in the evening increases rectal body temperature and delays occurrence of reduction in core body temperature. This increases slow wave sleep in healthy female older adult clients and has been shown to be an effective treatment for insomnia (Liao, 2002).
- Because of the aging process, more moisture is needed; client's skin can be rehydrated with lotions and fluids (Lueckenotte, 2000).
- Older adults with incontinence need meticulous skin care to reduce skin irritation from urine and feces (see Chapter 15).

- Older adults with limited mobility need assistance in perineal care. Using a side-lying position increases client's comfort and provides nurse with opportunity to provide perineal care and inspect surrounding skin as well.

Home Care Considerations

- In the home setting, set up equipment according to established routines. Client is best resource for what works in terms of convenience and saving time.
- Clients at risk for falls need to have grab bars installed around tub and may have bathroom floor carpeted. Client also may use portable shower seat.
- Type of bath chosen depends on assessment of the home, availability of running water, and condition of bathing facilities.
- If beds do not have side rails, positioning may be accomplished with pillows or by placing bed against wall.
- Never leave bathing client unattended. Adhesive strips on bottom of tub or shower, handrails, chairs, or stools in tub or shower will further protect client.
- Determine if there is need to have home care aide or other assistance after discharge. Contact social service or appropriate department within hospital to obtain referral to home care agency.

Long-Term Care Considerations

- Tubs in long-term care settings frequently come equipped with electronic thermometers to measure water temperature. The tubs also have hydraulic lifts to assist residents into the tub.
- Skin-related problems in long-term care settings may include methicillin-resistant *Staphylococcus aureus* (MRSA) infections, pressure ulcers, circulatory ulcers, dermatitis, skin cancers, herpes zoster (shingles) (Lueckenotte, 2000).
- Residents in long-term care facilities should be encouraged to do as much personal care as possible and to wear their own street clothes (Sorrentino, 1999).

SKILL 14-2 Oral Hygiene

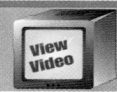

Maintenance of an adequate level of daily oral hygiene, including brushing, flossing, and rinsing, is essential for the prevention and control of plaque-associated oral diseases. In addition to preventing inflammation and infection, oral hygiene promotes comfort, nutrition, and verbal communication. Brushing cleanses the teeth of food particles, plaque (the cause of dental caries), and bacteria; massages the gums; and relieves discomfort from unpleasant odors and tastes. Flossing removes tartar that collects at the gum line. Rinsing removes dislodged food particles and excess toothpaste. Recent research has shown that twice daily rinsing with an essential oil–containing mouth rinse (e.g., Cool

BOX 14-2 Procedural Guideline
Cleaning dentures

DELEGATION CONSIDERATIONS
The skill of cleaning dentures can be delegated to assistive personnel.

EQUIPMENT
Soft-bristled toothbrush or denture toothbrush, emesis basin or sink, denture dentifrice or toothpaste, denture adhesive (optional), glass of water, 4 × 4 inch gauze, washcloth, denture cup, disposable gloves.

ASSESSMENT
1. Determine if client can clean dentures independently or requires assistance. Dentures need to be cleansed as often as natural teeth.
2. Fill emesis basin with tepid water. (If using sink, place washcloth in bottom of sink, and fill sink with approximately 1 inch of water.)
3. Apply disposable gloves.
4. Remove dentures: If client is unable to do this independently, grasp upper plate at front with thumb and index finger wrapped in gauze, and pull downward. Gently lift lower denture from jaw, and rotate one side downward to remove from client's mouth. Place dentures in emesis basin or sink.
5. Apply dentifrice or toothpaste to denture, and brush surfaces of dentures (see illustration). Hold dentures close to water. Hold brush horizontally, and use back-and-forth motion to cleanse biting surfaces. Use short strokes from top of denture to biting surfaces to clean outer teeth surfaces. Hold brush vertically, and use short strokes to clean inner

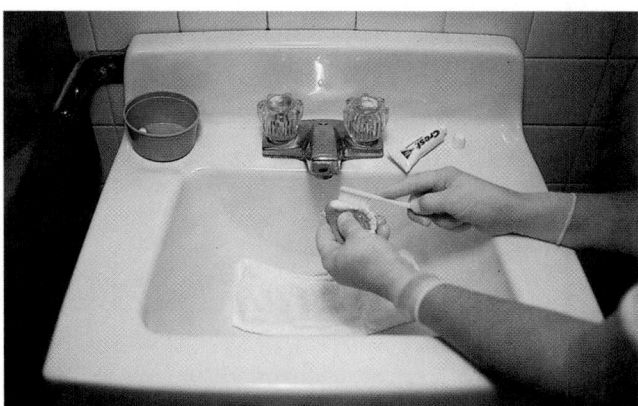

STEP **5** Brushing surface of denture.

teeth surfaces. Hold brush horizontally, and use back-and-forth motion to clean undersurface of dentures.
6. Rinse dentures thoroughly in tepid water.
7. Some clients use an adhesive to seal dentures in place. Apply a thin layer to undersurface before inserting.
8. If client needs assistance with insertion of dentures, moisten upper denture and press firmly to seal it in place. Then insert moistened lower denture. Ask if denture feels comfortable.
9. Some clients prefer to store their dentures to give the gums a rest and to reduce risk of infection. Store in tepid water in denture cup. Keep denture cup in a secure place and labeled with client's name to prevent loss.
10. Dispose of supplies. Remove and discard gloves.

Mint Listerine Antiseptic, Pfizer Healthcare) is an effective adjunct and at least as good as daily flossing in reducing plaque and gingivitis (Bauroth and others, 2003).

When a client becomes ill, many factors influence the need for oral hygiene. The nurse offers oral hygiene assistance as required, from preparing needed supplies to actually brushing the client's teeth. The nurse's responsibility also includes determining the frequency with which clients require oral hygiene. Frequency of care should be based on the condition of the oral cavity and the client's level of comfort. Oral hygiene may be required as often as every 1 to 2 hours.

Clients who wear dentures should be encouraged to continue to care for them and to provide this care as frequently as with natural teeth. Routine denture care reduces the risk of gingival infection. However, when clients are unable to care for their own dentures, the nurse must provide this care (Box 14-2). Dentures are the client's personal property and should be handled with care because they can be easily broken. Dentures should be stored in an enclosed, labeled cup for soaking or when dentures are not worn, such as during surgery or diagnostic procedures. Once clients are returned from their procedure, most prefer to have their dentures inserted as soon as possible.

DELEGATION CONSIDERATIONS

The skill of oral hygiene (including toothbrushing, flossing, and rinsing) and denture care may be delegated to assistive personnel. The nurse should assess a client's gag reflex if there is any question that the client is at risk for aspiration. The nurses provides assistive personnel with information, assistance, and direction, including:

* Having assistive personnel report any changes in oral mucosa (e.g., client's report of oral discomfort)

EQUIPMENT

- ❑ Soft-bristled toothbrush (hard toothbrush damages enamel and gums)
- ❑ Nonabrasive fluoride toothpaste (abrasive toothpastes wear down enamel)
- ❑ Dental floss
- ❑ Tongue depressor
- ❑ Water glass with cool water
- ❑ 20 ml essential oil–antiseptic mouth rinse
- ❑ Emesis basin or curved kidney basin
- ❑ Face towel
- ❑ Paper towels
- ❑ Disposable gloves

STEP	RATIONALE

■ ASSESSMENT

1. Perform hand hygiene, and apply disposable gloves.

2. Instruct client not to bite down. Then, using a tongue depressor, inspect integrity of lips, teeth, buccal mucosa, gums, palate, and tongue (see Chapter 18).

3. Identify presence of common oral problems:
   a. *Dental caries*—chalky white discoloration of tooth or presence of brown or black discoloration
   b. *Gingivitis*—inflammation of gums
   c. *Periodontitis*—receding gum lines, inflammation, gaps between teeth
   d. *Halitosis*—bad breath
   e. *Cheilosis*—cracking of lips
   f. *Stomatitis*—inflammation of the mouth

4. Remove gloves, and perform hand hygiene.

5. Assess risk for oral hygiene problems:

   a. Dehydration, inability to take fluids or food by mouth (NPO)

   b. Presence of nasogastric or oxygen tubes; mouth breathers

   c. Chemotherapeutic drugs

   d. Radiation therapy to head and neck

   e. Presence of artificial airway (e.g., endotracheal tube)
   f. Blood-clotting disorders (e.g., leukemia, aplastic anemia)
   g. Oral surgery, trauma to mouth

   h. Aging
   i. Chemical injury

Rationale column:

Reduces transmission of microorganisms. Gloves prevent contact with microorganisms in blood or saliva.

Determines status of client's oral cavity and extent of need for oral hygiene.

Helps determine type of hygiene client requires and information client requires for self-care.

Prevents spread of microorganisms.

Certain conditions increase likelihood of impaired oral cavity integrity and need for preventive care.

Causes excess drying and fragility of mucous membranes and lips; increases accumulation of secretions on tongue and gums.

Causes drying of mucosa.

Drugs kill mucous membrane cells more rapidly than they are replaced, resulting in stomatitis and sore formation (McKenry and Salerno, 2001).

Reduces salivary flow and lowers pH of saliva; can cause soreness, dryness, mild erythema, swollen mucosa, dysphagia, taste changes, and possible oral infection.

Increases irritation to gums and mucosa. Excess secretions accumulate on teeth and tongue.

Predisposes to inflammation and bleeding of gums.

Break in mucosa increases risk of infection. Vigorous brushing can disrupt suture lines.

With advancing age, mucosa becomes thin and less elastic.

Results from irritants such as alcohol, tobacco, acidic foods, or side effects of medications (e.g., antibiotics, steroids, antidepressants).

STEP	RATIONALE

j. Diabetes mellitus

Poorly controlled diabetes results in high glucose levels in the saliva, which can help bacteria to thrive (American Diabetes Association, 2003). Clients are prone to dryness of mouth, gingivitis, periodontal disease, and loss of teeth.

6. Determine client's oral hygiene practices and willingness to attend to hygiene needs:

Identifies errors in client's technique, deficiencies in preventive oral hygiene, and client's level of knowledge regarding dental care.

a. Frequency of toothbrushing and flossing
b. Type of toothpaste, mouth rinse used
c. Last dental visit
d. Frequency of dental visits
e. Type of mouthwash or moistening preparation

Lemon-glycerine preparations can be detrimental. Glycerine is an astringent that dries and shrinks mucous membranes and gums. Lemon exhausts salivary reflex and can erode tooth enamel (Adams, 1996; Fitch and others, 1999). Mouthwash provides pleasant aftertaste but can dry mucosa after extended use if it has an alcohol base. An essential oil–antiseptic mouthwash such as Cool Mint Listerine can be effective in reducing plaque and gingivitis (Bauroth and others, 2003).

7. Assess client's ability to grasp and manipulate toothbrush. Assessment determines level of assistance required from nurse.

Older adult clients or persons with musculoskeletal or nervous system alterations may be unable to hold toothbrush with firm grip or manipulate brush.

NURSING DIAGNOSES
- Impaired oral mucous membrane
- Bathing/hygiene self-care deficit
- Deficient knowledge regarding oral hygiene care
- Risk for infection

Related factors are individualized based on client's condition or needs.

PLANNING
1. Expected outcomes following completion of procedure:
   - Client expresses feeling of cleanliness.
   - Oral cavity structures have normal characteristics.
   - Oral mucosa is moist, intact, and of normal color.
   - Gums are pink, firm, and adherent to neck of teeth.
   - Teeth are clean, smooth, and shiny.
   - Tongue is pink and without secretions or coating.
   - Client describes correct oral hygiene techniques and necessary frequency.
   - Client makes choices regarding hygiene procedure and assists by flossing and brushing.
2. Prepare equipment at bedside.
3. Explain procedure to client, and discuss preferences regarding use of hygienic aids.

Hygiene measures remove secretions and thickened mucosa. If client had degree of alteration before brushing, condition should not be worse after brushing. Mucosa, tongue, and gums are moist and intact. Teeth are clean.

Demonstrates understanding of nurse's instructions.

Client is able to manage self-care.

Some clients feel uncomfortable about having the nurse care for their basic needs. Client involvement with procedure minimizes anxiety.

IMPLEMENTATION
1. Place paper towels on over-bed table, and arrange other equipment within easy reach.
2. Raise bed to comfortable working position. Raise head of bed (if allowed), and lower side rail. Move client or help client move closer. Side-lying position can be used.
3. Place paper towel over client's chest.

Creates organized workspace.

Raising bed and positioning client prevent nurse from straining muscles. Semi-Fowler's position helps prevent client from choking or aspirating.

Prevents soiling of client's gown.

STEP	RATIONALE

4. Apply gloves.

5. Apply enough toothpaste to brush to cover length of bristles (American Dental Association, 2003). Hold brush over emesis basin. Pour small amount of water over toothpaste.

6. Client may assist by brushing. Hold toothbrush bristles at 45-degree angle to gum line (see illustration). Be sure tips of bristles rest against and penetrate under gum line. Brush inner and outer surfaces of upper and lower teeth by brushing from gum to crown of each tooth. Clean biting surfaces of teeth by holding top of bristles parallel with teeth and brushing gently back and forth (see illustration). Brush sides of teeth by moving bristles back and forth (see illustration).

Prevents contact with microorganisms or blood in saliva. Moisture aids in distribution of toothpaste over tooth surfaces.

Angle allows brush to reach all tooth surfaces and to clean under gum line where plaque and tartar accumulate. Back-and-forth motion dislodges food particles caught between teeth and along chewing surfaces.

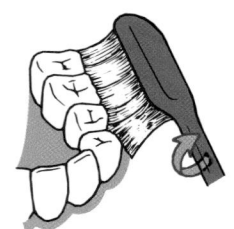
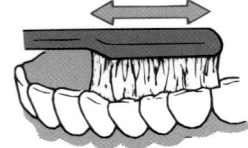
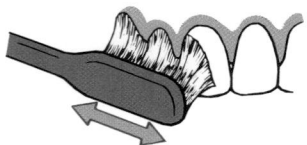

STEP **6** Directions of brush for toothbrushing.

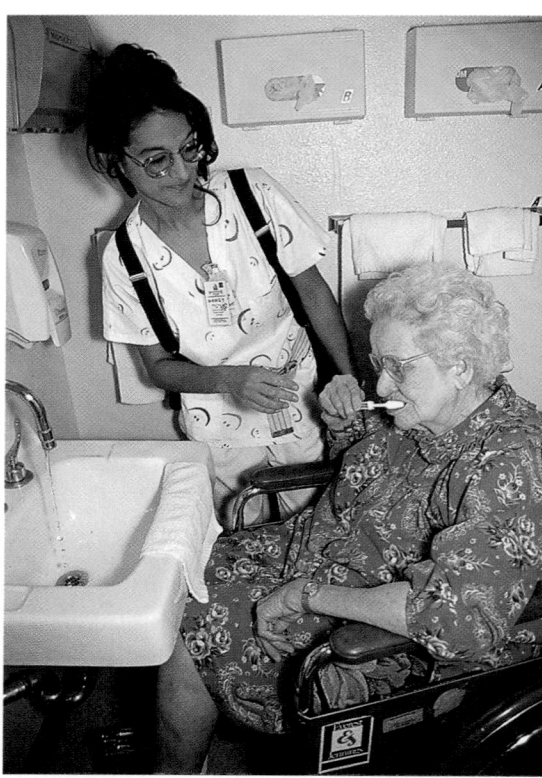

STEP **8** Nurse observes client's toothbrushing technique.

7. Have client hold brush at 45-degree angle and lightly brush over surface and sides of tongue. Avoid initiating gag reflex.

8. Allow client to rinse mouth thoroughly with water by taking several sips of water (may use straw), swishing water across all tooth surfaces, and spitting into emesis basin. Use this time to teach client importance of brushing teeth twice a day (see illustration).

9. Have client rinse teeth with antiseptic mouth rinse for 30 seconds. Then have client spit rinse into emesis basin.

Microorganisms collect and grow on tongue's surface and contribute to bad breath. Gagging may cause aspiration of toothpaste.

Rinsing removes food particles. The American Dental Association (2003) recommends persons brush their teeth twice a day with fluoride toothpaste.

Use of an essential oil–antiseptic mouth rinse a minimum of twice daily is at least as effective as flossing daily in reducing plaque and gingivitis (Bauroth and others, 2003).

STEP	**RATIONALE**
10. Assist in wiping client's mouth.	Promotes sense of comfort.
11. Allow client to floss. Floss between all teeth. Hold floss against tooth while moving floss up and down sides of teeth. Instruct client in importance of daily flossing (see illustration).	Removes plaque and prevents gum disease. American Dental Association (2003) recommends flossing once daily to remove decay-causing bacteria between teeth and under gum line.

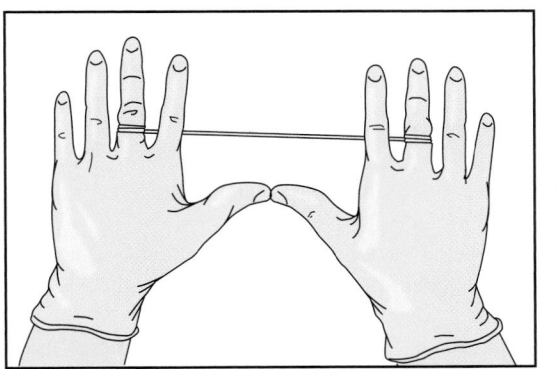

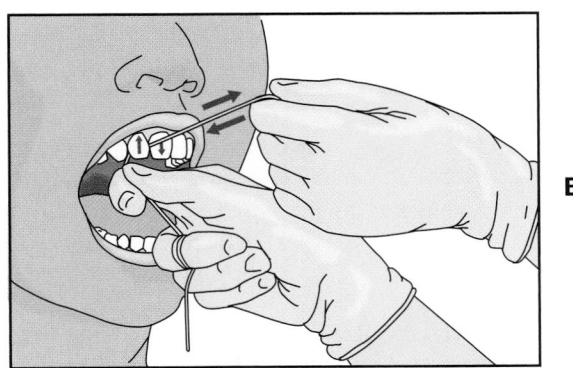

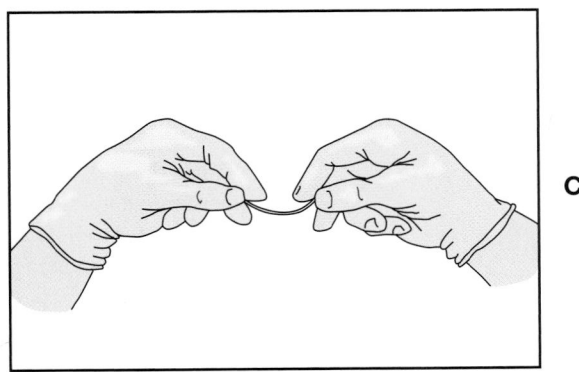

STEP **11** Flossing. **A,** Dental floss is held between the middle fingers to floss the upper teeth. **B,** Floss is moved in up-and-down motions between the teeth. Floss is moved up and down from the crown to the gum line. **C,** Floss is held with the index fingers to floss the lower teeth.

STEP	RATIONALE
12. Allow client to rinse mouth thoroughly with cool water and spit into emesis basin. Assist in wiping client's mouth.	Rinsing removes plaque and tartar from oral cavity.
13. Assist client to comfortable position, remove emesis basin and bedside table, raise side rail, if appropriate, and lower bed to original position.	Provides for client comfort and safety.
14. Wipe off over-bed table, discard soiled linen and paper towels in appropriate containers, remove soiled gloves, and return equipment to proper place.	Proper disposal of soiled equipment prevents spread of infection.
15. Perform hand hygiene.	Reduces transmission of microorganisms.

EVALUATION

1. Ask client if any area of oral cavity feels uncomfortable or irritated.	Pain indicates more chronic problem.
2. Apply gloves, and inspect condition of oral cavity.	Determines effectiveness of hygiene and rinsing.
3. Ask client to describe proper hygiene techniques and recommended frequency.	Evaluates client's learning.
4. Observe client brushing and flossing.	Evaluates client' ability to use correct technique.

Recording and Reporting

- Record procedure on flow sheet. Note condition of oral cavity in nurses' notes.
- Report bleeding, pain, or presence of lesions to nurse in charge or physician.

Unexpected Outcomes	Related Interventions
1. Mucosa is dry and inflamed. Tongue has thick coating.	• Increase client's hydration. • Increase frequency of tongue brushing. • Apply moisturizing lubricant to client's lips.
2. Gum margins are retracted from teeth, with localized areas of inflammation. Bleeding occurs around gum margins.	• Report findings because client may have an underlying bleeding tendency. • Switch to a soft-bristled toothbrush. • Avoid vigorous brushing and flossing.
3. Mucosa becomes inflamed from repeated chemotherapy administration, and sores develop.	• Assess condition of oral cavity every 4 hours. • Use a soft-bristled toothbrush or sponge at least every 8 hours. • Rinse the mouth with a solution of one half hydrogen peroxide and one half normal saline every 12 hours. • Administer topical analgesic medications as prescribed. • Assist client in using artificial saliva as needed and as ordered (McKenry and Salerno, 2001).
4. Teeth show signs of dental caries.	• Refer client to dentist.

Teaching Considerations

- Educate clients about methods to prevent tooth decay (e.g., reduce intake of carbohydrates, especially sweet snacks between meals; brush within 30 minutes of eating sweets; rinse mouth thoroughly with water or eat acid-containing fruit such as an apple; use fluoridated water) (Fellona and DeVore, 1999).
- Educate clients to visit a dentist regularly (twice a year) for professional cleansings and oral exams (American Dental Association, 2003).
- Replace toothbrush every 3 or 4 months or sooner if bristles become frayed (American Dental Association, 2003).

Pediatric Considerations

* As soon as teething begins, clean an infant's gum pads and teeth with a small piece of gauze twice a day (after breakfast and after the last meal of the day). This practice eliminates decay-producing plaque.
* Teach parents that a bottle given to a child at bedtime should contain only water. Falling asleep with a bottle of milk or juice or while breast-feeding bathes the teeth in a carbohydrate-rich fluid that can cause cavities and tooth discoloration.
* Parents and caregivers need to be responsible for the child's oral hygiene for about the first 8 years, because the child does not develop the neural patterns and muscular coordination needed for performing mouth care until that age.
* Flossing can be done more easily with two persons. One person holds the child with his or her head resting on their lap while the other individual flosses the child's teeth.
* Unless problems occur earlier, dental visits should begin about age 2. After the first visit, dental checkups every 6 months are encouraged (Hockenberry and others, 2003).

Gerontological Considerations

* A number of normal age-related changes occur in the oral cavity. Thinning of the oral mucosa and decreased vascularity of the gingivae predispose older adults to injury and periodontal disease. Loss of tissue elasticity and decreased mass and strength of the muscles make chewing more difficult. Resorption of the alveolar bone can loosen natural teeth.
* The number of taste buds declines with advancing age. In an attempt to enhance the taste of food, the older adult may choose salty and sugary foods, which erode tooth enamel and expose dentin (Pettigrew, 1989).
* Plaque retention is a problem in older adults, worsened by existing teeth restorations, missing teeth, gingival recession, and wearing of removable prosthesis. Older adults have difficulty removing plaque because of diminished manual dexterity, impaired vision, or associated debilitating conditions (Simons and others, 2001).

Home Care Considerations

* During the initial admission visit, document the condition of the client's mouth, teeth, and gums, thus providing a baseline for assessment of the client's ability to comply with special diets and fluid intake and to carry out oral hygiene practices.

SKILL 14-3 Performing Mouth Care for the Unconscious or Debilitated Client

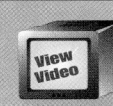

Unconscious or debilitated clients pose challenges because of their risk for having alterations of the oral cavity. The absence of saliva movement and production in the unconscious or orally intubated (artificial airway) client has serious implications. If left undisturbed for as little as 3 days, plaque can become a host for hundreds of gram-negative bacteria (Marsh and Martin, 1992). These bacteria can cause infection in the oral cavity and directly enter the bloodstream of the vascular mucosa to cause systemic disease. Critically ill clients with endotracheal tubes and who are on mechanical ventilation are at high risk for ventilator-associated pneumonia if saliva is aspirated into the tracheobronchial tree. Pathogens found in plaque that have the potential for causing pneumonia include *Staphylococcus aureus* and *Pseudomonas aeruginosa.*

The critically ill client faces the same risk factors for oral problems as other clients, such as dehydration, mouth breathing, chemical injury to the mucosa, and oral trauma. Some clients require mouth care as often as every 1 to 2 hours until the mucosa returns to normal. Many clients have no gag reflex as a result of change in consciousness or a neurological injury. Proper oral hygiene requires keeping the oral mucosa moist and removing secretions that can lead to infection. Preventing deterioration of oral health is an important part of nursing care of the unconscious or debilitated client.

Research has resulted in improved standards for oral care of the critically ill (Stiefel and others, 2000). Foam stick applicators, a popular substitute for the toothbrush, have been found to stimulate the mucosal tissues but are ineffective in removing debris from the teeth (Grap and others, 2003). A pediatric-size toothbrush is more effective in removing plaque and tartar and fits better around an endotracheal tube. Hydrogen peroxide, once used routinely in intensive care units (ICUs) for mouth care, removes debris and is antiinfective but if not diluted can easily cause burns of the mucosa (Grap and others, 2003).

DELEGATION CONSIDERATIONS

The skill of providing mouth care to an unconscious or debilitated client can be delegated to assistive personnel. However, the nurse must first assess the client's gag reflex. The nurse provides assistive personnel with information, assistance, and direction, including:

- Informing assistive personnel of the proper way to position clients for mouth care
- Making sure assistive personnel are proficient in use of oral suction catheter for clearing oral secretions (see Skill 24-1)
- Informing assistive personnel of signs of impaired integrity of oral mucosa to report to nurse
- Instructing assistive personnel to inform nurse if possible aspiration is suspected

EQUIPMENT

- ❏ Small pediatric soft-bristled toothbrush
- ❏ Sponge toothette for edentulous client
- ❏ Fluoridated toothpaste
- ❏ Tongue blade
- ❏ Oral airway (optional)
- ❏ Small bulb syringe or portable suction device with catheter
- ❏ Oral airway (uncooperative client or client who shows bite reflex)
- ❏ Vaseline lip lubricant or water-based lubricant
- ❏ Cup of water
- ❏ Face towel
- ❏ Paper towels
- ❏ Emesis basin
- ❏ Disposable gloves

STEP	RATIONALE

ASSESSMENT

1. Perform hand hygiene, and apply disposable gloves.	Reduces transmission of microorganisms in blood or saliva.
2. Test for presence of gag reflex by placing tongue blade on back half of tongue.	Reveals whether client is at risk for aspiration.

- *Critical Decision Point*
  Clients with impaired gag reflex require oral care as well. The nurse must determine the type of suction apparatus needed at the bedside to protect the client's airway against aspiration.

3. Inspect condition of oral cavity (see Chapter 18).	Determines condition of oral cavity and need for hygiene.
4. Remove gloves. Perform hand hygiene.	Prevents spread of infection.
5. Assess client's risk for oral hygiene problems (see Skill 14-2).	Certain conditions increase likelihood of alterations in integrity of oral cavity structures. May require more frequent care.

NURSING DIAGNOSES

- Impaired oral mucous membrane
- Risk for aspiration

Related factors are individualized based on client's condition or needs.

PLANNING

1. Expected outcomes following completion of procedure:	
• Buccal mucosa and tongue are pink, moist, and intact. Gums are moist and intact. Teeth are cleaner, smooth, and shiny. Tongue is pink and without coating. Lips are moist, smooth, and without cracks.	Degree of improvement in condition of oral cavity structures will depend on extent of secretions or changes that existed before care.
• Debilitated client expresses feeling of cleanliness.	Comfort achieved.
• Oral pharynx remains patent.	Secretions removed, thus avoiding aspiration.
2. Unless contraindicated (e.g., head injury, neck trauma), lower side rail and position client on side (Sims' position) with head turned well toward dependent side and head of bed lowered. Raise side rail.	Allows secretions to drain from mouth instead of collecting in back of pharynx. Prevents aspiration.
3. Explain procedure to client, even if client is unconscious.	Allows debilitated client to anticipate procedure without anxiety. Unconscious client may retain ability to hear.
4. Perform hand hygiene, and apply disposable gloves.	Reduces transfer of microorganisms.
5. Place paper towels on over-bed table, and arrange equipment. If needed, turn on suction machine, and connect tubing to suction catheter.	Prevents soiling of tabletop. Equipment prepared in advance ensures smooth, safe procedure.
6. Pull curtain around bed, or close room door.	Provides privacy.

STEP	RATIONALE

▌ IMPLEMENTATION

1. Raise bed to its highest horizontal level; lower side rail.

   Use of good body mechanics with bed in high position prevents injury.

2. Position client on side close to side of bed; keep client's head turned toward mattress.

   Proper positioning of head prevents aspiration.

3. Remove dentures or partial plates if present.

   Allows for thorough cleansing of prosthetics later. Provides clearer access to oral cavity.

4. Place towel under client's head and emesis basin under chin.

   Prevents soiling of bed linen.

5. If client is uncooperative or having difficulty keeping mouth open, insert an oral airway. Insert upside down, then turn the airway sideways and then over tongue to keep teeth apart. Insert when client is relaxed, if possible. Do not use force (see illustration).

   Prevents client from biting down on nurse's fingers and provides access to oral cavity.

- *Critical Decision Point*

  Never place fingers into the mouth of an unconscious or debilitated client. The normal client response is to bite down.

6. Brush teeth with toothpaste using an up-and-down gentle motion. Clean chewing and inner tooth surfaces first. Clean outer tooth surfaces. Brush roof of mouth, gums, and inside cheeks. Gently brush tongue but avoid stimulating gag reflex (if present). Moisten brush with water to rinse. (Bulb syringe may also be used to rinse.) Repeat rinse several times.

   Brushing action removes food particles between teeth and along chewing surfaces. Swabbing helps remove secretions and crusts from mucosa and moistens mucosa. Repeated rinsing removes all debris.

7. For clients without teeth, use a toothette moistened in water or normal saline to clean oral cavity.

   Less traumatic to mucosa of gums.

8. Suction secretions as they accumulate, if necessary.

   Suction removes secretions and fluid that can collect in posterior pharynx. Reduces risk of aspiration.

9. Apply thin layer of water-soluble jelly to lips (see illustration).

   Lubricates lips to prevent drying and cracking.

10. Inform client that procedure is completed.

   Provides meaningful stimulation to unconscious or less responsive client.

11. Raise side rails as appropriate. Remove gloves, and dispose in proper receptacle.

   Prevents transmission of microorganisms.

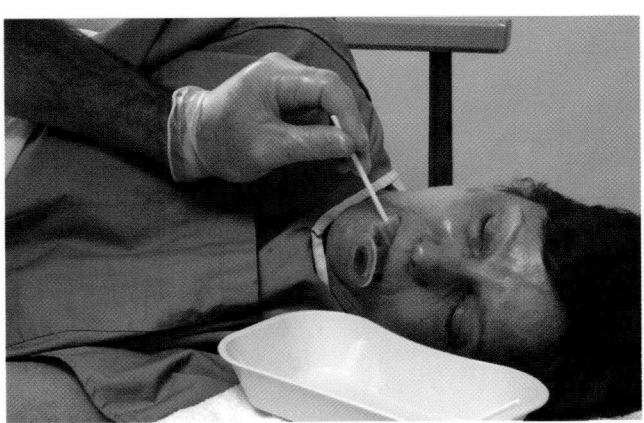

STEP **5** Cleansing around oral airway.

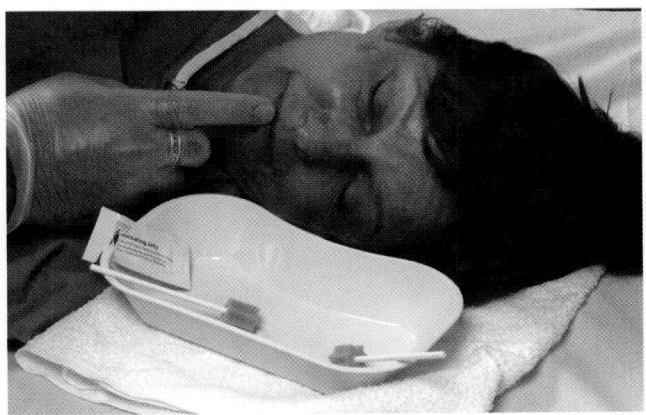

STEP **9** Application of water-soluble moisturizer to lips.

STEP	RATIONALE
12. Lower side rails. Reposition client comfortably, and return bed and side rail to original position.	Maintains client's comfort and safety.
14. Clean equipment, and return to its proper place. Place soiled linen in proper receptacle.	Proper disposal of soiled equipment prevents spread of infection.
15. Perform hand hygiene.	Reduces transmission of microorganisms.

EVALUATION

1. Apply gloves, and inspect oral cavity.	Determines efficacy of cleansing. Once thick secretions are removed, underlying inflammation or lesions may be revealed.
2. Ask debilitated client if mouth feels clean.	Evaluates level of comfort.
3. Assess client's respirations on an ongoing basis.	Ensures early recognition of aspiration.

Recording and Reporting

* Record procedure on flow sheet. Chart in nurses' notes client's ability to cooperate and whether suction is necessary for oral care.
* Record in nurses' notes any pertinent observations (e.g., presence of gag reflex, presence of bleeding gums, dry mucosa, ulcerations, crusts on tongue).
* Report any unusual findings to nurse in charge or physician.

Unexpected Outcomes	Related Interventions
1. Secretions or crusts remain on mucosa, tongue, or gums.	• More frequent oral hygiene is needed.
2. Localized inflammation of gums or mucosa is present.	• More frequent oral hygiene with soft-bristled toothbrush is needed. • Apply Oral Balance moisturizing gel to mucosa and massage (Fitch and others, 1999). • Chemotherapy and radiation can cause stomatitis. Clients should rinse mouth before and after meals and at bedtime using normal saline or solution of $\frac{1}{2}$ to 1 teaspoon of salt or baking soda to 1 pint of tepid water.
3. Lips are cracked or inflamed.	• Apply moisturizing gel or water-soluble lubricant to lips.
4. Client aspirates secretions.	• If present, suction oral airway as secretions accumulate to maintain patent airway (see Chapter 24). • Elevate client's head of bed to facilitate breathing. • Be prepared to have chest x-ray examination performed following physician's order.

Teaching Considerations

* Family members may care for debilitated client in the home. Instruction in mouth care is needed so that family understands how to protect client from aspirating, while thoroughly cleansing oral cavity. Observe family caregiver perform mouth care procedure.

Home Care Considerations

* Irrigate oral cavity with bulb syringe; if unavailable, substitute gravy baster or large syringe. Caution family caregiver against instilling a large amount of solution.

* Encourage primary caregiver to cleanse client's mouth at least twice a day. If client breathes through mouth, a soft-bristled toothbrush or gauze or soft linen wrapped around tongue blade, moistened, and used every 1 to 2 hours will keep mouth moist and fresh.
* A solution to use for oral care, available at most pharmacies, is carbamide peroxide.

SKILL 14-4 Hair Care (Combing and Shaving)

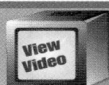

A person's appearance and sense of well-being are influenced by how the hair looks and feels. Brushing, combing, and shampooing are basic measures for all clients unable to provide self-care. Male clients should be offered the opportunity to shave or be shaved when their condition allows. Most men prefer to shave themselves. Men without beards usually shave daily. Some religions and cultures forbid cutting or shaving any body hair (Galanti, 1991). Most hospitals have beauty shops where clients can go for professional hair care.

Fever, malnutrition, emotional stress, and depression affect the condition of the hair. Diaphoresis leaves the hair oily and unmanageable. Excessively dry or oily hair may be associated with hormone changes. Dry, brittle hair occurs with aging and excessive use of shampoo.

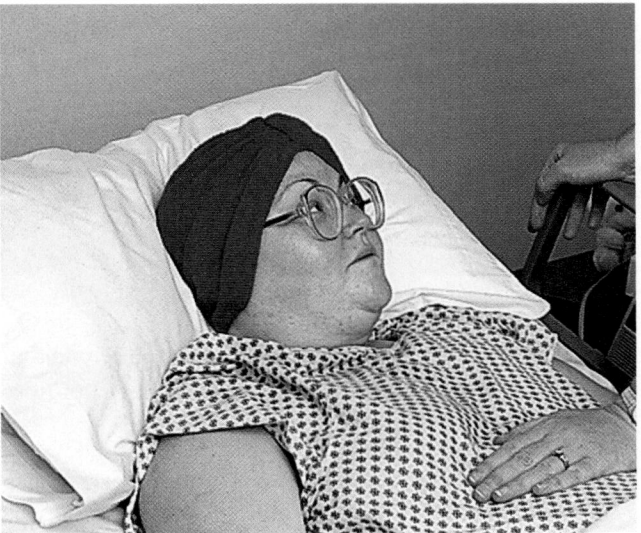

Figure **14-3** Clients may choose to wear a turban because of hair loss.

Certain chemotherapy agents and radiation therapy may cause loss of hair (alopecia). Many clients choose to wear a wig; however, some choose to wear hair scarves or turbans (Figure 14-3). The average growth of healthy hair is ½ inch per month. Table 14-2 describes common hair and scalp conditions and nursing interventions.

The frequency of shampooing depends on the condition of the hair and the person's daily routines and cultural preferences. Hair condition may have gender and racial variations. Coarse, curly hair, seen, for example, in African-American clients, does not retain moisture as other types of hair. Shampooing may be necessary only once a week (Crute, 1997). Dry hair, which commonly results from aging and protein deficiency, requires less frequent shampooing than oily hair or the hair of people who exercise actively.

The nurse should remind hospitalized clients that staying in bed, excess perspiration, or treatments that leave blood or solutions in the hair may require more frequent shampoos. In a hospital setting it may be necessary to transport a client by stretcher to a special facility where a spray nozzle and sink are available for shampooing.

Clients who are allowed to sit in a chair usually can be shampooed in front of a sink. The individual should be positioned facing away from the sink, with the head and neck hyperextended over the sink's edge. The nurse also checks to be sure that neck hyperextension is not contraindicated by the client's condition. Caution is needed with clients who have suffered neck injuries, because flexion and hyperextension of the neck could cause further injury. In addition, clients with positional vertigo may not be able to tolerate neck hyperextension if it increases their dizziness. A folded towel placed under the neck on the edge of the sink provides added comfort. If the client cannot sit in a chair or be transferred to a stretcher, shampooing must be done with the client in bed (Box 14-3). This may be done after the bath (common in the care of infants) or later as a separate procedure.

TABLE 14-2   COMMON HAIR AND SCALP CONDITIONS

PROBLEM	IMPLICATIONS	INTERVENTIONS
Dandruff—Scaling of the scalp accompanied by itching; in severe cases, dandruff on eyebrows.	Dandruff causes embarrassment; if dandruff enters eyes, conjunctivitis may develop.	Shampoo regularly with medicated shampoo; in severe cases seek physician's advice.
Ticks—Small gray-brown parasites that burrow into skin and suck blood.	Ticks transmit several diseases, including Rocky Mountain spotted fever, Lyme disease, and tularemia.	Do not pull ticks from skin because sucking apparatus remains and may become infected; placing drop of oil or ether on tick or covering it with petrolatum eases removal; oil suffocates tick.

Continued

TABLE 14-2   **COMMON HAIR AND SCALP CONDITIONS—CONT'D**

PROBLEM	IMPLICATIONS	INTERVENTIONS
Pediculosis capitis (head lice)—Tiny grayish/brown/white parasitic insects that attach to hair strands; about size of a sesame seed; nits or eggs look like oval particles attached at an angle to hair shaft; bites or pustules may be observed behind ears and at hairline.	Head lice are difficult to remove and if not treated may spread to furniture and other people.	Check entire scalp. Use medicated shampoo for eliminating lice or permethrin (Nix) available as a crème rinse. **Caution against use of products containing Lindane, because the ingredient is toxic and known to cause adverse reactions** (National Pediculosis Assn, 2001). Remove client's clothing before treatment, and apply new clothing following treatment. Repeat treatment according to product directions. Check the hair for nits, and comb with a nit comb for 2 to 3 days until sure all lice and nits have been removed. Manual removal of lice is best option when treatment has failed. Vacuum infested areas of home.
Pediculosis corporis (body lice)—Tend to cling to clothing so may not be easily seen; body lice suck blood and lay eggs on clothing and furniture.	Client itches constantly; scratches on skin may become infected; hemorrhagic spots may appear on skin where lice are sucking blood. May spread to other people.	Client should bathe or shower thoroughly; after skin is dried, apply lotion for eliminating lice; after 12 to 24 hours another bath or shower should be taken; bag infested clothing or linen until laundered. Vacuum items that cannot be washed.
Pediculosis pubis (crab lice)—Found in pubic hair; crab lice are grayish white with red legs.	Lice may spread through bed linen, clothing, or furniture or sexual contact.	Shave hair off affected area; cleanse as for body lice; if lice were sexually transmitted, partner must be notified.
Alopecia—Balding patches in periphery of hairline; hair becomes brittle and broken; caused by improper use of hair curlers and picks, tight braiding, hot styling tools, certain diseases.	Patches of uneven hair growth and loss alter client's appearance.	Offer clients access to scarves, hairpieces, or wigs. Stop hair care practices that damage hair.

BOX 14-3 Procedural Guideline
Shampooing hair of bed-bound client

DELEGATION CONSIDERATIONS

The skill of shampooing the hair of bed-bound clients can be delegated to assistive personnel. The nurse provides assistive personnel with information, assistance, and direction, including:

- Informing assistive personnel of the proper way to position client with head or neck mobility restriction
- Clarifying assistive personnel's knowledge of care for lice, stressing steps to take to prevent transmission to other clients

EQUIPMENT

Disposable gloves, bath towels, washcloths, shampoo and hair conditioner (optional), water pitcher, plastic shampoo trough, washbasin, bath blanket, waterproof pad, clean comb and brush, hair dryer (optional), disposable gown (optional)

ASSESSMENT

1. Before washing client's hair, determine that there are no contraindications to procedure. Certain medical conditions, such as head and neck injuries, spinal cord injuries, and arthritis, could place client at risk for injury during shampooing because of positioning and manipulation of client's head and neck.

2. Apply disposable gloves, and inspect the hair and scalp before beginning shampoo. Assess for presence of lice (see Table 14-2). This determines if special shampoos or treatments are necessary (e.g., dandruff, lice, removal of blood). If lice are present, caregivers should wear disposable gown and gloves during procedure.

3. Place waterproof pad under client's shoulders, neck, and head. Position client supine, with head and shoulders at top edge of bed. Place plastic trough under client's head and washbasin at end of trough (see illustration). Be sure trough spout extends beyond edge of mattress.

4. Place rolled towel under client's neck and bath towel over client's shoulders.

5. Brush and comb client's hair.

6. Obtain warm water.

7. Ask client to hold face towel or washcloth over eyes.

8. Slowly pour water from pitcher over hair until it is completely wet (see illustration). If hair contains matted blood, apply gloves, apply hydrogen peroxide to dis-

BOX 14-3 Procedural Guideline
Shampooing hair of bed-bound client—cont'd

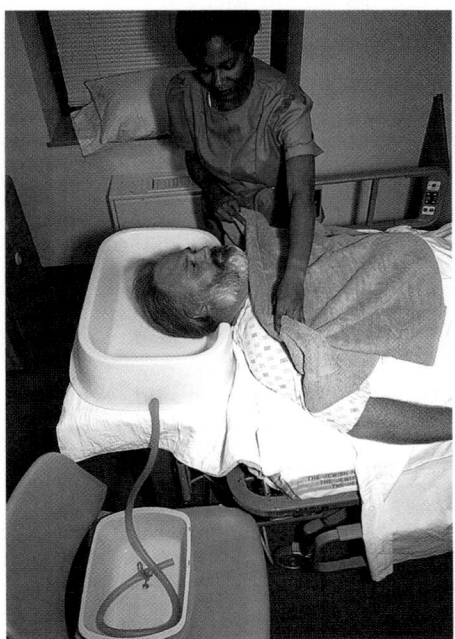

STEP **3** Client with waterproof pad under shoulders, neck, and head.

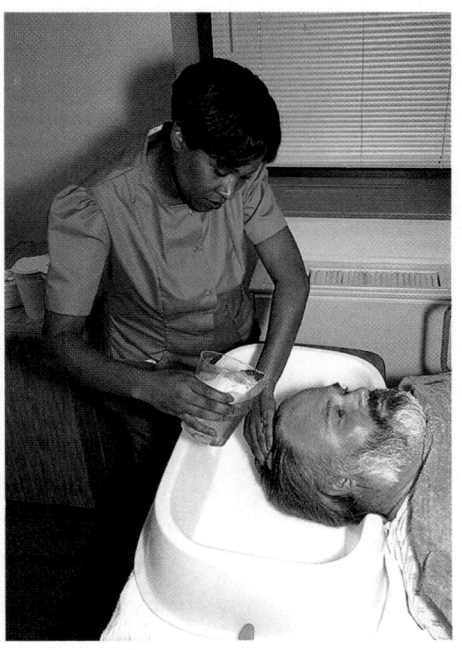

STEP **8** Pour water over hair

solve clots, and then rinse hair with saline. Apply small amount of shampoo.

9. Work up lather with both hands. Start at hairline, and work toward back of neck. Lift head slightly with one hand to wash back of head. Shampoo sides of head. Massage scalp by applying pressure with fingertips.

10. Rinse hair with water. Make sure water drains into basin. Repeat rinsing until hair is free of soap.

11. Apply conditioner or cream rinse if requested, and rinse hair thoroughly.

12. Wrap client's head in bath towel. Dry client's face with cloth used to protect eyes. Dry off any moisture along neck or shoulders.

13. Dry client's hair and scalp. Use second towel if first becomes saturated.

14. Comb hair to remove tangles, and dry with dryer if desired.

15. Apply oil preparation or conditioning product to hair, if desired by client.

16. Variation for clients with coarse, curly hair: Condition hair after washing. To untangle hair, use the wide teeth of a comb. Beginning at the nape of the neck, comb small subsections of the hair starting at the hair ends. Continue to work through small sections until hair is free of tangles (Crute, 1997).

17. Assist client to comfortable position, and complete styling of hair.

DELEGATION CONSIDERATIONS

The skill of hair care can be delegated to assistive personnel. The nurse provides assistive personnel with information, assistance, and direction, including:

- Informing assistive personnel of proper way to position client with head or neck mobility restriction
- Reviewing any procedures for use of medicated shampoo for lice, stressing the steps to take to prevent transmission to other clients

EQUIPMENT

- ❑ Wide-tooth comb
- ❑ Hairbrush
- ❑ Conditioner (optional)
- ❑ Disposable razor: razor with new blade, disposable gloves (optional), bath towel(s), mirror, washcloth, washbasin, shaving cream or soap, aftershave lotion (if client desires)
- ❑ Electric razor: razor (with clean cutting heads), bath towel, skin or beard conditioner, mirror, aftershave lotion (if client desires)
- ❑ Mustache care: scissors, brush or comb, bath towel, gooseneck lamp or overhead light, mirror

STEP	RATIONALE

ASSESSMENT

1. Inspect condition of hair and scalp. Inspect for presence of any infestation (e.g., pediculosis). NOTE: Apply disposable gloves if infestation is suspected.

   Findings may indicate need for medicated applications or shampoo.

2. Assess client's hair care and shaving product preferences (e.g., shampoo, aftershave lotion, skin conditioner).

   Influences approach to grooming. Promotes client's independence through decision making.

3. Before shaving, assess if client has bleeding tendency. Review medical history or laboratory values (e.g., platelet counts, prothrombin time).

   Determines need to use electric razor for client's safety.

• *Critical Decision Point*
Clients receiving anticoagulant therapy should use an electric razor.

4. Assess client's ability to manipulate razor.

   Determines level of assistance required.

NURSING DIAGNOSES

- Dressing/grooming self-care deficit
- Impaired physical mobility

- Risk for injury

Related factors are individualized based on client's condition or needs.

PLANNING

1. Expected outcomes following completion of procedure:
   - Client expresses sense of comfort with hair and scalp grooming.

     Scalp stimulated and areas of matted or tangled hair removed.
   - Client expresses sense of comfort, with sensation of face feeling clean and refreshed.

     Hair and soap lather are removed.
   - Skin surface is smooth, well hydrated, and free of cuts.

     Client is free from injury.
   - Client assists with procedure.

     Participation provides sense of control.

2. While performing procedure, ask client to explain steps he or she uses to comb hair and/or shave. Ask client to indicate if becomes uncomfortable.

   Client can become apprehensive about hair being pulled or skin being accidentally cut.

3. Position client sitting in chair or in bed with head elevated 45 to 90 degrees (as tolerated).

   Elevation of head of bed makes it easier to access all sides of head and face.

4. Arrange supplies at bedside table, and adjust lighting. Perform hand hygiene.

   Easy access to supplies prevents interruption of procedure. Lighting provides clear view of client's face.

IMPLEMENTATION

COMBING AND BRUSHING HAIR

1. Part the hair into two sections, then separate hair into two more sections (see illustration).

   Brushing and combing are more effective when small areas of hair are groomed at any one time.

2. Brush or comb from the scalp toward the hair ends.

   Minimizes pulling.

3. Moisten hair lightly with water, conditioner, or an alcohol-free detangle product before combing.

   Makes hair easier to comb.

4. Move fingers through hair to loosen any larger tangles.

   Lessens pulling.

5. Using a wide-tooth comb, start on either side of the head, and insert the comb with the teeth upward to the hair near the scalp. Comb through the hair in a circular motion by turning the wrist while lifting up and out. Continue until all hair is combed through, and then comb into place to shape and style.

   Move comb evenly through hair without pulling.

STEP	RATIONALE

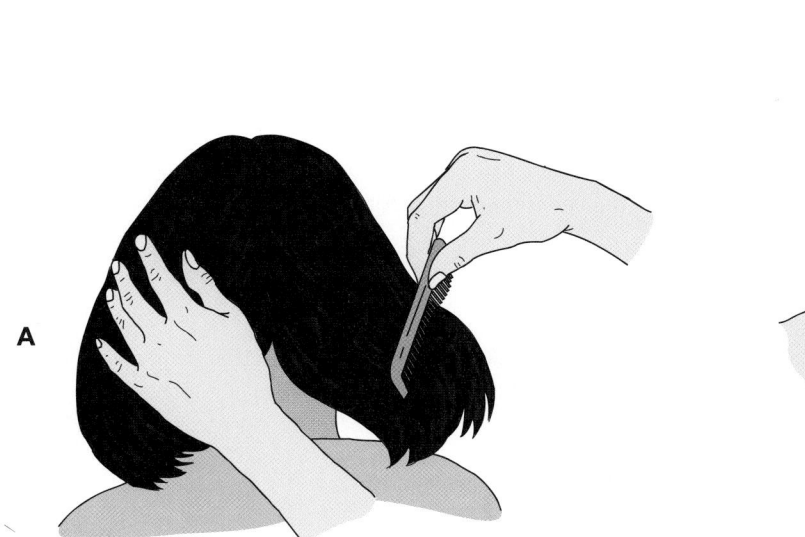

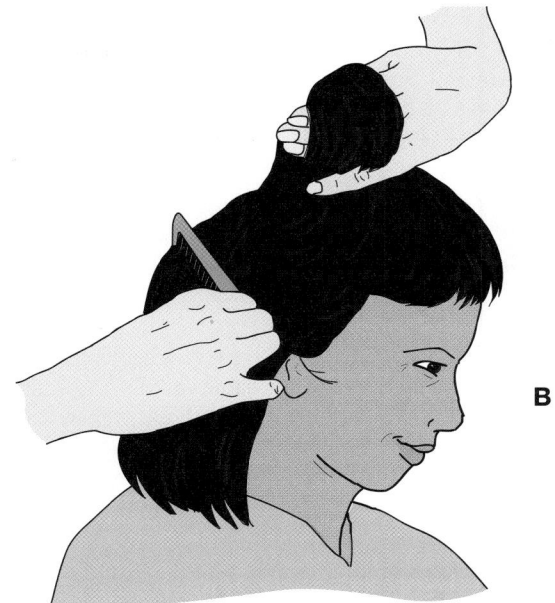

STEP 1 Parting hair. **A,** Part hair down the middle, and divide it into two main sections. **B,** Then part the main section into two smaller sections.

SHAVING WITH DISPOSABLE RAZOR

1. Place bath towel over client's chest and shoulders.
   Prevents shaving cream or water from soiling gown.
2. Run warm water in washbasin. Check water temperature.
   Warm water will soften beard. Proper temperature prevents accidental burns.
3. Place washcloth in basin, and wring out thoroughly. Apply cloth over client's entire face for several seconds.
   Warm cloth helps soften skin and beard. Sensation of warmth can be relaxing.

• *Critical Decision Point*
  If client has sores, open lesions, or a tendency to bleed, the nurse should apply disposable gloves.

4. Apply shaving cream or soap to client's face. Smooth cream evenly over sides of face, chin, and under nose.
   Cream creates additional softening effect and lubricates skin for application of razor.
5. Hold razor in dominant hand at 45-degree angle to the client's skin. Begin by shaving across one side of client's face using short, firm strokes in direction hair grows (see illustration). Use nondominant hand to gently pull skin taut while shaving. Check with client, and ask if he feels comfortable.
   Technique facilitates shaving of facial hair. Short downward strokes work best over upper lip. Holding skin taut prevents razor cuts and discomfort during shaving. Client is best resource to confirm if shaving technique causes discomfort.

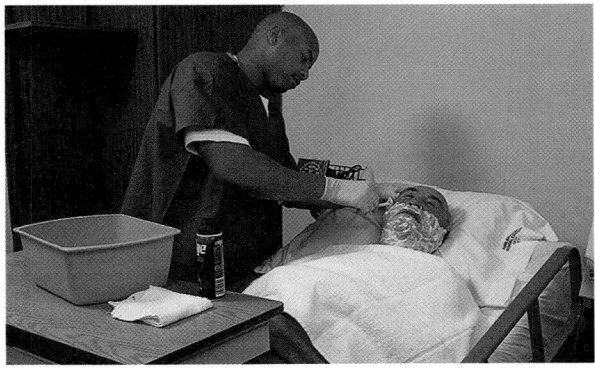

STEP 5 Shaving a client using short, firm strokes.

STEP	RATIONALE
6. Dip razor blade in water as shaving cream accumulates on blade's edge.	Keeps cutting surface of razor blade clean.
7. After all facial hair is shaved, rinse face thoroughly with moistened washcloth.	Prevents accumulation of shaving cream, which can cause drying of skin.
8. Dry face thoroughly, and apply aftershave lotion if desired.	Retained moisture may cause chapping of skin.
9. Assist client to comfortable position.	
10. Return equipment to proper place. Discard soiled linen in hamper. Perform hand hygiene.	Maintains cleanliness of client's environment and reduces transmission of infection.

ELECTRIC RAZOR

1. Perform step 1 for disposable razor.	
2. Apply skin conditioner or preshave preparation.	Softens skin and beard to reduce friction from razor head.
3. Turn razor on, and begin by shaving across side of face. Gently hold skin taut while shaving over skin's surface. Use gentle downward stroke of razor in direction of hair growth.	Prevents pulling of beard and skin.
4. After completing shave, apply aftershave lotion as desired.	Stimulates and lubricates skin.
5. Perform steps 9 and 10 for disposable razor.	

MUSTACHE AND BEARD CARE

1. Perform step 1 for disposable razor.	
2. If necessary, gently comb mustache or beard.	Straightens hair that requires trimming.
3. Allow client to use mirror and direct areas to trim with scissors.	Allows client to make decisions about care; maintains sense of independence.

EVALUATION

1. Ask client how hair and scalp feel.	Evaluates client's satisfaction with grooming
2. Inspect condition of shaved area and skin underneath beard or mustache.	Nurse looks for areas of localized bleeding from cuts and for areas of dryness.
3. Ask client if face feels clean and comfortable.	Evaluates level of client's comfort.
4. Ask if client is satisfied with degree of participation.	Client maintains sense of control.

Recording and Reporting

- It is not necessary to record shaving procedure unless it is included on the agency's checklist. However, record any complications such as bleeding in nurses' notes.

Unexpected Outcomes	Related Interventions
1. Client senses tangles or discomfort in scalp.	• Inspect scalp area. Repeat brushing/combing as needed.
2. Small isolated nicks or cuts may appear on skin.	• Obtain a new disposable razor, or change the blade. If razor is reusable, be sure to clean according to agency policy. • Change technique so as to glide razor over the client's skin.
3. Skin surface may appear dry.	• This is a result of soap drying skin; use a moisturizing shaving foam. • Apply moisturizing lotion to client's skin after shave.

Teaching Considerations

- Shaving is a simple procedure that can be taught to a family member. Instruct primary caregiver in safety precautions for shaving, especially if client is receiving anticoagulant therapy.
- Instruct family member in technique to follow in the event the client is accidentally nicked.

Pediatric Considerations

- Usually the facial hair of adolescents does not grow quickly, and thus a shave might not be necessary each day.
- Adolescents who shave should be asked about the frequency and allowed to perform activity as desired. Family members may wish to be involved in shaving their adolescent child if the child is unable to perform the activity.
- Young girls with long hair may not tolerate brushing tangles out of hair. Tangling occurs easily in children restricted to bed. Once tangles are removed, it may be helpful to braid the hair.

- Children with lice should be isolated for 24 hours after effective therapy and when no live lice are seen. It is important for families to understand that head lice are not a sign of poor hygiene. All clothing and linens must be washed in hot water or, if not washable, must be bagged for a minimum of 10 days.

Gerontological Considerations

- Usually the facial hair of older clients does not grow quickly, and a shave might not be necessary each day.

Home Care Considerations

- Provide adequate towels around client's neck to avoid spilling shaving cream or water on chest or bed.
- Provide adequate lighting for procedure.
- Perform procedure in comfortable setting, such as bathroom or bedroom.

SKILL 14-5 Performing Nail and Foot Care

View Video

Feet and nails often require special care to prevent infection, odors, pain, and injury to soft tissues. Often people are unaware of foot or nail problems until discomfort or pain occurs. Common foot and nail problems are listed in Table 14-3. For proper foot and nail care, clients should be instructed to protect the feet from injury, keep the feet clean and dry, and wear appropriate footwear. The nurse instructs clients in the proper way to inspect the feet for lesions, dryness, or signs of infection. To maintain and promote foot and nail health, clients should visit a podiatrist when necessary. This is especially important for clients with peripheral vascular diseases, diabetes mellitus, older adults, and clients whose immune system is suppressed.

Clients most at risk for developing serious foot problems are those with peripheral neuropathy and peripheral vascular disease. These two disorders, commonly found in clients

with diabetes, cause a reduction in blood flow to the extremities and a loss of sensory, motor, and autonomic nerve function. As a result, a client is unable to feel heat and cold, pain, pressure, and position of the foot. A person could have a tack or stone in his or her shoe and walk on it all day without perceiving a foreign object in the shoe. The reduction in blood flow impairs healing and promotes risk for infection. Diabetic clients often develop foot ulcers as a result of direct causes that include deformities such as heel spurs and bunions, repetitive stresses from abnormal gait patterns, direct trauma, and improper foot wear (Strauss, 2001). If foot ulcers do not heal, they can quickly become infected and lead to gangrene and, in turn, amputation.

Nail and foot care should be included in a client's daily hygiene; the best time is during the client's bath. Many agencies requires a physician's order before a nurse can trim nails.

TABLE 14-3   COMMON FOOT AND NAIL PROBLEMS

CONDITION	CHARACTERISTICS	IMPLICATIONS	INTERVENTIONS
Callus Callus on sole of foot.	Thickened portion of epidermis, consisting of mass of horny, keratotic cells; usually flat, painless, and found on undersurface of foot or on palm of hand; caused by local friction or pressure.	Foot calluses may cause discomfort when wearing tight-fitting shoes.	Advise client to wear gloves when using tools or objects that may create friction on palms; wear comfortable shoes. Soak callus in warm water (*exception:* diabetic client) and Epsom salts to soften cell layers. Use pumice stone to remove callus after it softens. Applications of creams or lotions can reduce re-formation. Use of orthotic devices (e.g., foam insoles, cushioning devices) redistributes weight and pressure away from callus area.
Corns Corn.	Keratosis caused by friction and pressure from shoes; mainly on toes, over bony prominence; usually cone-shaped, round, and raised. Calluses with painful core.	Conical shape compresses underlying dermis, making it thin and tender. Pain is aggravated by tight-fitting shoes. Clients may suffer alteration in gait because of pain.	Surgical removal may be necessary, depending on severity of pain and size of corn. Use oval corn pads carefully, because they increase pressure on toes and reduce circulation.
Plantar warts Plantar warts.	Fungating lesions on sole of foot caused by papillomavirus.	Warts may be contagious, are painful, and make walking difficult.	Refer client to podiatrist.
Athlete's foot (tinea pedis) Tinea pedis.	Fungal infection of foot; scaliness and cracking of skin between toes and on soles of feet; small blisters containing fluid may appear, apparently induced by constricting footwear.	Athlete's foot can spread to other body parts, especially hands. It is contagious and frequently recurs.	Feet should be well ventilated. Drying feet well after bathing and applying powder help prevent infection. Wearing clean socks or stockings reduces incidence. Physician may order application of griseofulvin, miconazole nitrate, or tolnaftate.
Ingrown nails Ingrown toenail.	Toenail or fingernail growing inward into soft tissue around nail; results from improper nail trimming, poor shoe fit, or heredity.	Ingrown nails can cause localized pain when pressure is applied.	Treatment is frequent warm soaks (*exception:* diabetic client) in antiseptic solution and removal of portion of nail that has grown into skin. Instruct client on proper nail-trimming techniques. Refer to podiatrist.
Paronychia Paronychia.	Inflammation of tissue surrounding nail after hangnail or other injury; occurs in people who frequently have their hands in water; common in diabetic clients.	Area can become infected.	Treatment is warm compresses or soaks (**EXCEPTION:** diabetic client) and local application of antibiotic ointments. Paronychia can be prevented by careful manicuring.
Foot odors	Result of excess perspiration promoting microorganism growth. Faulty foot hygiene or improper footwear may also contribute.		Frequent washing, use of foot deodorants and powders, and clean footwear will pre-

DELEGATION CONSIDERATIONS

The skill of nail and foot care of the nondiabetic client and clients without circulatory compromise can be delegated to assistive personnel. The nurse provides assistive personnel with information, assistance, and direction, including:

- Informing and assisting care provider in proper way to use nail clippers (NOTE: Many agencies do not allow assistive personnel or even RNs to use nail clippers; consult agency policy)
- Cautioning assistive personnel to use warm water
- Instructing assistive personnel to report any changes that may indicate inflammation or injury

EQUIPMENT

- ❑ Washbasin
- ❑ Emesis basin
- ❑ Washcloth
- ❑ Bath or face towel
- ❑ Nail clippers (check agency policy)
- ❑ Orange stick (optional)
- ❑ Emery board or nail file
- ❑ Body lotion
- ❑ Disposable bath mat
- ❑ Paper towels

STEP	RATIONALE

▮ ASSESSMENT

1. Inspect all surfaces of fingers, toes, feet, and nails. Pay particular attention to areas of dryness, inflammation, or cracking. Also inspect areas between toes, heels, and soles of feet. Inspect socks for stains.

   Integrity of feet and nails determines frequency and level of hygiene required. Heels, soles, and sides of feet are prone to irritation from ill-fitting shoes. Socks may become stained from bleeding or draining ulcer.

2. Assess color and temperature of toes, feet, and fingers. Assess capillary refill of nails. Palpate radial and ulnar pulse of each hand and dorsalis pedis pulse of foot; note character of pulses.

   Assesses adequacy of blood flow to extremities. Circulatory alterations may change integrity of nails and increase client's chance of localized infection when break in skin integrity occurs (Strauss and others, 1998).

3. Observe client's walking gait. Have client walk down hall or walk straight line while wearing comfortable shoes or slippers (if able).

   Painful disorders of feet can cause limping or unnatural gait (Armstrong and Lavery, 1998).

4. Ask female clients about whether they use nail polish and polish remover frequently.

   Chemicals in these products can cause excessive dryness.

5. Assess type of footwear worn by clients: Are socks worn? Are shoes tight or ill fitting? Are garters or knee-high nylons worn? Is footwear clean?

   Types of shoes and footwear may predispose client to foot and nail problems (e.g., infection, areas of friction, ulcerations).

6. Identify client's risk for foot or nail problems:

   Certain conditions increase likelihood of foot or nail problems.

   a. Older adult

   Poor vision, lack of coordination, or inability to bend over contribute to difficulty among older adults in performing foot and nail care. Normal physiological changes of aging also result in dry, brittle nails.

   b. Diabetes

   Vascular changes associated with diabetes reduce blood flow to peripheral tissues. Break in skin integrity places diabetic at high risk for skin infection.

   c. Heart failure, renal disease

   Both conditions can increase tissue edema, particularly in dependent areas (e.g., feet). Edema reduces blood flow to neighboring tissues.

   d. Cerebrovascular accident, stroke

   Presence of residual foot or leg weakness or paralysis results in altered walking patterns. Altered gait pattern causes increased friction and pressure on feet.

7. Assess type of home remedies clients use for existing foot problems:

   Certain preparations or applications may cause more injury to soft tissue then initial foot problem.

   a. Over-the-counter liquid preparations to remove corns or warts

   Liquid preparations can cause burns and ulcerations.

   b. Cutting of corns or calluses with razor blade or scissors

   Cutting of corns or calluses may result in infection caused by break in skin integrity.

   c. Use of oval corn pads

   Oval pads may exert pressure on toes, thereby decreasing circulation to surrounding tissues.

   d. Application of adhesive tape

   Skin of older adult is thin and delicate and prone to tearing when adhesive tape is removed.

STEP	RATIONALE
8. Assess client's ability to care for nails or feet: visual alterations, fatigue, musculoskeletal weakness.	Extent of client's ability to perform self-care determines degree of assistance required from nurse.
9. Assess client's knowledge of foot and nail care practices.	Level of client's knowledge determines client's need for health teaching.

NURSING DIAGNOSES

- Ineffective tissue perfusion
- Dressing/grooming self-care deficit
- Impaired physical mobility

- Impaired skin integrity
- Deficient knowledge regarding foot and nail care
- Risk for infection

Related factors are individualized based on client's condition or needs.

PLANNING

1. Expected outcomes following completion of procedure:	
• Nails are smooth. Cuticles and tissues surrounding nail are clear and of normal color. Surfaces of feet are smooth.	Excess skin layers are removed. Nail integrity and cleanliness are maintained.
• Client walks freely, without pain or unusual gait.	Sources of pressure or irritation are removed (Slovenkai, 1998).
• Client explains or demonstrates nail care correctly.	Client learns skill.
2. Explain procedure to client, including fact that proper soaking requires several minutes in warm water.	Client must be willing to place fingers and feet in basins for 10 to 20 minutes. Client may become anxious or fatigued.
3. Obtain physician's order for cutting nails (required by most agencies).	Client's skin may be accidentally cut. Certain clients are more at risk for infection, depending on their medical condition.

IMPLEMENTATION

1. Perform hand hygiene. Arrange equipment on over-bed table.	Easy access to equipment prevents delays.
2. Pull curtain around bed, or close room door (if desired).	Maintaining client's privacy reduces anxiety.
3. Assist ambulatory client with sitting in bedside chair. Help bedfast client to supine position with head of bed elevated. Place disposable bath mat on floor under client's feet, or place towel on mattress.	Sitting in chair facilitates immersing feet in basin. Bath mat protects feet from exposure to soil or debris.
4. Fill washbasin with warm water. Test water temperature.	Warm water softens nails and thickened epidermal cells, reduces inflammation of skin, and promotes local circulation. Proper water temperature prevents burns and injury (Armstrong and Lavery, 1998).
5. Place basin on bath mat or towel, and help client place feet in basin. Place call light within client's reach.	Clients with muscular weakness or tremors may have difficulty positioning feet. Client's safety is maintained.

• Critical Decision Point

The American Diabetes Association (1999) does not recommend soaking of a diabetic client's feet, due to risk of infection.

6. Adjust over-bed table to low position, and place it over client's lap. (Client may sit in chair or lie in bed.)	Easy access prevents accidental spills.
7. Fill emesis basin with warm water, and place basin on paper towels on over-bed table.	Warm water softens nails and thickened epidermal cells.
8. Instruct client to place fingers in emesis basin and place arms in comfortable position.	Prolonged positioning can cause discomfort unless normal anatomical alignment is maintained.
9. Allow client's feet and fingernails to soak for 10 to 20 minutes. Rewarm water after 10 minutes.	Softening of corns, calluses, and cuticles ensures easy removal of dead cells and easy manipulation of cuticle.

STEP	RATIONALE

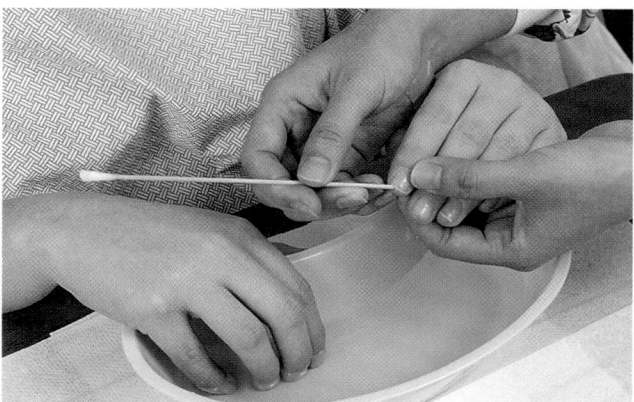

STEP **10** Cleanse under fingernails.

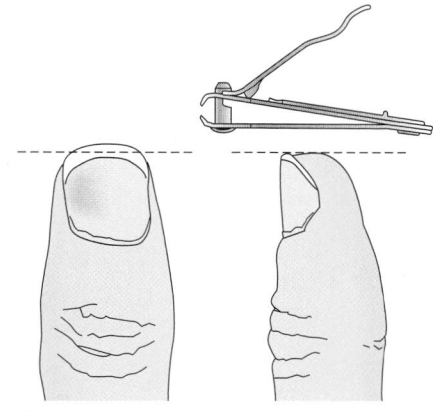

STEP **11** Clip fingernails straight across. Use a nail clipper.

10. Clean gently under fingernails with orange stick or end of wooden applicator stick while fingers are immersed (see illustration). Remove emesis basin and dry fingers thoroughly.

11. With nail clippers, clip fingernails straight across and even with tops of fingers (see illustration). Shape nails with emery board or file.

Orange stick removes debris under nails that harbors microorganisms. Thorough drying impedes fungal growth and prevents maceration of tissues.

Cutting straight across prevents splitting of nail margins and formation of sharp nail spikes that can irritate lateral nail margins. Filing prevents cutting nail too close to nail bed (Strauss and others, 1998).

• *Critical Decision Point*
If client is diabetic or has circulatory problems, do not cut nails. File only.

12. Push cuticle back gently with orange stick.
13. Move over-bed table away from client.
14. Apply disposable gloves, and scrub callused areas of feet with washcloth.
15. Clean gently under nails with orange stick. Remove feet from basin, and dry thoroughly.
16. Clean and trim toenails using procedures in steps 11 and 12. Do not file corners of toenails.
17. Apply lotion to feet and hands, and assist client back to bed and into comfortable position.

Pushing back cuticles reduces incidence of inflamed cuticles.
Provides easier access to feet.
Gloves prevent transmission of fungal infection. Friction removes dead skin layers.
Removal of debris and excess moisture reduces chances of infection.
Shaping corners of toenails may damage tissues (Strauss and others, 1998).
Lotion lubricates dry skin by helping to retain moisture.

• *Critical Decision Point*
The American Diabetes Association (2003) does not recommend lotion between toes of clients with diabetes. Moisture can cause maceration and skin breakdown.

18. Remove disposable gloves, and place in receptacle. Clean and return equipment and supplies to proper place. Dispose of soiled linen in hamper. Perform hand hygiene.

Reduces transmission of infection.

STEP	RATIONALE
EVALUATION	
1. Inspect nails, areas between toes, and surrounding skin surfaces.	Inspection enables nurse to evaluate condition of skin and nails and allows nurse to note any remaining rough nail edges.
2. Ask client to explain or demonstrate nail care.	Demonstration allows nurse to evaluate client's level of learning techniques.
3. Observe client's walk after toenail care.	Observation allows nurse to evaluate level of comfort and mobility achieved.

Recording and Reporting

- Record procedure and observations in nurses' notes (e.g., breaks in skin, inflammation, ulcerations).
- Report any breaks in skin or ulcerations to nurse in charge or physician.

Unexpected Outcomes	Related Interventions
1. Nails discolored, rough, and concave or irregular in shape.	• Continue hygiene practice because a single hygiene measure will not improve nail condition.
2. Cuticles and surrounding tissues may be inflamed and tender to touch. Localized areas of tenderness may occur on feet with calluses or corns at point of friction.	• Repeated nail care is needed. • Change in footwear or corrective foot surgery may be needed for permanent improvement in calluses or corns. • Referral to podiatrist may be needed.
3. Ulcerations involving toes or feet may remain.	• Institute wound care policies (see Chapter 37). • Consult with wound care specialist and/or podiatrist.
4. Client unable to explain or perform foot care.	• Repeat client teaching and demonstration of foot care. Consider including family caregiver in instruction. • Use return demonstration to document client/family learning.
5. Client complains of pain while walking and has unsteady gait.	• Pressure or irritation on foot is still present. Special footwear may be required, or client may need referral to podiatrist.
6. Toenails are long and cannot be cut.	• Refer client to podiatrist.

Teaching Considerations

- Instruct diabetic clients or clients with peripheral vascular disease in the following precautions (American Diabetes Association, 1999, 2003):
  - Examine the feet daily, including top, bottom, sides, and between toes of each foot. A mirror can be very useful. Have clients look for new onset of redness, swelling, breaks in the skin, blisters, calluses, and macerated areas (Strauss, 2001).
  - Wash the feet daily. Wash gently, but really wash them with soap and warm water and washcloth. Gently pat dry with a clean, soft, absorbent towel. Do not put lotion between the toes.
  - Minor cuts should be washed immediately and dried thoroughly. Only mild antiseptics (e.g., Neosporin ointment) should be applied to the skin. Avoid iodine or merbromin because they can be very irritating to tissues.
  - Do not cut corns or calluses or use commercial removers. Consult a physician or podiatrist. Have at least one thorough foot examination each year.
  - If the feet perspire, apply a bland foot powder.
  - If dryness is noted along the feet or between the toes, apply lanolin, baby oil, or even corn oil, and rub gently into the skin.
  - File toenails straight across and square; do not use scissors or clippers. Consult a podiatrist.

- Do not use over-the-counter preparations to treat athlete's foot or ingrown nails.
- Avoid wearing elastic stockings, knee-high hose, or constricting garters. Shoes should be long enough, wide enough, and deep enough to cover feet without rubbing, causing pressure, or constricting any part of them. Buy shoes at end of day when feet are slightly swollen. Wear clean socks you plan to use with the shoes. Soles of shoes should be flexible and nonslipping. Shoes should have porous uppers and be sturdy, closed in, and not restrictive to feet (Slovenkai, 1998).
- Check inside your shoes before you put them on. Something may have fallen (or crawled) into them. Feel inside of each shoe with your hand to make sure nothing is inside. Check inside of shoes daily for pebbles, foreign objects, and tears in inner liner (Osterman and Stuck, 1990).
- Wear clean socks or stockings daily. Socks should be dry and free of holes or darns.
- Never walk barefoot.

Pediatric Considerations
- Assessment and clipping of nails of children should be done to prevent them from scratching themselves. Appropriate-size clippers should be used when clipping the nails of infants and small children. Do not use scissors.

Gerontological Considerations
- Changes in aging skin include thinning of epidermis and subcutaneous fat and dryness because of decreased activity of oil and sweat glands. These changes can be seen in the feet. In addition, nails become opaque, tough, scaly, brittle, and hypertrophied.
- A lifetime of limited exercise can result in laxity of foot ligaments and musculature and lead to instability and impaired mobility.
- Common foot problems of older adults include heel pain caused by tearing of plantar fascia and foot musculature, metatarsalgia (pain beneath metatarsal head), hammer toes and claw toes, corns and calluses, pathological nail conditions (e.g., ingrown toenails, fungal infections), arthritis, and neuropathies that cause diminished sensation in foot (Lueckenotte, 2000).
- Older persons are also more vulnerable to bunions because feet tend to spread with aging. Young people are rarely affected, although bunions sometimes occur in individuals as young as 10 to 14 years of age (Lueckenotte, 2000).

Home Care Considerations
- Alternative therapies: moleskin applied to areas of feet that are under friction is less likely to cause local pressure than corn pads; spot adhesive bandages can guard corns against friction but do not have padding to protect against pressure; wrapping small pieces of lamb's wool around toes reduces irritation of soft corns between toes (Beuscher, 1998).
- In the home assess use of bathroom sink for soaking client's hands and tub for soaking feet.

SKILL 14-6 Care of the Client's Environment

When caring for clients who need to remain in or near their bed for an extended period, it is important to try to make that environment as comfortable as possible. A calm, comfortable restorative environment can be maintained in a hospital, extended care facility, or the client's home. Rooms should be comfortable, safe, and large enough to allow clients, visitors, and care providers to move about freely. The care provider should be able to control temperature, ventilation, noise, and odors easily.

A room in a typical hospital, extended care, or long-term care facility contains the following basic pieces of furniture: over-bed table, bedside stand, storage space, chairs, lights, and bed with call light. These furnishings provide a setting for the client to rest, as well as safe and convenient access to all client care supplies. Behind each bed is a wall unit that may contain various power outlets and receptacles for connecting oxygen and suction equipment. In most hospitals a sphygmomanometer with cuff is attached to the wall. Intensive care unit rooms often have poles extending from the ceiling on which to hang IV fluid bags. The room is generally designed so that all necessary supplies and equipment are easily accessible for the nurse's and physician's use.

When care is provided in the client's home, special equipment and adaptations to the client's home may be necessary. If a client is to receive home oxygen, then oxygen tanks are needed, and with some oxygen equipment, the client may need additional electrical wiring in the home. Clients and their families may need to order a hospital bed and over-bed table so that physical care can be given easily. In addition, the client's bathroom is adapted with safety equipment for ease in toileting and getting into and out of the tub and shower.

ROOM EQUIPMENT

Chairs

Most hospital rooms contain an armless, straight-back chair and an upholstered lounge chair with arms. When clients are recovering from surgery or illnesses resulting in abdominal pain, they often prefer the straight-back chair because less effort is needed to get into or out of it. Straight-back chairs are convenient when temporarily transferring the client from the bed, for example, during bed making. The straight-back chair is also easier to maneuver than the heavy lounge chair. However, the straight-back chair may be more uncomfortable and less safe for certain clients than the deeper lounge chair. The lounge chair often has a deeper seat and may require more effort on the part of the client to sit comfortably.

Lights

Each room has an over-bed light that focuses on the client's bed. The light controls are usually on the call light apparatus or nearby wall switch. Each room also has a floor or table lamp. Special examination lights may extend over the bed from the wall or ceiling. These lights are useful during procedures such as a dressing change. They are often moveable and should be positioned for easy reach but moved aside when not in use. Portable lamps provide extra illumination for bedside procedures. These are especially useful to focus light on hard-to-reach areas, for example, during urinary catheter insertion.

A call light is at each client's bedside (Figure 14-4). When a client presses a button located on the side rail of the bed or at the end of an extension cord, a light goes on at the nurses' station or outside the client's room. The call light signal indicates that a client needs assistance and is "calling" the nurse. The light usually triggers a light outside the client's room so that any staff member can see the light and respond to the client's call. In some hospitals the call light system is wired into a portable telephone system, allowing each nurse to personally respond when their client calls. In addition to call lights, many hospitals have intercom systems that allow clients to talk to a staff person at the nurses' station. Many hospital units also have emergency signal lights, particularly in the client's bathroom, which nurses use to call for assistance when clients are in trouble. Clients may also be instructed to use the emergency signal lights if an emergency situation arises when they are in the bathroom alone.

Over-Bed Tables

The over-bed table is a long, narrow table with wheels. It can be adjusted to various heights over the client's bed or chair. It usually contains two storage drawers. The table provides ideal working space for the nurse and serves as a surface on which to place meal trays, toiletry items, and objects frequently used by the client.

Bedside Stand

The bedside stand or table is a small table or cabinet located next to the bed. It is used to store the client's personal articles and hygiene equipment such as the bath basin, towels, or an emesis basin. Each table usually contains a drawer above and

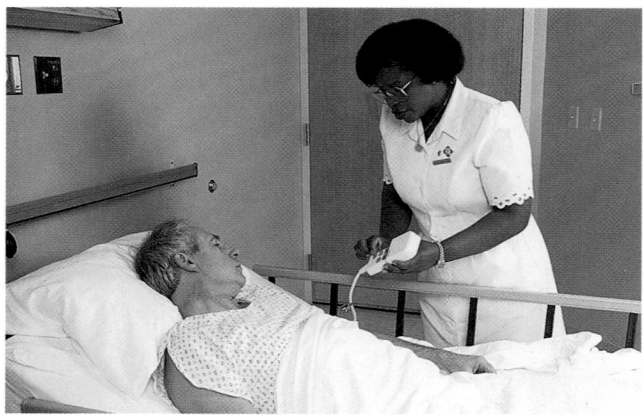

FIGURE **14-4** Nurse teaching client how to use intercom to nurses' station.

a cupboard below. The telephone, water pitcher, facial tissues, and drinking cup are commonly placed on the bedside table.

Beds

Because the bed is the piece of equipment used most by the client, it should be designed for comfort and safety, and it should be adaptable to various positions. The typical hospital bed consists of a firm mattress on a metal frame that can be raised and lowered horizontally. The frame is divided into three sections so that the operator can raise and lower the head and foot of the bed separately, in addition to inclining the entire bed with the head up or down. Table 14-4 lists common bed positions. Most beds are powered by electric motors.

Hospital beds come in two different lengths. Standard length is approximately 6 feet (a longer bed is available for taller clients). Each bed sits on four rollers, or casters, that allow the nurse to move the bed easily. Often clients who are critically ill or who are immobilized in traction are transported to different locations, such as the radiology department, in bed. There are beds in which scales are incorporated to facilitate routine weighing of a client.

The position of a bed is usually changed by electric controls built into the side of the bed, at the foot of the bed, or on a bedside cable. Clients can thus raise or lower sections of the bed without expending much energy. It is important for nurses to instruct clients in the proper use of the controls and to caution them against positions that might cause harm. A hospital bed is usually 65 to 70 cm (26 to 28 inches) above the floor at its lowest level. In the home most beds are 50 to 55 cm (20 to 22 inches) high. The greater height of a hospital bed prevents undue musculoskeletal strain on the nurse and the client. It is unnecessary for the nurse to reach across or bend down while caring for clients, and clients can move from the bed to a chair with minimal stress on hips and knees.

Beds contain a number of safety features. Locks located on the wheels, casters, or at the center of the bed frame (Figure 14-5) should be used whenever the bed is stationary to prevent accidental movement during performance of a procedure (e.g., transferring the client from bed to a stretcher). Side rails (either four or two depending on bed design), located on both sides of a bed, help clients position themselves and provide upper extremity support as a client gets out of bed. Caution must be used in raising side rails. Research suggests that the risk of client falls is greater when side rails on both sides of the bed are raised because clients try to climb over the rails to exit the bed. Raising only one rail (when there are only two) or three (when there are four rails) gives clients an exit route if they are able to move independently. Use of all side rails is considered a physical restraint (see Chapter 4). Side rails are adjustable metal frames that can be raised and lowered by pushing or pulling a knob. When a side rail has been lowered, the nurse never leaves the bedside with the client still in bed. Each bed also has a special headboard that is removable. This feature is important in emergency situations when the medical team must have easy access to the client's head during cardiopulmonary resuscitation (see Chapter 26).

TABLE 14-4   COMMON BED POSITIONS

POSITION	DESCRIPTION	USES
Fowler's	Head of bed raised to angle of 45 to 90 degrees or more; semisitting position (knees raise on most beds approximately 15 degrees).	Preferred while client eats; used during nasogastric tube insertion and nasotracheal suction; promotes lung expansion.
Semi-Fowler's	Head of bed raised approximately 30 to 45 degrees; incline is less than Fowler's position (knees raise on most beds approximately 15 degrees). Intensive care beds have circular measuring device on side of bed to indicate exact elevation angle.	Promotes lung expansion; relieves strain on abdominal muscles.
Trendelenburg's	Entire bed frame tilted, with head of bed down.	For postural drainage; facilitates venous return in clients with poor peripheral perfusion.
Reverse Trendelenburg's	Entire bed frame tilted, with foot of bed down.	Used infrequently; promotes gastric emptying and prevents esophageal reflux.
Flat	Entire bed frame parallel with floor.	For clients with vertebral injuries and in cervical traction. Position used for clients who are hypotensive, and generally preferred by clients for sleeping.

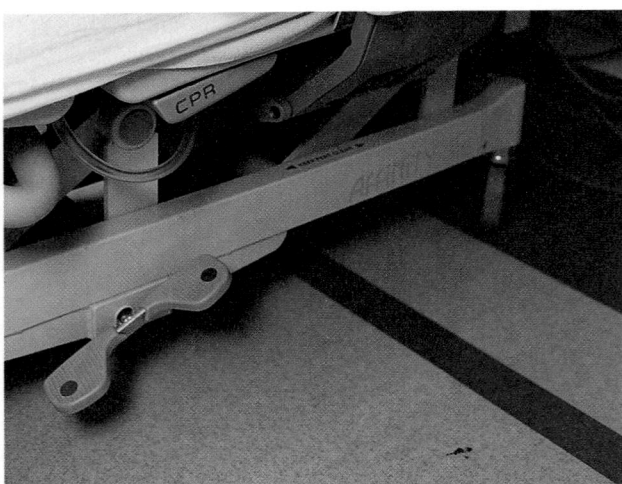

FIGURE **14-5** Lock on bed wheels.

Mattresses

Most beds have firm, water-repellent mattresses. A mattress should have an even surface for the client's comfort. A rubber or plastic surface permits easy cleaning. Special mattresses provide extra comfort and support for clients and relieve pressure on bony prominences. Chapter 13 reviews a variety of special mattresses and support surfaces and indications for their use.

Special Equipment

There is special equipment that may be added to a bed or room. Examples include bed boards and IV poles. The nurse is responsible for knowing how to use all equipment safely.

Skill Performance Guidelines

1. Keep the environment as comfortable as possible. Depending on a client's age and physical condition, room temperature should be maintained between 20° C and 23° C (68° F and 74° F). Infants, older adults, and the acutely ill may need a warmer temperature. However, certain critically ill clients require cooler room temperatures to lower the body's metabolic demands. Controlling drafts and eliminating lingering odors from draining wounds, vomitus, bedpans, or urinals will also improve a client's comfort. Hospitals now prohibit smoking in clients' rooms.
2. Control extraneous noises in a client's room. Ill clients are sensitive to noises in a hospital environment. A nurse should try to control noise level by handling equipment properly; making sure equipment is in proper working order; controlling voice volume; and, unless contraindicated, closing the client's room door.
3. Make the environment as safe as possible. Keep all personal care items within the client's reach. When the head of the bed is raised, the bedside stand is usually not within easy reach and must be moved forward. If the client must leave the bed to go to the bathroom, be sure there are no objects obstructing the way.

4. Make the environment personal for the client. A picture of family members, some get well cards, or a small radio may help the client to relax. However, do not clutter the client's room with unnecessary equipment and supplies. Whenever possible, remove equipment and supplies after treatments are complete.
5. Be sure the client is easily accessible to the health care team. Often a client will have numerous IV lines and drainage tubes connected to portable poles and suction machines. At times of emergency, the health care team must reach the client easily and quickly. Keep IV poles and portable equipment in positions that do not obstruct access to the client.

Making an Unoccupied Bed

Clients spend much of their time in bed, eating, bathing, using bedpans or urinals, and undergoing numerous therapeutic procedures. It is essential that the nurse keep the bed as clean and comfortable as possible. Frequent inspections are necessary to be sure that the linen is clean, dry, and wrinkle free. Bed linen that becomes wet or soiled should be changed immediately.

Whenever possible the nurse should make the bed while it is unoccupied. Having the client get out of bed is an ideal way to promote ambulation. The nurse usually makes a bed in the morning after the client's bed bath or while the client is up bathing and showering. Another convenient time for bed making is when the client is out of the room for tests or procedures.

By making an unoccupied bed the nurse can ensure that the linen is smooth and free of wrinkles. It is also easier to insert any extra waterproof pads or special mattresses (see Chapter 13) when bed is unoccupied (Box 14-4).

Making an Occupied Bed

At times it is necessary to make a bed that is occupied by a client. The client may be too weak to get out of bed; the illness may prohibit sitting up; or the client may be restricted to bed because of postprocedure precautions, traction, or heavy body or leg casts. If a client is confined to bed, bed making should be done in a way that conserves time and the client's energy. In addition, the nurse must know what position the client can safely assume while the bed linens are changed. The nurse also tries to keep the client as comfortable as possible. In cases where a client experiences severe pain, an analgesic administered 30 to 60 minutes before the procedure is helpful in controlling pain and maintaining comfort.

Even though the client is unable to get out of bed, the nurse encourages self-help as much as possible. For example, the client can turn, assist in moving up in bed, or hold top sheets while linen is applied. These activities help maintain the client's strength and mobility and allow participation in hygiene care.

Making an occupied bed poses some difficulties. It is harder to prevent transfer of organisms from soiled linens to clean linens and to keep newly applied linen smooth and wrinkle-free. The procedure can be done quickly, however, if the nurse is organized.

BOX 14-4 Procedural Guideline
Making an unoccupied bed

DELEGATION CONSIDERATIONS

The skill of making an unoccupied bed can be delegated to assistive personnel. Inform assistive personnel of any position or activity restrictions that apply to client's ability to get out of bed.

EQUIPMENT

Linen bag, mattress pad (change only when soiled), bottom sheet (flat or fitted), drawsheet (optional), top sheet, blanket, bedspread, waterproof pads (optional), pillowcases, bedside chair or table, disposable gloves (if linen is soiled), washcloth, antiseptic cleanser

ASSESSMENT

1. Determine if client has been incontinent or if excess drainage is on linen. Gloves will be necessary.
2. Assess activity orders or restrictions in mobility/positioning in planning if client can get out of bed for procedure. Assist to bedside chair or recliner.
3. Lower side rails on both sides of bed, and raise bed to comfortable working position.
4. Remove soiled linen, and place in laundry bag. Avoid shaking or fanning linen.
5. Reposition mattress, and wipe off any moisture using a washcloth moistened in antiseptic solution (consult agency housekeeping guidelines). Dry thoroughly.
6. Apply all bottom linen on one side of bed before moving to opposite side.
7. Be sure fitted sheet is placed smoothly over mattress. To apply a flat unfitted sheet, allow about 25 cm (10 inches) to hang over mattress edge. Lower hem of sheet should lie seam down, even with bottom edge of mattress. Pull remaining top portion of sheet over top edge of mattress. While standing at head of bed, miter top corner of bottom sheet (see Skill 14-6, step 14).
8. Tuck remaining portion of unfitted sheet under mattress.
9. Optional: Apply drawsheet, laying center fold along middle of bed lengthwise. Smooth drawsheet over mattress, and tuck excess edge under mattress, keeping palms down.
10. Move to opposite side of bed, and spread bottom sheet smoothly over edge of mattress from head to foot of bed.
11. Apply fitted sheet smoothly over each mattress corner. For an unfitted sheet, miter top corner of bottom sheet (see step 8), making sure corner is taut.
12. Grasp remaining edge of unfitted bottom sheet, and tuck tightly under mattress while moving from head to foot of bed. Smooth folded drawsheet over bottom sheet, and tuck under mattress, first at middle, then at top, and then at bottom.
13. If needed, apply waterproof pad over bottom sheet or drawsheet.
14. Place top sheet over bed with vertical center fold lengthwise down middle of bed. Open sheet out from head to foot, being sure top edge of sheet is even with top edge of mattress.
15. Make horizontal toe pleat; stand at foot of bed, and fanfold in sheet 5 to 10 cm (2 to 4 inches) across bed. Pull sheet up from bottom to make fold approximately 15 cm (6 inches) from bottom edge of mattress.
16. Tuck in remaining portion of sheet under foot of mattress. Then place blanket over bed with top edge parallel to top edge of sheet and 15 to 20 cm (6 to 8 inches) down from edge of sheet. (Optional: Apply additional spread over bed.)
17. Make cuff by turning edge of top sheet down over top edge of blanket and spread.
18. Standing on one side at foot of bed, lift mattress corner slightly with one hand, and with other hand tuck top sheet, blanket, and spread under mattress. Be sure toe pleats are not pulled out.
19. Make modified mitered corner with top sheet, blanket, and spread. After triangular fold is made, do not tuck tip of triangle (see illustration).
20. Go to other side of bed. Spread sheet, blanket, and spread out evenly. Make cuff with top sheet and blanket. Make modified corner at foot of bed.
21. Apply clean pillowcase.
22. Place call light within client's reach on bed rail or pillow, and return bed to height allowing for client transfer. Assist client to bed.
23. Arrange client's room. Remove and discard supplies. Perform hand hygiene.

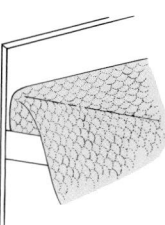

STEP 19 Modified mitered corner.

DELEGATION CONSIDERATIONS

The skill of making an occupied bed can be delegated to assistive personnel. The nurse provides assistive personnel with information, assistance, and direction, including:

- Reviewing any precautions or activity restrictions for the client
- Making sure assistive personnel know what to do if wound drainage, dressing material, drainage tubes, or IV tubing becomes dislodged or is found in the linens
- Instructing assistive personnel in what to do if client becomes fatigued

EQUIPMENT (Figure 14-6)

- ❏ Linen bag(s)
- ❏ Mattress pad (needs to be changed only when soiled)
- ❏ Bottom sheet (flat or fitted)
- ❏ Drawsheet
- ❏ Top sheet
- ❏ Blanket
- ❏ Bedspread
- ❏ Waterproof pads
- ❏ Bath blanket (optional)
- ❏ Pillowcases
- ❏ Bedside chair or table
- ❏ Disposable gloves (optional)
- ❏ Towel
- ❏ Disinfectant

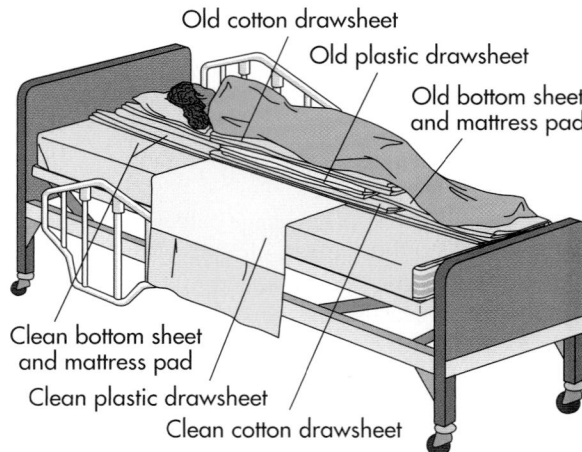

FIGURE **14-6** Equipment for making occupied bed. Type of linen may vary. (From Sorrentino SA, *Mosby's textbook for nursing assistants,* ed 5, St. Louis, 2000, Mosby.)

STEP	RATIONALE

ASSESSMENT

1. Assess potential for client incontinence or for excess drainage on bed linen from drainage tubes or wounds.
2. Check client's chart for orders or specific precautions concerning movement and positioning.

Determines need for protective waterproof pads or extra bath blankets on bed.
Ensures client safety and use of proper body mechanics.

NURSING DIAGNOSES

- Activity intolerance
- Impaired physical mobility
- Pain (acute, chronic)

- Bathing/hygiene self-care deficit
- Impaired skin integrity and risk for

Related factors are individualized based on client's condition or needs.

PLANNING

1. Expected outcomes following completion of procedure:
   - Client's skin remains free from breakdown.
   - Client expresses feeling of relaxation and comfort.
   - There are no areas of redness from bed linen irritation.
2. Explain procedure to the client, noting that the client will be asked to turn on side and roll over linen.

Bed linen is smooth and without wrinkles.

Client's skin free of pressure
Minimizes anxiety and promotes cooperation.

STEP	RATIONALE

IMPLEMENTATION

1. Perform hand hygiene, and apply gloves (gloves are worn only if linen is soiled or there is risk for contact with body secretions).

Reduces transmission of microorganisms.

2. Assemble equipment, and arrange on bedside chair or table. Remove unnecessary equipment such as a dietary tray or items used for hygiene.

Assembling all equipment provides for smooth procedure and assists in increasing client's comfort. Placing linen on clean surface minimizes spread of infection.

3. Draw room curtain around bed, or close door.

Maintains client's privacy.

4. Adjust bed height to comfortable working position. Lower head of bed, if tolerated by client. Lower side rail on nurse's side; leave far side rail up. Remove call light.

Minimizes strain on back. It is easier to remove and apply linen evenly to bed in flat position. Provides easy access to bed and linen.

5. Loosen top linen at foot of bed.

Makes linen easier to remove.

6. Remove bedspread and blanket separately, leaving client covered with top sheet. If spread and blanket are soiled, place them in linen bag. Keep soiled linen away from uniform.

Reduces transmission of microorganisms.

7. If blanket and spread are clean and are to be reused, fold each in quarters, and place over bottom of bed or on back of chair.

Folding method facilitates replacement and prevents wrinkles.

8. Cover client with bath blanket in the following manner: unfold bath blanket over top sheet. Ask client to hold top edge of bath blanket. If client is unable to help, tuck top of bath blanket under shoulder. Grasp top sheet under bath blanket at client's shoulders, and bring sheet down to foot of bed. Remove sheet, and discard in linen bag.

Bath blanket provides warmth and keeps body parts covered during linen removal.

9. With assistance from another nurse, slide mattress toward head of bed.

If mattress slides toward foot of bed when head of bed is raised, it is difficult to tuck in linen. In addition, it is uncomfortable for the client because the client's feet may be pressed against or hang over the foot of the bed.

10. Assist client to a side-lying position on the far side of the bed, facing away from the nurse. Be sure side rail in front of client is up. Adjust pillow under client's head. Check that any tubing is not being pulled.

Turning client onto side provides space for placement of clean linen. Side rail ensures client's safety from forward falls from the bed surface and helps client in moving.

11. Loosen all bottom linens. Then fanfold bottom sheet, drawsheet, and any pads toward and under client. Tuck edges of bottom linen just under client's buttocks, back, and shoulders. Do not fanfold mattress pad if it is to be reused (see illustration).

Provides maximum workspace for placing clean linen. Later, when client turns to other side, soiled linen can be removed easily.

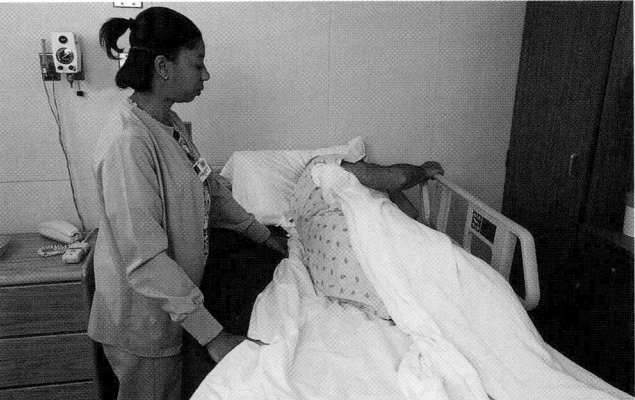

STEP **11** Old linen tucked alongside client.

STEP	**RATIONALE**

12. Wipe off any moisture on exposed mattress with towel and appropriate disinfectant.

13. Apply clean linen to exposed half of bed:
    a. Place clean mattress pad on bed by folding it lengthwise with center crease in middle of bed. Fanfold top layer over mattress. (If pad is reused, simply smooth out any wrinkles.)
    b. Unfold bottom sheet lengthwise so that center crease is situated lengthwise along center of bed. Fanfold sheet's top layer toward center of bed alongside the client (see illustration). Smooth bottom layer of sheet over mattress, and bring edge over closest side of mattress. Allow edge of sheet to hang about 25 cm (10 inches) over mattress edge. Lower hem of bottom sheet should lie seam down and even with bottom edge of mattress.

14. Miter top corner of flat bottom sheet at head of bed:
    a. Face head of bed diagonally. Place hand away from head of bed under top corner of mattress, near mattress edge, and lift.
    b. With other hand, tuck top edge of bottom sheet smoothly under mattress so that side edges of sheet above and below mattress would meet if brought together.
    c. Face side of bed, and pick up top edge of sheet at approximately 45 cm (18 inches) from top of mattress (see illustration).
    d. Lift sheet, and lay it on top of mattress to form a neat triangular fold, with lower base of triangle even with mattress side edge (see illustration).

Reduces transmission of microorganisms.

Applying linen over bed in successive layers minimizes energy and time used in bed making.

Proper positioning of linen on one side ensures that adequate linen will be available to cover opposite side of bed. Keeping seam edges down eliminates irritation to client's skin.

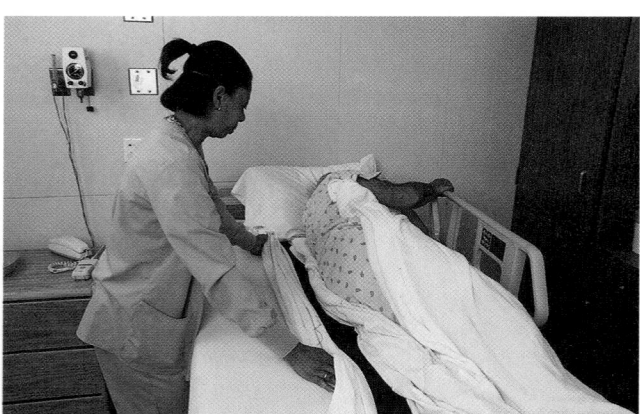
STEP **13b** Clean linen applied to bed.

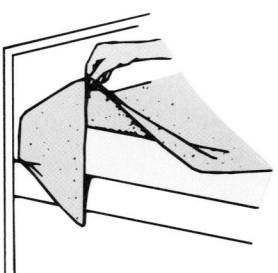
STEP **14c** Top edge of sheet picked up.

STEP	RATIONALE

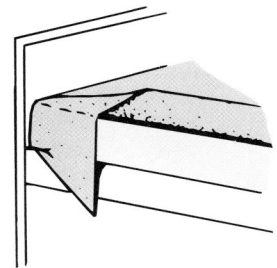

STEP 14d Sheet on top of mattress in triangular fold.

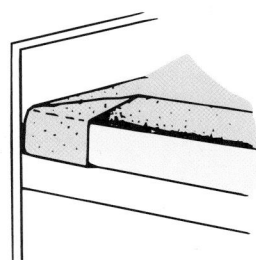

STEP 14e Lower edge of sheet tucked under mattress.

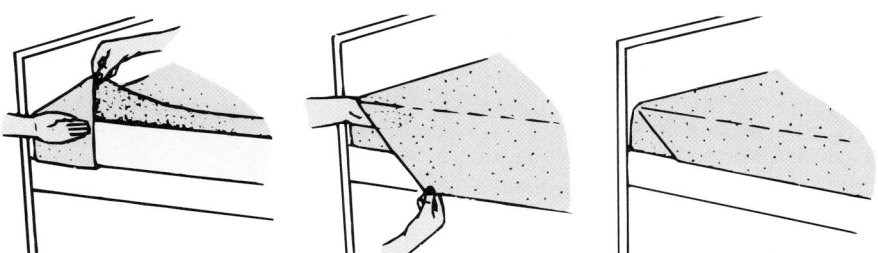

STEP 14f Triangular fold placed over side of mattress.

   e. Tuck lower edge of sheet, which is hanging free below the mattress, under mattress. Tuck with palms down, without pulling triangular fold (see illustration).

   f. Hold portion of sheet covering side of mattress in place with one hand. With the other hand, pick up top of triangular linen fold, and bring it down over side of mattress (see illustration). Tuck this portion under mattress (see illustrations).

15. Tuck remaining portion of sheet under mattress, moving toward foot of bed. Keep linen smooth.

16. *(Optional)* Open drawsheet so that it unfolds in half. Lay center fold along middle of bed lengthwise, and position sheet so that it will be under the client's buttocks and torso (see illustration). Fanfold top layer toward client, with edge along client's back. Smooth bottom layer out over mattress, and tuck excess edge under mattress (keep palms down).

Mitered corner cannot be loosened easily even if client moves frequently in bed.

Folds of linen are source of irritation and pressure.

Drawsheet is used to lift and reposition client. Placement under client's torso distributes most of client's body weight over sheet.

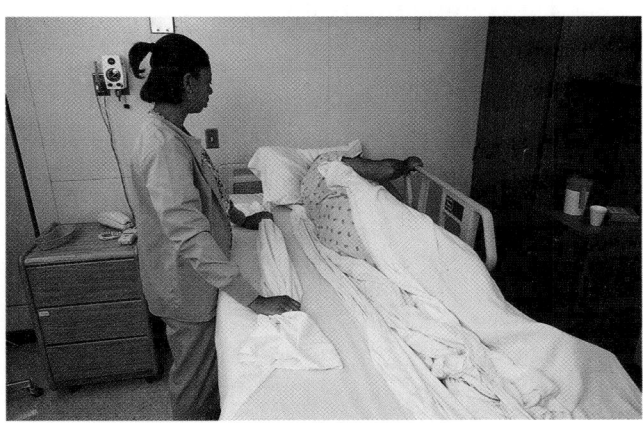

STEP 16 Placement of optional drawsheet.

STEP	RATIONALE

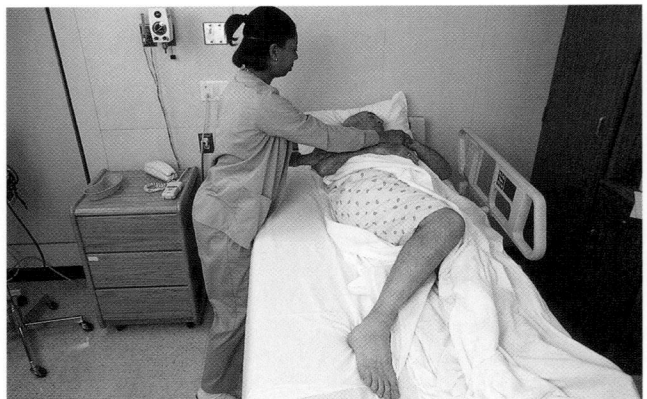

STEP **18** Client rolling over layers of linen.

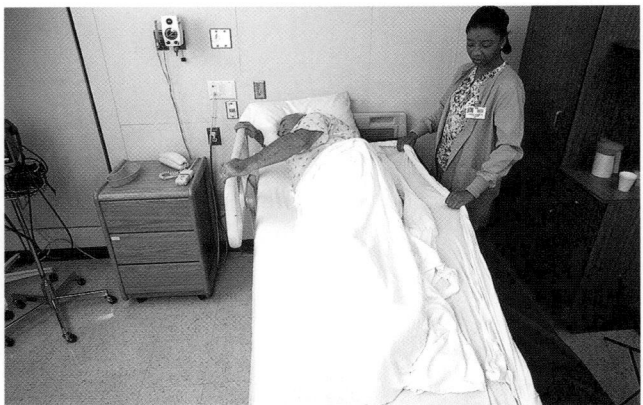

STEP **19** Loosen edges of soiled linen.

17. Place waterproof pad over drawsheet, with centerfold against client's side. Fanfold top layer toward client.

Protects bed linen from being soiled.

18. Have client roll slowly toward you, over the layers of linen (see illustration). Raise side rail on working side, and go to other side.

Positions client for removal and placement of linens. Maintains client's safety and body alignment during turning.

19. Lower side rail. Assist client in positioning on other side, over folds of linen. Loosen edges of soiled linen from under mattress (see illustration).

Exposes opposite side of bed for removal of soiled linen and placement of clean linen. Makes linen easier to remove.

20. Remove soiled linen by folding it into a bundle or square. Hold it away from uniform. Discard in linen bag if close by. Do not leave client alone with side rail down. If necessary, wipe mattress with antiseptic solution, and dry mattress surface before applying new linen. Remove gloves if worn, and dispose of them properly.

Reduces transmission of microorganisms. Ensures client safety.

21. Pull clean, fanfolded linen smoothly over edge of mattress from head to foot of bed.

Smooth linen will not irritate client's skin.

22. Assist client in rolling back into supine position. Reposition pillow.

Maintains client's comfort.

23. Miter top corner of bottom sheet (see step 14). When tucking corner, be sure that sheet is smooth and free of wrinkles.

Wrinkles and folds can cause irritation to skin.

24. Facing side of bed, grasp remaining edge of bottom sheet. Lean back; keep back straight; and pull while tucking excess linen under mattress. Proceed from head to foot of bed. (Avoid lifting mattress during tucking to ensure fit.)

Proper use of body mechanics while tucking linen prevents injury.

25. Smooth fanfolded drawsheet out over bottom sheet. Grasp edge of sheet with palms down; lean back; and tuck sheet under mattress. Tuck from middle to top and then to bottom.

Tucking first at top or bottom may pull sheet sideways, causing poor fit. A smooth-fitting sheet reduces the risk of pressure against the skin from rolled linen.

26. Place top sheet over client with center fold lengthwise down middle of bed. Open sheet from head to foot, and unfold over client.

Sheet should be equally distributed over bed by correctly positioning center fold.

27. Ask client to hold clean top sheet, or tuck sheet around client's shoulders. Remove bath blanket and discard in linen bag.

Sheet prevents exposure of body parts. Having client hold sheet encourages client participation in care.

STEP	**RATIONALE**

28. Place blanket on bed, unfolding it so that crease runs lengthwise along middle of bed. Unfold blanket to cover client. Top edge should be parallel with edge of top sheet and 15 to 20 cm (6 to 8 inches) from top sheet's edge.

Blanket should be placed to cover client completely and provide adequate warmth.

29. Place spread over bed according to step 28. Be sure that top edge of spread extends about 2.5 cm (1 inch) above blanket's edge. Tuck top edge of spread over and under top edge of blanket.

Gives bed neat appearance and provides extra warmth.

30. Make cuff by turning edge of top sheet down over top edge of blanket and spread.

Protects client's face from rubbing against blanket or spread.

31. Standing on one side at foot of bed, lift mattress corner slightly with one hand, and tuck top linens under mattress. Top sheet and blanket are tucked under together. Be sure that linens are loose enough to allow movement of client's feet. Making a horizontal toe pleat is an option.

Makes neat-appearing bed. Pressure ulcers can develop on client's toes and heels from feet rubbing against tight-fitting bed sheets.

32. Make modified mitered corner with top sheet, blanket, and spread (see illustration):
    a. Pick up side edge of top sheet, blanket, and spread approximately 45 cm (18 inches) from foot of mattress. Lift linen to form triangular fold, and lay it on bed.
    b. Tuck lower edge of sheet, which is hanging free below mattress, under mattress. Do not pull triangular fold.

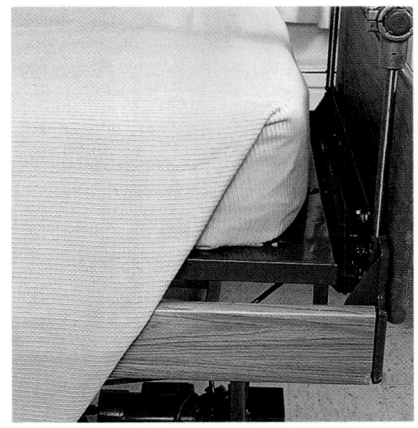

STEP **32** Modified mitered corner.

    c. Pick up triangular fold, and bring it down over mattress while holding linen in place alongside mattress. Do not tuck tip of triangle.

Secures top linen but keeps even edge of blanket and top sheet draped over mattress.

33. Raise side rail. Move to other side of bed and lower side rail. Spread sheet, blanket, and bedspread out evenly. Fold top edge of spread over blanket, and make cuff with top sheet (see step 30); make modified mitered corner at foot of bed (see step 32).

Side rail protects client from accidental falls.

34. Change pillowcase:
    a. Have client raise head. While supporting neck with one hand, remove pillow. Allow client to lower head.

Support of neck muscles prevents injury during flexion and extension of neck.

    b. Remove soiled case by grasping pillow at open end with one hand and pulling case back over pillow with the other hand. Discard case in linen bag.

Pillows slide out easily, thus minimizing contact with soiled linen.

    c. Grasp clean pillowcase at center of closed end. Gather case, turning it inside out over the hand holding it. With the same hand, pick up middle of one end of the pillow. Pull pillowcase down over pillow with the other hand.

Eases sliding of pillowcase over pillow.

    d. Be sure pillow corners fit evenly into corners of pillowcase. Place pillow under client's head.

Poorly fitting case constricts fluffing and expansion of pillow and interferes with client comfort.

STEP	RATIONALE
35. Place call light within client's reach, and return bed to comfortable position.	Ensures client safety and comfort.
36. Open room curtains, and rearrange furniture. Place personal items within easy reach on over-bed table or bedside stand. Return bed to a comfortable height.	Promotes sense of well-being.
37. Discard dirty linen in hamper or chute, and perform hand hygiene.	Prevents transmission of microorganisms.

EVALUATION

1. Ask if client feels comfortable.	Bed linens clean and smooth.
2. Inspect skin for areas of irritation.	Skin free of injury.
3. Observe client for signs of fatigue, dyspnea, pain, or discomfort.	Provides nurse with data about client's level of activity tolerance and ability to participate in other procedures.

Recording and Reporting

- Making an occupied bed need not be recorded. However, make a note in nurses notes if client tolerates procedure poorly.

Unexpected Outcomes	Related Interventions
1. Client feels discomfort from linen folds.	• Tighten sheets. • Change client's position frequently.
2. Client's skin is reddened and shows signs of breakdown.	• Institute skin care measures, or apply appropriate support surface to reduce risk of pressure ulcer (see Chapters 13 and 15). • Change client's position frequently.

Teaching Considerations

- Explain steps of procedure involving client's participation.

Home Care Considerations

- Family caregiver should be encouraged to have another family member or friend assist with turning client if an occupied bed must be made. Encourage use of fitted sheets.

FOCUS on CLINICAL PRACTICE

Mrs. Giles is a 67-year-old woman who has had Parkinson's disease for 8 years. She has the three cardinal symptoms of the disease: muscle rigidity, slow movement, and tremors of both upper extremities and hands. Her fingers are abducted and flexed, and she shows tremors during any intentional movement, for example when she tries to use an eating utensil or when she tries to brush her teeth. She is able to feed herself but has difficulty chewing and swallowing. She needs assistance to get in and out of bed and walks with short hesitant steps. After any activity she tires easily. Mrs. Giles cares for herself at home and is actively engaged in decisions about her care. Her sister visits her several times during the week to offer any assistance.

1. Mrs. Giles tells you that she likes to help with her bath. Which type of bath would be most appropriate for Mrs. Giles?
   A. Complete bed bath
   B. Sponge bath at sink
   C. Tub bath
   D. Shower
2. Describe three ways a nurse can manage a client's fatigue while giving a complete bed bath.

3. Which aspect of oral hygiene assessment is most likely to reveal a potential problem for Mrs. Giles?
   A. Inspection of oral cavity
   B. Identification of the risk factor of age
   C. Ability to manipulate a standard toothbrush
   D. Self-care practices at home
4. If Mrs. Giles has difficulty flossing her teeth, what option might you suggest for reducing plaque and gum inflammation?
5. Mrs. Giles tells you that she has trouble washing her feet, which become very dry. Her sister offers to help with foot care. List three suggestions for how the sister should examine Mrs. Giles's feet on a regular basis.
6. Safety is an important part of foot and nail care. Which of the following statements is (are) true?
   A. All patients must soak their feet for 10 minutes before nail care.
   B. Testing the temperature of the water used for soaking is important especially for clients with reduced sensation.
   C. Cut nails to follow the angle of the fingertips.
   D. When a client is a diabetic, file the nails only, do not cut the nails.

NCLEX REVIEW QUESTIONS

1. Understanding the physiological mechanisms of skin integrity helps to explain the principles of bathing. One of the purposes of regular bathing is:
   1. To restore the skin's normal pH to a base coating
   2. To remove resident bacteria that normally cause disease
   3. To cleanse and remove the outer skin of dead skin cells
   4. To promote the maturation of new skin cells
2. Which of the following clients require special precautions when the nurse shampoos the hair?
   1. Diabetic and hypertensive clients
   2. Clients with hearing deficits
   3. Immobile and exercise-intolerant clients
   4. Clients with neck injuries and vertigo
3. Mr. Martin is a 50-year-old contractor admitted to the hospital for ketoacidosis. He has had difficulty controlling his diabetes for the last 2 months. The factor that increases the risk of oral infection in a diabetic client is:
   1. Thinning of mucosa
   2. Increased glucose levels in the saliva
   3. Erosion of tooth enamel
   4. Lowering of salivary pH

4. An unconscious client presents the risk of having alterations of the oral cavity due to:
   1. A buildup of gram-negative bacteria in the oral cavity
   2. Impaired gag reflex
   3. Increase in salivary movement
   4. Loss of sensation of taste
5. Mrs. Snider is an 88-year-old client diagnosed with dementia. She frequently becomes very agitated and even becomes aggressive with caregivers. The best approach for bathing Mrs. Snider would be:
   1. To assist her with a shower
   2. Provide a complete bed bath
   3. Avoid bathing until she becomes more relaxed
   4. Provide a thermal bath in bed
6. Jessica Wilson is a 12-year-old client who comes to the local health clinic. Jessica's mother tells the nurse that her daughter has been scratching excessively. Upon closer examination the nurse notes scratches on Jessica's skin and is able to detect body lice. The nurse will recommend which of the following for Jessica's care?
   1. Throwing away items in Jessica's bedroom that cannot be washed
   2. Use a body shampoo containing Lindane
   3. Bag infested clothing until laundered
   4. Take a medicated bath every 4 to 5 days

References

Adams R: Qualified nurses lack adequate knowledge of oral health, resulting in inadequate oral care of patients on mechanical ventilation, *J Adv Nurs* 24:552, 1996.

Agency for Health Care Policy and Research: *Pressure ulcers in adults: prediction and prevention*, Pub Nos 92-0047, 92-0050, Rockville, Md, 1992, Public Health Service, U.S. Department of Health and Human Services.

American Dental Association: *Oral health topics*, http://www.ada.org/public/topics/cleaning.oasp, accessed October 5, 2003.

American Diabetes Association: Position statement on preventive foot care in people with diabetes: clinical practice recommendations 1999, *Diabetes Care* 22 (Suppl 1):1, 1999.

American Diabetes Association: *Diabetes forecast: the foot care top ten tips*, http://www.diabetes.org/diabetes-forecast/may2003/feet.jsp, accessed October 11, 2003.

American Society of Health-System Pharmacists: Clinical practice guidelines for sustained neuromuscular blockade in the adult critically ill patient, *Am J Health Syst Pharm* 59(2):179, 2002.

Armstrong DG, Lavery LA: Diabetic foot ulcers: prevention, diagnosis and classification, *Am Fam Physician* 57(6):1425, 1998.

Beighton D and others: The influence of specific foods and oral hygiene on the microflora of fissures and smooth surfaces of molar teeth: a 5-day study, *Caries Res* 33(5):349, 1999.

Beuscher TL: Community outreach foot care for the elderly: a winning proposition, *Home Healthc Nurse* 16(1):37, 1998.

Crute S, editor: *Health and healing for African-Americans*, Emmaus, Pa, 1997, Rodale Press.

Fellona MO, DeVore LR: Oral health services in primary care nursing centers: opportunities for dental hygiene and nursing collaboration, *J Dent Hyg* 73(2):69, 1999.

Fitch JA and others: Oral care in the adult intensive care unit, *Am J Crit Care* 8(2):314, 1999.

Galanti G: *Caring for patients from different cultures*, Philadelphia, 1991, University of Pennsylvania Press.

Hockenberry MJ and others: *Wong's nursing care of infants and children*, ed 7, St. Louis, 2003, Mosby.

Ignatavicius DD, Workman, ML: *Medical-surgical nursing*, ed 4, Philadelphia, WB Saunders, 2002.

Lueckenotte AG: *Gerontologic nursing*, ed 2, St. Louis, 2000, Mosby.

Marsh P, Martin M: *Oral microbiology*, ed 3, London, 1992, Chapman Hall.

McKenry LM, Salerno E: *Mosby's pharmacology in nursing*, ed 21, St. Louis, 2001, Mosby.

National Pediculosis Association: *Child care provider's guide to controlling head lice*, 2001, www.headlice.org.

Osterman HM, Stuck FM: The aging foot, *Orthop Nurs* 9:43, 1990.

Pettigrew D: Investing in mouth care, *Geriatr Nurs* 10:22, 1989.

Skewes SM: No more bed baths! *RN* 57(1):34, 1994.

Slovenkai NP: Getting and keeping a leg up on diabetes-related foot problems, *J Musculoskel Med* 15(12):46, 1998.

Sorrentino SA: *Assisting with patient care*, St. Louis, 1999, Mosby.

Strauss MB, Hart JD, Winant DM: Preventive foot care: a user friendly system for patients and physicians, *Postgrad Med* 103(5):233, 1998.

Strauss MB: Diabetic foot problems: keys to effective, aggressive prevention. *Consultant* 41(14):1693, 2001.

Research References

Bauroth K and others: The efficacy of an essential oil antiseptic mouthwash vs. dental flossing in controlling interproximal gingivitis: a comparative study, *J Am Dental Assoc* 144(3):359, 2003.

Dunn JC and others: Bathing: pleasure or pain? *J Gerontol Nurs* 28(11):6, 2002.

Grap MJ and others: Oral care interventions in critical care: frequency and documentation, *Am J Crit Care* 12(2):114, 2003.

Guralnik J and others: Occurrence and predictors of pressure sores in the national health and nutrition examination survey follow up, *J Am Geriatr Soc* 36:807, 1988.

Hardy M: A pilot study of the diagnosis and treatment of impaired skin integrity: dry skin in older persons, *Nurs Diagn* 1(2):57, 1996.

Liao W: Effects of passive body heating on body temperature and sleep regulation in the elderly: a systematic review, *Int J Nurs Stud* 39:803, 2002.

Olson B: The effects of massage for prevention of pressure ulcers, *Decubitus* 2(4):32, 1989.

Sheppard CM, Brenner PS: The effects of bathing and skin care practices on skin quality and satisfaction with an innovative product, *J Gerontol Nurs* 26(10):36, 2000.

Simons D and others: Relationship between oral hygiene practices and oral status in dentate elderly people living in residential homes, *Community Dent Oral Epidemiol* 29(6):464, 2001.

Stiefel KA and others. Improving oral hygiene for the seriously ill patient: implementing research-based practice, *Medsurg Nurs* 9(1):40, 2000.

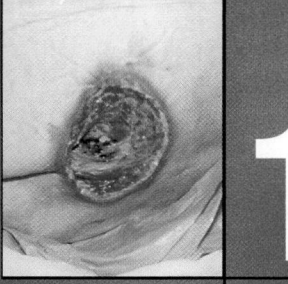

15

Pressure Ulcer Care

15-1 Risk Assessment, Skin Assessment, and Prevention Strategies

15-2 Treatment of Pressure Ulcers

MEDIA RESOURCES

Evolve Site *evolve*
http://evolve.elsevier.com/Perry/skills
- Weblinks
- Video clips
- Mosby's Nursing Skills Video Exercises

Mosby's Nursing Skills Videos/CD-ROM
- *Preventing and Treating Pressure Ulcers Video:*
  Assessing risk, use of the Braden Scale for Predicting Pressure Sore Risk, elements of the comprehensive assessment, stages of pressure ulcer formation; preventive measures, skin inspection, skin care, positioning in the 30-degree lateral position, position changes, pressure-relief devices, air flotation mattress, elbow protector, and foam foot stabilizer; treatment of pressure ulcers, dressing change, inspection of wound, measuring wound, application of prescribed medications, irrigation

OBJECTIVES

Mastery of content in this chaper will enable the nurse to:

- Describe guidelines to implement for prevention of pressure ulcers.
- Identify risk factors for development of pressure ulcers.
- Identify outcome criteria for clients at risk for pressure ulcers or impaired skin integrity.
- Discuss the use of risk assessment scores commonly used in assessment of pressure ulcer risk.
- Describe client characteristics, as well as the characteristics of pressure ulcer itself, to include in an assessment.
- Discuss indications for the use of topical agents in the treatment of pressure ulcers.
- Use topical agents correctly in the management of a pressure ulcer.
- Discuss teaching needs of the client and family regarding pressure ulcers.

KEY TERMS

Debridement	Pressure ulcer
Erythema	Reactive hyperemia
Eschar	Risk assessment tool
Exudate	Shear
Ischemia	Slough
Maceration	Topical agents
Necrosis	Undermining

Pressure ulcers are areas of localized tissue destruction caused by the compression of soft tissue over a bony prominence and an external surface for a prolonged period of time (Wound Ostomy and Continence Nurses Society [WOCN], 2003). Inaccurately called decubitus ulcers or bed sores by some, it was once thought that a person needed to be bed bound to develop these ulcers. It is now known that pressure ulcers occur from any position that causes soft tissue compression. Compression of soft tissue interferes with the blood flow to the tissue; if this compression continues for a prolonged period of time, the tissue dies from lack of blood flow, or ischemia. Ischemia develops when pressure on the skin is greater than the pressure inside the vessels, causing the vessels to collapse, preventing the blood from reaching the tissue. The tissue dies from ischemic injury. Initially, ischemia may be evident by skin discoloration such as redness and warmth in clients with light skin or purple and warmth in clients with darkly pigmented skin. If pressure is unrelieved or repeated, tissues will continue to break down relative to the client's general health and tolerance for pressure. This pressure, if not relieved, can cause irreversible tissue damage in as little as 90 minutes (Kosiak, 1959).

Pressure points over bony prominences where pressure ulcers can occur are shown in Figure 15-1. The most common sites are the sacrum, coccyx, ischial tuberosities, greater trochanters, elbows, heels, scapulas, ileal crests, and lateral and medial malleoli (Ayello and others, 2004). Pressure ulcers can occur on any area of skin subjected to pressure. Non-bony locations in which pressure ulcers can occur include the nares, usually related to pressure caused from nasogastric (NG) tubes or oxygen cannulas; the ears, resulting from an oxygen cannula; or the genitalia, with ulcers resulting from Foley catheter tension.

Other factors such as incontinence, friction and shear, immobility, and poor nutrition can contribute to pressure ulcer formation. Moisture from incontinence softens the skin, allowing the skin to become susceptible to breakdown. Friction, the mechanical force of two surfaces moving over each other, causes surface damage such as blisters. Shear is any tension that stretches the skin during turning or moving in bed. This force causes reduced blood flow to the tissues. Immobility prevents the client from the ability to change and control body position, thus increasing the pressure over bony prominences. It is strongly suspected that malnutrition contributes to the development of pressure ulcers (Colwell, 2004; WOCN, 2003). In addition, this circulatory impairment often is compounded by the altered body metabolism and negative nitrogen balance that commonly occur in immobilized clients.

Pressure ulcers pose serious risks to a client's health. A break in the skin, seen in stages II to IV pressure ulcers (Table 15-1), eliminates the body's first line of defense against infection.

When an ulcer extends into the subcutaneous tissues, protein- and electrolyte-rich body fluids are lost through the wound. A pressure ulcer can prolong morbidity and interfere with the rehabilitative and supportive care the client receives.

The numbers of clients who develop pressure ulcers is significant. Reports vary as to the number of clients who are at risk for and develop pressure ulcers. Clients are now older and sicker; they are hospitalized for shorter periods of time and are discharged to home or intermediate or long-term care facilities at a more acute stage of illness (Pieper, 2000). These changes will contribute to an increased number of clients at risk for and developing pressure ulcers. It is thus critical that nurses respond with an aggressive preventive approach. It is imperative that the nurse identify the factors that place the client at risk for the development of pressure ulcers. Once the factors are identified, interventions can be instituted to reduce or relieve the negative effects of each factor. When a pressure ulcer develops, the nurse must explore the factors that contributed to the skin breakdown, vigorously attempt to minimize the effects of these variables, and propose wound care treatment using current wound healing principles in the management of the ulcer (see Chapters 37 and 38).

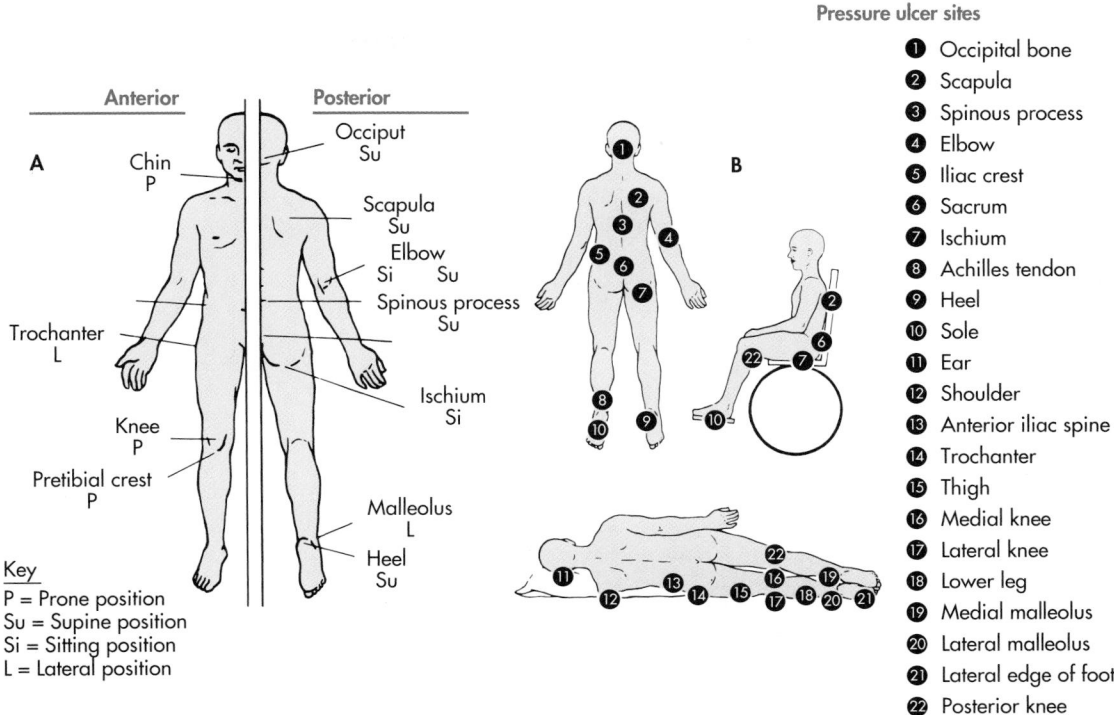

FIGURE 15-1 A, Bony prominences most frequently underlying pressure sores. **B,** Pressure ulcer sites. (From Trelease CC: Developing standards for wound care, *Ostomy Wound Manage* 26:50, 1988.)

Evidence-Based Practice Trends

Risk assessments should be performed on entry to a health care setting and repeated when there is a significant change in the client's health status or on a regularly scheduled basis (Figure 15-2). This schedule of assessment should be based upon the acuity of the client (Ayello and Braden, 2002). When looking at the overall score on the Braden scale the client will fall within one of these categories: mild risk, 16 to 18; moderate risk, 13 to 14; high risk, 9 or less (Braden and Bergstrom, 1994). These risk scores should be used to plan care, by looking at the individual risk factors that place the client at risk and developing a care plan to decrease or eliminate the identified risk factors.

In the acute care setting, pressure ulcers usually develop within the first 2 weeks of hospitalization (Langemo and others, 1989), and 15% of elderly will develop pressure ulcers within the first week of hospitalization (Lyder and others, 2001). Therefore clients in high-risk settings, it is important to target prevention efforts to minimize risk (WOCN, 2003).

Interventions that will reduce the risk associated with pressure ulcer development will be indicated by the findings of the risk assessment. The client who is found to be incontinent of stool and urine will require a plan that will include the use of a perineal cleanser and a skin barrier. Absorbent products that will wick the drainage away from the skin should be used. For patients who are at risk for skin breakdown related to immobility, the plan of care should consider the use a pressure-reduction surface, a turning schedule, and regular skin assessments (WOCN, 2003).

The treatment plan for a client with a pressure ulcer should include elimination or reduction of the factors that have caused the pressure ulcer. Topical care is planned based upon the principle of moist wound healing. A moist wound environment will support the growth of new tissue. If the wound is not free of necrotic tissue, topical wound care should be chosen that will clean the wound bed of devitalized tissue. Wound healing in a client with a pressure ulcer will be enhanced if the client has an adequate nutritional status, as well as control over such conditions as diabetes and cardiovascular and pulmonary disease (Waldrop and Doughty, 2000).

Skill Performance Guidelines

1. The amount and duration of pressure must be reduced to prevent ischemic tissue injury. Frequently turn and position the client to relieve pressure from the superficial capillaries and allow tissues to compensate for temporary ischemia. Classic research (Kosiak, 1959) and subsequent research (Langemo and others, 1989) found that tissue ischemia begins within 1 to 2 hours after onset of pressure in paraplegic animals. Turning clients at a minimum of every 1 to 2 hours and properly positioning them will help minimize formation of pressure ulcers (see Chapter 10).

TABLE 15-1   STAGING OF PRESSURE ULCERS

STAGING DEFINITION

STAGE I

A stage I pressure ulcer is an observable pressure-related alteration of intact skin whose indicators as compared to an adjacent or opposite area on the body may include changes in one or more of the following:
- Skin temperature (warmth or coolness)
- Tissue consistency (firm or boggy feel)
- Sensation (pain, itching)

The ulcer appears as a defined area of persistent redness in a lightly pigmented skin, whereas in darker skin tones, the ulcer may appear with persistent red, blue, or purple hues.

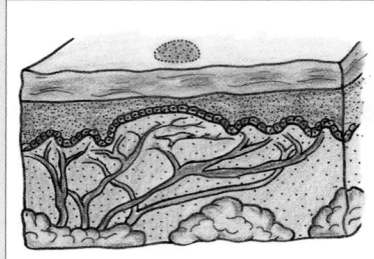 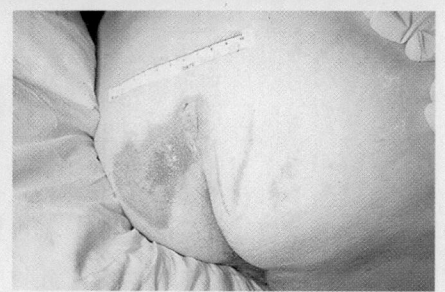

STAGE II

Partial-thickness skin loss involving epidermis and/or dermis or both. The ulcer is superficial and presents clinically as an abrasion, blister, or shallow crater.

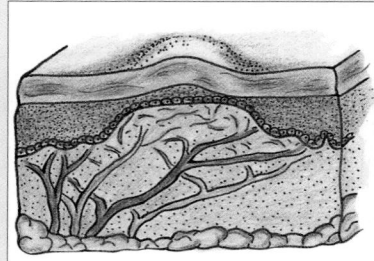 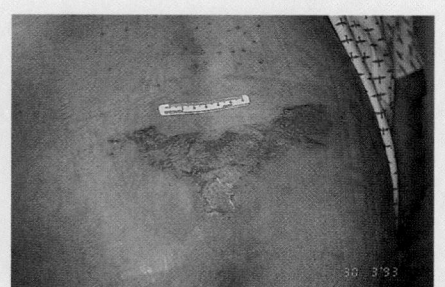

STAGE III

Full-thickness skin loss involving damage to, or necrosis of, subcutaneous tissue that may extend down to, but not through, underlying fascia. The ulcer presents clinically as a deep crater with or without undermining of adjacent tissue.

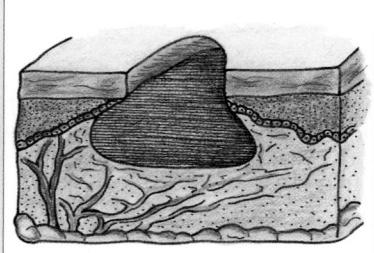 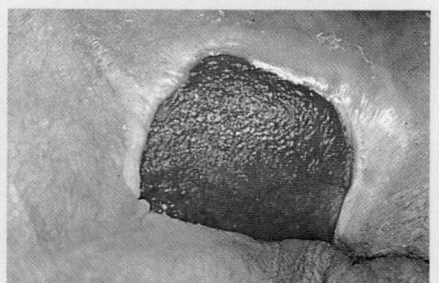

STAGE IV

Full-thickness skin loss with extensive destruction, tissue necrosis, or damage to muscle, bone, or supporting structures (e.g., tendon, joint capsule). Undermining and sinus tracts may also be associated with stage IV pressure ulcers.

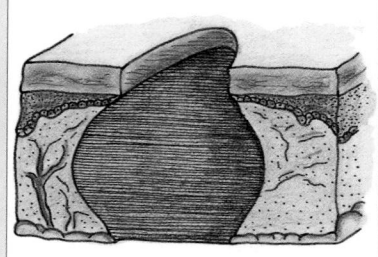 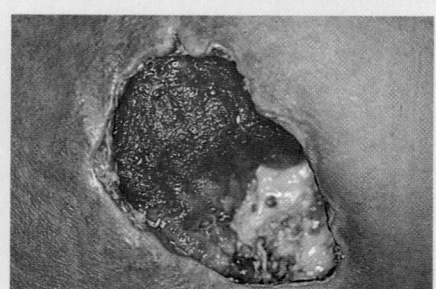

STAGING DEFINITIONS RECOGNIZE THE FOLLOWING LIMITATIONS:

Assessment of stage I pressure ulcers may be difficult in clients with darkly pigmented skin. When eschar is present, accurate staging of the pressure ulcer is not possible until the eschar has sloughed or the wound has been debrided.

Data from National Pressure Ulcer Advisory Panel: Pressure ulcer prevalence, cost and risk assessment: consensus development conference statement, *Decubitus* 2(2):24,1989; National Pressure Ulcer Advisory Panel, 2003.

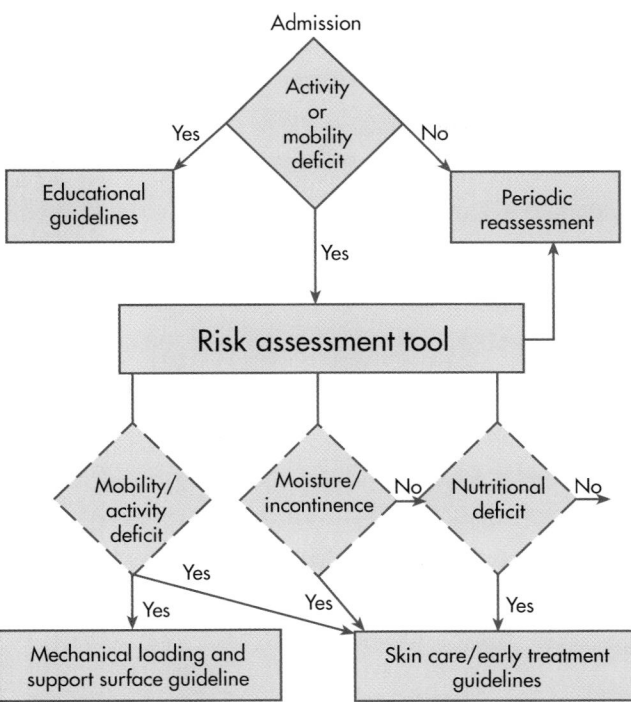

Admission

Activity or mobility deficit

Yes — Educational guidelines

No — Periodic reassessment

Yes

Risk assessment tool

Mobility/ activity deficit

Moisture/ incontinence — No — Nutritional deficit — No

Yes

Yes

Yes

Yes

Mechanical loading and support surface guideline

Skin care/early treatment guidelines

FIGURE 15-2 Risk assessment tool. (Modified from Panel for the Prediction and Prevention of Pressure Ulcers in Adults: *Pressure ulcers in adults: prediction and prevention,* Clinical practice guideline No. 3, Pub No. 92-0047, Rockville, Md, 1992, Agency for Health Care Policy and Research, Public Health Service, U.S. Department of Health and Human Services.)

2. Specialized beds, overlays, and mattresses (see Chapter 13) distribute pressure on dependent body parts more evenly. By distributing pressure evenly over the client's body surface, less pressure will be applied at the skin level. Clients at high risk for pressure ulcer formation should be placed on these devices as soon as possible. Consider the use of a chair cushion to reduce pressure when the client is seated. Think about the use of the above interventions for the immobile client who cannot independently reposition.

3. Clients who are incontinent of stool or urine should be cleansed as soon as possible. Skin moisture and wetness from incontinence can be a risk factor for skin breakdown (Newman and others, 2001). Areas subjected to repeated episodes of incontinence should be protected with a barrier ointment or barrier paste.

4. Institute interventions to minimize friction and shear. Use lift sheets when repositioning the client because this will reduce the amount of rubbing of the skin against the sheets. Raise the head of the bed no more than 30 degrees (unless medically contraindicated) to prevent sliding and shear injury (WOCN, 2003).

5. Adequate nutrition is important in the prevention and treatment of pressure ulcers (WOCN, 2003). A diet high in protein with enough calories, vitamins, and minerals can maintain normal tissue status and promote healing. With tissue injury, more calories and substrates are needed for healing; deficiencies in any nutrients may result in impaired or delayed healing. Protein needs are especially increased (Stotts, 2000). Monitoring the nutritional status should be part of the total assessment (WOCN, 2003).

6. If a client develops a pressure ulcer, the ulcer should be routinely assessed to determine progress toward healing. Interventions to support healing will be based upon the assessment.

SKILL 15-1   Risk Assessment, Skin Assessment, and Prevention Strategies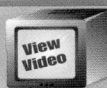

The goal in preventing the development of pressure ulcers is early identification of the at-risk client and the implementation of prevention strategies. In 1992 the Agency for Health Care Policy and Research (AHCPR, 1992) panel developed clinical guidelines for pressure ulcer prevention and treatment of pressure ulcers. These guidelines have served to assist the health care provider in planning and implementing care for both prevention and treatment of the client with a pressure ulcer (Bergstrom and others, 1994). In 2003 the Wound, Ostomy and Continence Nurses Society developed the *Guideline for Prevention and Management of Pressure Ulcers.* Much like the process used to develop the AHCPR guidelines, a panel of experts performed extensive searches on available literature on pressure ulcers. The panel then established a level of evidence rating that provides the best available evidence in the prevention and management of pressure ulcers. This guideline has

been accepted by the guideline resource component of the Agency for Healthcare Research and Quality, which has replaced the AHCPR. The overall management goals suggested by the WOCN Society (2003) include:

1. Identify individuals at risk for developing pressure ulcers and initiate an early prevention program
2. Implement appropriate strategies/plans to:
   a. Attain/maintain intact skin
   b. Prevent complications
   c. Promptly identify or manage complications
   d. Involve the client and caregiver in self-management
3. Implement cost-effective strategies/plans that prevent and treat pressure ulcers

The WOCN Society 2003 panel recommended that a risk assessment should be performed on entry to a health care set-

TABLE 15-2   BRADEN SCALE FOR PREDICTING PRESSURE ULCER RISK*

SENSORY PERCEPTION

Ability to respond meaningfully to pressure-related discomfort	1. *Completely limited:* Unresponsive (does not moan, flinch, or grasp) to painful stimuli due to diminished level of consciousness or sedation. OR Limited ability to feel pain over most of body.	2. *Very limited:* Responds only to painful stimuli. Cannot communicate discomfort except by moaning or restlessness. OR Has a sensory impairment that limits the ability to feel pain or discomfort over half of body.	3. *Slightly limited:* Responds to verbal commands but cannot always communicate discomfort or need to be turned. OR Has some sensory impairment which limits ability to feel pain or discomfort in 1 or 2 extremities.	4. *No impairment:* Responds to verbal commands. Has no sensory deficit that would limit ability to feel or voice pain or discomfort.

MOISTURE

Degree to which skin is exposed to moisture	1. *Constantly moist:* Skin is kept moist almost constantly by perspiration, urine, etc. Dampness is detected every time client is moved or turned.	2. *Very moist:* Skin is often, but not always, moist. Linen must be changed at least once a shift.	3. *Occasionally moist:* Skin is occasionally moist, requiring an extra linen change approximately once a day.	4. *Rarely moist:* Skin is usually dry, linen requires changing only at routine intervals.

ACTIVITY

Degree of physical activity	1. *Bedfast:* Confined to bed.	2. *Chairfast:* Ability to walk severely limited or nonexistent. Cannot bear own weight and/or must be assisted into chair or wheelchair.	3. *Walks occasionally:* Walks occasionally during day, but for very short distances, with or without assistance. Spends majority of each shift in bed or chair.	4. *Walks frequently:* Walks outside the room at least twice a day and inside room at least once every 2 hours during waking hours.

MOBILITY

Ability to change and control body position	1. *Completely immobile:* Does not make even slight changes in body or extremity position without assistance.	2. *Very limited:* Makes occasional slight changes in body or extremity position but unable to make frequent or significant changes independently.	3. *Slightly limited:* Makes frequent though slight changes in body or extremity position independently.	4. *No limitations:* Makes major and frequent changes in position without assistance.

NUTRITION

Usual food intake pattern	1. *Very poor:* Never eats a complete meal. Rarely eats more than one third of any food offered. Eats 2 servings or less of protein (meat or dairy products) per day. Takes fluids poorly. Does not take a liquid dietary supplement. OR Is NPO and/or maintained on clear liquids or IVs for more than 5 days.	2. *Probably inadequate:* Rarely eats a complete meal and generally eats only about half of any food offered. Protein intake includes only 3 servings of meat or dairy products per day. Occasionally will take a dietary supplement. OR Receives less than optimal amount of liquid diet or tube feeding.	3. *Adequate:* Eats over half of most meals. Eats a total of 4 servings of protein (meat, dairy products) each day. Occasionally will refuse a meal, but will usually take a supplement when offered. OR Is on a tube-feeding or TPN regimen that probably meets most of nutritional needs.	4. *Excellent:* Eats most of every meal. Never refuses a meal. Usually eats a total of 4 or more servings of meat and dairy products. Occasionally eats between meals. Does not require supplementation.

FRICTION AND SHEAR

	1. *Problem:* Requires moderate to maximum assistance in moving. Complete lifting without sliding against sheets is impossible. Frequently slides down in bed or chair; repositioning with maximal assistance. Spasticity, contractions, or agitation leads to almost constant friction.	2. *Potential problem:* Moves feebly or requires minimal assistance. During a move skin probably slides to some extent against sheets, chair, restraints, or other devices. Maintains relatively good position in chair or bed most of the time but occasionally slides down.	3. *No apparent problem:* Moves in bed and in chair independently and has sufficient muscle strength to sit up completely during move. Maintains good position in bed or chair.	

From Barbara Braden, PhD, RN, Creighton University School of Nursing, Omaha, Neb.

*Score client in each of the six subscales. Maximum score is 23, indicating little or no risk. A score of ≤16 indicates "at risk"; ≤9 indicates high risk.

ting and repeated on a regularly scheduled basis or when there is a significant change in the individual's condition. For example, if a client who was ambulatory becomes bed bound because of a surgical procedure, this person will potentially be at higher risk for skin breakdown than when first admitted when ambulatory. The Society suggested the use of risk assessment tools such as the Braden scale or the Norton scale. The earliest reported scale, in 1962, was the Norton scale, which has the following five risk factors: physical condition, mental state, activity, mobility, and incontinence (Norton and others, 1975). The Braden scale (Table 15-2) has the following six parameters: sensory perception (recognition of pressure), friction and shear, ability to change and control body position, skin moisture, nutritional intake, and physical activity (Ayello and Braden, 2002; Bergstrom and others, 1987). Risk cutoff scores may also vary for specific client populations (Table 15-3). It is important to understand how to interpret the meaning of the client's total score on whatever scale you use.

Skin and bony prominences should be inspected at least daily. Devices, shoes, socks, heel and elbow protectors should be removed for the skin inspection. All bony prominences should be inspected including back of head, shoulders, rib cage, elbows, hips, ischium, sacrum, knees, ankles, and heels (see Figure 15-1). Any reddened or discolored areas should be palpated with a gloved finger to determine if

TABLE 15-3   PRESSURE ULCER BRADEN RISK CUTOFF SCORES BY CLIENT POPULATION

CLIENT POPULATION	RISK CUT SCORES
General population	≤16
Intensive care unit patients	≤15
Older adult patients	≤18
Black and Latino patients	≤18

Data from Braden BJ, Bergstrom N: Clinical utility of the Braden scale for predicting pressure sore risk, *Decubitus* 2(3):44, 1989; Bergstrom N, Braden BJ: Predictive validity of the Braden scale among black and white subjects, *Nurs Res* 51(6): 398-403, 2002; Lyder CH and others: The Braden scale for pressure ulcer risk: evaluating the predictive validity in black and Latino/Hispanic elders, *Appl Nurs Res* 12(2):60, 1999.

the erythema blanches. As skin is exposed to pressure, the area that is compressed becomes ischemic. When the pressure is relieved in a short period of time, blood flow can return and cause the area to become reddened. This phenomenon is called reactive hyperemia, the return of the blood to the area. If when palpating an area of reactive hyperemia the area does not blanch (turn lighter in color when pressed with a gloved finger), this may be an indication that there is tissue damage. Areas of nonreactive hyperemia should be noted in the skin assessment as potential sites for skin breakdown.

DELEGATION CONSIDERATIONS

The skill of assessment of pressure ulcer risk is the responsibility of the nurse. However, certain aspects of the client's care may be delegated to assistive personnel. The nurse should instruct assistive personnel to report to the nurse:

- Any redness or break in client's skin
- Any abrasion from assistive devices

EQUIPMENT

- ❑ Risk assessment tool
- ❑ Documentation record
- ❑ Pressure-reduction mattress, bed, and/or chair cushion
- ❑ Positioning aids
- ❑ Gloves

STEP	**RATIONALE**

ASSESSMENT

1. Identify any client characteristics that might be risk factors for pressure ulcer formation.

    a. Paralysis, or immobilization caused by restrictive devices

    b. Sensory loss (e.g., hemiplegia, spinal cord injury)

    c. Circulatory disorders (e.g., diabetes mellitus)

    d. Fever

    e. Anemia

    f. Malnutrition

Determines need to administer preventive care and identifies specific factors placing client at risk.

Client is unable to turn or reposition independently to relieve pressure.

When sensory loss is present, the client feels no discomfort from pressure and does not independently change position.

Disorders reduce perfusion of skin's tissue layers.

Increases metabolic demands of tissues. Accompanying diaphoresis leaves skin moist.

Decreased hemoglobin reduces oxygen-carrying capacity of blood and amount of oxygen available to tissues.

Inadequate nutrition can lead to weight loss, muscle atrophy, and reduced tissue mass. Severe protein deficiency makes tissue more susceptible to breakdown (Sager, 2002). Poor protein, vitamin, mineral, and caloric intake limits wound-healing capabilities.

STEP	RATIONALE
g. Incontinence	Skin becomes exposed to moist environment containing bacteria. Moisture causes skin maceration.
h. Heavy sedation and anesthesia	Client is not mentally alert and does not turn or change position independently. Sedation can also alter sensory perception.
i. Age	There is a loss of dermal thickness in the older individual, impairing the ability to distribute pressure (Pieper, 2000). Neonates and very young children are at high risk with the head being the most common site of pressure ulcer occurrence (WOCN, 2003).
j. Dehydration	Results in decreased skin elasticity and turgor.
k. Edema	Edematous tissues are less tolerant of pressure, friction, and shear.
l. Existing pressure ulcers	Limits surfaces available for position changes, placing available tissues at increased risk.
m. History of pressure ulcer	Tensile strength of the skin from a previously healed pressure ulcer is about 80%; therefore this area cannot tolerate pressure as much as undamaged skin (Waldrop and Doughty, 2000).
2. Select one of the risk assessment tools. Perform the risk assessment on entry to the health care setting, and repeat on a regularly scheduled basis or when there is a significant change in the individual's condition (WOCN, 2003).	A valid and reliable risk assessment tool should be used to evaluate client's risk for developing a pressure ulcer. Using the risk assessment will identify risk factors that can contribute to the potential for skin breakdown and pinpoint specific areas to target interventions to decrease the risk of skin breakdown.
3. Obtain risk score (see Tables 15-2, 15-3, and 15-4), and evaluate its meaning based on client's unique characteristics.	The risk cutoff score will depend on the instrument used. In addition, the score involves identifying the risk factors that contributed to the score and minimizing those specific deficits.

TABLE 15-4 GUIDELINES FOR PRESSURE ULCER RISK ASSESSMENT

LEVEL OF CARE	INITIAL	REASSESSMENT
Acute care	On admission	• At least every 48 hours • Whenever a major change in client's condition occurs • Intervals will vary depending upon how rapidly client's condition is changing
Long-term care	On admission	• Weekly for first 4 weeks after admission • Routinely on quarterly basis • Whenever the client's condition changes or deteriorates
Home care	On admission	• Every RN visit

Modified from Ayello EA, Braden B: How and why to do pressure ulcer risk assessment, *Adv Wound Care* 15(3):125, 2002.

STEP	RATIONALE
4. Asses condition of client's skin over regions of pressure (see Figure 15-1). Body weight against bony prominences places underlying skin at risk for breakdown. Look for areas of:	Inspect skin and bony prominences at least daily. Any skin changes should be documented, including a description of skin changes and any action taken (WOCN, 2003).
a. Skin discoloration (redness in light-tone skin; purplish or bluish in darkly pigmented skin), temperature changes (warmth or coolness) (Bennett, 1995; Henderson and others, 1997), tissue consistency (firm or boggy feel), and/or sensations (Ayello and others, 2004; Lyder and others, (2001). See Box 15-1 for cultural considerations in assessing clients with darkly pigmented skin.	May indicate that tissue was under pressure; hyperemia is a normal physiological response to hypoxemia in tissues.
b. Blanching	If an area of redness blanches (lightens in color), this indicates that the tissue should not be at risk for skin breakdown. Tissue that does not blanch when palpated may indicate that there is ischemic injury.
c. Pallor and mottling	Persistent hypoxia in tissues that were under pressure; an abnormal physiological response.
d. Absence of superficial skin layers	Represents early pressure ulcer formation, usually a partial-thickness wound.

BOX 15-1   Cultural Considerations for Skin Assessment for Pressure Ulcers: The Client With Darkly Pigmented Skin

Clients with darkly pigmented skin cannot be assessed for pressure ulcer risk by examining only skin color. Follow these recommended guidelines:

ASSESS LOCALIZED SKIN COLOR CHANGES

Any of the following may appear:
- Skin color changes are different from usual skin tone.
- Color is darker than surrounding skin—purplish, bluish, eggplant.

Importance of lighting for skin assessment:
- Use natural or halogen light.
- Avoid fluorescent lamps, which can give the skin a bluish tone.
- Avoid wearing tinted lenses when assessing skin color.

TISSUE CONSISTENCY
- Assess for edema, swelling.
- Assess for firm or boggy feel.

SENSATION
- Assess for pain or changes in skin sensation such as itching.

SKIN TEMPERATURE
- Initially skin in the area of pressure ulcer may feel warmer than surrounding skin.
- Subsequently skin may feel cooler than surrounding skin.
- Feel areas of skin that are not involved in or around a pressure point to serve as a point of temperature reference.

Data from Bennett MA: Report of the Task Force on the Implications for Darkly Pigmented Intact Skin in the Prediction and Prevention of Pressure Ulcers, *Adv Wound Care* 8(6):34, 1995; Henderson CT and others: Draft definition of stage I pressure ulcers: inclusion of persons with darkly pigmented skin, *Adv Wound Care* 10(5):16, 1997.

STEP	RATIONALE
e. Skin temperature	Palpation of differences in temperature between the area of a stage I pressure ulcer and adjacent skin area may be an initial indicator of ischemia (Sprigle and others, 2001).
5. Assess client for additional areas of potential pressure.	Clients at high risk have multiple sites for pressure necrosis, in addition to bony prominences.
a. Nares: NG tube, oxygen cannula	
b. Tongue and lips: oral airway, endotracheal (ET) tube	
c. Ears: oxygen cannula, pillow	
e. Drainage tubes	Stress against tissue at exit site.
f. Wound drainage	Wound drainage is caustic to skin and underlying tissues, thereby increasing risk for skin breakdown.
g. Indwelling urethral (Foley) catheter	For female clients, the catheter can put pressure on the labia, especially when edematous. For male clients, pressure from a catheter not properly anchored can put pressure on the tip of the penis and urethra.
h. Orthopedic and positioning devices	Improperly fitted or applied devices have the potential to cause pressure on adjacent skin and underlying tissue.

• *Critical Decision Point*
Inspect skin around and beneath orthopedic devices, such as cervical collar, braces, or cast.
Note for redness or warmth in areas where devices can rub against the skin.

STEP	RATIONALE
6. Observe client for preferred positions when in bed or chair.	Preferred positions result in weight of body being placed on certain bony prominences. Presence of contractures may result in pressure exerted in unexpected places.
7. Observe ability of client to initiate and assist with position changes.	Potential for friction and shear increases when client is completely dependent on others for position changes.
8. Assess client and caregiver understanding of risks for the development of pressure ulcers.	Determines baseline knowledge for pressure ulcer risk and identifies areas for client teaching.

NURSING DIAGNOSES

- Risk for impaired skin integrity
- Impaired skin integrity
- Imbalanced nutrition: less than body requirements
- Ineffective tissue perfusion
- Impaired physical mobility
- Deficient knowledge related to pressure ulcer prevention

Related factors are individualized based on client's condition or needs

PLANNING

1. Expected outcomes following completion of procedure:	
• No change from baseline skin assessment.	The systematic use of a risk assessment scale will identify risk factors and target prevention efforts.
• Skin is intact with no evidence of erythema or no signs of breakdown.	Prevention strategies reduce risk factors.
2. Explain procedure(s) and purpose to client and caregiver.	Relieves anxiety and provides opportunity for education.
3. Perform hand hygiene, and prepare equipment and supplies.	Reduces transmission of microorganisms.

STEP	RATIONALE

BOX 15-2   Interventions: Prevention of Pressure Ulcers

1. Assess individual risk for developing pressure ulcers.
   - A. Select and use a risk assessment tool, the Braden and Norton scales have been the ones most extensively studied.
   - B. Risk assessment should be performed on entry to a health care setting and repeated on a regularly scheduled basis or when there is a significant change in a client's condition.
2. Identify all individual risk factors (incontinence, nutritional status, immobility, friction and shear, and high-risk groups such as older adults, very young children, spinal cord injury population).
3. Assess and inspect skin at least daily. Note all pressure points, document results.
4. Institute prevention interventions as indicated by the findings of the risk assessment:
   - A. Assess and treat incontinence: Clean and dry skin after each incontinent episode using a pH balanced cleanser. Use incontinence skin barriers as needed to protect and maintain skin integrity. Select underpads, diapers, or briefs that are absorbent to wick incontinence away from the skin. Consider a pouching system or collection device to contain urine or stool and to protect the skin from the effluent.

   - B. Use turning or lift sheets or devices to turn or transfer clients.
   - C. Maintain the head of bed at or below 30 degrees or at the lowest level of elevation to decrease shear/friction.
   - D. Schedule regular and frequent turning and repositioning for bed and chair bound clients. Turn at least every 2 to 4 hours.
   - E. Place "at risk" individuals on pressure-reduction surface and not on an ordinary hospital mattress. Consult with trained health care professionals who have specific knowledge and expertise in this area.
   - F. Relieve pressure under heels by using pillows or other devices.
   - G. Maintain adequate nutrition that is compatible with the client's wishes or condition to maximize the potential for healing.
   - H. Educate the client/caregiver about the causes and risk factors for pressure ulcer development and ways to minimize risk.

Modified from Wound Ostomy and Continence Nurses Society: *Guideline for prevention and management of pressure ulcers,* WOCN clinical practice guidelines series, Glenview, Ill, 2003.

IMPLEMENTATION

STEP	RATIONALE
1. Implement the recommendations adapted from the Wound, Ostomy and Continence Nurses Society's *Guideline for Prevention and Management of Pressure Ulcers* (2003) (Box 15-2).	Reduce risk of client for developing a pressure ulcer.
2. Close room door or bedside curtain.	Maintains client privacy.
3. If client has open, draining wounds, use disposable gloves.	Use of standard precautions prevents accidental exposure to body fluids.
4. Assist client with changing position. Use the following positions (see Chapters 10 and 11):	Avoid positions that place client directly on an area of existing skin breakdown. It may be helpful to use a schedule for position changes.
a. Supine	Protects shoulders, trochanter, and malleolus.
b. Prone	Used only in clients who can tolerate; breathing difficulty is normal.

STEP	RATIONALE

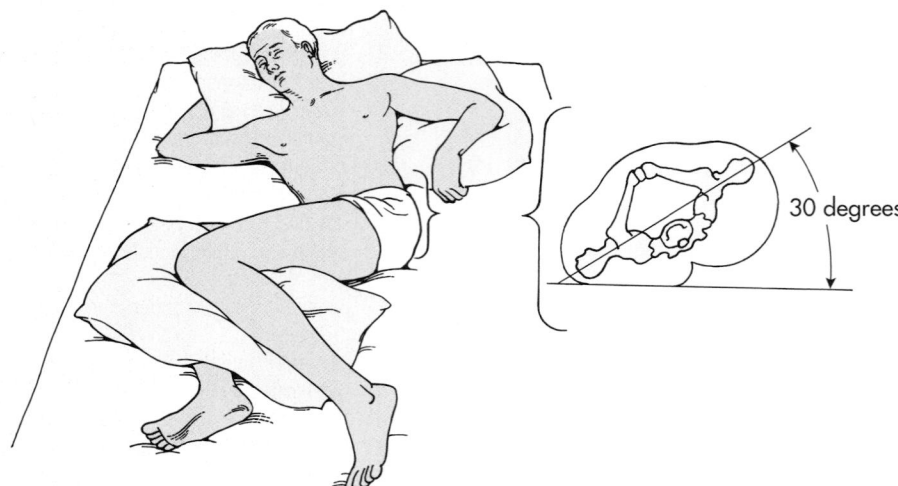

STEP 4c 30-degree lateral position.

c. 30-degree lateral (see illustration)	Achieved with one pillow under shoulder and one pillow under leg on the same side. The 30-degree lateral position should provide pressure relief from the sacrum and the trochanter (WOCN, 2003).

- **Critical Decision Point**

  When repositioning the client, observe for skin discoloration in area that was under pressure. In light-skinned clients, redness from initial flushing is expected. In darkly pigmented clients, skin may appear purplish or bluish (Bennett, 1995; Henderson and others, 1997). Bennett also suggests using natural or halogen light sources when assessing for discoloration on clients with darkly pigmented skin. Avoid using fluorescent lighting because it can give a bluish tint to skin that can interfere with accurate assessment of skin coloring (see Box 15-1).

5. Palpate any area of discoloration or mottling. Note if the involved area blanches with palpation or remains discolored or red. Nonblanchable erythema or skin temperature changes may be an important early indicator of a stage I pressure ulcer (see Table 15-1).	Early detection of pressure indicates need for more frequent position changes or the use of a pressure-relief device.
6. Do not massage any reddened or discolored pressure points.	Areas of nonblanchable erythema or discolored areas may indicate that deeper tissue damage is present. Massage in this area may worsen the inflammation by damaging underlying damaged blood vessels.
7. When positioning the client in bed, keep the head of the bed at a 30-degree angle or lower if the client's medical condition allows.	Pressure is reduced to the sacral area when the head of the bed is not at a high elevation.

- **Critical Decision Point**

  If client requires a pressure-reduction surface for the bed, an appropriate pressure-reduction surface should also be considered for the chair.

8. Remove gloves, discard appropriately, and perform hand hygiene.	Reduces spread of microorganisms.

STEP	**RATIONALE**

EVALUATION

1. Observe a client's skin for areas at risk for change in color or texture.

Enables nurse to evaluate success of prevention techniques.

2. Observe tolerance of client for position change.

Position changes may interfere with client's sleep and rest pattern.

3. Compare subsequent risk assessment scores.

Provides ongoing comparison of client's risk level to facilitate appropriateness of plan of care.

Recording and Reporting

- Record client's risk score.
- Record skin assessment.
- Describe positions, turning intervals, pressure-reducing devices, and other prevention measures. Note client's response to the interventions.
- Report need for additional consultations for the high-risk client.

Unexpected Outcomes	**Related Interventions**
1. Skin becomes mottled, reddened, purplish, or bluish.	• Document and communicate interval for reevaluation of risk assessment score. • Obtain physician's order (when needed) for identified consults such as wound ostomy and continence nurse, dietitian, clinical nurse specialist (CNS), and physical therapist. Reevaluate position changes.
2. Client reports sense of fatigue and inability to sleep.	• Modify client's positioning and turning schedule to promote sleep.
3. Areas under pressure develop persistent discoloration, induration, or temperature changes.	• Document and communicate interval for reevaluation of risk assessment score. • Obtain physician's order (when needed) for identified consults such as wound ostomy and continence nurse, dietitian, CNS, and physical therapist.

Teaching Considerations

- Assist client (and family) with understanding multiple factors involved in preventing and treating pressure ulcers.
- Explain and demonstrate positioning options to achieve pressure relief.
- Explain the purpose and maintenance of pressure-reduction devices.
- When teaching clients to change position for pressure relief, suggest using television programming and commercial intervals or a watch with an alarm as reminders.

Gerontological Considerations

- In older adults, a risk score of 18 may be the prediction of pressure ulcer risk on the Braden scale (Bergstrom and others,1998; Pieper, 2000).
- Sitting posture and position need to be reevaluated because body weight and muscle tone change with age.

- In the older client, the dermis demonstrates decreased thickness, causing thinning of the skin, especially over the legs and forearms. There is less subcutaneous tissue, leading to less padding protection over bony prominences, and the time for epidermal regeneration is diminished, leading to slower healing (Lyder, 2004).

Home Care Considerations

- Identify community resources, such as neighbors and relatives, for assistance should client need help with position changes, including after a fall.
- Pressure-relief maneuvers must be customized to the independent client. The individual may find a watch with a timer, even or odd hours, and television commercials helpful in remembering to complete pressure-relief techniques.
- Home care clients older than 60 years old should be closely monitored for pressure ulcer development if they

have any of the following risk factors: wheelchair dependence, incontinence, anemia, fracture, oxygen use, skin drainage, or adult child as primary caregiver (Langemo and Baranosk, 2003).

- Remind the client and the caregiver that position changes must be done while a client is sitting in a chair. Consider shifts every 15 minutes. Small shifts such as moving or repositioning the legs can relieve pressure over bony prominences (WOCN, 2003).

SKILL 15-2   Treatment of Pressure Ulcers

Treatment of clients with pressure ulcers requires a holistic approach to the client. A thorough assessment of the client, the client's ability to heal, and a good understanding of the identified goal for the client's overall care must be determined before implementing topical pressure ulcer treatment. The first principle of managing a client with a pressure ulcer should be to relieve or control the contributing factors. Therefore the first assessment made is to determine the etiology of the pressure ulcer. Once the cause of the pressure ulcer is determined, steps must be taken to control or eliminate those factors. For example, if the ulcer is related to unrelieved pressure, the appropriate pressure-reduction surface might be chosen, a turning schedule developed, or the appropriate chair pad is chosen. The next assessment is to determine the client's wound healing abilities: cardiovascular and pulmonary function, nutritional status, and other conditions that are known to deter wound healing, such as diabetes, steroid administration, and immunosuppression (Rolstad and others, 2000).

The principle that guides the selection and use of topical dressings is to provide a wound environment that will support wound healing (Jones and others, 2004). A wound that is free from necrotic tissue and infection and is maintained in a moist environment is the optimal wound environment for healing. Interventions and dressings that support a clean, moist wound bed are appropriate. An important assessment before initiating wound therapy is a thorough assessment of the wound and the periwound skin. This assessment will assist in planning the appropriate care for the client with a pressure ulcer.

No specific studies demonstrate the benefit of using one cleanser over another for pressure ulcers. In the majority of cases, water or saline is sufficient for cleansing a clean wound (WOCN, 2003). When the wound is contaminated with debris or necrotic tissue or heavy drainage, a commercial cleanser that is noncytotoxic to healthy tissue (e.g., Sur Cleans) can be used. If the tissue in the wound is devitalized, debridement should be considered. Debridement, the removal of devitalized tissue, can be accomplished by the choice of dressing, the use of enzyme preparations, or surgical or laser techniques. The choice of the type of debridement will depend upon the condition of the wound, the type of devitalized tissue, and the pain tolerance of the client.

Wound dressings are chosen to meet the characteristics of the wound bed (Baranoski and Ayello, 2004). The choice of a wound dressing will depend upon the type of wound tissue in the base of the wound, the amount of wound drainage, the presence or absence of infection, the location of the wound, the size of the wound, the ease of use, the cost-effectiveness, and comfort for the client. Categories of wound dressings include transparent films, hydrocolloids, hydrogels, foams, calcium alginates, gauze, and antimicrobial dressings. The use of dressings in the management of a pressure ulcer will change as the wound characteristics change; thus frequent wound evaluation is key.

Advanced wound care products that are used in select cases include growth factors, electrical stimulation, hyperbaric therapy, negative pressure therapy, normothermic therapy, and tissue-engineered skin substitutes. Growth factors occur naturally in wound fluid and may stimulate both granulation and epithelialization when applied topically. Pulsed electrical stimulation is a procedure that can be performed by physical therapists with the goal of increased wound healing. Hyperbaric oxygen therapy uses increased amounts of pressurized oxygen delivered to clients in a variety of specialized methods. Negative pressure therapy (such as the vacuum-assisted wound closure [VAC]) applies suction to remove excess fluid from the wound bed. The VAC works via a tubing system placed into a foam dressing placed into the wound and covered with a semiocclusive dressing. This therapy is thought to support the proliferation of granulation tissue. Normothermic therapy provides warmth to the wound bed and is thought to increase blood flow to the healing wound. Tissue-engineered skin substitutes develop living cells that can be placed over a clean wound bed to facilitate wound closure. Advanced wound therapies can play an important role in pressure ulcer healing but should be used after consultation with a wound care expert.

DELEGATION CONSIDERATIONS

This skill is the responsibility of the nurse. However, certain aspects of the client's care may be delegated to assistive personnel. The nurse should instruct assistive personnel to report any wound drainage that might be found on linens or intact skin, which would indicate the need to change the dressing or to use an alternative dressing.

EQUIPMENT

- ❏ Disposable gloves (clean)
- ❏ Goggles and cover gown
- ❏ Plastic bag for dressing disposal
- ❏ Measuring device
- ❏ Cotton-tipped applicators
- ❏ Topical agent (as ordered)
- ❏ Cleansing agent (as ordered)
- ❏ Sterile solution container
- ❏ Washbasin, washcloths, towels
- ❏ Dressing of choice
- ❏ Hypoallergenic tape (if needed)
- ❏ Documentation records

STEP	RATIONALE

ASSESSMENT

1. Assess the client's level of comfort and need for pain medication (Dallan and others, 2004).

The dressing change should not be a traumatic event for the client; the majority of clients with pressure ulcers report pain at dressing change (Szor and Bourguignon, 1999).

2. Determine if client has allergies to topical agents.

Topical agents contain elements that may cause localized skin reactions.

3. Review the order for topical agent or dressing.

Ensures that proper medication and treatment are administered.

- **Critical Decision Point**

  Determine if the order is consistent with established wound care guidelines and outcomes for the client. If the order is not consistent with guidelines or varies from the identified outcome for the client, review the order with the health care team.

4. Close room door or bedside curtains. Perform hand hygiene, and apply clean gloves.

Provides privacy.
Reduces transmission of microorganisms and prevents accidental exposure to body fluids.

5. Position client to allow dressing removal, and position plastic bag for dressing disposal.

Area should be accessible for dressing change. Proper disposal of old dressing promotes proper handling of contaminated waste.

6. Assess each of the client's pressure ulcer(s) and surrounding skin to determine ulcer characteristics, including the stage (see Table 15-1).

Staging is a way of assessing a pressure ulcer, based on the depth of tissue destruction. The nurse must be able to see the type of tissue at the base of the pressure ulcer. Therefore a pressure ulcer that is covered with necrotic tissue (eschar, which is black, hard necrotic tissue) or slough (yellow, stringy necrotic tissue) cannot be staged (National Pressure Ulcer Advisory Panel [NPUAP], 1995, 2000).

- **Critical Decision Point**

  To correctly stage a pressure ulcer, the nurse must be able to see the base of the wound. Therefore pressure ulcers that are covered with necrotic tissue cannot be staged until the eschar is debrided (NPUAP, 1998). The nurse would document that the ulcer is unstageable.

7. Assess the type of tissue in the wound bed. Color type will indicate the type of tissue. Black tissue is necrotic tissue, yellow tissue is slough, and red tissue is granulation tissue. Chart the approximate amount of each tissue found in the wound bed.

The approximate percentage of each type of tissue in the wound will provide critical information on the progress of wound healing and the choice of dressing. A wound with a high percentage of black tissue will require debridement, yellow tissue or slough tissue may indicate the presence of an infection, and granulation tissue will indicate a wound moving toward healing.

STEP	**RATIONALE**

8. Wounds should be assessed on a frequent basis. Consider using an assessment tool such as the Bates-Jensen Pressure Sore Status Tool (PSST) (1990) (Figure 15-3). Reassess the wound at each dressing change to determine whether modifications are needed (WOCN, 2003).

Changes in the appearance of a wound can indicate that the topical therapy should be adjusted to continue to move the wound toward healing.

BATES-JENSEN WOUND ASSESSMENT TOOL   NAME _____

Complete the rating sheet to assess pressure sore status. Evaluate each item by picking the response that best describes the wound and entering the score in the item score column for the appropriate date.

Location: Anatomic site. Circle, identify right (**R**) or left (**L**) and use "**X**" to mark site on body diagrams:

_____ Sacrum & coccyx   _____ Lateral ankle
_____ Trochanter   _____ Medial ankle
_____ Ischial tuberosity   _____ Heel   Other Site _____

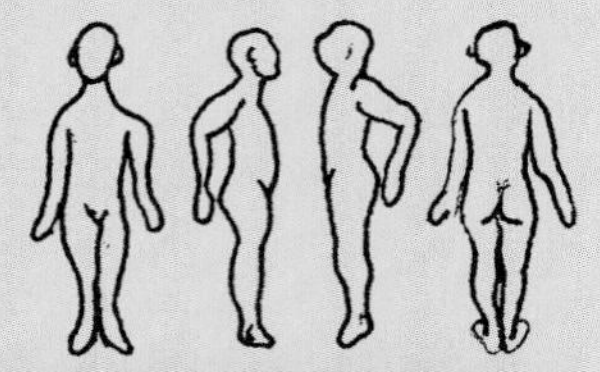

Shape: Overall wound pattern; assess by observing perimeter and depth.
Circle and <u>date</u> appropriate description:

_____ Irregular   _____ Linear or elongated
_____ Round/oval   _____ Bowl/boat
_____ Square/rectangle _____ Butterfly   Other Shape _____

Item	Assessment	Date	Date	Date
		Score	Score	Score
1. **Size**	1 = Length x width < 4 sq cm 2 = Length x width 4-16 sq cm 3 = Length x width 16.1-36 sq cm 4 = Length x width 36.1-80 sq cm 5 = Length x width > 80 sq cm			
2. **Depth**	1 = Non-blanchable erythema on intact skin 2 = Partial thickness skin loss involving epidermis &/or dermis 3 = Full thickness skin loss involving damage or necrosis of subcutaneous tissue; may extend down to but not through underlying fascia; &/or mixed partial & full thickness &/or tissue layers obscured by granulation tissue 4 = Obscured by necrosis 5 = Full thickness skin loss with extensive destruction, tissue necrosis or damage to muscle, bone or supporting structures			
3. **Edges**	1 = Indistinct, diffuse, none clearly visible 2 = Distinct, outline clearly visible, attached, even with wound base 3 = Well-defined, not attached to wound base 4 = Well-defined, not attached to base, rolled under, thickened 5 = Well-defined, fibrotic, scarred or hyperkeratotic			
4. **Under-mining**	1 = None present 2 = Undermining < 2 cm in any area 3 = Undermining 2-4 cm involving < 50% wound margins 4 = Undermining 2-4 cm involving > 50% wound margins 5 = Undermining > 4 cm in any area or tunneling in any area			
5. **Necrotic Tissue Type**	1 = None visible 2 = White/grey non-viable tissue &/or non-adherent yellow slough 3 = Loosely adherent yellow slough 4 = Adherent, soft, black eschar 5 = Firmly adherent, hard, black eschar			
6. **Necrotic Tissue Amount**	1 = None visible 2 = < 25% of wound bed covered 3 = 25% to 50% of wound covered 4 = > 50% and < 75% of wound covered 5 = 75% to 100% of wound covered			

© 2001 Barbara Bates-Jensen

FIGURE 15-3 Bates-Jensen Wound Assessment Tool. (Courtesy Barbara Bates-Jensen.)

STEP	RATIONALE

Item	Assessment	Date	Date	Date
		Score	Score	Score
7. **Exudate Type**	1 = None 2 = Bloody 3 = Serosanguineous: thin, watery, pale red/pink 4 = Serous: thin, watery, clear 5 = Purulent: thin or thick, opaque, tan/yellow with or without odor			
8. **Exudate Amount**	1 = None 2 = Scant 3 = Small 4 = Moderate 5 = Large			
9. **Skin Color Surrounding Wound**	1 = Pink or normal for ethnic group 2 = Bright red &/or blanches to touch 3 = White or grey pallor or hypopigmented 4 = Dark red or purple &/or non-blanchable 5 = Black or hyperpigmented			
10. **Peripheral Tissue Edema**	1 = No swelling or edema 2 = Non-pitting edema extends < 4 cm around wound 3 = Non-pitting edema extends ≥ 4 cm around wound 4 = Pitting edema extends < 4 cm around wound 5 = Crepitus &/or pitting edema extends ≥ 4 cm			
11. **Peripheral Tissue Induration**	1 = None present 2 = Induration < 2 cm around wound 3 = Induration 2-4 cm extending < 50% around wound 4 = Induration 2-4 cm extending ≥ 50% around wound 5 = Induration > 4 cm in any area around wound			
12. **Granulation Tissue**	1 = Skin intact or partial thickness wound 2 = Bright, beefy red; 75% to 100% of wound filled &/or tissue overgrowth 3 = Bright, beefy red; < 75% & > 25% of wound filled 4 = Pink, &/or dull, dusky red &/or fills ≤ 25% of wound 5 = No granulation tissue present			
13. **Epithelialization**	1 = 100% wound covered, surface intact 2 = 75% to < 100% wound covered &/or epithelial tissue extends > 0.5 cm into wound bed 3 = 50% to < 75% wound covered &/or epithelial tissue extends to < 0.5 cm into wound bed 4 = 25% to < 50% wound covered 5 = < 25% wound covered			
TOTAL SCORE				
SIGNATURE				

WOUND STATUS CONTINUUM

1   5   10 **13** 15   20   25   30   35   40   45   50   55   **60**

←——————————————————————————————→

TISSUE   WOUND   WOUND
HEALTH   REGENERATION   DEGENERATION

Plot the total score on the Wound Status Continuum by putting an "X" on the line and the date beneath the line. Plot multiple scores with their dates to see-at-a-glance regeneration or degeneration of the wound.
© 2001 Barbara Bates-Jensen

FIGURE 15-3, cont'd For legend, see facing page.   *Continued*

| STEP | RATIONALE |

WOUND ASSESSMENT TOOL

Instructions for use
General Guidelines:

Fill out the attached rating sheet to assess a pressure sore's status after reading the definitions and methods of assessment described below. Evaluate once a week and whenever a change occurs in the wound. Rate according to each item by picking the response that best describes the wound and entering that score in the item score column for the appropriate date. When you have rated the pressure sore on all items, determine the total score by adding together the 13-item scores. The HIGHER the total score, the more severe the pressure sore status. Plot total score on the Pressure Sore Status Continuum to determine progress.

Specific Instructions:

1.   **Size**: Use ruler to measure the longest and widest aspect of the wound surface in centimeters; multiply length x width.

2.   **Depth**: Pick the depth, thickness, most appropriate to the wound using these additional descriptions:
      1 = tissues damaged but no break in skin surface.
      2 = superficial, abrasion, blister or shallow crater. Even with, &/or elevated above skin surface (e.g., hyperplasia).
      3 = deep crater with or without undermining of adjacent tissue.
      4 = visualization of tissue layers not possible due to necrosis.
      5 = supporting structures include tendon, joint capsule.

3.   **Edges**: Use this guide:

Indistinct, diffuse	=	unable to clearly distinguish wound outline.
Attached	=	even or flush with wound base, <u>no</u> sides or walls present; flat.
Not attached	=	sides or walls <u>are</u> present; floor or base of wound is deeper than edge.
Rolled under, thickened	=	soft to firm and flexible to touch.
Hyperkeratosis	=	callous-like tissue formation around wound & at edges.
Fibrotic, scarred	=	hard, rigid to touch.

4.   **Undermining**: Assess by inserting a cotton tipped applicator under the wound edge; advance it as far as it will go without using undue force; raise the tip of the applicator so it may be seen or felt on the surface of the skin; mark the surface with a pen; measure the distance from the mark on the skin to the edge of the wound. Continue process around the wound. Then use a transparent metric measuring guide with concentric circles divided into 4 (25%) pie-shaped quadrants to help determine percent of wound involved.

5.   **Necrotic Tissue Type**: Pick the type of necrotic tissue that is <u>predominant</u> in the wound according to color, consistency and adherence using this guide:

White/gray non-viable tissue	=	may appear prior to wound opening; skin surface is white or gray.
Non-adherent, yellow slough	=	thin, mucinous substance; scattered throughout wound bed; easily separated from wound tissue.
Loosely adherent, yellow slough	=	thick, stringy, clumps of debris; attached to wound tissue.
Adherent, soft, black eschar	=	soggy tissue; strongly attached to tissue in center or base of wound.
Firmly adherent, hard/black eschar	=	firm, crusty tissue; strongly attached to wound base <u>and</u> edges (like a hard scab).

© 2001 Barbara Bates-Jensen

FIGURE 15-3, cont'd Bates-Jensen Wound Assessment Tool. (Courtesy Barbara Bates-Jensen.)

STEP	RATIONALE

6. **Necrotic Tissue Amount**: Use a transparent metric measuring guide with concentric circles divided into 4 (25%) pie-shaped quadrants to help determine percent of wound involved.

7. **Exudate Type**: Some dressings interact with wound drainage to produce a gel or trap liquid. Before assessing exudate type, gently cleanse wound with normal saline or water. Pick the exudate type that is <u>predominant</u> in the wound according to color and consistency, using this guide:

Bloody	=	thin, bright red
Serosanguineous	=	thin, watery pale red to pink
Serous	=	thin, watery, clear
Purulent	=	thin or thick, opaque tan to yellow
Foul purulent	=	thick, opaque yellow to green with offensive odor

8. **Exudate Amount**: Use a transparent metric measuring guide with concentric circles divided into 4 (25%) pie-shaped quadrants to determine percent of dressing involved with exudate. Use this guide:

None	=	wound tissues dry.
Scant	=	wound tissues moist; no measurable exudate.
Small	=	wound tissues wet; moisture evenly distributed in wound; drainage involves $\leq$ 25% dressing.
Moderate	=	wound tissues saturated; drainage may or may not be evenly distributed in wound; drainage involves > 25% to $\leq$ 75% dressing.
Large	=	wound tissues bathed in fluid; drainage freely expressed; may or may not be evenly distributed in wound; drainage involves > 75% of dressing.

9. **Skin Color Surrounding Wound**: Assess tissues within 4 cm of wound edge. Dark-skinned persons show the colors "bright red" and "dark red" as a deepening of normal ethnic skin color or a purple hue. As healing occurs in dark-skinned persons, the new skin is pink and may never darken.

10. **Peripheral Tissue Edema**: Assess tissues within 4 cm of wound edge. Non-pitting edema appears as skin that is shiny and taut. Identify pitting edema by firmly pressing a finger down into the tissues and waiting for 5 seconds, on release of pressure, tissues fail to resume previous position and an indentation appears. Crepitus is accumulation of air or gas in tissues. Use a transparent metric measuring guide to determine how far edema extends beyond wound.

11. **Peripheral Tissue Induration**: Assess tissues within 4 cm of wound edge. Induration is abnormal firmness of tissues with margins. Assess by gently pinching the tissues. Induration results in an inability to pinch the tissues. Use a transparent metric measuring guide with concentric circles divided into 4 (25%) pie-shaped quadrants to determine percent of wound and area involved.

12. **Granulation Tissue**: Granulation tissue is the growth of small blood vessels and connective tissue to fill in full thickness wounds. Tissue is healthy when bright, beefy red, shiny and granular with a velvety appearance. Poor vascular supply appears as pale pink or blanched to dull, dusky red color.

13. **Epithelialization**: Epithelialization is the process of epidermal resurfacing and appears as pink or red skin. In partial thickness wounds it can occur throughout the wound bed as well as from the wound edges. In full thickness wounds it occurs from the edges only. Use a transparent metric measuring guide with concentric circles divided into 4 (25%) pie-shaped quadrants to help determine percent of wound involved and to measure the distance the epithelial tissue extends into the wound.

© 2001 Barbara Bates-Jensen

FIGURE 15-3, cont'd   For legend, see facing page.

STEP	RATIONALE
a. Note color, temperature, edema, moisture, and condition of skin around the ulcer. Remember to modify the assessment technique based on the client's individual skin color (see Box 15-1).	Skin condition at the ulcer edge may indicate progressive tissue damage. Maceration on the periwound skin may show the need to alter the choice of the wound dressing.
b. Measure the wound dimensions. Measure using a wound measurement guide (see illustration); measure two dimensions, length and width per the facility's protocol.	Consistency in how the wound is measured is important for determining wound progress.

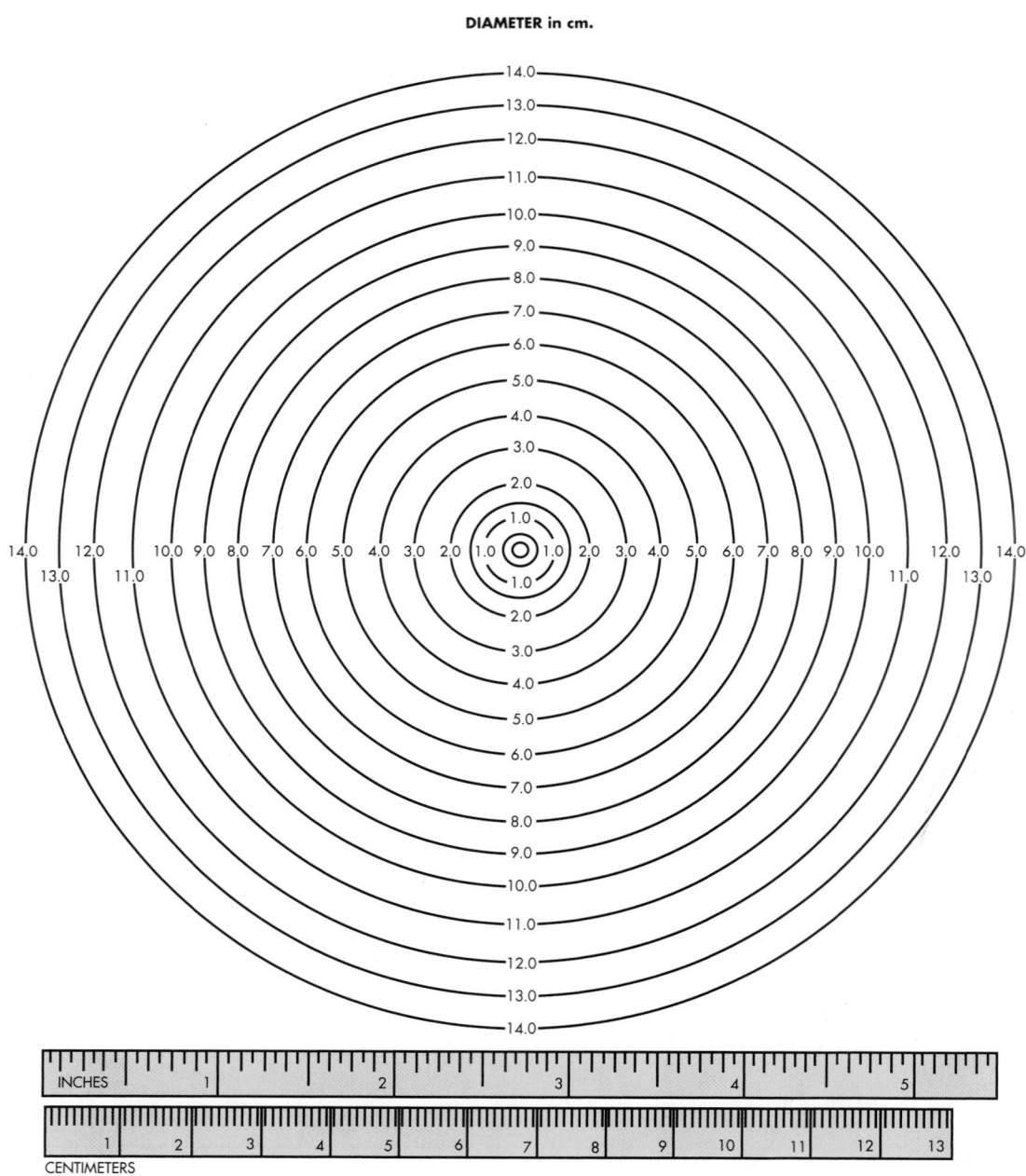

DIAMETER in cm.

DISCARD AFTER USE

STEP 8b Measuring guide. Center over wound to be measured. (Modified from Maklebust J, Sieggreen M: *Pressure ulcers: guidelines for prevention and nursing management*, ed 2, Springhouse, Pa, 1996, Springhouse.)

STEP	**RATIONALE**
c. Measure the depth of the pressure ulcer using a sterile, cotton-tipped applicator or other device that will allow measurement of wound depth. Place the applicator *gently* into the pressure ulcer until it touches the bottom. Mark the place on the applicator where it reaches the top of the wound, and then remove the applicator from the ulcer. Measure the distance from the tip of the applicator to the mark using a measuring tape or ruler to determine the depth of the pressure ulcer.	Depth measure is important for determining the amount of tissue loss.
d. Measure depth of undermining tissue. Use a cotton-tipped applicator, and gently probe under skin edges.	Undermining represents the loss of the underlying tissue (see illustration). Undermining may indicate progressive tissue necrosis, or the ongoing injury from shearing.

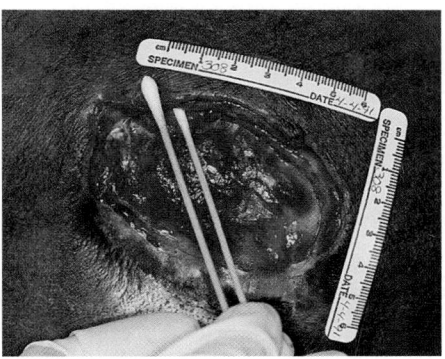

STEP 8d Measuring depth of undermining of skin.

9. Remove gloves, discard appropriately, and perform hand hygiene.	Reduces transmission of microorganisms. Repeated hand washing is necessary as nurse assesses different pressure areas. Different wounds may be contaminated by different organisms. Failure to repeatedly perform hand hygiene can cause cross-wound contamination.
10. Assessment of the entire client is necessary in developing a pressure ulcer treatment plan. Include in this assessment the identification of complications and comorbid conditions, a nutritional assessment, an assessment of pain, a psychosocial assessment, and an evaluation of the individual's risks for additional pressure ulcers.	

• *Critical Decision Point*
When malnutrition is suspected, consider a nutritional consult to modify client's diet to promote wound healing.

11. Educate clients and caregivers about prevention, treatment, and factors contributing to the recurrence of pressure ulcers (AHCPR, 1994; WOCN, 2003).	Explanations relieve anxiety and promote cooperation during procedure. The client and caregiver must partner with the health care providers to prevent further skin breakdown.

STEP	RATIONALE

NURSING DIAGNOSES

- Impaired skin integrity
- Pain (acute, chronic)
- Imbalanced nutrition: less than body requirements

- Ineffective tissue perfusion
- Impaired physical mobility
- Deficient knowledge regarding pressure ulcer treatment plan

Related factors are individualized based on client's condition or needs.

PLANNING

1. Expected outcomes following completion of procedure:
   - Ulcer drainage decreases.

   Less drainage from the ulcer reflects a decrease in the inflammatory process and progress toward healing.

   - Granulation tissue is present in wound base.

   Evidence that wound is moving toward healing.

   - Skin surrounding ulcer remains healthy and intact.

   No additional damage is noted; the dressing that is used is appropriate to contain wound drainage.

   - Nutrition is adequate to compensate for wound fluid losses and wound repair (see illustration).

   Nutritional therapy provides adequate protein to support wound healing.

   - Client's overall skin is protected from further breakdown.

   Client may remain at risk for further breakdown while existing ulcer heals.

2. Explain procedure to client and family. Individualize the teaching plan for older adult clients, taking into account the normal aging changes that affect learning.

   Preparatory explanations relieve anxiety, correct any misconceptions about the ulcer and its treatment, and offer an opportunity for client and family education.

3. Prepare the following necessary equipment and supplies:
   a. Washbasin, warm water, soap, washcloth, and bath towel.

   Used to bathe surrounding skin.

   b. Normal saline or other wound-cleansing agent in sterile solution container.

   Ulcer surface must be cleansed before the application of topical agents and a new dressing.

- *Critical Decision Point*

  Use only noncytotoxic agents to clean ulcers, such as Sur Cleans.

   c. Prescribed topical agent:
      (1) Enzymatic agents: Make sure the manufacturer's specific directions for the frequency of application is followed
      OR

      Enzymes debride dead tissue to clean ulcer surface.

      (2) Topical antibiotics

      Topical antibiotics are used to decrease the bioburden of the wound and should be considered for use if no healing is noted after 2 to 4 weeks of optimal care (AHCPR, 1994; WOCN, 2003).

- *Critical Decision Point*

  If using an enzymatic debriding agent, do not use wound-cleansing agents with metals.

STEP	RATIONALE

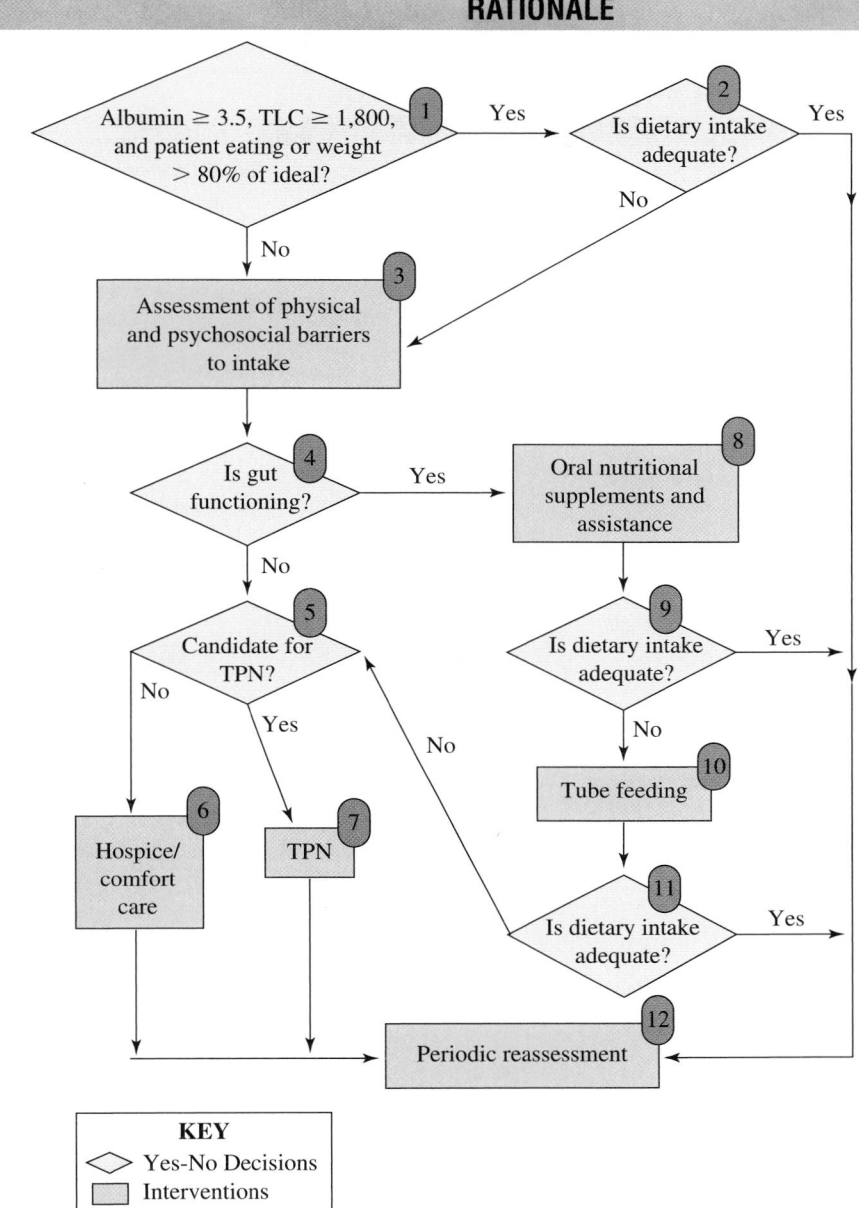

STEP 2 Nutritional assessment and support. (From Bergstrom N and others: *Treatment of pressure ulcers,* AHCPR Pub No. 95-0652, Rockville, Md, 1994, Agency for Health Care Policy and Research, Public Health Service, U.S. Department of Health and Human Services.)

d. Dressing (Table 15-5) (see also Chapter 38).

    (1) Select an appropriate dressing based on the pressure ulcer characteristics, purpose for which the dressing is intended, and client care setting.

    (2) Gauze.

The dressing should maintain a moist environment for the wound while keeping the surrounding skin dry (AHCPR, 1994).

Use as a moist dressing; squeeze excessive saline from gauze, and apply over wound.

Can be used to deliver solution to a wound.

Can be used as topper dressing when using enzymatic agent or topical antibiotics.

STEP	RATIONALE

TABLE 15-5 TREATMENT OPTIONS BY ULCER STAGE

ULCER STAGE	ULCER STATUS	DRESSING	COMMENTS*	EXPECTED CHANGE	ADJUVANTS
I	Intact	None	Allows visual assessment.	Resolves slowly without epidermal loss over 7 to 14 days.	Turning schedule. Support hydration. Nutritional support.
		Transparent dressing	Protects from shear. Do not use in the presence of excessive moisture.		
		Hydrocolloid	May not allow visual assessment.		Pressure-reduction mattress or chair cushion.
II	Clean	Composite film	Limits shear.	Heals through re-epithelialization.	See previous stage.
		Hydrocolloid	Change when seal of dressing breaks, maximal wear time 7 days.		Manage incontinence.
		Hydrogel	Provides a moist environment.		
III	Clean	Hydrocolloid	See stage II Clean.	Heals through granulation and re-epithelialization.	See previous stages.
		Hydrogel foam	Apply over wound to protect and absorb moisture.		Evaluate pressure-relief needs.
		Calcium alginate	Use when there is significant exudate. Cover with secondary dressing.		
		Gauze	Use with normal saline or other prescribed solution. Wring out excess solution, unfold to make contact with wound.		
		Growth factors	Use with gauze per manufacturer's instructions.		
IV	Clean	Hydrogel	See stage III Clean.	Heals through granulation and re-epithelialization.	Surgical consult may be necessary for closure. See stages I, II, and III.
		Calcium alginate	See stage III Clean.		
	Eschar	Gauze	See stage III Clean. Fill all dead space with gauze.		
		Growth factors	Use with gauze.		
		Adherent film	Will facilitate softening of eschar.	Eschar will lift at the edges as healing progresses.	See previous stages. Surgical consult may be considered for debridement.
		Hydrocolloid	Will facilitate softening of eschar.		
		Gauze plus ordered solution	Will deliver solution and wick wound drainage.		May be considered for slow debridement.
		Enzymes			
		None	Rarely, if eschar is dry and intact, no dressing is used, allowing eschar to act as physiological cover.		

*As with *all* occlusive dressings, wounds should *not* be clinically infected.

STEP	RATIONALE

• *Critical Decision Point*

Make sure the dressing's absorbency is adequate for the amount of wound drainage. Check that wound does not dry out or that surrounding skin does not become macerated.

| (3)   Transparent dressing. | Applied over superficial ulcers and skin subjected to friction. Maintains a moist environment. |

• *Critical Decision Point*

Transparent membrane dressings can also be used for autolytic debridement of noninfected pressure ulcers.

| (4)   Hydrocolloid dressing. | Maintains moist environment to facilitate wound healing while protecting the wound base. |

• *Critical Decision Point*

Hydrocolloid can also be used to protect skin from friction and shear injury. Some of the brands have custom shapes available for specific anatomical parts, such as heels, elbows, and sacrum.

(5) Hydrogel.	Maintains moist environment to facilitate wound healing. Available in a sheet or in a tube.
(6) Calcium alginate.	Highly absorbent of wound exudate in heavily draining wounds.
(7) Foam.	Protective and will prevent wound dehydration; also absorbs small to moderate amounts of drainage.
e. Hypoallergenic tape or adhesive dressing sheet.	Used to secure nonadherent dressing. Prevents skin irritation and tearing.

IMPLEMENTATION

1. Assemble needed supplies at beside. Close room door or bedside curtains. Perform hand hygiene, and apply gloves. Open sterile packages and topical solution containers. (Goggles and moisture-proof cover gown should be worn if potential for contamination from spray exists when cleansing the wound.)	Maintains client privacy. Supplies should be ready for easy application so that nurse can use supplies without contaminating them; reduces transmission of microorganisms.
2. Remove bed linen and client's gown to expose ulcer and surrounding skin. Keep remaining body parts draped.	Prevents unnecessary exposure of body parts.
3. Gently wash skin surrounding ulcer with warm water and soap.	Cleansing of skin surface reduces bacteria.
4. Rinse area thoroughly with water.	Soap can be irritating to skin.
5. Gently dry skin thoroughly by patting lightly with towel.	Retained moisture causes maceration of skin layers.
6. Perform hand hygiene and change gloves.	Aseptic technique must be maintained during cleansing, measuring, and application of dressings. Refer to institutional policy regarding use of clean or sterile gloves.
7. Cleanse ulcer thoroughly with normal saline or prescribed wound-cleansing agent.	Wound should be cleansed at each dressing change, minimizing the trauma to the wound (WOCN, 2003).
8. Whirlpool treatments may be used to assist with wound debridement. Keep the wound directly away from the water jets.	Removes wound debris. Previously applied enzymes may require soaking for removal. Whirlpool should not be used on clean granulating wounds.

STEP	RATIONALE
9. Apply topical agents, if prescribed. **a.** Enzymes:	Follow manufacturer's directions for frequency of application. Be aware of what solutions inactivate the enzymes, and avoid their use in wound cleaning.
(1) Using a wooden tongue blade, apply a small amount of enzyme debridement ointment directly to the necrotic areas on the base of pressure ulcer. Avoid getting the enzyme on the surrounding skin. The amount of enzyme should be the same as the amount of butter you would spread on bread. A thick layer of ointment is not necessary; a thin layer absorbs and acts more effectively. Do not apply enzyme to surrounding skin.	Proper distribution of ointment ensures effective action. Some enzymes can cause burning, paresthesia, and dermatitis to surrounding skin.
(2) Place gauze dressing directly over ulcer, and tape it in place. Follow specific manufacturer's recommendation for type of dressing material to use to cover a pressure ulcer when using enzymatic agent.	Protects wound and prevents removal of ointment during turning or repositioning.
(3) If using an antibiotic solution, apply per order, and cover with gauze pad. Generally applied every 12 hours.	
b. Hydrogel agents: **(1)** Cover surface of ulcer with hydrogel using applicator or gloved hand.	Provides a moist environment..
(2) Apply a secondary dressing, such as dry gauze, hydrocolloid, or transparent dressing over gel to completely cover ulcer.	Holds hydrogel against wound surface because hydrogel amphorous form (in tube) or sheet form does not adhere to the wound and requires a secondary dressing to hold it in place.
c. Calcium alginates: **(1)** Pack wound with alginate using applicator or gloved hand.	Use in heavily draining wounds.
(2) Apply a secondary dressing, such as dry gauze, foam, or hydrocolloid over alginate.	Holds alginate against wound surface.
10. Reposition client comfortably off pressure ulcer.	Avoids accidental removal of dressings.
11. Remove gloves, and dispose of soiled supplies. Perform hand hygiene.	Reduces transmission of microorganisms.

EVALUATION

1. Observe skin surrounding ulcer for inflammation, edema, and tenderness.	A clean pressure ulcer should show evidence of movement toward healing within 2 to 4 weeks.
2. Inspect dressings and exposed ulcers, observing for drainage, foul odor, and tissue necrosis. Monitor client for signs and symptoms of infection, including fever and elevated white blood cell (WBC) count.	Ulcers can become infected.
3. Compare subsequent ulcer measurements.	Allows comparison of serial measurements to assess wound healing.
4. Use one of the scales designed to measure wound healing, such as the PUSH Scale (Table 15-6) (NPUAP, 2004) (Thomas and others, 1997) or the PSST (Bates-Jensen, 1990).	Provides a standard method of data collection that will demonstrate wound progress or lack thereof.

- *Critical Decision Point*
  Deterioration of the client's or the ulcer's condition indicates the need for reevaluation of the treatment plan (AHCPR, 1994).

STEP	RATIONALE

TABLE 15-6   PUSH TOOL 3.0

Patient Initials:_____   Study ID#:_____
Study Day #:_____   Date:_____

DIRECTIONS:

Observe and measure the pressure ulcer. Categorize the ulcer with respect to surface area, exudate, and type of wound tissue. Record a sub-score for each of these ulcer characteristics. Add the sub-scores to obtain the total score. A comparison of total scores measured over time provides an indication of the improvement or deterioration in pressure ulcer healing.

Length	0	1	2	3	4	5	
	0 cm^2	$<0.3 \text{ cm}^2$	$0.3–0.6 \text{ cm}^2$	$0.7–1.0 \text{ cm}^2$	$1.1–2.0 \text{ cm}^2$	$2.1–3.0 \text{ cm}^2$	
Width	6	7	8	9	10		Sub-score ___
	$3.1–4.0 \text{ cm}^2$	$4.1–8.0 \text{ cm}^2$	$8.1–12.0 \text{ cm}^2$	$12.1–24.0 \text{ cm}^2$	$>24.0 \text{ cm}^2$		
Exudate amount	0	1	2	3			Sub-score ___
	None	Light	Moderate	Heavy			
Tissue type	0	1	2	3	4		Sub-score ___
	Closed	Epithelial tissue	Granulation tissue	Slough	Necrotic tissue		
							Total score ___

Length × Width: Measure the greatest length (head to toe) and the greatest width (side to side) using a centimeter ruler. Multiply these two measurements (length × centimeter ruler and always use the same method each time the ulcer is measured.

Exudate amount: Estimate the amount of exudate (drainage) present after removal of the dressing and before applying any topical agent to the ulcer. Estimate the exudate (drainage) as none, light, moderate, or heavy.

Tissue type: This refers to the types of tissue that are present in the wound (ulcer) bed. Score as a "4" if there is any necrotic tissue present. Score as a "3" if there is any amount of slough present and necrotic tissue is absent. Score as a "2" if the wound is clean and contains granulation tissue. A superficial wound that is re-epithelizing is scored as a "1". When the wound is closed, score as a "0".

4—Necrotic Tissue (Eschar): black, brown, or tan tissue that adheres firmly to the wound bed or ulcer edges and may be either firmer or softer than surrounding skin.

3—Slough: yellow or white tissue that adheres to the ulcer bed in strings or thick clumps, or is mucinous.

2—Granulation Tissue: pink or beefy red tissue with a shiny, moist, granular appearance.

1—Epithelial Tissue: for superficial ulcers, new pink or shiny tissue (skin) that grows in from the edges or as islands on the ulcer surface.

0—Closed/Resurfaced: the wound is completely covered with epithelium (new skin).

Version 3.0: 2004 National Pressure Ulcer Advisory Panel.

Recording and Reporting

- Record appearance of ulcer in client's record.
- Describe type of topical agent used, dressing applied, and client's response.
- Report any deterioration in ulcer appearance to nurse in charge or physician.

Unexpected Outcomes	Related Interventions
1. Skin surrounding ulcer becomes macerated.	• Reduce exposure of surrounding skin to topical agents and moisture. • Select a dressing that has increased moisture-absorbing capacity.
2. Ulcer becomes deeper with increased drainage and/or development of necrotic tissue.	• Review current wound care management. • Consult with multidisciplinary team regarding changes in wound care regimen. • Obtain wound cultures (see Chapter 44).
3. Pressure ulcer extends beyond original margins.	• Monitor for systemic signs and symptoms of poor wound healing, such as abnormal laboratory results (WBC, hemoglobin/hematocrit, serum albumin, serum prealbumin, total proteins), weight loss, and fluid imbalances. • Assess and revise current turning schedule. • Consider further pressure-relieving devices.

Teaching Considerations

- Discuss treatment, and identify individual(s) who will assist with care at home.
- Discuss process of wound healing and expected wound appearance, for example, client's and support persons' perception about appearance of the pressure ulcer. An eschar may look like a scab that indicates wound healing to the client or support persons.
- Discuss with client and support persons perceptions about size of pressure ulcer. Lay people may think that a "bedsore" is small, about the size of a wedding ring. Some of the larger wounds, especially after debridement, may be very troublesome to the client and support persons.
- Discuss with client and support persons perceptions about treatment. Client and support persons may believe it is cruel for staff to keep turning and positioning the client every 2 hours. They may misunderstand some dressing change techniques such as pulling out the dried gauze dressing used for mechanical debridement.
- Identify the signs, symptoms, and four stages of ulcers to report to the health care team.
- Review prevention guidelines to halt further breakdown.
- Discuss options for maintaining good nutrition.

Gerontological Considerations

- Wound healing may be slower in the older adult (Baranoski and Ayello, 2004).
- The normal reduction in the Langerhans cells in the older adult's epidermis causes a decrease in T-cell function and immunity.
- Because older skin has a slower and less intense inflammatory reaction, older clients must be monitored more closely for altered responses to skin irritants.

Home Care Considerations

- Consider caregiver time when selecting a dressing. In the home care setting, caregivers may choose more expensive dressing materials to reduce the frequency of dressing changes (AHCPR, 1994).
- Cost can also be a factor. Some clients have more time than financial resources. They may choose a less expensive treatment option such as dressing material, especially if there is no third-party reimbursement. Another example might be teaching the family to make a normal saline solution rather than buying it premade.
- Identify clean storage area for dressing supplies. Determine availability of required supplies. Discuss need for home care nurse.
- Discuss need for home pressure-reducing surface or bed. Identify adaptive equipment needed to care for client at home.
- Medicare regulations limit reimbursement of some types of pressure-reduction equipment in the treatment of pressure ulcers.

Long-Term Care Considerations

- Rehabilitation units may use a variety of position-relief devices and beds.
- Clients may be discharged to long-term care facilities that specialize in pressure ulcer and wound care.

FOCUS *on* CLINICAL PRACTICE

Ms. Malles, a 72-year-old Hispanic woman, is transferred from the medical intensive care unit (ICU) to the general medicine unit following a cerebral vascular accident. Her significant past medical history includes hypertension and diabetes. She has right-sided weakness and is unable to independently move from side to side. She never verbally communicates with any staff members. She is a small woman approximately 5 feet 3 inches tall and 103 pounds. She is wearing a diaper, due to loose stools the frequency of which has been reported to be at least every 6 hours, and has a Foley catheter in place.

1. You will be performing a risk assessment to identify if Ms. Malles is at risk for pressure ulcer development. After reading the above scenario, what factors may contribute to the potential for skin breakdown?
2. The tool that you will be using is the Braden Scale for Predicting Pressure Sore Risk. This tool will provide you with the following information:
   A. The type of dressing that would be most appropriate for Ms. Malles's pressure ulcers, the frequency of use, and the method for application
   B. Specific risk factors that place Ms. Malles at risk for skin breakdown
   C. The type of treatment that would most appropriate for management of Ms. Malles's diabetes
   D. The best method to manage Ms. Malles's nutritional deficits
   Explain your choice.
3. As you assess Ms. Malles, evaluating the moisture subscale of the Braden scale, which of the descriptors would be most appropriate?
   A. 1—Constantly moist: Skin is kept moist almost constantly by perspiration, urine, etc. Dampness is detected every time patient is moved or turned.
   B. 2—Very moist: Skin is often, but not always, moist. Linen must be changed at least once a shift.
   C. 3—Occasionally moist: Skin is occasionally moist, requiring an extra linen change approximately once a day.
   D. 4—Rarely moist: Skin usually dry, linen requires changing only at routine intervals.
   Explain your choice.
4. The use of the Braden Scale for Predicting Pressure Sore Risk will provide you with measurements of the length and depth of any existing pressure ulcers.
   A. True
   B. False
   Explain your choice.

NCLEX REVIEW QUESTIONS

1. You are working on a surgical unit providing care to clients who have recently undergone major abdominal procedures. How often should a pressure ulcer risk assessment be performed for the clients on this unit?
   1. Every day of their hospital stay
   2. Upon admission to the unit on a regularly scheduled basis, and as their condition changes
   3. Every other day until the fifth postoperative day
   4. Only if indicated by the presence of pressure ulcers
2. You have assessed a client for the risk of developing a pressure ulcer using the Braden scale. The subscale related to mobility demonstrates that the client is completely immobile, does not make even slight changes in body or extremity position without assistance. What would be an appropriate intervention to prevent pressure ulcers in this client?
   1. Use a moisture barrier ointment at least 3 times per day.
   2. Consult with the wound clinical nurse specialist about the most appropriate bed surface to reduce pressure.
   3. Order a nutrition consult to be sure that the client has adequate vitamin and mineral intake.
   4. Consult with the physical therapy staff to determine exercises to increase muscle strength.
3. Upon assessing the client's skin integrity, an ulcer is noted over the sacral area. This ulcer is approximately 2 cm in width and 3 cm in length. The base of the

ulcer is covered with dark, hard, adherent tissue. What stage is this pressure ulcer?
1. Stage II, a partial-thickness ulcer
2. Stage III, a full-thickness ulcer because of the involvement of all tissue layers
3. Stage IV, a full-thickness ulcer that must be involving supporting tissue because of the hard dark tissue that is defined as eschar
4. This pressure ulcer cannot be staged because you must be able to see the wound base to assess the depth of tissue destruction.

4. The order for managing your client with a pressure ulcer is to use a hydrocolloid dressing. What is the rationale for using a hydrocolloid dressing?
1. Hydrocolloid dressings provide an antibiotic solution to decrease surface bacteria.
2. Hydrocolloid dressings protect the wound base and provide a moist environment.
3. Hydrocolloid dressings can be changed several times per day without damaging the wound bed.
4. Hydrocolloid dressings contain a debriding agent to clean a wound environment.

References

AHCPR Panel for the Prediction and Prevention of Pressure Ulcers in Adults: *Pressure ulcers in adults: prediction and prevention,* Clinical practice guideline No. 3, Pub No. 92-0047, Rockville, Md, 1992, Public Health Service, U.S. Department of Health and Human Services.

AHCPR Panel for the Treatment of Pressure Ulcers in Adults: *Treatment of pressure ulcers,* Clinical practice guideline No.15, Pub No. 95-0653, Rockville, Md, 1994, Public Health Service, U.S. Department of Health and Human Services.

Ayello EA, Braden B: How and why do pressure ulcer risk assessment, *Adv Wound Care* 15(3):125, 2002.

Ayello EA and others: Pressure ulcers. In Baranoski S, Ayello EA, editors: *Wound care essentials: practice principles,* Philadelphia, 2004, Lippincott, Williams.

Baranoski S, Ayello EA: Wound treatment options. In Baranoski S, Ayello EA, editors: *Wound care essentials: practice principles,* Philadelphia, 2004, Lippincott, Williams.

Bates-Jensen B: New pressure ulcer status tool, *Decubitus* 3(3):14, 1990.

Bennett MA: Report of the Task Force on the Implications for Darkly Pigmented Intact Skin in the Prediction and Prevention of Pressure Ulcers, *Adv Wound Care* 8(6):34, 1995.

Bergstrom N and others: *Treatment of pressure ulcers.* AHCPR Pub No. 95-0652, Rockville, Md, 1994, Agency for Health Care Policy and Research, Public Health Service, U.S. Department of Health and Human Services,

Braden BJ, Bergstrom N: Clinical utility of the Braden scale for predicting pressure sore risk, *Decubitus* 2(3):44, 1989.

Colwell J: Pressure ulcers. In Elkin MK and others, editors: *Nursing interventions and clinical skills,* St. Louis, 2004, Mosby.

Dallan LE and others: Pain management and wounds. In Baranoski S, Ayello EA, editors: *Wound care essentials: practice principles,* Philadelphia, 2004, Lippincott, Williams.

Henderson CT and others: Draft definition of stage I pressure ulcers: inclusion of persons with darkly pigmented skin, *Adv Wound Care* 10(5):16, 1997.

Jones V and others: Acute and chronic wound healing: pressure ulcers. In Baranoski S, Ayello EA, editors: *Wound care essentials: practice principles,* Philadelphia, 2004, Lippincott, Williams.

Langemo D, Baranoski S: Key points on caring for pressure ulcer in home care, *Home Healthc Nurse* 21(5):309, 2003.

Lyder CH: Regulation and wound care. In Baranoski S, Ayello EA, editors: *Wound care essentials: practice principles,* Philadelphia, 2004, Lippincott, Williams.

National Pressure Ulcer Advisory Panel: Pressure ulcer prevalence, cost and risk assessment: consensus development conference statement, *Decubitus* 2(2):24,1989.

National Pressure Ulcer Advisory Panel (NPUAP): *Facts about reverse staging,* 2000, NPUAP position statement, www.npuap.org, 2003, accessed Feb 6, 2005.

National Pressure Ulcer Advisory Panel (NPUAP): *NPUAP staging report,* 2003, www.npuap.org, accessed Feb 6, 2005.

Norton D and others: *An investigation of geriatric nursing problems in hospital, 1962,* reissue, Edinburgh, 1975, Churchill Livingstone.

Pieper B: Mechanical forces: pressure, shear and friction. In Byrant RA, editor: *Acute and chronic wounds, nursing management,* ed 2, St. Louis, 2000, Mosby.

Rolstad BS and others: Principles of wound management. In Byrant RA, editor: *Acute and chronic wounds, nursing management,* ed 2, St. Louis, 2000, Mosby.

Sager P: Nutritional care to prevent and heal pressure ulcers, *Isr Med Assoc J* 4(9):713, 2002.

Stotts N: Nutritional assessment and support. In Byrant RA, editor: *Acute and chronic wounds, nursing management,* ed 2, St. Louis, 2000, Mosby.

Thomas DR and others: Pressure ulcer scale for healing: derivation and validation of the PUSH tool, *Adv Wound Care* 10(5):96, 1997.

Waldrop J, Doughty D: Wound healing physiology. In Byrant RA, editor: *Acute and chronic wounds, nursing management,* ed 2, St. Louis, 2000, Mosby.

Wound, Ostomy and Continence Nurses Society: *Guideline for prevention and management of pressure ulcers,* WOCN clinical practice guidelines series, Glenview, Ill, 2003 The Association.

Research References

Bergstrom N, Braden, BJ: Predictive validity of the Braden Scale among black and white subjects, *Nurs Res* 51(6): 398, 2002.

Bergstrom N, Demuth PJ, Braden BJ: A clinical trial of the Braden scale for predicting pressure sore risk, *Nurs Clin North Am* 22(2):417, 1987.

Bergstrom N and others: Predicting pressure ulcer risk: a multisite study of the predictive validity of the Braden scale, *Nur Res* 47(5):261, 1998.

Braden BJ, Bergstrom N: Predictive utility of the Braden scale for predicting pressure sore risk, *Res Nurs Health* 17:459, 1994.

Kosiak M: Etiology and pathology of decubitus ulcers, *Arch Phys Med Rehabil* 40:62, 1959.

Langemo DK and others: Incidence of pressure sores in acute care, rehabilitation, extended care, home health, and hospice in one locale, *Decubitus* 2(2):42, 1989.

Lyder CH and others. Quality of care for hospitalized Medicare patients at risk for pressure ulcers, *Arch Intern Med* 161:1549, 2001.

Lyder CH and others: The Braden scale for pressure ulcer risk: evaluating the predictive validity in black and Latino/Hispanic elders, *Appl Nurs Res* 12(2):60, 1999.

Newman DK and others: Moisture control and incontinence management. In Krasner DL and others. *Chronic wound care: a clinical source book for healthcare professionals,* ed 3, Wayne, Pa, 2001, HMP Communications.

Sprigle S and others: Clinical skin temperature measurement to predict incipient pressure ulcers, *Adv Skin Wound Care* 14(3):133, 2001.

Szor JK, Bourguignon C: Description of pressure ulcer pain at rest and dressing change, *J Wound Ostomy Continence Nurs* 26(3):115, 1999.

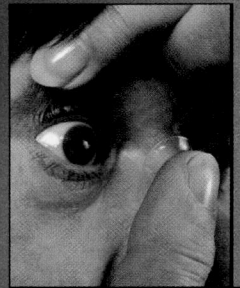

16

Care of Eye and Ear Prostheses

MEDIA RESOURCES

Evolve Site *evolve*
http://evolve.elsevier.com/Perry/skills
• Weblinks

OBJECTIVES

Mastery of content in this chaper will enable the nurse to:

- Explain why proper care of prostheses is important to a client's self-esteem.
- Identify guidelines used in caring for contact lenses, hearing aids, and artificial eyes.
- Explain differences in the care of soft and rigid contact lenses.
- Correctly remove, store, clean, and insert a contact lens.
- Explain the rationale for maintaining aseptic technique during care of an artificial eye.
- Explain differences in irrigation procedures for removing exudates and chemicals.
- Describe techniques that determine whether a hearing aid functions properly.
- Correctly remove, clean, and reinsert a hearing aid.

KEY TERMS

Audiologist

Cerumen

Contact lens

Enucleation

Extended wear

Myopia

Ocularist

Ophthalmologist

Optometrist

Presbycusis

Prosthesis

Refractive error

Many clients rely on artificial devices, known as prostheses, to replace or restore function to diseased or lost body parts. Eyeglasses and contact lenses help to restore visual loss, and hearing aids can improve sound reception. A client may also depend on a prosthetic device to maintain an attractive appearance. Artificial eyes in particular help clients maintain a normal appearance when an eye has been lost as a result of injury or disease. Any prosthesis must fit and work properly if the client is to function optimally within his or her environment. Breakage or loss may result in serious impairment that can put the client at risk for injury, interfere with communication, isolate the client socially, and increase client dependence and thereby threaten self-esteem. Understandably, clients can be especially sensitive about care of contact lenses, hearing aids, or artificial eyes.

Prosthetic devices must be cleaned regularly to ensure function and prevent injury. Most clients have an established routine for cleaning their prostheses. When clients are unable to care for themselves, the nurse must understand the correct way to clean, handle, and store contact lenses, hearing aids, and artificial eyes. Clients usually show great interest in the manner in which the nurse performs cleaning and maintenance procedures. Careful handling of prostheses is vital to avoid damage to these devices or to the clients' eyes or ears.

Evidence-Based Practice Trends

Up to 80% of contact lens wear complications can be attributed to poor compliance (Ky and others, 1998). Noncompliance patterns have not been correlated with economic or social factors such as age or gender (de Andrade Sobrinho and Carvalho, 2003). However, some have found that the complexity of the cleaning regimens is related (Rakow, 2003) and that continued client education in proper cleaning may help increase compliance (Fan and others, 2002). Given these findings, nurses should consider verifying care instructions provided by the client, take care to understand complex cleaning regimens, and address client needs for knowledge.

The orbital implant, which provides a surface for the cosmetic prosthesis or "artificial eye," may be equipped with a peg for securing the prosthesis. Although the peg enhances transfer of eye movement to the prosthesis, its presence increases risk for eye infection (Lin and others, 2002). Consequently, researchers are exploring alternatives such as magnetic attachment of the prosthesis to the implant (Murray and others, 2000). The nurse should be particularly alert for signs of infection in a pegged orbital implant.

Often cool tap water is recommended for emergency eye flushing because it is effective and immediately available for first aid. Nevertheless, controversy remains over the best solution for irrigating the eye in a health care setting (Kompa and others, 2002; Kuckelkorn and others, 2002; Ramponi, 2000). When faced with a choice of normal intravenous (IV) solutions, lactated Ringer's is more effective than normal saline in restoring pH after a chemical burn to the eye (Kuckelkorn and others, 2002). A Morgan lens is a device similar in shape and placement to an artificial eye that connects via tubing to a source of irrigation solution. Solution flows beneath the lens to wash the eye (Ramponi, 2000). Use of a Morgan lens has been criticized because it fails to expose the insides of the eyelids to irrigation solution (Kuckelkorn and others, 2002). Nurses should continue to teach clients to flush the eyes with cool tap water in an emergency.

Skill Performance Guidelines

1. Let the client be a resource in the care of each device. Although it is the nurse's responsibility to ensure clients do not damage the devices or injure themselves, clients familiar with their devices are likely to have an established routine and helpful tips.
2. Always protect the device from breakage. In addition to the client dependence caused by loss of the prosthesis, replacement or repair can be very expensive.
3. When a sensory loss exists, use techniques that facilitate interaction with the client. Be sensitive to the degree of loss that may remain when a device is used.
4. Encourage clients to express feelings related to reliance on an artificial device for function or appearance. The nurse can be supportive and can teach clients and their families methods for interacting more effectively.

SKILL 16-1 Taking Care of Contact Lenses

A contact lens is a thin, concave disk that fits directly over the cornea of the eye. It is transparent over at least the pupil and may be colorless or tinted. Contact lenses are designed to correct refractive errors of the eye or abnormalities in the cornea's shape that distort vision. They are relatively easy to apply and remove.

All modern contact lenses are gas (oxygen) permeable and adhere to the cornea by surface tension. There are two basic types of contact lenses in use today: rigid gas permeable (RGP) and soft. They differ primarily in size, flexibility, and durability. Rigid contact lenses are made of firm, durable plastic and are smaller than the cornea. Soft contact lenses are made of a flexible hydrogel plastic and cover the entire cornea and a small rim of the sclera. There are many different kinds of both RGP and soft lenses to accommodate client needs for comfort, vision correction, and convenience. Specific lenses have prescribed wear and replacement schedules.

The wear schedule determines how long the lens may be kept in the eye after insertion. Most contact lens wearers use daily wear lenses (American Optometric Association, 2003). Clients wear these lenses only while awake and then discard them or clean them for reinsertion. Others use extended wear lenses, which are worn continuously for several days before removal and may be soft or RGP. Although the limit for extended wear lenses is usually 6 nights, certain soft lenses have been approved for continuous wear up to 30 nights (U.S. Food and Drug Administration, 2001).

The replacement schedule determines how long the lens may be used before it is discarded. Conventional soft and RGP lenses are relatively durable and are replaced only when they show wear or the client's needs change. Most soft contact lenses, however, are replaced according to a specific schedule. Daily replacement lenses are disposed of each night and a fresh pair inserted the next day. The most popular type of soft lens is discarded after 1 to 2 weeks of daily or extended wear. This type of soft lens is often called "disposable," even though some are cleaned and reused during their short lives. "Frequent" or "planned" replacement lenses are replaced every 1 to several months depending on the model.

It is important to remember that all lenses must be removed periodically to prevent infection and corneal damage and that proper cleaning is necessary before reinserting a lens. As contact lenses are worn, secretions and foreign matter adhere to the lens surfaces. This material distorts vision, irritates the eye, and increases the risk for infection and injury. Pain, tearing, discomfort, and redness of the conjunctivae may be symptoms of excessive wear or improper cleaning. Persistence of symptoms even after lens removal is abnormal, however, and may indicate serious ocular damage (Suchecki and others, 2003).

An estimated 30 million Americans wear contact lenses today (American Optometric Association, 2003). It is extremely important that nurses determine whether clients wear contact lenses, particularly when clients are admitted to hospitals or agencies in unresponsive or confused states. If a seriously ill client is wearing contact lenses and this fact goes undetected, severe corneal injury can result (Crowston and others, 1996).

Care of contact lenses includes removal, cleaning and storage, and insertion. Clients usually have a prescribed method for caring for their lenses. When it is necessary for the nurse to assist with lens care, the client's preferences should be considered and manufacturer or prescriber clarification sought as needed.

DELEGATION CONSIDERATIONS

This skill may be delegated to assistive personnel. Before delegating this skill, the nurse must:

- Instruct assistive personnel in caring for the client's specific type of contact lens, including cleaning solutions and routine, wear schedule, and replacement schedule
- Instruct assistive personnel to report eye pain or discomfort, redness, swelling, tearing, or drainage
- Reinforce the importance of careful handling of the lens to prevent damage and injury

EQUIPMENT

- ❑ Bath towels or waterproof pads (2)
- ❑ Sterile saline solution
- ❑ Sterile lens care solution(s) for cleaning, disinfecting, and rinsing
- ❑ Sterile wetting or conditioning solution (depends on care regimen)
- ❑ Sterile enzyme solution (depends on care regimen)
- ❑ Clean lens storage container
- ❑ Suction cup (optional)
- ❑ Powder-free, disposable gloves

STEP	RATIONALE

ASSESSMENT

1. Stand at client's side. Inspect eye, or ask client if contact lens is in place.

Lenses are generally comfortable to wear, and client may forget they are in place.

• *Critical Decision Point*
Unconscious or confused clients entering the health care setting should be carefully assessed; lenses are often difficult to detect if colorless (untinted).

2. Ask if client is able to manipulate and hold contact lens and whether eyeglasses are available.

Determines level of assistance required in care.

3. Ask if client feels any eye discomfort, and determine length of time client normally wears lenses and length of time since last insertion.

Scratched lens can cause corneal irritation and abrasion. Accumulation of dust or debris between lens and cornea causes irritation. Continuous wearing of certain types of lenses can irritate cornea.

4. Assess client's knowledge of and routines for cleaning and disinfecting lenses.

Determines compliance with and knowledge of self-care.

5. Assess client for any unusual visual signs/symptoms (reduced visual acuity, blurred vision, halos, photophobia).

May indicate underlying visual alteration or injury or need to clean lens or change lens prescription.

6. Assess types of medications prescribed for client: sedatives, hypnotics, muscle relaxants, antihistamines, anticholinergics, and antidepressants.

Sedatives, hypnotics, and muscle relaxants reduce blink reflex and thus reduce lubrication of cornea. Antihistamines, anticholinergics, and antidepressants can reduce tear production.

NURSING DIAGNOSES

- Bathing/hygiene self-care deficit
- Deficient knowledge regarding contact lens care
- Pain (acute, chronic)
- Risk for infection

- Risk for injury
- Disturbed sensory perception (visual)
- Risk for situational low self-esteem

Related factors are individualized based on client's condition or needs.

PLANNING

1. Expected outcomes following completion of procedure:
   - Client verbalizes comfort after removal and/or reinsertion of lenses.

Lenses are removed or inserted properly.

   - Client's eyes show no signs of ocular infection (e.g., redness, pain, swelling, discharge, blurred vision, photophobia) or injury (e.g., irritation, foreign body sensation, tearing).

Indicates that there is no infection or injury from removal or insertion of lenses.

   - Client verbalizes improved visual perception after lens cleaning.

Lenses cleaned and positioned correctly.

   - Client demonstrates the proper techniques for removing, cleaning, and reinserting lenses.

Learning is achieved.

2. Discuss procedure with client.

Client can assist in planning by explaining technique that may aid removal and insertion. Reduces client anxiety.

3. Ensure fingernails of care provider are short and smooth.

Nails may scratch or tear lens.

4. Assemble supplies at bedside. Place towel over work area.

Provides easy access to supplies. Towel catches lens if accidentally dropped and avoids breakage, scratching, and tearing.

5. Check expiration date and condition of each solution. Discard any solutions that have expired or become cloudy or discolored.

Failure to use fresh, sterile solutions may result in infection or irritation.

STEP	RATIONALE

- *Critical Decision Point*

   Use only solutions and methods recommended by lens manufacturer or vision care specialist. Some solutions are incompatible with others and with certain lenses. Specific solutions must be used as directed to be effective.

6. Have client assume supine or sitting position in bed or chair.	Provides easy access for nurse while retracting eyelids and manipulating lenses.

IMPLEMENTATION

1. **Removing Lenses**	
a. Perform hand hygiene. Apply snug, powder-free, disposable gloves.	Reduces transmission of microorganisms. Powder may irritate eye. Snug gloves help prevent touching eye accidentally.
b. Place towel just below client's face.	Catches lens if one should accidentally fall from eye.
c. Removal of soft lens:	
(1) Add 2 to 3 drops of sterile saline solution to client's eye.	Lubricates eye to facilitate lens removal.
(2) Ask the client to look up.	Exposes lower eyeball to which lens will be displaced.
(3) Using middle finger of dominant hand, gently retract lower lid.	Exposes lower eyeball to which lens will be displaced.
(4) With pad of index finger of same hand, slide lens off cornea down onto lower sclera.	Positions lens for easy grasping. Use of finger pad rather than fingernail prevents injury to cornea and damage to lens.
(5) Use thumb of same hand to gently pinch lens together and lift away.	Air enters underneath lens to release suction and causes lens to fold. Protects lens from damage.

- *Critical Decision Point*

   If lens edges stick together, place lens in palm and soak thoroughly with sterile saline solution. Gently roll lens with index finger in back-and-forth motion. If necessary, soak lens in storage solution, which may return lens to normal shape.

d. Removal of rigid lens:	
(1) Inspect the eye to be sure lens is positioned directly over cornea.	Correct position of lens allows easy and safe removal from eye.

- *Critical Decision Point*

   If lens is not positioned directly over cornea, have client close eyelid, place index and middle fingers of one hand on eyelid just beside the lens and beneath, and gently attempt to massage lens back into place. If lens is not repositioned easily, an immediate referral to the ophthalmologist should be made.

(2) Place index finger on outer corner of client's eye, and draw skin gently back toward ear.	Tightens eyelid against eyeball.
(3) Ask client to open eye wide.	Lid margins must clear top and bottom of lens until the blink.

- *Critical Decision Point*

   For clients unable to open eye or blink on command, a lens suction cup can be used to remove lens from eye. Gently apply suction cup to lens surface and lift out.

(4) Ask client to blink. Do not release pressure on eyelid until blink is completed.	Eyelid catches edge of lens and dislodges it.

STEP	RATIONALE

- **Critical Decision Point**
  If lens fails to dislodge, gently retract eyelids beyond edges of lens. Press lower eyelid gently against lower edge of lens to dislodge lens.

(5) Allow both eyelids to close slightly, and grasp lens as it rises from eye. Cup lens in hand.	Positions lens for removal. Protects lens from breakage.
2. Clean and store lens (see step 6).	Lenses must be cleaned after removal to protect lens and prevent eye infection.

- **Critical Decision Point**
  Disposable lenses due for replacement may be discarded.

3. Repeat step 1c or 1d and step 2 for other lens.	
4. Assess eyes for redness, tearing, and pain.	Signs/symptoms may indicate corneal abrasion.
5. Dispose of towel, remove gloves, and perform hand hygiene.	Reduces transmission of microorganisms.
6. **Typical Cleaning and Disinfecting of Contact Lenses (verify specific method for lenses)**	
a. Apply 1 or 2 drops of cleaning solution to lens in palm of hand. Using index finger (soft lenses) or little finger (rigid lenses), rub lens gently but thoroughly on both sides for 20 to 30 seconds.	Removes secretions and foreign materials adhering to lens surfaces.

- **Critical Decision Point**
  Do not touch or scratch lens with fingernail.

b. Holding lens over emesis basin, rinse thoroughly with recommended rinsing solution.	Removes debris and cleaning solution from lens surfaces.

- **Critical Decision Point**
  Do not use tap water for cleaning, rinsing, or storage. Tap water contains microbes and may be absorbed into the lens, making it uncomfortable to wear.

c. Place lens in proper storage case compartment: "R" for right lens and "L" for left (see illustration). Rigid lenses should be inside up.	Lens prescription may differ for each eye. Placing lens with concave side up makes safe removal easier.
d. Fill with recommended disinfectant or storage solution.	Disinfects and conditions lens, protects from contamination.

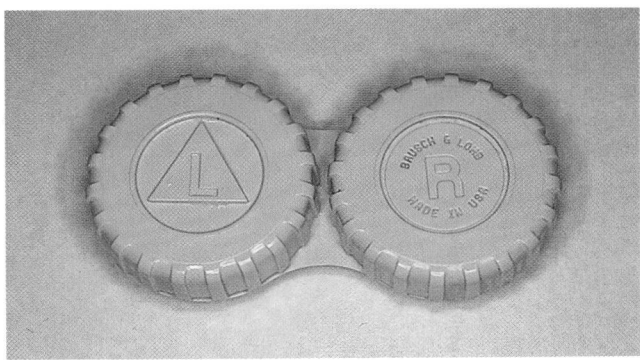

STEP 6c Contact lens storage case.

STEP	RATIONALE

e. Secure cover(s) over storage case. Label case with client's name, identification number, and room number.

Proper storage prevents cracking, tearing, breakage, scratching, discoloration, and loss.

• *Critical Decision Point*

Periodic cleaning with enzymatic cleaner and/or heat disinfecting may be part of the prescribed regimen. Follow prescriber's instructions and schedules.

7. **Inserting Lenses**

   a. Perform hand hygiene. Apply snug, powder-free, disposable gloves.

   b. Place towel just below client's face.

Reduces transmission of microorganisms. Powder may irritate eye. Snug gloves help prevent touching eye accidentally.
Catches lens if accidentally dropped and avoids scratching and tearing.

   c. Insertion of soft lens:

     (1) Remove right lens from storage case, and rinse with recommended rinsing solution; inspect lens for foreign materials, tears, and other damage.

Always begin with right lens to avoid placing wrong lens in eye. Removes disinfectant solution. A damaged or dirty lens may irritate or damage eye.

     (2) Hold lens on tip of index finger of dominant hand with concave side up.

Positions lens for inspection and placement against cornea.

     (3) Inspect lens from side at eye level to ensure that lens is not inverted (see illustration).

Soft lens is inverted (inside out) if rim curves outward forming a lip; it is in proper position if rim curves upward.

     (4) Using middle or index finger of opposite hand, retract upper lid until iris is exposed. Using middle finger of the hand holding the lens, pull down lower lid (see illustration).

Separating lids as much as possible allows room for lens to completely contact cornea without touching lids or lashes.

     (5) Instruct client to look straight ahead and focus on an object in the distance. Gently place lens directly on cornea, and release lids slowly, starting with lower lid.

Helps client keep eye still. Prevents lens being dislodged by eyelids.

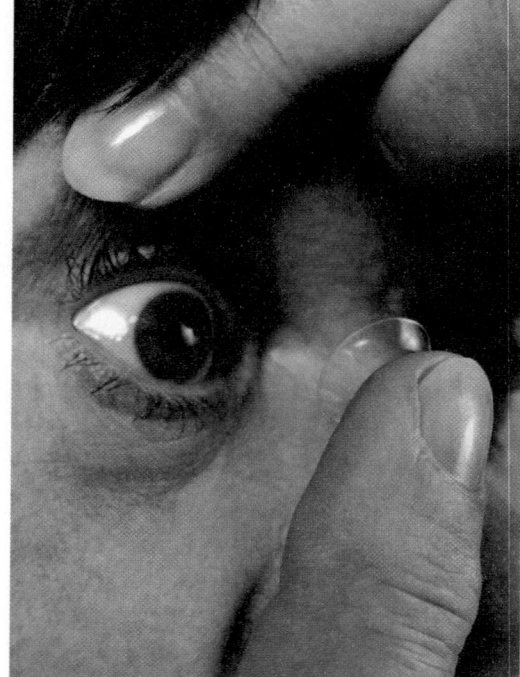

STEP **7c(4)** Correct position of hands for soft lens insertion.

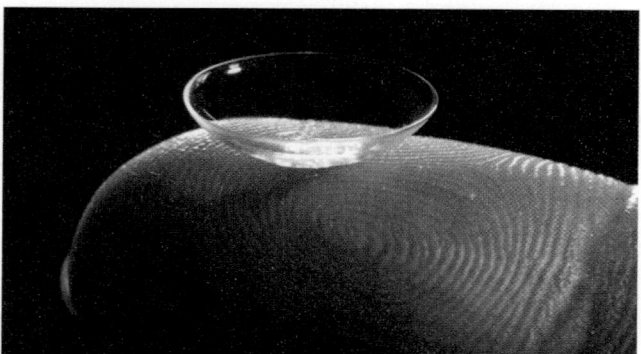

STEP **7c(3)** Correct position of soft lens before insertion.

STEP	**RATIONALE**

d. Insertion of rigid lens:

(1) Remove right lens from storage case; attempt to lift lens straight up (see illustration).

Always begin with right lens to avoid placing wrong lens in eye. Sliding lens out of case can cause scratches on the surface.

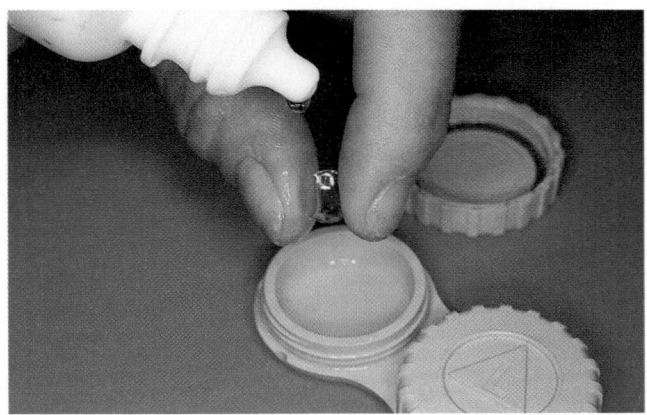

STEP **7d(1)** Removal of rigid lens from storage case.

(2) Hold lens on tip of index finger of dominant hand with concave side up.

Positions lens for placement against cornea.

(3) Inspect the lens to ensure that it is moist, clean, clear, and free of chips or cracks.

A damaged or dirty lens may damage or irritate eye.

(4) Wet the lens surfaces using a few drops of prescribed wetting solution.

Cushions and lubricates lens to protect cornea.

(5) Using middle or index finger of opposite hand, retract upper lid until iris is exposed. Using middle finger of the hand holding the lens, pull down lower lid (see illustration).

Separating lids as much as possible allows room for lens to completely contact cornea without touching lids or lashes.

(6) Instruct client to look straight ahead and focus on an object in the distance (see illustration). Gently place lens directly on cornea, and release lids slowly, starting with lower lid.

Helps client keep eye still. Prevents lens being dislodged by eyelids.

(7) Ask client to close eyes briefly and to avoid blinking.

Helps to secure position of lens.

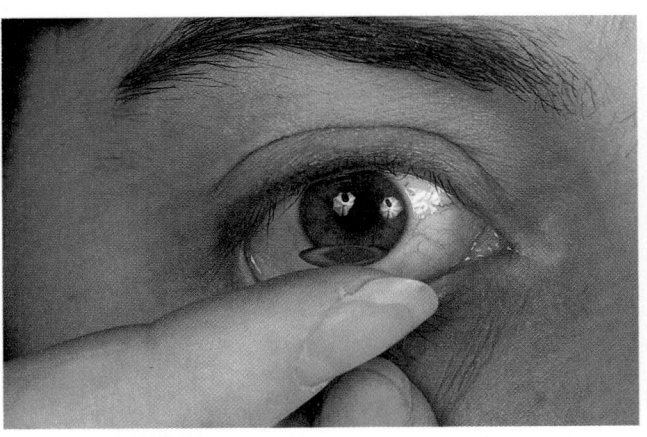

STEP **7d(5)** Hand position for rigid lens insertion.

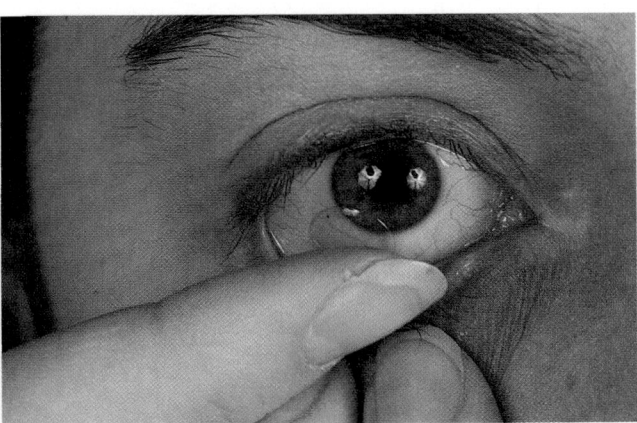

STEP **7d(6)** Instruct client to look straight ahead and focus on an object in the distance.

STEP	RATIONALE
8. Inspect eye to ensure lens is on cornea.	Incorrectly positioned lens cannot correct vision and may damage eye.

• **Critical Decision Point**
  If lens is on sclera rather than cornea, ask client to slowly close eye and look toward the lens. Gentle pressure on the eyelid may help to center the lens on the cornea.

STEP	RATIONALE
9. Ask client to blink a few times.	Ensures lens is centered, free of trapped air, and comfortable.
10. Ask client to cover other eye with hand and report if vision is clear and lens is comfortable.	Determines whether lens is properly positioned over cornea.
11. Repeat step 7c or 7d and steps 8 through 10 for left eye.	
12. Discard solution from storage case, and rinse case thoroughly with sterile lens storage solution. Sterilize or replace case as recommended by manufacturer. Allow case to air dry. Dispose of towel, remove gloves, and perform hand hygiene.	Lens cases have been shown to harbor harmful microbes and microbial toxins (Clark and others, 1994; Fulk and others, 1997). Reduces transmission of microorganisms.

EVALUATION

1. After lenses are removed, inspect eye for redness, pain, swelling of eyelids or conjunctivae, discharge, or excess tearing.	Signs/symptoms indicate corneal irritation or abrasion.
2. Ask client if lens feels comfortable after removal and reinsertion of lenses.	Client may experience discomfort if debris is trapped between lens and cornea or if eye has been injured.
3. Inspect eye, over time, for signs of ocular infection or injury.	Demonstrates efficacy of lens care over time.
4. Ask client to cover each eye alternately and report if vision is clear.	Verifies proper lens cleaning and positioning.
5. Observe client removing, cleaning, and reinserting lenses.	Demonstrates client's understanding of techniques.

Recording and Reporting

• Record in nurses' notes procedure, time, solutions, and lens storage location.
• If client goes to surgery or other special procedure, record whether contact lenses are in eyes or stored at client's bedside.
• Record and report any signs or symptoms of alterations in vision, infection, or injury.
• Record and report uncorrected problems with removal or insertion of lenses.

Unexpected Outcomes	Related Interventions
1. Burning, pain, or foreign body sensation	• Remove lenses. • Clean and disinfect lenses. • Rest eyes. • If symptoms continue, refer to ophthalmologist.
2. Blurred vision	• Ensure lens is over cornea. Reposition using gentle pressure on eyelid as necessary. • Ensure that lens is in correct eye. • Remove and clean lens and reinsert. • Ensure that soft lens is not inverted on insertion. • If symptoms continue, refer to ophthalmologist.

Unexpected Outcomes	Related Interventions
3. Redness, discharge, swelling, or excessive tearing.	• Remove lenses. • Refer to ophthalmologist.
4. Client lacks knowledge and/or skills to perform lens care properly.	• Teach family caregiver appropriate skills of cleaning, disinfecting, inserting, and removing lenses. • Provide written instructions and brochures with needed information.

Teaching Considerations

- Emphasize following prescribed lens care to avoid damage to lens and/or eye. Advise client against using saliva, homemade saline solution, tap water, or expired or cloudy solutions. Advise client to avoid touching bottle tips to skin, eye, lashes, lenses, or other surfaces. Sterile, normal saline may be used to store lenses in an emergency but must be followed by prescribed lens treatments before reinsertion.
- Clients with contact lenses should visit their vision care specialist (ophthalmologist or optometrist) at least annually.
- Teach client *RSVP*: *R*edness, *S*ensitivity, *V*ision problems, and *P*ain. If *RSVP* persists after lens removal and reinsertion, contact the vision care specialist (Lewis and others, 2000).
- Caution client to use aerosol products (e.g., hair spray, cologne, deodorants) only before lenses are inserted and to avoid exposure to noxious or irritating vapors or fumes.
- Advise client to wash hands with mild soap before handling lenses. Lotion, oil, perfume, or deodorant in hand cleansers may damage lens or irritate eye. Alcohol-based hand rubs do not remove lotions, oils, or other substances from hands.
- Apply makeup after lenses are inserted and use only water-based, fiber-free eye makeup.
- Client should use only eye drops or medications approved by vision care specialist.
- Client should remove lenses for sleeping, sunbathing, swimming, and showering unless otherwise instructed.

Pediatric Considerations

- Even in children, some conditions, such as absence of a natural lens or extreme refractive errors, are best addressed with contact lenses.
- Parents and older children can learn how to care for lenses.

Gerontological Considerations

- Clients and caregivers should be alert for and report signs of visual changes such as loss of night vision, changes in functional ability, decreased socialization, increased frequency in bumping into objects, slowness when descending stairs.

Home Care Considerations

- Labels on lens solutions, cases, and eye medications may be difficult for the client to read when lenses are removed for cleaning and disinfection. Caregivers should ensure that labeling is adequate for the client with uncorrected vision.

Long-Term Care Considerations

- Periodic procedures such as enzymatic cleaning, lens replacement, lens case sterilization and replacement, and vision care specialist evaluations must be accommodated.

SKILL 16-2 Taking Care of an Artificial Eye

As a result of tumor, infection, congenital blindness, or severe trauma to the eye, clients may undergo enucleation, the complete surgical removal of the eyeball. During this surgical procedure a spherical implant is placed in the orbit to maintain the natural eye structure and provide support for a cosmetic prosthesis. The muscles and other tissues of the eye are sewn around the implant, holding it in place. The implant therefore is not visible (Figure 16-1). Modern implants are made of hydroxyapatite, a porous material that allows the tissues of the eye to grow into the sphere (Perry, 1991). Like a healthy eye, this integrated implant moves as the companion eye moves.

A concave cosmetic prosthesis is placed over the implant, resulting in a nearly normal appearance. Some implants are fitted with a peg that secures and optimally transfers implant movement to the prosthesis. The prosthesis, the artificial eye, is glass or plastic and colored to match the companion eye.

Prostheses are relatively easy to remove and insert and are usually worn day and night. Cleaning with sterile saline or soap and water is done at intervals of up to a year based on ocularist recommendations and the client's preference (Kolberg Ocular Prosthetics, 2004).

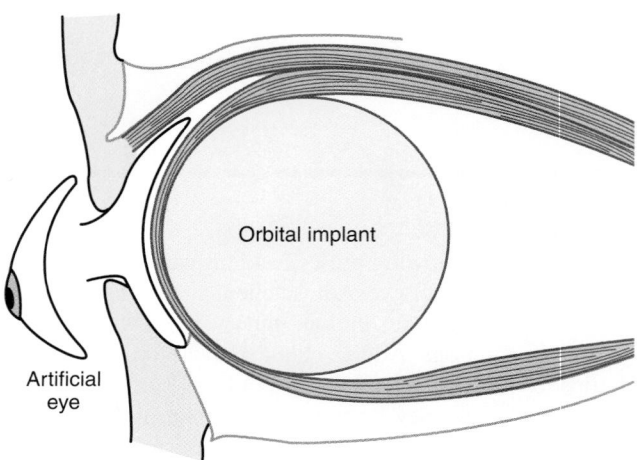

FIGURE 16-1 Side view of orbital implant, artificial eye removed.

DELEGATION CONSIDERATIONS

This skill may be delegated to assistive personnel. Before delegating this skill, the nurse must:
- Instruct assistive personnel to report eye pain or discomfort, inflammation, drainage, or odor
- Reinforce the importance of careful handling of the prosthesis to prevent damage or injury

EQUIPMENT

- ❏ Bath towels or waterproof pads (2)
- ❏ Sterile saline for washing prosthesis
- ❏ Irrigation bulb or large syringe (without needle)
- ❏ Sterile saline, 30 to 180 ml, 90° to 100° F (about 32° to 38° C)
- ❏ Emesis basin
- ❏ 4 × 4 inch gauze pads
- ❏ Disposable gloves
- ❏ Facial tissues (optional)
- ❏ Washbasin with warm water and mild soap (optional)
- ❏ Suction device (or medicine dropper bulb) (optional)
- ❏ Covered plastic storage case (optional)

STEP	RATIONALE

ASSESSMENT

1. Ask client or inspect eyes to determine which is artificial.

Implant imparts movement to prosthesis and can make distinguishing it difficult. Artificial eye pupil will not react to changes in light.

2. Assess client's frequency and method of cleaning and length of time since last cleaning.

Determines compliance with and knowledge of self-care. Establishes time of next anticipated removal and cleaning.

- **Critical Decision Point**

  Unless advised by the client's eye care practitioner, the prosthesis is usually not removed unless the client experiences discomfort because excessive handling may cause irritation and increased secretions (Kolberg Ocular Prosthetics, 2004).

STEP	**RATIONALE**

3. Assess client's ability to remove, clean, and reinsert prosthesis.

Determines level of assistance required during care.

4. Before and after removal of prosthesis, assess eyelids and socket for inflammation, tenderness, swelling, drainage, or odor. Pay particular attention to the implant peg if present. Assess client's pain or other symptoms.

Signs/symptoms may indicate infection or injury. Infection can spread easily to neighboring eye, underlying sinuses, or brain tissue. The implant peg is a common site of infection (Lin and others, 2002).

NURSING DIAGNOSES

- Bathing/hygiene self-care deficit
- Deficient knowledge regarding eye prosthesis care
- Pain (acute, chronic)
- Risk for infection

- Risk for injury
- Disturbed sensory perception (visual)
- Risk for situational low self-esteem

Related factors are individualized based on client's condition or needs.

PLANNING

1. Expected outcomes following completion of procedure:
   - Client verbalizes feelings regarding prosthesis removal and care.
   - Client verbalizes that prosthetic eye fits comfortably.
   - Client's eyelid margins are clean and of normal pink color, with lashes turned away from prosthesis.
   - Client demonstrates no signs of infection, such as inflammation, tenderness, or discharge from socket or eyelid margins.
   - Client demonstrates the proper techniques for removing, cleaning, and reinserting prosthesis.

Client senses trust from level of acceptance conveyed by nurse.
Prosthesis is inserted correctly.
Eyelids are cleaned and positioned correctly.

Eyelid margins and socket are free of infection.

Learning is achieved.

2. Discuss procedure with client.

Allows client opportunity to suggest further ideas about procedure.

3. Assemble supplies at bedside. Place one towel over work area.

Provides easy access to supplies. Towel catches prosthesis if accidentally dropped and avoids breakage or scratching.

4. Assist client to sitting or supine position with head elevated. Provide privacy.

Position facilitates removal of prosthesis with less chance of breakage. Privacy supports positive body image.

IMPLEMENTATION

1. Perform hand hygiene. Apply disposable gloves.
2. Place towel just below client's face.

Reduces transmission of microorganisms.
Catches prosthesis if accidentally dropped and avoids breakage or scratching. Absorbs excess irrigation fluid.

3. With thumb of dominant hand, gently retract lower eyelid against lower orbital ridge (see illustration).

Exposes lower edge of prosthesis.

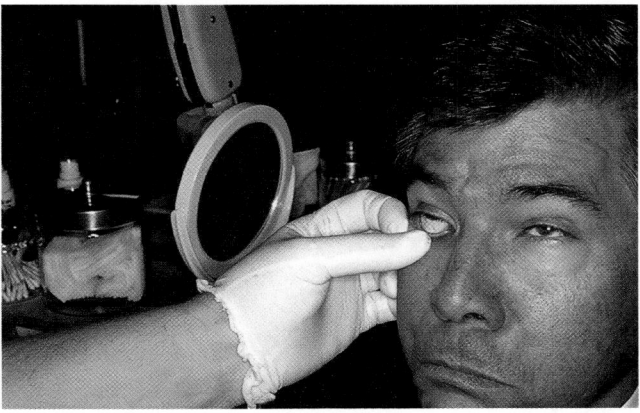

STEP **3** Retraction of lower lid to aid removal of eye prosthesis.

STEP	RATIONALE
4. Exert slight pressure below eyelid, and slide prosthesis out (see illustration).	Breaks suction, causing prosthesis to rise and slide out of socket.

• *Critical Decision Point*
  If prosthesis does not slide out, use moistened suction device to apply direct suction to prosthesis (Kolberg Ocular Prosthetics, 2004).

STEP	RATIONALE
5. Note presence and orientation of colored dot at margin of prosthesis.	A colored dot usually indicates "up" on an artificial eye.
6. Place prosthesis in palm of hand.	Protects prosthesis from breakage.
7. Clean prosthesis:	
a. Wash with mild soap and warm water or plain saline solution by rubbing well between thumb and index finger.	Tears, secretions, and microorganisms may have collected on surface of prosthesis. Soap is less irritating than detergents.
b. Polish with moistened facial tissues or gauze if necessary.	Removes stubborn deposits.
c. Rinse well under running tap water or saline solution (see illustration).	Removes soap and residue.
8. Inspect prosthesis for rough edges or surfaces. Set aside on towel.	Damaged prosthesis may injure eye socket.
9. If prosthesis will not be reinserted immediately, store in sterile saline in a labeled case in a documented location.	Proper storage prevents damage, infection, and loss (Kolberg Ocular Prosthetics, 2004).
10. Clean eyelid margins and socket:	
a. Wash and rinse eyelid margins with mild soap and water. Wipe from inner to outer canthus using a clean section of cloth with each wipe.	Prevents secretions from entering nasolacrimal duct.
b. Retract upper and lower eyelid margins with thumb and index finger.	Exposes eye socket.
c. Gently irrigate socket with sterile saline solution. Note presence of discharge or odor.	Removes secretions and residual soap. Purulent discharge or odor may indicate infection.
d. Remove excess moisture with gauze pads by wiping from inner to outer canthus.	Removes moisture that can harbor microorganisms. Prevents fluid from entering nasolacrimal duct.
11. Moisten prosthesis in water or sterile saline.	Lubrication makes insertion easier.

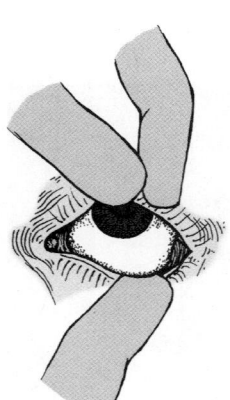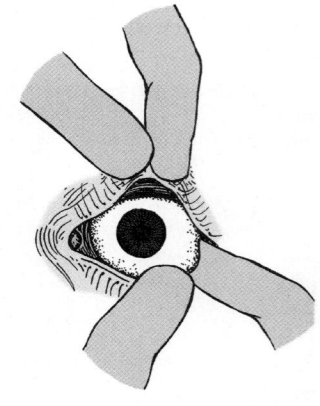

STEP 4 Exertion of pressure below eyelid and removal of prosthesis.

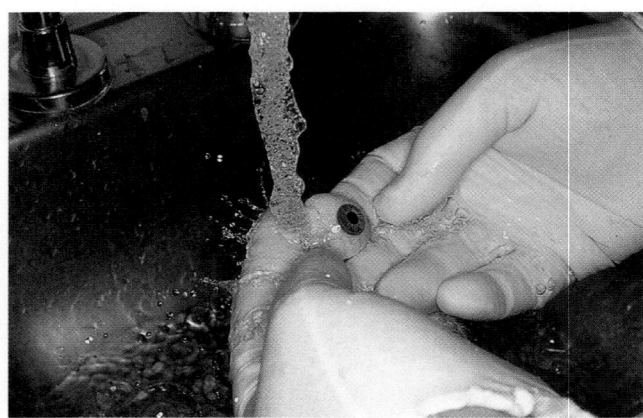

STEP 7c Rinsing of eye prosthesis.

STEP	RATIONALE
12. Retract client's upper eyelid with index finger or thumb of nondominant hand.	Exposes socket.
13. With dominant hand, hold prosthesis so that iris faces outward and colored dot is properly oriented.	Ensures proper orientation.
14. Gently slide prosthesis up under upper eyelid and then push down lower lid to allow prosthesis to slip into place (see illustration).	Reverses removal steps. Guides prosthesis into position.

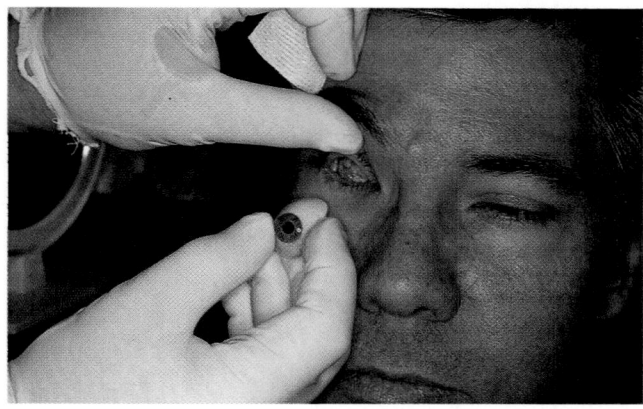

STEP **14** Replacement of eye prosthesis into eye socket.

- **Critical Decision Point**

  Do not force prosthesis into socket. For a pegged implant, center the depression on the back of the prosthesis over the peg while inserting.

15. Blot excess moisture from eye with gauze or tissue.	Wiping from inner to outer canthus may dislodge prosthesis.
16. Dispose of soiled supplies, remove gloves, and perform hand hygiene.	Reduces transmission of microorganisms.

EVALUATION

1. Ask client about feelings regarding prosthesis removal and care.	Provides opportunity to express disturbances in or acceptance of body image.
2. Ask client if prosthesis fits comfortably.	Verifies proper cleaning and positioning.
3. Inspect eyelids and socket for signs of infection, injury, or lashes turned toward prosthesis.	Verifies proper positioning. Demonstrates efficacy of care over time.
4. Observe client removing, cleaning, and reinserting prosthesis.	Demonstrates client's understanding of techniques.

Recording and Reporting

- Record removal of prosthesis and storage location if not reinserted after cleaning.
- Record and report any signs or symptoms of infection or injury.

•

Unexpected Outcomes	Related Interventions
1. Discomfort or pain	• Reposition prosthesis. • If sensation remains, remove prosthesis and inspect for any sharp or rough edges. • If sensation remains, remove prosthesis, provide client with eye patch, and refer to eye care specialist.
2. Inflammation	• Remove prosthesis, clean, and store. • Irrigate eye socket, and provide client with eye patch until inflammation subsides.
3. Excessive, purulent, or foul drainage	• Remove prosthesis, clean, and store until infection resolves. • Immediately refer to physician. • Be prepared to collect sample of exudate for culture.
4. Excessive tearing or clear discharge (often due to low humidity)	• Consider using artificial tears or special prosthesis lubricant. • Arrange consultation with ocularist.
5. Excessive itching (often due to accumulations of protein secretions)	• Remove, clean, and reinsert prosthesis. • Consult ocularist for antihistamine eye drops and polishing of prosthesis.
6. Client lacks knowledge and/or skills to perform prosthesis care properly.	• Teach client and home care provider prosthesis care skills. • Provide written instructions and brochures with needed information.

Teaching Considerations

- Advise client against using alcohol, solvents, or other chemicals to clean the prosthesis because they may damage the plastic or irritate the eye (Kolberg Ocular Prosthetics, 2004).
- Encourage client to protect the companion eye with polycarbonate safety lenses.
- Encourage client to visit ocularist annually for cleaning and polishing of the prosthesis.
- If rubbing the prosthetic eye, rub toward the nose. Wiping away from the nose may cause the eye to dislodge.
- Wear a protective patch or goggles when swimming, diving, or water skiing, or remove the prosthesis and store it.

Pediatric Considerations

- Retinoblastoma is a cancer that develops in young children typically under 5 years of age. Commonly one or rarely both eyes will be enucleated as part of the treatment (Retinoblastoma Society, 2003). These children, even infants and toddlers, may be fitted with an artificial eye. Parents must be taught how to care for the prosthesis until the child is able to independently perform care.
- Children may cause the eye to accidentally dislodge. Children who are able to understand should be made aware of this possibility so they do not become frightened if it occurs. Contact sports should be avoided, or protective eyewear should be worn during these activities (Hockenberry and others, 2003).

Gerontological Considerations

- Visual changes that normally occur with aging will continue to occur in the companion eye. Consequently, the older client should be assessed for such changes as decreased visual acuity, delayed dark-light adaptation, and impaired night vision and color perception.

Home Care Considerations

- If a client becomes disabled and suffers an inability to perform self-care measures on a regular basis, be sure the prosthesis is cleaned regularly to prevent infection.
- Assess client's home for safety hazards (see Chapter 41), and determine need for special precautions given client's limited field of vision.

Long-Term Care Considerations

- Accommodate need for periodic cleaning.

SKILL 16-3 Eye Irrigation

Eye irrigation is performed to flush out exudates, irritating solutions, or foreign particles. It is often performed in an emergency attempt to preserve vision. When a chemical or irritating substance contaminates the eyes, irrigate immediately with copious amounts of cool water for at least 15 min-utes to minimize corneal damage (U.S. National Library of Medicine, 2003). Users of contact lenses or artificial eyes may need eye irrigation to flush out particles of dust or fibers from the eye or socket.

DELEGATION CONSIDERATIONS
The skill of eye irrigation should not be delegated to assistive personnel.

EQUIPMENT
❏ Bath towel or waterproof pad
❏ Prescribed irrigation solution, usually 30 to 180 ml at 90° to 100° F (about 32° to 38° C)
❏ Sterile basin or bag for solution
❏ Soft bulb syringe, eyedropper, or IV tubing
❏ Emesis basin
❏ 4 × 4 inch gauze pads
❏ Disposable gloves

STEP	RATIONALE

ASSESSMENT

1. Assess reason for eye irrigation.

Determines the amount and type of solution and the immediacy of the need for treatment.

2. Assess the eye for redness, tearing, discharge, and swelling. Ask the client about symptoms of itching, burning, pain, blurred vision, or photophobia.

Establishes baseline signs and symptoms.

3. Assess client's ability to cooperate.

Determines level of assistance needed.

• **Critical Decision Point**
Spasm of the eyelid or pain may make opening the eye difficult. Topical anesthetic eye drops or additional assistance may be necessary (Kuckelkorn and others, 2002).

NURSING DIAGNOSES
• Risk for injury
• Pain (acute)

• Risk for infection
• Disturbed sensory perception (visual)

Related factors are individualized based on client's condition or needs.

PLANNING

1. Expected outcomes following completion of procedure:
   • Client demonstrates minimal anxiety during irrigation.
   • Client verbalizes reduced burning or itching and improved visual acuity after irrigation.
   • Client maintains normal pupillary reaction and eye movement after irrigation.
2. Discuss procedure with client.
3. Assemble supplies at bedside.
4. Assist client to side-lying position on side of affected eye or supine position for simultaneous irrigation of both eyes.

Potential for anxiety is high during emergency.
Reflects effectiveness of procedure in removing irritant.

Reflects effectiveness of procedure in minimizing exposure to irritant.
Decreases client anxiety.
Provides easy access to supplies.
Position facilitates flow of solution from inner to outer canthus, preventing contamination of unaffected eye and nasolacrimal duct.

STEP	RATIONALE

IMPLEMENTATION

1. Perform hand hygiene. Apply disposable gloves.

   Reduces transmission of microorganisms. Protects hands from chemical irritants.

2. Remove any contact lens if possible.

   Contact lens may have absorbed irritant, or it may prevent a thorough irrigation. Lens may be lost if flushed out by irrigation.

• *Critical Decision Point*

In an emergency such as first aid for a chemical burn, do not delay by removing client's contact lens before irrigation (U.S. Library of Medicine, 2003). Advise client to consult prescriber before reusing contact lens.

3. Place towel just below client's face and emesis basin just below client's cheek.

   Catches irrigation fluid.

4. Clean visible secretions or foreign material from eyelids and lashes, wiping from inner to outer canthus.

   Minimizes transfer of material into eye during irrigation. Prevents secretions from entering nasolacrimal duct.

5. Gently retract eyelids. Hold open by applying pressure to orbit, not to eyeball.

   Exposes eye and minimizes blinking.

6. Hold solution-filled bulb, dropper, or tubing approximately 1 inch (2.5 cm) from inner canthus.

   Eye may be injured by direct contact with irrigation equipment.

7. Ask client to look toward brow. Gently irrigate with a steady stream toward the lower conjunctival sac (see illustration).

   Minimizes force of stream on cornea. Flushes irritant out of eye and away from other eye and nasolacrimal duct.

8. Reinforce the importance of the procedure, and encourage client using calm, confident, soft voice.

   Reduces anxiety.

9. Allow client to blink periodically.

   Moves irritant from upper conjunctival sac.

10. Continue for prescribed volume and/or time or until secretions have been cleared.

    Ensures complete removal of irritant.

11. Blot excess moisture from eyelids and face with gauze or towel.

    Removes moisture that may contain microbes or irritant. Promotes client comfort.

12. Dispose of soiled supplies, remove gloves, and perform hand hygiene.

    Reduces transmission of microorganisms.

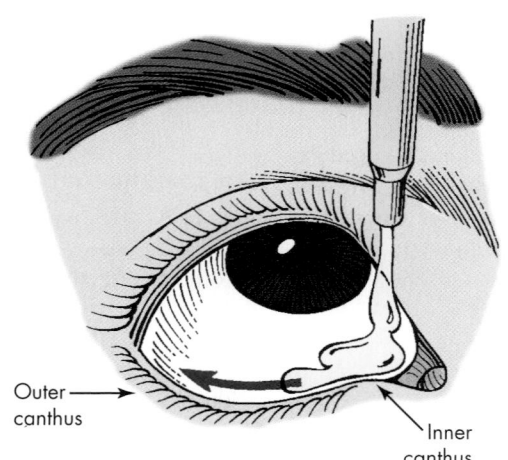

STEP 7 Irrigation of eye from inner to outer canthus.

Outer canthus

Inner canthus

STEP	RATIONALE

EVALUATION

1. Observe for verbal and nonverbal signs of anxiety during irrigation.

   Verifies client is adequately comforted.

2. Assess client's comfort level after irrigation.

   Verifies effective removal of irritant.

3. Inspect eye for reaction to light, accommodation, and eye movement.

   Impaired reaction to light, accommodation, or movement may indicate injury.

Recording and Reporting

- Record in nurses' notes condition of eye, type and amount of irrigation solution, duration of irrigation, and client's report of pain and visual symptoms.
- Report continuing symptoms of pain or blurred vision.

Unexpected Outcomes	Related Interventions
1. Anxiety	• Reinforce rationale for irrigation. • Allow client to close eye periodically during irrigation. • Instruct client to take slow, deep breaths. • Seek extra assistance as needed to prevent injury.
2. Pain or foreign body sensation	• Advise client to close eye and avoid eye movement. • Immediately notify physician or eye care practitioner.

Teaching Considerations

- Assist client with identifying potential hazards at home and work and taking steps to prevent accidents, such as use of safety goggles while working with dust or chemicals.
- Review first aid procedures for eye emergencies with client and/or caregiver.

Pediatric Considerations

- A child with a foreign body or chemical in the eye may panic. It may be necessary to restrain the child to safely and quickly irrigate the eye.

Home Care Considerations

- If a child or adult needing continuing irrigations is unable to perform them independently, teach the caregiver to perform eye irrigation.

SKILL 16-4 Taking Care of Hearing Aids

Hearing is vital for normal communication and orientation to sounds in the environment. For people with hearing loss, hearing aids may improve the ability to hear and understand spoken words. A hearing aid is a small, battery-powered, electronic device that amplifies sound. All parts of the hearing aid work together. The microphone changes sound waves to electrical signals. These signals pass through the amplifier and are made louder. The receiver changes the amplified electrical signals back into sound waves. Finally, the amplified sound waves are channeled into the ear through the hearing aid earmold (air conduction) or as vibrations through the skull (bone conduction) (Boys Town National Research Hospital, 2004). These prostheses are limited by the function of the ear structures.

For clients with profound damage to the structures of the inner ear (sensorineural deafness), a cochlear implant may be surgically placed. This internal implant receives signals from a separate external processor and transmits them electrically to the auditory nerve. The external processor looks similar to a conventional hearing aid and has a microphone but does not produce sound (Advanced Bionics Corporation, 2003).

Conventional hearing aids may be analog or digital. Digital technology converts the microphone signal to binary code before it is amplified (Unitron Hearing, 2003). This allows the signal to be analyzed to remove background noise and automatically adjust volume. Some hearing aids are programmable by the audiologist to amplify some sound frequencies more than others. Clients often experience greater hearing loss at higher frequencies; in speech this represents consonant sounds like *p, k, f, th,* and *s.* A programmable aid can accommodate differences in hearing loss and help make speech understandable. *Programmable* may also be used to refer to a client's ability to set the aid for different listening situations, or "programs," such as music, conversation, or telephone.

There are many styles of hearing aids to accommodate client needs for comfort, appearance, amplification, and versatility. Smaller, in-the-canal (ITC) and completely-in-canal (CIC) hearing aids are most discreet but tend to accumulate the most cerumen and may be difficult to handle because of their size (Figure 16-2). In-the-ear (ITE) aids are larger and can hold more internal circuitry and external controls (Figure 16-3). All of the circuitry for these hearing aids is contained within the custom-made, rigid ear mold. The circuitry for behind-the-ear (BTE) or postaural aids is better protected from earwax, and the separate earmold may be easily adjusted to changes in ear shape (Figure 16-4). With any style, controls for adjusting volume and programs may be on the aid itself or on a separate remote control. The circuitry and battery pack may also be separate and worn at the chest or waist or even on eyeglasses.

It can be a challenge to adjust one's communication style to accommodate a client with a hearing impairment. Use the client as a resource for communication techniques that are generally helpful. Briefly, be sure that the client can see your face, speak slowly in a normal tone, and rephrase rather than

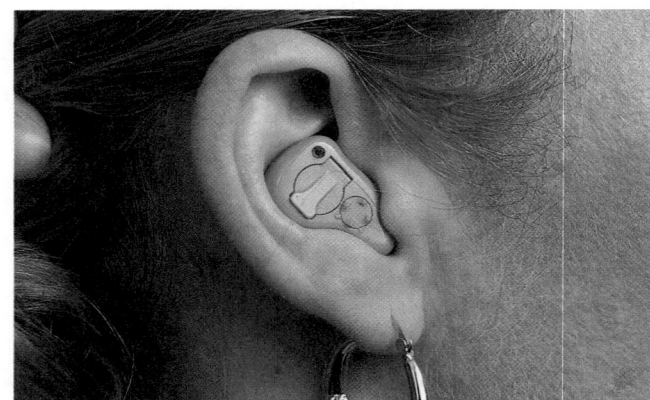

FIGURE **16-3** In-the-ear (ITE) hearing aid.

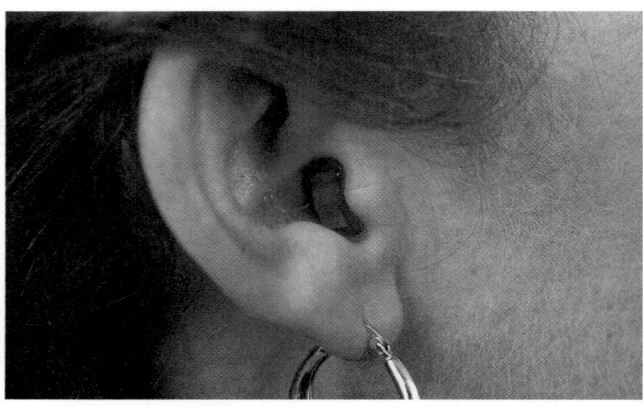

FIGURE **16-2** Completely-in-canal (CIC) hearing aid.

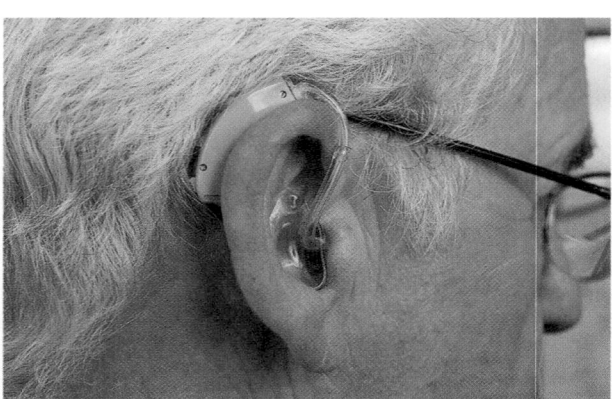

FIGURE **16-4** Behind-the-ear (BTE) hearing aid.

repeat if the client cannot understand you. Ask the facility's telecommunications department about assistive devices and adjunct services for hearing-impaired clients (Lucas and Matthews-Flint, 2001). Also, remember that the client may be unable to hear alerts such as fire alarms or overhead announcements (Sommer and Sommer, 2002).

Hearing aids are usually worn only while the client is awake and are cleaned as needed after removal. Anyone caring for a client with a hearing aid should know that the device is delicate and must be protected from moisture, heat, and breakage.

DELEGATION CONSIDERATIONS

This skill may be delegated to assistive personnel. Before delegating this skill, the nurse must:

- Instruct assistive personnel to report ear pain, inflammation, drainage, odor, or changes in hearing.
- Review alternate ways to communicate with the client while the aid is not in use.
- Reinforce the importance of careful handling of the aid to prevent damage or injury.

EQUIPMENT

- ❑ Bath towels (2)
- ❑ Facial tissues
- ❑ Wax loop
- ❑ Storage case
- ❑ Wash cloth
- ❑ Warm water and soap
- ❑ Spare battery, size depends on aid (optional)
- ❑ Dryer, desiccant or electronic (optional)
- ❑ Disposable gloves (if drainage present)

STEP	RATIONALE
ASSESSMENT	
1. Determine whether client can hear clearly with use of aid. With your back to the client, ask a question slowly and clearly in a normal tone of voice.	Confused facial expression, reaction incongruent with the conversation, verbalization of inability to hear, or movement to better see the nurse's face indicate uncompensated impairment or a malfunctioning hearing aid. Prevents lip-reading.
2. Ask if client is able to manipulate and hold hearing aid, or observe client insert aid independently.	Determines level of assistance required in care.
3. Assess client's knowledge of and routines for cleaning and caring for hearing aid.	Determines compliance with and knowledge of self-care.
4. Assess client for any unusual physical or auditory signs/symptoms (pain, itching, redness, discharge, odor, tinnitus, decreased acuity).	May indicate injury, infection, or cerumen accumulation.
5. Assess client for perceived ability to deal with situations and events such as conversing in a group, going to a social event, being in a lecture audience, or talking on the phone.	May indicate situational low self-esteem related to functional impairment.
NURSING DIAGNOSES	
• Bathing/hygiene self-care deficit	• Risk for injury
• Impaired verbal communication	• Risk for situational low self-esteem
• Deficient knowledge regarding hearing aid care	• Disturbed sensory perception (auditory)

Related factors are individualized based on client's condition or needs.

PLANNING	
1. Expected outcomes following completion of procedure:	
• Client verbalizes comfort after removal and reinsertion of hearing aid.	Hearing aid is removed or inserted properly and positioned correctly.
• Client responds appropriately to normal conversation and environmental sounds.	Hearing aid and batteries are operational. Aid is secure and unobstructed.
• Client demonstrates proper care of hearing aid.	Learning is achieved.
2. Discuss procedure with client. Explain all steps before removing aid.	Client can assist in planning by explaining additional tips for care. Client may be confused or anxious if verbal instructions are given after removal of hearing aid.

STEP	RATIONALE
3. Assemble supplies at bedside. Place towel over work area.	Provides easy access to supplies. Towel catches aid if accidentally dropped and avoids breakage.
4. Have client assume supine, side-lying, or sitting position in bed or chair.	Provides easy access for nurse. Promotes client comfort.

IMPLEMENTATION

1. Removing and Cleaning Hearing Aid

a. Perform hand hygiene. Apply disposable gloves if drainage is present.	Reduces transmission of microorganisms.
b. Turn hearing aid volume off. Grasp aid securely, and gently remove device following natural ear contour.	Prevents feedback (whistling) during removal. Prevents dropping hearing aid. Prevents injury to ear.

• *Critical Decision Point*

Some ITC and CIC devices have no volume control but may be turned off by opening the battery door. Ask client if this is necessary. CIC devices have a clear plastic, fiber handle for removal. Firmly grasp handle, and gently pull straight out.

c. Hold aid over towel, and wipe exterior with tissue to remove cerumen.	Prevents breakage if dropped. Cerumen may irritate canal and interfere with fit.
d. Inspect all openings in aid for accumulated cerumen. Carefully remove cerumen with wax loop or other device supplied with the hearing aid.	Cerumen may block sound from receiver. Cerumen may block pressure equalization channel and create feeling of ear pressure. Makeshift tools may damage hearing aid.

• *Critical Decision Point*

The pressure equalization channel is a tiny hole through the entire length of the earmold and should be clear for the entire length. The receiver points into the ear through another opening. It is easily damaged. NEVER insert anything into the receiver port!

e. Inspect earmold for rough edges.	May irritate ear canal.
f. Open battery door, and place hearing aid in labeled storage container.	Allows drying of internal components. Protects against breakage and loss.

• *Critical Decision Point*

Regular storage with desiccant or in an electronic dryer will extend hearing aid and battery life (Ear Technology Corporation, 2003).

g. Repeat steps 1b through 1f for other aid.	
h. Assess ear for redness, tenderness, discharge, or odor.	Signs may indicate injury or infection.
i. Place towel beneath client's ear(s). Wash ear canal(s) with washcloth moistened in soap and water. Rinse and dry.	Absorbs excess water. Removes cerumen from ear canal. Removes soap residue and water that may harbor microbes or damage aid.
j. Dispose of towels, remove gloves, and perform hand hygiene.	Reduces transmission of microorganisms.

2. Inserting Hearing Aid

a. Perform hand hygiene.	Reduces transmission of microorganisms.
b. Remove hearing aid from storage case, and check battery.	
(1) Close battery door.	Door must be closed to turn on hearing aid.
(2) Turn volume slowly to high.	Prevents damage to hearing aid.
(3) Cup hand over hearing aid and listen for feedback (whistle or squeal).	Feedback occurs when hearing aid is working but not in correct position.

STEP	RATIONALE
c. Turn hearing aid volume off.	Prevents feedback (whistling) during insertion.

• *Critical Decision Point*
Some ITC and CIC devices have no volume control but may be turned off by opening the battery door. Ask the client if this is necessary.

STEP	RATIONALE
d. Identify hearing aid as either right (marked "R" or red color coded) or left (marked "L" or blue color coded).	Proper orientation prevents damage and injury.
e. Hold hearing aid with thumb and index finger of dominant hand. Insert pointed end of earmold into ear canal. Follow natural ear contours to guide aid into place.	Prevents dropping. Proper positioning prevents injury. Pulling on ear may distort canal and make insertion more difficult (Lucas and Matthews-Flint, 2001).
f. Anchor any separate pieces, as in case of BTE aid or body aid.	Prevents pieces from falling and breaking.
g. Slowly turn on volume to comfortable level for client.	Gradual adjustment prevents discomfort and injury to ear.
h. Close and store case. Perform hand hygiene.	Preserves desiccant. Prevents loss. Reduces transmission of microorganisms.

EVALUATION

1. Assess client's comfort level after removal or insertion.	Verifies proper technique and positioning.
2. Observe client during normal conversation and in response to environmental sounds.	Verifies aid is operational, correctly positioned, unobstructed, and effective.
3. Observe client removing, cleaning, and reinserting hearing aid.	Demonstrates client's understanding of techniques.

Recording and Reporting

- Record removal of hearing aid and storage location if not reinserted after cleaning.
- Record client's preferred communication techniques.
- Record and report any signs or symptoms of infection or injury or sudden decrease in hearing acuity.

Unexpected Outcomes	Related Interventions
1. Whistling or squealing from inserted aid	• Reposition hearing aid. • Reduce volume if adjustable. • Assess ear for inflammation or blockage.
2. Inability to understand conversations or hear environmental sounds	• Check function, type, and placement of battery, and replace battery if indicated. • Increase volume if adjustable. • Inspect aid and ear canal for cerumen blockage. • Refer to audiologist for reassessment.
3. Discomfort or pain	• Remove aid, and inspect for sharp or rough edges. Refer to provider for repair. • Assess ear for signs of injury or infection. • Confirm R or L. Reposition hearing aid. • If sensation remains, remove aid, and report to physician.

Continued

Unexpected Outcomes	Related Interventions
4. Inflammation	• Remove aid, clean, and store until inflammation subsides. • Clean ear canal.
5. Drainage or odor	• Remove aid, clean, and store until infection resolves. • Refer to physician. • Be prepared to collect sample of exudate for culture.
6. Client lacks knowledge and/or skills to perform hearing aid care properly.	• Teach client and home care provider hearing aid care skills. • Provide written instructions and brochures with needed information.

Teaching Considerations

*   Advise client to protect the hearing aid from water, alcohol, hairspray or cologne, perspiration, rain, and snow. Advise client to avoid exposing the hearing aid to extremes of temperature.
*   Encourage client to store hearing aids and batteries with desiccant or in an electronic dryer to prolong life, minimize repairs, and preserve batteries.
*   Dogs in particular are attracted to the smell of used hearing aids. Advise the client to protect the hearing aids and their pets by properly storing the aids out of reach.
*   Batteries are toxic if swallowed; keep them away from pets and children.
*   Encourage the client to visit hearing aid specialist or audiologist at least annually.
*   Encourage clients to identify helpful communication tips and teach them to others. Many clients find facial cues informative. Speakers should:
    *   Face the client, stay within 3 to 4 feet away, and keep hands away from the mouth
    *   Get the client's attention before speaking
    *   Rephrase rather than repeat when the client cannot understand
    *   Reduce background noise or move to a quiet area

Pediatric Considerations

*   Children are more often fitted with BTE hearing aids because the ear canal is still growing.
*   The aid can be made less conspicuous with hair styling or become a statement of fashion and personality with a brightly-colored or transparent case.
*   Parents must be taught how to care for the hearing aid until the child is able to independently perform care. Parent should learn to store batteries out of the reach of children.
*   Assistance may be needed by the child to prevent acoustic feedback (whistling), which they may be unable

to hear. This usually can be eliminated by removing and reinserting the device and making sure no hair is caught between the ear mold and canal, or lowering the volume of the device (Hockenberry and others, 2003).

Gerontological Considerations

*   The small size of some hearing aids may make them difficult to manipulate, particularly for individuals with decreased dexterity or visual acuity. The audiologist should be consulted to identify an aid that accommodates the client's particular need.
*   Presbycusis is a loss of ability to hear or discriminate sounds due to aging. Clients often experience greater hearing loss at higher frequencies; in speech this represents consonant sounds like *p, k, f, th,* and *s.* In English these are the sounds by which words are recognized. Consequently, clients with presbycusis may first complain that they can hear but they have difficulty understanding speech. A programmable hearing aid may selectively amplify higher frequencies and provide relief to this client.
*   Clients and caregivers should be alert for and report signs of decreased auditory acuity such as inappropriate responses to questions, inattentiveness, decreased socialization, difficulty following oral instructions, or monopolizing conversation.

Home Care Considerations

*   Assess willingness and ability of caregiver to perform necessary care of hearing aid.
*   Assess client's home, and determine need for special precautions given client's limited hearing.

Long-Term Care Considerations

*   Accommodate need for regular reassessment and hearing aid maintenance.

FOCUS on CLINICAL PRACTICE

Mr. Ojo is a 19-year-old Hispanic-American college student being admitted to the emergency department with complaints of severe pain in his ankle after a fall during soccer practice. While taking his history, you discover that Mr. Ojo is severely myopic (near sighted) and an RGP contact lens wearer.

1. In preparing to assist with contact lens care, what data will you be collecting in your examination of Mr. Ojo's eyes?
2. During the examination you ask Mr. Ojo to alternately cover each eye and read lines from a visual acuity chart. The primary purpose of this activity is to:
   A. Establish baseline visual acuity for comparison with periodic examinations during hospitalization.
   B. Develop the therapeutic relationship by demonstrating recognition of the importance of Mr. Ojo's vision to his self-esteem.
   C. Determine the presence of a correctly placed contact lens in each eye.
   D. Distract Mr. Ojo while you inspect each eye for corneal abrasions.
   Explain your choice.
3. Mr. Ojo demonstrates markedly decreased visual acuity in his left eye. A contact lens is visible over the cornea in the right eye but not in the left. You decide to:
   A. Document that the left contact lens was probably dislodged during the fall.

B. Ask the client whether he has experienced this sort of vision change in the past.
C. Carefully inspect the left sclera and report if the lens is not visible.
D. Immediately schedule a consultation with the staff ophthalmologist.
Explain your choice.
4. The left contact lens was visualized over the sclera and successfully removed by the client. Mr. Ojo does not have his lens case or solutions with him. Which of the following action(s) would be appropriate at this point?
   A. Allow Mr. Ojo to hold the contact lens in his mouth to keep it moist until his preferred lens wetting solution can be transferred from the hospital pharmacy.
   B. Store the contact lens in a labeled, sterile container of saline.
   C. Ask Mr. Ojo to remove the right contact lens so that they can be stored together in the same container to prevent loss.
   D. After he removes the second lens, assist Mr. Ojo by completing his admission and consent forms for him.
   Explain your choice(s).

NCLEX REVIEW QUESTIONS

1. A client who wears contact lenses for 20/150 vision in each eye is scheduled for hand surgery. The client's hand will be in a cast for 6 weeks. A nurse developing a plan of care for this client documents the most appropriate nursing diagnosis as:
   1. Anxiety
   2. Self-care deficit
   3. Alteration in nutrition
   4. Sensory perceptual alterations
2. A client is being discharged following care for severe conjunctivitis related to noncompliance with the prescribed lens care regimen. The client statement that indicates a need for further teaching is:
   1. "I should discard my open lens care solutions when I get home."
   2. "Cloudy solutions should be discarded even if they haven't expired."

3. "Plain soap is the best thing for washing my hands before I touch my contacts."
4. "I'm switching to disposable contacts so I won't have to worry about getting another infection."
3. A client is being discharged home unable to care for her artificial eye. The client statement that indicates a need for further teaching is:
   1. "I will clean the eye at least once a week."
   2. "I don't have to use sterile solutions for cleaning the eye."
   3. "The colored dot is there to show me which way to put it in."
   4. "Rubbing alcohol and fingernail polish remover are bad for the eye."

Continued

NCLEX REVIEW QUESTIONS

4. A nurse is performing an assessment on a client with an artificial eye. Identification of the natural eye would be confirmed by the presence of:
   1. Tears
   2. Movement
   3. Accommodation
   4. Appearance of veins

5. A fellow nurse in an acute care setting splashes rubbing alcohol into his right eye. He is a contact lens wearer. The initial nursing action would be to:
   1. Carefully remove the contact lens.
   2. Gently cover the eye with a comfortable patch.
   3. Test the pH of the secretions with litmus paper.
   4. Irrigate the eye with water or prescribed solution.

6. A nurse is caring for a client who is hearing impaired. Communication will be best facilitated by:
   1. Speaking loudly
   2. Speaking normally
   3. Speaking frequently
   4. Speaking directly into the impaired ear

7. The following statement made by a client with a new hearing aid indicates a need for further teaching:
   1. "My desiccant will help my hearing aids last longer."
   2. "Earwax is normal, but if I notice a lot more of it, I'll let you know."
   3. "I'll put in my hearing aids before I get dressed so my ears can begin to adjust."
   4. "It may take some time before I'm able to use the hearing aids in all situations."

References

Advanced Bionics Corporation: *Hearing health: hearing loss,* 2003, http://www.bionicear.com, retrieved January 10, 2004.

American Optometric Association: *Eye conditions and concerns: contact lens—facts and stats,* 2003, http://www.aoa.org/, retrieved January 6, 2004.

Boys Town National Research Hospital: *About hearing aids: hearing aids and how they work,* http://www.boystownhospital.org/parents/hearing_aids/how.asp, retrieved January 10, 2004.

Ear Technology Corporation: *Why condition your hearing aids with Dry and Store?,* 2003, http://www.dryandstore.com, retrieved January 10, 2004.

Hockenberry MJ and others: *Wong's nursing care of infants and children,* ed 7, St. Louis, 2003, Mosby.

Kolberg Ocular Prosthetics: *Artificial eye information and patient support page,* 2004, http://www.artificialeye.net, retrieved January 10, 2004.

Kuckelkorn R and others: Emergency treatment of chemical and thermal eye burns, *ACTA Ophthalmol Scand* 80:4, 2002.

Lewis S and others: *Medical-surgical nursing: assessment and management of clinical problems,* ed 5, St. Louis, 2000, Mosby.

Lucas LJ, Matthews-Flint LJ: Photo guide: sound advice about hearing aids, *Nursing* 31(2):59, 2001.

Perry AC: Advances in enucleation, *Ophthal Plast Reconstr Surg* 4:173, 1991.

Rakow PL: Current contact lens care systems, *Ophthalmol Clin North Am* 16(3):415, 2003.

Ramponi D: Go with the flow during an eye emergency, *Nursing* 30(8):54, 2000.

Retinoblastoma Society: *The Retinoblastoma Society: fighting eye cancer in children,* 2003, http://www.rbsociety.org.uk, retrieved January 10, 2004.

Sommer SL, Sommer N: When your patient is hearing impaired, *RN* 65(12):28, 2002.

Suchecki JK and others: Contact lens complications, *Ophthalmol Clin North Am* 16(3):471, 2003.

Unitron Hearing: *Digital technology: analog versus digital,* 2003, http://www.unitronhearing.us/ICCUS/professionals/products_us.htm, retrieved January 10, 2004.

U.S. Food and Drug Administration: *FDA approves 30-night continuous wear contact lenses,* 2001, http://www.fda.gov/bbs/topics/ANSWERS/2001/ ANS01109.html, retrieved January 7, 2004.

U.S. National Library of Medicine: Medline Plus: *Eye emergencies,* 2003, http://www.nlm.nih.gov/medlineplus/ency/article/000054.htm, retrieved January 10, 2004.

Research References

Clark BJ and others: Microbial contamination of cases used for storing contact lenses, *J Infect* 28(3):293, 1994.

Crowston J and others: Contact lens care in the unconscious, *J Trauma* 40(4):640, 1996.

de Andrade Sobrinho MV, Carvalho RA: Do the economic and social factors play an important role in relation to the compliance of contact lenses care routines? *Eye Contact Lens* 29(4):210, 2003.

Fan DSP and others: Health belief and health practice in contact lens wear—a dichotomy? *CLAO J* 28:36, 2002.

Fulk GW and others: Endotoxin concentration in contact lens storage cases, *J Am Optom Assoc* 68(5):296, 1997.

Kompa S and others: Comparison of emergency eye-wash products in burned porcine eyes, *Graefes Arch Clin Exp Ophthalmol* 240(4):308, 2002.

Ky W and others: Clinical survey of lens care in contact lens patients, *CLAO J* 24(4):216, 1998.

Lin CJ and others: Complications of motility peg placement for porous hydroxyapatite orbital implants, *Br J Ophthalmol* 86(4):394, 2002.

Murray TG and others: Design of a magnetically integrated microporous implant, *Arch Ophthalmol* 118:1259, 2000.

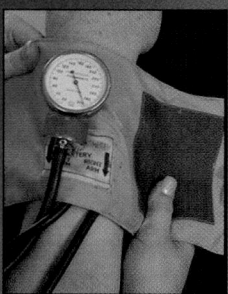

17

Vital Signs

MEDIA RESOURCES

Evolve Site *evolve*

http://evolve.elsevier.com/Perry/skills
- Weblinks
- Video clips
- Mosby's Nursing Skills Video Exercises

Mosby's Nursing Skills Videos/CD-ROM
- *Measurements Video: Vital signs; temperature:* oral, axillary, and rectal, using both glass and electronic thermometers; pulse: radial and apical; rate, rhythm, and quality; how to locate the apical pulse and the point of maximal/maximum impulse; respiration: rate, rhythm, and effort; blood pressure: one-step and two-step methods

OBJECTIVES

Mastery of content in this chaper will enable the nurse to:

- Identify when it is appropriate to assess each vital sign.
- Correctly assess a client's oral, rectal, axillary, and tympanic membrane temperatures.
- Correctly record vital signs.
- Identify factors to assess in determining potential alterations in body temperature.
- Discuss factors in selecting temperature measurement sites.
- Correctly assess a client's radial and apical pulse.
- Identify factors to assess in determining potential alterations in pulse character.
- Explain implications of a pulse deficit.
- Correctly assess a client's respirations.
- Identify factors to assess in determining potential alterations in respirations.
- Correctly measure a client's blood pressure using techniques of auscultation and palpation.
- Discuss benefits and disadvantages of using an automatic blood pressure machine.
- Discuss factors in selecting an extremity to measure blood pressure.
- Identify factors to assess in determining potential alterations in BP.
- Correctly assess a client's oxygenation status using pulse oximetry.
- Identify factors to assess in determining potential alterations in oxygen saturation.

KEY TERMS

Antipyretic	Orthopnea
Apical pulse	Orthostatic hypotension
Axillary	Oximetry
Bradycardia	Oxygen saturation
Bradypnea	Postural hypotension
Cardiac output (CO)	Premature ventricular
Centigrade	contraction (PVC)
Core temperature	Pulse deficit
Diastolic pressure	S_1
Dyspnea	S_2
Dysrhythmia	Sphygmomanometer
Fahrenheit	Stroke volume (SV)
Febrile	Systolic pressure
Fever	Tachycardia
Heatstroke	Tachypnea
Hypertension	Thermoregulation
Hyperthermia	Tympanic
Hypotension	Vasoconstriction
Hypothermia	Vasodilation

Temperature, pulse, blood pressure (BP), oxygen saturation, and respiration are the most frequent measurements obtained by health care practitioners. These measurements can indicate if the circulatory, pulmonary, neurological, and endocrine body systems are functioning normally. Because of their importance as indicators of the body's physiological status and response to physical, environmental, and psychological stressors, they are referred to as vital signs. Vital signs may reveal sudden changes in a client's condition, as well as changes that occur progressively over time. Any difference between a client's normal baseline measurement and present vital signs can indicate the need for nursing therapies and necessary medical interventions.

Pain assessment is considered a fifth vital sign in many health care settings. There are few clients who do not experience some level of discomfort or pain. Frequently pain is the symptom that leads clients to seek health care. For this reason, assessment of a client's pain status is critical to understanding a client's clinical status and progress. Assessment of a client's level of comfort and pain is frequently done with some vital sign measurements. Chapter 6 summarizes pain assessment.

Vital signs are included in a routine physical assessment (see Chapter 18). The nurse's findings aid in determining whether it is necessary to assess specific body systems more thoroughly. For example, during a routine vital sign measurement the nurse notes an abnormal respiratory rate; the nurse then auscultates lung sounds. In addition, vital sign assessment may be limited to measurement of a single vital sign for the purpose of reviewing a specific aspect of a client's condition. For example, following administration of an antipyretic medication, the nurse measures the client's temperature to evaluate the drug's effects. Part of the nurse's clinical judgment involves deciding which vital sign to measure, when measurements should be made, and the frequency of assessment (Box 17-1). The nurse should always obtain a baseline measurement of vital signs upon first con-

---

BOX 17-1   When to Take Vital Signs

1. On a client's admission to a health care facility
2. In a hospital or care facility on a routine schedule according to a physician's order or institution's standards of practice
3. When assessing the client during home health visits
4. Before and after a surgical or invasive diagnostic procedure
5. Before and after the administration of medications or application of therapies that affect cardiovascular, respiratory, and temperature control functions
6. When the client's general physical condition changes (e.g., loss of consciousness, increased severity of pain)
7. Before, during, and after nursing interventions influencing a vital sign (e.g., before and after a client previously on bed rest ambulates, before and after the client performs range-of-motion exercises)
8. When the client reports specific symptoms of physical distress (e.g., feeling "funny" or "different")

tact with a client to provide a means for comparison with subsequent vital sign measurements.

Evidenced-Based Practice Trends

Research supports the use of a variety of methods to measure body temperature. Chemical dot thermometers are beneficial as screening measures, especially in infants and young children (Molton and others, 2001). In addition, the chemical dot thermometer was effective in screening temperatures in orally intubated clients (Potter and others, 2003). However, a follow-up measurement with an electronic thermometer is used to confirm temperature measurements made with a chemical dot thermometer when treatment decisions are involved.

Recommendations for the classification of high blood pressure have changed (Joint National Committee, 2003), making it more important to obtain an accurate blood pressure. One of the major contributors to blood pressure measurement error is an improperly fitting blood pressure cuff. The prevalence of adults with a large arm circumference is over 40% (Fonseca-Reyes and others, 2003), indicating that a "standard adult" cuff is not appropriate for these individuals (Graves and others, 2003). Overestimation of a blood pressure from a cuff that is too small has been well researched (Graves, 2001), yet nurses, physicians, and other health care providers continue to ignore the data (Armstrong, 2002). Nurses must advocate for the availability of a variety of blood pressure cuff sizes at their facility and appropriately assess arm or leg circumference before applying a blood pressure cuff.

Cultural Considerations

- Provide privacy when performing apical pulse, especially for traditional female clients and elders from Asian, Middle Eastern, Hispanic, and African cultures.
  - Use gender-congruent providers or family members to take rectal temperatures and touch the client's chest.
  - Procedures that are normally noninvasive can produce anxiety because of cultural variables of touch, privacy, and gender.
- Consult the physician and family decision maker regarding giving information to the client about abnormal vital signs.
  - Collectivistic cultures (e.g., Hispanics, Africans, and Asians) demonstrate their caring for ill members by protecting them from bad news about their health and well-being.
    - Document this information in the client's chart.
    - Communicate the family decision to the physician (Pacquiao, 2003).
- Determine the client's understanding of new procedures being done.
  - Use an interpreter if needed, and demonstrate the procedure to promote client's understanding.

Skill Performance Guidelines

1. The nurse caring for a client is responsible for vital signs measurement. Although measurement of select vital signs can be delegated to assistive personnel, the nurse must analyze and interpret their significance and make decisions about appropriate interventions.
2. Equipment used to measure vital signs must be functional and chosen based on a client's condition and physical characteristics to ensure accurate findings.
3. Knowing the standard range for all vital signs enables the nurse to detect deviations.
4. A client's usual range for vital signs may differ from the standard range for age or physical state. Acceptable values for a client serve as a baseline for comparing later findings; thus a nurse detects changes in condition over time.
5. The nurse knows the client's medical history, therapies, and prescribed medications. Some illnesses or treatments cause predictable vital sign changes. Most medications affect at least one of the vital signs.
6. The nurse controls or minimizes environmental factors that may affect vital signs. Measuring a client's BP after exercise or an emotional upset may yield values that are not clear indicators of the client's current status.
7. An organized, systematic (step-by-step) approach when taking vital signs ensures accuracy of findings.
8. Based on the client's condition, the nurse collaborates with the physician to decide the minimum frequency of vital sign assessment. The nurse may judge independently if more frequent assessments are needed. If a client's physical condition begins to worsen, the nurse takes vital signs more often, sometimes as often as every 5 to 10 minutes. After a client returns from surgery or a major diagnostic examination, such as cardiac catheterization, frequent measurements are taken until the vital signs stabilize back to the acceptable range before the procedure. Changes or trends in vital signs are useful in making therapeutic decisions for client care.
9. The nurse analyzes results of vital sign measurements and incorporates all the clinical findings about a client in determining nursing diagnoses. Vital signs are not assessed in isolation. The nurse assesses physical signs or symptoms, as well as vital signs, to be aware of the client's ongoing health status.
10. The nurse verifies and communicates significant changes in vital signs. Baseline measurements allow a nurse to identify changes in vital signs. When vital signs appear abnormal, it may help to have another nurse repeat the measurement. The nurse informs the physician when vital signs become abnormal and reports any changes to the nurse in charge.
11. In an outpatient setting, vital signs are taken before the health care provider examines the client.

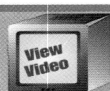

SKILL 17-1 Measuring Body Temperature

Body temperature is the difference between the amount of heat produced by the body processes and the amount of heat lost to the external environment. The core temperature, or temperature of the deep body tissues, is under control of the hypothalamus and is maintained within a narrow range. Skin or body surface temperature rises and falls as the temperature of the surrounding environment changes and can fluctuate dramatically.

The body tissues and cells function best within a relatively narrow temperature range, from 36° C to 38° C (96.8° F to 100.4° F), but no single temperature is normal for all people. An acceptable temperature range for adults depends on age, gender, range of physical activity, and state of health (Figure 17-1).

Many factors affect body temperature. Physiological and behavioral control mechanisms act to maintain a constant core temperature. For example, the mechanism of peripheral vasodilation increases blood flow to the skin, which increases the amount of heat radiated to the environment. Control mechanisms have failed when heat produced by the body is not equal to heat lost to the environment. For example, clients who lack sweat gland function are unable to tolerate warm temperatures because they cannot cool themselves adequately. Fever occurs when heat loss mechanisms are unable to keep pace with excess heat production, resulting in an abnormal rise in body temperature. When an individual has a febrile condition, pyrexia, the nurse initiates temperature-control measures such as controlling environmental temperatures, removing external coverings, and administering ordered antipyretics to achieve better temperature control.

The measurement of body temperature is aimed at obtaining a representative average temperature of core body tissues. Average usual temperature varies depending on the measurement site used. Research findings from numerous studies are contradictory; however, it is generally accepted that rectal temperatures are usually 0.5° C (0.9° F) higher than oral temperatures, and axillary and tympanic temperatures are usually 0.5° C (0.9° F) lower than oral temperatures. Sites reflecting core temperature are more reliable indicators of body temperature than sites reflecting surface temperatures (Box 17-2).

To ensure accurate temperature readings each site must be measured correctly. The same site should be used when repeated measurements are necessary or temperature measurements are compared over time. Each site has advantages and disadvantages (Box 17-3). The nurse determines the safest and most accurate site for the client.

Two types of thermometers are commonly available to measure body temperature: electronic and chemical dot single use or reusable. Each type has advantages and limitations (Box 17-4). The mercury-in-glass thermometer, a stan-

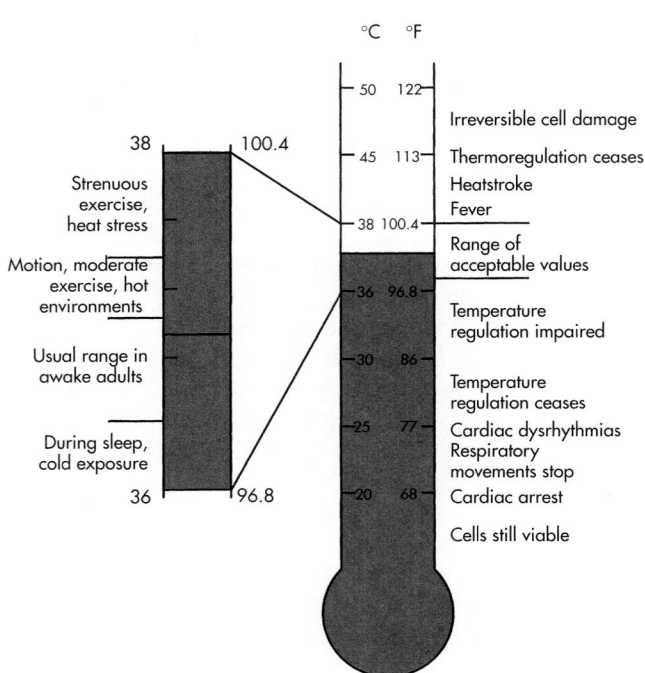

FIGURE 17-1 Ranges of normal temperature values and physiological consequences of abnormal body temperature. (Modified from Thibodeau GA, Patton KT: *Anatomy and physiology*, ed 5, St. Louis, 2003, Mosby.)

BOX 17-2 Core and Surface Temperature Measurement Sites

CORE SITE	SURFACE SITE
Rectum	Skin
Tympanic membrane	Oral cavity
Esophagus	Axilla
Pulmonary artery	
Urinary bladder	

dard device for temperature measurement for nearly 100 years, has been eliminated from most health care facilities because of the environmental hazards of mercury-containing medical devices. However, mercury-in-glass thermometers may be found in client's homes.

The electronic thermometer consists of a rechargeable, battery-powered display unit, a thin wire cord, and a temperature-processing probe covered by a disposable plastic sheath (Figure 17-2). The electronic thermometer has become the most common type found within health care settings. Separate probes are available for oral and rectal use. The oral probe has a blue tip, and the rectal probe has a red tip. Electronic thermometers are designed to provide

BOX 17-3   Advantages and Limitations of Select Temperature Measurement Sites

ORAL

Advantages

Easily accessible—requires no position change
Comfortable for client
Provides accurate surface temperature reading
Reflects rapid change in core temperature
Shown to be reliable route to measure temperature in intubated clients (Fallis, 2000)

Limitations

Causes delay in measurement if client recently ingested hot/cold fluids or foods, smoked, or receive oxygen by mask/cannula
Should not be used with clients who have had oral surgery, trauma, history of epilepsy, or shaking chills
Should not be used with infants, small children, or confused, unconscious, or uncooperative clients
Risk of body fluid exposure

Tympanic Membrane Sensor

Advantages

Easily accessible site
Minimal client repositioning required; can be obtained without disturbing, waking, or repositioning client
Can be used for clients with tachypnea without affecting breathing
Provides accurate core reading because eardrum is close to hypothalamus; sensitive to core temperature changes
Very rapid measurement (2 to 5 seconds)
Unaffected by oral intake of food or fluids or smoking
Can be used in newborns to reduce infant handling and heat loss (Bailey and Rose, 2001)

Limitations

More variability of measurement than with other core temperature devices
Requires removal of hearing aids before measurement
Requires disposable sensor cover with only one size available
Otitis media and cerumen impaction can distort readings (Guiliano and others, 2000)
Should not be used with clients who have had surgery of the ear or tympanic membrane
Does not accurately measure core temperature changes during and after exercise
Cannot obtain continuous measurement
Affected by ambient temperature devices such as incubators, radiant warmers, and facial fans (Guiliano and others, 2000)

RECTAL

Advantages

Argued to be more reliable when oral temperature cannot be obtained

Limitations

May lag behind core temperature during rapid temperature changes (Guiliano and others, 2000)
Should not be used for clients with diarrhea, clients who have had rectal surgery, rectal disorders, bleeding tendencies, or diarrhea
Requires positioning and may be source of client embarrassment and anxiety
Risk of body fluid exposure
Requires lubrication
Should not be used for routine vital signs in newborns

AXILLA

Advantages

Safe and inexpensive
Can be used with newborns and unconscious clients

Limitations

Long measurement time
Requires continuous positioning by nurse
Measurement lags behind core temperature during rapid temperature changes
Not recommended to detect fever in infants and young children
Requires exposure of thorax, which can result in temperature loss, especially in newborns

SKIN

Advantages

Inexpensive
Provides continuous reading
Safe and noninvasive
Can be used for neonates

Limitations

Measurement lags behind other sites during temperature changes, especially during hyperthermia
Diaphoresis or sweat can impair adhesion
Can be affected by environmental temperature

4-second predictive temperatures and 3-minute standard temperatures. In day-to-day clinical situations, the 4-second predictive is most commonly used.

Another form of electronic thermometer is used exclusively for tympanic temperature. An otoscope-like speculum with an infrared sensor tip detects heat radiated from the tympanic membrane of the ear (Figure 17-3). Within 2 to 5 seconds after placement in the auditory canal and depressing the scan button, a value appears on the display unit. A sound signals when the peak temperature reading has been measured.

Chemical dot single-use or reusable thermometers are disposable thin strips of plastic with a temperature sensor at one end. The sensor consists of a matrix of chemically impregnated dots that are formulated to change color at different temperatures. In the Celsius version there are 50 dots,

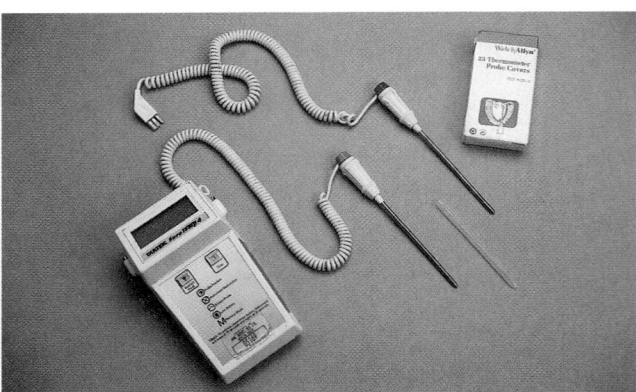

FIGURE **17-2** Electronic thermometer with disposable plastic sheath.

BOX 17-4 Advantages and Limitations of Types of Thermometers

CHEMICAL THERMOMETER

Advantages

Disposable, easy to store
Used for clients in isolation
Useful for screening temperatures, especially for infants and during invasive procedures (e.g., during surgery)

Limitations

Can be difficult to read
Has been shown to underestimate and overestimate temperature (Potter and others, 2003)
Not appropriate for monitoring temperature therapies

ELECTRONIC THERMOMETER

Advantages

Plastic sheath unbreakable; ideal for children
Very rapid measurement

Limitations

Probe or sensor covers are expensive

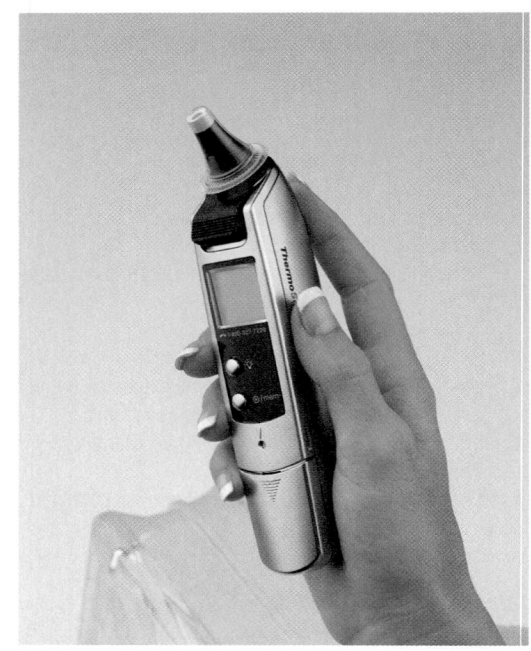

FIGURE **17-3** Tympanic membrane thermometer. (Photo courtesy Welch Allyn.)

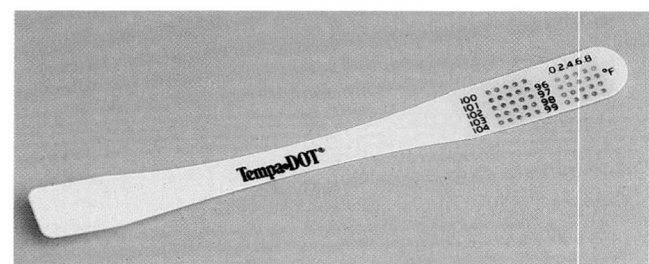

FIGURE **17-4** Disposable, single-use thermometer.

each representing temperature increments of 0.1° C over a range of 35.5° C to 40.4° C. The Fahrenheit version has 45 dots with increments of 0.2° F and a range of 96.0° F to 104.8° F. Chemical dots on the thermometer change color to reflect temperature reading, usually within 60 seconds. Most are designed for single use (Figure 17-4). In one brand that can be reused for a single client the chemical dots return to the original color within a few seconds. The chemical dots thermometers are most commonly used for oral temperatures. They can also be used at axillary or rectal sites, covered by a plastic sheath at the latter, with a placement time of 3 minutes.

DELEGATION CONSIDERATIONS

The skill of temperature measurement can be delegated to assistive personnel. Before delegating this skill the nurse may:

- Inform assistive personnel if any precautions are needed in positioning the client during measurement
- Instruct assistive personnel of appropriate route and device to measure temperature
- Provide assistive personnel the frequency of temperature measurement for select client
- Determine that assistive personnel are aware of the client's previous temperature measures
- Instruct assistive personnel in the need to report abnormalities that should be reconfirmed by the nurse

EQUIPMENT

- ❑ Appropriate thermometer
- ❑ Soft tissue
- ❑ Lubricant (for rectal measurements only)
- ❑ Pen, pencil, vital sign flow sheet or record form
- ❑ Disposable gloves, plastic thermometer sleeve, disposable probe or sensor cover
- ❑ Towel

STEP	RATIONALE

ASSESSMENT

1. Determine need to measure client's body temperature:

    a. Note client's risks for temperature alterations: expected or diagnosed infection, open wounds or burns, white blood cell count below 5000 or above 12,000, immunosuppressive drug therapy, injury to hypothalamus, exposure to temperature extremes, blood product infusion, hypothermia or hyperthermia therapy, or postoperative status.

    Certain conditions place clients at risk for temperature alterations and may require more frequent temperature measurement and nursing assessment.

    b. Assess for signs and symptoms that may accompany temperature alteration:

    Fever: (depending on stage) pale or flushed skin; skin warm or hot to touch; skin dry or diaphoretic; dry mucous membranes; shivering with chills; piloerection or "gooseflesh" of skin; tachycardia; malaise with muscle or joint pain; nausea, vomiting, or diarrhea; feeling hot or cold; restlessness.

    Physical signs and symptoms may alert nurse to alteration in body temperature.
    Hyperthermia: Decreased skin turgor, tachycardia; hypotension; decreased venous filling; concentrated urine.
    Heatstroke: Hot, dry skin; tachycardia; hypotension; excessive thirst; muscle cramps; visual disturbances; confusion or delirium.
    Hypothermia: Pale skin; skin cool or cold to touch; bradycardia and dysrhythmias; uncontrollable shivering; reduced level of consciousness; shallow respirations.

2. Assess for factors that normally influence temperature:

    Allows nurse to accurately assess for presence and significance of temperature alteration.

    a. Age

    Older adults have a narrower range of temperature than do younger adults.

- **Critical Decision Point**

    No single temperature is normal for all people. A temperature within an acceptable range in an adult may reflect a fever in an older adult. Undeveloped temperature control mechanisms in infants and children can cause temperature to rise and fall rapidly.

    b. Exercise

    Muscle activity raises heat production.

    c. Hormones

    Women have wider temperature fluctuations than men because of menstrual cycle hormonal changes (Sund-Levander and others, 2002); body temperature change can vary during menopause.

    d. Stress

    Stress elevates temperature.

    e. Environmental temperature

    Infants and older adults are more sensitive to environmental temperature changes.

STEP	RATIONALE
f. Medications	Drugs may impair or promote sweating, vasoconstriction, vasodilation, or interfere with the ability of the hypothalamus to regulate temperature.
g. Daily fluctuations	Body temperature normally changes 0.5 to 1° C during a 24-hour period. Temperature is lowest during early morning. Most clients have maximum temperature elevation around 6 PM; temperature falls gradually during night.
3. Assess site most appropriate for client's temperature measurement (see Box 17-3):	Determines if client's status contraindicates selection of a specific method or site.
• *Critical Decision Point* *Know contraindications for each site.*	
a. Oral **b.** Rectum **c.** Axilla **d.** Tympanic membrane	
4. Determine previous baseline temperature and measurement site (if available) from client's record.	Allows nurse to assess for change in condition. Provides comparison with future temperature measurements.

NURSING DIAGNOSES

* Risk for imbalanced body temperature
* Hyperthermia
* Ineffective thermoregulation
* Hypothermia

Related factors are individualized based on client's condition or needs.

PLANNING

1. Expected outcomes following completion of procedure: • Body temperature is within acceptable range for client's age-group.	Thermoregulation is maintained.
• Body temperature returns to baseline range following therapies for abnormal temperature.	Nurse controls for environmental factors that could alter temperature.
2. Explain to client the way temperature will be measured and importance of maintaining proper position until reading is complete.	Promotes client cooperation and increases compliance. Clients are often curious about their temperatures and should be cautioned against prematurely removing the thermometer to read results.

IMPLEMENTATION

1. Perform hand hygiene.	Reduces transmission of microorganisms.
2. Assist client to comfortable position that provides easy access to temperature measurement site.	Ensures both client's comfort and accuracy of temperature reading.
3. Obtain temperature reading.	
a. Oral temperature measurement with electronic thermometer	
(1) Apply disposable gloves (optional).	Use of an oral probe cover, which can be removed without physical contact, minimizes need to wear gloves.
(2) Remove thermometer pack from charging unit. Attach oral thermometer probe stem (blue tip) to thermometer unit. Grasp top of probe stem, being careful not to apply pressure on the ejection button.	Charging provides battery power. Ejection button releases plastic cover from probe stem.

STEP	RATIONALE

(3) Slide disposable plastic probe cover over thermometer probe stem until cover locks in place (see illustration).

Soft plastic cover will not break in client's mouth and prevents transmission of microorganisms between clients.

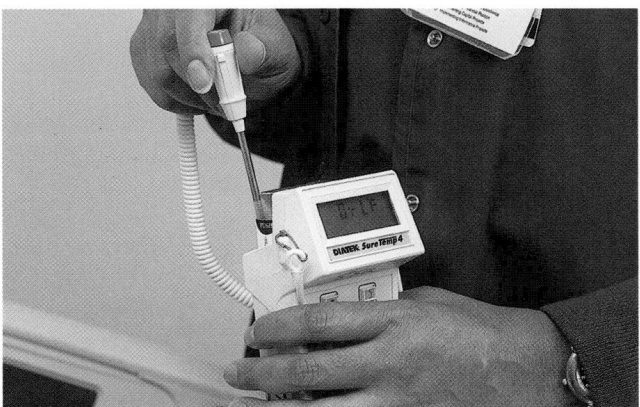

STEP **3a(3)** Nurse inserts electronic thermometer probe stem into probe cover. Cover snaps in place.

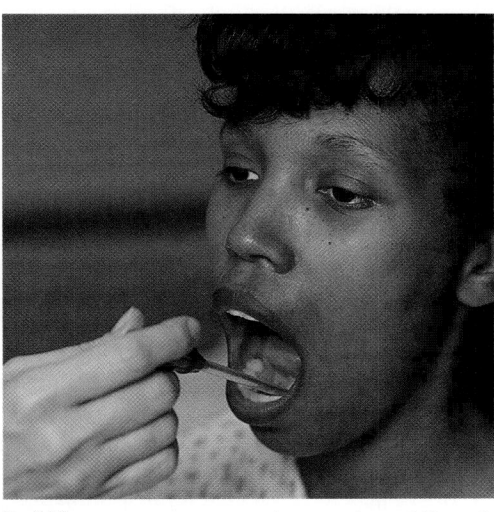

STEP **3a(4)** Probe under tongue in posterior sublingual pocket.

(4) Ask client to open mouth; then gently place thermometer probe under tongue in posterior sublingual pocket lateral to center of lower jaw (see illustration).

Heat from superficial blood vessels in sublingual pocket produces temperature reading. With electronic thermometer, temperatures in right and left posterior sublingual pocket are significantly higher than in area under front of tongue.

(5) Ask client to hold thermometer probe with lips closed.

Maintains proper position of thermometer during recording.

(6) Leave thermometer probe in place until audible signal indicates completion and client's temperature appears on digital display; remove thermometer probe from under client's tongue.

Probe must stay in place until signal occurs to ensure accurate reading.

(7) Push ejection button on thermometer probe stem to discard plastic probe cover into an appropriate receptacle.

Reduces transmission of microorganisms.

(8) Return thermometer probe stem to storage position of thermometer unit.

Returning thermometer probe stem automatically causes digital reading to disappear. Storage position protects stem.

(9) If gloves worn, remove and dispose in appropriate receptacle. Perform hand hygiene.

Reduces transmission of microorganisms.

(10) Return thermometer to charger.

Maintains battery charge of thermometer unit.

b. Rectal temperature measurement with electronic thermometer

(1) Draw curtain around bed and/or close room door. Assist client to side-lying Sims' position with upper leg flexed. Move aside bed linen to expose only anal area. Keep client's upper body and lower extremities covered with sheet or blanket.

Maintains client's privacy, minimizes embarrassment, and promotes comfort.

(2) Apply disposable gloves.

Maintains standard precautions when exposed to items soiled with body fluid.

STEP	**RATIONALE**

(3) Remove thermometer pack from charging unit. Attach rectal thermometer probe stem (red tip) to thermometer unit. Grasp top of probe stem, being careful not to apply pressure on the ejection button.

Ejection button releases plastic cover from probe stem.

(4) Slide disposable plastic probe cover over thermometer probe stem until cover locks in place.

Probe cover prevents transmission of microorganisms between clients.

(5) Squeeze liberal portion of lubricant on tissue. Dip thermometer's blunt end into lubricant, covering 2.5 to 3.5 cm (1 to 1½ inches) for adult.

Lubrication minimizes trauma to rectal mucosa during insertion. Tissue avoids contamination of remaining lubricant in container.

(6) With nondominant hand, separate client's buttocks to expose anus. Ask client to breathe slowly and relax.

Fully exposes anus for thermometer insertion. Relaxes anal sphincter for easier thermometer insertion.

(7) Gently insert thermometer into anus in direction of umbilicus 3.5 cm (1½ inches) for adult. Do not force thermometer.

Ensures adequate exposure against blood vessels in rectal wall.

(8) If resistance is felt during insertion, withdraw immediately. Never force thermometer.

Prevents trauma to mucosa.

(9) Once positioned, hold thermometer probe in place until audible signal indicates completion and client's temperature appears on digital display; remove thermometer probe from anus (see illustration).

Probe must stay in place until signal occurs to ensure accurate reading.

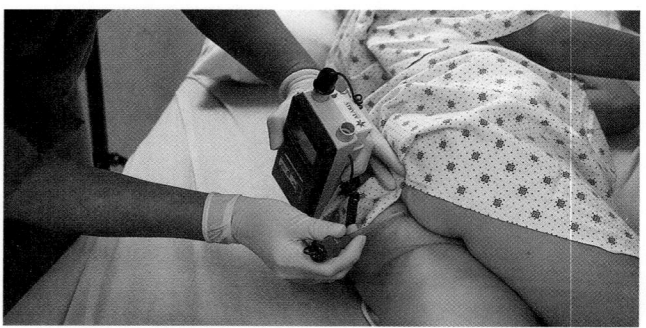

STEP 3b(9) Probe removed smoothly from anus.

(10) Push ejection button on thermometer stem to discard plastic probe cover into an appropriate receptacle.

Reduces transmission of microorganisms.

(11) Return thermometer stem to storage position of recording unit.

Returning thermometer stem automatically causes digital reading to disappear.

(12) Wipe client's anal area with soft tissue to remove lubricant or feces, and discard tissue. Assist client in assuming a comfortable position.

Provides for comfort and hygiene.

(13) Remove and dispose of gloves in appropriate receptacle. Perform hand hygiene.

Reduces transmission of microorganisms.

(14) Return thermometer to charger.

Maintains battery charge of thermometer unit.

c. Axillary temperature measurement with electronic thermometer

(1) Draw curtain around bed and/or close room door. Assist client to supine or sitting position. Move clothing or gown away from shoulder and arm.

Maintains client's privacy, minimizes embarrassment, and promotes comfort. Exposes axilla for correct thermometer probe placement.

STEP	RATIONALE
(2) Remove thermometer pack from charging unit. Attach oral thermometer probe stem (blue tip) to thermometer unit. Grasp top of thermometer probe stem, being careful not to apply pressure on the ejection button.	Ejection button releases plastic cover from probe stem.
(3) Slide disposable plastic probe cover over thermometer stem until cover locks in place.	Probe cover prevents transmission of microorganisms between clients.
(4) Raise client's arm away from torso. Inspect for skin lesions and excessive perspiration; if needed, dry axilla.	May interfere with accurate reading.

- **Critical Decision Point**
  Do not use axilla if skin lesions are present because local temperature may be altered and area may be painful to touch.

STEP	RATIONALE
(5) Insert thermometer probe into center of axilla, lower arm over probe, and place arm across client's chest.	Maintains proper position of thermometer against blood vessels in axilla.
(6) Once positioned, hold thermometer probe in place until audible signal indicates completion and client's temperature appears on digital display; remove thermometer probe from axilla.	Thermometer probe must stay in place until signal occurs to ensure accurate reading.
(7) Push ejection button on thermometer stem to discard plastic probe cover into appropriate receptacle.	Reduces transmission of microorganisms.
(8) Return thermometer stem to storage position of recording unit.	Returning thermometer stem to storage position automatically causes digital reading to disappear. Protects stem from damage.
(9) Assist client in assuming a comfortable position, replacing linen or gown.	Restores comfort and sense of well-being.
(10) Perform hand hygiene.	Reduces transmission of microorganisms.
(11) Return thermometer to charger.	Maintains battery charge of thermometer unit.
d. Tympanic membrane temperature with electronic thermometer	
(1) Assist client in assuming comfortable position with head turned toward side, away from nurse. If client lies on one side, use upper ear.	Ensures comfort and facilitates exposure of auditory canal for accurate temperature measurement. Heat trapped in ear facing down will cause false high temperature reading (Bailey and Rose, 2001).
(2) Note if there is an obvious presence of earwax in the client's ear canal.	Lens cover of speculum must not be impeded by earwax to ensure clear optical pathway. Switch to other ear or select alternative measurement site.
(3) Remove thermometer handheld unit from charging base, being careful not to apply pressure to the ejection button.	Removal of handheld unit from base prepares it to measure temperature. Ejection button releases plastic probe cover from thermometer tip.
(4) Slide disposable speculum cover over the otoscope-like lens tip until it locks in place. Be careful not to touch lens cover.	Soft plastic probe cover prevents transmission of microorganisms between clients. Lens cover must be unimpeded by dust, fingerprints, or earwax to ensure clear optical pathway.
(5) If holding handheld unit with right hand, obtain temperature from client's right ear; left-handed persons should obtain temperature from client's left ear.	Facilitates correct angle of approach for a better probe position and seal.

STEP	RATIONALE

(6) Insert speculum into ear canal following manufacturer's instructions for tympanic probe positioning:

(a) Pull ear pinna backward, up, and out for an adult. For children less than 2 years of age, point covered probe toward midpoint between eyebrow and sideburns (Hockenberry and others, 2003) (see illustration).

(b) Move thermometer in a figure-eight pattern.

(c) Fit speculum tip snug in canal, and do not move.

(d) Point speculum tip toward nose.

Correct positioning of probe with respect to ear canal allows maximum exposure of tympanic membrane. The ear tug straightens the external auditory canal, allowing maximum exposure of tympanic membrane. Some manufacturers recommend movement of speculum tip in a figure-eight pattern that allows sensor to detect maximum tympanic membrane heat radiation. Gentle pressure seals ear canal from ambient air temperature, which can alter readings as much as 2.8° C or 5° F.

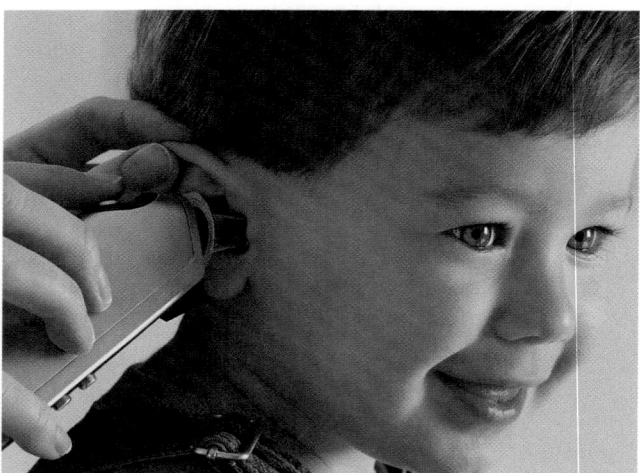

STEP 3d(6) Tympanic membrane thermometer with probe cover placed in child's ear. (Photo courtesy Welch Allyn.)

(7) As soon as probe is in place, depress scan button on handheld unit. Leave thermometer probe in place until audible signal occurs and client's temperature appears on digital display.

(8) Carefully remove speculum from auditory meatus. Push ejection button on handheld unit to discard speculum cover into appropriate receptacle.

(9) If temperature is abnormal or second reading is necessary, replace probe cover, and wait 2 to 3 minutes before repeating in same ear or repeat measurement in other ear. Consider an alternative site or instrument.

(10) Return handheld unit to thermometer base.

(11) Assist client in assuming a comfortable position.

(12) Perform hand hygiene.

4. Inform client of temperature reading, and record measurement.

Depression of scan button causes infrared energy to be detected. Otoscope tip must stay in place until signal occurs to ensure accurate reading. Signal indicates infrared energy has been detected.

Reduces transmission of microorganisms. Automatically causes digital reading to disappear.

Lens cover must be free of cerumen to maintain optical path. Time allows ear canal to regain usual temperature (Guiliano and others, 2000).

Protects sensor tip from damage.

Restores comfort and sense of well-being.

Reduces transmission of microorganisms.

Promotes participation in care and understanding of health status.

EVALUATION

1. If temperature is assessed for the first time, establish temperature as baseline if it is within acceptable range.

Used to compare future temperature measurements.

2. Compare temperature reading with client's previous baseline and acceptable temperature range for client's age-group.

Body temperature fluctuates within narrow range; comparison reveals presence of abnormality. Improper placement or movement of thermometer can cause inaccuracies. Second measurement confirms initial findings of abnormal body temperature.

3. If client has fever, temperature should be taken approximately 30 minutes after administering antipyretics, and every 4 hours until temperature stabilizes.

Will determine if temperature begins to fall in response to therapy.

Recording and Reporting

- Record temperature and route on vital sign flow sheet (Figure 17-5) or record form.
- Record in nurses' notes any signs or symptoms of temperature alterations.
- Report abnormal findings to nurse in charge or physician.

Unexpected Outcomes	Related Interventions
1. Body temperature is 1° C or more above acceptable range.	• Initiate measures to lower body temperature. 　• Cool room environment. 　• Reduce external covering on client's body to promote heat loss, but do not induce shivering. 　• Keep clothing and bed linen dry. 　• Apply hypothermia blanket as ordered (see Chapter 40). 　• Limit physical activity and sources of emotional stress. 　• Administer antipyretics as ordered. 　• Increase fluid intake to at least 3 L daily (unless contraindicated). 　• Initiate measure to stimulate appetite, and provide nutrients to meet increased energy needs (see Chapter 29). • Prevent or control spread of infection. 　• Wound care (see Chapter 37) 　• Pulmonary hygiene (see Chapter 23) 　• Adequate urinary elimination (see Chapter 32)
2. Body temperature is 1° C or more below acceptable range.	• Initiate measures to increase body temperature. 　• Heat room environment. 　• Cover client with warm blankets. 　• Apply hyperthermia blankets if ordered (see Chapter 40). 　• Close room doors or control drafts. 　• Encourage warm liquids.
3. No temperature obtained.	• Reassess correct placement of temperature probe or sensor. • Chose alternative temperature measurement site. • Obtain alternative temperature measurement device.

Teaching Considerations

- Identify client's ability to initiate preventive health measures and recognize alteration in body temperature. Educate clients and family members about measures to prevent body temperature alterations.
- Educate clients about risk factors for hypothermia and frostbite: fatigue; malnutrition; hypoxemia; cold, wet clothing; alcohol intoxication.
- Educate clients about risk factors for heatstroke: strenuous exercise in hot humid weather; tight-fitting clothing in hot environments; exercising in poorly ventilated areas; sudden exposures to hot climates; poor fluid intake before, during, and after exercise.
- Educate clients regarding the importance of taking and continuing antibiotics as directed until course of treatment for infection is completed.

VITAL SIGN / I & O / PAIN RECORD

DATE _____

HOUR	00	01	02	03	04	05	06	07	08	09	10	11	12	13	14	15	16	17	18	19	20	21	22	23
TEMP: R = Rectal A = Axillary T = Tympanic			T 36^8						T 37^2				T 37^2				T 37^4							
METHOD																								
PULSE			82/AP						84/AP				86/AP				80/AP							
RESPIRATION			16						16		18		20				16							

BP	SYSTOLIC / DIASTOLIC																							
			R 140 / 80						R 146 / 80		R 140 / 78		R 146 / 82				R 140 / 80							

FREQUENT VITAL SIGNS	TIME	BP	PULSE	RESP	TEMP	TIME	BP	PULSE	RESP	TEMP	TIME	BP	PULSE	RESP	TEMP	TIME	BP	PULSE	RESP	TEMP

WEIGHT — SCALE KEY: ☐ BED ☐ STANDING ☐ W/CHAIR ☐ SLING   **WT** _____ ☐ LB ☐ KG

PAIN

PAIN RATING SCALES

☐ Verbal

0 1 2 3 4 5 6 7 8 9 10
No pain — Moderate pain — Worst possible pain

☐ Faces

0 2 4 6 8 10

☐ Non-verbal

0 1 2 3 4 5 6 7 8 9 10
Sleeping/Calm · Grimacing w/movement · Moaning w/movement · Restless · Constant moaning w/o stimuli

LOCATION	TARGET	00	01	02	03	04	05	06	07	08	09	10	11	12	13	14	15	16	17	18	19	20	21	22	23
X = SITE 1 O = SITE 2	PAIN INTENSITY 10 / 5 / 0																								
TYPE *SEE KEY																									
INTERVENTION *SEE KEY																									
RELIEF ACCEPTABLE (Y / N)																									
LEVEL OF CONSCIOUSNESS																									

KEY

TYPE OF PAIN:

Aching	**B**urning	**CS**-Crushing	**R**adiating	**TH**robbing
ACute	**CO**nstant	**D**ull	**S**harp	Other: _____
AGitation	**C**ramping	**H**eavy	**ST**-Stabbing	
ANxiety	**CR**-Chronic	**I**ntermittent	**T**ender	

INTERVENTION:

1 - Medication	5 - Heat	9 - Prayer
2 - Relaxation	6 - Cold	10 - Massage
3 - Touch	7 - Pastoral care	11 - Other
4 - Guided imagery	8 - Music	_____

LEVEL OF CONSCIOUSNESS: 1 = Wide awake   2 = Drowsy   3 = Dozing intermittently   4 = Only awakens when aroused   5 = Difficult to arouse

SIGNATURE/TITLE	HRS WORKED	SIGNATURE/TITLE	HRS WORKED	SIGNATURE/TITLE	HRS WORKED

31000130

ADDRESSOGRAPH / LABEL

SSM HEALTH·CARE

VITAL SIGN / I & O / PAIN RECORD

SLM-1000-035 (6/2000) 10 FRONT

FIGURE 17-5 Temperature, pulse, and respiration recording on vital sign flow sheet. (Courtesy St. Mary's Health Center, St. Louis.) Form courtesy SSM Health Care, St. Mary's Health Center, St. Louis, Mo. (*Pain Rating Scale from McCaffery M, Pasero C: *Pain clinical manual,* ed 2, St. Louis, 1999, Mosby; **Wong-Baker FACES Pain Rating Scale from Hockenberry MJ and others: *Wong's nursing care of infants and children,* ed 7, St. Louis, 2003, Mosby.)

Pediatric Considerations

- Infants and young children may lose more heat to environmental losses because of their increased surface area/volume ratios. Neonates and infants less than 6 months old may suffer from cold stress that may go undetected and will place greater oxygen demands on the infant in an attempt to regulate their temperature.
  - Critically ill children may have cool skin but a high core temperature because of poor perfusion to the skin. Children at risk may be monitored using a Foley temperature probe or central lines with thermometers.
  - Tympanic temperatures can be used in healthy preterm neonates (Bailey and Rose, 2001).
- Axillary temperatures may be used for screening purposes but cannot be relied on to detect fevers in infants and young children. Alternative methods may include rectal temperatures for appropriate clients or temperatures taken with an ear-based sensor.
- Children may assume prone position for rectal temperature measurement.
- Temperature is best taken as the last vital sign with children who cry or become restless.

Gerontological Considerations

- The temperature of older adults is at the lower end of the acceptable temperature range: 36° C (96.8° F).
- Temperatures considered within normal range may reflect a fever in an older adult (Sund-Levander and others, 2002).

- Edentulous adults or older adults with poor muscle control may be unable to close their mouth tightly enough to obtain accurate oral temperature readings.
- Older adults are very sensitive to environmental temperature changes because their thermoregulatory systems are not as efficient.
- With aging, cerumen tends to be drier and cilia become stiff, contributing to buildup of cerumen impaction, which can interfere with accurate tympanic temperature measurement.
- A decrease in sweat gland reactivity in the older adult results in a higher threshold for sweating at high temperatures, which can lead to hyperthermia (Maas and others, 2001).
- With aging, a loss of subcutaneous fat reduces the insulating capacity of the skin.
  - Older adults are at high risk for hypothermia because of diminished sensation to cold, abnormal vasoconstrictor responses, and impaired shivering.

Home Care Considerations

- Assess temperature and ventilation of client's environment to determine existence of any environmental conditions that may influence client's temperature.
- Assess presence of mercury-in-glass thermometers, and suggest to client and caregiver alternative temperature measurement devices for home use.
- Educate client and caregiver about mercury hazards and proper disposal of any mercury-containing devices.

SKILL 17-2 Assessing Radial Pulse

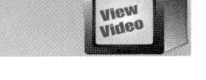

The ejection of blood from the heart distends the walls of the aorta. Because of the force of the blood exiting the heart, aortic distention creates a pulse wave that travels rapidly toward the extremities. When the pulse wave reaches a peripheral artery, it can be felt by palpating the artery lightly against underlying bone or muscle. The pulse is the palpable bounding of the blood flow. The number of pulsing sensations occurring in 1 minute is the pulse rate.

Assessing the client's peripheral pulse sites offers valuable data for determining the integrity of the cardiovascular system. Pulse rate, rhythm, and strength indirectly evaluate the heart's cardiac output (CO). An abnormally slow, rapid, or irregular pulse may indicate the heart's inability to deliver an adequate cardiac output; a pulse deficit may be present (see Box 17-5). The strength or amplitude of a pulse reflects the volume of blood ejected against the arterial wall with each heart contraction, also called stroke volume (SV). If the heart's stroke volume decreases, the pulse often becomes weak and difficult to

palpate. In contrast, a full bounding pulse is an indication of increased stroke volume.

The integrity of peripheral pulses indicates the status of blood perfusion to the area distributed by the pulse (Table 17-1). For example, assessment of the right femoral pulse determines whether blood flow to the right leg is adequate. If a peripheral pulse distal to an injured or treated area of an extremity feels weak on palpation, the volume of blood reaching tissues below the affected area may be inadequate and surgical intervention may be needed.

The radial artery pulse is the most common peripheral site for pulse rate assessment (Figure 17-6). The carotid artery site is also commonly used when the radial pulse is weak or difficult to palpate. Assessment of other peripheral pulse sites, such as the brachial or femoral artery, is unnecessary when routinely obtaining vital signs. Other peripheral pulses are assessed when a complete physical is conducted or when the radial artery is not available for assessment because of surgery, trauma, or impaired blood flow.

TABLE 17-1 PULSE SITES

SITE	LOCATION	RATIONALE FOR SELECTION
Temporal	Over temporal bone of the head, above and lateral to the eye	Easily accessible site to assess pulse in children
Carotid	Along medial edge of sternocleidomastoid muscle in the neck	Easily accessible site to assess character of peripheral pulse; used during physiological shock or cardiac arrest when other sites are not palpable
Apical	Fourth to fifth intercostal space at left midclavicular line	Site for auscultation of heart sounds
Brachial	Groove between biceps and triceps muscles at the antecubital fossa	Site used to auscultate upper extremity blood pressure; assesses status of circulation to lower arm
Radial	Radial or thumb side of forearm at the wrist	Common site to assess character of peripheral pulse; assesses status of circulation to hand
Ulnar	Ulnar side of forearm at the wrist	Site used to assess status of circulation to ulnar side of hand; used to perform Allen's test
Femoral	Below the inguinal ligament, midway between symphysis pubis and anterior superior iliac spine	Site used to assess character of pulse during physiological shock or cardiac arrest when other pulses are not palpable; assesses status of circulation to the leg
Popliteal	Behind the knee in popliteal fossa	Site used to auscultate lower extremity blood pressure; assesses status of circulation to the lower leg
Posterior tibial	Inner side of each ankle, below medial malleolus	Site used to assess status of circulation to the foot
Dorsalis pedis	Along top of foot between extension tendons of great and first toe	Site used to assess status of circulation to the foot

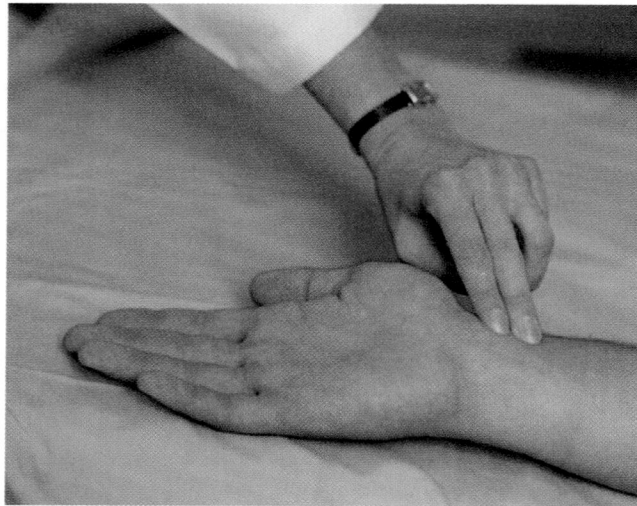

FIGURE **17-6** Location of right radial pulse site.

DELEGATION CONSIDERATIONS

The skill of radial pulse measurement can be delegated to assistive personnel unless the client is considered unstable or the nurse is evaluating a response to a treatment or medication. Before delegating this skill the nurse must:

- Inform assistive personnel of client history or risk for abnormally slow, rapid, or irregular pulse
- Provide assistive personnel the frequency of pulse measurement for select client
- Determine that assistive personnel are aware of the client's usual baseline pulse rate
- Instruct assistive personnel to report any abnormalities that should be reconfirmed by the nurse

EQUIPMENT

- ❑ Wristwatch with second hand or digital display
- ❑ Pen, pencil, vital sign flow sheet or record form

STEP	RATIONALE

ASSESSMENT

1. Determine need to assess radial pulse:

   a. Note risk factors for alterations in pulse.

   Certain conditions place clients at risk for pulse alterations: a history of heart disease, cardiac dysrhythmia, onset of sudden chest pain or acute pain from any site, invasive cardiovascular diagnostic tests, surgery, sudden infusion of large volume of intravenous (IV) fluid, internal or external hemorrhage, or administration of medications that alter cardiac function. A history of peripheral vascular disease can alter pulse rate and quality.

   b. Assess for signs and symptoms of altered SV and CO, such as presence of dyspnea, fatigue, chest pain, orthopnea, syncope, palpitations (person's unpleasant awareness of heartbeat), jugular venous distention, edema of dependent body parts, cyanosis or pallor of skin (see Chapter 18).

   Physical signs and symptoms may indicate alteration in cardiac function, which affects radial pulse rate and rhythm.

   c. Assess for signs and symptoms of peripheral vascular disease such as pale, cool extremities; thin, shiny skin with decreased hair growth; thickened nails (see Skill 18-6).

   Physical signs and symptoms may indicate alteration in local arterial blood flow.

2. Assess for factors that influence radial pulse rate and rhythm: age, exercise, position changes, fluid balance, medications, temperature, sympathetic stimulation.

   Allows nurse to accurately assess presence and significance of pulse alterations.

3. Determine client's previous baseline pulse rate (if available) from client's record.

   Allows nurse to assess for change in condition. Provides comparison with future pulse measurements.

NURSING DIAGNOSES

- Activity intolerance
- Ineffective tissue perfusion

- Deficient fluid volume
- Decreased cardiac output

Related factors are individualized based on client's condition and needs.

PLANNING

1. Expected outcomes following completion of procedure:
   - Radial pulse is palpable, within acceptable range for client's age.

   Adults average 60 to 100 beats per minute.

   - Rhythm is regular.

   Cardiac status is stable.

   - Radial pulse is strong, firm, and elastic.

   Radial artery is patent.

2. Explain to client that radial pulse rate (HR) is to be assessed. Encourage client to relax as much as possible. If client has been active, wait 5 to 10 minutes before assessing pulse.

   Anxiety or activity can cause elevation in heart rate. Radial pulse rate should be assessed at rest to allow for objective comparison of values.

IMPLEMENTATION

1. Perform hand hygiene.

   Reduces transmission of microorganisms.

2. If necessary, draw curtain around bed and/or close door.

   Maintains privacy and minimizes embarrassment.

3. Assist client with assuming a supine or sitting position.

   Provides easy access to pulse sites.

STEP	RATIONALE

4. If client is supine, place client's forearm straight along-side or across lower chest or upper abdomen with wrist extended straight (see illustration). If client is sitting, bend client's elbow 90 degrees, and support lower arm on chair or on nurse's arm. Slightly extend or flex wrist with palm down until strongest pulse is noted.

Relaxed position of lower arm and extension of wrist permits full exposure of artery to palpation.

5. Place tips of first two or middle three fingers of hand over groove along radial or thumb side of client's inner wrist (see illustration).

Fingertips are most sensitive parts of hand to palpate arterial pulsation. Nurse's thumb has pulsation that may interfere with accuracy.

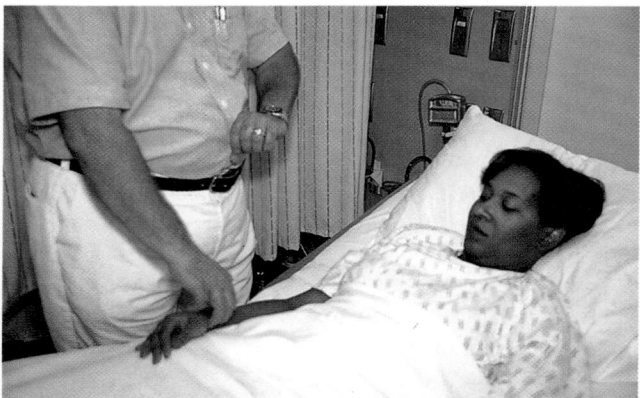

STEP 4 Pulse check with client's forearm at side with wrist extended.

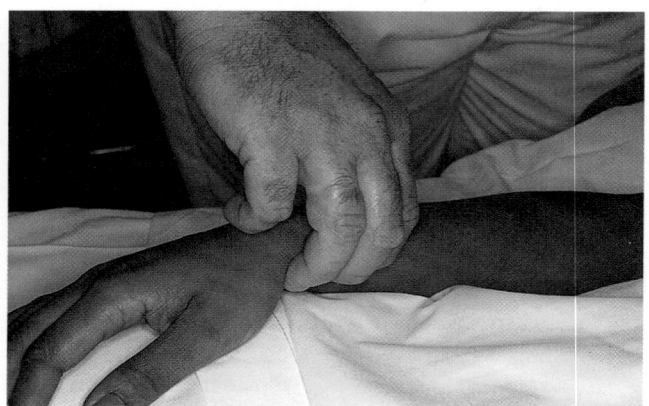

STEP 5 Hand placement for pulse check.

6. Lightly compress against radius, obliterate pulse initially, and then relax pressure so pulse becomes easily palpable.

Pulse is more accurately assessed with moderate pressure. Too much pressure occludes pulse and impairs blood flow.

7. Determine strength of pulse. Note whether thrust of vessel against fingertips is bounding, strong, weak, or thready.

Strength reflects volume of blood ejected against arterial wall with each heart contraction.

8. After pulse can be felt regularly, look at watch's second hand and begin to count rate: when sweep hand hits number on dial, start counting with zero, then one, two, and so on.

Rate is determined accurately only after nurse is ensured pulse can be palpated. Timing begins with zero. Count of one is first beat palpated after timing begins.

9. If pulse is regular, count rate for 30 seconds and multiply total by 2.

A 30-second count is accurate for rapid, slow, or regular pulse rates.

10. If pulse is irregular, count rate for a full 60 seconds. Assess frequency and pattern of irregularity.

Inefficient contraction of heart fails to transmit pulse wave, interfering with CO, resulting in irregular pulse. Longer time period ensures accurate count.

11. When pulse is irregular, compare radial pulses bilaterally.

A marked inequality may indicate arterial flow is compromised to one extremity and action should be taken.

- **Critical Decision Point**
  If pulse is irregular, assess for pulse deficit (see Box 17-5), which may indicate alterations in CO.

12. Assist client in returning to comfortable position.

Promotes comfort and sense of well-being.

13. Discuss findings with client as needed.

Promotes participation in care and understanding of health status.

14. Perform hand hygiene.

Reduces transmission of microorganisms.

STEP	RATIONALE

EVALUATION

1. If pulse is assessed for the first time, establish radial pulse as baseline if it is within acceptable range.

   Used to compare future pulse assessments.

2. Compare pulse rate and character with client's previous baseline and acceptable range for client's age.

   Allows nurse to assess for change in client's condition and for presence of cardiac alteration.

Recording and Reporting

- Record pulse rate and site assessed on vital sign flow sheet (see Figure 17-5), record, or nurses' notes.
- Record any accompanying signs and symptoms of pulse alterations.
- Report abnormal findings to nurse in charge or physician.

Unexpected Outcomes	Related Interventions
1. Pulse rate for an adult is over 100 beats per minute (tachycardia).	• Identify related data, including pain, fear or anxiety, recent exercise, low BP, blood loss, elevated temperature, or inadequate oxygenation. • Observe for symptoms associated with abnormal cardiac function: · Dyspnea, fatigue, chest pain, orthopnea, syncope, palpitations, jugular vein distention, edema of body parts, cyanosis or pallor of the skin
2. Weak or difficult to palpate radial pulse.	• Observe for symptoms associated with altered tissue perfusion: · Pallor · Cyanosis · Cold extremity • Assess for swelling in surrounding tissues or any encumbrance (e.g., dressing or cast) that may impede blood flow. • Obtain Doppler or ultrasound stethoscope to detect low-velocity blood flow. • Assess both radial pulses, and compare findings. • Have another nurse assess pulse.
3. Pulse rate for an adult is under 60 beats per minute (bradycardia).	• Auscultate the apical pulse (see Skill 17-3). • Confer with physician, and be prepared to order/obtain an electrocardiogram.
4. Pulse is irregular.	• Auscultate the apical pulse (see Skill 17-3). • Assess for pulse deficit (see Box 17-5).

Teaching Considerations

- Clients taking certain prescribed cardiotonic or antidysrhythmic medications should learn to assess their own pulse rates to detect side effects of medications. Clients undergoing cardiac rehabilitation should learn to assess their own pulse rates to determine their response to exercise.
- Monitoring carotid pulse rate is taught to clients taking heart medications or starting a prescribed exercise regimen.

Pediatric Considerations

- An accurate pulse can be taken radially in children over 2 years of age (Hockenberry and others, 2003).
- Children often have a sinus dysrhythmia, which is an irregular heartbeat that speeds up with inspiration and slows down with expiration. Breath holding in a child affects pulse rate.

Gerontological Considerations

- It is often difficult to palpate the pulse of an older adult or obese client. A Doppler ultrasound stethoscope provides a more accurate reading.
- The arteries of an older adult may feel stiff and knotty because of decreased elasticity.

- The older adult has a decreased heart rate at rest (Ebersole and Hess, 2001).
- Once elevated, the pulse rate of an older adult takes longer to return to normal resting rate (Lueckenotte, 2000).

SKILL 17-3 Assessing Apical Pulse

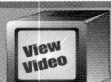

Each ventricular contraction of the heart ejects approximately 60 to 70 ml (stroke volume) of blood into the aorta. The heart rate is the number of ejections occurring in 1 minute. The volume of blood pumped by the heart during 1 minute is the cardiac output. The cardiac output equals the product of the amount of blood pumped by the ventricle per stroke, or the stroke volume, and the heart rate for 1 minute. The apical pulse is the most reliable noninvasive way to assess cardiac function. The apical pulse rate is the assessment of the number and quality of apical sounds in 1 minute. Each apical pulse is the combination of two sounds, S_1 and S_2. S_1 is the sound of the tricuspid and mitral valves closing at the end of ventricular filling, just before systolic contraction begins. S_2 is the sound of the pulmonic and aortic valves closing at the end of the systolic contraction.

A stethoscope is used to auscultate sound waves of the apical pulse (Figure 17-7). It is a closed cylinder that amplifies sound waves as they reach the body's surface. The five major parts of the stethoscope are the earpieces, binaurals, tubing, bell, and diaphragm.

The plastic or rubber earpieces should fit snugly and comfortably in the nurse's ears. Binaurals should be angled and strong enough so the earpieces stay firmly in place without causing discomfort. The earpieces follow the contour of the ear canal, pointing toward the face when the stethoscope is in place.

The polyvinyl tubing should be flexible and 30 to 40 cm (12 to 18 inches) in length; longer tubing decreases sound transmission. The tubing should be thick walled and moderately rigid to eliminate transmission of environmental noise and to prevent kinking.

The chestpiece consists of a bell and diaphragm that are rotated into position depending on which part the nurse chooses to use. To test, lightly tap to determine which side is functioning.

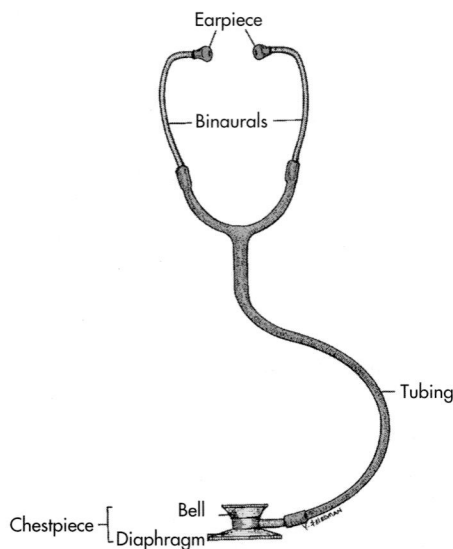

FIGURE 17-7 Acoustic stethoscope.

The diaphragm is a circular flat-surfaced portion of the chestpiece covered with a plastic disk. It transmits high-pitched sounds created by high-velocity movement of air and blood. The diaphragm is positioned to make a tight seal against the client's skin. Enough pressure is exerted to complete the seal and should leave a temporary red ring on the client's skin when the diaphragm is removed.

The bell is the cone-shaped portion of the chestpiece usually surrounded by a rubber ring to avoid chilling the client. It transmits low-pitched sounds created by the low-velocity movement of blood. The bell is held lightly against the skin for sound amplification.

DELEGATION CONSIDERATIONS

Often the apical pulse is measured when the nurse suspects an irregularity in the radial pulse or the client's condition warrants a more accurate assessment. In this situation, delegation of pulse assessment is inappropriate. When measurement of apical pulse is a routine practice, it can be delegated to assistive personnel. Before delegating this skill the nurse must:

* Inform assistive personnel of client history or risk for abnormally slow, rapid, or irregular pulse
* Provide assistive personnel the frequency of pulse measurement for select client
* Determine that assistive personnel are aware of the client's usual baseline pulse rate
* Instruct assistive personnel to report any abnormality in rate or rhythm that should be reconfirmed by the nurse

EQUIPMENT

* ❏ Stethoscope
* ❏ Wristwatch with second hand or digital display
* ❏ Pen, pencil, vital sign flow sheet or record form
* ❏ Alcohol swab

STEP	RATIONALE

ASSESSMENT

1. Determine need to assess apical pulse:
   a. Note risk factors for alterations in apical pulse.

   Certain conditions place clients at risk for pulse alterations: heart disease, cardiac dysrhythmias, onset of sudden chest pain or acute pain from any site, invasive cardiovascular diagnostic tests, surgery, sudden infusion of large volume of IV fluid, internal or external hemorrhage, and administration of medications that alter heart function.

   b. Assess for signs and symptoms of altered stroke volume and cardiac output such as dyspnea, fatigue, chest pain, orthopnea, syncope, palpitations, jugular venous distention, edema of dependent body parts, cyanosis or pallor of skin.

   Physical signs and symptoms may indicate alteration in cardiac output or stroke volume.

2. Assess for factors that normally influence apical pulse rate and rhythm:

   Allows nurse to accurately assess presence and significance of pulse alterations.

   a. Age

   Infant's heart rate at birth ranges from 100 to 160 beats per minute at rest; by age 2, pulse rate slows to 90 to 140 beats per minute; by adolescence, rate varies between 60 and 90 beats per minute and remains so throughout adulthood; no changes occur in older adults at rest and in absence of disease.

   b. Exercise

   Physical activity requires an increase in CO that is met by an increased HR and SV; a well-conditioned client may have a slower-than-usual resting HR and returns more quickly to resting rate after exercise.

   c. Position changes

   Heart rate increases temporarily when changing from lying to sitting or standing position.

   d. Medications

   Antidysrhythmics, sympathomimetics, and cardiotonics affect rate and rhythm of pulse; large doses of narcotic analgesics can slow HR; general anesthetics slow HR; central nervous system stimulants such as caffeine can increase HR.

   e. Temperature

   Fever or exposure to warm environments increases HR; HR declines with hypothermia.

   f. Sympathetic stimulation

   Emotional stress, anxiety, or fear results in stimulation of the sympathetic nervous system, which increases HR.

3. Determine previous baseline apical rate (if available) from client's record.

   Allows nurse to assess for change in condition. Provides comparison with future apical pulse measurements.

STEP	RATIONALE

NURSING DIAGNOSES

- Ineffective tissue perfusion
- Decreased cardiac output

Related factors are individualized based on client's condition or needs.

PLANNING

1. Expected outcomes following completion of procedure:
   - Apical heart rate is within acceptable range.
   - Rhythm is regular.
2. Explain to client that apical pulse rate is to be assessed. Encourage client to relax as much as possible. Ask client not to speak while assessing pulse. If client has been active, wait 5 to 10 minutes before assessing pulse.

Adults average 60 to 100 beats per minute.
Cardiovascular status is stable.
Anxiety or activity can cause elevation in HR. Client's speech interferes with nurse's ability to hear sounds when apical pulse is measured. Apical pulse rate should be assessed at rest to allow for objective comparison of values.

IMPLEMENTATION

1. Perform hand hygiene.
2. Draw curtain around bed and/or close door.
3. Assist client to supine or sitting position. Move aside bed linen and gown to expose sternum and left side of chest.
4. Locate anatomical landmarks to identify the point of maximal impulse (PMI), also called the apical impulse (see Chapter 18). Heart is located behind and to left of sternum with base at top and apex at bottom. Find Angle of Louis just below suprasternal notch between sternal body and manubrium; it can be felt as a bony prominence (see illustrations). Slip fingers down each side of angle to find second intercostal space (ICS). Carefully move fingers down left side of sternum to fifth ICS and laterally to the left midclavicular line (MCL). A light tap felt within an area 1 to 2 cm ($\frac{1}{2}$ to 1 inch) of the PMI is reflected from the apex of the heart.
5. Place diaphragm of stethoscope in palm of hand for 5 to 10 seconds.
6. Place diaphragm of stethoscope over PMI at the fifth ICS, at the left MCL, and auscultate for normal S_1 and S_2 heart sounds (heard as "lub-dub") (see illustrations).
7. When S_1 and S_2 are heard with regularity, use watch's second hand and begin to count rate: when sweep hand hits number on dial, start counting with zero, then one, two, and so on.
8. If apical rate is regular, count for 30 seconds and multiply by 2.
9. If heart rate is irregular, or client is receiving cardiovascular medication, count for a full 1 minute (60 seconds).
10. Note regularity of any dysrhythmia (S_1 and S_2 occurring early or late after previous sequence of sounds; e.g., every third or every fourth beat is skipped).
11. Replace client's gown and bed linen; assist client in returning to comfortable position.
12. Discuss findings with client as needed.

13. Perform hand hygiene.
14. Clean earpieces and diaphragm of stethoscope with alcohol swab routinely after each use.

Reduces transmission of microorganisms.
Maintains privacy and minimizes embarrassment.
Exposes portion of chest wall for selection of auscultatory site.
Use of anatomical landmarks allows correct placement of stethoscope over apex of heart. This position enhances ability to hear heart sounds clearly. If unable to palpate the PMI, reposition client on left side. In the presence of serious heart disease, the PMI may be located to the left of the MCL or at the sixth ICS.

Warming of metal or plastic diaphragm prevents client from being startled and promotes comfort.
Allow stethoscope tubing to extend straight without kinks that would distort sound transmission. Normal sounds S_1 and S_2 are high pitched and best heard with the diaphragm.
Apical rate is determined accurately only after nurse is able to auscultate sounds clearly. Timing begins with zero. Count of one is first sound auscultated after timing begins.

Regular apical rate can be assessed within 30 seconds.

Irregular rate is more accurately assessed when measured over longer interval.
Regular occurrence of dysrhythmia within 1 minute may indicate inefficient contraction of heart and alteration in cardiac output.
Restores comfort and promotes sense of well-being.

Promotes participation in care and understanding of health status.
Reduces transmission of microorganisms.
Stethoscopes are frequently contaminated with microorganisms. Regular disinfection can control nosocomial infections.

STEP	RATIONALE

A
B
B
D

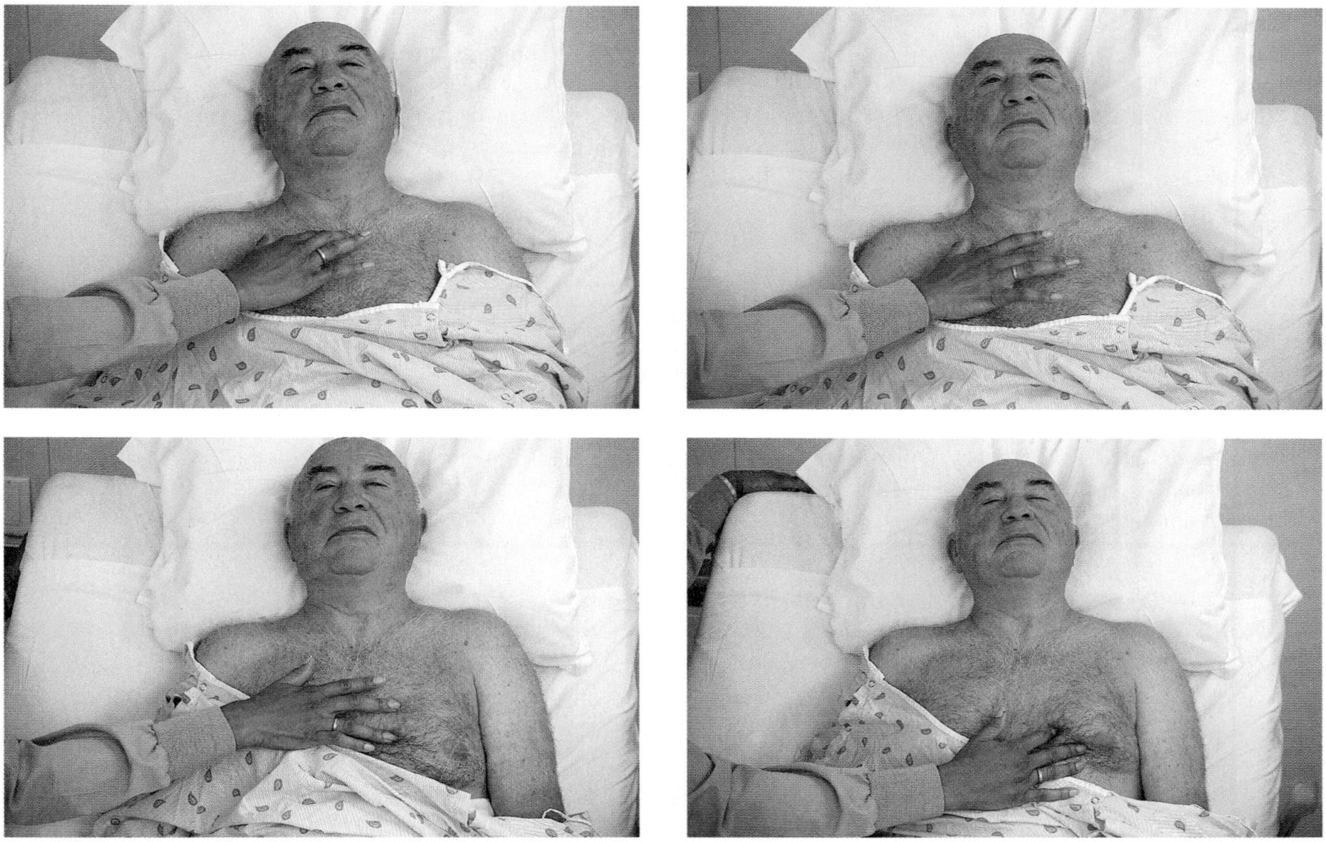

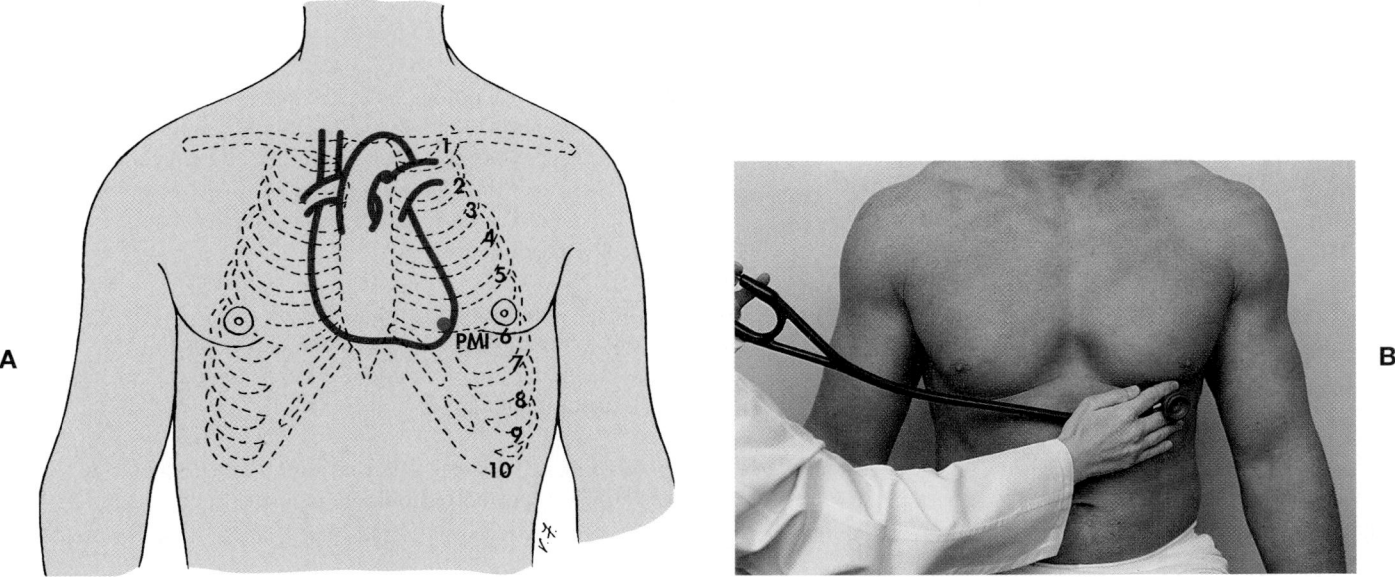

STEP 4 **A,** Nurse locates sternal notch. **B,** Nurse locates second intercostal space. **C,** Nurse locates fifth intercostal space. **D,** Nurse locates PMI at intercostal space at the midclavicular line.

A
B

STEP 6 **A,** Location of PMI in adult. **B,** Stethoscope over PMI.

STEP	RATIONALE

EVALUATION

1. If pulse is assessed for the first time, establish apical rate as baseline if it is within an acceptable range.

   Used to compare future pulse assessments.

2. Compare apical rate and character with client's previous baseline and acceptable range of heart rate for client's age.

   Allows nurse to assess for change in client's condition and for presence of cardiac alteration.

- *Critical Decision Point*
  If apical rate is abnormal or irregular, repeat measurement or have another nurse conduct measurement. Original measurement may result from error by assessor. Second measurement confirms initial findings of abnormal HR.

Recording and Reporting

- Record apical rate and rhythm on vital sign flow sheet (see Figure 17-5), record, or nurses' notes.
- Record any signs or symptoms of alterations in CO in nurses' notes.
- Report abnormal findings to nurse in charge or physician.

Unexpected Outcomes	Related Interventions
1. Apical rate over 100 (tachycardia).	• Identify related data, including pain, fear or anxiety, recent exercise, low BP, blood loss, elevated temperature or inadequate oxygenation. • Observe for symptoms associated with abnormal cardiac function. · Dyspnea, fatigue, chest pain, orthopnea, syncope, palpitations, jugular vein distention, edema of body parts, cyanosis or pallor of the skin.

2. Apical rate under 60 (bradycardia).	• Observe for symptoms associated with altered tissue perfusion.
	    · Pallor
	    · Cyanosis
	    · Cold extremity
	• Have another nurse assess apical pulse.
	• Report findings to nurse in charge and/or physician. It may be necessary to withhold prescribed medications that alter heart rate and regularity, such as digoxin and antiarrhythmics, until the physician can evaluate the need to alter the dosage.

3. Irregular apical rhythm indicating a potential for inefficient ventricular ejection and poor CO.	• Assess for pulse deficit (Box 17-5). • Report findings to nurse in charge and/or physician. • An electrocardiogram may be ordered to detect cardiac conduction alteration.
4. Occasional premature ventricular contractions (PVCs) are common in most persons. However, frequency of PVCs increases with heart disease. Nurse will hear premature sequence of S_1 and S_2 and then short pause before normal S_1 and S_2 return.	• Numerous PVCs or PVCs that alternate with a normal heartbeat repeatedly should be reported to physician.

BOX 17-5 Procedural Guideline
Assessing apical-radial pulse

An inefficient contraction of the heart that fails to transmit a pulse wave to the peripheral pulse site creates a pulse deficit. Pulse deficits are frequently associated with dysrhythmias and warn of potential alteration of cardiac output. To assess for a pulse deficit, the nurse and a colleague assess a peripheral pulse rate and the apical pulse rate simultaneously and compare the measurements. The difference between the rates is the pulse deficit.

DELEGATION CONSIDERATIONS

The skill of radial pulse palpation may be delegated to assistive personnel while the nurse assesses the apical pulse. However, the nurse is responsible for determining the presence of a pulse deficit and follow-up assessments.

EQUIPMENT

Stethoscope; watch with second hand or digital display; pen, pencil, vital sign flow sheet or record form; alcohol swab

ASSESSMENT

1. Determine need to assess for pulse deficit. Clients with irregular heart rate and signs and symptoms such as dyspnea, fatigue, chest pain, and palpitations may indicate decreased cardiac output.
2. Perform hand hygiene.

3. Draw curtain around bed and/or close door.
4. Assist client to supine or sitting position. Move aside bed linen and gown to expose sternum and left side of chest.
5. Locate apical and radial pulse sites. If two nurses are available, one nurse auscultates the apical pulse (see Skill 17-3) and one nurse palpates the radial pulse (see Skill 17-2).
6. The nurse measuring the radial pulse and holding the watch states "start" to ensure that the pulse rate is measured simultaneously.
7. Both nurses count the pulse rate for 60 seconds simultaneously. The count ends when the nurse taking the radial pulse states "stop." Sixty seconds is required when a discrepancy between the pulse sites is expected or the rhythm is irregular.
8. Subtract the radial rate from the apical rate to obtain the pulse deficit. The pulse deficit reflects the number of ineffective cardiac contractions in 1 minute.
9. If a pulse deficit is noted, assess for other signs and symptoms of decreased cardiac output.
10. Discuss findings with client as needed.
11. Perform hand hygiene; clean earpieces and diaphragm of stethoscope with alcohol swab routinely after each use.
12. Record the apical pulse, the radial pulse and site, and the pulse deficit in the nurses' notes. Inform the nurse in charge or physician of the presence of a pulse deficit.

Teaching Considerations

- Caregivers of clients taking certain prescribed cardiotonic or antidysrhythmic medications should learn to assess apical pulse rates to detect side effects of medications.

Pediatric Considerations

- Point of maximal impulse of an infant is usually located at the third to fourth ICS near the left sternal border.
- In infants and children less than 2 years an apical pulse is more reliable and should be counted for a full minute because of possible irregularities in rhythm (Hockenberry and others, 2003).
- Breath holding in an infant or child affects apical pulse rate.

Gerontological Considerations

- The PMI may be difficult to palpate in an older adult because the anterior-posterior diameter of the chest increases with age, and the heart becomes repositioned as a result of left ventricular enlargement.
- When assessing older adult women with sagging breast tissue, gently lift the breast tissue and place the stethoscope at the fifth ICS or the lower edge of the breast.
- Heart sound may be muffled or difficult to hear in older adults because of an increase in air space in the lungs.

Home Care Considerations

- Assess home environment to determine which room affords a quiet environment for auscultation of apical rate.

SKILL 17-4 Assessing Respirations

The mechanism of respiration exchanges oxygen (O_2) and carbon dioxide (CO_2) between cells of the body and the atmosphere. Three processes are involved in respiration: *ventilation,* mechanical movement of gases into and out of the lungs; *diffusion,* movement of O_2 and CO_2 between the alveoli and the red blood cells; and *perfusion,* distribution of red blood cells to and from the pulmonary capillaries. The nurse directly assesses ventilation by observing the rate, depth, and rhythm of respiratory movements. Accurate assessment of respiration depends on recognizing normal thoracic and abdominal movements. Normal breathing is active and passive. On inspiration the diaphragm contracts, causing abdominal organs to move downward and forward, thereby increasing the vertical size of the chest cavity. At the same time, the ribs lift upward and outward and the sternum lifts outward to aid the transverse expansion of the lungs. On expiration the diaphragm relaxes upward, the ribs and sternum return to their relaxed position, and the abdominal organs return to their original position (Figure 17-8). During quiet breathing the chest wall gently rises and falls. More energy is required during inspiration than during expiration. Little energy is needed to expire air out of the lungs. Expiration is an active process only during exercise, voluntary hyperventilation, and certain disease states.

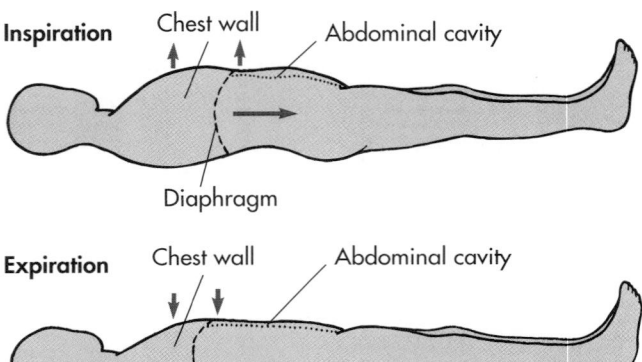

FIGURE 17-8 Illustration of diaphragmatic and chest wall movement during inspiration and expiration.

DELEGATION CONSIDERATIONS

The skill of respiration measurement can be delegated to assistive personnel unless the client is considered unstable. Before delegating this skill the nurse must:

- Inform assistive personnel if the client is at risk for increased or decreased respiratory rate or irregular respirations
- Provide assistive personnel the frequency of measurement for specific client
- Inform assistive personnel of the usual values for the client
- Instruct assistive personnel of the need to report any abnormalities that should be reconfirmed by the nurse

EQUIPMENT

- ❏ Wristwatch with second hand or digital display
- ❏ Pen, pencil, vital sign flow sheet or record form

STEP	RATIONALE

■ ASSESSMENT

1. Determine need to assess client's respirations:
   a. Note risk factors for respiratory alterations.

Conditions that place client at risk for ventilatory alterations detected by changes in respiratory rate, depth, and rhythm: fever, pain and anxiety, diseases of chest wall or muscles, constrictive chest or abdominal dressings, presence of abdominal incisions, gastric distention, chronic pulmonary disease (emphysema, bronchitis, asthma), traumatic injury to chest wall with or without collapse of underlying lung tissue, presence of a chest tube, respiratory infection (pneumonia, acute bronchitis), pulmonary edema and emboli, head injury with damage to brain stem, and anemia.

   b. Assess for signs and symptoms of respiratory alterations, such as bluish or cyanotic appearance of nail beds, lips, mucous membranes, and skin; restlessness, irritability, confusion, reduced level of consciousness; pain during inspiration; labored or difficult breathing; orthopnea; use of accessory muscles; adventitious breath sounds (Chapter 18), inability to breathe spontaneously; thick, frothy, blood-tinged, or copious sputum produced on coughing.

Physical signs and symptoms may indicate alterations in respiratory status related to ventilation.

2. Assess for factors that influence character of respirations:

Allows nurse to accurately assess for presence and significance of respiratory alterations.

   a. Exercise

Respirations increase in rate and depth to meet the need for additional oxygen and rid the body of CO_2.

   b. Anxiety

Respirations increase in rate and depth as a result of stimulation by the sympathetic nervous system.

   c. Acute pain

Pain alters rate and rhythm of respirations; breaths become shallow. Client may inhibit or splint chest wall movement when pain is in area of chest or abdomen.

   d. Smoking

Chronic smoking changes pulmonary airways, resulting in an increased respiratory rate at rest when not smoking.

   e. Medications

Narcotic analgesics, general anesthetics, and sedative hypnotics depress rate and depth; amphetamines and cocaine may increase rate and depth, bronchodilators cause dilation of airways that ultimately can slow respiratory rate.

   f. Body position

Standing or sitting erect promotes full ventilatory movement and lung expansion; stooped or slumped posture impairs ventilatory movement; lying flat prevents full chest expansion.

   g. Neurological injury

Damage to the brain stem impairs the respiratory center and inhibits rate and rhythm.

STEP	RATIONALE

    h. Hemoglobin function

Decreased hemoglobin levels lower the amount of oxygen carried in the blood, which results in increased respiratory rate to increase oxygen delivery. An increase in altitude lowers the amount of saturated hemoglobin, which increases respiratory rate and depth.

3. Assess pertinent laboratory values:
    a. Arterial blood gases (ABGs) (values may vary slightly among institutions) normal ranges are:
       pH 7.35 to 7.45
       $PaCO_2$ 35 to 45 mm Hg
       PaO_2 80 to 100 mm Hg
       SaO_2 94% to 98%

Arterial blood gases measure arterial blood pH, partial pressure of O_2 and CO_2, and arterial O_2 saturation, which reflects client's oxygenation status.

    b. Pulse oximetry (SpO_2): normal SpO_2 90% to 100%; 85% to 89% may be acceptable for certain chronic disease conditions; less than 85% is abnormal (Skill 17-6).

SpO_2 less than 85% is often accompanied by changes in respiratory rate, depth, and rhythm.

    c. Complete blood count (CBC): normal CBC for adults (values may vary within institutions): hemoglobin: 14 to 18 g/100 ml, males; 12 to 16 g/100 ml, females. Hematocrit: 40% to 54%, males; 38% to 47%, females. Red blood cell count: 4.6 to 6.2 million/mm^3, males; 4.2 to 5.4 million/mm^3, females.

Complete blood count measures red blood cell count, volume of red blood cells, and concentration of hemoglobin, which reflects client's capacity to carry O_2.

4. Determine previous baseline respiratory rate (if available) from client's record.

Allows nurse to assess for change in condition. Provides comparison with future respiratory measurements.

NURSING DIAGNOSES

- Activity intolerance
- Ineffective airway clearance
- Impaired gas exchange

- Ineffective breathing pattern
- Impaired spontaneous ventilation

Related factors are individualized based on client's condition or needs.

PLANNING

1. Expected outcomes following completion of procedure:
- Respiratory rate is within acceptable range.
- Respirations are regular and of normal depth.

Adults average 12 to 20 respirations per minute.
Respiratory status is stable.

2. If client has been active, wait 5 to 10 minutes before assessing respirations.

Exercise increases respiratory rate and depth. Respirations should be assessed at rest to allow for objective comparison of values.

3. Assess respirations after pulse measurement in adult.

Inconspicuous assessment of respirations immediately after pulse assessment prevents client from consciously or unintentionally altering rate and depth of breathing.

4. Be sure client is in comfortable position, preferably sitting or lying with the head of the bed elevated 45 to 60 degrees.

Sitting erect promotes full ventilatory movement. Position of discomfort may cause client to breathe more rapidly.

- *Critical Decision Point*
Clients with difficulty breathing (dyspnea), such as those with congestive heart failure or abdominal ascites or in late stages of pregnancy should be assessed in the position of greatest comfort. Repositioning may increase the work of breathing, which will increase respiratory rate.

STEP	RATIONALE

IMPLEMENTATION

1. Draw curtain around bed and/or close door. Perform hand hygiene.

Maintains privacy. Prevents transmission of microorganisms.

2. Be sure client's chest is visible. If necessary, move bed linen or gown.

Ensures clear view of chest wall and abdominal movements.

3. Place client's arm in relaxed position across the abdomen or lower chest, or place nurse's hand directly over client's upper abdomen (see illustration).

A similar position used during pulse assessment allows respiratory rate assessment to be inconspicuous. Client's or nurse's hand rises and falls during respiratory cycle.

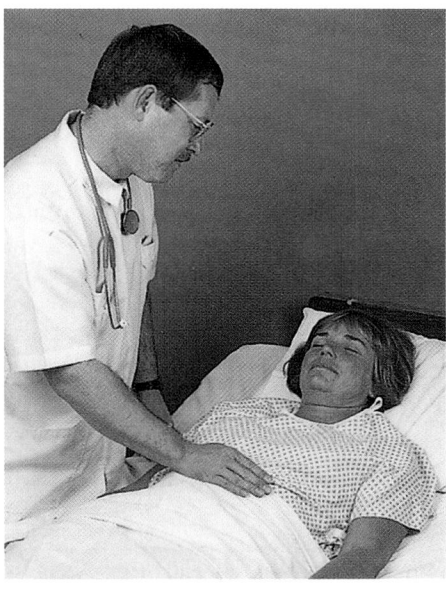

STEP 3 Nurse's hand over client's abdomen to check respiration.

4. Observe complete respiratory cycle (one inspiration and one expiration).

Rate is accurately determined only after nurse has viewed respiratory cycle.

5. After cycle is observed, look at watch's second hand and begin to count rate: when sweep hand hits number on dial, begin time frame, counting one with first full respiratory cycle.

Timing begins with count of one. Respirations occur more slowly than pulse; thus timing does not begin with zero.

6. If rhythm is regular, count number of respirations in 30 seconds and multiply by 2. If rhythm is irregular, less than 12, or greater than 20, count for 1 full minute.

Respiratory rate is equivalent to number of respirations per minute. Suspected irregularities require assessment for at least 1 minute (Table 17-2).

7. Note depth of respirations, subjectively assessed by observing degree of chest wall movement while counting rate. Nurse can also objectively assess depth by palpating chest wall excursion or auscultating the posterior thorax after rate has been counted (Chapter 18). Depth is described as shallow, normal, or deep.

Character of ventilatory movement may reveal specific disease state restricting volume of air from moving into and out of the lungs.

8. Note rhythm of ventilatory cycle. Normal breathing is regular and uninterrupted. Sighing should not be confused with abnormal rhythm. Periodically people unconsciously take single deep breaths or sighs to expand small airways prone to collapse.

Character of ventilations can reveal specific types of alterations.

9. Replace bed linen and client's gown.

Restores comfort and promotes sense of well-being.

10. Perform hand hygiene.

Reduces transmission of microorganisms.

11. Discuss findings with client as needed.

Promotes participation in care and understanding of health status.

STEP	RATIONALE

EVALUATION

1. If respirations are assessed for the first time, establish rate, rhythm, and depth as baseline if within acceptable range.
2. Compare respirations with client's previous baseline and usual rate, rhythm, and depth.
3. Correlate respiratory rate, depth, and rhythm with data obtained from pulse oximetry and arterial blood gas measurements if available.

- Used to compare future respiratory assessment.

- Allows nurse to assess for changes in client's condition and for presence of respiratory alterations.
- Evaluation of ventilation, perfusion, and diffusion are interrelated.

TABLE 17-2 ALTERATIONS IN BREATHING PATTERN

ALTERATION	DESCRIPTION
Bradypnea	Rate of breathing is regular but abnormally slow (less than 12 breaths per minute).
Tachypnea	Rate of breathing is regular but abnormally rapid (greater than 20 breaths per minute).
Hyperpnea	Respirations are increased in depth; occurs normally during exercise.
Hyperventilation	Rate and depth of respirations increase. Hypocarbia, an abnormally low level of carbon dioxide in the blood, may occur.
Hypoventilation	Respiratory rate is abnormally low; depth of ventilation may be depressed. Hypercarbia, an abnormally elevated level of carbon dioxide in the blood, may occur.
Apnea	Respirations cease for several seconds. Persistent cessation results in respiratory arrest.
Cheyne-Stokes respiration	Respiratory rate and depth are irregular, characterized by alternating periods of apnea and hyperventilation. Respiratory cycle begins with slow, shallow breaths that gradually increase to abnormal rate and depth. The pattern reverses, breathing slows and becomes shallow, climaxing in apnea before respiration resumes.
Kussmaul's respiration	Respirations are abnormally deep, regular, and increased in rate. Common in diabetic ketoacidosis.
Biot's respiration	Respirations are abnormally shallow for two to three breaths followed by irregular period of apnea.

Recording and Reporting

- Record respiratory rate on vital sign flow sheet or record (see Figure 17-5). Record abnormal depth and rhythm in narrative form in nurses' notes.
- Measurement of respiratory rate after administration of specific therapies is documented in narrative form in the nurses' notes.
- Indicate type and amount of oxygen therapy, if used, in nurses' notes.
- Report abnormal findings to nurse in charge or physician.

Unexpected Outcomes	Related Interventions
1. Respiratory rate is below 12 (bradypnea) or above 20 (tachypnea). Rhythm may be irregular (see Table 17-2). Depth of respirations increased or decreased.	• Assess for conditions that restrict full expansion of chest wall. • Position client in a comfortable Fowler's or high-Fowler's position. • Check for tight dressings. • Maintain patency of any existing artificial airway. • Notify physician if alteration continues, and be prepared to initiate oxygen therapy as needed. An ABG test or chest x-ray examination may be ordered to evaluate nature of respiratory problem.
2. Client demonstrates Kussmaul's, Cheyne-Stokes, or Biot's respirations (see Table 17-2).	• Notify physician, and anticipate immediate therapy will be ordered.

Teaching Considerations

- Clients who demonstrate decreased ventilation may benefit from being taught deep breathing and coughing exercises (see Chapter 22).
- Instruct family caregiver to contact home care nurse or physician if unusual fluctuations in respiratory rate occur.

Pediatric Considerations

- Assessment of respiratory rate should be done before other vital signs or assessments if able to view movement of chest wall or abdomen. This may allow assessment of rate and rhythm before the child becomes anxious due to stranger anxiety or fear of other assessment procedures.
- Acceptable average respiratory rate (breaths per minute) for newborns is 35 to 40; infant (6 months to 1 year) is 30 to 50; toddler (2 years) is 25; and children from 3 to 12 years range from 18 to 23 (Hockenberry and others, 2003).
- Infant's respirations are primarily diaphragmatic and thus observed by abdominal movement.
- Infants tend to breathe less regularly.
- Nurse can simply observe infant or young child while chest and abdomen are exposed.

- A young child may breathe slowly for a few seconds and then suddenly breathe more rapidly.
- Cardiorespiratory monitors may be used for infants or newborns that are at risk for respiratory compromise or arrest.

Gerontological Considerations

- Aging causes ossification of costal cartilage and downward slant of ribs, resulting in more rigid rib cage, which reduces chest wall expansion. Kyphosis and scoliosis that can occur in older adults may also restrict chest expansion.
- Depth of respirations tends to decrease with aging (Sheahan and Musialowski, 2001).
- The change in lung function with aging results in respiratory rates that are generally higher in older adults with a range of 16 to 25 breaths per minute (Lueckenotte, 2000).
- Older adults may depend more on accessory abdominal muscles during respiration than weakened thoracic muscles.

Home Care Considerations

- Assess for environmental factors in the home that may influence client's respiratory rate such as secondhand smoke, poor ventilation, or gas fumes.

SKILL 17-5 Assessing Arterial Blood Pressure

Blood pressure is the force exerted by the blood against the vessel walls. During a normal cardiac cycle, BP reaches a peak that is followed by a trough, or low point, in the cycle. The peak pressure occurs when the heart's ventricular contraction, or systole, forces blood under high pressure into the aorta. When the ventricles relax, the blood remaining in the arteries exerts a minimum or diastolic pressure. Diastolic pressure is the minimal pressure exerted against the arterial wall at all times.

The standard unit for measuring BP is millimeters of mercury (mm Hg). The measurement indicates the height to which the BP can sustain the column of mercury. The most common technique of measuring BP is auscultation using a sphygmomanometer and stethoscope. As the sphygmomanometer cuff is deflated, the five different sounds heard over an artery are called Korotkoff phases. The sound in each phase has unique characteristics (Figure 17-9). Blood pressure is recorded with the systolic reading (first Korotkoff sound) before the diastolic (beginning of the fifth Korotkoff sound) (Beevers and others, 2001b). The difference between systolic pressure and diastolic pressure is the pulse pressure. For a BP of 120/80, the pulse pressure is 40.

Blood pressure reflects various interrelated hemodynamic factors within the circulatory system: cardiac output, peripheral resistance, blood volume, blood viscosity, and vessel wall elasticity. Blood pressure has a direct relation-

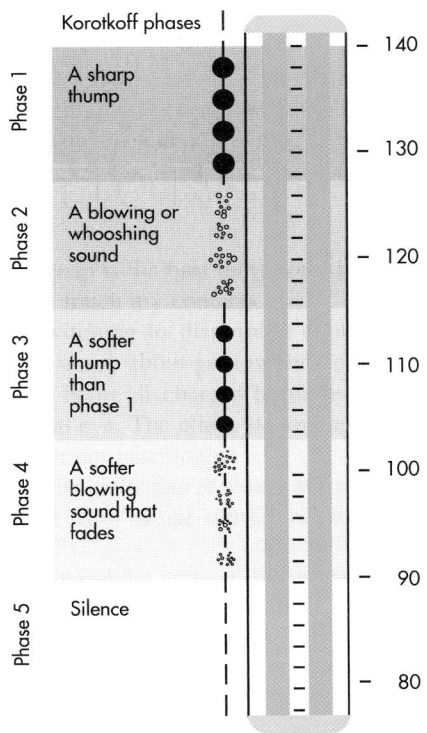

FIGURE 17-9 The sounds auscultated during blood pressure measurement can be differentiated into five Korotkoff phases. In this example, the blood pressure is 140/90 mm Hg.

ship to cardiac output (CO) and peripheral vascular resistance (R):

$$BP = CO \times R$$

As CO increases, more blood is pumped into the arterial system, causing systolic BP to rise. When the size of the arteries and arterioles decreases, the resistance to blood flow increases, causing the BP to rise. In contrast, as vessels dilate and vascular resistance falls, BP drops. The volume of blood circulating within the vascular system affects BP. Normally blood volume remains constant: 5000 ml in an adult. However, if volume increases, such as after a rapid IV infusion, pressure exerted against arterial walls rises. When circulating blood volume falls, as in the case of hemorrhage or dehydration, BP falls. When the thickness or viscosity of the blood increases, the heart must contract more forcefully to move the blood through the circulatory system and BP rises. When vessel walls are elastic, they are easily distensible and can accommodate changes in pressure. Arteriosclerotic vessels lose their elasticity, no longer yield to pressure, and the BP rises.

HYPERTENSION

Hypertension is a major factor underlying death from heart attack and stroke in the United States and Canada. The Joint National Committee on Prevention, Detection, Evaluation, and Treatment of High Blood Pressure (2003) has set criteria for determining categories of hypertension (Table 17-3). Prehypertension is a designation for clients at high risk of developing hypertension. In these clients early intervention by adoption of healthy lifestyles could reduce the risk or prevent hypertension. Hypertension is defined as systolic blood pressure (SBP) of 140 mm Hg or greater, diastolic blood pressure (DBP) of 90 mm Hg or greater, or taking antihypertensive medication (Joint National Committee, 2003). The diagnosis of hypertension in adults is made on the average of two or more readings taken at each of two or more visits after an initial screening.

One BP recording revealing a high SBP or DBP does not qualify as a diagnosis of hypertension. However, if the nurse assesses a high reading (for example, 150/90 mm Hg), the client should be encouraged to return for another checkup within 2 months (Table 17-4).

HYPOTENSION

Hypotension is generally considered present when the systolic blood pressure falls to 90 mm Hg or below. Although some adults have a low blood pressure normally, for the majority of people, low blood pressure is an abnormal finding associated with illness (e.g., hemorrhage or myocardial infarction). Orthostatic hypotension, also referred to as postural hypotension, occurs when a normotensive person develops symptoms (e.g., light-headedness or dizziness) and low blood pressure when rising to an upright position (see Chapter 11). In severe cases, loss of consciousness may occur. Normally, when a healthy individual changes from a lying to sitting or standing position, the peripheral blood vessels in the legs constrict, the heart rate and contractility increase, and blood pressure re-

TABLE 17-3 CLASSIFICATION OF BLOOD PRESSURE FOR ADULTS AGE 18 YEARS AND OLDER*

CATEGORY	SYSTOLIC (mm Hg)		DIASTOLIC (mm Hg)
Normal	<120	and	<80
Prehypertension	120-139	or	80-89
Stage 1	140-159	or	90-99
Stage 2	≥160	or	≥100

From The seventh report of the Joint National Committee on Prevention, Detection, Evaluation and Treatment of High Blood Pressure, *JAMA* 289:2560, 2003.

*Based on the average of two or more readings taken at each of two or more visits after an initial screening. Client is not taking antihypertensive drugs and not acutely ill. When systolic and diastolic blood pressures fall into different categories, the higher category should be selected to classify the individual's blood pressure status. For example, 160/92 mm Hg should be classified as stage 2 hypertension.

TABLE 17-4 RECOMMENDATIONS FOR BLOOD PRESSURE FOLLOW-UP

INITIAL BLOOD PRESSURE	FOLLOW-UP RECOMMENDED*
Normal	Recheck in 2 years.
Prehypertension	Recheck in 1 year.†
Stage 1 hypertension	Confirm within 2 months.†
Stage 2 hypertension	Evaluate or refer to source of care within 1 month. For those with higher pressure (e.g., >180/110 mm Hg), evaluate and treat immediately or within 1 week, depending on clinical situation and complications.

*Modify the scheduling of follow-up according to reliable information about past BP measurements, other cardiovascular risk factors, or target organ damage.

†Provide advice about lifestyle modifications.

mains adequate to perfuse the heart and brain. Orthostatic changes in vital signs are good indicators of blood volume depletion. Some medications can cause orthostatic hypotension if misused, especially in young clients and older adults.

BLOOD PRESSURE EQUIPMENT

Arterial blood pressure may be measured either directly (invasively) or indirectly (noninvasively). The direct method requires electronic monitoring equipment and the insertion of a thin catheter into an artery. The risks of invasive blood pressure monitoring require use in an intensive care setting.

The more common noninvasive method requires use of the sphygmomanometer and stethoscope (Box 17-6). A sphygmomanometer includes a pressure manometer, an occlusive cloth or disposable vinyl cuff that encloses an inflatable rubber bladder, and a pressure bulb with a release valve that inflates the bladder (Figure 17-11). There are two types of manometers: aneroid and mercury. The aneroid manometer has a glass-enclosed circular gauge containing a needle that registers millimeter calibrations. Metal parts in the aneroid manometer are subject to temperature expansion

BOX 17-6 Procedural Guideline
Noninvasive automatic blood pressure measurement

Many different styles of electronic blood pressure machines are available to determine BP automatically (Figure 17-10). Electronic BP machines rely on an electronic sensor to detect the vibrations caused by the rush of blood through an artery. When the cuff is deflated, one style of BP machine determines the initial burst of oscillations and translates the information into a systolic pressure reading. The diastolic measurement is made when the oscillations are lowest, just before they stop. Other styles of electronic BP machines record the mean blood pressure and compute the systolic and diastolic BP from a programmed formula (Yucha, 2001). Although electronic BP machines are fast and free the care provider for other activities, the nurse must consider the advantages and limitations of electronic BP machines (Box 17-7). The devices are used when frequent assessment is required, such as in critically ill or potentially unstable clients, during or after invasive procedures, or when therapies require frequent monitoring.

DELEGATION CONSIDERATIONS
The use of an electronic BP machine can be delegated to assistive personnel unless the client is considered unstable. Before delegating this skill the nurse must:
- Provide assistive personnel the frequency of blood pressure measurement for select client
- Determine that assistive personnel are aware of the usual values for the client
- Inform assistive personnel if the client has alterations affecting the appropriate limb for blood pressure measurement
- Inform assistive personnel of appropriate-size blood pressure cuff for designated extremity
- Instruct assistive personnel of the need to report any abnormalities that should be reconfirmed by the nurse

EQUIPMENT
Electronic BP machine, BP cuff of appropriate size as recommended by manufacturer

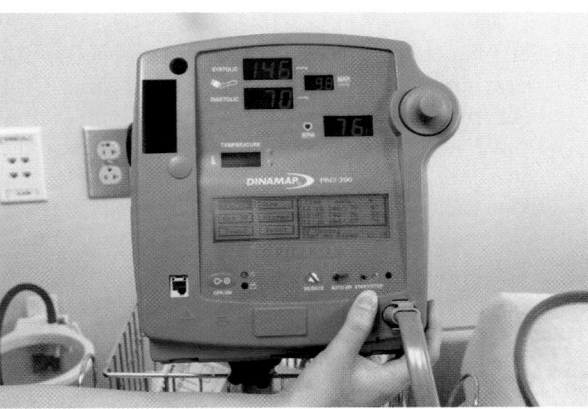

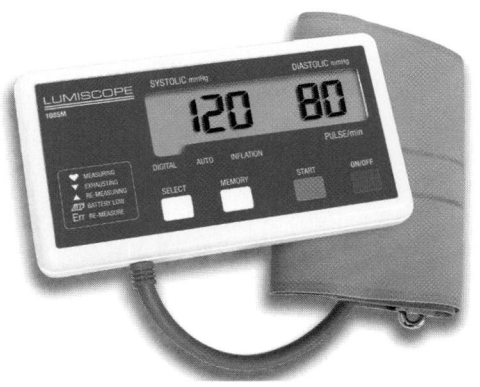

FIGURE **17-10** Variety of noninvasive electronic blood pressure machines. (Photo courtesy the Lumiscope Company.)

BOX 17-7   Advantages and Limitations of Electronic BP Machines

ADVANTAGES

Ease of use.
Efficient when frequent repeated measurements are indicated.
Ability to use a stethoscope not required.
Allows BP to be recorded more frequently, as often as every 15 seconds with accuracy (Yarrows and others, 2001).

LIMITATIONS

Expensive.
Requires source of electricity.
Requires space to position machine.
Sensitive to outside motion interference and cannot be used in clients with seizures, tremors, or shivers.
Not accurate for hypotensive clients or in conditions with reduced blood flow (e.g., hypothermia) (Anwar and White, 2001).
Accuracy standards for electronic blood pressure machine manufacturers are voluntary (Jones and others, 2003).
Vulnerable to error in clinical circumstances (Jones and others, 2003):
- Arrhythmias
- Older adults
- Obese extremity

Continued

BOX 17-6 Procedural Guideline
Noninvasive automatic blood pressure measurement—cont'd

ASSESSMENT

1. Determine the appropriateness of using electronic BP measurement. Clients with irregular heart rate, peripheral vascular disease, seizures, tremors, and shivering are not candidates for this device.
2. Determine best site for cuff placement (see Skill 17-5, step 3)
3. Assist client to comfortable position, either lying or sitting. Plug in device to electrical outlet and place device near client, ensuring that connector hose, between cuff and machine, will reach.
4. Locate on/off switch, and turn on machine to enable device to self-test computer systems.
5. Select appropriate cuff size for client extremity (see Figure 17-11) and appropriate cuff for machine. Electronic BP cuff and machine must be matched by manufacturer and cannot be interchanged.
6. Expose upper arm fully by removing constricting clothing, which ensures proper cuff application. Do not place blood pressure cuff over clothing
7. Prepare BP cuff by manually squeezing all the air out of the cuff and connecting cuff to connector hose.
8. Wrap flattened cuff snugly around extremity, verifying that only one finger can fit between cuff and client's skin. Make sure the "artery" arrow marked on the outside of the cuff is correctly placed (see illustration).
9. Verify that connector hose between cuff and machine is not kinked. Kinking prevents proper inflation and deflation of cuff.

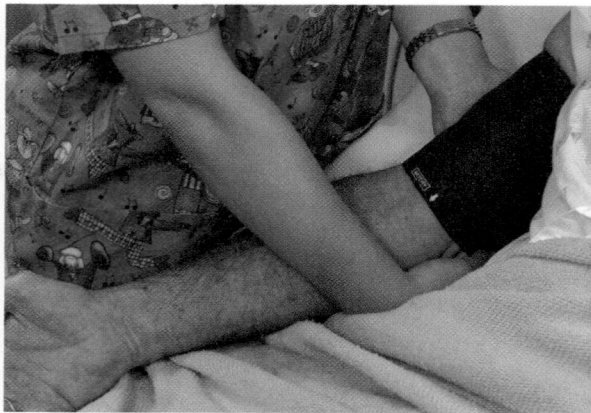

STEP **8** Aligning BP cuff arrow with brachial artery.

10. Following manufacturer's directions, set the frequency control for automatic or manual, then press start button. The first BP measurement will pump the cuff to a peak pressure of about 180 mm Hg. After this pressure is reached, the machine begins a deflation sequence that determines the BP. The first reading determines the peak pressure inflation for additional measurements.
11. When deflation is complete, digital display will provide most recent values and flash time in minutes that has elapsed since the measurement occurred.

• *Critical Decision Point*
If unable to obtain BP with electronic device, verify machine connections (e.g., plugged into working electrical outlet, hose-cuff connections tight, machine on, correct cuff). Repeat electronic blood pressure; if unable to obtain, use auscultatory technique (Skill 17-5).

12. Set frequency of BP measurements, upper and lower alarm limits for systolic, diastolic, and mean BP readings. Intervals between BP measurements can be set from 1 to 90 minutes. The nurse determines frequency and alarm limits based on client's acceptable range of blood pressure, nursing judgment, and physician order.
13. Additional readings, which may be needed for unstable clients, can be obtained at any time by pressing the start button. Pressing the cancel button immediately deflates the cuff.
14. If frequent BP measurements are required, cuff may be left in place. Remove cuff every 2 hours to assess underlying skin integrity and if possible, alternate blood pressure sites. Clients with abnormal bleeding tendencies are at risk for microvascular rupture from repeated inflations. When electronic BP machine no longer used, clean BP cuff according to facility policy to reduce transmission of microorganisms.
15. Discuss findings with client. Perform hand hygiene.
16. Compare electronic BP readings with auscultatory BP measurements to verify the accuracy of electronic BP device.
17. Record BP and site assessed on vital sign flow sheet (see Figure 17-5) or nurses' notes; record any signs or symptoms of BP alterations in narrative form in nurses' notes; report abnormal findings to nurse in charge or physician.

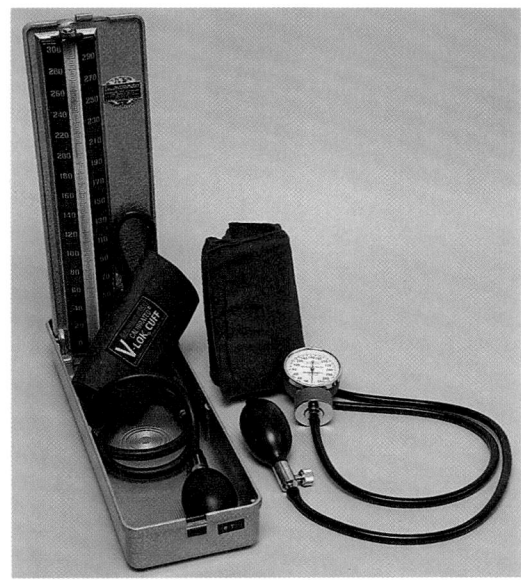

FIGURE **17-11** Mercury and aneroid sphygmomanometers.

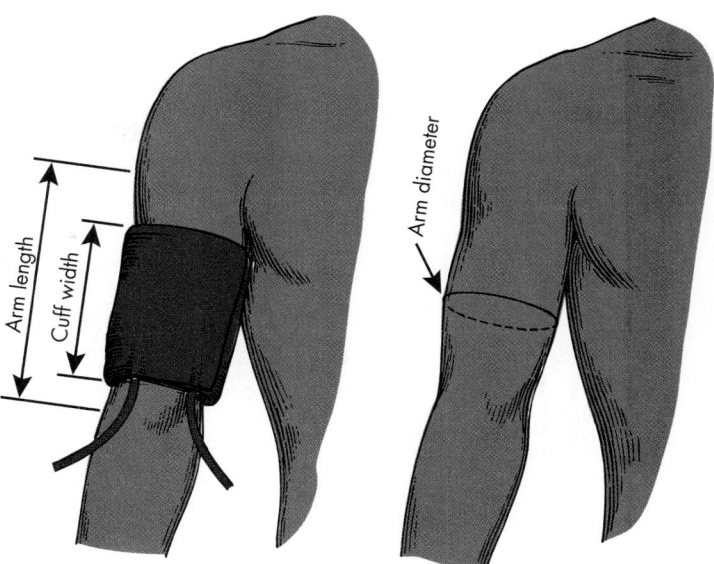

FIGURE **17-12** Guidelines for proper blood pressure cuff size. Cuff width = 20% more than upper arm diameter, or 40% of circumference and two thirds of upper arm length.

and contraction and must be recalibrated at least every 6 months to verify their accuracy (Jones and others, 2003). Before using the aneroid manometer, the nurse must be sure the needle points to zero.

The mercury manometer, once the gold standard for measuring blood pressure, is less commonly found because it is an upright tube containing mercury, a hazardous substance. Many municipalities have prohibited the sale or use of mercury-containing devices. However, some facilities or nursing units may have mercury manometers. Pressure created by inflation of the bladder moves the column of mercury up the tube against the force of gravity. Millimeter calibrations mark the height of the mercury column. To ensure accurate readings, the mercury column should fall freely when pressure is released and always be at zero when the cuff is deflated. Mercury manometers may be wall mounted or portable. Accurate readings are obtained by looking at the height or meniscus level of the mercury at eye level. Looking up or down at the mercury results in distorted readings.

The release valves of both mercury and aneroid sphygmomanometers should be clean and freely moveable in either direction. The valve, when closed, should hold the mercury or pressure constant. A sticky valve makes pressure cuff deflation hard to regulate. The pressure bulb and tubing should be airtight.

Cloth or disposable vinyl compression cuffs contain an inflatable bladder and come in several different sizes. The size selected is proportional to the circumference of the limb being assessed (Figure 17-12). Ideally the width of the cuff should be 40% of the circumference (or 20% wider than the diameter) of the midpoint of the limb on which the cuff is to be used. The bladder enclosed within the cuff should encircle at least 80%

TABLE 17-5 COMMON MISTAKES IN BLOOD PRESSURE ASSESSMENT	
ERROR	**EFFECT**
Bladder or cuff too wide	False low reading
Bladder or cuff too narrow or too short	False high reading
Cuff wrapped too loosely or unevenly	False high reading
Deflating cuff too slowly	False high diastolic reading
Deflating cuff too quickly	False low systolic and false high diastolic reading
Arm below heart level	False high reading
Arm above heart level	False low reading
Arm not supported	False high reading
Stethoscope that fits poorly or impairment of the examiner's hearing, causing sounds to be muffled	False low systolic and false high diastolic reading
Stethoscope applied too firmly against antecubital fossa	False low diastolic reading
Inflating too slowly	False high diastolic reading
Repeating assessments too quickly	False low systolic reading
Inaccurate inflation level	False low systolic reading
Multiple examiners using different Korotkoff sounds for diastolic readings	False high systolic and false low diastolic reading

of the upper arm (Joint National Committee, 2003). Many adults require a large adult cuff. A regular-size cuff holds a bladder in the width of 12 to 13 cm (4.8 to 5.2 inches) and the length of 22 to 23 cm (8.5 to 9 inches). An improperly fitting cuff produces inaccurate BP readings (Table 17-5).

DELEGATION CONSIDERATIONS

The skill of blood pressure measurement can be delegated to assistive personnel unless the client is considered unstable. Before delegating this skill the nurse must:

- Inform assistive personnel of frequency of blood pressure measurement for select client
- Determine that assistive personnel are aware of the usual values for the client
- Inform assistive personnel if the client has alterations affecting the appropriate limb for blood pressure measurement
- Provide assistive personnel the appropriate-size blood pressure cuff for designated extremity
- Notify assistive personnel if the client is at risk for orthostatic hypotension
- Instruct assistive personnel of the need to report any abnormalities that should be reconfirmed by the nurse

EQUIPMENT

- ❏ Aneroid sphygmomanometer
- ❏ Cloth or disposable vinyl pressure cuff of appropriate size for client's extremity
- ❏ Stethoscope
- ❏ Alcohol swab
- ❏ Pen, pencil, vital sign flow sheet or record form

STEP	RATIONALE

ASSESSMENT

1. Determine need to assess client's BP:

   a. Note risk factors for alteration in BP.

   Certain conditions place clients at risk for BP alteration: history of cardiovascular disease, renal disease, diabetes, circulatory shock (hypovolemic, septic, cardiogenic, or neurogenic), acute or chronic pain, rapid IV infusion of fluids or blood products, increased intracranial pressure, postoperative, toxemia of pregnancy.

   b. Assess for signs and symptoms of BP alterations: Hypertension is often asymptomatic until pressure is very high. In clients at risk for high blood pressure (HBP), assess for headache (usually occipital), flushing of face, nosebleed, and fatigue in older adults. Hypotension is associated with dizziness; mental confusion; restlessness; pale, dusky, or cyanotic skin and mucous membranes; cool, mottled skin over extremities.

   Physical signs and symptoms may indicate alterations in BP.

2. Assess for factors that influence BP:

   a. Age

   Normal average BP varies throughout life (see Pediatric and Gerontological Considerations).

   b. Gender

   During and after menopause women can have higher blood pressures than men of same age.

   c. Daily (diurnal) variation

   Blood pressure varies throughout day; pressure is lowest in early morning, rises during morning and afternoon, and peaks in late afternoon or evening (Beevers and others, 2001a). Blood pressure can drop 10% to 20% during nighttime sleep (Joint National Committee, 2003).

   d. Position

   Blood pressure can fall as person moves from lying to sitting or standing position; normally, postural variations are minimal.

   e. Exercise

   Increases in oxygen demand by the body for activity increase BP.

   f. Weight

   Obesity is an independent predictor of hypertension (Thomas and others, 2002).

STEP	RATIONALE
g. Sympathetic stimulation	Pain, anxiety, or fear stimulates the sympathetic nervous system to increase HR, CO, and vascular resistance, causing BP to rise. Anxiety raises BP as much as 30 mm Hg (Beevers and others, 2001b).
h. Medications	Antihypertensives, diuretics, beta-adrenergic blockers, vasodilators, calcium channel blockers, angiotensin-converting enzyme (ACE) inhibitors, and antidysrhythmics lower BP; narcotic analgesics and general anesthetics can also cause hypotension.
i. Smoking	Smoking results in vasoconstriction, a narrowing of blood vessels. BP rises acutely and returns to baseline in about 15 minutes after stopping smoking (Joint National Committee, 2003).
j. Ethnicity	Rate of hypertension is higher in urban African-Americans than in European-Americans. African-Americans tend to develop more severe hypertension at an earlier age and have twice the risk for the complications of hypertension. Hypertension-related deaths are also higher among African-Americans.
3. Determine best site for BP assessment. Avoid applying cuff to extremity when intravenous fluids are infusing, an arteriovenous shunt or fistula is present, breast or axillary surgery has been performed on that side, or if extremity has been traumatized, diseased, or requires a cast or bulky bandage. The lower extremities may be used when the brachial arteries are inaccessible.	Inappropriate site selection may result in poor amplification of sounds, causing inaccurate readings. Application of pressure from inflated bladder temporarily impairs blood flow and can further compromise circulation in extremity that already has impaired blood flow.
4. Determine previous baseline BP and site (if available) from client's record.	Allows nurse to assess for change in condition. Provides comparison with future BP measurements.

NURSING DIAGNOSES

- Ineffective tissue perfusion
- Deficient fluid volume
- Decreased cardiac output

- Excess fluid volume
- Deficient knowledge regarding medication adherence for BP control

Related factors are individualized based on client's condition or needs.

PLANNING

1. Expected outcomes following completion of procedure: • Blood pressure is within acceptable range for client's age.	Cardiovascular status is stable.
2. Explain to client that BP is to be assessed. Have client rest at least 5 minutes before measuring lying or sitting blood pressure and rest 1 minute before measuring standing (Joint National Committee, 2003). Ask client not to speak when BP is being measured (Joint National Committee, 2003).	Reduces anxiety that can falsely elevate readings. Exercise can cause false elevations in BP as well. Talking to a client when the BP is being assessed increases readings 10% to 40% (Thomas and others, 2002).
3. Be sure client has not ingested caffeine or smoked for 30 minutes before assessment of BP (Joint National Committee, 2003).	Caffeine or nicotine can cause false elevations in blood pressure. Smoking increases blood pressure immediately and lasts up to 15 minutes. The effects of coffee or caffeine increase blood pressure up to 3 hours (Pickering, 2001).
4. Have client assume sitting or lying position. Be sure room is warm, quiet, and relaxing.	Maintains client's comfort during measurement. The client's perceptions that the physical or interpersonal environment is stressful affect the BP measurement (Thomas and others, 2002).

STEP	RATIONALE
5. Select appropriate cuff size (see Figure 17-11).	Use of improper-size cuff can cause false low or false high reading (see Table 17-5).
6. Perform hand hygiene.	Reduces transmission of microorganisms.

IMPLEMENTATION

ASSESSING BLOOD PRESSURE BY AUSCULTATION: UPPER EXTREMITIES

1. With client sitting or lying, position client's forearm, supported if needed at heart level, with palm turned up (see illustration). If sitting, client should be instructed to keep feet flat on floor without legs crossed.	If arm is extended and not supported, client may perform isometric exercise that can increase diastolic pressure 10% (Beevers and others, 2001a). Placement of arm above the level of the heart causes false low reading. Even in the supporting position a diastolic pressure effort up to 3 to 4 mm Hg can occur for each 5-cm change in heart level (Netea, 2003). Leg crossing can falsely increase systolic and diastolic blood pressure (Keele-Smith and Price-Daniels, 2001).

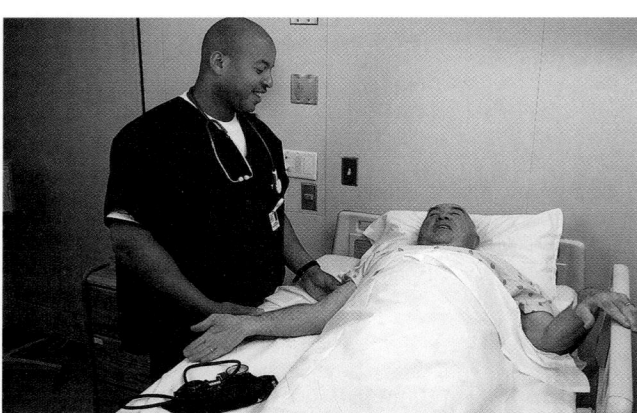

STEP **1** Client's forearm supported on bed.

2. Expose upper arm fully by removing constricting clothing.	Ensures proper cuff application. Do not place blood pressure cuff over clothing.
3. Palpate brachial artery (see illustration *A*). Position cuff 2.5 cm (1 inch) above site of brachial pulsation (antecubital space). Apply bladder of cuff above artery by centering arrows marked on cuff over artery (see illustration *B*). If there are not any center arrows on cuff, estimate the center of the bladder and place this center over artery. With cuff fully deflated, wrap cuff evenly and snugly around upper arm (see illustration *C*).	Inflating bladder directly over brachial artery ensures proper pressure is applied during inflation. Loose-fitting cuff causes false high readings.
4. Position manometer vertically at eye level. Observer should be no farther than 1 m (approximately 1 yard) away (Beevers and others, 2001b).	Looking up or down at the scale can result in distorted readings.

STEP	**RATIONALE**

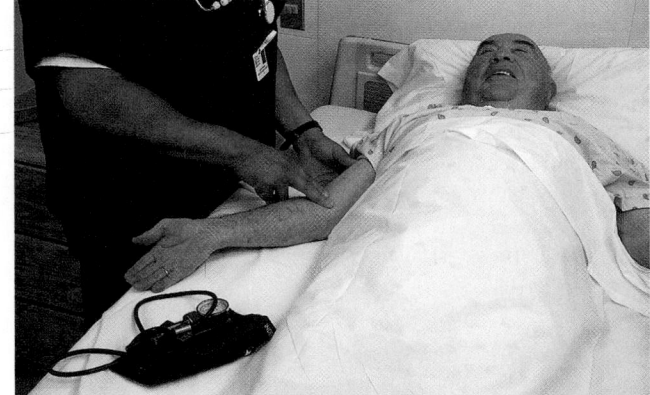

A

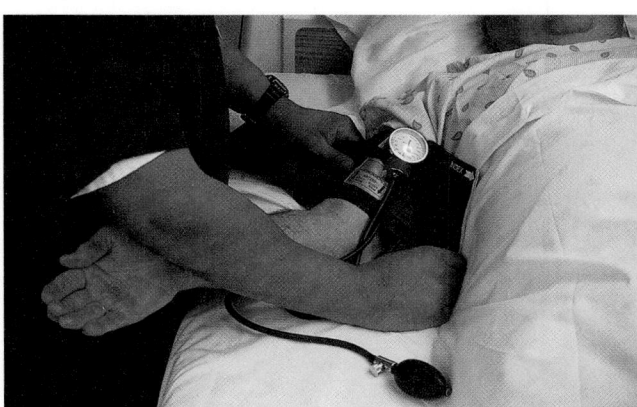

B

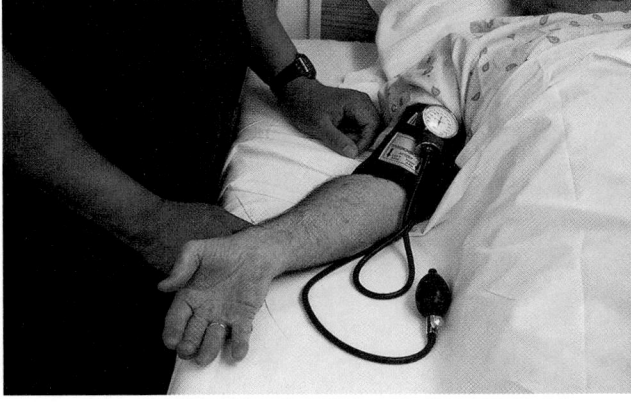

C

STEP **3** **A,** Nurse palpating client's brachial artery. **B,** Center bladder of cuff above artery. **C,** Blood pressure cuff wrapped around upper arm.

5. Measure blood pressure.
   a. Two-step method
      (1) Relocate brachial pulse. Palpate artery distal to the cuff with fingertips of nondominant hand while inflating cuff. Note point at which pulse disappears, and continue to inflate cuff to a pressure 30 mm Hg above that point. Note the pressure reading. Slowly deflate cuff, and note point when pulse reappears. Deflate cuff fully and wait 30 seconds.
      (2) Place stethoscope earpieces in ears and be sure sounds are clear, not muffled.

Estimating systolic pressure prevents false-low readings, which may result in the presence of an auscultatory gap. Maximal inflation point for accurate reading can be determined by palpation. If unable to palpate artery because of weakened pulse, an ultrasonic stethoscope can be used. Deflating cuff prevents venous congestion and false high readings.

Each earpiece should follow angle of ear canal to facilitate hearing.

STEP	RATIONALE

(3) Relocate brachial artery and place the bell or diaphragm of stethoscope over it. Do not allow chestpiece to touch cuff or clothing (see illustration).

Proper stethoscope placement ensures optimal sound reception. Stethoscope improperly positioned causes muffled sounds that often result in false low systolic and false high diastolic readings. The bell will give better sound reproduction, whereas the diaphragm is easier to secure with fingers and covers a larger area (Beevers and others, 2001b).

(4) Close valve of pressure bulb clockwise until tight.

Tightening of valve prevents air leak during inflation.

(5) Quickly inflate cuff to 30 mm Hg above client's estimated systolic pressure (see illustration).

Rapid inflation ensures accurate measurement of systolic pressure.

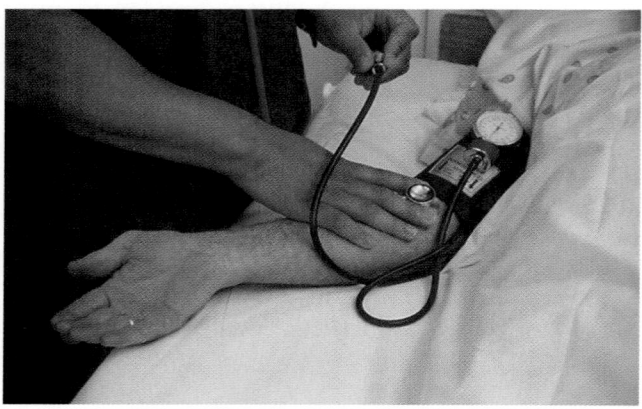

STEP **5a(3)** Stethoscope over brachial artery to measure BP.

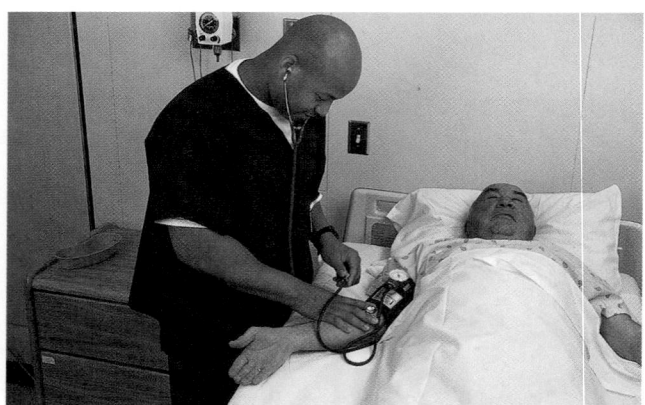

STEP **5a(5)** Inflating BP cuff.

(6) Slowly release pressure bulb valve, and allow manometer needle to fall at rate of 2 to 3 mm Hg/sec. Make sure there are no extraneous sounds.

Too rapid or slow a decline can cause inaccurate readings. Noise interferes with precise hearing of Korotkoff phases.

(7) Note point on manometer when first clear sound is heard. The sound will slowly increase in intensity.

First Korotkoff sound reflects systolic blood pressure.

(8) Continue to deflate cuff gradually, noting point at which sound disappears in adults. Note pressure to nearest 2 mm Hg. Listen for 20 to 30 mm Hg after the last sound, and then allow remaining air to escape quickly.

Beginning of the fifth Korotkoff sound is recommended as indication of diastolic pressure in adults (Joint National Committee, 2003). Fourth Korotkoff sound involves distinct muffling of sounds and is recommended as indication of diastolic pressure in children.

b. One-step method

(1) Place stethoscope earpieces in ears, and be sure sounds are clear, not muffled.

Earpieces should follow angle of ear canal to facilitate hearing.

(2) Relocate brachial artery, and place bell or diaphragm of stethoscope over it. Do not allow chestpiece to touch cuff or clothing.

Proper stethoscope placement ensures optimal sound reception.

(3) Close valve of pressure bulb clockwise until tight. Quickly inflate cuff to 30 mm Hg above client's usual systolic pressure.

Tightening of valve prevents air leak during inflation. Inflation above systolic level ensures accurate measurement of systolic pressure.

(4) Slowly release pressure bulb valve and allow manometer needle to fall at rate of 2 to 3 mm Hg/sec. Note point on manometer when first clear sound is heard. The sound will slowly increase in intensity.

Too rapid or slow a decline in mercury level can cause inaccurate readings.

The first Korotkoff sound reflects systolic pressure.

STEP	RATIONALE

   (5) Continue to deflate cuff gradually, noting point at which sound disappears in adults. Note pressure to nearest 2 mm Hg. Listen for 10 to 20 mm Hg after the last sound, and then allow remaining air to escape quickly.

Beginning of the fifth Korotkoff sound is recommended as indication of diastolic pressure in adults (Joint National Committee, 2003). Fourth Korotkoff sound involves distinct muffling of sounds and is recommended as indication of diastolic pressure in children.

6. The Joint National Committee (2003) recommends the average of two sets of BP measurements, 2 minutes apart. Use the second set of blood pressure measurements as your baseline.

Two sets of BP measurements help to prevent false positives based on a client's sympathetic response (alert reaction). Averaging minimizes the effect of anxiety, which often causes a first reading to be higher than subsequent measures (Joint National Committee, 2003).

7. Remove cuff from client's arm unless measurement must be repeated.

Continuous cuff inflation causes arterial occlusion, resulting in numbness and tingling of client's arm.

8. If this is first assessment of client, repeat procedure on other arm.

Comparison of BP in both arms detects circulatory problems. (Normal difference of 5 to 10 mm Hg exists between arms.)

9. Assist client in returning to comfortable position, and cover upper arm if previously clothed.

Restores comfort and provides sense of well-being.

10. Discuss findings with client as needed.

Promotes participation in care and understanding of health status. Makes client accountable for follow-up assessment.

11. Perform hand hygiene. Clean earpieces and diaphragm of stethoscope with alcohol swab as needed (optional).

Reduces transmission of microorganisms.
Controls transmission of microorganisms when nurses share stethoscope.

ASSESSING BLOOD PRESSURE BY AUSCULTATION: LOWER EXTREMITIES

1. Assist client to prone position. If unable to assume position, assist client to supine position with knee slightly flexed.

Prone position provides best access to popliteal artery.

2. Move aside bed linen and any constrictive clothing from leg.

Ensures proper cuff positioning.

3. Locate popliteal artery behind knee.

Artery palpation site lies just below client's thigh, in back of knee in popliteal space.

4. Apply large leg cuff 2.5 cm (1 inch) above popliteal artery around posterior aspect of middle thigh. Center arrows marked on cuff over artery (see illustration).

Proper cuff size is necessary for accurate reading. Cuff must be wide and long enough to allow for larger girth of the thigh. Narrow cuff causes false high readings.

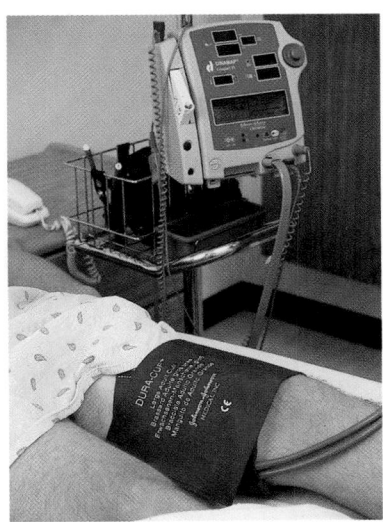

STEP 4 Blood pressure cuff applied around thigh.

STEP	RATIONALE
5. Position manometer vertically at eye level. Observer should be no farther than 1 m (approximately 1 yard) away (Beevers and others, 2001b).	Looking up or down at the scale can result in distorted readings.
6. Using the popliteal artery, follow step 5b of one-step method for auscultation of upper extremity.	
7. If this is first assessment of client, repeat procedure on other leg.	Comparison of BP in both legs detects circulatory problems.
8. Assist client in returning to comfortable position, and cover leg if previously clothed.	Restores comfort and promotes sense of well-being.
9. Discuss findings with client as needed.	Promotes participation in care and understanding of health status. Makes client accountable for follow-up assessment. Systolic blood pressure in the legs is usually higher by 10 to 40 mm Hg than in the brachial artery, but diastolic blood pressure is the same.
10. Perform hand hygiene. Clean earpieces and diaphragm of stethoscope with alcohol swab as needed *(optional)*.	Reduces transmission of microorganisms. Controls transmission of microorganisms when nurses share stethoscope.

ASSESSING BLOOD PRESSURE BY PALPATION

1. Follow steps 1 through 4 of auscultation method for upper extremity.
2. Locate and then continually palpate either brachial or radial artery with fingertips of one hand. Inflate cuff to a pressure 30 mm Hg above point at which pulse can no longer be palpated. *Optional:* Palpatation of popliteal artery can also be done with leg cuff.

                                            Ensures accurate detection of true systolic pressure once pressure valve is released.

- *Critical Decision Point*
  If unable to palpate artery because of weakened pulse, a Doppler ultrasonic stethoscope can also be used (see illustration).

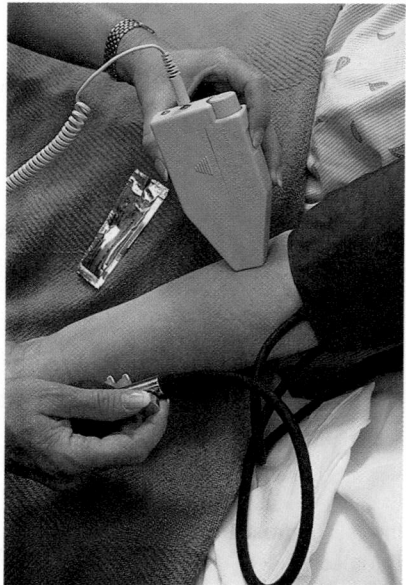

STEP **2** Doppler ultrasonic stethoscope over brachial artery to measure BP.

STEP	RATIONALE
3. Slowly release valve and deflate cuff, allowing manometer needle to fall at rate of 2 mm Hg/sec. Note point on manometer when pulse is again palpable.	Too rapid or slow a decline can result in inaccurate readings. Palpation can identify the systolic pressure only.
4. Deflate cuff rapidly and completely. Remove cuff from client's extremity unless measurement must be repeated.	Continuous cuff inflation causes arterial occlusion, resulting in numbness and tingling of client's arm.
6. Assist client in returning to comfortable position and cover upper arm if previously clothed.	Restores comfort and promotes sense of well-being.
7. Discuss findings with client as needed.	Promotes participation in care and understanding of health status.
8. Perform hand hygiene.	Reduces transmission of microorganisms.

EVALUATION

1. If BP is assessed for the first time, establish BP as baseline if it is within acceptable range.	Used to compare future BP measurements.
2. Compare BP reading with client's previous baseline and usual BP for client's age.	Allows nurse to assess for change in condition. Provides comparison with future BP measurements.

Recording and Reporting

- Record BP and site assessed on vital sign flow sheet (see Figure 17-5) or nurses' notes.
- Record any signs or symptoms of BP alterations in narrative form in nurses' notes.
- Report abnormal findings to nurse in charge or physician.

Unexpected Outcomes	Related Interventions

1. Blood pressure is above acceptable range.	• Repeat measurement.
	  • Verify correct blood pressure cuff size.
	  • Have RN colleague repeat measurement in 1 to 2 minutes.
	  • Assess BP in other arm or extremity, and compare findings.
	• Observe for related symptoms that are not apparent unless BP is extremely high.
	  • Headache (usual occipital)
	  • Facial flushing
	  • Nosebleed
	  • Fatigue in older client
	• Implement medical orders.
	  • Administer antihypertensive medications as ordered.
	  • If no medications ordered, report BP to nurse in change or physician to initiate appropriate evaluation and treatment.

2. Blood pressure is hypotensive, and blood pressure is not sufficient for adequate perfusion and oxygenation of tissues.	• Compare BP value to baseline. A systolic reading of 90 mm Hg can be an acceptable value for some clients.
	• Position client in a supine position to enhance circulation, and restrict activity that may decrease BP further.
	• Observe for symptoms associated with hypotension related to decreased cardiac output.
	  • Tachycardia
	  • Weak, thready pulse
	  • Weakness, dizziness, confusion
	  • Cool, pale, dusky, or cyanotic skin

Unexpected Outcomes	Related Interventions
	• Observe for factors that would contribute to a low BP. • Hemorrhage • Dilation of blood vessels resulting from hyperthermia, anesthesia, or medication side effects • Increase rate of IV infusion, or administer vasoconstricting drugs if ordered. • Report BP to nurse in charge or physician to initiate appropriate evaluation and treatment.
3. Blood pressure inaudible or difficult to obtain.	• Determine that no immediate crisis is present by obtaining pulse and respiratory rate. • Use alternative sites or procedures to obtain blood pressure. • Auscultate BP in lower extremity. • Use a Doppler ultrasonic instrument. • Implement palpation method to obtain systolic blood pressure.
4. Client experiences orthostatic hypotension.	• Maintain client safety. • Return client to safe position in bed or chair. • Restrict activity that may drop BP further.
5. A difference of more than 20 mm Hg systolic or diastolic between BP measurements on upper extremities.	• Report abnormal findings to nurse in charge or physician (Beevers and others, 2001a).

Teaching Considerations

- Educate client about risks for hypertension. Persons with family history of hypertension, premature heart disease, lipidemia, or renal disease are at significant risk. Obesity, cigarette smoking, heavy alcohol consumption, high blood cholesterol and triglyceride levels, and continued exposure to stress from psychosocial and environmental conditions are factors linked to hypertension (Joint National Committee, 2003).
- Primary prevention of hypertension includes lifestyle modifications (e.g., lose weight, exercise daily, reduce sodium and saturated fat intake, and maintain adequate intake of dietary potassium and calcium). Cigarette smoking is a powerful risk factor, and tobacco should be avoided in any form (Joint National Committee, 2003).
- Instruct primary caregiver to take BP at same time each day and after client has had a brief rest. Take BP sitting or lying down; use same position and arm each time pressure is taken.
- Instruct primary caregiver that if the pressure is difficult to hear, it may be that the cuff is too loose, not big enough, or too narrow; the stethoscope is not over arterial pulse; cuff was deflated too quickly or too slowly; or cuff was not pumped high enough for systolic readings.

Pediatric Considerations

- Blood pressure is not a routine part of assessment in children under 3 years.
- Blood pressure measurement can frighten children. Prepare child for squeezing feeling of inflated BP cuff by comparing sensation to elastic band on finger or a tight hug on the arm.
- Obtain BP in child before anxiety-producing tests or procedures are performed. At times it may be unrealistic to wait 5 minutes to assess BP. In emergency situations, do not wait.
- Accuracy of blood pressure will be affected by the cuff size selected for use. Measure the arm circumference at the midpoint between the elbow and shoulder, or select the cuff width that is two thirds of the upper arm.
- When a child reaches adolescence, BP varies by body size. The level of a child or adolescent BP is assessed with respect to body size and age. Heavier and taller children have a higher BP than smaller children of the same age. During adolescence, BP continues to vary according to body size. Normal range for 10- to 17-year-olds at the 90th percentile is 124 to 136/77 to 84 for boys and 124 to 127/63 to 74 for girls (Hockenberry and others, 2003).
- Korotkoff sounds are difficult to hear in children because of low frequency and amplitude. A pediatric stethoscope bell can be helpful.

Gerontological Considerations

- Older adults, especially frail older adults, have lost upper arm mass, requiring special attention to selection of BP cuff size.
- Skin of older adults is more fragile and susceptible to cuff pressure when BP measurements are frequent. More frequent assessment of skin under cuff or rotation of BP sites is recommended.
- Older adults have an increase in systolic pressure related to decreased vessel elasticity (Lueckenotte, 2000).
- Older adults often experience a fall in BP after eating.
- Older adults are instructed to change position slowly and wait after each change to avoid postural hypotension and prevent injuries.

Home Care Considerations

- Assess home noise level to determine the room that will provide the quietest environment for assessing BP.
- Instruct client on the importance of an appropriate-size blood pressure cuff for home use.
- Assess family's financial ability to afford a sphygmomanometer for performing BP evaluations on a regular basis. Validated electronic devices or aneroid sphygmomanometers that have proven to be accurate according to standard testing are recommended, along with appropriate-size cuffs. Finger monitors are inaccurate (Joint National Committee, 2003).

SKILL 17-6   Measuring Oxygen Saturation (Pulse Oximetry)

Pulse oximetry is the noninvasive measurement of arterial blood oxygen saturation—the percent to which hemoglobin is filled with oxygen. A pulse oximeter is a probe with a light-emitting diode (LED) connected by cable to an oximeter. Light waves emitted by the LED are absorbed and then reflected back by oxygenated and deoxygenated hemoglobin molecules. The reflected light is processed by the oximeter, which calculates pulse oxygen saturation (SpO_2). SpO_2 is a reliable estimate of arterial oxygen saturation (SaO_2) (Grap, 2002). For this reason, the use of oximetry can judiciously reduce the need to collect ABG specimens for oxygen saturation analysis. In adults the oximeter probe can be applied to the earlobe, finger, toe, or bridge of the nose, because a highly vascular area is needed to detect the degree of change in the transmitted light (Box 17-8).

The measurement of SpO_2 is simple, painless, and has few of the risks associated with more invasive measurements of SaO_2 such as arterial blood gas sampling. However, the measurement of SpO_2 is affected by factors that affect light transmission, such as outside light sources or client motion. Avoid direct sunlight or fluorescent lighting when using an oximeter. Light reflection from hemoglobin molecules can be influenced by carbon monoxide in the blood, jaundice, and intravascular dyes. Conditions that decrease arterial blood flow, such as peripheral vascular disease, hypothermia, pharmacological vasoconstrictors, hypotension, or peripheral edema, affect accurate determination of SpO_2.

Because light reflected from hemoglobin molecules is processed to determine SpO_2, any abnormality in the type or amount of hemoglobin affects oxygen saturation and SpO_2

BOX 17-8   Characteristics of Pulse Oximeter Sensor Probes and Sites

REUSABLE PROBE

Digit Probe

Easy to apply, conforms to various sizes.

Earlobe

Clip-on smaller and lighter though more positional than digit probe.
Yields strong correlation with SaO_2.
Research suggests greater accuracy at lower saturations (Grap, 2002).
Good when uncontrollable or rhythmic movements (e.g., hand tremors), exercise are present.
Vascular bed least affected by decreased blood flow (Grap, 2002).

DISPOSABLE SENSOR PAD

Can be applied to a variety of sites: earlobe of adult, nose bridge, palm or sole of infant.
Less restrictive for continuous SpO_2 monitoring.
Expensive.
Contains latex.
Skin under adhesive may become moist and harbor pathogens.
Available in variety of sizes; pad can be matched to infant weight.

values. The more hemoglobin that is saturated by oxygen, the higher the oxygen saturation. Normally SpO_2 is greater than 90%. Pulse oximetry is clinically indicated in clients who have an unstable oxygen status or are at risk for impaired gas exchange.

DELEGATION CONSIDERATIONS

The skill of oxygen saturation measurement can be delegated to assistive personnel. Before delegating this skill the nurse must:

* Provide assistive personnel the frequency of oxygen saturation measurements
* Instruct assistive personnel to notify the nurse immediately of any reading lower than SpO_2 of 90%
* Determine that assistive personnel are aware of factors than can falsely lower $SpO2$
* Caution assistive personnel to *not* use pulse oximetry as assessment of heart rate because an irregular rhythm may not be detected

EQUIPMENT

* ❏ Oximeter
* ❏ Oximeter probe appropriate for client and recommended by oximeter manufacturer
* ❏ Acetone or nail polish remover
* ❏ Pen, pencil, vital sign flow sheet or record form

STEP	RATIONALE

ASSESSMENT

1. Determine need to measure client's oxygen saturation:
   a. Identify risk factors for alteration of oxygen saturation.

   Oxygen saturation monitoring is indicated for clients at risk for decreased oxygen saturation: acute or chronic compromised respiratory function, recovery from general anesthesia or conscious sedation, traumatic injury to chest wall with or without collapse of underlying lung tissue, ventilator dependence, changes in supplemental O_2 therapy, or activity intolerance (Grap, 2002).

   b. Assess for signs and symptoms of alterations in oxygen saturation: altered respiratory rate, depth, or rhythm; adventitious breath sounds (Chapter 18); cyanotic appearance of nail beds, lips, mucous membranes, and skin; restlessness, irritability, confusion; reduced level of consciousness; labored or difficulty breathing.

   Physical signs and symptoms may indicate abnormal oxygen saturation.

2. Assess for factors that influence measurement of SpO_2, such as oxygen therapy, respiratory therapy such as postural drainage and percussion, hemoglobin level, hypotension, temperature, and medications such as bronchodilators.

   Allows nurse to accurately assess oxygen saturation variations. Peripheral vasoconstriction related to hypothermia can interfere with SpO_2 determination.

3. Review client's medical record for physician's order, or consult agency's procedure manual for standard of care for measurement of SpO_2.

   Medical order may be required to assess oxygen saturation with pulse oximetry.

4. Determine previous baseline SpO_2 (if available) from client's record.

   Baseline information provides basis for comparison and assists in assessment of current status and evaluation of interventions.

5. Determine most appropriate client-specific site (e.g., finger, earlobe, bridge of nose) for sensor probe placement by measuring capillary refill (Chapter 18). If capillary refill less than 3 seconds, select alternative site.
   a. Site must have adequate local circulation and be free of moisture.
   b. Artificial nails and certain nail polish colors will alter readings (Grap, 2002); place probe on finger free of polish or artificial nail.
   c. If client has tremors or is likely to move, use earlobe.

   Sensor requires pulsating vascular bed to identify hemoglobin molecules that absorb emitted light. Changes in SpO_2 are reflected in the circulation of finger capillary bed within 30 seconds and the capillary bed of earlobe within 5 to 10 seconds. Moisture impedes ability of sensor to detect SpO_2 levels. Motion artifact is most common cause of inaccurate readings.

STEP	RATIONALE

d. If client is obese, clip-on probe may not fit properly; obtain a single use (tape-on) probe.

NURSING DIAGNOSES

- Activity intolerance
- Impaired gas exchange
- Dysfunctional ventilatory weaning response

- Ineffective breathing pattern
- Impaired spontaneous ventilation
- Ineffective airway clearance

Related factors are individualized based on client's condition or needs.

PLANNING

1. Expected outcomes following completion of procedure:
   - Client's SpO_2 remains between 90% and 100%.
   - Client's oxygenation therapies are adjusted without requiring invasive assessment measures.
2. Obtain appropriate equipment, and place at bedside.

3. Explain purpose of procedure to client and how oxygen saturation will be measured.

Indicates adequate oxygenation.
Oximetry provides accurate SpO_2 measurement.

Mixing probes from different manufacturers can result in burn injury to client. If client has a latex sensitivity or latex allergy, avoid adhesive sensor that contains latex.
Promotes client cooperation and increases compliance.

IMPLEMENTATION

1. Perform hand hygiene.
2. Position client comfortably. If finger is chosen as monitoring site, support lower arm. Instruct client to breathe normally.
3. If finger is to be used, remove fingernail polish with acetone or polish remover from digit to be assessed.

4. Attach sensor to monitoring site (see illustration). Instruct client that clip-on probe will feel like a clothespin on the finger but will not hurt.

Reduces transmission of microorganisms.
Ensures probe positioning and decreases motion artifact that interferes with SpO_2 determination. Prevents large fluctuations in minute ventilation and possible changes in SpO_2.
Opaque coatings decrease light transmission; nail polish containing blue pigment can absorb light emissions and falsely alter saturation.
Select sensor site based on peripheral circulation and extremity temperature. Peripheral vasoconstriction can alter SpO_2. Pressure of sensor's spring tension on a finger or earlobe may be uncomfortable.

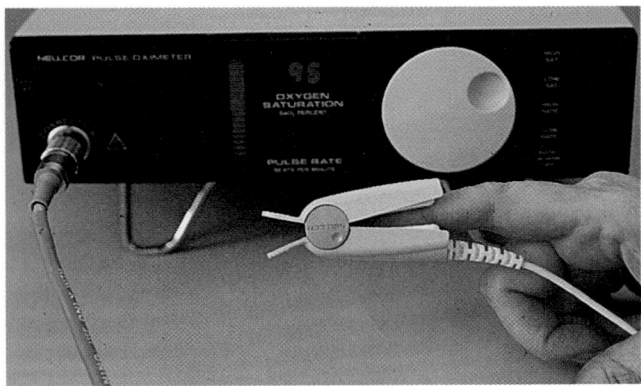

STEP **4** Oximeter sensor attached to finger.

STEP	RATIONALE

- *Critical Decision Point*

  Do not attach probe to finger, ear, or bridge of nose if area is edematous or skin integrity is compromised. Do not attach sensor to fingers that are hypothermic. Select ear or bridge of nose if adult client has a history of peripheral vascular disease. Do not use disposable adhesive sensors if client is allergic to latex. Do not place sensor on same extremity as electronic BP cuff because blood flow to finger will be temporarily interrupted when cuff inflates and cause inaccurate reading that can trigger alarms.

5. Once sensor is in place, turn on oximeter by activating power. Observe pulse waveform/intensity display and audible beep. Correlate oximeter pulse rate with client's radial pulse.

   Pulse waveform/intensity display enables detection of valid pulse or presence of interfering signal. Pitch of audible beep is proportional to SpO_2 value. Double checking pulse rate ensures oximeter accuracy.

- *Critical Decision Point*

  If oximeter pulse rate, client's radial pulse, and apical pulse are different, reevaluate oximeter probe placement and reassess pulse rates.

6. Inform client that oximeter alarm will sound if sensor falls off or if client moves sensor.

7. Leave sensor in place until oximeter readout reaches constant value and pulse display reaches full strength during each cardiac cycle. Read SpO_2 on digital display.

   Reading may take 10 to 30 seconds, depending on site selected.

8. Discuss findings with client as needed, and record findings.

   Promotes participation in care and understanding of health status.

9. If continuous SpO_2 monitoring is planned, verify SpO_2 alarm limits, which are preset by the manufacturer at a low of 85% and a high of 100%. Limits for SpO_2 and pulse rate should be determined as indicated by client's condition. Verify that alarms are on. Assess skin integrity under sensor every 2 hours. Relocate sensor at least every 4 hours and more frequently if skin integrity is altered or tissue perfusion compromised.

   Alarms must be set at appropriate limits and volumes to avoid frightening clients and visitors. Spring tension of sensor or sensitivity to disposable sensor adhesive can cause skin irritation and lead to disruption of skin integrity.

10. Remove probe, and turn oximeter power off. Store sensor in appropriate location.

    Batteries can be depleted if oximeter left on. Sensors are expensive and vulnerable to damage.

11. Assist client in returning to comfortable position.

    Restores comfort and promotes sense of well-being.

12. Perform hand hygiene.

    Reduces transmission of microorganisms.

EVALUATION

1. If oxygen saturation is assessed for the first time, establish SpO_2 as baseline if it is within acceptable range.

   Used to compare future assessments of oxygen saturation.

2. Compare SpO_2 with client's previous baseline and acceptable SpO_2. Note use of oxygen therapy.

   Allows nurse to assess for change in client's condition and presence of respiratory alteration.

3. During continuous monitoring, assess skin integrity underneath probe at least every 2 hours, based on client's peripheral circulation.

   Prevents tissue ischemia.

STEP	RATIONALE

Recording and Reporting

- Record SpO_2 on vital sign flow sheet (see Figure 17-5), record, or nurses' notes.
- Record type and amount of oxygen therapy used by client during assessment.
- Assessment of O_2 saturation after administration of specific therapies should be documented in narrative form in nurses' notes.
- Record any signs and symptoms of oxygen desaturation in nurses' notes.
- Report abnormal findings to nurse in charge or physician.
- Correlate SpO_2 with SaO_2 obtained from arterial blood gas measurements if available to verify the reliability of noninvasive assessment.
- Record in nurses' notes client's use of continuous or intermittent pulse oximetry to document use of equipment for third-party payers.

Unexpected Outcomes	Related Interventions
1. SaO_2 is less than 90%.	• Reposition probe and reevaluate. If SaO_2 is unacceptable, notify physician. An arterial blood gas level may be obtained to validate oximetry reading. • Promote oxygenation. • Position client in high-Fowler's or semi-Fowler's position. • Implement measures to reduce energy consumption. • Verify appropriate oxygen delivery system and liter flow; administer oxygen according to physician's orders.
2. Pulse waveform/intensity display is dampened or irregular.	• Locate different peripheral vascular bed, and reposition pulse oximeter probe. • Use another sensor if available. • Protect sensor from room light by covering sensor site with opaque covering or washcloth.
3. Pulse rate indicated on oximeter is less than radial or apical pulse rate.	• Check and/or change sensor site. • Clients who have cold hands or peripheral vascular disease may have decreased blood flow to extremity. • Excessive spring pressure by sensor can constrict blood flow. • Assess apical and radial pulse along with other signs and symptoms that would indicate compromised cardiac status or decreased peripheral blood flow.

Teaching Considerations

- Teach client significance of monitoring oxygen saturation.
- Teach client signs and symptoms of hypoxemia: headache, somnolence, confusion, dusky color, shortness of breath, dyspnea.
- Teach client effect of high-risk behaviors, such as cigarette smoking, on oxygen saturation.

Pediatric Considerations

- Placement recommendation for infants is to secure probe to the great toe, secure wire to foot, and cover foot with a snugly fitting sock. Placement recommendations for the child is to secure on the index finger and secure wire to hand (Hockenberry and others, 2003).
- Earlobe and bridge-of-nose sensors are not used for infants and toddlers.
- Sensors can be affected by heat and light sources. Sensors should be covered when used during phototherapy or with radiant warmers (Hockenberry and others, 2003).

Gerontological Considerations

- Identifying an acceptable pulse oximeter probe site may be difficult in older adults because of likelihood of peripheral vascular disease, decreased carbon dioxide level, cold-induced vasoconstriction, and anemia.

- Older adults require more frequent assessment of skin under sensor site because of tissue fragility and decreased elasticity caused by aging.

Home Care Considerations
- Pulse oximetry is used in home care to noninvasively monitor oxygen therapy or changes in oxygen therapy.

FOCUS *on* CLINICAL PRACTICE

You have been assigned to admit Ms. Coburn, a 16-year-old high school student who has just returned from the postoperative recovery unit after closed reduction of right radial fracture sustained during a volleyball game. Ms. Coburn is awake but sleepy, and there is a cast on the right arm and an IV in the left antecubital space. Ms. Coburn's fingers extend outside of the cast.

1. Which routine postoperative vital signs can you assign to the nursing assistant? What directions do you provide the nursing assistant regarding obtaining vital signs for this client?

2. The nursing assistant reports that the blood pressure for Ms. Coburn is 86/60 mm Hg. You note that preoperatively the emergency department nurse recorded a blood pressure of 138/82 mm Hg. What might explain the differences in blood pressure values? What interventions do you consider at this time?

3. After an hour Ms. Coburn is quietly sleeping. The nursing assistant reports that the oximeter sensor on her right finger has triggered the alarm. You note a dampened wave form, an SpO$_2$ value of 88%, and a heart rate of 52. What are your priority nursing actions?

NCLEX REVIEW QUESTIONS

1. Which two temperature sites will provide a core temperature measurement?
   1. Rectal and oral
   2. Tympanic and skin
   3. Skin and oral
   4. Tympanic and rectal

2. A mother brings her infant son to the pediatric clinic and states she has been obtaining his temperature using a chemical strip attached to his leg. She is concerned that his temperature is 97.8° C. What is your priority nursing action?
   1. Inform the mother of the correct placement of chemical dot thermometers.
   2. Notify the nurse in charge or physician.
   3. Obtain a temperature using a tympanic thermometer on the infant.
   4. Obtain pulse rate, respiratory rate, and oxygen saturation on the infant.

3. A postoperative client complains of fatigue, dizziness, and feeling warm. You delegate vital signs to the nursing assistant, who reports a temperature of 102.3° C and heart rate of 124. What is (are) your priority nursing action(s)?
   1. Obtain apical heart rate, and repeat the temperature assessment using a rectal thermometer.

2. Contact the laboratory to obtain blood cultures as previously ordered by the physician.
   3. Conduct a complete assessment of the client, then contact the physician.
   4. Remove extra clothing and bed covers, and evaluate the client's complaints.

4. In delegating a pulse rate you inform the nursing assistant that a 60-second count is required. What condition would cause you to make this request?
   1. Bradycardia
   2. Regular rate
   3. Tachycardia
   4. Irregular rate

5. A young football player is admitted to your unit with an IV in the right hand and the left arm splinted to his chest following surgery for a broken left collar bone. You assess the left radial pulse and note it is weak and thready. What is your priority nursing intervention?
   1. Assess right radial pulse for symmetry.
   2. Check the tightness of the splint.
   3. Ask the client to move his fingers to encourage circulation.
   4. Notify the nurse in charge.

NCLEX REVIEW QUESTIONS

6. An older adult will be discharged soon after a myocardial infarction. You will be teaching him to take his own pulse rate. Which artery will he be palpating?
   1. Radial
   2. brachial
   3. carotid
   4. Popliteal

7. In which situation can the assessment of the apical pulse be delegated to a nursing assistant?
   1. When the client is having chest discomfort
   2. During a procedure to drain the lung of fluid
   3. Upon admission to the hospital
   4. During routine vital sign measurement

8. Which of the following activities will decrease heart rate?
   1. Crossing the legs
   2. Standing up
   3. Drinking cold fluids
   4. Sleeping

9. Why is the PMI used during apical heart rate assessment?
   1. It is near the angle of Louis.
   2. It reflects the cardiac apex.
   3. It is easy to locate.
   4. It reflects the S_2 heart sound.

10. Vital signs are obtained by the nursing assistant from a known hypertensive client. BP is 145/84 mm Hg, radial pulse is 88 beats per minute, apical pulse is 80 beats per minute, tympanic temperature is 97.8° F, and respiratory rate is 16 breaths per minute. What is your priority nursing action?
    1. Calculate and record pulse pressure and pulse deficit.
    2. Assess for related symptoms of hypertension.
    3. Ask the nursing assistant for help in obtaining apical-radial pulse.
    4. Assess for orthostatic hypotension.

11. One cause of decreased respiratory rate is:
    1. Smoking
    2. Exercise
    3. Decreased hemoglobin
    4. Narcotic analgesics

12. What effect does increased age have on respiratory assessment?
    1. Increased depth of respirations
    2. Decreased use of abdominal muscles
    3. Increased presence of apnea
    4. Decrease in chest expansion

13. A hypertensive client has a blood pressure of 164/92 mm Hg. What is the pulse pressure?
    1. 12   3. 72
    2. 24   4. 266

14. What is the effect of a blood pressure cuff that is too small for a client's arm?
    1. Produces false low systolic pressure
    2. Produces false high systolic pressure
    3. Is uncomfortable when inflated
    4. Has no effect

15. When completing an assessment, the client is nervously talking while the blood pressure is obtained. What is the priority nursing action?
    1. Reassure client, and document the client's anxiety in the nurse's notes.
    2. Ask the client to remain silent, and repeat the blood pressure measurement in the other arm.
    3. Repeat the blood pressure measurement again at the end of the assessment after the client has been resting quietly.
    4. Request that another nurse obtain the blood pressure.

16. When is the diastolic blood pressure measurement determined in a healthy adult?
    1. When the pulse is no longer felt at the end of palpation
    2. When the fifth Korotkoff sound is diminished
    3. When the aneroid needle can fall freely without bouncing
    4. When the fourth Korotkoff sound has changed character

17. The nurse observes the nursing assistant obtaining a blood pressure with an aneroid sphygmomanometer. Within 25 seconds the nursing assistant has inflated the cuff, 20 mm Hg higher each time. What action should the nurse take?
    1. Compare the blood pressure value obtained with the client's baseline.
    2. Demonstrate the one-step blood pressure technique on the client's other arm.
    3. Record the blood pressure.
    4. Notify the nurse in charge.

18. The postoperative client has vital signs ordered every 15 minutes for an hour. The nursing assistant applies an electronic blood pressure cuff on the client's left arm and informs you of the first two readings: 122/68 mm Hg, 144/90 mm Hg. What action should you take?
    1. Ask the nursing assistant to reposition the blood pressure cuff.
    2. Assess the blood pressure using the auscultatory technique.
    3. Retake the client's blood pressure observing the electronic device.
    4. Check the hose-to-cuff connections for kinking.

NCLEX REVIEW QUESTIONS

19. Following a client's nebulizer treatment by the respiratory therapist, the pulse oximetry waveform intensity display is weak and reads 89%. The client states his breathing is improved after the treatment. What action should you take?
    1. Reposition the oximeter sensor.
    2. Cover the sensor with a cloth to eliminate extraneous light.
    3. Locate a different vascular bed for sensor.
    4. Assess apical and radial pulse to evaluate cardiovascular status.

20. What is one advantage of an earlobe pulse oximetry sensor?
    1. Available in a variety of sizes
    2. Can be used for infants
    3. Easily positioned for continuous measurements
    4. Least affected by decreased blood flow

References

Anwar YA, White WB: Ambulatory monitoring of the blood pressure: devices, analysis and clinical utility. In White WB, editor: *Blood pressure monitoring in cardiovascular medicine and therapeutics,* Totowa, NJ, 2001, Humana Press.

Beevers G and others: ABC's of hypertension. I. Blood pressure measurement, *Br Med J* 322(7292):981, 2001a.

Beevers G and others: ABC's of hypertension. II. Blood pressure measurement, *Br Med J* 322(7293):1043, 2001b.

Ebersole P, Hess P: *Geriatric nursing and healthy aging,* St. Louis, 2001, Mosby.

Grap MJ: Pulse oximetry, *Crit Care Nurse* 22(3):69, 2002.

Hockenberry MJ and others: *Wong's nursing care of infants and children,* ed 7, St. Louis, 2003, Mosby.

Joint National Committee: The seventh report of the Joint National Committee on Prevention, Detection, Evaluation and Treatment of High Blood Pressure, *JAMA* 289:2560, 2003.

Jones DW and others: Measuring blood pressure accurately, *JAMA* 289(8):1027, 2003.

Lueckenotte AG: *Gerontologic nursing,* ed 2, St. Louis, 2000, Mosby.

Maas ML and others: *Nursing care of older adults,* St. Louis, 2001, Mosby.

Pacquiao DF: Cultural competence in ethical decision-making. In Andrews M, Boyle J: *Transcultural concepts in nursing care,* Philadelphia, 2003, Lippincott.

Pickering TG: Self-monitoring of blood pressure. In White WB, editor: *Blood pressure monitoring in cardiovascular medicine and therapeutics,* Totowa, NJ, 2001, Humana Press.

Sheahan SL, Musialowski R: Clinical implications of respiratory system changes in aging, *J Gerontol Nur* 27(5):26, 2001.

Thibodeau GA, Patton KT: *Anatomy and physiology,* ed 5, St. Louis, 2003, Mosby.

Research References

Armstrong RS: Nurses' knowledge of error in blood pressure measurement technique, *Int J Nurs Pract* 8:118, 2002.

Bailey J, Rose P: Axillary and tympanic membrane temperature recording in the pre-term neonate: a comparative study, *J Adv Nurs* 34(4):465, 2001.

Fallis WM: Oral measurement of temperature in orally intubated critical care clients: state of the science review, *Am J Crit Care* 9(5):334, 2000.

Fonseca-Reyes S and others: Effect of standard cuff on blood pressure readings in clients with obese arms: how frequent are arms of a "large circumference"? *Blood Press Monit* 8(3):101, 2003.

Graves JW: Prevalence of blood pressure cuff sizes in a referral practice of 430 consecutive adult hypertensives, *Blood Press Monit* 6(1):17, 2001.

Graves JW and others: The changing distribution of arm circumferences in NHANES III and NHANES 2000 and its impact on the utility of the "standard adult" blood pressure cuff, *Blood Press Monit* 8(6):223, 2003.

Guiliano KK and others: Temperature measurement in critically ill adults: a comparison of tympanic and oral methods, *Am J Crit Care* 9(4):254, 2000.

Keele-Smith R, Price-Daniels C: Effects of crossing legs on blood pressure measurement, *Clin Nurs Res* 10(2):202, 2001.

Molton AH and others: Temperature taking in children, *J Child Health Care* 5(1):5, 2001.

Netea RT and others: Both body and arm position significantly influence blood pressure measurement, *J Hum Hypertens* 17(7):459, 2003.

Potter P and others: Evaluation of chemical dot thermometers for measuring body temperature of orally intubated clients, *Am J Crit Care* 12(5):403, 2003.

Sund-Levander and others: Norma oral, rectal, tympanic and axillary body temperature in adult men and women: a systematic literature review, *Scand J Caring Sci* 16:112, 2002.

Thomas SA and others: A review of nursing research on blood pressure, *J Nurs Scholarsh* 34(4):313, 2002.

Yarrows SA and others: Rapid oscillometric blood pressure measurement compared to conventional oscillometric measurement, *Blood Press Monit* 6(3):145, 2001.

Yucha CB: Ambulatory blood pressure monitoring: measurement implications for research, *J Nurs Meas* 9(1):49, 2001.

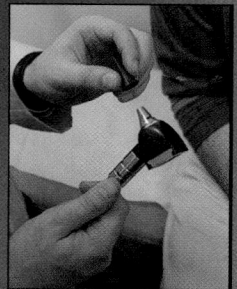

18

Health History and Physical Examination

MEDIA RESOURCES

Evolve Site *evolve*

http://evolve.elsevier.com/Perry/skills
- Weblinks
- Mosby's Nursing Skills Video Exercises

Mosby's Nursing Skills Videos/CD-ROM
- *Measurements Video:* Height and weight; intake and output; vital signs

OBJECTIVES

Mastery of content in this chaper will enable the nurse to:

- Discuss the purposes of physical assessment.
- Describe the techniques used with each assessment skill.
- Describe proper positioning for the client during each phase of the examination.
- Describe how to conduct a physical examination on clients from diverse cultures.
- List techniques to promote the client's physical and psychological comfort during an examination.
- Make environmental preparations before an assessment.
- Identify information to collect from the nursing history before a physical assessment.
- Discuss normal physical findings for clients across the life span.
- Discuss ways to incorporate health promotion and health teaching into an assessment.
- Identify self-screening assessments commonly performed by clients.
- Successfully complete a history and physical assessment.
- Document assessment findings on appropriate forms.
- Communicate abnormal findings to appropriate personnel.

KEY TERMS

Atrophy	Edema
Auscultation	Erythema
Bruit	Friction rub
Cardiomegaly	Inspection
Cerumen	Intercostal space
Conjunctiva	Nares
Costovertebral angle	Olfaction
(CVA) tenderness	Orthostatic hypotension
Crackles	Pallor
Cyanosis	Palpation
Dorsum	Percussion

Clients undergo periodic systematic physical assessments on a regular basis during health care encounters. In acute care settings a brief shift assessment is done at the beginning of each shift to identify changes in the client's status compared with the previous assessment. This routine physical assessment takes 10 to 15 minutes and reveals information that supplements the database for the client. In nursing homes and home care settings similar assessments are done weekly or monthly and more frequently when a change in health status occurs.

A more comprehensive assessment is done on admission to a health care agency. This assessment involves a detailed review of a client's condition, with the nurse collecting a nurs-

ing history and performing a behavioral and physical examination. The health history involves an interview with a client to gather subjective data about any presenting conditions. A physical assessment is a head-to-toe review of each body system that offers objective information about the client. The client's condition and response affect the extent of the examination. Once data are gathered, the nurse groups significant findings into patterns of data that reveal actual or potential nursing diagnoses (Table 18-1). Each abnormal finding directs the nurse to gather additional data. Information gathered during an initial assessment and examination provides the baseline measurement for a client's functional abilities and serves as a comparison for future assessment findings. In addition, the information helps the nurse select the best nursing measures to manage the client's health problems.

Nurses are often the first to detect changes in clients' conditions, regardless of the setting. For this reason the ability to think critically and interpret client behaviors and physiological changes is essential. The skills of physical assessment are powerful tools with which to detect subtle as well as obvious changes in a client's health.

Assessment Techniques

Inspection, palpation, percussion, auscultation, and olfaction are assessment techniques that enable the nurse to collect a broad range of physical data about clients. Inspection is the process of visual examination of body parts. An experienced nurse learns to make many observations, almost simultaneously, while becoming very perceptive of abnormalities. The secret is to always pay attention to the client. Watch all movements and look carefully at any body part being inspected. It is important to recognize normal physical characteristics of clients of all ages before trying to distinguish abnormal findings.

Experience is needed to recognize normal variations among clients, as well as ranges of normal for individual clients. Cultural diversity is also recognized as one of the factors that influences both normal variations and potential alterations. It is extremely important for the nurse to methodically take the time necessary to carefully assess each body part. If the nurse becomes hurried, significant signs may be overlooked, and incorrect conclusions may be made about a client's condition.

Inspection requires good lighting and full exposure of body parts. Each area is inspected for size, shape, color, symmetry, position, and the presence of abnormalities. If possible, each area inspected is compared with the same area on the opposite side of the body. When necessary, use additional light, such as a penlight, to inspect body cavities such as the mouth and throat. Do not hurry. Pay attention to detail. Verify and clarify all abnormalities with subjective client data. In other words, ask the client for further information about each abnormality or change.

Palpation involves use of the sense of touch. Through palpation the hands can make delicate and sensitive measurements of specific physical signs, including resistance,

TABLE 18-1	DEVELOPMENT OF INDIVIDUALIZED NURSING DIAGNOSES		
ASSESSMENT METHOD	**FINDINGS**	**PATTERNS**	**NURSING DIAGNOSIS**
Inspection of skin	Skin along sacral area is intact. There is 3-cm area of redness around coccyx; skin blanches on palpation. No skin lesions are observed.	There is pressure area around coccyx.	Risk for impaired skin integrity
Palpation of skin	Skin is moist from diaphoresis. There is tenderness to palpation around sacral area. There is good skin turgor.	Skin moisture promotes maceration.	
Historical data	Client suffered fractured left leg. Client is immobilized due to left leg traction.	Continued pressure is exerted over sacrum.	

resilience, roughness, texture, temperature, and mobility. Palpation is often used with or after visual inspection. The nurse uses different parts of the hand to detect specific characteristics. For example, the dorsum (back) of the hand is sensitive to temperature variations. The pads of the fingertips detect subtle changes in texture, shape, size, consistency, and pulsation of body parts. The palm of the hand is especially sensitive to vibration. The nurse measures position, consistency, and turgor by lightly grasping the body part with the fingertips.

Assist the client to be relaxed and position the client comfortably because muscle tension during palpation impairs the nurse's ability to palpate correctly. Asking the client to take slow, deep breaths enhances muscle relaxation. Tender areas are palpated last. The nurse asks the client to point out areas that are more sensitive and notes any nonverbal signs of discomfort. Clients appreciate warm hands, short fingernails, and a gentle approach. Palpation may be either light or deep and is controlled by the amount of pressure applied with the fingers or hand. Light palpation precedes deep palpation. The nurse must consider the client's condition, the area being palpated, and the reason for using palpation. For example, when a client is admitted to the emergency department following an automobile accident the nurse should consider the factors surrounding the client's injury and inspect the chest wall carefully before performing any palpation around the area of the ribs.

To palpate, the nurse applies pressure slowly, gently, and deliberately, depressing about 1 cm ($\frac{1}{2}$ inch) (Figure 18-1, *A*). Tender areas are examined further using light intermittent pressure. After light palpation, deeper palpation may be used to examine the condition of organs (Figure 18-1, *B*). The nurse depresses the area being examined approximately 2 cm (1 inch). Caution is the rule. Bimanual palpation involves one hand placed over the other while pressure is applied. The upper hand exerts downward pressure as the other hand feels the subtle characteristics of underlying organs and masses. The nursing student seeks the assistance of a qualified instructor before attempting deep palpation.

Percussion involves tapping the body with the fingertips to evaluate the size, borders, and consistency of body organs

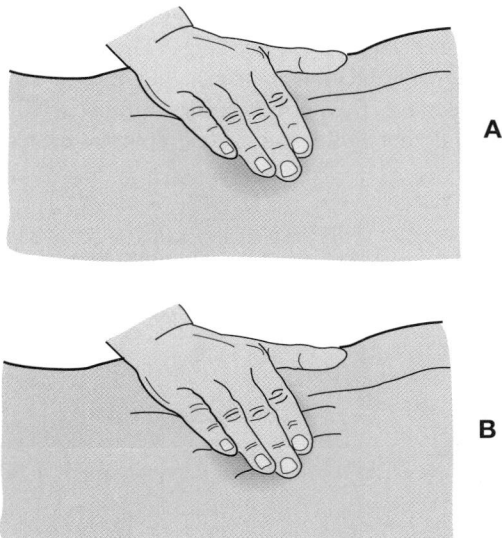

FIGURE **18-1** **A,** During light palpation, gentle pressure against underlying skin and tissues can be used to detect areas of irregularity and tenderness. **B,** During deep palpation, depress tissue to assess condition of underlying organs.

and to discover fluid in body cavities (Figure 18-2). It requires practice and skill. Percussion helps identify the location, size, and density of underlying structures. The nurse strikes the body's surface with a finger to create a vibration, and sound waves are heard as percussion tones arising from vibrations in body tissues (Seidel and others, 2003). The character of sound depends on the density of underlying tissues. For example, the normal lung transmits sounds with high intensity and low pitch, whereas the solid liver transmits a high-pitched sound of soft intensity.

There are two methods of percussion: direct and indirect. The direct method involves striking the body surface directly with one or two fingers. The indirect technique is performed by placing the middle finger of the examiner's nondominant hand firmly against the body surface. With palm and fingers remaining off the skin, the tip of the middle finger of the dominant hand strikes the base of the distal joint of the finger. The examiner uses a quick, sharp stroke, keeping the forearm stationary. The wrist remains relaxed to deliver the proper blow. Once the finger has struck, the wrist snaps back. If the blow is not sharp, if the hand is held loosely, or if the palm rests on the body surface, the sound is softened and the nurse cannot detect the presence of underlying structures. A light, quick blow produces the clearest sounds. Table 18-2 describes the five different percussion sounds.

Auscultation is listening to sounds produced by the body with a stethoscope. To auscultate correctly, listen in a quiet environment both for the presence of sound and its characteristics. The nurse is more successful in auscultation after knowing normal sounds from each body structure, including the passage of blood through an artery, heart sounds, and movement of air through the lungs. These sounds vary according to the location in which they can most easily be heard. Likewise, the nurse becomes familiar with areas that normally do not emit sounds. It is important for a student to listen to many normal sounds in order to recognize abnormal sounds when they arise.

To auscultate, the nurse needs good hearing acuity, a good stethoscope, and knowledge of how to use the stethoscope properly (Box 18-1). Nurses with hearing disorders may purchase stethoscopes with greater sound amplification and may need to ask colleagues to verify some findings through auscultation. It is more effective to place the stethoscope directly on client's naked skin because clothing obscures and changes sound.

Through auscultation the nurse notes the following characteristics of sound:

Frequency—Number of sound wave cycles generated per second by a vibrating object. The higher the frequency, the higher the pitch of a sound and vice versa.
Loudness—Amplitude of a sound wave. Auscultated sounds are described as loud or soft.

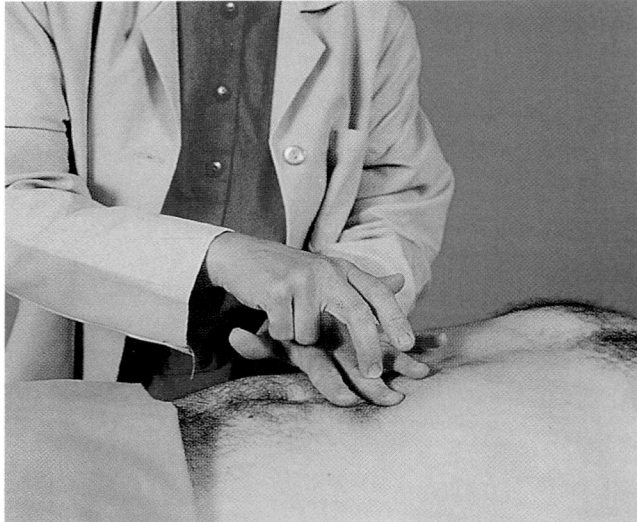

FIGURE **18-2** Indirect percussion of the abdomen. (From Barkauskas VH and others: *Health and physical assessment,* ed 2, St. Louis, 1998, Mosby.)

BOX 18-1 Learning to Use a Stethoscope

1. Place earpieces in both ears with tips of earpieces turned toward the face. *Lightly* blow into the stethoscope's diaphragm. Again place earpieces in both ears, this time with ends turned toward the back of the head. *Lightly* blow into the stethoscope's diaphragm. The earpiece should follow the contour of the ear canal. After learning the right fit for the loudest sound, wear the stethoscope the same way each time.
2. Put the stethoscope on and *lightly* blow into the diaphragm. If sound is barely audible, *lightly* blow into the bell. Sound is carried through only one part of the chestpiece at a time. If sound is greatly amplified through the diaphragm, the diaphragm is in position for use. If sound is barely audible through the diaphragm, the bell is in position for use.
3. Listen while moving the diaphragm lightly over the hair on your arm. The bristling sound created by rubbing of hair against the diaphragm mimics a sound heard in the lungs. Also, always be sure to keep the diaphragm stationary and firm to reduce extraneous sounds.
4. Place the stethoscope on and gently tap tubing. The sound can distract from being able to hear sounds created by body organs. Always avoid stretching or moving the tubing; it should hang freely.

TABLE 18-2 SOUNDS PRODUCED BY PERCUSSION

SOUND	INTENSITY	PITCH	DURATION	QUALITY	COMMON LOCATION
Tympany	Loud	High	Moderate	Drumlike	Enclosed, air-containing space; gastric air bubble, puffed-out cheek
Resonance	Moderate to loud	Low	Long	Hollow	Normal lung
Hyperresonance	Very loud	Very low	Longer than resonance	Booming	Emphysematous lung
Dullness	Soft to moderate	High	Moderate	Thudlike	Liver, spleen, gallbladder
Flatness	Soft	High	Short	Flat	Muscle

Quality—Sounds of similar frequency and loudness from different sources. Terms such as blowing or gurgling describe quality of sound.

Duration—Length of time that sound vibrations last. Duration of sound is short, medium, or long. Layers of soft tissue dampen the duration of sounds from deep internal organs.

A nurse cannot be successful at auscultation without knowing how to use a stethoscope properly. Chapter 17 describes the parts of the acoustic stethoscope and use of the bell and diaphragm.

Olfaction uses the sense of smell to detect abnormalities that go unrecognized by any other means. Some alterations in body function and certain bacteria create characteristic odors (Table 18-3).

Preparation for Assessment

The shift assessment begins the moment the nurse sees the client and continues with each care encounter. It is important to have as much awareness as possible of the client's health history and the reason for care. The nurse is alert for any changes or problems that may have developed since the last assessment.

Preparation of the environment, equipment, and client promotes a smooth assessment. To promote client comfort and efficiency it is essential to provide privacy for the client (e.g., a separate room; curtains or dividers to enclose the client's bed; or in the home, a bedroom can be used); a warm, comfortable temperature; a loose-fitting gown or pajamas for the client; adequate direct lighting; control of outside noises; and precautions to prevent interruptions by visitors or other health care personnel. The bed should be at the nurse's waist level if possible.

Preparing the Client

To facilitate an accurate assessment, the nurse prepares the client both physically and psychologically. A tense, anxious client may have difficulty understanding or following directions or cooperating with the nurse's instructions. To prepare the client:

1. Provide for the client's physical comfort by allowing the opportunity to empty the bowel or bladder (a good time to collect needed specimens).
2. Provide privacy.
3. Minimize client's anxiety and fear by conveying an open, receptive, and professional approach. The nurse thoroughly explains what will be done, what the client should expect to feel, and how the client can cooperate, using simple terms.
4. Provide access to body parts while draping areas that need not be exposed.
5. Eliminate drafts, control room temperature, and provide warm blankets.
6. Help the client assume positions during the assessment (Table 18-4) so that body parts are accessible and the client stays comfortable. A client's ability to assume positions will depend on physical strength and limitations. Some positions are uncomfortable or embarrassing; keep a client in position no longer than is necessary.
7. Pace assessment according to the client's physical and emotional tolerance.
8. Use a relaxed voice tone and facial expressions to put client at ease.
9. Encourage the client to ask questions and report discomfort felt during the examination.
10. Have a family member or a third person of the client's gender in the room during assessment of genitalia.

TABLE 18-3   ASSESSMENT OF CHARACTERISTIC ODORS

ODOR	SITE OR SOURCE	POTENTIAL CAUSES
Alcohol	Oral cavity	Ingestion of alcohol; diabetes
Ammonia	Urine	Urinary tract infection
Body odor	Skin, particularly in areas where body parts rub together (e.g., under arms, breasts, perineal area)	Poor hygiene, excess perspiration (hyperhidrosis), foul-smelling perspiration (bromhidrosis)
Feces	Wound site	Wound abscess
	Vomitus	Undigested food
	Rectal area	Bowel obstruction
		Fecal incontinence
Foul-smelling stools in infant	Stool	Malabsorption syndrome
Halitosis	Oral cavity	Poor dental and oral hygiene, gum disease
Sweet, fruity ketones	Oral cavity	Diabetic acidosis
Stale urine	Skin	Uremic acidosis
Sweet, heavy, thick odor	Draining wound	*Pseudomonas* (bacterial) infection
Musty odor	Casted body part	Infection inside cast
Fetid, sweet odor	Tracheostomy or mucus secretions	Infection of bronchial tree (*Pseudomonas* bacteria)

TABLE 18-4   POSITIONS FOR PHYSICAL ASSESSMENT

POSITION	AREAS ASSESSED	RATIONALE	LIMITATIONS
Sitting	Head and neck, back, posterior thorax and lungs, anterior thorax and lungs, breasts, axillae, heart, vital signs, and upper extremities	Sitting upright provides full expansion of lungs and provides better visualization of symmetry of upper body parts.	Physically weakened or a developmentally disabled client may be unable to sit. Examiner should use supine position with head of bed elevated instead.
Supine	Head and neck, anterior thorax and lungs, breasts, axillae, heart, abdomen, extremities, pulses	This is most normally relaxed position. It provides easy access to pulse sites.	If client becomes short of breath easily, examiner may need to raise head of bed.
Dorsal recumbent	Head and neck, anterior thorax and lungs, breasts, axillae, heart, abdomen	Position is used for abdominal assessment because it promotes relaxation of abdominal muscles.	Clients with painful disorders are more comfortable with knees flexed.
Lithotomy	Female genitalia and genital tract	This position provides maximal exposure of genitalia and facilitates insertion of vaginal speculum.	Lithotomy position is embarrassing and uncomfortable, so examiner minimizes time that client spends in it. Client is kept well draped. Clients with arthritis or other joint deformities may be unable to tolerate the position.
Sims'	Rectum and vagina	Flexion of hip and knee improves exposure of rectal area.	Joint deformities may hinder client's ability to bend hip and knee.
Prone	Musculoskeletal system	This position is used only to assess extension of hip joint.	This position is poorly tolerated in clients with respiratory difficulties.
Lateral recumbent	Heart	This position aids in detecting murmurs.	This position is poorly tolerated in clients with respiratory difficulties.
Knee-chest	Rectum	This position provides maximal exposure of rectal area.	This position is embarrassing and uncomfortable. Clients with arthritis or other joint deformities may be unable to assume position.

This prevents the client from accusing the nurse of behaving in an unethical manner.

Physical Assessment of Various Age-Groups
Children and Adolescents

1. Routine examinations of children have a focus on health promotion and illness prevention, particularly for care of well children with competent parenting and no serious health problems (Hockenberry and others, 2003). The focus is on growth and development, sensory screening, dental examination, and behavioral assessment.
2. It is helpful to gain a child's trust before doing any type of an examination. Talk and play with the child first. It also helps to perform parts of the examination that can be done visually before actually touching the child.
3. Children will feel safer during an examination if it is initiated from the periphery and then moves to the central. Examine the extremities before moving to the chest, for example.
4. Children who are chronically ill, disabled, in foster care, or foreign-born adopted may require additional assessment because of their unique health risks.
5. When obtaining histories of infants and children, gather all or part of the information from parents or guardians.

6. Parents may think they are being tested or judged by the examiner. Offer support during examination, and do not pass judgment.

7. Call children by their preferred name, and address parents as "Mr. and Mrs. Brown" rather than by first names.

8. Open-ended questions often allow parents to share more information and to describe more of the child's problems.

9. Older children and adolescents tend to respond best when treated as adults and individuals and often can provide details about their health history and severity of symptoms.

10. The adolescent has a right to confidentiality. After talking with parents about historical information, the nurse arranges to be alone with the adolescent to speak further privately and to perform the examination.

Older Adults

1. Do not assume that aging is always accompanied by illness or disability. Most older adults are able to adapt to change and maintain functional independence (Lueckenotte, 2000).

2. Allow extra time and be patient, relaxed, and unhurried with older adults.

3. Provide adequate space for an examination, particularly if the client uses a mobility aid.

4. Plan the history and examination, taking into account the older adult's energy level, physical limitations, pace, and adaptability. More than one session may be needed to complete the assessment (Lueckenotte, 2000).

5. Measure performance under the most favorable conditions. Take advantage of natural opportunities for assessment (e.g., during bathing, grooming, mealtime) (Lueckenotte, 2000).

6. Sequence an examination to keep position changes to a minimum. Be efficient throughout the examination to limit client movement.

7. Be sure an examination of an older adult includes review of mental status.

Cultural Considerations

The nurse can conduct an accurate and complete assessment only after considering how a client's cultural background influences the approach to the examination. The client's race, gender, age, and cultural beliefs often influence assessment findings and examination approaches to use. A client's health beliefs, use of alternative therapies, nutritional habits, relationships with family, and comfort with close physical contact during an assessment must also be considered.

- Learn how to use open-ended questions to assess sociocultural and religious values that influence health/illness beliefs and practices.
  - Communicate respect through proper use of distance, attention, eye contact, tone, and loudness of voice.
  - Use a professional interpreter familiar with the client's culture and language.
  - Allow time for responses.

- Observe language and communication patterns of clients.
  - Work with the established family hierarchy as identified by the client.
  - Develop knowledge of words that are offensive to the culture. For example, words such as *vagina, penis,* and *breasts* are referred to as parts of a female or male among Southeast Asian groups.
- Assess meaning of symptoms to the client and family.
  - Jot down client's own words to describe these meanings.
- Obtain prior knowledge of health risks common to the cultural group.
  - Certain diseases are prevalent in some groups, for example, malaria among Africans and Asians and parasitic worms among migrants from the Third World.
- Integrate knowledge of cultural differences in growth and development, physical characteristics, and norms in interpreting assessment data.
  - Physical parameters such as skin and mucosal color, hair texture/color, and height and weight are influenced by biological/racial characteristics.
  - Recognize Mongolian spots common among infants and children of color as physiological differences in skin pigmentation rather than bruising.
  - Develop awareness of healing modalities used by some cultures, especially Asians, that may leave the skin discolored or scratched, such as cupping, coining, and pinching.
    - These treatments are used to expel bad wind and restore balance in cold conditions.
    - In cupping, the skin appears reddened initially because of the application of heated cups, which changes to bruised or discolored circular spots after a few days. The skin returns to normal color after a week.
    - In coining, heated oil is rubbed on the skin, and the edge of a coin is scratched against the skin, leaving superficial scratch marks on the chest and back.
    - After rubbing the skin with warm oil, it is pinched symmetrically and appears reddened after the treatment (Andrews, 2003).
- Provide privacy to the client during the health history and physical examination.
  - It is not unusual for clients from ethnocultural groups to ask for a family member to be present during the examination to interpret for them or provide moral support.
  - Accommodate client's request for presence of family member.
  - Weigh carefully questions to be asked in the presence of the family member because clients from collectivistic groups may provide only safe answers in the presence of family members.
  - Use gender-congruent providers to perform the physical assessment.
  - Ask permission before you touch the client (Box 18-2).
  - Drape the client thoroughly, and use the bedside screen or curtains.

BOX 18-2 Cultural Awareness of Touch During Physical Examination

Physical contact with a client can convey a variety of meanings, depending on the client's cultural background. Consider these guidelines, but remember that each client is an individual and may respond differently.

HISPANICS

Highly tactile
Very modest (men and women)
May ask for health care provider of same gender
Women may refuse to be examined by male health care provider

ASIANS/PACIFIC ISLANDERS

Avoid touching (patting head is strictly taboo)
Touching during an argument equals loss of control (shame)
Public display of affection toward members of same gender is permissible (but not toward members of opposite gender)

AFRICAN-AMERICANS

May not like to be touched without permission
May exercise level of distrust or caution initially in care provider

NATIVE AMERICANS

Shake hands lightly
May not like to be touched without permission
Nonverbal communication is important

Data from Lueckenotte A: *Gerontologic nursing*, ed 2, St. Louis, 2000, Mosby; Seidel HM and others: *Mosby's guide to physical examination*, ed 5, St. Louis, 2003, Mosby.

Evidenced-Based Practice Trends

Health Promotion: Screening for Skin Cancer

There are three major types of skin cancer: basal cell carcinoma, squamous cell carcinoma, and the most serious form of skin cancer, melanoma. According to the American Cancer Society (ACS) (2004), approximately 55,100 people will be diagnosed with melanoma in 2004. Cancerous melanomas start as small, molelike growths that increase in size, change color, become ulcerated, and bleed. The client should be instructed to conduct a complete monthly self-examination of the skin, noting moles, blemishes, and birthmarks. All skin surfaces should be inspected. A simple ABCD rule (ACS, 2004) outlines warning signals (see Box 18-4, p. 552):

A is for Asymmetry.
B is for Border irregularity; edges are ragged, notched, or blurred.
C is for Color; pigmentation is not uniform; variation in the shading/multiple color—blue black, or variegated (Lapka, 2000).
D is for Diameter; greater than 6 mm (about the size of a pencil eraser).

The client should report to his or her health care provider any change in skin lesions or a sore that does not heal.

The nurse should instruct the client to prevent skin cancer by avoiding overexposure to the sun: wear wide-brimmed hats and long sleeves, apply broad-spectrum sunscreens with SPF of 15 or greater to protect against UVB and UVA rays approximately 15 minutes before going into the sun and after swimming or perspiring, avoid tanning under the direct sun at midday (10 AM to 4 PM), and do not use indoor sunlamps, tanning parlors, or tanning pills. Medications such as oral contraceptives, antibiotics, immunosuppressive agents, antiinflammatories, and antihypertensives can make the skin more sensitive to the sun (Lapka, 2000). Special care should be taken to protect children from the sun, because severe sunburns in childhood may greatly increase the risk of melanoma later in life (ACS, 2004).

Skill Performance Guidelines

1. Set priorities for assessment based on a client's presenting signs and symptoms or health care needs. For example, a client who develops sudden shortness of breath should first undergo an assessment of the lungs and thorax. If a client is acutely ill, the nurse may choose to assess only the involved body systems. The nurse's judgment is needed to ensure that an examination is relevant and inclusive.

2. Organize the examination. Compare both sides of the body for symmetry. If a client becomes fatigued, offer rest periods. Perform painful procedures near the end of the examination.

3. Use a head-to-toe approach. Follow the sequence of inspection, palpation, percussion, and auscultation (except for during the abdominal assessment). This sequence facilitates an effective assessment.

4. Encourage the client to be an active participant. Clients are usually knowledgeable about their physical condition. Often the client can let the nurse know when certain findings are normal or when actual changes have occurred.

5. Follow standard precautions for infection control. Assessments may require the nurse to have contact with body fluids and discharge. When there are breaks in the skin, lesions, or wounds, or when having contact with mucous membranes, gloves must be worn. In some circumstances the nurse must wear a gown.

6. Consider the possibility of latex allergy. The incidence of serious allergic reaction to latex has increased dramatically (Seidel and others, 2003) (see Chapter 8).

7. Record quick notes to facilitate accurate documentation.

8. Continue to use assessment skills during each client contact, including activities such as bathing, administration of medications, or other therapies or while conversing with a client.

9. Integrate health promotion and education into physical assessment activities. There are "teachable moments" when the nurse can share findings and educate clients about health promotion.

10. Record summary of the assessment using appropriate medical terminology and in the sequence that findings are gathered. Use commonly accepted medical abbreviations to keep notes concise.

SKILL 18-1 General Survey

The general survey begins a review of the client's primary health problems, and it includes assessment of the client's vital signs, height and weight, general behavior, and appearance. The survey provides information about characteristics of an illness, a client's hygiene, skin condition and body image, emotional state, recent changes in weight, and developmental status. The survey can reveal important information about the client's behavior that can influence how the nurse communicates instructions to the client and continues the assessment.

DELEGATION CONSIDERATIONS

The general survey should not be delegated to assistive personnel. The following activities may be delegated to assistive personnel:

- Measuring height and weight
- Oral intake
- Urinary output
- Vital signs (not the initial set, but subsequent measurements if client is stable)
- Reporting a client's subjective signs and symptoms

All monitoring data must be reported to the nurse.

EQUIPMENT

- ❏ Stethoscope
- ❏ Sphygmomanometer and cuff
- ❏ Thermometer
- ❏ Digital watch or wristwatch with second hand
- ❏ Tape measure
- ❏ Clean nonlatex gloves

STEP	RATIONALE

ASSESSMENT

1. Note if client has had any acute distress: difficulty breathing, pain, anxiety. If such signs are present, defer general survey until later.

Signs establish priorities regarding what part of the examination to conduct first.

- *Critical Decision Point*
  Findings may change the direction of the examination. Any client in acute distress will require an immediate assessment of the body system(s) affected.

2. Review graphic sheet for temperature, pulse, respirations, and blood pressure, and consider factors or conditions that may alter reading of vital signs (see Chapter 17).

Provides baseline and historical data regarding client's vital signs.

3. Determine client's primary language. If need for an interpreter is identified, it is best to obtain services of professional interpreter rather than a family member. Have the interpreter translate verbatim if possible.

Facilitates the presence of an interpreter familiar with medical terminology. If possible, have interpreters of the same gender and one who is older.

4. Reconfirm (after reviewing history) primary reason client has sought health care.

Keeps assessment focused on client to ensure that client's expectations are addressed.

5. Identify client's normal height and weight. If a sudden gain or loss in weight has occurred, determine amount of weight change and period of time in which it occurred. Assess if client has recently been dieting or following an exercise program.

Generally, weight of 10% to 20% above standard indicates excess body fat (Moore, 2001); however, fluid retention is one factor that must be ruled out. A person's weight can fluctuate daily because of fluid loss or retention (1 L of water weighs 1 kg, or 2.2 pounds).

STEP	RATIONALE
6. Review client's past fluid intake and output (I&O) records.	Fluid and electrolyte balance maintains health and function in all body systems. Intake includes all liquids taken orally, by feeding tube, and parenterally. Liquid output includes urine, diarrhea stool, fistulas, vomitus, drainage from gastric suction, and drainage from postsurgical tubes, such as chest tubes or Jackson-Pratt drains.
7. Identify client's general perceptions about personal health.	Assessment of client's general appearance coupled with client's own perceptions may reveal specific problem areas.
8. Assess for evidence of latex allergy, which may include contact dermatitis or systemic reactions. Ask if client has risk factors such as food allergies (papaya, avocado, banana, peach, kiwi, tomato); high latex exposure (housekeepers, food handlers, health care worker); or must avoid products containing latex (rubber bands, adhesive tape, certain paints or carpets).	Gloves will be worn during certain aspects of the assessment. Repeated exposure may result in more serious reactions, including asthma, itching, and anaphylaxis (Seidel and others, 2003). These are a few risk factors for latex allergy.

NURSING DIAGNOSES

- Imbalanced nutrition: less than body requirements or more than body requirements
- Deficient fluid volume or excess fluid volume
- Anxiety
- Bathing/hygiene self-care deficit
- Fear

- Impaired bed mobility
- Impaired skin integrity
- Ineffective breathing pattern
- Impaired physical mobility
- Ineffective peripheral tissue perfusion
- Pain (acute, chronic)

Related factors are individualized based on client's condition or needs.

PLANNING

1. Expected outcomes following completion of procedure:	
• Client demonstrates alert, cooperative behavior without evidence of physical or emotional distress during assessment.	Nurse uses calm and confident approach during assessment. Client has no abnormal findings.
• Client provides appropriate subjective data related to physical condition.	Client able to cooperate with assessment.
2. *Prepare client:* Tell the client you will be doing a routine process to check for areas of concern. Ask client to tell you if any area you examine hurts when touched.	Understanding promotes client's cooperation. Pain is an important finding during assessment.

IMPLEMENTATION

1. Throughout assessment note client's verbal and nonverbal behaviors. Determine the level of consciousness and orientation by observing and talking to client (Box 18-3).	Behaviors may reflect specific physical abnormalities. Dementia and level of consciousness influences ability to cooperate.
2. Obtain temperature, pulse, respirations, and blood pressure unless taken within last 3 hours or a serious potential change is noted (e.g., change in level of consciousness or difficulty breathing) (see Chapter 17). Inform client of vital signs.	Vital signs provide important information regarding physiological changes in relation to oxygenation and circulation (Elkin and others, 2004).
3. Observe the following aspects of appearance: gender, race, and age. Note the client's physical features.	Gender influences type of examination performed and manner in which assessments are made. Different physical characteristics and predisposition to illnesses are related to gender and race.

STEP	RATIONALE

BOX 18-3 Symptoms That May Indicate Dementia

LEARNING AND RETAINING NEW INFORMATION

Trouble remembering recent conversations, events, and appointments
Frequently misplaces objects

LANGUAGE

Increasing difficulty with expressing self
Difficulty following conversations

HANDLING COMPLEX TASKS

Difficulty following a complex train of thought
Difficulty performing tasks that require many steps

BEHAVIOR

Appears more passive and less responsive
More irritable and suspicious than usual
Misinterprets visual and auditory stimuli

REASONING ABILITY

Unable to develop plan to address problems at work or home
Displays uncharacteristic disregard for rules of social conduct

SPATIAL ABILITY AND ORIENTATION

Difficulty driving
Difficulty in organizing objects around the house
Difficulty finding way around familiar places

Data from Agency for Health Care Policy and Research: *Recognition and initial assessment of Alzheimer's disease and related dementias,* Rockville, Md, 1996, Agency for Health Care Policy and Research.

---

4. If uncertain whether client understands a question, rephrase or ask a similar question.

   Inappropriate response from a client may be caused by language or deterioration of mental status, preoccupation with illness, or decreased hearing acuity.

5. If a client's responses are inappropriate, ask short, to-the-point questions regarding information the client should know, for example: "Tell me your name." "What is the name of this place?" "Tell me where you live." "What day is this?" "What month is this?" or "What season of the year is this?"

   Measures client's orientation to person, place and time. This may be noted in documentation as "Oriented × 3." If disoriented in any way, include subjective and/or objective data rather than just documenting "disoriented."

6. If client is unable to respond to questions of orientation, offer simple commands, for example, "Squeeze my fingers" or "Move your toes."

   Levels of consciousness exist along a continuum including full responsiveness, inability to consciously initiate meaningful behaviors, and unresponsiveness to stimuli.

STEP	RATIONALE

7. Assess posture and position, noting alignment of shoulders and hips while client stands and/or sits. Observe whether the client has a slumped, erect, or bent posture (see illustration).

May reveal musculoskeletal problem, mood, or presence of pain.

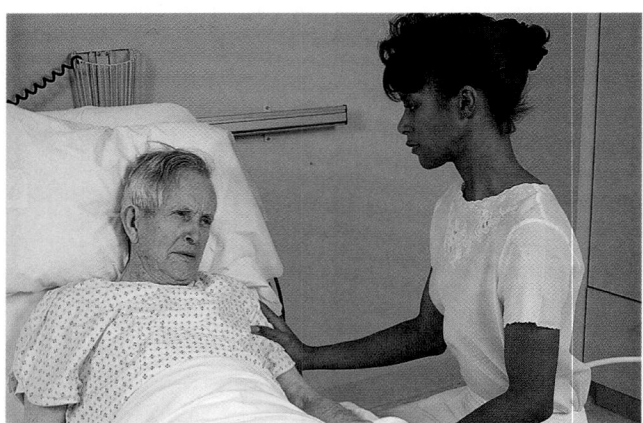

STEP **7** Observe client's position and posture.

    a. Observe body movements. Are they purposeful? Are there tremors of the extremities? Are any body parts immobile?

May indicate neurological or muscular problem or emotional stress.

    b. Note if movements are coordinated or uncoordinated.

8. Assess speech. Is it understandable and moderately paced? Is there an association with the person's thoughts?

Alterations may reflect neurological impairment, injury or impairment of mouth, improperly fitting dentures, or differences in dialect and language.

9. Observe hygiene and grooming for presence or absence of makeup, type of clothes (hospital or personal), and cleanliness.

Grooming may reflect activity level before examination, resources available to purchase grooming supplies, client's mood, and self-care practices. May also reflect culture, lifestyle, economic status, and personal preferences.

    a. Observe the color, distribution, quantity, thickness, texture, and lubrication of hair.

Changes in hair distribution may reflect hormonal changes, changes from aging, poor nutrition, or use of certain hair care products.

    b. Inspect the condition of nails.

Changes may indicate inadequate nutrition or grooming practices, nervous habits, or systemic diseases.

    c. Assess the presence or absence of body odor.

Body odor may result from physical exercise, deficient hygiene, or physical or mental abnormalities. Inadequate oral hygiene or unhealthy teeth may cause bad breath.

10. Assess the eyes.

    a. Inspect position of eyes, color, condition of conjunctiva, and movement.

Asymmetrical positioning or eye movement may reflect trauma or tumor growths. Differences in color may be congenital; changes in color of conjunctiva may be due to local infection or symptomatic of another abnormality (e.g., pale conjunctiva is associated with anemia).

    b. Assess client's near vision (ability to read newspaper or magazines) and far vision (follow movement, ability to read the clock, television, or signs at a distance).

If client has visual acuity or visual field loss, make adjustments to support self-care measures (e.g., feeding, bathing and hygiene, dressing) and teaching.

STEP	**RATIONALE**

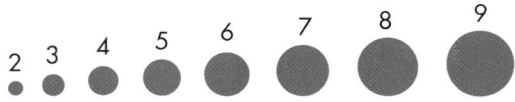

STEP **10c** Pupil sizes in millimeters.

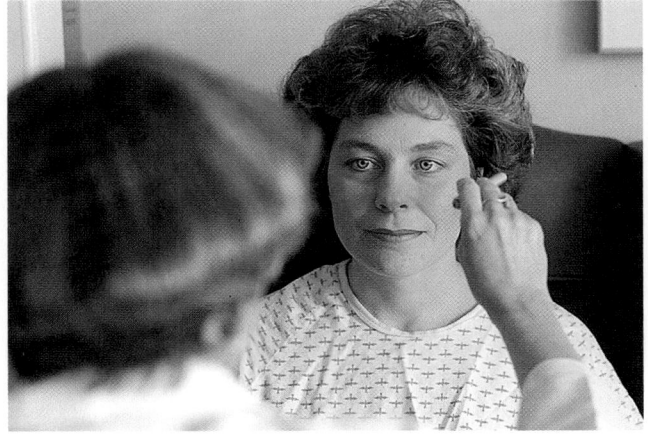
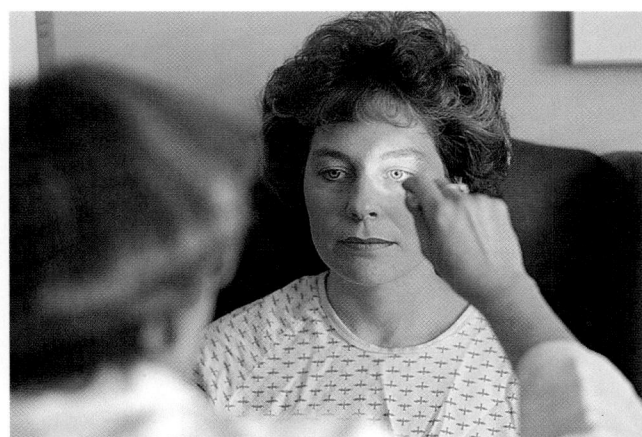

A   B

STEP **10d** **A,** Holding penlight to side of client's face. **B,** Illumination of pupil causes pupillary constriction.

c. Inspect pupils for size, shape, and equality (see illustration).

Normal pupils are round, clear, and equal in size and shape.

d. Test pupillary reflexes. To test reaction to light, dim room lights. If lights can not be dimmed, cup hand over eye to temporarily shield the light. As client looks straight ahead, move penlight from side of client's face and direct light on pupil. Observe pupillary response of both eyes, noting briskness and equality of reflex (see illustrations).

Darkened room normally ensures brisk response of pupils to light. Pupil that is illuminated constricts. Pupil in other eye should constrict equally (consensual light reflex).

11. Assess hearing. Note the client's response to questions and the presence/use of a hearing aid. If hearing loss is suspected, test by asking client to repeat random words spoken by the nurse. Use one- or two-syllable words. Repeat, gradually increasing voice intensity until client correctly repeats the numbers.

Seidel and others (2003) report that clients normally hear numbers clearly when whispered, responding correctly at least 50% of the time. For client with obvious hearing impairment, speak clearly and concisely, stand so that client can see face, and toward client's good ear, speak in low pitch, and avoid yelling.

• **Critical Decision Point**

If hearing deficit is present, inspect client's ears. Impaired hearing may be due to impacted cerumen, external otitis, or swelling in ear canal due to allergic reactions to materials in hearing aids.

12. Inspect nose externally for shape, skin color, alignment, and presence of deformity or inflammation. Note color of mucosa and any lesions, discharge, swelling, or presence of bleeding.

13. In clients with a nasogastric, nasointestinal, or nasotracheal tube, inspect nares for excoriation or inflammation. Stabilize tube as needed.

Character of discharge and inflammation indicate allergy or infection. Perforation and erosion of the septum and puffiness and/or increased vascularity of the mucosa can indicate habitual use of intranasal cocaine and opioids.

Swallowing or coughing causes movement of tubes against nares, and pressure against tissues and mucosa can result in tissue erosion.

STEP	RATIONALE

14. Assess the mouth. Use a tongue blade to lightly depress the tongue. Illuminate the oral cavity with a pen light. Inspect oral mucosa, tongue, teeth, and gums for hydration, discoloration, and obvious lesions (see illustration). Determine if client wears dentures or retainers and if they are comfortable. Dentures should be removed to properly visualize and palpate gums.

Ill-fitting dentures and retainers chronically irritate mucosa and gums and may pose risk for mouth cancer.

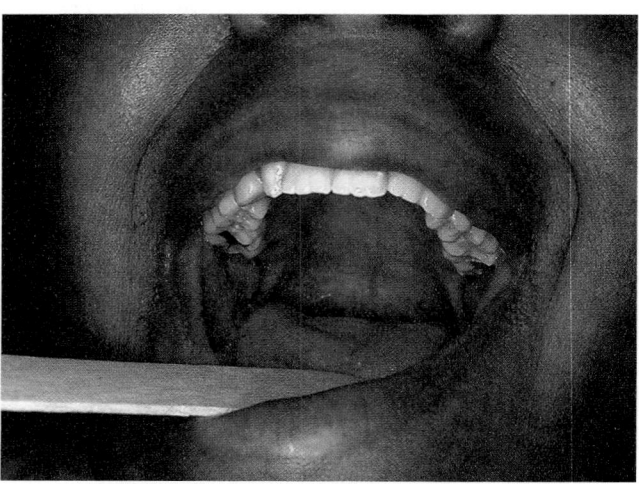

STEP **14** Inspect mouth.

15. During the examination inspect exposed areas of the skin and ask if client has noted any changes in the skin, including:
  a. Pruritus, oozing, bleeding
  b. Change in the appearance of a mole, bump or nodule; a change in sensation; itchiness, tenderness, or pain
  c. Petechiae (tiny, pinpoint-size, red or purple spots on the skin caused by small hemorrhages in the skin layers).

Incidence of melanoma, an aggressive form of skin cancer, has increased significantly. It is more than 10 times higher in whites than in African-Americans (ACS, 2003). The cancer can spread to other parts of the body quickly. Early detection and prompt treatment are critical (Box 18-4).

Petechiae may indicate serious blood clotting disorder, drug reaction, or liver disease.

BOX 18-4   **Malignant Melanoma**

MNEMONICS

The ABCD Rule of Melanoma (ACS, 2004)

Here is a simple way to remember the characteristics that should alert you to the possibility of malignant melanoma.

A   *A*symmetry of lesion
B   *B*orders: irregular
C   *C*olor: blue/black or variegated
D   *D*iameter > 6 mm

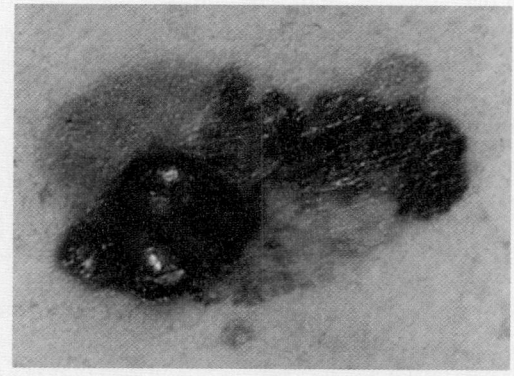

Malignant melanoma. (From Zitelli B, Davis H: *Atlas of pediatric physical diagnosis*, ed 3, St. Louis, 1997, Mosby.)

STEP	RATIONALE

TABLE 18-5   SKIN COLOR VARIATIONS

COLOR	CONDITION	CAUSES	ASSESSMENT LOCATIONS
Bluish (cyanosis)	Increased amount of deoxygenated hemoglobin (associated with hypoxia)	Heart or lung disease, cold environment	Nail beds, lips, base of tongue, skin (severe cases)
Pallor (decrease in color)	Reduced amount of oxyhemoglobin	Anemia	Face, conjunctivae, nail beds, palms of hands
	Reduced visibility of oxyhemoglobin resulting from decreased blood flow	Shock	Skin, nail beds, conjunctivae, lips
Loss of pigmentation	Vitiligo	Congenital or autoimmune condition causing lack of pigment	Patchy areas on skin over face, hands, arms
Yellow-orange (jaundice)	Increased deposit of bilirubin in tissues	Liver disease, destruction of red blood cells	Sclera, mucous membranes, skin
Red (erythema)	Increased visibility of oxyhemoglobin caused by dilation or increased blood flow	Fever, direct trauma, blushing, alcohol intake	Face, area of trauma, sacrum, shoulders, other common sites for pressure ulcers
Tan-brown	Increased amount of melanin	Suntan, pregnancy	Areas exposed to sun: face, arms; areolae, nipples

16. Inspect skin surfaces, comparing color of symmetrical body parts. Scan the entire body, noting areas unexposed to sun. Look for any patches or areas of skin color variation.

Changes in color can be indicative of pathological alterations (Table 18-5).

• Critical Decision Point

Be alert for basal cell carcinomas, often seen in sun-exposed areas. Frequently these occur in a background of sun-damaged skin.

17. Carefully inspect color of face, oral mucosa, lips, conjunctiva, sclera, and nail beds.

Nurse can more readily identify abnormalities in areas of body where melanin production is lowest.

• Critical Decision Point

When assessing the skin of a client with bandages, cast, restraints, or other restrictive devices, note areas of pallor and decreased temperature, which may indicate impaired circulation. Immediate release of pressure from the restrictive device may be necessary.

18. Use ungloved fingertips to palpate skin surfaces to feel moisture of intact skin.

Moisture is directly related to degree of hydration and condition of outer lipid layer of the skin surface. Older adults are prone to xerosis, which is evident as dry, scaly skin (Lueckenotte, 2000).

    a. Stroke skin surfaces lightly with fingertips to detect texture of skin's surface. Note whether skin is smooth or rough, thick or thin, tight or supple and if localized areas of hardness or lesions are present.

Localized texture changes result from trauma, surgical wounds, or lesions.

    b. Palpate any areas that appear irregular in texture.

Allows nurse to detect localized areas of hardness and/or tenderness within subcutaneous skin layers.

• Critical Decision Point

If client receives routine injections (e.g., insulin, heparin), localized areas of hardness may be found over injection sites. Develop a plan to rotate injection sites systematically. Local skin changes from repeated injections can be prevented by site rotation (Ahern and Mazur, 2001).

STEP	RATIONALE

19. While wearing clean gloves, inspect character of any secretions; note color, odor, amount, and consistency (e.g., thin and watery, thick and oily).

Character of secretions from skin lesions helps to indicate type of lesion.

20. Using dorsum (back) of hand, palpate for temperature of skin surfaces. If nurse is wearing a glove, remove temporarily.) Compare symmetrical body parts. Compare upper and lower body parts. Note distinct temperature differences. Note localized areas of warmth.

Increased or decreased skin temperature reflects increase or decrease in blood flow. Skin on dorsum of hand is thin, which allows detection of subtle temperature changes. A stage I pressure ulcer may cause warmth and erythema (redness) of an area. The temperature of the environment and anxiety may also affect skin temperature.

21. Assess skin turgor by grasping fold of skin on the sternal area or forearm with the fingertips. Release skinfold, and note ease and speed with which skin returns to place (see illustration).

With reduced turgor, skin remains suspended or "tented" for a few seconds before slowly returning to place. This indicates decreased elasticity and possible dehydration (Elkin and others, 2004). With altered turgor it is essential to provide measures for prevention of pressure ulcers.

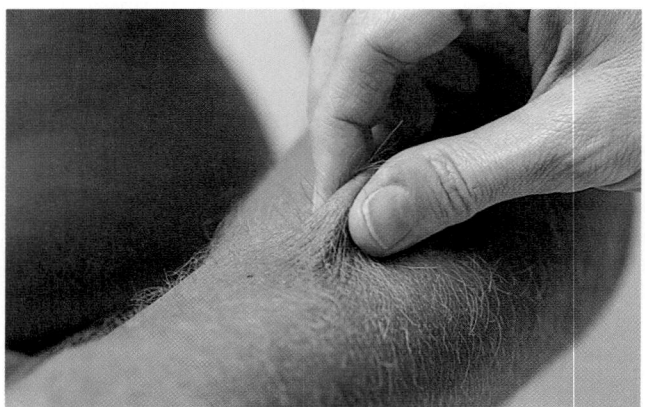

STEP **21** Checking skin turgor.

22. Assess condition of skin for pressure areas, paying particular attention to regions of pressure (e.g., sacrum, greater trochanter, heels, occipital area, clavicles). If areas of redness are noted, place fingertip over area and apply gentle pressure, then release.

Normal reactive hyperemia (redness) is visible effect of localized vasodilation, body's normal response to lack of blood flow to underlying tissue. Affected area of skin will blanch with fingertip pressure.

• *Critical Decision Point*
Evidence of normal reactive hyperemia on pressure points should result in repositioning of client and development of turning schedule if client is dependent (see Chapter 15).

23. When any lesion is detected, use adequate lighting to inspect its color, location, texture, size, shape, type (Box 18-5). Note also grouping (e.g., clustered, linear) and distribution (localized or generalized).

Certain skin lesions can be identified by a characteristic pattern of features.

   a. Gently palpate any lesion to determine mobility, contour (flat, raised, or depressed), and consistency (soft or hard). If lesion is moist or draining, apply disposable gloves before palpation.

Gentle palpation prevents accidental rupture of underlying cysts. Gloves reduce transmission of microorganisms.

   b. Note if client reports tenderness during palpation.

Tenderness may be indicative of inflammation or pressure on body part.

   c. Measure size of lesion (height, width, depth) with centimeter ruler.

Provides for baseline to assess changes in lesion over time.

STEP	RATIONALE

BOX 18-5   Types of Primary Skin Lesions

Macule: Flat, nonpalpable change in skin color, smaller than 1 cm (e.g., freckle, petechia)

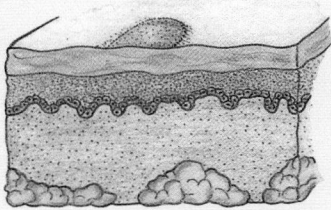

Vesicle: Circumscribed elevation of skin filled with serous fluid, smaller than 1 cm (e.g., herpes simplex, chickenpox)

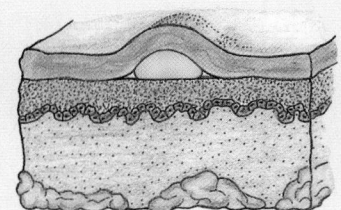

Papule: Palpable, circumscribed, solid elevation in skin, smaller than 1 cm (e.g., elevated nevus)

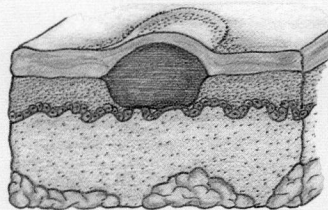

Pustule: Circumscribed elevation of skin similar to vesicle but filled with pus, varies in size (e.g., acne, staphylococcal infection)

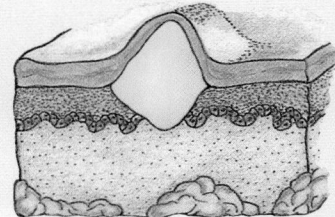

Nodule: Elevated solid mass, deeper and firmer than papule, 1 to 2 cm (e.g., wart)

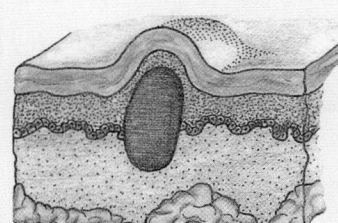

Ulcer: Deep loss of skin surface that may extend to dermis and frequently bleeds and scars, varies in size (e.g., venous stasis ulcer)

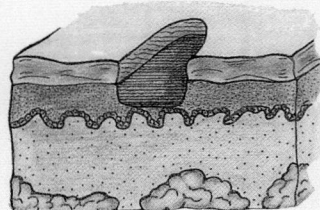

Tumor: Solid mass that may extend deep through subcutaneous tissue, larger than 1 to 2 cm (e.g., epithelioma)

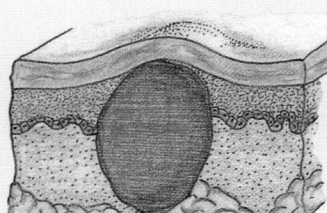

Atrophy: Thinning of skin with loss of normal skin furrow with skin appearing shiny and translucent, varies in size (e.g., arterial insufficiency)

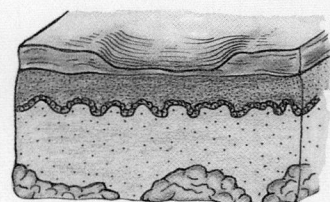

Wheal: Irregularly shaped, elevated area or superficial localized edema, varies in size (e.g., hive, mosquito bite)

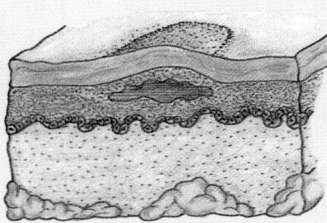

STEP	RATIONALE

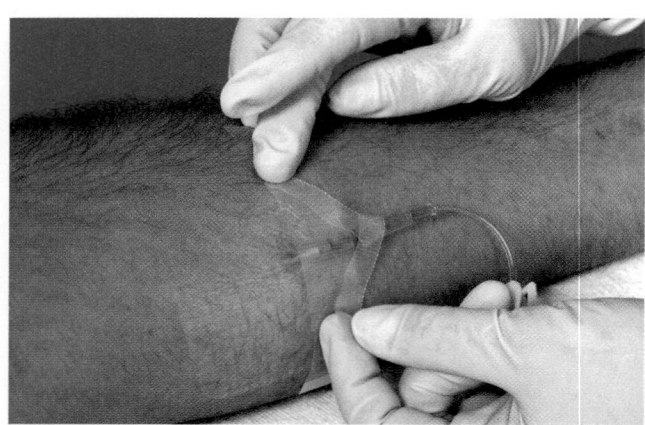

A   B

STEP **24** **A** and **B,** Palpating IV site for tenderness.

24. Using clean gloves, inspect and palpate any intravenous (IV) site (see illustrations) for evidence of inflammation (redness, heat, swelling, drainage, or tenderness) or infiltration (puffiness, pallor, and coolness). Note when site is due to be changed.

Presence of infiltration or phlebitis requires IV to be discontinued (see Chapter 27). Agency policy dictates frequency of site change.

25. Use the "six rights" to check IV fluids and medications, including type of fluids and rate of infusion. Note expiration date of fluids and tubing.

Infusion rate that is too rapid may result in fluid volume excess; a rate too slow can result in inadequate fluid replacement. Changing the fluids and tubing according to agency policy helps prevent IV-related infections.

26. Assess affect and mood: note if verbal expressions match nonverbal behavior and if appropriate to situation.

Reflects client's mental status, consciousness, feelings, and emotional status.

27. Observe client interaction with spouse or partner, older adult child, or caregiver. Be alert for indications of fear, hesitancy to report health status, or willingness to let caregiver control assessment interview. Does partner or caregiver have a history of violence, alcoholism, or drug abuse? Is the person unemployed, ill, or frustrated with caring for client? Note if client has any obvious physical injuries.

Abuse may first be suspected in clients who have suffered obvious physical injury or neglect, show signs of malnutrition, or have bruises on the extremities or trunk. Partners or caregivers may have history of abusive or addictive behaviors.

● *Critical Decision Point*
Be discreet in how interview is handled. Direct questions about abuse must be asked in private. It may be necessary to delay assessment to a later time, when the partner or caregiver is not present. Asking a partner or caregiver to leave during an assessment may create an awkward situation.

STEP	**RATIONALE**

28. Observe for signs of abuse:

   a. *For a child:* Blood on underclothing, pain in genital area, difficulty sitting or walking.

Indicative of child sexual abuse.

   b. *For a female client:* Injury or trauma inconsistent with reported cause, obvious injuries to face or neck (black eyes, broken nose, lip lacerations, broken teeth, strangulation marks, burns).

Indicates domestic abuse.

   c. *For an older adult:* Injury or trauma inconsistent with reported cause, injuries in unusual locations (such as neck or genitalia), pattern injuries (left when an object with which a person is struck leaves an imprint), parallel injuries (such as bilateral bruises on the upper arms suggesting the client was held and shaken), and burns (shaped like a cigarette, iron, rope, or immersion with a clear line of demarcation).

Prolonged interval between injury and time medical care was sought are signs indicative of older adult abuse or neglect (Gray-Vickrey, 2001).

- *Critical Decision Point*

   A pattern of findings indicating abuse usually mandates a report to a social service center (refer to state guidelines). Nurse should obtain immediate consultation with physician, social worker, and other support staff to facilitate placement in a safer environment.

EVALUATION

1. Observe throughout the assessment for evidence of physical or emotional distress.

Interaction during assessment can reveal emotional problems. Maneuvers used during physical examination can reveal presence of physical problems.

2. Compare assessment findings with previous observations.

Determines if change has occurred.

3. Ask the client if there is information about physical condition that has not been discussed.

Clients may feel they are bothering the nurse by asking questions unless the opportunity for questions is provided.

Recording and Reporting

- Record client's vital signs on vital sign flow sheet.
- Record description of alterations in client's general appearance.
- Describe client's behaviors using objective terminology. Include client's self-report of signs and symptoms.
- Report abnormalities and acute symptoms to nurse in charge or physician.

Unexpected Outcomes	**Related Interventions**
1. Client demonstrates acute distress (e.g., respiratory distress, acute pain, severe anxiety).	• Respond immediately to identified need (repositioning, oxygen, or medication as appropriate). • Obtain vital signs. • Notify physician.
2. Client has abnormal skin condition (dry texture, reduced turgor, lesions).	• Identify contributing factors, and prevent continued irritation or damage as appropriate (see Chapter 15).
3. Client is unwilling or unable to provide adequate information relating to identified concerns.	• Seek information from family members if present. • Review client's record for baseline data.

Teaching Considerations

- During general survey, inform client about normal range of vital signs for age and physical condition and normal weight for height and body frame.
- Explain that it is best to weigh self in the morning after voiding and before food or drink is taken.
- If client is on established diet, discuss any problems client has in diet preparation or food selection. The best form of weight reduction is to achieve gradual weight loss by increasing exercise and decreasing caloric intake. Refer to clinical dietitian for specific information.
- Explain the common visual changes associated with aging include reduced acuity (presbyopia), loss of or reduction in peripheral vision, reduced tearing, sensitivity to glare or bright lights.
- Teach the visually impaired client and family that adjustments in how rooms are arranged at home will aid in safe ambulation. Self-help aids are also available to assist client with functioning independently with daily living activities.

Pediatric Considerations

- Measurement of physical growth is a key element in evaluation of a child's health status. These physical growth parameters include height, length, weight, skinfold thickness, and arm and head circumference (Hockenberry and others, 2003).
- Infants are weighed nude. Children may be weighed in light underclothes or gown.
- A child's interactions with parents provide valuable information regarding the child's behavior.

Gerontological Considerations

- An older adult's presenting signs and symptoms can be deceiving. An older adult has a diminished physiological reserve that may mask the usual, or "classic," signs and symptoms of a disease. In older adults signs and symptoms are often blunted or atypical (Lueckenotte, 2000).

- Nutritional problems are frequently noted in older adults. Skipping meals is a common practice. The amount of nutrition becomes questionable. The following factors pose risks for malnutrition in older adults: limited income, loneliness, abuse of alcohol and other central nervous system depressants, forgetfulness, inability to feed self, reduced strength and mobility, and decreased vision (Moore, 2001).
- Common skin changes with aging include dryness, wrinkling, reduced elasticity, and "liver spots" in areas exposed to sun. Common lesions include seborrheic keratosis (pigmented macular-papular lesion that can be warty, scaly, or greasy); cherry angioma (bright, ruby-red or purplish papular lesion); skin tags (soft pinkish-tan to light-brown pedunculated lesions); and senile lentigines (gray-brown irregular macular lesions on sun-exposed areas) (Lueckenotte, 2000). Inspection of the feet is critically important in the presence of impaired circulation, impaired vision, and diabetes. Common podiatric conditions include ulceration, fungal infection, calluses, bunions, and plantar warts (Lueckenotte, 2000).

Home Care Considerations

- In the home the focus of an examination may be on the client's ability to perform basic self-care tasks.

Long-Term Care Considerations

- The minimum data set (MDS) is a tool that includes a comprehensive assessment of residents in the long-term care setting. It is meant to provide a total picture of a resident and to provide an ongoing comprehensive assessment of each resident, emphasizing functional ability and both a physical and a psychosocial profile. Only an RN can function as the assessment coordinator (Lueckenotte, 2000). Contributions are made by all members of health team.

SKILL 18-2 Assessing the Thorax and Lungs

Assessment of respiratory function is one of the most critical assessments because alterations can quickly become life threatening. Routine shift assessment is essential because changes in respiration can occur quickly as a result of a variety of factors, including immobility, infection, and fluid overload. Alteration in pulmonary function usually affects other body systems. For example, reduced blood oxygena-

tion can cause changes in mental alertness because of the brain's sensitivity to lowered oxygen levels. Thus the nurse must carefully assess findings from all body systems when determining the nature of pulmonary problems.

Shift assessment of the lungs includes auscultation, which assesses the movement of air through the tracheobronchial tree. Recognizing the sounds created by normal

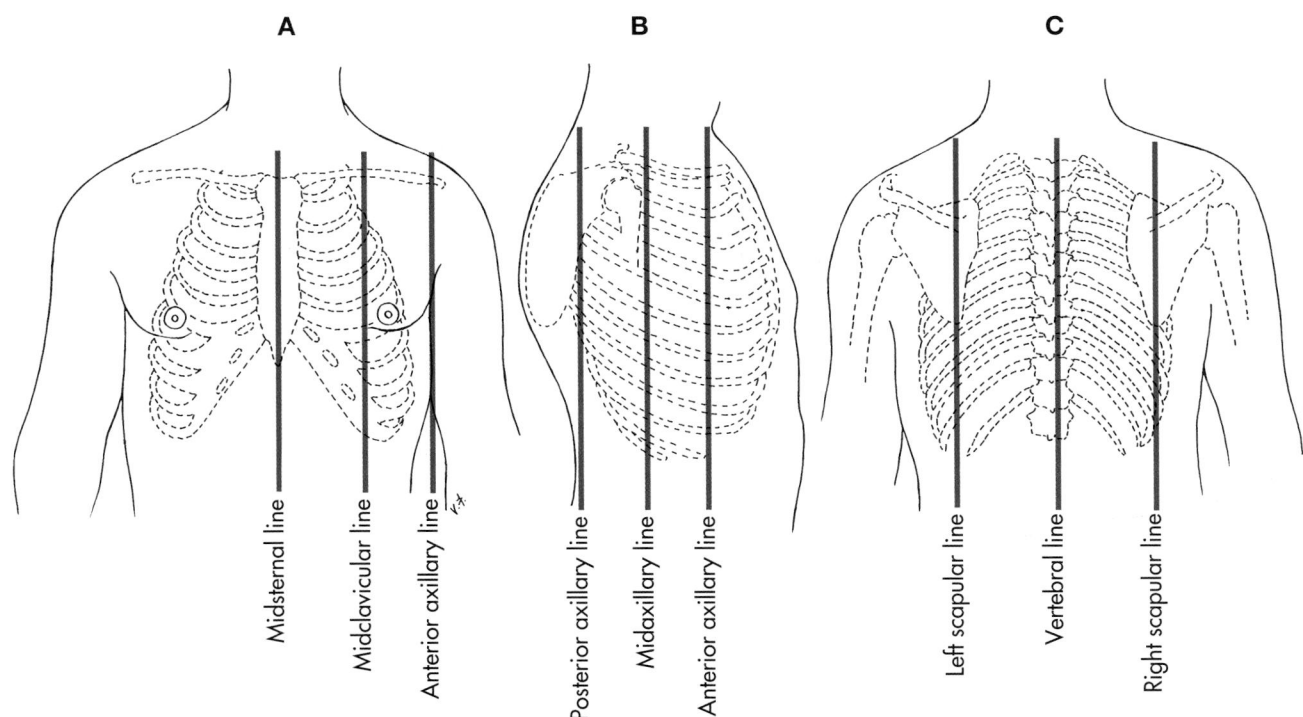

FIGURE **18-3** Anatomical landmarks of chest wall. **A,** Posterior view. **B,** Lateral view. **C,** Anterior view.

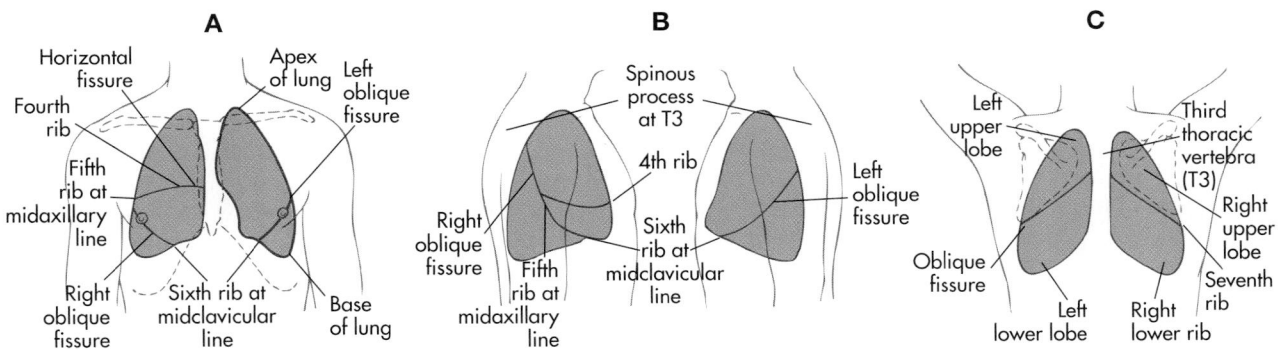

FIGURE **18-4** Position of lung lobes in relation to anatomical landmarks. **A,** Anterior. **B,** Lateral. **C,** Posterior.

airflow allows the nurse to detect sounds caused by obstruction of the airways. Assessment also includes inspection, palpation, and percussion.

To perform a lung assessment accurately, the nurse needs to be familiar with the anatomical landmarks of the chest wall (Figure 18-3). This assists in identifying the location of findings in relation to the location of the lobes of the lung (Figure 18-4) and the position of each rib. To locate the position of each rib anteriorly, the nurse begins by finding the Angle of Louis at the manubriosternal junction. The angle is a visible and palpable protrusion of the sternum at the point at which the second rib articulates with the sternum. The nurse counts the ribs and intercostal spaces from this point.

The number of each intercostal space corresponds to that of the rib just above it. Intercostal spaces are not always visible and are difficult to palpate in some individuals.

Examination of the lungs and thorax is most effective when the client is undressed to the waist. Begin with the client sitting for assessment of the posterior and lateral chest. The client may sit or lie down for examination of the anterior chest. A female client may keep a gown draped loosely over her chest while the posterior chest is examined. Good lighting is essential. The nurse needs to assess the client's ability to tolerate position changes and level of distress. Often a client confined to bed rest or the client with chest pain has limited lung expansion.

DELEGATION CONSIDERATIONS

The skill of assessing the lungs and thorax should not be delegated to assistive personnel. The following activities may be delegated:

- Measuring the client's respirations after stability has been determined
- Reporting respiratory distress, difficulty breathing, and changes in rate and depth

EQUIPMENT

- ❏ Stethoscope
- ❏ Disposable gloves

STEP	RATIONALE

ASSESSMENT

1. Assess history of tobacco or marijuana use, including type of tobacco, duration, and amount in pack years. (Pack years equal number of years smoking times the number of packs per day.) If client has quit, determine the length of time since smoking stopped.

Smoking is a risk factor for lung cancer, heart disease, and chronic lung disease (emphysema and chronic bronchitis). Smoking is responsible for 87% of all lung cancers in the United States (ACS, 2004).

2. Ask if client experiences any of the following: *persistent cough* (productive or nonproductive), *sputum production*, chest pain, shortness of breath, orthopnea, dyspnea during exertion or at rest, activity intolerance, or *recurrent attacks of pneumonia or bronchitis.*

Symptoms of respiratory alterations may help nurse localize objective physical findings. (Warning signals for lung cancer are in italic type.)

3. Determine if client works in environment containing pollutants (e.g., asbestos, arsenic, coal dust) or requiring exposure to radiation. Does client have exposure to sidestream cigarette smoke?

Clients with chronic respiratory disease, particularly asthma, have symptoms aggravated by change in temperature and humidity, irritating fumes or smoke, emotional stress, and physical exertion.

4. Review history for known or suspected human immunodeficiency virus (HIV) infection, substance abuse, low income, residence in nursing home, or recent immigration to United States.

These are risk factors for tuberculosis.

5. Ask if client has history of persistent cough, hemoptysis, unexplained weight loss, fatigue, night sweats, and/or fever.

Signs and symptoms for both tuberculosis and HIV infection.

6. Does client have history of chronic hoarseness?

Hoarseness may indicate laryngeal disorder or abuse of cocaine or opioids (sniffing).

7. Assess for history of allergies to pollen, dust, or other airborne irritants, as well as to any foods, drugs, or chemical substances.

Symptoms client demonstrates may be caused by allergic response to allergen: choking feeling, bronchospasm with respiratory stridor, wheezing on auscultation, dyspnea, cyanosis, and diaphoresis.

8. Review family history for cancer, tuberculosis, allergies, or chronic obstructive pulmonary disease (COPD).

Familial history places client at risk for lung disease.

NURSING DIAGNOSES

- Ineffective airway clearance
- Ineffective breathing pattern
- Impaired gas exchange

- Pain (acute, chronic)
- Fatigue
- Risk for infection

Related factors are individualized based on client's condition or needs.

PLANNING

1. Expected outcomes following completion of procedure:
   - Respirations are passive, diaphragmatic or costal, and regular (12 to 20 per minute in adult) with symmetrical expansion.

   Characteristics of normal respirations.

   - Breath sounds are clear to auscultation and equal bilaterally.

   Air flows without interference or obstruction. Corresponding sites side to side should sound the same.

STEP	**RATIONALE**

- Client is able to describe factors that predispose to lung disease.
- Client assumes appropriate posture for best ventilation.

Awareness of risks can improve compliance with healthful behavior.
Client can learn about benefits of good posture as examination maneuvers are performed.

IMPLEMENTATION

1. Position client sitting upright. For bedridden client, elevate head of bed 45 to 90 degrees.

   Promotes full lung expansion during examination.

   a. If unable to tolerate sitting, supine position and side-lying positions are used.

   Clients with chronic respiratory disease will likely need to sit up throughout the examination because of shortness of breath. Assistance of another caregiver may be required to position unresponsive clients.

   b. Remove gown or drape first from posterior chest, keeping legs covered. As examination progresses, remove gown from area being examined.

   Avoids unnecessary exposure and provides full visibility of thorax. Allows direct placement of diaphragm or bell on the client's skin, which enhances clarity of sounds.

   c. Explain all steps of procedure, encouraging client to relax and breathe normally through the mouth.

   Anxiety may alter respiratory function. Breathing through the mouth decreases extraneous sounds from air passing through the nose.

2. **Posterior thorax:** If possible, stand behind client to inspect thorax for shape, deformities, position of the spine, slope of the ribs, retraction of intercostal spaces during inspiration, and bulging of intercostal spaces during expiration.

   Allows for identification of any factors that may impair chest expansion and any symptoms of respiratory distress. In a child, shape of chest is almost circular, with anteroposterior (AP) diameter in 1:1 ratio. In adult, chest is twice as wide (lateral) as deep (anterior/posterior) with 2:1 lateral: anterior/posterior diameter. Chronic lung disease results in 1:1 ratio. This is referred to as a "barrel chest." Clients with breathing problems assume postures that improve ventilation.

- *Critical Decision Point*
  Localized chest pain may be evidenced by the client holding the chest wall during breathing. Assess the nature of pain, including onset, severity, precipitating factors, quality, region, and radiation.

3. Determine the rate and rhythm of breathing (see Chapter 17). Have client relaxed.

   This is a good time to count respirations, with client unaware of inspection. Awareness could alter respirations.

4. Systematically palpate posterior chest wall, costal spaces, and intercostal spaces, noting any masses, pulsations, unusual movement, or areas of localized tenderness (see illustration). If suspicious mass or swollen area is detected, palpate for size, shape, and typical qualities of lesion (see Skill 18-1). Do not palpate painful areas deeply.

   Palpation assesses further characteristics and confirms or supplements findings from inspection. Localized swelling or tenderness may indicate trauma to ribs or underlying cartilage. A fractured rib fragment could be displaced.

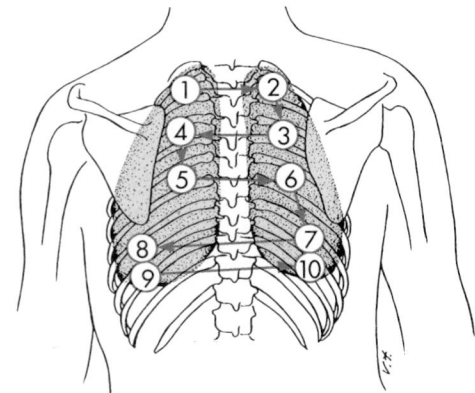

STEP 4 Pattern for assessment of posterior thorax.

STEP	RATIONALE

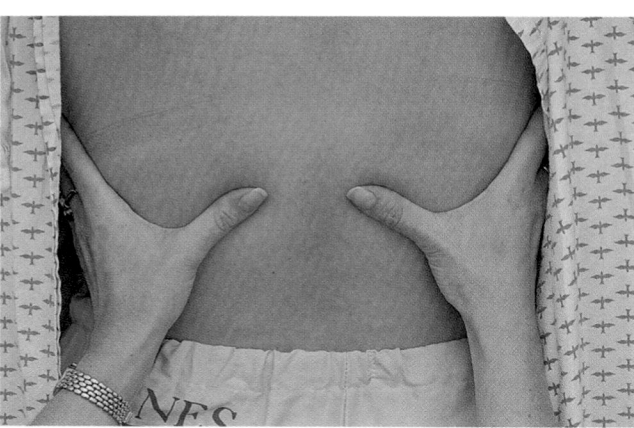

A   **B**

STEP 5 A, Position of hands for palpation of posterior thorax excursion. **B,** As client inhales, movement of chest excursion separates nurse's thumbs.

5. Standing behind client, place thumbs along the spinal processes at the tenth rib, with the palms lightly contacting the posterolateral surfaces (see illustration *A*). The nurse's thumbs should be about 2 inches (5 cm) apart, with the thumbs pointing toward the spine and the fingers pointing laterally. Press hands toward client's spine to form small skinfold between thumbs. After exhalation, client takes deep breath. Note movement of thumbs (see illustration *B*), and note symmetry of chest wall movement. Normally symmetrical separation of the thumbs occurs during chest excursion.

Palpation of chest excursion assesses depth of client's breathing. This technique is good measure to evaluate client's ability to perform deep-breathing exercises (see Chapter 35). Limited movement on one side may indicate that client is voluntarily splinting during ventilation because of pain. Avoid allowing the hands to slide over the skin, which gives a false measure of excursion.

6. Ask client to fold arms forward across chest. Percuss the posterior chest wall moving from side to side and top to bottom following the same pattern as with palpation (see step 4). Using indirect percussion, percuss intercostal spaces over symmetrical areas of the lungs. Compare percussion notes for all lung lobes.

Position separates scapulas to expose more lung tissue to assessment. Determines density of underlying lung tissue.

7. Auscultate breath sounds. Have client take slow deep breaths with the mouth slightly open. For adult, place diaphragm of stethoscope firmly on chest wall over intercostal spaces (see illustration). Listen to entire inspiration and expiration at each stethoscope position. (See pattern in step 4.) Systematically compare breath sounds over right and left sides. If sounds are faint, ask client to breathe a little deeper temporarily.

Assesses movement of air through tracheobronchial tree (Table 18-6). Recognition of normal airflow sounds allows detection of sounds caused by mucus or airway obstruction. Sounds are characterized by length of inspiratory and expiratory phases.

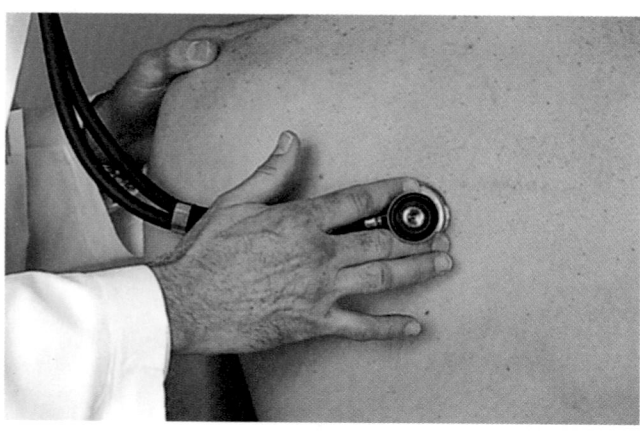

STEP 7 Use of diaphragm of stethoscope to auscultate breath sounds. (From Seidel HM and others: *Mosby's guide to physical examination,* ed 5, St. Louis, 2003, Mosby.)

STEP	RATIONALE

TABLE 18-6   NORMAL BREATH SOUNDS

DESCRIPTION	LOCATION	ORIGIN
VESICULAR		
Vesicular sounds are soft, breezy, and low pitched. Inspiratory phase is 3 times longer than expiratory phase.	Best heard over lung's periphery (except over scapula)	Created by air moving through smaller airways
BRONCHOVESICULAR		
Bronchovesicular sounds are medium pitched and blowing sounds of medium intensity. Inspiratory phase is equal to expiratory phase.	Best heard posteriorly between scapulas and anteriorly over bronchioles lateral to sternum at first and second intercostal spaces	Created by air moving through large airways
BRONCHIAL		
Bronchial sounds are loud and high pitched with hollow quality. Expiration lasts longer than inspiration (3:2 ratio).	Best heard over trachea	Created by air moving through trachea close to chest wall

8. **Lateral thorax:** Instruct client to raise arms, and inspect chest wall for same characteristics as reviewed for posterior chest.

Improves access to lateral thoracic structures.

9. Extend palpation, percussion, and auscultation of posterior thorax to lateral sides of chest, except for excursion measurement (see illustration).

Allows for location of abnormalities in lateral lung fields.

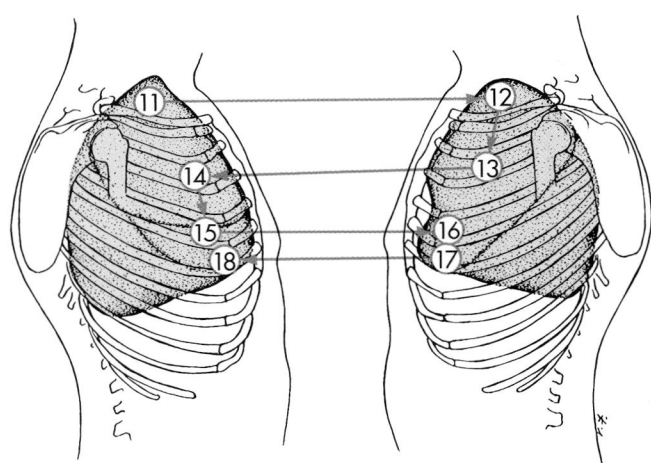

STEP **9** Pattern for assessment of lateral thorax.

10. **Anterior thorax:** Inspect accessory muscles of breathing: sternocleidomastoid, trapezius, and abdominal muscles, noting effort to breathe.

Extent to which accessory muscles are used reveals degree of effort to breathe. Generally these muscles are not used for breathing.

11. Inspect width or spread of angle made by costal margins and tip of sternum. Angle is usually larger than 90 degrees between margins.

Indicates congenital, acquired, or traumatic alterations that may influence client's chest expansion.

12. Observe the client's breathing pattern, observing symmetry and degree of chest wall and abdominal movement. Respiratory rate and rhythm are more often assessed on the anterior chest wall.

Assesses client's effort to breathe; symmetrical, passive movement indicates no respiratory distress.

STEP	RATIONALE

13. Palpate anterior thoracic muscles and ribs for lumps, masses, tenderness, or unusual movement following pattern across and down (see illustration).

Localized swelling or tenderness may indicate trauma to underlying ribs or cartilage.

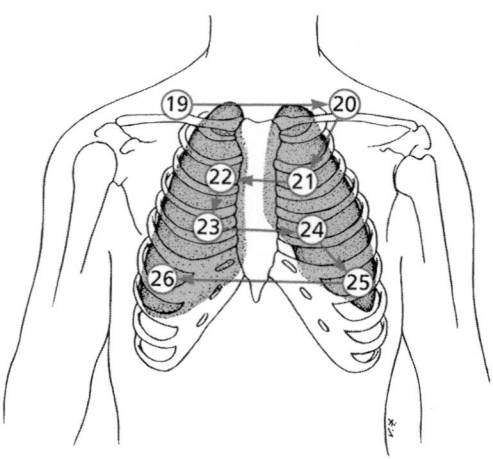

STEP **13** Pattern for assessing anterior chest.

14. Palpate anterior chest excursion. Place hands over each lateral rib cage, with thumbs approximately 5 cm (2 inches) apart and angled along each costal margin. As client inhales deeply, thumbs should symmetrically move apart.

Assesses depth of client's breathing and ability to perform deep-breathing exercises. Certain abnormalities are evident if expansion is not symmetrical.

15. Percuss anterior thorax between intercostal spaces with client lying or sitting (procedure is easier if client lies down). Begin above clavicles; move across and then down as during palpation.

Lying position facilitates ability to deliver sharp blow to chest wall to elicit clear sound. Percussion over anterior thorax enables nurse to locate position of liver, heart, and lung. Normal lung is resonant. Underlying liver, heart, and stomach create percussion notes different from that of lung (see illustration).

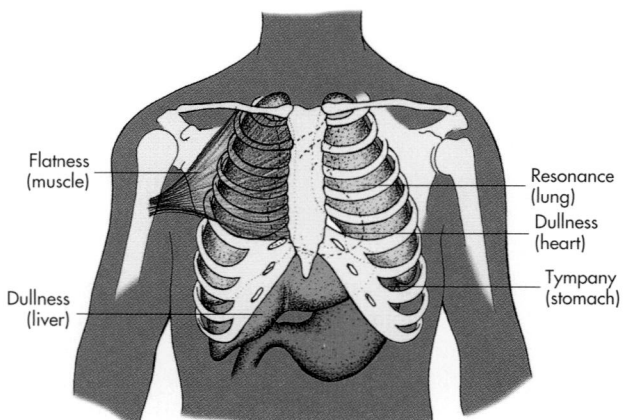

STEP **15** Variations in percussion notes in normal thorax and upper abdomen.

16. With client sitting, auscultate anterior thorax following same pattern as for percussion. If adventitious sounds are auscultated (Table 18-7), have client cough. Listen with stethoscope to determine if sound has disappeared.

Using a systematic pattern of assessment comparing sides helps to identify abnormal sounds. Rhonchi often are eliminated or altered by coughing. Crackles and wheezes are not.

STEP	RATIONALE

TABLE 18-7   ADVENTITIOUS BREATH SOUNDS

SOUND	SITE AUSCULTATED	CAUSE	CHARACTER
Crackles	Most commonly heard in dependent lobes: right and left lung bases	Random, sudden reinflation of groups of alveoli; also related to increase in fluid in small airways	Fine crackles are high-pitched fine, short, interrupted crackling sounds heard during end of inspiration, usually not cleared with coughing Medium crackles are lower, more moist sounds heard during middle of inspiration; not cleared with coughing Coarse crackles are loud bubbly noise heard during inspiration; not cleared with coughing
Rhonchi	Primarily heard over trachea and bronchi; if loud enough, can be heard over most lung fields	Muscular spasm, fluid, or mucus in larger airways cause turbulence	Loud, low-pitched, rumbling coarse sounds heard most often during inspiration or expiration; may be cleared by coughing
Wheezes	Can be heard over all lung fields	High-velocity airflow through severely narrowed bronchus	High-pitched, continuous musical sounds like a squeak heard continuously during inspiration or expiration; usually louder on expiration; do not clear with coughing
Pleural friction rub	Heard over anterior lateral lung field (if client is sitting upright)	Inflamed pleura, parietal pleura rubbing against visceral pleura	Dry, grating quality heard best during inspiration; does not clear with coughing; heard loudest over lower lateral anterior surface

EVALUATION

1. Compare findings with normal assessment characteristics for thorax and lungs.	Determines presence of abnormalities.
2. Have client identify factors leading to lung disease.	Demonstrates learning.

Recording and Reporting

- Record observations and findings in nurses' notes or assessment flow sheet.
- Record respiratory rate and character on vital signs flow sheet.
- Record amount, color, consistency and odor of mucus.
- Report abnormalities to nurse in charge or physician.

Unexpected Outcomes	Related Interventions
1. Client has productive cough, and mucus is purulent.	• Obtain a specimen. • Auscultate lungs for abnormal sounds.
2. Posturing is observed, with client leaning over table or splinting side of chest with hand. Indicates breathing difficulties (chronic lung disease and pain, respectively).	• Assist client into a position to improve lung expansion (e.g., high-Fowler's position).
3. Respirations are rapid or slow and irregular (see Chapter 17), and bulging of intercostal spaces may be present.	• Position client. • Auscultate lungs for abnormal sounds. • Notify physician.
4. Chest excursion is reduced. Depth of breathing is reduced by pain, postural deformity, or fatigue.	• Reposition client. • Administer analgesic if appropriate.
5. Percussion note is dull or flat over lung tissue. Dullness occurs over the scapula, ribs, sternum, or spine. Dullness over lung tissue may be created by presence of fluid.	• Have client cough and deep breathe. • Notify physician. • Obtain chest x-ray examination if needed.
6. Abnormal breath sounds (adventitious sounds) are auscultated over one or both lungs.	• Have client cough to determine if clear. • Notify physician
7. Client is unfamiliar with risks for lung disease.	• Education is necessary.
8. Client does not assume preferred posture for optimal ventilation.	• This is difficult to change quickly; may require exercise and further discussion.

Teaching Considerations
- Educate clients about risks of cigarette smoking. Cigarette smoking alone causes approximately 30% of all cancer deaths. Individuals who stop smoking live longer than those who continue to smoke. The probability of these individuals dying from lung cancer or other related causes continues to decline with further abstinence (ACS, 2004).
- Explain to clients that exposure to radiation, arsenic, and asbestos from occupational, medical, and environmental sources, air pollution, tuberculosis, and passive smoke contribute significantly to lung cancer.
- Discuss with clients the warning signs of lung cancer such as a persistent cough, sputum streaked with blood, chest pains, and recurrent attacks of pneumonia or bronchitis.

Pediatric Considerations
- In children, observe for retractions during assessment of the thorax. Retractions are signs of respiratory distress and may involve the intercostals, suprasternal or supraclavicular (Hockenberry and others, 2003).

- Children younger than age 7 exhibit noticeable abdominal or diaphragmatic movement.
- Nasal flaring is a significant finding of respiratory distress in infants.
- Use bell to auscultate breath sounds in children. Breath sounds are louder in children because of their thin chest walls.
- Head bobbing in a sleeping or exhausted infant is a sign of dyspnea (Hockenberry and others, 2003).

Gerontological Considerations
- Older adults have a costal angle (anteriorly) of slightly less than 90 degrees. The anteroposterior diameter may be increased from kyphosis.
- In older adults chest expansion is reduced because of calcification of rib cartilage and partial contraction of inspiratory muscles.
- Older adults should be vaccinated against the flu in the early fall (Lueckenotte, 2000).
- Chest contour is abnormal, with anteroposterior diameter in 1:1 ratio. Barrel-shaped chest may be caused by aging.

SKILL 18-3 Assessing the Heart and Neck Vessels

A client who has signs or symptoms of heart (cardiac) problems, such as chest pain, may be suffering a life-threatening condition requiring immediate attention. In this situation, the nurse acts quickly and decides on the portions of the examination that are absolutely necessary. When a client's condition is stable, a more thorough assessment can reveal baseline heart function and any risks for heart disease. Clients tend to seek information about heart disease because it remains a leading cause of death in the United States. The heart and neck vessels can be assessed together because the two systems work in unison and are in close proximity.

The nurse may begin assessment of the heart after examining the lungs because the client is already in a suitable position with the chest exposed. Assessment then proceeds to the neck vessels. The nurse uses inspection, palpation, and auscultation during the examination.

DELEGATION CONSIDERATIONS

Comprehensive heart and neck vessel assessment should not be delegated to assistive personnel. Assistive personnel can be trained to count apical pulse and peripheral pulses after the nurse's initial assessment. Assessment of peripheral pulses is important for all staff to know, particularly in specialty areas such as vascular surgery and orthopedics, where the skill is performed frequently. The staff member must be familiarized with the importance of measuring peripheral pulses in specific clients. Assistive personnel need to be instructed to recognize temperature and color changes along with changes in peripheral pulses.

EQUIPMENT

❑ Stethoscope
❑ Doppler stethoscope (optional)
❑ Conducting gel (if a Doppler is used)

STEP	RATIONALE

ASSESSMENT

1. Assess client for history of smoking, alcohol intake, caffeine intake (coffee, tea, soft drinks, chocolate), use of "recreational" drugs, exercise habits, and dietary patterns and intake.

    These can contribute to risk factors for cardiovascular disease.

2. Determine if client is taking medications for cardiovascular function (e.g., antidysrhythmics, antihypertensives, antianginals) and if client knows their purpose, dosage, and side effects.

    Allows nurse to assess client's compliance with and understanding of drug therapies. Medications for cardiovascular function cannot be taken intermittently.

3. Ask if client has experienced dyspnea, chest pain or discomfort, palpitations, excess fatigue, cough, leg pain or cramps, edema of the feet, cyanosis, fainting, and orthopnea. Ask if symptoms occur at rest or during exercise.

    These are the cardinal symptoms of heart disease. Cardiovascular function may be adequate during rest but not during exercise.

4. If client reports chest pain, determine onset (sudden or gradual), precipitating factors, quality, region, severity, and if it radiates. Anginal pain is usually a deep pressure or ache that is substernal and diffuse, radiating to one or both arms, neck, or jaw.

    Symptoms may reveal myocardial infarction or coronary artery disease.

5. Assess family history for heart disease, diabetes, high cholesterol levels, hypertension, stroke, or rheumatic heart disease.

    Family history of heart problems increases risk for heart and vascular disease, as do these other factors.

6. Ask client about a history of heart trouble (e.g., heart failure, congenital heart disease, coronary artery disease, dysrhythmias, murmurs), heart surgery, or vascular disease (hypertension, phlebitis, varicose veins).

    Knowledge reveals client's level of understanding of condition. A preexisting condition influences examination techniques used by nurse and expected findings.

STEP	RATIONALE

NURSING DIAGNOSES

- Activity intolerance
- Ineffective peripheral tissue perfusion
- Deficient knowledge regarding risks for heart disease

- Pain (acute, chronic)
- Decreased cardiac output

Related factors are individualized based on client's condition or needs.

PLANNING

1. Expected outcomes following completion of procedure:
   - Heart rate is 60 to 100 beats per minute (adolescent through adult) and without extra sounds or murmurs.
   - Point of maximal impulse (PMI) is palpable at fifth intercostal space at left midclavicular line in adult.
   - Client describes changes in own behavior that reduce risks for heart disease and/or may improve cardiovascular function.
   - Client describes schedule, dosage, purpose, and benefits of medications being taken for cardiovascular function.
   - Blood pressure is within normal limits for client (see Chapter 17).
   - Carotid pulse is localized, strong, elastic, and equal bilaterally. No change occurs during inspiration or expiration. No carotid bruit present.
   - Jugular veins distend when client lies supine and flatten when client is in sitting position.

Indicates normal rhythm and rate, normal sinus rhythm (NSR).

Indicates normal heart position.

Information may improve client's health care habits.

Information related to health benefits may improve compliance with therapy.

Normal cardiovascular function.

Vessel is patent.

Venous pressure is normal.

IMPLEMENTATION

1. Assist client to be as relaxed and comfortable as possible.

2. Have client assume semi-Fowler's or supine position.

3. Explain procedure. Avoid facial gestures reflecting concern.
4. Be sure that room is quiet.
5. Form a mental image of the exact location of the heart (see illustration). The base of the heart is the upper portion, and the apex is the bottom tip. The surface of the right ventricle constitutes most of the heart's anterior surface.

An anxious or uncomfortable client can have mild tachycardia that may lead the nurse to confounding findings.
Provides adequate visibility and access to left thorax and mediastinum. Client with heart disease often experiences shortness of breath while lying flat.
Client with previously normal cardiac history may become anxious if nurse shows concern.
Subtle, low-pitched heart sounds are difficult to hear.
Visualization improves ability to assess findings accurately and determines possible source of abnormalities.

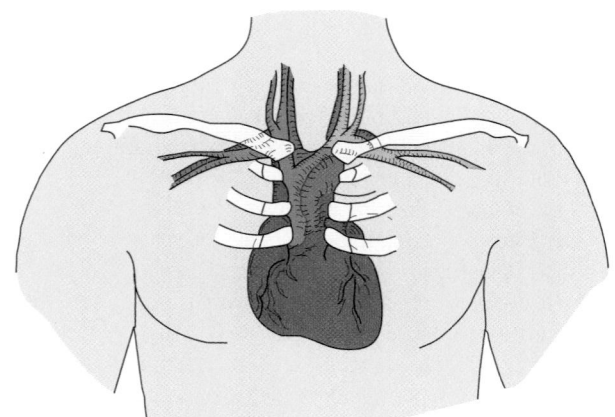

STEP 5 Anatomical position of the heart.

STEP	**RATIONALE**

6. Find the angle of Louis, felt as a ridge just below the suprasternal notch (between the sternal body and manubrium). Slip fingers down each side of angle to feel adjacent ribs. The intercostal spaces are just below each rib.

Anatomical point used to locate intercostal spaces to assess corresponding heart sounds.

7. Find the following anatomical landmarks (see illustration):

   a. The aortic area is at the second intercostal space, right of the client's sternum (*1*).

   b. The pulmonic area is at the second intercostal space, left of the client's sternum (*2*).

   c. The second pulmonic area is found by moving down left side of sternum to the third intercostal space (*3*), also referred to as Erb's point.

   d. The tricuspid area (*4*) is located at the fourth left intercostal space along the sternum.

   e. The mitral area is found by moving fingers laterally to client's left to locate fifth intercostal space at left midclavicular line (*5*).

   f. The epigastric area (*6*) is at the inferior tip of the sternum.

Familiarity with landmarks allows nurse to describe findings more clearly and ultimately may improve assessment.

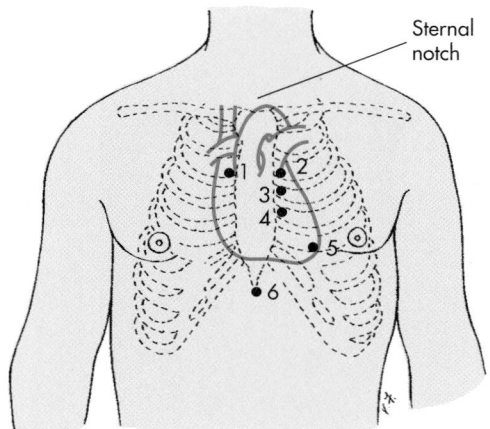

Sternal notch

STEP 7 Areas for examination of the heart (note location of bony landmarks).

8. Stand to the client's right to inspect and palpate the precordium with the client supine. Note any visible pulsations and more exaggerated lifts at the anatomical landmarks. Inspect closely at the area of the apex. Palpate for pulsations (using the proximal halves of the four fingers together and then alternating with ball of hand) at all anatomical landmarks.

May reveal size and symmetry of the heart. The apical impulse is normally visible at the midclavicular line in the fifth intercostal space. The apical impulse (PMI) may become visible only when the client sits up, bringing the heart closer to the anterior wall. It is easily obscured by obesity. Normally no pulsations or vibrations can be felt in the second, third, or fourth intercostal spaces.

● *Critical Decision Point*

Presence of a palpable thrill is not normal and may indicate a disruption of blood flow caused by a defect in closure of a heart valve or atrial septal defect. Report to physician.

STEP	RATIONALE

9. Locate the PMI by palpating with fingertips along fifth intercostal space in midclavicular line (see illustration). Note a light, brief pulsation in an area 1 to 2 cm (½ to 1 inch) in diameter at the apex.

In the presence of serious heart disease, the PMI will be located to the left of the midclavicular line related to enlarged left ventricle. In chronic lung disease the PMI may be to the right of the midclavicular line as a result of right ventricular enlargement.

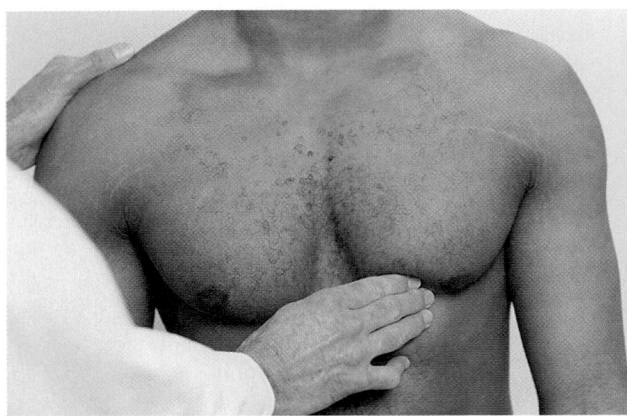

STEP **9** Palpation of PMI. (From Seidel HM and others: *Mosby's guide to physical examination,* ed 5, St. Louis, 2003, Mosby.)

- **Critical Decision Point**
  A stronger than expected impulse may be a heave or lift, which may indicate increased cardiac output or left ventricular hypertrophy.

10. If palpating PMI is difficult, turn client onto left side.

Maneuver moves the heart closer to the chest wall.

11. Inspect the epigastric area and palpate the abdominal aorta. Note a localized strong beat.

Rules out reduced blood flow or diffuse pulse, which may indicate a number of abnormalities.

12. Auscultate heart sounds. Begin by having client sit up and lean slightly forward; then have client lie supine, and end the examination with client in a left lateral recumbent position (see illustrations). In a female client it may be necessary to lift the left breast to hear heart sounds more effectively.

Different positions help to clarify type of sounds heard. Sitting position is best to hear high-pitched murmurs (if present). Supine is a common position to hear all sounds. Left lateral recumbent is the best position to hear low-pitched sounds.

13. While auscultating sounds at each anatomical landmark, ask client not to speak but to breathe comfortably. Begin with the diaphragm of the stethoscope; then alternate with the bell. Use very light pressure for the bell. Inch the stethoscope along; avoid jumping from one area to another. Do not try to hear all heart sounds at once.

Auscultation requires the examiner to isolate each heart sound at all auscultation sites.

   a. Begin at the apex or PMI; then move systematically to the tricuspid area, second pulmonic area, and pulmonic and aortic areas. (NOTE: Some examiners use reverse sequence.) Listen for the S_1 at each site. It sounds like "lub." S_1 is best heard at the apex and is simultaneous with the carotid pulse.

At normal slow rates S_1 is high pitched and dull in quality and sounds like a "lub." This sound precedes the systolic phase of heart contraction.

   b. Listen for S_2 at each site. It precedes the diastolic phase and sounds like "dub." This sound is best heard at the aortic area. Heart sounds will vary by pitch, loudness, and duration, depending on the auscultatory site (Table 18-8).

Normal sounds S_1 and S_2 are high pitched and best heard with diaphragm.

STEP	RATIONALE

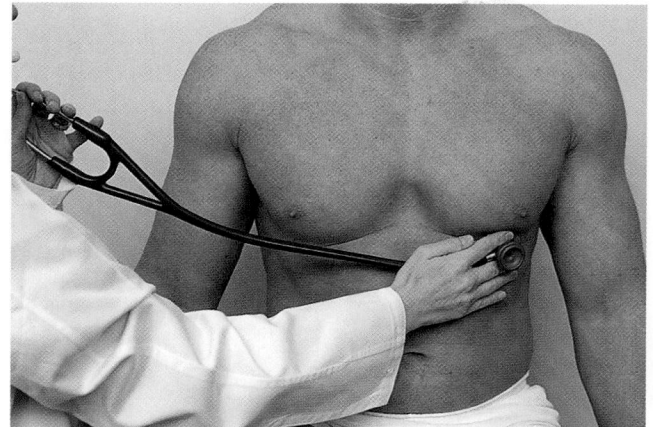

A

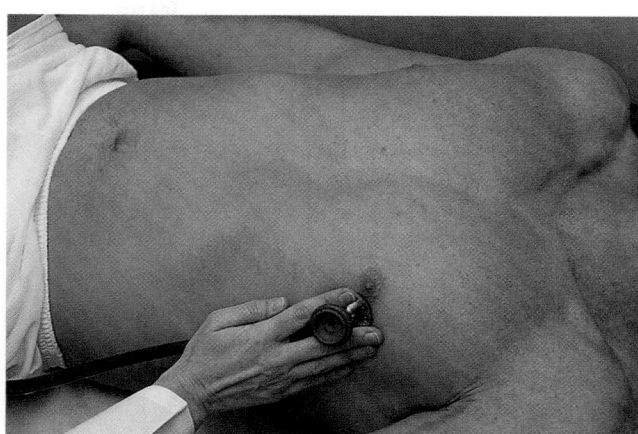

B

C

STEP 12 Client positions for auscultation of heart sounds. **A,** Sitting. **B,** Supine. **C,** Left lateral. (From Seidel HM and others: *Mosby's guide to physical examination,* ed 5, St. Louis, 2003, Mosby.)

TABLE 18-8   HEART SOUNDS ACCORDING TO AUSCULTATORY AREA

	AORTIC	PULMONIC	SECOND PULMONIC	MITRAL	TRICUSPID
Pitch	$S_1 < S_2$	$S_1 < S_2$	$S_1 < S_2$	$S_1 < S_2$	$S_1 < S_2$
Loudness	$S_1 < S_2$	$S_1 < S_2$	$S_1 < S_2$*	$S_1 > S_2$†	$S_1 > S_2$
Duration and others	$S_1 > S_2$	$S_1 > S_2$	$S_1 > S_2$	$S_1 > S_2$	$S_1 > S_2$

Modified from Seidel HM and others: *Mosby's guide to physical examination,* ed 5, St. Louis, 2003, Mosby.

*S_1 is relatively louder in second pulmonic area than in aortic area.

†S_1 may be louder in mitral area than in tricuspid area.

c. After both sounds are heard clearly as "lub-dub," count each combination of S_1 and S_2 as one heartbeat. Count the number of beats for 1 minute.

d. Assess heart rhythm by noting the time between S_1 and S_2 (systole) and then the time between S_2 and the next S_1 (diastole). Listen to the full cycle at each auscultation area. Note regular intervals between each sequence of beats. There should be a distinct pause between S_1 and S_2.

Determines apical pulse rate.

Failure of heart to beat at regular intervals is a dysrhythmia, which interferes with heart's ability to pump effectively.

STEP	RATIONALE

TABLE 18-9   COMMON TYPES OF DYSRHYTHMIAS

DEFINITION	CAUSE
Sinus dysrhythmia: Pulse rate changes during respiration, increasing at peak of inspiration and declining during expiration.	Blood is momentarily trapped in lungs during inspiration, causing fall in heart's stroke volume.
Sinus tachycardia: Pulse rhythm is regular, but rate is accelerated to more than 100 beats/min.	Exercise, emotional stress, and caffeine or alcohol ingestion are common factors that cause increased firing of sinoatrial node.
Sinus bradycardia: Pulse rhythm is regular, but rate is slower than normal at 40-60 beats/min.	Sinoatrial node fires less frequently. This is common in well-conditioned athletes and with use of antidysrhythmic medications.
Premature ventricular contraction: Premature beat occurs before regularly expected heart contraction.	Ventricle contracts prematurely because of electrical impulse bypassing normal conduction pathway. It may occur so early that it is difficult to detect as second beat. It may be followed by a pause.
Atrial fibrillation: Rapid, random contractions of atria cause irregular ventricular beats at 130-150 beats/min.	Atria discharge very rapidly, with some impulses not reaching ventricles. This condition occurs in rheumatic heart disease and mitral stenosis. It causes reduced cardiac output.

e.   When heart rate is irregular, compare apical and radial pulses (Table 18-9). Auscultate the apical pulse, and then immediately palpate the radial pulse. A colleague can assess the radial pulse while you assess the apical pulse.

Determines if a pulse deficit (radial pulse is slower than apical) exists. Deficit indicates that ineffective contractions of the heart fail to send pulse waves to the periphery.

14. Continue to auscultate for extra heart sounds at each site. If any abnormal sounds are heard, note pitch, loudness, duration, and timing (when in relation to the cardiac cycle). Note location on the chest wall.

Abnormal sounds include murmurs. Characteristics of murmurs help to identify contributing factors.

a.   Use the bell of the stethoscope, and listen for low-pitched extra heart sounds such as S_3 and S_4 gallops, clicks, and rubs. S_3, or a ventricular gallop, occurs just after S_2 at the end of ventricular diastole. It may sound like "lub-dub-ee" or "Ken-tuc-ky." S_4, or an atrial gallop, occurs just before S_1 or ventricular systole. It sounds like "dee-lub-dub" or "Ten-nes-see."

Gallops may be caused by premature rushes of blood into a ventricle that is stiff or dilated or an atrial contraction pushing against a ventricle that is not accepting blood.

b.   Listen for clicks as short, high-pitched extra sounds.

Clicks are caused by abnormalities such as mitral valve prolapse or prosthetic valves.

c.   With client leaning forward or lying on the left side, listen for friction rubs as squeaky or rubbing sounds. Instruct client to hold breath as you continue to listen.

Rubs may result from lungs or inflamed visceral and parietal layers of the pericardium of the heart rubbing against one another. If the sound is present only while the client is breathing, the origin of the rub is pulmonary rather than cardiac.

15. Auscultate for heart murmurs over each of the auscultation sites.

Murmurs are sustained swishing or blowing sounds heard at the beginning, middle, or end of systole or diastole. They are caused by increased blood flow through a normal valve, forward flow through a stenotic valve or into a dilated vessel or chamber, or backward flow through a valve that fails to close.

16. When a murmur is detected, listen carefully to note where the murmur can be heard best. Note the intensity of the murmur.

Intensity is related to rate of blood flow through the heart or the amount of blood regurgitated. A thrill is a continuous palpable sensation like the purring of a cat. A thrust is the upward lift felt when palpating the chest wall.

17. Note if the murmur is low, medium, or high in pitch, using the bell for low-pitched sounds.

Pitch depends on velocity of blood flow through the valves.

18. Assess carotid arteries: Have client remain in sitting position.

Allows easier mobility of neck to expose artery for inspection and palpation.

19. Inspect neck on both sides for obvious pulsations of artery. Ask client to turn head slightly away from artery being examined. Sometimes pulse wave can be seen.

Carotids are the only sites to assess quality of pulse wave (see illustration). Experience is required to evaluate wave in relation to events of cardiac cycle.

STEP	RATIONALE

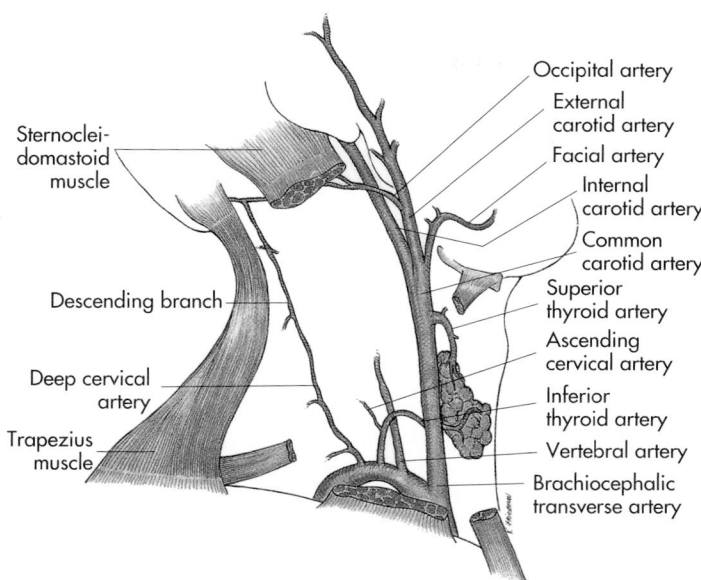

STEP **19** Anatomical position of carotid artery.

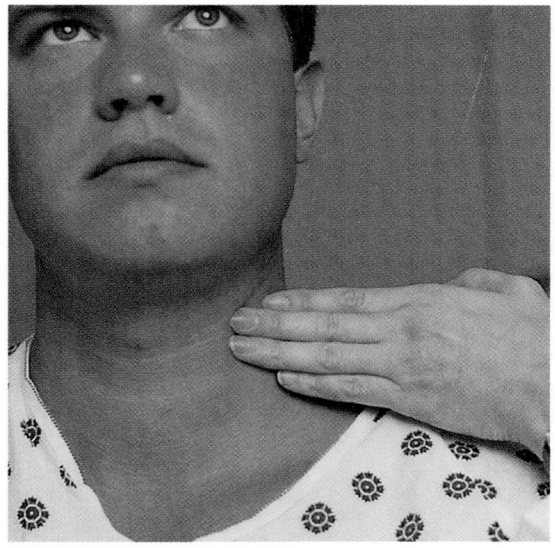

STEP **20** Palpate each carotid artery separately.

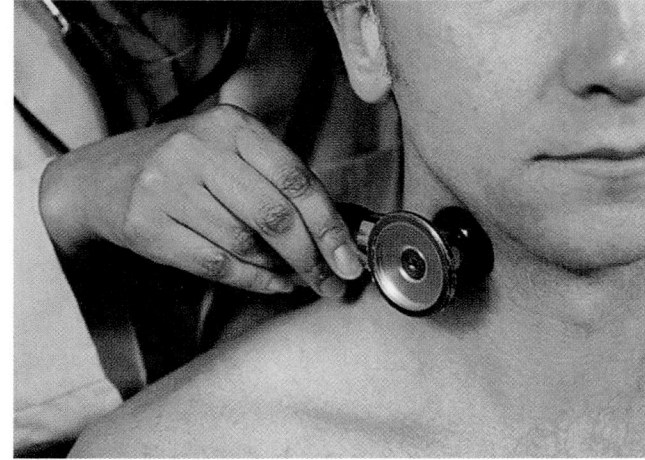

STEP **21** Auscultation for carotid artery bruit. (From Barkauskas VH and others: *Health and physical assessment,* ed 2, St. Louis, 1998, Mosby.)

20. Palpate each carotid artery separately with index and middle fingers around medial edge of sternocleidomastoid muscle. Ask client to raise chin slightly, keeping the head straight (see illustration). Note rate and rhythm, strength, and elasticity of artery. Also note if pulse changes as client inspires and expires.

21. Place bell of stethoscope over each carotid artery, auscultating for blowing sound (bruit) (see illustration). Ask the client to hold a breath for a few heartbeats so that respiratory sounds will not interfere with auscultation (Seidel and other, 2003).

If both arteries were occluded simultaneously, client could lose consciousness from reduced circulation to brain. Turning head improves access to artery. Change may indicate a sinus dysrhythmia.

Narrowing of carotid artery's lumen by arteriosclerotic plaques causes disturbance in blood flow. Blood passing through narrowed section creates turbulence and emits blowing or swishing sound.

STEP	RATIONALE

- **Critical Decision Point**
  Do not vigorously palpate or massage the artery. Stimulation of carotid sinus may cause a reflex drop in heart rate and blood pressure.

22. To assess venous pressure have client assume a supine position. Then raise the head of the bed 45-degrees. Avoiding neck hyperextension or flexion. Locate the highest point along the internal jugular vein where a pulsation can be seen (tangential lighting helps). Locate the sternal angle with a centimeter ruler and measure the vertical distance between the sternal angle and the meniscus of the internal jugular vein (see illustration).

Normal veins are flat when client is sitting, and pulsations become evident as client's head is lowered. A height of pulsation greater than 2.5 cm indicates fluid overload.

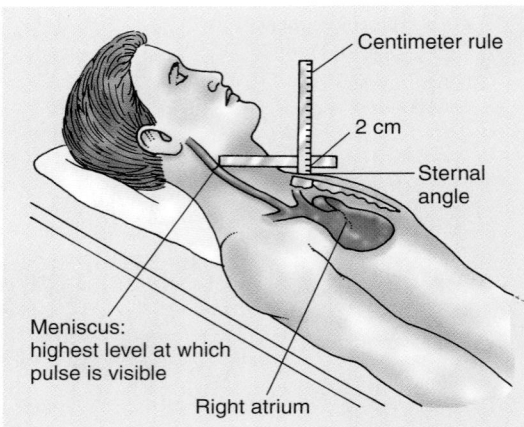

STEP 22 Position for assessment of jugular vein distention. (Modified from Thompson JM and others: *Mosby's manual of clinical nursing,* ed 5, St. Louis, 2001, Mosby.)

EVALUATION

1. Compare findings with normal assessment characteristics of heart and vascular system.
2. If heart sounds are not audible, or if pulses are not palpable, ask another nurse to confirm assessment.
3. Ask client to describe behaviors that increase risk for heart and vascular disease.

Determines presence of abnormalities.

Abnormal assessment findings should be validated by another professional nurse.

Demonstrates learning.

Recording and Reporting

- Record all findings for heart and vascular assessment in nurses' notes or flow sheet.
- Record any instruction provided to client and client's response.
- Report immediately to physician any irregularities in heart function and indications of impaired arterial blood flow.
- Clients with dysrhythmias or pulse deficits may require an electrocardiogram or Holter monitor per physician's order.

Unexpected Outcomes	Related Interventions
1. Abnormal findings that are new to the assessment data require physician notification. These include: ■ Pulsations, vibrations, or both are palpable. These are result of valvular problem, murmur, or both. ■ Point of maximal impulse is found to left of mid-clavicular line, which is the result of cardiomegaly. ■ Extra heart sounds S_3 or S_4 are auscultated. Extra sounds indicate atrial or ventricular gallop. ■ Murmur is auscultated. Impaired blood flow through heart may indicate need for immediate medical attention. Some murmurs are benign. ■ Jugular venous pressure is elevated. This is a sign of right-sided heart failure.	• Notify physician.
2. Heart rate is irregular, with rate less than 60 beats per minute or more than 100 beats per minute.	• Check blood pressure. If low, dysrhythmia may be contributing to inadequate cardiac output. • Observe for sensations or reports of dizziness or feeling "faint." • Notify physician.
3. Pulse deficit is noted. There is risk for inadequate cardiac output.	• Obtain vital signs. • Notify physician.
4. Client is unable to explain risks for heart or vascular disease.	• Additional education is needed.

Teaching Considerations

- Explain risk factors for heart disease: high dietary intake of saturated fat or cholesterol, lack of regular aerobic exercise, smoking, excess weight, stressful lifestyle, hypertension, and family history of heart disease.
- Refer client (if appropriate) to resources available for controlling or reducing risks (e.g., nutritional counseling, exercise class, and stress reduction programs).
- Explain that research shows clinical benefit from reducing dietary intake of cholesterol and saturated fats. Tell client that about 70% to 75% of saturated fatty acids come from meats, poultry, fish, and dairy products and that the one-step diet recommended by the National Institutes of Health includes an intake of total fat less than 30% of calories, saturated fatty acids less than 10% of calories, and cholesterol less than 300 mg/100 ml (Moore, 2001).
- Encourage client to have regular measurement of total blood cholesterol levels and triglycerides. Desirable levels are less than 200 mg/100 ml. More than one cholesterol measurement is needed to assess the blood cholesterol level accurately. Low-density lipoprotein (LDL) cholesterol is the major component of atherosclerotic plaques. Separate measurement of LDL cholesterol is wise in a client with high total blood cholesterol levels. An LDL cholesterol level of less than 100 mg/100 ml is the goal; a level of 160 mg/100 ml or higher indicates high risk.
- Advise client to avoid cigarette smoking because nicotine causes vasoconstriction.

- Advise client to quit smoking because this lowers the risk for coronary heart disease and coronary vascular disease (ACS, 2004).

Pediatric Considerations

- Perform cardiac assessment on infant or toddler while quiet, before more uncomfortable procedures.
- Point of maximal impulse is at third or fourth intercostal space at left midclavicular line in infant or child.
- It is not uncommon for children to have third heart sounds (S_3). Sinus arrhythmia occurs normally in many children (Hockenberry and others, 2003).
- Children have louder, higher-pitched heart sounds because of their thin chest walls.

Gerontological Considerations

- Point of maximal impulse may be difficult to find in an older adult because anteroposterior diameter of the chest deepens.
- Accidental massage of the carotid sinus during palpation of the carotid artery can be a particular problem for older adults, causing a sudden drop in heart rate from vagal nerve stimulation (Lueckenotte, 2000).
- Older adults with hypertension may benefit from regular monitoring of blood pressure (daily, weekly, or monthly). Home monitoring kits are available. Teach client how to use them correctly.

SKILL 18-4 Assessing the Abdomen

Abdominal assessment is complex because of the multiple organs located within and near the abdominal cavity. This area of the body is associated with many health complaints, and many people are embarrassed by bowel or bladder dysfunction, reproductive or urinary elimination problems. Abdominal pain is one of the most common symptoms clients report when seeking medical care. Abdominal pain could be caused by alterations in organs such as the stomach, gallbladder, or intestines; or the pain may be the result of spinal or muscular injury. An accurate assessment requires matching the client's history with a careful assessment of the location of physical symptoms (Table 18-10).

To perform an effective abdominal assessment the nurse needs a detailed knowledge of the underlying structures involved, including the lower pelvis, kidneys, rectum, genitalia, liver, gallbladder, stomach, spleen, intestines, and reproductive organs (Figure 18-5). An abdominal assessment is routine after abdominal surgery and for any client who has undergone invasive diagnostic tests of the gastrointestinal tract (see Chapter 44).

The order of an abdominal assessment differs from that of other assessments. The nurse begins with inspection and follows with auscultation. It is important to auscultate before palpation and percussion since these maneuvers may alter the frequency and character of bowel sounds.

TABLE 18-10 COMMON CAUSES FOR ABDOMINAL PAIN

CONDUCTION	PHYSICAL ALTERATION	PHYSICAL SIGNS AND SYMPTOMS
Appendicitis	Obstruction of the appendix associated with inflammation, perforation, and peritonitis.	Sharp pain directly over the irritated peritoneum 2-12 hours after onset. Often pain localizes at McBurney's point in the right lower quadrant between the anterior iliac crest and the umbilicus. Associated with rebound tenderness.
Cholecystitis	Obstruction of the cystic duct causing inflammation or distention of the gallbladder.	*Murphy's sign:* Apply gentle pressure below the right subcostal arch and below the liver margin. Sharp pain and inspiratory arrest occur when the client takes a deep breath (Seidel and others, 2003).
Constipation	Symptom of infrequent bowel movements. Disruption in normal bowel pattern, defecation may occur with narcotic use or inadequate fiber and fluid intake.	Generalized discomfort accompanied by distention and palpation of a hard mass in the left lower quadrant. Nausea and vomiting may begin after several days.
Crohn's disease	A chronic inflammatory lesion of the ileum. Cause is unknown.	Steady colicky pain in the right lower quadrant, with cramping, tenderness, flatulence, nausea, fever, and diarrhea. Often associated with bloody stools, weight loss, weakness, and fatigue.
Gastroenteritis	Inflammation of the stomach and intestinal tract.	Generalized abdominal discomfort accompanied by nausea, vomiting, diarrhea.
Intestinal obstruction	Blockage of the lumen of the intestine.	Colicky pain, nausea, vomiting, constipation, and abdominal distention. Bowel sounds are hyperactive with a rushing sound or absence of bowel sounds.
Pancreatitis	Inflammation of the pancreas associated with alcoholism and gallbladder disease.	Steady epigastric pain close to the umbilicus radiates to the back. Associated with abdominal rigidity and vomiting. Pain is unrelieved by vomiting.
Paralytic ileus	Obstruction of the small bowel that occurs after abdominal surgery or use of anticholinergic medications.	Generalized severe abdominal distention, nausea, and vomiting. Decreased/absent bowel sounds.
Peptic ulcers (gastric and duodenal)	Damage of gastrointestinal (GI) mucosa at any area of the GI tract. May be caused by bacterial infection or nonsteroidal antiinflammatory drugs. Believed to be unrelated to stress. Aggravated by smoking and excessive alcohol use.	*Gastric ulcer:* Dull epigastric pain, localized midline. Early satiety; not usually relieved by food or antacids. *Duodenal ulcer:* Pain is episodic in nature, lasting 30 minutes to 2 hours. Pain is located midline epigastric region, may radiate around costal border to back; described as aching, burning, or gnawing. Typically occurs 1-3 hours after meals and at night (12 midnight to 3 AM). Often relieved by food/antacid. *Both:* dyspepsia syndrome: complaints of fullness, epigastric discomfort, vague feeling of nausea, abdominal distention and bloating; anorexia; weight loss (Phipps and others, 2003).

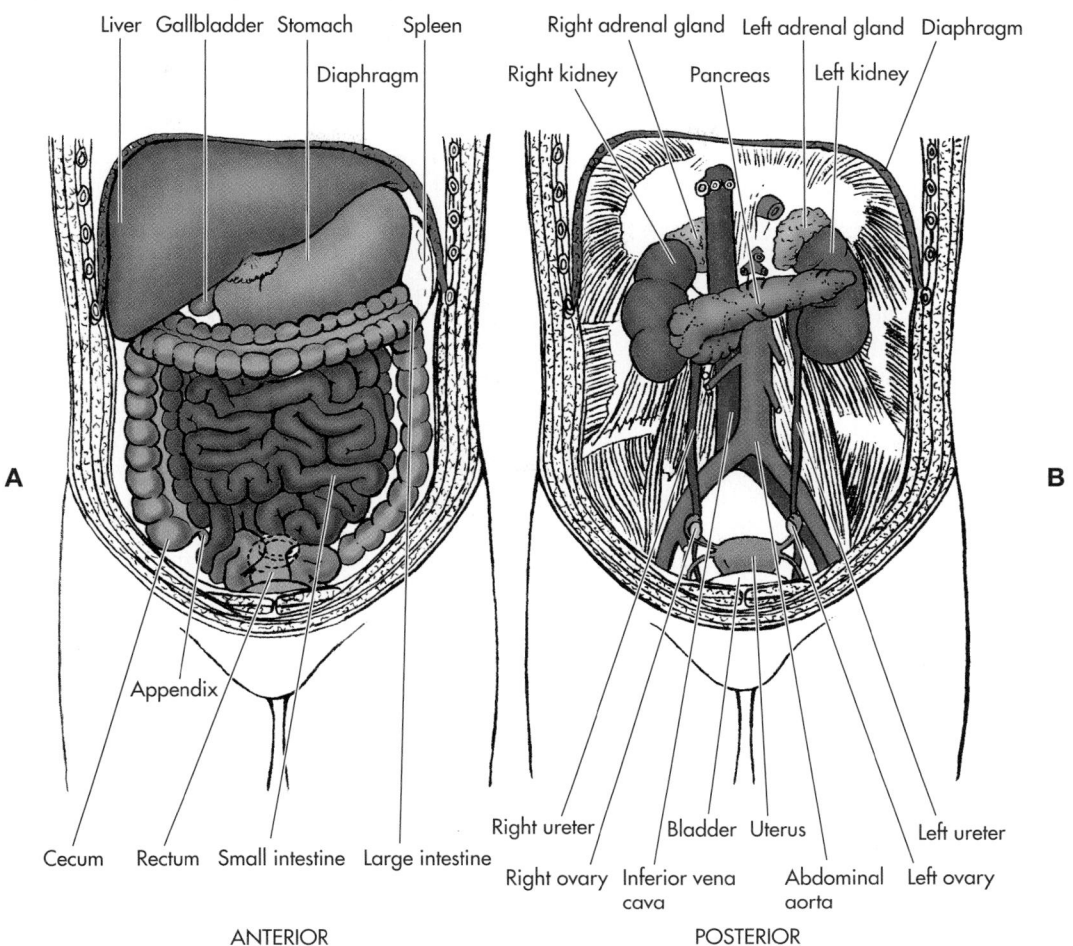

FIGURE 18-5 Location of organs in the abdomen. **A,** Anterior. **B,** Posterior. (Modified from Daly S: *Mosby's expert ten minute physical examinations,* St. Louis, 1997, Mosby.)

DELEGATION CONSIDERATIONS

This skill should not be delegated to assistive personnel. However, assistive personnel should know to report the development of abdominal pain or changes in the client's bowel habits or dietary intake.

EQUIPMENT

- ❑ Stethoscope
- ❑ Tape measure
- ❑ Examination light
- ❑ Marking pen

STEP	RATIONALE

▍ASSESSMENT

1. If client has abdominal or low back pain, assess the character of pain in detail (location, onset, frequency, precipitating factors, aggravating factors, type of pain, severity, course).

2. Carefully observe client's movement and position, such as lying still with knees drawn up, moving restlessly to find a comfortable position, or lying on one side or sitting with knees drawn up to chest.

Knowing pattern of characteristics of pain helps determine its source, which is then confirmed during examination.

Positions assumed by the client may reveal nature and source of pain. Movement aggravates the pain of peritonitis, so clients will lie still.

Acute pancreatitis pain is worsened by lying supine; may be lessened by flexed knee, curved-back position (Phipps and others, 2003).

Clients with appendicitis often lie on side or back with knees flexed in an attempt to decrease muscle strain on the abdominal wall (Phipps and others, 2003).

STEP	RATIONALE
3. Assess client's normal bowel habits: frequency of stools; character of stools; recent changes in character of stools; measures used to promote elimination, such as laxatives, enemas, dietary intake; and eating and drinking habits.	These data, compared with information from physical assessment, may help to identify cause and nature of elimination problems.
4. Determine if client has had abdominal surgery, trauma, or diagnostic tests of the gastrointestinal tract.	Surgical or traumatic alterations of abdominal organs may cause adhesions in expected areas (e.g., position of underlying organs). Diagnostic tests may change character of stool.
5. Determine whether client has had any nausea, vomiting, or cramping, especially in last 24 hours.	Changes may indicate alterations in upper gastrointestinal tract (e.g., stomach or gallbladder) or lower colon.
6. Assess for difficulty in swallowing, belching, flatulence, bloody emesis (hematemesis), black or tarry stools (melena), heartburn, diarrhea, or constipation.	Indicative of gastrointestinal alterations.
7. Determine if client takes antiinflammatory medications (e.g., aspirin, steroids, and nonsteroidal antiinflammatory drugs), or antibiotics.	These pharmacological agents may cause gastrointestinal upset or bleeding.
8. Inquire about family history of cancer, kidney disease, alcoholism, hypertension, or heart disease.	Data may reveal risk for significant abdominal alterations. Chronic alcohol ingestion can cause gastrointestinal and liver problems.
9. Determine if female client is pregnant.	Pregnancy may cause nausea and vomiting, as well as changes in abdominal shape and contour.
10. Review client's history for health care occupation, hemodialysis, intravenous drug use, household or sexual contact with hepatitis B virus (HBV) carrier, sexually active heterosexual person (more than one sex partner in previous 6 months), sexually active homosexual or bisexual man, international traveler in area of high HBV prevalence.	These are risk factors for HBV exposure. Abdominal findings for hepatitis include jaundice, hepatomegaly, anorexia, abdominal and gastric discomfort, tea-colored urine, and clay-colored stools (Seidel and others, 2003).

NURSING DIAGNOSES

- Imbalanced nutrition: less than body requirements
- Imbalanced nutrition: more than body requirements
- Constipation
- Diarrhea
- Pain (acute, chronic)
- Anxiety

Related factors are individualized based on client's condition or needs.

PLANNING

1. Expected outcomes following completion of procedure:	
• Abdomen is soft and symmetrical with smooth and even contour. No mass, distention, or tenderness is palpable. No forceful visible pulsations are noted.	Normal findings.
• Bowel sounds are active and audible in all four quadrants.	Indicates normal peristaltic activity.
• No costovertebral angle (CVA) tenderness is present.	No inflammation of kidney.
• Client denies discomfort or worsening of existing discomfort following examination.	Nurse uses proper examination procedures.
• Client is able to list warning signs of colon cancer.	Demonstrates learning.

IMPLEMENTATION

1. Prepare client:	
a. Ask if client needs to empty bladder or defecate.	Palpation of full bladder can cause discomfort and feeling of urgency and make it difficult for client to relax.
b. Keep upper chest and legs draped.	Maintains client's comfort during examination, promoting relaxation.
c. Be sure that room is warm.	Promotes client's comfort.

STEP	**RATIONALE**

d. Expose area from just above the xiphoid process down to the symphysis pubis.

Provides full visualization of abdomen.

e. Have client lie supine or in a dorsal recumbent position with arms down at sides and knees slightly bent. A small pillow may be placed under client's knees.

Placing the arms under the head or keeping knees fully extended can cause the abdominal muscles to tighten. Tightening of muscles prevents adequate palpation.

- *Critical Decision Point*
  Observe respirations as position is changed. If abdomen is distended, lying flat may result in increased respiratory difficulty due to pressure on the diaphragm (Daly, 1997).

f. Maintain conversation during assessment except during auscultation. Explain steps calmly and slowly.

Client's ability to relax during assessment improves accuracy of findings. Talking will prevent clear detection of bowel sounds.

g. Ask client to point to tender areas.

Painful areas are assessed last. Manipulation of body part can increase client's pain and anxiety and make remainder of assessment difficult to complete.

2. Identify landmarks that divide abdominal region into quadrants. Boundary is from the tip of xiphoid process to symphysis pubis with line crossing and intersecting the umbilicus, dividing abdomen into four equal sections (see illustration).

Location of findings by common reference point helps successive examiners to confirm findings and locate abnormalities.

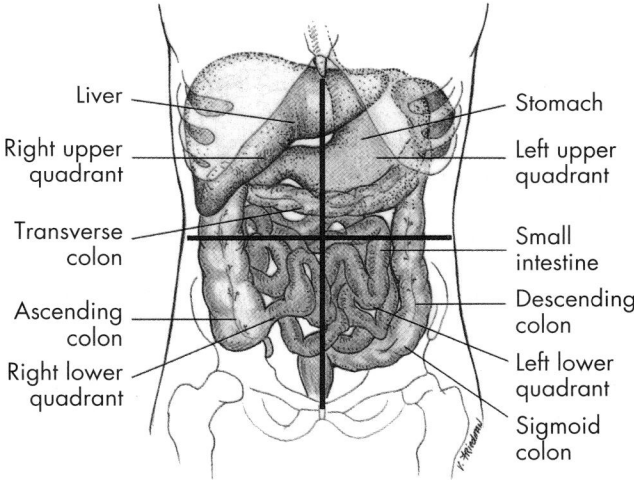

Liver — Right upper quadrant — Transverse colon — Ascending colon — Right lower quadrant

Stomach — Left upper quadrant — Small intestine — Descending colon — Left lower quadrant — Sigmoid colon

STEP 2 Division of abdomen into quadrants.

3. Inspect skin of abdomen's surface for color, scars, venous patterns, rashes, lesions, silvery white striae (stretch marks), and artificial openings. Observe lesions for characteristics described in Skill 18-1.

Scars reveal evidence that client has had past trauma or surgery. Striae indicate stretching of tissue from growth, obesity, pregnancy, ascites, or edema. Venous patterns may reflect liver disease (portal hypertension). Artificial openings indicate bowel or urinary diversion (see Chapter 34).

4. If bruising is noted, ask if client self-administers injections (e.g., heparin or insulin).

Frequent injections can cause bruising and hardening of underlying tissues.

- *Critical Decision Point*
  Bruising may also indicate physical abuse, accidental injury, or bleeding disorders.

STEP	RATIONALE

5. Inspect the contour, symmetry, and surface motion of the abdomen. Note any masses, bulging, or distention. (Flat abdomen forms a horizontal plane from xiphoid process to symphysis pubis. Round abdomen protrudes in convex sphere from horizontal plane. Concave abdomen sinks into muscular wall. All are normal.)

Changes in symmetry or contour may reveal underlying masses, fluid collection, or gaseous distention. An everted umbilicus (protruding outward) may indicate distention. A hernia can also cause the umbilicus to protrude upward.

6. If abdomen appears distended, note if distention is generalized. Look at the flanks on each side.

Distention may be caused by the nine F's (fat, flatus, feces, fluids, fibroid, full bladder, false pregnancy, fatal tumor, and fetus) (Seidel and others, 2003). If gas causes distention, flanks do not bulge. If fluid causes distention, flanks bulge. Tumor may cause a more unilateral bulging or distention. Pregnancy causes symmetrical bulge in lower abdomen.

7. If distention is suspected, measure size of abdominal girth by placing tape measure around abdomen at level of umbilicus (see illustration). Use the marking pen to indicate where tape measure was applied.

Consecutive measurements will show any increase or decrease in abdominal distention. All subsequent measurements are taken at same level of umbilicus to provide objective means to evaluate changes. A water-based pen can be used to make a mark on abdomen for subsequent measurements.

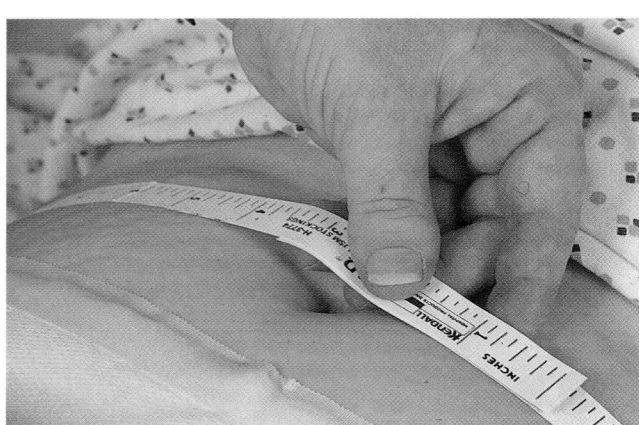

STEP **7** Measuring abdominal girth at the level of the umbilicus.

8. If nasogastric or intestinal tube is connected to suction, turn off momentarily.

Sound of suction machine obscures bowel sounds.

9. Auscultate bowel sounds by placing the diaphragm of the stethoscope lightly over each of the four abdominal quadrants. Ask client not to talk. Listen until repeated gurgling or bubbling sounds are heard in each quadrant (minimum of once in 5 to 20 seconds). Describe sounds as normal, hyperactive, hypoactive, or absent. Listen 5 minutes over each quadrant before deciding that bowel sounds are absent.

Normal bowel sounds occur irregularly every 5 to 15 seconds. Absence of sounds indicate cessation of gastric motility. Hyperactive bowel sounds not related to hunger or a recent meal may indicate diarrhea or early intestinal obstruction. Hypoactive or absent bowel sounds may indicate paralytic ileus or peritonitis. It is common for bowel sounds to be hypoactive postoperatively for 24 hours or more, especially following abdominal surgery.

• **Critical Decision Point**
Paralytic ileus may be accompanied by nausea and vomiting, increasing distention, and inability to pass flatus.

10. Place the bell of the stethoscope over the epigastric region of the abdomen and each quadrant. Auscultate for vascular (whooshing) sounds.

Determines presence of turbulent blood flow (bruit) through thoracic or abdominal aorta.

STEP	RATIONALE

- *Critical Decision Point*
  If aortic bruit is auscultated, suggesting presence of an aneurysm, stop assessment and notify physician immediately. Do not percuss or palpate a suspected area where a bruit is heard.

11. With client supine, gently percuss each of four abdominal quadrants systematically. Note areas of tympany and dullness.

12. To determine if distention is caused by fluid or air, percuss for a fluid wave:
    a. Ask another person to assist by pressing gently and firmly at the midline of the abdomen (see illustration).
    b. Place your fingertips along both sides of the lower abdomen in the lumbar region. Thrust quickly into the client's side with your dominant hand, keeping the nondominant hand in place.
    c. Feel for a fluid wave with the nondominant hand.

Reveals presence of air or fluid in stomach and intestines. Normal percussion is tympanic because of swallowed air in gastrointestinal tract. Presence of fluid or underlying masses is revealed by dull percussion.

If no fluid wave is felt, the distention is caused by air. Presence of a fluid wave indicates ascites, found in cirrhosis, peritonitis, metastatic carcinoma, ovarian carcinoma, and pancreatitis. Ascites from liver congestion is often accompanied by jaundice, pruritus, dependent edema, and enlarged superficial abdominal veins (Phipps and others, 2003).

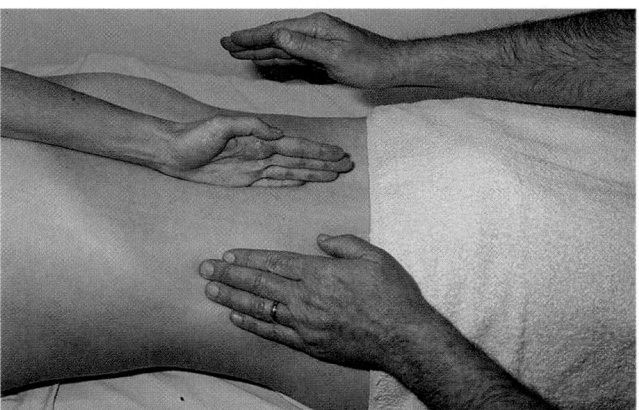

STEP **12a** Testing for fluid wave. (From Seidel HM and others: *Mosby's guide to physical examination,* ed 5, St. Louis, 2003, Mosby.)

13. Ask client if abdomen feels unusually tight, and determine if this is a recent development.

Continued sensation of fullness helps to detect distention. A feeling of fullness after a heavy meal causes only temporary distention. Tightness is not felt with obesity.

STEP	RATIONALE

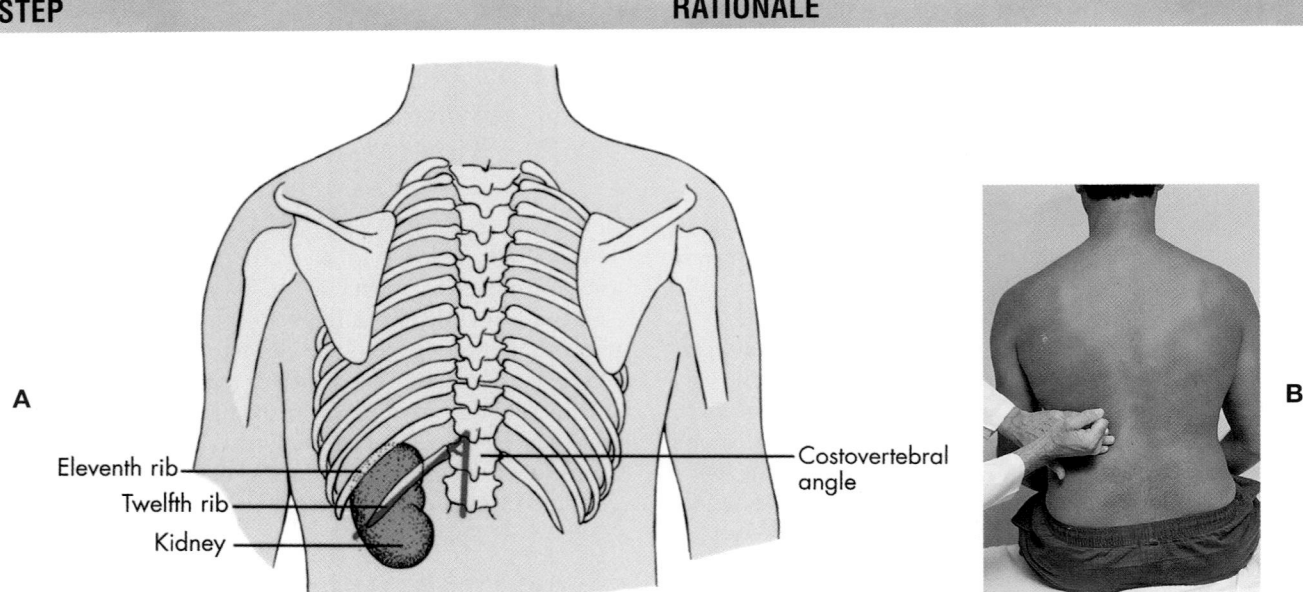

STEP 14 A, Position of kidney in relation to costovertebral angle. **B,** Percussion of the kidney for costovertebral angle (CVA) tenderness. (From Seidel HM and others: *Mosby's guide to physical examination,* ed 5, St. Louis, 2003, Mosby.)

14. With client sitting, gently but firmly percuss over each costovertebral angle along scapular lines (see illustration *A*). Use ulnar surface of fist to percuss directly against client's skin or indirectly by placing nondominant hand flat against costovertebral angle and percuss with dominant hand (see illustration *B*). Note if client experiences pain.

    Determines presence of kidney inflammation.

15. Lightly palpate over each abdominal quadrant, laying the palm of the hand with fingers extended and approximated lightly on the abdomen. Keep the palm and forearm horizontal. The pads of the fingertips depress the skin approximately 1 cm (½ inch) in a gentle dipping motion (see illustration).

    Detects areas of localized tenderness, degree of tenderness, and presence and character of underlying masses. Palpation of sensitive area causes guarding (voluntary tightening of underlying abdominal muscles).

    a. Note muscular resistance, distention, tenderness, and superficial masses or organs while observing client's face for signs of discomfort.

    Client's verbal and nonverbal cues may indicate discomfort from tenderness. Firm abdomen may indicate active obstruction with fluid or gas building up.

    b. Note if abdomen is firm or soft to touch.

    Soft abdomen is normal or reveals that obstruction is resolving.

16. Just below umbilicus and above symphysis pubis, palpate for a smooth, rounded mass. While applying light pressure, ask if client has sensation of need to void.

    Detects presence of dome of distended bladder.

- *Critical Decision Point*

    Routinely check for distended bladder if client has been unable to void, client has been incontinent, or an indwelling Foley catheter is not draining well.

STEP	RATIONALE

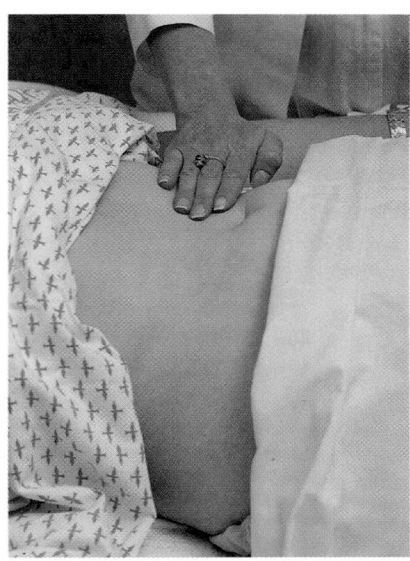

STEP **15** Light palpation of the abdomen.

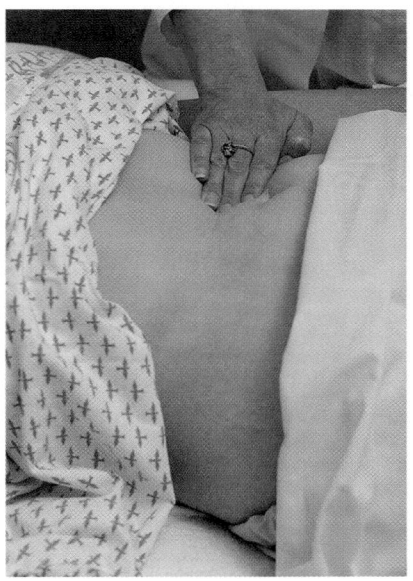

STEP **19** Deep palpation of the abdomen.

17. If masses are palpated, note size, location, shape, consistency, tenderness, mobility, and texture.

Descriptive characteristics help to reveal type of mass.

18. When tenderness is present, press one hand slowly and deeply into the involved area and then let go quickly. Note if pain is aggravated.

Tests for rebound tenderness. Results are positive if pain increases and indicates peritoneal irritation (Seidel and others, 2003).

19. Perform deep palpation, being sure the client is relaxed. Depress the palm and fingers approximately 2.5 to 7.5 cm (1 to 3 inches) into the abdomen (see illustration).

Detects less obvious masses and delineates abdominal organs.

EVALUATION

1. Compare assessment findings with normal assessment characteristics of abdomen.

Determines presence of abnormalities.

2. Ask client to describe signs and symptoms of colon cancer.

Demonstrates learning.

Recording and Reporting

- Record results of assessment in nurses' notes or flow sheet.
- Record content of any client instruction.
- Report serious abnormalities, such as absent bowel sounds, presence of mass, or acute pain, to nurse in charge and physician.

Unexpected Outcomes	Related Interventions
1. Abdomen is asymmetrical, with palpable mass, and dull to percussion.	• Report to the physician because findings may indicate enlarged liver, spleen, or tumor.
2. Abdomen protrudes symmetrically, with skin taut; client complains of tightness; and/or bowel sounds are absent. Gastrointestinal motility has ceased. Client is vomiting.	• Keep client on nothing by mouth (NPO) status, and encourage ambulation. • Notify physician. • Gastric decompression following insertion of nasogastric tube may become necessary.
3. Hyperactive bowel sounds are evident with gastrointestinal motility. Commonly they result from anxiety, diarrhea, overuse of laxatives, inflammation of the bowel, or reaction of the intestines to certain foods.	• Client may need to be NPO. • Client may need antidiarrheal medication.
4. Rebound abdominal tenderness is found.	• Avoid palpating area. • Notify physician if this is a new finding. • Place client on NPO status.
5. Bladder is palpable over symphysis pubis. Bladder is distended.	• Facilitate voiding. • If unable to void, urinary catheterization may be necessary
6. Internal organs (liver, spleen) are enlarged.	• Notify physician. • Do not continue to palpate area. • Place client on NPO status.
7. Abdominal girth is increased, accompanied by a fluid wave. Fluid has built up within peritoneal cavity.	• Notify physician. • Place client on NPO status.
8. Client is unable to describe signs and symptoms of colon cancer.	• Additional education is necessary.

Teaching Considerations

- Explain signs of colon cancer, including long-term progressive weight loss (late symptom), change in bowel habits, and blood in stools.
- Explain that factors such as diet, regular exercise, limited use of over-the-counter drugs causing constipation, establishment of regular elimination schedule, and good fluid intake promote normal bowel elimination (see Chapter 33).
- Caution client about dangers of excessive use of laxatives or enemas.
- If client has acute pain, explain activities or positions to avoid.
- If client is a health care worker or has contact with blood or body fluids of affected persons, encourage client to receive series of three hepatitis B vaccine doses.

Pediatric Considerations

- Most common palpable mass in child is feces, usually felt in right lower quadrant (Hockenberry and others, 2003).
- Have a child stand erect and then lie supine during inspection of abdominal surface. Normal abdomen of infants and young children is cylindrical in erect position and flat in supine position.
- In infants and children skin is usually taut and without wrinkles or creases.
- Children may perceive superficial palpation as tickling. Drawing attention to their laughter may only cause it to increase. Have the child help by placing their hand on top of yours, or have them place their hand on their abdomen with their fingers separated and then palpate between their fingers.

Gerontological Considerations

- Older adult often lacks abdominal tone; underlying organs are more easily palpable.
- A weakened intestinal musculature and decreased peristalsis affect the large intestine.
- Constipation along with nausea, flatulence, and heartburn are common.

- Stress to older adults importance of adequate fluid intake, regular exercise, and a diet with at least four servings daily of fresh fruit and vegetables and high-fiber foods to promote normal defecation.

SKILL 18-5 Musculoskeletal, Neurological, and Peripheral Vascular Assessment

The nurse uses the skills of inspection and palpation during the musculoskeletal, neurological, and peripheral vascular assessments. Initial assessment of the musculoskeletal and neurological systems involve a general inspection of gait, posture, and body position. A more thorough assessment of major bone, joint, and muscle groups and the nervous system is indicated in the presence of abnormalities or as required by client's condition. Much of the assessment can be performed while the nurse examines other body systems; for example, while assessing head and neck structures, the nurse can also assess neck range of motion (ROM) and examine select cranial nerves. It is effective for the nurse to integrate these assessments into routine activities of care, for example, while bathing or positioning the client. Assessment of these systems is especially important when the client reports pain, loss of sensation, or impairment of joint and/or muscle function. The integrity of the peripheral vascular system is assessed by noting the adequacy of blood flow to the extremities, accomplished by measuring arterial pulses and inspecting the condition of the skin and nails.

Prolonged illness or immobility may result in muscle weakness and atrophy. Hospitalized clients may experience neurovascular dysfunction as a result of high or low blood pressure or constriction of the extremities with dressings or a cast.

Inadequate tissue perfusion results in an inadequate delivery of oxygen and nutrients to cells, a condition called ischemia. This can be caused by constriction of vessels or by occlusion (blockage) from clot formation. The effects of ischemia depend on the duration of the problem and the metabolic needs of the tissues. Ischemia results in pain. If lack of oxygen to tissues is unrelieved, tissue necrosis (death) occurs. An embolus is a blood clot that breaks loose and travels through the circulation. If the clot obstructs circulation to the lungs or the brain, it can be life threatening.

DELEGATION CONSIDERATIONS

Assessment of musculoskeletal and neurological function should not be delegated to assistive personnel. However, assistive personnel should recognize clients' problems with gait and ROM. Assistive personnel should be instructed to report any problems noted in ROM or muscle strength and to know to take precautions during ROM exercises to avoid forcing a joint beyond the client's current ROM. Assistive personnel should be informed of clients at risk for falls and should be provided with instructions for clients with muscular weakness who require special assistance with transfer and ambulation. Assessment of peripheral vascular function should not be delegated to assistive personnel. However, assistive personnel should be taught to recognize temperature and color changes in the extremities along with changes in peripheral pulses.

EQUIPMENT

- ❏ Cotton balls or cotton tipped applicators
- ❏ Doppler and conducting gel
- ❏ Penlight
- ❏ Opposite tip of cotton swab or tongue blade broken in half
- ❏ Tape measure
- ❏ Tongue blade

STEP	RATIONALE

ASSESSMENT

1. Review client history for heavy alcohol use; cigarette smoking; constant dieting; calcium intake less than 500 mg daily; thin and light body frame; nulliparous status; menopause before age 45; postmenopause status; family history of osteoporosis; or white, Asian, Native American, or northern European ancestry. Assess for excessive caffeine intake; advanced age; history of fractures/falls; chronic diseases (Cushing's, hyperthyroidism and hypothyroidism, malabsorption/malnutrition disorders, neoplasms); long-term use of corticosteroids, methotrexate, phenytoin, heparin, and aluminum-containing antacids (Peterson, 2001).

   These are risk factors for osteoporosis.

2. Ask client whether he or she has been screened for osteoporosis.

   Women age 65 and older should be screened routinely for osteoporosis (U.S. Preventive Services Task Force, 2003).
   Men should be screened as well; they are equally at risk for development of osteoporosis as they age (Kessenich, 2000).

3. Ask client to describe history of bone, muscle, or joint function (e.g., recent fall, trauma, lifting heavy objects, bone or joint disease with sudden or gradual onset) and location of alteration.

   Assists in assessing nature of musculoskeletal problem.
   Osteoporosis-related fractures occur in half of all postmenopausal women; of those, 25% will have vertebral deformities, and 15% will suffer from hip fractures (U.S. Preventive Services Task Force, 2003).

4. Assess nature and extent of client's musculoskeletal pain: location, duration, severity, predisposing and aggravating factors, relieving factors, and type of pain. If pain or cramping is reported in the lower extremities, ask if it is relieved or aggravated by walking. Assess the distance walked and characteristics of pain before, during, and after activity.

   Alterations in bone, joints, or muscle are frequently accompanied by pain, which has implications not only for comfort but also ability to perform activities of daily living. Pain caused by certain vascular conditions tends to increase with activity.

5. Assess client's normal activity pattern, including type of exercise routinely performed.

   Provides baseline in assessment. Sedentary lifestyle and lack of appropriate exercise increases bone loss and risk of fractures (Peterson, 2001).

6. Determine how client's alteration influences ability to perform activities of daily living (e.g., bathing, feeding, dressing, toileting, and ambulating) and social functions (e.g., household chores, work, recreation, sexual activities).

   Level of nursing care is determined by extent to which client can perform self-care. Type and degree of restriction in continuing social activities influence topics for client education and ability of nurse to identify alternative ways to maintain function.

7. Assess for a decrease in height in women older than 50 by subtracting current height from recall of maximum adult height.

   Measurement may be useful screening tool to predict osteoporosis. A loss of height is frequently the first clinical sign of osteoporosis (Pachucki-Hyde, 2001).

8. Determine if client is taking analgesics, antipsychotics, antidepressants, or nervous system stimulants.

   These medications can alter level of consciousness or cause behavioral changes.

9. Assess client's use of alcohol, sedative-hypnotics, or recreational drugs.

   Abuse can cause tremors, ataxia, and changes in peripheral nerve function.

10. Determine if client has recent history of seizures/convulsions: clarify sequence of events (aura, fall to ground, motor activity, loss of consciousness); character of any symptoms; and relationship of seizure to time of day, fatigue, or emotional stress.

    Seizure activity often originates from central nervous system alteration. Characteristics of seizure help determine its origin.

STEP	RATIONALE
11. Screen client for headache, tremors, dizziness, vertigo, numbness or tingling of body part, visual changes, weakness, pain, or changes in speech.	These symptoms frequently originate from alterations in central nervous system or peripheral nervous system function. Identification of specific patterns may aid in diagnosis of pathological condition.
12. Discuss with spouse, family member, or friends any recent changes in client's behavior (e.g., increased irritability, mood swings, memory loss, change in energy level).	Behavioral changes may result from intracranial pathological states.
13. Assess client for history of change in vision, hearing, smell, taste, or touch.	Major sensory nerves originate from brain stem. These symptoms may help to localize nature of problem.
14. If an older client displays sudden acute confusion (delirium), review history for drug toxicity (anticholinergics, diuretics, digoxin, cimetidine, sedatives, antihypertensives, antiarrhythmics), serious infections, metabolic disturbances, heart failure, and severe anemia.	One of the most common mental disorders in older persons.
15. Review past history for head or spinal cord injury, hypertension, or psychiatric disorders.	Factors may cause neurological symptoms or behavioral changes to develop, focusing assessment on possible cause.
16. Determine if client experiences leg cramps, numbness or tingling in extremities, sensation of cold hands or feet, pain in legs, or swelling or cyanosis of feet, ankles, or hand.	These signs and symptoms indicate vascular disease.
17. If client experiences leg pain or cramping in lower extremities, ask if it is relieved or aggravated by walking or standing for long periods or during sleep.	Relationship of symptoms to exercise can clarify whether problem is vascular or musculoskeletal. Pain caused by vascular condition tends to increase with activity. Musculoskeletal pain is not usually relieved when exercise ends.
18. Ask women if they wear tight-fitting garters or hosiery and sit or lie in bed with legs crossed.	Tight hosiery around lower extremities and crossing legs can impair venous return.
19. Reconsider previous heart risk factors (e.g., smoking, exercise, nutritional problems).	These predispose client to vascular disease.
20. Assess medical history for heart disease, hypertension, phlebitis, diabetes, or varicose veins.	Circulatory and vascular disorders influence findings gathered during examination.

NURSING DIAGNOSES

- Activity intolerance
- Disturbed body image
- Risk for injury
- Impaired physical mobility
- Impaired walking

- Pain (acute, chronic)
- Risk for trauma
- Ineffective peripheral tissue perfusion
- Risk for peripheral neurovascular dysfunction

Related factors are individualized based on client's condition or needs.

PLANNING

1. Expected outcomes following completion of procedure: • Client demonstrates erect posture, strong grasp, steady gait, with arms swinging freely at side.	Indicates normal alignment, gait, and neuromuscular muscle strength.
• There is bilateral symmetry of extremities in length, circumference, alignment, position, and skinfolds (Seidel and others, 2003).	
• Full active ROM is present in all joints with good muscle tone and absence of contractures, spasticity, or muscular weakness.	Indicates normal ROM of joints.
• Client will be alert and oriented to person, place, and time. Behavior and appearance appropriate for condition/situation.	Indicates normal cerebral function.

STEP	RATIONALE
• Client demonstrates: pupils equal, reactive, respond to light and accommodation (PERRLA), direct and consensual; external ocular muscles (EOMs) intact; facial sensation intact; symmetrical facial expressions; soft palate and uvula midline and rise upon phonation; gag reflex intact; speech clear without hoarseness; swallows without difficulty.	Indicates normal functioning of cranial nerves III, IV, VI, V, VII, IX, and X.
• Client is able to distinguish between sharp and dull sensations and light touch on symmetrical areas of extremities. Able to distinguish vibratory sensations on symmetrical distal joints of toes and fingers. Position sense intact to lower extremities.	Indicates normal function of sensory nerves.
• Gait coordinated, steady with appropriate stance and swing phases. Romberg test negative.	Indicates normal cerebellar and motor system functioning.
• Peripheral pulses are equal and strong (2+), extremities are warm and pink, with capillary refill less than 2 seconds. There is no dependent edema.	Peripheral circulation intact.

IMPLEMENTATION

1. Prepare client:

   a. Integrate musculoskeletal and neurological assessments during other portions of physical assessment or during nursing care.

   Nurse can conduct assessment of the musculoskeletal and neurological systems as client moves in bed, rises from chair, or goes through movements required during complete physical examination. Integration saves time for both nurse and client.

   b. Plan time for short rest periods during assessment.

   Movement of body parts and various maneuvers may fatigue client. It is especially important to consider rest periods with older adult and very ill clients.

2. Musculoskeletal assessment

   a. Observe ability to use arms and hands for grasping objects (see illustration).

   Assesses coordination and muscle strength.

   b. Assess muscle strength of upper extremities by applying gradual increase in pressure to muscle group.

   Upper and lower extremity on client's dominant side is normally stronger than that on nondominant side. Pain, rather than weakness, may cause reduced muscle strength; however, long-term pain can lead to muscle weakening.

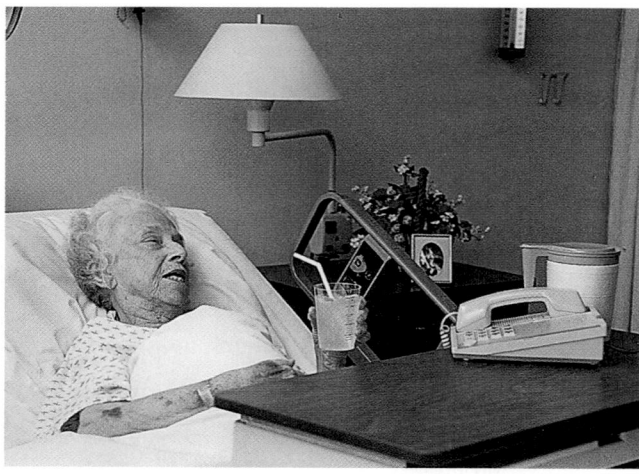

STEP **2a** Observe use of arms and hands.

STEP	**RATIONALE**

c. To assess hand grasp strength, cross your hands, and have the client grasp the fingers of both of your hands and squeeze them as hard as possible. To avoid discomfort, you may cross index and middle fingers (see illustration).

It is common for the client's dominant hand to be slightly stronger than the nondominant hand. By crossing hands client's right hand grasps your right hand.

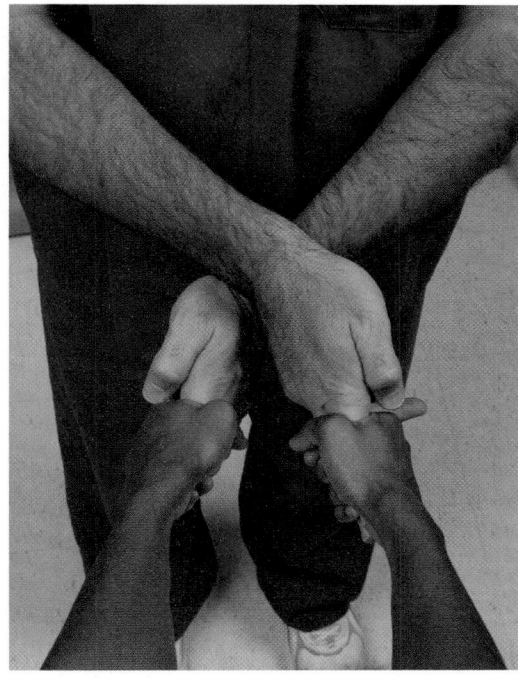

STEP **2c** Assessing strength of hand grasps, comparing sides.

d. Have client resist pressure applied by attempting to move against resistance (e.g., flex elbow). Have client maintain resistance until told to stop. Compare symmetrical muscle groups. Note weakness, and compare right with left.

Compares symmetrical muscle groups for strength on the following scale. Rate muscle strength on scale of 0 to 5: Grade as follows:
0—No voluntary contraction
1—Slight contractility, no movement
2—Full range of motion, passive
3—Full range of motion, active
4—Full range of motion against gravity, some resistance
5—Full range of motion against gravity, full resistance
Indicates degree of atrophy.

e. If muscle weakness is identified, measure muscle size with tape measure placed around body of muscle. Compare with same muscle on opposite side of body.

f. Observe body alignment for sitting, supine, prone, or standing positions. Muscles and joints should be exposed and free to move to allow for accurate measurement.

Each joint or muscle group may require different position for measurement.

g. Inspect gait as client walks and stands. Observe for foot dragging, shuffling or limping, balance, presence of obvious deformity in lower extremities, and position of the trunk in relation to the legs.

Gait is more natural if client is unaware of nurse's observation. The observations may indicate a neuromusculoskeletal disorder.

STEP	**RATIONALE**

h. Stand behind client, and observe postural alignment (position of hips relative to shoulders). Look sideways at cervical, thoracic, and lumbar curves (see illustration).

Abnormal curves of posture include lordosis (swayback, increased lumbar curvature), kyphosis (hunchback, exaggerated posterior curvature of thoracic spine), and scoliosis (lateral spinal curvature). Postural changes may indicate muscular, bone, or joint deformity; pain; or muscular fatigue. Head should be held erect.

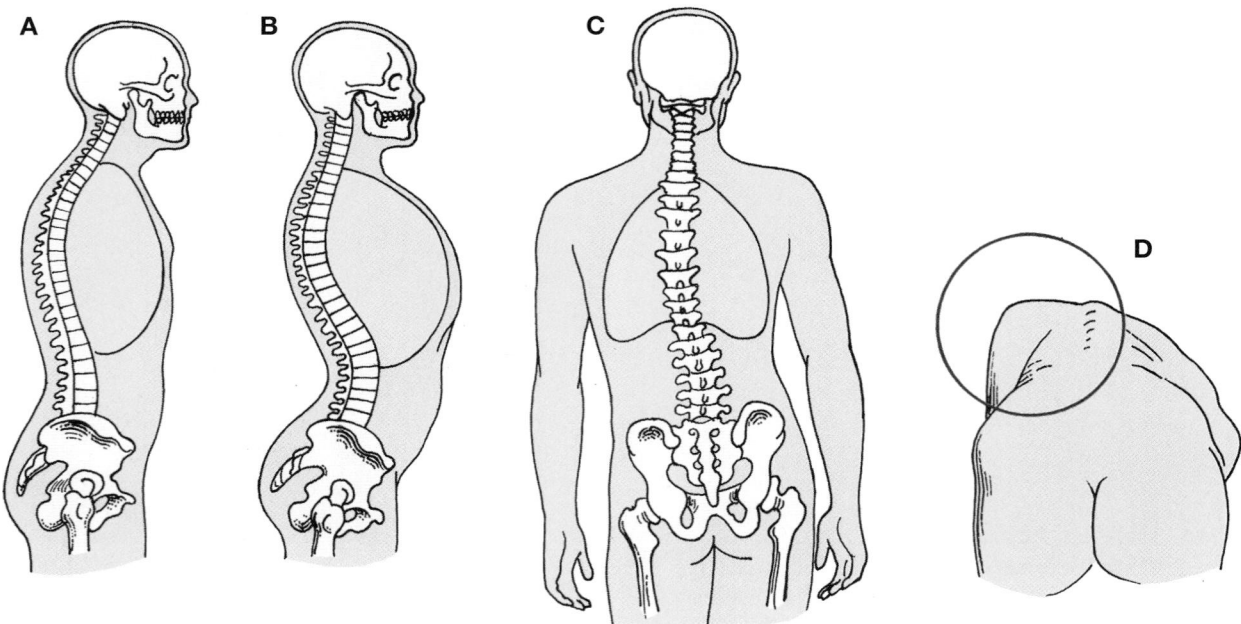

STEP 2h Spinal deformities. **A,** Kyphosis. **B,** Lordosis. **C,** Scoliosis. **D,** Scoliosis with client bending forward.

i. Make a general observation of the extremities. Look at overall size, gross deformity, bony enlargement, alignment, and symmetry.

General review helps to pinpoint areas requiring in-depth assessment.

j. Gently palpate bones, joints, and surrounding tissues where client reports pain. Note any heat, tenderness, edema, or resistance to pressure.

May reveal changes resulting from trauma or chronic disease. Do not attempt to move joint when fracture is suspected or when joint is apparently "frozen" by lack of movement over a long period of time.

k. Ask client to put major joint through its full ROM (Table 18-11). Observe equality of motion in same body parts:

Assessment of client's normal ROM provides baseline for assessing later changes after surgery or inactivity. Clients with deformities, reduced mobility, joint fixation, or weakness may require passive motion assessment.

(1) Active motion (client needs no support or assistance and is able to move joint independently): Instruct client in moving each joint through its normal range. It may be necessary to demonstrate movements and ask client to mimic your movements.

Identifies muscle strength, as well as detecting altered strength or limited range of motion.

(2) Passive motion (joint has full ROM but client does not have the strength to move it independently): Have client relax and move the same joints passively until the end of the range is felt. Support extremity at joint. Do not force the joint if there is pain or muscle spasm.

Determines ability to perform joint motion in the presence of muscle weakness. Forcing joint may cause injury and pain.

STEP	RATIONALE

TABLE 18-11   ASSESSING RANGE OF MOTION (ROM)*

BODY PART	ASSESSMENT PROCEDURE	ROM
UPPER EXTREMITIES		
Shoulders	Raise both arms to a vertical position level with sides of the head.	Flexion.
	Place both hands behind the neck, with elbows out to the sides.	External rotation and abduction.
	Place both hands behind the small of the back (internal rotation).	Internal rotation.
	Have client make small circles with hands with arms extended at shoulder level.	Circumduction.
Elbows	Bend and straighten the elbows.	Flexion and extension.
	Place hands at waist with elbows flexed.	Internal rotation.
Wrist	Bend and straighten wrist.	Flexion and extension.
	Bend wrist to radial then ulnar side.	Radial and ulnar deviation.
	Turn palm upward, then downward.	Supination and pronation.
Hand	Make a fist with both hands.	Flexion and extension.
	Extend and spread fingers and thumb.	Adduction and abduction.
LOWER EXTREMITIES		
Hips (with client supine)	With knees extended, raise one leg upward.	Flexion: Expect 90 degrees.
	Repeat with knee flexed.	Abduction: Expect 45 degrees.
	Swing legs laterally.	Adduction: Expect 30 degrees.
	With knee flexed, hold the ankle, and rotate the leg inward and outward.	Internal and external rotation: Expect 40-45 degrees.
Knees (with client sitting)	Raise the foot, keeping the knee in place.	Extension: Expect full extension and up to 15 degrees hyperextension.
Ankle	With foot held off the floor, point toes, then bring toes back toward the knee.	Plantar flexion: Expect 45 degrees. Dorsiflexion: Expect 20 degrees.
	Turn foot inward and then outward.	Inversion and eversion: Expect to reach 5 degrees.
Toes	Bend toes down and back.	Expect to reach 40 degrees.

*This may be done actively by the client (AROM) or passively by the nurse (PROM).

l. Palpate joint for swelling, stiffness, tenderness, and heat; note any redness.

Indicates acute or chronic inflammation. Range of motion may cause pain or injury.

m. Assess muscle tone in major muscle groups. Normal tone causes mild, even resistance to movement through entire ROM.

If muscle has increased tone (hypertonicity), any sudden movement of joint is met with considerable resistance. Hypotonic muscle moves without resistance. Muscle feels flabby.

3. Neurological assessment

a. Assess level of consciousness and orientation by asking client to identify name, location, day of week, and year; note behavior and appearance.

A fully conscious client responds to questions spontaneously. As consciousness lowers, may show irritability, shortened attention span, or an unwillingness to cooperate. As consciousness deteriorates, client becomes disoriented to name, time, and place. Behavior and appearance reveal information about the client's mental status.

b. Assess cranial nerves:
   (1) CN III (oculomotor), IV (trochlear), VI (abducens) by assessing extraocular movement EOM functioning. Ask client to follow movement of nurse's finger through the six cardinal positions of gaze; measure pupillary reaction to light reflex and accommodation with use of penlight (see Skill 18-1).

These cranial nerves are most likely to be affected by increasing intracranial pressure (ICP). ICP causes change in response of pupil or size of pupil; pupils may change shape (more oval); react sluggishly. ICP impairs movements of EOMs.

STEP	RATIONALE
(2) CN V (trigeminal) by applying light sensation with a cotton ball to symmetrical areas of face.	Sensations should be symmetrical; unilateral decrease or loss of sensation may be due to CN V lesion or in higher sensory pathways.
(3) CN VII (facial) by noting facial symmetry. Have client frown, smile, puff out cheeks, and raise eyebrows.	Expressions should be symmetrical; drooping of upper and lower face may be caused by Bell's palsy; asymmetry may be caused by cerebrovascular accident (CVA).
(4) CN IX (glossopharyngeal) and CN X (vagus) by having client speak and swallow. Ask client to say "ah" while using tongue blade and penlight. Check for midline uvula and symmetrical rise of uvula and soft palate. Use tongue blade, and place on posterior tongue to elicit gag reflex.	Damage to CN IX causes impaired swallowing; damage to CN X causes loss of gag reflex, hoarseness, nasal voice. A unilateral paralysis may be observed when palate fails to rise and uvula pulls toward normal side.
c. Sensory assessment of extremities	
(1) *Pain:* Ask client to indicate when sharp or dull sensation is felt as you alternately apply sharp and blunt ends of tongue blade to skin surface. Apply in symmetrical areas of extremities.	Client should be able to distinguish sharp or dull sensations. Impaired sensations may indicate disorders of the spinal cord or of peripheral nerve roots.
(2) *Light touch:* Apply light wisp of cotton to different points along skin's surface in symmetrical areas of extremities.	Client should be able to distinguish when touched.
(3) *Vibration:* Apply stem of vibrating tuning fork to distal joints of toes and fingers. Have client voice when and where vibration is felt and when sensation stops.	Loss of vibratory sensation occurs with peripheral neuropathy.
(4) *Position:* Grasp finger or toe, holding it by its sides with your thumb and index finger. Alter moving finger or toe up and down. Ask client to state when finger is up or down. Repeat with toes.	Client should be able to distinguish movements of a few millimeters. Decreased/absent position sense may occur in spinal anesthesia, paralysis, or other neurological disorders.
d. Motor and cerebellar function	
(1) *Gait:* Have client walk across the room, turn, and come back. Note use of assistive devices.	Neurological and musculoskeletal disorders may impair gait and balance.
(2) *Romberg test:* Have client stand with feet together, arm at sides, both with eyes open and eyes closed (for 20 to 30 seconds). Protect client's safety by standing at side; observe for swaying.	Romberg test should be negative; slight swaying is considered normal.
4. Peripheral vascular assessment	
a. Inspect lower extremities for changes in color and condition of the skin (Table 18-12). Note skin and nail texture, hair distribution, venous patterns, edema, and scars or ulcers. Compare skin color lying and standing.	Changes may reflect impaired peripheral circulation.
b. Palpate edematous areas, noting mobility, consistency, and tenderness.	Assists in determining extent of edema.

STEP	RATIONALE

TABLE 18-12	COMPARISON OF VENOUS AND ARTERIAL INSUFFICIENCY	
ASSESSMENT	**ARTERIAL**	**VENOUS**
Pain	Burning, throbbing, cramping, increases with exercise	Aching, increases in evening and with dependent position
Paresthesia	Numbness, tingling, decreased sensation	None
Temperature/color	Cool to touch, pale when elevated; dusky red when extremity is lowered	Normal to touch; normal, flushed, or cyanotic
Capillary refill	>2 seconds	Not applicable
Pulses	Diminished or absent	Present
Skin changes	Thin, shiny skin; decreased hair growth; thickened nails	Brown pigmentation around ankles
Ulcerations	Deep, well defined at site of trauma or tips of toes	Shallow ulcers around ankles (chronic venous stasis); edema apparent

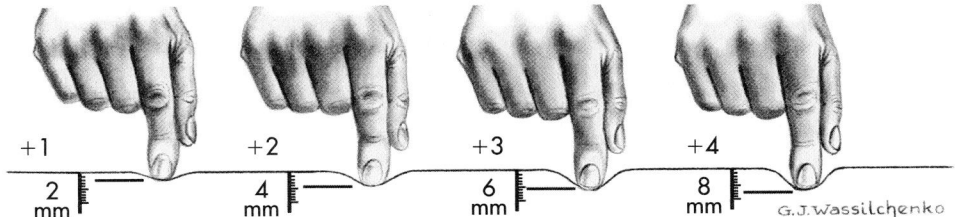

STEP **4c** Pitting edema. (From Seidel HM and others: *Mosby's guide to physical examination,* ed 5, St. Louis, 2003, Mosby.)

c. Assess for pitting edema by pressing area firmly with thumb for 5 seconds, then releasing. Depth of indentation determines severity (see illustration).
2 mm: 1 + edema
4 mm: 2 + edema
6 mm: 3 + edema
8 mm: 4 + edema
    A tape measure may be used to measure the circumference of the extremity.

Unilateral edema of affected leg is one of the most reliable physical findings of deep vein thrombosis (DVT) (Day, 2003).
Edema results from fluid in tissues. Inadequate venous return causes edema in the sacrum if client is confined to bed or in the feet and ankles if sitting.

d. Assess capillary refill by grasping client's fingernail or toenail and noting color of nail bed. Next, apply gentle, firm pressure to the nail bed. Release quickly, watching for color change. Circulation is restored and normally returns to pink color in less than 2 seconds.

Cold environmental temperature, with vasoconstriction, and vascular disease can delay refill. Local pressure from a cast or bandage may also deter refill.

e. Ask if the client experiences pain or tenderness, and then palpate for heat, firmness, or localized swelling of the calf muscle, which are signs of phlebitis or DVT.

Clients who have been immobilized for several days and those who have bone or joint disease, surgical correction of joint or bone, or pain are at risk for altered tissue perfusion (Breen, 2000). Some clients have DVT and only complain of calf pain (Urbano, 2001).

• **Critical Decision Point**
If there is a strong suspicion of DVT, testing for Homans' sign is contraindicated. If a clot is present, it may become dislodged from its original site during this test. This could result in a pulmonary embolism.

STEP	RATIONALE

f. If calf appears normal, test for Homans' sign by supporting the leg while flexing the foot in dorsiflexion. Ask if the client experiences pain in the calf.

If pain is apparent, a positive Homans' sign is noted, and the possibility of deep vein thrombosis needs to be considered. However, Homans' sign is absent in nearly half of known cases and may be present in other conditions as well (Breen, 2000; Day, 2003).

- **Critical Decision Point**

Homans' sign is no longer considerered a reliable indicator for the presence or absence of DVT (Breen, 2000; Day, 2003; Urbano, 2001) and should not be considered a reliable parameter. Trauma to the vein or muscle, reduced mobility, and increased blood clotting are reliable risk factors. If calf is swollen, tender, or red, notify client's physician for further assessment and evaluation.

g. Starting at the most distal part of each extremity, palpate each peripheral artery for equality, comparing side to side; elasticity of vessel wall: depress and release artery, noting ease with which it springs back to shape and strength of pulse (force of blood against arterial wall) using the following rating scale (Seidel and others, 2003):

0	No pulse palpable
1+	Pulse is difficult to palpate, weak and thready, and easy to obliterate
2+	Stronger than 1+, easy to palpate, normal pulse
3+	Easy to palpate and not easily obliterated
4+	Strong, bounds against fingertips, and cannot be obliterated

Comparison of both arteries allows nurse to determine any localized obstruction or disturbance in blood flow. Pulses should be symmetrical side to side. If asymmetry is noted, look for other factors related to impaired circulation.

h. Palpate radial pulse by lightly placing tips of first and second fingers in groove formed along radial side of forearm, lateral to flexor tendon of wrist (see illustration).

Pulse is relatively superficial and should not require deep palpation.

i. Palpate ulnar pulse by placing fingertips along ulnar side of forearm (see illustration).

Palpated when arterial insufficiency to hand is expected or when nurse assesses effects that radial occlusion (e.g., during arterial blood gas sampling) might have on circulation to hand (see Chapter 43).

j. Palpate brachial pulse by locating groove between biceps and triceps muscles above elbow at antecubital fossa (see illustration). Place tips of first two fingers in muscle groove.

Artery runs along medial side of extended arm, requiring moderate palpation.

k. Have client lie supine with feet relaxed, and palpate dorsalis pedis pulse. Gently place fingertips between great and first toe; slowly move fingers along groove between extensor tendons of great and first toe until pulse is palpable (see illustration).

Artery lies superficially and does not require deep palpation. Pulse may be congenitally absent.

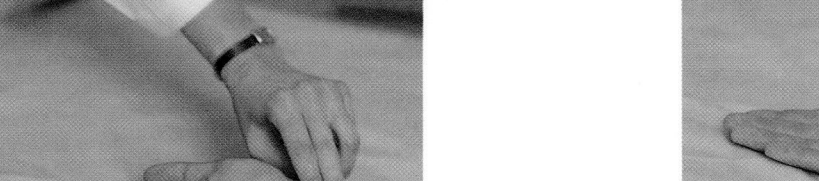

| **STEP** | **RATIONALE** |

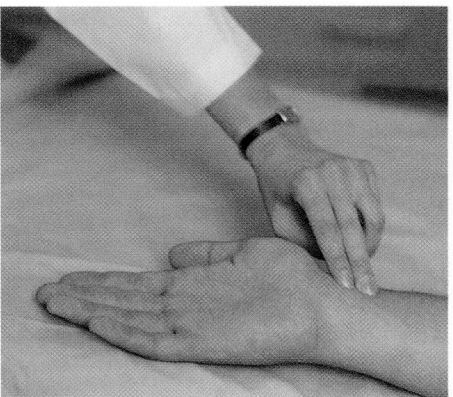

STEP **4h** Palpation of radial pulse.

STEP **4i** Palpation of ulnar pulse.

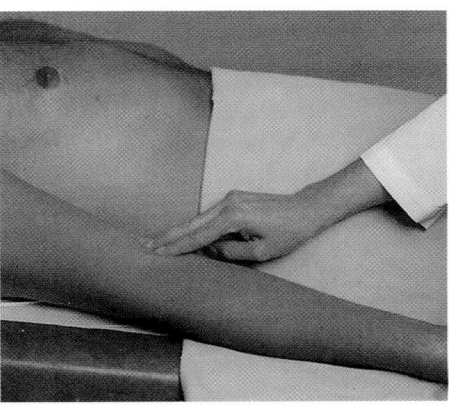

STEP **4j** Palpation of brachial pulse.

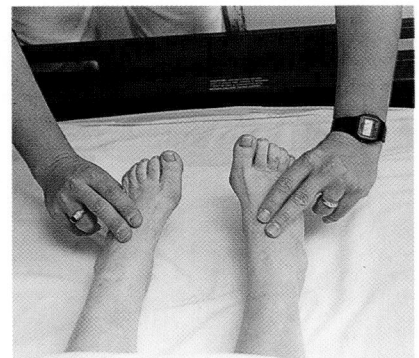

STEP **4k** Palpation of dorsalis pedis pulses.

l. If the dorsalis pedis pulse is difficult to palpate, or it is not palpable, use a Doppler instrument over the pulse site:
    (1) Apply conducting gel to the client's skin over the pulse site or onto transducer tip of probe.
    (2) Turn Doppler on. Gently apply ultrasound probe to the skin, altering angle until pulsation is audible. Adjust volume as needed (see illustration).

m. Palpate posterior tibial pulse by having client relax and slightly extend feet. Place fingertips behind and below medial malleolus (ankle bone) (see illustration).

Doppler amplifies sounds, allowing nurse to hear low-velocity blood flow through peripheral arteries.

Artery is easily palpable with foot relaxed.

STEP	RATIONALE

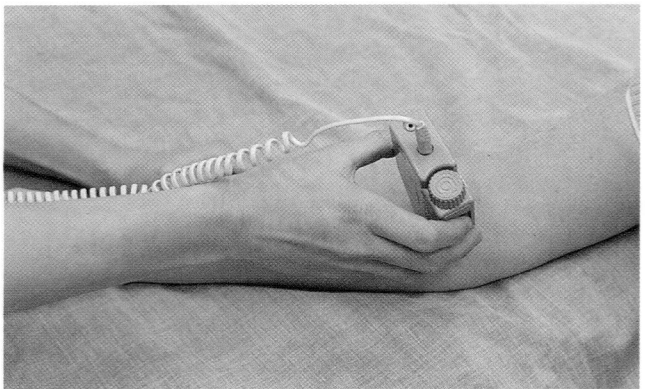

STEP **4l(2)** Use of Doppler for brachial pulse.

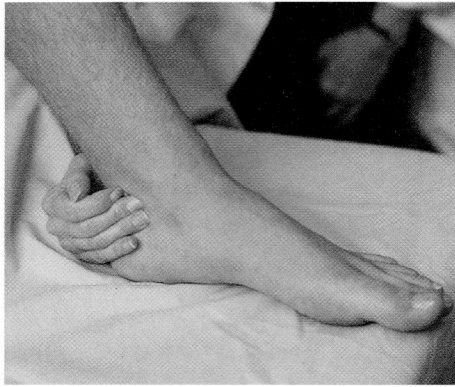

STEP **4m** Palpation of posterior tibial pulse.

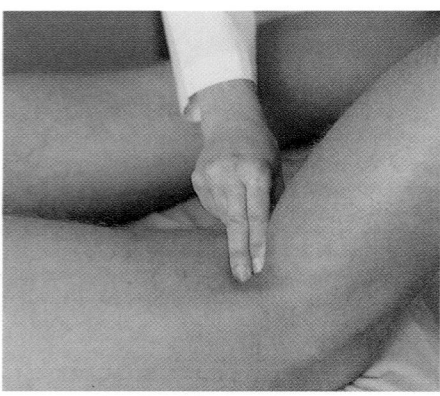

STEP **4n** Palpation of popliteal pulse with client prone.

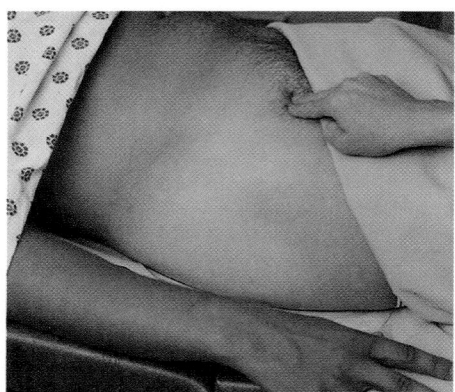

STEP **4o** Palpation of femoral pulse.

n. Palpate popliteal pulse by having client slightly flex knee with foot resting on table or bed. Instruct client to keep leg muscles relaxed. Palpate deeply into popliteal fossa with fingers of both hands placed just lateral to midline. Client may also lie prone to achieve exposure of artery (see illustration).

Flexion of knee and muscle relaxation improve accessibility of artery. Popliteal pulse is one of the more difficult pulses to palpate.

o. With client supine, palpate femoral pulse by placing first two fingers over inguinal area below inguinal ligament, midway between pubic symphysis and anterosuperior iliac spine (see illustration). If drainage or secretions are present, apply gloves.

Supine position prevents flexion in groin area, which interferes with artery access.

p. In clients with back pain or surgery, a cerebrovascular accident, or spinal cord compression it is appropriate to monitor deep tendon reflexes (DTRs) (McHugh and McHugh, 1990). This is not typically part of the routine shift assessment and will not be discussed here.

Muscle spasticity and hyperactive reflexes may result from disorders such as stroke and paralysis. Diminished DTRs and muscle weakness may suggest lower motor neuron disorders such as amyotrophic lateral sclerosis (ALS) or Guillain-Barré syndrome.

STEP	RATIONALE

▌EVALUATION

1. Compare muscle strength and range of motion with previous shift assessment.

2. Compare neurological status with previous shift assessment.

3. Compare pulses and capillary refill bilaterally with previous shift assessment.

4. Compare presence and extent of edema with previous shift assessment.

5. Evaluate level of client's discomfort following procedure.

Determines presence of abnormalities.

Determines if manipulation of musculoskeletal structures intensifies client's discomfort.

Recording and Reporting

* Record all findings in nurses' notes or appropriate assessment flow sheet.
* Report to nurse in charge or physician acute pain or sudden muscle weakness, which may be indicative of condition requiring immediate treatment.
* Report changes in peripheral circulation evidenced by edema or diminished or absent pulses or capillary refill, which may indicate circulatory compromise that can result in permanent nerve damage or tissue death if untreated.

Unexpected Outcomes	Related Interventions
1. Joints are prominent, swollen, and tender with nodules or overgrowth of bone in distal joints, indicating signs of arthritis.	• Instruct client in proper ROM. • Determine client's knowledge regarding antiinflammatory medications.
2. Reduced ROM in one or more major joints—shoulder, elbow, wrist, fingers, knee, hip.	• Assess further for pain during movement, with joint unstable, stiff, painful, or swollen or with obvious deformity. • Notify physician. • Reduce mobility in extremity until cause of abnormal joint motion is determined.
3. Client demonstrates weakness in one or more major muscle groups, or gait demonstrates unsteady balance with shuffling or stumbling of feet.	• Place client on fall precautions. • Promote client safety when ambulating (see Chapter 11). • Notify physician.
4. Client has changes in mental status and pupillary response or other neurological deficits.	• Notify physician. • Continue to monitor client closely.
5. Previously palpable dorsalis pedis pulses are diminished or absent, indicating circulatory compromise.	• Notify physician. • Elevate extremity.
6. Client's lower extremities have pale, cool, thin, and shiny skin, with reduced hair growth and thickened nails, indicating chronic arterial insufficiency.	• Instruct client on proper foot care. • Refer to podiatrist for nail trimming. • Inspect feet for signs of impaired skin integrity.

Teaching Considerations

- Instruct client about correct postural alignment. Consult with physical therapist to provide client with exercises for improving posture.
- To reduce bone demineralization, instruct older adult client on a proper weight-bearing exercise program (e.g., walking, low-impact aerobics) to be followed 3 or more times a week.
- Encourage intake of calcium to meet the recommended daily allowance. Increased vitamin D will aid calcium absorption. Recommendations for daily calcium supplements: men and premenopausal women and postmenopausal women on estrogen, 1000 mg; postmenopausal women on no estrogen, 1500 mg; men and women over 65, 1500 mg.
- Explain to clients with low back pain that they can benefit from modification of worker risk factors (e.g., lifting heavy weights, use of protective equipment), regular aerobic exercise, exercises that strengthen the back and increase trunk flexibility, and learning how to lift properly.
- Explain to family/friends the neurological implications of any behavioral or mental impairments shown by client.
- Explain measures to ensure safety (e.g., use of ambulation aids or safety bars in bathrooms or stairways) for clients with sensory or motor impairments.

Pediatric Considerations

- Infants must be carefully examined for musculoskeletal anomalies resulting from genetic or fetal insults. An examination includes review of posture, generalized movement, symmetry and skin creases of the extremities, muscle strength, and hip alignment.
- Normally the back of a newborn is rounded or C-shaped from the thoracic and pelvic curves.

- Scoliosis, lateral curvature of the spine, is an important childhood problem, especially in females, apparent at puberty. (For closer examination, have child stand erect, wearing only underclothes. Observe from behind, looking for asymmetry of shoulders and hips. Then observe from the back as the child bends forward.) Uneven dress hems or pant leg hems or uneven fit of clothing at the waist may be noted.
- Watching a child during play can reveal information about musculoskeletal function.

Gerontological Considerations

- Instruct older adults about fall prevention. Modifications can be made in the home environment to reduce the risk of falls (see Chapter 41).
- Instruct older adults and those with osteoporosis on proper body mechanics, as well as range-of-motion and moderate weight-bearing exercises (e.g., swimming, walking) to minimize trauma and subsequent fracture of bones.
- Older adult's gait normally has smaller steps and a wider base of support.
- Functional assessment is a measurement of older person's ability to perform basic self-care tasks (Lueckenotte, 2000). When client is unable to perform self-care easily, determine the need for assistive devices (e.g., zippers on clothing instead of buttons, elevation of chairs to minimize bending of knees and hips). Creativity by the nurse is often needed (Baird, 2003; Kee, 2000).
- Instruct older adult client to pace activities to compensate for loss in muscle strength.
- Older adults tend to assume a stooped, forward-bent posture, with hips and knees somewhat flexed and arms bent at the elbows and the level of the arms raised.

SKILL 18-6 Assessing Intake and Output

Measuring and recording I&O during a 24-hour period helps to complete the assessment database for fluid and electrolyte balance. The nurse is responsible for recording all intake (liquids taken orally, by feeding tube, and parenterally) and all output (urine, diarrhea, vomitus, gastric suction, and drainage from surgical tubes). When possible, assistance from the alert client or family facilitates accuracy, independence, and a sense of participation in the plan of care.

Monitoring I&O may be an independent or a dependent nursing intervention. Keeping records of I&O is appropriate if a client has a fever, has edema, is receiving intravenous or diuretic therapy, or is placed on restricted fluids.

It is also important when a client has electrolyte losses associated with vomiting, diarrhea, gastrointestinal drainage, or extensive open wounds such as burns. General monitoring of I&O should be evaluated for all clients, although measuring and documentation on the chart is not required in some situations.

When indicated, I&O is totaled and evaluated at the end of each shift or at specified times, usually 8 hours. Significant alterations are apparent by comparing 24-hour totals over several days. Because fluid imbalance may occur at any time, awareness of I&O should be maintained for all clients, even when documentation is not required.

DELEGATION CONSIDERATIONS

Evaluation of I&O totals at the end of each shift, comparing 24-hour totals over several days, and monitoring and recording of intravenous therapy, wound or chest tube drainage, and tube feedings should not be delegated to assistive personnel. The following skills may be delegated:

* Measuring and recording oral intake
* Measuring and recording urinary output and wound drainage device output (see Skill 37-3)

Emphasize the importance of standard precautions relating to body fluids, accuracy in measuring and recording I&O, and the use of the metric system with standard containers. Clarify information that should be reported, including significant alteration in intake or changes in color, amount, or odor of output. Caution assistive personnel to be sensitive to the privacy needs of the client.

EQUIPMENT

- ❑ Sign alerting all personnel of I&O measurement
- ❑ Daily I&O record
- ❑ Graduated measuring container
- ❑ Bedpan, urinal, bedside commode, or urine "hat" (a receptacle that fits under the toilet seat)
- ❑ Disposable clean gloves

STEP	RATIONALE

ASSESSMENT

1. Identify clients with conditions that can increase fluid loss:

   a. Fever

   b. Diarrhea and/or vomiting

   c. Surgical wound drainage or chest tube drainage

   d. Gastric suction

   e. Major burns

   f. Severe trauma (especially crushing injuries)

   g. Endocrine imbalance
      (1) Cushing's disease

      (2) Addison's disease

      (3) Diabetic ketoacidosis

2. Identify clients with the following conditions: clients with impaired swallowing, unconscious clients, clients with impaired mobility.

3. Identify clients who are taking medications that can influence fluid balance, including diuretics and steroids.

4. Assess signs and symptoms of dehydration and fluid overload (e.g., bradycardia versus tachycardia, hypotension versus hypertension, reduced skin turgor versus edema).

Rationale column:

Prolonged fever diminishes body fluids by increasing insensible water losses from lungs through increased respiratory rate and from diaphoresis.

Diarrhea and vomiting may lead to fluid and electrolyte imbalances, especially in the very young and frail older adults. Loss of potassium and chloride ions and excretion of hydrogen ions alter acid-base balance.

Wound drainage represents plasma or whole blood loss. If significant amounts are lost, fluid loss must be replaced.

Hydrochloric acid, potassium, and fluids from the stomach are removed.

Fluid volume loss is directly proportional to amount and depth of injury. Major fluid shifts can occur at specific intervals following severe burns.

Hyperkalemia results from release of intracellular potassium from injured cells.

Corticosteroids can cause sodium and water retention with potassium excretion.

Deficiency of corticosteroids causes sodium and water excretion.

Osmotic diuresis from increased blood glucose levels causes fluid volume deficit.

These clients have risk of insufficient fluid intake.

Synthetic steroid preparations such as prednisone can cause fluid retention, whereas diuretics may cause a fluid deficit.

Signs of dehydration result from reduction of fluid within tissues and circulatory system. Compensation for overhydration results in a fluid shift into tissues, causing edema.

STEP	RATIONALE

5. Weigh clients daily, and observe for dehydration or fluid volume excess.

Kidneys attempt to excrete excess fluid during periods of overhydration and conserve body water during periods of dehydration.

• *Critical Decision Point*
Daily weights must be obtained with the same scale, same time of day, and with comparable articles of clothing.

6. Monitor laboratory reports:

Clients' condition and therapies such as parenteral fluid replacement can alter laboratory values.

   a. Urine specific gravity (normal is 1.010 to 1.030)

Increased hematocrit suggests dehydration.

   b. Hematocrit (Hct) (normal range is 38% to 47% for females and 40% to 54% for males).

Low hematocrit suggests blood loss/hemorrhage.

7. Assess client and family's knowledge of the purpose and process of I&O measurement.

Improves cooperation in reporting intake and output to nurse.

NURSING DIAGNOSES

- Deficient fluid volume
- Excess fluid volume
- Urinary retention

- Urinary incontinence (functional, stress, reflex, or urge)
- Diarrhea

Related factors are individualized based on client's condition or needs.

PLANNING

1. Expected outcomes following completion of procedure:
   - Oral intake is 600 to 900 ml greater than output and at least 1500 ml per 24 hours.
   - Weight remains within 2% of baseline.
   - Hematocrit and urine specific gravity are within normal limits (WNL).
2. Post sign alerting personnel that I&O measurement is required.
3. Place I&O record in established location at the bedside or at the door.

Normal oral intake maintained.

Normal hydration achieved without fluid alterations.

Ensures that all sources of intake and output will be measured by staff.

IMPLEMENTATION

1. Explain to client and family the reasons I&O are important.

Encouraging fluids is a nursing responsibility. Any client not restricted in total fluid intake should be encouraged to consume at least 1500 ml/day. Postoperative clients are frequently prescribed clear liquid diets and advanced to solid fluids as the nurse determines that they are able to tolerate it.

2. Measure and record all intake of fluid:
      a. Liquids with meals, gelatin, custards, ice cream, Popsicles, sherbets, ice chips (recorded as 50% of measured volume [e.g., 100 ml of ice chips equals 50 ml of water]).
      b. Liquid medicines such as antacids are counted as fluid intake, as are fluids with medications.
      c. Tube feedings (see Chapter 30).
      d. Parenteral fluids, blood components, and total parenteral nutrition solutions (see Chapter 31).

Provides comprehensive and accurate assessment.

STEP	RATIONALE

- **Critical Decision Point**
  Intake should be recorded as soon as it is measured to maintain accuracy. If more than one client is in the same room, each must have urine receptacles labeled with name and bed location.

3. Instruct client and family to call nurse to empty contents of urinal, urine hat, or commode each time it is used (see illustration). Incontinence, vomiting, and excessive perspiration also need to be monitored and reported to the nurse.

   Urine leakage on a pad can be weighed (1 ml of urine weighs 1 g), and the number of pads used in 24 hours can be counted.

4. Inform client and family that Foley catheter drainage bag and wound, gastric, or chest tube drainage are closely monitored, measured, and recorded and that the nurse or assistive personnel are responsible for this. Each client must have a graduated container clearly marked with name and bed location and used only for the client indicated.

   Prevents client or family from disrupting drainage systems.

5. Apply disposable gloves. Measure drainage at the end of the shift, using appropriate containers and noting color and characteristics. If splashing is anticipated, wear mask, eye protection, and/or gown.

   Provides comprehensive and accurate assessment over standard time frames. Prevents transmission of infection.

   a. Urine drainage is measured using a "hat" into which client voids or a graduated container (see illustration).

   b. Observe color and characteristics of urine in Foley tubing. Sometimes hourly urine output is measured using a special device (see illustration).

   Drainage in the tubing is representative of current output. Characteristics of drainage in the bag are often very noticeably different based on changes over time.

   c. Chest tube drainage is measured by marking and recording the time on the collection chamber at specified intervals (see illustration) (see Chapter 25).

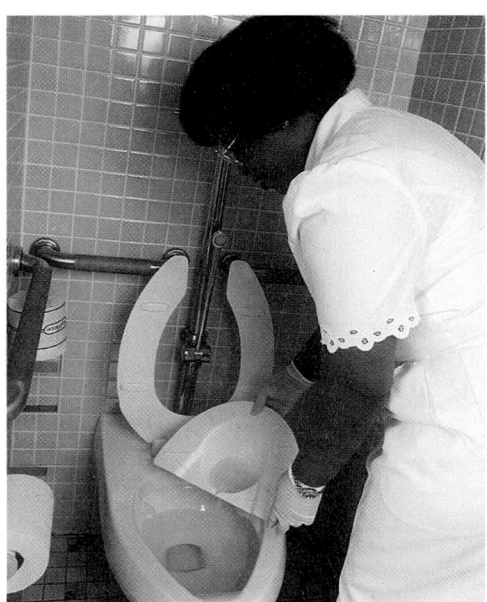

STEP **5a** Measuring and emptying the urine "hat."

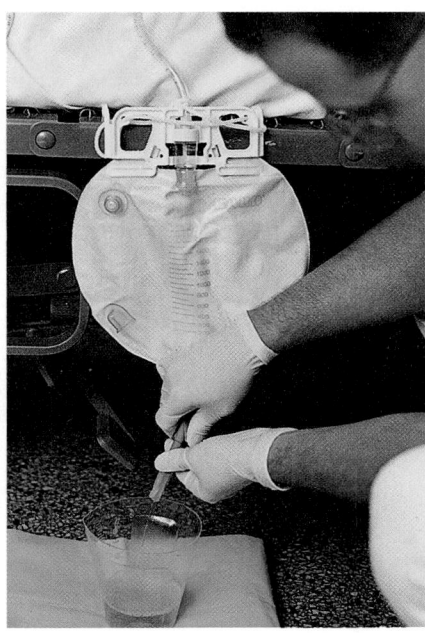

STEP **5b** Device for monitoring hourly urine output.

STEP	RATIONALE

- **Critical Decision Point**

  Chest tube drainage is emptied ONLY when container is nearly full. A closed system is necessary to maintain lung reexpansion.

- **Critical Decision Point**

  In adults, urine output less than 30 ml/hr can indicate decreased renal perfusion and should be reported. When output is low, a special device that facilitates measuring hourly output should be used.

d. Measure Jackson-Pratt Hemovac drainage using a medicine cup (see illustration).   Drainage is usually less than 30 ml in volume.

e. Measure gastric drainage or larger drainage pouches with graduated cup with a 240-ml capacity (see illustration).

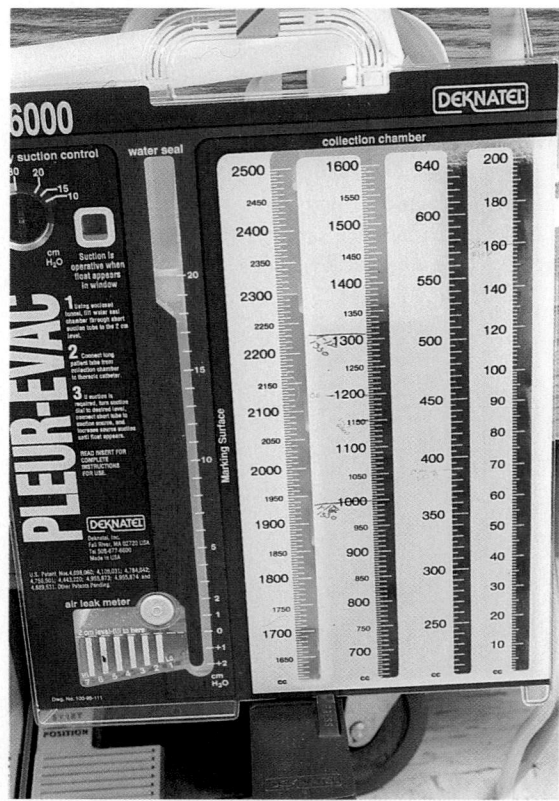

STEP **6a** Collection chamber for measuring chest tube drainage.

STEP	RATIONALE

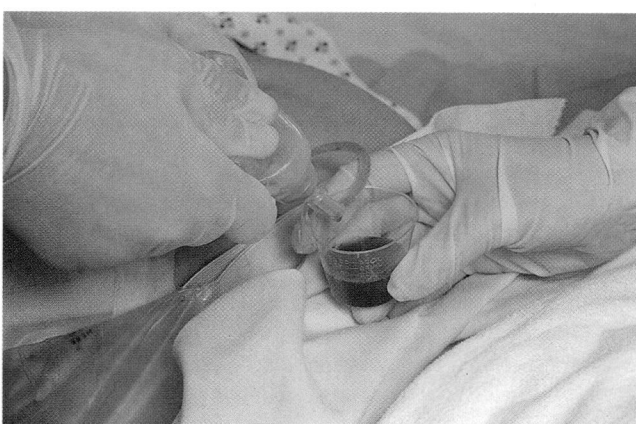

STEP **6b** Measuring wound drainage through a Jackson-Pratt drain.

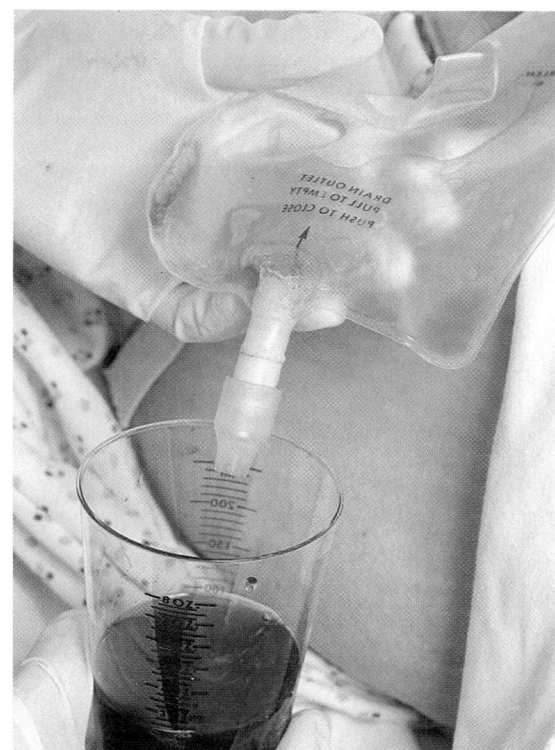

STEP **6c** Measuring drainage from large drainage pouch.

EVALUATION

1. Observe condition of skin and mucous membranes.	Condition reflects hydration status.
2. Observe color, characteristics, and amount of urine and wound drainage.	Presence of sudden increase in bright red blood may indicate hemorrhage, which can lead to hypovolemic shock.
3. Note I&O balance or imbalance (see Table 18-13).	Indicates client's overall fluid status.

TABLE 18-13   ASSESSING FOR FLUID IMBALANCES

FLUID VOLUME DEFICIT	FLUID VOLUME EXCESS
• Output greater than intake	• Intake greater than output
• Decreased blood pressure	• Crackles (pulmonary edema)
• Increased pulse	• Bounding pulse
• Fever	
• Flat neck veins when supine	• Jugular venous distention (JVD)
• Slow venous filling of dependent hands	
• Rapid weight loss >5%	• Rapid weight gain
• Dry mouth	
• Dry skin	
• Tenting	• Pitting edema

Recording and Reporting

- At specified time according to agency policy calculate total intake and output on the specified intake and output record at the bedside or at the door.
- Document the total on the client's record (Figure 18-6).
- Report immediately to physician any urine output less than 30 ml/hr or significant changes in daily weight, which suggest fluid volume deficit or excess.

Unexpected Outcomes	Related Interventions
1. Prolonged fluid loss without adequate replacement of fluid as evidenced by output greater than intake, weight loss greater than 2% over 24 to 48 hours, and an increased hematocrit value.	• Obtain frequent vital signs. • Observe for orthostatic hypotension when sitting client up in bed or assisting with ambulation (see Chapters 11 and 17). • Administer fluid replacement as ordered. • Notify physician of changes in client's physical assessment status.
2. Chemical or physiological imbalance results in fluid retention evidenced by intake greater than output.	• Notify physician. • Weigh client. • Place client on fluid restrictions. • Administer diuretics as ordered.

Teaching Considerations

- Some clients who are able to ambulate need to be reminded of need to measure and record all liquid intake and output.
- Severely ill or disoriented clients may be unable to understand reasons for I&O measurement or participate in measuring and recording. Family members often are able to help maintain accurate records.
- Clients who have fluid restriction (e.g., renal failure, congestive heart failure) may need strict I&O because fluid imbalance can quickly result in serious physiological changes.

Pediatric Considerations

- Infants and young children have a greater need for water and are more vulnerable to alterations in fluid and electrolyte balance from conditions such as vomiting and diarrhea (Hockenberry and others, 2003).
- Measuring output in infants may be done by weighing diapers; 1 g of diaper weight is equal to 1 ml of urine.
- Infants need to ingest a greater amount of fluid per kilogram of body weight than do older children (Hockenberry and others, 2003).

Gerontological Considerations

- With age, bladder capacity decreases, the prevalence of involuntary bladder contractions increases, and more urine is produced at night (Lueckenotte, 2000).
- Urinary incontinence is not a function of age and should be thoroughly evaluated (Lueckenotte, 2000).
- Clients with chronic illness and/or older than age 60 are at greater risk of fluid and electrolyte imbalances secondary to gastroenteritis.
- Older adults are more susceptible to fluid and electrolyte imbalances with prolonged fever.

Home Care Considerations

- Have client and caregiver practice measuring I&O correctly using I&O chart and available containers. Provide more appropriate measuring devices if needed.
- Instruct client and caregiver regarding daily weights as an important adjunct to monitoring I&O. Stress the importance of using the same scale, same time of day, and similar clothing.

VITAL SIGN / I & O / PAIN RECORD

Date _____ **INTAKE**   KEY: **C**ontinent / **I**ncontinent   **OUTPUT**

To Count:	Parenteral				Oral / Tube Feedings			Urine		Other				
Type:					Oral	TF	Flush							BM
To Count:					Amt	Amt	Amt	Amt	Amt	Amt	Amt	Amt	Amt	Amt/Freq
2300					120									
2400								325		Chest Tube 75				
0100	50													
0200														
0300														
0400														
0500														
0600														
8 hr Sub Totals	50				120			325	75					

8 hr Total Parenteral _____   8 hr total Oral/tube _____

To Count:					8 hr Shift Intake	**770**				8 hr Shift's Output		**400**		
0700					650									
0800								500						
0900														
1000	50									75				
1100														
1200														
1300														
1400														
8 hr Sub Totals	50				650			500	75					

8 hr Total Parenteral _____   8 hr total Oral/tube _____

To Count:					8 hr Shift Intake	**700**				8 hr Shift's Output		**575**		
1500					650			600						
1600														
1700										75				
1800														
1900	50													
2000														
2100														
2200														
8 hr Sub Totals	50				650			600	75					

8 hr Total Parenteral _____   8 hr total Oral/tube _____

8 hr Shift Intake **700**   8 hr Shift's Output **675**

Twenty-four hour Total	**1570**	**Twenty-four hour Total**	**1650**

FLUID EQUIVALENTS

1 oz	30cc	8 oz (1 cup)	240cc
4 oz (1/2 cup)	120cc	12 oz (soda-1 can)	360cc
6 oz (3/4 cup)	180cc		

ADDRESSOGRAPH / LABEL

SSM
HEALTH · CARE

VITAL SIGN / I & O / PAIN RECORD

SLM-1000-035 (6/2000) 10 BACK

FIGURE **18-6** Intake and output summary. (Courtesy SSM Health Care, St. Mary's Health Center, St. Louis, Mo.)

FOCUS on CLINICAL PRACTICE

You are caring for Mrs. Williams, a 63-year-old retired schoolteacher who underwent a hysterectomy for uterine cancer. This is her first postoperative day on your clinical unit. The night nurse reported that client had an "uneventful" night. She has an IV, abdominal dressing, Foley catheter to gravity, and a perineal pad in place.

1. What body systems would you assess for this client?
   (a) Describe key elements in these assessments.
2. Upon auscultation of her posterior lung field bases, you hear a crackling noise upon inspiration. What is this sound, and what does it indicate? What nursing diagnosis would be priority at this time?
3. You next assess her cardiac status, and she has a heart rate of 86 beats per minute, rhythm regular. You know that this is considered:
   A. Normal
   B. Bradycardia
   C. Tachycardia
   D. Abnormal
4. Mrs. Williams complains of abdominal incisional pain and requests pain medication. After you administer the medication, you inspect and then auscultate her ab-

domen. After listening for 60 seconds at a site below and to the right of the umbilicus you are unable to hear bowel sounds. What is the best assessment of this situation?
   A. Your client has peritonitis.
   B. You need to listen longer.
   C. You are not listening in the right place.
   D. Your client has a partial bowel obstruction.
5. While assisting Mrs. Williams with the bath, you note unilateral leg swelling; she states that her calf is tender to the touch. What is your assessment of the situation?
   A. Your client has muscle fatigue.
   B. Your client should not be concerned—all clients have this symptom after surgery.
   C. Your client has developed a phlebitis.
   D. Your client should have a Homans' sign test performed as soon as possible to check for deep vein thrombosis.
6. Mrs. Williams is to be evaluated for osteoporosis before discharge. Which specific questions would you ask to ascertain her risk? What physical examination techniques would you employ?

NCLEX REVIEW QUESTIONS

1. You are conducting the general survey of an adult client. The general survey includes:
   1. Appearance and behavior
   2. Obtaining peripheral pulses
   3. Observing specific body systems
   4. Conducting a detailed history
2. You are teaching the client to inspect all skin surfaces and to report pigmented skin lesions that:
   1. Are symmetrical
   2. Have regular borders
   3. Are blue/black or variegated in color
   4. Are less than 6 mm in diameter
3. You are auscultating the client's lung fields. The systematic pattern you use for comparison is:
   1. Side to side
   2. Top to bottom
   3. Anterior to posterior
   4. Interspace to interspace

4. When palpating the client's posterior thorax, you palpate for:
   1. Presence of fremitus
   2. Presence of breath sounds
   3. Use of accessory muscles
   4. Symmetry of chest excursion
5. The client's respiratory assessment reveals loud, low-pitched, rumbling sounds heard primarily over the bronchi. The nurse interprets these sounds as:
   1. Normal
   2. Crackles
   3. Rhonchi
   4. Wheezes
6. While auscultating heart sounds, you document that S_2 is heard best at the base. This sound correlates with closure of the:
   1. Aortic and mitral valves
   2. Tricuspid and mitral valves
   3. Aortic and pulmonic valves
   4. Tricuspid and pulmonic valves

NCLEX REVIEW QUESTIONS

7. This cardiac dysrhythmia is characterized by a regular pulse rhythm but at a rate that is slower than normal. This is called:
   1. Sinus bradycardia
   2. Sinus tachycardia
   3. Atrial fibrillation
   4. Premature ventricular contraction

8. You are assessing a client's capillary refill. To perform this examination, you:
   1. Inspect for bulging of tissues at the nail base
   2. Palpate the chest wall for vibrations while the client says "ninety-nine"
   3. Compare the anteroposterior diameter of the chest with the lateral diameter of the chest
   4. Observe the amount of time it takes for normal color to return to fingernail after pressure has been applied for a few seconds

9. In performing the abdominal assessment, the primary reason you auscultate before palpation is to:
   1. Prevent distortion of vascular sounds
   2. Prevent distortion of the bowel sound
   3. Determine any areas of tenderness or pain
   4. Allow the client to relax and be comfortable

10. You are performing an abdominal assessment and auscultate an abdominal bruit. Your next line of action is to:
    1. Measure abdominal girth
    2. Check for rebound tenderness
    3. Proceed with percussion and palpation
    4. Notify the physician immediately

11. The client is being assessed for shoulder range-of-joint movement. You ask the client to place both hands behind the small of the back, evaluating the movement of:
    1. Flexion
    2. Extension
    3. Internal rotation
    4. External rotation

12. You ask the client to smile, frown, and raise and lower the eyebrows; these actions test cranial nerve:
    1. III—oculomotor
    2. V—trigeminal
    3. VII—facial
    4. IX—glossopharyngeal

13. When testing sensory pathways, you:
    1. Use a predictable order
    2. Perform each test quickly
    3. Compare symmetrical areas
    4. Ensure that the client's eyes remain open

14. To assess the client's dorsalis pedis pulse, you would palpate:
    1. Behind the knee
    2. Over the lateral malleolus
    3. In the groove behind the medial malleolus
    4. Lateral to the extensor tendon of the great toe

15. Your older adult female client presents with a history of vomiting and diarrhea. Assessment findings reveal lethargy, inelastic skin turgor, dry mucous membranes, weight loss of 5 pounds in 3 days, hematocrit 51%, and urine specific gravity 1.035. Based on this information, your priority nursing diagnosis is:
    1. Fatigue
    2. Excess fluid volume
    3. Deficient fluid volume
    4. Imbalanced nutrition, less than body requirements

References

Ahren J, Mazur ML: Site rotation, *Diabetes Forecast* 54(4):66, 2001.

Andrews M.: The influence of cultural and health belief systems on health care practices. In Andrews M, Boyle J: *Transcultural concepts in nursing care,* Philadelphia, 2003, Lippincott.

Breen P: DVT: what every nurse should know, *RN* 63(4):58, 2000.

Daly S: *Expert 10 minute physical examinations,* St. Louis, 1997, Mosby.

Day MW: Recognizing and management: DVT—deep vein thrombosis, *Nursing* 33(5):36, 2003.

Elkin M and others: *Nursing interventions and clinical skills,* ed 2, St. Louis, 2000, Mosby.

Elkin M and others: *Nursing interventions and clinical skills,* ed 3, St. Louis, 2004, Mosby.

Gray-Vickrey P: Protecting the older adult, *Nurs manage* 32(10):36, 2001.

Hockenberry MJ and others: *Wong's nursing care of infants and children,* ed 7, St. Louis, 2003, Mosby.

Kee C: Osteoarthritis: manageable scourge of aging, *Nurs Clin North Am* 35(1):199, 2000.

Kessenich CR: Update on osteoporosis in elderly men, *Geriatr Nurs* 21(5):242, 2000.

Lapka DV: Skin cancer, *RN* 63(7):32, 2000.

Lueckenotte A: *Gerontologic nursing,* ed 2, St. Louis, 2000, Mosby.

McHugh J, McHugh W: How to assess deep tendon reflexes, *Nursing* 20(8):62,1990.

Moore MC: *Pocket guide to nutritional care*, ed 4, St. Louis, 2001, Mosby.

Pachuki-Hyde L: Assessment of risk factor for treatment and prevention of osteoporosis, *Nurs Clin North Am* 36(3):401, 2001.

Peterson JA: Osteoporosis overview, *Geriatr Nurs* 22(1):17, 2001.

Phipps WJ and others: *Medical-surgical nursing: health and illness perspectives*, ed 7, St. Louis, 2003, Mosby.

Potter P, Perry A: *Fundamentals of nursing*, ed 6, St. Louis, 2004, Mosby.

Seidel HM and others: *Mosby's guide to physical examination,* ed 5, St. Louis, 2003, Mosby.

Urbano FL: Homan's sign in the diagnosis of deep vein thrombosis, *Hosp Physician* 37(3):22, 2001.

Research References

Agency for Health Care Policy and Research: *Recognition and initial assessment of Alzheimer's disease and related dementias,* Rockville, Md, 1996, Agency for Health Care Policy and Research.

American Cancer Society: *Cancer facts and figures 2004,* Atlanta, 2004, The Society.

Baird CL: Holding on self-caring with osteoarthritis, *J Gerontol Nurs* 29(6):32, 2003.

U.S. Preventive Services Task Force: Screening for osteoporosis in postmenopausal women: recommendations and rationale, *Am J Nurs* 103(1):73,2003.

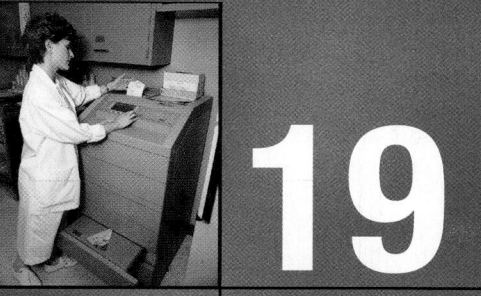

19

Preparing for Medication Administration

MEDIA RESOURCES

Evolve Site *evolve*

http://evolve.elsevier.com/Perry/skills
- Weblinks
- Mosby's Nursing Skills Video Exercises

Mosby's Nursing Skills Videos/CD-ROM
- *Safe Medication Administration Video:* The Six Rights of Medication Administration, common errors; oral medication administration: preparation of liquid medications, pills and tablets, using the unit-dose system; documenting medications, what to do if patient refuses medication, what to do when patient asks for medication at time when medication cannot be given

OBJECTIVES

Mastery of content in this chaper will enable the nurse to:

- Discuss the JCAHO's National Patient Safety Goals for medication administration.
- Identify guidelines for safe administration of medications.
- Describe the most common factors contributing to medication errors.
- Discuss common types of medication actions.
- Identify the system of measurement for a given prescribed medication.
- Calculate medication doses.
- Describe two methods for delivering medications to the nursing unit.
- Describe the six rights of medication administration.
- Explain cultural variations to consider in medication administration.
- Identify steps to take in reporting medication errors.

KEY TERMS

Adverse drug reactions (ADRs)
Anaphylaxis
Duration of action
Floor stock
Idiosyncratic reaction
Medication administration record (MAR)
Medication dependence
Medication polymorphism
Medication tolerance
NPO
Onset of medication action
Over-the-counter (OTC) medication

Parenteral
Peak action
Peak concentration
Plateau
Polypharmacy
prn
Side effect
Summation
Synergistic reaction
Therapeutic effect
Toxic effects
Trough concentration
Unit-dose system
Verbal order

During the year 2000 the Institute of Medicine (IOM) published the book *To Err Is Human: Building a Safer Health System* (IOM, 2000). The book created a new national awareness of problems within the health care system. It reported that estimates suggest 98,000 people die in any given year from medical errors that occur in hospitals. This means that more people die from medical errors than from motor vehicle accidents, breast cancer, acquired immunodeficiency syndrome (AIDS), and workplace injuries. Medication-related errors for hospitalized clients cost roughly $2 billion annually. The IOM sets forth a national agenda for reducing medical errors and improving patient safety through the design of a safer health system. One essential recommendation made by the IOM is to develop standards for patient safety

to establish minimum levels of performance and set expectations for health professionals (IOM, 2003).

The Joint Commission on Accreditation of Healthcare Organizations (JCAHO) is an organization that provides accreditation services to hospitals across the United States. Improving client safety is a commitment of JCAHO. The organization's accreditation program is a risk-reduction activity in that compliance with its standards is intended to reduce the risk of adverse outcomes for clients (JCAHO, 2004c). The JCAHO established in July of 2002 its first set of National Patient Safety Goals for improving the safety of patient care in health care organizations. All JCAHO-accredited health care organizations are surveyed for implementation of the goals and requirements. Each year a new set of goals is published. Failure of an organization to comply with the safety goal requirements can lead to penalties and delayed accreditation approval. Box 19-1 lists the National Patient Safety Goals for medication administration during 2004 and 2005.

All professional nurses should take seriously the implications involved in the administration of medications. Safe and accurate administration of medications is one of the nurse's most important responsibilities when caring for clients. The nurse's judgment is critical to confirm that the right medication is given to a client, that it is administered properly, and that appropriate observations and measurements are made to evaluate the medication's effect and the client's response. Safe medication administration requires the synthesis of knowledge, experience, and excellent critical thinking attitudes and standards.

The RN and LPN in many states are empowered to administer medications under the direction of a licensed physician. Advanced practice nurses (APNs) have some prescriptive authority in almost every state, but the degree of required physician involvement varies. Nurses are personally responsible—legally, morally, and ethically—for every drug administered, no matter who prescribes them (McKenry and Salerno, 2004). Medication administration, including the evaluation of client responses, cannot be delegated to assistive personnel. However, assistive personnel should be instructed to report specific client complaints or unusual client behaviors/responses that may be related to either a drug's intended effect or possible side effects.

Pharmacological Concepts
Medication Names

A medication may have as many as three different names. The chemical name provides an exact description of the medication's composition and molecular structure. A chemical name such as *N*-acetyl-para-aminophenol, commonly known as Tylenol, is rarely used in clinical practice. A manufacturer who first develops a medication gives the generic name of a medication. Acetaminophen is an example of the generic name for Tylenol. The generic name becomes the official name that is listed in official publications such as the *United States Pharmacopeia (USP)*. The trade name or brand name of a medication is the name used to market the

---

BOX 19-1   JCAHO National Patient Safety Goals—With Implications for Medication Administration

2004

- Improve the accuracy of patient identification.
  - Use at least two patient identifiers (neither to be patient's room number) when taking blood samples or administering medications or blood products.
- Improve the effectiveness of communication among caregivers.
  - Verbal or telephone orders require a verification "read-back" of the complete order or test result by the person receiving the order/test result.
  - Standardize abbreviations, acronyms, and symbols, including a list of abbreviations, acronyms, and symbols not to use.
- Improve the safety of using high-alert medications.
  - Remove concentrated electrolytes from patient care units.
  - Standardize and limit the number of drug concentrations available in the organization.
- Improve the safety of using infusion pumps.
  - Ensure free-flow protection on all general use and patient-controlled analgesia intravenous infusion pumps.

2005 (INCLUDES 2004 PLUS NEW GOAL REQUIREMENTS)

- Improve the accuracy of patient identification (see 2004).
  - Develop a plan for implementing bar code technology for patient identification and for matching patients to their medications.

- Improve the effectiveness of communication among caregivers (see 2004).
- Improve the safety of using medications (see 2004).
  - Restrict intravenous drug preparation to the pharmacy, and/or use commercially available premixed intravenous fluids.
  - Identify a list of look-alike/sound-alike drug pairs used in the organization, and take action to prevent errors involving interchange of these drugs.
- Improve the safety of using infusion pumps (see 2004).
  - Perform an independent double-check whenever programming or reprogramming infusion pumps.
- Accurately and completely reconcile medications and other treatments across the continuum of care.
  - On admission to agency and with patient involvement, obtain and document a complete list of patient's medications and other treatments. Reconcile the medications and treatments with those at the previous setting of care.
  - For each patient identify a licensed independent practitioner responsible for coordinating the patient's care and reconciling medications and other treatments.

Modified from Joint Commission on Accreditation of Healthcare Organizations: *JCAHO National Patient Safety Goals,* www.jcaho.org/accredited+organizations/patient+safety, accessed May 22, 2004c.

---

medication. The trade name has the symbol™ at the upper right of the name, indicating the manufacturer has trademarked the medication name (e.g., Panadol™, Tempra™, Tylenol™.

The IOM has recommended that the Food and Drug Administration (FDA) give increased attention to the safe use of medications (IOM, 2003). This includes developing standards for the design of medication packaging and labeling. In addition, the IOM recommends identifying and correcting potential sound-alike and look-alike confusion with medication names. Medication manufacturers have chosen names that are easy to pronounce, spell, and remember so that laypersons will recognize trade names. However, many drug companies produce the same medication, so similarities in trade names can be confusing. Hospital and clinic pharmacies try to consistently dispense medications with the same trade names so nurses can become familiar with them. However, nurses find medications under a variety of different names and must be careful to obtain the exact name and spelling before administering a medication.

Classification

Nurses learn to categorize medications with similar characteristics by their class. Medication classification indicates the effect of a medication on a body system, the symptoms the medication relieves, or the medication's de-

sired effect. For example, clients who have type 2 diabetes often take oral medications to lower their blood glucose level. This class of medication is called oral hypoglycemic agents. Other examples of medication classifications include antiinfectives, antihypertensives, and analgesics. One medication may be part of more than one classification. For example, aspirin is an analgesic, an antipyretic, and an antiinflammatory medication.

Medication Forms

Medications are available in a variety of forms or preparations. The form of the medication determines its route of administration. The composition of a medication is designed to enhance its absorption and metabolism. Many medications are made in several forms (Table 19-1). When administering a medication, the nurse must be certain to use the proper form.

Types of Medication Action

When administering medications, the nurse should be aware that a medication always has a desired or therapeutic effect. However, because of a medication's chemical makeup and physiological action, it can produce more than one effect. A client may not respond in the same way to each successive dose of a medication. The different types of effects are summarized below.

TABLE 19-1 FORMS OF MEDICATION BY ROUTE OF ADMINISTRATION

MEDICATION FORMS COMMONLY PREPARED FOR ADMINISTRATION BY ORAL ROUTE

Solid Forms

Caplet	Solid dosage form for oral use; shaped like a capsule and coated for ease of swallowing.
Capsule	Medication encased in a gelatin shell.
Tablet	Powdered medication compressed into hard disk or cylinder.
Enteric coated	Tablet that is coated so that it does not dissolve in stomach; meant for intestinal absorption.

Liquid Forms

Elixir	Clear fluid containing water and alcohol; designed for oral use; usually has sweetener added.
Extract	Concentrated medication form made by removing the active portion of medication from its other components.
Glycerite	Solution of medication combined with glycerin for external use.
Solution	Liquid preparation that may be used orally, parenterally, or externally; can also be instilled into body organ or cavity (e.g., bladder irrigation); must be sterile for parenteral use.
Suspension	Finely dissolved particles in a liquid medium; when left standing, particles settle to bottom of container; not used intravenously.
Syrup	Medication dissolved in a concentrated sugar solution.

Other Oral Forms and Terms Associated With Oral Preparations

Troche (lozenge)	Flat, round dosage form containing medication that dissolves in mouth; not meant for ingestion.
Aerosol	Aqueous medication sprayed and absorbed in the mouth and upper airway; not meant for ingestion.
Sustained release	Tablet or capsule that contains small particles of a medication coated with material that requires a varying amount of time to dissolve.

MEDICATION FORMS COMMONLY PREPARED FOR ADMINISTRATION BY TOPICAL ROUTE

Ointment (salve or cream)	Semisolid, externally applied preparation, usually containing one or more medications.
Liniment	Oily liquid.
Lotion	Emollient liquid that can be clear solution, suspension, or emulsion.
Paste	Medication preparation that is thicker than ointment; absorbed through the skin more slowly than ointment.
Transdermal patch	Disk or patch embedded with a medication that is absorbed through the skin over a designated period of time.

MEDICATION FORMS COMMONLY PREPARED FOR ADMINISTRATION BY PARENTERAL ROUTE

Solution	Preparation that contains water with one or more dissolved compounds. The solution must be sterile.
Powder	Particles of medication that are reconstituted with water, dissolved, and administered parenterally. The solution must be sterile.

MEDICATION FORMS COMMONLY PREPARED FOR INSTILLATION INTO BODY CAVITIES

Suppository	Solid dosage form mixed with gelatin and shaped in the form of a pellet for insertion into a body cavity (rectum or vagina). The suppository melts when it reaches body temperature and is then absorbed.
Intraocular disk	Disk (similar to a contact lens) embedded with a medication that is inserted into the client's eye. The medication is absorbed over a designated period of time.

Therapeutic Effects

The therapeutic effect is the intended or desired physiological response of a medication. Each medication has a desired therapeutic effect for which it is prescribed. For example, the nurse administers morphine sulfate, an analgesic, to relieve a client's pain. A single medication may have many therapeutic effects. For example, aspirin is administered to relieve pain, to reduce a fever, and to reduce inflammation of swollen tissues. Thus it is important for the nurse to know the exact therapeutic effect for which a medication is prescribed. This allows the nurse to properly teach the client about the medication's intended effect and to accurately evaluate the medication's desired effect.

Side Effects/Adverse Reactions

Medications can react in the body to produce unpredictable and sometimes unexplainable responses (McKenry and Salerno, 2004). No medication is totally safe and absolutely free of nontherapeutic effects. Side effects are usually predictable and oftentimes unavoidable secondary effects produced by a drug at the usual therapeutic drug dose. Side effects may be harmless or injurious. In the example of codeine phosphate, administered for analgesia, drowsiness and constipation are common side effects. The intensity of side effects is often dose dependent (McKenry and Salerno, 2004). If the side effects are serious enough to outweigh the beneficial effects of a medication's therapeutic action, the prescriber may discontinue the medication. Clients may stop taking medications because of side effects. The most commonly reported side effects are anorexia, nausea, vomiting, dizziness, drowsiness, dry mouth, abdominal gas, constipation, and diarrhea. Any side effect should be reported to a physician and pharmacist to ensure that they are not incorrectly interpreted as a more serious adverse medication reaction.

Adverse medication reactions (ADRs) are unintended, undesirable, and often unpredictable drug effects. An ADR can create abnormal symptoms that may result in a client's disability. An iatrogenic ADR creates an illness resulting from a medication and thus leads to prolonged hospitalization (Arnold, 1998). Early clinical recognition of ADRs is the important first step in identifying nontherapeutic effects of medications (Arnold, 1998). Sometimes ADRs are immediately apparent, whereas at other times they may take weeks or months to develop (McKenry and Salerno, 2004). A nurse must be alert to assess any unusual individual responses to drugs, especially with newly released medications. The nurse must understand that there is a continuum of ADRs, ranging from mild, expected side effects to fatal allergic and toxic effects. Prompt recognition and reporting of ADRs can prevent serious injury to clients. Box 19-2 highlights clients most at risk for ADRs. Although no client is totally risk free from having an ADR, clients falling into one or more risk categories require close monitoring (Arnold, 1998). Each health care agency has specific policies for reporting ADRs.

Toxic Effects. Toxicity basically refers to the degree to which something becomes poisonous. A toxic drug effect develops after prolonged intake of high doses of medication, after ingestion of medications intended for external application, or when a medication accumulates in the blood because of impaired metabolism or excretion. Toxic effects may be lethal, depending on the medication's action. For example, morphine acts on the central nervous system to relieve pain by producing a combination of depressing and stimulating effects. Toxic levels of morphine cause severe respiratory depression and can lead to death if unrecognized or not treated appropriately.

Idiosyncratic Reactions. Medications may cause unpredictable effects, such as an idiosyncratic reaction, in which a client overreacts or underreacts to a medication or has a reaction different from normal. Predicting which clients will have an idiosyncratic response is impossible. For example, Ativan, an antianxiety medication, when given to an older adult may cause agitation and delirium.

Allergic Reactions. An allergic reaction is another unpredictable response to a medication. Exposure to an initial dose of a medication causes a client to become sensitized immunologically. With repeated administration, the client develops an allergic response to the medication, its chemical preservatives, or a metabolite. The medication or chemical

---

BOX 19-2 Clients at Increased Risk for Adverse Medication Reactions

- Clients taking a medication for the first time
- Very young and elderly
- Women
- Clients taking more than four to five medications (polypharmacy)
- Clients extremely underweight or overweight
- Clients with renal and/or hepatic disease
- Clients with altered blood flow conditions
- Clients with a past history of an ADR
- Clients with depression or anxiety
- Clients with sensory deprivation or overload
- Clients who abuse alcohol, nicotine, or street medications
- Clients who treat selves with over-the-counter medications

Modified from Arnold GJ: Clinical recognition of adverse medication reactions: obstacles and opportunities for the nursing profession, *J Nurs Care Qual* 13(2):45, 1998.

---

acts as an antigen, which causes antibodies to be produced. An allergic reaction may be mild or severe. Allergic symptoms vary, depending on the client and the medication. Among the different classes of medications, antibiotics cause a high incidence of allergic reactions. Common, mild allergy symptoms are summarized in Table 19-2. Severe or anaphylactic reactions are characterized by sudden constriction of bronchiolar muscles, edema of the pharynx and larynx, severe wheezing, and shortness of breath. The client may become severely hypotensive, necessitating emergency resuscitation measures. Anaphylaxis can be fatal.

A client with a known history of an allergy to a medication should avoid exposure to that medication in the future. It is common practice for clients who are hospitalized or in extended treatment facilities and who have a known medication allergy to have allergy information recorded in a clearly identifiable place that is easily seen by all those involved in the client's care. In many institutions this information is often recorded on the front of the client's medical record, in the medication administration record (MAR), or on a specially designed label or sticker that is applied to the front of the client's chart. Clients are also given a color-coded allergy identification band to wear around the wrist. Client allergies should always be recorded in the client's MAR. Clients cared for in other settings (e.g., home, community clinics) and who have a known history of an allergy to a medication or substance should be encouraged to wear an identification bracelet or medical alert medal, which alerts all health care providers to the allergies in case the client is found unconscious (Figure 19-1).

Medication Tolerance and Dependence. Medication tolerance exists when there is a decreased physiological response after repeated administration of a medication or a chemically related substance (McKenry and Salerno, 2004). It is usually noted clinically when clients receive the same medication for long periods of time and require higher doses

TABLE 19-2 MILD ALLERGIC REACTIONS

SYMPTOM	DESCRIPTION
Urticaria (hives)	Raised, irregularly shaped skin eruptions with varying sizes and shapes; eruptions have reddened margins and pale centers.
Eczema (rash)	Small, raised vesicles that are usually reddened; often distributed over the entire body.
Pruritus	Itching of the skin; accompanies most rashes.
Rhinitis	Inflammation of mucous membranes lining the nose, causing swelling and a clear watery discharge.
Wheezing	Constriction of smooth muscles surrounding bronchioles, which decreases the diameter of airways. Occurs primarily on inspiration because of severely narrowed airways. The development of edema in pharynx and larynx further obstructs airflow.
Angioedema	An acute, painless, dermal, subcutaneous, or submucosal swelling of short duration involving the face, neck, lips, larynx, hands, feet, genitalia, or viscera.
Fever	Abnormal elevation of body temperature above 37° C (98.6° F)

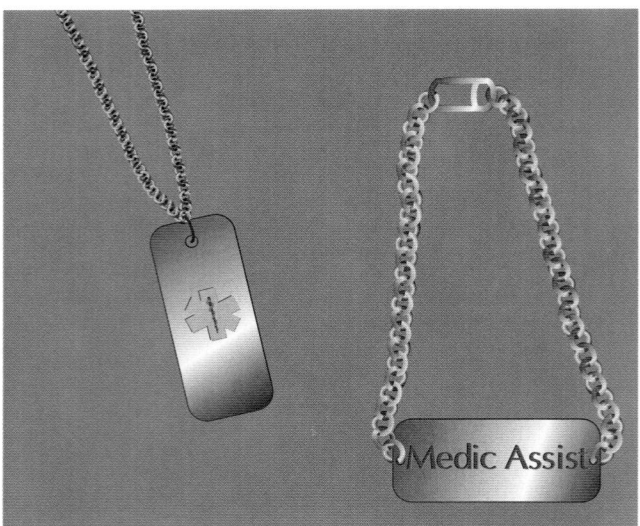

FIGURE **19-1** Medical alert bracelet and medal.

to produce the desired therapeutic effect. Medications known to produce tolerance include opium alkaloids (e.g., morphine), nitrites, and barbiturates. Generally clients hospitalized for acute episodes of illness do not develop tolerance. It may take a month or even longer for this phenomenon to occur (McCaffery and Pasero, 1999). Cross-tolerance may occur following tolerance to a medication. In cross-tolerance a client develops tolerance to pharmacologically similar drugs and drugs that act at the same receptor sites (McKenry and Salerno, 2004).

Medication tolerance is not the same as medication dependence. Two types of medication dependence exist: psychological (or addiction) and physical. In psychological dependence the client desires the medication for some benefit other than the intended effect. The individual believes a desirable effect will result when taking the medication. An example is the medication marijuana, which many individuals use to cause relaxation. Physical dependence involves a physiological adaptation to a medication that manifests itself by intense physical disturbance when the medication is withdrawn. An example is the repeated use of codeine for reducing mild to moderate pain. When clients receive medications for a short term (such as for postoperative pain), dependence is rare (McCaffery and Pasero, 1999). If a client is dependent or tolerant to alcohol, a higher-than-usual medication dose may be required for the desired effect of the medication.

Medication Interactions. When one medication modifies the action of another medication, a medication interaction occurs. Medication interactions are common in individuals taking many medications. A medication may potentiate or diminish the action of other medications and may alter the way in which another medication is absorbed, metabolized, or eliminated from the body. This is a common problem in older adults, who tend to have multiple physicians prescribe a variety of medications without discontinuing any previous medications.

A medication interaction is sometimes desirable. Often a physician orders combination medication therapy to create a medication interaction for therapeutic benefit. For example, a client with moderate hypertension typically receives several medications, such as diuretics and vasodilators, that act together to keep blood pressure at a desirable level.

Summation occurs when the combined effect of two drugs produces a result that equals the sum of the individual effects of each drug (McKenry and Salerno, 2004). For example, codeine and aspirin both act as analgesics. When the two drugs are given together, they provide an additive or greater pain relief than when either one is used alone. The combination allows the administration of a lower dose of each drug with less risk of adverse reactions.

When two medications are given simultaneously, they can have a synergistic effect. With a synergistic reaction the physiological action of the two medications in combination is greater than the effect of the medications when given separately. For example, alcohol is a central nervous system depressant that has a synergistic effect on antihistamines, antidepressants, and narcotic analgesics.

Medication Dose Responses

After the nurse administers a medication, it undergoes absorption, distribution, metabolism, and excretion (Figure 19-2). These are pharmacokinetic processes that determine how much of the administered dose reaches the site of ac-

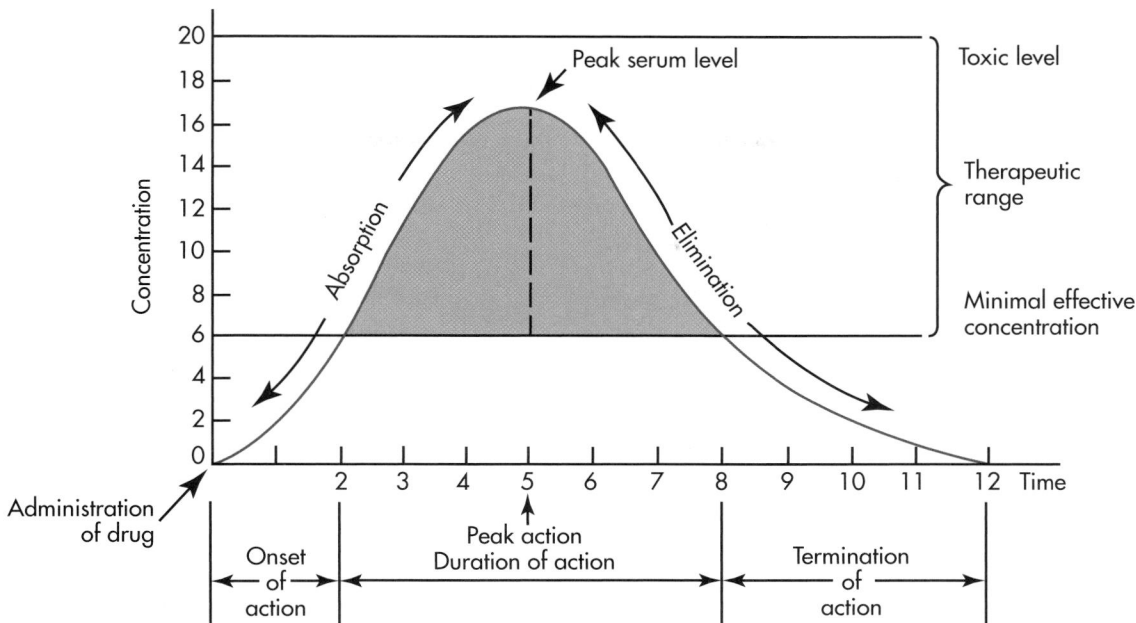

FIGURE 19-2 Plasma level profile of a drug. (From McKenry LM, Salerno E: *Mosby's pharmacology in nursing,* ed 20, St. Louis, 1998, Mosby.)

tion. These processes are influenced by factors such as body surface area, body water content, body fat content, and protein stores.

When certain medications are prescribed, the goal is to achieve a constant medication blood level within a safe therapeutic range. Repeated doses are required to achieve a constant therapeutic concentration of a medication because a portion of the medication is always being excreted. The highest serum concentration or peak concentration of medication usually occurs just before the last of the medication is absorbed (McKenry and Salerno, 2004). After peaking, the serum medication concentration falls progressively. With intravenous infusions, the peak concentration occurs quickly, but the serum level also begins to fall immediately. The point at which the lowest amount of drug is detected in the serum is the trough concentration.

Some medications (e.g., vancomycin) are dosed based on peak and trough serum levels. The trough level is generally drawn 30 minutes before the drug is administered, and the peak level is drawn whenever the drug reaches its peak concentration (varies with drug pharmacokinetics). Precise coordination with the laboratory is essential for obtaining meaningful information. These data allow physicians to modify medication dosages.

The client and nurse must follow regular dosage schedules and administer prescribed doses at correct intervals. Knowledge of the following time intervals of medication action helps to anticipate a medication's effect:

1. *Onset of medication action*—Period of time it takes after a medication is administered for it to produce a therapeutic effect

TABLE 19-3	ROUTES OF MEDICATION ADMINISTRATION
ROUTE	**DESCRIPTION**
NONPARENTERAL	
Oral	By mouth
Sublingual	Under the tongue
Topical	On the skin (as a cream or patch) and eye/ear drops
Suppository	Into the rectum or vagina
PARENTERAL	
Intramuscular (IM)	Into a muscle
Subcutaneous (Sub-Q)	Into the subcutaneous tissue of the skin
Intradermal (ID)	Into the dermis of the skin
Intrathecal	Into the subarachnoid space
Intravenous (IV)	Into a vein

2. *Peak action*—Time it takes for a medication to reach its highest effective peak concentration.
3. *Duration of action*—Length of time during which the medication is present in a concentration great enough to produce a therapeutic effect
4. *Plateau*—Blood serum concentration reached and maintained after repeated, fixed doses

Routes of Administration

The route prescribed for administering a medication depends on its properties and desired effect and on the client's physical and mental condition (Table 19-3). The nurse is often the best person to judge a medication route. Thus the nurse collaborates with the prescriber in determining the best route for a client's medical condition. Table 19-4 summarizes the factors that influence the choice of administration routes.

Medication Distribution

Medication distribution is the responsibility of the institution or community pharmacy. Pharmacists provide the medications, but nurses distribute or administer medications to clients. Institutions providing nursing care have a special area for stocking and dispensing medications. Special medication rooms, portable locked carts, computerized medication cabinets, and individual storage units next to clients' rooms are examples of storage areas. Nurses must make sure that medication storage areas are locked when unattended.

The standard for medication distribution is the unit-dose system. The system uses portable carts containing a drawer with a 24-hour supply of medications for each client. The unit dose is the ordered dose of medication the client receives at one time. Each tablet or capsule is wrapped in a foil or paper container. Liquid doses come in prepackaged foil or paper cups. At a designated time each day the pharmacist refills the drawers in the unit-dose cart with a fresh supply. The cart may also contain limited amounts of prn and stock medications for special situations. The advantage to unit-dose dispensing of medications is that it reduces medication costs and errors.

Automated medication dispensing systems (AMDS) are used successfully throughout the country (Figure 19-3). The systems are designed to achieve computerized control of unit-dose medication dispensing throughout a health care institution (Novek and others, 2000). All procedures connected to an AMDS are controlled electronically via a client's profile. A client name and his or her drug profile order must be accessed before the AMDS will dispense a medication. Each nurse has a security code allowing access to the system. In these systems the nurse selects the desired medication, dosage, and

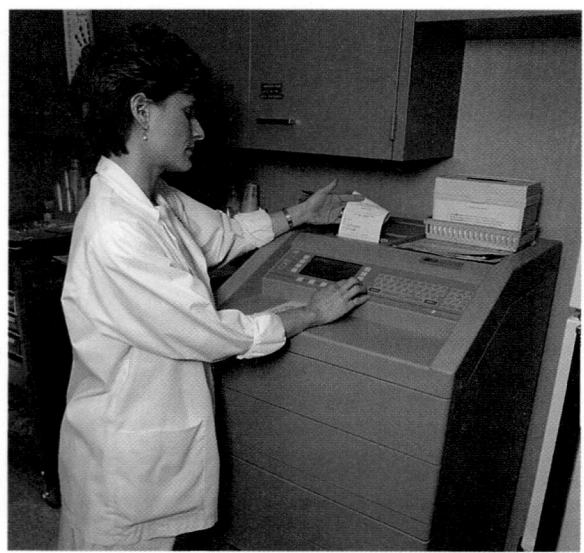

FIGURE 19-3 Automated medication dispensing system.

route from a list displayed on the computer screen. The system causes the drawer containing the medication to open, records it, and charges it to the client. Frequently these systems are linked to computer software programs in the pharmacy that can help to detect dosage errors and incompatible medications or send alerts regarding clients' medication allergies. An AMDS is not foolproof. The system has mechanical moving parts, electronics, and software that can fail. Errors can occur with an AMDS system, including errors by pharmacy on order entry and cabinet loading or by nursing on the retrieval of medications from the cabinet.

Some medications (e.g., aspirin, antacids, laxatives) may be distributed as floor stock. With this system, medications are available in large multidose containers. Medications that are appropriate for floor stock are often those that are routinely prescribed or prescribed on an as-needed (prn) basis. This type of system of medication dispensing has been associated with a high rate of medication errors and is not commonly used today.

Systems of Medication Measurement

The proper administration of medication depends on the nurse's ability to compute medication doses accurately and measure medications correctly. A careless mistake in placing a decimal point or adding a zero to a dose can lead to a fatal error. The prescriber and client depend on the nurse to check the dose before administering a medication. The most common system used in the measurement of medications is the metric system. The apothecary and household measurement systems can also be used.

Metric System

As a decimal system, the metric system is the most logically organized of the measurement systems. Metric units can be easily converted and computed through simple multiplication and division. Each basic unit of measure is organized into units of 10. Multiplying or dividing by 10 forms secondary units. In multiplication the decimal point moves to the right; in division the decimal moves to the left.

$$10 \text{ mg} \times 10 = 100 \text{ mg}$$
$$10 \text{ mg} \div 10 = 1 \text{ mg}$$

The basic units of measure in the metric system are the meter (length), the liter (volume), and the gram (weight). For medication calculations the nurse uses primarily volume and weight units. In the metric system small or large letters are used to designate the basic units. For example:

$$\text{Gram} = g \text{ or } Gm$$
$$\text{Liter} = l \text{ or } L$$

Small letters are abbreviations for subdivisions of major units:

$$\text{Milligram} = mg$$
$$\text{Millimeter} = mm$$
$$\text{The one exception: Milliliter} = ml \text{ or } mL$$

A system of Latin prefixes designates subdivision of the basic units: deci- ($\frac{1}{10}$ or 0.1), centi- ($\frac{1}{100}$ or 0.01), and milli- ($\frac{1}{1000}$ or

TABLE 19-4   **FACTORS INFLUENCING CHOICE OF ADMINISTRATION ROUTES**

ADVANTAGES BY ROUTE	DISADVANTAGES/CONTRAINDICATIONS
ORAL, BUCCAL, SUBLINGUAL	
Easy and comfortable to administer, convenient, economical; may produce local or systemic effects. Rarely causes anxiety for client.	Avoid giving to clients with alterations in gastrointestinal function (e.g., nausea and vomiting), reduced motility (after general anesthesia or inflammation of bowel), and surgical resection of portion of gastrointestinal tract. Some medications are destroyed by gastric secretions. Oral administration is contraindicated in clients who are NPO and unable to swallow (e.g., clients with neuromuscular disorders, esophageal strictures, and lesions of the mouth). Oral medications cannot be given when client has gastric suction and are contraindicated in clients before some tests or surgery. An unconscious or confused client may be unable or unwilling to swallow or hold medication under the tongue. Oral medications may irritate the lining of the gastrointestinal tract, discolor teeth, or have an unpleasant taste.
PARENTERAL (SUB-Q, IM, IV, INTRADERMAL, INTRATHECAL, EPIDURAL)	
Routes provide means of administration when oral medications are contraindicated. More rapid absorption occurs than with topical or oral routes.	Risk of introducing infection, medications are expensive, and these routes are avoided in clients with bleeding tendencies. Risk of tissue damage with Sub-Q injections.
IV infusion provides medication delivery when client is critically ill. If peripheral perfusion is poor, IV route is preferred over injections.	IV and IM infusions are rapidly absorbed, requiring close monitoring.
Intrathecal route allows medications that cannot pass through the blood-brain barrier to enter cerebrospinal fluid.	All parenteral routes cause considerable anxiety in many clients, especially children.
Epidural provides excellent pain control.	Limits mobility during administration. Risk of infection.
SKIN	
Topical	
Topical skin applications provide primarily local effect. Route is painless. Limited side effects occur.	Extensive applications may require dressings that can be bulky for a client when maneuvering. Do not apply to skin if abrasions are present. Medications can be absorbed by person applying it if gloves are not worn.
Transdermal	
Transdermal applications provide prolonged systemic effects, with limited side effects.	Application leaves oily or pasty substance on skin and may soil clothing. Client may have sensitivity to adhesive.
MUCOUS MEMBRANES (INCLUDES EYES, EARS, NOSE, VAGINAL, RECTAL, BUCCAL, AND SUBLINGUAL ROUTES)	
Therapeutic effects are provided by local application to involved sites. Aqueous solutions are readily absorbed and capable of causing systemic effects.	Mucous membranes are highly sensitive to some medication concentrations.
Mucous membranes provide route of administration when oral medications are contraindicated.	Insertion of rectal and vaginal medications often causes embarrassment. Rectal suppositories are contraindicated if clients have had rectal surgery or if active rectal bleeding is present. If eardrum is ruptured, otic medications may be contraindicated.
INHALATION	
Inhalation provides rapid relief for local respiratory problems. Route provides easy access for introduction of general anesthetic gases.	Some local agents can cause serious systemic effects. If clients unable to administer inhaler correctly, medication will be ineffective. Difficult to learn for older adults and children.
INTRAOCULAR DISK	
Route is advantageous in that it does not require frequent administration like eye drops. The client can also wear disk when sleeping or swimming. Dry eyes do not affect medication delivery.	Local reactions can occur such as tearing, itchiness, or redness of the eyes. Client must be taught how to insert disk into and remove from the eye. Client may be anxious about doing this. Medication can be expensive. Medication is contraindicated in clients with infections of the eye.

0.001). Greek prefixes designate multiples of the basic units: deka- (10), hecto- (100), and kilo- (1000). For example:

$$1 \text{ gram} = 1000 \text{ milligrams (mg)}$$

When writing medication dosages in metric units, prescribers and nurses use either fractions or multiples of a unit. Fractions should be converted to decimal form. A zero must be placed in front of the decimal to prevent error. For example:

500 mg or 0.5 g, not ½ g or .5 g

10 ml or 0.01 L, not ¹⁄₁₀₀ L or .01 L

Trailing zeroes should not be used when writing metric dosages (e.g., 14.0 mg) (Armitage and Knapman, 2003). A trailing zero has been found to be associated with dosage errors. For example, 10.0 mg could be confused for a dose of 100 mg. A zero to the right of the decimal should not be used. Always use a zero before a decimal point.

Apothecary System

The apothecary system of measurement is one of the oldest systems of measurement. It is seldom used; however, some drug companies still include apothecary measures in addition to metric. The basic units of measure in the apothecary system include weight (grains) and volume (minims, drams, and ounces). The measures used in this system are approximates, and a 10% variance has become acceptable in preparation and administration of most medications. The apothecary system often uses roman numerals and fractions. The symbol "ss" is used for the fraction ½. Unlike the metric system, in the apothecary system the abbreviation or symbol for a unit of measure is written before the amount or quantity. For example:

gr 15 or gr xv

Household Measurements

Household measures are familiar to most people and are used when more accurate systems of measure are unnecessary. For example, household measures are commonly used in the home when administering liquids such as cough medicine, antacids, and laxatives. Included in household measures are drops, teaspoons, tablespoons, cups, and glasses for volume; and ounces and pounds for weight.

Medication Administration

Standards are those actions that ensure safe nursing practice. To ensure safe medication administration the nurse should follow a nursing standard called the *six rights of medication administration*. All medication errors can be linked, in some way, to an inconsistency in adhering to the six rights (Box 19-3).

Right Medication

A medication order is required for any medication to be administered by a nurse. Types of orders based on frequency and/or urgency of medication administration include standing or routine, prn orders, stat orders, and single one-time orders. Each order must include the client's name, the drug ordered, dosage, route of administration, and time of administration.

BOX 19-3   The Six Rights of Medication Administration

1. The *right* medication
2. The *right* dose
3. The *right* client
4. The *right* route
5. The *right* time
6. The *right* documentation

BOX 19-4   Prohibited Abbreviations

ABBREVIATION	PREFERRED TERM
U (for unit)	Write out the word "unit"
IU (for international unit)	Write out "international unit"
QD (once daily)	Write "daily"
QOD (once every other day)	Write "every other day"
MS (morphine sulfate)	Write "morphine sulfate"
MgSO$_4$ (magnesium sulfate)	Write "magnesium sulfate"
HS (for half strength)	Write out "half strength"
SC or SQ (for subcutaneous)	Write "sub-Q" or "SubQ")
D/C (for discharge)	Write "discharge"
cc (for cubic centimeters)	Write "ml"

Modified from Joint Commission on Accreditation of Healthcare Organizations: *FAQs about the 2004 National Patient Safety Goals,* www.jcaho.org/accredited+organizations/patient+safety, accessed May 18, 2004.

The JCAHO now discourages the use of range orders for prn medications. An example of a range order is morphine sulfate 2 to 6 mg IV push q2-4 hr prn for pain. Range orders are often unclear and have been the source of medication errors. The JCAHO recommends that organizations develop practice guidelines that define how range orders can be implemented (Rich, 2002). An example of a practice guideline might be "Increase the dose 50% to 100% if pain is moderate to severe."

The nurse should know the nurse practice act and institutional policies regarding which providers, other than physicians, may prescribe medications. In addition, nurses should know the proper abbreviations that can be used when writing and transcribing medication orders. Each organization has a list of acceptable abbreviations. The Joint Commission on Accreditation of Healthcare Organizations (2004b) has identified a list of prohibited or "dangerous" abbreviations that when used frequently lead to error. The goal of JCAHO was to have all health care organizations discontinue use of these abbreviations by the end of 2004. It is likely more abbreviations will be added to this list over time. Box 19-4 lists the prohibited abbreviations effective in 2004.

There are some hospitals instituting physician order entry, a program that allows physicians to electronically enter an ordered medication. The process eliminates written orders. However, most institutions still use a written order system. Written orders must be transcribed either by hand or electronically on an MAR (Figure 19-4). The nurse or a designated unit secretary writes the prescriber's complete order on the MAR. The transcribed order includes the client's full name; date the order is written; date the medication order expires (if applicable); medication name, dose, and frequency (time ordered), and route of administration. The transcriber makes sure the client's room and bed number (which are usually pre-

Room: 3700-03

Patient: PDM, Pharmacy
Birth: 11/30/79 Admit: 01/01/00
MRN: 2000403 Acct: 900015
A Doctor: Jim Smith

Age: 20 y Ht: 5 ft 2 in Wt: 125.2 lbs
Metric: Ht: 1 m 57 cm Wt: 56.79 kg

≡ⅼⅼ Saint Francis
ᆿⅼ⊏ Medical Center

MEDICATION ADMINISTRATION RECORD

Date: 01/18/00 – 01/19/00

ADEs/Nondrug allergies: Latex – Zosyn – Amoxicillin –
Insulins – Darvocet – Lugols soln. – Antihi +

Medication	0800	0900	1000	1100	1200	1300	1400	1500	1600	1700	1800	1900	2000	2100	2200	2300	2400	0100	0200	0300	0400	0500	0600	0700
P00014 Bacitracin ointment AKA: Bacitracin ointment Dose: Apply STRGH: 30 gm/tube TID Topical: Right lower leg For external use only Testing			RL 10																					
P00029 Insulin/human regular AKA: Humulin R Dose: 15 units Strgh: 1 ml = 100 units AC Sub–Q	RL 0730																							
P00030 Fexofenadine 60 mg/psuedo 120 mg AKA: Allegra–D Sr Tab Dose: 1 tab STRGH: 60/120/tab BID Oral Auto Sub: 1 Allegra–D Tab bid For Claritin–D 12 hr and 24 hr Per P&T Comm			RL 10																					
P00036 Aspirin AKA: Aspirin 325 mg Tab Dose: 2 tab 650 mg STRGH: 325 mg/tab q3–4h Oral Testing						RL 1315																		
P00039 Haloperidol tablet AKA: Haldol 0.5 mg tab Dose: 1 mg STRGH: 1 mg/tab QHS Oral																								
P00035 Zolpidem AKA: Ambien 5 mg tab Dose: 5 mg STRGH: 5/tab QHS PRN Oral MR × 1 Testing																								

Circle = Dose not given
Initials = Dose given Page: 01 (continued)
Deltoid = R.D., L.D.
Vastus Lateralis = R.V.L., L.V.L.
Lower Abdominal = R.L.A., L.L.A.
Anterior Gluteal = R.A.G., L.A.G.
Posterior Gluteal = R.P.G., L.P.G.

0800	0900	1000	1100	1200	1300	1400	1500	1600	1700	1800	1900	2000	2100	2200	2300	2400	0100	0200	0300	0400	0500	0600	0700

Initials and signature	Initials and signature	Initials and signature
Rita Lassater RL		
Initials and signature	Initials and signature	Initials and signature
Initials and signature	Initials and signature	Initials and signature

FIGURE 19-4 Medication administration record (MAR). (Courtesy Saint Francis Medical Center.)

TABLE 19-5 COMMON ABBREVIATIONS AND SYMBOLS RELATED TO MEDICATION ADMINISTRATION*

Abbreviation	Unabbreviated Form	Meaning	Abbreviation	Unabbreviated Form	Meaning
ac	ante cibum	before meals	PM	post meridiem	after noon
ad lib	ad libitum	freely	PO	per os	by mouth, orally
AM	ante meridiem	morning	prn	pro re nata	according to necessity
bid	bid in die	twice each day	pt	patient	patient
c̄	cum	with	q	quaque	every
caps	capsule	capsule	qh	quaque hora	every hour
clt	client	client	q4h, q4°	every 4 hours	every 4 hours around-the-clock
elix	elixir	elixir			
g, gm	gram	1000 milligrams	qid	quater in die	four times each day
gr	grain	60 milligrams	qs	quantum satis	sufficient quantity
gtt	guttae	drops	Ⓡ	right	right
h, hr	hora	hour	℞	recipe	take
IM	intramuscular	into a muscle	s̄	sine	without
IV	intravenous	into a vein	SL	sub lingua	under the tongue
IVPB	IV piggyback	secondary IV line	SOS	si opus sit	if it is necessary, one dose only
kg	kilogram	2.2 pounds			
KVO	keep vein open	very slow infusion rate	stat	statim	at once
Ⓛ	left	left	Sub-Q, subQ	subcutaneous	into subcutaneous tissue
L	liter	liter			
mcg	microgram	one millionth of a gram	tbsp	tablespoon	tablespoon (15 mL)
mg	milligram	one thousandth of a gram	tid	ter in die	three times a day
			TO	telephone order	order received over the telephone
mEq	milliequivalent	the number of grams of solute dissolved in one milliliter of a *normal* solution	tsp	teaspoon	teaspoon (4 or 5 mL)
			VO	verbal order	order received verbally
min or m	minim	minim (¹⁄₁₅ or ¹⁄₁₆ mL)	i, ii	one, two	one, two (as in "gr i," "gr ii,")
ml, mL	milliliter	one thousandth of a liter			
ng	nanogram	one bilionth of a liter	℥		ounce of fluid once	ounce (30 mililiters)
ō	no or none	no or none	×	times	as in two times a week
os	os	mouth	=	equal to	equal to
OTC	over-the-counter	nonprescription drug	↑, ↗	increase or increasing	increase or increasing
pc	post cibum	after meals	↓, ↙	decrease or decreasing	decrease or decreasing

*It is recommended that certain abbreviations be abandoned if they are found to be confusing.

stamped on the order form) are accurate on the form. With unit-dose systems, only one transcription is necessary, limiting the opportunity for errors. When transcribing orders in written form, the nurse should be sure names, dosages, symbols, and abbreviations are legible and not smudged (Table 19-5). When the nurse is checking an order transcribed by the unit secretary, every element of the order is to be checked for accuracy and legibility. An RN is responsible for checking and initialing all transcribed orders against the original orders

A verbal order is a medication or treatment order received by the nurse in the presence of the prescriber. Verbal orders should be limited to emergency situations when the prescriber has no time to write the order. When a nurse takes a verbal order, he or she must read back the complete order

to the independent practitioner who made the order. This verification process is required by the JCAHO (2004c). Verbal orders are entered into the client's medical record by the nurse and transcribed the same way as if the prescriber wrote the order (Figure 19-5). The name of the prescriber is written next to that of the nurse.

Telephone orders are medication orders given over the phone, usually after the nurse updates the prescriber about a change in a client's condition. A telephone order is transcribed the same as a verbal order and requires a read-back by the person receiving the order. Institutional and state regulations require verbal and telephone orders to be signed by the provider or prescriber within 24 hours. Therefore it is important to limit their use as much as possible.

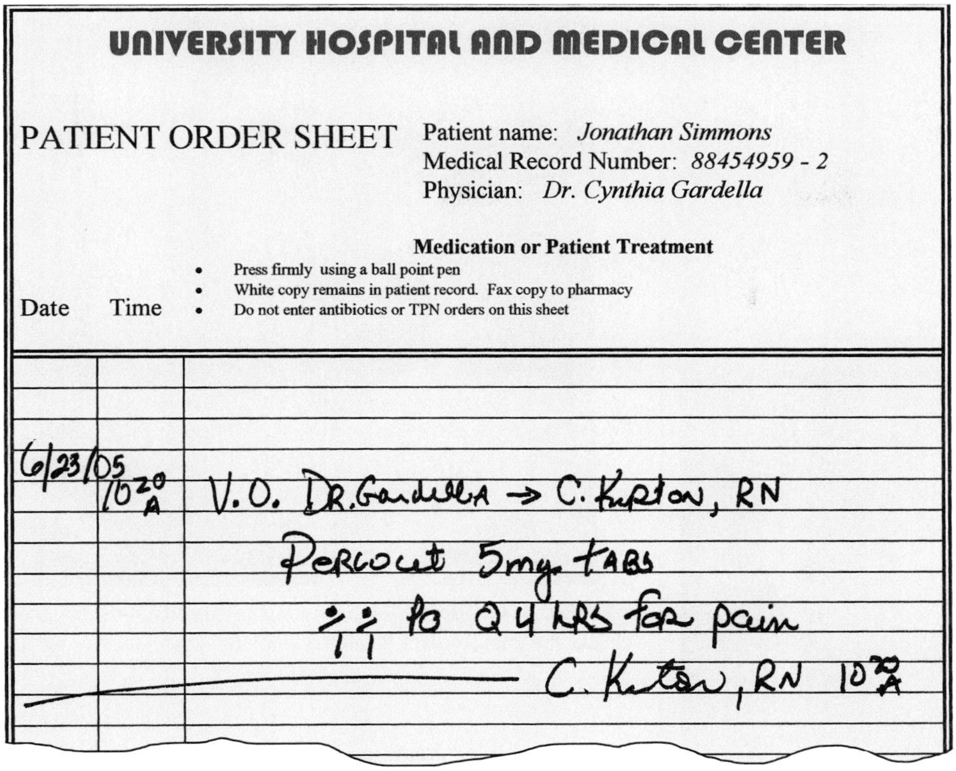
UNIVERSITY HOSPITAL AND MEDICAL CENTER

PATIENT ORDER SHEET

Patient name: *Jonathan Simmons*
Medical Record Number: *88454959 - 2*
Physician: *Dr. Cynthia Gardella*

Medication or Patient Treatment

- Press firmly using a ball point pen
- White copy remains in patient record. Fax copy to pharmacy
- Do not enter antibiotics or TPN orders on this sheet

Date	Time	
6/23/05	10[20] A	V.O. Dr. Gardella → C. Kirton, RN
		Percocet 5mg tabs
		ii po Q 4 hrs for pain
		C. Kirton, RN 10[20] A

FIGURE **19-5** Example of a verbal order.

When medications are first ordered, the nurse compares the medication recording form or computer order screen with the prescriber's written orders. When administering medications, the nurse compares the label of the medication container with the medication form. The nurse does this *3 times:* (1) before removing the container from the drawer or shelf, (2) as the amount of medication ordered is removed from the container, and (3) before returning the container to storage. With unit-dose prepackaged medications, the nurse checks the label with the medicine form a third time even though there is no permanent container. Unit-dose medications may be checked before opening at the client's beside.

Nurses administer only the medications they prepare from what is provided by the pharmacy. If an error occurs, the nurse who administers the medication is responsible for the error. If a client questions the medication a nurse prepares, it is important not to ignore these concerns. An alert client will know whether a medication is different from those received before. The nurse should withhold the medication until the preparation can be rechecked against the order.

If a medication order seems incorrect or inappropriate, the nurse consults the prescriber. For example, if a prescribed medication name does not seem appropriate for the client's known condition, the nurse should check. Similarly, if a dosage seems out of range of normal, the nurse should confirm the correct ordered dosage.

Right Dose

The unit dose system is designed to minimize errors. However, when a medication must be prepared from a larger volume or strength than needed or when the prescriber orders a system of measurement different from what the pharmacy supplies, the chance of error increases. When performing medication calculations or conversions, the nurse should have another qualified nurse check the calculated doses. Agency policies differ, but most require a nurse to verify prepared doses of anticoagulant, insulin, and IV push medications prepared by another nurse.

After calculating doses, the nurse prepares the medication using standard measurement devices. Graduated cups, syringes, and scaled droppers can be used for accurate measurement. At home, clients should use kitchen measuring spoons and not regular tablespoons, which vary in volume.

At times it is necessary to administer a portion of a tablet to ensure accurate dosage. When it is necessary to break a scored tablet, the break should be even. A scored tablet may be cut in half by using a knife-edge or a cutting device. Tablets that do not break evenly are discarded. The two halves are given in successive doses if the second half is repackaged and labeled. In some cases, tablets can be crushed for administration. The nurse then mixes the tablet in the client's food. A crushing device should always be cleaned completely between uses to eliminate any particles of medication being accidentally given to another client. This is critically important because a client might be allergic to the medication previously crushed. Crushed medications should be mixed with very small amounts of food or liquid. Do not use the client's favorite food or liquid because the medication may alter the taste and decrease the client's desire for them. Never crush medications that are to be given sublingually or that are enteric coated or time released.

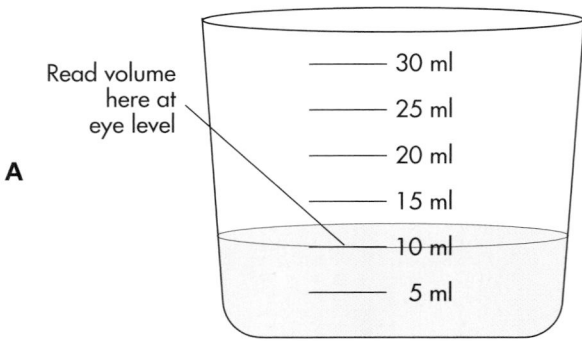

A

Read volume here at eye level

30 ml
25 ml
20 ml
15 ml
10 ml
5 ml

B

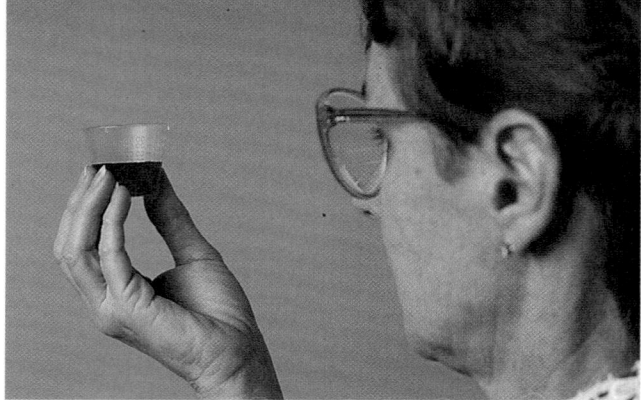

FIGURE **19-6 A,** Pour the desired volume of liquid so that the base of the meniscus is level with line on scale. **B,** Nurse looks at base of meniscus to confirm volume poured.

Key principles for the nurse to observe when using measuring receptacles:

1. Medications poured into medication cups should be done so at eye level. This allows the nurse to accurately see the desired amount. The amount of poured liquid should be even with the base of the meniscus (Figure 19-6).
2. Pour liquid medications away from a label to ensure that liquid will not run down a label, making it difficult to read.
3. Medications drawn into syringes (without a needle) should be drawn slowly to prevent air bubbles from entering the syringe. Air displaces medications and may lead to inaccurate measurement of doses.

Right Client

Once a nurse is prepared to administer a medication, the client's identification band (ID bracelet) is checked against the MAR (Figure 19-7), and the client is asked to state his or her full name. "Please state your name," is the best question to ask for the client's name. Do not enter a room and state the client's name for him, "Mr. Miles, here is your medication." This assumes that the client, by acknowledging your presence, is indeed who you say he is. If an identification bracelet becomes smudged or illegible or is missing, the nurse must acquire a new one for the client.

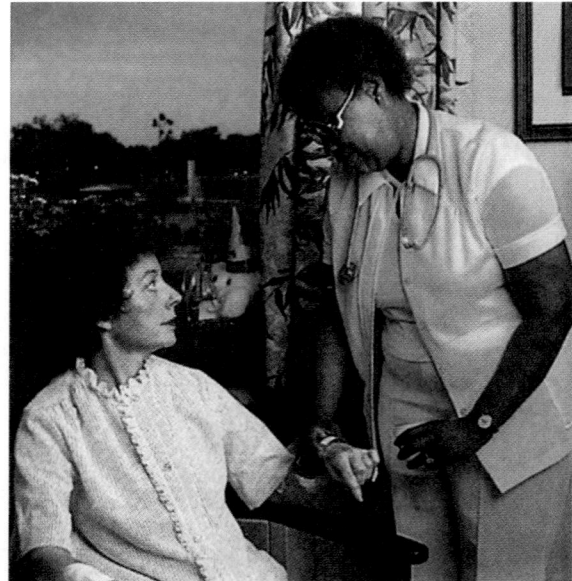

FIGURE **19-7** Before administering any medications the nurse checks the client's identification and allergy bracelets.

There will be situations when clients are confused or unresponsive. The nurse then compares the medical record number on the MAR with the client's ID bracelet. If the client is a child, parents or legal guardians can be used to identify the child. The practice of checking clients' identification is invaluable in preventing errors, especially when caring for multiple clients. It is also essential even after caring for the same client for several days. If a client questions the practice of identification verification, explain that this is a routine practice for making sure clients receive the correct medication. In many hospitals a new system of bar coding is being used to help identify the right client.

Right Route

The prescriber's order must designate a route of administration. If the route of administration is missing, or if the specified route is not the recommended route, the nurse must consult the prescriber immediately. The nurse can make clinical judgments in recommending a route; for example, when a client is nauseated, the nurse can recommend the prescriber order a Tylenol suppository for pain instead of a Tylenol capsule. When an injection is administered, the nurse must use only preparations intended for parenteral use. Injection of a liquid intended for oral use can produce local complications, such as sterile abscess, or fatal systemic effects. Medication companies label parenteral medication "for injectable use only."

Right Time

The nurse must know why a medication is ordered for certain times of the day and whether the time schedule can be altered. For example, two medications are ordered, one q8h (every 8 hours) and the other tid (3 times a day). Both medications are to be given 3 times within a 24-hour period. The prescriber intends the q8h medication to be given around the clock to maintain a therapeutic blood level of the drug. In contrast, the tid medication is given during the waking hours and offers a bit more flexibility. Dosing intervals are derived for treating the ideal "average" client; therefore drug therapy regimens must be reassessed continually for an individual client's needs (McKenry and Salerno, 2004). Each agency has a recommended time schedule for medications ordered at frequent intervals. *All routinely ordered medications should be given within 30 minutes before or after the scheduled time;* however, nursing judgment may allow some variance, depending on the medication involved. For example, it is always important to administer antibiotics within the 30-minute time frame. It is also important to administer a drug within 30 minutes when the drug is ordered before, with, or after a meal. Exempt from the 30-minute standard are stat or one-time-only drug orders, such as those given before diagnostic tests or surgery and those medications given at more frequent intervals, such as every 2 hours. In contrast to the 30-minute standard, some institutions follow a 60-minute standard before or after scheduled times for drugs that are administered during waking hours and do not require maintaining constant therapeutic blood levels.

A medication may also be ordered for special circumstances. A preoperative medication may be ordered "stat" (to be given immediately); "now," which means as soon as available, usually within an hour; or "on call," which means the operating room or treatment area will notify the nurse when it is the appropriate time. A medication may be ordered AC (before meals) or PC (after meals). Insulin and oral hypoglycemic agents should be given at a precise interval before a meal.

Some medications require the nurse's clinical judgment in determining the right administration time. A medication that is ordered prn (*pro re nata*) is intended to be given according to circumstances or when needed. For example, when a prn analgesic is ordered "q3-4h prn," the nurse needs to assess the characteristics and severity of the pain to determine when to administer within the 3- to 4-hour time span or longer. In the case of a stool softener, for example, an order for sodium docusate "prn daily" requires the nurse to assess the character of a client's stool daily.

Right Documentation

This right has been added to the traditional five rights of medication administration by several authors (Aschenbrenner and others, 2002). Medication safety is enhanced through accurate documentation. Nurses must ensure that the appropriate documentation exists before and after giving medications. Written orders and medication forms should clearly reflect the client's name, the name of the ordered medication, and the medication dosage, route, and frequency. If any of these pieces of information is missing, the nurse must contact the prescriber to verify the order. After a medication is administered, the name of the ordered medication, the time of administration, and the dosage, route, and frequency must be recorded as soon as possible. Accurate documentation serves as a way for health care providers to communicate with each other and to prevent an accidental dose from being administered to a client.

Evidence-Based Practice Trends

The Joint Commission on Accreditation of Healthcare Organizations (2004a) has defined a medication error as any preventable event that may cause inappropriate medication use or jeopardize patient safety. Medication errors are unfortunately common in health care settings. In a random sample of 36 health care institutions (hospitals and skilled nursing facilities) in Georgia and Colorado, Barker and others (2002) identified the most common types of medication errors. The most frequent errors by category were wrong time (43%), omission (30%), wrong dose (17%), and unauthorized drug (4%). Seven percent of the errors were judged potentially harmful to clients. Additional sources of errors include IV rate too fast, delivering too much medication; missed doses; wrong route; and wrong medication delivered due to misidentification of the client (Benner and others, 2002). With the prevalence of drug errors being high, it is imperative for nurses to understand factors that can contribute to errors so that those factors can be avoided as much as possible. For example, the risk of adverse drug error rises as the number of different drugs a client receives is increased, and if a client starts a new drug while being hospitalized (Armitage and Knapman, 2003). In addition, distractions and interruptions within a busy health care setting are believed to be associated with errors. In these situations, nurses must focus more attention on the process of drug preparation and administration to avoid careless mistakes. A nurse must be attentive to what is required to correctly prepare and administer a medication.

In many cases, drug errors arise as a result of failure of nurses to follow policy (Keill and Johnson, 1993). However, some policies can promote unthinking rather than a rigorous problem-solving approach. Nurses must make clinical judgments when administering medications and not simply give drugs automatically. This means thorough client assessment and review of the pharmacokinetics and purpose of a medication is critical for safe medication administration.

Preparation of Medications

The nurse performs several steps before actual administration of medications: interpreting medication labels, conversion of measurement units within a system or between systems, and calculation of medication doses. It is important to remember: *Medications ordered in units and milliequivalents are not convertible to metric, apothecary, or household measurements.*

Interpreting Medication Labels

Medication labels include seven basic pieces of information: the trade name of the medication in large letters, the generic name in smaller letters, the form of the medication, the dose, the expiration date, the lot number, and the name of the manufacturer (Figure 19-8). The trade name given by the manufacturer often suggests the action of the medication. It is im-

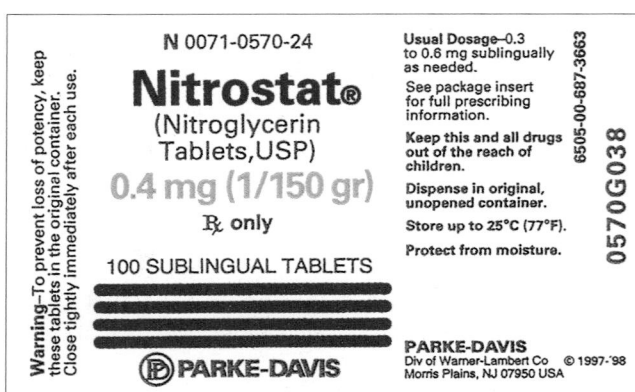

FIGURE **19-8** Interpreting a medication label. (Courtesy Warner-Lambert Company.)

BOX 19-5 **Approximate Equivalents**

1 gr* = 60 mg
1 g = 1000 mg = 16 gr*
1000 mcg = 1 mg
1000 g = 1 kg = 2.2 lb*
1 mL or ml = 15-16 minims* = 15 drops (gtt)
4-5 ml =1 fluidram* = 1 tsp†
15-16 ml = 3 tsp = 1 tbsp†
30 ml = 1 fluid oz† = 2 tbsp
240 ml = 8 fluid oz* = 1 cup†
1000 ml = 1 L

*Apothecary measure.
†Household measure.

portant to read a label carefully, uninterrupted, especially if you are required to administer only a portion of the medication made available.

Conversions

Medications are not always dispensed in the unit of measure in which they are ordered. Medication companies package and bottle certain standard equivalents. The nurse often must convert available units of volume and weight to desired doses or vice versa. The nurse must know approximate equivalents in all of the measurement systems or make use of conversion tables (Box 19-5). An example follows:

The nurse receives an order: ceftazidime 1 g IV.
The pharmacy supplies ceftazidime in 500-mg vials.
Because the medication dose on the medication label is in milligrams, conversion should be from grams to milligrams.
To convert gram to milligrams, move the decimal point three spaces to the right.

$$1 \text{ g} = 1000 \text{ mg}$$

Once this information is known, the nurse can move to the next step: dose calculations.

Dose Calculations

Dose calculations are necessary when the dose on the medication label differs from the dose ordered. There are several methods for calculating doses. The most common methods are ratio-proportion or use of a formula. The following basic formula can be applied when preparing solid or liquid forms of medication:

$$\frac{\text{Dose ordered}}{\text{Dose on hand}} \times \text{Amount on hand} = \text{Amount to administer}$$

The dose ordered is the amount of medication prescribed. The dose on hand is the weight or volume of medication available in units supplied by the pharmacy; it may be written on the medication label as the contents of a tablet or cap-

sule or as the amount of medication dissolved per unit volume of liquid. The amount on hand is the basic unit or quantity of the medication that contains the dose on hand. For solid medications the amount on hand may be one capsule; for liquids the amount may be 1 ml or 1 L depending on the container. The amount to administer is the actual amount the nurse will administer.

Example: The prescriber orders morphine sulfate 2 mg IV. Thus the dose ordered is 2 mg. The medication is available in a vial containing 10 mg per milliliter. Thus the dose on hand is 10 mg in an amount on hand of 1 ml.

$$\frac{2 \text{ mg}}{10 \text{ mg}} \times 1 \text{ ml} = \text{Volume in milliliters to administer}$$

To simplify the ²/₁₀ fraction, divide numerator and denominator by 2.

$$\frac{1}{5} \times 1 \text{ ml} = \frac{1}{5} \text{ ml to administer}$$

Syringes are calibrated in decimals; ⅕ equals 0.2. Prepare 0.2 ml of morphine.

The formula also applies to solid dose forms.
Example: The prescriber orders 0.125 mg orally (PO) of digoxin. The medication is available in tablets containing 0.25 mg.

$$\frac{0.125 \text{ mg}}{0.250 \text{ mg}} \times 1 \text{ tablet} = \text{Number of tablets to administer}$$

The fraction $^{0.125}/_{0.250}$ equals ½ or 0.5. Therefore

0.5 tablet = 0.5 or ½ tablet to be administered

Dimensional analysis is becoming a popular method for dose calculation because it involves simple multiplication and division and does not require algebra (Box 19-6). The following examples apply the use of dimensional analysis.

Example 1
When the dose ordered has the same label as the dose available:
Dose ordered: 0.5 g
Tablets available: 0.25 g per tablet
Step 1. The starting factor is 0.5 g.

BOX 19-6   Dimensional Analysis

Step 1. Identify the starting factor (amount ordered), which is the first item of the equation, and the answer label (tablets, capsules, or ml), which is the last item.

Step 2. Identify appropriate equivalents with a 1:1 ratio (e.g., 1 g = 1000 mg). Set up the equation so that labels can be canceled; for example, if mg is in the numerator, mg must be in the denominator to cancel.

Step 3. Solve the equation.
   a. Cancel labels first; the answer label should not cancel.
   b. Reduce numbers to lowest terms.
   c. Multiply/divide to solve equation.
   d. Reduce answer to lowest terms, convert to decimal, and round to a measurable quantity.

$$\text{Starting factor} \times \frac{\text{Equivalent}}{\text{Equivalent}} = \text{Answer label}$$

The answer label is tablets; that is, How many tablets should be given?

Step 2. Formulate the conversion equation:
The equivalent needed is 1 tablet = 0.25 g.

$$\frac{0.5 \text{ g}}{1} \times \frac{1 \text{ tab}}{0.25 \text{ g}} = ?$$

Cancel labels (g).
NOTE: If properly written, all labels except the answer label will cancel.

Step 3. Solve the equation:
Reduce the numerical values, and multiply the numerators and the denominators.

$$\frac{\overset{2}{\cancel{0.5 \text{ g}}}}{1} \times \frac{1 \text{ tab}}{\cancel{0.25 \text{ g}}} = 2 \text{ tabs}$$

Example 2

When the dose ordered has a different label than the dose available:

Dose ordered: 0.5 g
Tablets available: 250 mg per tablet

Step 1. The starting factor is 0.5 g.
The answer label is tablets; that is, How many tablets should be given?

Step 2. Formulate the conversion equation:
The equivalents needed are 1 g = 1000 mg and 1 tab = 250 mg.

$$\frac{0.5 \text{ g}}{1} \times \frac{1000 \text{ mg}}{1 \text{ g}} \times \frac{1 \text{ tab}}{250 \text{ g}} = ?$$

Cancel labels (g, mg).

Step 3. Solve the equation:
Reduce the values, and multiply the numerators and the denominators.

$$\cancel{0.5 \text{ g}} \times \frac{\overset{4}{\cancel{1000 \text{ mg}}}}{\underset{2}{\cancel{1 \text{ g}}}} \times \frac{1 \text{ tab}}{\cancel{250 \text{ g}}} = \frac{4}{2} = 2 \text{ tabs}$$

Example 3

When the dose ordered is available in a liquid form:

Dose ordered: Keflex 250 mg PO
Available: 125 mg per 5 ml

Step 1. The starting factor is 250 mg.
The answer label is ml.

Step 2. Formulate the conversion equation:

$$\frac{250 \text{ mg}}{1} \times \frac{5 \text{ ml}}{125 \text{ mg}} = \text{ml}$$

Cancel labels (mg).

Step 3. Solve the equation:
Reduce and multiply.

$$\frac{\overset{2}{\cancel{250 \text{ mg}}}}{1} \times \frac{5 \text{ ml}}{\cancel{125 \text{ mg}}} = 10 \text{ ml}$$

Example 4

When dose is ordered based on body surface area (commonly done for pediatric doses). The body surface area is estimated on the basis of weight, using standard charts or nomogram. The formula is a ratio of the child's body surface area compared with the body surface area of an average adult (1.7 square meters, or 1.7 m²).

$$\text{Child's dose} = \frac{\text{Surface area of child}}{1.7 \text{ m}^2} \times \text{Normal adult dose}$$

The physician orders ampicillin for a child weighing 12 kg, and the nomogram chart shows that the body surface area is 0.54 m². The normal single dose is 250 mg.

1. $\text{Child's dose} = \dfrac{0.54 \text{ m}^2}{1.7 \text{ m}^2} \times 250 \text{ mg}$

2. The m² units cancel out and can be ignored.

3. $\text{Child's dose} = \dfrac{0.54}{1.7} \times 250 \text{ mg}$

$$0.3 \times 250 \text{ mg} = 75 \text{ mg}$$
$$\text{Child's dose} = 75 \text{ mg}$$

Pediatric Doses. Children vary in age, weight, and the ability to absorb, metabolize, and excrete medications. Children's doses are usually lower than those of adults, and caution is needed in preparing medications. In addition, a standard medication dose is nearly nonexistent in pediatrics (McKenry and Salerno, 2004). Medications may or may not be prepared and packaged in doses appropriate for children. Preparing appropriate doses often requires calculation based on body weight or body surface area. A child's parents may be helpful in determining the best way to give a child medication. Sometimes it is more effective to have the parent give the medication as the nurse stands by. However, many institutions have protocols that require that only the nurse administer the drug to the child.

Older Adult Dosages. Older adults require special consideration during medication administration. In addition to

BOX 19-7 Altered Pharmacokinetics in Older Adults

Absorption	↑ Gastric pH
	↓ Intestinal blood flow
Distribution	↓ Lean body mass
	↑ Adipose (fat) stores
	↓ Total body water
	↓ Serum albumin
Metabolism	↓ Liver size
	↓ Liver blood flow
	↓ Liver functions (microsomal enzyme activity)
Excretion	↓ Kidney function

BOX 19-8 Commonly Prescribed Medications for Older Adults

- Aminoglycoside antibiotics (e.g., gentamicin)
- Analgesics, opioids
- Anticholinergics, antispasmodics
- Anticoagulants
- Antihypertensives
- Aspirin, aspirin-containing products
- Digoxin, digitalis preparations
- Diuretics (e.g., thiazides, furosemide)
- Hypnotics/sedatives (e.g., flurazepam, triazolam)
- H₂ receptor antagonists (e.g., ranitidine)
- Nonsteroidal antiinflammatory drugs
- Tricyclic antidepressants

From McKenry LM, Salerno E: *Mosby's pharmacology in nursing,* ed 21, Mosby, St. Louis, 2001.

physiological changes of aging, behavioral and economic factors influence an older person's use of medications. Box 19-7 summarizes how medication pharmacokinetics are altered in older adults. A common problem for older adult clients is polypharmacy, the use of a number of different medications, prescribed or not, for one or more health problems (McKenry and Salerno, 2004). Some of the medications taken may have similar effects. Polypharmacy increases the chances of medication interactions occurring. These interactions can be mistaken as medication toxicity, an increase in disease severity or suboptimal treatment, or an apparently unrelated event (Lueckenotte, 2000). The nurse, physician, and pharmacist share the responsibility of reducing or eliminating the adverse risk factors associated with various medication regimens older adults typically receive. The nurse must conduct a thorough assessment of the client's health status, current medication regimen (including OTC drugs and herbal products), the reason for existing and proposed medications, and any environmental factors that can influence accurate and safe medication administration by the client and caregivers. Although there are no standardized dosages for older adults, the nurse must recognize physiological changes in the client that influence dosages prescribed. Frequently physicians will lower recommended adult dosages to treat older adult clients. The potent medications available to treat older adults often have a narrow index between effectiveness and toxicity (McKenry and Salerno, 2004). The medications most commonly prescribed for older adults, and that therefore commonly cause problems for older adults, are listed in Box 19-8.

Nursing Process in Medication Administration

Medication administration should be done in a safe and orderly manner. Application of the nursing process ensures that critical thinking and clinical judgment are integrated into the client's care.

Assessment

Nursing assessment relating to medication therapy involves client assessment and medication review. The nurse determines if a client has a history of medication allergies. The

hospitalized client's medical record should be clearly marked with a list of allergies, and the client should have an allergy band. A client should never be given a medication to which he or she is known to be allergic.

A careful assessment of the client's physiological status is also important. How is the client tolerating food or liquids by mouth? Does the client have abnormal laboratory values suggesting a change in renal or liver function? Does the client's blood pressure or pulse rate contraindicate administration of a medication? Is the client becoming less responsive at times, making him or her prone to aspiration of a liquid medication? These are just examples of conditions the nurse considers when helping to judge the appropriateness of a medication and/or the route for administration. Nursing assessment also reveals if it is necessary to withhold a prescribed medication. Any withheld medication should be reported to the prescriber.

Assessing the client's current medication history is useful when attempting to determine the reason for the client's presenting signs and symptoms. This is especially true in urgent situations. In clinic and medical office settings, nurses ask clients to bring a list of their current medications for review. Review of current medications also allows the nurse to simultaneously assess the client's knowledge level necessary for safe self-administration of medications. Does the client know the medication's dosage schedule, purpose, common side effects, and actions to take when side effects develop?

In the home care setting, nursing assessment also includes a review of the environment where the client self-administers medications (see Chapter 41). Are medications stored safely away from children? Are there facilities to adequately prepare the medications? Does the client use a system to assist in organizing medications and remembering dosage schedules? Is there a mechanism to dispose of biomedical equipment (e.g., needles and syringes)? The nurse also determines the family member's or significant other's ability to assist with medication administration.

A medication review requires the nurse to methodically consider what is known about each medication. A nurse should have an understanding of a medication's purpose, action, normal dosage and route, time interval for action, expected side effects, and the specific reason for why a client has the medication prescribed. Nursing implications for administering each medication safely will depend on the type of medication being given (e.g., all antihypertensives should require a blood pressure measurement before administration). When in doubt about medication information, the nurse checks available medication references or the pharmacy.

Planning

When administering medications, three basic goals should be met:

1. The client achieves the medication's therapeutic effect.
2. The client experiences no complications related to the prescribed medication and the method of administration.
3. Client and family will understand how to self-administer medications safely.

Implementation

The principles of safe and effective medication preparation and administration must be followed for each client.

Preadministration Activities

1. Minimize distractions during medication preparation—ask colleagues to not interrupt you, close the door of the medication room, and do not try to perform other tasks while preparing a medication.
2. Make sure you have a written order for every medication for which you assume responsibility for administering. Ensure that a medication order has not expired. Follow institutional policy for medication order renewal.
3. Make sure that the information on the medication computer sheet or MAR corresponds exactly with the prescriber's written order and with the medication container label.
4. Read the label on the medication container and compare it with the MAR at least 3 times: when removing the drug from the supply drawer, when placing the medication in a administration cup/syringe, and just before administering the medication to the client.
5. Follow guidelines described earlier for medication calculation. *Remember: Take your time with all calculations, and have another nurse check the calculation.*
6. Review any preadministration assessments (e.g., vital signs, review of laboratory results).
7. Use good medical aseptic technique; perform hand hygiene before preparing a dose of medication. Avoid touching tablets and capsules. Use sterile technique for parenteral medications (Chapter 21).
8. Use correct equipment when preparing a medication.
9. To avoid common errors do not prepare medications from containers with labels that are unmarked or illegible; do not give medications that have changed from clear to cloudy or have changed color; discard a liquid

medication if sediment can be seen in the bottom of its container, unless the medication is a suspension; and always check the medication expiration date.

Medication Administration

1. Follow the *six rights* of medication administration. Never administer a medication prepared by another nurse.
2. When entering the room, inform the client of each medication's name and its purpose. This is a good time to review any medication information that will be necessary for the client to know for self-administration.
3. Tablets and capsules should be kept in their wrappers and opened at the client's bedside. This allows you to review each medication with the client. Respect the client's right to refuse a medication. If a client refuses medication, never return unwrapped medication to a container; discard it. If the medication wrapper remains intact, the medication may be returned to the client's unit-dose drawer. When medication is refused, determine the reason for it, and take action accordingly. Refusal of medications must be documented and the prescriber notified within 24 hours.
4. There can be interactions between medications and certain foods or beverages. Know what is compatible. Milk and grapefruit juice are examples of liquids that can alter the absorption of medications. It is always safe to offer water with oral medications. In the home setting clients should know to never take alcohol with medications. Of the more than 100 most commonly prescribed drugs, more than half contain at least one ingredient known to interact adversely with alcohol (McKenry and Salerno, 2004).
5. Remain with the client as the client takes the medication. Provide assistance if necessary (e.g., for the client who is weak and unable to administer eye drops). Do not leave medications at a client's bedside without a prescriber's order to do so.

Postadministration Activities

1. After administering a medication, record the following information on the MAR or other appropriate form (e.g., nurses' notes) required by the institution:

   - Medication name
   - Dose
   - Route of administration
   - Time of administration
   - Any unexpected client responses (see evaluation)
   - Pertinent data or assessment collected at time of administration
   - Signature and title of nurse administering medication

2. If the client refuses a medication, document the reason for refusal in the nurses' notes. The MAR may require a special symbol that indicates that the client refused the medication.

Evaluation

Once a medication is administered, the nurse is responsible for critically evaluating what is known about the client's condition, how the medication is expected to affect the client, and how the client actually responds. This means the nurse is looking for therapeutic effects, as well as adverse outcomes. Should adverse outcomes develop, the nurse recognizes the clinical signs and responds quickly.

1. Monitor client's physical response to the medication (e.g., vital signs, urine output, relief of pain or other symptoms).
2. Monitor client's behavioral responses to the medication (e.g., level of anxiety, agitation, consciousness).
3. Observe injection sites for bruises, inflammation, localized pain, numbness, or bleeding.
4. Determine client's understanding of medication therapy and ability to self-administer medication.

Special Considerations When Administering Medications

Children

When the nurse is administering medications to a child, the parents can be a valuable resource. Nearly all parents have administered medications to their children and can describe the approaches that work. Parents can also offer information regarding the child's reaction to similar experiences if the child has been previously hospitalized or has been given medications in a practitioner's office (Hockenberry and others, 2003). It may be less traumatic to the child if a parent gives the medication under the nurse's supervision (consult agency policy). Typically children require extra psychological preparation and patience when parenteral medications are administered. Children rarely become accustomed to the discomfort of an injection.

Older Adults

McKenry and Salerno (2004) recommend that nurses make geriatric medication therapy as simple as possible. Conferring with the prescriber may help to limit the number of medications a client is taking. The nurse should also work closely with family caregivers to determine if medication schedules are best suited to the client's typical routine.

Nurses should suspect medications as a cause whenever they notice a change in an older adult client's behavior, particularly restlessness, irritability, and confusion. These symptoms are characteristic of medication toxicity (McKenry and Salerno, 2004). Instructing assistive personnel to alert the nurse to any changes in client behavior is prudent. What is frequently described as "senility" is often medication-induced lethargy or confusion.

Environmental, Genetic, and Cultural Factors

Recent studies suggest that ethnicity affects how individuals react to medications (Kudzma, 1999). When individuals show a variation in response to a medication, it is called medication polymorphism. Factors that contribute to polymorphism are environmental, genetic, and cultural. Environmental factors affect a medication's half-life and assimilation. For example, diet can affect medication absorption. If a client eats a high-fat diet, certain medications may work more effectively than others. The Japanese typically eat diets high in sodium chloride, which often makes antihypertensive medications less effective.

Culturally, a client's values and beliefs affect medication response. Medication adherence is significantly influenced by a client's level of education, prior experience with medication therapy, and the family's influence on actions. In Japan, for example, nausea, vomiting, and bowel changes related to medication use are underreported because it is not acceptable to complain about gastrointestinal problems. Often a person's cultural background results in the use of herbal and homeopathic remedies that can alter response to a medication. Although most practitioners do not consider ethnicity when prescribing medications, Kudzma (1999) predicts this will change.

Special Handling of Medications
Controlled Substances

Any medication that has the potential for abuse is handled differently than other medications. These medications are called controlled substances and are often referred to as narcotics. Narcotics delivered to a nursing unit are kept in a locked cabinet. At the beginning of each shift, two registered nurses must count all of the narcotics in the locked cabinet and record the count on a narcotic administration record. Automated medication dispensing systems make counting narcotics unnecessary because these systems automatically count and record the nurse's electronic signature as the dose is dispensed. Any discrepancies found in a narcotic count are investigated by RNs. Any narcotics unaccounted for must be reported to the nurse manager or supervisor immediately.

When administering narcotics to a client, the nurse follows these general guidelines:

1. Before obtaining the narcotic, check the narcotic administration record for the number of narcotics left in stock. Compare this number with the actual supply available. If it is correct, obtain the desired dose of narcotic. If the count is incorrect, notify the nurse manager, and follow institutional policy.
2. Count the remaining supply. The following information is often recorded on the narcotic administration sheet after removal of your dose:

   - Client's name
   - Prescribing physician
   - Client's medical record number
   - Dose of the medication ordered
   - Number of tablets (or injectables) remaining
   - Nurse's signature

3. Administer the narcotic according to policy.
4. If the narcotic cannot be given to the client (e.g., client refuses, medication is contaminated, vital signs change) or not all is used, the medication must be "wasted."

Narcotic wasting often requires that another nurse witness the administering nurse discard the medication according to hospital policy. When narcotics are wasted, this information is recorded on the narcotic administration form or another designated form. The witnessing nurse records on that form a signature indicating the medication has been discarded properly. In electronic systems the information is recorded in the computer.

Medication Errors

A medication error may cause or lead to inappropriate medication use or client harm while the medication is in the control of a health care professional. Medication errors include inaccurate prescribing, administration of the wrong medication, route, and time interval, as well as administering extra doses or failing to administer a medication. Medication errors can be related to professional practice, health care product design, or procedures and systems such as product labeling and distribution. When an error occurs, the client's safety and well-being become the top priority. The nurse assesses and examines the client's condition and notifies the physician or prescriber of the incident as soon as possible. Once the client is stable, the nurse reports the incident to the appropriate person in the institution (e.g., manager or supervisor).

The nurse is also responsible for preparing a written incident report that usually must be filed within 24 hours of the incident. The report includes client identifying information; the location and time of the incident; an accurate, factual description of what occurred and what was done; and the signature of the nurse involved. The incident report is not a permanent part of the medical record and should not be referred to in the record. This is to legally protect the health care professional and institution. Institutions use incident reports to track incident patterns and to initiate quality improvement programs as needed. Depending on the circumstances and the severity of the outcome, the nurse or institution may be responsible for reporting the incident to the Joint Commission on Accreditation of Healthcare Organizations, MedWatch (FDA's Medical Products Reporting Program), or U.S. Pharmacopeia's Medication Errors Reporting Program (Morris, 1999).

It is good risk management to report all medication errors, including mistakes that do not cause obvious or immediate harm or near misses. A nurse should feel comfortable in reporting an error and not fear repercussions from managerial staff. Even when a client suffers no harm from a medication error, the institution can still learn why the mistake occurred and what can be done to avoid similar errors in the future. Prevention is the key. Box 19-9 lists steps to take in preventing medication errors.

Client and Family Teaching

A properly informed client is more likely to take medications correctly than one who is unsure about the purpose of a medication and how it will affect his or her daily lifestyle. The nurse provides information about the purpose of medications, their actions, side effects, dosage schedules, actions to take in case of side or toxic effects, and administra-

---

BOX 19-9   Steps to Take in Preventing Medication Errors

- Follow the six rights of medication administration.
- Be sure to read labels at least 3 times (comparing MAR with label): before, during, and after administering the medication.
- Use at least two patient identifiers (e.g., name band, client pronouncing name) whenever administering a medication.
- Do not allow any other activity to interrupt your administration of medication to a client.
- Double-check all calculations, and verify with another nurse.
- Do not interpret illegible hand writing; clarify with prescriber.
- Question unusually large or small doses.
- Document all medications as soon as they are given.
- When you have made an error, reflect on what went wrong; ask how you could have prevented the error.
- Evaluate the context or situation in which a medication error occurred. This helps to determine if nurses have the necessary resources for safe medication administration.
- When repeated medication errors occur within a work area, identify and analyze the factors that may have caused the errors, and take corrective action.
- Attend in-service programs that focus on the medications you commonly administer.

---

tion guidelines. It is never too early to begin instruction. When a client receives an order for a new medication, the nurse covers a comprehensive range of information about the medication. If a client has been receiving a medication, the nurse assesses the client's knowledge base, current administration practices, and fills in where gaps or misunderstandings exist. When teaching clients it is best to include persons who may become involved in their care (e.g., family, friends, partners) or who are available should a client become ill at home.

Taking prescribed medications routinely can become a challenge, depending on a person's lifestyle and the number of medications prescribed. When providing instruction, have the client or family member repeat the name and use for each medication plus the dosing instructions. Have the client demonstrate preparing and setting up a medication. Use of teaching pamphlets or medication information leaflets can help to reinforce important information. Determine if the client requires a compliance aid or memory cue. This is especially important in older adults. Medication dose containers, organized by the hours and days of the week, can be very useful. In the event clients miss a dose of medication, they need to know how to adjust their medication schedule safely.

Teaching Clients About Side Effects

All medications have side effects. The nurse teaches the client and family members about side effects associated with each medication prescribed, focusing on the side effects that are the *most likely* to occur early after administration. For example, some antibiotics cause hypersensitivity and should be used with caution for clients who have liver or kidney disease. Hypersensitivity reactions are likely to occur shortly after taking a few doses of an antibiotic. Other side effects tend to occur after long-term antibiotic administration. Teach clients about side effects in terms of things they can see, feel, touch, or hear. For example, thrombocytopenia, a reduction in the number of platelets in the blood, can be a side effect of a medication. The client cannot see, touch, or hear thrombocytopenia. However, thrombocytopenia can cause bleeding, and there are ways the client can look for evidence of bleeding in any part of the body (e.g., bruising of the skin, blood in urine or stool, nosebleeds). Be sure to teach the client what to do about side effects when they are discovered. Also, encourage clients to listen and adhere to instructions provided by their local pharmacist.

Teaching Medication Safety

Evaluating the effectiveness of teaching ensures that the client can administer medications in a safe manner. Have clients describe their medication schedules, and then have a discussion that allows them to ask questions and clarify their understanding:

- Why are you taking this medication?
- How often do you take this medication?
- How much do you take?
- What side effects can occur?
- What do you do when side effects occur?

Another method to evaluate client understanding of medications is to create medication cards with the name of the medication on the front of the card and all pertinent medication information on the back of the card. The nurse flashes the card in front of the client and asks the client to read the name of the medication. This also ensures that the client can read the name of the medication. If the client correctly identifies the name of the medication, further discussion about medication doses and side effects can be conducted.

It may be helpful to have actual medication bottles labeled with the medication name available at a teaching session. Medication bottles often have fine print and may not be easily read by the client with impaired visual acuity. This would be the time to discover visual limitations so that a larger print label can be provided.

The nurse also evaluates the client's sensory, motor, and cognitive functions, which, when impaired, may affect the client's ability to safely self-administer medications. This includes the ability to open medication containers, prepare a dose in a syringe, or read a label. When impairments are assessed, family members, friends, or home care aides may be available to assist with medication administration.

FOCUS *on* CLINICAL PRACTICE

Mr. Stacy is a 60-year-old client who has been diagnosed with type 2 diabetes for 5 years. In the past, his blood sugar has been managed by weight loss and diet. He now takes glipizide (Glucotrol XL) 10 mg PO daily with breakfast. He is also hypertensive and takes furosemide (Lasix) 40 mg PO daily and prazosin (Minipress) 0.5 mg PO bid. Mr. Stacy is admitted to the hospital with pneumonia. He is started on an antibiotic azithromycin, 500 mg PO the first day and 250 mg daily thereafter. He asks the nurse about the antibiotic, because he is allergic to penicillin and has not taken azithromycin in the past. Mr. Stacy is alert and interested in learning about his medications.

1. Administering both Lasix and Minipress to Mr. Stacy is designed to cause what effect?
   A. A toxic effect
   B. An idiosyncratic effect
   C. A side effect
   D. A synergistic effect
2. Mr. Stacy is prescribed to receive four different oral medications. List three conditions that contraindicate the administration of oral medications.

3. Which of the following conditions places Mr. Stacy at risk for having an allergic reaction to azithromycin?
   A. History of diabetes
   B. Age
   C. First-time administration
   D. Diabetic diet
4. As the nurse begins to prepare Minipress, he notes that the drug is available in 0.25 mg-tablets. Use the ratio-proportion formula to determine the correct amount to administer to Mr. Stacy.
5. Medication safety is important for the nurse to consider each time a medication is prepared and administered. Answer the following questions about medication safety:
   A. How many rights of medication administration should be followed when administering medications?
   B. How many times should the nurse read a medication label during the administration process?
   C. When should the nurse document a medication?

NCLEX REVIEW QUESTIONS

1. Which of the following accurately describes a medication side effect?
   1. Unpredictable
   2. Usually avoidable
   3. Related to dose
   4. Usually lethal
2. The serum trough level of a medication is best described as:
   1. The serum level achieved just before the last of the medication is absorbed
   2. The point at which the lowest amount of drug is detected in the serum
   3. Blood serum concentration reached and maintained after repeated, fixed doses
   4. The serum level achieved after the last dose of a 24-hour cycle.
3. A topical medication is best described as a drug administered:
   1. Into the dermis of the skin
   2. Under the tongue
   3. Inhaled
   4. On the skin
4. Mrs. Ramirez has asked for a pain medication to relieve the discomfort from her abdominal incision. She has experienced nausea since this morning. Mrs. Ramirez is on a soft diet. She last received a dose of her ordered oral analgesic 4 hours ago. The medication, hydrocodone 10 mg PO is ordered q4h prn. Which of the following "rights" of drug administration most likely will challenge the nurse caring for Mrs. Ramirez?
   1. Right route
   2. Right patient
   3. Right dose
   4. Right time

References

Armitage G, Knapman H: Adverse events in drug administration: a literature review, *J Nurs Manag* 11:130, 2003.

Arnold GJ: Clinical recognition of adverse medication reactions: obstacles and opportunities for the nursing profession, *J Nurs Care Qual* 13(2):45, 1998.

Aschenbrenner DS and others: *Drug therapy in nursing,* Philadelphia, 2002, Lippincott.

Hockenberry MJ and others: *Wong's nursing care of infants and children,* ed 7, St. Louis, 2003, Mosby.

Institute of Medicine, Kohn LT, Corrigan J, Donaldson MS, editors, Committee on Quality of Health Care in America: *To err is human: building a safer health system,* Washington, DC, 2000, National Academy Press.

Institute of Medicine: www.iom.edu, accessed November 1, 2003.

Joint Commission on Accreditation of Healthcare Organizations: *Comprehensive Accreditation manual for hospitals,* Oakbrook Terrace, Ill, 2004a, The Commission.

Joint Commission on Accreditation of Healthcare Organizations: *FAQs about the 2004 National Patient Safety Goals,* www. jcaho.org/accredited+organizatins/patient+safety, accessed May 18, 2004b.

Joint Commission on Accreditation of Healthcare Organizations: *JCAHO National Patient Safety Goals,* www.jcaho.org/accredited +organizations/patient+safety, accessed May 22, 2004c.

Keill P, Johnson T: Shifting gears: improving delivery of medications, *J Nurs Qual Assur* 7(2):24, 1993.

Kudzma EC: Culturally competent medication administration, *Am J Nurs* 99(8):46, 1999.

Lueckenotte AG: *Gerontologic nursing,* ed 2, St. Louis, 2000, Mosby.

McCaffery M, Pasero C: *Pain,* ed 2, St. Louis, 1999, Mosby.

McKenry LM, Salerno E: *Mosby's pharmacology in nursing,* ed 22, St. Louis, 2004, Mosby.

Morris MR: Preventing med errors, *RN* 62(9):69, 1999.

Rich DS: Ask the Joint Commission, *Hosp Pharm* 37(6):1, 2002.

Research References

Barker KN and others: Medication errors observed in 36 health care facilities, *Arch Intern Med* 162:1897, 2002.

Benner P and others: Individual, practice, and system causes of errors in nursing, *J Nurs Adm* 32(10):509, 2002.

Novek J and others: Nurses' perceptions of the reliability of an automated medication dispensing system, *J Nurs Care Qual* 14(2): 1, 2000.

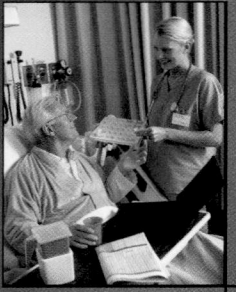

20

Oral and Topical Medications

MEDIA RESOURCES

Evolve Site *evolve*

http://evolve.elsevier.com/Perry/skills
- Weblinks
- Video clips
- Mosby's Nursing Skills Video Exercises

Mosby's Nursing Skills Videos/CD-ROM
- *Nonparenteral Medications Video:* Topical medications, application of estrogen patch and nitroglycerin paste; eye medications: eye drops and ointment; eardrops; use of metered-dose inhaler; insertion of rectal suppository

OBJECTIVES

Mastery of content in this chapter will enable the nurse to:

- Correctly administer a medication by oral, nasogastric, skin (topical), ophthalmic, otic, nasal, inhaled, vaginal, and rectal routes.
- Correctly administer medications for irrigation and instillation.
- Identify guidelines for administering oral, nasogastric, skin (topical), ophthalmic, otic, nasal, inhaled, vaginal, and rectal medications.
- Describe factors to assess before administering medications.
- Differentiate types of topical administrations that require sterile technique and those that require clean medical aseptic technique.
- Instruct clients in proper use of metered-dose inhalers (MDIs) and small-volume nebulizers.
- Identify conditions contraindicating the administration of medications.
- Prepare a teaching plan regarding medication use for a selected client.

KEY TERMS

Anaphylaxis	Nebulizer
Anesthetics	Nitroglycerin
Antianginal	Ointment
Cerumen	Ophthalmic
Cycloplegic	Orifice
Dermatitis	Otic
Dermatological	Overdose
Eczema	Pruritus
Glaucoma	Suppository
Lotion	Suspension
Metered-dose inhaler (MDI)	Sympathomimetic
Mydriatics	Topical
Nares	Transdermal
Nasal	Vertigo

The easiest and most desirable way to administer medications is by mouth. Clients usually are able to ingest or self-administer oral drugs with a minimum of problems. Situations, however, may arise that contraindicate the client's receiving medications by mouth, such as the presence of gastrointestinal alterations, the inability of a client to swallow food or fluids, and the use of gastric suction. If a nasogastric tube is present, the nurse must first ensure that the medications are appropriate for tube administration, and that the tube is in the correct position before medications are given. Some medication formulations should not be crushed.

Topical administration of medications involves applying drugs locally to skin, mucous membranes, or tissue membranes. The nurse applies medications to the skin by painting, spraying, or spreading medication over an area, applying moist dressings, soaking body parts in solution, or giving medicated baths. Adhesive-backed medicated disks can also be applied to the skin to provide a continuous release of medication over several hours or days. Systemic effects from topical agents can occur if the skin is thin, if the drug concentration is high, or if contact with the skin is prolonged. Topical administration avoids puncturing skin and lessens the risk of infection and tissue injury that may occur with injections. However, topical application can also cause localized reactions, and rotation of sites decreases the risk of severity of the reaction.

Drugs applied to membranes such as the cornea of the eye or rectal mucosa are absorbed quickly because of the membrane's vascularity. Mucous and other tissue membranes differ in their sensitivity to medications. The cornea of the eye, for example, is extremely sensitive to chemicals. Clients commonly experience burning sensations during administration of eye and nose drops. Medications are generally less irritating to vaginal or rectal mucosa.

Medications for topical use can be administered in the following ways:

1. *Direct application of liquid*—eye drops, gargling, swabbing the throat.
2. *Inserting drug into a body cavity*—suppository insertion into rectum or vagina or creams and foams inserted into the vagina.
3. *Instillation of fluid into body cavity (fluid is retained)*—ear drops, nose drops, bladder and rectal instillation.
4. *Irrigation of body cavity (fluid is not retained)*—flushing eye, ear, vagina, bladder, or rectum with medicated fluid.
5. *Spraying*—instillation into nose or throat.
6. *Inhalation of medicated aerosol spray*—distributes medication throughout the nasal passages and tracheobronchial airway. There are two types of devices designed for this purpose: metered-dose inhalers (MDIs) and small-volume nebulizers.
7. *Direct application to skin or mucosa*—lotion, ointment, cream, powder, spray, patch, and disk.
8. *Sublingual*—medication placed under the tongue and allowed to dissolve.
9. *Buccal*—medication placed between the upper or lower molar teeth and cheek area and allowed to dissolve.

Evidenced-Based Practice Trends

When administering oral and topical medications, nurses must keep patient safety uppermost in mind. The U.S. Pharmacopeia reported that one of the most common medication errors was administration of an improper dosage, strength, or quantity of a drug (Drug watch, 2001). When preparing to give oral or topical medications, it is essential that the nurse follow the "six rights" to ensure client safety and optimal results from medication therapy (see Chapter 19). Another means of ensuring client safety is to determine the correct position of a nasogastric tube before administering fluids or medications. The traditional nursing practices of auscultating the epigastrium for air inserted through the tube or observing the client for the presence or absence of respiratory symptoms cannot be relied upon as primary methods of assessing proper nasogastric tube placement. The appearance and color of gastric contents, as well as pH, are more reliable indicators for ensuring proper placement, next to x-ray studies (Metheny and Titler, 2001).

Nurses must also ensure that clients are able to self-administer medications properly. For example, studies have shown that many patients have demonstrated poor technique with metered-dose inhalers (MDIs). One study showed that only 21% of patients who used inhalers performed all the self-administration steps correctly (Shrestha and others, 1996). Nurses need to be knowledgeable about self-administration of medications to perform patient teaching and to demonstrate skills effectively.

Cultural Considerations

When giving oral and topical medications to clients of different cultures, it is important to incorporate cultural practices that are unique to the client. In some instances these cultural practices may affect only the method of administration; they do not alter the medication's effectiveness. However, there are times when cultural preferences, such as dietary preferences, timing of medication administration, or adherence to the medication regimen, may be in conflict with the medication order. It is important for the nurse to carefully determine when cultural preferences can be safely integrated into the administration of oral and topical medications.

- Some cultural groups such as Haitians, Southeast Asians, and Sudanese have a tendency to share medications and would discontinue Western medications as soon as symptoms are resolved (Holcomb and others, 1996; Kemp and Rasbridge, 2001).
- When giving oral medications to Hindus and Muslims, use the right hand, not the left (Al-Shahri, 2002). The right hand is considered clean; the left hand is seen as dirty.
- Southeast Asians believe that Western medicines are too strong and may stop taking them once symptoms are relieved (Nowak, 2003).
  - Emphasize the importance of completing a prescribed regimen.
  - Develop client and family awareness of dangers associated with taking medications without medical supervision.
  - Encourage client and family to ask questions without making any value judgment.
- Obtain the client's consent before instilling eye and ear medications or performing ear irrigations.

- Among Africans and Southeast Asians touching the head of the client by a nonrelative is believed to predispose loss of one's spirit and power (Mashaba, 2002; Orque, 1983).
- Assess the meaning of the illness and the healing modalities used by different cultural groups.
  - Latinos believe that asthma is a cold disease and would prefer medications with colors symbolizing hot properties, such as orange casing for inhalers.
  - Ma Huang, a common herb used to treat asthma and allergies among Chinese, can potentiate actions of decongestants, beta 2 agonists, and theophylline products (Wang, 2003).
  - Puerto Ricans may use cathartics and emetics to relieve asthma that is believed to be caused by mucus clogging the lungs (George, 2001).

Skill Performance Guidelines

1. Assess client's sensory function, including sight, hearing, touch, and physical coordination. Sensory and coordination deficits may impair client ability to see medications, open prescription bottles, and read labels at home.
2. Clients often receive more than one oral medication at a time. The nurse evaluates each medication for potential drug-drug or drug-food interactions. Always consult with the pharmacist when in doubt.
3. Always assess for drug allergies. If the client reports having an allergy, ask about what type of reaction occurred.
4. Evaluate whether medication can be taken with food. Some drugs require an empty stomach to enhance absorption. Other drugs can irritate the stomach lining and should always be taken with food.
5. For all medications administered, gather information pertinent to the drug(s) ordered: purpose, normal dosage and route, common side effects, time of onset and peak action, nursing implications.
6. For all medications administered, review prescriber's order for client's name, name of drug, strength, time of administration, and site of application.
7. Administration of some medications requires specific nursing actions. For example, the nurse should monitor the client's apical pulse and serum drug levels before administering digoxin.
8. Know potential local and systemic effects of all topically applied medications.
9. If clients are mentally and physically able, prepare the clients for discharge by instructing them on self-administration techniques. Include family members and/or caregivers if possible.
10. Check the expiration date for all medications.

SKILL 20-1 Administering Oral Medications

The easiest and most desirable way to administer medications is by mouth. The majority of medications the nurse administers are given by this route. The nurse usually prepares the medications in an area designed for medication preparation or at the unit-dose cart.

DELEGATION CONSIDERATIONS

The skill of administering oral medications should not be delegated to assistive personnel. However, because other aspects of care, are delegated, the nurse must:

- Instruct assistive personnel about potential side effects of medications and to report their occurrence
- Instruct assistive personnel to inform the nurse if client's symptoms (e.g., pain, itching) continue after the medication was given

EQUIPMENT

- ❏ Medication cart or tray
- ❏ Disposable medication cups
- ❏ Glass of water, juice, or preferred liquid
- ❏ Drinking straw
- ❏ Pill-crushing or cutting device (optional)
- ❏ Paper towels
- ❏ Medication administration record (MAR)

STEP	RATIONALE

ASSESSMENT

1. Assess for any contraindications to client receiving oral medication: Is client suffering from nausea/vomiting? Is client diagnosed as having bowel inflammation or reduced peristalsis? Has client had recent gastrointestinal surgery? Does client have gastric suction? Is the client restricted to nothing by mouth (NPO)? What is the client's level of consciousness?

2. Assess risk for aspiration (see Skill 29-2). Is client able to swallow? Assess client's swallow, cough, and gag reflexes. Determine the client's ability to swallow oral medications safely (Box 20-1).

Alterations in gastrointestinal function interfere with drug absorption, distribution, and excretion. Clients with gastrointestinal suction might not receive benefit from the medication because it may be suctioned from gastrointestinal tract before it can be absorbed. Clients with altered levels of consciousness may not be able to swallow oral medications.

Aspiration occurs when food, fluid, or medication intended for gastrointestinal administration is inadvertently administered into the respiratory tract. Clients with altered ability to swallow oral medications are at higher risk for aspiration.

BOX 20-1 Dysphagia

Dysphagia, or difficulty in swallowing, may lead to aspiration. A variety of signs and symptoms may be associated with dysphagia:

- Choking while eating or drinking
- Frequent need to clear the throat
- Unusually intense chewing, or repeated swallowing of one bite of food
- Drooling or leakage of food from the mouth
- Coughing during or after meals
- Holding pockets of food in the cheeks
- Gurgly voice quality after eating (listen as the client says "Ah")
- Increased congestion or secretions after eating or drinking
- Impaired breathing

The client's swallow, cough, and gag reflexes must be carefully assessed. Swallowing can be assessed at the bedside by placing the thumb and index finger on both sides of the client's Adam's apple and feeling for elevation of the larynx when the client tries to swallow. The elevation should be symmetrical. See Chapter 35 on proper techniques of coughing. If the client has intact swallow and cough reflexes, then assess the gag reflex by gently stroking the back of the throat on each side with a tongue blade. The nurse should also watch how and where food and liquids are placed in the client's mouth, how the food bolus is chewed or moved before it is swallowed, and how well the tongue moves the food bolus to the back of the throat. Then observe for any oral residue after the swallow.

If swallowing difficulties are suspected or detected, a referral to a speech pathologist is needed for definitive diagnosis. Dysphagia that is not recognized or managed may lead to aspiration pneumonia.

Data from Galvin TJ: Dysphagia: going down and staying down, *Am J Nurs* 101(1):37, 2001; Mahan LK, Escott-Stump S: *Krause's food, nutrition, and diet therapy,* ed 11, Philadelphia, 2004, WB Saunders; Terrado M and others: an overview, *Medsurg Nurs* 10(5):233, 2001.

STEP	RATIONALE

- **Critical Decision Point**

  Clients with neuromuscular disorders, esophageal strictures, lesions of the mouth, and those who are unresponsive or comatose and cannot swallow or with high risk for aspiration should not receive medications by the oral route. The nurse should request that the prescriber order the medication by an alternate route (e.g., intravenously). When contraindication exists to the client receiving oral medications, or if in doubt about the client's ability to safely swallow the medication, temporarily withhold the medication and inform the prescriber.

3. Assess client's medical history, history of allergies, medication history, and diet history. Drug allergies should be listed on each page of the MAR and prominently displayed on the client's medical record.

   These factors can influence how certain drugs act. Information also reflects client's need for medications. Medication history may reveal past problems with medication administration.

4. Gather and review physical assessment findings and laboratory data that may influence drug administration, such as vital signs, and renal and liver function studies.

   Physical examination or laboratory data may contraindicate drug administration. Renal and liver function status will affect metabolism and excretion of the medication (Lilley and others, 2005).

5. Assess client's knowledge regarding health and medication use. Consider drug use problems such as drug tolerance, noncompliance, abuse, addiction, or dependence.

   Determines client's need for drug education. Also assists in identifying client's adherence to drug therapy at home. If substance abuse problem is suspected, refer client to appropriate health care professional.

6. Assess client's preferences for fluids.

   Offering fluids during drug administration is an excellent way to increase client's fluid intake. Fluids ease swallowing and facilitate absorption from the gastrointestinal tract. However, fluid restrictions must be maintained if ordered.

7. Assess whether the medication can be administered with the preferred fluid.

   Some fluids may interfere with absorption of the medication. For example, taking tetracyclines with milk products greatly reduces their absorption (Lilley and others, 2005).

8. Check accuracy and completeness of each MAR with prescriber's written medication order. Check client's name, drug name and dosage, route of administration, and time for administration. Compare MAR with medication label. Incomplete or unclear orders should be clarified with the prescriber before implementation.

   The order sheet is the most reliable source and only legal record of drugs client is to receive. Ensures client receives correct medication.

9. After confirming order, recopy or reprint any portion of the MAR that is illegible.

   Soiled or illegible MAR forms can be a source of drug error.

NURSING DIAGNOSES

- Deficient knowledge regarding drug actions and purpose and self-administration
- Impaired swallowing
- Noncompliance regarding drug regimen

- Health-seeking behaviors (self-care)
- Ineffective therapeutic regimen management
- Risk for aspiration

Related factors are individualized based on client's condition or needs.

PLANNING

1. Expected outcomes following completion of procedure:
   - Client experiences desired medication effect within period of onset of medication.

     Drug has exerted its therapeutic action.

   - Client denies any gastrointestinal discomfort or symptoms of alterations.

     Oral medications can irritate gastrointestinal mucosa.

   - Client explains purpose of medication and drug dose schedule.

     Demonstrates understanding of drug therapy.

STEP	RATIONALE
2. Explain procedure to client. Be specific if client wishes to self-administer medications.	Makes client a participant in care and minimizes anxiety. Begins client teaching regarding medications. Enables client to self-administer drug if physically able.

■ IMPLEMENTATION

1. Prepare medications:

a. Perform hand hygiene.	Reduces transfer of microorganisms.
b. Arrange medication tray and cups in medication preparation area, or move medication cart to position outside client's room.	Organization of equipment saves time and reduces error.
c. Unlock medicine drawer or cart.	Medications are safeguarded when locked in cabinet or cart.
d. Prepare medications for one client at a time. Keep all pages of MAR for one client together.	Prevents preparation errors.
e. Select correct drug from stock supply or unit-dose drawer. Compare label of medication with MAR (see illustration).	Reading label first time and comparing it against transcribed order reduces errors.
f. Calculate drug dose as necessary. Double-check calculation.	Double-checking reduces risk of error.
g. To prepare tablets or capsules from a floor-stock bottle, pour required number into bottle cap, and transfer medication to medication cup. Do not touch medication with fingers. Extra tablets or capsules may be returned to bottle.	Drugs are very expensive; avoid waste. Tablets that are not prescored cannot be broken into equal halves, and the result will be an inaccurate dose.

- *Critical Decision Point*

  Medications that need to be broken to administer half the dosage can be broken, using a gloved hand, or cut with a cutting device (see illustration step 1g). Tablets that are to be broken in half must be prescored. Prescored tablets are identified by a manufactured line that transverses the center of the tablet.

h. To prepare unit-dose tablets or capsules, place packaged tablet or capsule directly into medicine cup. (Do not remove wrapper.)	Wrapper maintains cleanliness of medications and identifies drug name and dose.

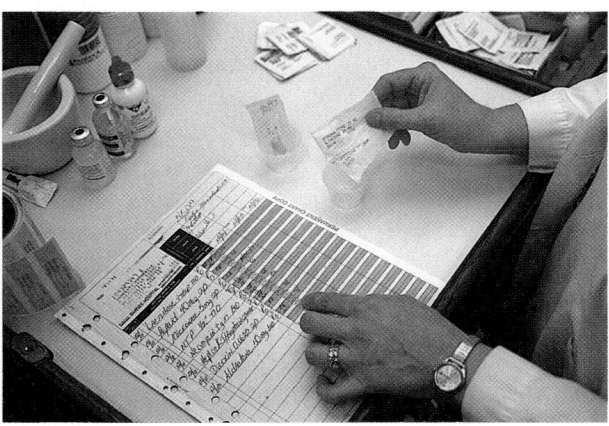

STEP 1e The nurse checks the label of the medication with the transcribed medication order on the MAR.

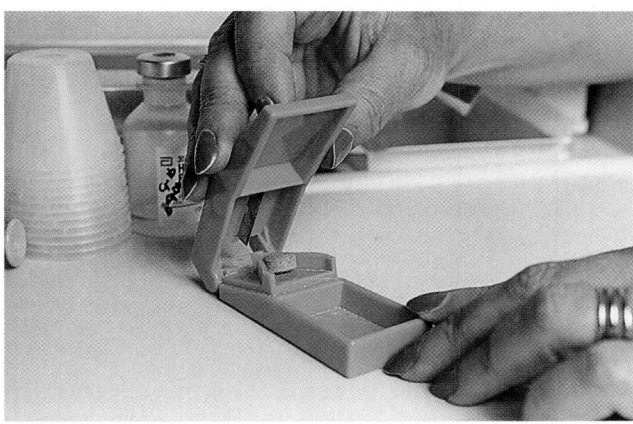

STEP 1g Tablet is placed in a cutting device and cut in half.

STEP	**RATIONALE**

- **Critical Decision Point**

  If preparing narcotics, check narcotics record for previous drug count and compare with supply available, and maintain adherence to controlled substance laws.

  i. All tablets or capsules to be given to client at same time may be placed in one medicine cup except for those requiring preadministration assessments (e.g., pulse rate or blood pressure).

  Keeping medications that require preadministration assessments separate from others make it easier for the nurse to withhold drugs as necessary.

  j. If client has difficulty swallowing, use pill-crushing device such as a mortar and pestle to crush pills (see illustration). If a pill-crushing device is not available, place tablet between two medication cups and grind with a blunt instrument. Mix ground tablet in small amount of soft food (custard or applesauce).

  Large tablets can be difficult to swallow. Ground tablet mixed with palatable soft food is usually easier to swallow.

- **Critical Decision Point**

  Not all drugs can be crushed (e.g., capsules, enteric-coated and long-acting/slow-release drugs). The coating of these drugs is designed to protect the stomach from irritation or protect the drug from destruction from stomach acids. Consult with pharmacist when in doubt (Miller and Miller, 2000).

  k. Prepare liquids:

  (1) Gently shake container. If medication is in a unit-dose container with the correct amount to administer, no further preparation is needed. If medication is in a multidose bottle, remove bottle cap from container, and place cap upside down on work surface.

  Prevents contamination of inside of cap.

  (2) Hold bottle with label against palm of hand while pouring.

  Spilled liquid will not drip and soil or fade label.

  (3) Hold medication cup at eye level, and fill to desired level on scale. Scale should be even with fluid level at its surface or base of meniscus, not edges (see illustration).

  Ensures accuracy of measurement.

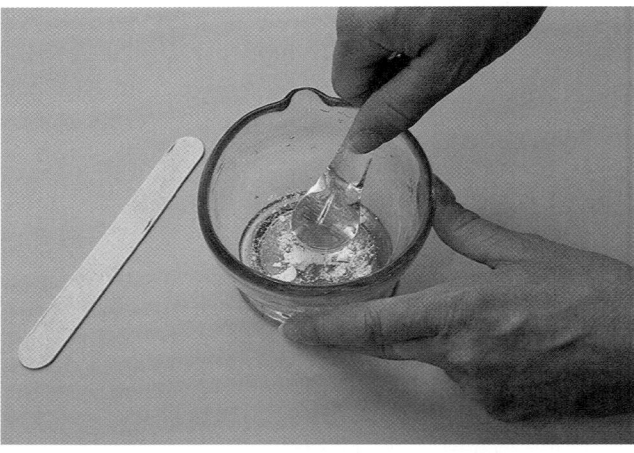

STEP **1j** Pill placed in mortar for crushing.

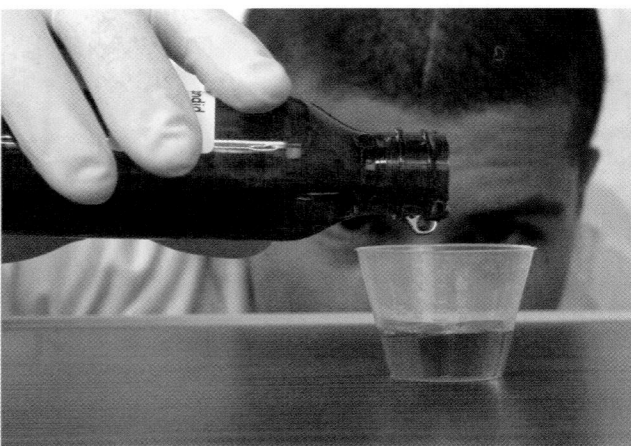

STEP **1k(3)** Pour the desired volume of liquid so that base of meniscus is level with line on scale.

STEP	RATIONALE

(4) Discard any excess liquid into sink. Wipe lip and neck of bottle with paper towel, and recap the bottle.

Prevents contamination of bottle's contents and prevents bottle cap from sticking.

(5) For small doses of liquid medications, draw liquid into a calibrated oral syringe. Do not use a hypodermic syringe or a syringe with a needle or syringe cap.

Using a calibrated oral syringe allows for accurate measuring of small doses of liquid medications.

• Critical Decision Point
Only syringes specifically designed for oral use should be used for administering liquid medications. If hypodermic syringes are used, the medication may be inadvertently administered parenterally, or the syringe cap or needle, if not removed from the syringe before administration, may become dislodged and accidentally aspirated when the syringe plunger is pressed (Institute for Safe Medicine Practices [ISMP], 2001).

l. Check expiration date on all medications.

Medications used past expiration date may be inactive or harmful to client.

m. When preparing narcotics, check narcotic record for previous drug count and compare with supply available.

Controlled substance laws require careful monitoring of dispensed narcotics.

n. Compare MAR with prepared drugs and continue.

Reading label a second time reduces errors.

o. Return stock containers or unused unit-dose medications to shelf or drawer and read label again.

Third check of label reduces administration errors.

p. Do not leave drugs unattended.

Nurse is responsible for safekeeping of drugs.

2. Administer medications:

a. Take medications to client at correct time. Identify client by comparing name on MAR with name on client's identification bracelet. Ask client to state name. Replace any missing or faded identification bracelets.

Identification bracelets are made at time of client's admission and are the most reliable source of identification. Ensures correct client receives medication. At least two patient identifiers (neither to be the patient's room number) are to be used whenever administering medications (JCAHO, 2004).

b. Explain purpose of each medication and its action to client. Allow client to ask any questions about drugs.

Client has right to be informed, and client's understanding of purpose of each medication improves compliance with drug therapy.

• Critical Decision Point
If client refuses medication, withhold medication and notify prescriber.

c. Assist client to a seated or side-lying position if sitting is contraindicated by client's condition.

Decreases risk of aspiration during swallowing.

• Critical Decision Point
Check the client's swallow, cough, and gag reflexes (see Box 20-1) if in doubt about client's ability to manage oral medications. Withhold medication if swallow, cough, or gag reflex is impaired, and notify physician.

d. For tablets: Client may wish to hold solid medications in hand or cup before placing in mouth. Offer water or juice to help client swallow medications.

Client can become familiar with medications by seeing each drug. Choice of fluid promotes client's comfort and can improve fluid intake.

STEP	RATIONALE

   e. **For sublingual-administered medications:** Have client place medication under tongue and allow it to dissolve completely (see illustration). Caution client against swallowing tablet.

Drug is absorbed through blood vessels of undersurface of tongue. If swallowed, drug is destroyed by gastric juices or so rapidly detoxified by liver that therapeutic blood levels are not attained.

   f. **For buccal-administered medications:** Have client place medication in mouth against mucous membranes until it dissolves (see illustration).

- **Critical Decision Point**
  Avoid administering liquids until buccal/sublingual medication has dissolved.

   g. Caution client against chewing or swallowing lozenges.

Drug acts through slow absorption through oral mucosa, not gastric mucosa.

   h. **For powdered medications:** Mix with liquids at bedside, and give to client to drink.

When prepared in advance, powdered drugs may thicken and even harden, making swallowing difficult.

   i. Give effervescent powders and tablets immediately after dissolving.

Effervescence improves unpleasant taste of drug and often relieves gastrointestinal problems.

   j. If client is unable to hold medications, place medication cup to the lips and gently introduce each drug into the mouth, one at a time. Do not rush.

Administering single tablet or capsule eases swallowing and decreases risk of aspiration.

   k. If tablet or capsule falls to the floor, discard it and repeat preparation.

Drug is contaminated when it touches floor.

   l. Stay until client has completely swallowed each medication. Ask client to open mouth if uncertain whether medication has been swallowed.

Nurse is responsible for ensuring that client receives ordered dosage. If left unattended, client may not take dose or may save drugs, causing risk to health.

   m. For highly acidic medications (e.g., aspirin), offer client nonfat snack (e.g., crackers) if not contraindicated by client's condition.

Reduces gastric irritation. The fat content of foods may delay absorption of the medication.

   n. Assist client in returning to comfortable position.

Maintains client's comfort.

   o. Dispose of soiled supplies, and perform hand hygiene.

Reduces transmission of microorganisms.

3. Record administration of medication on MAR. Return MAR to appropriate file for next administration time.

Timely recording reduces medication errors. The MAR is used as reference for when next dose is due. Loss can lead to administration error.

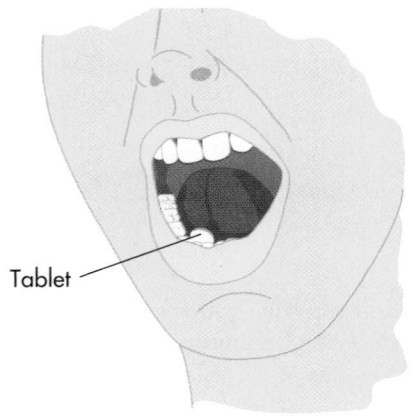

STEP 2e Sublingual administration of a tablet.

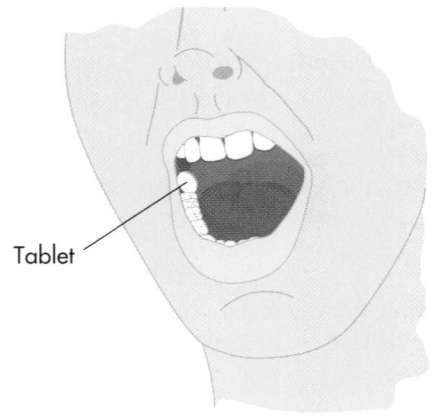

STEP 2f Buccal administration of a tablet.

STEP	RATIONALE

▌ EVALUATION

1. Return within an appropriate time to evaluate client's response to medications.
2. Ask client or family member to identify drug name and explain purpose, action, dose schedule, and potential side effects of drug.

Evaluates drug's therapeutic benefit and can detect onset of side effects or allergic reactions.

Determines level of knowledge gained by client and family.

Recording and Reporting

- Record actual time each drug was administered on MAR immediately after administration. Include initials or signature. Do not chart medication administration until *after* it is given to client.
- If drug is withheld, record reason in nurses' notes. Circle time the drug normally would have been given on MAR (or follow institution's policy for noting withheld doses).
- Report adverse effects/client response and/or withheld drugs to nurse in charge or physician. Depending on medication, immediate prescriber notification may be required.

Unexpected Outcomes	Related Interventions
1. Client exhibits adverse effects (side effect, toxic effect, allergic reaction)	• Withhold further doses. • Notify prescriber and pharmacy. • Symptoms such as urticaria, rash, pruritus, rhinitis, and wheezing may indicate an allergic reaction.
2. Client is unable to explain drug information.	• Further assess the client's or family member's knowledge of medications and guidelines for drug safety. • Further instruction is necessary.
3. Client refuses medication.	• Assess why client is refusing medication. • Do not force client to take medications. • Notify prescriber. • Record refused medication and why.

Teaching Considerations

- Instruct client on specific information pertaining to drug regimen (purpose, action, dose, dosage intervals, side effects, foods to avoid or take with drugs).
- All clients should learn the basic guidelines for drug safety (see Chapter 41).

Pediatric Considerations

- Liquid forms of medication are safer to swallow to avoid aspiration of small pills.
- Bitter or distasteful oral preparation will be rejected by the child. Mix the drug with a small amount (about 1 tsp) of a sweet-tasting substance, such as jam, applesauce, sherbet, ice cream, or fruit puree. Do not use honey in infants because of the risk of botulism. The nurse can also offer the child juice or an ice pop after medication administration. Do not place medication in an essential food item, such as milk or formula; the child may refuse the food at a later time. Give a "chaser" of water, juice, or flavored ice pop after the drug.

- Measure small amount of liquid medications using a plastic calibrated oral dosing syringe or a hollow-handled medicine spoon. Amounts less than a teaspoon are impossible to measure accurately with a molded medicine cup (Hockenberry and others, 2003).

Gerontological Considerations

- Physiological changes of aging influence how oral medications are distributed, absorbed, and excreted. Common changes include loss of elasticity in oral mucosa; reduction in parotid gland secretion, causing dry mouth; delayed esophageal clearance, impaired swallowing; reduction in gastric acidity and stomach peristalsis, increased susceptibility to highly acidic drugs; reduced liver function, resulting in altered drug metabolism and potentially increasing drug toxicity; and, lastly, reduced renal function and reduced colon motility, slowing drug excretion.
- Rinse client's oral cavity frequently with tepid water, floss daily, and brush gently.

- Administer a full glass of water (unless restricted) with medications to aid passage of the drug. Give client time to swallow.
- Older adults may have several health problems or chronic conditions that require the use of multiple drugs, often prescribed by different health care providers. This polypharmacy creates a high risk for drug interactions and adverse reactions. Note if there is a potential for drug interactions, and administer drugs at a different time, if possible.
- The most common adverse reactions that may occur in older adults are lethargy, sedation, falls, confusion, constipation, and gastrointestinal upset.
- When instructing about the medication regimen, include client's spouse or another family member. If possible,

provide a written medication schedule for client to follow at home. Keep in mind that large print may be helpful in written materials if vision is impaired (Ebersole and others, 2004).

Home Care Considerations
- When measuring liquid medications at home, clients should use kitchen measuring spoons, not eating utensil spoons that may vary in volume.
- See Skill 41-3, Medication and Medical Device Safety, and Skill 42-6, Teaching Clients Self-Medication Administration.

SKILL 20-2 Administering Medications by Nasogastric Tube

Clients with nasogastric tubes often receive nothing by mouth. Oral medications that need to be administered to these clients can be given by nasogastric tube. Most commonly, oral medications are given through small-bore feeding tubes. Medications should not be administered into nasogastric/intestinal tubes that are inserted for decompression. To administer medications by a nasogastric tube, the nurse modifies the form of a tablet to be administered by crushing and dissolving it. Medications may also be available in liquid form. Generally, sustained-release, chewable, long-acting, or enteric-coated tablets

and capsules are not administered by gastric tubes. Consult with the hospital pharmacy when in doubt. It is essential to verify correct placement of a nasogastric tube before administering medications.

Some clients may have a percutaneous endoscopic gastrostomy (PEG) tube inserted. PEG tubes are used when long-term enteral feeding is necessary. If medications are ordered to be given through the PEG tube, follow the same steps as for giving medications through a nasogastric tube (see Chapter 30).

DELEGATION CONSIDERATIONS
The skill of administering medications by nasogastric tube should not be delegated to assistive personnel. However, because certain aspects of a client's care may be delegated to assistive personnel, the nurse must:
- Instruct assistive personnel about potential side effects of medications and to report their occurrence

EQUIPMENT
- ❏ 60-ml syringe: catheter tip for large-bore tubes; Luer-Lok tip for small-bore tubes
- ❏ Gastric pH test tape (scale of 0.0 to 11.0 or 14.0 preferred)
- ❏ Graduated container
- ❏ Water
- ❏ Medication to be administered
- ❏ Pill crusher if medication in tablet form
- ❏ Medication administration record
- ❏ Disposable gloves

STEP	RATIONALE

ASSESSMENT

1. Assess for any contraindications to client receiving medication enterally. Has the client been diagnosed as having bowel inflammation or reduced peristalsis? Has client had recent gastrointestinal surgery? Does client have gastric suction? Can the suction be temporarily turned off?

Alterations in gastrointestinal function interfere with drug distribution, absorption, and excretion. Clients with gastrointestinal suction should not receive medications via nasogastric tube because it may be suctioned from gastrointestinal tract before it can be absorbed.

STEP	RATIONALE

- *Critical Decision Point*

  Always review client's postoperative orders for gastric tube care. Manipulation and irrigation of tube or instillation of medication may be contraindicated.

2. Assess client's medical history, history of allergies, medication history, and diet history.

These factors can influence how certain drugs act. Information also reflects client's need for medications. Medication history may reveal past problems with medication administration.

3. Gather and review physical assessment and laboratory data that may influence drug administration, such as vital signs, and renal and liver function studies.

Physical examination or laboratory data may contraindicate drug administration. Renal and liver function status will affect metabolism and excretion of the medication (Lilley and others, 2005).

- *Critical Decision Point*

  If contraindications exist, withhold medication and inform the prescriber of your findings.

4. Before administration of medications verify placement of the gastric tube (see Skill 30-2).

Reduces the risk of aspiration.

NURSING DIAGNOSES
- Impaired swallowing
- Feeding self-care deficit

- Risk for aspiration

Related factors are individualized based on client's condition or needs.

PLANNING
1. Expected outcomes following completion of procedure:
   - Client experiences desired medication effect within period of onset of medication.

   Drug has exerted its therapeutic action.

   - Client's feeding tube remains patent after administration of medication.

   A patent nasogastric tube indicates passage of medication into stomach, ensuring proper absorption. A blocked tube can later interfere with irrigation and fluid instillation.

2. Check accuracy and completeness of each MAR with prescriber's written medication order. Check client's name, drug name and dosage, route of administration, and time for administration. Compare MAR with medication label.

The order sheet is the most reliable source and only legal record of drugs client is to receive. Ensures client receives correct medication.

3. Explain procedure to client, including description of medication to be instilled into nasogastric tube.

Makes client a participant in care and minimizes anxiety. Begins client teaching regarding medications.

IMPLEMENTATION
1. Perform hand hygiene.

Reduces transfer of microorganisms.

2. Prepare medications for instillation into feeding tube. Check label against MAR three times (see Skill 20-1). Fill graduated container with 50 to 100 ml of tepid water.

Adequate preparation saves nursing time. Ensures client receives correct medication.

STEP	RATIONALE

• *Critical Decision Point*

Whenever possible, liquid medications are preferred to crushed tablets, but if tablets must be crushed, the tubing must be flushed before and after the medication to prevent the drug from adhering to the inside of the tube (Lewis and others, 2004). In addition, concentrated medications need to be thoroughly diluted. Never add crushed medications directly to the tube feeding.

STEP	RATIONALE
a. Crush tablets using a pill-crushing device such as a mortar and pestle to grind pills into a fine powder. If a pill-crushing device is not available, place tablet between two medication cups and grind with a blunt instrument. Dissolve in at least 30 ml of warm water.	
b. *Capsules:* Ensure that contents of capsule (granules or gelatin) can be expressed from the covering (consult with pharmacist). Open capsule or pierce gelcap with sterile needle and empty contents into 30 ml of warm water. Gelcaps can also be dissolved in warm water.	Ensures contents of tablets or capsules are a fine powder or solution so as not to occlude nasogastric tube.
3. Check client's identification bracelet, and client to state name.	Ensures correct client receives medication. At least two patient identifiers (neither to be the patient's room number) are to be used whenever administering medications (JCAHO, 2004).
4. Prepare client by placing the client in a high-Fowler's position (if not contraindicated by client's medical condition).	Reduces risk of aspiration.
5. Apply clean gloves.	Reduces transfer of microorganisms.
6. Check placement of feeding tube (see Skill 30-2, p. 1021) by observing gastric contents and checking pH of aspirate contents.	Ensures proper tube placement and reduces the risk of introducing fluids into the respiratory tract (Metheny and Titler, 2001).
7. Check for gastric residual (see illustration). Connect syringe to end of nasogastric tube, then pull back evenly to aspirate gastric contents. Return aspirated contents to stomach unless the volume exceeds 100 ml (or as defined by agency policy), then flush tubing with at least 30 ml of water.	Residual volume indicates if gastric emptying is delayed. Return of aspirate prevents fluid and electrolyte imbalance. Irrigation clears tubing (Ignatavicius and Workman, 2002).

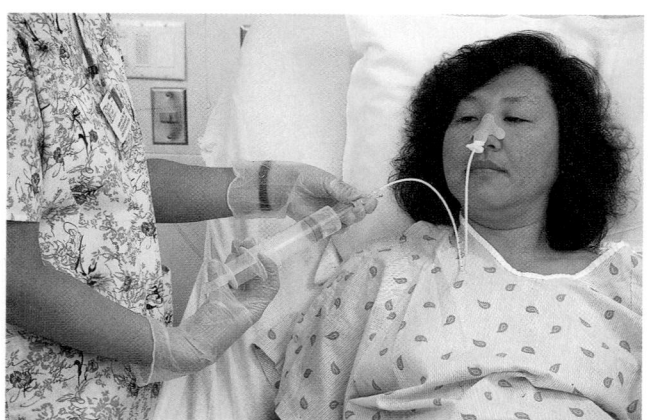

STEP 7 Nurse pulls back on syringe to aspirate stomach contents.

STEP	RATIONALE

- **Critical Decision Point**

  If large-volume aspirate is found (e.g., 100 ml or more), return aspirate to client, withhold medication, and notify client's health care provider. Large-volume aspirates (e.g., 100 to 150 ml) indicate delayed gastric emptying, which may contribute to gastric distention, esophageal reflux, and vomiting, all of which place the client at risk for aspiration (Mahan and Escott-Stump, 2004).

STEP	RATIONALE
8. Pinch nasogastric tube, and remove syringe. Draw up 30 ml of water in syringe. Reinsert tip of syringe into nasogastric tube, and flush tube. Pinch nasogastric tube again.	Pinching nasogastric tube prevents leakage or spillage of stomach contents. Flushing ensures tube is patent.
9. Remove bulb or plunger of syringe.	Removal of bulb or plunger prepares syringe for delivery of medications.
10. Administer first dose of dissolved medication by pouring into syringe.	

- **Critical Decision Point**

  If water or medication does not flow freely, a gentle push with bulb of Asepto syringe or plunger of Toomey syringe may facilitate flow of fluid.

STEP	RATIONALE
a. If only one dose of medication is given, flush with 30 ml of water.	Maintains patency of nasogastric tube.
b. To administer more than one medication, give each separately, and flush between medications with 10 ml of water.	Keeping the medications separate allows for accurate identification of medication if a dose is spilled. In addition, some medications may not be compatible with each other, which could cause clogging of tube (Phipps and others, 2003).
c. Follow last dose of medication with 30 to 60 ml of water.	Maintains patency of nasogastric tube. Ensures passage of medication into stomach (Phipps and others, 2003).
11. When a tube feeding is not being administered, clamp the proximal end of the feeding tube, and cap end of tube.	Prevents air from entering the stomach between medication doses.
12. When continuous tube feeding is being administered by an infusion pump:	
a. Follow medication administration steps 1 to 9, then stop the feeding for 1 hour (check agency policy).	Allows for adequate absorption of medication, and avoids potential drug-food interaction between medication and enteral feeding (Ignatavicius and Workman, 2002).
13. Assist client to comfortable position, but keep the head of the bed elevated for 1 hour after the medication is given.	Prevents aspiration (Ignatavicius and Workman, 2002).
14. Remove gloves, dispose of soiled supplies, and rinse graduated container and syringe with tap water. Perform hand hygiene.	Reduces transmission of microorganisms.

EVALUATION

STEP	RATIONALE
1. Return within 30 minutes to evaluate client's response to medications.	By monitoring client's response, nurse assesses drug's therapeutic benefit and can detect onset of side effects or allergic reactions.

Recording and Reporting

- Record in nurses' notes method used to check placement of nasogastric tube, volume of stomach aspirate, and pH of stomach aspirate (see Chapter 30).
- Record actual time each drug was administered on MAR immediately after administration. Include initials or signature. Do not chart medication administration until *after* it is given to client.
- Record total amount of fluid used for medication administration on proper intake/output sheet.
- If drug is withheld, record reason in nurses' notes. Circle time the drug normally would have been given on MAR (or follow institution's policy for noting withheld doses).
- Report adverse effects/client response and/or withheld drugs to nurse in charge or physician. Depending on medication, immediate prescriber notification may be required.

Unexpected Outcomes	Related Interventions
1. Client exhibits signs of aspiration of administered medications/fluids, which include respiratory distress, changes in vital signs, or changes in oxygen saturation.	• Stop all medications/fluids through the tube. • Elevate the head of the bed, and stay with the client. • Assess vital signs and breath sounds while another staff member notifies the client's physician.
2. Client does not receive medication as prescribed because of a blocked nasogastric tube.	• Requires interventions to unclog tube to ensure drug delivery (Box 20-2).
3. Client exhibits adverse effects (side effect, toxic effect, allergic reaction).	• Withhold further doses. • Always notify prescriber and pharmacy when the client exhibits adverse effects. • Symptoms such as urticaria, rash, pruritus, rhinitis, and wheezing may indicate an allergic reaction.

BOX 20-2   Unclogging a Blocked Feeding Tube

- Prevent tube from becoming blocked by flushing it with at least 30 ml of tepid water before and after administering each dose of medication, before and after checking gastric residual volumes, and every 4 to 6 hours around the clock.
- If a tube becomes blocked, first try to irrigate it gently with tepid water.
- If irrigation with water is not effective, obtain an order for a pancrelipase tablet (such as Viokase) and follow manufacturer's guidelines for irrigation of the tube. In addition, a declogging stylus may be used.
- The tube may have to be removed and a new one reinserted if the medication is urgent.

Modified from Lewis SM and others: *Medical-surgical nursing: assessment and management of clinical problems,* ed 6, St. Louis, 2004, Mosby.

Teaching Considerations

- In the home setting, provide instruction so clients/family members can administer medications safely.
  - Instruct client or family on how to store medications and tube feeding supplements (see Chapter 30).
  - Teach client or family how to verify correct placement of tube before medication or tube feeding administration.
  - Instruct family about the importance of consistent irrigation of feeding tube following medication administration.
  - Provide client and family resources to determine which medications can be crushed, how to obtain medications that may be crushed, or how to obtain liquid formulations of medications.

Pediatric Considerations

- Volumes for instillation of medications or for irrigation of nasogastric tubes may be smaller. Check agency policy (Miller and Miller, 2000).

Gerontological Considerations

- Older adults with visual impairment may need assistance or magnifiers to determine the accurate volume of medication.

SKILL 20-3 Administering Skin Applications

Many locally applied drugs such as lotions, patches, pastes, and ointments can create systemic and local effects if absorbed through the skin. To protect from accidental exposure, the nurse should apply these drugs using gloves and applicators. If the client's skin is intact, the nurse uses clean technique when applying lotions, patches, and ointments. If the client has an open wound, sterile technique is essential.

Skin encrustations and dead tissue harbor microorganisms and block contact of medications with the tissues to be treated. Simply applying new medications over previously applied drugs does little to prevent infection or offer therapeutic benefit. The nurse cleans the skin thoroughly before applying medications by washing the area gently with soap and water, soaking an involved site, or locally debriding tissue. Each type of medication, whether an ointment, lotion, powder, or patch, should be applied in a specific way to ensure proper penetration and absorption.

DELEGATION CONSIDERATIONS

The skill of administering skin (topical) medications should not be delegated to assistive personnel. However, some institutions may permit assistive personnel to apply some forms of topical agents, such as lotions, ointment, and powders, to irritated skin or for the protection of the perineum, during morning care. Check agency policies. The nurse must instruct assistive personnel about the expected therapeutic effects and potential side effects of medications and to report their occurrence.

- If assistive personnel are permitted to apply topical agents, ensure that the correct method and site of application is understood, and ensure the six rights of medication administration.

EQUIPMENT

- ❏ Clean gloves (for intact skin) or sterile gloves (for nonintact skin)
- ❏ Ordered agent (powder, cream, lotion, ointment, spray, patch)
- ❏ Cotton-tipped applicators or tongue blades (optional)
- ❏ Basin of warm water, washcloth, towel, nondrying soap
- ❏ Sterile dressing, tape (if needed)
- ❏ Medication administration record

STEP	RATIONALE

ASSESSMENT

1. Assess condition of client's skin. First wash site thoroughly with mild, nondrying soap and warm water, rinse, and dry. Be sure any previously applied medication or debris is removed. Also remove any blood, body fluids, secretions, or excretions. Assess for symptoms of skin irritation such as pruritus or burning.

Cleansing site thoroughly allows nurse to obtain a proper assessment of skin surface. Assessment provides baseline to determine change in condition of skin after therapy. Application of certain topical agents can lessen or aggravate these symptoms.

STEP	RATIONALE
2. Further inspect the condition of the skin or membranes. Do not administer topical medications to skin whose integrity is altered, unless indicated.	Break in skin integrity can affect drug absorption and actions.
3. Determine whether client has known allergy to topical agent. Ask if client has had reaction to a cream or lotion applied to the skin.	Allergic contact dermatitis is relatively common and can worsen dermatological condition. In addition, some clients may be allergic to preservatives or fragrances in topical medications.
4. Determine amount of topical agent required for application by assessing affected area, reviewing prescriber's order, and reading application directions carefully (a thin, even layer is usually adequate).	An excessive amount of topical agent can cause chemical irritation of skin, negate drug's effectiveness, and/or cause adverse systemic effects, such as decreased white cell counts.
5. Assess client's knowledge of action and purpose of medication being given and interest in treating health problem.	Reveals client's level of understanding and whether instruction is necessary.
6. Determine if client is physically able to apply medication by assessing fine grasp, hand strength, reach, and coordination.	Necessary if client is to self-administer drug in the home.

NURSING DIAGNOSES

- Impaired skin integrity
- Ineffective therapeutic regimen management
- Deficient knowledge regarding medication application

- Pain (acute, chronic)
- Impaired physical mobility

Related factors are individualized based on client's condition or needs.

PLANNING

1. Expected outcomes following completion of procedure:	
• Client is able to identify drug and describe action, purpose, dose, side effects, and schedule of medication.	Demonstrates learning.
• Client is able to apply medication without assistance on prescribed schedule.	Demonstrates learning and compliance.
• With repeated applications, skin becomes clear, without inflammation or drainage from lesions.	Existing lesions heal and/or disappear as a result of medication's therapeutic action.
2. Check accuracy and completeness of each MAR with prescriber's written medication order. Check client's name, drug name and dosage, route of administration, and time for administration. Compare MAR with medication label three times during preparation of medication.	The order sheet is the most reliable source and only legal record of drugs client is to receive. Ensures client receives correct medication.
3. Check client's identification bracelet, and ask name.	Ensures correct client receives medication. At least two patient identifiers (neither to be the patient's room number) are to be used whenever administering medications (JCAHO, 2004).
4. Explain procedure to client, including description of skin area to be treated.	Makes client a participant in care and minimizes anxiety.

IMPLEMENTATION

1. Perform hand hygiene and arrange supplies at bedside. If skin is broken (e.g., wound), use sterile gloves; otherwise apply clean gloves.	Reduces transmission of infection. Sterile gloves are used when applying agents to open noninfectious skin lesions. Topical agents are not usually premeasured in medication room. The use of gloves also prevents absorption of the medication into the nurse's skin.
2. Close room curtain or door, and position client comfortably. Remove gown or bed linen so as to keep unaffected skin areas draped.	Provides client privacy and easy access to area being treated. Promotes client's comfort.

STEP	RATIONALE

3. Apply topical agent.
   a. Technique for applying creams, ointments, and oil-based lotions:

      (1) Place required amount of medication in palm of gloved hand and soften by rubbing briskly between hands.

      Softening of topical agent makes it easier to spread on skin.

      (2) Once medication is softened, spread it evenly over skin surface, using long, even strokes that follow direction of hair growth. Apply to the thickness specified by manufacturer's instructions.

      Ensures even distribution and sufficient dosage of medication. Technique prevents irritation of hair follicles.

      (3) Explain to client that skin may feel greasy after application.

      Ointments often contain oils.

   b. Technique for applying nitroglycerin (an antianginal) ointment:

      (1) Apply desired number of inches of ointment over paper measuring guide (see illustration).

      Ensures correct dose of medication. Antianginal (nitroglycerin) ointments are usually ordered in inches and can be measured on small sheets of paper marked off in $\frac{1}{2}$-inch markings. Unit-dose packages are available. (**Warning:** One package equals 1 inch; smaller amount should not be measured from this package.)

      (2) Remove previous dose paper. Wipe off residual medication with tissue.

      Prevents overdose that can occur with multiple dose papers left in place.

      (3) Antianginal medication may be applied to the chest area, back, upper arm, or legs. Do not apply on hairy surfaces or over scar tissue.

      If client complains of headaches, apply ointment farther from head. Application on hairy surfaces or scar tissue may interfere with absorption.

      (4) Rotate site when applying nitroglycerin pastes.

      Prevents skin irritation.

      (5) Apply ointment to skin surface by holding edge or back of the paper measuring guide and placing ointment and wrapper directly on the skin (see illustration). Do not rub or massage ointment into skin.

      Minimizes chance of ointment covering gloves and later touching nurse's hands. Medication is designed to absorb slowly over several hours; massaging may increase absorption rate.

      (6) Date and initial paper, and note time.

      Prevents missing doses.

      (7) Secure ointment and paper with a transparent dressing or strip of tape. Plastic wrap may be used as an occlusive dressing.

      Prevents staining of clothing or inadvertent removal of the medication (McConnell, 2001).

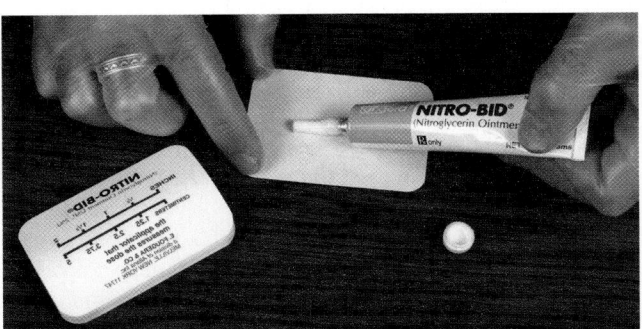

STEP 3b(1) Ointment spread in inches over measuring guide.

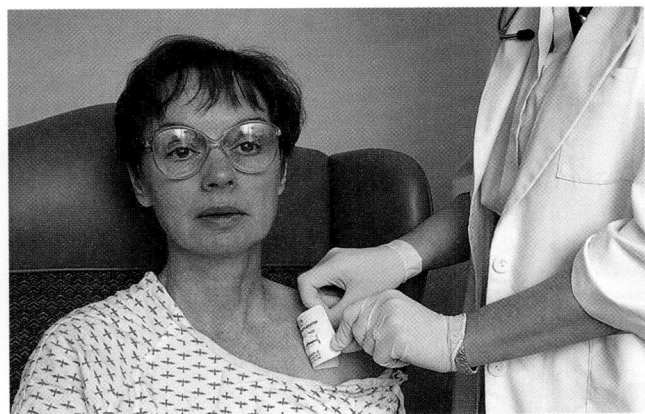

STEP 3b(5) Nurse applies wrapper with medication on client's skin.

STEP	**RATIONALE**

c. A variety of medications are available as transdermal (skin) patches (see illustration). Technique for applying a transdermal patch:

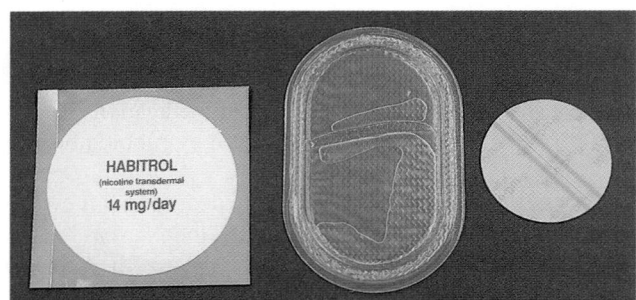

STEP **3c** Examples of transdermal (skin) patches

(1) Locate and remove old patch before applying a new one. If necessary, cleanse the area.

Failure to remove the old patch can result in drug overdose if a new patch is applied and the old patch remains on. Cleansing the area may be necessary to remove traces of the older dose and adhesive, which may irritate the skin.

(2) Date and initial the outer side of the patch before applying it, and note time. Use a soft-tip or felt-tip marker pen.

Visual reminder prevents missing or extra doses. It is better to write on the patch before it is applied to the client's skin. Take care not to damage the patch with a sharp pen.

(3) Choose a clean, dry area of the body that is free of hair. Some patches have specific instructions for placement locations (e.g., Testoderm scrotal patches).

Increases absorption. Proper placement ensures correct delivery of drug.

• ***Critical Decision Point***

Do not attempt to apply the patch on skin that is oily, burned, broken out, cut, or irritated in any way.

(4) Carefully remove the patch from its protective covering. Hold the patch by the edge; do not touch the adhesive edges.

Touching only the edges ensures that the patch will adhere and that the medication dose has not been changed. The protective covering must be removed to allow the medication to be absorbed through the skin.

(5) Immediately apply the patch, pressing firmly with the palm of one hand for 10 seconds. Make sure it sticks well, especially around the edges. Apply overlay if provided with patch.

Sufficient pressure is needed to ensure that the adhesive will keep the patch on the skin surface.

(6) When the next dose is due, remove the old patch, and choose a different site. Do not apply to previously used sites for at least 1 week.

Rotation of sites reduces skin irritation from medication and adhesive.

• ***Critical Decision Point***

It is recommended that nitroglycerin transdermal patches be removed after 10 to 12 hours to allow for a nitrate-free interval and reduce the chance of tolerance to the medication. Check with the client's prescriber (Lilley and others, 2005).

(7) Dispose of patches by folding in half with sticky sides together. Throw the patch in the trash away from children and pets. Some agencies require the patch to be cut before disposal.

Proper disposal protects others from accidental exposure to medication (Lee and Phillips, 2002).

STEP	**RATIONALE**

d. Technique for applying aerosolized medication (spray):

   (1) Shake container vigorously.

Mixes contents and propellant to ensure distribution of fine, even spray.

   (2) Read container's label for distance recommended to hold spray away from area (usually 6 to 12 inches, 15 to 30 cm).

Proper distance ensures fine spray hits skin surface. Holding container too close results in thin, watery distribution.

   (3) If neck or upper chest is to be sprayed, ask client to turn face away from spray or briefly cover face with towel.

Prevents inhalation of spray.

   (4) Spray medication evenly over affected site (in some cases spray is timed for select period of seconds).

Entire affected area of skin should be covered with thin spray.

e. Technique for applying a suspension-based lotion:

   (1) Shake container vigorously.

Mixes powder throughout liquid to form well-mixed suspension.

   (2) Apply small amount of lotion to small gauze dressing or pad, and apply to skin by stroking evenly in direction of hair growth.

Method of application leaves protective film of powder on skin after water base of suspension dries. Technique prevents irritation to hair follicles.

   (3) Explain to client that area will feel cool and dry.

Water evaporates to leave thin layer of powder.

f. Technique for applying a powder:

   (1) Be sure skin surface is thoroughly dry.

Minimizes caking and crusting of powder.

   (2) Fully spread apart any skin folds such as between toes or under axilla and dry with a towel.

Fully exposes skin surface for application.

   (3) Dust skin site lightly with dispenser so that area is covered with fine, thin layer of powder.

A thin layer of powder has slight lubricating properties to reduce friction and promote drying (Lilley and others, 2005).

4. Cover skin area with dressing if ordered by physician.

May help prevent agent from being rubbed off skin. Protects clothing from being stained.

5. Assist client to comfortable position, reapply gown, and cover with bed linen as desired.

Provides for client's sense of well-being.

6. Remove gloves, dispose of soiled supplies in receptacle especially designated for such articles, and perform hand hygiene.

Keeps client's environment neat and reduces transmission of infection and/or residual medication to children, pets, or others.

EVALUATION

1. Ask the client or significant other to name the medication and its action, purpose, dose, schedule, and side effects.

Evaluates learning.

2. Have client keep a diary of doses taken.

Confirm compliance with prescribed therapy.

3. Observe client apply lotion, ointment, or patch.

Return demonstration measures learning.

4. Inspect condition of skin between applications.

Determines if skin condition improves.

Recording and Reporting

- Describe condition of skin before topical agent application in nurses' notes.
- Record actual time each drug was administered, type of agent applied, strength, and site of application in nurses' notes and on MAR immediately after administration. Include initials or signature. Do not chart medication administration until *after* it is given to client.
- If drug is withheld, record reason in nurses' notes. Circle time drug normally would have been given on MAR (or follow institution's policy for noting withheld doses).
- Report adverse effects/client response and/or withheld drugs to nurse in charge or physician. Depending on medication, immediate prescriber notification may be required.
- Report any abnormalities in condition of skin to nurse in charge or physician.

Unexpected Outcomes	Related Interventions
1. Skin site may appear inflamed and edematous with blistering and oozing of fluid from lesions. These signs are indicative of subacute inflammation or eczema that can develop if skin lesions are getting worse.	• Notify prescriber; alternative therapies may be needed.
2. Client continues to complain of pruritus and tenderness. Indicates slow or impaired healing.	• Notify prescriber; alternative therapies may be needed.
3. Client is unable to explain information about drug or does not administer as prescribed.	• Identify possible reasons for noncompliance. • Reinstruction is necessary, or client is unable to learn. • Offer client or family opportunity to apply topical agent during next application and to ask questions. • Reexplore client's health beliefs and resources.

Teaching Considerations

• If skin is inflamed, instruct clients to use only warm water rinse without soap for cleansing.
• When applying creams or ointments, warn clients not to pat or vigorously rub skin. This may cause irritation.
• When applying powders, take care that the client does not inhale the powdered medication.
• Include a family member or friend when possible during instruction about topical application of medications.
• When instructing client, be sure lighting is adequate and area to be treated is well exposed.
• Have client demonstrate the application technique to ensure effective therapy and compliance (Lilley and others, 2005).

Gerontological Considerations

• Many changes occur in the skin of the older adult client. The nurse should be aware of these changes when applying topical medications so that proper application can occur. For example, the older adult client's skin is often subject to increased capillary fragility, which can lead to bruising. The nurse handles the skin gently when applying an ointment. Table 20-1 lists common age-related skin changes and assessment findings.

Home Care Considerations

• Instruct client to wrap applicators, used patches, and similar materials and dispose into cardboard or plastic disposable containers. Careful disposal is necessary to ensure the safety of client, other adults, pets, and children.

TABLE 20-1   EFFECT OF AGING ON THE INTEGUMENTARY SYSTEM

CHANGES	ASSESSMENT FINDINGS
Decreased subcutaneous fat, muscle laxity, degeneration of elastic fibers, collagen stiffening	Increased wrinkling, sagging breast and abdomen, redundant flesh around eyes, slowness of skin to flatten when pinched together (tenting)
Decreased extracellular water, surface lipids, and sebaceous gland activity	Dry, flaking skin with possible signs of excoriation caused by pruritus
Increased capillary fragility and permeability	Evidence of bruising
Increased melanocytes in basal layer with pigment accumulation	Senile lentigines on face and back of hands
Diminished blood supply	Decrease in rosy appearance of skin and mucous membranes; cool to touch; diminished awareness of pain, touch, temperature, and peripheral vibration
Decrease in skin cell proliferative capacity	Diminished rate of wound healing

Modified from Lewis SM and others: *Medical-surgical nursing: assessment and management of clinical problems,* ed 6, St. Louis, 2004, Mosby.

SKILL 20-4 Administering Eye Medications

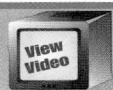

Common eye (ophthalmic) medications used by clients are drops and ointments, including over-the-counter preparations such as artificial tears and vasoconstrictors (e.g., Visine and Murine). However, many clients receive prescribed ophthalmic drugs for eye conditions such as glaucoma and infections and following cataract extraction. In addition, a third type of delivery system, the intraocular disk, is used. Medications delivered by disk resemble a contact lens, but the disk is placed in the conjunctival sac, not the cornea, and it remains in place for up to 1 week.

The eye is the most sensitive organ to which the nurse applies medications. The cornea is richly supplied with sensitive nerve fibers. Care must be taken to prevent instilling medication directly onto the cornea. The conjunctival sac is much less sensitive and thus a more appropriate site for medication instillation.

Any client receiving topical eye medications should learn correct self-administration of the medication, especially clients with glaucoma, who must often undergo lifelong medication administration for control of their disease. Nurses can easily instruct clients while administering medications. At times it may become necessary for family members to learn how to administer eye medications. This is particularly true immediately after eye surgery, when a client's vision is so impaired that it is difficult to assemble needed supplies and handle applicators correctly.

Eye medications come in a variety of concentrations. Instilling the wrong concentration may cause local irritation of eyes, as well as systemic effects. Certain eye medications, such as mydriatics and cycloplegics, temporarily blur a client's vision. Use of the wrong drug concentration can prolong these undesirable effects.

DELEGATION CONSIDERATIONS

The skill of administering eye medications should not be delegated to assistive personnel. However, because certain aspects of a client's care may be delegated to assistive personnel, the nurse must:

- Instruct assistive personnel about potential side effects of medications and to report their occurrence
- Instruct care providers in the potential for temporary visual impairment after administration of eye medications

EQUIPMENT

- ❑ Medication bottle with sterile eye dropper, ointment tube, or medicated intraocular disk
- ❑ Cotton ball or tissue
- ❑ Washbasin filled with warm water and washcloth
- ❑ Eye patch and tape (optional)
- ❑ Clean gloves
- ❑ Medication administration record (MAR)

STEP	RATIONALE

ASSESSMENT

1. Review prescriber's medication order for number of drops (if a liquid) and eye (right, left, or both) to receive medication.

Ensures correct administration of medication.

2. Assess condition of external eye structures (may also be done just before drug instillation.)

Provides baseline to later determine if local response to medications occurs. Also indicates need to clean eye before drug application.

3. Determine whether client has any known allergies to eye medications. Also ask if client has allergy to latex.

Protects client from risk of allergic drug response. Latex allergy requires use of nonlatex gloves.

4. Determine whether client has any symptoms of visual alterations.

Certain eye medications act to either lessen or increase these symptoms. Nurse must be able to recognize change in client's condition.

5. Assess client's level of consciousness and ability to follow directions.

If client becomes restless or combative during procedure, a greater risk of accidental eye injury exists.

6. Assess client's knowledge regarding drug therapy and desire to self-administer medication.

Client's level of understanding may indicate need for health teaching. Motivation influences teaching approach.

7. Assess client's ability to manipulate and hold dropper.

Reflects client's ability to learn to self-administer drug.

STEP	RATIONALE

NURSING DIAGNOSES

- Deficient knowledge regarding drug actions, purpose, and self-administration
- Health-seeking behaviors (self-care)
- Pain (acute or chronic)

- Disturbed sensory perception (visual)
- Impaired physical mobility
- Risk for injury

Related factors are individualized based on client's condition or needs.

PLANNING

1. Expected outcomes following completion of procedure:
   - Client experiences desired effect of medication.
   - Client denies discomfort.
   - Client experiences no side effects, and symptoms (e.g., irritation) are relieved.
   - Client is able to discuss information about medication and technique correctly.
   - Client demonstrates self-instillation of eye drops.

   Drug is administered correctly without injury to client.
   Drug is administered correctly without injury to client.
   Drug is distributed and absorbed properly.

   Demonstrates learning.

   Demonstrates learning.

2. Check accuracy and completeness of each MAR with prescriber's written medication order. Check client's name, drug name and dosage, route of administration, and time for administration. Compare MAR with label of eye medication three times during preparation of medication.

   The order sheet is the most reliable source and only legal record of drugs client is to receive. Ensures right drug is administered.

3. Check client's identification bracelet, and ask name.

   Ensures correct client receives medication. At least two patient identifiers (neither to be the patient's room number) are to be used whenever administering medications (JCAHO, 2004).

4. Explain procedure to client.

   Relieves anxiety about medication being instilled into eye.

IMPLEMENTATION

1. Perform hand hygiene, and arrange supplies at bedside; apply clean gloves.

   Reduces transmission of microorganisms; ensures a smooth, orderly procedure.

   a. If eye drops are stored in refrigerator, rewarm to room temperature before administering.

   Reduces irritation to eye due to cold temperature of solution.

2. Ask client to lie supine or sit back in chair with head slightly hyperextended.

   Position provides easy access to eye for medication instillation and minimizes drainage of medication through tear duct.

- *Critical Decision Point*
  Do not hyperextend the neck of a client with cervical spine injury.

STEP	**RATIONALE**

3. If crusts or drainage are present along eyelid margins or inner canthus, gently wash away. Soak any crusts that are dried and difficult to remove by applying damp washcloth or cotton ball over eye for a few minutes. Always wipe clean from inner to outer canthus (see illustration).

Crusts or drainage harbor microorganisms. Soaking allows easy removal and prevents pressure from being applied directly over eye. Cleansing from inner to outer canthus avoids entrance of microorganisms into lacrimal duct.

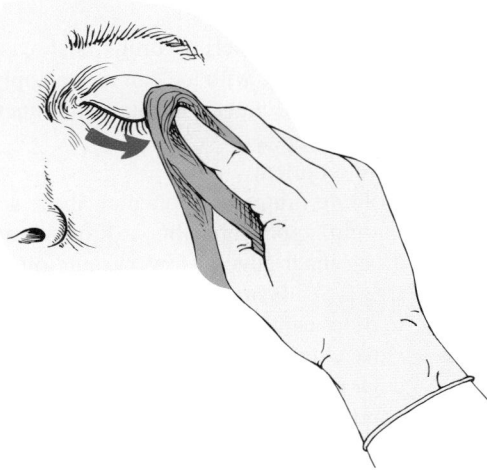

STEP **3** Cleanse eye, washing from inner to outer canthus before administering drops or ointment.

4. Hold cotton ball or clean tissue in nondominant hand on client's cheekbone just below lower eyelid.

Cotton or tissue absorbs medication that escapes eye.

5. With tissue or cotton resting below lower lid, gently press downward with thumb or forefinger against bony orbit. Never press directly against client's eyeball.

Technique exposes lower conjunctival sac. Retraction against bony orbit prevents pressure and trauma to eyeball and prevents fingers from touching eye. Pressure to the eyeball may cause damage.

6. Ask client to look at ceiling and explain steps to client.

Action moves sensitive cornea up and away from conjunctival sac and reduces stimulation of blink reflex. Explanation facilitates the client's cooperation with the procedure.

   a. Instill eye drops:

     (1) With dominant hand resting on client's forehead, hold filled medication eye dropper approximately 1 to 2 cm ($\frac{1}{2}$ to $\frac{3}{4}$ inch) above conjunctival sac (see illustration).

Helps prevent accidental contact of eye dropper with eye structures, thus reducing risk of injury to eye and transfer of infection to dropper. Ophthalmic medications are sterile.

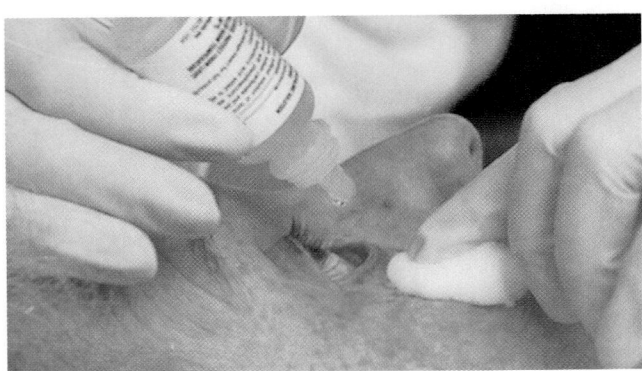

STEP **6a(1)** Eye dropper held above conjunctival sac.

STEP	RATIONALE

    (2) Drop prescribed number of medication drops into conjunctival sac.

Conjunctival sac normally holds 1 or 2 drops. Provides even distribution of medication across eye.

    (3) If client blinks or closes eye, or if drops fall on outer lid margins, repeat procedure.

Therapeutic effect of drug is obtained only when drops enter conjunctival sac.

    (4) After instilling drops, ask client to close eye gently.

Helps to distribute medication. Squinting or squeezing of eyelids forces medication from conjunctival sac.

    (5) When administering drugs that cause systemic effects, with a clean tissue apply gentle pressure to client's nasolacrimal duct for 30 to 60 seconds.

Prevents overflow of medication into nasal and pharyngeal passages. Prevents absorption into systemic circulation.

  b. Instill eye ointment:

    (1) Holding ointment applicator above lower lid margin, apply thin ribbon of ointment evenly along inner edge of lower eyelid on conjunctiva (see illustration) from the inner canthus to outer canthus.

Distributes medication evenly across eye and lid margin.

    (2) Have client close eye and rub lid lightly in circular motion with cotton ball, if rubbing is not contraindicated.

Further distributes medication without traumatizing eye.

  c. Intraocular disk

    (1) Application:

      (a) Perform hand hygiene, and apply gloves.

Reduces transmission of microorganisms.

      (b) Open package containing the disk. Gently press your fingertip against the disk so that it adheres to your finger. (NOTE: It may be necessary to moisten gloved finger with sterile saline.) Position the convex side of the disk on your fingertip.

Allows nurse to inspect disk for damage or deformity. Prepares disk for proper administration.

      (c) With your other hand, gently pull the client's lower eyelid away from his eye. Ask client to look up.

Prepares conjunctival sac for receiving medicated disk.

      (d) Place the disk in the conjunctival sac, so that it floats on the sclera between the iris and lower eyelid (see illustration).

Ensures delivery of medication.

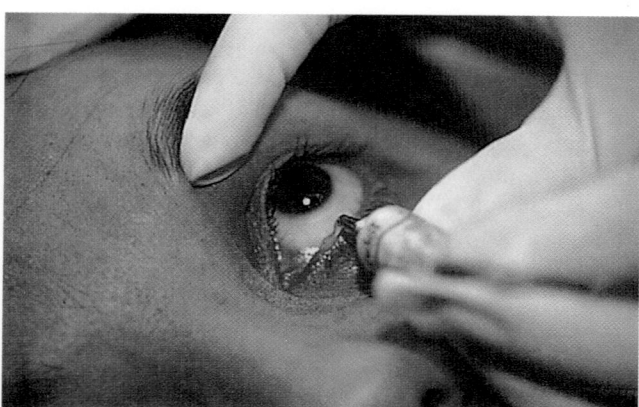

STEP **6b(1)** Nurse applies ointment along the lower eyelid from the inner to outer canthus.

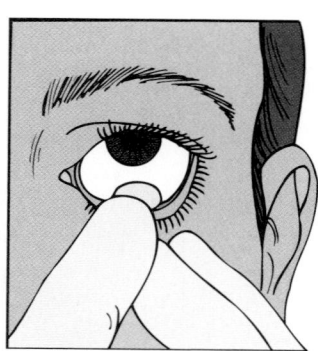

STEP **6c(1)d** Place intraocular disk in the conjunctival sac between the iris and the lower eyelid.

STEP	RATIONALE

(e) Pull the client's lower eyelid out and over the disk (see illustration).

Ensures accurate medication delivery.

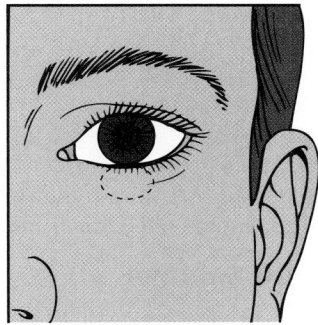

STEP **6c(1)e** Gently pull the client's lower eyelid over the disk.

• *Critical Decision Point*
You should not be able to see the disk at this time. Repeat step (e) if you can see the disk.

(2) Removal:
    (a) Perform hand hygiene, and apply gloves.
    (b) Explain procedure to client.
    (c) Gently pull on the client's lower eyelid to expose the disk.
    (d) Using your forefinger and thumb of your opposite hand, pinch the disk, and lift it out of the client's eye (see illustration).

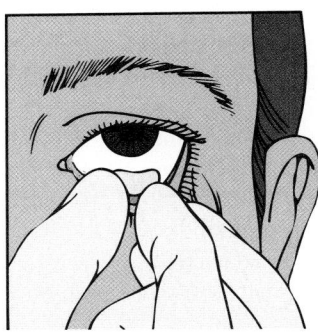

STEP **6c(2)d** Carefully pinch the disk to remove it from the client's eye.

7. If excess medication is on eyelid, gently wipe it from inner to outer canthus.
8. If client had eye patch, apply clean one by placing it over affected eye so entire eye is covered. Tape securely without applying pressure to eye.
9. Assist client to comfortable position.
10. Remove gloves, dispose of soiled supplies in proper receptacle, and perform hand hygiene.
11. Clients experienced in self-instillation may be allowed to give drops under nurse's supervision (check agency policy).

Promotes comfort and prevents trauma to eye.

Clean eye patch reduces chance of infection.

Provides for client's sense of well-being.
Maintains neat environment at bedside and reduces transmission of microorganisms.

STEP	RATIONALE
EVALUATION	
1. Note client's response to instillation; ask if any discomfort was felt.	Determines if procedure was performed correctly and safely.
2. Observe response to medication by assessing visual changes, asking if symptoms are relieved, and noting any side effects.	Evaluates effects of medication.
3. Ask client to discuss drug's purpose, action, side effects, and technique of administration.	Determines client's level of understanding.
4. Have client demonstrate self-administration of next dose.	Provides feedback regarding competency with skill.

Recording and Reporting

- Record drug, concentration, number of drops, time of administration, and eye (left, right, or both) that received medication on MAR immediately after administration. Include initials or signature. Do not chart medication administration until *after* it is given to the client.
- If drug is withheld, record reason in nurses' notes. Circle time the drug normally would have been given on MAR (or follow institution's policy for noting withheld doses).
- Record appearance of eye in nurses' notes.
- Report adverse effects/client response and/or withheld drugs to nurse in charge or physician. Depending on medication, immediate prescriber notification may be required.

Unexpected Outcomes	Related Interventions
1. Client complains of burning or pain or experiences local side effects (e.g., headache, bloodshot eyes, local eye irritation). The drug concentration and the client's sensitivity both influence the chances of side effects developing.	• Eye drops may have been instilled onto the cornea, or the dropper touched the surface of the eye. • Notify prescriber for a possible adjustment in medication type and dosage.
2. Client experiences systemic effects from drops (e.g., increased heart rate and blood pressure from epinephrine, decreased heart rate and blood pressure from timolol). • Systemic absorption through tear duct can cause potentially dangerous effects. • Ophthalmic anesthetics and antibiotics may cause the same type of adverse reactions as systemically administered drugs (e.g., anaphylaxis).	• Notify prescriber immediately. • Remain with client. • Withhold further doses.
3. Client is unable to discuss information about medication correctly.	• Reinstruction is needed, or client is unable to learn. • Discuss with family member or caregiver.
4. Client is unable to instill eye drops.	• Further practice is necessary. • Clients who will be administering drugs at home should demonstrate instillation until performed correctly. • Instruct family member as needed.

Teaching Considerations

- Warn clients receiving mydriatics that vision will be temporarily blurred. Wearing sunglasses will reduce photophobia. If necessary, arrangement may need to be made for someone else to drive the client home from an office or clinic visit.
- Clients who receive medications that paralyze the ciliary muscles of the eye (e.g., scopolamine, Isopto-Hyoscine, atropine, Isopto Atropine, and cycloplegics) should temporarily not drive or attempt to perform any activity that requires acute vision.
- Many clients lack confidence in their ability to instill drops without supervision. Others are unable to manipulate the dropper or are unable to see. The nurse teaches others, such as a family member, to instill drops into client's eye.

Pediatric Considerations

- When instilling drops in an infant or young child, have parent gently restrain child's head with child in parent's lap. Be sure that child's hands do not interfere with instillation.
- Infants often clench the eyes tightly to avoid eye drops. To administer drops in an uncooperative infant, with the head gently restrained, place the drops at the nasal corner where the lids meet. When the child opens the eye the medication will flow into the eye.
- Eye ointments are easily placed into the sleeping child's eye (Hockenberry and others, 2003).

Gerontological Considerations

- Before discharging older adult client, nurse evaluates client's ability to perform all the necessary steps for the administration of eye drops and ointments.

- Nurse teaches family members of clients unable to perform the necessary skills. Clients without this type of assistance should be evaluated for home care nursing.

Home Care Considerations

- Clients with chronic health care problems should consult with their health care provider before using over-the-counter eye medications.
- When using over-the-counter eye drops, clients should not share medications with other family members. Risk of infection transmission is high. In addition, clients should be instructed to follow manufacturer's instructions carefully for dosing.

SKILL 20-5 Administering Ear Drops

When administering ear (otic) medications the nurse should be aware of certain safety precautions. Internal ear structures are very sensitive to temperature extremes. Failure to instill a solution at room temperature can cause vertigo (severe dizziness) or nausea and debilitate a client for several minutes. Although structures of the outer ear are not sterile, use sterile drops and solutions in case the eardrum is ruptured.

Entrance of nonsterile solutions into the middle ear can cause serious infection. A final precaution is to avoid forcing any solution into the ear. The nurse must not occlude the ear canal with a medicine dropper, because this can cause pressure within the canal during instillation and subsequent injury to the eardrum. If these precautions are followed, instillation of ear drops is a safe and effective therapy.

DELEGATION CONSIDERATIONS

The skill of administering ear medications should not be delegated to assistive personnel. However, because certain aspects of the client's care, such as hygiene and vital signs, may be delegated to an assistive personnel, the nurse must:

- Instruct assistive personnel about potential side effects of medications and to report their occurrence
- Instruct assistive personnel to report any dizziness or light-headedness to the nurse for further assessment

EQUIPMENT

- ❑ Medication bottle with dropper
- ❑ Cotton-tipped applicator
- ❑ Cotton ball (optional)
- ❑ Clean gloves (optional, only if client has drainage)
- ❑ Medication administration record (MAR)

STEP	RATIONALE

ASSESSMENT

1. Review prescriber's medication order for number of drops to instill and which ear (right, left, or both) is to receive medication.

2. Assess condition of external ear structures and canal (see Chapter 18).

Ensures safe and correct administration of medication.

Provides baseline to later determine if local response to medication occurs, whether client's condition improves, or whether it will be necessary to clean ear before instilling medication.

STEP	RATIONALE
3. Determine whether client has symptoms of discomfort and/or hearing impairment.	Disorders of external ear can be painful. Occlusion of external ear canal by swelling, drainage, or cerumen can impair hearing acuity. These conditions may change after drug instillation and require ongoing monitoring.
4. Assess client's level of consciousness and ability to follow instructions.	Client must lie still during drug administration. Sudden movements can cause injury from ear dropper.
5. Assess client's level of knowledge regarding drug therapy and motivation to self-administer medication.	Client's knowledge level determines whether health teaching is required. Motivation influences teaching approach.
6. Assess client's ability to grasp and manipulate dropper.	Determines client's ability to self-administer drug.

NURSING DIAGNOSES

- Deficient knowledge regarding drug actions and purpose
- Health-seeking behaviors (self-care)
- Pain (acute or chronic)

- Disturbed sensory perception (auditory)
- Impaired physical mobility
- Risk for injury

Related factors are individualized based on client's condition or needs.

PLANNING

1. Expected outcomes following completion of procedure:	
• Client denies discomfort during administration.	Procedure is performed correctly without injury to client.
• Ear canal becomes clear, without drainage, excess cerumen, or inflammation, as medication is repeatedly instilled.	Drug action is effective.
• Client's hearing acuity improves.	This response occurs only if hearing loss was caused by obstruction in external ear canal.
• Client is able to explain steps for instilling ear drops and demonstrates technique for administration.	Cognitive and psychomotor learning occurs.
2. Check accuracy and completeness of each MAR with prescriber's written medication order. Check client's name, drug name and dosage, route of administration, and time for administration. Compare MAR with label of ear medication three times during drug preparation.	The order sheet is the most reliable source and only legal record of drugs client is to receive. Ensures right drug is administered.
3. Check client's identification bracelet, and ask name.	Ensures correct client receives medication. At least two patient identifiers (neither to be the patient's room number) are to be used whenever administering medications (JCAHO, 2004).
4. Explain each step of procedure to client, allowing for questions.	Reduces client anxiety; timing of instruction enhances learning.

IMPLEMENTATION

1. Perform hand hygiene, and arrange supplies at bedside. Apply clean gloves (if drainage is present).	Reduces transmission of microorganisms; helps nurse perform procedure smoothly.
2. Warm medication by running warm water over the bottle (without damaging the label directions or allowing water to get into the bottle).	Prevents nausea and vertigo that may occur if the medication is too cold.
3. Have client assume side-lying position (if not contraindicated by client's condition) with ear to be treated facing up, or client may sit in chair or at the bedside. The nurse should stabilize the client's head with his or her hand.	Position provides easy access to ear for instillation of medication. Ear canal is in position to receive medication. Stabilizing the head promotes safety during instillation with a dropper.

STEP	**RATIONALE**

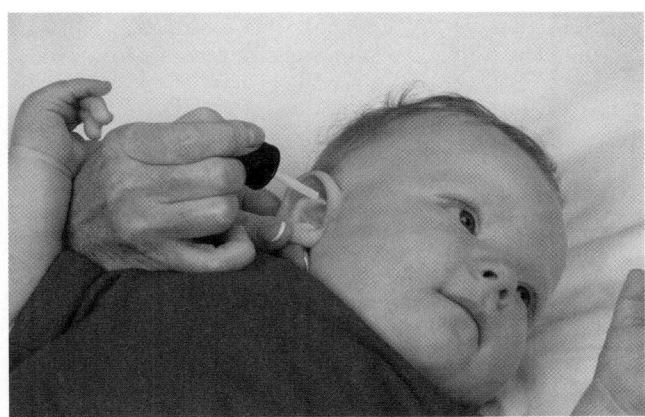

STEP **4** **A,** Pull the pinna up and back for adults and children over age 3. **B,** Pull the pinna down and back for children age 3 or less.

4. For adults and children over age 3, gently pull the pinna up and back; in children age 3 or less, the pinna should be pulled down and back (see illustrations) (Lilley and others, 2005).

Straightening of ear canal provides direct access to deeper external ear structures. Developmental differences in younger children and infants necessitate different methods of doing this.

5. If cerumen or drainage occludes outermost portion of ear canal, wipe out gently with cotton-tipped applicator (see illustration).

Cerumen and drainage harbor microorganisms and can block distribution of medication.

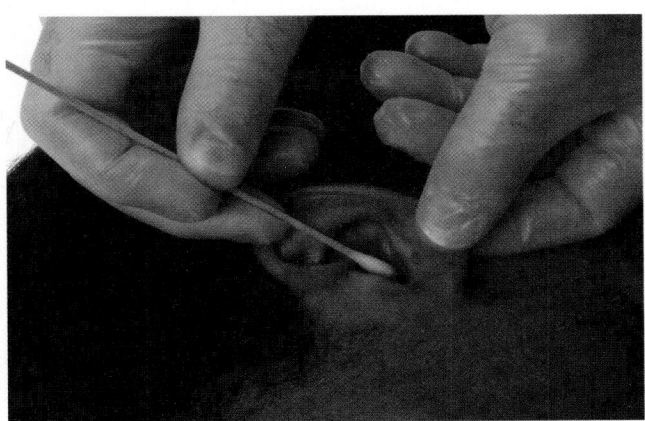

STEP **5** Always cleanse only outer canal. Do not push secretions into ear.

- **Critical Decision Point**
  Do not use the cotton-tipped applicator to force wax inward to block or occlude canal.

6. Instill prescribed drops holding dropper 1 cm (½ inch) above ear canal (see illustration for step 4).

Forceful instillation of drops into occluded canal can cause injury to eardrum.

STEP	RATIONALE
7. Ask client to remain in side-lying position for 5 to 10 minutes. Apply gentle massage or pressure to tragus of ear with finger (see illustration).	Allows complete distribution of medication. Pressure and massage moves medication inward.

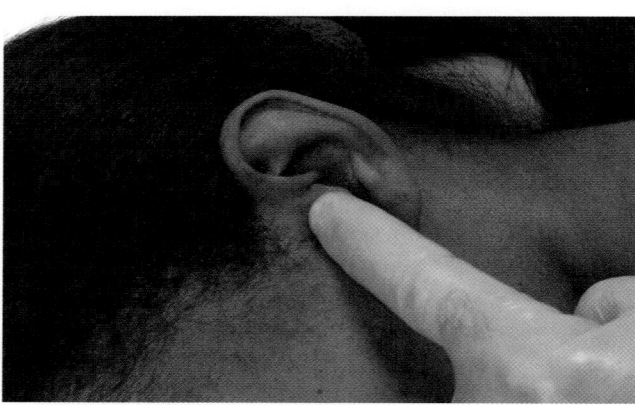

STEP **7** Nurse applies pressure to tragus of ear after instilling drops.

- *Critical Decision Point*

  If medication is ordered for both ears, ask the client to stay in the side-lying position for at least 10 minutes after the dose before turning to the other side.

STEP	RATIONALE
8. At times, the prescriber orders insertion of portion of cotton ball into outermost part of canal. Do not press cotton into canal.	Inserting cotton into outer canal prevents escape of medication when client sits or stands. Cotton should not block canal to impair hearing.
9. Remove cotton after 15 minutes.	Time period promotes drug distribution and absorption.
10. Dispose of soiled supplies, remove gloves, and perform hand hygiene.	Reduces transmission of microorganisms.
12. Assist client to comfortable position after drops are absorbed.	Restores comfort.

EVALUATION

1. Ask client if any discomfort is felt during instillation.	Determines if procedure is performed correctly and reveals severity of symptoms.
2. Evaluate condition of external ear between drug instillations.	Determines response to medication.
3. Evaluate client's hearing acuity.	Hearing may change after drug administration.
4. Ask client to explain technique for instilling ear drops and purpose of medication.	Evaluates degree of learning.
5. Have client demonstrate self-administration of next dose.	Provides feedback regarding competency with skill.

Recording and Reporting

- Record drug, concentration, number of drops, time administered, and ear (left, right, or both) into which drops instilled on MAR immediately after administration. Include initials or signature. Do not chart medication administration until *after* it is given to client.
- If drug is withheld, record reason in nurses' notes. Circle time the drug normally would have been given on MAR (or follow institution's policy for noting withheld doses).
- Record condition of ear canal in nurses' notes.
- Report any sudden change in client's hearing acuity.
- Report adverse effects/client response and/or withheld drugs to nurse in charge or physician. Depending on medication, immediate prescriber notification may be required.

Unexpected Outcomes	Related Interventions
1. Ear canal is inflamed, swollen, tender to palpation. Drainage is present.	• Symptoms of continuing ear infection are present; notify prescriber.
2. Client's hearing acuity continues to be reduced.	• Obstruction within ear canal is unrelieved. Notify prescriber.
3. Ear canal is occluded by cerumen.	• Wax has become impacted in the canal. Ear irrigation may be necessary to remove wax impaction.
4. Client is unable to explain drug information and steps for drug instillation.	• Nurse must repeat instructions, or client is unable to learn. • Include family or caregivers when instructing.
5. Client has difficulty self-administering ear drops.	• Reinstruction is needed. Have client demonstrate instillation of ear drops until performed.

Teaching Considerations
- Instruct client in proper way to cleanse ears and to avoid use of sharp objects in ear canal.
- Teach the signs of hearing loss and the need for frequent follow-ups to parents with children who have chronic otitis media.

Pediatric Considerations
- For children younger than 3 years of age gently pull the pinna of the ear downward and straight back. Ensure that parents and/or caregivers are aware of the proper method of administration.
- Infants or young children should be restrained in supine position with head turned to expose affected ear. Hold child in this position until the drug has time to be absorbed.

- Cotton pledgets may be used to prevent medication from flowing out of external canal. They should be inserted loose enough to allow any discharge to exit from ear. To prevent cotton from absorbing medication in ear, premoisten cotton with a few drops of medication (Hockenberry and others, 2003).

Gerontological Considerations
- Some older adults experience excessive accumulation of cerumen in the ear. This should be removed before administration of medication.

SKILL 20-6 Administering Ear Irrigations

Medications used to irrigate or wash out a body cavity such as the ear (otic) are delivered through a stream of solution. The common indications for irrigation of the external ear are presence of a foreign body, local inflammation of the canal, and accumulation of cerumen. Irrigations should be done with liquid warmed to body temperature to avoid vertigo (dizziness) or nausea in clients (Phipps and others, 2003). The greatest danger during administration of ear irrigation is rupture of the tympanic membrane. Fluids must not be instilled under pressure or with the ear canal occluded by the irrigating device.

DELEGATION CONSIDERATIONS

The skill of ear irrigation should not be delegated to assistive personnel. However, because certain aspects of the client's care, such as hygiene and vital signs, may be delegated to an assistive personnel, the nurse must:

- Instruct assistive personnel about potential side effects of ear irrigation and to report their occurrence
- Instruct assistive personnel to report any dizziness or light-headedness to the nurse for further assessment

EQUIPMENT

- ❏ Clean disposable gloves
- ❏ Otoscope (optional)
- ❏ Irrigation syringe
- ❏ Basin
- ❏ Towel
- ❏ Cotton balls
- ❏ Prescribed irrigation solution warmed to body temperature, or mineral oil, or over-the-counter softener
- ❏ Medication administration record (MAR)

STEP	RATIONALE

ASSESSMENT

1. Review prescriber's medication order, including solution to be instilled and the affected ear(s) (right, left, or both) to receive irrigation.

Ensures safe and correct administration of medication.

2. Review medical record for history of ruptured tympanic membrane, or visualize client's tympanic membrane using an otoscope.

Ruptured membrane contraindicates irrigation.

3. Inspect the pinna and external auditory meatus for redness, swelling, drainage, abrasions, and presence of cerumen or foreign objects.

Findings provide baseline to monitor effects of medication or solution.

  a. Always attempt to remove foreign objects in the ear by first simply straightening the ear canal.

This may cause the object to fall out.

  b. If vegetable matter (such as a dried bean or pea) is occluded in the canal, do not perform an irrigation.

Children often place vegetable matter in the ear. The material can swell on contact with water and cause further damage to the canal.

4. Ask if client is experiencing discomfort. Note client's ability to hear clearly.

Pain is symptomatic of external ear infection or inflammation. Occlusion of auditory canal by cerumen or foreign object can impair hearing.

5. Review client's knowledge of purpose for irrigation and of normal care of the ears.

May indicate need for instruction regarding hygiene.

NURSING DIAGNOSES

- Deficient knowledge regarding purpose for irrigation
- Pain (acute or chronic)

- Disturbed sensory perception (auditory)
- Risk for injury

Related factors are individualized based on client's condition or needs.

PLANNING

1. Expected outcomes following completion of procedure:
   - Client denies pain during instillation.
   - Client hears conversation more clearly.
   - Client is able to discuss purpose of irrigation and describe correct ear care techniques.
   - Skin overlying meatus and canal becomes clear, without redness, swelling, tenderness, or discharge. Canal is clear of cerumen and foreign material.

Fluid is properly instilled.
Obstruction in ear canal is resolved.
Feedback reflects client's learning.

Inflammation, irritation, and occlusion of canal are relieved.

2. Check accuracy and completeness of each MAR with prescriber's written medication or procedure order. Check client's name, drug name and dosage, route of administration, and time for administration. Compare MAR with label of ear irrigation solution.

The order sheet is the most reliable source and only legal record of drugs or procedure the client is to receive. Ensures client receives correct medication.

STEP	RATIONALE

3. If client is found to have impacted cerumen, instill 1 to 2 drops of mineral oil or over-the-counter softener into ear twice a day for 2 to 3 days before irrigation.

Loosens cerumen and ensures easier removal during irrigation.

4. Check client's identification by reading identification bracelet and asking name.

Ensures correct client receives medication. At least two patient identifiers (neither to be the patient's room number) are to be used whenever administering medications (JCAHO, 2004).

5. Explain procedure. Warn that the irrigation may cause sensation of dizziness, ear fullness, and warmth.

Prepares client to anticipate effects of irrigation and promotes cooperation.

IMPLEMENTATION

1. Perform hand hygiene, arrange supplies at bedside, and apply gloves.

Reduces transfer of microorganisms; helps nurse to perform procedure smoothly.

2. Close curtain or room door.

Maintains privacy.

3. Assist client to a sitting or lying position with head turned toward affected ear. Place towel under client's head and shoulder, and have client, if able, hold basin under affected ear.

Position minimizes leakage of fluids around neck and facial area. Solution will flow from ear canal to basin.

4. Pour irrigating solution into basin.

5. Gently clean auricle and outer ear canal with moistened cotton applicator. Do *not* force drainage or cerumen into the ear canal.

Prevents infected material from reentering ear canal. Forceful instillation of solution into occluded canal can cause injury to eardrum

6. Fill irrigating syringe with solution (approximately 50 ml).

Enough fluid is needed to provide a steady irrigating stream.

7. For adults and children over age 3, gently pull pinna up and back; in children age 3 or less, pinna should be pulled down and back (Lilley and others, 2005).

Straightening of ear canal provides direct access to deeper external ear structures. Developmental differences in younger children and infants necessitate different techniques. Allows fluid to flow through length of canal.

8. Slowly instill irrigating solution by holding tip of syringe 1 cm (½ inch) above opening to ear canal. The fluid should be directed toward the superior aspect of ear canal. Allow fluid to drain out during instillation into the basin. Continue until canal is cleansed or solution is used (see illustration).

Slow instillation prevents buildup of pressure in ear canal and ensures contact of solution with all canal surfaces.

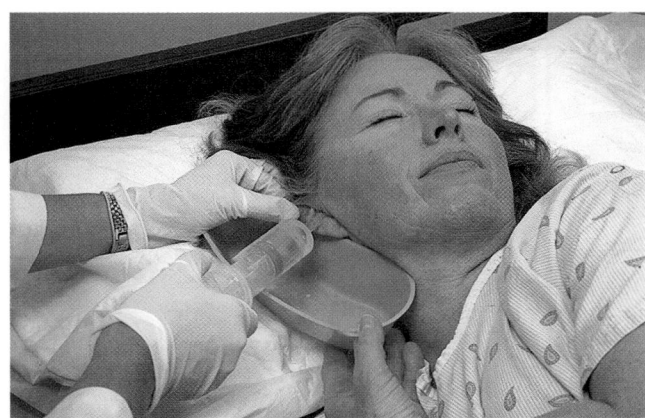

STEP **8** Tip of syringe does not occlude ear canal during irrigation.

9. Do *not* occlude ear canal with tip of syringe.

Buildup of fluid in ear canal under forced pressure could cause rupture of tympanic membrane.

10. Dry outer ear canal with cotton ball. Leave cotton loosely in place for 5 to 10 minutes.

Maintains comfort. Absorbs excess moisture in ear canal.

STEP	RATIONALE
11. Assist client to a sitting position.	Maintains comfort.
12. Remove gloves, dispose of supplies, and perform hand hygiene.	Reduces transmission of infection.

EVALUATION

1. Ask client if discomfort is noted during instillation of solution.	Fluid instilled improperly under pressure causes discomfort.
2. Reinspect condition of meatus and canal.	Determines if solution relieves symptoms and removes foreign materials.
3. Measure client's hearing acuity.	Determines if conduction deafness is relieved.
4. Ask client to describe purpose of irrigation and proper techniques for ear care.	Reflects client's understanding of procedure and proper hygiene.

Recording and Reporting

- Record in nurses' notes and/or MAR, the procedure, amount of solution instilled, time of administration, and ear receiving irrigation. Include initials or signature. Do not chart medication administration until *after* it is given to client.
- Record appearance of external ear and client's hearing acuity in nurses' notes.
- If drug is withheld, record reason in nurses' notes. Circle time the drug normally would have been given on MAR (or follow institution's policy for noting withheld doses).
- Report adverse effects/client response and/or withheld drugs to nurse in charge or physician. Depending on medication, immediate prescriber notification may be required.

Unexpected Outcomes	Related Interventions
1. Client experiences increased ear pain.	• Rupture of eardrum may have occurred. Stop irrigations immediately, and notify prescriber immediately.
2. Ear canal remains occluded with cerumen.	• Repeat irrigation is required.
3. Foreign body remains in ear canal.	• Refer client to an otolaryngologist if a foreign object remains after irrigation.
4. Client is unable to explain ear care practices.	• Reinstruction is necessary. • Include family members or caregivers if possible.

Teaching Considerations

- Instruct client that cerumen has an antibacterial effect that maintains an acid pH in the auditory canal.
- Instruct clients to clean ears daily with a washcloth, soap, and warm water.
- Warn clients against placing objects (including cotton swabs) in ears.

Pediatric Considerations

- When cleansing the ear of a small child, be certain child's head is immobilized to prevent puncturing eardrum. It may be necessary to have child's parent participate in this procedure.

Home Care Considerations

- Instruct client to use a clean bulb syringe for irrigation. Mineral oil drops or over-the-counter otic preparations may be used to facilitate removal of cerumen, but client should be instructed to consult a health care provider if problems continue (Ignatavicius and Workman, 2002).

SKILL 20-7 Administering Nasal Instillations

Clients with nasal sinus alterations may receive drugs by spray, drops, or tampons. The most commonly administered form of nasal instillation is a decongestant spray or drops used to relieve sinus congestion and cold symptoms. Many over-the-counter nose drops contain sympathomimetic drugs (such as Afrin or Neo-Synephrine). These drugs are relatively safe when administered nasally because only small doses are needed. However, the drugs can enter the systemic circulation by way of the nasal mucosa or gastrointestinal tract if an excess amount is swallowed.

Repeated use of sprays can worsen nasal congestion because of a rebound effect. It is easy for a client to self-administer sprays. The client can be placed in a seated position with the head in a slightly hyperextended position.

Nasal drops (prescribed) often contain antibiotics for the treatment of sinus infections. Proper positioning of clients during instillation of drops is essential for medication to reach the affected sinus. The client should be instructed to lie in the supine position with head tilted back.

DELEGATION CONSIDERATIONS

The skill of administering nasal medications should not be delegated to assistive personnel. However certain aspects of the client's care, such as hygiene and vital signs, may be delegated. Before delegation the nurse should:

* Instruct assistive personnel about potential side effects of medications and to report their occurrence
* Instruct assistive personnel to report any bloody nasal drainage

EQUIPMENT

❑ Prepared medication with clean dropper or spray container
❑ Facial tissue
❑ Small pillow (optional)
❑ Washcloth (optional)
❑ Gloves
❑ Medication administration record (MAR)

STEP	RATIONALE

ASSESSMENT

1. For nasal drops, determine which sinus is affected by referring to medical record.

2. Assess client's history of hypertension, heart disease, diabetes, and hyperthyroidism.

3. Inspect condition of nose and sinuses. Palpate sinuses for tenderness. Note type of drainage, if present.

4. Assess client's knowledge regarding use of nasal instillations and technique for instillation and willingness to learn self-administration.

Affects client's position during drug instillation.

These conditions can contraindicate use of decongestants that stimulate the central nervous system. Side effects of transient hypertension, tachycardia, palpitations, and headache may occur.

Provides baseline to monitor effects of medication. Presence of discharge interferes with drug absorption. Clear nasal discharge indicates sinus problem. Yellow or greenish discharge indicates infection.

May require health teaching regarding use of drugs. Motivation influences teaching approach.

NURSING DIAGNOSES

* Deficient knowledge regarding drug action and purpose
* Pain (acute or chronic)

* Health-seeking behaviors (self-care)
* Risk for injury

Related factors are individualized based on client's condition or needs.

PLANNING

1. Expected outcomes following completion of procedure:
   * Client is able to breathe with ease through nose.
   * Client's nasal sinuses become clear, moist, pink, without drainage after repeated instillations (applies to antiinfective medications).
   * Client is able to explain medication's purpose and administers nasal instillations correctly.

Nasal congestion has been relieved.
Inflammation of mucosa has been relieved.

Feedback reflects client's learning.

STEP	RATIONALE
2. Check accuracy and completeness of each MAR with prescriber's written medication order. Check client's name, drug name and dosage, route of administration, and time for administration. Compare MAR with label of nasal medication three times during preparation of medication.	The order sheet is the most reliable source and only legal record of drugs client is to receive. Ensures right drug is administered.
3. Check client's identification bracelet, and ask name.	Ensures correct client receives medication. At least two patient identifiers (neither to be the patient's room number) are to be used whenever administering medications (JCAHO, 2004).
4. Explain procedure to client regarding positioning and sensations to expect, such as burning or stinging of mucosa or choking sensation as medication trickles into throat.	Helps client anticipate experience of procedure to reduce anxiety.

IMPLEMENTATION

1. Perform hand hygiene. Arrange supplies and medications at bedside. Apply gloves.	Reduces transmission of microorganisms; ensures smooth, orderly procedure.
2. Instruct client to clear or blow nose gently unless contraindicated (e.g., risk of increased intracranial pressure or nosebleeds).	Removes mucus and secretions that can block distribution of medication.

3. Administer nasal drops:
  a. Assist client to supine position.
  b. Position head properly:
   (1) For access to posterior pharynx, tilt client's head backward.
   (2) For access to ethmoid or sphenoid sinus, tilt head back over edge of bed, or place small pillow under client's shoulder and tilt head back (see illustration).
   (3) For access to frontal and maxillary sinus, tilt head back over edge of bed or pillow with head turned toward side to be treated (see illustration).
  c. Support client's head with nondominant hand.
	Proper positioning provides access to specific nasal passages.
	
	Position allows medication to drain into affected sinus.
	
	Prevents straining of neck muscles.

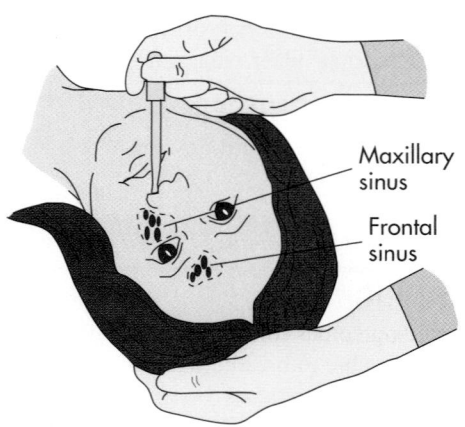

STEP 3b(2) Position for instilling nose drops into ethmoid or sphenoid sinus.

Ethmoid sinuses

Sphenoid sinus

Maxillary sinus

Frontal sinus

STEP 3b(3) Position for instilling nose drops into frontal and maxillary sinus.

STEP	RATIONALE
d. Instruct client to breathe through mouth.	Mouth breathing reduces chance of aspirating nasal drops into trachea and lungs.
e. Hold dropper 1 cm ($\frac{1}{2}$ inch) above nares, and instill prescribed number of drops toward midline of ethmoid bone.	Avoids contamination of dropper. Instilling toward ethmoid bone facilitates distribution of medication over nasal mucosa.
f. Have client remain in supine position 5 minutes.	Prevents premature loss of medication through nares.
g. Offer facial tissue to blot runny nose, but caution client against blowing nose for several minutes.	Allows maximal amount of medication to be absorbed.
4. Assist client to a comfortable position after drug is absorbed.	Restores comfort.
5. Dispose of soiled supplies in proper container, and perform hand hygiene.	Maintains neat, orderly environment. Reduces spread of microorganisms.

EVALUATION

1. Observe client for onset of side effects 15 to 30 minutes after administration.	Drugs absorbed through mucosa can cause systemic reaction.
2. Ask if client is able to breathe through nose after decongestant administration. May be necessary to have client occlude one nostril at a time and breathe deeply.	Determines effectiveness of decongestant medication.
3. Reinspect condition of nasal passages between instillations.	Condition of mucosa reveals response to medication.
4. Ask client to describe risks of overuse of decongestants and methods for administration.	Feedback ensures that client can self-administer drugs properly.
5. Have client demonstrate self-medication.	Feedback demonstrates learning.

Recording and Reporting

- Record medication administration on MAR immediately after administration, including drug name, concentration, number of drops; nostril into which drug was instilled; and time of administration. Include initials or signature. Do not chart medication administration until *after* it is given to client.
- If drug is withheld, record reason in nurses' notes. Circle time the drug normally would have been given on MAR (or follow institution's policy for noting withheld doses).
- Record client's response in nurses' notes.
- Report any unusual systemic effects or adverse effects/client response and/or withheld drugs to nurse in charge or physician. Depending on medication, immediate prescriber notification may be required.

Unexpected Outcomes	Related Interventions
1. Client is unable to breathe easily through nasal passages. Mucosa appears swollen, and congestion is unrelieved.	• Client may be experiencing rebound effect, or medication may not be effective. • Stop medication use, and notify prescriber. May need to consider alternative therapy.
2. Nasal mucosa remains inflamed and tender, with discharge from nares.	• Inflammatory or infectious process remains. May need to consider alternative therapy.
3. Client complains of sinus headache. Sinuses remain congested.	• May need to consider alternative therapy.
4. Client is unable to explain technique and risks of drug therapy.	• Further explanation is required. • Include family members or caregiver when possible.
5. Client is unable to self-administer medication.	• Reinstruction is necessary. • Include family members or caregiver when possible.

Teaching Considerations

- Instruct clients that each family member should have a different dropper or spray applicator. Applicators should be washed or rinsed after each use.
- Use over-the-counter nasal sprays or nose drops for only one illness; bottles become easily contaminated with bacteria.
- Caution clients against overuse of nasal spray decongestants because they can cause rebound effect, worsening of mucosal swelling. Risk increases as more drug is used.

Pediatric Considerations

- Positioning child with head extended over edge of bed or pillow facilitates smooth instillation of nasal drops. Instruct child or parent to remain in this position for at least 1 minute to ensure that drops come into contact with affected tissue.
- Infants are nose breathers, and the possible congestion caused by nasal medications may inhibit their sucking. Nose drops, if ordered, should be administered 20 to 30 minutes before feedings (James and others, 2002).

SKILL 20-8   Using Metered-Dose Inhalers

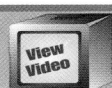

Inhaled medications are usually designed to produce local effects; for example, bronchodilators open narrowed bronchioles, and mucolytic agents liquefy thick mucous secretions. However, because these medications are absorbed rapidly through the pulmonary circulation, some have the potential for producing systemic side effects (e.g., isoproterenol [Isuprel] dilates bronchioles but can also cause cardiac dysrhythmias).

Clients who receive drugs by inhalation frequently suffer from chronic respiratory disease. Drugs administered by inhalation provide control of airway hyperactivity or constriction. Because clients depend on these medications for disease control, they must learn about the medications and how to administer them safely. Metered-dose inhalers (MDIs) and small-volume nebulizers (see Skill 20-9) are two devices that deliver medications.

MDIs are handheld devices that disperse medications through an aerosol spray, mist, or fine powder to penetrate lung airways (Figure 20-1). The deeper passages of the respiratory tract provide a large surface area for drug absorption. The alveolar-capillary network absorbs medication rapidly.

Drugs can be administered by MDIs in high concentrations with few side effects. An MDI delivers a measured dose of the drug with each push of a canister. Approximately 5 to 10 pounds of pressure must be used to activate the aerosol. This may be a problem for older clients because hand strength diminishes with age. Because use of a metered-dose inhaler requires coordination during the breathing cycle, many clients spray only the back of their throats and fail to receive a full dose. The inhaler must be depressed to expel medication just as the client inhales. This ensures the medication reaches the lower airways. Poor coordination can be solved by the use of spacer devices (Aerochamber, Inspirease) or the use of a breath-activated MDI, such as the Maxair Autoinhaler (Togger and Brenner, 2001). Box 20-3 summarizes common problems in using an inhaler.

BOX 20-3   Common Problems in Using an Inhaler

1. Not taking the medication as *prescribed,* but taking either too much or too little.
2. Incorrect activation. This usually occurs through pressing the canister *before* taking a breath.
3. Both should be done simultaneously so that the drug can be carried down to the lungs with the breath Forgetting to shake the inhaler. The drug is in a suspension, and therefore particles may settle. If the inhaler is not shaken, it may not deliver the correct dose of the drug.
4. Not waiting long enough between puffs. The whole process should be repeated to take the second puff, otherwise an incorrect dose may be delivered, or the drug may not penetrate into the lungs.
5. Failure to clean the valve. Particles may jam up the valve in the mouthpiece unless it is cleaned occasionally. This is a frequent cause of failure to get 200 puffs from one inhaler.
6. Failure to observe whether the inhaler is actually releasing a spray. If it is not, this should be checked with the pharmacist.

FIGURE **20-1 A,** Metered-dose inhaler (MDI). **B,** Automated MDI. **C,** "Disk-type" MDI that delivers powdered medication.

DELEGATION CONSIDERATIONS

The skill of administering MDI medications should not be delegated to assistive personnel. However, other aspects of the client's care may be delegated. Before delegation the nurse must:

- Instruct assistive personnel about potential side effects of medications and to report their occurrence
- Instruct the care provider to report paroxysmal coughing, audible wheezing, and client's report of breathlessness or difficulty breathing.

EQUIPMENT

- ❑ Metered-dose inhaler with medication canister
- ❑ Stethoscope
- ❑ Spacer device, such as Aerochamber or Inspirease (optional)
- ❑ Facial tissues (optional)
- ❑ Washbasin or sink with warm water
- ❑ Paper towel
- ❑ Medication administration record (MAR)

STEP	RATIONALE

ASSESSMENT

1. Assess respiratory pattern, and auscultate breath sounds.

2. Assess client's readiness to learn: client asks questions about medication, disease, or complications; requests education in use of inhaler; is mentally alert; participates in own care.

3. Assess client's ability to learn: client should not be fatigued, in pain, or in respiratory distress; assess level of understanding of technical vocabulary terms.

4. Assess client's knowledge and understanding of disease and purpose and action of prescribed medications.

5. Assess client's ability to hold, manipulate, and depress canister and inhaler.

6. Assess drug schedule and number of inhalations prescribed for each dose.

7. If previously instructed in self-administration of inhaled medicine, assess client's technique in using an inhaler.

Establishes baseline of airway status for comparison during and after treatment.

Affects client's ability to understand explanations and actively participate in teaching process.

Mental or physical limitations affect client's ability to learn and methods nurse uses for instruction.

Knowledge of disease is essential for client to realistically understand use of inhaler.

Any impairment of grasp or presence of hand tremors interferes with client's ability to depress canister within inhaler.

Influences explanations nurse provides for use of inhaler.

Nurse's instruction may require only simple reinforcement, depending on client's level of dexterity.

NURSING DIAGNOSES

- Activity intolerance
- Health-seeking behaviors (self-care)
- Ineffective breathing pattern
- Risk for injury

- Deficient knowledge regarding use of MDI
- Impaired gas exchange
- Ineffective therapeutic regimen management

Related factors are individualized based on client's condition or needs.

PLANNING

1. Expected outcomes following completion of procedure:
   - Client describes techniques for use of MDI.
   - Client correctly self-administers metered dose.
   - Client's breathing pattern improves, and airways become less restricted.
   - Client's gas exchange is adequate.

2. Check accuracy and completeness of each MAR with prescriber's written medication order. Check client's name, drug name and dosage, route of administration, and time for administration. Compare MAR with medication label three times during medication preparation.

3. Check client's identification bracelet and ask name.

Ensures compliance with therapeutic regimen.

Demonstrates learning.

Demonstrates proper administration and therapeutic effect of medication.

Demonstrates proper administration and therapeutic effect of medication.

The order sheet is the most reliable source and only legal record of drugs client is to receive. Ensures client receives correct medication.

Ensures correct client receives medication. At least two patient identifiers (neither to be the patient's room number) are to be used whenever administering medications (JCAHO, 2004).

STEP	**RATIONALE**
4. Explain procedure to client. Be specific if client wishes to self-administer drug. Explain where and how to set up in the home.	Makes client a participant in care and minimizes anxiety.
5. Provide adequate time for teaching session.	Prevents interruptions. Instruction should occur when client is receptive.

IMPLEMENTATION

1. Perform hand hygiene, and arrange equipment needed.	Reduces transfer of microorganisms and saves time.
2. Allow client opportunity to manipulate inhaler, canister, and spacer device. Explain and demonstrate how canister fits into inhaler.	Client must be familiar with how to use equipment.

• *Critical Decision Point*

If the client is using an MDI that is new or has not been used for several days (with or without a spacer), push a "test spray" into the air before administering the dose (Mayo Clinic, 2003).

3. Explain what metered dose is, and warn client about overuse of inhaler, including drug side effects.	Client must not arbitrarily administer excessive inhalations because of risk of serious side effects and/or tolerance developing to medications. If drug is given in recommended doses, side effects are uncommon.
4. Explain steps for administering inhaled dose of medication (demonstrate steps when possible):	Use of simple, step-by-step explanations allows client to ask questions at any point during procedure.
a. Remove mouthpiece cover from inhaler.	
b. Shake inhaler well for 2 to 5 seconds (five or six shakes).	Ensures mixing of medication in canister.
c. Hold inhaler in dominant hand.	
d. Instruct client to position inhaler in one of two ways:	
(1) Place inhaler in mouth with opening toward back of throat, closing lips tightly around it (see illustration).	

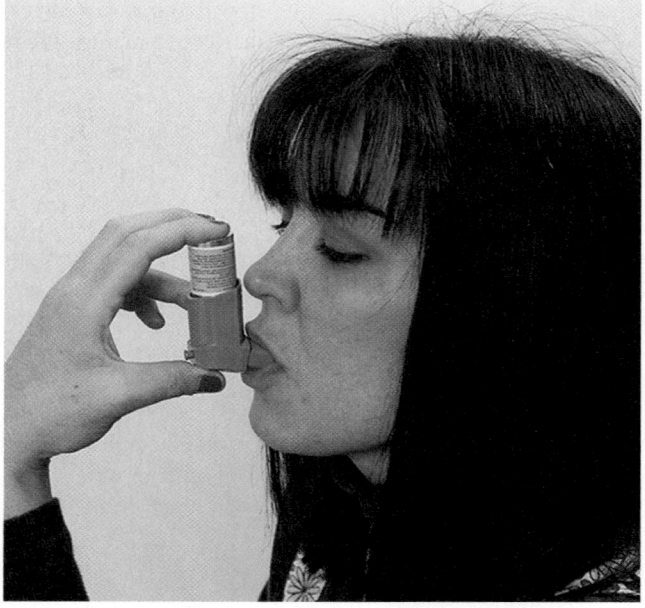

STEP 4d(1) One technique for use of the inhaler. The client opens lips and places inhaler in mouth with opening toward back of throat.

STEP	RATIONALE
(2) Position the device 2 to 4 cm (1 to 2 inches) in front of widely opened mouth (see illustration), with opening of inhaler toward back of throat. Lips should not touch the inhaler.	Directs aerosol spray toward airway. Positioning the mouthpiece 2 to 4 cm from the mouth is considered the best way to deliver the medication without a spacer.

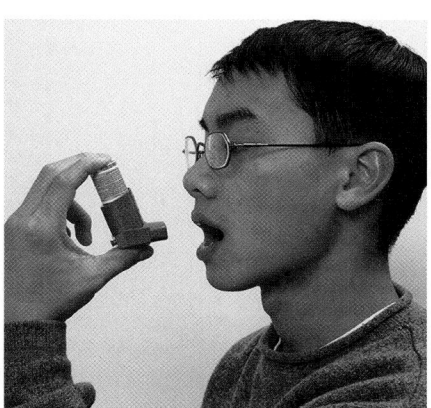

STEP 4d(2) One technique for use of the inhaler. The client positions the mouthpiece 2 to 4 cm (1 to 2 inches) from the widely open mouth. This is considered the best way to deliver the medication without a spacer.

STEP	RATIONALE
e. Have client take a deep breath and exhale completely.	Prepares client's airway to receive the medication.
f. With inhaler properly positioned, have client hold inhaler with thumb at the mouthpiece and the index finger and middle finger at the top (Lilley and others, 2005).	Proper hand position ensures proper activation of metered-dose inhaler.
g. Instruct client to tilt head back slightly, inhale slowly and deeply through mouth, and depress medication canister fully.	Medication is distributed to airways during inhalation. Inhalation through mouth rather than nose draws medication more effectively into airways.
h. Breathe in slowly for 2 to 3 seconds, then hold breath for approximately 10 seconds.	Allows tiny drops of aerosol spray to reach deeper branches of airways.
i. Remove the MDI from the mouth before exhaling, then exhale slowly through nose or pursed lips.	Keeps small airways open during exhalation.
5. Explain steps to administer inhaled dose of medication using a spacer device (demonstrate when possible):	
a. Remove mouthpiece cover from metered-dose inhaler and mouthpiece of spacer device.	Inhaler fits into end of spacer device.
b. Insert MDI into end of spacer device.	A spacer device traps medication released from MDI; client then inhales the drug from the device. These devices improve delivery of correct dose of inhaled medication (Togger and Brenner, 2001).
c. Shake inhaler well for 2 to 5 seconds (five or six shakes).	Ensures mixing of medication in canister.
d. Place spacer device mouthpiece in mouth and close lips. Do not insert beyond raised lip on mouthpiece. Avoid covering small exhalation slots with the lips.	Medication should not escape through mouth.

STEP	RATIONALE

e. Breathe normally through spacer device mouthpiece (see illustration).

Allows client to relax before delivering medication.

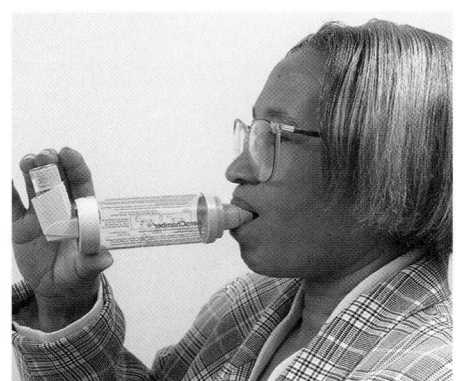

STEP **5e** Using a spacer device with an MDI.

f. Depress medication canister, spraying one puff into spacer device.

Emits spray that allows finer particles to be inhaled. Large droplets are retained in spacer device.

g. Breathe in slowly and fully (for 5 seconds).

Ensures particles of medication are distributed to deeper airways.

h. Hold full breath for 10 seconds.

Ensures full drug distribution.

6. Instruct client to wait 20 to 30 seconds between inhalations (if it is the same medication), or 2 to 5 minutes between inhalations if the medications are different.

Drugs must be inhaled sequentially. If bronchodilators are administered with inhaled steroids, the bronchodilators should be given first in order to allow the airway passages to be more open for the second medication.

7. Instruct client against repeating inhalations before next scheduled dose (see Box 20-3).

Drugs are prescribed at intervals during day to provide constant drug levels and minimize side effects. Beta-adrenergic MDIs are used either on an "as needed" basis or regularly every 4 to 6 hours.

8. Explain that client may feel gagging sensation in throat caused by droplets of medication on pharynx or tongue.

Results when inhalant is sprayed and inhaled incorrectly.

9. For daily cleaning, instruct client to remove the medication canister, rinse the inhaler and cap with warm running water, and ensure the inhaler is completely dry before reuse. Twice weekly, the L-shaped mouthpiece should be washed with mild dishwashing soap and warm water, rinsed, and dried well (National Heart, Lung, and Blood Institute, 1995).

Removes residual medication.

10. Ask if client has any questions.

Clarifies misconceptions or misunderstanding.

11. Perform hand hygiene, and assist client to comfortable position.

Reduces the spread of microorganisms and promotes client comfort.

EVALUATION

1. Have client explain and demonstrate steps in use of inhaler.

Return demonstration provides feedback for measuring client's learning.

2. Ask client to explain drug schedule.

Improves likelihood of compliance with therapy.

3. Ask client to describe side effects of medication and criteria for calling physician.

Allows client to recognize signs of overuse and need to seek medical support when drugs are ineffective.

4. After medication administration, assess client's respirations and breath sounds, and assess peak flow measures if ordered.

Determines status of breathing pattern and adequacy of ventilation/gas exchange.

Recording and Reporting

*   Record actual time each drug was administered, dosage, and concentration on MAR immediately after administration. Include initials or signature. Do not chart medication administration until *after* it is given to client.
*   If drug is withheld, record reason in nurses' notes. Circle time the drug normally would have been given on MAR (or follow institution's policy for noting withheld doses).
*   Record client's response to the medication, including pulse, respirations, breath sounds assessed, and any adverse effects.
*   Document what skills were taught and client's ability to perform them.
*   Report adverse effects/client response and/or withheld drugs to nurse in charge or physician. Depending on medication, immediate prescriber notification may be required.

Unexpected Outcomes	Related Interventions
1. Client's respirations are rapid and shallow, breath sounds indicate wheezing.	• May need to reassess type of medication and/or delivery method. • Notify prescriber.
2. Client experiences paroxysms of coughing. Aerosolized particles can irritate posterior pharynx.	• May need to reassess type of medication and/or delivery method. • Notify prescriber.
3. Client needs a bronchodilator more than every 4 hours.	• May indicate respiratory problems. • Reassessment of type of medication and delivery methods needed. • Notify prescriber.
4. Client experiences cardiac dysrhythmias (light-headedness, syncope), especially if receiving beta-adrenergics.	• Withhold all further doses of medication. • Notify prescriber for reassessment of type of medication and delivery method.
5. Client may not be able to self-administer medication properly.	• Alternative delivery routes or devices may need to be explored.
6. Client is unable to explain technique and risks of drug therapy.	• Further teaching may be required. • Include family members or caregivers when possible.

Teaching Considerations

*   Client may need supervised practice for several different steps of procedure before being able to perform each skill independently. Clients may have difficulty with timing inspiration with medication dispersal without proper instruction (Togger and Brenner, 2001).
*   Teach client how to determine fullness of canisters, using displacement in water technique (Figure 20-2).
*   Do not try to teach client how to use an inhaler during an episode of shortness of breath. Client's attention span will be very poor.
*   Ensure that the client knows that inhaled corticosteroids are for maintenance therapy for the treatment of asthma and not appropriate for the acute relief of bronchoconstriction (Ignatavicius and Workman, 2002).
*   Ensure that the client knows the proper sequence and spacing of medications if two different types of inhalers

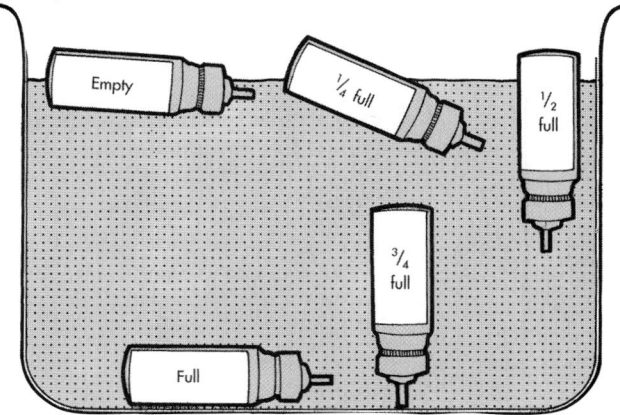

FIGURE 20-2 A simple method of estimating amount left in the inhalant canister is to place it in a container filled with water. The position the canister takes in the water determines the amount of inhalant remaining.

(i.e., bronchodilator and inhaled steroid) are due to be given at the same time (Lilley and others, 2005).

- Teach clients to use small handheld peak flowmeters to monitor response to therapy when bronchodilators or bronchospasm prevention drugs (steroids) are prescribed (Ignatavicius and Workman, 2002).
- Teach the client to rinse his or her mouth with water after the use of inhaled corticosteroids in order to prevent oropharyngeal candidiasis (Lewis and others, 2004).
- Teach client to cleanse valve after each use.

Pediatric Considerations

- Because of difficulty coordinating actuation and inhalation, the use of a spacer device is recommended for young children (Gallagher, 2002).
- Bronchodilators are used often in children, but use with extreme caution and monitor for adverse effects such as tremors, restlessness, dizziness, gastrointestinal upset, and tachycardia (Lilley and others, 2005).

- Educate child and parent about the need to use inhaler during school hours. Help family find resources within the school or day care facility. Keep in mind that many school systems do not permit self-administration of MDIs. Follow the school's policy regarding having the MDI available for use during school hours. A physician's order may be necessary.

Gerontological Considerations

- Older adult clients may be unable to depress medication canister because of weakened grasp or may be unable to coordinate actuation of the canister with inhalation. The use of a spacer device may be necessary.

Home Care Considerations

- Remind clients to carry prescribed inhalers to use as immediate treatment in case of an acute asthma attack.

SKILL 20-9 Using Small-Volume Nebulizers

Nebulization is a process of adding medications or moisture to inspired air by mixing particles of various sizes with air. Adding moisture to the respiratory system through nebulization may improve clearance of pulmonary secretions. Medications such as bronchodilators, mucolytics, and corticosteroids are often administered by nebulization.

Small-volume nebulizers provide medications in an aerosolized form that can be inhaled by the client into the tracheobronchial tree and possibly into the bloodstream

through the alveoli. As a result, systemic effects from the medications may occur.

Clients who receive drugs by inhalation frequently suffer from chronic lung disease. Drugs administered by inhalation provide control of airway hyperactivity or constriction. Because clients depend on these medications for disease control, they must learn how they work and how to administer them safely.

DELEGATION CONSIDERATIONS

The skill of administering medications by nebulizer should not be delegated to assistive personnel. However, aspects of the client's care may be delegated. Before delegation the nurse must:

- Instruct assistive personnel about potential side effects of medications and to report their occurrence
- Instruct care provider to report paroxysmal coughing, ineffective breathing patterns, and other respiratory difficulties

EQUIPMENT

- ❑ Medication ordered and diluent (if needed)
- ❑ Nebulizer bottle and tubing assembly
- ❑ Small-volume nebulizer machine (often called handheld nebulizer or simply nebulizer)
- ❑ Stethoscope
- ❑ Medication administration record (MAR)

STEP	RATIONALE

▌ ASSESSMENT

1. Assess client's medical history, history of allergies, medication and diet history.
2. Assess client's ability to assemble, hold, and manipulate the nebulizer equipment.

These factors can influence how certain drugs act. Information also reflects client's need for medications.

Any impairment of grasp or presence of hand tremors interferes with client's ability to use the equipment.

STEP	RATIONALE

• **Critical Decision Point**
If client is unable to hold the nebulizer mouthpiece during the treatment, use an aerosol mask in place of the mouthpiece. Such masks are also used for children. This ensures proper deposition of medication.

3. Assess drug ordered, including amount, type and amount of diluent (if unit dose is not available), and frequency.

Legal order for medication therapy must be complete. Unit-dose medications do not require dilution; however, a diluent may be used along with a unit-dose medication if a different percentage of drug is desired.

4. Assess pulse, respirations, breath sounds, and peak flow measurement (if ordered) before beginning treatment.

Establishes a baseline for comparison during and after treatment.

NURSING DIAGNOSES
- Activity intolerance
- Health-seeking behaviors (self-care)
- Ineffective therapeutic regimen management
- Risk for injury

- Deficient knowledge regarding use of small-volume nebulizers
- Impaired gas exchange
- Ineffective breathing pattern

Related factors are individualized based on client's condition or needs.

PLANNING
1. Expected outcomes following completion of procedure:
   - Client's breathing patterns are effective.

   Demonstrates proper administration and therapeutic effect of medication.

   - Client's gas exchange is adequate.

   Demonstrates proper administration and therapeutic effect of medication.

   - Client describes techniques for use of small-volume nebulizers.

   Increases likelihood of compliance with therapeutic regimen.

   - Client correctly self-administers medication using small-volume nebulizer.

   Demonstrates learning.

2. Check accuracy and completeness of each MAR with prescriber's written medication order. Check client's name, drug name and dosage, route of administration, and time for administration. Compare MAR with medication label.

   The order sheet is the most reliable source and only legal record of drugs client is to receive. Ensures client receives correct medication.

3. Check client's identification bracelet, and ask name.

   Ensures correct client receives medication. At least two patient identifiers (neither to be the patient's room number) are to be used whenever administering medications (JCAHO, 2004).

4. Explain procedure to client. Be specific if client wishes to self-administer drug.

   Makes client a participant in care and minimizes anxiety. Begins client teaching regarding medications. Enables client to self-administer drug if physically able and motivated.

IMPLEMENTATION
1. Perform hand hygiene, and arrange equipment needed.

   Reduces transfer of microorganisms and saves time.

2. Explain the use of the nebulizer, and warn client of possible drug side effects.

   Helps to make client more knowledgeable about treatment and medication.

3. Assemble nebulizer equipment per manufacturer's directions.

   Assembly may vary slightly with different manufacturers. Proper assembly ensures safe delivery of medication.

STEP	**RATIONALE**

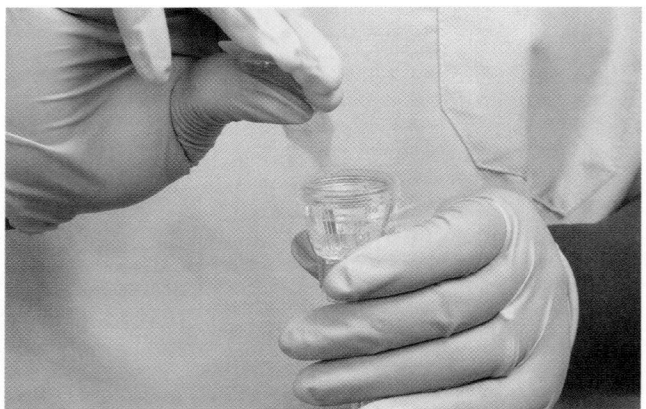

STEP 4 Add prescribed medication (and diluent, if needed) to nebulizer cup.

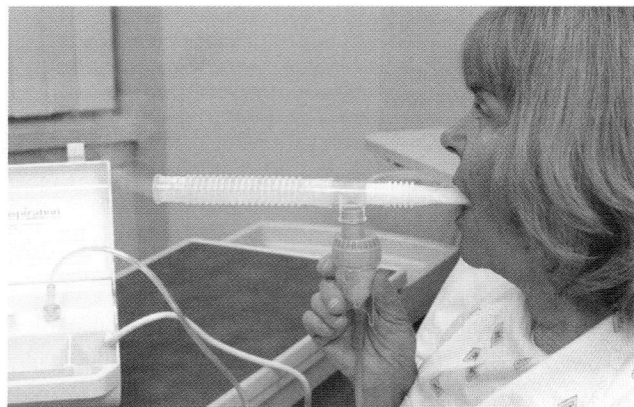

STEP 5 Nebulizer mouthpiece placed between client's lips.

4. Add prescribed medication and diluent (if needed) to nebulizer cup (see illustration).	Ensures proper dose and delivery of ordered medication.
5. Have client hold mouthpiece between lips with gentle pressure (see illustration). **a.** If client is a child or infant or an adult who is fatigued, who cannot follow instructions, or who is unable to follow instructions, use a face mask.	Use of a face mask does not require client to remember to hold mouthpiece correctly. Correct delivery ensures sufficient deposition of medication.
b. Use special adapters for clients with a tracheostomy.	
6. Have client take a deep breath, slowly, to a volume slightly greater than normal. Encourage a brief, end-inspiratory pause. Then have the client exhale passively.	Promotes greater deposition of medication in the airways.
a. If client is dyspneic, encourage client to hold every fourth or fifth breath for 5 to 10 seconds.	Improves effectiveness of medication.
7. Turn on the small-volume nebulizer machine, and ensure that a sufficient mist is formed.	Verifies that the equipment is working properly during delivery of medication.
a. Tap the nebulizer cup occasionally during treatment and toward the end of the treatment.	Releases droplets that may be clinging to the side of the cup, thus allowing for renebulization of the solution.
b. Remind client to repeat the breathing pattern described in step 6 until the drug is completely nebulized.	Maximizes effectiveness of medication.
(1) Some practitioners set a timed limit as the length of the treatment rather than waiting for the medication to completely nebulize.	
c. Monitor client's pulse during procedure, especially if beta-adrenergic blockers are used.	Enables nurse to observe for potential side effects of medications.
8. When medication is completely nebulized, turn off machine, and store tubing assembly per institution policy.	Proper storage reduces transfer of microorganisms.
a. Shake the nebulizer bottle, attempting to remove all remaining solution. NEVER rinse with tap water.	Tap water may contain microorganisms.
9. If steroids are nebulized, encourage client to rinse mouth and gargle with warm water after nebulizer treatment.	Removes medication residue from oral cavity and helps to prevent thrush, a possible side effect of steroid therapy.
10. After medication administration, assess client's respirations and breath sounds, and assess peak flow measures if ordered.	Determines status of breathing pattern and adequacy of ventilation/gas exchange.

STEP	RATIONALE
11. Perform hand hygiene, and assist client to comfortable position.	Reduces the spread of microorganisms and promotes client comfort.

- **Critical Decision Point**
  Some respiratory medications can cause systemic effects such as restlessness, nervousness, and palpitations. Administer these medications with caution to clients with cardiac disease because of the possibility of hypertension, arrhythmias, or coronary insufficiency. If severe bronchospasm occurs during treatment, discontinue drug immediately and notify physician.

EVALUATION

1. Assess client's pulse, respiratory rate and pattern, breath sounds, and peak flow measurement (if ordered) after procedure.	Allows comparison with baseline data and evaluation of effectiveness of procedure.
2. Have client explain and demonstrate steps in use of small-volume nebulizer.	Return demonstration provides feedback for measuring client's learning.
3. Ask client to explain drug schedule.	Improves likelihood of compliance with therapy.
4. Ask client to describe side effects of medication and criteria for calling physician.	Allows client to recognize signs of overuse and need to seek medical support when drugs are ineffective.

Recording and Reporting

- Record drug used, dosage and concentration, and time and date of administration on MAR immediately after administration. Include initials or signature. Do not chart medication administration until *after* it is given to client.
- Record client's response to the medication, including pulse, respirations, and breath sounds assessed.
- If drug is withheld, record reason in nurses' notes. Circle time the drug normally would have been given on MAR (or follow institution's policy for noting withheld doses).
- Document what skills were taught and client's ability to perform them.
- Report adverse effects/client response and/or withheld drugs to nurse in charge or physician. Depending on medication, immediate prescriber notification may be required.

Unexpected Outcomes	Related Interventions
1. Client's breathing pattern is ineffective; respirations are rapid and shallow; breath sounds indicate wheezing.	• May need to reassess type of medication and/or delivery method. • Notify prescriber.
2. Client experiences paroxysms of coughing. Aerosolized particles can irritate posterior pharynx.	• May need to reassess type of medication and/or delivery method. • Notify prescriber.
3. Client experiences cardiac dysrhythmias (light-headedness, syncope), especially if receiving beta-adrenergics.	• Withhold all further doses of medication. • Notify prescriber for reassessment of type of medication and delivery method.
4. Client may not be able to self-administer medication properly.	• Alternative delivery routes or devices may need to be explored.
5. Client is unable to explain technique and risks of drug therapy.	• Further teaching may be required. • Include family members or caregivers when possible.

Teaching Considerations

*   When teaching self-administration, do not try to teach client how to use a nebulizer during an episode of shortness of breath. Client's attention span will be very poor.
*   Teach client that length of treatment is usually 10 to 15 minutes, if equipment is working properly and correct medication and diluent are used. If treatment time is prolonged, check nebulizer or compressor function.
*   Use all the medication in nebulizer cup for each treatment. Teach client not to store medication in nebulizer for later use (James and others, 2002).
*   Review all steps of the procedure with client before discharge, and ask client to demonstrate the proper technique. Reinforce teaching as needed.
*   Advise clients taking long-acting beta-agonists, which are used for long-term control of symptoms, about possible adverse effects: nervousness, restlessness, tremor, headache, nausea, rapid or pounding heart, and dizziness. Emphasize that the drug should only be taken as ordered so that a tolerance to the drug is not developed.
*   Teach clients to use small handheld peak flowmeters to monitor response to therapy when bronchodilators or bronchospasm prevention drugs (steroids) are prescribed (Ignatavicius and Workman, 2002).
*   Teach the client to rinse his or her mouth with water after the use of inhaled corticosteroids to prevent oropharyngeal candidiasis (Lewis and others, 2004).
*   Teach client to change the filter according to the machine manufacturer's directions.

Pediatric Considerations

*   A mask may be used for the nebulizer treatment if child is too young to hold mouthpiece correctly for the duration of the treatment (James and others, 2002).
*   Instruct child to breathe normally with mouth open to provide a direct route to the airways for the medication.
*   Educate child and parent about the need to use nebulizer during school or day care hours. Help family find resources within the school or day care facility. Follow the school's policy regarding having the nebulizer and medication available for use during school hours. A physician's order may be necessary.

Home Care Considerations

*   When at home, nebulizer parts should be rinsed after each use with clear water and air dried. In addition, parts should be cleaned daily with warm, soapy water, rinsed, and allowed to dry.
*   Once a week, nebulizer parts should be soaked in a solution of vinegar and water (one part white vinegar to four parts water) for 30 minutes, rinsed thoroughly with clean water, and air dried. Nebulizer parts should never be stored until totally dried. Wet equipment encourages growth of bacteria and mold (James and others, 2002).
*   Follow manufacturer's recommendations for maintenance of small-volume nebulizer machine, including changing the filters when they become discolored (grayish).

SKILL 20-10 Administering Vaginal Instillations

Female clients can often develop vaginal infections that require topical application of antiinfective agents. Vaginal medications are available in foam, jelly, cream, or suppository form. Medicated irrigations or douches can also be given. However, their excessive use can lead to vaginal irritation.

Vaginal suppositories are oval shaped and come individually packaged in foil wrappers. They are larger and more oval than rectal suppositories. (Figure 20-3 provides a comparison with rectal suppositories.) Storage in a refrigerator prevents the solid suppositories from melting. A suppository is inserted into the vagina with an applicator or a gloved hand. After insertion, body temperature causes the suppository to melt, and the medication is then distributed. Foam, jellies, and creams are administered with an inserter or applicator. Clients often prefer administering their own vaginal medications and should be given privacy to do so. After instillation of the drug, a client may wish to wear a perineal pad to collect excess drainage. Because vaginal medications are frequently given to treat infection, any discharge may be foul smelling. Good aseptic technique should be followed, and the client should be offered frequent opportunities to maintain perineal hygiene (see Skill 14-1, p. 382).

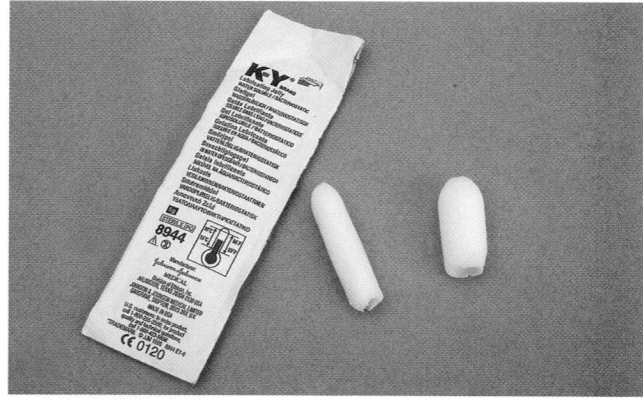

FIGURE 20-3 Vaginal suppositories *(right)* are larger and more oval than rectal suppositories *(left)*.

DELEGATION CONSIDERATIONS

The skill of vaginal instillations should not be delegated to assistive personnel. However, certain aspects of the client's care, such as hygiene and vital signs, may be delegated. Before delegation the nurse should:

- Instruct assistive personnel about potential side effects of medications and to report their occurrence
- Instruct assistive personnel to report any change in comfort level, new or increased vaginal discharge or bleeding to the nurse for further assessment

EQUIPMENT

- ❑ Vaginal cream, foam, jelly, tablet, or suppository, or irrigating solution
- ❑ Applicators (if needed)
- ❑ Disposable gloves
- ❑ Tissues
- ❑ Towels and/or washcloths
- ❑ Perineal pad
- ❑ Drape or sheet
- ❑ Water-soluble lubricants
- ❑ Bedpan
- ❑ Irrigation or douche container (if needed)
- ❑ Medication administration record (MAR)

STEP	RATIONALE
ASSESSMENT	
1. Review prescriber's order, including client's name, drug name, form (foam, jelly, cream, tablet, suppository, or irrigating solution), route, dosage, and time of administration.	Ensures safe and correct administration of medication.
2. Review pertinent information related to medication, including action, purpose, side effects, and nursing implications.	Allows nurse to administer drug properly and to monitor client's response.
3. Ask if client is experiencing any symptoms of pruritus, burning, or discomfort.	Assesses for symptoms of vaginal irritation.
4. Have client void.	Empties bladder and promotes comfort during insertion.
5. Assess client's ability to manipulate applicator, suppository, or irrigation equipment, and to properly position self to insert medication (may be done just before insertion).	Mobility restriction indicates level of assistance required from nurse.
6. Review client's knowledge of purpose of drug therapy and interest in self-administering medication.	May indicate need for health teaching. Understanding influences compliance with therapy.
NURSING DIAGNOSES	
• Deficient knowledge regarding vaginal medication administration	• Health-seeking behaviors (self-care)
• Impaired physical mobility	• Noncompliance with drug therapy
• Sexual dysfunction	• Pain (acute or chronic)

Related factors are individualized based on client's condition or needs.

PLANNING	
1. Expected outcomes following completion of procedure:	
• Vaginal tissues are pink and smooth. Genitalia are clear and without discharge.	Tissues take on normal characteristics.
• Client denies symptoms of discomfort and expresses relief from symptoms of infection/inflammation. A small amount of discharge may be seen that is the color of medication exiting from vaginal canal.	Inflammation or infection has resolved. When suppository or cream becomes distributed, small amount may escape from the vaginal orifice.
• Client is able to discuss information about prescribed drug.	Feedback reflects client's learning.
• Client self-administers suppository, medication, or irrigation.	Demonstrates learning.

STEP	RATIONALE
2. Check accuracy and completeness of each MAR with prescriber's written medication order. Check client's name, drug name and dosage, route of administration, and time for administration. Compare MAR with medication label three times during preparation of medication.	The order sheet is the most reliable source and only legal record of drugs client is to receive. Ensures right medication is administered.
3. Check client's identification bracelet, and ask name.	Ensures correct client receives medication. At least two patient identifiers (neither to be the patient's room number) are to be used whenever administering medications (JCAHO, 2004).
4. Explain procedure to client. Be specific if client plans on self-administering medication.	Promotes client's understanding. Enables client to self-administer drug if physically able.

IMPLEMENTATION

STEP	RATIONALE
1. Close room curtain or door.	Provides privacy.
2. Perform hand hygiene, arrange supplies at bedside, and apply clean gloves.	Reduces transfer of microorganisms; helps nurse perform procedure smoothly.
3. Assist client with lying in dorsal recumbent position. Clients with restricted mobility in knees or hips may lie supine with legs abducted.	Position provides easy access to and good exposure of vaginal canal. Dependent position also allows suppository to dissolve in vagina without escaping.
4. Keep abdomen and lower extremities draped.	Minimizes client's embarrassment by limiting exposure.
5. Be sure vaginal orifice is well-illuminated by room light. Otherwise, position portable gooseneck lamp.	Proper insertion requires visualization of external genitalia if not self-administered.
6. Inspect condition of external genitalia and vaginal canal (Chapter 18).	Provides baseline to monitor effect of medication.
7. For suppository insertion:	
a. Remove suppository from wrapper, and apply liberal amount of water-soluble lubricant to smooth or rounded end (see illustration). Be sure that suppository is at room temperature. Lubricate gloved index finger of dominant hand.	Lubrication reduces friction against mucosal surfaces during insertion. Use of petroleum jelly may leave a residue that harbors bacteria and yeast fungi.
b. With nondominant gloved hand, gently separate labial folds in the front-to-back direction.	Exposes vaginal orifice.
c. Insert rounded end of suppository along posterior wall of vaginal canal entire length of finger (7.5 to 10 cm or 3 to 4 inches) (see illustration).	Proper placement of suppository ensures equal distribution of medication along walls of vaginal cavity.

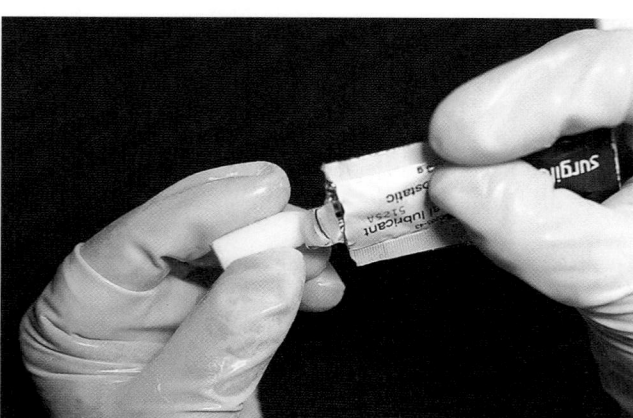

STEP **7a** Lubricate tip of suppository.

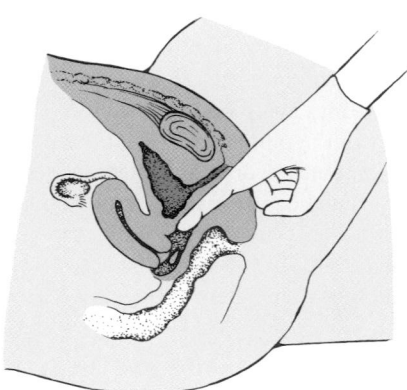

STEP **7c** Angle of vaginal suppository insertion.

STEP	RATIONALE
d. Withdraw finger, and wipe away remaining lubricant from around orifice and labia with a tissue or cloth.	Maintains comfort.
8. For application of cream or foam:	
a. Fill cream or foam applicator following package directions.	Dose is instilled based on volume in applicator.
b. With nondominant gloved hand, gently separate labial folds.	Exposes vaginal orifice.
c. With dominant gloved hand, insert applicator approximately 5 to 7.5 cm (2 to 3 inches). Push applicator plunger to deposit medication into vagina (see illustration).	Allows equal distribution of medication along vaginal walls.

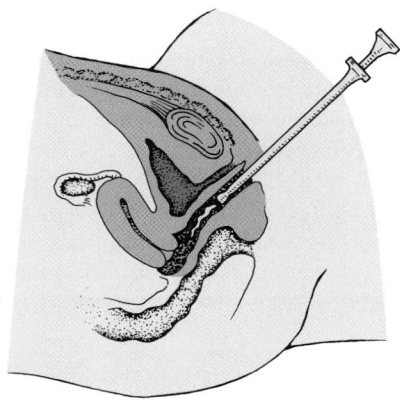

STEP **8c** Applicator inserted into vaginal canal. Plunger pushed to instill medication.

STEP	RATIONALE
d. Withdraw applicator and place on paper towel. Wipe off residual cream from labia or vaginal orifice with a tissue or cloth.	Maintains client comfort. Residual cream on applicator may contain microorganisms.
9. For irrigation and douche:	
a. Place client on bedpan with absorbent pad underneath.	Allows hips to be higher than shoulders and solution reaches posterior wall of vagina. Bedpan collects solution.
b. Be sure fluid is at body temperature. Run fluid through container nozzle (priming the tubing).	Body temperature promotes client comfort. Priming tubing removes air and moistens the nozzle tip.
c. Gently separate labial folds, and direct nozzle toward sacrum, following the floor of the vagina.	Correct angle allows nozzle access into the vagina.
d. Raise container approximately 30 to 50 cm (12 to 20 inches) above level of vagina. Insert nozzle 7 to 10 cm (3 to 4 inches). Allow solution to flow while rotating nozzle. Administer all the irrigating solution.	Rotating nozzle allows irrigation of all areas in vagina.
e. Withdraw nozzle, and assist client to a comfortable sitting position.	Remaining solution drains by gravity.
f. Allow client to remain on bedpan for a few minutes. Cleanse perineum with soap and water.	Ensures all solution drains from vagina. Provides comfort for the client.
g. Assist client off bedpan. Dry perineal area.	
10. Instruct client who received suppository, cream, or tablet to remain on her back for at least 10 minutes.	Allows melting and spreading of the medication throughout vaginal cavity and prevents loss through the orifice.
11. If applicator is used, wash with soap and warm water, rinse, and store for future use.	Vaginal cavity is not sterile. Soap and water assist in removal of bacteria and residual cream from applicator.
12. Offer perineal pad when client resumes ambulation.	Provides client comfort.
13. Discard gloves by turning them inside out, and dispose of gloves and other soiled equipment in appropriate receptacle. Perform hand hygiene.	Reduces transmission of microorganisms.

STEP	RATIONALE

▌ EVALUATION

1. Don gloves. Inspect condition of vaginal canal and external genitalia between applications. Assess vaginal discharge, if present.

Determines whether vaginal medication effectively reduced irritation or inflammation of tissues.

2. Question client regarding continued pruritus, burning, discomfort, or discharge.

Determines whether symptoms are relieved.

3. Ask client to discuss purpose, action, and side effects of medication.

Reflects client's understanding of drug therapy.

4. Have client demonstrate administration of next dose.

Reflects learning of technique.

Recording and Reporting

- Record appearance of vaginal canal and genitalia in nurses' notes, and report any unusual findings.
- Record actual time each drug (or solution if vaginal instillation) was administered on MAR immediately after administration. Include initials or signature. Do not chart medication administration until *after* it is given to client.
- If drug is withheld, record reason in nurses' notes. Circle time the drug normally would have been given on MAR (or follow institution's policy for noting withheld doses).
- If symptoms do not disappear, or if they get worse, report to prescriber.
- Report adverse effects/client response and/or withheld drugs to nurse in charge or physician.

Unexpected Outcomes	Related Interventions
1. A thick, white, patchy, curdlike discharge is clinging to vaginal walls. Vaginal walls appear bright pink or inflamed.	• Possible signs of yeast infection. Continue medication administration, and report if symptoms continue or appear to get worse.
2. Client reports localized pruritus and burning.	• Results of infection or inflammation, but may be a possible side effect of some medications (such as miconazole). • Monitor symptoms; report if they are worse.
3. Client is unable to discuss drug therapy correctly.	• Requires repeated instruction, or client is unable to learn. • Include family members or caregiver when appropriate.
4. Client is unable to self-administer medications.	• Reinstruction is necessary.

Teaching Considerations

- Teach client value of and technique for regular perineal hygiene.
- Encourage client to take *all* of the medication as prescribed, for the prescribed amount of time, to ensure effectiveness of the treatment.
- Women taking antifungal medications for the treatment of vaginal infections should abstain from sexual intercourse until the treatment is completed and the infection is resolved. Women should be told to continue to take the medication even if actively menstruating. Clients should notify the physician if symptoms persist past the treatment time period (Lilley and others, 2005).
- Many women prefer to self-administer vaginal irrigations and medications. Ensure that the client is able to perform the procedure correctly.

SKILL 20-11 Administering Rectal Suppositories

A variety of medications may be given rectally. Drugs administered rectally exert either a local effect on gastrointestinal mucosa, such as promoting defecation, or exert systemic effects, such as relieving nausea or providing analgesia. The rectal route is not as reliable as oral or parenteral routes in terms of drug absorption and distribution. However, the medications are relatively safe, because they rarely cause local irritation or side effects. Rectal medications are contraindicated in clients with rectal surgery or active rectal bleeding.

Rectal suppositories differ in shape from vaginal suppositories, being thinner and bullet shaped. (See Figure 20-3 for comparison with vaginal suppositories.) The rounded end prevents anal trauma during insertion. When the nurse administers the suppository, placing it past the internal anal sphincter and against the rectal mucosa is important. Improper placement can result in expulsion of the suppository before the medication dissolves and is absorbed into the mucosa. If a client prefers to self-administer a suppository, the nurse should give specific instructions so that the medication is deposited correctly. Do not cut the suppository into sections to divide the dosage; the active drug may not be distributed evenly within the suppository, and the result may be an inaccurate dose (Lilley and others, 2005).

DELEGATION CONSIDERATIONS

The skill of rectal medication administration should not be delegated to assistive personnel. However, certain aspects of the client's care may be delegated. Before delegation the nurse must:

- Instruct assistive personnel about expected fecal discharge or bowel movement and to report occurrence to the nurse
- Instruct assistive personnel about potential side effects of medications and to report their occurrence
- Instruct assistive personnel about informing nurse of any rectal discharge, pain, or bleeding

EQUIPMENT

- ❑ Rectal suppository
- ❑ Lubricating jelly (water soluble)
- ❑ Clean gloves
- ❑ Tissue
- ❑ Drape
- ❑ Medication administration record (MAR)

STEP	RATIONALE

ASSESSMENT

1. Review prescriber's order, including client's name, drug name, dosage, form, route, and time of administration.

2. Review pertinent information related to medication, including action, purpose, side effects, and nursing implications.

3. Review medical record for history of rectal surgery or bleeding.

Ensures safe and correct administration of medication.

Allows nurse to administer drug properly and to monitor client's response.

Conditions contraindicate use of suppository.

- *Critical Decision Point*

  Generally, a rectal suppository is contraindicated with the presence of active rectal bleeding. Unless the suppository is for constipation, placing a medication in a rectum filled with feces may result in poor absorption of the medication, or it may be prematurely expelled with defecation.

4. Review any presenting signs and symptoms of gastrointestinal alterations (e.g., constipation or diarrhea).

5. Assess client's ability to hold suppository and to position self to insert medication.

6. Review client's knowledge of purpose of drug therapy and interest in self-administering suppository.

Conditions may indicate use of suppository.

Mobility restriction indicates need for nurse to assist with drug administration.

May indicate need for health teaching. Level of motivation influences teaching approach.

STEP	RATIONALE

◼ NURSING DIAGNOSES

- Constipation
- Health-seeking behaviors (self-care)
- Pain (acute or chronic)

- Deficient knowledge regarding suppository administration
- Impaired physical mobility

Related factors are individualized based on client's condition or needs.

◼ PLANNING

1. Expected outcomes following completion of the procedure:
   - Client reports relief or reduction in symptoms for which medication is prescribed.
   - Client describes purpose of medication.
   - Client self-administers suppository.
2. Check accuracy and completeness of each MAR with prescriber's written medication order. Check client's name, drug name and dosage, route of administration, and time for administration. Compare MAR with medication label three times during preparation of medication.
3. Check client's identification bracelet, and ask name.

4. Explain procedure to client. Be specific if client wishes to self-administer drug.

Drug acts effectively.

Feedback reflects client's learning.
Demonstrates learning.
The order sheet is the most reliable source and only legal record of drugs client is to receive. Ensures right medication is administered.

Ensures correct client receives medication. At least two patient identifiers (neither to be the patient's room number) are to be used whenever administering medications (JCAHO, 2004).
Promotes client's understanding and cooperation. Enables client to self-administer drug safely if physically able and motivated.

◼ IMPLEMENTATION

1. Close room curtain or door.
2. Perform hand hygiene, arrange supplies at bedside, and apply gloves.
3. Assist client in assuming a left side-lying Sims' position with upper leg flexed upward.

Maintains privacy and minimizes embarrassment.
Reduces transfer of microorganisms, helps nurse perform procedure smoothly.
Position exposes anus and helps client to relax external anal sphincter. Left side lessens the likelihood of the suppository or feces being expelled.

- **Critical Decision Point**

  If client has mobility impairment that prevents a left side-lying Sims' position, assist client to a left lateral position. Obtain assistance from another health care provider to help client turn, and use pillows under client's upper arm and leg for support and comfort.

4. Keep client draped with only anal area exposed.
5. Examine condition of anus externally, and palpate rectal walls as needed (e.g., if impaction is suspected) (see Chapter 18). Dispose of gloves by turning them inside out and placing them in proper receptacle if they become soiled.

Maintains privacy and facilitates relaxation.
Determines presence of active rectal bleeding. Palpation determines whether rectum is filled with feces, which may interfere with suppository placement. Reduces transmission of infection.

- **Critical Decision Point**

  Do not palpate client's rectum if client has had rectal surgery. Generally, rectal suppository is contraindicated in the presence of active rectal bleeding and diarrhea (Lilley and others, 2005).

6. Apply new pair of disposable gloves (if previous gloves were soiled and discarded).

Minimizes contact with fecal material to reduce transmission of infection.

STEP	**RATIONALE**
7. Remove suppository from foil wrapper, and lubricate rounded end with water-soluble lubricant. Lubricate gloved index finger of dominant hand. If client has hemorrhoids, use liberal amount of lubricant, and handle area gently.	Lubrication reduces friction as suppository enters rectal canal.
8. Ask client to take slow deep breaths through mouth and to relax anal sphincter.	Forcing suppository through constricted sphincter causes pain.
9. Retract client's buttocks with nondominant hand. With gloved index finger of dominant hand, insert suppository gently through anus, past internal sphincter, and against rectal wall, 10 cm (4 inches) (see illustration).	Suppository must be placed against rectal mucosa for eventual absorption and therapeutic action.

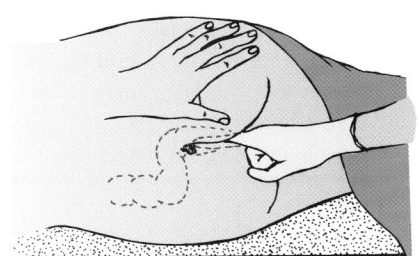

STEP **9** Insert rectal suppository past sphincter and against rectal wall.

- *Critical Decision Point*
  Suppository should not be inserted into a mass of fecal material; medication effectiveness will be reduced.

10. Withdraw finger, and wipe client's anal area.	Provides comfort.
11. Discard gloves by turning them inside out, and dispose of in appropriate receptacle.	Reduces transfer of microorganisms.
12. Ask client to remain flat or on side for 5 minutes.	Prevents expulsion of suppository.
13. If suppository contains laxative or fecal softener, place call light within reach so client can obtain assistance to reach bedpan or toilet.	Ability to call for assistance provides client with sense of control over elimination.
14. If the suppository was given for constipation, remind the client *not* to flush the commode after the bowel movement.	Allows staff to evaluate results of the suppository.
15. Perform hand hygiene, and dispose of gloves and other equipment.	Reduces risk of transfer of infection.

- *Critical Decision Point*
  Suppositories may be given through a colostomy (not ileostomy) if ordered. Use a small amount of water-soluble lubricant for insertion.

EVALUATION

1. Return within 5 minutes to determine if suppository was expelled.	Determines if drug is properly distributed. Reinsertion may be necessary.
2. Ask if client experienced localized anal or rectal discomfort during insertion.	Determines whether insertion of suppository was irritating.

STEP	RATIONALE
3. Evaluate client for relief of symptoms for which medication was prescribed to relieve or eliminate (within time expected action of drug occurs).	Determines medication's effectiveness.
4. Ask client to explain purpose of medication.	Reflects client's understanding of drug therapy.
5. Have client demonstrate administration of next dose of medication.	Demonstration measures learning.

Recording and Reporting

- Record actual time each drug was administered on MAR immediately after administration. Include initials or signature. Do not chart medication administration until *after* it is given to client.
- If drug is withheld, record reason in nurses' notes. Circle time the drug normally would have been given on MAR (or follow institution's policy for noting withheld doses).
- Record client's response to medication, including any unusual reactions.
- Report adverse effects/client response and/or withheld drugs to nurse in charge or physician. Depending on medication, immediate prescriber notification may be required.

Unexpected Outcomes	Related Interventions
1. Side effects of specific medication develops.	• May require alternative therapy.
2. Symptoms previously reported are unrelieved.	• May require alternative therapy.
3. Client reports rectal pain during insertion.	• Suppository may need more lubrication. • Rectal route may not be suitable; assess and notify prescriber.
4. Client is unable to explain purpose of drug therapy.	• Reinstruction is necessary, or client is unwilling or unable to learn. • Include family members or caregiver as appropriate.
5. Client is unable to self-administer medication.	• Reinstruction is necessary.

Teaching Considerations

- If client chooses to self-administer suppositories, teach principles and techniques of infection control to prevent contact with and spread of fecal material.
- Long-term use of laxatives often results in decreased bowel tone and may result in dependency. Client should be taught nonpharmacological measures (fiber and fluid intake, dietary habits) to promote healthy bowel elimination (Lilley and others, 2005).

Pediatric Considerations

- With children, it may be necessary to gently hold or tape the buttocks together for 5 to 10 minutes to relieve pressure on the anal sphincter until the urge to expel the suppository is gone (Hockenberry and others, 2003).

Gerontological Considerations

- Older adult clients with loss of sphincter control may have difficulty retaining suppository.

FOCUS on CLINICAL PRACTICE

Mrs. Brown, a 72-year-old African-American woman, has been admitted to the hospital for weight loss and weakness following the flu. She is widowed, lives with her daughter's family, and has helped with the care of her grandchildren. She has a history of hypertension and asthma, osteoarthritis in her hands, and an area of a second-degree burn on her left forearm that she says was caused when she spilled boiling water in the kitchen.

Medication orders include:

- IV D_5 ½ NS at 75 ml/hr
- Hydrochlorothiazide 25 mg every AM PO (diuretic)
- Diltiazem SR capsule, 60 mg bid PO (calcium channel blocker)
- Flovent (fluticasone propionate) MDI 220 mcg/actuation every 12 hours (inhaled corticosteroid)
- Proventil (albuterol) MDI every 4 hours (inhaled bronchodilator)
- Ibuprofen (Motrin) 600 mg every 8 hours 12.5 mg daily PO (nonsteroidal antiinflammatory drug)
- Silver sulfadiazine (Silvadene) cream to burned area bid, then cover with gauze

1. What should you assess before giving her medications?
2. Mrs. Brown asks if you could crush her medications. Which PO medications, if any, cannot be crushed? Explain.

3. At 1200 the Flovent is due. You decide to observe as she gives herself the MDI dose, and you note that she has trouble pressing the canister while she inhales.
   A. What could you suggest to help her?
   B. What should be done after she has finished taking the Flovent?
   C. If she was experiencing an episode of bronchospasm, which inhaler is appropriate to use? Explain.
4. While she is in the hospital, you demonstrate to her how to dress her arm wound. She is able to explain the procedure to you. Three days after she is discharged, a home care nurse visits to check her progress and finds that the jar of Silvadene is almost empty. It was supposed to last for 2 weeks. When the dressing is removed from the arm, the nurse notes that the ointment is caked onto the wound. Mrs. K.L. explains that she did not want to "waste" the medication by washing it off.

   What should be reemphasized regarding her wound care?

NCLEX REVIEW QUESTIONS

1. The proper way to measure liquid cough elixir for a child is to use a/an:
   1. Teaspoon
   2. Syringe *with* a needle attached
   3. Syringe *without* a needle attached
   4. Oral-dosing syringe
2. One of your clients says he prefers to chew rather than swallow his pills. One of the medications is an extended-release tablet. Which of the following is an appropriate action in response to his request?
   1. Break the tablet into halves or quarters.
   2. Allow him to chew the tablet if he prefers.
   3. The tablet should not be crushed, broken, or chewed.
   4. Use a mortar and pestle to crush the tablet.
3. Which is appropriate when administering medications through a nasogastric tube?
   1. Verify tube placement after medications are given.
   2. Mix all crushed medications together, and give all at once.

3. Flush tube with a minimal amount of water after giving medications.
   4. Flush tube with 30 to 60 ml of water after the last dose of medication.
4. If a nasogastric tube appears to be clogged, what should be done first?
   1. Notify the physician.
   2. Attempt to irrigate it gently with tepid water.
   3. Attempt to flush the tube with cranberry juice.
   4. Remove the tube immediately, and replace it.
5. Which of the following is appropriate when applying topical medications to an open wound?
   1. Use clean gloves when applying medication.
   2. Use sterile gloves when applying medication.
   3. Previously applied medication should remain on the wound surface.
   4. Be sure to apply a thick layer of medication over the wound.

Continued

NCLEX REVIEW QUESTIONS

6. The client demonstrates understanding of the use of transdermal patches when he states:
   1. "I will apply the patch to a different area each time."
   2. "I need to leave the old patch on to make sure I receive all the medicine."
   3. "If I get a headache from this medicine, I will cut the patch in half."
   4. "It does not matter where I throw away the old patch because the medicine is gone."

7. What is the best method for reducing systemic effects after administering eye drops?
   1. Wipe off excess liquid immediately after instilling drops.
   2. Have the client close the eye tightly after instilling drops.
   3. Have the client close the eye; then move the eye around to help distribute the medication.
   4. Apply gentle pressure to the client's nasolacrimal duct for 30 to 60 seconds after giving the drops.

8. The nurse is preparing to give eye drops to a client. Which of the following is correct?
   1. The drops should be instilled directly onto the cornea for best effect.
   2. The drops should be instilled into the conjunctival sac.
   3. The client should look down while the drops are administered.
   4. As soon as the drops are given, the client should be instructed to wipe his or her eye.

9. What is the proper technique for administering ear drops to a 2-year-old child?
   1. Administer the drops without pulling on the ear lobe.
   2. Straighten the ear canal by pulling the lobe upward and back.
   3. Straighten the ear canal by pulling the auricle down and back.
   4. Straighten the ear canal by pulling the auricle upward and outward.

10. What is the best way to warm ear drops before instillation?
   1. Allow them to sit at room temperature for at least 2 hours.
   2. Run warm water over the medication bottle.
   3. Heat for 15 seconds in a microwave oven on low power.
   4. Rub the bottle between your hands for 45 seconds.

11. Which of the following is an indication for ear irrigations?
   1. Vertigo
   2. Removal of cerumen
   3. Ruptured tympanic membrane
   4. Middle ear infection

12. When performing an ear irrigation, the nurse inserts the tip of the irrigating syringe as follows:
   1. Place the tip of the syringe into the ear canal to occlude it and reduce fluid backflow.
   2. Hold the tip of the syringe 2 inches above the opening to the ear canal.
   3. Hold the tip of the syringe 1 cm ($\frac{1}{2}$ inch) above the opening to the ear canal.
   4. Hold the tip of the syringe so that the fluid is directed toward the lower aspect of the ear canal.

13. Overuse of decongestant nose drops can result in:
   1. The development of a subclinical sinus infection
   2. Decreased drainage from the nares
   3. Excessive drying of the nasal mucosa
   4. Increased congestion and swollen mucosa

14. When is the best time to give nose drops to an infant who is bottle-fed?
   1. Just before feeding
   2. Just after feeding
   3. 20 to 30 minutes before feeding
   4. Timing of nose drops does not matter.

15. A client with asthma is to begin medication therapy with a metered-dose inhaler. What is an important reminder to include during your teaching sessions with her?
   1. Repeat subsequent puffs, if ordered, after 5 minutes.
   2. Inhale slowly while pressing down to release the medication.
   3. Inhale quickly while pressing down to release the medication.
   4. Administer the inhaler while holding it 3 to 4 inches away from her mouth.

16. Which intervention would help to improve self-administration of medication with a metered-dose inhaler?
   1. Teach the client to press the canister before taking a breath.
   2. Teach the client to avoid shaking the metered-dose inhaler before using it.
   3. Provide a spacer device for clients who have trouble pressing the canister.
   4. Instruct the client to hold his or her breath for at least 30 seconds after the inhaler is given.

NCLEX REVIEW QUESTIONS

17. During administration of medications with a small-volume nebulizer the nurse should monitor the client's:
    1. Respirations
    2. Breath sounds
    3. Pulse rate
    4. Capillary refill

18. Which of the following is correct when teaching a client regarding use of a small-volume nebulizer?
    1. Bronchodilators can be taken whenever the client feels a need for them.
    2. Clients should rinse their mouths with water after receiving inhaled steroids.
    3. Nebulizer parts should be washed with vinegar and water solution after each use.
    4. If the medication is not completely used with a treatment, it can be saved in the nebulizer cup for the next treatment.

19. Which of the following is correct when teaching the client about using vaginal medications?
    1. These medications are best given in the morning, after voiding.
    2. After administration, she should remain on her back for at least 10 minutes.
    3. Use petroleum jelly to lubricate suppositories if needed.
    4. The medication can be stopped once symptoms are gone.

20. Which position is the ideal position for receiving vaginal instillations?
    1. Left lateral
    2. Right lateral
    3. Dorsal recumbent
    4. Sims' position

21. Which technique is correct regarding the administration of rectal suppositories?
    1. Have the client lie on his or her right side unless contraindicated.
    2. Have the client hold his or her breath during insertion of the suppository.
    3. Lubricate the suppository with a small amount of petroleum-based lubricant.
    4. Encourage the client to lie on his or her left side for 15 to 20 minutes after insertion.

22. Contraindications to rectal suppositories include:
    1. Diarrhea
    2. Constipation
    3. Nausea
    4. Hemorrhoids

References

Al-Shahri MZ: Culturally sensitive caring for Saudi patients, *J Transcult Nurs* 13(2):133, 2002.

Ebersole P and others: *Toward healthy aging,* ed 6, St. Louis, 2004, Mosby.

Gallagher C: Childhood asthma: tools that help parents manage it, *Am J Nurs* 102(8):71, 2002.

Galvin TJ: Dysphagia: going down and staying down, *Am J Nurs* 101(1):37, 2001.

George M: The challenge of culturally competent health care: application for asthma, *Heart Lung* 30(5):392, 2001.

Hockenberry MJ and others: *Wong's nursing care of infants and children,* ed 7, St. Louis, 2003, Mosby.

Holcomb LD and others: Haitian-Americans: implications for nursing care, *J Community Health Nurs* 13(4):249, 1996.

Ignatavicius DD, Workman ML: *Medical-surgical nursing: critical thinking for collaborative care,* ed 4, Philadelphia, 2002, WB Saunders.

Institute for Safe Medicine Practices: Hazard alert! Asphyxiation possible with syringe tip caps, *ISMP medication safety alert,* August 2001, http://www.ismp.org/MSAarticles/Hypodermic.html, retrieved July 11, 2004.

James S and others: *Nursing care of children,* ed 2, Philadelphia, 2002, WB Saunders.

Joint Commission on the Accreditation of Healthcare Organizations: 2005 National patient safety goals, *2005 Critical access hospitals' national patient safety goals,* www.jacho.org/accredited+organizations/patientsafety/npsg.htm, accessed July 2004.

Lee M, Phillips J: Transdermal patches: high risk for error? *FDA safety page—drug topics,* April 1, 2002, http://www.fda.gov/cder/drug/MedErrors/transdermal.pdf, retrieved July 11, 2004.

Lewis SM and others: *Medical-surgical nursing: assessment and management of clinical problems,* ed 6, St. Louis, 2004, Mosby.

Lilley LL and others: *Pharmacology and the nursing process,* ed 4, St. Louis, 2005, Mosby.

Mahan LK, Escott-Stump S: *Krause's food, nutrition, and diet therapy,* ed 11, Philadelphia, 2004, WB Saunders.

Mashaba G: South African culturally based health-illness patterns and humanistic care practices. In Leininger M, McFarland M: *Transcultural nursing,* New York, 2002, McGraw-Hill.

Mayo Clinic: Metered-dose inhalers: how to use them properly, *Asthma health center,* March 6, 2003, www.mayoclinic.com, retrieved July 11, 2004.

McConnell EA: Clinical do's and don'ts: applying nitroglycerin ointment, *Nursing* 31(6):17, 2001.

Miller D, Miller H: To crush or not to crush, *Nursing* 30(2):51, 2000.

National Heart, Lung, and Blood Institute: *Nurses: partners in asthma care,* NIH Pub No. 95-3308, October 1994, www.nhlbi. nih.gov/health/prof/lung/asthma/nurs_gde.htm, retrieved July 11, 2004.

Nowak T: People of Vietnamese heritage. In Purnell L, Paulanka B: *Transcultural healthcare,* Philadelphia, 2003, FA Davis.

Orque MS: Nursing care of the South Vietnamese patients. In Orque MS and others, editors: *Ethnic nursing care,* St. Louis, 1983, Mosby.

Phipps WJ and others: *Medical-surgical nursing: health and illness perspectives,* ed 7, St. Louis, 2003, Mosby.

Terrado M and others: Dysphagia: an overview, *Medsurg Nurs* 10(5):233, 2001.

Togger DA, Brenner PS: Metered dose inhalers, *Am J Nurs* 101(10):26, 2001.

Wang Y: People of Chinese heritage. In Purnell L, Paulanka B: *Transcultural healthcare,* Philadelphia, 2003, FA Davis.

Research References

Drug watch: most med errors made during administration, *Am J Nurs* 101(3):25, 2001.

Kemp C, Rasbridge LD: *J Hosp Palliat Nurs* 3(3):110, 2001.

Metheny NA, Titler MG: Assessing placement of feeding tubes, *Am J Nurs* 101(5):36, 2001.

Shrestha M and others: Metered-dose inhaler technique of patients in an urban ED: prevalence of incorrect technique and attempt at education, *Am J Emerg Med* 14(4):380, 1996.

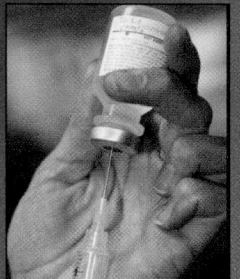

21

Parenteral Medications

MEDIA RESOURCES

Evolve Site *evolve*

http://evolve.elsevier.com/Perry/skills

- Weblinks
- Video clips
- Mosby's Nursing Skills Video Exercises

Mosby's Nursing Skills Videos/CD-ROM

- *Injections Video:* Preparing injections from an ampule and vial, how to break ampule/open vial, use of syringe and needle to withdraw medication, and changing needle for injection; preparing insulin, types of insulin and drawing up more than one type; intradermal injections, site identification and marking skin for allergy/TB testing; subcutaneous injections, site identification/needle length; intramuscular injections, including site identification/Z-track method
- *Intravenous Medications Video:* Adding medication to IV fluid containers; administering medications by IV bolus; administering IV medications by IV mini-infusion pumps

OBJECTIVES

Mastery of content in this chaper will enable the nurse to:

- Correctly prepare injectable medications from a vial and an ampule.
- Identify advantages, disadvantages, and risks of administering medications by each injection route.
- Explain the importance of selecting the proper size syringe and needle for an injection.
- Discuss factors to consider when selecting injection sites.
- Discuss ways to promote client comfort while administering an injection.
- Correctly administer intradermal, subcutaneous, and intramuscular injections.
- Correctly add medications to intravenous fluid containers.
- Compare the risks of three different intravenous routes.
- Correctly administer an intravenous infusion by intravenous piggyback, large-volume infusion, or bolus through a hanging intravenous line or a saline lock.
- Initiate, maintain, and discontinue a continuous subcutaneous medication.

KEY TERMS

Air embolus	Induration
Ampule	Infiltration
Anaphylactic reaction	Infusion
Aqueous	Injection
Aspirate	Intradermal (ID) injection
Bolus	Intramuscular (IM) injection
Compatibility	Intravenous (IV) injection
Continuous subcutaneous	Parenteral
infusion (CSQI or CSCI)	Phlebitis
Diluent	Piggyback infusion
Extravasation	Saline lock
Heparin lock	Subcutaneous (Sub-Q) injection
Hypodermoclysis	Vial
Incompatibility	Z-track method

Parenteral injections are used to instill medications into body tissues. The procedures for administering parenteral medications are invasive and thus pose greater risks than those associated with administering oral or topical medications. Injected drugs act more quickly than oral medications because they reach the bloodstream either directly or by rapid absorption through the tissues. Thus the client's response to parenteral medications and change in condition can occur rapidly. The nurse must closely monitor the client's response, be aware of potential adverse or allergic reactions, and understand the risk for infection once a needle enters the skin or a port of the intravenous system. The nurse uses strict aseptic technique whenever preparing and administering injections. Infection can originate from a variety of sources (Table 21-1).

Parenteral drugs can be administered through four different routes:

1. *Subcutaneous (Sub-Q) injection*—injection into tissues just below the dermis of the skin
2. *Intramuscular (IM) injection*—injection into the body of a muscle
3. *Intradermal (ID) injection*—injection into the dermis just under the epidermis
4. *Intravenous (IV) injection or infusion*—injection into a vein

Each type of injection requires a certain set of skills to make certain that the medication reaches the proper location. Failure to inject a medication correctly can result in complications such as a drug response that is too rapid or too slow, nerve injury with associated pain, localized bleeding, tissue necrosis, and sterile abscess.

Parenteral injections are delivered to a client by using a needle and a syringe. Needles and syringes come in a variety of sizes. The nurse determines the appropriate size of syringe and length of needle based on the type of medication to be delivered, the volume of solution to be delivered, and the medication route. Most syringes come with needleless systems. These safety systems help prevent needle-stick injuries. A variety of electronic infusion pumps are used to deliver intravenous or continuous Sub-Q infusions. Infusion pumps ensure a constant and accurate delivery of medication.

Syringes

A syringe consists of a cylindrical barrel, a tip designed to fit the hub of a hypodermic needle or a needleless device, and a plunger (Figure 21-1). Syringes are single-use and disposable. They are packaged separately, in a paper wrapper or rigid plastic container. Syringes may come with or without a sterile needle or with a needleless device and are classified as non–Luer-Lok or Luer-Lok. Non–Luer-Lok syringes use needles that slip onto the tip. Luer-Lok syringes (Figure 21-2, *A*) require special needles or needleless devices that are twisted onto the tip and lock themselves in place. The Luer-Lok design prevents the accidental removal of the needle from the syringe.

Syringes come in various sizes, ranging from 1 to 60 ml in capacity (Figure 21-2). The nurse, using knowledge about

TABLE 21-1   PREVENTING INFECTION DURING AN INJECTION

PRINCIPLE	TECHNIQUE
Prevent contamination of solution.	Add date, time, and initials to vials when opened. A multidose vial, properly labeled, can be used up to 30 days. Swab top of opened or unopened multidose vials with alcohol before piercing.
Prevent needle contamination.	Avoid letting needle touch contaminated surface: outer edges of ampule or vial, outer surface of needle cap, nurse's hands, countertop, or table surface.
Prepare skin.	Wash grossly contaminated sites with soap and water. Before giving an injection, use an alcohol swab to clean site; swab from center of site and move outward approximately 5 cm from center (2 inches).
Before handling any equipment, hand washing is essential to reduce the transfer of microorganisms.	Perform hand hygiene for a minimum of 15 seconds.

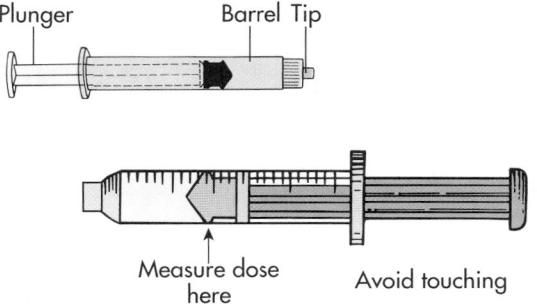

FIGURE **21-1** Parts of a syringe.

the medication prescribed, the types of syringes, and the location of an injection, determines which is the most appropriate to use. The nurse uses syringes from 1 to 30 ml to administer certain IV drugs and to add medications to IV solutions. Syringes from 1 to 5 ml are usually used for injections. A 1- to 3-ml syringe is adequate for IM and Sub-Q injections (see Figure 21-2, *A*). Some syringes have two scales along the barrel. One scale is divided into minims and the other into tenths of a milliliter. The tuberculin syringe (Figure 21-2, *B*) has a long, thin barrel with a preattached thin needle. The syringe, calibrated in sixteenths of a minim and hundredths of a milliliter, has a capacity of 1 ml. The nurse uses a tuberculin syringe to prepare small amounts of medication such as small, precise doses for infants or young children.

Insulin syringes (Figure 21-2, *C* and *D*) hold 0.3 ml, 0.5 ml, or 1 ml, come with a preattached needle, and are calibrated in units. Insulin syringes that hold 0.3 ml and 0.5 ml are known as low-dose syringes (30 units per 0.3 ml or 50 units per 0.5 ml) and are easier to read. These syringes are often used by people with visual problems and in children diagnosed with diabetes. Insulin syringes in the United States and Canada are U-100s, designed for use with U-100-strength insulin. Each milliliter of solution contains 100 units of insulin. Before use, the nurse carefully examines the syringe to determine which measurement scale is marked on the syringe and to ensure that the correct syringe is being used to prepare the ordered medication.

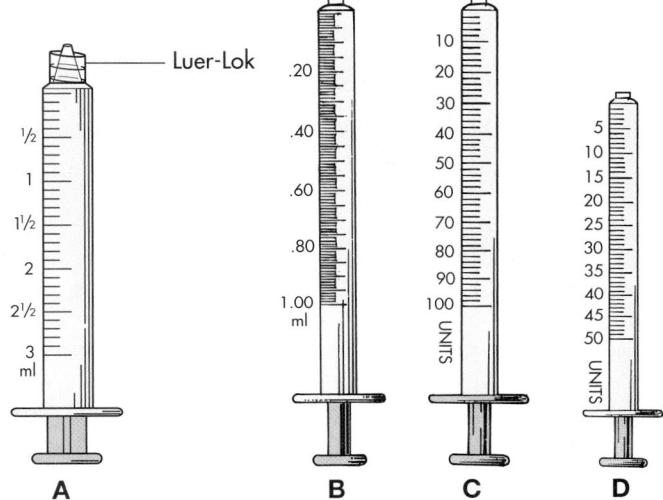

FIGURE **21-2** Types of syringes. **A,** Luer-Lok syringe with 3-ml capacity is marked in 0.1 (tenths). **B,** Tuberculin syringe marked in 0.01 (hundredths) for doses of less than 1 ml. **C,** Insulin syringe marked in units (100). **D,** Insulin syringe marked in units (50).

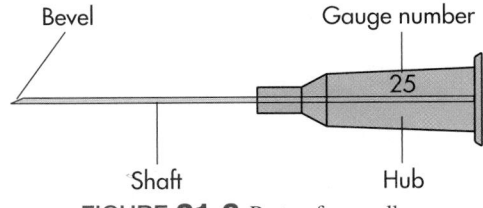

FIGURE **21-3** Parts of a needle.

Needles

Needles come packaged in individual sheaths to allow flexibility in choosing the right needle for a client. Some needles are preattached to standard-size syringes.

A needle has three parts: the hub, which fits onto the tip of a syringe; the shaft, which connects to the hub; and the bevel, or slanted tip (Figure 21-3). Some needles come with filters that are used in special situations. A filter needle should never

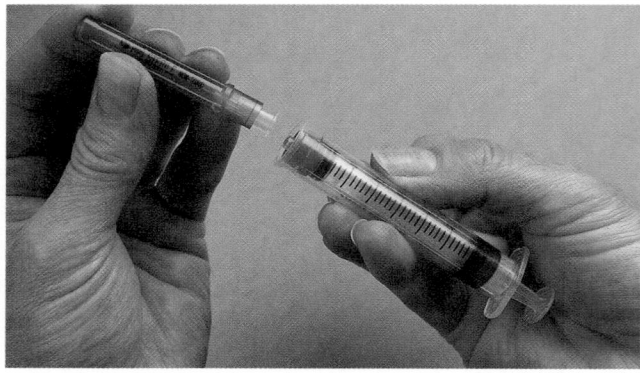

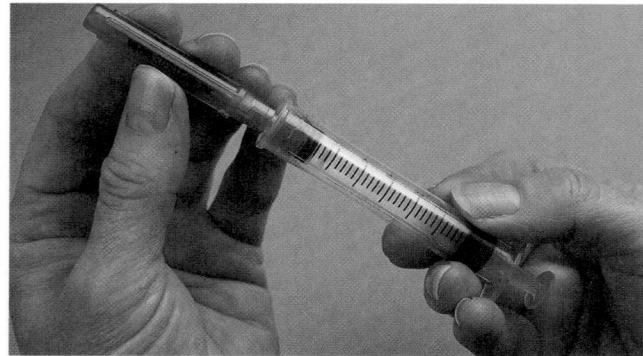

FIGURE **21-4** **A,** Capped needle placed on syringe tip. **B,** Needle secured.

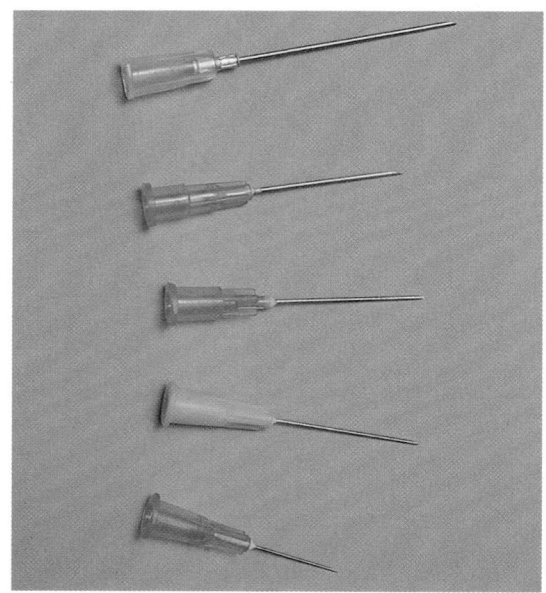

FIGURE **21-5** Needles. *Top to bottom:* 19 gauge, 1½-inch length; 20 gauge, 1-inch length; 21 gauge, 1-inch length; 23 gauge, 1-inch length; and 25 gauge, ⅝-inch length.

be used when administering a medication. The needle hub, shaft, and bevel must remain sterile at all times. To prevent contamination, the nurse places the needle onto the syringe with the cap intact, using gentle force (Figure 21-4).

Needle Features

The tip of a needle, or the bevel, is always slanted. The bevel creates a narrow slit when injected into tissue. The slit quickly closes when the needle is removed to prevent leakage of medication, blood, or serum. Longer beveled tips are sharper and narrower, which minimizes discomfort when tissue is entered for an Sub-Q or IM injection.

Needles vary in length from ⅜ inch to 3 inches (Figure 21-5). The nurse chooses the needle length according to the client's size and weight and the type of tissue into which the drug is to be injected. A child or slender adult generally requires a shorter needle. The nurse uses a longer needle (1 inch to 1½ inches) for IM injections and a shorter needle (⅜ to ⅝ inch) for Sub-Q or ID injections. As the needle gauge gets smaller, the needle diameter becomes larger. The selection of a gauge depends on the viscosity of fluid to be injected or infused. The rationale for needle selection is included in each skill.

Disposable Injection Units

Disposable single-dose prefilled syringes are available for some medications. With these syringes the nurse does not need to prepare medication doses, except perhaps to expel portions of unneeded medication.

The Carpuject Syringe System includes reusable plastic syringe holders and disposable, prefilled, sterile, glass cartridge units (Figure 21-6). The nurse places the cartridge, Luer tip first, into the plastic syringe holder. Following manufacturer's instructions, the nurse turns the plunger rod to the left (clockwise) and the lock to the right (counterclockwise) until it "clicks." The nurse checks for air bubbles in the syringe. Finally, the nurse removes the needle guard and advances the plunger to expel air and excess medication, as with a regular syringe. The glass cartridge may be used with needleless systems or safety needles. After the medication is given, the glass cartridge is easily and safely disposed of in a puncture-proof and leak-proof receptacle. This design reduces the risk of needle-stick injury.

Protecting Yourself From Needle-Stick Injury

The most frequent route of exposure to blood-borne disease is from needle-stick injuries (American Nurses Association, 2002; Perry and others, 2003). Exposure to blood-borne pathogens is one of the deadliest hazards nurses are exposed to on a daily basis. However, over 80% of needle-stick injuries can be prevented with the implementation of safe needle devices (American Nurses Association, 2002). The Needlestick Safety and Prevention Act is a federal law that became effective in April 2001. This federal law mandates health care facilities to use safe needle devices to reduce the frequency of needle-stick injury. One type of safe needle device is the safety syringe, which is equipped with a plastic guard or shield that slips over the needle as it is withdrawn from the skin (Figure 21-7, *A* and *B*). Another type of safety device can be found on needleless IV line connection systems (Figure 21-7, *C, D,* and *E*). Box 21-1 lists recommendations for health care workers to use to decrease the risk of needle-stick injuries.

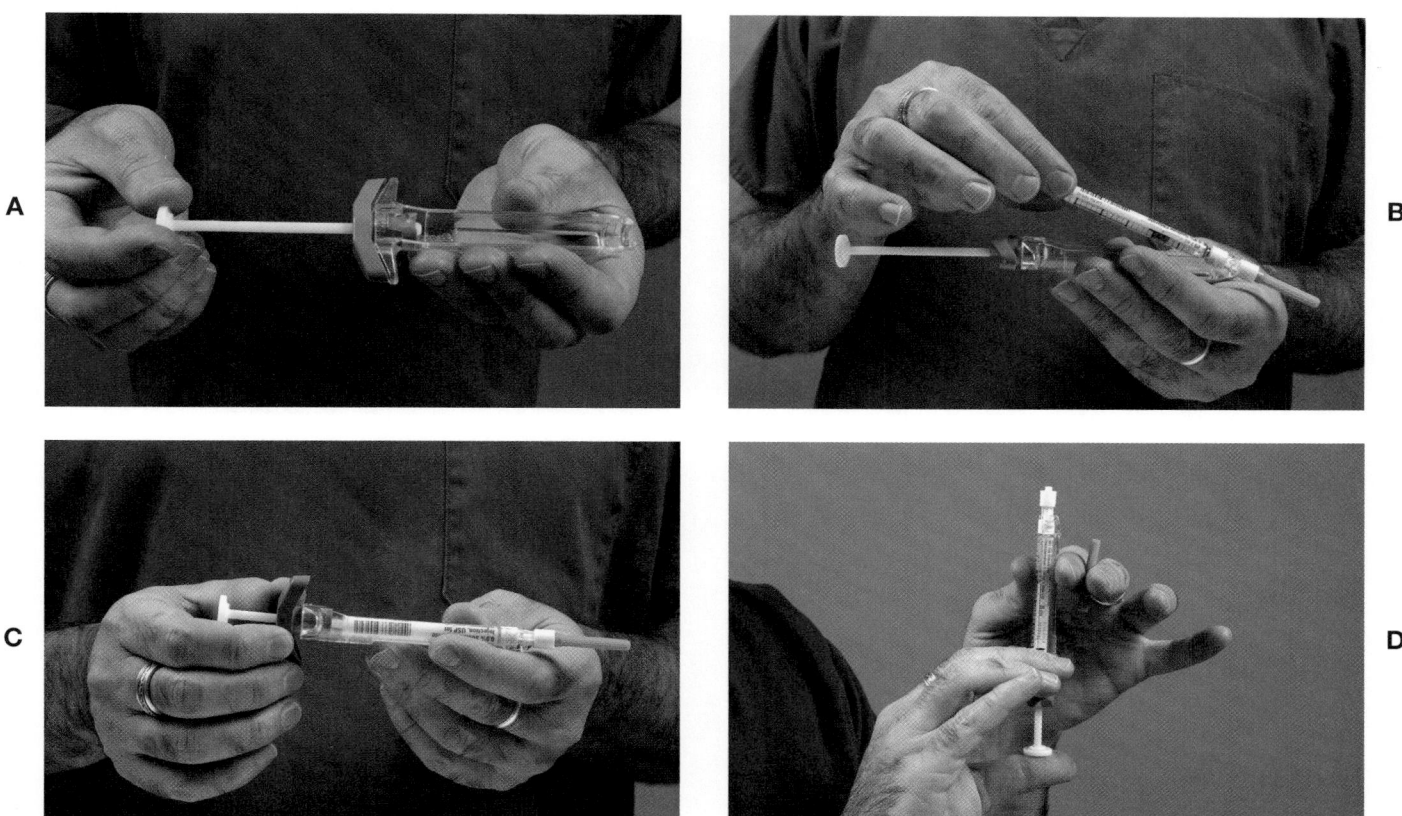

FIGURE **21-6** **A,** Carpuject syringe holder and prefilled sterile cartridge with needle. **B,** Assembling the Carpuject. **C,** The cartridge slides into the syringe barrel, turns, and locks at the needle end. The plunger then screws into the cartridge end. **D,** Nurse expells excess medication to gauge accurate dose.

Evidence-Based Practice Trends

Administering intramuscular injections is a responsibility of the professional nurse. It is associated with several complications, including contracture of skeletal muscles, abscesses at the injection site, nerve injury, pain, and hematoma (Chan, 2001; Nicoll and Hesby, 2002; Sparks, 2001). Unsafe intramuscular injection practices cause more than 1.3 million deaths and cost more than $535 million in direct medical costs (Nicoll and Hesby, 2002). Therefore nurses should administer an IM injection only when necessary, and the nurse must ensure that every IM injection is given safely (World Health Organization [WHO], 2004).

Certain scientific reasons justify the need for an IM injection (Nicoll and Hesby, 2002); for example, some medications, such as vitamin K, can only be administered IM. Consideration of the medication's onset of action, intensity of effect, and duration may also be used to determine the need for an IM injection. For example, some IM medications are in depot formulations. These medications provide a slow, sustained release over an extended period of time (e.g., over days or weeks). These medications must be given IM in order for the client to experience the desired effect of the medication.

Once the nurse determines the IM injection is necessary, the nurse selects the correct site for injection. The injection site used for IM injections is the most predictive factor associated with complications (Nicoll and Hesby, 2002). To avoid these complications, the nurse assesses the client's age, the medication type, and the medication volume in selecting the appropriate injection site. The dorsogluteal site has been a traditional site for intramuscular injection. However, studies have demonstrated the exact location of the sciatic nerve varies from one person to another. If a needle hits the sciatic nerve, the client may experience permanent or partial paralysis of the involved leg. Therefore the dorsogluteal site **should not** be used as a site for IM injections (Nicoll and Hesby, 2002).

The preferred injection sites for infants are the vastus lateralis or ventrogluteal, and the preferred sites for toddlers are the deltoid, ventrogluteal, and vastus lateralis. Preferred injection sites for preschoolers and older children include the deltoid or ventrogluteal, and the preferred sites for adults are the ventrogluteal or deltoid (Hockenberry and others, 2003; Nicoll and Hesby, 2002). Medications that are known to be irritating or are in an oily solution should be given in the ventrogluteal, whereas vaccines should be administered in the vastus lateralis in infants and young children and in the deltoid in older children and adults. Volumes of 2 ml or less may be given in the deltoid site, whereas volumes of 2 to 5 ml should be given in the ventrogluteal site (Nicoll and Hesby, 2002).

In addition, to reduce pain associated with intramuscular injections, nurses may apply manual pressure to the injection site before administering the injection (Chung and oth-

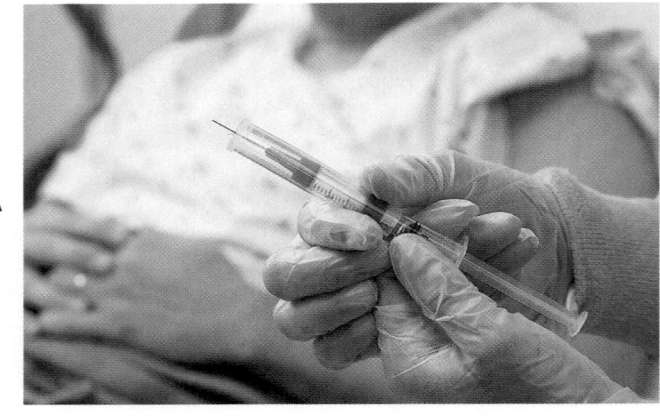

A

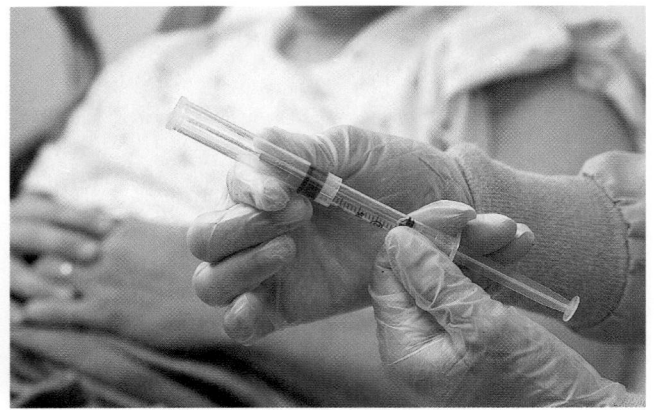

B

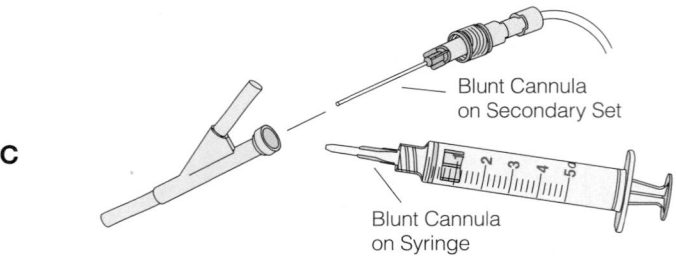

C

Blunt Cannula
on Secondary Set

Blunt Cannula
on Syringe

Prepierced Septum Y-site

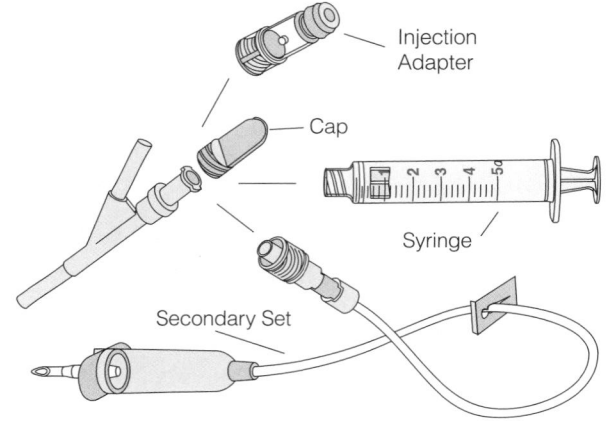

Injection
Adapter

Cap

Syringe

Secondary Set

Capped Luer Y-site

D

FIGURE **21-7** **A,** Protective syringe shown with sheath partially retracted. **B,** Sheath pulled and locked over needle. **C,** Prepierced Septum Y-site. **D,** Capped Luer Y-site. **E,** Valved Connector Y-site. (**C, D,** and **E** from Health Devices Needlestick-Prevention Device Selection Guide, Plymouth Meeting, Pa, 2000, ECRT.)

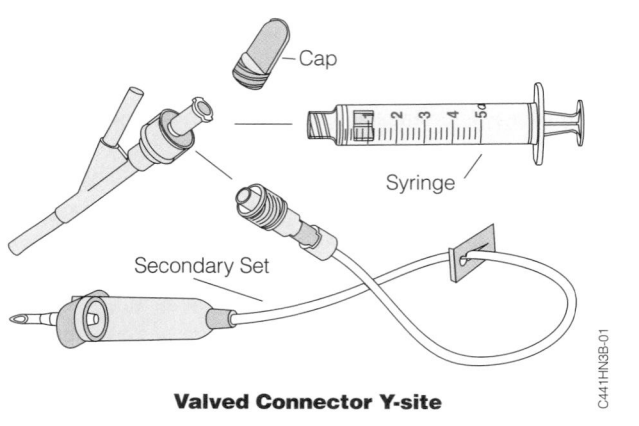

Cap

Syringe

Secondary Set

Valved Connector Y-site

E

C441HN3B-01

ers, 2002) and use distraction when administering the injection (Sparks, 2001). To reduce pain and bruising associated with subcutaneous heparin and low-molecular-weight heparin, the nurse may apply ice to the site for 5 minutes before the injection (Kuzu and Ucar, 2001), and the nurse should administer the injection over 30 seconds (Chan, 2001).

Cultural Considerations

Some cultural groups such as Hispanics and Arabs believe that parenteral medications are more effective than oral medications (Luna, 2002), and as a result client education often needs to focus on and emphasize the importance of oral medications as well. When cultural groups readily accept parenteral medications, it is important to remember to ask the client and/or family members which extremity is preferred. For example, Muslims and Hindus designate which hand is used for doing clean and dirty tasks (Ross, 2001).

When preparing to give parenteral medications, avoid removing articles from the extremities without the consent of the client/and or family members. Among Hmongs, strings are tied to the wrists, ankles, neck, and waist as protective spiritual items for the severely ill client (Johnson, 2002). In

BOX 21-1   Recommendations for the Prevention of Needle-Stick Injuries

1. Avoid using needles when effective needleless systems or Sharps with Engineered Sharps Injury Protection (SESIP) safety devices are available.
2. Do not recap needles.
3. Plan safe handling and disposal of needles before beginning a procedure that requires the use of a needle.
4. Immediately dispose of used needles, needleless systems, and SESIP into puncture-proof and leak-proof sharps disposal containers.
5. Maintain a sharps injury log that includes:
   a. Type and brand of device involved in the incident
   b. Location of the incident (e.g., department or work area)
   c. Description of the incident
   d. Methods to maintain privacy of employees who have experienced sharps injuries
6. Participate in educational offerings regarding blood-borne pathogens, and follow recommendations for infection prevention, including receiving the hepatitis B vaccine.
7. Report all needle-stick and sharps-related injuries immediately, according to institutional policies to ensure the receipt of appropriate follow-up care.
8. Participate in the selection and evaluation of needleless systems and devices with safety features within your place of employment whenever possible.
9. Support legislation that promotes the safe use of needles and sharps.

Data from Occupational Safety and Health Administration: Occupational exposure to blood borne pathogens, needlestick, and other sharps injuries: final rule, *Federal Register,* CFR 29, part 1910 (*Federal Register* 66:5317, Jan 18, 2001), available at www.osha.gov/pls/oshaweb/owadisp.show_document?p_table=STANDARDS&p_id=10051.

addition, privacy issues may have greater importance with some cultural groups. Muslims, Hindus, and Orthodox Jewish women avoid the exposure of the lower torso and the legs. It is important to use gender-congruent caregivers to administer injections to these clients.

Some older clients from Asian cultures may not readily accept invasive procedures because of their belief in holistic healing. When these situations arise, it is necessary to provide culturally appropriate teaching about the purpose and expected effects of these treatments. The nurse or client's cultural caregiver must explain that the procedure does not allow for the spirit and power of the individual to escape from the body when punctured (Miller, 1995). Adequate explanations before parenteral medication therapy may assist in resolving or minimizing any anxieties associated with blood loss, exchange of body fluids, etc. Africans and Southeast Asians believe that the blood is part of the individual's life force (Mashaba, 2002; Orque, 1983).

When using some of the high-tech infusion pumps, provide culturally appropriate explanations, and demonstrate how the pumps work. Many clients from developing countries may not have knowledge of Western technology. Include family members when giving explanations, and give instructions about when and how to call for help with the equipment.

Skill Performance Guidelines

1. Use strict aseptic technique during all steps of medication preparation and administration.
2. To prevent contamination and maintain sterility of a syringe, hold only the outside of the syringe barrel and the handle on the plunger. Avoid touching the tip of the needle, the inside of the barrel, the shaft of the plunger, or the needle with an unsterile object.
3. Know the volume and characteristics of the medication to be administered. Injecting too large a volume of medication can cause adverse effects, extreme pain, and local tissue damage.
4. Identify the bony prominences and anatomical structures that outline the chosen injection sites. Correct identification of the specific muscle mass will prevent injury to major nerves and blood vessels located near the injection site.
5. Insert the needle at the proper angle to deliver medication into the correct tissue (Figure 21-8).
6. Before injecting an intramuscular medication, aspirate by pulling back on the plunger to ensure that the needle has not pierced a vein or artery. Injection directly into a blood vessel can cause a rapid drug response. If blood is aspirated, remove the needle, dispose of the syringe and medication, and prepare a new dose of medication.
7. Attempt to minimize the client's discomfort when giving an injection by:
   - Using sharp beveled needles in the shortest length and smallest gauge possible.
   - Changing the needle if liquid medication has coated the shaft of the needle.
   - Positioning and flexing client's limbs appropriately to reduce muscular tension.
   - Diverting the client's attention from the injection procedure.
   - Inserting the needle smoothly and quickly. Do not hesitate, and slowly push the needle into tissue.
   - Injecting the medication slowly but smoothly to reduce pain.
   - Holding the syringe steady once the needle is in the tissue to prevent tissue damage.
   - Withdrawing the needle smoothly at the same angle used for insertion.
   - Gently applying an antiseptic pad (e.g., alcohol) or a dry, sterile gauze pad to the site
   - Applying gentle pressure at the injection site.
   - Rotating injection sites to prevent the formation of indurations and abscesses.
8. Use the guidelines for administering medications, including the six rights of medication administration, listed in Chapter 19, when giving parenteral medications.
9. Do not recap needles after administering injections, and dispose of all needles in an appropriate puncture-proof and leak-proof container (Occupational Safety and Health Administration [OSHA], 2001).

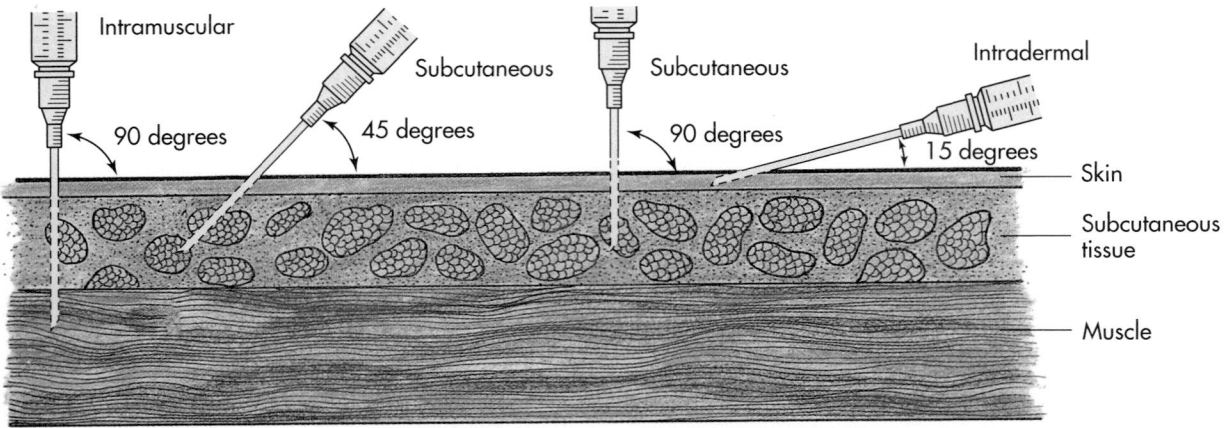

FIGURE **21-8** Comparison of the angles of insertion of IM (90 degrees), Sub-Q (45 to 90 degrees), and ID (15 degrees) injections.

SKILL 21-1 Preparing Injections From Ampules and Vials

Ampules contain single doses of injectable medication in a liquid form. They are available in sizes from 1 to 10 ml or more (Figure 21-9, *A*). An ampule is made of glass with a constricted neck that must be snapped off to allow access to the medication. A colored ring around the neck indicates where the ampule is prescored to be broken easily. Medications are easily withdrawn from the ampule by aspirating the fluid with a filter needle and syringe. Filter needles are used when preparing medications from glass ampules to prevent glass particles from

being drawn into the syringe with the medication (Nicoll and Hesby, 2002). The fluid enters the syringe because pulling on the plunger creates a vacuum in the syringe barrel.

A vial is a plastic or glass container with a rubber seal at the top (Figure 21-9, *B*). A vial that is entered and then discarded, regardless of the amount of medication used, is called a single-dose vial. A vial that can be entered into several times and contains several doses of medication is called a multidose vial. The date that multidose vials are opened

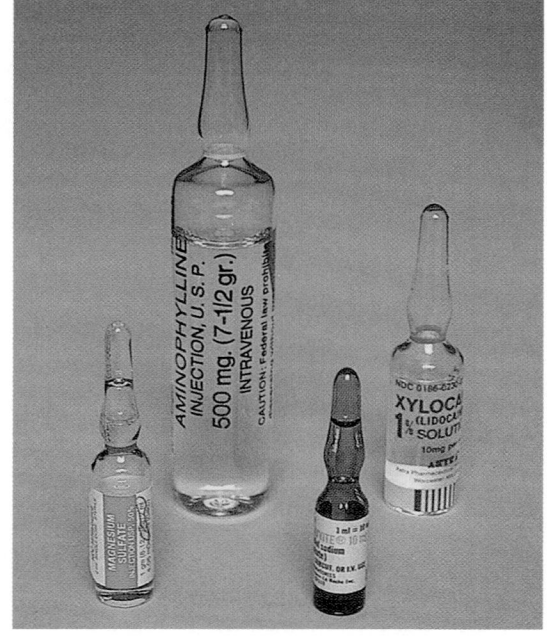

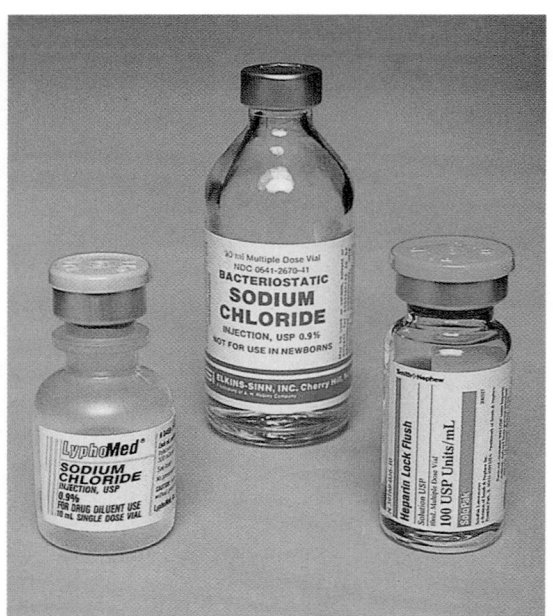

FIGURE **21-9** **A,** Medication in ampules. **B,** Medication in vials.

should be written on the label. Institutional policies vary on how long opened multidose vials can be used. Vials that have exceeded the time allowed by institutional policy should not be used and must be properly disposed.

A metal or plastic cap protects the vial's rubber seal. It is removed when the nurse is first preparing the vial for use. Vials contain liquid or dry forms of medications; drugs that are unstable in solution are packaged in a dry powder form. The vial label specifies the amount of diluent to be used to dissolve the powdered drug to prepare a desired drug concentration. Some vials contain a diluent solution in one chamber and a powdered substance in another chamber. The two chambers are separated by a rubber stopper. Before preparing the medication, the nurse pushes on the upper chamber, which dislodges the rubber stopper and allows the powder and the diluent to be mixed. Unlike the ampule, the vial is a closed system, and air must be injected into the container to permit easy withdrawal of the solution. Some medications, even when in a vial, may need to be drawn up with a filter needle because of the nature of the drug. Institutional policies will indicate which drugs should be prepared with a filter needle.

DELEGATION CONSIDERATIONS

The skill of preparing injections from ampules and vials should not be delegated to assistive personnel.

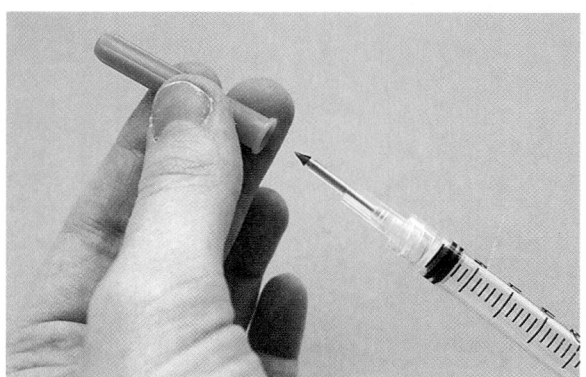

FIGURE **21-10** Syringe with needleless adaptor.

EQUIPMENT
Medication in an Ampule
- ❏ Syringe, filter needle, and needle or needleless system device
- ❏ Small gauze pad or unopened alcohol swab

Medication in a Vial
- ❏ Syringe
- ❏ Needles
- ❏ Blunt-tip vial access cannula (if needleless system used) (Figure 21-10)
- ❏ Filter needle (if indicated)
- ❏ Needle for drawing up medication and needle for injection (if needed)
- ❏ Small gauze pad or alcohol swab
- ❏ Diluent (e.g., normal saline or sterile water) (if indicated)

Both
- ❏ Medication administration record (MAR) or computer printout

STEP	RATIONALE
ASSESSMENT	
1. Verify client's name, name of medication, dose, route of administration, and time of administration on MAR against medication order.	Ensures correct administration of medication.
2. Assess the client's body build, muscle size, and weight and the desired route of administration.	Determines type and size of syringe and needles to be used for injection.
3. Check name of medication on vial/ampule label against MAR.	Ensures client receives correct medication.
4. Check medication's expiration date printed on vial or ampule.	Medications that have expired should not be used because the potency of medications changes when the medications become outdated.
PLANNING	
1. Expected outcomes following completion of procedure: • Proper dose is prepared. No air bubbles are present within syringe barrel.	Air bubbles displace medication. Elimination of air ensures medication dose is accurate.
2. Check medication administration record or computer printout.	Verifies orders.
IMPLEMENTATION	
1. Perform hand hygiene.	Reduces transmission of microorganisms.
2. Assemble medication and supplies at work area in medicine area.	Organization saves time and reduces the risk for error.

STEP	RATIONALE

3. Ampule preparation:
   a. Tap top of ampule lightly and quickly with finger until fluid moves from neck of ampule (see illustration).
   b. Place small gauze pad or unopened alcohol swab around neck of ampule (see illustration).

   c. Snap neck of ampule quickly and firmly away from hands (see illustration).

Dislodges any fluid that collects above neck of ampule. All solution moves into lower chamber.

Placing pad around neck of ampule protects nurse's fingers from trauma as glass tip is broken off. *Do not use opened alcohol swab to wrap around top of ampule because alcohol may leak into ampule.*

Protects nurse's fingers and face from being cut by glass.

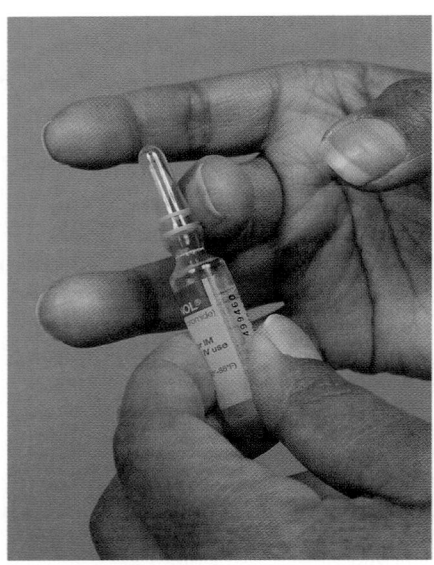

STEP 3a Tapping moves fluid down neck.

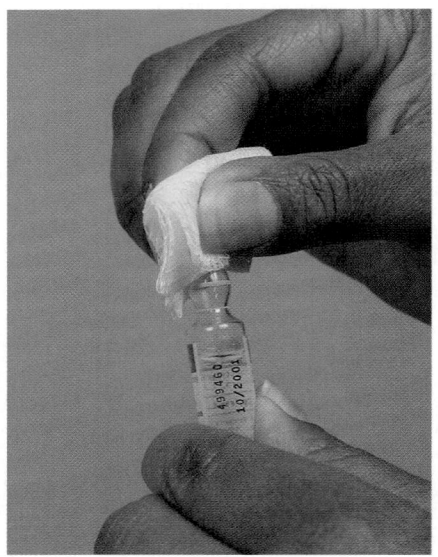

STEP 3b Gauze pad placed around neck of ampule.

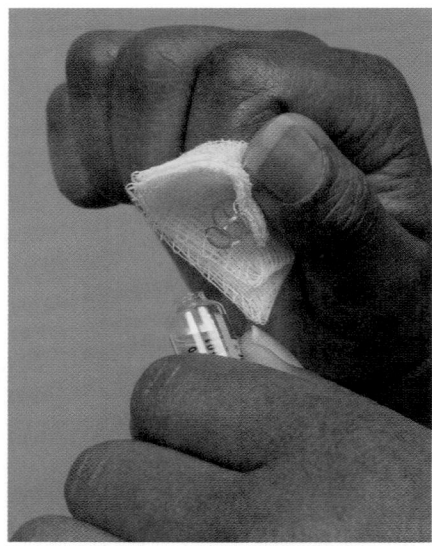

STEP 3c Neck snapped away from hands.

STEP	RATIONALE
d. Draw up medication quickly, using a filter needle long enough to reach bottom of ampule.	System is open to airborne contaminants. Needle must be long enough to access medication for preparation. Filter needles are used to filter out glass fragments (Nicoll and Hesby, 2002).
e. Hold ampule upside down, or set it on a flat surface. Insert filter needle into center of ampule opening. Do not allow needle tip or shaft to touch rim of ampule.	Broken rim of ampule is considered contaminated. When ampule is inverted, solution dribbles out of ampule if needle tip or shaft touches rim of ampule.
f. Aspirate medication into syringe by gently pulling back on plunger (see illustrations).	Withdrawal of plunger creates negative pressure within syringe barrel, which pulls fluid into syringe.
g. Keep needle tip under surface of liquid. Tip ampule to bring all fluid within reach of the needle.	Prevents aspiration of air bubbles.
h. If air bubbles are aspirated, do not expel air into ampule.	Expelling air creates pressure that may force fluid out of ampule, and medication will be lost.
i. To expel excess air bubbles, remove needle from ampule. Hold syringe with needle pointing up. Tap side of syringe to cause bubbles to rise toward needle. Draw back slightly on plunger, and then push plunger upward to eject air. **Do not eject fluid.**	Withdrawing plunger too far will remove it from barrel. Holding syringe vertically allows air bubbles to rise to top of barrel and fluid to settle in bottom of barrel. Pulling back on plunger allows fluid within needle to enter barrel so fluid is not expelled. Air at top of barrel and within needle is then expelled.
j. If syringe contains excess fluid, use sink for disposal. Hold syringe vertically with needle tip up and slanted slightly toward sink. Slowly eject excess fluid into sink. Recheck volume of medication in syringe by holding it vertically.	Medication is safely dispersed into sink. Position of needle allows medication to be expelled without its flowing down needle shaft and onto nurse's hand. Rechecking fluid level ensures proper dose.
k. Cover needle with its safety sheath or cap. Replace filter needle with needle for injection.	Prevents contamination of needle. Filter needles cannot be used for injection.

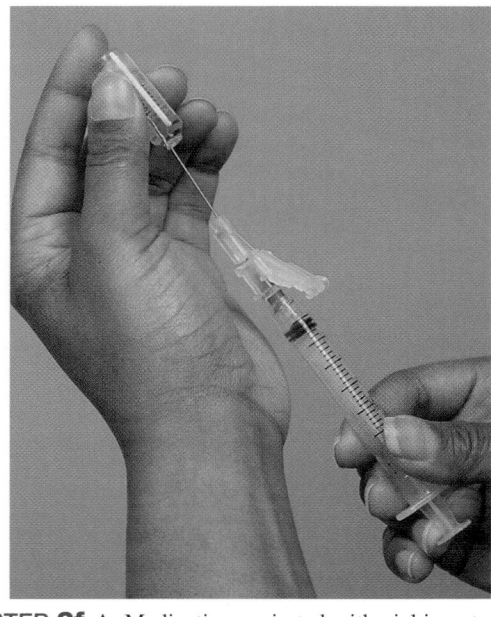 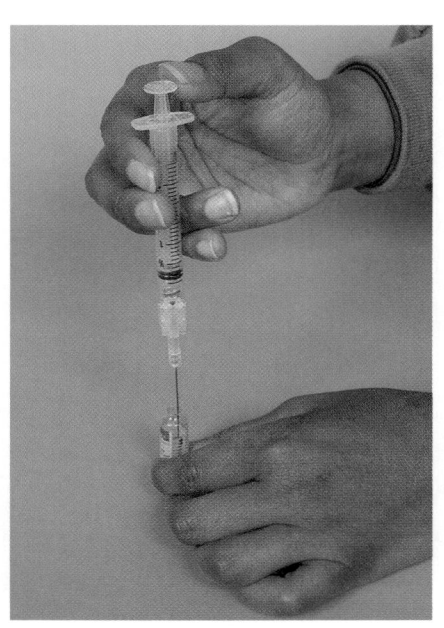

STEP 3f A, Medication aspirated with vial inverted. **B,** Medication aspirated with vial on flat surface.

STEP	RATIONALE

4. **Vial containing a solution:**

   a. Remove cap covering top of unused vial to expose rubber seal. If using a multidose vial that has been opened, cap is already removed. Firmly and briskly wipe surface of rubber seal with alcohol swab, and allow it to dry.

   Vials come packaged with cap that cannot be replaced after removal. Not all drug manufacturers guarantee that rubber seals of unused vials are sterile. Therefore, rubber seals must be swabbed with alcohol before drawing up medication. Allowing alcohol to dry prevents alcohol from coating needle and mixing with medication.

   b. Pick up syringe, and remove cap covering needleless vial access device. Pull back on plunger to draw amount of air into syringe equivalent to volume of medication to be aspirated from vial.

   Air must first be injected into vial to prevent buildup of negative pressure in vial when aspirating medication.

- *Critical Decision Point*
  Some medications and some institutions require that a filter needle be used when preparing medications from a vial. Check agency policy to determine if use of filter needle is indicated (Nicoll and Hesby, 2002; Rodger and King, 2000).

   c. With vial on flat surface, insert needleless vial access device or tip of safety filter needle with beveled tip entering first through center of rubber seal (see illustration).

   Center of seal is thinner and easier to penetrate. Inserting the needle with the bevel up prevents coring of rubber seal, which could enter vial or needle (Nicoll and Hesby, 2002).

   d. Inject air into the vial's airspace, holding on to plunger with firm pressure. Hold plunger with firm pressure, plunger may be forced backward by air pressure within vial.

   Air must be injected before aspirating fluid. Injecting into vial's airspace prevents formation of bubbles and inaccuracy in dose.

   e. Invert vial while keeping firm hold on syringe and plunger (see illustration). Hold vial between thumb and middle fingers of nondominant hand. Grasp end of syringe barrel and plunger with thumb and forefinger of dominant hand to counteract pressure in vial.

   Inverting vial allows fluid to settle in lower half of container. Position of hands prevents forceful movement of plunger and permits easy manipulation of syringe.

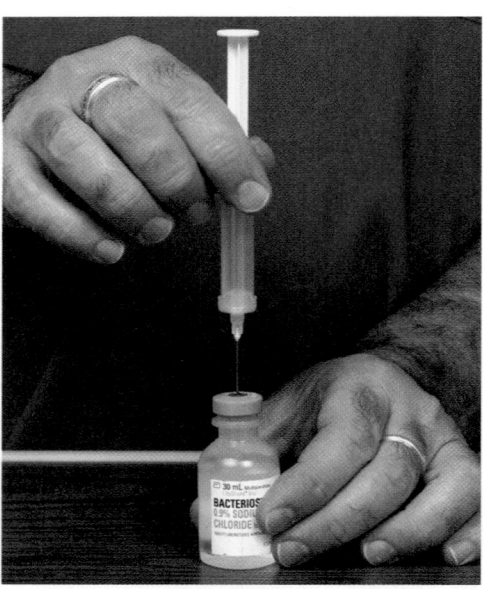

STEP **4c** Insert needle's adapter through center of diaphragm.

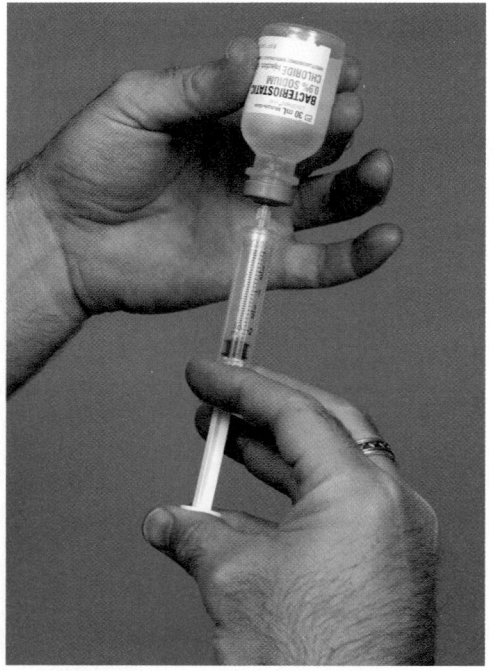

STEP **4e** Withdraw fluid with vial inserted.

STEP	**RATIONALE**
f. Keep tip of needleless vial access device or filter needle below fluid level.	Prevents aspiration of air.
g. Allow air pressure from the vial to fill syringe gradually with medication. If necessary, pull back slightly on plunger to obtain correct amount of medication.	Positive pressure within vial forces fluid into syringe. Pulling back too quickly or forcefully on the plunger will pull unwanted air into the syringe.
h. When desired volume has been obtained, position needleless vial access device or filter needle into vial's airspace; tap side of syringe barrel carefully to dislodge any air bubbles. Eject any air remaining at top of syringe into vial.	Forcefully striking barrel while needle is inserted in vial may bend needle. Accumulation of air displaces medication and causes dose errors.

● *Critical Decision Point*

Do not withdraw the last drops in a vial to reduce the likelihood of withdrawing foreign particles into the syringe (Nicoll and Hesby, 2002).

i. Remove needleless vial access device or filter needle from vial by pulling back on barrel of syringe.	Pulling plunger rather than barrel causes plunger to separate from barrel, resulting in loss of medication.
j. Hold syringe at eye level, at 90-degree angle, to ensure correct volume and absence of air bubbles. Remove any remaining air by tapping barrel to dislodge any air bubbles (see illustration). Draw back slightly on plunger; then push plunger upward to eject air. Do not eject fluid. Recheck volume of medication.	Holding syringe vertically allows air to rise to top of barrel and fluid to settle in bottom of barrel. Pulling back on plunger allows fluid within needle to enter barrel so fluid is not expelled. Air at top of barrel and within needle is then expelled.

● *Critical Decision Point*

When preparing medication from single-dose vial, do not assume that volume listed on label is total volume in vial. Some manufacturers provide small amount of extra liquid, expecting loss during preparation. Be sure to draw up only desired volume.

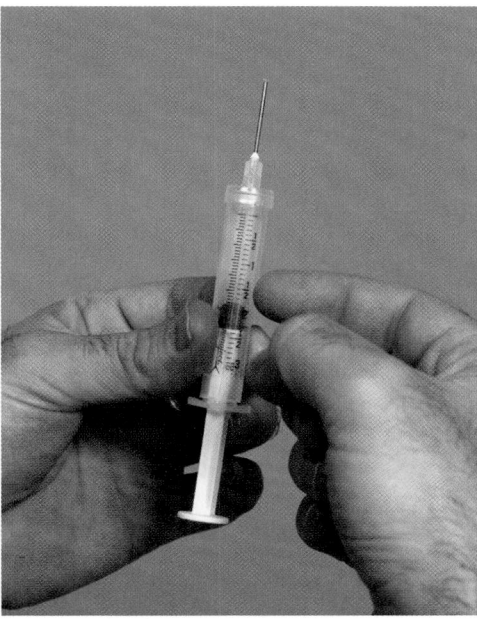

STEP 4j Hold syringe upright; tap barrel to dislodge air bubbles.

STEP	RATIONALE
k. If medication is to be injected into client's tissue, change needleless vial access device or filter needle for a needle of appropriate gauge and length according to route of medication.	A needleless vial access device must be changed for a needle because it cannot pierce the skin. Filter needles cannot be used for injections (Nicoll and Hesby, 2002).
l. For multidose vial, make label that includes date of opening, mixing (if necessary), concentration of drug per milliliter, and nurse's initials.	Ensures that future doses will be prepared correctly. Some drugs must be discarded after certain number of days after opening or mixing of vial.
5. Vial containing a powder (reconstituting medications):	
a. Remove cap covering vial of powdered medication and cap covering vial of proper diluent. Firmly swab both rubber seals with alcohol swab, and allow alcohol to dry.	Vials come packaged with cap that cannot be replaced after removal. Not all drug manufacturers guarantee that rubber seals of unused vials are sterile. Therefore rubber seals must be swabbed with alcohol before drawing up medication. Allowing alcohol to dry prevents alcohol from coating needle and mixing with medication.
b. Draw up diluent into syringe following steps 4b to j.	Prepares diluent for injection into vial containing powdered medication.
c. Insert tip of needleless vial access device through center of rubber seal of vial of powdered medication. Inject diluent into vial. Remove needleless device from vial and cover with its cap.	Diluent begins to dissolve and reconstitute medication. Maintaining sterility of needleless vial access device and syringe allows syringe to be used to draw up medication once it is reconstituted.
d. Mix medication thoroughly. Roll in palms. Do not shake.	Ensures proper dispersal of medication throughout solution.
e. Reconstituted medication in vial is ready to be drawn into syringe. Read label carefully to determine concentration after reconstitution.	Once diluent has been added, concentration of medication (mg/ml) determines amount to be given.
f. Draw up medication into syringe following steps 4b to 4l.	

- **Critical Decision Point**
Some institutions require that medications prepared for parenteral administration be verified for accuracy by another nurse. Check individual institution guidelines before administering medication.

6. Dispose of soiled supplies. Place broken ampule and/or used vials and used needle in puncture-proof and leakproof container. Clean work area, and perform hand hygiene.	Proper disposal of glass and needle prevents accidental injury to staff (OSHA, 2001). Controls transmission of infection.

EVALUATION

1. Compare dose in syringe with desired dose.	Ensures that accurate dose has been prepared.

Unexpected Outcomes	Related Interventions
1. Air bubbles remain within syringe barrel.	• Expel air from syringe, and add medication to syringe until correct dose is prepared.
2. Excess or insufficient volume of medication is prepared.	• Correct amount of medication in syringe before administering to ensure correct dose of medication is given.

SKILL 21-2 Mixing Parenteral Medications in One Syringe

Occasionally the nurse must mix medications from two vials or from a vial and an ampule. Mixing compatible medications avoids the need to give a client more than one injection at a time. Medication compatibility is determined by referring to a compatibility chart. Compatibility charts are found in various drug reference guides or are posted within client care areas. A pharmacist or drug handbook should always be consulted when a nurse is unsure about the compatibility of medications. When mixing medications, the nurse must remember how to correctly aspirate fluid from each type of container. When using multidose vials, the nurse must not contaminate the vial's contents with medication from another vial or ampule.

Mixing medications from a vial and an ampule is simple because adding air to withdraw medication from an ampule is unnecessary. The nurse prepares medications from the vial first and then, using the same syringe and a safety filter needle, withdraws medication from the ampule. Mixing medications from two vials is somewhat more complicated because air must be added to both vials.

Special consideration must be given to the proper preparation of insulin, which comes in vials. Insulin is the hormone used to treat high blood glucose levels most frequently associated with diabetes. Often clients with diabetes receive a combination of different types of insulin to control their blood glucose levels. Regular insulin is a rapid- or short-acting solution that can be given subcutaneously, intravenously, or intramuscularly. Other types of insulin contain the addition of a protein that slows absorption. Intermediate- or long-acting insulin preparations cannot be given intravenously or intramuscularly.

Some insulins can be mixed in the same syringe. However, when insulins are mixed, chemical changes may occur either immediately or over time. This can result in a

client response to insulin that is different than the response that would occur if the insulins had been given separately. Box 21-2 lists recommendations from the American Diabetes Association for mixing insulins.

BOX 21-2 Recommendations for Mixing Insulins

- Clients whose blood sugar levels are well controlled on a mixed insulin dose should maintain their individual routine when preparing and administering their insulin.
- Insulin should not be mixed with any other medications or diluent unless approved by the prescribing physician or advanced practice nurse.
- Insulin glargine should not be mixed with any other forms of insulin.
- Commercially available premixed insulins may be used if the ratio of the insulins within the vial matches the client's current insulin requirements.
- Injections that mix NPH and short-acting insulins may be administered immediately or they may be stored for future use.
- Rapid-acting insulin may be mixed with NPH, Lente, and Ultralente.
- Mixtures of rapid-acting insulin with either an intermediate- or long-acting insulin should be injected within 15 minutes before a meal.
- Short-acting and Lente insulins should not be mixed unless the client's blood sugar levels are currently under control with this mixture.
- Phosphate-buffered insulins (e.g., NPH) should not be mixed with Lente insulins. If they are mixed, a precipitate may form and the time of onset and peak action of the insulins will change.
- Insulin formulations may change. Follow manufacturer's guidelines if the manufacturer's guidelines conflict with the American Diabetes Association Guidelines.

Modified from American Diabetes Association: Insulin administration: position statement, *Diabetes Care* 27(suppl 1):S106, 2004.

DELEGATION CONSIDERATIONS

The skill of mixing medications from two vials or a vial and an ampule should not be delegated to assistive personnel.

EQUIPMENT

- ❏ Single-dose or multidose vials and ampules containing medications
- ❏ Syringe with needleless vial access device or filter needle and syringe
- ❏ Extra needle for injection
- ❏ Alcohol swab
- ❏ Puncture-proof container for disposing of syringes, needles, and glass
- ❏ Medication administration record (MAR) or computer printout

STEP	RATIONALE

ASSESSMENT

1. Verify client's name, name of medication, dose, route of administration, and time of administration on MAR against medication order.

2. Assess client's body build, muscle size, and weight and desired route of medication administration.

3. Check name of medication on vial/ampule label against MAR.

4. Consider medications to be mixed, compatibility of medications, and type of injection.

5. Check medication's expiration date printed on vial or ampule.

Verifies order.

Determines type and size of syringe and needles for injection.

Ensures client receives correct medication.

Determines if medications can be mixed, order of drawing up medications, and size of syringe.

Medications that have expired should not be used because the potency of medications changes when the medications become outdated.

PLANNING

1. Expected outcomes following completion of procedure:
   - Combined medications equal correct dose. No air bubbles are present in syringe barrel.

Indicates medication is prepared correctly.

IMPLEMENTATION

1. Perform hand hygiene.

2. Assemble medication and supplies at work area in medication preparation area.

3. **Mixing medications from two vials:**
   a. Take syringe with needleless vial access device or filter needle, and aspirate volume of air equivalent to first dose of medication (vial A).

   b. Inject air into vial A, making sure needleless device or filter needle does not touch solution (Figure 21-11, *A*).

   c. Holding on to plunger, withdraw needleless vial access device or filter needle and syringe from vial A. Aspirate air equivalent to second dose of medication (vial B).

   d. Insert needleless vial access device or filter needle into vial B, inject air, and then withdraw proper volume of medication from vial (Figure 21-11, *B*).

   e. Withdraw needleless access device or filter needle and syringe from vial B. Ensure that proper volume has been obtained.

Reduces transmission of microorganisms.
Organization saves time and reduces risk of error.

Air must be introduced into vial to create positive pressure needed to withdraw solution.

Prevents cross contamination.

If plunger is not held in place, injected air may escape from vial A. Air is injected into vial B to create positive pressure needed to withdraw desired dose.

First portion of dose has been prepared.

Ensures correct dose is prepared.

FIGURE **21-11 A,** Injecting air into vial A. **B,** Injecting air into vial B and withdrawing dose. **C,** Withdrawing medication from vial A; medications are now mixed.

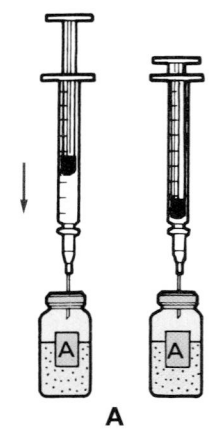

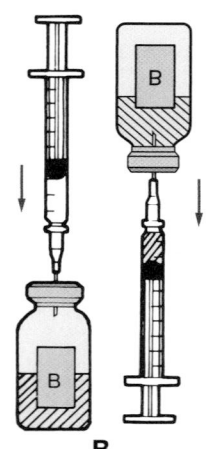

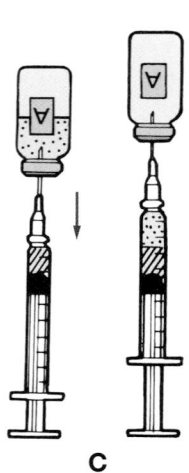

A   **B**   **C**

STEP	RATIONALE

f. Determine at which point on syringe scale combined volume of medications should measure.

Prevents accidental withdrawal of too much medication from second vial.

g. Insert needleless access device or filter needle into vial A, being careful not to push plunger and expel medication into vial. Invert vial, and carefully withdraw the correct amount of medication into syringe (Figure 21-11, *C*).

Positive pressure within vial A allows fluid to fill syringe without need to aspirate.

h. Withdraw needleless access device or filter needle, and expel any excess air or fluid from syringe. Check fluid level in syringe. Medications are now mixed.

Air bubbles should not be injected into tissues. Excess fluid causes incorrect dose.

• *Critical Decision Point*

If too much medication is withdrawn from second vial, discard syringe and start over. Do not push medication back into vial.

i. Change needleless access device for appropriate-size needle if medication is being injected. Replace filter needle with needleless system or with appropriate-size needle according to route of medication. Keep needleless device or needle capped until administration time.

A needleless vial access device must be changed for a needle if medication is to pierce the skin. Filter needles cannot be used for injections (Nicoll and Hesby, 2002).

j. Dispose of soiled needleless access device or filter needle and supplies in proper receptacles.

Controls spread of infection and prevents needle-stick injuries (OSHA, 2001).

k. Perform hand hygiene.

Reduces transmission of infection.

4. **Mixing insulin:**

a. If mixing rapid- or short-acting insulin with intermediate- or long-acting insulin, take insulin syringe and aspirate volume of air equivalent to dose to be withdrawn from cloudy insulin first (see illustration). If two modified forms of insulin are mixed, it makes no difference which vial is prepared first.

Air must be introduced into vial to create pressure needed to withdraw solution.

• *Critical Decision Point*

If long-acting insulin glargine (Lantus) is ordered, note this a clear insulin which should not be mixed with other insulin.

b. Inject air into vial of intermediate- or long-acting insulin. Be sure that needle does not touch solution.

Prevents cross contamination.

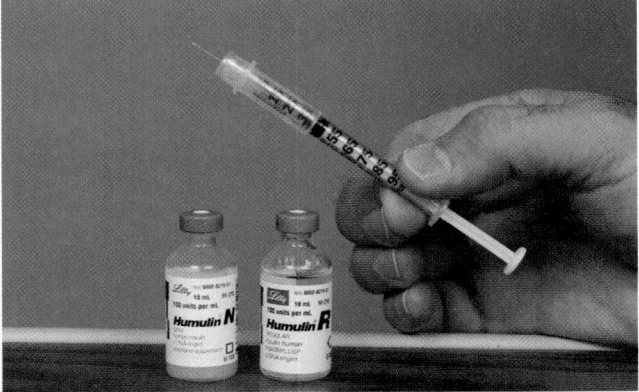

STEP **4a** Vials of intermediate- or long-acting insulin and rapid- or short-acting insulin and syringe with air aspirated.

STEP	RATIONALE
c. Withdraw needle and syringe from vial without aspirating medication. Aspirate air equivalent to dose to be withdrawn from rapid- or short-acting insulin.	Air will be injected into vial to withdraw desired dose.
d. Insert needle into vial of rapid- or short-acting insulin, inject air, and then fill syringe with correct insulin dose (see illustration).	First portion of dose has been prepared. Always fill syringe with rapid- or short-acting insulin first to prevent contamination of the rapid- or short-acting insulin with intermediate- or long-acting insulin.
e. Withdraw needle and syringe from vial by pulling on barrel; remove any air bubbles, and check dose.	Prevents accidental pulling of plunger, which may cause loss of medication. Ensures correct dose prepared.

- **Critical Decision Point**
  Some institutions require insulin doses to be verified by another nurse for accuracy. If indicated by institutional policy, have dose of clear insulin verified before proceeding with mixing of insulin at this time. Have dose verified after the medications are mixed as well.

f. Determine at which point on syringe scale combined units of insulin should measure by adding the number of units of both insulins together (e.g., 5 units Regular + 12 units NPH = 17 units total).	Prevents accidental withdrawal of too much insulin from second vial.
g. Insert needle into vial of intermediate- or long-acting insulin. Be careful not to push plunger and expel medication into vial. Invert vial, and carefully withdraw desired amount of insulin into syringe (see illustration).	Positive pressure within vial of intermediate- or long-acting insulin allows fluid to fill syringe without need to aspirate.
h. Withdraw needle, and check fluid level in syringe. Keep needle of prepared syringe sheathed or capped until administering medication.	Ensures accurate dose. Inaccurate doses of insulin can cause serious hypoglycemia or hyperglycemia. Keeping needle capped or sheathed keeps needle sterile for insulin administration.

- **Critical Decision Point**
  Administer mixture of insulins within 5 minutes of preparation. Rapid- or short-acting insulin can bind with intermediate- or long-acting insulin, thus reducing the action of the more rapid-acting insulin (Strowig, 2001).

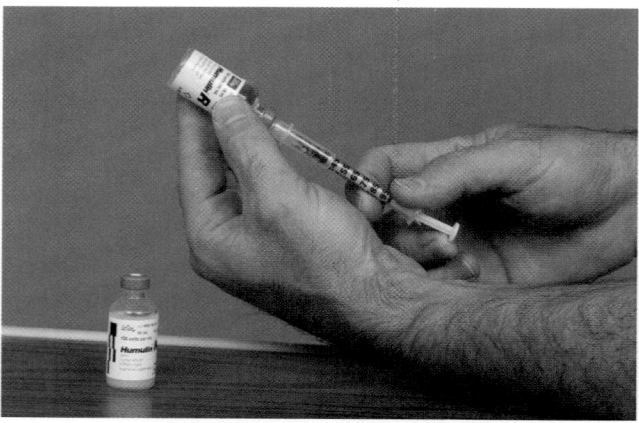

STEP **4d** Withdrawal of regular insulin.

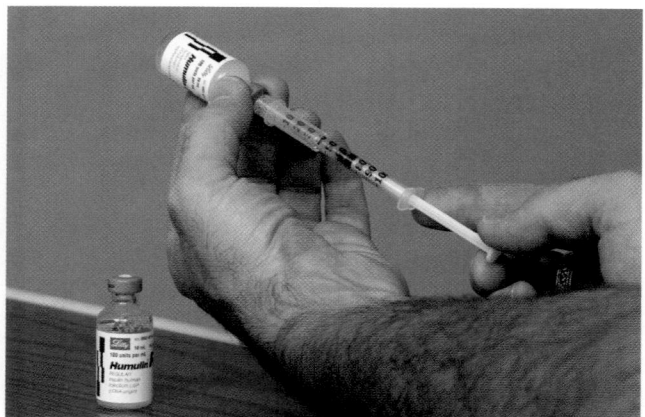

STEP **4g** Withdrawal of modified insulin.

STEP	RATIONALE

i. Dispose of soiled supplies in proper receptacle.	Controls spread of infection.
j. Perform hand hygiene.	Reduces transmission of infection.
5. Mixing medications from a vial and an ampule:	
a. Prepare medication from vial first, following steps 4a to j in Skill 21-1.	Medication administration from vial requires insertion of air into vial. Therefore vial medication is prepared first.
b. Determine at which point on syringe scale combined volume of medication should measure.	Prevents accidental withdrawal of too much medication from ampule.

● *Critical Decision Point*
If needleless vial access device was used in preparing medication from vial, change needleless system to filter needle.

c. Prepare medication from ampule, following steps 3a to i in Skill 21-1.	Ensures appropriate amount of medication prepared.
d. Withdraw filter needle from ampule, and verify fluid level in syringe. Change filter needle to appropriate needleless device or needle with appropriate gauge. Keep needleless device or needle sheathed or capped until administering medication.	Ensures accurate dose. Keeping needle or needleless device capped maintains sterility for medication administration.
e. Dispose of soiled supplies in proper receptacle.	Controls spread of infection.
f. Perform hand hygiene.	Reduces transmission of infection.

EVALUATION

1. Check syringe carefully for total combined dose of medications.	Accurate dose ensures safe medication administration.

● *Critical Decision Point*
Administer mixture of insulins within 5 to 15 minutes of preparation. Short-acting and regular insulins bind with intermediate- and long-acting insulins, reducing the action of regular insulin.

Unexpected Outcomes	Related Interventions
1. Air bubbles remain in syringe barrel.	● Expel air from syringe, and add medication to syringe until correct dose is prepared.
2. Excess or insufficient volume of medication is prepared.	● Be sure correct amount of medication is in syringe before administering to ensure correct dose of medication is given.

Teaching Considerations

● Because insulin is essential to life, all clients with type 1 diabetes and some clients with type 2 diabetes must be able to prepare and inject insulin as ordered (see Chapter 42).

● Assess client's ability to mix insulin by having client complete a return demonstration of insulin preparation. Insulin can be prescribed in premixed formulations. The nurse should communicate if the client is unable to mix insulin accurately and should discuss changing the client's insulin type to a premixed formula with the client's health care provider.

Pediatric Considerations

● Children of about 8 or 9 years should be able to prepare and administer their own injections, including insulin.

● Children may need participation/supervision of a parent or legal guardian through adolescence.

● The nurse assesses the pediatric client's physical readiness, psychological readiness, and development in activities of daily living before teaching the client how to prepare and self-administer injections, such as insulin.

● Family education is essential to successful disease management and medication administration in the pediatric client, especially when the preparation and administration of medications in a syringe are required.

Gerontological Considerations

- Physiological changes in the older adult, such as decreased peripheral vision, presbyopia, and reduction in the power of skeletal and voluntary muscle contractions, may make it difficult for clients to prepare and self-administer injections.
- The nurse assesses the older client's physical readiness, psychological readiness, and development in activities of daily living before teaching a client how to prepare and self-administer injections, such as insulin.
- Clients unable to perform the task may be assisted by family members, a visiting nurse, or home health attendants.

Home Care Considerations

- Some clients may prefer to use their syringe more than once. Many studies have shown that it is both safe and practical for the syringe to be used more than once if the client desires as long as the syringe is not contaminated when used and is recapped after each use. Insulin preparations have bacteriostatic additives that inhibit growth of bacteria commonly found on the skin (American Diabetes Association [ADA], 2004a).
- At home, insulin may be premixed and stored. Sometimes, this can lead to an alteration of the insulin's peak and duration. Therefore, if insulins are premixed, the prescriber needs to assess the effect of premixing insulins on control of blood glucose levels. In addition, the client must be taught to ensure consistency in insulin preparation and careful blood glucose monitoring (ADA, 2004a).
- Refer to Home Care Considerations in Skill 21-4, for syringe disposal guidelines for the home care setting.

SKILL 21-3 Administering Intradermal Injections

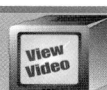

The nurse typically gives intradermal injections for skin testing, for example, in tuberculin screening and allergy tests. Because these medications are potent, they are injected into the dermis, where blood supply is reduced and drug absorption occurs slowly. A client may have an anaphylactic reaction if the medications enter the client's circulation too rapidly. For clients with a history of numerous allergies, the physician may perform skin testing.

Skin testing often requires the nurse to visually inspect the test site; therefore intradermal sites should be free of lesions and injuries and should be relatively hairless. The inner forearm and upper back are ideal locations.

To administer an injection intradermally the nurse uses a tuberculin or small syringe with a short ($\frac{3}{8}$ to $\frac{5}{8}$ inch), fine gauge (25 to 27) needle. The angle of insertion for an intradermal injection is 5 to 15 degrees (see Figure 21-8). Only small amounts of medication (0.01 to 0.1 ml) are injected intradermally. If a bleb does not appear, or if the site bleeds after needle withdrawal, the medication may have entered subcutaneous tissues. In this situation skin test results will not be valid.

DELEGATION CONSIDERATIONS

Administering intradermal injections should not be delegated to assistive personnel. Other aspects of the client's care, such as hygiene, measuring vital signs, or assisting with activity, may be delegated to assistive personnel, and the nurse should instruct assistive personnel about the following:

- Potential medication side effects and to report their occurrence to the nurse
- Any impact of medication on client's physical status, vital signs, or level of consciousness (e.g., sedation)
- Any change in the client's condition

EQUIPMENT

- ❏ 1-ml tuberculin syringe with preattached 26- or 27-gauge needle
- ❏ Small gauze pad and/or alcohol swab
- ❏ Vial or ampule of skin test solution
- ❏ Disposable gloves
- ❏ Medication administration record or computer printout
- ❏ Skin pencil (optional)

STEP	RATIONALE

◾ ASSESSMENT

1. Review prescriber's medication order for client's name, drug name, dose, time, and route of administration against MAR.

Ensures safe and correct administration of medication by verifying order.

STEP	RATIONALE
2. Collect drug reference information regarding expected reaction when testing skin with specific allergen or medication and appropriate time to read site.	Type of reaction depends on client's ability to mount a cell-mediated immune response. Knowledge of expected and adverse reactions to skin testing helps the nurse determine future assessment criteria, including what symptoms to monitor for and how frequently and when to reassess client.
3. Assess client's history of allergies, type of substance, and normal allergic reaction.	Nurse should not administer any substance to which client is known to be allergic.
4. Assess client's knowledge of purpose and reactions of skin testing.	Reveals need for client instruction.
5. Check name of medication on vial/ampule label against MAR.	Ensures client receives correct medication.
6. Check medication's expiration date.	Medications that have expired should not be used because the potency of the medications changes when medications become outdated.

NURSING DIAGNOSES

- Anxiety
- Fear

- Health-seeking behaviors regarding disease screening practices
- Deficient knowledge regarding skin testing

Related factors are individualized based on client's condition or needs.

PLANNING

1. Expected outcomes following completion of procedure:	
• Client experiences very mild burning sensation during injection but no discomfort after injection.	Normal reaction to medication deposited in dermis.
• Small, light-colored bleb approximately 6 mm (¼ inch) in diameter forms at site and gradually disappears. Minimal bruising may be present.	Medication is in dermis and is eventually absorbed. Bruising is result of minor bleeding from capillaries.
• Client is able to identify signs of a skin reaction and their significance.	Demonstrates learning.
2. Perform hand hygiene.	Reduces transfer of microorganisms.
3. Prepare correct dose from vial or ampule (see Skill 21-1). Check dose carefully.	Ensures that medication is sterile and dose is accurate.
4. Identify client by checking identification bracelet and asking client's name. Compare with medication administration record.	Ensures that correct client receives ordered drug. At least two client identifiers (neither to be the client's room number) are to be used when administering medications (JCAHO, 2004).
5. Explain steps of procedure, and tell client that injection will cause a slight burning or sting.	Helps minimize client's anxiety.

IMPLEMENTATION

1. Close room curtain or door.	Provides privacy.
2. Select appropriate injection site. Inspect skin surface over sites for bruises, inflammation, or edema. Note lesions or discolorations of skin. If possible, select site three to four finger widths below antecubital space and one hand width above wrist (Centers for Disease Control and Prevention [CDC], 2004). If forearm cannot be used, inspect the upper back. If necessary, sites appropriate for subcutaneous injections (see Figure 21-12) can be used.	Injection sites should be free of abnormalities that may interfere with drug absorption. An intradermal site should be clear so that results of skin test can be seen and interpreted correctly.
3. Assist client to comfortable position. Extend and support elbow and forearm on flat surface if using arm.	Stabilizes injection site for easiest accessibility.

STEP	RATIONALE
4. Perform hand hygiene, and apply disposable gloves.	Follows Centers for Disease Control and Prevention (CDC) recommendations to prevent accidental exposure to blood and body fluids (OSHA, 2001).
5. Cleanse site with an antiseptic swab. Apply swab at center of the site, and rotate outward in a circular direction for about 5 cm (2 inches).	Mechanical action of swab removes secretions containing microorganisms.
6. Hold swab or square of sterile gauze between third and fourth fingers of nondominant hand.	Gauze or swab remains readily accessible when needle is withdrawn.
7. Remove needle cap or sheath from needle by pulling it straight off.	Keeping needle from touching sides of cap prevents contamination.
8. Hold syringe between thumb and forefinger of dominant hand with bevel of needle pointing up.	Smooth injection requires proper manipulation of syringe parts. With bevel up, medication is less likely to be deposited into tissues below dermis.
9. With nondominant hand, stretch skin over site with forefinger or thumb.	Needle pierces tight skin more easily.
10. With needle almost against client's skin, insert it slowly at 5- to 15-degree angle until resistance is felt. Then advance needle through epidermis to approximately 3 mm (1/8 inch) below skin surface. Needle tip can be seen through skin (see illustration).	Ensures that needle tip is in dermis. Inaccurate results will be obtained if needle is not injected at correct angle and depth (CDC, 2004).
11. Inject medication slowly. Normally resistance is felt. If not, needle is too deep; remove and begin again.	Slow injection minimizes discomfort at site. Dermal layer is tight and does not expand easily when solution is injected.

- **Critical Decision Point**

  It is not necessary to aspirate because dermis is relatively avascular.

12. While injecting medication, notice that small bleb approximately 6 mm (1/4 inch) in diameter (resembling mosquito bite) appears on skin's surface (see illustration).	Bleb indicates that medication is deposited in dermis.
13. Withdraw needle while applying alcohol swab or gauze gently over site.	Support of tissue around injection site minimizes discomfort during needle withdrawal. Dry gauze may minimize client discomfort associated with alcohol on nonintact skin.
14. Do not massage site or apply bandage to site.	Massage or pressure to site may disperse medication into underlying tissue layers and alter test results.
15. Assist client to comfortable position.	Gives client sense of well-being.

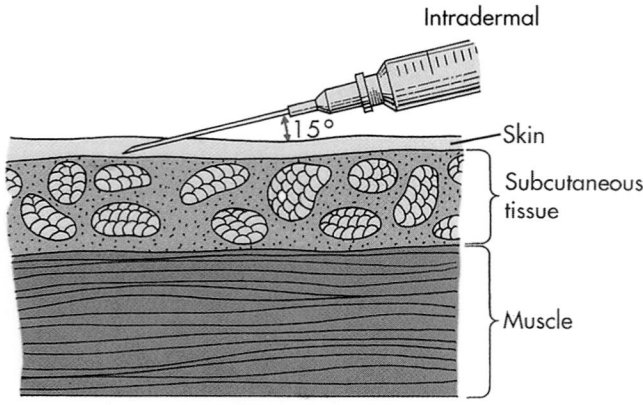

STEP **10** Intradermal needle tip inserted into dermis.

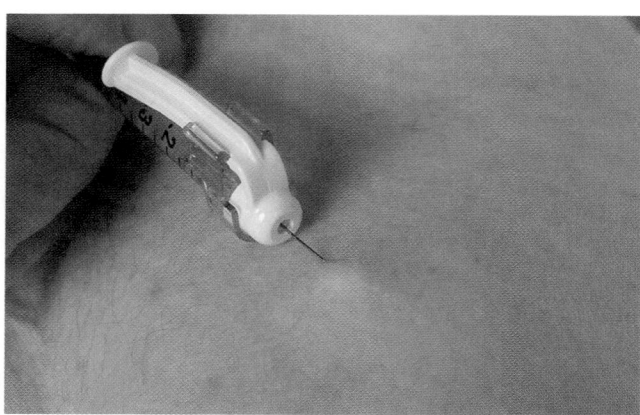

STEP **12** Injection creates small bleb.

STEP	**RATIONALE**
16. Discard uncapped needle or needle enclosed in safety shield and attached syringe in puncture-proof and leak-proof receptacle.	Prevents injury to clients and health care personnel. Capping of needles places the health care worker at risk for a needle-stick injury. Safety shields protect against needle sticks.
17. Remove gloves, and perform hand hygiene.	Reduces transmission of microorganisms.
18. Use skin pencil, and draw circle around perimeter of injection site. Read site within appropriate amount of time, designated by type of medication or skin test given.	The results of skin testing are determined at various times, based on the type of medication used or the type of skin testing. Refer to the manufacturer's directions to determine when to read the test's results.

- **Critical Decision Point**
  Read tuberculin (TB) test at 48 to 72 hours. Positive TB reaction is indicated by induration (hard, dense, raised area) of skin around injection site of:
  - *15 mm or more in clients with no known risk factors for TB*
  - *10 mm or more in clients who are recent immigrants; injection drug users; residents and employees of high-risk settings; clients with certain chronic illnesses; children less than 4 years of age; and infants, children, and adolescents exposed to high-risk adults*
  - *5 mm or more in clients who are human immunodeficiency virus (HIV) positive, immunocompromised clients, or clients recently exposed to TB (CDC, 2004)*

EVALUATION

1. Stay with client, and observe for any allergic reactions.	Severe anaphylactic reaction is characterized by dyspnea, wheezing, and circulatory collapse and requires immediate attention.
2. Inspect bleb. *Optional:* Use skin pencil to draw circle around perimeter of injection site.	Site must be read at various intervals to determine test results. Pencil mark makes site easy to find.
3. Ask client to discuss implications of skin testing and signs of hypersensitivity.	Client's ability to recognize signs of skin testing helps to ensure timely reporting of results.

Recording and Reporting

- Record amount and type of testing substance and date and time on MAR.
- Record area of injection and appearance of skin in nurses' notes.
- Report any undesirable effects from medication to client's health care provider, and document adverse effects according to institutional policy.

Unexpected Outcomes	**Related Interventions**
1. Raised, reddened, or hard zone forms around test site (induration), indicating sensitivity to injected allergen (positive test for tuberculin skin testing).	• Document results, and notify client's health care provider.
2. Onset of allergic reaction develops within minutes.	• Follow institutional policy or guidelines for appropriate response to allergic reactions, and notify client's health care provider.
3. Client is unable to explain purpose or signs of skin testing.	• Provide further instruction, or recognize client is unable to learn at this time.

Teaching Considerations

- Instruct client not to squeeze medication out of injection site.
- Teach clients that negative skin tests may not rule out allergies, especially when low concentrations of medication are used.
- Client should wear medical identification band listing all substances to which client is allergic.
- Caution client not to wash off markings around injection site.
- When clients are tested in a clinic or other outpatient setting, have them call in results of skin tests if a follow-up appointment is not made.
- Explain to client how to observe for skin reactions.

Pediatric Considerations

- Only amounts up to 0.5 ml can be administered intradermally to small children (Hockenberry and others, 2003).

- Children who are exposed to persons with confirmed or suspected infectious TB should be tested for TB immediately following exposure (American Academy of Pediatrics, 2000).
- Children who are exposed to high-risk individuals (e.g., HIV-infected, homeless, incarcerated) should be tested for TB every 2 to 3 years (American Academy of Pediatrics, 2000).

Gerontological Considerations

- The skin becomes less elastic during physiological changes in the older adult. Therefore the skin must be held taut to ensure the intradermal injection is administered correctly.

SKILL 21-4 Administering Subcutaneous Injections

A Sub-Q injection involves depositing medication into the loose connective tissue underlying the dermis. Subcutaneous tissue is not as richly supplied with blood vessels as muscles; thus drugs are not absorbed as quickly as those given IM. Anything affecting local blood flow to tissues, such as physical exercise or the local application of hot or cold compresses, influences the rate of drug absorption. Conditions such as circulatory shock or occlusive vascular disease impair client's blood flow and thus contraindicate Sub-Q injections.

Drugs given subcutaneously are isotonic, nonirritating, nonviscous, and water soluble. Examples of drugs given by this route are epinephrine, insulin, allergy medications, narcotics, and heparin. Only small doses of medications (0.5 to 1 ml) should be given subcutaneously. The tissue is sensitive to irritating solutions and large volumes of medications. Medications collecting within the tissues can cause sterile abscesses, which appear as hardened, painful lumps.

The best sites for Sub-Q injections include vascular areas around the outer aspect of the upper arms, the abdomen from below the costal margins to the iliac crests, and the anterior aspect of the thighs (Figure 21-12). These areas are easily accessible, especially for clients who must self-administer subcutaneous injections, such as insulin. They also are large enough areas so that multiple injections may be rotated within each anatomical location.

Injection sites should be free of infection, skin lesions, scars, bony prominences, and large underlying muscles or nerves. Rotation prevents the formation of lipohypertrophy or lipoatrophy in the skin. Body weight and the amount of adipose tissue influence the nurse's choice of needle length and angle of needle insertion. Generally a 25-gauge $\frac{1}{2}$- to $\frac{5}{8}$-inch

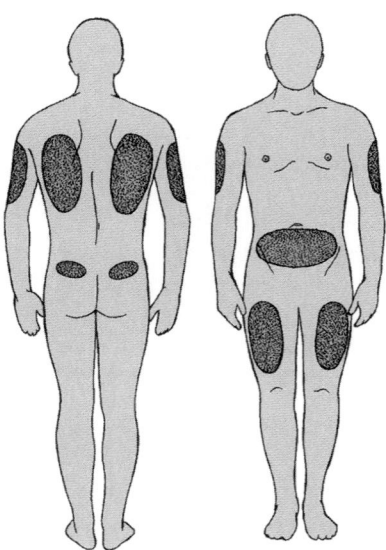

FIGURE **21-12** Common sites for subcutaneous injections.

needle with a medium bevel inserted at a 45- to 90-degree angle (Figure 21-13) deposits medication into the subcutaneous tissue of a normal-size client. If a client is obese, the nurse often pinches the tissue and uses a needle long enough to insert through the fatty tissue at the base of the skinfold; the angle of injection is 90 degrees. Cachectic clients may have insufficient tissue for Sub-Q injections. The upper abdomen is the best injection site for clients with little peripheral subcutaneous tissue. The preferred needle length is one half the width of the skinfold. To ensure that the medication reaches subcuta-

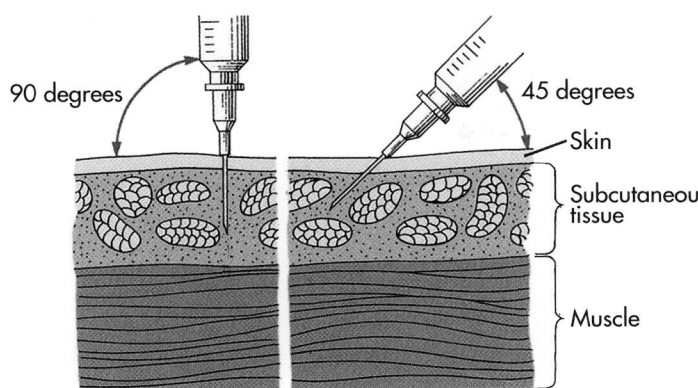

FIGURE 21-13 Subcutaneous injection. Angle and needle length depend on the thickness of skinfold.

neous tissue, the nurse pinches the subcutaneous tissue to prevent injecting the medication into the muscle. The syringe is inserted at a 45- to 90-degree angle depending on how much subcutaneous tissue is pinched (Pope, 2002).

Aspiration of any medication, including heparin and insulin, after injecting a Sub-Q injection is not necessary. Piercing a blood vessel in a Sub-Q injection is very rare and may cause hematoma formation (ADA, 2004; McConnell, 2000).

Special Considerations for Administration of Insulin

Insulin is the hormone used to treat diabetes mellitus. Clients' blood glucose levels may elevate whenever they experience unusual stress (e.g., hospitalization or trauma). Insulin may be used to treat hyperglycemia in these situations as well. Clients often receive a combination of different types of insulin to control their blood glucose levels. Rotation of injection from major site to major site (e.g., rotating from abdomen to upper arms to thighs from one injection to the next), once a common practice for clients who use insulin, is no longer necessary because the newer human insulins carry a much lower risk for hypertrophy. Therefore, clients can choose one anatomical area (e.g., the abdomen) and systematically rotate sites within that region. This helps maintain consistency in insulin absorption from day to day. Once all potential sites within an area are used, the client may choose either to move to another anatomical site (e.g., the thigh) or to start the rotation pattern over in the same anatomical area. (ADA, 2004a). Absorption rates of insulin vary based on the injection site. Insulin is absorbed the quickest in the abdomen, followed by the arms, thighs, and buttocks (Caffrey, 2003).

An important nursing consideration with insulin administration is the timing of injections. When planning insulin injection times, the nurse must determine when the client will eat or be fed next, as well as the client's current blood glucose level. Also, the peak action and duration of the client's insulin must be determined when developing an effective diabetes management plan. Table 21-2 compares the onsets, peaks, and durations of various insulin preparations. Box 21-3 provides general guidelines for insulin administration.

Special Considerations for Administration of Heparin

Heparin therapy is used to provide therapeutic anticoagulation to reduce the risk of thrombus formation. It is administered subcutaneously or intravenously. Heparin suppresses clot formation. Therefore clients receiving heparin are at risk for bleeding. Nurses should be alert for signs of bleeding (e.g., bleeding gums, hematemesis, hematuria, or melena) in clients who receive long-term anticoagulation therapy. Coagulation blood tests (e.g., activated partial thromboplastin time [APTT] or partial thromboplastin time [PTT]) are used in monitoring the desired therapeutic range for IV heparin therapy.

Before administering heparin, the nurse assesses for preexisting conditions that may contraindicate the use of heparin, including threatened abortion, cerebral or aortic aneurysm, cerebrovascular hemorrhage, severe hypertension, blood dyscrasias, and recent ophthalmic surgery or neurosurgery. In addition, the nurse assesses for conditions in which increased risk of hemorrhage is present: recent childbirth, severe diabetes, severe renal disease, liver disease, severe trauma, vasculitis, and active ulcers or lesions of the gastrointestinal (GI), genitourinary (GU), or respiratory tract. The client's current medication regimen must be assessed for possible drug interactions with heparin. Drugs that interact with heparin include aspirin, nonsteroidal antiinflammatory drugs (NSAIDs), cephalosporins, antithyroid agents, probenecid, and thrombolytics (McKenry and Salerno, 2003).

Low-molecular-weight (LMW) heparins (e.g., enoxaparin) have been found to be more effective than heparin in some clients (McKenry and Salerno, 2003). LMW heparins have a longer half-life, requiring less laboratory monitoring. These medications often come from the manufacturer in a prepared syringe. To minimize the pain and bruising associated with LMW heparin, it is given Sub-Q on the right or left side of the abdomen, at least 2 inches away from the umbilicus; this area is commonly referred to as a client's "love handles" (Aventis, 2003). Some of the prefilled syringes have a safety device included. The manufacturer's guidelines should be consulted when determining how to activate the safety device after medication administration.

TABLE 21-2 COMPARISON OF INSULIN PREPARATIONS

INSULIN TYPE*	ONSET (HOURS)	PEAK EFFECT (HOURS)	DURATION OF ACTION (HOURS)
RAPID-ACTING			
Insulin lispro (Humalog)	¼	1	4
Regular insulin**	½-1	2-4	5-7
Prompt insulin zinc suspension (Semilente)	1-3	2-8	12-16
INTERMEDIATE-ACTING			
Insulin zinc suspension (Lente insulin)	1-3	8-12	18-28
Isophane insulin suspension (NPH)	3-4	6-12	18-28
COMBINATION INSULINS			
Isophane insulin suspension (70%) plus regular insulin (30%) (Humulin 70/30 or Novolin 70/30)	½	4-8	24
Isophane human insulin (50%) and regular insulin (50%) (Humulin 50/50)	½	3	22-24
LONG-ACTING			
Extended insulin zinc suspension (Ultralente)	4-6	18-24	36
Protamine zinc insulin suspension (PZI)	4-6	14-24	36
Insulin glargine (Lantus)***	1	None	24
MIXED INSULINS			

Humulin 70/30 (70% NPH; 30% regular insulin)
Novolin 70/30 (70% NPH; 30% regular insulin)
Humalog Mix 75/25 (75% Lispro Protamine susp; 25% Lispro insulin)
Novolog Mix 70/30 (75% NPH; 25% insulin aspart)

Modified from McKenry LM, Salerno E: *Pharmacology in nursing,* revised ed 21, St. Louis, 2003, Mosby.

*All above insulins are available in 100-unit strengths. Beef, pork, beef-pork, and human insulins are available in rapid-acting insulins and the two insulins listed under intermediate-acting.
**This is the only insulin for IV use. Intravenously, the onset of action is within 10 to 30 minutes, peak effect within 15 to 30 minutes, and duration of action within 30 minutes to 1 hour.
***Cannot be mixed with other insulins.

BOX 21-3 General Guidelines for Insulin Administration

- Vials of insulin not in use should be refrigerated. Vials of insulin being used may be kept at room temperature to reduce irritation at the injection site.
- Inspect insulin vials before each use for changes (e.g., clumping, frosting, precipitation, or change in clarity or color) that may indicate a loss in potency.
- Insulin species or types should not be interchanged unless approved by the client's prescriber.
- Rapid-acting insulin should be injected within 15 minutes before a meal. The most commonly recommended interval between injection of short-acting insulin and a meal is 30 minutes.
- Preferred injection sites include the upper arm, anterior and lateral aspects of the thigh, buttocks, and abdomen avoiding a 2-inch radius around the navel. Site selection should be based on anticipated rate of absorption. Insulin absorbs quickest in the abdomen, followed by the arms, thighs, and buttocks.
- The client should self-administer insulin whenever possible. The developmental level of a child should be taken into consideration when determining the appropriate age for self-administration. Generally, self-administration of insulin should not be delayed beyond adolescence.
- Clients who use insulin should self-monitor their blood sugars whenever possible.
- Various changes in client status may necessitate the need for a different insulin dose. Health professionals should obtain information about blood glucose values whenever clients need help adjusting their insulin during times of illness or stress.
- All clients who take insulin should carry at least 15 g carbohydrate to be eaten or taken in liquid form in the event of a hypoglycemic reaction (e.g., 4 ounces juice, 8 ounces milk).
- Significant others need to be taught how to administer insulin and glucagon for situations in which the client is unable to self-administer insulin or is unable to ingest oral carbohydrates during hypoglycemia.

Modified from American Diabetes Association: Insulin administration: position statement, *Diabetes Care* 27(suppl 1):S106, 2004.

DELEGATION CONSIDERATIONS

Administering subcutaneous injections should not be delegated to assistive personnel. Other aspects of the client's care may be delegated to assistive personnel, and the nurse should instruct assistive personnel about the following:

- Any unexpected drug reactions to report or client's report of pain at injection site
- Report any impact of the medication on the client's vital signs or level of consciousness
- Report any change in the client's condition

EQUIPMENT

- ❑ Syringe (1 to 3 ml)
- ❑ Needle (25 to 27 gauge, ⅜ to ⅝ inch)
- ❑ Alcohol swab
- ❑ Small gauze pad (optional)
- ❑ Medication ampule or vial
- ❑ Disposable gloves
- ❑ Medication administration record (MAR) or computer printout

STEP	RATIONALE

ASSESSMENT

1. Review provider's medication order for client's name, drug name, dose, time, and route of administration against MAR.
2. Gather drug reference information pertinent to drug(s) ordered: action, purpose, time of onset and peak action, normal dosage, side effects, and nursing implications.
3. Review medical record and assess for factors that may contraindicate Sub-Q injections, such as circulatory shock or reduced local tissue perfusion.
4. Assess contraindications for oral medications: unconscious or confused client, client who is unable to swallow or has gastrointestinal disturbances, presence of gastric suction.
5. Assess client's medical history, history of allergies, and medication history.

6. Assess adequacy of client's adipose tissue.

7. Assess client's knowledge regarding medication to be received.
8. Observe client's verbal and nonverbal responses toward injection.

Ensures safe and correct administration of medication by verifying order.

Nurse must be able to anticipate drug's effects and observe client's response. Allows nurse to judge appropriateness of therapy as client's condition changes.
Reduced tissue perfusion interferes with drug absorption and distribution.

Contraindicates use of oral medications (i.e., analgesics); therefore parenteral route is more desirable. Some medications, such as heparin or insulin, are not absorbed from the gastrointestinal tract.
May influence how drug acts. Information also indicates client's need for medication or contraindications for medication use.
Physiological changes of aging or client illness may influence amount of subcutaneous tissue a client possesses. This influences methods for administering injections.
Information may pose implications for client education. Assessment may also reveal drug use problems at home.
Injections can be painful. Clients may experience considerable anxiety while anticipating injection, which can increase pain. Allows nurse to plan approach.

NURSING DIAGNOSES

- Anxiety
- Fear
- Ineffective health maintenance

- Deficient knowledge regarding medication administration or drug therapy
- Pain (acute)

Related factors are individualized based on client's condition or needs.

PLANNING

1. Expected outcomes following completion of procedure:
   - Client experiences no pain or mild burning at injection site.

   - Desired effect of medication achieved with no signs of allergies or undesired effects.
   - Client explains purpose, dosage, and effects of medication.

Injection given correctly. Subcutaneous medications are usually nonirritating to tissues, but displacement of tissues or medication may cause mild burning.
Drug action is effective.

Demonstrates learning.

STEP	RATIONALE
2. Check medication administration record or computer printout.	Verifies correct medication.
3. Check medication's expiration date printed on vial or ampule.	Medications that have expired should not be used because the potency of medications changes when the medications became outdated.
4. Prepare correct medication dose from ampule or vial (see Skill 21-1 or 21-2). Check dose carefully.	Ensures that medication is sterile and dose is accurate. Preparation techniques differ for ampule and vial.
5. Identify client by checking identification bracelet and asking client's name. Compare with medication administration record.	Ensures that correct client is receiving medication. At least two client identifiers (neither to be the client's room number) are to be used whenever administering medications (JCAHO, 2004).
6. Explain procedure to client, and proceed in calm, confident manner.	Helps client anticipate nurse's actions. Calm approach minimizes client's anxiety.

IMPLEMENTATION

1. Close room curtains or door.	Provides privacy.
2. Perform hand hygiene, and apply disposable gloves.	Follows Centers for Disease Control and Prevention recommendations to prevent accidental exposure to blood and body fluids (OSHA, 2001).
3. Keep sheet or gown draped over body parts not requiring exposure.	Respects client's dignity while area to be injected is exposed.
4. Select appropriate injection site. Inspect skin's surface over site for bruises, inflammation, or edema. Palpate site for masses, edema, or tenderness. NOTE:	Injection site should be free of lesions that might interfere with drug absorption.
• When administering heparin subcutaneously, use abdominal injection sites.	Anticoagulant may cause local bleeding and bruising when injected into areas such as arms and legs, which are involved in muscular activity.
• When administering LMW heparin subcutaneously, choose a site on the right or left side of the abdomen, at least 2 inches away from the umbilicus.	Injecting LMW heparin on the side of the abdomen will help decrease pain and bruising at the injection site (Aventis, 2003).
• When administering insulin, rotate the injection site within the same anatomical area (e.g., the abdomen), and systematically rotate sites within that area. Once all potential sites within that area are used, the client may choose either to move to another anatomical site (e.g., the thigh) or to start the rotation pattern over in the same anatomical area.	Rotating insulin sites within the same anatomical area helps maintain consistency in insulin absorption from day to day (ADA, 2004a).

• *Critical Decision Point*

Applying ice to the injection site for 5 minutes before and after the injection may decrease the client's perception of pain (Kuzu and Ucar, 2001).

5. Be sure that needle size is correct by grasping skinfold at site with thumb and forefinger. Measure skinfold from top to bottom; be sure that needle is approximately half this length.	Subcutaneous injections can be inadvertently given in the muscle, especially in the abdomen and thigh sites. Appropriate size of needle ensures that medication will be injected into subcutaneous tissue as ordered.
6. Assist client to comfortable position. Instruct client to relax arm, leg, or abdomen, depending on site chosen for injection. Talk with client about subject of interest.	Relaxation of area minimizes discomfort during injection. Promoting client's comfort through positioning and distraction helps reduce anxiety.
7. Re-locate site using anatomical landmarks.	Accurate injection of medication requires insertion in correct site to avoid injury to underlying nerves, bone, or blood vessels.

STEP	**RATIONALE**

8. Cleanse site with antiseptic swab (see illustration). Apply swab at center of site, and rotate outward in circular direction for about 5 cm (2 inches).

Mechanical action of swab removes secretions containing microorganisms.

9. Hold swab or square of sterile gauze between third and fourth fingers of nondominant hand.

Swab or gauze remains readily accessible for when needle is withdrawn.

10. Remove needle cap or sheath from needle by pulling it straight off.

Preventing needle from touching sides of cap prevents contamination.

11. Hold syringe between thumb and forefinger of dominant hand as if grasping a dart, holding syringe across tops of fingertips (see illustration).

Quick, smooth injection requires proper manipulation of syringe parts.

12. Administer injection:
   a. For average-size client, spread skin tightly across injection site, or pinch skin with nondominant hand.

   Needle penetrates tight skin more easily than loose skin. Pinching skin elevates subcutaneous tissue.

   b. Inject needle quickly and firmly at 45- to 90-degree angle. (Then release skin, if pinched.)

   Quick, firm insertion minimizes discomfort. (Injecting medication into compressed tissue irritates nerve fibers.)

   c. For obese client, pinch skin at site and inject needle at 90-degree angle below tissue fold.

   Obese clients have fatty layer of tissue above subcutaneous layer.

13. After needle enters site, grasp lower end of syringe barrel with nondominant hand. Move dominant hand to end of plunger, and slowly inject medication. Avoid moving syringe (see illustration).

Properly performed injection requires smooth manipulation of syringe parts. Movement of syringe may displace needle and cause discomfort.

- *Critical Decision Point*
  Applying ice to the injection site for 5 minutes before and after the injection may decrease the client's perception of pain (Kuzu and Ucar, 2001).

- *Critical Decision Point*
  Aspiration after injecting a Sub-Q medication is not necessary. Piercing a blood vessel in an Sub-Q injection is very rare (Stephens, 2003). Aspiration after injecting heparin and insulin is not recommended (ADA, 2004; McConnell, 2000).

14. Withdraw needle quickly while placing antiseptic swab or sterile gauze gently above or over site.

Supporting tissues around injection site minimizes discomfort during needle withdrawal. Dry gauze may minimize client discomfort associated with alcohol on nonintact skin.

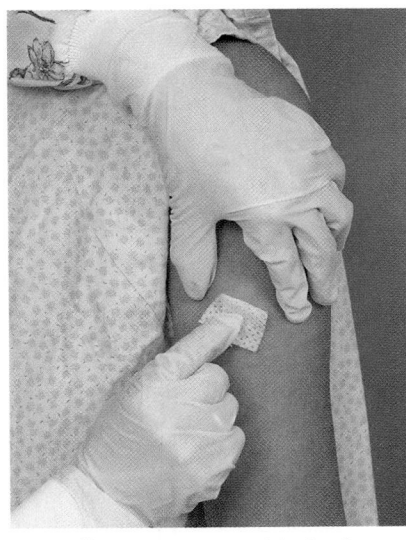

STEP **8** Cleansing site with circular motion.

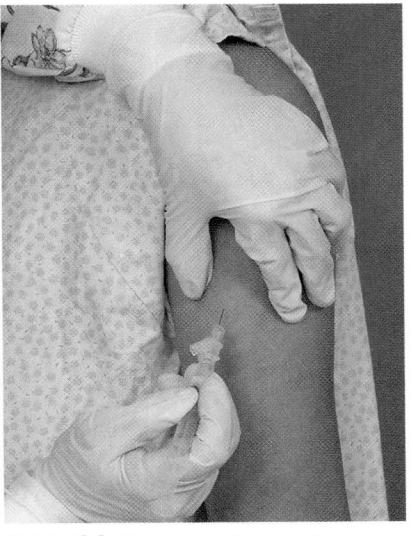

STEP **11** Holding syringe as if grasping a dart.

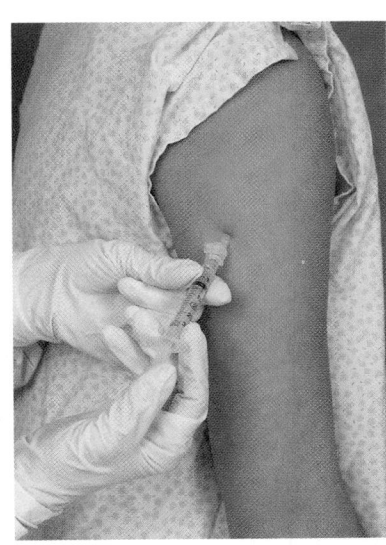

STEP **13** Inject medication slowly.

STEP	RATIONALE
15. Apply gentle pressure to site. *Do not massage site.* (If heparin is given, press alcohol swab or gauze continuously to site for 30 to 60 seconds.)	Aids absorption. Massage can damage underlying tissue.
16. Assist client to comfortable position.	Gives client sense of well-being.
17. Discard uncapped needle or needle enclosed in safety shield (see illustrations) and attached syringe into a puncture-proof and leak-proof receptacle.	Prevents injury to client and health care personnel. Recapping needles increases risk of needle-stick injury (OSHA, 2001).

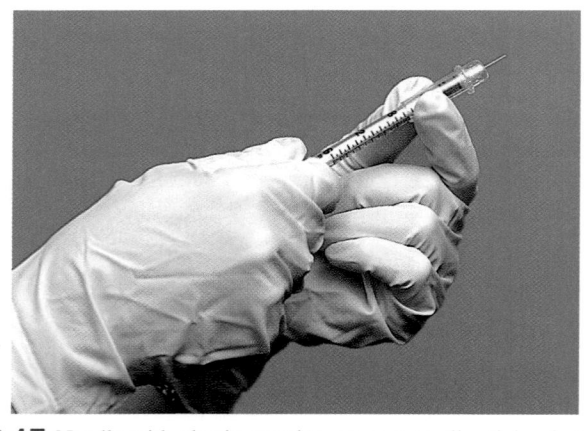 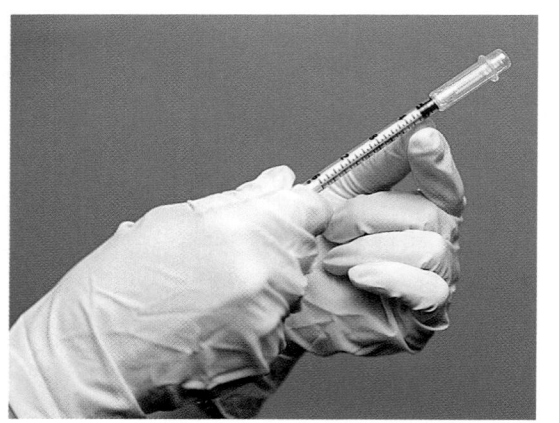

STEP 17 Needle with plastic guard to prevent needle sticks. **A,** Position of guard before injection. **B,** After injection the guard locks in place, covering the needle.

18. Dispose of used supplies, remove gloves, and perform hand hygiene.	Reduces transmission of microorganisms.

EVALUATION

1. Return to room, and ask if client feels any acute pain, burning, numbness, or tingling at injection site.	Continued discomfort may indicate injury to underlying bones or nerves.
2. Observe client's response to medication at times that correlate with the medication's onset, peak, and duration.	Determines efficacy of drug and allows evaluation of undesirable side effects.
3. Ask client to explain purpose and effects of medication.	Evaluates client's understanding of information taught.

Recording and Reporting

- Immediately after administration, chart medication dose, route, site, time, and date given on MAR to record care provided and prevent future drug administration errors. Correctly sign MAR according to institutional policy.
- Record client's response to medication.
- Report any undesirable effects from medication to client's health care provider, and document adverse effects according to institutional policy.

Unexpected Outcomes	Related Interventions
1. Client complains of localized pain or continued burning at injection site, indicating potential injury to nerve or vessels.	• Assess injection site for abscess formation. • Monitor client's heart rate, respirations, blood pressure, and temperature. • Notify client's health provider, and do not reuse site (Gilsenan, 2000).
2. Client displays signs of adverse reaction, including urticaria, eczema, pruritus, wheezing, and dyspnea.	• Follow institutional policy or guidelines for appropriate response to allergic reactions, and notify client's health care provider immediately.

Teaching Considerations

*   Instruct client to wear medical identification bracelet indicating important medical information, including diseases client has (e.g., diabetes) and allergies.
*   Clients who require daily injections will need to learn techniques of self-administration (see Skill 42-4). A family member or a significant other should also be taught injection techniques.
*   Clients with hypertrophy of skin due to repeated insulin injections (common with beef or pork insulin formulations) should be taught to avoid site until problem resolves.

Pediatric Considerations

*   Only amounts up to 0.5 ml may be administered subcutaneously to small children (Hockenberry and others, 2003).

Gerontological Considerations

*   Aging clients have reduced subcutaneous skinfold thickness, and skin is less elastic than that of younger clients. The upper abdominal site is the best site to use when the client has little subcutaneous tissue.

Home Care Considerations

*   Improper discarding of used needles and sharps in the home setting poses a health risk to the public and waste workers. Several options for safe sharps disposal at home exist. For example, clients can take their own sharps containers from home to collection sites, such as a doctor's office, a hospital, or a pharmacy. Mail-back programs, where clients mail their used syringes to a collection site, are available. Special devices that destroy the needle on the syringe, rendering it safe for disposal, are also available. If the client is unable to implement any of these options, needles and other sharps may be disposed of in a hard plastic or metal container with a tightly sealed lid (e.g., empty detergent bottle or coffee can). Pamphlets for safe home disposal of sharps can be found on the website of the Environmental Protection Agency (EPA) (2004).
*   Most insulin preparations have bacteriostatic properties that inhibit the growth of bacteria found on the skin. Therefore clients with diabetes may reuse their syringes at home if desired and if they are able to perform safe recapping of the needle. Syringes should be discarded when the needles become dull, bent, or contact any surface other than the skin. Wiping the needle off with alcohol is not recommended, because that may remove the silicon coating on the needle that makes injections less painful. Clients with poor personal hygiene, an acute illness, and open wounds on hands or clients who are immunocompromised should not reuse syringes (ADA, 2004a).
*   Pain during insulin injections may be decreased at home by injecting insulin at room temperature, waiting for alcohol to dry before injecting insulin, relaxing muscles around the injection site, and injecting the needle quickly (ADA, 2004a).

SKILL 21-5   Administering Intramuscular Injections

An injection given by the IM route deposits medication into deep muscle tissue. Because muscles have a rich blood supply, injections given IM absorb faster when compared to the Sub-Q route, which has a poor vascular supply (McKenry and Salerno, 2003). However, an increased risk of injecting drugs directly into blood vessels exists. As with Sub-Q injections, any factor that interferes with local tissue blood flow affects the rate and extent of drug absorption.

The nurse uses a longer and larger-gauge needle to pass through Sub-Q tissue and penetrate deep muscle tissue (see Figure 21-8). The viscosity of the medication, the injection site, and the client's weight and amount of adipose tissue influence needle size selection. The needle gauge is often determined by the length of the needle. Most immunizations and parenteral medications mixed in aqueous solutions can be administered using a 22- to 27-gauge needle. However, medications that are in an oil-based solution or medications that are more viscous are administered with an 18- to 25-gauge needle (Nicoll and Hesby, 2002).

An older adult or cachectic client may require a shorter, smaller-gauge needle because of muscle atrophy. Infants less than 4 months of age require a $\frac{5}{8}$-inch needle. For infants older than 4 months, a 1-inch needle is acceptable. In all infants the vastus lateralis or ventrogluteal sites are preferred (Hockenberry and others 2003). For well-developed children through adolescence a $\frac{5}{8}$-inch needle is used for deltoid injections, and a 1-inch needle is used for the ventrogluteal injections (Hockenberry and others, 2003).

When estimating the needle length necessary for IM injections into the vastus lateralis or deltoid muscle, the nurse grasps the muscle between the thumb and index finger. A needle length that is about half the distance between the two fingers is selected. When using the vastus lateralis, the nurse grasps the subcutaneous tissue between the thumb and index finger and uses a needle that is slightly greater than half the distance between the two fingers. Average needle lengths for children range from $\frac{5}{8}$ to 1 inch, whereas needles for adults range from 1 to $1\frac{1}{2}$ inches (Nicoll and Hesby, 2002).

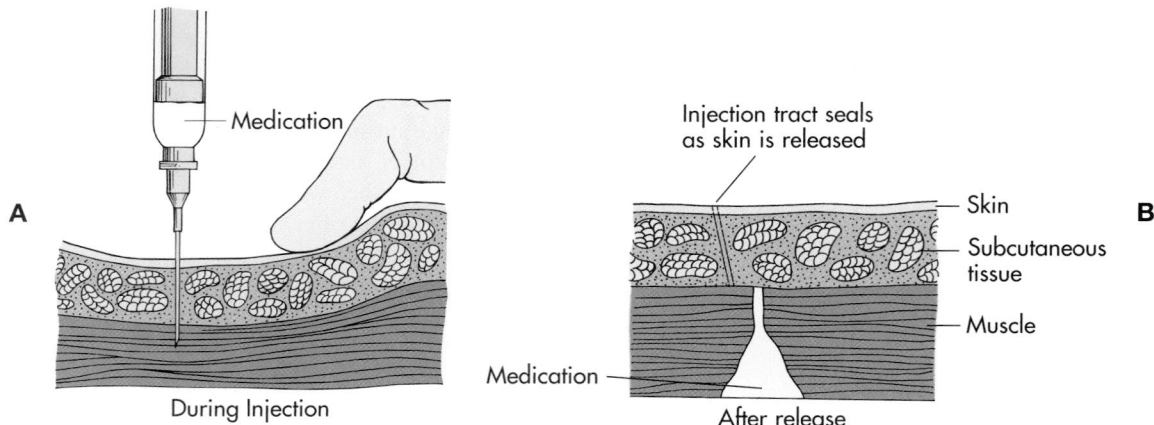

FIGURE **21-14** **A,** Pulling on overlying skin during IM injection moves tissue to prevent later tracking. **B,** The Z-track left after injection prevents the deposit of medication through sensitive tissue.

Intramuscular injections should be administered so that the needle is perpendicular to the client's body and as close to a 90-degree angle as possible (Katsma and Katsma, 2000; Nicoll and Hesby, 2002). Intramuscular injection sites should also be rotated to decrease the risk of hypertrophy. Emaciated muscles absorb medication poorly and should be avoided when possible.

Muscle is less sensitive to irritating and viscous drugs. A normal, well-developed adult client can safely tolerate as much as 5 ml of medication in larger muscles such as the ventrogluteal (Nicoll and Hesby, 2002). Infants should receive no more than 1 ml of medication intramuscularly, and small infants may only tolerate 0.5 ml. Depending on the child's size, a toddler may receive 1 to 2 ml of medication intramuscularly. Preschool and older children may have 2 to 3 ml, and the adolescent can have 3 to 5 ml injected into the muscle (Hockenberry and others, 2003).

The Z-track method is recommended for IM injections. The Z-track technique, pulling the skin either downward or laterally before injection, reduces leakage of medication into subcutaneous tissue and minimizes pain (Nicoll and Hesby, 2002). The nurse attaches the appropriate size needle to the syringe. Then the nurse selects an IM site, preferably in a large, deep muscle, such as the ventrogluteal. The overlying skin and subcutaneous tissues are pulled approximately 2.5 to 3.5 cm (1 to 1½ inches) down or laterally to the side with the ulnar side of the nondominant hand. The skin is held in this position until the injection has been administered. Once the medication is injected, the needle remains inserted for 10 seconds to allow the medication to disperse evenly. The nurse then releases the skin after withdrawing the needle, which leaves a zigzag path that seals the needle track wherever tissue planes slide across each other (Figure 21-14). The drug is less likely to escape from the muscle tissue.

Ventrogluteal Muscle

The ventrogluteal muscle involves the gluteus medius and minimus. It is situated deep and away from major nerves and blood vessels and is a safe site for all clients. Research has shown that injuries such as fibrosis, nerve damage, abscess, tissue necrosis, muscle contraction, gangrene, and pain have been associated with all the common IM sites except the ventrogluteal site (Nicoll and Hesby, 2002). Therefore the ventrogluteal site is a preferred injection site for infants, especially for administration of irritating or oily solutions, children, and adults (Hockenberry and others, 2003; Nicoll and Hesby, 2002).

The nurse locates the muscle by placing the heel of the hand over the greater trochanter of the client's hip with the wrist almost perpendicular to the femur. The right hand is used for the left hip, and the left hand is used for the right hip. The nurse points the thumb toward the client's groin, points the index finger to the anterior superior iliac spine, and extends the middle finger back along the iliac crest toward the buttock. The index finger, the middle finger, and the iliac crest form a V-shaped triangle, and the injection site is the center of the triangle (Figure 21-15).

Vastus Lateralis Muscle

The vastus lateralis muscle is another injection site used in the adult client and is the preferred site for administration of biologicals (e.g., immunizations) to infants (Nicoll and Hesby, 2002). The muscle is thick and well developed. It is located on the anterior lateral aspect of the thigh; in an adult it extends from a handbreadth above the knee to a handbreadth below the greater trochanter of the femur (Figure 21-16). The middle third of the muscle is the suggested site for injection. The width of the muscle usually extends from the midline of the thigh to the midline of the thigh's outer side.

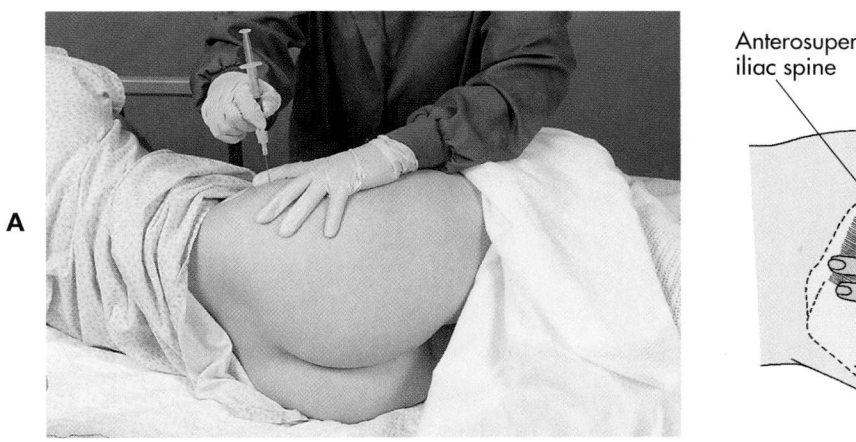 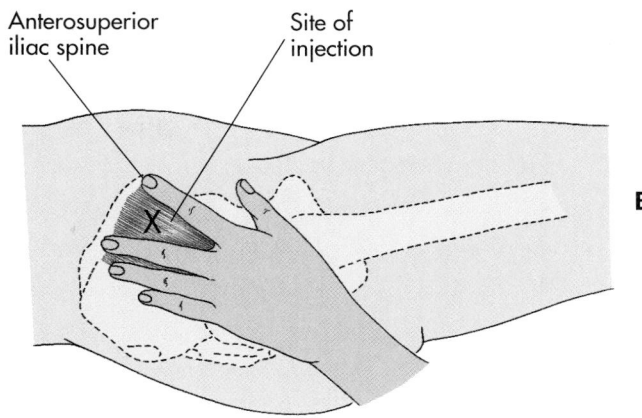

FIGURE **21-15** **A,** Injection site for ventrogluteal muscle avoids major nerves and blood vessels. **B,** Anatomical view of ventrogluteal muscle injection site.

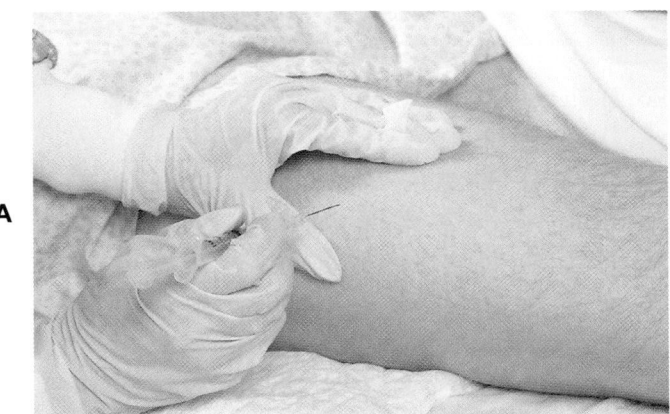 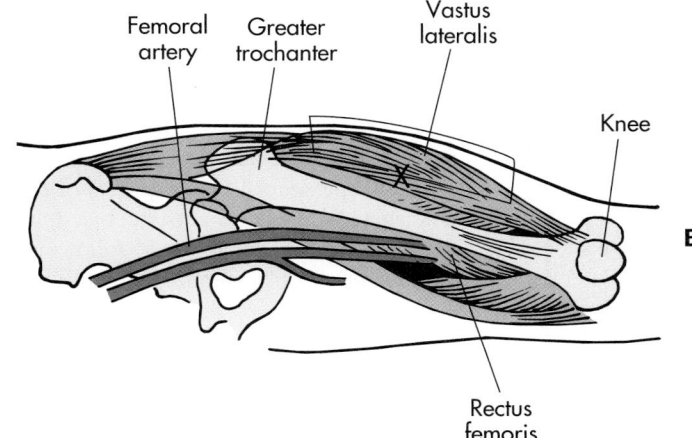

FIGURE **21-16** **A,** Giving IM injection in vastus lateralis site. **B,** Landmarks for vastus lateralis site.

Deltoid Muscle

Although the deltoid site is easily accessible, the muscle is not well developed in many adults. This site also has a potential for injury because the axillary nerve lies beneath the deltoid. The radial, brachial, and ulnar nerves and the brachial artery lie within the upper arm under the triceps and along the humerus (Figure 21-17, *A*). Therefore, nurses should use this site only for small medication volumes (0.5 to 1 ml), and for administration of routine immunizations in toddlers, older children, and adults (Nicoll and Hesby, 2002). This site may also be used when other sites are inaccessible because of dressings or casts.

To locate the deltoid muscle, the nurse fully exposes the client's upper arm and shoulder. A tight-fitting sleeve should not be rolled up. The nurse instructs the client to relax the arm at the side and flex the elbow by placing the hand on the hip or relaxing the lower arm across the abdomen or lap. The client may sit, stand, or lie down (Figure 21-17, *B*). The nurse

palpates the lower edge of the acromion process, which forms the base of a triangle in line with the midpoint of the lateral aspect of the upper arm. The injection site is in the center of the triangle, about 3 to 5 cm (1 to 2 inches) below the acromion process (see Figure 21-17, *A*). The nurse may also locate the site by placing four fingers across the deltoid muscle, with the top finger along the acromion process. The injection site is then three finger widths below the acromion process.

Dorsogluteal Muscle

The dorsogluteal muscle has been a traditional site for intramuscular injections. However, studies have demonstrated the exact location of the sciatic nerve varies from one person to another. If a needle hits the sciatic nerve, the client may experience permanent or partial paralysis of the involved leg. Therefore, this site should **not** be used for IM injections (Nicoll and Hesby, 2002).

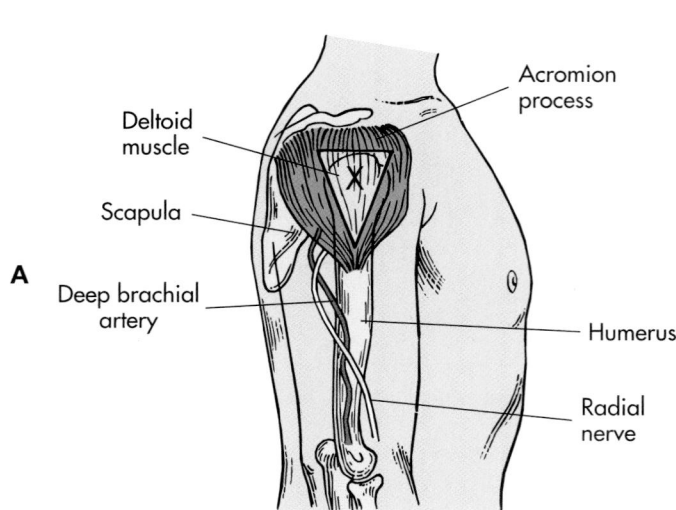 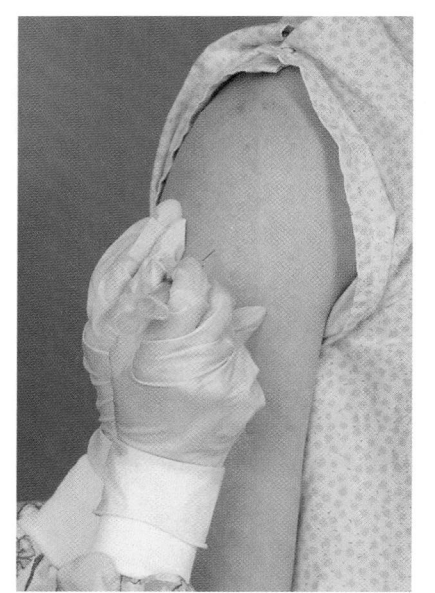

FIGURE 21-17 **A,** Landmarks for deltoid site. **B,** Giving IM injection in deltoid site.

DELEGATION CONSIDERATIONS

The skill of administering intramuscular medications should not be delegated to assistive personnel. Other aspects of the client's care may be delegated to assistive personnel, and the nurse should instruct assistive personnel about the following:

- Potential medication side effects to report or client's report of pain at the injection site
- Any impact of the medication on the client's physical status, vital signs, or level of consciousness (e.g., sedation) to report

EQUIPMENT

- ❑ Syringe with vial access device or filter needle: 2 to 3 ml for adult; 0.5 to 1 ml for infants and small children
- ❑ Needle, length corresponding to site of injection and age of client according to the following guidelines (Nicoll and Hesby, 2002):
- ❑ Infants and children: ⅝ to 1 inch (based on size of child)
- ❑ Vastus lateralis (adults): 1 to 1½ inch
- ❑ Deltoid (adults): 1 to 1½ inch
- ❑ Ventrogluteal (adults): 1½ inch
- ❑ Alcohol swab
- ❑ 2 × 2 gauze pad (optional)
- ❑ Medication ampule or vial
- ❑ Disposable gloves
- ❑ Medication administration record or computer printout

STEP	RATIONALE

ASSESSMENT

1. Review provider's medication order for client's name, drug name, dose, time, and route of administration against the MAR.

2. Gather drug reference information pertinent to drug(s) ordered: action, purpose, time of onset and peak action, normal dose, common side effects, nursing implications.

3. Review medical record or assess for factors that may contraindicate IM injection, for example, muscle atrophy, reduced blood flow, or circulatory shock.

Ensures safe and correct administration of medication by verifying order.

Nurse must be able to anticipate drug's effects and observe client's response. Allows nurse to judge appropriateness of therapy as client's condition changes.

Atrophied muscle absorbs medication poorly. Factors interfering with blood flow to muscles impair drug absorption (McKenry and Salerno, 2003).

- *Critical Decision Point*
  Consider calling prescriber for alternate route of medication administration. Because of the documented adverse effects of IM injections, other routes of medication injection are safer, and the IM route should only be used if the injection is justified (Nicoll and Hesby, 2002).

STEP	RATIONALE
4. Assess client's medical history, history of allergies, and medication history.	May influence action of certain drugs. Information also indicates client's need for medication.
5. Assess client's knowledge regarding medication and dosage schedule.	Information may pose implications for client education.
6. Observe client's verbal and nonverbal responses toward receiving injection.	Injections can be painful. Clients may experience considerable anxiety or fear while anticipating injection, which can increase pain. Allows nurse to plan approach.

NURSING DIAGNOSES

- Anxiety
- Fear
- Pain (acute)

- Deficient knowledge regarding medication administration or drug therapy

Related factors are individualized based on client's condition or needs.

PLANNING

1. Expected outcomes following completion of procedure:	
• Client experiences temporary mild burning at injection site.	Insertion of needle and/or injection of medications into tissues may cause discomfort.
• Desired effect of medication is achieved, with no allergies or undesired effects.	Drug administered properly. Drug action is normal.
• Client explains purpose and effects of medication.	Demonstrates learning.
• Client demonstrates no behaviors reflecting anxiety.	Anticipatory guidance relieves anxiety.
2. Check the name of medication on vial/ampule label against MAR.	Ensures client receives correct medication.
3. Prepare correct dose from ampule or vial (see Skill 21-1 or 21-2). Check dose carefully.	Ensures that medication is sterile and dose is accurate.
4. Remove vial access device or filter needle on syringe, and replace with needle for injection.	Vial access devices and filter needles cannot be used for IM injection.
5. For adults, select a 1- to 1½-inch, 22- to 27-gauge needle for medications prepared in aqueous solutions. If medications are viscous or in oil-based solutions, select an 18- to 25-gauge 1- to 1½-inch needle. For children select a ⅝- to 1-inch needle.	Needle must be long enough to reach muscle. Needles less than 1½ inches in length may not reach the muscle, especially in women (Engstrom and others, 2000; Katsma and Katsma, 2000).
6. Identify client by checking identification bracelet and asking client's name. Compare with medication administration record.	Ensures that correct client is receiving medication. At least two client identifiers (neither to be the client's room number) are to be used when administering medications (JCAHO, 2004).
7. Explain procedure, location of injection site, and how positioning lessens discomfort. Proceed in calm manner.	Allows client to anticipate injection so as to lessen anxiety.

IMPLEMENTATION

1. Close room curtains and/or door.	Provides client privacy.
2. Perform hand hygiene, and apply gloves.	Follows Centers for Disease Control and Prevention recommendations to prevent accidental exposure to blood and body fluids (OSHA, 2001).
3. Keep sheet or gown draped over body parts not requiring exposure.	Maintains client's dignity.
4. Select appropriate injection site by assessing size and integrity of muscle. Palpate for areas of tenderness or hardness. Note presence of bruising or area of infection.	The ventrogluteal site is the preferred site for all infants, children, and adults unless there are contraindications to this site. For example, the hepatitis-B vaccine should be administered in the deltoid in all clients greater than 12 months of age. In infants less than 12 months, the vastus lateralis should be used (Nicoll and Hesby, 2002).

STEP	RATIONALE

• *Critical Decision Point*

When choosing an injection site, do not use an area that is bruised, has indurations, has muscular atrophy, has reduced blood flow, or has signs associated with infection.

5. Assist client to comfortable position, depending on site chosen: ventrogluteal—client lies on side or back, flexes knee and hip on side to be injected; vastus lateralis—client lies flat, supine, with knee slightly flexed; deltoid—client may sit or lie flat with hand on hip or lower arm flexed but relaxed across abdomen or lap (Box 21-4).

Position that reduces strain on muscle minimizes discomfort of injection.

> **BOX 21-4 Positioning Client for Comfort With Intramuscular Injection**
>
> • To administer injection to a client in the side-lying position: Have the client flex the knee then move the knee forward, creating a 20-degree angle at the hip, allowing the knee to rest on the bed.
> • Giving an injection to a client in the supine position: Have the client flex the knee on the side where the injection is to be administered.

• *Critical Decision Point*

Ensure that client's position for injection is not contraindicated by medical condition (e.g., circulatory shock).

6. Re-locate site using anatomical landmarks.

Injection into correct anatomical site prevents injury to nerves, bones, and blood vessels.

7. Cleanse site with antiseptic swab. Apply swab to center of site, and rotate outward in circular direction for about 5 cm (2 inches).

Mechanical action of swab removes secretions containing microorganisms.

8. Hold swab or square of sterile gauze between third and fourth fingers of nondominant hand.

Swab or gauze remains readily accessible for when needle is withdrawn.

9. Position nondominant hand just below site, and pull the skin approximately 2.5 to 3.5 cm down or laterally with ulnar side of hand to administer in a Z-track. Hold this position until medication is injected.

Reduces discomfort and incidence of lesions.

• *Critical Decision Point*

If the client's muscle mass is small, grasp the body of the muscle between the thumb and fingers. This ensures that the medication reaches the muscle mass (Hockenberry and others, 2003; Nicoll and Hesby, 2002).

10. Place needle cap or sheath from needle in between thumb and index finger of nondominant hand. Hold barrel in dominant hand, and pull cap straight off.

Preventing needle from touching sides of cap prevents contamination.

11. Hold syringe between thumb and forefinger of dominant hand as if holding a dart. Hold it with palm down with needle perpendicular to the client's body.

Quick, smooth injection requires proper manipulation of syringe.

12. Administer injection:
    a. Inject needle quickly perpendicular to the client's body, as close to a 90-degree angle as possible.

Smooth, quick injection lessens pain. Angle ensures that medication reaches muscle mass (Katsma and Katsma, 2000; Nicoll and Hesby, 2002).

    b. After needle enters site, grasp lower end of syringe barrel with nondominant hand (while still holding skin back) to stabilize syringe. Continue to hold skin tightly with nondominant hand. Move dominant hand to end of plunger. Avoid moving syringe.

Smooth manipulation of syringe parts reduces discomfort from needle movement. Skin must remain pulled until after drug is injected to ensure Z-track administration.

STEP	RATIONALE
c. Pull back on plunger 5 to 10 seconds. If no blood appears, inject medication slowly at a rate of 1 ml/10 sec.	Aspiration of blood into syringe indicates accidental intravenous (IV) placement of needle. Intramuscular medications are not for IV use. Slow injection allows the muscle fibers to stretch and accommodate to the injected volume, which reduces pain and tissue trauma (Nicoll and Hesby, 2002).

- *Critical Decision Point*
  If blood appears in syringe, remove needle, and dispose of medication and syringe properly. Repeat preparation procedure.

d. Wait 10 seconds, then smoothly and steadily withdraw needle and release skin while placing antiseptic swab or dry gauze gently above or over injection.	Support of tissues around injection site minimizes discomfort during needle withdrawal. Dry gauze may minimize client discomfort associated with alcohol on nonintact skin.
13. Apply gentle pressure. *Do not massage site.*	Massage can damage underlying tissue.
14. For ventrogluteal and vastus lateralis sites, encourage leg exercises.	Promotes drug absorption.
15. Discard uncapped needle or needle enclosed in safety shield and attached syringe into puncture-proof and leak proof receptacle.	Prevents injury to client and health care personnel. Recapping needles increases risk of needle-stick injury (OSHA, 2001).
16. Dispose of soiled supplies, remove gloves, and perform hand hygiene.	Reduces transmission of microorganisms.

EVALUATION

1. Return to room, and ask if client feels any acute pain, burning, numbness, or tingling at injection site.	Continued discomfort may indicate injury to underlying bones or nerves.
2. Inspect site; note any bruising or induration.	Bruising or induration indicates complication associated with injection. Document findings, and notify health care provider. Apply warm compress to site.
3. Observe client's response to medication at times that correlate with the medication's onset, peak, and duration.	Intramuscular medications are absorbed quickly; undesired effects may also develop rapidly. Nurse's observations determine efficacy of drug action.
4. Ask client to explain purpose and effects of medication.	Evaluates client's understanding of information taught.

Recording and Reporting

- Immediately chart medication, dose, route, site, time, and date administered on MAR to record care provided and prevent future drug administration errors. Correctly sign MAR according to institutional policy.
- Record client's response to medication if indicated (for example, response to pain medication).
- Document and report any undesirable effects from medication to client's health care provider. Be aware that possible allergic reactions may not appear for several hours after a medication is given, especially when the client is receiving the medication for the first time.

Unexpected Outcomes	Related Interventions
1. While administering injection, it feels as though the needle has hit a bone.	• Pull back on the syringe about ¼ inch, being careful not to pull needle out of skin. Continue with medication administration (Gilsenan, 2000).
2. Client complains of localized pain or continued burning at injection site, indicating potential injury to nerve or vessels.	• Assess injection site for abscess formation. Monitor client's heart rate, respirations, blood pressure, and temperature. Notify client's health care provider, and do not reuse site (Gilsenan, 2000).
3. Client displays signs of adverse reaction, including urticaria, eczema, pruritus, wheezing, and dyspnea.	• Follow institutional policy or guidelines for appropriate response to allergic reactions, and notify client's health care provider immediately.

Teaching Considerations

• Clients who require regular injections, for example, vitamin B₁₂, will need to learn techniques of self-administration (see Skills 41-1 and 42-4). A family member or significant other should also be taught injection techniques and the importance of rotating sites to decrease the risk for hypertrophy.

• Instruct client and family member or significant other to observe injection sites for complications and to report complications to a health care provider immediately.

• Instruct client and family member or significant other to observe for effectiveness of medication and adverse reactions. Client or caregiver should report ineffectiveness of medication and adverse reactions to the health care provider.

• Have client perform several return demonstrations of preparing medications from vial or ampule and of injection technique.

Pediatric Considerations

• If muscle mass is well-developed in toddlers and older children, the deltoid muscle may be used for immunizations only. If there is any question about the development of the deltoid muscle in these children, then the vastus lateralis should be used (Nicoll and Hesby, 2002).

• Children may be extremely anxious or fearful of needles. Assistance with proper positioning and holding of the child may be necessary. Distraction, such as blowing bubbles and stroking the skin around the injection site before giving the injection, can help alleviate the child's anxiety (Sparks, 2001).

• If possible, apply EMLA cream to site at least 1 hour and up to 3 hours before IM injection (AstraZeneca, 2000) or a vapocoolant spray just before injection (Hockenberry and others, 2003) to decrease pain. These agents reduce pain from the piercing of the tissue from the needle. However, these agents do not absorb into the muscle, and the child may experience pain from the medication entering the muscle (Hockenberry and others, 2003).

Gerontological Considerations

• Older clients are more likely to have muscle atrophy. Therefore the nurse must carefully assess the injection site and may need to grasp the muscle between the thumb and fingers.

Home Care Considerations

• Because it is extremely difficult for a client to self-administer an IM injection in the vastus lateralis, a significant other should be taught to identify and administer injections in this site.

• Adult clients who require frequent injections can be taught to apply EMLA cream to the chosen injection site before administering the injection. Adults wishing to use EMLA cream should apply a "dollop" (about half of a 5-g tube) directly on the skin at least 60 minutes before administering the injection. The client needs to cover the area with an occlusive dressing. The dressing and EMLA cream should be removed, and the site should be cleaned with alcohol before the medication is given (AstraZeneca, 2000).

• Improper discarding of used needles and sharps in the home setting poses a health risk to the public and waste workers. Several options for safe sharps disposal at home exist. For example, clients can take their own sharps containers from home to collection sites, such as a doctor's office, a hospital, or a pharmacy. Mail-back programs, where clients mail their used syringes to a collection site, are available. Special devices that destroy the needle on the syringe, rendering it safe for disposal, are also available. If the client is unable to implement any of these options, needles and other sharps may be disposed of in a hard plastic or metal container with a tightly sealed lid (e.g., empty detergent bottle or coffee can). Pamphlets for safe home disposal of sharps can be found on the Environmental Protection Agency's website (2004).

• See Skills 41-1 and 42-4.

SKILL 21-6 Adding Medications to Intravenous Fluid Containers

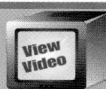

Medications given intravenously enter the venous circulation directly, causing rapid effects. The nurse must observe the client closely for symptoms of adverse reactions. Special attention is given to dose calculation and drug preparation. The nurse carefully checks the six rights of safe drug administration and is aware of the desired action and potential side effects of each medication.

Mixing drugs in large volumes of fluids is relatively safe and easy. The nurse or pharmacist dilutes IV medications in volumes of 50 to 1000 ml of compatible IV fluids such as normal saline, dextrose and water, or lactated Ringer's solution. In many hospital settings the pharmacy adds drugs to primary containers of IV solutions to ensure asepsis and minimize medication errors. The pharmacist may use special plastic caps to seal containers previously mixed. Vitamins and potassium chloride are two types of drugs commonly added to IV fluids.

Many parenteral medications are highly alkaline and irritating to muscle and subcutaneous tissue. Thus the IV route is best to minimize client discomfort. The nurse administers drugs intravenously by five methods:

1. As mixtures within large volumes of IV fluids
2. By piggyback infusion of a solution containing the prescribed medication and a small volume of fluid (50 ml, 100 ml) through an adjoining container or existing IV line (see Skill 21-7)
3. By volume-control administration device, in which a small container, holding 50 to 150 ml of fluid, is attached below the primary infusion bag (see Skill 21-7)
4. By various electronic infusion devices (see Skill 21-7)
5. By injection of a bolus or small volume of medication through an existing IV infusion line or heparin or saline IV lock (see Skill 21-8)

In all the methods, the client has either an existing IV infusion line or an IV access site in the form of a heparin lock or a saline lock. In most institutions and settings there are policies that identify the medications that nurses are allowed to administer intravenously.

DELEGATION CONSIDERATIONS

The skill of adding medications to intravenous fluid containers should not be delegated to assistive personnel. Other aspects of the client's care may be delegated to assistive personnel, and the nurse should instruct assistive personnel about the following:

- Expected actions of the medications to report
- To report any changes in the client's status, vital signs, or level of comfort
- To report any client complaints of moisture or discomfort around IV insertion site

EQUIPMENT

- ❏ Vial or ampule of prescribed medication
- ❏ Syringe of appropriate size (1 to 20 ml)
- ❏ Sterile needle (1 to 1½ inch, 19 to 21 gauge) with special filters if indicated
- ❏ Correct diluent if indicated (e.g., sterile water, normal saline)
- ❏ Sterile IV fluid container (bag or bottle, 50 to 1000 ml in volume)
- ❏ Alcohol or antiseptic swab
- ❏ Label to attach to IV bag or bottle
- ❏ Medication administration record (MAR) or computer printout

STEP	RATIONALE

ASSESSMENT

1. Check provider's order, including the client's name, drug name, dose, time, route, and appropriate type and amount of IV solution to use against the MAR.

2. Collect medication reference information necessary to administer drug safely, including action, purpose, side effects, normal dose, rate of administration, time of peak onset, and nursing implications.

3. When more than one medication is to be added to IV solution, assess for compatibility of medications. Check institutional reference for drug compatibility list.

4. Assess client's systemic fluid balance, as reflected by skin hydration and turgor, body weight, pulse, blood pressure, and electrolyte laboratory values.

5. Assess client's history of drug allergies, type of substance, and normal reaction.

Client's overall physical condition and compatibilities of ordered medication dictate type of IV solution used to ensure safe and accurate drug administration. Verifies correct medication.

Allows nurse to give drug safely and to monitor client's response to therapy.

Drug incompatibility often becomes apparent when drugs are mixed together. Chemical reactions that occur result in clouding or crystallization of IV fluids.

Danger of continuous IV infusions, especially in older adults or children, is that fluids may infuse too rapidly, causing circulatory overload (Hockenberry and others, 2003).

Intravenous administration of drugs causes rapid effects. Allergic response can be immediate.

STEP	**RATIONALE**
6. Perform hand hygiene.	Reduces transfer of microorganisms
7. Assess IV insertion site for signs of infiltration or phlebitis (see Chapter 27). Presence of complication will require IV to be restarted.	An intact, properly functioning site ensures that medication is given safely.

NURSING DIAGNOSES

- Deficient knowledge regarding medication therapy
- Risk for imbalanced fluid volume

Related factors are individualized based on client's condition or needs.

PLANNING

1. Expected outcomes following completion of procedure:	
• Desired effect of medication is achieved, with no signs of allergies or undesired effects.	Drug prepared and administered properly.
• Client develops no signs or symptoms of fluid volume excess.	Intravenous rate is correctly maintained.
• Intravenous site remains free of swelling or inflammation.	Fluid was delivered without infusion site complications.
• Client will explain purpose and side effects of medication.	Demonstrates learning.
2. Check name of medication on vial/ampule label against MAR.	Ensures client receives correct medication.
3. Assemble supplies in medication area.	Ensures orderly procedure with less chance of supply contamination.
4. Prepare prescribed medication from vial or ampule (see Skill 21-1). (If filter needle is used, replace it with regular needle before injecting medication into IV fluid container.)	Different techniques are used for each type of container.
5. Identify client by reading identification band and asking name. Compare with medication administration record.	Ensures that correct client receives ordered medication. At least two client identifiers (neither to be the client's room number) are to be used when administering medications (JCAHO, 2004).
6. Prepare client by explaining that medication is to be given through existing IV line or one to be started. Explain that no discomfort should be felt during drug infusion. Encourage client to report symptoms of discomfort.	Most IV medications do not cause discomfort when diluted. However, some medications, such as potassium chloride, can be irritating. Pain at insertion site may be early indication of infiltration.

IMPLEMENTATION

1. Perform hand hygiene.	Reduces transfer of microorganisms.
2. **To add medication to new container:**	
a. *Solution in a bag:* Locate medication injection port on plastic IV solution bag. Port has small rubber stopper at end. Do not select port for IV tubing insertion or air vent.	Medication injection port is self-sealing to prevent introduction of microorganisms after repeated use.
b. *Solution in a bottle:* Locate injection site on IV solution bottle, which is often covered by a metal or plastic cap.	Accidental injection of medication through main tubing port or air vent can alter pressure within bottle and cause fluid leaks through air vent. Cap seals bottle to maintain its sterility.
c. Wipe off port or injection site with alcohol or antiseptic swab.	Reduces risk of introducing microorganisms into bag during needle insertion.
d. Remove needle cap or sheath from syringe, and insert needle or needleless adapter of syringe through center of injection port or site; inject medication.	Injection of needle into sides of port may produce leak and lead to fluid contamination.
e. Withdraw syringe from bag or bottle.	Open tubing port in bottle provides direct route for microorganisms to enter solution. Bags have self-sealing port.

STEP	**RATIONALE**

    f. Mix medication and IV solution by holding bag or bottle and turning it gently end to end.

Allows even distribution of medication.

    g. Complete medication label with name and dose of medication, date, time, and nurse's initials. Stick it on bottle or bag (see illustration). *Optional* (check institution's policy): Apply a flow strip that identifies the time that the solution was hung and intervals indicating fluid levels.

Label can be easily read during infusion of solution. Informs nurses and physicians of contents of bag or bottle.

• *Critical Decision Point*

Do not use felt-tip markers on plastic IV bag surface. The ink can penetrate the plastic and leak into the IV solution.

    h. Spike bag or bottle with IV tubing, prime IV tubing if necessary, and hang (see Chapter 27). Regulate infusion at ordered rate.

Ensures medication is given over appropriate amount of time.

3. **To add medication to existing container:**

• *Critical Decision Point*

Because there is no way to know exactly how much IV fluid is in an existing hanging IV container, there is no way for the nurse to determine the exact concentration of the medication in the IV solution. Therefore it is recommended that medications should be added to new containers whenever possible.

    a. Prepare vented IV bottle or plastic bag:

      (1) Check volume of solution remaining in bottle or bag.

Proper minimal volume (see drug insert) is needed to dilute medication adequately.

      (2) Close off IV infusion clamp.

Prevents medication from directly entering circulation as it is injected into bag or bottle.

      (3) Wipe off medication port with an alcohol or antiseptic swab (see illustration).

Mechanically removes microorganisms that could enter container during needle insertion.

      (4) Insert syringe needle through injection port, and inject medication (see illustration).

Injection port is self-sealing and prevents fluid leaks.

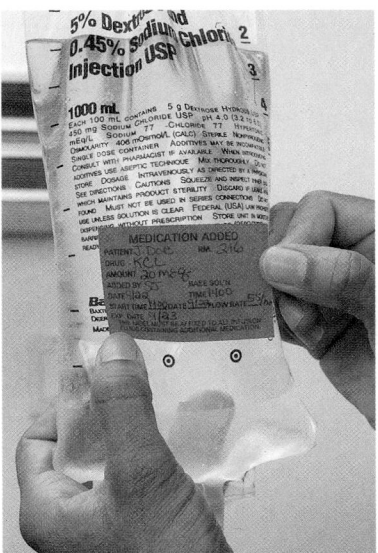
STEP **2g** Label affixed to IV bag.

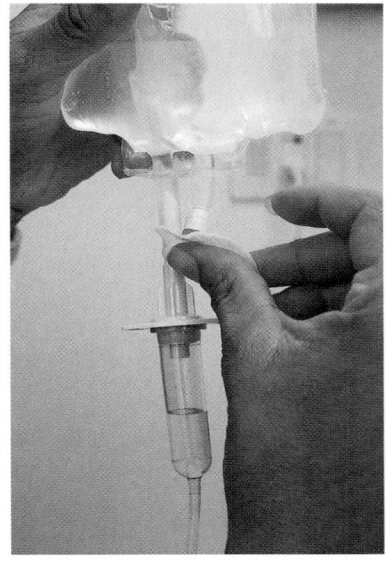
STEP **3a(3)** Injection port cleansed with alcohol.

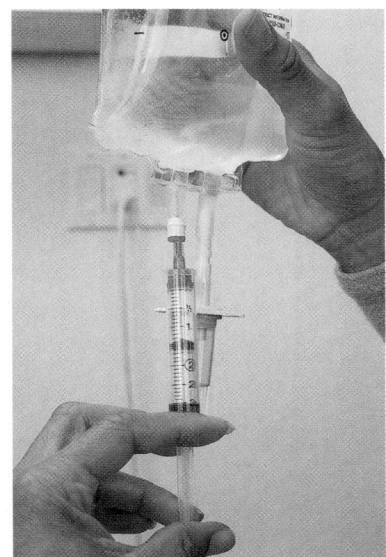
STEP **3a(4)** Medication injected through port.

STEP	RATIONALE
(5) Lower bag or bottle from IV pole, and gently mix. Rehang bag.	Ensures medication is evenly distributed.
b. Complete medication label, and stick it to bag or bottle.	Informs nurses and physicians of contents of bag or bottle.
c. Regulate infusion to desired rate.	Ensures medication is given over the appropriate amount of time.

• **Critical Decision Point**
Some medications, for example, potassium chloride boluses, can cause serious adverse reactions, including cardiac dysrhythmias. These IV medications should be infused on an IV pump. Check institutional policies for which IV medications require administration on an IV pump.

4. Properly dispose of equipment and supplies. Do not cap needle of syringe. Specially sheathed needles are discarded as a unit with needle covered.	Proper disposal of needle prevents injury to nurse and client. Capping of needles increases risk of needle-stick injuries (OSHA, 2001).
5. Perform hand hygiene.	Reduces transmission of microorganisms.

EVALUATION

1. Observe client for signs or symptoms of drug reaction.	Intravenous medications can cause rapid effects.
2. Assess IV insertion site and rate of infusion every 1 to 2 hours or as directed by institutional policy.	Over time IV site may become infiltrated or needle may become malpositioned. Flow rate may change according to client's position or volume left in container.
3. Observe IV site for signs or symptoms of infiltration or phlebitis.	Infiltrated drugs can injure tissue. Phlebitis indicates need to restart IV.
4. Observe for signs and symptoms of fluid volume excess.	Rapid uncontrolled infusion can cause circulatory overload.
5. Have client explain purpose and effects of drug therapy.	Demonstrates learning.

Recording and Reporting

- Record solution and medication added to parenteral fluid on appropriate form (Figure 21-18).
- Report any adverse effects to client's health care provider, and document adverse effects according to institutional policy.

Unexpected Outcomes	Related Interventions
1. Client has adverse reaction to medication.	• Follow institutional policy or guidelines for the appropriate response to and reporting of adverse drug reactions. • Notify client's health care provider of adverse effects immediately.
2. Client develops signs of fluid volume excess (e.g., abnormal breath sounds [crackles], blood pressure changes, jugular venous distention, edema, shortness of breath, intake greater than output).	• Stop IV infusion. • Notify client's health care provider of fluid excess immediately.
3. Intravenous site becomes swollen, warm, reddened, and tender to touch (see Chapter 27), indicating phlebitis.	• Stop IV infusion, and discontinue IV. • Treat IV site as indicated by institutional policy. • Insert new IV site if continuation of IV therapy is indicated.

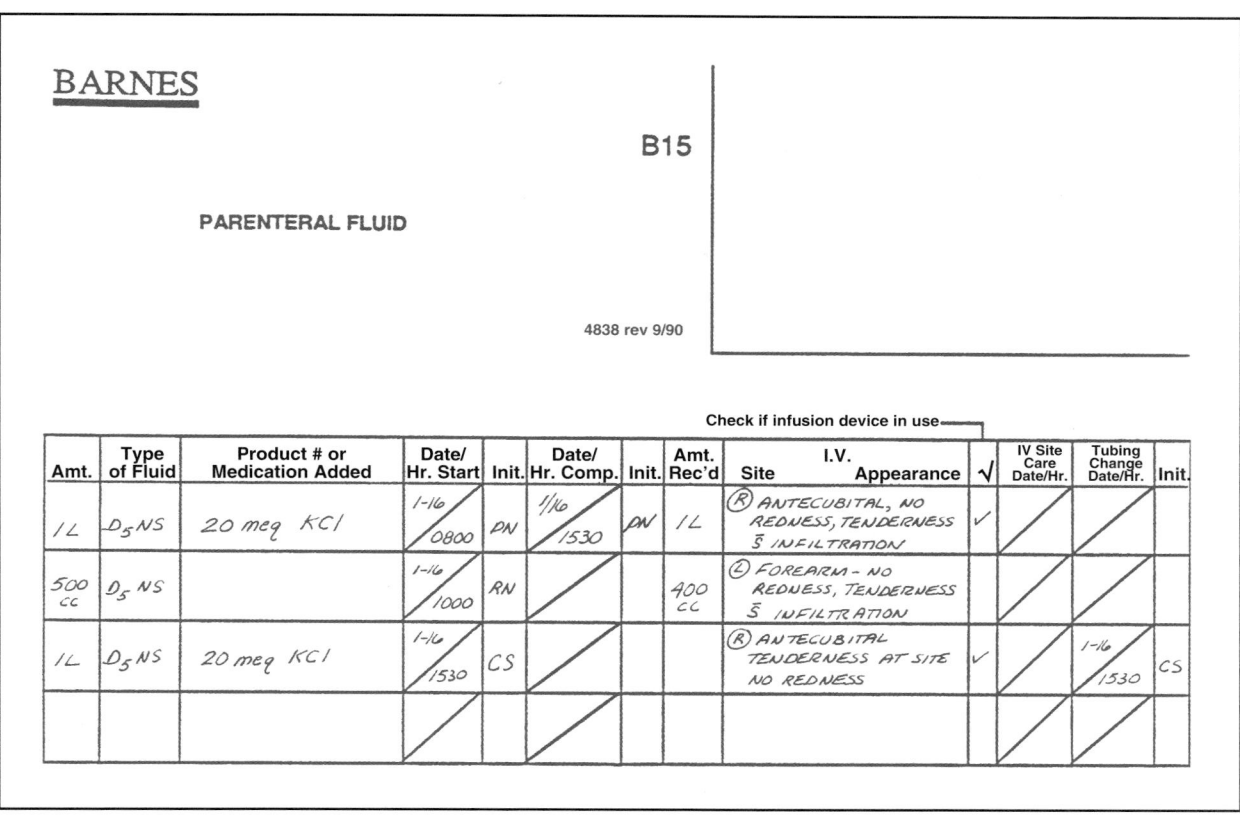

FIGURE **21-18** Example of documentation form for parenteral fluids.

Unexpected Outcomes	**Related Interventions**
4. Intravenous site becomes cool, pale, and swollen (see Chapter 27), indicating infiltration.	• Stop IV infusion, and discontinue IV. • Assess and measure site to determine extent of infiltration and to determine client's range of motion and sensation on the affected extremity. • Estimate amount of infiltrated fluid by determining when site was last assessed and how fast the IV fluid was infusing. • Document the infiltration. • Notify the client's health care provider for follow-up care. • Provide IV extravasation care (e.g., injecting phentolamine [Regitine] around the IV infiltration site) as ordered by health care provider or as indicated by institutional policy. • Do not routinely apply hot or cold compresses, exercise affected extremity, or elevate extremity without first consulting prescriber, pharmacist, or institutional policy for extravasation care. Rapid absorption of IV medications and fluids may cause underlying tissue damage (Fabian, 2000).

Teaching Considerations

- Clients or caregivers who will be expected to perform this skill should be taught both how to prepare the medication in a syringe and how to mix the medication in the IV solution. Allow plenty of time for learning, reinforcement, and return demonstration to ensure the medication can be prepared accurately.

Pediatric Considerations

- To prevent the risk of infusing too much IV solution to children, usually IV bags that hold no more than 500 ml of fluid are used and are used with an infusion pump to regulate the rate fluid infusion (Hockenberry and others, 2003).

Gerontological Considerations

- Older adults are at a higher risk for medication toxicity because of the altered pharmacokinetics of medications and the effects of polypharmacy. Therefore nurses should carefully monitor the response of the older adult to IV medication therapy (McKenry and Salerno, 2003).

- Older adults are at a higher risk for developing fluid volume overload, especially when receiving large amounts of IV fluids. Nurses should carefully assess the older adult for signs of fluid volume overload and heart failure (e.g., intake greater than output, peripheral edema, shortness of breath).

Home Care Considerations

- Clients or their caregivers should keep a record of medications that are mixed and when they are given at home. Records should include the name of the medications being mixed, the solution they are mixed in, and when they are infused.
- Clients or their caregivers can discard IV tubing with their regular garbage. If the tubing has needles or sharp points, they should be cut off and placed in a sharps container before discarding the tubing.

SKILL 21-7 Administering Intravenous Medications by Intermittent Infusion Sets and Miniinfusion Pumps

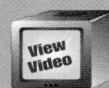

Administering drugs by intermittent infusion is a method in which the nurse dilutes IV medications in small volumes of solution and administers them over a short period. Administering drugs by this method reduces the risk of rapid drug-dose infusion and provides greater comfort and independence for the client. Clients receiving drugs by intermittent infusion have an established IV line that is kept patent by intermittent flushes of normal saline.

Intermittent infusion of drugs can be administered in several ways:

1. *Piggyback.* A piggyback is a small (25 to 250 ml) IV bag or bottle connected to short tubing lines that connect to the *upper* Y-port of a primary infusion line or to an intermittent venous access (Figure 21-19). The piggyback tubing is a microdrip or macrodrip system (see Chapter 27). The set is called a "piggyback" because the small bag or bottle is set *higher* than the primary infusion bag or bottle. In the piggyback setup the main line does not infuse when a compatible piggybacked medication is infusing. The port of the primary IV line contains a back-check valve that automatically stops the flow of the primary infusion once the piggyback infusion flows. After the piggyback solution infuses and the solution within the tubing falls below the level of the primary infusion drip chamber, the back-check valve opens and the primary infusion again flows.

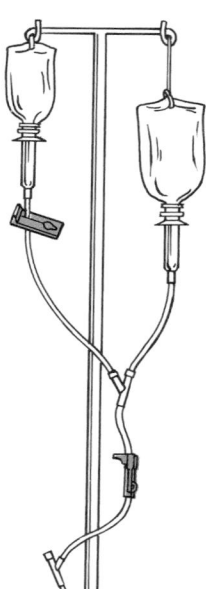

FIGURE 21-19 Piggyback infusion set.

2. *Tandem.* A tandem setup is a small (25–100 ml) IV bag or bottle connected to a short tubing line to the lower Y-port of a primary infusion line or to an intermittent venous access. The tandem set is placed at

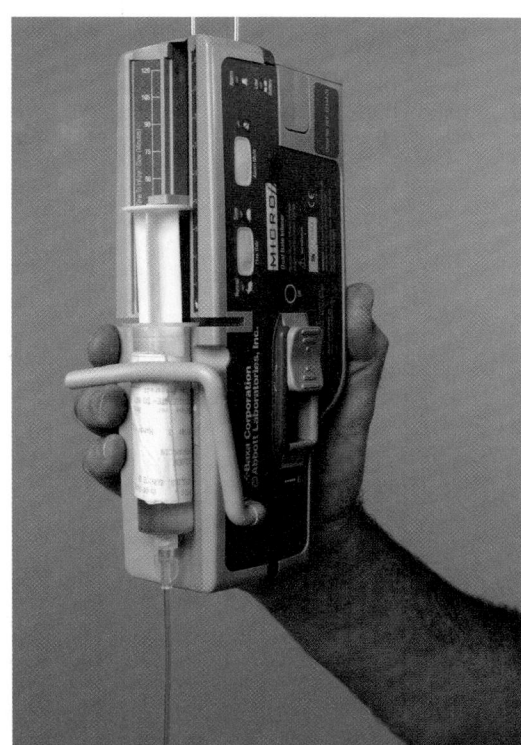

FIGURE **21-20** Miniinfusion pump.

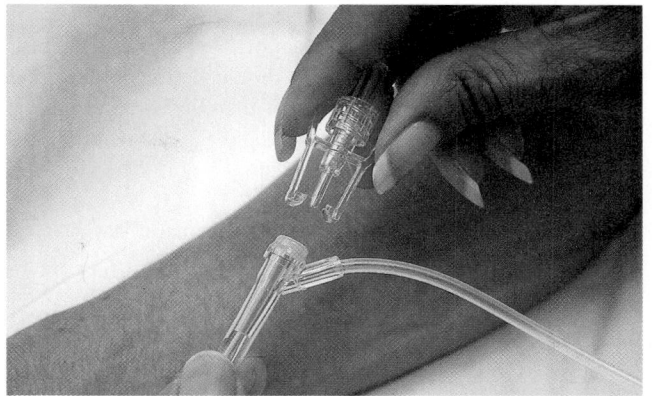

A

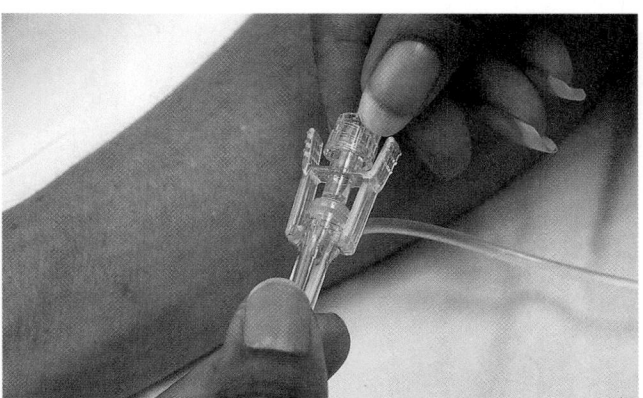

B

FIGURE **21-21 A,** Needleless lever lock cannula system.
B, Blunt-ended cannula inserts into port and locks.

the same height as the primary infusion bag or bottle. In the tandem setup the tandem and the main line infuse simultaneously. The nurse must monitor the tandem setup closely. If the tandem setup is not immediately clamped when the medication is infused, the IV solution from the primary line will back up into the tandem line.

3. *Volume-control administration.* Volume-control administration (e.g., Volutrol, Buretrol, Pediatrol) sets are small (50 to 150 ml) containers that attach just below the primary infusion bag or bottle. The set is attached and filled in a manner similar to that used with a regular IV infusion. However, the priming of the set is different, depending on the type of filter (floating valve or membrane) within the set. Follow the package directions for priming sets.

4. *Miniinfusion pump.* The miniinfusion pump allows medications to be given in very small amounts of fluid (5 to 60 ml) within controlled infusion times using standard syringes. It is powered by either electricity or batteries (Figure 21-20).

The Needle Safety and Prevention Act of 2001 has resulted in more institutions using manufactured needleless systems (Figure 21-21) or systems with catheter ports or Y connector sites designed to contain a needle housed in a protective covering. Needleless infusion lines allow a direct connection with the IV line via a recessed connection port or a blunt-ended cannula or shielded needle device, eliminating the risk of exposure to an IV needle (OSHA, 2001).

DELEGATION CONSIDERATIONS

Administering intravenous medications by intermittent infusion sets and miniinfusion pumps should not be delegated to assistive personnel. Other aspects of the client's care may be delegated to the assistive personnel, and the nurse should instruct assistive personnel to immediately report the following:

- Any unexpected drug reactions
- Client's report of any discomfort at infusion site
- Changes in client status or vital signs

EQUIPMENT

- ❏ Antiseptic swab
- ❏ IV pole or rack
- ❏ Medication administration record (MAR) or computer printout

- ❏ Medication label, if needed (Many IV medications are premixed and dispensed from pharmacy and arrive on the nursing unit with medication label already affixed.)

  Piggyback, Tandem, or Miniinfusion Pump
- ❏ Medication prepared in labeled infusion bag
- ❏ Short microdrip or macrodrip tubing set for piggyback with needleless device or stopcock
- ❏ Needle, 21 to 23 gauge, only if needleless system is not available; use needleless system whenever possible (OSHA, 2001).
- ❏ Miniinfusion pump
- ❏ Adhesive tape (optional)

  Volume-Control Administration Set
- ❏ Volutrol or Buretrol, Pediatrol
- ❏ Infusion tubing (may have needleless system attachment)
- ❏ Syringe (1 to 20 ml)
- ❏ Vial or ampule of ordered medication

STEP	RATIONALE

ASSESSMENT

1. Check provider's order to determine type of IV solution to be used, type of medication, dose, route, and time of administration.

2. Collect drug reference information necessary to administer drug safely, including how quickly to infuse the medication and its action, purpose, side effects, normal dose, time of peak onset, and nursing implications.

3. Assess compatibility of drug with existing IV solution.

Client's overall physical condition dictates type of IV solution used. Ensures safe and accurate drug administration.

Allows nurse to give drug safely and to monitor client's response to therapy.

Drugs that are incompatible with IV solutions may result in clouding or crystallization of solution in IV tubing, which may harm the client.

- **Critical Decision Point**

  Never administer IV medications through tubing that is infusing blood, blood products, or parenteral nutrition solutions.

4. Assess patency of client's existing IV infusion line or saline lock (see Chapter 27).

Intravenous line must be patent, and fluids must infuse easily for medication to reach venous circulation effectively.

- **Critical Decision Point**

  If the client's IV site is saline locked, cleanse the port with alcohol, and assess the patency of the IV line by flushing it with 2 to 3 ml of sterile normal saline. Attach appropriate IV tubing to the saline lock, and administer the medication via piggyback, miniinfusion, or volume-control administration set. When the infusion is completed, disconnect the tubing, cleanse the port with alcohol, and flush the IV line with 2 to 3 ml sterile normal saline. Maintain sterility of IV tubing between intermittent infusions. Optional: Cleanse port with antiseptic swab and flush with heparin solution if indicated by agency policy after final normal saline flush.

5. Perform hand hygiene. Assess IV insertion site for signs of infiltration or phlebitis: redness, pallor, swelling, and tenderness on palpation.

6. Assess client's history of drug allergies.

7. Assess client's understanding of purpose of drug therapy.

Confirmation of placement of IV needle or catheter and integrity of surrounding tissues ensures that medication is administered safely.

Effects of medications can develop rapidly after IV infusion. Nurse should be aware of clients at risk and not administer the medication if the client has an allergy to it.

May reveal need for education.

STEP	RATIONALE

NURSING DIAGNOSES

- Deficient knowledge regarding drug therapy
- Risk for ineffective health maintenance

- Risk for imbalanced fluid volume

Related factors are individualized based on client's condition or needs.

PLANNING

1. Expected outcomes following completion of procedure:
   - Drug infuses without adverse reactions.
   - Medication infuses within desired period.
   - Intravenous site remains intact without signs of swelling or inflammation or symptoms of tenderness at site.
   - Client is able to explain drug purpose, action, side effects, and dosage.
   - Client's serum drug level reveals therapeutic laboratory value attained without renal or hepatic toxicity.
2. Assemble supplies at bedside.

Drug was given safely with desired therapeutic effect.
Intravenous line remains patent.
Fluid infuses into vein rather than tissues.

Demonstrates learning.

Therapeutic effect of medication achieved without signs of adverse reactions.
Drug preparation usually is not required. Nurse may assemble infusion tubing and bag of medication in medication area or client's room.

IMPLEMENTATION

1. Perform hand hygiene.
2. Check client's identification by looking at arm bracelet and asking client's name.

3. Explain purpose of medication and side effects to client. Explain that medication is to be given through existing IV line. Encourage client to report symptoms of discomfort at site.
4. Administer infusion:
   a. **Piggyback infusion through existing line:**
      (1) Prepare medication by checking label on small infusion bag against MAR.
      (2) Connect infusion tubing to medication bag (see Chapter 27). Squeeze drip chamber, and fill half full. Allow solution to fill tubing by opening regulator flow clamp. Once tubing is full, close clamp, and cap end of tubing.

Reduces transmission of microorganisms.
Ensures drug is administered to correct client. At least two client identifiers (neither to be client's room number) are to be used when administering medications (JCAHO, 2004).
Keeps client informed of treatment. Clients who can verbalize pain at the IV site can help detect IV infiltrations early, lessening damage to surrounding tissues.

Infusion tubing should be filled with solution and free of air bubbles to prevent air embolus.

STEP	RATIONALE

(3) Hang piggyback medication bag (see illustration) above level of primary fluid bag. (Hook may be used to lower main bag.)

Height of fluid bag affects rate of flow to client. Ensures medication will infuse correctly.

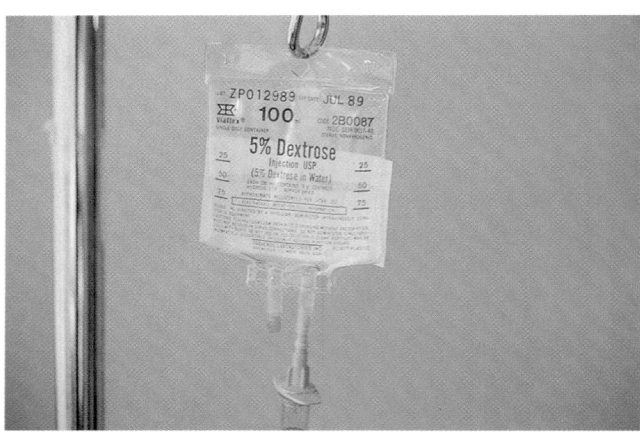

STEP **4a(3)** Small volume minibag for piggyback infusion.

(4) Connect tubing of piggyback to appropriate connector on primary infusion line:

Establishes route for IV medication to enter main IV line.

  (a) *Needleless system:* Wipe off needleless port on main IV line, and insert tip of piggyback infusion tubing. Lock into place as indicated by manufacturer of needleless system.

Needleless connections should be used whenever possible to prevent accidental needle-stick injuries (OSHA, 2001).

  (b) *Stopcock:* Wipe off stopcock port with alcohol swab, and connect tubing. Turn stopcock to open position.

Stopcock eliminates need for needle.

  (c) *Tubing port:* Connect sterile 21- to 23-gauge needle to end of piggyback infusion tubing, remove cap, cleanse injection port on main IV line, and insert needle through center of port. Consider placing a piece of tape at the junction where the needle enters the IV port to secure the medication line to the main IV line.

Prevents introduction of microorganisms during needle insertion.

(5) Regulate flow rate of medication solution by adjusting regulator clamp or IV pump infusion rate. Rate of flow should be determined by institutional policy. If a policy does not exist, consult a pharmacist or a drug manual. (Usually medications are recommended to infuse within 20 to 90 minutes.)

Provides slow, safe, intermittent infusion of medication and maintains therapeutic blood levels.

(6) Perform hand hygiene.

Prevents spread of microorganisms.

(7) After medication has infused, check flow rate of primary infusion. If stopcock is used, turn stopcock to the off position.

Back-check valve prevents infusion of primary line while medication is infusing. Primary infusion will automatically begin to flow when piggyback infusion is empty. Checking flow rate ensures proper administration of IV fluids.

STEP	RATIONALE
(8) Regulate main infusion line to desired rate, if necessary.	Infusion of piggyback may interfere with main line infusion rate.
(9) Leave IV piggyback bag and tubing in place for future drug administration, or discard in appropriate containers. If needle used, discard in sharps container.	Establishment of IV piggyback line produces route for microorganisms to enter main line. Repeated changes in tubing increase risk of infection transmission Check agency policy and procedure for frequency of IV tubing changes.
b. Volume-control administration set (e.g., Volutrol):	
(1) Prepare medication from vial or ampule (see Skill 21-1). Check name of drug on medication label against MAR.	Ensures right dose of medication is prepared and ensures sterility of medication.
(2) Fill volume-control administration set with desired amount of fluid (50 to 100 ml) by opening clamp between volume-control administration set and main IV bag (see illustration).	Dilution of IV medication reduces risk of infusion that is too rapid.
(3) Close clamp, and check to be sure clamp on air vent of volume-control administration chamber is open.	Prevents additional leakage of fluid into volume-control administration set. Air vent allows fluid in administration set to exit at regulated rate.
(4) Clean injection port on top of volume-control administration set with antiseptic swab.	Prevents introduction of microorganisms during needle insertion.
(5) Remove needle cap or sheath, and insert syringe needle through port, then inject medication (see illustrations). Gently rotate volume-control administration chamber between hands.	Rotating mixes medication with solution in volume-control administration set to ensure equal distribution.
(6) Regulate IV infusion rate to allow medication to infuse in time recommended by institutional policy, a pharmacist, or a medication reference manual.	For optimal therapeutic effect, medication should infuse in prescribed time interval.

A   B

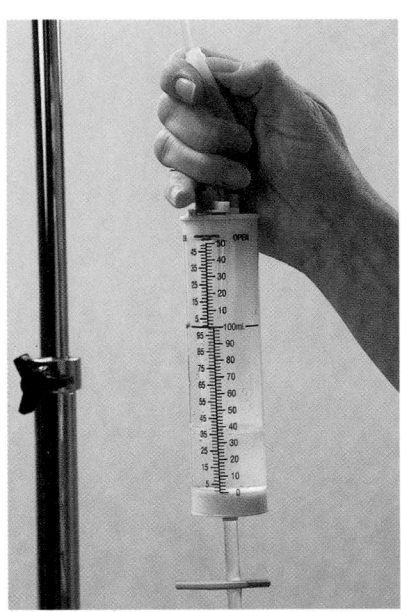

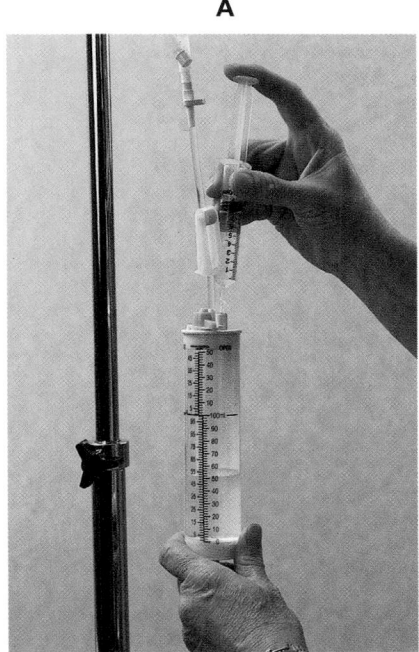

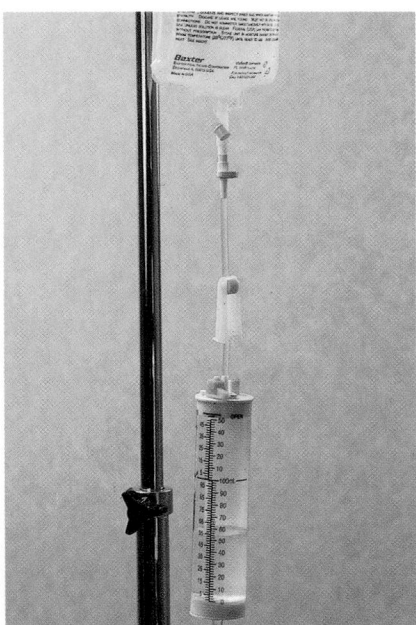

STEP **4b(2)** Filling volume-control administration device.

STEP **4b(5)** **A,** Medication injected into device. **B,** Prepared device.

STEP	RATIONALE
(7) Label volume-control administration chamber with name of medication, dosage, total volume including diluent, and time of administration.	Alerts nurses to medication being infused. Prevents other medications from being added to volume-control administration chamber.
(8) Dispose of uncapped needle or needle enclosed in safety shield and syringe in proper container. Perform hand hygiene.	Prevents accidental needle sticks and prevents spread of microorganisms.
(9) After medication has infused, be sure main IV solution is infusing as ordered, or disconnect IV tubing from IV, and flush IV lock per agency policy.	Ensures accurate infusion of continuous intravenous fluids. Flushing IV lock maintains patent IV site.
(10) Place sterile cap on end of volume-control administration set for future use, or discard set in appropriate containers.	If tubing set is to be reused, sterility must be maintained.
c. Administer medication using miniinfuser pump:	
(1) Check label on prefilled syringe for drug name and compare with MAR, then connect prefilled syringe to miniinfuser tubing.	Ensures client receives correct medication. Special tubing designed to fit syringe delivers medication to main IV line.
(2) Carefully apply pressure to syringe plunger, allowing tubing to fill with medication.	Ensures tubing is free of air bubbles to prevent air embolus.
(3) Hang infusion pump with syringe on IV pole alongside main IV bag.	
(4) Place syringe into miniinfusion pump (follow product directions). Be sure that syringe is secured (see illustration).	Syringe must be securely placed into miniinfuser to deliver medication.
(5) Connect miniinfusion tubing to main IV line:	Establishes route for IV medication to enter main IV line.
(a) *Needleless system:* Wipe off needleless port on main IV line, and insert tip of miniinfuser tubing. Lock into place as indicated by manufacturer of needleless system.	Needleless connections should be used whenever possible to prevent accidental needle-stick injuries (OSHA, 2001).

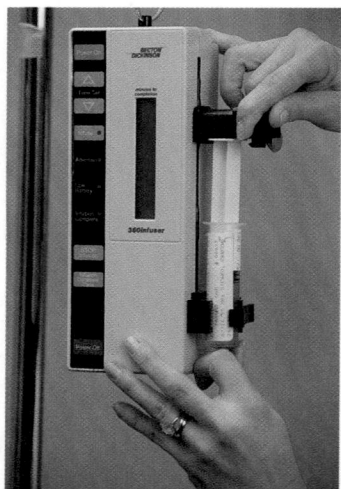

STEP **4c(4)** Ensure syringe is secure after placing it into mini-infusion pump.

STEP	RATIONALE
(b) *Stopcock:* Wipe off stopcock port with alcohol swab, and connect tubing. Turn stopcock to open position.	Stopcock eliminates need for needle.
(c) *Tubing port:* Connect sterile 21- to 23-gauge needle to miniinfuser tubing, remove cap, cleanse injection port on main IV line or saline lock, and insert needle through center of port. Consider placing tape where IV tubing enters port to keep connection secured.	Cleansing reduces transmission of microorganisms. Only use needles if needleless system is not available.
(6) Set pump to deliver medication within time recommended by institutional policy, a pharmacist, or a medication reference manual. Usually medications are recommended to infuse over 20 to 90 minutes. Press button on pump to begin infusion. *Optional:* Set alarm.	Pump automatically delivers medication at safe, constant rate based on volume in syringe. Alarm indicates completion of infusion.
(7) After medication has infused, check flow regulator on primary infusion. Infusion should continue to flow when pump stops. Regulate main infusion line to desired rate as needed. If stopcock is used, turn off miniinfusion line.	Checking flow rate ensures proper administration of IV fluids.
(8) Leave miniinfuser pump and tubing at the bedside for future drug administration, or dispose of supplies appropriately.	Miniinfuser pump tubing must remain sterile for future uses.
5. Perform hand hygiene.	Reduces transmission of microorganisms.

EVALUATION

1. Observe client for signs or symptoms of adverse reaction.	Intravenous medications act rapidly.
2. During the infusion, periodically check infusion rate of IV site.	Intravenous line must remain patent for proper drug administration.
3. Observe IV site for signs or symptoms of infiltration or phlebitis.	Infiltrated drugs can injure tissue. Development of infiltration necessitates discontinuing infusion and possibly initiating IV extravasation care. Phlebitis indicates need to restart IV.
4. Observe for signs and symptoms of fluid volume excess.	Rapid uncontrolled infusion can cause circulatory overload.
5. Ask client to explain purpose and side effects of medication.	Evaluates client's understanding of instruction.

Recording and Reporting

- Immediately record drug, dose, route, and time administered on MAR or computer printout to record care provided and prevent future drug administration errors. Correctly sign MAR according to institutional policy.
- Record volume of fluid in medication bag or Volutrol on intake and output (I&O) form to monitor total fluid intake.
- Report any adverse reactions to client's health care provider. Client's response may indicate need for additional medical therapy.

Unexpected Outcomes	Related Interventions
1. Client develops adverse drug reaction.	• Stop medication infusion immediately, and follow institutional policy or guidelines for appropriate response and reporting of adverse drug reactions. • Notify client's health care provider of adverse effects immediately.
2. Medication does not infuse over desired period.	• Can result from improper calculation of flow rate, malpositioning of IV needle at insertion site, or infiltration. • Determine reason, and take corrective action as indicated (e.g., correct flow rate, reposition IV, discontinue and restart IV).
3. Intravenous site becomes swollen, warm, reddened, and tender to touch (see Chapter 27), indicating phlebitis.	• Stop IV infusion, and discontinue IV. • Notify prescriber. • Treat IV site as indicated by institutional policy, and insert new IV site if continuation of IV therapy is indicated.
4. Intravenous site becomes cool, pale, and swollen (see Chapter 27), indicating signs of infiltration.	• Stop IV infusion immediately. • Provide extravasation care as indicated by institutional policy or prescriber. • See other related interventions for infiltration in Skill 21-6.

Teaching Considerations

- Review all intravenous medications with the client and significant others whenever possible. Include why the client is receiving the medication and potential adverse effects, including allergic responses.
- Teach the client and/or significant other that the rate of infusion must not be increased or decreased without consulting the prescriber. IV medications must be infused at a specified rate to achieve their desired effect and to avoid adverse effects.
- Teach the client and/or significant others to report any adverse effects immediately to the nurse.

Pediatric Considerations

- Infants and young children are more vulnerable to alterations in fluid balance, and they do not adjust as quickly as older children and adults do to changes in fluid balance. Therefore monitor intake and output carefully in infants and small children when they are receiving intravenous medications to assess their fluid balance (Hockenberry and others, 2003).

Gerontological Considerations

- Older clients are at a risk for developing toxicity to drugs. They also tend to have multiple medications prescribed, which can lead to many drug-drug interactions. Because medications administered intravenously have an immediate effect on the client, nurses must carefully and frequently assess this population for drug interactions, adverse effects, and toxic effects of all medications the older client receives (McKenry and Salerno, 2003).

Home Care Considerations

- Nurses must teach clients or significant others who administer intravenous medications at home every step of medication administration. The nurse should have the client or significant other perform several return demonstrations of medication administration before allowing the client or significant other to perform this skill independently. In addition, clients and significant others must be taught signs of complications of intravenous medication administration, such as phlebitis and infiltration, as well as what to do if a complication should arise at home.

SKILL 21-8 Administering Medications by Intravenous Bolus

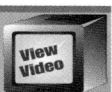

An IV bolus involves introducing a concentrated dose of a drug directly into the systemic circulation. An IV bolus may be given directly into a vein, into an existing IV line through an injection port, or through a saline or heparin lock. A saline lock consists of an indwelling needle or catheter attached to a plastic tube with a sealed injection port on the end. Institutional policy dictates which medications the nurse may give by IV push. The advantages and disadvantages to administering IV push medications are summarized in Box 21-5.

The IV bolus allows no time to correct errors. Therefore nurses should be very careful in calculating the correct amount of the medication to give. They may be required to have their calculations verified by another nurse. In addition, a bolus may cause direct irritation to the lining of blood vessels. Thus the nurse must be sure that the IV catheter or needle is correctly positioned in the client's vein. An IV bolus should never be given if the insertion site appears puffy or edematous or if the fluid from a connecting IV line cannot flow at the proper rate. Accidental injection of a medication into tissues surrounding a vein can cause pain, necrotic sloughing of tissues, and abscesses.

Administering an IV push medication too quickly can cause serious negative client outcomes, including death. The Institute for Safe Medication Practices (2003) has identified the following three strategies to reduce harm from rapid IV push medications:

- Nurses should have information regarding IV push times readily available to them.
- Less concentrated solutions should be used whenever possible.
- Avoid using terms in orders such as *IV push* or *IV bolus* with medications that should be administered over 1 minute or longer.

The rate of administration of IV push drugs varies from drug to drug. Therefore the nurse must verify a medication's rate of administration with institutional guidelines before administering a drug. If institutional guidelines are not available, then the nurse uses a medication manual to determine the appropriate rate of administration.

The Needlestick Safety and Prevention Act of 2001 has resulted in more institutions using manufactured needleless systems. Needleless systems allow the syringe containing the IV push medication to connect directly with the IV line via a recessed connection port or a blunt-ended cannula or shielded needle device, eliminating the risk of exposure to an IV needle. Needleless systems should be used whenever possible in implementing this skill (OSHA, 2001).

BOX 21-5   Advantages and Disadvantages of the Intravenous Push Method

ADVANTAGES

- Rapid onset of medication's effects, which is especially helpful in clients experiencing critical or emergent alterations in health.
- Small amount of nursing time is required to prepare an IV push.
- Doses of medications are easily controlled. Therefore dosages of short-acting medications can be titrated based on the client's individual requirements and responses to the drug therapy.
- IV push medications can be given one after another very quickly, avoiding the larger amounts of time that would be required if the medications had to be given by IV piggyback.
- IV push medications provide a more accurate dose of medication delivered because no medication is left in IV tubing (Skokal, 2000).

DISADVANTAGES

- Higher risk of side effects and adverse reactions; a temporary brief "toxicity" may occur because the medication peaks quickly with this route.
- If the medication is given very quickly (e.g., within 1 minute or less), there is little or no opportunity to stop the injection if an allergic reaction occurs.
- Increased risk of phlebitis, especially if a highly concentrated medication is given or a small peripheral vein is used.
- *Not all medications can be delivered IV push.*
- Speed shock, a systemic reaction to a medication when given too quickly, can occur, especially in clients with preexisting liver, renal, or cardiac problems (Skokal, 2000).

DELEGATION CONSIDERATIONS

Administering medications by intravenous bolus should not be delegated to assistive personnel. Other aspects of the client's care may be delegated to assistive personnel, and the nurse should instruct assistive personnel about the following:

- Potential medication side effects or drug reactions and to report their occurrence to the nurse.
- Report any unexpected drug reactions to the nurse
- Report discomfort at infusion site as soon as possible
- Obtain any required vital signs and report these findings to the nurse

EQUIPMENT

- ❑ Watch with second hand
- ❑ Medication administration record or computer printout
- ❑ Disposable gloves
- ❑ Antiseptic swab
  Intravenous Push (Existing Line)
- ❑ Medication in vial or ampule
- ❑ Syringe
- ❑ Needleless device or sterile needle (21 to 25 gauge)
  Intravenous Push (Intravenous Lock)
- ❑ Medication in vial or ampule
- ❑ Syringe
- ❑ Vial of appropriate flush solution (saline most common, but heparin may also be used; if heparin is used, most common concentration is 10 to 100 units/ml; check agency policy)
- ❑ Needleless device or sterile needle (21 to 25 gauge)

STEP	RATIONALE

ASSESSMENT

1. Check physician's order for type of medication, dose, time, and route of administration.

Ensures safe and accurate drug administration.

- *Critical Decision Point*

Some IV medications can only be pushed safely when the client is being continuously monitored for dysrhythmias, blood pressure changes, or other adverse effects. Therefore some medications can only be pushed in specific areas within a health care agency. Confirm institutional guidelines regarding requirements for special monitoring, and verify these requirements are available before giving medication (Zurlinden, 2002).

2. Collect drug reference information necessary to administer drug safely, including action, purpose, side effects, normal dose, time of peak onset, how slowly to give the medication, and nursing implications, such as the need to dilute the medication or administer it through a filter.

Allows nurse to give drug safely and to monitor client's response to therapy.

3. If drug is to be given through existing IV line, determine compatibility of medication with IV fluids and any additives within IV solution.

Intravenous medication may not be compatible with IV solution and/or additives.

4. Perform hand hygiene. Assess condition of IV or saline (heparin) lock insertion site for signs of infiltration or phlebitis.

Drug should not be administered if site is edematous or inflamed.

5. Check client's history of drug allergies.

Intravenous bolus delivers drug rapidly. Allergic reaction could prove fatal.

6. Assess client's understanding of purpose of drug therapy.

May reveal need for education.

NURSING DIAGNOSES

- Deficient knowledge regarding medication therapy

- Acute pain

Related factors are individualized based on client's condition or needs.

STEP	RATIONALE

PLANNING

1. Expected outcomes following completion of procedure:
   * Drug infuses without adverse reactions occurring.
   * Intravenous site remains clear, without swelling.
   * Client will explain purpose and side effects of medication.
2. Assemble supplies in medication room.
3. Check name of medication on vial/ampule against MAR.
4. Prepare medication from vial or ampule (see Skill 21-1 or 21-2).

Drug is given safely.
Medication infuses without complications to IV site.
Demonstrates learning.

Ensures sterile preparation of medications.
Ensures client receives correct medication.
Ensures that medication is sterile and correctly prepared.

* *Critical Decision Point*

   Some IV medications require dilution before administration. Verify with agency policy. If a small amount of medication is given (e.g., less than 1 ml), dilute medication in 5 to 10 ml of normal saline or sterile water so that the medication does not collect in the "dead spaces" (e.g., Y-site injection port, IV cap) of the IV delivery system.

5. Explain procedure to client. Encourage client to report symptoms of discomfort at IV site.

Informs client of planned therapies, keeps client involved in care, and helps identify possible infiltration early.

IMPLEMENTATION

1. Perform hand hygiene.
2. Check client's identification by looking at arm bracelet and asking name. Compare with medication administration record.
3. Put on disposable gloves.

Reduces transmission of microorganisms.
Ensures that drug is administered to correct client. At least two client identifiers (neither to be client's room number) are to be used when administering medications (JCAHO, 2004).
Follows Centers for Disease Control and Prevention recommendations to prevent accidental exposure to blood and body fluids (OSHA, 2001).

4. **Intravenous push (existing line):**
   a. Select injection port of IV tubing closest to client. Whenever possible, injection port should be a stopcock or other needleless component.
   b. Clean off injection port with antiseptic swab. Allow to dry.
   c. Connect syringe to IV line: Insert needleless blunt cannula tip of syringe or a small-gauge needle containing drug through center of port (see illustration).
   d. Occlude IV line by pinching tubing just above injection port (see illustration). Pull back gently on syringe's plunger to aspirate for blood return.

Follows provisions of the Needle Safety and Prevention Act of 2001 (OSHA, 2001).

Prevents introduction of microorganisms during needle insertion.
Prevents introduction of microorganisms. Prevents damage to port diaphragm.

Final check ensures that medication is being delivered into bloodstream.

STEP	RATIONALE

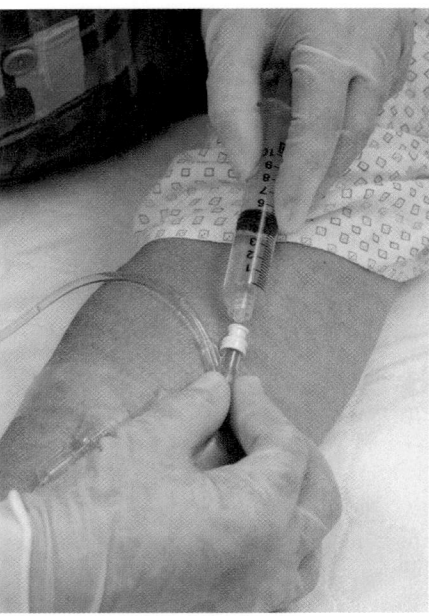

STEP **4c** Connecting syringe to IV line with needleless blunt cannula tip.

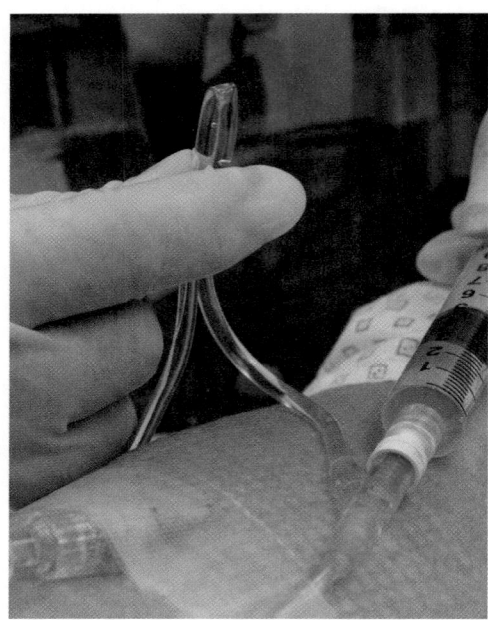

STEP **4d** Occluding IV tubing above injection port.

- **Critical Decision Point**

  In some cases, especially with a smaller gauge IV needle, blood return may not be aspirated, even if IV is patent. If IV site does not show signs of infiltration, and IV fluid is infusing without difficulty, proceed with IV push.

e. Release tubing, and inject medication within amount of time recommended by institutional policy, pharmacist, or medication reference manual. Use a watch to time administrations (see illustration). Intravenous line may be pinched while pushing medication and released when not pushing medication. Allow IV fluids to infuse when not pushing medication.

Ensures safe drug infusion. Rapid injection of IV drug can be fatal. Allowing IV fluids to infuse while pushing IV drug will enable medication to be delivered to client at prescribed rate.

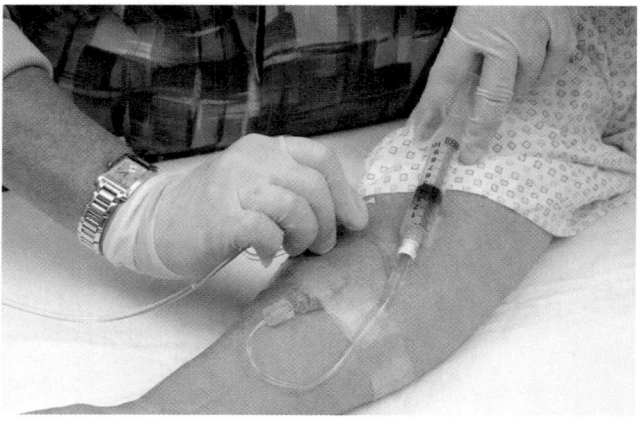

STEP **4e** Using a watch to time an IV push medication.

STEP	**RATIONALE**

• *Critical Decision Point*

If IV medication is incompatible with IV fluids, stop the IV fluids, clamp the IV line, flush with 10 ml of normal saline or sterile water, give the IV bolus over the appropriate amount of time, flush with another 10 ml of normal saline or sterile water at the same rate as the medication was administered, and then restart the IV fluids at the prescribed rate. This allows the nurse to give IV push medication through the existing line without creating potential risks associated with IV incompatibilities. If IV that is currently hanging is a medication (e.g., ranitidine), disconnect IV and administer IV push medication as outlined in step 5 to avoid giving a sudden bolus of the medication in the existing IV line to the client. Verify institutional policy regarding the stopping of IV fluids or continuous IV medications. If unable to stop IV infusion, start a new IV site (see Chapter 27), and administer medication using the IV push (IV lock) method.

STEP	**RATIONALE**
f. After injecting medication, withdraw syringe, and recheck fluid infusion rate.	Injection of bolus may alter rate of fluid infusion. Rapid fluid infusion can cause circulatory fluid overload.
5. Intravenous push (intravenous lock):	
a. Prepare flush solutions according to hospital policy.	
(1) Saline flush method (preferred method):	
• Prepare two syringes filled with 2 to 3 ml of normal saline (0.9%).	Normal saline has been found to be effective in keeping IV locks patent and is compatible with a wide range of medications.
(2) Heparin flush method (traditional method):	
• Prepare one syringe with ordered amount of heparin flush solution.	
• Prepare two syringes with 2 to 3 ml of normal saline (0.9%).	
b. Administer medication:	
(1) Clean lock's injection port with antiseptic swab.	Cleaning prevents introduction of microorganisms during needle insertion.
(2) Insert syringe with normal saline 0.9% through injection port of IV lock (see illustrations).	
(3) Pull back gently on syringe plunger, and check for blood return.	Indicates if needle or catheter is in vein.

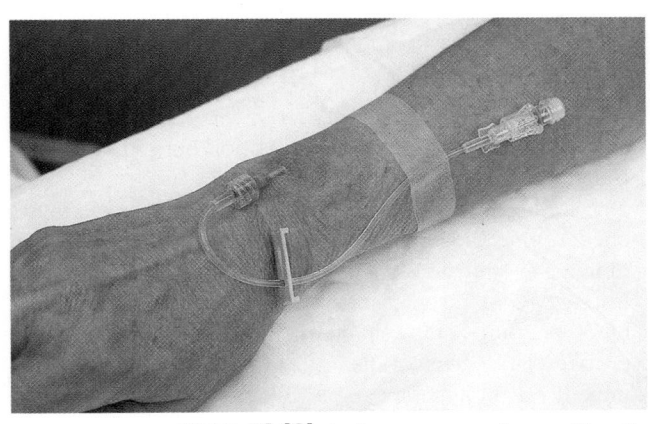
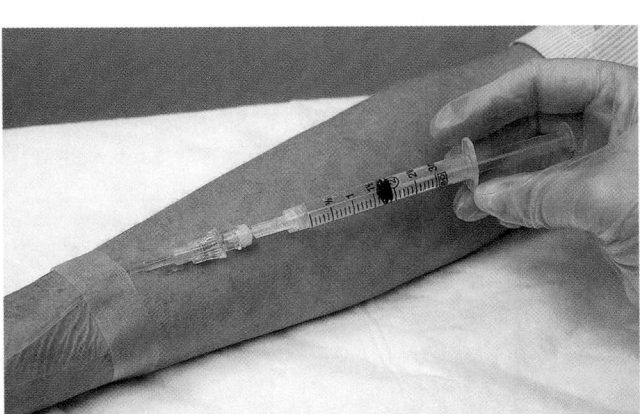

STEP **5b(2)** **A,** Intravenous catheter with saline lock adapter. **B,** Syringe inserted into injection port.

STEP	RATIONALE

- **Critical Decision Point**

In some cases, especially with a smaller gauge IV needle, blood return may not be aspirated, even if IV is patent. If IV site does not show signs of infiltration, and IV flushes without difficulty, proceed with IV push.

(4) Flush IV site with normal saline by pushing slowly on plunger.	Cleans needle and reservoir of blood. Flushing without difficulty indicates patent IV.

- **Critical Decision Point**

Closely observe the area of skin above the IV catheter. Note any puffiness or swelling as the IV site is flushed, which could indicate infiltration into the vein, requiring removal of catheter.

(5) Remove saline-filled syringe.	
(6) Clean lock's injection port with antiseptic swab.	Prevents transmission of infection.
(7) Insert syringe containing prepared medication through injection port of IV lock.	
(8) Inject medication within amount of time recommended by institutional policy, pharmacist, or medication reference manual. Use a watch to time administration.	Many medication errors are associated with IV pushes being administered too quickly. Following guidelines for IV push rates promotes client safety (Karch and Karch, 2003).
(9) After administering medication, withdraw syringe.	
(10) Clean lock's injection site with antiseptic swab.	Prevents transmission of infection.
(11) Flush injection port.	
(a) Attach syringe with normal saline, and inject normal saline flush at the same rate the medication was delivered.	Irrigation with saline prevents occlusion of IV access device and ensures all medication delivered. Flushing IV site at same rate as medication ensures that any medication remaining within IV needle is delivered at the correct rate.
(b) *Heparin flush option:* After instilling saline, attach syringe containing heparin flush. Inject heparin slowly, and then remove syringe.	Maintains patency of IV needle by inhibiting clot formation. *SASH method: S*aline, *A*dministration of medication, *S*aline, *H*eparin.
6. Dispose of uncapped needles and syringes in puncture-proof and leak-proof container.	Prevents accidental needle-stick injuries and follows CDC guidelines for disposal of sharps (OSHA, 2001).
7. Remove gloves, and perform hand hygiene.	Reduces transmission of microorganisms.

EVALUATION

1. Observe client closely for adverse reactions during administration and for several minutes thereafter.	Intravenous medications act rapidly.
2. Observe IV site during injection for sudden swelling.	Determines development of infiltration into tissues surrounding vein.
3. Assess client's status after giving medication to evaluate the effectiveness of the medication.	Some IV bolus medications can cause rapid changes in the client's physiological status. Some drugs require careful monitoring and assessment and possibly future laboratory testing (e.g., vasopressors and antiarrhythmics require blood pressure and heart rate monitoring, whereas heparin requires laboratory studies after administration to determine if it is in a therapeutic level).
4. Ask client to explain drug's purpose and side effects.	Evaluates learning.

Recording and Reporting

- Immediately record drug, dose, route, and time administered on MAR or computer printout to record care provided and prevent future drug administration errors. Correctly sign MAR according to institutional policy.
- Report any adverse reactions to client's health care provider. Client's response may indicate need for additional medical therapy.

Unexpected Outcomes	Related Interventions
1. Client develops adverse reaction to medication.	• Stop delivering medication immediately, and follow institutional policy or guidelines for appropriate response and reporting of adverse drug reactions. • Notify client's health care provider of adverse effects immediately.
2. Intravenous site becomes cool, pale, and swollen (see Chapter 27), indicating signs of infiltration.	• Stop IV infusion immediately. • Provide extravasation care as indicated by institutional policy or prescriber. • See other related interventions for infiltration in Skill 21-6.
3. Client is unable to explain medication information.	• Client requires reinstruction, or is unable to learn at this time.

Teaching Considerations

- Teach client and/or significant other that effects of IV push medications take place very quickly. Explain reasons for giving medication slowly, and teach signs of adverse effects.

Pediatric Considerations

- Many practical problems exist when administering IV push medications to neonates, infants, and small children. The therapeutic dosage for these clients is often so small that it can be difficult to accurately prepare the prescribed dose, even with a tuberculin syringe. These drugs need to be infused very slowly and in small volumes because of the risk for fluid volume overload (Hockenberry and others, 2003). Therefore, to maintain client safety, the nurse must carefully follow institutional policies when administering medications via IV bolus to this population.

Gerontological Considerations

- Although all body systems are affected by the aging process, the central nervous system and cardiovascular system seem to be the most affected. To reduce the risk for adverse effects of IV push drugs, smaller dosages are often prescribed (McKenry and Salerno, 2003). Older clients may better tolerate IV push medications if they are given over longer periods of time as well.

Home Care Considerations

- Medications are being ordered more frequently to be given IV push in the home setting. Nurses, pharmacists, and physicians need to collaborate closely in the care of these clients. Nurses need to ensure that the clients or significant others can give the IV push medication safely. Adequate eyesight and manual dexterity are needed to manipulate the syringe. Medications need to be clearly labeled. Clients need to understand their venous access device, how fast to give the medications, and what to flush their access device with before and after the medication is administered. Clients also need to know how to safely store their medications and whom to contact in case of an emergency (Skokal, 2000).

SKILL 21-9 Administering Continuous Subcutaneous Medications

The continuous subcutaneous infusion (CSQI or CSCI) route of medication administration is often used as an alternative to IV (e.g., IV bolus) or injection (e.g., IM, Sub-Q) routes of medication administration. This route is mainly used for the administration of medications for pain management (e.g., opioids) and insulin. This route has also been effectively used with terbutaline to stop preterm labor (Elliott and others, 2001). One factor that determines the infusion rate of medications delivered with CSQI is related to how quickly the medication can be absorbed. Most clients can absorb 2 to 3 ml/hr of medication (Pasero, 2002). As the rate of infusion increases, absorption of the medication decreases.

Continuous subcutaneous infusion is used in many settings, including the home, because it enables clients to manage their illness and/or pain without the risks and expenses involved with IV medication administration. For example, when used for pain management, this route is relatively easy to learn and understand. It has been associated with improved pain control in many populations, including clients in hospice settings (Pasero, 2002) and in children from 2 weeks to 18 years of age (Dietrich and Tobias, 2003).

When CSQI is used for diabetes management, clients receive intense diabetes self-management education provided by certified diabetes educators or insulin pump trainers who are provided by the insulin pump manufacturer. People with diabetes who use insulin pumps generally require 25% less insulin when using a pump because they absorb their insulin more efficiently (Olohan and Zappitelli, 2003). Box 21-6 summarizes benefits associated with the use of CSQI in clients requiring pain management. Selection criteria for clients considering an insulin pump are listed in Box 21-7.

The procedure to initiate and discontinue CSQI therapy is similar regardless of the type of medication that is being delivered. However, nursing assessment and interventions vary depending on the medication's classification and desired effect. For example, in pain management, the advanced practice nurse, physician, or pharmacist determines the drug dose based on how much pain medication the client uses in 24 hours. An equianalgesic chart is used to convert IV, IM, and oral (PO) medication doses to Sub-Q doses (Pasero, 2002). The nurse evaluates the effectiveness of the medication by assessing the client's pain. Alternatively, if the client is receiving insulin, the advanced practice nurse, physician, or pharmacist reviews how much insulin the client requires in a 24-hour period and the response to insulin in determining the appropriate basal (or continuous) rate and a sliding scale for the client to use before eating. The effectiveness of insulin therapy is evaluated by assessing the client's blood glucose levels, weight gain, and occurrences of hypoglycemia or hyperglycemia (Weissberg-Benchell and others, 2003).

A small-gauge (25 to 27) winged or butterfly IV needle is used to deliver medications through CSQI. Alternatively, a special commercially prepared Teflon cannula may be used. Although Teflon needles are generally more expensive, they tend to be more comfortable for the client, have lower rates of complications when compared with winged IV needles, and are associated with fewer needle-stick injuries (Dawkins and others, 2000; Torre, 2002). The choice of needle type is based on institutional guidelines or client preference. The needle used should be of the shortest length and the smallest gauge necessary to establish and maintain the infusion.

Anatomical sites for subcutaneous injections (see Figure 21-12) and the upper chest may be used for medication administration by this route. Site selection depends on the client's activity level and the type of medication delivered. For example, pain medications given to ambulatory clients are best delivered in the upper chest. This allows the client to move

---

BOX 21-6 Benefits Associated With Pain Management Delivered by Continuous Subcutaneous Infusion

- Can be used in clients with poor venous access.
- Provides pain relief to clients who are unable to tolerate oral pain medications.
- Allows client to be more mobile.
- Onset of action takes about 20 minutes.
- Provides better pain control than IM injections.
- Costs are almost half of costs associated with IV infusions.

Modified from Pasero C: Subcutaneous opioid infusion, *Am J Nurs* 102(7):61, 2002.

BOX 21-7 Selection Criteria for Clients Using Insulin Pumps

- Possesses strong motivation and commitment to use diabetes management skills
- Requires or desires improved control of blood sugar levels
- Requires greater flexibility than allowed by traditional insulin injection schedules
- Is willing to participate in a formal diabetes education program
- Possesses strong critical thinking and problem-solving skills
- Accepts responsibilities associated with the self-management of diabetes
- Is able to perform self-blood glucose monitoring and to operate the insulin pump
- Displays effective coping patterns
- Has support systems available
- Secures financial resources to cover costs associated with CSQI

Data from American Diabetes Association: Continuous subcutaneous insulin infusion, *Diabetes Care* 27(S1):S110, 2004; Lenhard MJ, Reeves GD: Continuous subcutaneous insulin infusion: a comprehensive review of insulin pump therapy, *Arch Intern Med* 161(19):2293, 2001.

freely. Insulin is absorbed most consistently in the abdomen, thus a site in the abdomen away from the belt line is the preferred site for insulin administration. Sites should be free from irritation, away from bony prominences and the waistline, and rotated at least every 72 hours or whenever complications (e.g., infection, leaking) occur (MedTronic MiniMed, 2004).

Medications given by the CSQI route require a computerized pump with safety features, including lockout intervals and warning alarms. A variety of medication pumps are currently available (Figure 21-22). If used at home, clients should be able to give themselves loading doses and boluses of the medication when needed. Ideally, medication pumps should be chosen for each individual, based on the medication being delivered and the client's needs. Other factors used in the selection process of the appropriate pump include the availability and cost of the pump and its supplies. When possible, clients using CSQI at home should be offered a selection of pumps and be allowed to choose the one that they find the easiest to use.

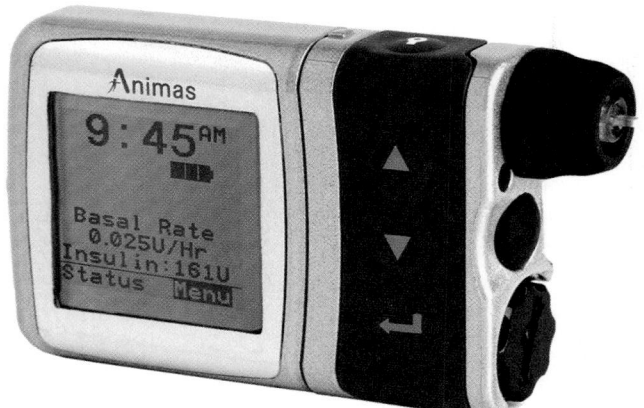

FIGURE **21-22** Insulin infusion pump.

DELEGATION CONSIDERATIONS

The skill of administering continuous subcutaneous medications should not be delegated to assistive personnel. Other aspects of the client's care may be delegated to assistive personnel, and the nurse should instruct assistive personnel about the following:

- Potential medication side effects or drug reactions and to report their occurrence to the nurse
- Complications (e.g., leaking, redness, discomfort) at the insertion site
- To report any change in client's status or vital signs

EQUIPMENT

Initiation of CSQI Therapy
- ❑ Clean, nonsterile gloves
- ❑ Alcohol swab
- ❑ Antibacterial skin prep such as chlorhexidine
- ❑ Small- (25- to 27-) gauge winged IV catheter with attached tubing or catheter designed especially for CSQI (e.g., Sof-set)
- ❑ Infusion pump
- ❑ Occlusive, transparent dressing
- ❑ Tape
- ❑ Medication in appropriate syringe or container

Discontinuing CSQI
- ❑ Clean, nonsterile gloves
- ❑ 2 × 2 gauze dressing and tape or adhesive bandage
- ❑ Alcohol swab and chlorhexidine (optional)

STEP	RATIONALE

ASSESSMENT

1. Check physician's order for client's name, drug name, type of medication, dosage, and route of administration against MAR.

2. Collect drug reference information necessary to administer drug safely, including action, purpose, side effects, safe dosage range, and nursing implications. Verify that medication can be given through this route.

3. Assess client's medical history, drug allergies, and medication history.

4. Assess for factors that may contraindicate CSQI, such as circulatory shock or reduced local tissue perfusion.

5. Assess adequacy of client's adipose tissue to determine appropriate site.

Ensures safe and accurate drug administration.

Allows nurse to give drug safely using this route and to monitor client's response to therapy.

Indicates client's need for medication, contraindications for medication use, and risk for drug interactions.

Reduced tissue perfusion interferes with drug absorption and distribution.

Physiological changes of aging or client illness may influence amount of subcutaneous tissue a client possesses. This influences choice of catheter insertion site.

STEP	RATIONALE
6. Assess client's knowledge regarding medication to be received and readiness to learn self-administration. (NOTE: When administering analgesia, assess client's level of pain using a scale of 0 to 10.)	Information poses implications for approach to client education.
7. Assess client's symptoms before initiating medication therapy (e.g., assess pain severity if analgesic is to be given, assess blood glucose levels if insulin is to be started).	Provides nurse with assessment data that will be used to evaluate desired effect of medication in the future.

NURSING DIAGNOSES

- Anxiety
- Fear
- Ineffective health maintenance
- Risk for infection

- Risk for injury
- Deficient knowledge regarding CSQI therapy
- Pain (acute, chronic)

Related factors are individualized based on client's condition or needs.

PLANNING

1. Expected outcomes following completion of procedure:	
• Needle insertion site remains free from infection.	Risk for infection at needle insertion site is a potential complication of CSQI therapy (Weissberg-Benchell and others, 2003).
• Desired effect of medication achieved with no signs of allergies or undesired effects.	Medication is delivered effectively.
• Client explains purpose, dosage, and effects of medication and verbalizes understanding of CSQI therapy.	Demonstrates learning.
2. Check name of medication on label on syringe or container against MAR.	Ensures client receives correct medication.
3. Prepare correct medication dose from vial or ampule (see Skill 21-1 or 21-2), or check dose on prefilled syringe, and prime tubing with medication.	Ensures that medication is sterile and dose is accurate.
4. Obtain and program medication administration pump.	Needed for safe medication infusion.
5. Explain procedure to client, and proceed in calm, confident manner.	Involves client in care and eases anxiety.

IMPLEMENTATION

1. Provide for privacy.	Respects client's dignity.
2. Perform hand hygiene.	Reduces transmission of microorganisms.
3. **To initiate CSQI:**	
a. Select appropriate injection site. Most common sites used are subclavicular, abdomen, upper arms, or thighs.	Site must be free from irritation and not over bony prominences.
b. Assist client to comfortable position.	Eases pain associated with insertion of needle.
c. Put on clean, nonsterile gloves.	Follows CDC recommendations to prevent accidental exposure to blood and body fluids (OSHA, 2001).

- **Critical Decision Point**
  Clients managing CSQI at home may use an antibacterial soap (e.g., Hibiclens, PhisoHex) instead of alcohol and chlorhexidine to cleanse insertion site.

STEP	RATIONALE
d. Cleanse injection site with alcohol using a circular motion, followed by skin prep agent such as chlorhexidine using straight cleansing strokes. Allow both agents to dry.	Reduces risk of infection at insertion site.
e. Hold needle in dominant hand, and remove needle guard.	Prepares needle for insertion.
f. Gently pinch or lift up skin with nondominant hand.	Ensures needle will enter subcutaneous tissue.
g. Gently and firmly insert needle at a 45- to 90-degree angle (see illustration).	Decreases pain related to insertion of needle.

- **Critical Decision Point**
  Some prepackaged needles (e.g., Sof-Set, Sub-Q-Set) are inserted at a 90-degree angle. These needles are shorter than butterfly needles. Refer to manufacturer's directions.

h. Release skinfold, and apply tape over "wings" of needle.	Secures needle.

- **Critical Decision Point**
  Some cannulas have a sharp needle with a plastic catheter covering the needle. In this case, remove the needle, and leave the plastic catheter in the skin.

i. Place occlusive, transparent dressing over insertion site (see illustration).	Protects site from infection and allows nurse to assess site during medication infusion.
j. Attach tubing from needle to tubing from infusion pump.	Allows medication to be administered.
k. Turn infusion pump on.	Initiates medication therapy.
l. Dispose of any sharps in appropriate leak-proof, puncture-resistant container. Discard used supplies and perform hand hygiene.	Prevents injury to client and health care personnel (OSHA, 2001).
m. Assess site before leaving client, and instruct client to inform nurses if site becomes red or begins to leak.	A new site with a new needle must be initiated whenever erythema or leaking occurs (Pasero, 2002).

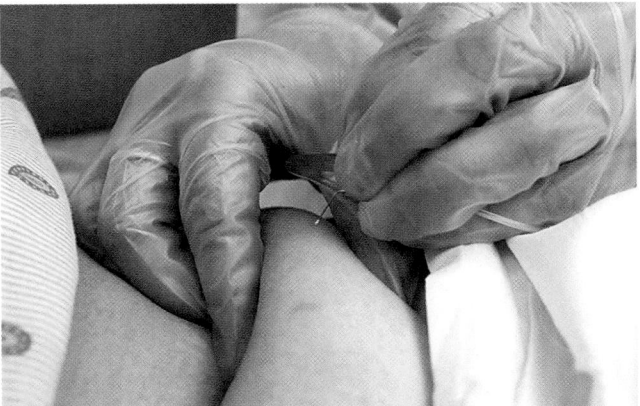

STEP 3g Insertion of butterfly needle into subcutaneous tissue of abdomen.

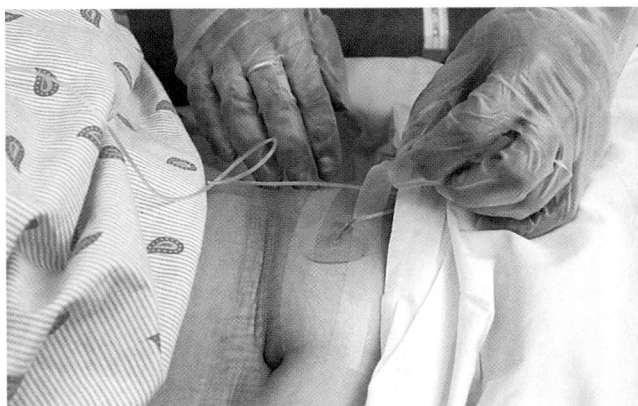

STEP 3i Securing insertion site.

STEP	RATIONALE

4. To discontinue CSQI:

a. Verify health care provider's order, and establish alternative method for medication administration if applicable.

b. Stop infusion pump.

c. Perform hand hygiene, and put on clean, nonsterile gloves.

d. Remove dressing without dislodging or removing the needle.

If medication will be required after discontinuing CSQI, a different medication and/or route may be necessary to continue to manage client's illness or pain.

Prevents spillage of medication.

Follows CDC recommendations to prevent accidental exposure to blood and body fluids (OSHA, 2001).

Exposes needle.

• *Critical Decision Point*

If site is infected or if included in institutional guidelines, cleanse site with alcohol and skin prep agent, such as chlorhexidine. Apply triple antibiotic cream to site if it is excoriated (Pasero, 2002).

e. Remove tape from the wings of needle, and pull needle out at the same angle it was inserted.

f. Apply pressure at site until no fluid leaks out of skin.

g. Apply 2 × 2 gauze dressing or adhesive bandage to site.

h. Discard used supplies, and perform hand hygiene.

Promotes comfort.

Dressing will stick to site if skin remains dry.

Prevents bacterial entry into puncture site.

Reduces transmission of microorganisms

• *Critical Decision Point*

If medication is a narcotic, follow institutional policy to document waste (Pasero, 2002).

EVALUATION

1. Evaluate client's response to medication.

Determines effect of therapy. Decreased or absent response to medication may indicate client is not receiving medication into subcutaneous tissue (e.g., pump malfunction, medication leaking at site).

2. Observe site at least every 4 hours for redness, pain, drainage, or swelling.

Indicates infection at insertion site.

Recording and Reporting

- Immediately after initiating CSQI, chart medication, dose, route, site, time, date, and type of medication pump in appropriate place in client's chart.
- Record client's response to medication and appearance of site every 4 hours or according to institutional policy.
- Report any adverse effects from medication or infection at insertion site to client's health care provider, and document according to institutional policy. Client's condition may indicate need for additional medical therapy.

Unexpected Outcomes	Related Interventions
1. Client complains of localized pain or burning at needle's insertion site, or site appears red, swollen, or is leaking.	• Symptoms indicate potential infection or needle is not securely in subcutaneous tissue. • Remove needle, and place new needle in a different site.
2. Client displays signs of allergic reaction to medication.	• Follow institutional policy or guidelines for appropriate response to allergic reactions, and notify client's health care provider immediately.
3. Continuous subcutaneous infusion becomes dislodged.	• Stop the infusion, apply pressure at the site until no fluid leaks out of skin, cover site with a 2 × 2 gauze dressing or adhesive bandage, and initiate a new site. • Assess client to determine effects of not receiving medication (e.g., assess pain level if client is receiving pain medication via CSQI). • Document dislodgement of CSQI, assessment findings, and nursing interventions in client's permanent record. Dislodgement of CSQI may necessitate notifying the client's primary care provider and/or documenting the event on an occurrence report per institutional policy.
4. Desired effect of medication not achieved.	• Follow established protocols for titration of medication, or notify client's health care provider for either change in dosage or medication.

Teaching Considerations

- Instruct client to wear medical identification bracelet indicating important medical information, including disease client has (e.g., diabetes) and allergies.
- Clients receiving insulin require intensive diabetes management instruction (Box 21-8).

Pediatric Considerations

- Insulin pump therapy has been successfully used in toddlers and preschoolers. Litton and others (2002) found that toddlers who were placed on an insulin pump achieved better glycemic control with fewer episodes of hypoglycemia. Parents of these young children experience higher levels of confidence and independence in diabetes management with appropriate education and guidance.
- Despite the barriers to CSQI in adolescents with diabetes (e.g., frequent blood glucose testing, wearing tight clothing, transferring responsibility of diabetes management from parent to child), insulin pumps offer more flexibility, and insulin dosage can be quickly changed based on the client's current situation (Plotnick and others, 2003). To achieve successful diabetes management, intensive education is required both for the client and the family, especially during the first few weeks after starting CSQI. The nurse must ensure clients and their families have all the information and skills necessary to use CSQI. The nurse also plays an important role in

---

BOX 21-8   **Educational Topics Essential for Clients Receiving Insulin With Continuous Subcutaneous Infusion**

- Blood sugar monitoring
- Meal planning and food choices
- Incorporating exercise into daily routine
- How to program and use the insulin pump
- Sick-day guidelines and management
- Treatment of hypoglycemia, including use of glucagon
- Treatment of hyperglycemia and prevention of diabetic ketoacidosis
- Prevention of infection, especially at site of infusion
- Problem-solving and decision-making skills
- Special considerations and precautions (e.g., what to do with pump when showering and sleeping)

Modified from American Association of Diabetes Educators: AADE position statement: education for continuous subcutaneous insulin infusion pump users, *Diabetes Educ* 29(1):97, 2003.

follow-up care, education, and the enhancement of problem-solving skills.

Gerontological Considerations

- CSQI is frequently used for the administration of pain medications in the terminally ill older adult client. CSQI can also be used to deliver isotonic IV solutions to dehydrated older adults. This is called hypodermoclysis therapy. This method of providing hydration avoids the need to transfer the client from home or long-term care facility to an acute care hospital. It appears to be well accepted by clients and offers a cost savings when compared with IV therapy (Slesak and others, 2003). It is less invasive, less expensive, and is well-tolerated (Dasgupta and others 2000). Fluids should infuse slowly (e.g., 30 ml/hr) during the first hour of hypodermoclysis. If the client remains comfortable, the rate of infusion may be increased. Usually infusion rates do not exceed 80 ml/hr. In general, hypodermoclysis should only be used to treat short-term reversible fluid deficits. It should also only be used if the client requires less than 3000 ml in a 24-hour period

(Mion and O'Connell, 2003). If long-term management is required, an IV access should be initiated.

Home Care Considerations

- When clients are going home using CSQI, the nurse should assess the client's readiness to learn before teaching how to administer medications using this route. A responsible caregiver should be included in the instructions. Clients and caregivers should understand the desired effect of the medication, side effects and adverse effects of the medication, operation of the pump, how to evaluate the effectiveness of the medication, when and how to assess and rotate injection sites, and when to call a health care provider for problems. They also need to determine where and how to obtain the required supplies (Olohan and Zappitelli, 2003).

FOCUS *on* CLINICAL PRACTICE

You are assigned to care for Mrs. Stevens, a 60-year-old retired teacher. Mrs. Stevens has been diagnosed with non-Hodgkin's lymphoma and has received her first round of chemotherapy. As a result of her chemotherapy, her white blood cell count is dropping, putting her at risk for developing an infection. The physician has ordered Neupogen (filgrastim) to be given Sub-Q every day for the next 2 weeks to help bring her white blood cell count back to normal levels. You have just received the order and are getting ready to start this medication.

1. What information would you need to know about the medication before you prepare it?
2. What information would you need to know about Mrs. Stevens before you administer the Neupogen?
3. The Neupogen arrives at your nursing unit in an ampule. What should you use to open the ampule?
   A. An opened alcohol swab around the neck of the ampule
   B. Clean gloves
   C. A gauze pad wrapped around the neck of the ampule
   Explain your choice:

4. You assess Mrs. Stevens and find that she weighs 60 kg (132 pounds). You complete the drug calculation and determine that she needs 1 ml of Neupogen. What size syringe and needle will you use to administer her injection?
   A. 3-ml syringe, 22-gauge 1-inch needle
   B. 50-unit insulin syringe, 28-gauge $\frac{1}{2}$-inch needle
   C. 1-ml syringe, 25-gauge 1$\frac{1}{2}$-inch needle
   D. 1-ml syringe, 25-gauge $\frac{5}{8}$-inch needle
   Explain your choice:
5. Four hours after her Neupogen injection, Mrs. Stevens begins to complain of bone pain, an adverse reaction to Neupogen. Her physician has ordered her to receive morphine sulfate 1 mg IV push. What do you need to know before you give the morphine? Select all that apply.
   A. If morphine needs to be diluted before you administer the medication
   B. How fast morphine can be given IV push
   C. Mrs. Stevens's allergies
   D. The compatibility of morphine and her maintenance IV
   Explain your answer:

NCLEX REVIEW QUESTIONS

1. When preparing a medication that needs to be reconstituted before administering, the nurse:
   1. Shakes the vial after the fluid is injected into the vial to mix it well
   2. Does not need to wipe the tops of vials with alcohol because the tops of the vials are sterile
   3. Injects the powder into the vial of diluent
   4. Evaluates the medication's concentration after the diluent and powder are mixed

2. When mixing two medications in one syringe when one medication is in a vial and the other is in an ampule, the nurse:
   1. Prepares the medication in the vial first
   2. Prepares the medication in the ampule first
   3. Draws all the medication out of both the ampule and the vial
   4. Inserts air into the ampule first

3. Which of the following assessment findings indicates a positive TB reaction in a client with no known risk factors for TB?
   1. A large area of redness and swelling at the injection site
   2. An induration of 18 mm
   3. Frequent, productive cough accompanied by a fever
   4. Sudden onset of shortness of breath and wheezing

4. You are caring for a client who is receiving heparin Sub-Q twice a day to prevent the development of deep vein thrombosis. The client is experiencing bruising around the injection sites. Which nursing intervention might be helpful in decreasing the bruising associated with the heparin injections?
   1. Distract the client when administering the injection.
   2. Massage the injection site after the injection.
   3. Administer the injection over 30 seconds.
   4. Help the client get into a comfortable position.

5. Which of the following symptoms may indicate that a client has sustained an injury to a nerve following an IM injection?
   1. Pain, numbness, and tingling at the injection site 2 hours after the injection
   2. Pain experienced during the injection
   3. Urticaria, eczema, wheezing, and dyspnea
   4. Nausea, vomiting, and diarrhea

6. Which of the following needle sizes would be the best for the nurse to use when administering an IM injection to an average-size, 30-year-old woman in the ventrogluteal site?
   1. 28-gauge, $\frac{5}{8}$ inch
   2. 22-gauge, $1\frac{1}{2}$ inch
   3. 25-gauge, 1 inch
   4. 16-gauge, $1\frac{1}{2}$ inch

7. While giving an intravenous infusion of a medication that has been added to an intravenous bag of fluids, the client's IV site becomes cool, pale, and swollen. Upon assessing these symptoms, the nurse knows the client is experiencing:
   1. Infiltration
   2. Phlebitis
   3. An allergic reaction to the medication
   4. Fluid volume excess

8. The nurse must administer 40 ml of ceftazidime, a third-generation cephalosporin, over 30 minutes. The nurse chooses to use a miniinfusion pump to deliver the medication because:
   1. Assistive personnel can assist in giving IV medications with miniinfusion pumps
   2. It eliminates the need to use needles during medication administration
   3. The nurse does not have the time to administer this medication via IV push
   4. The pump allows small amounts of fluid to be infused within a specified amount of time

9. Which of the following will not reduce the risks associated with IV push medication?
   1. Using medications that are in less concentrated solutions
   2. Having information about IV push times readily available
   3. Using the term *IV push* with medications that are to be given over more than 1 minute
   4. Establishing clear institutional guidelines about IV push times

10. Before administering an IV push medication, the nurse should:
    1. Assess the condition of the IV insertion site
    2. Always stop the maintenance IV fluids
    3. Tell the client that it will probably take a long time for the medication to work
    4. Ensure that the correct size filter needle is applied to the syringe

11. When initiating CSQI the nurse should:
    1. Insert the needle at a 15-degree angle
    2. Place a gauze dressing over the needle insertion site
    3. Put on sterile gloves
    4. Pinch the skin with the nondominant hand before inserting the needle

References

American Academy of Pediatrics: *2000 red book: report of the Committee on Infectious Diseases,* ed 25, Elk Grove Village, 2000, The Academy.

American Association of Diabetes Educators: AADE position statement: education for continuous subcutaneous insulin infusion pump users, *Diabetes Educ* 29(1):97, 2003.

American Diabetes Association: Insulin administration: position statement, *Diabetes Care* 27(suppl 1):S106, 2004a.

American Diabetes Association: Continuous subcutaneous insulin infusion, *Diabetes Care,* 27(suppl 1):S110, 2004b.

American Nurses Association: *American Nurses Association needlestick prevention guide: safe needles save lives,* 2002, www.nursingworld.org/needlestick/needleguide.pdf, retrieved March 9, 2004.

AstraZeneca: How to apply EMLA Cream, 2000, http://www.emla-us.com/apply/indexcream.htm, retrieved April 10, 2004.

Aventis: *Lovenox: enoxaparin sodium injection,* 2003, http://www.lovenox.com/, retrieved July 6, 2004.

Caffrey RM: Are all syringes created equal? *Am J Nurs* 103(6):46, 2003.

Centers for Disease Control and Prevention: *Mantoux tuberculin skin test facilitator guide,* 2004, www.cdc.gov/nchstp/tb/pubs/Mantoux/images/Mantoux.pdf, retrieved March 21, 2004.

Environmental Protection Agency: *New information about disposing of medical sharps,* 2004, http://www.epa.gov/epaoswer/other/medical/sharps.htm, retrieved April 7, 2004.

Fabian B: Intravenous complication: infiltration, *J Intraven Nurs* 23(4):229, 2000.

Gilsenan I: A practical guide to giving injections, *Nurs Times* 96(33):43, 2000.

Hockenberry MJ and others: *Wong's nursing care of infants and children,* ed 7, St. Louis, 2003, Mosby.

Institute for Safe Medication Practices: *How fast is too fast for IV push medications?* 2003, http://www.ismp.org/msaarticles/ismp%20safety%20alert%20-%20push%20drugs.doc, retrieved April 11, 2004.

Joint Commission on the Accreditation of Health Care Organizations: *2005 National Patient Safety Goals,* 2004, http:www.jcaho.org/accreditation&organization/patient&safety/05&hpsy/05-npsg-cah.htm, retrieved July, 2004.

Karch AM, Karch FE: Not so fast! *Am J Nurs* 103(8):71, 2003.

Luna L: Arab Muslims and culture care. In Leininger M, McFarland M: *Transcultural nursing,* New York, 2002, McGraw-Hill.

Mashaba G: South African culturally based health-illness patterns and humanistic care practices. In Leininger M, McFarland M: *Transcultural nursing,* New York, 2002, McGraw-Hill.

McConnell EA: Administering subcutaneous heparin, *Nursing* 36(6):17, 2000.

McKenry LM, Salerno, E: *Pharmacology in nursing,* revised ed 21, St. Louis, 2003, Mosby.

MedTronic MiniMed: *Pump infusion set overview,* 2004, http://www.minimed.com/patientfam/pf_ipt_pumpinfusion_overview.shtml, retrieved April 12, 2004.

Miller JA: Caring for Cambodian refuges in the emergency department, *J Emerg Nurs* 21(6):498, 1995.

Mion L, O'Connell A: Parenteral hydration and nutrition in the geriatric patient: clinical and ethical issues, *J Infus Nurs* 26(3):144, 2003.

Occupational Safety and Health Administration: Occupational exposure to blood borne pathogens, needlestick, and other sharps injuries: final rule, *Federal Register,* CFR 29, part 1910 (*Federal Register* 66:5317, Jan 18, 2001), available at www.osha.gov/pls/oshaweb/owadisp.show_document?p_table=STANDARDS&p_id=10051.

Olohan K, Zappitelli D: The insulin pump: making life with diabetes easier, *Am J Nurs* 103(4):48, 2003.

Orque MS: Nursing care of the South Vietnamese patients. In Orque MS, Bloch R, Monrroy LSA, editors: *Ethnic nursing care,* St. Louis, 1983, Mosby.

Pasero C: Subcutaneous opioid infusion, *Am J Nurs* 102(7):61, 2002.

Perry J and others: Nurses and needlesticks, then and now, *Nursing* 33(4):22, 2003.

Pope BA: How to administer subcutaneous and intramuscular injections, *Nursing* 32(1):50, 2002.

Ross HM: Islamic tradition at the end of life, *Medsurg Nurs* 10(2):83, 2001.

Skokal W: IV push at home? *RN* 63(10):26, 2000.

Stephens M: Subcutaneous injections, *Nurs Times* 99(36):29, 2003.

Strowig S: Insulin therapy, *RN* 64(9):38, 2001.

World Health Organization: *Injection safety,* 2004, www.who.int/injection_safety/en/, retrieved June 19, 2004.

Zurlinden J: Double check IV push, *Nurs Spectr* 15(25IL):16, 2002.

Research References

Chan H: Effects of injection duration on site-pain intensity and bruising associated with subcutaneous heparin, *J Adv Nurs* 35(6):882, 2001.

Chung JWY and others: An experimental study on the use of manual pressure to reduce pain in intramuscular injections, *J Clinical Nurs* 11(4):457, 2002.

Dasgupta M and others: Subcutaneous fluid infusion in a long-term care setting, *J Am Geriatr Soc* 48(7):795, 2000.

Dawkins L and others: A randomized trial of winged Vialon cannulae and metal butterfly needles, *Int J Palliat Nurs* 6(3):110, 2000.

Dietrich CC, Tobias JD: Subcutaneous fentanyl infusions in the pediatric population, *Am J Pain Manage* 13(4):146, 2003.

Elliott JP and others: Pregnancy prolongation in triplet pregnancies: oral vs. continuous subcutaneous terbutaline, *J Reprod Med* 46(11):975, 2001.

Engstrom JL and others: Procedures used to prepare and administer intramuscular injections: a study of infertility nurses, *J Obstet Gynecol Neonatal Nurs* 29(2):159, 2000.

Johnson SK: Hmong health beliefs and experiences in the Western health care system, *J Transcult Nurs* 13(2):126, 2002.

Katsma DL, Katsma R: The myth of the 90°-angle intramuscular injection, *Nurse Educ* 25(1):34, 2000.

Kuzu N, Ucar H: The effect of cold on the occurrence of bruising, haematoma and pain at the injection site in subcutaneous low molecular weight heparin, *Int J Nurs Stud* 38(1):51, 2001.

Lenhard MJ, Reeves GD: Continuous subcutaneous insulin infusion: a comprehensive review of insulin pump therapy, *Arch Intern Med* 161(19):2293, 2001.

Litton J and others: Insulin pump therapy in toddlers and preschool children with type 1 diabetes mellitus, *J Pediatr* 141(4):490, 2002.

Nicoll LH, Hesby A: Intramuscular injection: an integrative research review and guideline for evidence-based practice, *Appl Nurs Research* 16(2):149, 2002.

Plotnick L and others: Safety and effectiveness of insulin pump therapy in children and adolescents with type 1 diabetes, *Diabetes Care* 26(4):1142, 2003.

Rodger MA, King L: Drawing up and administering intramuscular injections: a review of the literature, *J Adv Nurs* 31(3):574, 2000.

Slesak G and others: Comparison of subcutaneous and intravenous rehydration in geriatric patients: a randomized trial, *J Am Geriatr Soc* 51(2):155, 2003.

Sparks L: Taking the "ouch" out of injections for children, *MCN Am J Matern Child Nurs* 26(2):72, 2001.

Torre MC: Subcutaneous infusion: non-metal cannulae vs. metal butterfly needles, *Br J Community Nurs* 7(7):365, 2002.

Weissberg-Benchell J and others: Insulin pump therapy: a meta analysis, *Diabetes Care* 26(4): 1079, 2003.

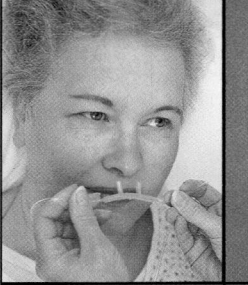

22

Oxygen Therapy

MEDIA RESOURCES

Evolve Site *evolve*

http://evolve.elsevier.com/Perry/skills
- Weblinks
- Video clips
- Mosby's Nursing Skills Video Exercises

Mosby's Nursing Skills Videos/CD-ROM
- *Oxygenation Video:* Oxygen safety; flow rates by nasal cannula and face mask; application of cannula and mask
- *Preoperative Nursing Care Video:* Incentive spirometry

OBJECTIVES

Mastery of content in this chaper will enable the nurse to:

- Discuss indications for oxygen therapy.
- Discuss methods for administering oxygen therapy.
- Demonstrate applying a nasal cannula and an oxygen mask.
- Demonstrate administering oxygen therapy to a client with an artificial airway.
- Demonstrate proper use of incentive spirometry.
- Demonstrate use of noninvasive ventilation using continuous positive airway pressure (CPAP) or bilevel positive airway pressure (BiPAP).
- Demonstrate administering mechanical ventilation.

KEY TERMS

Cyanosis	Oxygen mask
Hypercapnia	Oxygen therapy
Hypoxemia	Positive-pressure ventilation
Hypoxia	T tube
Incentive spirometry	Tidal volume
Nasal cannula	Tracheostomy collar
Noninvasive ventilation	

Oxygen therapy is the administration of supplemental oxygen (O_2) to a client to prevent or treat hypoxia. Hypoxia is a condition in which there is insufficient oxygen to meet the metabolic demands of the tissues and cells. Hypoxia results from hypoxemia, a deficiency of arterial blood oxygen. Hemoglobin is the carrier of respiratory gases, O_2 and carbon dioxide (CO_2). It combines with the gas to carry it to and from the cells. The presence of decreased hemoglobin levels reduces the amount of oxygen transported to the cells and CO_2 transported away from the cells. Hemoglobin levels and acid-base status have direct effects on oxygenation. A state of acidemia increases the ability of hemoglobin to release oxygen to the tissues. Alkalemia prevents the hemoglobin from easily releasing oxygen to the tissues.

Various disease states require the use of oxygen therapy to correct impaired gas exchange and the resultant hypoxemia. An example of such a disease state is pneumonia. Pneumonia results in impaired gas exchange because of fluid and secretions in the lung, causing a decrease in oxygen diffusion from the lungs to the arterial blood supply.

A client with chronic bronchitis, a form of chronic obstructive pulmonary disease (COPD), may have normal arterial oxygen levels during the day but may experience oxygen desaturation, a reduction in the arterial oxygen level, during sleep. These clients may require oxygen at night to prevent hypoxemia. A client with emphysema, another type of COPD, may experience low oxygen levels all the time or

in association with increased activity, a condition called exercise-induced hypoxia.

Clients with COPD may retain carbon dioxide and are at risk for developing CO_2 narcosis induced by administration of high levels of oxygen. Normally the chemoreceptors monitor CO_2 levels. In the individual with healthy lungs the chemoreceptors are sensitive to small changes in CO_2 levels and effectively regulate ventilation. When the CO_2 level rises to a certain level, the person inhales air. In certain clients with COPD who retain CO_2, the chemoreceptors are not sensitive to small changes in CO_2 and regulate ventilation poorly. Therefore in these clients, changes in the oxygen level stimulate changes in ventilation. If high levels of oxygen are administered, their stimulus to breathe is extinguished. Administration of oxygen therapy is not without possible complications.

Clients with cardiovascular disease, such as left ventricular failure, may not be able to supply oxygen to the tissues due to decreased cardiac output. Supplemental oxygen helps decrease the work of the left ventricle and increase oxygen delivery to the tissues.

Before administering oxygen assess the client for a temporary or permanent abnormal chest wall configuration. Temporary abnormalities that can affect ventilation and the delivery of oxygen include obesity, pregnancy, and chest trauma. Congenital musculoskeletal abnormalities such as kyphosis affect oxygenation because of decreased lung expansion.

The nursing assessment of a client requiring supplemental oxygen therapy may reveal many findings associated with hypoxia (Box 22-1). Presenting symptoms depend on the client's age, level of health, present disease process, and the presence of chronic illnesses. Anxiety, confusion, and restlessness are early signs of hypoxia. Additional assessment findings may reveal changes in baseline vital signs; the

---

BOX 22-1   Assessment of Signs and Symptoms Associated With Hypoxia

- Apprehension, anxiety, behavioral changes
- Decreased level of consciousness (LOC), confusion, drowsiness, altered concentration
- Increased pulse rate
- Increased rate and depth of respiration or irregular respiratory patterns
- Decreased lung sounds, adventitious lung sounds (e.g., crackles, wheezes)
- Elevated blood pressure evolving to decreased blood pressure
- Dyspnea
- Use of accessory muscles of respiration, rib retractions
- Cardiac dysrhythmias
- Pallor, cyanosis
- Increased fatigue
- Dizziness
- Clubbing of nails due to prolonged, chronic hypoxia

pulse may become rapid and irregular because of cardiac dysrhythmias (Jevon and Ewens, 2001).

Initially blood pressure is elevated. If hypoxia remains uncorrected, hypotension may develop. Respiratory rate and depth are increased. As hypoxia worsens, the client's activity tolerance decreases, and the client may become confused, with loss of short-term memory. Worsening of a hypoxic state may lead to a decreased level of consciousness and coma.

Cyanosis, a bluish discoloration of the skin and mucous membranes, is a late sign of hypoxia. Cyanosis is caused by vasoconstriction of the peripheral blood vessels or decreased oxyhemoglobin. It can be seen in clients who are very cold or have decreased peripheral circulation because of vascular disease and in those with a decreased level of circulating oxyhemoglobin. The nurse never assumes a lack of cyanosis means adequate oxygenation. Cyanosis caused by hypoxia is assessed in the oral mucosa, the conjunctiva of the eye, and around the lips, known as circumoral cyanosis.

Oxygen Systems

Oxygen therapy is inexpensive, widely available, and used in a variety of settings (Thomson and others, 2002). Clients with decreased tissue oxygenation can benefit from controlled oxygen administration. Oxygen is not a substitute for other treatment, however, and should be used only when indicated. Oxygen should be treated as a drug. It has dangerous side effects, such as atelectasis or oxygen toxicity or CO_2 retention in certain COPD clients (Thomson and others, 2002). As with any drug, the dosage or concentration of oxygen should be continuously monitored. The nurse should routinely check the physician's orders to verify that the client is receiving the prescribed oxygen concentration. The six rights of medication administration also pertain to oxygen administration (see Chapter 19).

The oxygen delivery system selected depends on the level of oxygen support the client needs, based on the severity of the hypoxia and the disease process. Other factors considered include the client's age, level of health and orientation level, the presence of an artificial airway, whether the setting is in the hospital or the home, the type of home environment, and the type of support and care given after discharge. Common oxygen delivery systems include nasal cannula; face mask, or noninvasive ventilation; and mechanical ventilation.

Oxygen is available in a number of systems. Oxygen provided in a hospital or institutional setting is a bulk liquid oxygen system designed to store the oxygen at a precise and safe temperature and deliver it as a gas through wall outlets in a client's room. An oxygen flowmeter is required to regulate the flow rate in liters per minute (Figure 22-1).

Compressed oxygen is available in gas cylinders and exists as a nonliquid gas stored at a precise temperature under high pressure and measured as pounds per square inch (psi). Oxygen cylinders used in hospital and institutional care settings include the large H cylinders and the smaller E cylinders, which have greater portability (Figure 22-2).

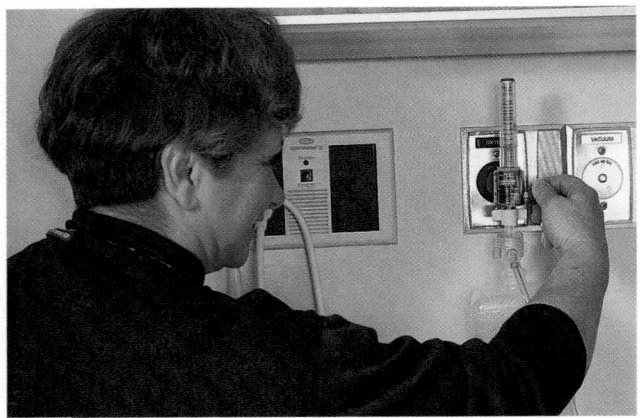

FIGURE 22-1 Flowmeter attached to oxygen source.

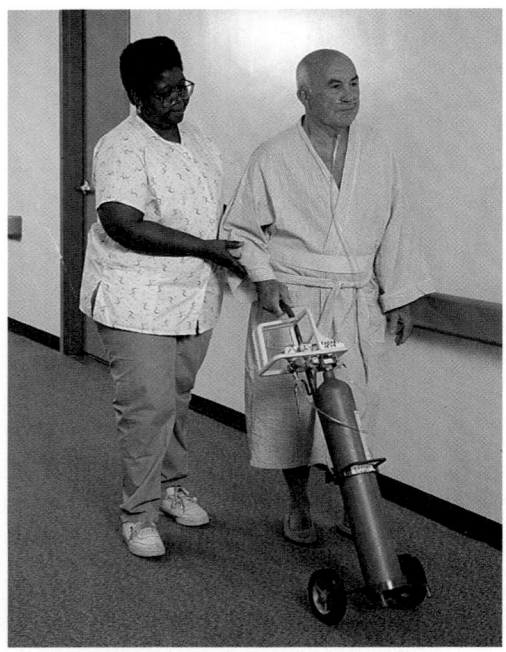

FIGURE 22-2 Smaller E tank for portability.

Evidence-Based Practice Trends

Oxygen remains one of the most effective therapeutic agents available (Thompson and others, 2002). While this therapy benefits hypoxemic clients with nonpulmonary problems and those with acute exacerbations of COPD, it also relieves pulmonary vasoconstriction and right heart workload and decreases myocardial ischemia. As a result, there is improved cardiac output. In addition, there is evidence that improved oxygen delivery to the lung enhances pulmonary defenses and assists mucociliary transport and mucous clearing (Bach and others, 2001).

A major concern in the administration of oxygen therapy to clients with acute exacerbations of COPD is resultant elevations in CO_2 levels (hypercarbia) and increased risk of respiratory failure. Administration of oxygen, even at low levels of 24% to 28%, may result in hypercarbia and should be used with caution (Snow and others, 2001). For long-term use, the best data available are from the 1980s Nocturnal Oxygen Therapy Trial, which noted that following acute exacerbations of COPD clients no longer required any oxygen therapy 3 weeks after discharge from a hospital or extended care facility (Bach and others, 2001).

Cultural Considerations

Orient clients and family members to the oxygen set-up and precautions to be observed. Clients and visitors with limited English proficiency may not be able to understand signs posted in the room. Safely accommodate valued practices of cultural groups when oxygen is used. For example, Hindus and Buddhists may burn incense to promote healing of ill members (Fadiman, 1997; Johnson, 2002). When oxygen is used in the home, designate areas where incense can be safely burned, and encourage family members to bring the ashes to the bedside. Jewish clients light candles during Sabbath and accept use of battery-operated candles while in the hospital (Robinson, 2000). Collaborate with family members and religious leaders on how to accommodate these practices during illness and recovery.

Skill Performance Guidelines

1. Know the client's normal range of vital signs and pulse oximetry. Hypoxia affects the client's vital signs and pulse oximetry values.
2. Know the client's usual behavioral pattern. The nurse, friends, and family may notice behavioral changes such as restlessness, agitation, anxiety, apprehension, and inability to concentrate.
3. Know the client's medical history. It is important to be aware of the client with COPD who retains carbon dioxide. High-inspired oxygen concentrations may result in severe side effects such as respiratory depression and oxygen toxicity.
4. Be aware of environmental conditions. Clients with chronic respiratory diseases have difficulty maintaining optimal oxygen levels in polluted environments. If a client is to receive home oxygen therapy, an environmental assessment is completed to determine respiratory hazards in the home such as the use of gas stoves or kerosene space heaters or the presence of smokers in the home.
5. Document the client's smoking history. Smoking damages the lungs' mucociliary clearance mechanism and paralyzes the ciliary action, resulting in a decreased ability to clear mucus from the airways. Mucus pools in the airways create an environment for the development of infections. Accumulation of mucus may lead to the development of chronic bronchitis. Long-term chronic bronchitis ultimately results in hypoxia.

6. Know the client's most recent hemoglobin values.
7. Know the client's past and current arterial blood gas (ABG) values.
8. Know the client's cardiac output. Estimate the cardiac output by the blood pressure. If the client is hypotensive, the cardiac output is low or inadequate, and oxygen delivery to the tissues will be reduced.
9. Oxygen is regarded as a medication. Increasing the oxygen liter flow rate for shortness of breath is similar to doubling heart, asthma, or other medications (Thompson and others, 2002).
10. It is important to provide education to the client and family about home oxygen therapy so that the client and family understand proper use of the equipment. Safety measures for oxygen use are very important (Box 22-2). These measures are taught to the client and caregivers to ensure proper use. In the hospital setting, an appropriate sign is used to alert caregivers and visitors that oxygen is in use (Figure 22-3).

BOX 22-2   Oxygen Safety Guidelines

- Oxygen is a medication and should not be adjusted without a physician's order.
- An "Oxygen in Use" sign must be placed on the client's door and in the client's room. If oxygen is used at home, a sign is placed on the door of the house.
- Oxygen delivery systems must be kept 10 feet from any open flames.
- Oxygen supports combustion; however, it will not explode.
- No smoking should be allowed on the premises.
- When oxygen cylinders are used, they must be secured so that they will not fall over. Oxygen cylinders are stored upright, chained, or in appropriate holders.
- Determine that all electrical equipment in the room is functioning correctly and is properly grounded (see Chapter 4). An electrical spark in the presence of oxygen can result in a serious fire.
- Check the oxygen level of portable tanks before transporting a client to ensure that there is enough oxygen in the tank.

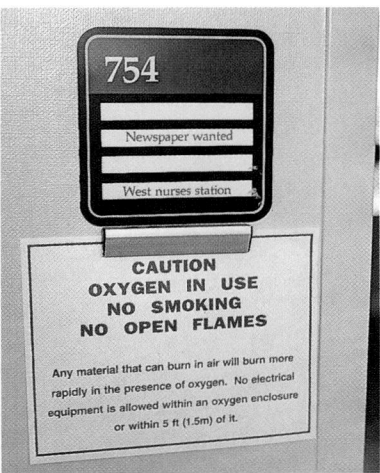

FIGURE **22-3** Proper display for "Oxygen in Use" sign.

SKILL 22-1 Applying a Nasal Cannula or Oxygen Mask

Nasal Cannula

A nasal cannula is a simple, comfortable device for delivering oxygen to a client (Figure 22-4). The two tips of the cannula, about 1.5 cm ($^1/_2$ inch) long, protrude from the center of a disposable tube and are inserted into the nostrils. Oxygen is delivered via the cannula at a flow rate from 1 to 6 L/min. Higher flow rates dry airway mucosa and do not increase the inspired oxygen concentration (FIO_2). Humidification is not used for rates less than 4 L/min. At flow rates greater than 4 L/min, humidification helps prevent drying of nasal and oral mucous membranes. Approximate FIO_2 can be estimated by the flow rate (Table 22-1). The delivered oxygen percentage will vary, depending on the rate and depth of the client's breathing.

A nasal cannula is an effective mechanism for oxygen delivery. It allows the client to breathe through the mouth or nose, is available for all age-groups, and is adequate for short-term or long-term use. Cannulas are inexpensive, disposable, generally comfortable, and easily accepted by most clients.

Oxygen Mask

An oxygen mask is shaped to fit snugly over the client's mouth and nose and is secured in place with a strap. The two primary types of masks are those delivering a low FIO_2 and those delivering a high FIO_2.

The simple face mask (Figure 22-5) is used for short-term oxygen therapy. It fits loosely and delivers oxygen concentrations from 40% to 60%. The mask is contraindicated for clients with carbon dioxide retention because retention can be worsened. The percentage of oxygen that can be delivered with a simple face mask depends on the liter flow and depth of respirations (see Table 22-1).

A plastic face mask with a reservoir bag (Figure 22-6) and a Venturi mask are capable of delivering higher concentrations of oxygen. When used as a nonrebreather, the plastic face mask with a reservoir bag can deliver from 60% to 100% oxygen at appropriate flow rates (see Table 22-1). This oxygen mask maintains a high-concentration oxygen supply in the reservoir bag. The nurse should frequently inspect the bag to make sure it is inflated. If it is deflated, the client may be breathing large amounts of exhaled carbon dioxide.

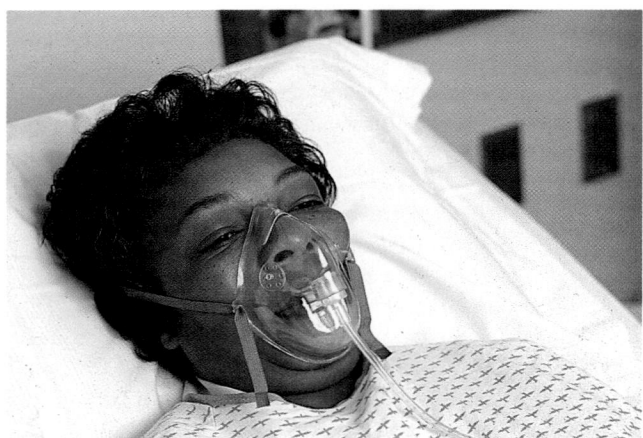

FIGURE **22-5** Simple face mask can deliver concentrations of 40% to 60% using flow rates of 5 to 10 L/min.

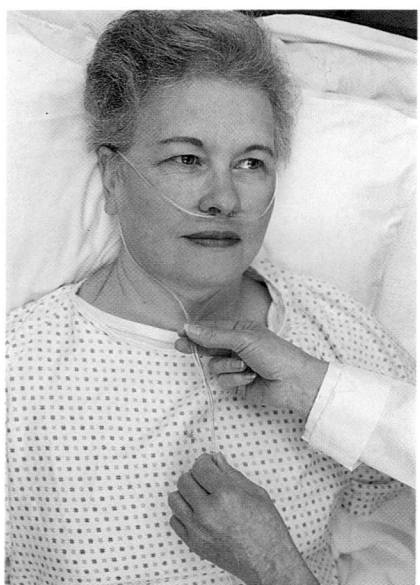

FIGURE **22-4** Nasal cannula is useful for low oxygen concentration (2 L/min) for clients with chronic lung disease.

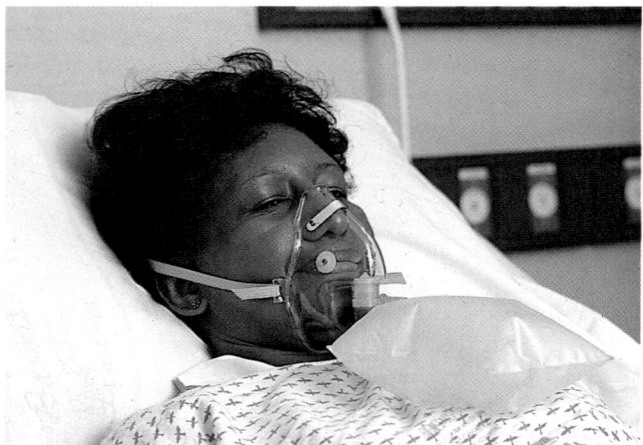

FIGURE **22-6** Partial rebreathing mask can deliver concentrations of 60% to 95% using flow rates of 6 to 10 L/min.

TABLE 22-1   OXYGEN DELIVERY SYSTEMS

DELIVERY SYSTEM	FIO$_2$* DELIVERED	ADVANTAGES	DISADVANTAGES
Nasal cannula	1 L/min: 24% 2 L/min: 28% 3 L/min: 32% 4 L/min: 36% 5 L/min: 40% 6 L/min: 44%	Safe and simple. Easily tolerated. Delivers low concentrations while allowing the client to eat, speak, and drink. Does not impede eating or talking. Inexpensive, disposable.	Unable to use with nasal obstruction. Drying to mucous membranes. Can dislodge easily. May cause skin irritation or breakdown. Client's breathing pattern will affect exact FIO$_2$.
Oximizer	1-15 L/min: 24%-60%	Higher concentrations without mask. Releases O$_2$ only on inhalation. Conserves O$_2$, increased portability. Does not require humidification.	Nasal reservoir may interfere with drinking from cup. May be cosmetically unappealing. Potential reservoir membrane failure. Client's breathing pattern will affect exact FIO$_2$.
Simple face mask	5-6 L/min: 40% 6-7 L/min: 50% 7-8 L/min: 60% > 8 L/min: 60%	Can assist in providing humidified oxygen.	Exact FIO$_2$ level is difficult to estimate. Requires high FIO$_2$ levels to prevent rebreathing of carbon dioxide. Client entrains room air through the side holes in the mask.
Venturi mask	4 L/min: 24%-28% 8 L/min: 35%-40% 12 L/min: 50%-60%	Controls the amount of specified oxygen concentration. Delivers percentage of FIO$_2$ from 24% to 60%. Does not dry mucous membranes. Delivers humidity with oxygen concentration.	Hot and confining, increased levels of humidification may irritate skin. A specific flow rate is necessary to deliver a specific FIO$_2$, and the FIO$_2$ can be decreased if the mask does not fit properly. Interferes with eating and talking.
Partial nonrebreather—bag should always remain partially inflated. Therefore flow rate must be high enough to prevent collapse of the bag.	6 L/min: 60% 7 L/min: 70% 8 L/min: 80% 9 L/min: 90% 10 L/min: 95%	Delivers increased FIO$_2$. It is useful for clients requiring a high concentration of oxygen (e.g., asthma, multiple trauma). Easily humidifies O$_2$. Does not dry mucous membranes.	No inspiratory valve, so exhaled air mixes with inspired air. Hot and confining, may irritate skin, tight seal necessary. Interferes with eating and talking. Bag may twist or kink.
Nonrebreather	6-15 L/min: 60%-100%	Valve closes during expiration, so exhaled air does enter reservoir and mix with inhaled air. Delivers highest possible FIO$_2$ without intubation. Does not dry mucous membranes.	Requires tight seal, difficult to maintain and uncomfortable. May irritate skin. Bag should not totally deflate.
Face tent	8-12 L/min: 28%-100%	Alternative to aerosol mask. Provides high humidity with oxygen.	Difficult to keep in place, and the FIO$_2$ cannot be controlled.
Oxygen hood—usually pediatric use	5-8 L/min: 28%-40% 8-12 L/min: 49%-85%	Provides warmed humidified oxygen at a specific temperature.	Flow rate of less than 5 L/min may lead to carbon dioxide narcosis.
Oxygen tent—usually pediatric use	10-15 L/min: up to 50%	Provides humidified oxygen and can provide a cool environment to control body temperature.	Can be isolating for the child because every time the tent is opened the oxygen and humidity levels change.

*FIO$_2$, Fraction of inspired oxygen concentration.

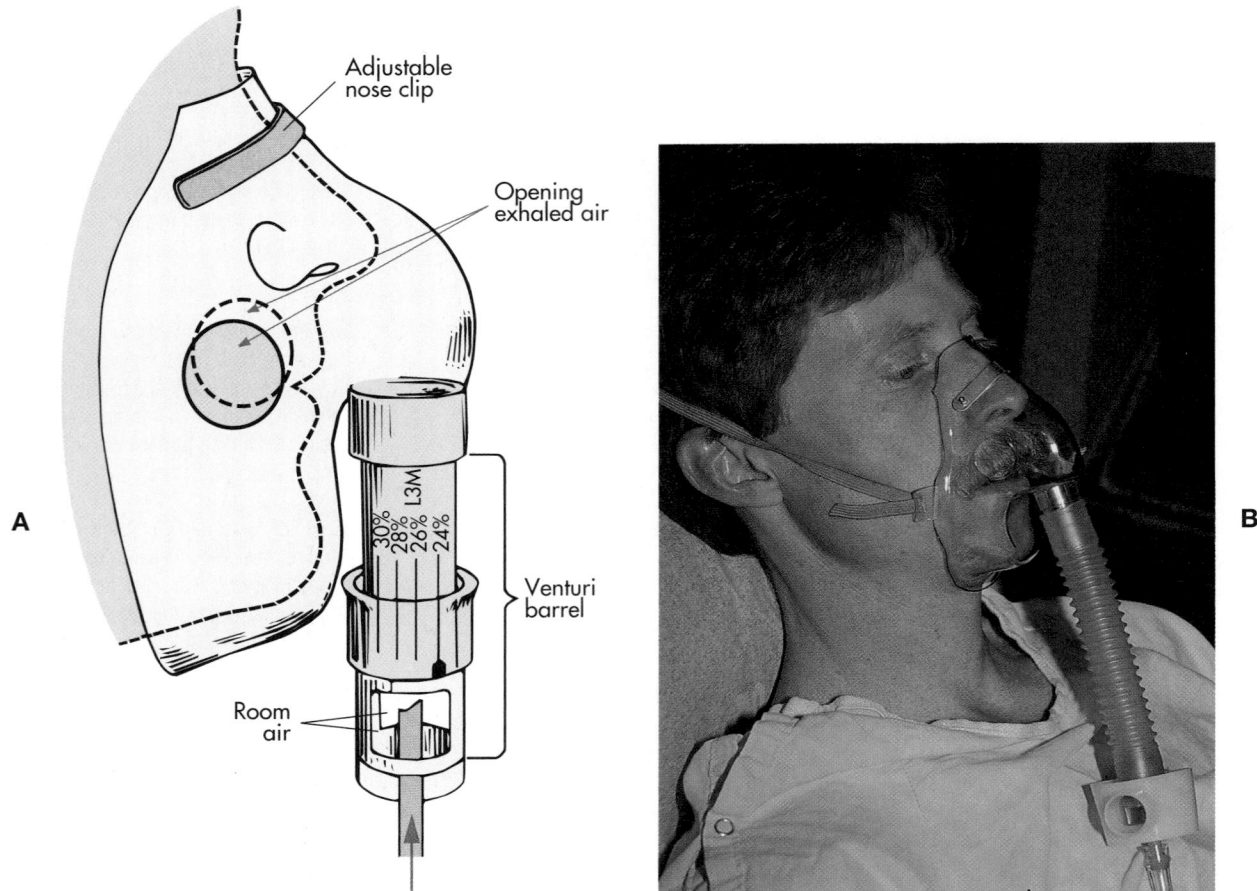

FIGURE **22-7** **A,** Turning Venturi barrel sets percentage of oxygen delivered from 24% to 50% at preset intervals. **B,** Venturi mask.

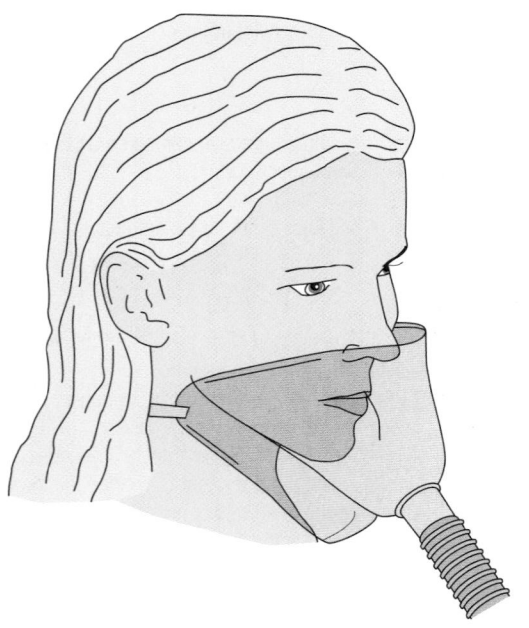

FIGURE **22-8** Face tent for oxygen delivery.

A Venturi mask is a cone-shaped device with entrainment ports of various sizes at the base of the mask (Figure 22-7). The entrainment ports are adjustable to permit regulation of FIO_2 from 24% to 60%. This mask is useful because it delivers a more precise concentration of oxygen to the client (see Table 22-1).

The face tent is a shieldlike device that fits under the client's chin and sweeps around the face (Figure 22-8). Oxygen concentrations of 28% to 100% may be delivered. If the device is used with compressed room air for aerosol purposes only, 21% oxygen is delivered. When higher oxygen concentrations are desired, the flow rate is set at 10 to 12 L/min. The actual concentration of oxygen delivered will be affected by the rate and depth of the client's respirations.

Oxygen hoods and tents are commonly used in the pediatric setting. These devices are able to provide high concentrations of humidified oxygen. This is particularly useful in the child with airway inflammation, epiglottitis (croup), or other respiratory tract infections.

DELEGATION CONSIDERATIONS

The placement of a cannula mask may be delegated to assistive personnel. The nurse is responsible for assessing the client's respiratory system, response to oxygen therapy, and setup of the oxygen therapy and liter flow. Before delegating this skill the nurse must:

* Discuss with assistive personnel how the system is set up and to report any differences to the nurse for further assessment
* Instruct assistive personnel to immediately report any vital sign changes or other unexpected outcomes associated with the oxygen delivery device.

EQUIPMENT

* ❑ Oxygen delivery device as ordered by physician
* ❑ Oxygen tubing
* ❑ Humidifier, if indicated
* ❑ Sterile water for humidifier
* ❑ Oxygen source
* ❑ Oxygen flowmeter
* ❑ Appropriate room signs

STEP	RATIONALE

ASSESSMENT

1. Assess client's respiratory status, including symmetry of chest wall expansion, respiratory rate and depth, sputum production, and lung sounds (see Chapter 18) and for signs and symptoms associated with hypoxia (see Box 22-1).

Decreased chest wall movement, crackles or decreased lung sounds, increased respiratory rate, increased sputum production, or hypoxia can indicate the need for noninvasive ventilation to improve oxygenation.

* **Critical Decision Point**

    Clients with sudden changes in their vital signs, level of consciousness, or behavior may be experiencing profound hypoxia. Clients who demonstrate subtle changes over time may have worsening of a chronic or existing condition or a new medical condition (Jevon and Ewens, 2001).

2. Observe for patent airway, and remove airway secretions by having client cough and expectorate mucous or by suctioning (see Chapter 24).

Secretions can plug the airway, decreasing the amount of oxygen that is available for gas exchange in the lungs.

3. If available, note client's most recent ABG results or pulse oximetry (SpO_2) value.

Objectively documents the client's pH, arterial oxygen, arterial CO_2, or arterial oxygen saturation.

* **Critical Decision Point**

    Note if the current oxygen therapy has been meeting the client's oxygenation needs. Determine what factors have changed, resulting in the new assessment findings.

4. Review client's medical record for the medical order for oxygen, noting delivery method, flow rate, and duration of oxygen therapy.

Ensures safe and accurate O_2 administration. Safe oxygen delivery includes the six rights of medication administration.

NURSING DIAGNOSES

* Impaired gas exchange
* Ineffective airway clearance

* Ineffective breathing pattern

Related factors are individualized based on client's condition or needs.

PLANNING

1. Expected outcomes following completion of procedure:
    * Client's signs of hypoxia are reduced or eliminated.
    * Client's vital signs will return to baseline.

Client demonstrates improved oxygenation.

When there is no underlying cardiovascular disease, clients may be able to adapt to decreased oxygen levels by increasing pulse and blood pressure. However, this is a short-term adaptive response, and once the signs of hypoxia are reduced or controlled, the client's vital signs should return to normal.

STEP	RATIONALE
• Client's work of breathing will decrease.	Hypoxia causes varying degrees of airway narrowing, which worsens as the hypoxia continues. With improved oxygenation, the client's airways are open, and the work of breathing decreases.
• Client will experience increased lung expansion.	Improved oxygenation can assist in resolving collapsed and constricted airways and improve work of breathing, and the client is able to improve lung expansion.
• Client's level of consciousness (LOC) will return to baseline.	In the presence of hypoxia or excessive carbon dioxide levels the client's level of consciousness is altered. Frequently clients are sleepy, confused, and may be difficult to arouse (Jevon and Ewens, 2001).
• Arterial blood gas values or oxygen saturation will return to normal or baseline.	Documents physiological response to oxygen therapy.
• Client's nares and nasal mucosa remain intact.	Oxygen cannula applied correctly.
2. Explain the procedure to client and family.	Increases compliance and cooperation of the client and family.

IMPLEMENTATION

STEP	RATIONALE
1. Perform hand hygiene.	Reduces transmission of microorganisms.
2. Attach oxygen delivery device (e.g., cannula, mask to oxygen tubing) and attach to humidified oxygen source adjusted to prescribed flow rate (see Figure 23-1), usually between 1 and 6 L/min.	Humidity prevents drying of nasal and oral mucous membranes and airway secretions. Ensures correct O_2 delivery.
3. Adjust elastic headband on face mask or nasal cannula so that a snug and comfortable fit is achieved (Figures 22-4 and 22-5).	Directs flow of oxygen into client's upper respiratory tract. Client is more likely to keep device in place if it fits comfortably.
4. Maintain sufficient slack on oxygen tubing and secure to client's clothes.	Allows client to turn head without causing mask to shift position or dislodge nasal cannula.
5. Observe for proper function of oxygen delivery device:	Ensures patency of delivery device and accuracy of prescribed oxygen flow rate.
a. *Nasal cannula:* Cannula is positioned properly in the nares.	Provides prescribed oxygen rate and reduces pressure on tips of nares.
b. *Nonrebreathing mask:* Apply mask over client's mouth and nose to form a tight seal. The valves on the mask close so exhaled air does not enter reservoir bag.	Does not allow exhaled air to be rebreathed. Valves on mask side ports permit exhalation, but close during inhalation to prevent inhaling room air.
c. *Partial rebreathing mask:* Apply mask over client's mouth and nose to form a tight seal. Ensure that the bag remains partially inflated.	Allows the exhaled air to mix with the inhaled air. Ports on the side of the mask permit most of the expired air to escape; however, the bag should remain partially inflated.
d. *Venturi mask:* Apply mask over client's mouth and nose to form a tight seal. Percentage of FIO_2 should correlate with flow rate (see Table 22-1).	Reduces carbon dioxide buildup.
e. *Face tent:* Apply tent under client's chin and over the mouth and nose. It will be loose, and a mist should always be present.	Excellent source of humidification; however, O_2 concentrations cannot be controlled.
6. Assess flowmeter and oxygen source for proper setup and prescribed flow rate.	Ensures delivery of prescribed oxygen therapy in conjunction with the specific cannula/mask.
7. Check cannula/mask every 8 hours. Keep humidification jar filled at all times.	Ensures patency of cannula and oxygen flow. Maintains inhalation of humidified oxygen.

STEP	RATIONALE
8. Monitor client's response to changes in the oxygen flow rate with pulse oximetry (see Chapter 17).	Continual monitoring with pulse oximetry should be available in all settings where acutely ill clients are managed and are on oxygen therapy. Changes in supplemental oxygen are based on individual client's oxygen saturation levels (Thompson and others, 2002).

• *Critical Decision Point*
Collaborate with physician for a plan of ongoing monitoring of oxygenation with ABG levels or trending pulse oximetry.

| 9. Perform hand hygiene. | Reduces transmission of microorganisms. |

EVALUATION

1. Observe for decreased anxiety, improved LOC and cognitive abilities, decreased fatigue, absence of dizziness, decreased respiratory rate, improved color, improved oxygen saturation, and returns to client's baseline vital signs.	Evaluates client's response to supplemental oxygen. As the client's oxygen level improves, so too should the vital signs, pulse oximetry, and other physical assessment parameters associated with decreased oxygen levels.
2. Monitor arterial blood gas levels, or observe pulse oximetry for oxygen saturation.	Documents client's level of oxygenation.
3. Assess adequacy of oxygen flow each shift.	Ensures patency of the oxygen delivery device.
4. Observe client's external ears, nares, and nasal mucous membranes for evidence of skin breakdown.	Oxygen therapy can cause drying of nasal mucosa. The delivery device can cause skin breakdown where the device comes in contact with the face, neck, and ears.

Recording and Reporting

• Record the respiratory assessment findings; method of oxygen delivery, flow rate, client's response; any adverse reactions or side effects; change in physician's orders.
• Report any unexpected outcome to physician or nurse in charge.

Unexpected Outcomes	Related Interventions
1. Client experiences skin irritation or breakdown (e.g., at ears, nares, or other pressure areas), drying of nasal and oral mucosa, sinus pain, or epistaxis.	• Increase humidification to oxygen delivery system. • Provide appropriate skin care.
2. Client experiences continued hypoxia.	• Obtain physician's orders for follow-up pulse oximetry monitoring or ABG determinations. • Notify the physician about the continued hypoxia. • Consider measures to improve airway patency, coughing techniques, oropharyngeal or oral-tracheal suctioning.
3. D y nasal and upper airway mucosa	• If oxygen flow rate is greater than 4 L/min, determine the need for humidification. • Assess the client's fluid status, and increase fluids if appropriate. • Provide frequent oral care. • Obtain physician order for use of sterile nasal saline intermittently.

Teaching Considerations

- If oxygen therapy is to continue after discharge, teach the client and family the importance of and rationale for oxygen therapy, how to use the oxygen delivery device, how to contact the supplier of medical equipment, and when to contact the health care provider.
- Discuss safety precautions for oxygen use (see Box 22-2) with the client and family.
- Discuss signs of oxygen toxicity and CO_2 retention (e.g., confusion, headache, decreased LOC, somnolence, CO_2 narcosis, respiratory arrest) that should be reported to the health care provider (see Box 22-1).

Pediatric Considerations

- Some infants and small children can tolerate nasal cannula. Secure the prongs of the cannula with Dermaclear tape or strips of transparent dressing over the child's cheek.
- Typically infants receive oxygen therapy via an oxygen hood. The hood is placed over the client's head, and may also include shoulders of a small infant. Sufficient room must exist between the curve of the hood and the client's neck to allow CO_2 to escape.
- Inspect toys placed in the tent for safety and suitability. Any source of sparks (e.g., from mechanical or electrical toys) is a potential fire hazard (Hockenberry, 2004).

- Provide comfort and reassurance to the child. Make sure the child is able to see someone nearby (Hockenberry, 2004).

Gerontological Considerations

- The client's arterial oxygen pressure (PO_2) falls 4 mm Hg per decade of life. A 70-year-old will have a normal arterial PO_2 between 75 and 80 mm Hg (Weilitz, 2000).
- Older adults may have a reduced oxygen-carrying capacity if they have a decreased hemoglobin level due to poor nutrition or other underlying illnesses.

Home Care Considerations

- Be sure that client is able to clearly see the flow rate and manipulate the settings (Eliopoulos, 1999).
- Oxygen tubing in the home setting is available in lengths of 15 m (50 feet).
- Oxygen-conserving devices that administer oxygen during inhalation are often used in the home care setting. These help reduce the use and cost of long-term oxygen therapy (Rice, 2000).

SKILL 22-2 Administering Oxygen Therapy to a Client With an Artificial Airway

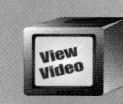

Clients with an artificial airway require constant humidification to the airway (see Chapter 24). An artificial airway bypasses the normal filtering and humidification process of the nose and mouth. The two devices that supply humidified gas to an artificial airway are a T tube and a tracheostomy collar.

The T tube, also called a Briggs adaptor, is a T-shaped device with a 15-mm ($3/5$-inch) connection that connects an oxygen source to an artificial airway such as an endotracheal (ET) tube or tracheostomy (Figure 22-9). The recommended flow rate is 10 L/min with a nebulizer set to the appropriate inspired oxygen concentration (FIO_2).

A tracheostomy collar is a curved device with an adjustable strap that fits around the client's neck (Figure 22-10). There are two ports: an exhalation port that remains patent at all times and the port that connects to the oxygen source with large-bore tubing. The flow rate is set at 10 L/min with a nebulizer set to the appropriate FIO_2 that provides humidification to the lower airways via the tracheostomy tube opening.

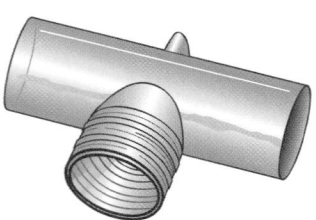

FIGURE **22-9** T tube.

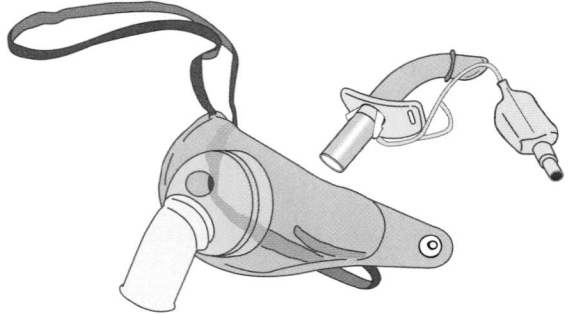

FIGURE **22-10** Tracheostomy collar.

DELEGATION CONSIDERATIONS

The placement of the oxygen device may be delegated to assistive personnel. However, the nurse is responsible for assessing the client's respiratory system, response to oxygen therapy, and setup of the oxygen therapy device and flow rate. Before delegating this skill the nurse must:

- Discuss with assistive personnel any client-specific variations for application of the T tube or tracheostomy collar (e.g., methods to avoid pressure or pulling on the artificial airway, methods for handling accumulated secretions in devices)
- Instruct assistive personnel to immediately report any unexpected outcomes, such as increase in anxiety, change in vital signs, and increased secretions, associated with the oxygen delivery device.

EQUIPMENT

- ❑ T tube or tracheostomy collar
- ❑ Large-bore oxygen tubing
- ❑ Nebulizer
- ❑ Sterile water for nebulizer
- ❑ Oxygen or gas source
- ❑ Gloves
- ❑ Goggles (if splash risk exists)
- ❑ Flowmeter
- ❑ "Oxygen in Use" sign

STEP	RATIONALE

ASSESSMENT

1. Assess client's respiratory status, including symmetry of chest wall expansion, respiratory rate and depth, sputum production, and lung sounds (see Chapter 18) and for signs and symptoms associated with hypoxia (see Box 22-1).

Decreased chest wall movement, crackles or decreased lung sounds, increased respiratory rate, increased sputum production, or signs of hypoxia may indicated worsening respiratory status and the need for other therapies.

- **Critical Decision Point**
  Clients with sudden changes in their vital signs, level of consciousness, or behavior may be experiencing profound hypoxia. Clients who demonstrate subtle changes over time may have worsening of a chronic or existing condition or a new medical condition (Jevon and Ewens, 2001).

2. Observe for patent airway, and remove airway secretions by suctioning (see Chapter 24).

Secretions can plug the airway, decreasing the amount of oxygen that is available for gas exchange in the lung. Secretions can also occlude the T tube or tracheostomy collar, impeding oxygen delivery to the client.

3. If available, note client's most recent ABG results or pulse oximetry (SpO_2).

Objectively documents the client's pH, arterial oxygen, arterial carbon dioxide (CO_2), or arterial oxygen saturation.

- **Critical Decision Point**
  Note if the current oxygen therapy has been meeting the client's oxygenation needs. Determine what factors have changed, resulting in the new assessment findings.

4. Review client's medical record for the medical order for oxygen, noting delivery method, flow rate, and duration of oxygen therapy.

Ensures safe and accurate O_2 administration.

NURSING DIAGNOSES

- Impaired gas exchange
- Ineffective airway clearance
- Ineffective breathing pattern

Related factors are individualized based on client's condition or needs.

STEP	RATIONALE

■ PLANNING

1. Expected outcomes following completion of procedure:
   - • Signs of hypoxia are reduced or eliminated.

     Client experiences improved oxygenation.
   - • Client's vital signs will return to baseline.

     When there is no underlying cardiovascular disease, clients may be able to adapt to decreased oxygen levels by increasing pulse and blood pressure. However, this is a short-term adaptive response, and once the signs of hypoxia are reduced or controlled, the client's vital signs should return to normal.
   - • Client's work of breathing will decrease.

     Hypoxia causes varying degrees of airway narrowing, which worsens as the hypoxia continues. With improved oxygenation, the client's airways are open, and the work of breathing decreases.
   - • Client will experience increased lung expansion.

     Improved oxygenation can assist in resolving collapsed and constricted airways and improve work of breathing, and the client is able to improve lung expansion.
   - • Client's LOC will return to baseline.

     In the presence of hypoxia or excessive carbon dioxide levels the client's level of consciousness is altered. Frequently clients are sleepy, confused, and may be difficult to arouse (Jevon and Ewens, 2001).
   - • Arterial blood gas values or arterial oxygen saturation will return to normal or baseline.

     Documents physiological response to oxygen therapy.
2. Explain the purpose of the T tube or tracheostomy collar to the client and family.

   Explanation decreases the client's anxiety and reduces oxygen consumption.

■ IMPLEMENTATION

1. Perform hand hygiene, apply gloves, apply goggles, and consider use of barrier gown.

   Reduces transmission of microorganisms and prevents contact with pulmonary secretions. Clients with excessive secretions or forceful productive coughs place the caregiver at risk for splash contact with pulmonary secretions.
2. Attach T tube or tracheostomy collar to large-bore oxygen tubing and to humidified room air or oxygen source, if indicated.

   Provides supplemental humidification to avoid drying of the airway.
3. If oxygen is ordered, adjust flow rate to 10 L/min or as ordered, adjust nebulizer to proper FIO_2 setting, and attach T tube or tracheostomy collar to endotracheal or tracheostomy tube.

   Flow rate ensures humidification; nebulizer regulates FIO_2.
4. Monitor client's response to changes in the oxygen flow rate with pulse oximetry (see Chapter 17).

   Monitoring with pulse oximetry allows for noninvasive, cost-effective trending of the client's arterial oxygen saturation and pulse rate (Thompson and others, 2002).

- • *Critical Decision Point*
  Collaborate with physician for plan of ongoing monitoring of oxygenation with ABG levels or trending pulse oximetry.

5. Observe that T tube does not pull on endotracheal or tracheostomy tube. Observe for secretions within T tube or tracheostomy collar, and suction as necessary (see Chapter 24).

   Pulling effect can increase client's discomfort and cause pressure to side of client's mouth or tracheal stoma. Maintains patent airway.
6. Observe oxygen tubing frequently for accumulation of fluid. If fluid is present, drain tube away from client, and discard fluid in proper receptacle.

   Excess water is medium for bacterial growth. Draining contaminated water into proper receptacle prevents contamination of entire humidifying unit.

STEP	RATIONALE
7. Set up suction equipment at client's bedside.	Client may experience increased airway secretions resulting from humidification.
8. Remove gloves and goggles; perform hand hygiene.	Reduces transmission of microorganisms and contamination with pulmonary secretions.

EVALUATION

1. Observe for decreased anxiety, improved LOC and cognitive abilities, decreased fatigue, absence of dizziness, decreased respiratory rate, improved color, improved oxygen saturation, and return to client's baseline vital signs.	Evaluates client's response to supplemental oxygen. As the client's oxygen level improves, so too should the vital signs, pulse oximetry, and other physical assessment parameters associated with decreased oxygen levels.
2. Observe the position of the oxygen delivery device to ensure that it is not pulling on the artificial airway.	Pulling on the artificial airway may result in damage to the oral cavity or stoma.
3. Monitor arterial blood gas levels or observe pulse oximetry.	Documents client's level of oxygenation.

Recording and Reporting

- Record the respiratory assessment findings; method of oxygen delivery, flow rate, client's response; any adverse reactions or side effects; change in physician's orders.
- Report any unexpected outcome to physician or nurse in charge.

Unexpected Outcomes	Related Interventions
1. Client experiences tracheal stoma irritation; thick, tenacious secretions; pressure areas on neck or near stoma site.	• Implement measures to maintain skin integrity (see Chapter 15). • Increase frequency of airway care. • Suction secretions from artificial airway and lungs as indicated.
2. Client experiences continued hypoxia.	• Determine if the cause of the continued hypoxia is the oxygen delivery device, plugging of the airway, the oxygen flow rate, or a new clinical problem. • Notify physician of continued or worsening hypoxia.

Teaching Considerations

- Teach the client and family alternative communication techniques (Chapter 2) to enhance communication with caregivers and to reduce frustration.
- Teach the client and family the importance of and rationale for the oxygen therapy.
- Teach the client and family safety precautions for oxygen use (see Box 22-2).
- Teach the client and family signs and symptoms of oxygen toxicity and CO_2 retention (e.g., confusion, headache, decreased LOC, somnolence) (see Box 22-1).

Home Care Considerations

- The client with an artificial airway who is at home may have a permanent tracheostomy, as well as a T tube or a tracheostomy collar.
- The client or caregiver should be physically able to perform tracheostomy care and suctioning techniques (see Chapter 24).

SKILL 22-3 Using Incentive Spirometry

Incentive spirometry assists the client in deep breathing. An incentive spirometer (IS) is most often used following abdominal or thoracic surgery to help reduce the incidence of postoperative pulmonary atelectasis. The use of IS is especially important in clients with underlying pulmonary diseases because of their risk for postoperative pneumonia (Snow and others, 2001). Postoperative deep breathing and coughing have been shown to be as effective as using an incentive spirometer when performed frequently.

The advantage of the IS is the device's visual feedback to clients about the depth of their breaths. The two types of spirometers are flow oriented and volume oriented. Flow-oriented ISs have one or more plastic chambers with freely movable, colored balls. As the client inhales slowly, the balls are elevated to a premarked area (Figure 22-11). The client's goal is to keep the balls elevated for as long as possible to ensure maximal sustained inhalation, not to snap the balls to the top of the chamber with a rapid, very brief, low-volume breath. Even if a very slow inspiration does not elevate the balls, this pattern may achieve greater lung expansion. The advantage of a flow-oriented IS is the slow, steady expansion of the lung.

Volume-oriented ISs have a bellows that the client must raise to a predetermined volume by inhaling slowly (Figure 22-12). An achievement light or counter is used to provide feedback to the client. Some devices have a marker that moves up as the client inhales. The advantage of the volume-oriented IS is that a known inspiratory volume can be achieved and measured with each breath.

The use of the IS encourages clients to breathe deeply and achieve their normal inspiratory capacity. Before surgery it is helpful to determine the client's baseline inspiratory capacity. An inspiratory volume one half to three quarters of baseline is an acceptable postoperative volume. Clients benefiting from incentive spirometry include those using it preoperatively, especially before abdominal, cardiac, or orthopedic surgery; clients with a history of smoking, pneumonia, or chronic respiratory disease; and clients with atelectasis.

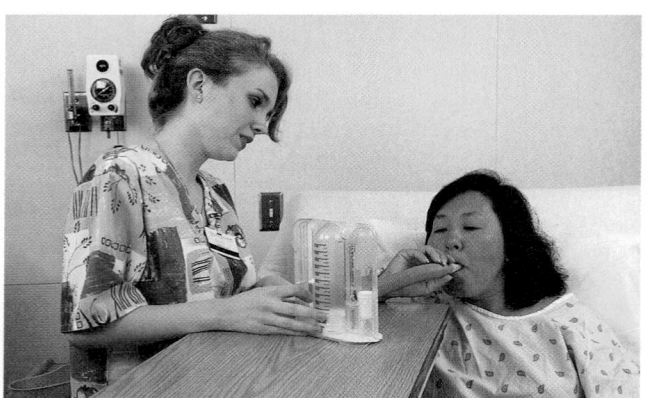

FIGURE **22-11** Flow-oriented incentive spirometer.

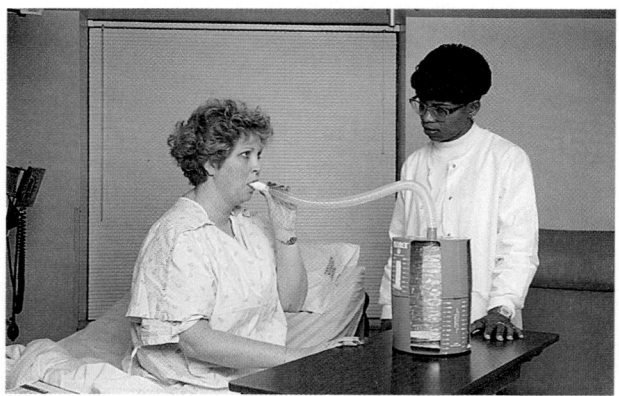

FIGURE **22-12** Volume-oriented incentive spirometer.

DELEGATION CONSIDERATIONS

This skill may be delegated to assistive personnel. The nurse is responsible for client assessment and monitoring and evaluating the client response. Before delegating this skill the nurse must:

- Inform assistive personnel of the client's target goal for spirometry
- Instruct assistive personnel to immediately inform the nurse regarding any unexpected outcomes, such as chest pain, excessive sputum production, and fever

EQUIPMENT

❑ Flow-oriented IS or volume-oriented IS

STEP	RATIONALE

ASSESSMENT

1. Identify clients who would benefit from incentive spirometry, especially those clients who have existing pulmonary disease, are overweight, or have other debilitating chronic illnesses (Bach and others, 2001).

Alerts health care personnel to those clients at risk for respiratory complications during illness or postoperatively.

● *Critical Decision Point*

Incentive spirometry is usually contraindicated in clients with flail chest. These clients require other respiratory maneuvers to correct asymmetrical chest wall motion. Clients who may experience difficulty with incentive spirometry include those who are confused, malnourished, or cognitively impaired and those who lack necessary motor skills.

2. Assess client's respiratory status, including symmetry of chest wall expansion, respiratory rate and depth, sputum production, and lung sounds (see Chapter 18).

Decreased chest wall movement, crackles or decreased lung sounds, increased respiratory rate, or increased sputum production can indicate a need for incentive spirometry to improve lung expansion.

3. Review the physician's order for incentive spirometry.

Health care institutions frequently require a medical order for incentive spirometry in order to receive third-party reimbursement for the spirometer.

NURSING DIAGNOSES

● Impaired gas exchange
● Ineffective airway clearance

● Ineffective breathing pattern

Related factors are individualized based on client's condition or needs.

PLANNING

1. Expected outcomes following completion of procedure:
   ● Client will demonstrate correct use of the IS.
   ● Client achieves target volume and number of repetitions per hour.
   ● Client has normal breath sounds.

Demonstrates learning.
Demonstrates increased lung expansion.

Incentive spirometry is designed to assist the client in deep breathing and managing airway secretions.

2. Explain the procedure to the client and family.

Understanding the purpose of incentive spirometry and its proper use will improve compliance with use.

3. Indicate to the client where on the spirometer is the target volume.

Clients are encouraged to "do better" with each breath and to meet or exceed the target volume. When clients have a visual target, they can gauge their improvement.

IMPLEMENTATION

1. Perform hand hygiene.

Reduces transmission of microorganisms.

2. Position client in a semi-Fowler's or high-Fowler's position.

Promotes optimal lung expansion during respiratory maneuver.

3. Instruct client to place lips completely over mouthpiece.

Showing client to correctly place mouthpiece is a reliable technique for teaching psychomotor skill and enables client to ask questions.

4. Instruct client to take a slow deep breath and maintain a constant flow, like pulling through a straw. When maximal inspiration is reached, client should hold breath for 2 to 5 seconds, and then exhale slowly.

Maintains maximal inspiration; reduces risk of progressive collapse of individual alveoli.

STEP	RATIONALE

- *Critical Decision Point*

  Clients with COPD may only be able to hold their breath for 2 to 3 seconds. Encourage clients to do their best and to try to extend the duration of breath holding. Allow clients to rest between IS breaths to prevent hyperventilation and fatigue.

5. Have client repeat the maneuver until goals are achieved.	Ensures correct use of the spirometer and client's understanding of use.
6. Perform hand hygiene.	Reduces transmission of microorganisms.

EVALUATION

1. Observe client's ability to use incentive spirometry by return demonstration.	Determines client's ability to perform breathing exercise correctly.
2. Assess if the client is able to achieve the target volume or frequency.	Measures compliance with therapy and lung expansion.
3. Auscultate chest during respiratory cycle.	Documents lung wall expansion, identifies any abnormal lung sounds, and determines if airways are clear.

Recording and Reporting

- Record the lung sounds before and after incentive spirometry, the frequency of use, the volumes achieved, and any adverse effects.
- Report any changes in respiratory assessment or client's inability to use IS.

Unexpected Outcomes	Related Interventions
1. Client is unable to achieve incentive spirometry target volume.	• Encourage client to attempt IS more frequently followed by rest periods. • Teach cough-control exercises. • Teach client how to splint and protect incision sites during deep breathing.
2. Client has decreased lung expansion and/or abnormal breath sounds.	• Teach client cough-control exercises. • Provide assistance with suctioning if clients cannot effectively cough up their secretions.

Teaching Considerations

- Teach client to examine sputum for consistency, amount, and color changes.
- Teach client the rationale for performing incentive spirometry and the impact on recovery.

Pediatric Considerations

- Incentive spirometry is not typically used in pediatrics except for the school-age child; the pediatric client needs the fine motor skills and ability to follow instructions to effectively use incentive spirometry (Hockenberry, 2004).
- Allowing the child to play with and try out the incentive spirometer assists in decreasing the child's anxiety and encourages participation in care.
- Use games or bubbles and balloons to encourage small children to take deep breaths. These activities can achieve the same goals as IS in some children.

Gerontological Considerations

- Older adults with chronic illnesses or arthritis may have difficulty coordinating the use of the IS. They may require additional time to demonstrate the procedure.
- Weakened respiratory muscles and decreased elastic recoil properties of the lungs affect client's ability to cough and deep breathe. Therefore it may take the older adult longer to achieve the target volume (Ebersole and Hess, 2002).

Home Care Considerations

- Have client return demonstrate correct procedure for use before discharge.

SKILL 22-4 Care of the Client Receiving Noninvasive Ventilation

Noninvasive ventilation (NIV) maintains positive airway pressure and improves alveolar ventilation without the need for an artificial airway. In addition, this mechanical ventilator alternative reduces and reverses atelectasis, improves oxygenation, reduces pulmonary edema, and improves cardiac function (Woodrow, 2003a). Continuous positive airway pressure keeps the terminal airways (alveoli) partially inflated, reducing the risk for atelectasis; and if atelectasis has occurred, positive pressure assists in reinflation. Because the alveoli remain partially inflated, there is continued exchange of respiratory gases, and as a result the client's oxygenation improves. In the cardiac client, NIV reduces pulmonary edema because the increased alveolar pressure forces interstitial fluid out of the lungs and back into the pulmonary circulation. In clients with altered cardiac function secondary to sleep apnea, NIV provides improved myocardial oxygenation and improved function.

In selected clients, such as those with postpolio syndrome and other neuromuscular diseases, congestive heart failure, sleep disorders, and pulmonary diseases, NIV may be the treatment of choice in supporting ventilation without the hazards associated with endotracheal intubation (Preston, 2001; Woodrow, 2003b). In addition, when NIV is used, there is a reduced risk for pneumonia, gastric aspiration, and ventilator dependency (Perkins, 2000).

This skill focus on two types of noninvasive ventilation: continuous positive airway pressure (CPAP) and bilevel positive airway pressure (BiPAP). CPAP has been available for many years and maintains a set positive airway pressure throughout the client's breathing cycle (Figure 22-13). Therefore a CPAP of 5 cm of water provides 5 cm of pressure during inspiration and expiration. It is very beneficial to the client with obstructive sleep apnea. During sleep the upper airway collapses and prevents normal airflow. When the airflow is interrupted, there is a drop in the client's oxygen saturation and frequent awakenings occur. CPAP uses continuous positive pressure to keep the airway open and prevent upper airway collapse. As a result the client breathes more normally, sleeps better, and has markedly reduced snoring. The usual CPAP pressure is 5 to 20 cm of water (Perkins, 2000). However, there are disadvantages to this device (Box 22-3).

BiPAP works by providing assistance during inspiration and preventing airway closure during expiration (see Figure 22-13). During inspiration BiPAP generates a preset positive pressure support, which increases the client's tidal volume and ultimately alveolar ventilation. This pressure support ends when the client initiates the expiratory phase; however, a CPAP is maintained within the airways throughout the expiratory phase (Preston, 2001). As a result there is an increase in the functional residual capacity (the amount of air

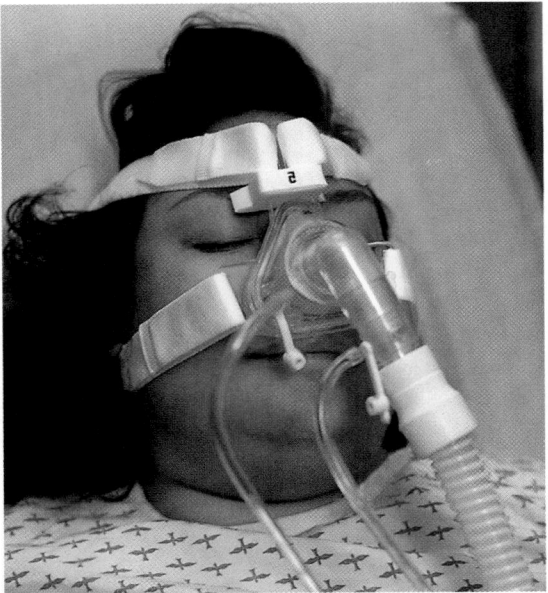

FIGURE **22-13** Mask suitable for either continuous positive airway pressure (CPAP) or bilevel positive airway pressure (BIPAP) device.

BOX 22-3 Problems Associated With Continuous Positive Airway Pressure (CPAP)

PROBLEM	CAUSE
Discomfort	Large tight-fitting mask that fits over client's nose. Oxygen flow rate causes dry mucous membranes.
Risks to skin integrity	Tight fit of the mask causes pressure and diaphoresis. Clients need to remove the mask to relieve pressure.
Hypercapnia	Although CPAP improves alveolar function, which increases carbon dioxide clearance from the blood, it also causes air trapping. In some clients this may cause a rise in carbon dioxide levels. Initially the client's ABG levels need to be monitored.
Gastric distention	CPAP forces more air into the stomach, which can cause distention and discomfort in some clients. In addition, severe gastric distention can impede diaphragmatic motion and reduce lung volumes.
Noise	Some clients may find the machine very noisy, not only interfering with sleep but also leisure activities, such as watching TV or listening to music.

Data from Perkins L, Shortall SP: Ventilation without intubation, *RN* 63(1):34, 2000; Woodrow P: Using non-invasive ventilation in acute wards, part I, *Nurs Stand* 18(1):39, 2003a.

remaining in the lungs at the end of expiration), reduced airway closure, reexpansion of atelectatic area, and improved oxygenation. BiPAP is delivered via a large face mask, so clients may find it uncomfortable and noisy as well (see Box 22-3).

The goals of noninvasive ventilation should include improved ventilation, improved sleep, enhanced quality of life, provision of an environment that enhances individual potential, reduction of morbidity, improvement of physical and physiological function, and cost-effectiveness (Perkins, 2000; Woodrow, 2003b). Clients and families who are candidates for noninvasive ventilation should be prepared for discharge by a multidisciplinary team including representatives of nursing, medicine, dietary service, social service, the home care nurse, and the home care durable medical equipment company.

DELEGATION CONSIDERATIONS

This skill should not be delegated to assistive personnel. However, certain aspects of client care may be delegated. The nurse is responsible for the assessment and evaluation of the client receiving noninvasive ventilation, as well as determining the safe functioning of the equipment. Before delegating aspects of care the nurse must:

- Instruct assistive personnel to immediately report any changes in client's pulse, blood pressure, respiratory rate, SpO_2, mental status, or skin color
- Instruct assistive personnel about any modification in care, such as hygiene, for example, how long the mask can be removed for oral care or any special skin care needs
- Instruct assistive personnel in the prescribed settings of the noninvasive ventilation equipment and to notify nurse of any change in settings or client comfort

EQUIPMENT

(NOTE: When device is used in the home, the home care equipment vendor provides the equipment.)
- ❏ Nasal mask/full face mask (with quick-release straps), or nasal pillows
- ❏ Oxygen source and tubing
- ❏ CPAP/BiPAP per physician order
- ❏ Humidification source, if needed
- ❏ Pressure generator (in institutional health care settings the client's room may have a pressure source)
- ❏ Delivery tubing
- ❏ Pulse oximetry
- ❏ Gloves
- ❏ Goggles (if splash risk exists)

STEP	RATIONALE

ASSESSMENT

1. Assess client's respiratory status, including symmetry of chest wall expansion, respiratory rate and depth, SpO_2, sputum production, and lung sounds (see Chapter 18). When possible ask client about dyspnea, and observe for signs and symptoms associated with hypoxia (see Box 22-1).

Decreased chest wall movement, crackles or decreased lung sounds, increased respiratory rate, increased sputum production, or hypoxia can indicate the need for noninvasive ventilation to improve oxygenation.

- **Critical Decision Point**
  Clients with sudden changes in their vital signs, level of consciousness, or behavior may be experiencing profound hypoxia. Clients who demonstrate subtle changes over time may have worsening of a chronic or existing condition or a new medical condition (Jevon and Ewens, 2001).

2. Observe client's ability to clear and remove airway secretions.

Secretions can plug the airway, decreasing the amount of oxygen that is available for gas exchange in the lung.

3. If available, note client's most recent ABG results or arterial oxygen saturation.

Objectively documents the client's pH, arterial oxygen, arterial CO_2, or arterial oxygen saturation.

STEP	**RATIONALE**

• *Critical Decision Point*
If the client is currently on NIV, evaluate if the therapy is meeting the client's oxygenation and ventilation needs. Determine what factors have changed, resulting in the new assessment findings.

4. Obtain vital signs before initiation of therapy.	Provides baseline data to compare desired or untoward vital sign changes resulting from the therapy.
5. Review client's medical record for the medical order for CPAP/BiPAP and appropriate settings.	Physician's order is needed for this therapy.

NURSING DIAGNOSES

- Impaired gas exchange
- Ineffective airway clearance

- Ineffective breathing pattern

Related factors are individualized based on client's condition or needs.

PLANNING

1. Expected outcomes following completion of procedure:	
• Client will have increased lung expansion.	Client experiences improved oxygenation and ventilation.
• Client will maintain ABG levels or oxygen saturation within normal range or at baseline.	Determines the need to change the machine settings using client assessment data.

• *Critical Decision Point*
When CPAP/BiPAP is first initiated, it is important to monitor ABGs in addition to pulse oximetry, especially in clients with COPD, pulmonary edema, or acute respiratory failure. This is done to observe for carbon dioxide retention (Perkins, 2000).

• Client experiences reduction in feelings of dyspnea and work of breathing.	In clients with acute conditions there should be improvement in dyspnea within 30 to 60 minutes (Soroksky and others, 2003; Woodrow, 2003b). Clients with chronic pulmonary diseases may require nocturnal CPAP/BiPAP indefinitely to achieve long-term benefits (Woodrow, 2003b).
• Client's vital signs and respiratory assessment parameters improve.	Reduced pulse and respiratory rate, improved mental status, improved skin color, and decreased use of accessory and abdominal muscles occurs because client's work of breathing decreases as the level of oxygenation improves (Perkins, 2000; Woodrow, 2003b).
2. Explain to client and family the purpose and reasons for CPAP/BiPAP	Helps reduce the sense of claustrophobia from the mask. In addition, information reduces anxiety and increases cooperation and compliance with the therapy (Woodrow, 2003a).

IMPLEMENTATION

1. Perform hand hygiene; apply gloves and goggles. Apply barrier gown if secretions are projectile.	Reduces transmission of microorganisms and exposure to pulmonary secretions.

STEP	RATIONALE

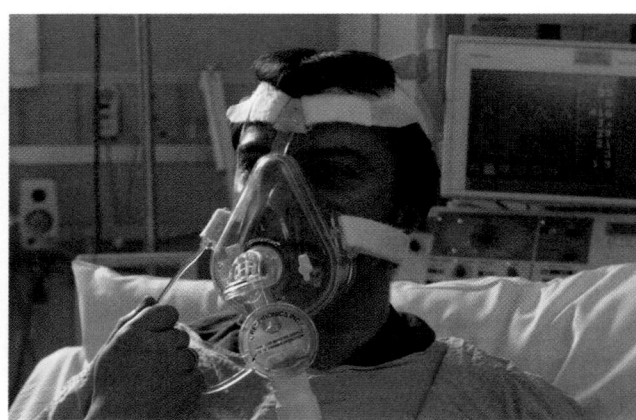

A   B

STEP 2 A, Mask sizing. **B,** Full-face mask with quick-release restraining straps.

2. Determine correct mask size. Masking charts are supplied to determine the correct size (S, M, L, XL) (see illustrations).

The mask should fit snugly over client's nose (CPAP) or nose and mouth (BiPAP), because a tight seal is needed to deliver the positive pressure. It is imperative that the mask have quick-release straps, so in the case of an emergency (e.g., vomiting, respiratory arrest) the mask can be quickly removed. This quick-release system also allows the client to remove the mask quickly when needed (Preston, 2001).

3. Connect CPAP/BiPAP device delivery tubing to pressure generator.

Ensures client is receiving proper noninvasive ventilation as ordered.

• **Critical Decision Point**
In some clients it may also be necessary to connect oxygen delivery source; however, this equipment is frequently used without oxygen.

4. Connect client to pulse oximetry.

It is important to continually monitor the client's level of oxygenation when noninvasive ventilation is initiated (Perkins, 2000).

5. Set CPAP/BiPAP initial settings:
   CPAP: 4 to 8 cm H_2O
   BiPAP:
   Inspiratory pressure usually set at 8 cm H_2O
   Expiratory pressure usually set at 4 cm H_2O
   (Preston, 2001)

These settings allow the health care team to determine initial client response. CPAP provides single positive pressure at the end of exhalation, which helps to keep the alveoli open at end-expiration.

BiPAP supplies pressures at both inhalation and exhalation. The inhalation pressure prevents airway closure, and the expiratory pressure helps to keep the alveoli open at end-expiration (Preston, 2001).

6. Perform frequent skin assessment to determine the presence of pressure, skin irritation, or skin breakdown.

A mask that is too tight increases the risk for skin breakdown over the bridge of the nose.

7. Dispose of supplies as appropriate, and perform hand hygiene.

Reduces transmission of microorganisms.

STEP	RATIONALE

EVALUATION

1. Evaluate client's response to noninvasive ventilation. Observe for decreased anxiety; improved LOC and cognitive abilities; decreased fatigue; absence of dizziness; decreased pulse, regular rhythm; decreased respiratory rate and work of breathing; return to normal blood pressure; improved color.

As hypoxia and hypercapnia are reduced or corrected, the client's physical assessment parameters improve.

2. Monitor ABG levels—observe pulse oximetry.

Documents client's level of oxygenation. When first initiating NIV, especially in clients with underlying COPD, it is important to obtain ABG levels after the first hour and every 2 to 6 hours during the first day because these client's may retain carbon dioxide (Perkins, 2000).

3. Observe skin integrity over the bridge of the client's nose.

A mask that is too tight causes skin breakdown, and frequent skin assessment is needed.

4. Monitor client and family's ability to manipulate device and face mask.

Determines client's ability to perform self-care and adhere to CPAP/BiPAP plan.

Recording and Reporting

- Record in progress notes:
  - Respiratory assessment findings
  - CPAP/BiPAP settings
  - Pulse oximetry
  - Client's response
  - Change in the physician's orders
- Report to nurse in charge or physician:
  - Sudden change in client's respiratory status
  - Worsening ABG levels or pulse oximetry value

Unexpected Outcomes	Related Interventions
1. Client experiences hypoxia.	• Notify physician. • Reassess client. • Determine correct settings and integrity of noninvasive ventilation system.
2. Client experiences hypercapnia.	• Notify physician. • Reassess client. • Determine correct settings and integrity of noninvasive ventilation system.
3. Client states a sense of smothering or claustrophobia.	• Reexplain system to client. • Demonstrate use of quick-release straps. • Have client demonstrate use of quick-release straps.

Teaching Considerations

- Teach the client and family the best hours to use the machine (e.g., bedtime, watching TV); usually the client is prescribed 6 to 8 hours of continual CPAP/BiPAP.
- Teach the client and family how to apply the mask and connect it to the machine and how to add oxygen if ordered.
- Instruct family to bring the machine, along with a list of correct settings, to the hospital any time the client is admitted (Perkins, 2000).
- When clients require home noninvasive ventilation, instruct complete care of the CPAP/BiPAP system. Skills include assembling the system, cleaning the system, and daily equipment maintenance (Perkins, 2000).

Home Care Considerations

- The durable medical equipment provider, the home care nurse, and the primary care nurse should develop a teaching plan to ensure that client and family have a complete working knowledge of the system before discharge.
- Instruct client and primary caregiver in what to do in case of respiratory distress or power failure. Check to determine availability of emergency batteries.

SKILL 22-5 Care of the Client on a Mechanical Ventilator

Clients requiring mechanical ventilation need support for ventilation and/or oxygenation. Clinical problems such as respiratory failure, exacerbation of chronic obstructive lung disease, spinal cord trauma, respiratory muscle paralysis, and pneumonia may require mechanical ventilation support. Clients receiving mechanical ventilation are most often cared for in an intensive care unit.

There are two types of mechanical ventilation: positive pressure and negative pressure. Positive-pressure ventilation is the usual method of ventilation. Positive-pressure ventilation delivers a positive pressure to inflate the lungs. There are multiple complications associated with positive-pressure ventilation: decreased cardiac output, aspiration, tension pneumothorax (see Chapter 25), bronchospasm, laryngeal trauma, sinusitis, and ventilator-associated pneumonia. In addition, as the length of time needed for mechanical ventilation increases, there is an increased risk of failure to wean from the ventilator (Grap and others, 2003). The nurse must be alert for these side effects. An artificial airway, such as an ET or a tracheostomy tube, is needed (see Chapter 24).

NIV is positive-pressure ventilation, in which the client is fitted with a facial mask (see Skill 22-4). This mode of ventilation delivers CPAP or BiPAP and is useful in clients with COPD.

Negative-pressure ventilation, is a noninvasive, negative-pressure ventilation technique that is used for clients with primary neuromuscular illnesses that interfere with normal respiratory muscle function, such as multiple sclerosis and muscular dystrophy (Preston, 2001). The client is fitted with a poncho or shell that is connected to the ventilator. Air is removed from between the client's chest wall and the interior wall of the poncho or shell, causing the client to inhale. The client using negative-pressure ventilation does not need an artificial airway.

This skill described in this chapter focuses on positive-pressure mechanical ventilation frequently used in acute, subacute, and in some selective home care settings. There are many types of positive-pressure mechanical ventilators available for acute care use. Mechanical ventilators are available in pressure-cycled and volume-cycled machines. Pressure-cycled ventilation delivers a specified pressure to the client, achieving a tidal volume, or amount of air, in milliliters per breath (Figure 22-14). Volume-cycled ventilation delivers a specified tidal volume. Volume-cycled ventilators are most often used in the clinical setting. Clients using pressure-cycled ventilators are at higher risk for development of pneumothorax, hypotension, and decreased cardiac output as a result of the ventilator's achieving the prescribed pressure without regard for lung compliance. Volume-cycled ventilators achieve tidal volume with preset pressure limits and are more sensitive to lung compliance. Time-cycled ventilators provide an inspiratory phase until a preset time is reached. This often results in varying tidal volumes.

Modes of Ventilation

There are many different modes of mechanical ventilation to support different conditions and physiological processes. Modes of ventilation include control mode (CM), continuous mandatory ventilation (CMV), synchronized intermittent mandatory ventilation (SIMV), and pressure support ventilation (PSV). The more frequently used modes of ventilation are CMV, SIMV, and PSV. They support oxygenation and provide varying levels of ventilatory support that can be adjusted to meet the client's needs (Table 22-2).

Continuous mandatory ventilation provides continuous ventilation to the client, maintaining the respiratory rate and tidal volume. Synchronized intermittent mandatory ventilation attempts to synchronize the ventilator breaths with the client's spontaneous breathing. This reduces competition between the ventilator and the client.

Pressure support ventilation is actually a spontaneous breathing mode, because the ventilator does not deliver a preset tidal volume or rate. It provides a preset pressure to augment the inspiratory process and helps overcome the initial work of breathing. It is used both for ventilation and to assist in weaning the client. Clients on PSV need to be assessed frequently for respiratory muscle fatigue and potential periods of apnea.

Positive end-expiratory pressure (PEEP) and CPAP are adjuncts to ventilation used to increase oxygenation. Positive end-expiratory pressure is positive airway pressure maintained at the end of exhalation. This allows more time for gas exchange and opens small airways and closed alveolar units, thus improving oxygenation. Continuous positive airway pressure is the maintenance of a positive airway pressure above atmospheric pressure during inspiration and expiration in the spontaneously breathing client. It improves oxygenation in the same manner as PEEP.

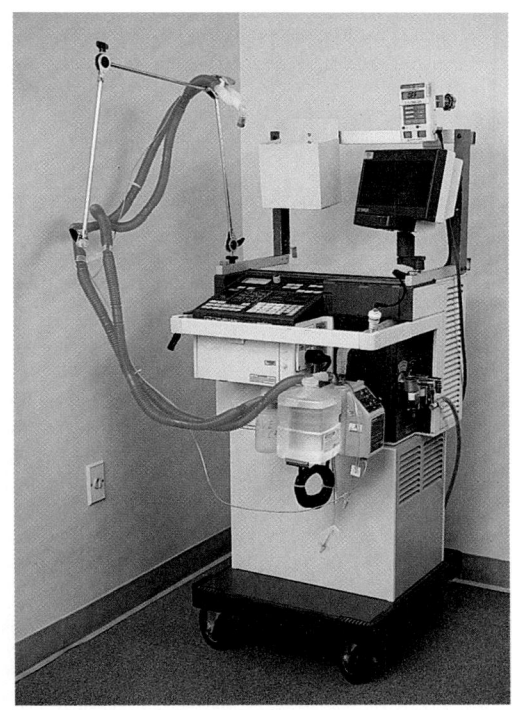

FIGURE 22-14 A mechanical ventilator. (From Sorrentino SA: *Mosby's textbook for nursing assistants*, ed 5, St. Louis, 2000, Mosby.)

TABLE 22-2   MODES OF MECHANICAL VENTILATION

MODE	DEFINITION	INDICATIONS	COMMENTS
Control mode (CM)	Preset tidal volume and preset rate delivered to the client regardless of the client's respiratory effort. Client cannot initiate breaths or change the ventilatory pattern.	Neuromuscular disease Drug overdose Reduction of work of breathing	Client may require sedation to reduce competition with the ventilator. Rarely used.
Continuous mandatory ventilation (CMV)	Preset tidal volume at preset rate is delivered to the client. The client can initiate breaths that are delivered at the preset tidal volume.	Reduction of work of breathing Respiratory muscle fatigue COPD Post anesthesia	Client may need sedation to reduce spontaneous breaths.
Synchronized intermittent mandatory ventilation (SIMV)	Preset tidal volume at preset rate is synchronized with the client's spontaneous breathing to reduce competition between machine-delivered and client-spontaneous breaths.	Primary ventilatory mode Used to wean clients from mechanical ventilation	Client synchrony with the ventilator is improved. Rates ≤6 breaths per minute can result in increased work of breathing.
Pressure support ventilation (PSV)	Provides positive pressure during the inspiratory cycle of a spontaneous inspiratory effort (Weilitz, 2000).	Weaning clients with COPD Primary ventilatory mode in higher pressures	There is no preset respiratory rate. The nurse must assess for respiratory muscle fatigue and periods of apnea. Decreases work of breathing by overcoming resistance of airway and ventilatory circuit.
Pressure controlled ventilation (PCV)	Uses minimal pressure to deliver acceptable tidal volumes. This may be calculated by measuring the compliance of the client/ventilator interface and calculating the acceptable tidal volume.	Useful in clients with obstructive airway diseases	Reduces risk of barotraumas from high pressure. Adjusts to the compliance of the client/ventilator interface and thus reduces the work of breathing.

TABLE 22-3 VENTILATOR PARAMETERS

PARAMETER	DEFINITION	VENTILATOR SETTING
Tidal volume (V_T)	Amount of air inspired and expired with each breath	8 to 15 ml/kg of ideal body weight (clients with nonrestrictive pulmonary diseases)
Respiratory rate (R or RR)	Number of breaths delivered per minute	10 to 16 breaths per minute
Fraction of inspired oxygen (FiO_2)	Amount of oxygen the client receives	Ideally less than 40% to maintain PaO_2 60 to 80 mm Hg
PEEP	Positive pressure applied at end-expiration to improve oxygenation	+3 to 5 cm H_2O may be used to approximate physiological PEEP*
		May require higher levels (>5 cm H_2O) in respiratory failure (e.g., adult respiratory disease syndrome)
Sigh	Larger than normal breath to provide hyperinflation; helps prevent atelectasis	Usually twice the tidal volume breath; about 10 to 15 ml/kg Rate is usually set at 10 to 15 times per hour
Sensitivity	Determines the inspiratory effort required to trigger the ventilator	Set to respond to an inspired volume of less than 1% of the client's tidal volume
Peak airway pressure	The maximal pressure level required to deliver the desired tidal volume	<40 cm H_2O
	Comparison of inspiratory (I) to expiratory (E) time	Normally set 1:1, 1:2, or 1:3
I:E ratio		*Example:* inspiration 2 seconds, expiration 4 seconds; then I:E = 1:2
Exhaled minute ventilation (V_E)	Measures the exhaled minute ventilations in liters	Alarm set at 15% greater than client's average V_E

*Some clinicians believe that the ET with inflated cuff creates a closed system with the ventilator and does not require 3 to 5 cm of PEEP.

Alarms and Settings

The mechanical ventilator has a number of settings to adjust the amount of oxygen delivered, the amount of tidal volume, the time for inspiration and expiration, and the pressure at which each breath is delivered. The tidal volume, the amount of air per breath, is usually set at 8 to 15 ml/kg of ideal body weight. If the client has a restrictive lung disease, such as pulmonary fibrosis, or a flail chest or recent thoracic surgery, the tidal volumes are usually set lower.

The respiratory rate is usually set at 10 to 16 breaths per minute. Initially the FiO_2 may be set at 100% and is quickly reduced to less than 40% based on client ABG levels. The goal of providing oxygenation is to maintain a PO_2 of greater than or equal to 60 mm Hg using an FiO_2 of 40% or less. Table 22-3 lists the ventilator parameters the nurse must become familiar with to care for a client on mechanical ventilation.

There are a number of alarms on the ventilator to ensure client safety. Each ventilator is a little different; however, the basic alarms are similar. Alarms common to all ventilators include high-pressure, low-pressure, low-exhaled volume, and oxygen alarms (Table 22-4). The nurse must know how to respond to the ventilator alarms and what nursing actions may be required to preserve the client's respiratory status. The two most frequent alarms are the high-pressure and low-pressure alarms. The high-pressure alarm is usually set at 10 to 15 cm greater than the peak airway pressure. When this alarm sounds, it indicates the ventilator has met resistance to delivering the tidal volume and requires more pressure to inflate the lungs. The client may have coughed during the inspiratory cycle, may need suctioning, or may have changed position. More acute problems that require immediate nursing intervention include the development of a pneumothorax or displacement of the ET or tracheostomy tube. The low-pressure alarm sounds when the ventilator has no resistance to inflating the lung. The client may be disconnected from the ventilator, or a leak has developed in the ventilator circuit.

Once the condition for which the client required mechanical ventilation is corrected, the weaning process is initiated. Weaning from mechanical ventilation is the gradual reduction of ventilation and oxygenation support until the client is breathing spontaneously and can be oxygenated with a low-flow oxygen device. Many clients who are unable to wean from the mechanical ventilator may be transferred to subacute nursing care for continued care or in preparation for home mechanical ventilation. Generally these clients are hemodynamically stable; however, they require continual ventilatory support.

The mechanical ventilator also has settings to regulate the temperature of the water in the humidifier, known as the cascade. The temperature of the heater in the cascade is set at or just below normal body temperature. This provides warm, moistened air for delivery to the airway. The cascade is a potential source of contamination of the ventilator circuit if the water that collects in the ventilator tubing is drained back into the cascade unit.

Home Mechanical Ventilation

The client on mechanical ventilation can be successfully managed in the home. Neuromuscular disease such as amyotrophic lateral sclerosis (ALS), muscular dystrophy, brain

TABLE 22-4 TROUBLESHOOTING MECHANICAL VENTILATION

VENTILATOR ALARM	POSSIBLE CAUSE	NURSING INTERVENTIONS
Sudden increase in peak airway pressure (high-pressure alarm)	Coughing Airway plugging Changes in client position Pneumothorax Incorrect ET position Kinked ventilator circuit Excessive water in ventilator circuit	Clear secretions by suctioning. Reposition client. Assess breath sounds and chest wall movement. Verify placement of ET. Assess breath sounds. Verify centimeter level of ET. Check circuit; unkink tubing. Drain ventilator tubing.
Gradual increase in peak airway pressure	Decreasing lung compliance Exacerbation of acute process	Evaluate breath sounds; suction. Check for reversible causes: airway plugging, bronchospasm.
Sudden decrease in peak airway pressure (low-pressure alarm)	Client disconnected from ventilator Leak in ventilator circuit	Check for disconnection. Evaluate circuit connections; tighten loose connections.
Change in minute ventilation or tidal volume	Leak in ET cuff	Check cuff seal.
Decrease	Airway secretions System leak Increased respiratory rate	Suction excessive secretions. Check circuit connections. Evaluate respiratory rate.
Increase	Hypoxia	Evaluate for signs of hypoxia. Evaluate need to obtain ABG sample or monitor pulse oximetry.
Change in respiratory rate	Client anxiety Increased metabolic demand Hypoxia	Reassure client. Evaluate body therapy, heart rate, and rhythm. Obtain ABG levels, or monitor pulse oximetry.

and spinal cord diseases, chest wall disease, central hypoventilation syndrome, and advanced COPD are just a few of the diseases for which clients are managed at home on mechanical ventilators. Many factors determine if a client and family are candidates for home ventilation. Assessment criteria include the desire of the client and family, the client's acceptance of ventilator dependence, the client's and family's ability to understand and perform daily care procedures, the home environment, personal resources, monetary resources, and resources and technologies for support in the community.

The goals of long-term ventilator care should include extension of life, enhancement of the quality of life, provision of an environment that enhances individual potential, reduction of morbidity, improvement of physical and physiological function, and cost-effectiveness. Clients and families who are candidates for home mechanical ventilation should be prepared for discharge by a multidisciplinary team including representatives of nursing, medicine, dietary service, social service, the home care nurse, and the home care durable medical equipment company. The nurse in the hospital must be familiar with the home ventilator to assist the client with discharge planning and education.

DELEGATION CONSIDERATIONS

The skill of administering mechanical ventilation should not be delegated to assistive personnel. However, certain aspects of the client's care, such as hygiene, intake and output, and vital signs, may be delegated to assistive personnel. Before delegating any component of care the nurse must:

- Instruct assistive personnel to report any change in the client's respiratory status, such as rapid breathing, not breathing in sequence with the ventilator, client indication of breathlessness.
- Instruct assistive personnel as to the expected pulse oximetry parameters and client's vital signs and to notify the nurse immediately for any change in these values.
- Instruct assistive personnel to immediately inform the nurse if any of the ventilator's alarms sound.

EQUIPMENT

- ❑ Appropriate mechanical ventilator
- ❑ Oxygen source
- ❑ Pulse oximetry (SpO_2) probe and monitor
- ❑ Capnography ($EtCO_2$) window and monitor
- ❑ Stethoscope
- ❑ 10-ml syringe
- ❑ Oral airway/bite block
- ❑ Manual resuscitation bag (bag-valve-mask) with oxygen connecting tubing and flowmeter
- ❑ Gloves
- ❑ Goggles (if splash risk exists)
- ❑ Suction equipment at bedside (in-line/individual catheters)
- ❑ Method for client communication
- ❑ Ventilator flow sheet to document ventilator changes and settings

STEP	RATIONALE

ASSESSMENT

1. Assess client's respiratory status, including symmetry of chest wall expansion, respiratory rate and depth, sputum production, and lung sounds (see Chapter 18), and for signs and symptoms associated with hypoxia (see Box 22-1).

Decreased chest wall movement, crackles or decreased lung sounds, increased respiratory rate, increased sputum production, or signs of worsening hypoxia can indicate a need for mechanical ventilation or changes in the current ventilator settings to improve oxygenation.

2. Check ventilator, $EtCO_2$, SpO_2, and ventilator and cardiac alarms at the beginning of each shift and periodically throughout care.

Verifies that the ventilator settings are as ordered by the physician.

3. Verify placement of artificial airway through auscultation of lung sounds and verification of distal tip marking on endotracheal tube. Determine that tube is securely placed (see Chapter 24).

Prevents migration of the tube into the right or left bronchus and accidental extubation.

   a. Auscultate over trachea for presence of air leak.

Cuff of artificial airway must be inflated to create a seal in order for positive-pressure ventilation to occur.

   b. Using minimal occlusive pressure, check inflation of cuff of artificial airway (see Chapter 24).

- **Critical Decision Point**

   When clients have a chest x-ray examination, placement of the artificial airway should also be verified.

4. Observe for patent airway and remove airway secretions by suctioning (see Chapter 24).

Secretions can plug the airway, decreasing the amount of oxygen that is available for gas exchange in the lung. Secretions can also occlude the T tube or tracheostomy collar, impeding oxygen delivery to the client.

5. If available, note client's most recent ABG results or pulse oximetry reading (SpO_2). Determine if any factors have changed during mechanical ventilation.

Objectively documents the client's pH, arterial oxygen, arterial CO_2, or arterial oxygen saturation.

6. Determine a method for communication with client. If possible, review previous communication techniques with client and family.

Clients with an artificial airway and mechanical ventilation cannot communicate verbally. In addition, some of these clients are too weak to use a note pad to communicate their needs. Therefore assessing for and determining communication needs before instituting mechanical ventilation is the ideal. However, each time the client has a new caregiver, communication preferences should be assessed.

STEP	**RATIONALE**
7. Review client's medical record for the medical order for mechanical ventilation, noting mode of ventilation, respiratory rate, oxygen setting, and tidal volume.	Mechanical ventilation and changes in the ventilator settings require a physician's order.

NURSING DIAGNOSES

- Impaired gas exchange
- Ineffective airway clearance
- Risk for infection
- Impaired verbal communication

- Ineffective breathing pattern
- Impaired spontaneous ventilation
- Dysfunctional ventilatory weaning response

Related factors are individualized based on client's condition or needs.

PLANNING

1. Expected outcomes following completion of procedure:	
• Client will have increased lung expansion.	Client experiences improved oxygenation and ventilation.
• Client will maintain ABG levels and oxygen saturation within normal range or at client baseline.	Determines the need to change the ventilator settings using client assessment data.
• Client's vital signs and respiratory assessment parameters improve.	Reduced pulse and respiratory rate, improved mental status, improved skin color, and decreased use of accessory and abdominal muscles occurs because client's work of breathing decreases as the level of oxygenation improves (Perkins, 2000; Woodrow, 2003b).
• Client experiences reduction in feelings of dyspnea and work of breathing.	As the pulmonary problem resolves, the client's perceptions of dyspnea and the actual work of breathing declines (Twibell and others, 2003).
• Client uses communication board, paper and pencil, or computer to state needs.	Appropriate communication system matches client's abilities.
2. Explain the ventilator system to the client and family and be sure to include the purpose of and reasons for initiation of mechanical ventilation.	Helps client to express fears and wishes. Plays a role in the weaning process (Moody and others, 1997).

IMPLEMENTATION

1. Perform hand hygiene; apply gloves and goggles. Apply barrier gown if secretions are projectile.	Reduces transmission of microorganisms and exposure to pulmonary secretions.
2. Attach mechanical ventilator to ET or tracheostomy tube. Observe for proper functioning of mechanical ventilator.	Ensures closed system, which enables the ventilator to exert appropriate pressure or volume to meet the client's oxygen demands.

- *Critical Decision Point*
  The mechanical ventilator requires programming of accurate settings before attaching to the client. This is most often the responsibility of the respiratory therapist; however, it may also be a collaborative responsibility of the nurse.

3. Verify that the ET or tracheostomy tube is properly positioned during an inspiratory and expiratory cycle by listening to both lungs and assessing chest wall symmetry.	Properly placed artificial airway will ensure that both lungs are equally ventilated. Improper airway placement may lead to unilateral lung ventilation.
4. Observe client for synchronization with mechanical ventilation and response to therapy.	Ensures client is comfortable using ventilator and has not experienced any adverse hemodynamic effects.
5. Monitor heart rate, blood pressure, respiratory rate, and cardiac rhythm.	Implementation of mechanical ventilation can result in decreased venous return and associated hemodynamic changes.
6. Secure ventilator tubing to the artificial airway; be sure that the tubing does not pull on tracheostomy or ET tube.	Provides connection of the artificial airway to the ventilator and prevents accidental dislodging of artificial airway.

STEP	RATIONALE
7. Note and mark the level of the ET at the lips or nares (see Chapter 24).	Provides a baseline for depth of tube placement.
8. Set up suction equipment (see Chapter 24).	Need to provide airway care and suctioning as needed of ET or tracheostomy tube to prevent plugging of the airway and to reduce the risk of infection.

• **Critical Decision Point**
Determine if the client will need an oral suction setup, as well as endotracheal suctioning.

STEP	RATIONALE
9. Position client to promote best oxygenation and ventilation, and monitor SpO_2 levels during and after positioning. Depending on client's oxygenation status, this position can be high-Fowler's, lateral, or even prone.	Positioning can affect oxygenation and ventilation. Some client's SpO_2 may drop during the position change and recover once the client is completely positioned. In other clients a change in position (e.g., high-Fowler's to lateral) may result in a sustained drop in SpO_2, thus indicating that the client in unable to tolerate that particular position at that time (Gawlinski and Dracup, 1998; Manning and others, 1999).
10. Collaborate with the physician frequently about the status of the client, the response to therapy, and ongoing monitoring.	Assesses oxygenation status and continued need for mechanical ventilation.
a. Monitor SpO_2 continuously.	Provides the nurse with the ability to continually assess oxygenation levels.
b. Monitor $EtCO_2$ continually and with serial ABG levels to detect possible overventilation or inadequate alveolar ventilation.	Overventilation causes respiratory alkalosis from decreased carbon dioxide. Inadequate alveolar ventilation may cause respiratory acidosis from increased carbon dioxide retention (Ahrens and others, 1999).
c. Obtain ABG levels with changes in client's condition or ventilator changes.	Provides more accurate measure of O_2 saturation and partial pressures of oxygen and carbon dioxide level.
11. Do hourly safety checks on client and ventilator system.	
a. Make sure the client can reach call light.	Provides mechanism for client to contact health care personnel.
b. Check the security of all ventilator connections; make sure alarms are all turned on, including both high- and low-pressure alarms and volume alarms.	Ensures continuous safe and proper functioning of the ventilator system. Enables the nurse to identify and correct problems in a timely manner.
c. Verify that all ventilator settings are correct and correspond to physician orders.	Maintains integrity of the system and ensures that all settings are consistent with physician orders.
d. Check and refill humidifier as needed. Check corrugated tubing for condensation and drain and appropriately discard liquid.	Do not return condensation to humidifier because of possible bacterial contamination.
e. When present, observe temperature gauges on the panel of the mechanical ventilator, making sure that gas is being delivered at the correct temperature. Desired ranges of inspired gas should be between 89.6° F (32° C) and 98.6° F (37° C).	The temperature of inspired gas can artificially alter the client's body temperature. As a result body temperature measurements may not reflect the client's condition.
12. Perform mouth care at least 4 times per 24 hours. Use a solution such as chlorhexidine, which is effective in reducing oral bacteria and the risk of ventilator-associated pneumonia (Munro and Grap, 2004).	Ventilator-associated pneumonia is common, and it is associated with microaspiration of oropharyngeal secretions. Frequent mouth care reduces client's risk for ventilator-associated pneumonia (Sole and others, 2003). Frequent oral care of at least 4 times per 24 hours may help in reducing the risk of pneumonias (Grap and others, 2003).

STEP	**RATIONALE**
13. Perform nursing activities to prevent hazards of immobility (e.g., assist client to change position, assist with range of joint motion, encourage independence and activity as tolerated by the client).	Maintaining activity avoids complications associated with decreased mobility. Assists in preventing complications such as pressure ulcers, pneumonia, deep vein thrombosis (DVT), and activity intolerance. Clients receiving mechanical ventilation need assistance with activity.
14. Keep client informed on progress, and plan for weaning from the mechanical ventilator.	Apprehension and anxiety can be potentiated when the client is ill informed about progress, changes in care, or changes in ventilator setting. Clients need information as well as emotional support to successfully tolerate and wean from mechanical ventilation (Twibell and others, 2003).
15. Remove gloves and goggles; perform hand hygiene.	Reduces transmission of microorganisms and exposure to pulmonary secretions.

▌ EVALUATION

1. Reassess and monitor client's response to mechanical ventilation every 2 to 4 hours.
   - **a.** *Neurological assessment:* LOC, orientation, sleepiness, changes in anxiety
   - **b.** *Pulmonary assessment:* lung sounds, airway clearance, work of breathing, breathing pattern, rate of respirations, SpO_2, $EtCO_2$
   - **c.** *Cardiovascular assessment:* vital signs, heart rhythm, heart sounds, lower extremity edema
2. Monitor ABG levels—observe pulse oximetry.
3. Observe integrity of client ventilator system.
4. Observe and evaluate effectiveness of the communication methods:
   - **a.** Ask client if needs and concerns are addressed.
   - **b.** Observe for signs of frustration (e.g., client shaking head in irritation, crying, withdrawal).
   - **c.** Observe client/family and health care personnel use communication methods.

Clients requiring mechanical ventilation may have unstable physiological status. It is important to perform key focused assessment frequently as the client's condition warrants.

Documents client's level of oxygenation and ventilation.
Ensures adequate delivery of mechanical ventilation.
Communication or lack of it can increase the client's frustration, sense of powerlessness, and confusion during mechanical ventilation and the weaning process (Twibell and others, 2003).

Recording and Reporting

- Record in progress notes:
  - Respiratory assessment findings
  - Mode of mechanical ventilation
  - Oxygen level, actual client tidal volume, ordered tidal volume, actual client respiratory rate, ordered respiratory rate, peak airway pressure
  - Client's response to mechanical ventilation
  - Level of the ET, any adverse reactions or side effects
  - Change in the physician's orders
- Report to nurse in charge or physician:
  - Sudden change in client's respiratory status
  - Ventilator-associated problems

Unexpected Outcomes	Related Interventions
1. Client experiences stiff, noncompliant lung; alveolar edema; pulmonary congestion; chest pain; intraalveolar hemorrhage; substernal chest pain; pneumothorax; continued decrease in blood pressure related to use of positive pressure.	• Notify physician. • Remain with client. • Conduct a complete cardiac and pulmonary assessment.
2. Client experiences hypoxia.	• Notify physician. • Assess client. • Assess integrity of ventilator system. • Expect ventilator change (increase PEEP levels).
3. Client experiences hypercapnia.	• Notify physician. • Assess client. • Assess integrity of ventilator system.
4. Tension pneumothorax as evidenced by sudden respiratory distress: air hunger, distended neck veins, tracheal/mediastinal shift, hypotension, and tachycardia.	• Remain with client, and remove client from ventilator and ventilate with bag-valve-mask (see Chapter 26). • Notify physician. • Ask assistive personnel to obtain chest tube insertion kit. • Ask additional personnel to obtain client vital signs.
5. Pressure alarm	• Assess for airway obstruction (e.g., secretions, client biting on endotracheal tube). • Remove obstruction (e.g., ET suctioning, inserting oral airway/bite block).
6. Low-volume alarm	• Assess integrity of the ventilator tubing, and reconnect if disconnected. • Check for airway displacement (e.g., extubation). • Assess integrity of the airway cuff (e.g., deflate and reinflate, and determine if seal is present) (see Chapter 24). • Remain with client, and remove client from ventilator and ventilate with bag-valve-mask.

Teaching Considerations

• Teach the client and family about the rationale for mechanical ventilation.
• Teach client and family about the alarms and what they mean.
• Teach client and family alternative communication techniques to reduce frustration and fear.

Pediatric Considerations

• There are increasing numbers of children on home mechanical ventilation. For this reason it is important to include the parent in the child's care as appropriate. Parents also need to be prepared that when a readmission to a hospital occurs, due to the chronic nature of the illness, the child may not be readmitted to an ICU, but rather remain on the general medical or surgical area.
• Once the child is stable on the mechanical ventilator, promote normal or near normal activities as the child's condition warrants (e.g., promote play, resume school activities, encourage mobility).

Gerontological Considerations

• Presence of underlying chronic illnesses increase client's risk for longer intensive care, hospital stays.
• Older adults may not be able to tolerate the usual sedative, antianxiety medications ordered. The prescribed dose should be altered based on client's baseline kidney and liver functions (Eliopoulos, 1999).

Home Care Considerations

• Clients requiring home mechanical ventilation need to be taught complete care of the mechanical ventilator system, suctioning, and artificial airway care. Skills include assembling the ventilator circuit, cleaning the circuit, and daily equipment maintenance (Rice, 2000).
• Use a checklist for ensuring consistency of care for the client on a ventilator.

- Evaluate the following areas during each visit: oxygen flow, alarm system, inspiratory pressure, high-pressure alarm, tidal volume setting, humidifier, respiratory rate, tubing, temperature, resuscitation bag, tracheostomy care, breath sounds, suctioning, and tubing changes.
- The durable medical equipment provider, the home care nurse, and the primary care nurse should develop a teaching plan to ensure that client and family have a complete working knowledge of the ventilator before discharge.

- Instruct client and primary caregiver in what to do in case of respiratory distress or power failure. Check to determine availability of emergency batteries.
- Instruct family in use of the bag-valve-mask (see Chapter 26).
- Clients who require long-term mechanical ventilation may be transferred to a chronic ventilator facility or a long-term ventilator dependency floor within the hospital. The purpose of such a transfer is to aggressively rehabilitate the client through physical therapy, occupational therapy, and speech therapy. The overall goal is to effectively wean client from the mechanical ventilator.

FOCUS on CLINICAL PRACTICE

You are caring for newly admitted Mr. Landon, who has a history of COPD that is well controlled. However, 2 weeks ago he developed an upper respiratory tract infection; he was treated with antibiotics. He completed his full course of antibiotics, but his symptoms continued. He has a 4-day history of high fever greater than 102.8° F, fatigue, productive coughing, worsening dyspnea, and decreased activity tolerance. His private physician does a complete examination, orders a chest x-ray examination, and obtains a sputum specimen. Preliminary chest x-ray results indicate right lower lobe pneumonia. Mr. Landon is admitted to a general medicine floor for treatment with intravenous (IV) antibiotics, supplemental oxygen, and pulmonary hygiene measures.

1. You observe him and notice that he is fatigued, has difficulty speaking, and in general looks very uncomfortable. You decide to do a focused assessment. What systems will you assess, and what information will you obtain? State your rationale for choosing these systems.
2. Mr. Landon is started on oxygen therapy via nasal cannula at 2 L/min. What is the approximate FiO_2 level, and what are the hazards for oxygen therapy in this client?
3. Mr. Landon continues to remove the cannula because of discomfort at the nares and ears from the device. What are the causes of this discomfort? What are your interventions?
4. One of the nurses suggests a partial rebreather mask for Mr. Landon's oxygen therapy. You do not think this is a good idea, and the rationale for your decision is:
   A. Increased inspired oxygen percentage
   B. Decreased carbon dioxide retention

C. Decreased inspired oxygen percentage
D. Increased carbon dioxide retention

5. As the day progresses, Mr. Landon is getting more breathless and fatigued. He is unable to clear his secretions effectively and needs nasotracheal suctioning. His level of consciousness is declining; he is difficult to arouse and at times appears confused and continually takes off his nasal cannula. His pulse oximetry value is 85%, ABG levels show slight acidemia with CO_2 retention. The doctors want to try Mr. Landon on BiPAP in the hopes of avoiding intubation and mechanical ventilation.
   A. What concerns do you have with Mr. Landon's confusion and initiation of BiPAP? What are your interventions?
   B. The physician orders hourly ABG measurements and continuous pulse oximetry. What is the rationale?
6. As you continue to assess Mr. Landon, what assessment parameters indicate a worsening status?
   A. Increased respiratory rate, decreased oxygen saturation, decreased carbon dioxide level, sleepiness
   B. Increased respiratory rate, decreased oxygen saturation, increased carbon dioxide level, sleepiness
   C. Decreased respiratory rate, decreased oxygen saturation, increased carbon dioxide level, alertness
   D. Decreased respiratory rate, increased oxygen saturation, decreased carbon dioxide level, alertness

NCLEX REVIEW QUESTIONS

1. Partial assessment of a dyspneic client would not include which of the following?
   1. Respiratory rate
   2. Sputum
   3. Chest x-ray
   4. Breathing pattern
2. 2 L/min of oxygen via nasal cannula or simple face mask is given to clients with underlying chronic obstructive lung disease in order to:
   1. Reduce the risk of oxygen toxicity
   2. Reduce the risk of carbon dioxide retention
   3. Increase pH level
   4. Increase diaphragmatic excursion
3. Humidification is added to oxygen therapy via nasal cannula oxygen in order to:
   1. Prevent drying of the nasal mucosa
   2. Liquefy pulmonary secretions
   3. Increase the client's cough
   4. Improve oxygenation
4. BiPAP differs from CPAP in that:
   1. Positive pressure is only given during inhalation
   2. Positive pressure is only given during exhalation
   3. It uses negative pressure during inhalation and exhalation
   4. It uses positive pressure during inhalation and exhalation
5. The use of noninvasive ventilation (CPAP or BiPAP) has the potential to cause carbon dioxide retention in selected clients. Which clients are at greatest risk for carbon dioxide retention?
   1. Clients with an underlying diagnosis of congestive heart failure
   2. Clients with an underlying diagnosis of pulmonary fibrosis
   3. Clients with an underlying diagnosis of chronic obstructive pulmonary disease
   4. Clients with an underlying diagnosis of pulmonary edema
6. Your client is on mechanical ventilation. Suddenly he develops severe respiratory distress, his vital signs change, his oxygen saturation suddenly declines, and his tracheal tube is no longer midline. You suspect a tension pneumothorax. Your immediate actions are to:
   1. Begin manual ventilation and obtain vital signs and pulse oximetry as soon as possible
   2. Keep the ventilator settings the same and notify physician
   3. Notify the physician
   4. Suction the client and obtain vital signs
7. Your client has a large amount of pulmonary secretions. Over the last hour you note that the secretions are thicker and the volume has increased. During the last 30 minutes, the pressure alarm on the mechanical ventilator has triggered repeatedly. What action is appropriate to correct this problem?
   1. Manually ventilate the client.
   2. Change the sensitivity setting on the ventilator.
   3. Suction the client's airway.
   4. Call the physician.

References

Ahrens T and others: Capnography: a key under-utilized technology, *Crit Care Nurs Clin North Am* 11(1):49, 1999.

Ebersole P, Hess P: *Toward healthy aging: Human needs and nursing response,* ed 6, St. Louis, 2002, Mosby.

Eliopoulos C: *Manual of gerontologic nursing,* ed 2, St. Louis, 1999, Mosby.

Fadiman A: *The spirit catches you and you fall down.* New York, 1997, Farrar, Straus & Giroux.

Hockenberry MJ: *Wong's clinical manual of pediatric nursing,* ed 6, St. Louis, 2004, Mosby.

Jevon P, Ewens B: Assessment of a breathless patient, *Nurs Stand* 15(16):48, 2001.

Perkins L, Shortall SP: Ventilation without intubation, *RN* 63(1):34, 2000.

Preston R: Introducing non-invasive positive pressure ventilation, *Nurs Stand* 15(26):42, 2001.

Rice R: *Manual of home health nursing procedures,* ed 2, St. Louis, 2000, Mosby.

Robinson G: *Essential Judaism: a complete guide to beliefs, customs and rituals,* New York, 2000, Pocket Books.

Weilitz PB: Respiratory system. In Lueckenotte AG: *Gerontologic nursing,* ed 2, St. Louis, 2000, Mosby.

Woodrow P: Using non-invasive ventilation in acute wards, part I, *Nurs Stand* 18(1):39, 2003a.

Woodrow P: Using non-invasive ventilation in acute wards, part II, *Nurs Stand* 18(2):41, 2003b.

Research References

Bach PB and others: Management of acute exacerbations of chronic obstructive pulmonary disease: a summary and appraisal of published evidence, *Ann Intern Med* 134(7):600, 2001.

Gawlinski A, Dracup K: Effect of positioning on SvO_2 in the critically ill patient with a low ejection fraction, *Nurs Res* 47(5):293, 1998.

Grap MJ and others: Oral care interventions in critical care: frequency and documentation *Am J Crit Care* 12(2):113, 2003.

Grap MJ and others: Collaborative practice: development, implementation, and evaluation of a weaning protocol for patients receiving mechanical ventilation, *Am J Crit Care* 12(5):454, 2003.

Johnson SK: Hmong health beliefs and experiences in the Western health care system, *J Transcult Nurs* 13(2):126, 2002.

Manning F and others: Effects of side lying on lung function in older individuals, *Phys Ther* 79(5):456, 1999.

Moody LE and others: Psychophysiologic predictors of weaning from mechanical ventilation in chronic bronchitis and emphysema, *Clin Nurs Res* 6(4):311, 1997.

Munro CL, Grap MJ: Oral health and care in the intensive care unit: state of the science, *Am J Crit Care* 13(1):25, 2004.

Sole ML and others: A multisite survey of suctioning techniques and airway management practices, *Am J Crit Care* 12(3):220, 2003

Snow V and others: The evidence base for management of acute exacerbations of COPD: clinical practice guideline, part I, *Chest* 119(4):1185, 2001.

Soroksky A, Stav D, Shipirer I: A pilot prospective, randomized, placebo-controlled trial of bilevel positive airway pressure in acute asthmatic attack, *Chest* 123(4):1018, 2003.

Thomson A and others: Oxygen therapy in acute medical care: the potential dangers of hyperoxia need to be recognised, *Br Med J* 324(7351):1406, 2002.

Twibell R and others: Subjective perceptions and physiological variables during weaning from mechanical ventilation, *Am J Crit Care* 12(2):101, 2003.

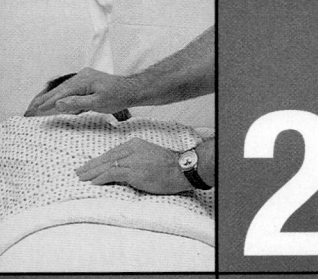

23

Performing Chest Physiotherapy

MEDIA RESOURCES

Evolve Site *evolve*

http://evolve.elsevier.com/Perry/skills
• Weblinks

/ **OBJECTIVES**

Mastery of content in this chaper will enable the nurse to:

- Assess the need to perform chest physiotherapy (CPT) maneuvers.
- Assess the need to modify or discontinue CPT maneuvers, including contraindications and individual variations.
- Explain how to prepare the client and family for the performance of each CPT maneuver.
- Identify goals for performing each CPT maneuver.
- Perform the outlined CPT maneuvers, including standard and modified versions.
- Describe expected and unexpected outcomes of each CPT maneuver.
- Describe discharge teaching and planning related to the use of each CPT maneuver in the home setting.

KEY TERMS

Chest physiotherapy (CPT)   Postural drainage (PD)
Cough   Shaking
Mucociliary transport   Vibration
Percussion

Chest physiotherapy (CPT) consists of physical chest wall maneuvers such as percussion, vibration and shaking, postural drainage (PD), and cough. Percussion is a rhythmical force provided by clapping the caregiver's cupped hands against the client's thorax. Percussion assists in loosening retained secretions from the airway. Vibration and shaking are performed with the goal of moving secretions from small distal airways into larger central airways. The caregiver contracts all muscles in the upper extremities and causes vibration while applying pressure to the client's chest wall. Shaking is a stronger bouncing maneuver, which also supplies a concurrent, compressive force to the chest wall (Frownfelter and Dean, 1996). Postural drainage is achieved by positioning the client so that the position of the lung segment to be drained allows gravity to have its greatest effect (Frownfelter and Dean, 1996).

Once CPT has mobilized the secretions into the large central airways, the secretions need to be coughed out or suctioned. Cough is achieved by taking a deep breath, closing the glottis to build up a back pressure, and then forcefully exhaling. During the expiratory phase of a cough, the airways are dynamically compressed, which results in a decrease in their cross-sectional area. Airway narrowing and forced exhalation results in an increase in the velocity of airflow in the large central airways, which propels the mucus up and out of the trachea

CPT and coughing maneuvers assist with airway clearance of mucus in clients with retained tracheobronchial se-

cretions (Jones and Rowe, 1999). Secretions accumulate in clients with bronchitis, asthma, cystic fibrosis (CF), pneumonia, and bronchiectasis. Surgical clients in the postoperative period can also have excess secretions due to pain and anesthesia. When secretions accumulate in the airway, it can result in mucous plugging, atelectasis, and lobar collapse. Chest physiotherapy is often used in combination with other therapeutic modalities, including antibiotics, smoking cessation, bronchodilators, mucolytic agents, and systemic hydration. These therapies along with CPT reduce mucus production and facilitate airway clearance. The goals of these therapies are to: (1) clear the airways of excessive secretions in order to reduce the work of breathing and (2) facilitate the client's ability to cough up secretions.

In the normal lung the mucociliary transport system is able to keep the airways clear of excessive mucus and inhaled particles. This system lines the internal lumen of the entire tracheobronchial tree and consists of a thin layer of mucus that is constantly being propelled toward the larynx by cells that have hairlike projections called cilia. Inhaled particles are trapped on the mucus, and the cilia act as a conveyor belt to sweep the mucus toward the throat, where it can be swallowed or removed by coughing. Airways normally remain clear, and mucus is constantly being cleared almost as fast as it is made. Normal mucus remains thin, white, and watery. When disease causes excessive sputum production, therapeutic interventions can help natural airway clearance mechanisms (cough and mucociliary transport) clear the airways of obstructing mucus.

In various disease states, mucus clearance slows down or the cilia are overwhelmed by production of excessively large quantities of mucus. The lung can no longer clear the mucus as fast as it is produced. Secretions stagnate in the airways, change color, and become thick and sticky. The cilia cannot remove large amounts of thick mucus from the lungs. In addition, many people with lung disease cannot cough effectively to clear airways. Therefore it becomes important to employ systemic hydration and other maneuvers to aid in clearing excess lung secretions. These therapies prevent mucus from stagnating and allow secretions to return to their normal thin, white, and watery consistency.

Adequate hydration is an important part of a client's lung clearance program. Fluids make the mucus thin and watery so that it can be mobilized, coughed up, and expectorated more easily. Unless contraindicated by other disease states, such as congestive heart failure or renal failure, fluids should be given along with CPT to assist in making mucus thin and watery. During an acute pulmonary illness, it often takes three or four CPT treatments a day and 2 L or more of fluid a day to mobilize and thin secretions. Hydration and CPT help to prevent the buildup of excessive secretions in the airway and reduce shortness of breath, decrease work of breathing, and improve gas exchange.

This chapter presents three CPT skills that can be implemented in the clinical and home settings. Although they are separate skills, they must be thought of as different components of CPT. All must be mastered if treatment is to be effective.

Evidence-Based Practice Trends

Chest physiotherapy is very effective in selected clients, such as those with cystic fibrosis. Newer studies compare the effectiveness of newer airway clearance methods (oscillating positive expiratory pressure devices (see Skill 23-2), high-frequency chest wall oscillators, and intrapulmonary compression ventilators) with standard manual chest physiotherapy, which was the gold standard for over 40 years (Gondor and others, 1999; Oermann and others, 2001; Varekojis and others, 2003). These studies demonstrate that chest physiotherapy and these newer devices are safe and effective modalities for the clearance of airway secretions. However, many of the mechanical devices are expensive and are not always available. What is important is that these studies show significant improvements in pulmonary function studies, 6-minute walk distance, and secretion production and clearance following CPT or use of these newer airway clearance methods, especially in clients with cystic fibrosis. More severely impaired clients with cystic fibrosis have better oxygenation during CPT if it is administered in conjunction with noninvasive ventilation (Holland and others, 2003).

Client satisfaction and compliance with CPT are also evaluated when using mechanical devices (Oermann and others, 2000; Varekojis and others, 2003). Despite the role of CPT as the cornerstone therapy for airway clearance in cystic fibrosis, it continues to be associated with concerns that limit client compliance and satisfaction. With the mechanical devices there is a greater degree of client independence and compliance because they can be self-administered (Oermann and others, 2000).

Skill Performance Guidelines

The nurse plans the client's care and subsequent selection of CPT skills based on specific assessment findings. The following guidelines help the nurse in physical assessment and subsequent decision making:

1. Know the client's normal range of vital signs. Conditions such as atelectasis and pneumonia requiring CPT can affect a client's vital signs. The degree of change is related to the level of hypoxia, overall cardiopulmonary status, and tolerance to the procedure.

2. Know the client's present medications. Some medications, particularly diuretics and antihypertensives, cause fluid and hemodynamic changes. These changes may decrease the client's tolerance of the positional changes. Steroid medications, age, and malnutrition increase the client's risk of pathological rib fractures and often contraindicate rib shaking.

BOX 23-1 Contraindications for Postural Drainage

Intracranial pressure (ICP) >20 mm Hg
Head and neck injury until stabilized (*)
Active hemorrhage with hemodynamic instability (*)
Recent spinal surgery (e.g., laminectomy) or acute spinal injury
Active hemoptysis (*)
Empyema
Bronchopleural fistula
Pulmonary edema associated with congestive heart failure
Large pleural effusions
Pulmonary embolism
Aged, confused, or anxious patients who are unable to tolerate position change
Rib fracture, with or without flail chest
Surgical wound or healing tissue

TRENDELENBURG POSITION IS CONTRAINDICATED FOR THE FOLLOWING:

Clients in whom increased ICP is to be avoided or ICP greater than 20 mm Hg
Uncontrolled hypertension
Distended abdomen
Esophageal surgery
Recent gross hemoptysis (*)
Uncontrolled airway at risk for aspiration

Modified from AARC clinical practice guideline: postural drainage therapy, *Respir Care* 36(12):1418, 1991.
*Indicates absolute contraindication.

---

3. Know the client's medical and surgical history. Certain conditions, such as increased intracranial pressure, spinal cord injuries, or abdominal aneurysm resection, contraindicate the positional changes of postural drainage (Box 23-1). Thoracic trauma may contraindicate percussion, vibration and shaking.

4. Know the client's level of cognitive function. Alteration in mental status can make it difficult or impossible for the client to cough and expectorate secretions. Participation in controlled cough techniques requires the client to understand and to follow instructions. Congenital or acquired cognitive limitations may alter the client's ability to learn and to participate in these techniques. If the client is unable to cough and expectorate secretions, be prepared to suction out the trachea and mainstem bronchi.

5. Be aware of the client's exercise tolerance. Chest physiotherapy maneuvers are fatiguing. When the client is not used to physical activity, initial tolerance of the maneuvers may be decreased. However, with gradual increases in activity and planned CPT, the client's tolerance of the procedure improves.

SKILL 23-1 Performing Postural Drainage

Postural drainage achieves gravitational clearance of airway secretions from specific bronchial segments by using several different body positions. Each position drains a specific corresponding section of the tracheobronchial tree, either from the upper, middle, or lower lung field, into the trachea. Coughing or suctioning can then remove secretions from the trachea. Figure 23-1 shows the anatomy of the upper, middle, and lower lobe bronchi. The images in Table 23-1 show the bronchial lobes and the corresponding body postures for drainage of each.

Areas are selected for drainage based on (1) knowledge of the client's condition and disease process, (2) physical assessment of the chest, (3) chest x-ray results, and (4) the extent of the pathological condition and lobe involvement based on the physical examination and chest x-ray findings.

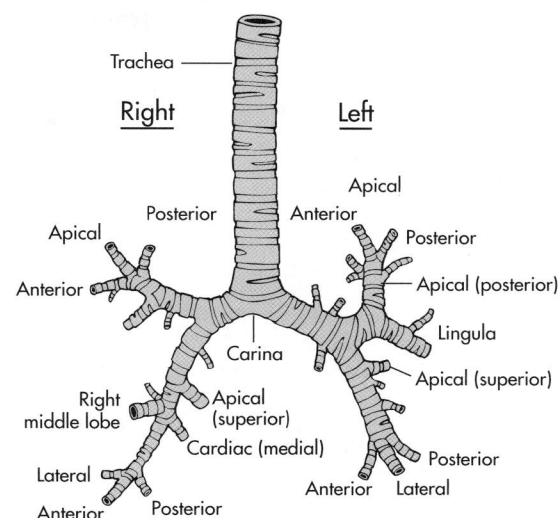

FIGURE **23-1** Tracheobronchial tree. (Modified from Frownfelter DL, Dean E: *Principles and practice of cardiopulmonary therapy,* ed 3, St. Louis, 1996, Mosby.)

DELEGATION CONSIDERATIONS

This skill may be delegated to appropriately trained assistive personnel in special situations. Following nursing assessment and review of x-ray results and a determination by the nurse that the client is stable and able to tolerate the procedure, the skill of performing postural drainage can be delegated to assistive personnel. Before delegating this skill the nurse must:

- Instruct assistive personnel to be alert for the client's tolerance of procedure, such as comfort level and changes in breathing pattern, and to immediately report changes to the nurse
- Instruct assistive personnel about specific client precautions related to disease or treatment
- Identify any positioning restrictions or problems unique to the client

EQUIPMENT

- ❏ Stethoscope
- ❏ Pulse oximeter
- ❏ Trendelenburg's hospital bed or tilt table
- ❏ Water in pitcher and glass
- ❏ Chair (for draining upper lobes)
- ❏ One to four pillows
- ❏ Tissues and paper bag
- ❏ Clear graduated screw-top container
- ❏ Suction equipment (if client unable to cough and clear own secretions)

TABLE 23-1 POSITIONS AND PROCEDURES FOR DRAINAGE, PERCUSSION, VIBRATION AND SHAKING

AREA AND PROCEDURE	ANATOMICAL AREA	POSITION OF CLIENT

LEFT AND RIGHT UPPER LOBE ANTERIOR APICAL BRONCHI

Have client sit in chair, or high Fowler, leaning back. Percuss and vibrate with heel of hands at shoulders and fingers over collarbones (clavicles) in front; can do both sides at same time. Note body posture and arm position of nurse. Nurse's back is kept straight, and elbows and knees are slightly flexed.

Direction of mucus flow through upper lobe anterior apical bronchi.

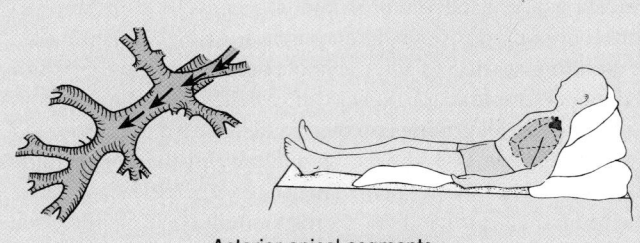

Anterior apical segments

Nurse positions hands for chest physiotherapy over left and right upper lobe anterior apical bronchi.

LEFT AND RIGHT UPPER LOBE POSTERIOR APICAL BRONCHI

Have client sit in chair, leaning forward on pillow or table. Percuss and vibrate with hands on either side of upper spine. Can do both sides at same time.

Direction of mucus flow through upper lobe posterior apical bronchi.

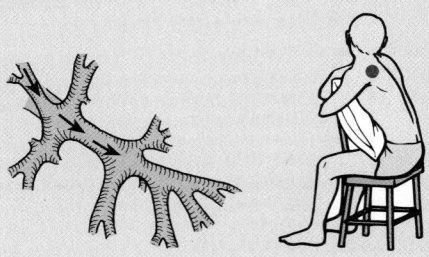

Posterior apical segments

Nurse positions hands for chest physiotherapy over left and right upper lobe posterior apical bronchi.

RIGHT AND LEFT ANTERIOR UPPER LOBE BRONCHI

Have client lie flat on back with small pillow under knees. Percuss and vibrate just below clavicle on either side of sternum.

Direction of mucus flow through anterior upper bronchi.

Left and right anterior lower lobe segments

Nurse positions hands for chest physiotherapy over right and left anterior upper lobe bronchi.

LEFT UPPER LOBE LINGULAR BRONCHUS

Have client lie on right side with arm over head in Trendelenburg's position, with foot of bed raised 30 cm (12 inches). Place pillow behind back, and roll client one-quarter turn onto pillow. Percuss and vibrate lateral to left nipple below axilla.

Direction of mucus flow through left upper lobe lingular bronchus.

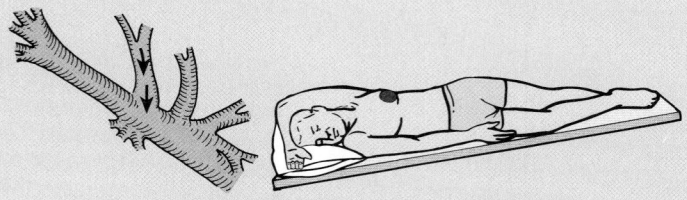

Left upper lobe lingular segment

Nurse positions hands for chest physiotherapy over left upper lobe lingular bronchus.

TABLE 23-1   **POSITIONS AND PROCEDURES FOR DRAINAGE, PERCUSSION, VIBRATION AND SHAKING — CONT'D**

AREA AND PROCEDURE	ANATOMICAL AREA	POSITION OF CLIENT

RIGHT MIDDLE LOBE BRONCHUS

Have client lie on left side or abdomen. Place pillow behind back and roll client one-quarter turn onto pillow. Percuss and vibrate to right nipple below axilla.

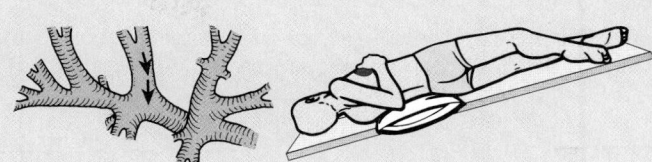

Right middle lobe segment

Direction of mucus flow through right middle lobe bronchus.

Nurse positions hands for chest physiotherapy over right middle lobe bronchus.

LEFT AND RIGHT ANTERIOR LOWER LOBE BRONCHI

Have client lie on back, with foot of bed elevated 45 to 50 cm (18 to 20 inches). Have knees bent on pillow. Percuss and vibrate over lower anterior ribs on both sides.

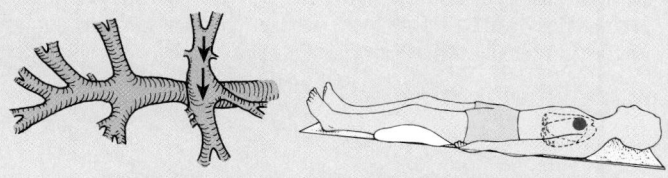

Left and right anterior upper lobe segments

Direction of mucus flow through anterior lower lobe bronchi.

Nurse positions hands for chest physiotherapy over left and right anterior lower lobe bronchi.

RIGHT LOWER LOBE LATERAL BRONCHUS

Have client lie on abdomen in Trendelenburg's position with foot of bed raised 45 to 50 cm (18 to 20 inches). Percuss and vibrate on left and right side of chest below shoulder blades (scapulas) posterior to midaxillary line.

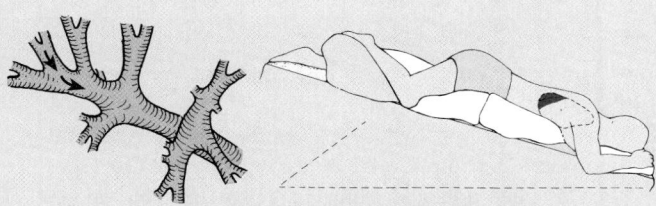

Left and right lower lateral lobe segments

Direction of mucus flow through right lower lobe lateral bronchus.

Nurse positions hands for chest physiotherapy over right lower lobe lateral bronchus.

LEFT LOWER LOBE LATERAL BRONCHUS

Have client lie on right side in Trendelenburg's position with foot of bed raised 45 to 50 cm (18 to 20 inches). Percuss and vibrate on left side of chest below scapulas posterior to midaxillary line.

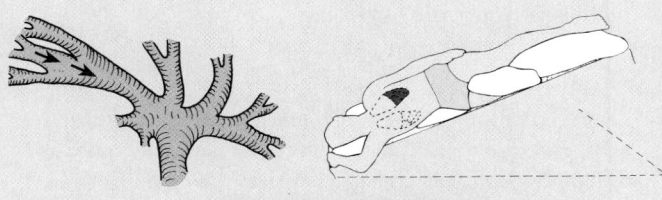

Left lower lobe lateral segment

Direction of mucus flow through left lower lobe lateral bronchus.

Nurse positions hands for chest physiotherapy over left lower lobe lateral bronchus.

Continued

TABLE 23-1   POSITIONS AND PROCEDURES FOR DRAINAGE, PERCUSSION, VIBRATION AND SHAKING — CONT'D

AREA AND PROCEDURE	ANATOMICAL AREA	POSITION OF CLIENT

RIGHT AND LEFT LOWER LOBE SUPERIOR BRONCHI

Have client lie flat on stomach with pillow under stomach. Percuss and vibrate below scapulas on either side of spine.

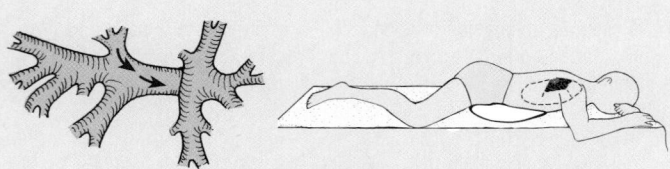

Right and left lower lobe superior segments

Direction of mucus flow through lower lobe superior bronchi.

Nurse positions hands for chest physiotherapy over right and left lower superior bronchi.

RIGHT AND LEFT POSTERIOR BASAL BRONCHI

Have client lie on stomach in Trendelenburg's position with foot of bed elevated 45 to 50 cm (18 to 20 inches). Percuss and vibrate over lower posterior ribs on either side of spine.

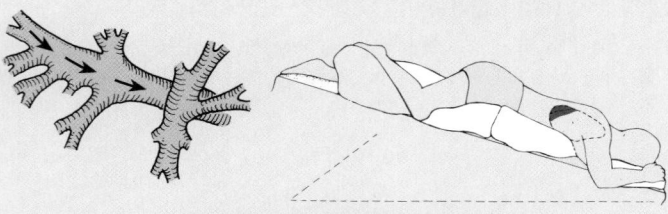

Right and left posterior segments

Direction of mucus flow through posterior basal bronchi.

Nurse positions hands for chest physiotherapy over right and left posterior lower lobe bronchi.

STEP	RATIONALE

ASSESSMENT

1. Assess client for history of decreased level of consciousness and muscle weakness, or disease processes, such as pneumonia and chronic obstructive pulmonary disease (COPD).

Conditions that pose risk for impaired airway clearance will require CPT.

- ### *Critical Decision Point*
  Contraindications to therapy may include contraindications to use of Trendelenburg's position or other postures that cause severe hypertension, severe hypoxemia, or severe shortness of breath. Procedure also contraindicated for head injuries; increased intracranial pressure; recent severe myocardial failure (see Box 23-1); lung hemorrhage; and certain surgical procedures, pain, or orthopedic traction.

2. Assess client and review medical record for signs and symptoms that indicate the need to perform postural drainage: x-ray film changes consistent with atelectasis, lobar collapse pneumonia, or bronchiectasis; ineffective coughing; thick, sticky, tenacious, and discolored secretions that are difficult to cough up; abnormal breath sounds, such as wheezing and rhonchi, or palpable fremitus.

X-ray film data and signs and symptoms indicate accumulation of pulmonary secretions and ineffective airway clearance.

STEP	**RATIONALE**
3. Identify which bronchial segments need to be drained by reviewing chest x-ray reports and performing auscultation over all lung fields to assess for decreased breath sounds, wheezes, and rhonchi. Palpate the chest wall over all lung fields in order to assess for increased or decreased fremitus and asymmetrical chest wall expansion.	Areas of lung congestion and postures for drainage will vary, depending on disease process, client condition, and clinical problems. Areas most in need of and responsive to postural drainage usually can be easily identified by presence of early inspiratory crackles and palpable crepitus, which indicate secretions in the airways. If airway is completely plugged, breath sounds and chest excursion decrease.
4. Assess vital signs and pulse oximetry.	Provides baseline to evaluate client's response to therapy.
5. Determine client's understanding of and ability to perform home postural drainage.	Allows nurse to identify potential need for instruction. Home care CPT is indicated in clients with chronic inability to clear lung secretions adequately, such as those with cystic fibrosis, chronic bronchitis, asthma, or bronchiectasis.

NURSING DIAGNOSES

- Ineffective airway clearance
- Deficient knowledge regarding postural drainage and airway clearance
- Ineffective breathing pattern
- Impaired gas exchange

Related factors are individualized based on client's condition or needs.

PLANNING

1. Expected outcomes following completion of procedures:	
• Lung sounds improve or become clear.	Airways are clear of retained secretions.
• Sputum is more easily expectorated or suctioned out on the trachea and mainstem bronchi.	CPT provides a mechanical stimulus to loosen secretions from the wall of the airway, and thus secretions are more easily expectorated.
• Secretions appear more normal in color and consistency.	Result of increased hydration.
• Dyspnea is decreased.	As secretions are removed, the client exchange of respiratory gases improves, and dyspnea gradually declines.
• Results of chest x-ray show improvements: lobar collapse and atelectasis are decreased or eliminated.	CPT improves atelectasis and facilitates the removal of secretions from the airways. As a result there is visual improvement on chest x-ray film.
2. Prepare client:	
a. Explain purpose and rationale for procedure. Explain positioning, sensations, how long it will take, and any discomforts or side effects.	Helps promote cooperation. Well-prepared client is usually more relaxed and comfortable, which is essential for effective drainage.
b. Encourage high fluid intake program unless contraindicated by other diseases and if physician approves. Maintain record of fluid intake and output.	Fluids thin secretions and make them easier to cough up. Clients need close monitoring and encouragement when first starting high fluid intake program.

- ***Critical Decision Point***
  Contraindications to high fluid intake are congestive heart failure and renal failure. When forcing fluids, build up daily intake gradually, and strive toward 8 to 12 8-oz glasses or until mucus is thin, white, and watery.

c. Plan treatments so they do not overlap with meals or tube feeding. Avoid postural drainage for 1 to 2 hours after meals or bolus tube feedings. Stop all continuous gastric tube feedings for 30 to 45 minutes before postural drainage. Check for residual feeding in client's stomach; if greater than 100 ml, hold treatment.	Postural drainage should be done when client's stomach is empty to avoid gastric reflux or vomiting and aspiration of stomach contents.

STEP	**RATIONALE**
d. Schedule treatments at appropriate times during day.	Postural drainage should be scheduled to obtain best results and should not conflict with other activities.
e. Have client remove any tight or restrictive clothing.	Helps client relax and promotes deep breathing.

IMPLEMENTATION

1. Perform hand hygiene, and apply gloves.	Reduces transmission of microorganisms.
2. Select congested areas to be drained based on assessment of all lung fields, clinical data, and chest x-ray data.	To be effective, treatment must be individualized to treat specific areas involved.
3. Place client in position to drain congested areas; first area selected may vary from client to client. (Refer to Table 23-1 for correct positioning to drain upper, middle, and lower lobe bronchi.) Help client assume position as needed. Teach client correct posture and arm and leg positioning. Place pillows for support and comfort. Drape client appropriately.	Specific positions are selected to drain each area involved. Proper client positioning promotes drainage of pulmonary secretions.
4. Have client maintain posture for 10 to 15 minutes.	In adults, draining each area takes time.
5. During 10 to 15 minutes of drainage in each posture, perform chest percussion and vibration and shaking (see Skill 23-3) over area being drained. Table 23-1 shows all postures and hand placement for percussion and vibration and shaking.	These maneuvers provide mechanical forces that aid in mobilization of airway secretions.
6. After 10 to 15 minutes of drainage in first posture, have client sit up and cough. If indicated, save expectorated secretions in a clear container. If client cannot cough, suctioning may need to be performed.	Any secretions mobilized into central airways should be removed by cough or suctioning before placing client into next drainage position. Coughing is most effective when client is sitting up and leaning forward.

- *Critical Decision Point*
  Sometimes client may experience transient dyspnea and fatigue because of irritation and bronchospasm from mobilizing secretions. These clients may benefit from an oscillating or vibrating device, such as an acapella device (see Skill 23-2). Dyspnea and bronchospasm usually subside after sputum is coughed up.

7. Have client rest briefly if necessary.	Short rest periods between postures can prevent fatigue and help client better tolerate therapy.
8. Have client take sips of water.	Keeping mouth moist aids in expectoration of secretions.
9. Repeat Steps 3 through 8 until all congested areas selected have been drained. Each treatment should not exceed 30 to 60 minutes.	Postural drainage is used only to drain areas involved and is based on individual assessment.
10. Perform hand hygiene.	Reduces transmission of microorganisms.

EVALUATION

1. Auscultate lung fields.	Clearance of secretions usually relieves gurgling, early inspiratory crackles, and palpable crepitus.
2. Inspect character and amount of sputum.	Determines if secretions are adequately thinned.
3. Review diagnostic reports, including sputum collections/cultures, chest x-ray films, and blood gas levels.	Provides objective data on improvements in lung function.
4. Obtain vital signs, pulse oximetry.	Procedure may result in dysrhythmias and decreases in oxygen saturation in some clients.
5. Have client explain purpose and procedure for postural drainage.	Evaluates client's understanding of procedure.

Recording and Reporting

- Record in nurses' notes pretherapy and posttherapy assessment of chest and chest x-ray findings; frequency and duration of treatment; postures used and bronchial segments drained; cough effectiveness; need for suctioning; color, amount, and consistency of sputum; hemoptysis or other unexpected outcomes; and client's tolerance and reactions.
- If client and family receive instruction in home care, chart instructions given, understanding of therapy, demonstration of skill, client acceptance of home care, barriers to learning and implementation, and referral for follow-up, that is, home care, rehabilitation, or pulmonary nurse specialist.

Unexpected Outcomes	Related Interventions
1. Client experiences severe dyspnea, bronchospasm, hypoxemia, hypercarbia, and/or is unable to tolerate treatment.	• Identify clients at risk such as (1) those with severe lung disease who have high $PaCO_2$ levels and/or who require high concentrations of oxygen and (2) those who are severely debilitated with altered mental status. • Discontinue or modify and shorten treatments. • Give bronchodilators 20 minutes before CPT. • Notify physician. • Suction and ventilate with bag-valve-mask as needed, and closely monitor arterial blood gas (ABG) levels, O_2 saturation, and vital signs.
2. Little to no secretions are obtained, and there is no improvement in chest assessment or chest x-ray results.	• Initially, increase treatments, and encourage and teach coughing exercises (there may be a lack of secretions, or they may be too thick to cough up). • Consult physician because client may need sputum culture, change in antibiotics, or a bronchoscopy to remove thick mucous plugs. • Improve hydration if dehydrated.
3. Hemoptysis occurs, or client develops acute hypotension, severe chest pain, vomiting, aspiration, and/or dysrhythmias.	• Stop therapy, and obtain vital signs. • Notify physician. • Remain calm, stay with client, call for help, and keep client comfortable, calm, warm, and quiet. • Assess for infection and erosion of blood vessel or airway wall. • If client vomits or aspirates, suction airway and place client on his or her side.
4. Client has difficulty tolerating treatment, and/or family is unable to learn technique for home use.	• Modify treatments by shortening duration or eliminating techniques that cause discomfort. • Consider trial use of chest vest because it is usually well tolerated and can be self-applied so client can use independently at home. • Use an oscillating or vibrating airway clearance mechanism, such as an acapella device (Skill 23-2) in conjunction with postural drainage.

Teaching Considerations

- Best times for treatments are (1) in morning before breakfast, when client can clear secretions that accumulate overnight, and (2) about 1 hour before bedtime, so that lungs are clear before sleeping and client has time after treatment to cough up any mobilized secretions. Frequency depends on need and client's tolerance and may vary from once daily to every 2 to 4 hours in an acute situation.
- If client is receiving inhaled bronchodilators or aerosol treatment, postural drainage should be done 20 minutes after such therapy. Plan for rest period after postural drainage.
- Do not schedule major activities (such as exercise or bath) right after chest therapy treatment, especially in clients with severe obstructive lung disease.
- Instruct client's family or primary caregiver to recognize when the client's respiratory status requires breathing exercises or postural drainage.
- Encourage primary caregiver or family member to encourage the client to participate in physical activities that will increase respiratory efficiency.
- Teach client and significant others how to assume postures at home. Some postures may need to be modified to meet individual needs; for example, side-lying Trendelenburg's position to drain lateral lower lobes may have to be done with client lying flat on side or in side-lying semi-Fowler's position if client is very short of breath.

Pediatric Considerations

- In the child with cystic fibrosis, chest physiotherapy is a cornerstone therapy and is usually performed at least twice daily, on rising in the morning and in the evening (Hockenberry and others, 2003). Many CF clients use the chest vest when at home so they are independent.
- Chest physiotherapy is not recommended during acute exacerbations of asthma.

Gerontological Considerations

- Postural drainage in older adults should be done while taking extra care and assessment. Change positions more slowly, and closely assess for any changes in oxygen saturation or vital signs with position changes.
- Older adults with chronic cardiac and pulmonary conditions may not tolerate a supine or side-lying position for CPT. In these positions clients experience decline in forced vital capacity (FVC) and subsequent decline in oxygen saturation (Manning and others, 1999).

Home Care Considerations

- Assess home environment for ventilation. Determine client's access to clean, fresh air. Assess the home for air conditioning and client's reaction to air conditioning.
- Discuss need for home postural drainage with family. Assess if they perceive need for home care and if any barriers exist to learning and implementing home program. If specialized home or outpatient follow-up is needed, refer client to pulmonary nurse specialist, pulmonary rehabilitation team, or home care personnel.
- Obtain foam wedge or multiple pillows for correct positioning (Rice, 2000).
- In home setting the Trendelenburg's position can be achieved in several ways. Select the most comfortable and practical method that best suits client:
  - Client can purchase slant board or make one out of old door or tabletop. Surface can be padded with foam or blankets.
  - Client's hips can be elevated with stack of old newspapers and pillows or foam wedge. These props tend to be uncomfortable and often flatten out because of client's body weight.
  - Wedge or stack of papers can be placed under bed board.

SKILL 23-2 Using an Acapella Device

DELEGATION CONSIDERATIONS

See Skill 23-1. This skill may be delegated to appropriately trained personnel in special circumstances. The nurse is responsible for determining that the procedure is appropriate and that the client is able to tolerate the procedure and evaluating the client's response to the procedure. Before delegating this procedure the nurse must:

- Instruct assistive personnel to be alert for the client's tolerance of procedure, such as comfort level and changes in breathing pattern, and to immediately report changes to the nurse
- Instruct assistive personnel about specific client precautions related to disease or treatment
- Identify any positioning restrictions or problems unique to the client

EQUIPMENT

- ❑ Stethoscope
- ❑ Pulse oximeter
- ❑ Trendelenburg's hospital bed or tilt table
- ❑ Water in pitcher and glass
- ❑ Chair (for draining upper lobes)
- ❑ One to four pillows
- ❑ Tissues and paper bag
- ❑ Clear graduated screw-top container
- ❑ Suction equipment (if client unable to cough and clear own secretions)
- ❑ Acapella device
- ❑ Client education materials

STEP	RATIONALE
1. Verify the need for a physician's order per agency's policy.	
2. Assess client for signs and symptoms indicating the need for this treatment.	This device combines resistive features of positive expiratory pressure and vibration to mobilize airway sectretions. Clients with chronic conditions, such as cystic fibrosis, appear to receive the greatest benefit of this type of treatment (Holland and others, 2003; Langenderfer, 1998). See Box 23-1, p. 798 for contraindications.
3. Assess client and family understanding of the device and procedure and explain and clarify procedure as needed.	
4. Prepare acapella device; initial setting: Turn acapella frequency adjustment dial counterclockwise to lowest resistance setting. As client improves or becomes more proficient adjust the proper resistance level upward by turning the dial clockwise.	This initial setting helps client to adjust to the device and benefit from the treatment.

- **Critical Decision Point**

Determine if aerosol drug therapy is ordered. If so, attach a neubulizer to the end of the acapella valve.

5. Instruct client to (Fink and Mahlmeister, 2002):	
a. Sit comfortably.	
b. Take in a breath that is larger than normal, but not to fill lungs completely.	
c. Place mouthpiece into the mouth, maintaining a tight seal.	
d. Hold breath for 2 to 3 seconds.	
e. To try not to cough and to exhale slowly for 3 to 4 seconds through the device, while it is vibrating.	Vibrations seem to reduce the viscosity of mucous and improves the client's ability to cough up and expectorate the secretions. (Langenderfer, 1998; Volsko and others, 2003).

- **Critical Decision Point**

If client cannot maintain an exhalation for this length of time, adjust the dial clockwise. Clockwise adjustment increases the resistance of the vibrating opening, which will allow the patient to exhale at a lower flow rate.

   f. Repeat cycle for 10 to 20 breaths as tolerated
   g. Remove mouthpiece and have client perform 2 to 3 "huffs": coughs
   h. Repeat steps a through gas ordered.
6. Auscultate lung fields
7. Obtain vital signs, pulse oximetry
8. Inspect color, character, and amount of sputum.

SKILL 23-3 Performing Percussion, Vibration, and Shaking

During postural drainage, physical maneuvers, such as percussion, vibration, and shaking, can be performed on the rib cage over lung tissue by a trained nurse, therapist, or family member. The techniques are done on specific parts of the rib cage over each area being drained. Normally the mucociliary escalator and cough transport can effectively clear airway secretions. When airway clearance is impaired in certain disease states, however, the techniques of percussion, vibration, and shaking combined with postural drainage help to clear mucus.

Percussion involves clapping the chest wall with cupped hands. If done correctly, it painlessly sets up vibrations in the chest to dislodge retained secretions. Vibration is a sustained contraction of the upper extremities of the caregiver. Vibration produces a downward vibrating pressure, done only during exhalation, with the flat part of the palm over the area being drained. Shaking is a more vigorous downward rocking motion on the rib cage done with the flat part of the hand during exhalation. These last two maneuvers are performed as the client exhales through pursed lips. They augment the natural movement of the rib cage during exhalation and assist with secretion clearance.

The natural expiratory movement of the chest wall involves (1) a decrease in the lateral and anteroposterior diameter of the lower ribs as they move downward and closer together and (2) a decrease in the anteroposterior diameter of the upper chest as the sternum, the clavicles, and the upper rib cage move downward. Pressure during vibration and shaking is always directed toward these natural expiratory movements of the rib cage. They are more effective if the client relaxes the rib cage muscles during exhalation and blows out using abdominal muscles. This relaxation during vibration and shaking enhances the rocking motion of the rib cage, makes vibration optimal, and assists in dislodging mucous plugs.

In diseases associated with mucus plugging, such as bronchitis and asthma, air is trapped behind obstructed airways, and the rib cage frequently becomes hyperinflated. The ribs can become somewhat fixed in their upward and outward position and lose their excursion and flexibility; vibration and shaking improves both. Vibration is better tolerated than percussion or shaking in the immediate postsurgical client, providing no other contraindications exist.

Before attempting to master these techniques, the nurse must know that each posture is associated with a general area of the rib cage to be percussed and vibrated. These postures and the specific areas are shown in Table 23-1. Generally, for any given posture the area to be percussed and vibrated can be thought of as that portion of the rib cage at the greatest vertical height. Areas that are never percussed or vibrated regardless of their vertical height include the clavicles, breast tissue, sternum, spine, waist, and abdomen. Percussion, vibration, and shaking should be performed only over the ribs.

DELEGATION CONSIDERATIONS

This skill may be delegated to assistive personnel. Before delegation the nurse must perform a respiratory assessment and review the client's chest x-ray film to determine that the client is stable, which areas of the lungs are affected, and specific positions for the client to assume. Before delegating this skill the nurse must:

* Instruct assistive personnel to be alert for the client's tolerance of procedure, to monitor vital signs, and to be alert to any client precautions related to disease or treatment
* Instruct assistive personnel to report any problems with tolerance of the procedure, pain, dyspnea, or changes in vital signs

EQUIPMENT

❑ Hospital bed or tilt table placed in Trendelenburg's position
❑ Chair (for upper lobes)
❑ One to four pillows
❑ Water pitcher and glass
❑ Tissues and paper bag
❑ Clear graduated screw-top container
❑ Mechanical vibrator or percussor (optional)
❑ Single layer of clothing
❑ Clean gloves
❑ Suction equipment (optional)

STEP	RATIONALE

ASSESSMENT

1. Assess breathing pattern, including muscles used for breathing, respiratory rate and depth, extent of excursion, and chest wall movement.

Certain disease states place client at risk for developing an ineffective breathing pattern. Rapid, shallow breathing with client using accessory muscles is seen in chronic obstructive lung disease, asthma, pain, hypoxemia, pneumonia, and atelectasis.

STEP	RATIONALE

2. Assess client and review medical record for signs and symptoms and conditions that indicate need to perform these skills (see Skill 23-1, Assessment).

When tolerated and not contraindicated, these techniques are done during postural drainage.

• *Critical Decision Point*
Percussion, vibration, and shaking may be contraindicated in certain situations, including rib fracture, fracture of other rib cage structures such as clavicle or sternum, pain, severe dyspnea, and severe osteoporosis, so nurse should obtain physician's order. Thin, frail clients with osteoporosis are most susceptible to injury and should be taught other secretion control measures (e.g., forceful coughing, humidification).

3. Identify and assess area of rib cage over bronchial segment being drained for pain, tenderness, abnormal configuration, abnormal excursion or chest wall movement during breathing, muscle tension.

Conditions may contraindicate procedure. Chest wall areas to be assessed and to receive percussion, vibration, and shaking vary with each postural drainage position (see Table 23-1).

4. Assess client's understanding and ability to cooperate with therapy, both in hospital and at home.

Assessment allows nurse to identify potential need for instruction of client, family, or significant others.

NURSING DIAGNOSES
- Ineffective airway clearance
- Ineffective breathing pattern
- Impaired gas exchange

- Deficient knowledge regarding the techniques of chest therapy

Related factors are individualized based on client's condition or needs.

PLANNING

1. Expected outcomes following completion of procedure:
   - Breathing pattern improves.
   - Sputum is more easily expectorated.

   Airways are clear of retained secretions.
   Vibration and shaking are mechanical stimuli to help loosen secretions from the wall of the airway and thus are more easily expectorated.

   - Secretions appear more normal in color and consistency. Over time they will decrease in volume.
   - Dyspnea is decreased.

   Hydration is successful in thinning secretions.

   As secretions are removed, the client exchange of respiratory gases improves, and dyspnea gradually declines.

   - Results of pulmonary function and blood gas studies improve.

   Reduced airway secretions promote proper transfer of oxygen to the pulmonary circulation, which is then delivered to the tissues. In turn there is greater excretion of carbon dioxide (CO_2) by the pulmonary system.

   - Body temperature, white blood cell count, and chest x-ray films are normal.

   No infectious process developing.

2. Prepare client:
   a. Explain procedure in detail: client's positioning, sensations, how it will be done, how long it will take, and any discomforts or side effects.

   Percussion, vibration, and shaking cannot be done effectively without client's cooperation.

   b. Encourage and help client to relax and deep breathe during procedure. Have client practice exhaling slowly through pursed lips while relaxing chest wall muscles. Client should blow out using abdominal muscles, not rib cage muscles.

   Percussion, vibration, and shaking are most effective if client breathes properly and works well with therapist. If done properly, these techniques should not cause pain or discomfort.

STEP	RATIONALE

IMPLEMENTATION

1. Perform hand hygiene and apply gloves.
2. With client placed in appropriate drainage position (see Skill 23-1, Implementation, steps 1 to 3), assess and identify chest wall area to be percussed and vibrated (see Table 23-1).

In general, for any given posture, rib cage area to be percussed and vibrated is in highest vertical position. Careful assessment of rib cage movement guides nurse in following natural movement during vibration and shaking.

3. Instruct client to relax by using one of these techniques: take slow, deep breaths, and exhale; use abdominal, diaphragmatic, or pursed-lip breathing.

Client should not lie passively but should relax and take deep breaths.

4. Use good body mechanics when clapping: elevate bed to comfortable working height, and stand close to bed with arms directly in front and knees slightly bent. Avoid bending over.

Use of good body mechanics avoids undue strain on therapist's back and legs.

5. Begin percussion on appropriate part of chest wall over draining area (see Table 23-1). Perform percussion for 3 to 5 minutes in each posture as tolerated. Always ask if client is experiencing any discomfort, such as undue pressure or stinging of the skin.

Percussion helps clear mucus and should be painless, because air in therapist's hand acts as cushion.

   a. Place hands side by side on chest wall over area to be drained. Hands should be cupped with fingers and thumbs held tightly together. Make sure that entire outer portion of hand makes contact with chest wall to avoid air leaks (see Table 23-1).

This hand position creates an air pocket that sends vibrations through the chest wall but is not painful.

   b. When clapping, most of arm movement should come from the elbow and wrist joints. Clapping can be done for 5 minutes without stopping or 2 to 3 minutes, alternating with vibration and shaking.

Using the larger muscles of the arms and shoulders improves endurance.

   c. Alternately clap chest with cupped hands to create rhythmic popping sound resembling galloping horse. Clapping can be done at moderate or fast speed; whichever is most comfortable and effective.

The popping sound comes from the air pocket that is formed between the hand and the chest wall.

6. Perform chest wall vibration and shaking over each area being drained. See Table 23-1 for correct hand position to use in each posture. Vibrations are usually done in sets of three followed by coughing so that any mobilized mucus can be expectorated.

Vibration and shaking during slow exhalation and coughing help to clear mucus.

   a. To perform vibration, gently place hands over area being drained, and have client take slow, deep breath through nose.

Slow inhalation helps relaxation.

   b. Gently resist chest wall as it rises during inhalation.
   c. Have client hold breath and then exhale through pursed lips, while contracting abdominal muscles and relaxing chest wall muscles. Chest wall should relax and fall.

Slight resistance on inhalation aids in expansion of rib cage.
Pursed-lip breathing makes exhalation easier. Relaxation of the chest wall makes vibrations more effective.

   d. While client is exhaling, gently push down and vibrate with flat part of hand.
   e. Repeat vibration three times, and then have client cascade cough by taking deep breath and doing series of small coughs until end of breath. Client should not inhale between coughs. Vibrate chest wall as client coughs. When applying pressure to ribs, always follow natural movement of rib cage. As client becomes comfortable and learns to relax rib cage during exhalation, chest wall movement and flexibility will increase. Allow client to sit up and cough as needed.

Vibrate only during exhalation so as to follow the natural downward movement of the rib cage.
Coughing with vibrations aids in clearing mucus.

STEP	RATIONALE
7. Assess client's tolerance of vibration and ability to relax chest wall and breathe properly as instructed.	Client's poor tolerance may necessitate discontinuing procedure.
8. Perform shaking with vibration.	Shaking helps to clear secretions from airway.
a. Place flat part of hand over area being drained. Maintain good body mechanics: lower bed so client is about at nurse's hip level; work with arms directly in front; maintain good leverage; do not lean over or strain back.	Proper positioning of therapist prevents strain on back muscles.
b. Have client inhale slowly through nose.	
c. During inhalation, apply light pressure on ribs and stretch skin so it is tight.	
d. Have client hold breath for 2 seconds.	
e. As client exhales, increase pressure. Maintain pressure while applying intermittent rocking motion on ribs. Pressure is directed toward following natural expiratory rib cage movement.	This helps to dislodge mucus. It may be better tolerated than postural drainage in postoperative clients (Frownfelter and Dean, 1996).
f. Client must exhale through pursed lips and relax chest wall muscles as much as possible.	If rib cage is relaxed, ribs can be rocked more vigorously in direction they naturally move.
g. Repeat shaking three times, have client inhale deeply, and then do rib shaking during cascade cough.	Coughing helps to clear mobilized secretions.
h. Perform a total of three or four sets of three vibrations and shaking and coughing in each posture as tolerated. Strength and frequency of vibration and shaking will vary: vibration requires all muscles in arm and shoulder to contract and tremble; shaking requires applying controlled pressure from shoulders and back while slightly leaning on chest; rocking motion is created by flexing and extending elbows using triceps.	
i. Suction if client is unable to cough up mucus (see Chapter 24).	
9. In each posture, complete vibration and shaking.	
10. If long-term therapy is needed, teach client and significant others the procedure for home use. If they cannot learn or use, refer for outpatient or home health follow-up.	Long-term use of these techniques can optimize airway clearance, reduce symptoms and infection, and improve chest mobility.

EVALUATION

1. Evaluate changes in chest assessment following procedure.	These maneuvers usually relieve signs of congestion, slow respiratory rate, and improve chest mobility and expansion.
2. Inspect character of mucus.	Inspection determines if mucus is adequately thinned.
3. Review diagnostic test results for pulmonary function.	This determines airway clearance and oxygenation status.
4. Observe caregiver during percussion, vibration, and shaking.	Return demonstration is an effective means to measure learning.

Recording and Reporting

- When treatment is in conjunction with postural drainage, record pretherapy and posttherapy pulmonary assessment and mobility status, client's ability to cooperate with therapy, client tolerance, duration of therapy, cough effectiveness, and sputum quality.
- Document client teaching, especially progress of client and family to independently perform percussion, vibration, and shaking.

Unexpected Outcomes	Related Interventions
1. Client experiences severe dyspnea with bronchospasm, hypoxemia, and hypercarbia.	• Identify clients at risk for this unexpected outcome such as those with impending respiratory failure. • Modify or stop therapy; they may only tolerate 3 to 5 minutes of CPT per hour. • Give bronchodilators before CPT.
2. Hemoptysis occurs.	• If severe, stop therapy, call physician, remain calm, stay with client, call for help, and keep client comfortable, calm, warm, and quiet.
3. Client experiences rib fractures, rib pain, and or chest wall pain.	• Notify physician and obtain a chest x-ray examination. Stop percussion, vibration, and rib shaking.
4. No secretions are obtained, and there is no improvement in chest examination or chest x-ray results.	• If still no change after several days of therapy, stop therapy. • Try increased hydration and suctioning if needed. • Teach controlled coughing exercises, and try mechanical devices if available.

Teaching Considerations

* Best times for treatments are (1) in the morning before breakfast, when client can clear secretions that accumulate overnight, and (2) about 1 hour before bedtime, so that lungs are clear before sleeping and client has time after treatment to cough up any mobilized secretions. Frequency depends on need and client's tolerance and may vary from once daily to every 2 to 4 hours in an acute situation.
* If client is receiving inhaled bronchodilators or aerosol treatment, postural drainage should be done 20 minutes after such therapy. Plan for rest period after postural drainage.
* Do not schedule major activities (such as exercise or bath) right after chest therapy treatment, especially in clients with severe obstructive lung disease.
* Instruct client's family or primary caregiver to recognize when the client's respiratory status requires breathing exercises or postural drainage.
* Encourage primary caregiver or family member to encourage the client to participate in physical activities that will increase respiratory efficiency.
* Teach client and significant others how to assume postures at home. Some postures may need to be modified to meet individual needs; for example, side-lying Trendelenburg's position to drain lateral lower lobes may have to be done with client lying flat on side or in side-lying semi-Fowler's position if client is very short of breath.

Pediatric Considerations

* Hand-held vibrators should be approved for use for a child in an oxygen-enriched environment (Hockenberry and others, 2003).
* Larger children may benefit from a more powerful vibrator (Hockenberry and others, 2003).

Gerontological Considerations

* Percussion, vibration, and shaking usually have to be done more gently in older adults.
* In frail older adults use a mechanical vibrator on low speed instead of manual percussion, vibration, and shaking.

Home Care Considerations

* Mechanical devices are sometimes used at home if (1) a trained therapist is not available or (2) client does not tolerate manual therapy. They are available through most home equipment companies.
* If home therapy is needed, instruct a family member in techniques of percussion, vibration, and shaking. Assess willingness to learn and follow through in home setting.

FOCUS *on* CLINICAL PRACTICE

Mr. Walker is a 69-year-old retired carpenter with a history of bronchitis, tobacco abuse, hypertension, and diabetes who was admitted to the hospital 3 days ago for colectomy to remove a colonic mass. Postoperatively he initially did well and was extubated in the recovery area and sent to the nursing division. Two day later he spiked a fever to 38.8° C and developed bilateral lower lobe atelectasis and lobar collapse of his right middle lobe.

1. Chest physiotherapy was ordered. What positions would you use?
2. Based on the chest x-ray findings, what would you expect to find on physical examination of the chest, and what additional signs and symptoms would you expect to see?

3. After 24 hours of aggressive CPT a chest x-ray examination was repeated. It showed a remarkable improvement with good expansion of the right middle lobe and markedly improved aeration of the lower lobes. Were the improvements in the x-ray examination a result of the CPT? What other clinical improvement would you expect?
4. What would you document regarding the CPT and clinical assessment?

NCLEX REVIEW QUESTIONS

1. Susan Davis was hospitalized with respiratory failure due to exacerbation of severe emphysema and bronchiectasis. Chest x-ray examination revealed good lung expansion except for left lower lobe collapse. She was febrile at 38.8° C and complained of increased shortness of breath and sputum production. What positions would you use for CPT in this client?
   1. Right side-lying Trendelenburg's
   2. Left side-lying Trendelenburg's
   3. Right side-lying flat
   4. Right side-lying Trendelenburg's with one-quarter turn back onto a pillow
2. Leroy Frank was admitted with recurrence of bilateral upper lobe lung abscesses due to tuberculosis. Chest computed tomography (CT) examination showed fluid- and air-filled abscesses in bilateral upper lobes

anteriorly. What positions would you use to drain these areas?
   1. Sitting up in a chair and leaning backward onto a pillow
   2. Sitting up in a chair and leaning forward onto a pillow or table
   3. Lying on back flat in bed
   4. Lying prone with bed flat
3. Research in the area of chest physiotherapy has shown CPT to have the most pronounced beneficial effects in clients with which of the following disease processes?
   1. Tuberculosis
   2. Pneumonia
   3. Cystic fibrosis
   4. Emphysema

References

AARC clinical practice guideline: postural drainage therapy, *Respir Care* 36(12):1418, 1991.

Fink JB, Mahlmeister MJ: High frequency oscillation of the airway and chest wall. *Resp Care,* 47(7):797, 2002.

Frownfelter DL, Dean E: *Principles and practice of cardiopulmonary therapy,* ed 3, St. Louis, 1996, Mosby.

Hockenberry MJ and others: *Wong's nursing care of infants and children,* ed 7, St. Louis, 2003, Mosby.

Jones AP, Rowe BH: Bronchopulmonary hygiene physical therapy in chronic obstructive pulmonary disease and bronchiectasis (Cochrane Review), *The Cochrane Library,* issue 3, Oxford, UK, 1999, Update Software.

Langenderfer B: Alternatives to percussion and postural drainage: a review of mucus clearance therapies—percussion and postural drainage, autogenic, positive expiratory pressure, flutter valve, intrapulmonary percussive ventilation, and high-frequency chest compression with the Thairapy Vest, *J Cardiopulmon Rehab,* 18(4):282, 1998.

Manning F and others: Effects of side lying on lung function in older individuals, *Phys Ther* 79(5):456, 1999.

Rice R: *Manual of home health nursing procedures,* ed 2, St. Louis, 2000, Mosby.

Volsko TA, DiFiore, JM, Chatburn RL: Performance comparison of two oscillating positive expiratory pressure devices: acapella versus flutter, *Resp Care* 48(2):124, 2003.

Research References

Gondor M and others: Comparison of flutter device and chest physical therapy in the treatment of cystic fibrosis pulmonary exacerbation, *Pediatr Pulmonol* 28:255, 1999.

Holland AE and others: Non-invasive ventilation assists chest physiotherapy in adults with acute exacerbations of cystic fibrosis, *Thorax* 58:880, 2003.

Oermann CM and others: Validation of an instrument measuring patient satisfaction with chest physiotherapy techniques in cystic fibrosis, *Chest* 118:92, 2000.

Oermann CM and others: Comparison of high-frequency chest wall oscillation and oscillating positive expiratory pressure in the home management of cystic fibrosis: a pilot study, *Pediatr Pulmonol* 32:372, 2001.

Varekojis SM and others: A comparison of the therapeutic effectiveness of and preference for postural drainage and percussion, intrapulmonary percussive ventilation, and high-frequency chest wall compression in hospitalized cystic fibrosis patients, *Respir Care* 48(1):24, 2003.

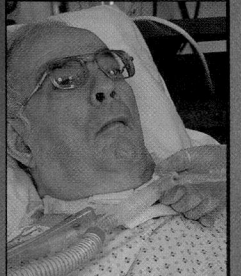

24

Airway Management

MEDIA RESOURCES

Evolve Site *evolve*
http://evolve.elsevier.com/Perry/skills
- Weblinks
- Video clips
- Mosby's Nursing Skills Video Exercises

Mosby's Nursing Skills Videos/CD-ROM
- *Oxygenation Video:* Tracheostomy care
- *Suctioning Video:* Preprocedure and postprocedure assessments; oropharyngeal suctioning; nasotracheal suctioning; suctioning and artificial airway

Many courses of action are available to promote an open or patent airway, which has the potential to become obstructed by mucus, mechanical obstruction (i.e., soft tissue in upper airway), or a foreign body. These actions may not require a physician's order, depending on the situation. The physician should be consulted if there are any concerns about the appropriateness of the intervention or when an airway obstruction is present, even when the obstruction was relieved by treatment.

Airway management involves maintaining the patency of the nose and upper airway, as well as the trachea and lower airway respiratory systems. Hydration, positioning, nutrition, chest therapy airway clearance techniques, mucous clearance device therapy, deep breathing, coughing, humidity, and aerosol therapy are noninvasive techniques that are helpful in maintaining a patent airway. For selected clients, medications such as antibiotics, bronchodilators, steroids, decongestants, antihistamines, and expectorants are adjuncts to these therapies.

When a client is unable to clear airway secretions with coughing, chest physiotherapy, or other noninvasive techniques, the client is unable to maintain a patent airway and is at risk for respiratory distress. More invasive measures, such as suctioning, directed at maintaining a patent airway are necessary, especially in the weak, confused, or critically ill client. This chapter focuses on nonemergent, invasive techniques to maintain airway patency, including artificial airways. The techniques discussed include suctioning the anatomical and artificial airways (endotracheal tube, tracheostomy tube), caring for clients with an endotracheal tube or a tracheostomy tube, and properly inflating the cuff on an artificial airway.

Evidence-Based Practice Trends

Preoxygenation and deep breathing, sometimes referred to as hyperventilation, assist in reducing suction-induced hypoxemia (Day and others, 2002). Preoxygenation is providing the client with a short-term increase in supplemental oxygen, such as increasing oxygen flow rate on nasal cannula or oxygen mask, increasing the percent of inspired oxygen of breaths delivered by the mechanical ventilator, or increasing oxygen flow rates to artificial airways. Preoxygenation should be used with caution in oxygen-sensitive clients, such as those with chronic heart and lung conditions and those with pneumonia. Hyperinflation is the process of providing 100% oxygen to the client before airway suctioning. It decreases the risk for atelectasis caused by negative pressure of suctioning (St. John, 1999). During preoxygenation a large proportion of resident lung gas is converted to 100% oxygen, which helps to offset changes in lung oxygen levels during suctioning (Akgul and Akyolcu, 2002; Wood, 1998).

Following suctioning, the client's oxygen must be readjusted as ordered by the physician to avoid increased risk of oxygen toxicity. In addition, there is also a risk for absorption atelectasis from prolonged administration of high concentrations of oxygen and increased carbon dioxide retention in clients with chronic obstructive lung diseases (Day and others, 2002).

The practice of normal saline instillation (NSI) into artificial airways to improve secretion removal is inconclusive. Clinical studies conducted to compare the results of suctioning following NSI with standard suctioning have not shown any clinical or significant results (Akgul and Akyolcu, 2002; Blackwood, 1999; Moore, 2003). There are anecdotal results supporting the theory that NSI stimulates the client to cough and as a result the airway secretions are loosened and dislodged. The practice of NSI has the potential of causing detrimental effects, such as decreased heart rate and hypotension, and as a result there is an adverse effect on the client's oxygen status (Wood, 1998).

There are psychosocial consequences of airway suctioning. Clients who remember the suctioning report it as painful, suffocating, or stressful. Clients recalled some of the physiological results of suctioning, such as tachycardia, confusion, shortness of breath, and dizziness (Leur, 2003).

Researchers developed a minimally invasive airway suctioning (MIAS) procedure in which the endotracheal tube was suctioned, and additional noninvasive measures, such as coughing, were used to improve airway clearance. These results noted no difference in complication or mortality rates of the study groups. However, once the clients' level of health returned, those clients who had the MAIS did not remember the sensations of pain, suffocation, or stress associated with the procedure (Leur and others, 2003).

Cultural Considerations

Communication is vital to all people in all cultures. Once a client has an artificial airway in place, communication is altered and clients, especially those from other cultures, feel frightened, frustrated, and vulnerable. In addition, the measures used to maintain airway patency are also new and frightening. Assess the meaning of oropharyngeal suctioning to the client and family members. Among Vietnamese, illness is believe to enter through the mouth, and they may interpret suctioning as introducing illness to the client (Shanahan and Brayshaw, 1995). Explain anticipated effects such as gagging and tearing, which can be very distressing to family members.

Provide culturally congruent explanations of the purpose and therapeutic effects of the procedure. Whenever possible provide demonstration as much as possible, and encourage client and family members to ask questions. If available, a professional interpreter is a valuable asset for explanation of procedures, especially those that are invasive and need to be repeated multiple times, such as suctioning and tracheostomy tube care. If an interpreter is not available, have a family or community member explain invasive procedures such as insertion of endotracheal tube or tracheostomy. Many clients from the Third World may not have any experience with the procedure. Encourage family members at the bedside to provide support for a client who has limited English proficiency. Collaborate with the family in providing alternative means of communication for the client.

tubes, a decreased level of consciousness, and a decreased swallowing ability.

4. Determine if the client has a history of nasal problems, such as nasal trauma, nasal polyps, deviated nasal septum, or chronic sinus. Allergy problems causing mucosal swelling may narrow nasal passages, which can affect the nurse's ability to easily pass a suction catheter.

5. Review the client's respiratory assessments. It is important to know what the client's condition has been for the past 4, 8, 12, 16, or 24 hours. These are relative baseline measurements that assist the nurse in distinguishing between gradual and acute changes in the client's status.

6. Perform a systematic respiratory assessment of upper and lower airways, including identifying respiratory rate, respiratory pattern, respiratory muscles used, breath sounds, ability to cough effectively, integrity of the rib cage, and the characteristics of sputum production.

7. Determine the type and frequency of intervention, based on assessment findings. Care that is appropriate for one day or shift can change, resulting in an increase or decrease in frequency of care or alterations in the type of intervention.

8. Identify and become familiar with the use of equipment available at the institution. Many types of artificial airways, suction catheters, and suction machines are available. Knowing how to operate the equipment before it is needed benefits both the nurse and the client.

9. Test all equipment before use. Have adequate supplies on hand at the bedside. Equipment must work properly to provide safe nursing care. Determine that the suction machine is generating adequate negative suction pressure (Table 24-1) and that there are suction catheters and appropriate equipment at the bedside.

10. Know the client's home care plan. Absence or interruption of certain therapies such as bronchodilators can place the client at risk for an obstructed airway

Skill Performance Guidelines

1. Know the client's normal range of vital signs and oxygen saturation levels. Baseline vital signs serve as a means to identify individual abnormalities and to recognize the onset of worsening of an illness.

2. Know the client's medical history. Smoking alters normal mucociliary clearance. Certain disorders such as chronic obstructive pulmonary diseases (including asthma and cystic fibrosis), pneumonia, thoracic surgery, chest trauma, and abdominal surgery place the client at increased risk for an obstructed airway.

3. Identify conditions that may increase the client's risk for aspiration of gastric contents into the lung, resulting in airway obstruction; these include the presence of enteral feeding tubes or other nasal or oral gastric

TABLE 24-1	VACUUM PRESSURE SETTINGS FOR SUCTIONING
AGE	**PRESSURE SETTING**
Preterm infants	40–60 mm Hg*
Infants	60–100 mm Hg*
Children	60–100 mm Hg*
Adults	80–120 mm Hg†
	More tenacious sputum may require more suction (up to 200 mm Hg†)

*Hockenberry MJ and others: *Wong's nursing care of infants and children*, ed 7, St. Louis, 2003, Mosby.
†Moore T: Suctioning techniques for the removal of respiratory secretions, *Nurs Stand* 18(9):47, 2003.

during the hospitalization or after discharge from the hospital.

11. Know the side effects of medications and other therapies. Some medications such as beta-adrenergic blockers have the side effect of bronchospasm. An adverse effect of narcotics and sedatives is respiratory depression. Similarly, too much oxygen can reduce the drive to breathe in clients with hypercapnia (elevated arterial carbon dioxide tension). Position changes may affect the client adversely. For example, in clients with impaired spinal cord innervations of the respiratory muscles, supine positions place the diaphragm at a mechanical disadvantage and increase the risk of aspiration.

SKILL 12-1 Performing Oropharyngeal Suctioning

Nurses use a Yankauer, or tonsillar tip, suction device to perform oropharyngeal suctioning (Figure 24-1). A Yankauer suction catheter is made of rigid, minimally flexible plastic. The tip of this suction catheter usually has one large and several small eyelets through which the mucus enters with application of negative pressure. The Yankauer suction catheter is angled to facilitate removal of pharyngeal secretions through the mouth. This catheter is used instead of a standard suction catheter when oral secretions are extremely copious and thick because it can handle large volumes of secretions better than a standard suction catheter (Vanderberg and others, 1999). The Yankauer suction catheter is not used to suction the nares because of its size.

The Yankauer suction device is useful in the removal of secretions from the mouth in clients after oral and maxillofacial surgery, trauma to the mouth, or neurovascular injury and cerebrovascular accident causing hemiparesis and drooling or impaired swallowing. Clients with artificial airways and impaired swallowing ability may require use of the Yankauer suction device to promote oral hygiene. Alert clients or assistive personnel can be easily taught how to use this apparatus and control the oral secretions.

Clients from other cultures need clear explanations and demonstration of the suction catheter. It is important to understand what this type of suctioning means to the client and

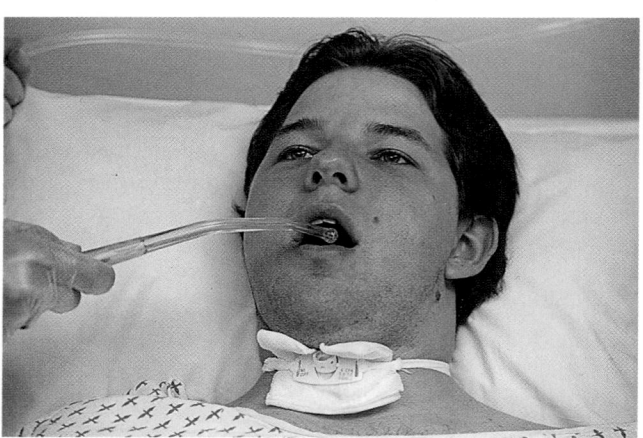

FIGURE **24-1** Oropharyngeal suctioning.

family members. When the client does not understand our language and culture, the client may interpret suctioning as introducing illness to the client (Shanahan and Brayshaw, 1995). Explain anticipated client effects, such as gagging and tearing from the eyes, which can be very distressing to family members.

DELEGATION CONSIDERATIONS

The skill of performing oropharyngeal (Yankauer) suctioning can be delegated to assistive personnel. Delegation of this skill for clients with oral or neck surgery should not be routinely delegated in the immediate postoperative period. If oropharyngeal suctioning is delegated to assistive personnel, the nurse must continually assess the client's respiratory status. The nurse must instruct assistive personnel:

- About appropriate suction limits for oropharyngeal suctioning for the particular client, for example, the appropriate suction pressure, expected frequency of suctioning, and the expected color and volume of secretions
- About the risks of applying excessive or inadequate suction pressure
- To avoid mouth sutures, avoid applying suction against sensitive tissues, and avoid dislodging tubes in the client's nose or mouth

EQUIPMENT

- ❑ Towel, cloth, or disposable paper drape
- ❑ Nonsterile gloves
- ❑ Yankauer or tonsillar tip suction catheter
- ❑ Face shield or mask
- ❑ Disposable cup or nonsterile basin
- ❑ Tap water or normal saline (about 100 ml)
- ❑ Suction equipment
- ❑ Connecting tubing (6 feet)
- ❑ Oral airway (if indicated)
- ❑ Washcloth (if indicated)

STEP	**RATIONALE**

■ ASSESSMENT

1. Observe for signs and symptoms associated with upper airway secretions requiring oropharyngeal suctioning: gurgling on inspiration or expiration, restlessness, obvious excess oral secretions, drooling, gastric secretions or vomitus in mouth, or coughing without clearing secretions from upper airway.

Physical signs and symptoms may indicate need to perform this procedure. Worsening status may result in total airway obstruction and hypoxia. The risk of aspiration of gastric contents and airway obstruction is increased in clients with vomiting, delayed gastric emptying, impaired esophageal sphincter control, hiatal hernia, impaired cough, impaired swallowing, or impaired gag reflex.

2. When ordered obtain client's oxygen saturation level via pulse oximetry (SpO_2) (see Chapter 17).

Provides an objective measure of the amount of oxygen saturation contained in the client's hemoglobin before oral suction. Also provides an early objective indication of worsening oxygenation status.

● *Critical Decision Point*

Signs and symptoms associated with hypoxia (low oxygen utilization at the cellular or tissue level), hypoxemia (low oxygen tension in the blood), or hypercapnia (elevated carbon dioxide tension in the blood) may also be present: apprehension, anxiety, audible lung sounds, decreased ability to concentrate, lethargy, decreased level of consciousness (especially acute), increased fatigue and dizziness, behavioral changes (especially irritability and restlessness), increased pulse rate, increased rate of breathing, decreased depth of breathing, elevated blood pressure, cardiac dysrhythmias, pallor, cyanosis, dyspnea, and use of accessory muscles for breathing (Wood, 1998).

3. Determine client's knowledge about use of the catheter.

Reveals need for client instruction.

4. Identify risk factors such as impaired cough or gag reflex, weakened respiratory muscles, impaired swallowing, and decreased level of consciousness, as well as the client's inability to manipulate and use the catheter device.

Risk factors may prevent client from protecting the airway from aspiration or from clearing secretions safely. Physical factors such as impaired mobility of the upper extremities prevent the client from using the catheter to help control oral secretions.

■ NURSING DIAGNOSES

- Ineffective airway clearance
- Risk for aspiration
- Ineffective breathing pattern
- Impaired swallowing

- Deficient knowledge regarding airway clearance techniques and devices
- Risk for infection
- Impaired gas exchange

Related factors are individualized based on client's condition or needs.

■ PLANNING

1. Expected outcomes following completion of procedure:
    - Upper airway (oral pharynx) is cleared of secretions.
    - No adventitious sounds are heard in client's pharynx on inspiration and expiration.
    - Drooling is diminished or absent.

    - Vomitus or gastric secretions are absent from mouth.

    - Pulse oximetry (SpO_2) improves or remains the same.

Suctioning is effective.

Presence of secretions in large upper airway produces noisy respirations.

Excessive drooling indicates that client is unable to handle oral secretions.

Gastric secretions retained in oral cavity increase client's risk for aspiration pneumonia.

Removal of secretions helps to improve oxygen saturation level. In clients with chronic pulmonary diseases, such as chronic obstructive pulmonary disease (COPD), the SpO_2 value may remain the same.

STEP	**RATIONALE**
2. Explain to client how the procedure will help clear airway secretions and relieve some breathing problems. Explain that coughing, gagging, or (less commonly) sneezing is normal and lasts only a few seconds. Encourage client to cough out secretions during procedure. Practice, if able. Splint surgical incisions, if necessary.	Gagging or coughing will occur only when the posterior pharynx is deeply suctioned or as a result of excess secretions. Coughing secretions out of lower airway or posterior pharynx will decrease the amount of suctioning required. Encourages cooperation and minimizes risks and associated anxiety.
3. Position client and, if necessary, place towel, cloth, or paper drape across client's neck and chest.	Promotes client comfort and removal of airway secretions. Towel protects client's gown and bed linen from contamination by secretions.

IMPLEMENTATION

1. Perform hand hygiene, and apply gloves. Apply mask or face shield.	Reduces transmission of microorganisms.
2. Fill cup or basin with approximately 100 ml of water or normal saline.	For cleansing catheter after suctioning.
3. Turn on suction equipment, set vacuum regulator to appropriate setting (see manufacturer's instructions).	Elevated pressure settings increase risk of trauma to the oral mucosa.
4. Connect one end of connecting tubing to suction machine and other to Yankauer suction catheter. Check that equipment is functioning properly by suctioning small amount of water or normal saline from cup or basin.	Prepares suction apparatus. Ensures equipment function and lubricates catheter.
5. Remove client's oxygen mask, if present. Nasal cannula may remain in place. Keep oxygen mask near client's face. Try removing the straps from around the client's head that hold the mask in place while leaving the mask in place until ready to suction client.	Allows access to mouth. Reduces chance of hypoxia.

• *Critical Decision Point*
Be prepared to quickly reapply supplemental oxygen if SpO$_2$ value falls or respiratory distress develops during or at the end of suctioning.

6. Insert catheter into mouth along gum line to pharynx. Move catheter around mouth until secretions are cleared. Encourage client to cough. Replace oxygen mask.	Catheter provides continuous suction. Take care not to allow suction tip to invaginate oral mucosal surfaces. Coughing moves secretions from lower airway into mouth and upper airway.
7. Rinse catheter with water in cup or basin until connecting tubing is cleared of secretions. Turn off suction. May need to wash face if secretions are present on client's skin.	Rinses catheter and reduces probability of transmission of microorganisms. Clean suction tubing enhances delivery of set suction pressure. Prevents skin breakdown.
8. Observe respiratory status. Repeat procedure, if indicated. May need to use standard suction catheter to reach into trachea if respiratory status not improved.	Directs nurse to continue or cease intervention or to choose another intervention.
9. Remove towel, cloth, or disposable drape, and place in trash or in laundry if soiled. Reposition client; Sims' position encourages drainage and should be used if client has decreased level of consciousness.	Reduces transmission of microorganisms. Facilitates drainage of oral secretions.
10. Discard remainder of water into appropriate receptacle. Rinse basin in warm soapy water, and dry with paper towels. Discard disposable cup into appropriate receptacle. Place catheter in clean dry area.	Reduces transmission of microorganisms and maintains medical asepsis. Moist environment encourages microorganism growth.

STEP	**RATIONALE**

- *Critical Decision Point*
  Catheter should be kept in nonairtight container such as brown paper or plastic bag attached to bed rail or in suction canister area. It should not be stored where it will come in contact with secretions or excretions or will contaminate clean supplies. Closure in an airtight container promotes bacterial growth.

11. Remove gloves and mask or face shield, and dispose of in appropriate receptacle. Perform hand hygiene.	Reduces transmission of microorganisms to other clients. Clean equipment should not be handled with contaminated gloves.
12. Position client, and provide oral hygiene as needed.	Promotes client's comfort.

EVALUATION

1. Compare assessment findings before and after procedure.	Identifies physiological response to the suction procedure.
2. Auscultate chest and airways for adventitious sounds.	Presence of lower airway adventitious sounds suggests a need for lower airway suctioning.
3. Obtain postsuction SpO$_2$ measure.	Provides objective postsuction data to compare with baseline and is another objective measure of the effectiveness of the suction procedure.
4. Observe client or family perform Yankauer suctioning.	Demonstrates learning.

Recording and Reporting

- Record the amount, consistency, color, and odor of secretions and the client's response to the procedure; document presuction and postsuction cardiopulmonary assessment.
- Record instruction to caregivers and ability to correctly perform procedure.

Unexpected Outcomes	**Related Interventions**
1. Worsening respiratory distress.	• Implement nasal, oropharyngeal, or tracheal suctioning. • Evaluate need for other means to protect airway (e.g., oral intubation, oral airway, positioning). • Provide supplemental oxygen. • Notify physician.
2. Return of bloody secretions.	• Assess oral cavity for trauma or sores. • Reduce the amount of suction pressure used. • Observe catheter tip for nicks, which can cause mucosal trauma. • Increase frequency of oral hygiene.

Teaching Considerations

- Instruct family or caregiver not to allow catheter to fall to the floor.
- Provide information regarding signs and symptoms of worsening respiratory status.
- Assess knowledge level of client, family, and primary caregiver to determine amount of instruction required and frequency of visits necessary to reach goals.

Pediatric Considerations

- Maintain healthy infant in supine position (American Academy of Pediatrics, 1996).
- Position infants with breathing problems or excessive vomitus in prone position (Hockenberry and others, 2003).
- Airways of infants and children are smaller than those of an adult; even small amounts of mucus can cause airway obstruction.

* Bulb syringe is used. Compress syringe before insertion to prevent forcing secretions into infant's bronchi (Hockenberry and others, 2003). If more forceful suctioning is required than that produced by a bulb syringe, it may be necessary to use mechanical suction.

Gerontological Considerations

* Clients with dysphagia may benefit from oral suctioning before, during, and after meals.
* Oral mucosa in older adults is fragile, and a lower suction pressure is needed.
* Older adults are prone to aspiration of oral secretions because of decreased cough and gag reflexes (Lueckenotte, 2000).

Long-Term and Home Care Considerations

* In the long-term care or home setting the secretion collection container is cleaned and disinfected or changed every 24 hours according to home care or institutional protocol. In many institutions the disposable secretion collection canister is sealed and disposed of in its entirety as biohazardous material.
* Assess home for the presence of respiratory irritants, including cigarette smoke, dust, pollen, and chemicals.

SKILL 24-2 Airway Suctioning

The major differences between oropharyngeal and tracheal airway suctioning are the depth suctioned and the potential for complications. Oropharyngeal suctioning only removes secretions from the back of the throat and requires clean technique. Tracheal airway suctioning extends into the lower airway and necessitates aseptic technique. Suctioning is necessary to remove respiratory secretions and maintain optimum ventilation and oxygenation in clients who are unable to independently remove these secretions (Moore, 2003). The nurse assesses the client to determine frequency and depth of suctioning. Some clients may require suctioning every hour or two, whereas others need to be suctioned only once or twice a day. How far to insert the suction catheter for tracheal suctioning depends on the size of the client, especially children.

If the secretions are only in the nose and mouth, then only the pharynx requires suctioning, although in most instances the nurse will suction both the pharynx and the trachea. Secretions should be suctioned from the pharynx as often as necessary. Secretions that are not removed are more likely to be aspirated into the lungs, increasing the risk for infection and respiratory failure.

Suctioning has many risks associated with performing the procedure. The most serious ones relate to hypoxemia, which may often result in cardiac dysrhythmias; laryngeal spasm; bradycardia, which is associated with stimulation of the vagus nerve; and nasal trauma and bleeding, which can develop from the suction catheter (Moore, 2003).

Nasopharyngeal and Nasotracheal Suctioning

Nasopharyngeal and nasotracheal suctioning assist in maintaining a patent airway by removing secretions from the pharynx or throat and the trachea. This type of suctioning is used when suctioning with a Yankauer device is ineffective or inappropriate or when the lower airway requires removal of secretions. It involves inserting a small rubber or soft plastic tube into the nares to the pharynx or trachea and then applying negative pressure to withdraw mucus.

Performing Artificial Airway Suctioning

Endotracheal (ET) tubes and tracheostomy ("trach") tubes (TT) are artificial airways inserted to relieve airway obstruction, provide a route for mechanical ventilation, permit easy access for secretion removal, and protect the airway from gross aspiration in clients with impaired cough or gag reflexes (Figure 24-2).

Endotracheal Tubes

Endotracheal intubation is a procedure performed by a physician or specially trained personnel (e.g., nurse, respiratory therapist, or rescue personnel). An ET tube is inserted through the nares (nasal ET tube) or the mouth (oral ET tube) past the epiglottis and vocal cords into the trachea.

It remains somewhat controversial as to how long ET tubes may be left in place; however, in most cases after 2 to 4 weeks a tracheostomy tube is inserted (St. John, 1999). ET tubes are usually made of plastic or rubber. Adult sizes of ET tubes have a cuff molded onto the tube to (1) prevent the aspiration of oral secretions or gastric contents into the lung and/or (2) obstruct the escape of air from mechanical ventilator breaths through the upper airway.

Tracheostomy Tubes

Although ET tubes are temporary, a tracheostomy tube can be temporary or permanent depending on the client's condition. A tracheostomy tube is inserted directly into the trachea through a small incision made in the client's

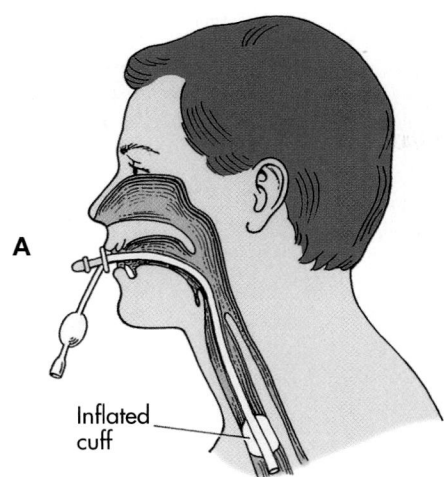

A

Inflated cuff

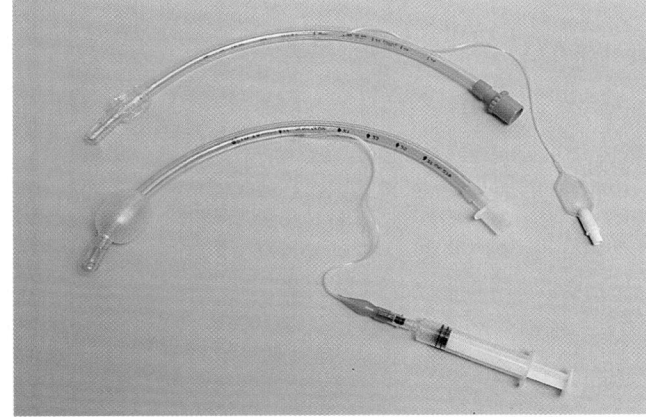

B

FIGURE **24-2** **A,** Endotracheal (ET) tube with inflated cuff.
B, ET tubes with uninflated and inflated cuffs and syringe for
inflation.

neck by the surgeon. Tracheostomy tubes are made of several different materials, including various polyvinyl chloride– or silicone-based plastics and stainless steel or metallic compounds. Metal tracheostomy tubes are thermal sensitive and must be protected from extreme heat and cold to prevent tissue injury in the client. Most metal and plastic tracheostomy tubes contain an inner cannula that can be temporarily withdrawn for cleaning airway-occluding mucus without removing the entire tracheostomy tube (see Skill 24-4).

A cuff on a tracheostomy tube serves the same purpose as one on an ET tube. Cuffs are made of a balloonlike inflatable plastic; usually they are manually inflated with air by the nurse or respiratory therapist (see Skill 24-5). Plastic-covered foam cuffs are self-air inflating if the inflation port is left open to the atmosphere.

Some institutions use a closed system suction catheter or in-line suction catheter device, which assist in minimizing infections, especially in critically ill or immunosuppressed clients (Zeitounss and others, 2003). Use of a closed system catheter (in-line) allows quicker lower airway suctioning without applying gloves or a mask and does not interrupt ventilation and oxygenation in critically ill clients. In addition, the nurse is protected from contamination by the client's secretions (see Box 24-1). With a closed system method the client's artificial airway is not disconnected from the mechanical ventilator (Paul-Allen and Ostrow, 2000).

DELEGATION CONSIDERATIONS

The skills of nasotracheal and artificial airway tube suctioning should not be routinely delegated to assistive personnel. When the client is assessed by the nurse to be stable, the skill of performing tracheostomy tube suctioning can be delegated to assistive personnel. These situations include clients with permanent tracheostomy tubes and clients receiving mechanical ventilation at home. Before delegating these skills, the nurse must:

* Discuss with assistive personnel any unique modifications of the skill, such as the need of supplemental oxygen or the use of a clean versus sterile suction technique
* Instruct assistive personnel about appropriate suction limits for suctioning tracheostomy tube and risks of applying excessive or inadequate suction pressure
* Instruct assistive personnel about signs and symptoms of hypoxemia, such as change in client's respiratory status, confusion, and restless, and to report these signs immediately to the nurse
* Instruct assistive personnel to report any change in secretion quality, quantity, and color

EQUIPMENT

❑ Appropriate-size suction catheter (smallest diameter that will remove secretions effectively) (Table 24-2)
❑ Nasal or oral airway (if indicated)
❑ Two sterile gloves or one sterile and one nonsterile glove
❑ Clean towel or paper drape
❑ Suction machine
❑ Mask or face shield
❑ Connecting tubing (6 feet)
❑ Small Y-adapter (if catheter does not have a suction control port)
❑ Water-soluble lubricant
❑ Sterile basin
❑ Sterile normal saline solution or water, about 100 ml
❑ Portable or wall suction apparatus

TABLE 24-2 EQUIPMENT GUIDELINES* FOR INTUBATION AND SUCTIONING

EQUIPMENT	INFANT (PREMATURE INFANT TO 1 YEAR)	SMALL CHILD (2-5 YEARS)	SCHOOL-AGE CHILD (6-12 YEARS)	ADOLESCENT TO ADULT
Airway:				
Oral	00–2	2–3	3–4	4–5
Nasal (French)	5–8	10–20	20–24	24–36
Handheld resuscitator size	Child	Child	Child/adult	Adult
Mask size	Premature infant/child	Child	Small adult	Adult
Laryngoscope blade size	0–1 (straight)	2 (straight)	2–3 (straight or curved)	4–5 (straight or curved)
Endotracheal tube size (mm)	2.5–4.0	4.0–5.0	5.0–6.5	7.0–9.0
Tracheostomy tube: Jackson size	000–1	1–2	3–4	4–10
Inner diameter (mm)	2.5–3.5	3.5–4.0	4.5–5.0	5.0–9.0
Suction catheter size (French)†	5–6	6–8	8–10	10–16

Data from St. John RE: Airway management, *Crit Care Nurse* 19(4):79, 1999.

*These guidelines should be used as an estimate only: actual sizes depend on the size and individual needs of the client.

†Catheter outer diameter should not exceed half the internal diameter of the tube.

STEP	RATIONALE

ASSESSMENT

1. Assess signs and symptoms of upper and lower airway obstruction requiring nasal or oral tracheal suctioning, including wheezes, crackles, or gurgling on inspiration or expiration; restlessness; ineffective coughing; unilateral, segmental, or lobar absent or diminished breath sounds (in absence of pneumonectomy or lobectomy); tachypnea; hypertension or hypotension; cyanosis; decreased level of consciousness, especially acute; or excess nasal secretions, drooling, or gastric secretions or vomitus in mouth (Moore, 2003).

Physical signs and symptoms result from decreased oxygen to tissues, as well as pooling of secretions in upper and lower airways. Assessment should be completed before and following the suction procedure (Moore, 2003).

2. Determine the presence of apprehension, anxiety, decreased ability to concentrate, lethargy, decreased level of consciousness (especially acute), increased fatigue, dizziness, behavioral changes (especially irritability), decreased oxygen saturation (from pulse oximetry), increased pulse rate, increased rate of breathing, decreased depth of breathing, elevated blood pressure, cardiac dysrhythmias, pallor, cyanosis, dyspnea, or use of accessory muscles.

Signs and symptoms associated with hypoxia (low oxygen at the cellular or tissue level), hypoxemia (low oxygen tension in the blood), or hypercapnia (elevated carbon dioxide tension in the blood). Clients report sensations of pain and discomfort with the suctioning procedure, and as a result anxiety may be present before suctioning. Anxiety and pain consume oxygen and in turn worsen the signs of hypoxia (Puntillo and others, 2002).

3. Assess for risk factors for upper or lower airway obstruction, including obstructive lung disease; pulmonary infections; impaired mobility; sedation; decreased level of consciousness; seizures; presence of feeding tube; decreased gag or cough reflex; decreased swallowing ability; allergies; sinus drainage; and head, neck, or chest tumors.

Presence of these risk factors may impair the client's ability to clear secretions from the airway and may necessitate nasopharyngeal or nasotracheal suctioning

4. Determine additional factors that normally influence upper or lower airway function: recent surgery, decreased level of consciousness, ineffective or absent cough, chemical neuromuscular blockade, neuromuscular diseases, congestive heart failure, pulmonary edema, adult respiratory distress syndrome, hyaline membrane disease, or diaphragmatic weakness or paralysis (Moore, 2003). Assess the following areas that may influence or affect airway function:

Allows nurse to identify clients at risk for airway obstruction needing ET or tracheostomy tube suctioning.

a. Fluid status

Fluid overload may increase amount of secretions. Dehydration promotes thicker secretions.

STEP	RATIONALE
b. Lack of humidity	The environment influences secretion formation and gas exchange, necessitating airway suctioning when the client cannot clear secretions effectively.
c. Infection (e.g., pneumonia)	Clients with respiratory infections are prone to increased secretions that are thicker and sometimes more difficult to expectorate.
d. Anatomy	Abnormal anatomy can impair normal drainage of secretions. For example, nasal swelling, deviated septum, or facial fractures may impair nasal drainage. Tumors in or around the lower airway may impair secretion removal by occluding or externally compressing the lumen of the airway.

5. Identify contraindications to nasotracheal suctioning:
   a. Facial trauma/surgery
   b. Bleeding disorders
   c. Nasal bleeding
   d. Epiglottitis or croup
   e. Laryngospasm
   f. Irritable airway
	These conditions are contraindications because the passage of a catheter through the nasal route can cause additional trauma, increase nasal bleeding, or cause severe bleeding in the presence of bleeding disorders. In the presence of epiglottitis, croup, laryngospasm, or irritable airway, the entrance of a suction catheter via the nasal route can cause intractable coughing, hypoxemia, and severe bronchospasm necessitating emergency intubation or tracheostomy (Moore, 2003).

6. Examine sputum microbiology data.	Certain bacteria are more easily transmitted or require isolation because of virulence or antibiotic resistance.
7. Assess client's understanding of procedure.	Reveals need for client instruction and encourages cooperation.

NURSING DIAGNOSES

- Deficient knowledge regarding airway clearance techniques and devices
- Ineffective breathing pattern
- Impaired spontaneous ventilation
- Risk for infection

- Ineffective airway clearance
- Impaired swallowing
- Impaired gas exchange
- Risk for aspiration

Related factors are individualized based on client's condition or needs.

PLANNING

1. Expected outcomes following completion of procedure: • Lower and upper airways demonstrate absent or diminished crackles, wheezes, and gurgles on inspiration and expiration; return of absent or diminished breath sounds; normalization of heart rate, blood pressure, respiratory rate and effort, pulse oximetry readings; absence of drooling, gastric secretions or vomitus in mouth, and nasal secretions.	Airways are cleared of secretions. In the presence of infection more secretions are produced; as infection improves, the amount of secretions and the need for suctioning diminish. When airway secretions are removed and oxygenation improves, the client's vital signs, pulse oximetry readings, and respiratory assessment findings improve.
• Client verbalizes easier breathing, if able.	Clear airway reduces work of breathing.
2. Explain to client how procedure will help clear airway and relieve breathing problems. Explain that temporary coughing, sneezing, gagging, or shortness of breath is normal during the procedure. Encourage client to cough out secretions. Practice coughing, if able. Splint surgical incisions, if necessary.	Encourages cooperation and minimizes risks, anxiety, and pain of procedure.
3. Explain importance of and encourage coughing during procedure.	Facilitates secretion removal and may reduce frequency and duration of future suctioning.
4. Assist client with assuming position comfortable for nurse and client (usually semi-Fowler's or sitting upright with head hyperextended, unless contraindicated).	Reduces stimulation of gag reflex, promotes client comfort and secretion drainage, prevents aspiration and nurse strain. Hyperextension facilitates insertion of catheter into trachea.
5. Place towel across client's chest, if needed.	Reduces transmission of microorganisms by protecting gown from secretions.

STEP	**RATIONALE**

IMPLEMENTATION

1. Perform hand hygiene, and apply face shield if splashing is likely.

Reduces transmission of microorganisms.

2. Connect one end of connecting tubing to suction machine, and place other end in convenient location near client. Turn suction device on, and set vacuum regulator to appropriate negative pressure.

Excessive negative pressure damages nasal pharyngeal and tracheal mucosa and can induce greater hypoxia.

3. If indicated, increase supplemental oxygen therapy to 100% or as ordered by physician. Encourage client deep breathing.

Hyperoxygenation provides some protection from suction-induced decline in oxygenation. Hyperoxygenation is most effective in the presence of hyperinflation, such as encouraging the client to deep breathe or increasing ventilator tidal volume settings (Moore, 2003).

- **Critical Decision Point**

  Oxygen must be readjusted as ordered by physician after procedure to avoid increased risk of oxygen toxicity and absorption, atelectasis from prolonged administration of high concentrations of oxygen, and increased carbon dioxide retention in clients with chronic obstructive lung diseases.

4. Prepare suction catheter.
   a. One-time-use catheter
      (1) Open suction kit or catheter with use of aseptic technique. If sterile drape is available, place it across client's chest or on the over-bed table. Do not allow the suction catheter to touch any nonsterile surfaces.

Maintains asepsis and reduces transmission of microorganisms.

      (2) Unwrap or open sterile basin, and place on bedside table. Be careful not to touch inside of basin. Fill with about 100 ml sterile normal saline solution or water (see illustration).

Saline or water is used to clean tubing after each suction pass.

      (3) Open lubricant. Squeeze small amount onto open sterile catheter package without touching package. NOTE: Lubricant is not necessary for artificial airway suctioning.

Prepares lubricant while maintaining sterility. Water-soluble lubricant is used to avoid lipoid aspiration pneumonia. Excessive lubricant can occlude catheter.

   b. Closed (in-line) suction catheter: Box 24-1.
5. Turn on suction device, and set regulator to appropriate pressure (see Table 24-1).

Excessive negative pressure can result in damage to the nasal pharyngeal and tracheal mucosa and can increase suction-induced hypoxia.

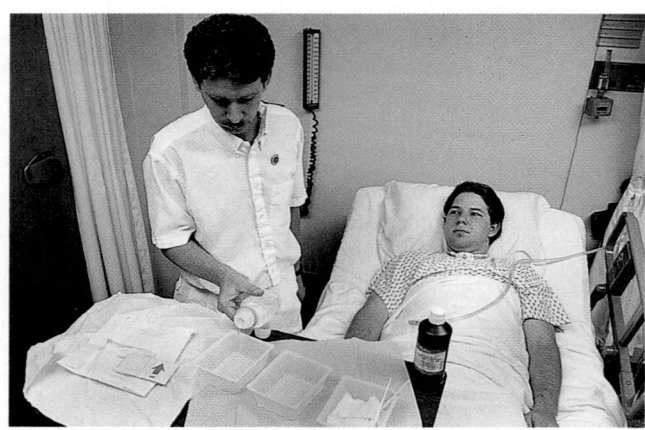

STEP **4a(2)** Pouring sterile saline into tray.

STEP	**RATIONALE**

6. Apply sterile glove to each hand, or apply nonsterile glove to nondominant hand and sterile glove to dominant hand.

Reduces transmission of microorganisms and allows nurse to maintain sterility of suction catheter.

7. Pick up suction catheter with dominant hand without touching nonsterile surfaces. Pick up connecting tubing with nondominant hand. Secure catheter to tubing (see illustration).

Maintains catheter sterility. Connects catheter to suction.

8. Check that equipment is functioning properly by suctioning small amount of normal saline solution from basin.

Ensures equipment function. Lubricates internal catheter and tubing.

9. Suction airway.
   a. Nasopharyngeal and nasotracheal suctioning.
      (1) Lightly coat distal 6 to 8 cm (2 to 3 inches) of catheter with water-soluble lubricant.

Lubricates catheter for easier insertion.

      (2) Remove oxygen delivery device, if applicable, with nondominant hand. Without applying suction and using dominant thumb and forefinger, gently but quickly insert catheter into nares during inhalation, and following natural course of the nares, slightly slant the catheter downward or through mouth. Do not force through nares (see illustration).

Application of suction pressure while introducing catheter into trachea increases risk of damage to mucosa and increases risk of hypoxia because of removal of entrained oxygen present in airways.

- **Critical Decision Point**
  Be sure to insert catheter during client inhalation, especially if inserting catheter into trachea, because epiglottis is open. Do not insert during swallowing, or catheter will most likely enter esophagus. Never apply suction during insertion. Client should cough. If client gags or becomes nauseated, catheter is most likely in esophagus and must be removed.

    (a) Nasopharyngeal suctioning (without applying suction): In adults, insert catheter about 16 cm; in older children, 8 to 12 cm (3 to 5 inches); in infants and young children, 4 to 8 cm (2 to 3 inches). Rule of thumb is to insert catheter distance from tip of nose (or mouth) to base of ear lobe.

Ensures that catheter tip is positioned correctly in pharynx for suctioning.

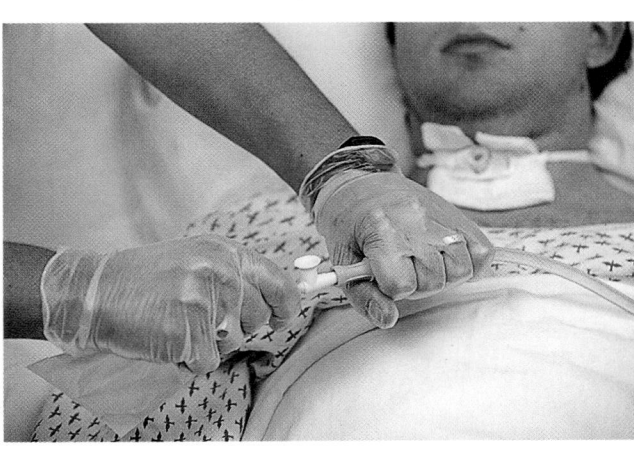

STEP 7 Attaching catheter to suction.

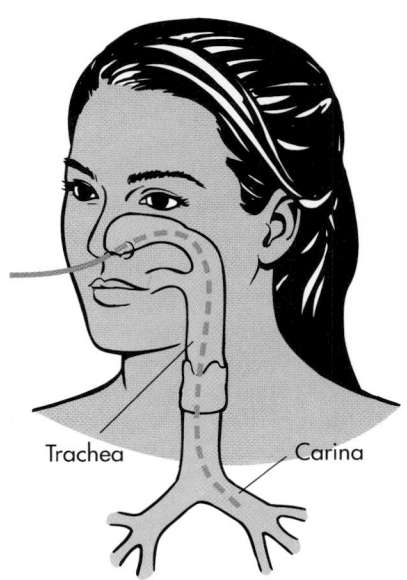

Trachea   Carina

STEP 9 Pathway for nasotracheal catheter progression.

STEP	RATIONALE

(b) Nasotracheal suctioning (without applying suction): In adults, insert catheter about 20 cm; in older children, 14 to 20 cm (5½ to 8 inches); and in young children and infants, 8 to 14 cm (3 to 5½ inches).

- *Critical Decision Point*
  When there is difficulty passing the catheter, ask client to cough or say "ahh," or try to advance the catheter during inspiration. Both these measures assist in opening the glottis to permit passage of the catheter into the trachea.

(1) Positioning: In some instances turning client's head to right helps nurse suction left mainstem bronchus; turning head to left helps nurse suction right mainstem bronchus. If resistance is felt after insertion of catheter for maximum recommended distance, catheter has probably hit carina. Pull catheter back 1 to 2 cm before applying suction.	Turning the client's head to the side elevates the bronchial passage on the opposite side.

- *Critical Decision Point*
  Use the nasal approach, and perform tracheal suctioning before pharyngeal suctioning whenever possible. The mouth and pharynx contain more bacteria than the trachea does. If copious oral secretions are present before beginning the procedure, suction mouth with oral suction device.

(3) Apply intermittent suction for up to 10 seconds (Moore, 2003) by placing and releasing nondominant thumb over vent of catheter and slowly withdrawing catheter while rotating it back and forth between dominant thumb and forefinger. Encourage client to cough and deep breathe. Replace oxygen device, if applicable.	Intermittent suction and rotation of catheter prevents injury to mucosa. If catheter "grabs" mucosa, remove thumb to release suction. Suctioning longer than 10 seconds can cause cardiopulmonary compromise, usually from hypoxemia or vagal overload.

- *Critical Decision Point*
  Monitor client's vital signs and oxygen saturation using pulse oximetry throughout suction procedure. If the client's pulse drops more than 20 beats per minute or increases more than 40 beats per minute, or if pulse oximetry falls below 90% or 5% from baseline, cease suctioning. Any deteriorating changes in the client's physiological status during suctioning requires termination of the procedure, hyperoxygenation, and other appropriate interventions (e.g., position change) (Moore, 2003).

STEP	**RATIONALE**
(4) Rinse catheter and connecting tubing with normal saline or water until cleared.	Secretions that remain in suction catheter or connecting tubing decrease suctioning efficiency.
(5) Assess for need to repeat suctioning procedure. Observe for alterations in cardiopulmonary status. When possible, allow adequate time (1 to 2 minutes) between suction passes for ventilation and oxygenation. Assist client with deep breathing and coughing.	Suctioning can induce hypoxemia, dysrhythmias, laryngospasm, and bronchospasm. Deep breathing reventilates and reoxygenates alveoli. Repeated passes clear the airway of excessive secretions but can also remove oxygen and may induce laryngospasm.
b. Artificial airway suctioning	
(1) Hyperinflate and/or hyperoxygenate client before suctioning, using manual resuscitation Ambu-bag connected to oxygen source or sigh mechanism on mechanical ventilator. Some mechanical ventilators have a button that when pushed delivers 100% oxygen for a few minutes and then resets to the previous value.	Hyperinflation decreases the risk for atelectasis caused by negative pressure of suctioning (St. John, 1999). Preoxygenation converts large proportion of resident lung gas to 100% oxygen to offset amount used in metabolic consumption while ventilator or oxygenation is interrupted, as well as to offset volume lost during suction procedure (Day and others, 2002; Wood, 1998).

- ### *Critical Decision Point*

   Caution is used when suctioning clients with a head injury. The suction procedure itself can cause elevations in intracranial pressure (ICP). This risk is reduced by presuctioning hyperventilation, which results in hypocarbia that in turn induces vasoconstriction. It is the vasoconstriction that reduces the potential increase in ICP. It is recommended that the introduction of a catheter be limited to two times with each suctioning procedure (Moore, 2003).

(2) If client is receiving mechanical ventilation, open swivel adapter, or if necessary remove oxygen or humidity delivery device with nondominant hand.	Exposes artificial airway.
(3) Without applying suction, gently but quickly insert catheter using dominant thumb and forefinger into artificial airway (it is best to try to time catheter insertion into the artificial airway with inspiration) until resistance is met or client coughs, then pull back 1 cm (½ inch).	Application of suction pressure while introducing catheter into trachea increases risk of damage to tracheal mucosa, as well as increased hypoxia related to removal of entrained oxygen present in airways. Pulling back stimulates cough and removes catheter from mucosal wall so that catheter is not resting against tracheal mucosa during suctioning.

- ### *Critical Decision Point*

   If unable to insert catheter past the end of the ET tube, the catheter is probably caught in the Murphy eye (i.e., side hole at the distal end of the ET tube that allows for collateral airflow in the event of tracheal mainstem intubation). If this happens, rotate the catheter to reposition it away from the Murphy eye, or withdraw it slightly and reinsert with the next inhalation. Usually the catheter meets resistance at the carina. One indication that the catheter is at the carina is acute onset of coughing, because the carina contains many cough receptors. The catheter should be pulled back 1 cm (½ inch).

STEP	RATIONALE
(4) Apply intermittent suction by placing and releasing nondominant thumb over vent of catheter; slowly withdraw catheter while rotating it back and forth between dominant thumb and forefinger (see illustration). Encourage client to cough. Watch for respiratory distress.	Intermittent suction and rotation of catheter prevent injury to tracheal mucosal lining. If catheter "grabs" mucosa, remove thumb to release suction.

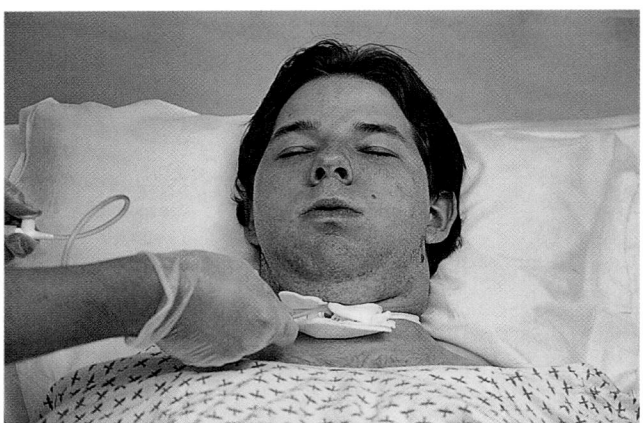

STEP **9b(4)** Suctioning tracheostomy.

- **Critical Decision Point**

  If client develops respiratory distress during the suction procedure, immediately withdraw catheter, and supply additional oxygen and breaths as needed. Oxygen can be administered directly through the catheter in an emergency. Disconnect suction, and attach oxygen at prescribed flow rate through the catheter.

STEP	RATIONALE
(5) If client is receiving mechanical ventilation, close swivel adapter, or replace oxygen delivery device.	Reestablishes artificial airway.
(6) Encourage client to deep breathe, if able. Some clients respond well to several manual breaths from the mechanical ventilator or bag-valve-mask.	Reoxygenates and reexpands alveoli. Suctioning can cause hypoxemia and atelectasis.
(7) Rinse catheter and connecting tubing with normal saline until clear. Use continuous suction.	Removes catheter secretions. Secretions left in tubing decrease suctioning efficiency and provide environment for microorganism growth.
(8) Assess client's cardiopulmonary status for secretion clearance. Repeat steps (1) through (7) once or twice more to clear secretions. Allow adequate time (at least 1 full minute) between suction passes.	Suctioning can induce dysrhythmias, hypoxia, and bronchospasm and impair cerebral circulation or adversely affect hemodynamic stability (Akgul and Akyolcu, 2002; Moore, 2003). Repeated passes with suction catheter clear airway of excessive secretions and promote improved oxygenation (Wood, 1998).
(9) When pharynx and trachea are sufficiently cleared of secretions, perform oropharyngeal suctioning to clear mouth of secretions. Do not suction nose again after suctioning mouth.	Removes upper airway secretions. More microorganisms are generally present in mouth. Upper airway is considered "clean" and lower airway is considered "sterile." Therefore the same catheter can be used to suction from sterile to clean areas (e.g., tracheal suctioning to oropharyngeal suctioning) but not from clean to sterile areas.

STEP	RATIONALE
10. When suctioning is completed, disconnect catheter from connecting tubing. Roll catheter around fingers of dominant hand. Pull glove off inside out so that catheter remains coiled in glove. Pull off other glove over first glove in same way to seal in contaminants. Discard in appropriate receptacle. Turn off suction device.	Reduces transmission of microorganisms.
11. Remove towel, place in laundry or appropriate receptacle, and reposition client. (Nurse may need to wear clean gloves for personal care.)	Reduces transmission of microorganisms. Promotes comfort.
12. If indicated, readjust oxygen to original level because client's blood oxygen level should have returned to baseline.	Prevents absorption atelectasis and oxygen toxicity while allowing client time to reoxygenate blood.
13. Discard remainder of normal saline into appropriate receptacle. If basin is disposable, discard into appropriate receptacle. If basin is reusable, rinse it out, and place it in soiled utility room.	Reduces transmission of microorganisms.
14. Remove face shield, and discard into appropriate receptacle. Perform hand hygiene.	
15. Place unopened suction kit on suction machine table or at head of bed.	Reduces transmission of microorganisms.
16. Assist client to a comfortable position, and provide oral hygiene as needed.	Provides immediate access to suction catheter for next procedure.

EVALUATION

1. Compare client's respiratory assessments before and after suctioning.	Identifies physiological effects of suction procedure to restore airway patency.
2. Ask client if breathing is easier and if congestion is decreased.	Provides subjective confirmation that airway obstruction is relieved with suctioning procedure.
3. Observe airway secretions.	Provides data to document presence or absence of respiratory tract infection.

Recording and Reporting

- Record the amount, consistency, color, and odor of secretions and client's response to suctioning. Document client's presuctioning and postsuctioning cardiopulmonary status.

Unexpected Outcomes	Related Interventions
1. Worsening respiratory status.	• Limit length of suctioning. • Determine need for more frequent suctioning, possibly of shorter duration. • Determine need for supplemental oxygen. Supply oxygen between suctioning passes. • Notify physician.
2. Return of bloody secretions.	• Determine amount of suction pressure used. May need to be decreased. • Consider performing suction correctly using intermittent suction and catheter rotation. • Evaluate suctioning frequency. • Provide more frequent oral hygiene.

Continued

Unexpected Outcomes	Related Interventions
3. Unable to pass suction catheter through nares at first attempt.	• Try other nares or oral route. • Insert nasal airway, especially if suctioning through client nares frequently (St. John, 1999). • Follow nares floor to avoid turbinates. • If obstruction is mucus, apply suction to relieve obstruction, but do not apply suction to mucosa. If obstruction is felt to be a blood clot, consult with physician. • Increase lubrication of catheter.
4. Paroxysms of coughing.	• Administer supplemental oxygen. • Allow client to rest between passes of suction catheter. • Consult with physician regarding need for inhaled bronchodilators or topical anesthetics.
5. No secretions obtained.	• Evaluate client's fluid status. • Assess for signs of infection. • Determine need for chest physiotherapy (see Chapter 23). • Assess adequacy of humidification on oxygen delivery device.

Teaching Considerations

• Instruct client that coughing may increase during the procedure.
• Explain why supplemental oxygen is given before suction.

Pediatric Considerations

• Small-diameter suction catheters required in pediatrics should be one-half the diameter of the child's tracheostomy tube (Hockenberry and others, 2003).
• Because of small diameter of suction catheter, thick secretions may be more difficult to remove.
• Distance suctioned should not be greater than 0.5 cm beyond the tip of the artificial airway. To determine distance, place catheter near a sample artificial airway (Hockenberry and others, 2003).
• Infant airways have less cartilage and may collapse easily, especially in premature infants or those with reactive airways.
• Suctioning should require no more than 5 seconds (Hockenberry and others, 2003).

Gerontological Considerations

• Older adults have lost some properties of elastic recoil and gas exchange.

• Capillaries of older adults are often fragile, predisposing client to bleeding problems.
• Older clients may have coronary artery disease, which places them at increased risk for cardiopulmonary compromise. In addition, older adults may be taking antiplatelet and/or anticoagulant medications such as aspirin or Coumadin for the prevention of coronary or cerebral artery occlusion.

Home Care Considerations

• Although most clients with airway clearance problems at home have a tracheostomy, some also require nasal pharyngeal suctioning. Catheters are often used for a 24-hour period and then cleaned and disinfected; or catheters are cleaned with soapy water after each use and discarded after 24 hours.
• In the home the secretion collection container is cleaned and disinfected or changed every 24 hours according to home care or institutional protocol.
• In the home setting stress the importance of brief intervals of applying suction pressure. Those performing suctioning should hold their breath during the application of negative suction pressure to help them remember to not suction too long.

BOX 24-1 Procedural Guideline
Closed (in-line) suction catheter

DELEGATION CONSIDERATIONS

The skill of airway suction with a closed (in-line) suction catheter should not be routinely delegated to assistive personnel. In special situations, such as suctioning a permanent tracheostomy, this procedure may be delegated to assistive personnel. The nurse is responsible for the cardiopulmonary assessment of the client and before delegation the nurse must:

- Instruct assistive personnel regarding any individualized aspects of client care that pertain to suctioning (e.g., position, duration of suction, pressure settings)
- Inform assistive personnel about expected quality, quantity, and color of secretions and to inform the nurse immediately if there are changes
- Inform assistive personnel about client's anticipated response to suction and to immediately report to the nurse changes in vital signs, complaints of pain, shortness of breath, confusion, or increased restlessness

EQUIPMENT

Closed system or in-line suction catheter; suction machine; 6 feet of connecting tubing; two clean gloves (optional), face shield

ASSESSMENT

1. Perform assessment as in Skill 24-2.
2. Explain the procedure to the client and the importance of coughing during the suctioning procedure.
3. Assist client with assuming a position of comfort for both client and nurse, usually semi- or high-Fowler's position. Place towel across the client's chest.
4. Perform hand hygiene, and attach suction.
   a. In many institutions the catheter is attached to the mechanical ventilator circuit by a respiratory therapist. If catheter is not already in place, open suction catheter package using aseptic technique, attach closed suction catheter to ventilator circuit by removing swivel adapter and placing closed suction catheter apparatus on ET or tracheostomy tube, and connect Y on mechanical ventilator circuit to closed suction catheter with flex tubing (see illustrations).
   b. Connect one end of connecting tubing to suction machine, and connect other to the end of a closed system or in-line suction catheter, if not already done. Turn suction device on, and set vacuum regulator to appropriate negative pressure (see manufacturer's directions). Many closed system suction catheters require slightly higher suction pressures; consult manufacturer's guidelines (Connelly and Stone, 1991).

5. Hyperinflate and/or hyperoxygenate client with bag-valve-mask or manual breathing mechanism on mechanical ventilator according to institution protocol and clinical status (usually 100% oxygen).
6. Unlock suction control mechanism if required by manufacturer. Open saline port, and attach saline syringe or vial.
7. Pick up suction catheter enclosed in plastic sleeve with dominant hand.

- **Critical Decision Point**
  The use of normal saline instillation with closed in-line suction catheters may not be appropriate for all clients and needs further investigation. Normal saline instillation in conjunction with endotracheal tube suctioning may lead to the dispersion of microorganisms into the lower respiratory tract (Fretag and others, 2003; Sole and others, 2002).

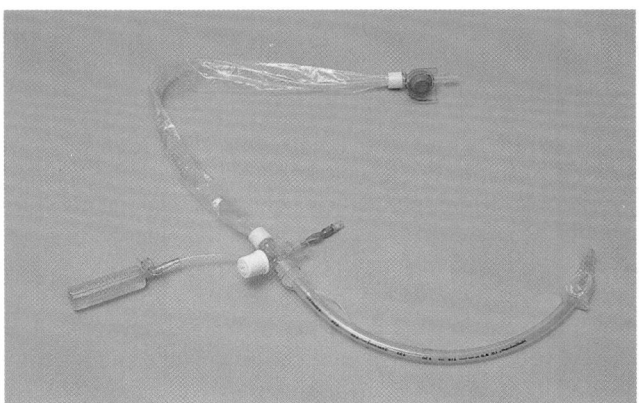

A

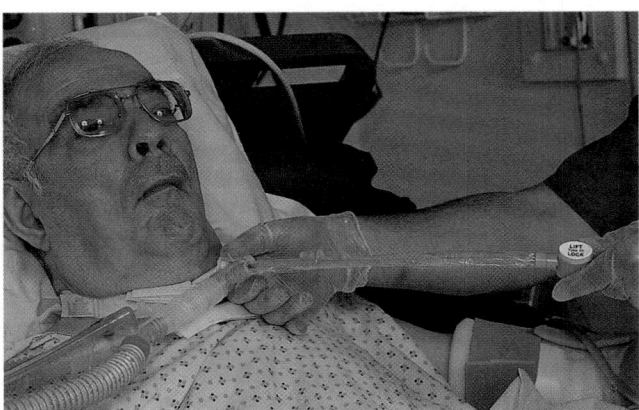

B

STEP 4a A, Closed system suction catheter attached to endotracheal tube. **B,** Suctioning tracheostomy with closed system suction catheter.

BOX 24-1 Procedural Guideline, cont'd
Closed (in-line) suction catheter

8. Insert catheter; use a repeating maneuver of pushing catheter and sliding (or pulling) plastic sleeve back between thumb and forefinger until resistance is felt or client coughs.

9. Encourage client to cough, and apply suction by squeezing on suction control mechanism while withdrawing catheter. It is difficult to apply intermittent pulses of suction and nearly impossible to rotate the catheter compared with a standard catheter. Be sure to withdraw catheter completely into plastic sheath so it does not obstruct airflow.

10. Reassess cardiopulmonary status, including pulse oximetry, to determine need for subsequent suctioning or complications. Repeat steps 5 through 9 one to two more times to clear secretions. Allow adequate time (at least 1 full minute) between suction passes for ventilation and reoxygenation.

11. When airway is clear, withdraw catheter completely into sheath. Be sure that colored indicator line on catheter is visible in the sheath. Squeeze vial or push syringe while applying suction to rinse inner lumen of catheter. Use at least 5 to 10 ml of saline to rinse the catheter until it is clear of retained secretions, which can cause bacterial growth and increase the risk of infection (Fretag and others, 2003). Lock suction mechanism, if applicable, and turn off suction.

12. If client requires oral or nasal suctioning, perform Skill 24-1 or 24-2 with separate standard suction catheter.

13. Reposition client.

14. Remove gloves and discard into appropriate receptacle, and perform hand hygiene.

15. Compare client's respiratory assessments before and after suctioning and observe airway secretions.

SKILL 24-3 Performing Endotracheal Tube Care

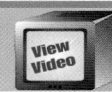
View Video

Endotracheal tubes (ETs) are used as short-term artificial airways to administer mechanical ventilation, relieve upper airway obstruction, protect against aspiration, and clear secretions. Routine care is needed to maintain correct position of the tube and to maintain good hygiene.

After insertion of an ET tube, the cuff is inflated. Preventing cuff-related problems is a critical component of nursing care and depends on securing the tube and inflating the cuff properly. In many institutions these functions are shared by nursing and respiratory therapy staff. An inadequately secured ET tube moves up and down the tracheobronchial tree. Allowing an ET tube to slip too far down into the lungs can prevent ventilation of a lung, usually the left lung (and sometimes the right upper lobe also) because of anatomical differences. Allowing an ET tube to slide too far up the tracheobronchial tree can allow air to escape through or damage the vocal cords and epiglottis or permit aspiration of upper airway secretions. Properly securing the ET tube prevents incidental extubation from coughing or pulling on the tube. In addition, movement of an ET tube can cause development of granulation tissue on the vocal cords, epiglottis, or trachea. Additional risks of movement of an artificial airway are tracheal stenosis, tracheomalacia, erosion of the innominate artery, and tracheoesophageal fistula, particularly when the cuff is overinflated. Risks for each of these complications can be reduced with proper nursing care.

After the tube is inserted and secured and the cuff is inflated (see Skill 24-5), the chief concern of the nurse is to maintain patency of the ET tube. In clients who cannot clear the airway of secretions, patency is achieved primarily through periodic suctioning of the artificial airway.

DELEGATION CONSIDERATIONS

This skill should not be delegated to assistive personnel. Assistive personnel may assist the nurse with endotracheal tube care. In addition, other aspects of care, such as vital signs, hygiene, and mobility, are delegated to assistive personnel. Before delegating any aspect of care of a client with an endotracheal tube, the nurse must:

* Instruct assistive personnel to immediately report to the nurse any signs of respiratory problems or increased airway secretions
* Instruct assistive personnel to immediately report to the nurse if the ET tube appears to have moved or become obstructed or dislodged
* Instruct assistive personnel in signs of hypoxia (e.g., irritability, restlessness, decreased pulse oximetry value, change in vital signs) and to immediately report these to the nurse for further assessment

EQUIPMENT

❑ Towel
❑ Endotracheal and oropharyngeal suction equipment
❑ 1- or 1½-inch wide adhesive or waterproof tape (do not use paper or silk tape) or commercial ET tube holder and mouthguard (follow manufacturer's instructions for securing)
❑ Nonsterile gloves (two pairs)
❑ Adhesive remover swab or acetone on cotton ball
❑ Mouthwash-soaked clean 4 × 4 inch gauze secured on tongue blade or sponge-tipped applicators
❑ Toothbrush, toothpaste (optional), and shaving supplies
❑ One wet and one soapy washcloth or paper towels
❑ Clean 2 × 2 inch gauze
❑ Tincture of benzoin, liquid adhesive, or skin prep pads
❑ Tongue blade (optional)
❑ Face shield, if indicated

STEP	RATIONALE

ASSESSMENT

1. Observe for signs and symptoms of need to perform ET tube care: soiled or loose tape; pressure sore on nares, lips, or corner of mouth; excess nasal or oral secretions; client moving tube with tongue, biting tube or tongue; tube repositioned by physician or other specially trained personnel; foul-smelling mouth.

Presence of ET tube impairs ability of client to swallow oral secretions. Client is also at increased risk for development of pressure areas from impaired circulation as tube is pulled or pressed against nasal or oral mucosa.

2. Observe for factors that increase risk of complications from ET tube: type and size of tube, movement of tube up and down trachea (in and out), duration of tube placement, cuff overinflation or underinflation, presence of facial trauma, malnutrition, and neck or thoracic radiation.

Nasal tube cannot be rotated from side to side like oral tube. Pressure sores are more likely. Tube moving up and down trachea predisposes client to develop tracheoesophageal fistula or tracheomalacia. The tube can become dislodged from the lower airway (incidental extubation), or it can enter mainstem bronchus. Cuff underinflation may allow aspiration, whereas cuff overinflation may cause ischemia or necrosis of tracheal tissue from obstruction of capillary bed. Client can "tongue" oral tube easily and dislodge it. Longer duration of intubation is associated with increased risk of lower airway complications, as is facial trauma. Tissue is more prone to breakdown in presence of malnutrition and radiation.

3. Determine proper ET tube depth as noted as centimeters to lip of gum line. This line is marked on the tube and recorded in the client's record at time of intubation.

Ensures that tube is a proper depth to adequately ventilate both lungs and that the tube is not to high to cause vocal cord damage or too low to result in right mainstem intubation in which only the right lung is ventilated (Day and others, 2002).

4. Assess client's knowledge of procedure.

Encourages cooperation, minimizes risks and anxiety. Identifies teaching needs.

NURSING DIAGNOSES

* Deficient knowledge regarding airway clearance techniques and devices
* Ineffective airway clearance
* Impaired spontaneous ventilation
* Risk for infection
* Ineffective breathing pattern

* Impaired skin integrity
* Impaired gas exchange
* Impaired swallowing
* Risk for aspiration

Related factors are individualized based on client's condition or needs.

STEP	RATIONALE

PLANNING

1. Expected outcomes following completion of procedure:
   - ET tube is maintained in correct position in client's trachea.
   - Client's skin around mouth and oral mucous membranes does not have pressure areas or other injury from biting: tube is repositioned on opposite side of mouth or center of mouth at least every 24 to 48 hours according to institution protocol (oral ET tube only). Oral airway, if used, is cleaned and reinserted to prevent biting of tongue or inner cheeks.
   - Endotracheal tube is resecured at proper depth as evidenced by the following: clean tape is firmly secured to cheeks, upper lip, or top of nose and tube only; depth of tube is same as when started or as ordered (same centimeter marking at gums or lips); bilateral breath sounds are equal.
2. Obtain assistance in this procedure.
3. Explain procedure and client's participation, including importance of the following: not biting or moving ET tube with tongue; trying not to cough when tape is off ET tube; keeping hands down and not pulling on tubing; removal of tape from face can be uncomfortable.
4. Assist client with assuming position comfortable for both nurse and client (usually supine or semi-Fowler's).
5. Place towel across chest.

Complications of lower airway and vocal cord trauma prevented.

Endotracheal tube does not place undue pressure against corners of mouth causing pressure area. Client is not able to bite inner cheeks or tongue.

Endotracheal tube care prevents movement of tube out of airway or into mainstem bronchus.

Reduces risk of incidental extubation of ET tube.

Reduces anxiety, encourages cooperation, and reduces risks.

Promotes client comfort; prevents nurse muscle strain.

Reduces transmission of organisms and protects client's gown and bed linen from contamination.

IMPLEMENTATION

1. Perform hand hygiene. Apply face shield if indicated.
2. Administer endotracheal, nasopharyngeal, and oropharyngeal suction (see Skills 24-1 and 24-2).
3. Connect oral suction catheter to suction source.
4. Prepare method to secure endotracheal tube.
   a. **Tape method.** Cut a piece of tape long enough to go completely around client's head from nares to nares plus 6 inches: adult, 30 to 60 cm (1 to 2 feet). Lay tape adhesive-side up on bedside table. Cut and lay 8 to 15 cm (3 to 6 inches) of tape, adhesive sides together, in center of long strip to prevent tape from sticking to hair. Smaller strip of tape should cover area between ears around back of head.
   b. **Commercially available endotracheal tube holder.** Open package per manufacturer's instructions. Set device aside with the head guard in place and the Velcro strips open.
5. Apply gloves. Instruct helper to apply pair of gloves and hold ET tube firmly at client's lips or nares. Note the number marking on the ET tube at the gum line.

Reduces transmission of microorganisms.

Removes secretions. Diminishes client's need to cough during procedure.

Prepares client for oropharyngeal suctioning.

Preparing tape ahead allows nurse to have one hand positioned on ET tube throughout procedure. Adhesive tape must encircle head below ears with sufficient tape left to wrap around tube.

Reduces transmission of microorganisms. Maintains proper tube position and prevents incidental extubation.

STEP	RATIONALE

• *Critical Decision Point*

Do not allow helper to hold the tube away from the lips or nares. Doing so allows too much "play" in the tube and increases the risk of tube movement and incidental extubation. Never let go of the ET tube, even for a moment. Client could move or cough, and the tube could become dislodged.

6. Remove old tape or device.	Provides nurse with access to skin under tape for assessment and hygiene. Reduces transmission of microorganisms.
a. **Tape.** Carefully remove tape from ET tube and client's face. If tape is difficult to remove, moisten with (soapy) wet washcloth, water, or adhesive tape remover. Discard tape in appropriate receptacle if nearby.	
b. **Commercially available device.** Remove Velcro strips from ET tube, and remove ET tube holder from client.	Commercial devices are latex free, fast, and convenient. These devices avoid the need for tape and the resultant skin breakdown and are easily applied in the presence of facial hair. The Velcro adhesive strips hold the ET tube in place and provide a marker to measure distance to client's lips or gums. These devices all permit access to client's mouth and lips for ease in oropharyngeal suctioning and oral hygiene.
7. Remove any secretions or adhesive from client's face.	Promotes hygiene. Adhesive can cause damage to skin. Prevents poor adhesion of new tape.
a. Use adhesive remover swab to remove excess adhesive left on face after tape removal. Wash adhesive remover from face.	
8. Remove oral airway or bite block, if present, and place on towel.	Provides access to and complete observation of client's oral cavity.

• *Critical Decision Point*

Do not remove oral airway if client is actively biting ET tube. Wait until tape is partially or completely secured to ET tube.

9. Clean mouth, gums, and teeth opposite ET tube with non–alcohol-based mouthwash solution and 4 × 4 inch gauze, sponge-tipped applicators, or saline swabs. Brush teeth as indicated. If necessary, administer oropharyngeal suctioning with Yankauer suction catheter.	Promotes hygiene and reduces risk of infection to teeth and gums. Alcohol-based mouthwashes dry oral mucosa (Lewis and others, 2000).
10. *Oral ET tube only:* Remembering "cm" ET tube marking at lips or gum line, with help of assistant move ET tube to opposite side or center of mouth. Do not change tube depth.	Prevents formation of pressure sores at sides of client's mouth. Ensures correct position of tube.
11. Repeat oral cleaning as in step 9 on opposite side of mouth.	Removes secretions from mouth and oral pharynx.
12. Clean face and neck with soapy washcloth, rinse, and dry. Shave male client as necessary (see Chapter 14).	Moisture and beard growth prevent adhesive tape adherence.
13. Pour small amount of skin protectant or liquid adhesive on clean 2 × 2 inch gauze, and dot on upper lip (oral ET tube) or across nose (nasal ET tube) and cheeks to ear. Allow to dry completely.	Protects skin from tape burns and makes more adherent.

STEP	RATIONALE

14. Secure ET tube
   a. **Tape method**
      (1) Slip tape under client's head and neck, adhesive side up. Take care not to twist tape or catch hair. Do not allow tape to stick to itself. It helps to gently stick tape to tongue blade, which serves as a guide. Then slide tongue blade under client's neck. Center tape so that double-faced tape extends around back of neck from ear to ear.

      Positions tape to secure ET tube in proper position.

      (2) On one side of face, secure tape from ear to nares (nasal ET tube) or over lip to ET tube (oral ET tube). Tear remaining tape in half lengthwise, forming two pieces that are $\frac{1}{2}$ to $\frac{3}{4}$ inch wide. Secure bottom half of tape across upper lip (oral ET tube) or across top of nose (nasal ET tube) to opposite ear (see illustration *A*). Wrap top half of tape around tube and up from bottom (see illustration *B*). Tape should encircle tube at least two times for security.

      Secures tape to face. Using top tape to wrap prevents downward drag on ET tube.

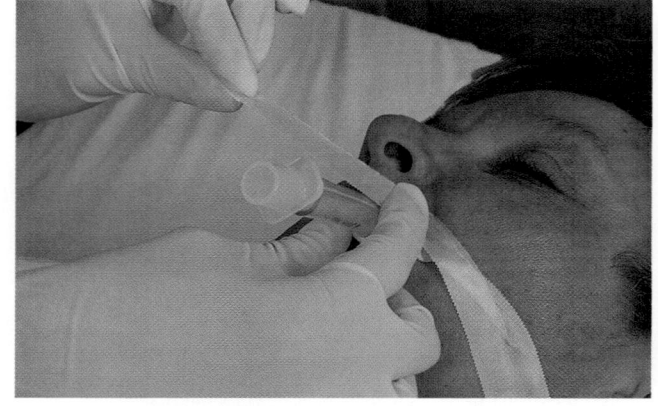
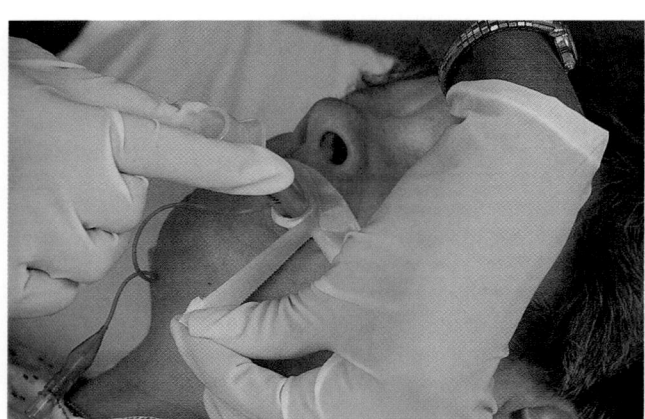

STEP 14a(2) **A,** Securing bottom half of tape across client's upper lip. **B,** Securing top half of tape around tube.

STEP	RATIONALE

(3) Gently pull other side of tape firmly to pick up slack, and secure to opposite side of face and ET tube the same as the first piece. NOTE: ET tube is secured. Assistant can release hold. (Nurse may want assistant to help reinsert oral airway.)

Secures tape to face and tube. Endotracheal tube should be at same depth at the lips or gum line (see illustration). Check earlier assessment for verification of tube depth in centimeters.

b. Commercially available device

(1) Thread ET tube through the opening designed to secure the ET tube. Be sure that the pilot balloon is accessible (see illustration).

Commercially available holders have a slit in the front of the holder designed to secure the ET tube.

(2) Place strips of ET holder under the client at the occipital region of the head.

(3) Verify that the ET tube is at the established depth using the lip or gum line marker as a guide.

Ensures that the ET tube remains at the correct depth as determined during assessment.

(4) Attach the Velcro strips at the base of the client's head. Leave 1 cm (½ inch) slack in the strips.

(5) Verify that tube is secure, it does not move forward from the client's mouth or backward down into the client's throat, and there are no pressure areas on the oral mucosa or the occipital region of the head.

The tube must be secure so that the position of the tube remains at the correct depth. The tube can be secured without being tight and causing pressure.

15. If not already done, remove and clean oral airway in warm soapy water, and rinse well. Hydrogen peroxide can aid in removal of crusted secretions. A mouthwash rinse will freshen client's mouth. Shake excess water from oral airway.

Promotes hygiene. Reduces transmission of microorganisms.

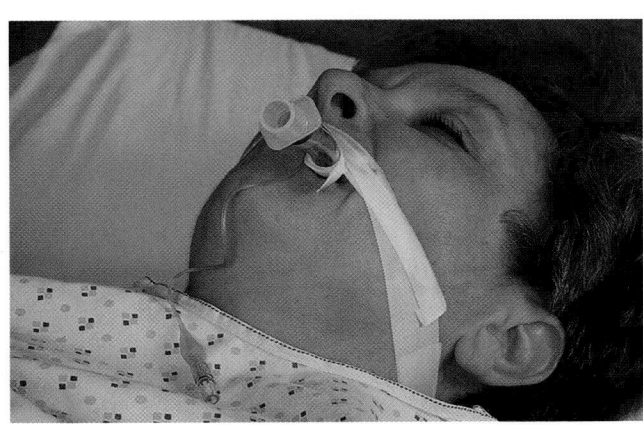

STEP **14a(3)** Tape securing endotracheal tube.

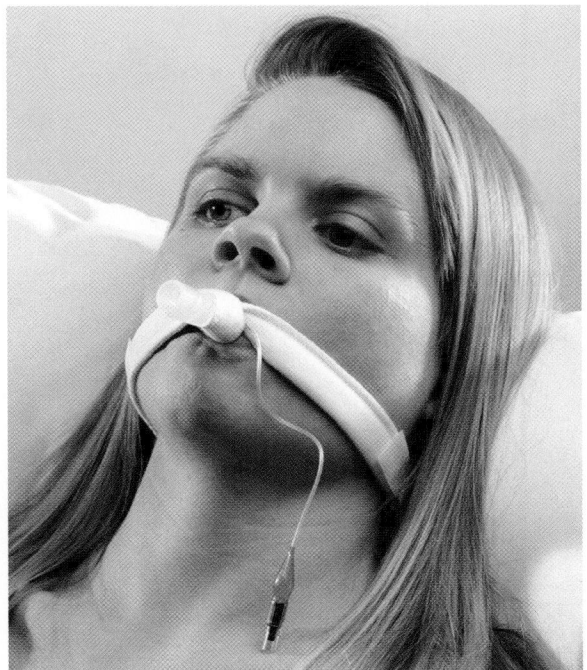

STEP **14b(1)** Endotracheal tube holder in place. (Courtesy Dale Medical Products, Plainesville, Mass.)

STEP	RATIONALE
16. Reinsert oral airway without pushing tongue into oropharynx, and secure with tape (see Chapter 26).	Prevents client from biting ET tube and allows access for oropharyngeal suctioning.
17. Discard soiled items in appropriate receptacle. Remove towel, and place in laundry.	Reduces transmission of microorganisms.
18. Reposition client.	Promotes comfort.
19. Remove gloves and face shield, discard in receptacle, and perform hand hygiene. Assistant is also to remove gloves and perform hand hygiene before leaving client's room. Place clean items (e.g., tincture of benzoin, mouthwash, excess swabs) in place of storage.	Reduces transmission of microorganisms. Contaminated gloves and hands should not touch clean items.

EVALUATION

1. Compare respiratory assessments before and after ET tube care.	Identifies any changes in presence and quality of breath sounds after procedure.
2. Observe depth and position of ET tube according to physician recommendation.	Position of ET tube should not be altered.
3. Assess security of tape by gently tugging at tube.	Tape should remain attached to face. Client may cough.
4. Assess skin around mouth and oral mucous membranes for intactness and pressure areas.	Tape should not tear skin. Pressure areas should be absent.

Recording and Reporting

- Record assessments before and after care, supplies used, client's tolerance of procedure, appropriate depth of ET tube, frequency of ET tube care, integrity of oral mucosa, pressure sore care as needed, and designated intervals.

Unexpected Outcomes	Related Interventions
1. Unexpected extubation.	• Remain with client. • Call for assistance. • Assess client for airway patency, spontaneous breathing, and vital signs • Prepare for reintubation.
2. Movement of endotracheal tube.	• Repeat taping procedure. • In very active clients without facial injury who are at risk for self-extubation, consider applying a second piece of tape around the back of the head but going *over* the ears.
3. Unequal breath sounds.	• Suction client. • Evaluate ET tube for proper depth before and after ET tube care. If ET tube is deeper or shallower, reposition tube only if allowed by institution and nurse has received appropriate instructions. • Notify physician, who may order chest x-ray film to verify placement, and then reposition ET tube.

Unexpected Outcomes	Related Interventions
4. Pressure areas from tube.	• Increase frequency of ET tube care. • Apply antimicrobial ointment per institutional protocol. • Align oxygen and humidity supply tubings so that they do not pull ET tube, creating pressure areas. • Monitor for infection. If skin tear is present on cheeks or over nose or upper lip, apply protective barrier such as stoma adhesive patch or hydrocolloid dressing, and apply tape to this.
5. Air escaping around tube (see Skill 24-5).	• Verify correct position of tube. If tube position is correct, assess proper cuff inflation. If tube position is incorrect, reposition according to protocol or notify physician (see Skill 24-5).

Teaching Considerations

- Instruct client and family not to manipulate the ET tube, tape, or ET tube holder. If the client is complaining or appears uncomfortable, instruct family to ask for the nurse.
- Inform the client and family that if the tube causes gagging to tell the nurse and interventions will be taken to reduce gagging. This may include repositioning of the tube and/or sedation.

Pediatric Considerations

- Neonatal and pediatric procedures for securing ET tubes and suctioning airways may vary (Hockenberry and others, 2003).

- Infant skin may be more prone to tearing when tape is removed (Hockenberry and others, 2003).
- Because of infants' delicate skin, skin prep may not be used before securing ET tube. ET tube holders are best used in this population.

Gerontological Considerations

- Older adult skin may be more prone to tearing when tape is removed.
- Older adults with tendency toward inadequate nutrition may be more prone to complications (e.g., infection, breakdown of oral mucosa).

SKILL 24-4 Performing Tracheostomy Care

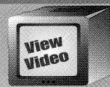

A tracheostomy tube can cause development of granulation tissue on the vocal cords, epiglottis, or trachea. Additional risks from movement of the artificial airway are tracheal stenosis, tracheomalacia, erosion of the innominate artery, and tracheoesophageal fistula, particularly when the cuff is overinflated. Risks for each of these complications can be reduced with proper nursing care. (See additional material related to cuff inflation in Skill 24-5.)

Some clients with a tracheostomy tube are able to cough secretions out of the tracheostomy tube completely, whereas others are able only to cough secretions up into the tracheostomy tube. The latter clients may not require suctioning when an inner cannula is present because it can be safely removed, cleaned, and reinserted.

A comprehensive plan and execution of care include properly securing the tube, inflating the cuff to an appropriate pressure, maintaining patency by suctioning, and encouraging communication and oral hygiene (Peers, 2003). The intubated client is unable to speak because placement of the ET and tracheostomy tube prevents normal airflow over and vibration of the vocal cords. When caring for an intubated client, the nurse is encouraged to use verbal and nonverbal communication skills to converse. Alphabet charts, pen and paper, slates or chalk boards, or magnetic pen doodle boards are some commonly used communication tools. There are many more simple to sophisticated communication devices that can be used. A speech therapist can assist the nurse in establishing effective communication.

DELEGATION CONSIDERATIONS

This skill should not be routinely delegated to assistive personnel. In some settings, clients who have well-established tracheostomy tubes may have the care delegated to assistive personnel. It is the responsibility of the nurse to assess and ensure that proper artificial airway care is provided. In addition, assistive personnel may perform other aspects of the client's care. The nurse should instruct assistive personnel about:

- Immediately reporting to the nurse any changes in the client's respiratory status, level of consciousness, confusion, restlessness or irritability, or change in level of comfort
- Immediately reporting any dislodgement or excessive movement of the tracheostomy tube
- Immediately reporting expected color of tracheal stoma and drainage

EQUIPMENT

- ❑ Bedside table
- ❑ Towel
- ❑ Tracheostomy suction supplies
- ❑ Sterile tracheostomy care kit, if available (be sure to collect supplies listed that are not available in kit) or three sterile 4 × 4 inch gauze pads
- ❑ Sterile cotton-tipped applicators
- ❑ Sterile tracheostomy dressing (precut and sewn surgical dressing)
- ❑ Sterile basin
- ❑ Small sterile brush (or disposable inner cannula)
- ❑ Roll of twill tape, tracheostomy ties, or tracheostomy holder
- ❑ Hydrogen peroxide
- ❑ Normal saline solution
- ❑ Scissors
- ❑ Sterile gloves (two)
- ❑ Face shield

STEP	RATIONALE

ASSESSMENT

1. Observe for signs and symptoms of need to perform tracheostomy care: excess peristomal secretions, excess intratracheal secretions, soiled or damp tracheostomy ties, soiled or damp tracheostomy dressing, diminished airflow through tracheostomy tube, or signs and symptoms of airway obstruction requiring suctioning (see Skill 24-2).

2. Observe for factors (e.g., hydration, humidity, infection, nutrition, ability to cough) that normally influence tracheostomy airway functioning.

3. Assess client's understanding of and ability to perform own tracheostomy care.

Signs and symptoms are related to presence of secretions at stoma site or within tracheostomy tube. The accompanying illustrations show a partially inflated cuff on an outer cannula, syringe used for cuff inflation, and an obturator that is used to insert outer cannula (see illustrations *A* and *B*).

Allows nurse to accurately assess need to perform tracheostomy care.

Allows nurse to identify potential need for instruction.

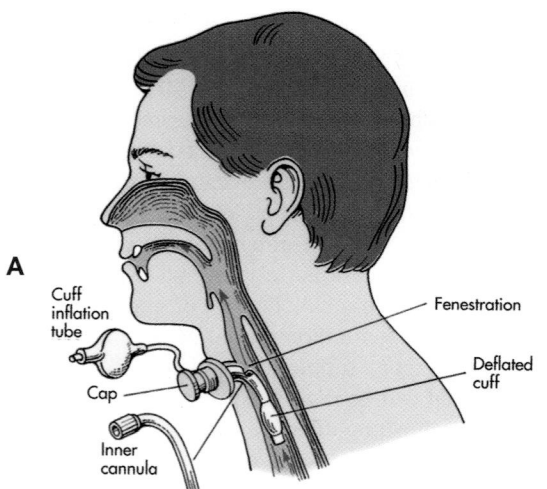

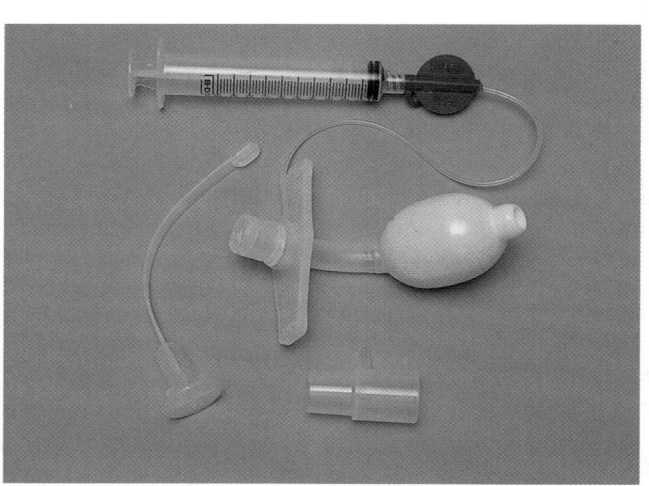

STEP 1 A, Tracheostomy tube (fenestrated) inserted with inner cannula removed, cuff deflated, and cap in place to allow speech. (Lewis SL and others: *Medical-surgical nursing: assessment and management of clinical problems,* ed 6, St. Louis, 2004, Mosby.) **B,** Tracheostomy tube with obturator for insertion and syringe for inflation of cuff.

STEP	**RATIONALE**
4. Check when tracheostomy care was last performed.	Tracheostomy care is provided at least every 8 to 12 hours and more often if indicated (e.g., increased airway secretions, infection [airway or stoma], increased secretions around stoma).

NURSING DIAGNOSES

- Deficient knowledge regarding airway clearance techniques and devices
- Ineffective airway clearance
- Ineffective breathing pattern
- Impaired gas exchange

- Impaired spontaneous ventilation
- Impaired swallowing
- Risk for aspiration
- Risk for infection

Related factors are individualized based on client's condition or needs.

PLANNING

1. Expected outcomes following completion of procedure: • Inner cannula and outer cannula of trach tube are free of secretions; ties are clean, secured snugly, and tied in double square knot.	Trach tube is patent and secure. Tracheostomy tube that is clear and free of secretions optimizes the amount of oxygen delivered to client and limits risk of infection from retained secretions.
• Stoma site is pink, does not bleed, and is free of secretions.	Indicates absence of infection at stoma site. Dry, intact tracheostomy stoma reduces risk of subsequent systemic infection.
2. Have another nurse or family member assist in this procedure.	Prevents accidental extubation of tracheostomy tube.
3. Explain procedure and client's participation.	Encourages cooperation, minimizes risks, and reduces anxiety.
4. Assist client to position comfortable for both nurse and client (usually supine or semi-Fowler's).	Promotes client comfort and prevents nurse muscle strain.
5. Place towel across client's chest.	Reduces transmission of microorganisms.

IMPLEMENTATION

1. Perform hand hygiene, and apply gloves and face shield if applicable.	Reduces transmission of microorganisms.
2. Suction tracheostomy (see Skill 24-2). Before removing gloves, remove soiled tracheostomy dressing, and discard in glove with coiled catheter.	Removes secretions to avoid occluding outer cannula while inner cannula is removed. Reduces need for client to cough.
3. While client is replenishing oxygen stores, prepare equipment on bedside table.	Prepares equipment and allows for smooth, organized completion of tracheostomy care.

   a. Open sterile tracheostomy kit. Open three 4 × 4 inch gauze packages using aseptic technique, and pour normal saline on one package and hydrogen peroxide on another. Leave third package dry. Open two cotton-tipped swab packages, and pour normal saline on one package and hydrogen peroxide on the other. Do not recap hydrogen peroxide and normal saline.

   b. Open sterile tracheostomy dressing package.

   c. Unwrap sterile basin, and pour about 0.5 to 2 cm (½ inch) hydrogen peroxide into it.

   d. Open small sterile brush package, and place aseptically into sterile basin.

STEP	RATIONALE

  e. Prepare length of twill tape long enough to go around client's neck two times, about 60 to 75 cm (24 to 30 inches) for an adult. Cut ends on diagonal. Lay aside in dry area.

   Cutting ends of tie on diagonal aids in inserting tie through eyelet.

  f. If using commercially available tracheostomy tube holder, open package according to manufacturer's directions.

4. Apply gloves. Keep dominant hand sterile throughout procedure.

   Reduces transmission of microorganisms.

5. Remove oxygen source. Apply oxygen source loosely over tracheostomy if client desaturates during procedure.

   Helps to reduce the amount of desaturation.

• *Critical Decision Point*

 For tracheostomy tube with no inner cannula or Kistner button, continue with step 8.

6. Tracheostomy With Inner Cannula Care

  a. While touching only the outer aspect of the tube, remove the inner cannula with nondominant hand. Drop inner cannula into hydrogen peroxide basin.

   Removes inner cannula for cleaning. Hydrogen peroxide loosens secretions from inner cannula.

  b. Place tracheostomy collar, T tube, or ventilator oxygen source over outer cannula (NOTE: T tube and ventilator oxygen devices cannot be attached to all outer cannulas when the inner cannula is removed.)

   Maintains supply of oxygen to client.

  c. To prevent oxygen desaturation in affected clients, quickly pick up inner cannula, and use small brush to remove secretions inside and outside inner cannula (see illustrations).

   Tracheostomy brush provides mechanical force to remove thick or dried secretions.

  d. Hold inner cannula over basin, and rinse with normal saline, using nondominant hand to pour normal saline.

   Removes secretions and hydrogen peroxide from inner cannula.

  e. Replace inner cannula, and secure "locking" mechanism (see illustration). Reapply ventilator or oxygen sources.

   Secures inner cannula and reestablishes oxygen supply.

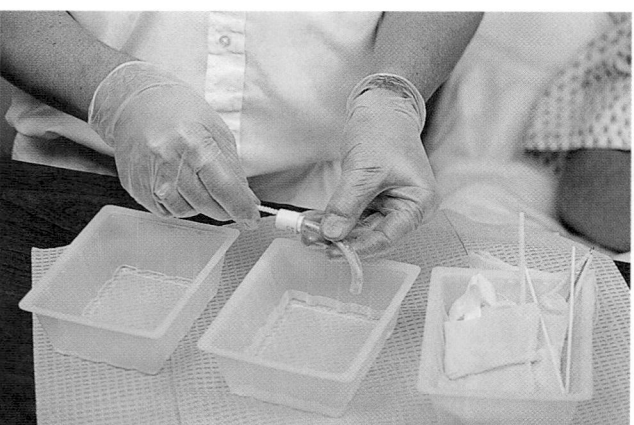

STEP **6c** Cleansing the tracheostomy inner cannula.

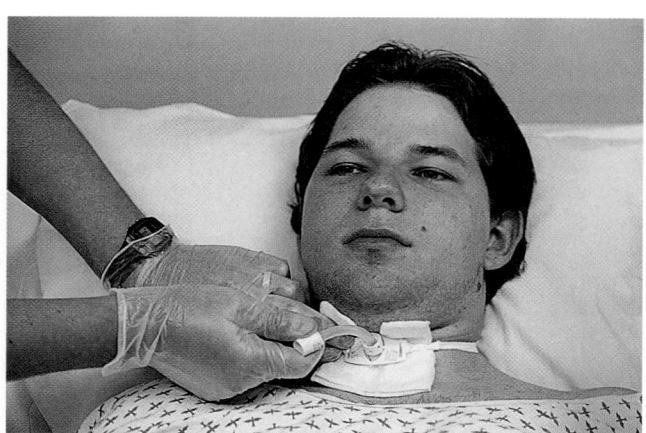

STEP **6e** Reinserting the inner cannula.

STEP	RATIONALE

7. Tracheostomy with disposable inner cannula
   a. Remove cannula from manufacturer's packaging.
   b. While touching only the outer aspect of the tube, withdraw inner cannula, and replace with new cannula. Lock into position.
   c. Dispose of contaminated cannula in appropriate receptacle, and apply ventilator or oxygen sources.

8. Using hydrogen peroxide–saturated cotton-tipped swabs and 4 × 4 inch gauze, clean exposed outer cannula surfaces and stoma under faceplate extending 5 to 10 cm (2 to 4 inches) in all directions from stoma (see illustration). Clean in circular motion from stoma site outward using dominant hand to handle sterile supplies.

Aseptically removes secretions from stoma site. Moving in outward circle pulls mucus and other contaminants from stoma to periphery.

9. Using normal saline–saturated cotton-tipped swabs and 4 × 4 inch gauze, rinse hydrogen peroxide from tracheostomy tube and skin surfaces.

Rinses hydrogen peroxide from surfaces. If not removed from skin, hydrogen peroxide can promote tissue injury.

10. Using dry 4 × 4 inch gauze, pat lightly at skin and exposed outer cannula surfaces.

Dry surfaces prohibit formation of moist environment for microorganism growth and skin excoriation.

11. Secure tracheostomy.
    a. Trach tie method
        (1) Instruct assistant, if available, to apply gloves and securely hold tracheostomy tube in place. With assistant holding tracheostomy tube, cut old ties.

Promotes hygiene and reduces transmission of microorganisms. Secures trach tube. Reduces risk of incidental extubation.

• *Critical Decision Point*
Assistant must not release hold on tracheostomy tube until new ties are firmly tied. If working without an assistant, do not cut old ties until new ties are in place and securely tied.

        (2) Take prepared tie and insert one end of tie through faceplate eyelet, and pull ends even (see illustration).
        (3) Slide both ends of tie behind the head and around neck to other eyelet, and insert one tie through second eyelet.
        (4) Pull snugly.

Ensures tracheostomy will not come out.

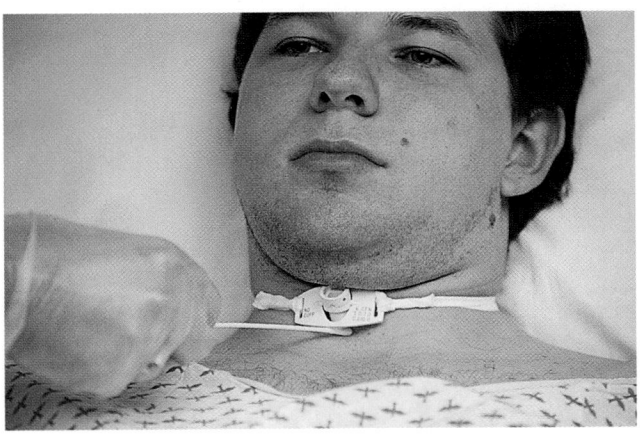

STEP **8** Cleansing around the stoma.

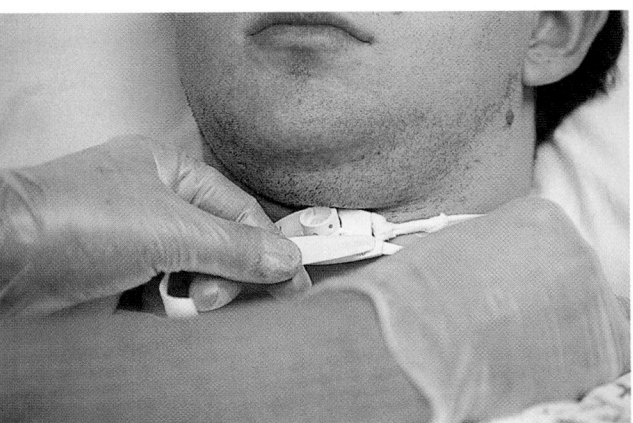

STEP **11a(2)** Replacing tracheostomy ties. Do not remove old tracheostomy ties until new ones are secure.

STEP	RATIONALE

    (5) Tie ends securely in double square knot, allowing space for only one loose or two snug finger widths in tie (see illustration).

    (6) Insert fresh tracheostomy dressing under clean ties and faceplate (see illustration).

  b. Trach tube holder method

    (1) While wearing gloves, maintain a secure hold on the tracheostomy tube. This can be done with an assistant or, when an assistant is not available, leave the old trach tube holder in place until the new device is secure.

    (2) Align strap under client's neck. Be sure that the Velcro attachments are positioned on either side of the tracheostomy tube.

    (3) Place narrow end of the ties under and through the faceplate eyelets. Pull ends even, and secure with the Velcro closures.

    (4) Verify that there is space for only one loose or two snug finger width(s) under neck strap (see illustration).

12. Position client comfortably, and assess respiratory status.

13. Replace any oxygen delivery sources.

14. Remove gloves and face shield, and discard in appropriate receptacle.

Rationale column:

One finger width of slack prevents ties from being too tight when tracheostomy dressing is in place and also prevents movement of trach tube in lower airway.

Absorbs drainage. Dressing prevents pressure on clavicle heads.

Promotes comfort. Some clients may require post–tracheostomy care suctioning.

Reduces transmission of microorganisms. Contaminated gloves should not touch clean supplies.

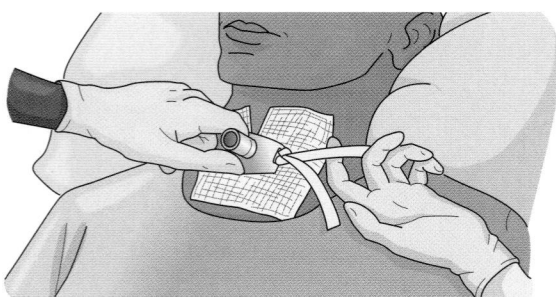

STEP 11a(5) Tracheostomy ties properly placed. (From Sorrentino SA: *Mosby's textbook for nursing assistants,* ed 5, St. Louis, 2000, Mosby.)

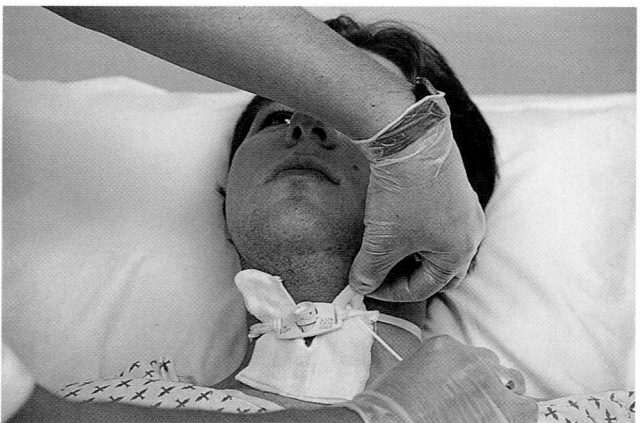

STEP 11a(6) Applying tracheostomy dressing.

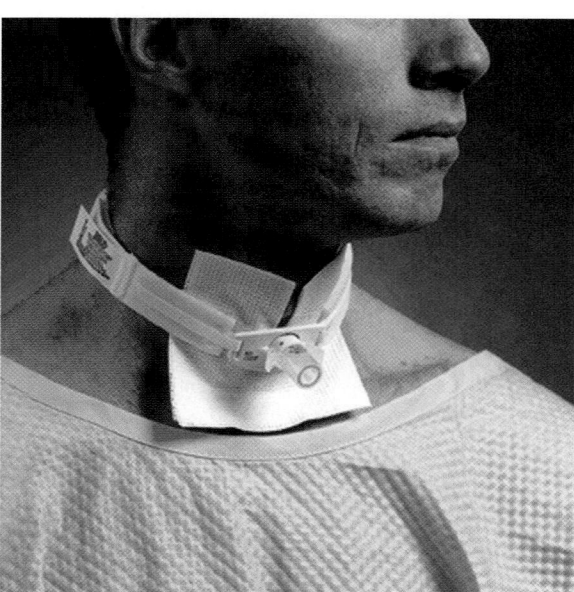

STEP 11b(4) Tracheostomy tube holder in place. (Courtesy Dale Medical Products, Plainesville, Mass.)

STEP	RATIONALE
15. Replace cap on hydrogen peroxide and normal saline bottles. Store reusable liquids and unused supplies in appropriate place.	Once opened, normal saline can be considered free of bacteria for 24 hours, after which it should be discarded.
16. Perform hand hygiene.	Reduces transmission of microorganisms among clients.

EVALUATION

1. Compare assessments before and after tracheostomy care.	Determines effectiveness of tracheostomy care.
2. Assess comfort of new tracheostomy ties.	Tracheostomy ties are uncomfortable and place client at risk for injury when they are too loose or too tight.
3. Inspect inner and outer cannulas for secretions.	Presence of secretions on cannulas indicates the need for more vigorous tracheostomy care.
4. Assess stoma for signs of infection or skin breakdown.	Broken skin places client at risk for infection. Stomal infection necessitates change in tracheostomy skin care plan.

Recording and Reporting

- Record respiratory assessments before and after care.
- Record the type and size of tracheostomy tube, frequency and extent of care, client tolerance, special care in event of stomatitis.

Unexpected Outcomes	Related Interventions
1. Excessively loose or tight tracheostomy ties/trach holder.	• Adjust ties, or apply new ties/trach holder.
2. Stomatitis.	• Increase frequency of tracheostomy care. • Consider intermittent application of heat to increase blood flow and promote healing. • Apply topical antibacterial solution, and allow it to dry and provide bacterial barrier. • Apply hydrocolloid or transparent dressing just under stoma to protect skin from breakdown. Consult with skin care specialist.
3. Pressure area around tracheostomy tube.	• Increase frequency of tracheostomy care, and keep dressing under faceplate at all times. • Consider using double dressing or applying hydrocolloid or stoma adhesive dressing around stoma.
4. Accidental decannulation.	• Call for assistance. • Replace old tracheostomy tube with new tube. Some experienced nurses or respiratory therapists may be able to quickly reinsert tracheostomy tube. • Keep spare tracheostomy tube of same size and kind at bedside in event of emergency replacement (Seay and others, 2002). • Same-size ET tube can be inserted in stoma in an emergency. • Insert suction catheter to confirm that the new tube is in the trachea (Seay and others, 2002). • Be prepared to manually ventilate clients in whom respiratory distress develops. • Notify physician.

Continued

Unexpected Outcomes	Related Interventions
5. Respiratory distress from mucous plug in cannula.	• Remove inner cannula, if applicable, for cleaning, or cannula can be suctioned. • Notify physician or specially trained personnel if tracheostomy tube requires replacement.

Teaching Considerations

• Different types of tracheostomy tubes have different faceplates. Some are rigid, others are not. Instruct caregivers not to lift up on rigid faceplates or they may dislodge tube.
• Some commercial tracheostomy tube holders require removal of excess tie material to fit properly.
• If long-term placement of tracheostomy is anticipated, nurse should plan to teach client and family tracheostomy care.
• Clients with new tracheostomy frequently have bloody secretions for 2 to 3 days after procedure and for 24 hours after each tracheostomy change.

Pediatric Considerations

• Children generally have shorter necks, so stoma may be more difficult to clean.
• Pediatric tracheostomy tubes (smaller than size 4) do not contain an inner cannula.
• Routine tracheostomy tube changes are carried out weekly after a tract has formed (Hockenberry and others, 2003).

Gerontological Considerations

• Older adults may have more fragile skin and may be more prone to skin breakdown from secretions or pressure (Lueckenotte, 2000).
• Older adults with impaired nutrition may not heal well.

SKILL 24-5 Inflating the Cuff on an Endotracheal or Tracheostomy Tube

The goals of correctly inflating the cuff on an artificial airway are to promote lung inflation for mechanical ventilation, to prevent aspiration of gastric contents, and at the same time to allow drainage of secretions that accumulate between the epiglottis and the cuff (Box 24-2). The amount of air inserted in the cuff is based on several factors; the two most important factors are the size of the client's trachea and the external diameter of the artificial airway. If two clients of approximately the same size are intubated—one with a size 6 and one with a size 8—the client with the larger tube (size 8) will require less air in the cuff. This is because the larger tube occludes more of the airway than the smaller tube does. If the cuff pressures are too high, permanent damage to the tracheal mucosa can occur (Peers, 2003).

There is no recommendation on a preferred method for cuff inflation. The minimal leak technique and the minimal occlusive technique are both acceptable methods (St. John, 1999) (Table 24-3).

BOX 24-2 Indications for Cuff Inflation

MECHANICAL VENTILATION

Continuous airway pressure
Positive end-expiratory pressure (PEEP)
Inability to meet ventilatory requirements with cuff down
Inability to meet oxygen requirements with cuff down

RISK OF ASPIRATING GASTRIC CONTENTS

Feeding tube, especially large bore, in stomach
Gastroesophageal reflux disease
Hiatal hernia
During and after meals
Impaired gastric emptying
Decreased gag reflex
Impaired swallowing

TABLE 24-3 ENDOTRACHEAL AND TRACHEOSTOMY CUFF INFLATION METHODS

INFLATION METHOD	PROCEDURE
Minimal occlusive technique	1. Inject air into the cuff until no airflow is auscultated over the trachea during the peak inflation pressure of a positive pressure breath. 2. Record the cuff volume.
Minimal leak technique	1. Inject air into the cuff until the air leak around the cuff is eliminated. 2. Remove a small amount of air from the cuff until a slight leak occurs (50 to 100 ml tidal volume decrease) at peak inflation pressure during a positive pressure breath. 3. Record the cuff volume.

From St. John RE: Airway management, *Crit Care Nurse* 19(4):79, 1999.

DELEGATION CONSIDERATIONS

The skill of inflating the cuff on an endotracheal or tracheostomy tube should not be delegated to assistive personnel. However, other aspects of care may be delegated to assistive personnel and the nurse should:

- Instruct assistive personnel to immediately report to the nurse any change in vital signs, respiratory status, confusion, restlessness, or discomfort
- Instruct assistive personnel to report to the nurse any indication of the artificial airway's moving or appearing loose

EQUIPMENT

- ❑ Endotracheal/tracheostomy suction apparatus (see Skill 24-2)
- ❑ Stethoscope
- ❑ 5- or 10-ml syringe
- ❑ Alcohol wipe
- ❑ Face shield, if indicated
- ❑ Gloves, if indicated

STEP	RATIONALE

ASSESSMENT

1. Observe for signs and symptoms of need to perform care, including gurgling on expiration, decreased exhaled tidal volume (mechanically ventilated client), spasmodic coughing, tense test balloon on tube, flaccid test balloon on tube, and unexpected phonation.

2. If client is discharged with a cuffed tracheostomy tube, determine caregiver's understanding of procedure.

Partially deflated cuff allows secretions to enter trachea and permits vocalization. High cuff pressure can result in necrosis, tracheomalacia, or tracheoesophageal fistula. Overinflated cuff may cause client to cough.

Identifies teaching needs.

NURSING DIAGNOSES

- Deficient knowledge regarding airway clearance techniques and devices
- Ineffective airway clearance
- Ineffective breathing pattern
- Impaired gas exchange

- Impaired spontaneous ventilation
- Impaired swallowing
- Risk for aspiration
- Risk for infection

Related factors are individualized based on client's condition or needs.

PLANNING

1. Expected outcomes following completion of procedure:
   - Mechanically ventilated clients receive prescribed tidal volume.
   - Minimal leak is auscultated at end inspiration.

   - No evidence of excessive phonation, aspiration of gastric or mouth contents, tracheoesophageal fistula, or tracheomalacia is found.

2. Explain procedure and how client can participate. Explain that some coughing during procedure is normal.

3. Assist client to position comfortable for nurse and client (usually semi-Fowler's).

Proper inflation of cuff ensures client receives tidal volume.

Allows drainage of secretions during inhalation when airway is at widest but prevents gross aspiration during exhalation when airway is narrower. Prevents continuous contact of tracheal mucosa with cuff.

Proper level of cuff inflation is consistently maintained. Aspiration and phonation can occur when cuff is underinflated. Tracheoesophageal fistula and tracheomalacia can occur when the cuff is overinflated.

Encourages cooperation, minimizes risks, and reduces anxiety.

Promotes client comfort, prevents nurse muscle strain, and facilitates drainage.

IMPLEMENTATION

1. Perform hand hygiene, and apply gloves and face shield, if indicated.

2. Suction secretions through ET or tracheostomy tube and also mouth.

3. Connect syringe to pilot balloon.

Reduces transmission of microorganisms.

Ensures patent airway and facilitates hearing airflow with stethoscope. Prevents aspiration of oral secretions when cuff is deflated.

Allows immediate access to equipment for adjusting cuff pressure.

STEP	RATIONALE
4. Place stethoscope in sternal notch or above tracheostomy tube, and listen for minimal amount of air leak at end of inspiration (see illustration).	Assesses proper cuff inflation.

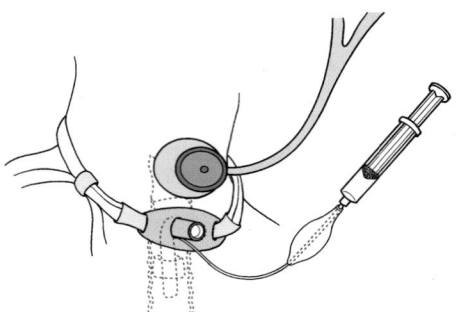

STEP **4** Inflating cuff on tracheostomy.

STEP	RATIONALE
5. If no air leak is heard, remove all air from cuff.	Releases excessive cuff pressure, which reduces capillary blood flow and increases risk of tissue necrosis.
6. Inflate cuff according to agency policy (see Table 24-3).	Inflates cuff to minimal leak. If air leak is audible with ear, air leak is too large. If no air leak is heard, cuff is overinflated.
7. If excessive air leak is heard, slowly add air as in step 6.	Air leak may prevent adequate lung expansion and increase risk of aspiration.
8. Remove stethoscope, and wipe diaphragm with alcohol wipe.	Reduces transmission of microorganisms.
9. Remove syringe, and discard into appropriate receptacle or store per policy. Do not leave attached to pilot balloon valve.	Reduces transmission of microorganisms.

- **Critical Decision Point**
  Leaving syringe in pilot balloon can cause valve to break or "stick open." When syringe is removed, air is lost from cuff.

STEP	RATIONALE
10. Reposition client.	Promotes comfort.
11. Remove gloves and face shield. Discard into appropriate receptacle. Perform hand hygiene.	Reduces transmission of microorganisms.

EVALUATION

1. Compare respiratory assessments before and after cuff care.	Determines effectiveness of cuff care procedure.
2. Observe exhaled tidal volume from mechanical ventilator.	Exhaled tidal volume should be not less than 50 ml of delivered tidal volume.
3. Auscultate for audible air leak.	Air leak should be heard only with stethoscope.
4. Observe for excessive phonation, presence of gastric secretions in airway secretions, or tracheoesophageal fistula.	Occurs with inadequate or excessive cuff inflation.

Recording and Reporting

- Record presence of minimal leak at end inspiration, volume of air injected into cuff, secretions obtained when suctioning, and frequency of cuff care. Documents safe cuff pressure levels.

Unexpected Outcomes	Related Interventions
1. Cuff pressure is excessive.	• Remove air from cuff. • Reinflate with appropriate minimal leak technique.
2. Excessive volume is required to inflate cuff.	• Notify physician. • Consider client may need insertion of larger tube.
3. Excessive air leak is heard.	• Reposition client or tubing. • Reinflate cuff if needed. • Prepare for insertion of new tube by physician or trained personnel if cuff ruptures. • Prepare to manually ventilate client if needed.
4. Cuff requires increased amounts of air to maintain minimal leak.	• Reassess position of tube. • Cuff of ET tube may be higher in trachea (where airway is wider) than previously. • Withdraw all air from cuff so pilot balloon is completely deflated (flat). • Remove syringe from pilot balloon. Watch to see if air reenters pilot balloon (cuff). If so, there is leak in cuff, and tube requires replacement. • Fill cuff appropriately.

Pediatric Considerations
• Pediatric tracheostomy tubes do not have cuffs.
• Neonatal and many pediatric ET tubes do not contain cuffs.

FOCUS on CLINICAL PRACTICE

You are assigned to care for Mrs. Karlowski, a 55-year-old bank manager. The only information you are given is that she has a history of chronic lung disease; a 1-week history of upper respiratory symptoms with shortness of breath; and a 2-day history of increasing fever, cough, malaise, nausea, and worsening shortness of breath.

1. What other information would you like to have about this client?
2. Mrs. Karlowski complains of secretions in her mouth. She feels that she can cough up the pulmonary secretions, but the secretions still remain in her mouth, and they make her nauseous. What intervention would you select to assist her in clearing oral secretions?
   A. Yankauer suctioning
   B. Naso tracheal suctioning
   C. Orotracheal suctioning
   Explain your choice.

3. As the day progresses, Mrs. Karlowski is becoming more fatigued, pulmonary crackles are worsening, and the sputum is thicker and progressively more difficult to clear. The client has an intravenous (IV) line and humidified source of oxygen present. However, coughing, deep breathing, and chest physical therapy are not efficient in maintaining a clear airway. As you, the charge nurse, and the physician discuss this client, what type of airway measures do you anticipate?
   A. Yankauer suctioning
   B. Nasotracheal suctioning
   C. Orotracheal suctioning
   Explain your choice.

Continued

FOCUS *on* CLINICAL PRACTICE

4. When performing airway management interventions the risk for nosocomial pneumonia is always present. What can you do to reduce this risk when using a suction technique to clear tracheal secretions? Check all that may apply.
   A. Perform hand hygiene.
   B. Use sterile suction technique.
   C. Use clean suction technique.
   D. Use humidified oxygen.
   E. All of the above.
   Explain your choice(s).

5. While suctioning Mrs. Karlowski, the returned sputum is thicker and is brown tinged. This is very different from earlier sputum. What action would you take? Select the correct choices.
   A. Notify physician or charge nurse.
   B. Decrease humidification.
   C. Increase fluids.
   D. Obtain artificial airway.
   E. Obtain sputum specimen.
   Explain your choice(s).

NCLEX REVIEW QUESTIONS

1. Mrs. Kline is hospitalized for acute pneumonia; she has a 10-year history of chronic lung disease and cannot clear her respiratory secretions. Before suctioning you observe restlessness, anxiety, confusion, increased heart rate, and elevated blood pressure. You would suspect:
   1. Hypoxia
   2. Hypocarbia
   3. Right-sided heart failure
   4. Left-sided heart failure

2. Mrs. Kline is able to cough, but not clear her airway. Which suctioning intervention is appropriate?
   1. Oropharyngeal
   2. Nasopharyngeal
   3. Endotracheal
   4. Tracheal

3. Hyperoxygenation before suctioning is done to:
   1. Compensate for the anticipated suction-induced hypocarbia
   2. Prevent atelectasis
   3. Control for suction-induced pain
   4. Control for suction-induced anxiety

4. When suctioning a client you suction the trachea before the oral pharynx because:
   1. Oral cavity is cleaner that the tracheal area and is suctioned last.
   2. Oral cavity is dirtier that the tracheal area and is suctioned first.
   3. Oral cavity is dirtier that the tracheal area and is suctioned last.
   4. Oral cavity is cleaner that the trachea and is suctioned first.

5. Secretions along the airway affect the client's ability to oxygenate because the secretions:
   1. Decrease airway size and decrease the work of breathing
   2. Decrease airway size and increase the work of breathing
   3. Increase airway size and increase the work of breathing
   4. Increase airway size and decrease the work of breathing

6. When caring for a client with an artificial airway whose pulse oximeter reading drops from 90% to 85% SpO_2, your first priority is to assess for:
   1. Presence of a pulse
   2. Presence of adequate blood pressure
   3. Presence of patent airway
   4. Presence of an oxygen supply

7. Mr. Jones has a well-established tracheostomy; he is hospitalized with worsening of his pulmonary disease and has an increased amount of thick yellow secretions. He develops respiratory distress, and you assess a nonpatent airway. Your first action is to:
   1. Notify the physician
   2. Call for help
   3. Suction the airway
   4. Administer cardiopulmonary resuscitation (CPR)

8. Humidification of an oxygen source has what effect on pulmonary secretions?
   1. Liquefies and thins secretions
   2. Solidifies and thins secretions
   3. Liquefies and thickens secretions
   4. No effect

References

American Academy of Pediatrics Taskforce on Infant Positioning and SIDS: Positioning and sudden infant death syndrome (SIDS): update, *Pediatrics* 98(6):1216, 1996.

Hockenberry MJ and others: *Wong's nursing care of infants and children,* ed 7, St. Louis, 2003, Mosby.

Lewis SL and others: *Medical-surgical nursing: assessment and management of clinical problems,* ed 5, St. Louis, 2000, Mosby.

Lueckenotte AG: *Gerontologic nursing,* ed 2, St. Louis, 2000, Mosby.

Moore T: Suctioning techniques for the removal of respiratory secretions, *Nurs Stand* 18(9):47, 2003.

Paul-Allen J, Ostrow CL: Survey of nursing practices with closed-system suctioning, *Am J Crit Care* 9(1):9, 2000.

Peers K: Cuff pressures, *Nurs Stand* 17(36):20, 2003.

St. John RE: Airway management, *Crit Care Nurse* 19(4):79, 1999.

Seay SJ and others: Tracheostomy emergencies: correcting accidental decannulation or displaced tracheostomy tube, *Am J Nurs* 102(3):59, 2002.

Sorrentino SA: *Mosby's textbook for nursing assistants,* ed 5, St. Louis, 2000, Mosby.

Research References

Akgul S, Akyolcu N: Effects of normal saline on endotracheal suctioning, *J Clin Nurs* 11(6):826, 2002.

Blackwood B: Normal saline instillation with endotracheal suctioning: primum non nocere (first do no harm), *J Adv Nurs* 29(4):928-934, 1999.

Connelly M, Stone K: Descriptive determination of negative airway pressure with closed system suctioning, *Heart Lung* 20(3):298, 1991.

Day T and others: Tracheal suctioning: an exploration of nurses' knowledge and competence in acute and high dependency ward areas, *J Adv Nurs* 39(1):35, 2002.

Fretag CC and others: Prolonged application of closed in-line suction catheters increase microbial colonization of lower respiratory tract bacterial growth on catheter surface, *Infection* 31(1):31, 2003.

Leur JP and others: Patient recollection of airway suctioning in the IU: routine versus a minimally invasive procedure, *Intensive Care Med* 29:433, 2003.

Puntillo KA and others: Practices and predictors of analgesic interventions for adults undergoing painful procedures, *Am J Crit Care* 11(5):415, 2002.

Shanahan M, Brayshaw SL: Are nurses aware of the differing health care needs of Vietnamese population? *J Adv Nurs* 22:456, 1995.

Sole ML and others: A multisite survey of suction techniques and airway management practices, *Am J Crit Care* 12(3):220, 2003.

Vanderberg JT and others: Large-diameter suction system reduces oropharyngeal evacuation time, *J Emerg Med* 17(6):941, 1999.

Wood CJ: Endotracheal suctioning: a literature review, *Intensive Crit Care Nurs* 14(9):124, 1998.

Zeitoun SS and others: A prospective randomized study of ventilator-associated pneumonia in patients using a closed vs. open suction system, *J Clin Nurs* 12(4):484, 2003.

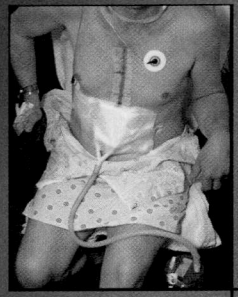

25

Closed Chest Drainage Systems

MEDIA RESOURCES

Evolve Site *evolve*

http://evolve.elsevier.com/Perry/skills
- Weblinks
- Video clips

OBJECTIVES

Mastery of content in this chaper will enable the nurse to:

- Explain the physiology of normal respiration.
- List three common sites for chest tube placement.
- List three conditions requiring chest tube insertion.
- Describe two closed chest drainage systems: water-seal and waterless systems.
- Describe principles and mechanisms of chest tube suction.
- Describe methods of troubleshooting chest tube systems.
- Discuss the nursing principles of care for clients with chest tubes.
- Describe autotransfusion.

KEY TERMS

Air leak	Parietal pleura
Atmospheric pressure	Pneumothorax
Chest tube	Positive pressure
Hemothorax	Subcutaneous emphysema
Intrapleural	Tidaling
Mediastinal shift	Visceral pleura
Negative pressure	

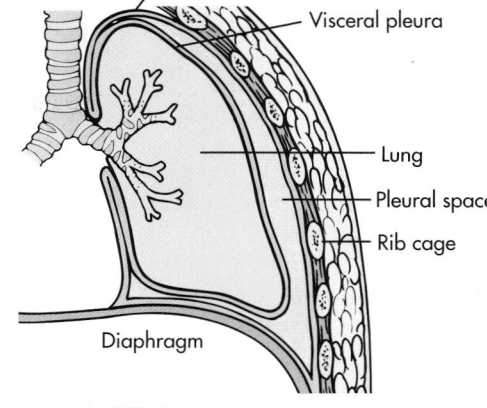

FIGURE **25-1** Partial structures of the lungs.

The chest cavity is a closed structure bound by muscle, bone, connective tissue, vascular structures, and the diaphragm. This cavity has three distinct sections, each sealed from the others: one section for each lung and a third section for the mediastinum, which surrounds structures such as the heart, esophagus, trachea, and great vessels.

The lungs are covered with a membrane called the visceral pleura. The interior chest wall is lined with another membrane, called the parietal pleura. The potential space between the visceral and parietal pleura is filled with approximately 4 ml of lubricating fluid and is called the pleural space (Figure 25-1). To expand the lungs, negative intrapleural pressure must be maintained. During inspiration the intercostal muscles pull outward and the diaphragm contracts and pulls down, thereby increasing the size of the chest cavity. This increase in size causes an increase in the amount of negative pressure (vacuum effect) being exerted in the intrapleural space.

Inspiration occurs when the increased negative pressure pulls the lungs against the enlarged chest cavity, expanding their size. The expanding lungs cause the intrapulmonic pressure to fall lower than atmospheric pressure. This increase in negative pressure within the lungs causes air to rush into the lungs until the intrapulmonic pressure is equal to the pressure in the atmosphere. When the chest cavity stops expanding and the lungs are full of air, the respiratory muscles and diaphragm relax, returning the chest cavity to its resting stage. At this time the intrapulmonic pressure is the same as the atmospheric pressure. During expiration a passive relaxation of the respiratory muscles causes the chest cavity space to decrease. This decrease in space causes the intrapulmonic pressure to increase, which allows the air to leave the lungs.

Trauma, disease, or surgery can result in air, blood, or fluid leaking into the intrapleural space, creating a positive pressure that collapses lung tissue. Small leaks may be absorbed spontaneously or may require interventions. The usual intervention is the insertion of a chest tube to remove air and fluids from the pleural space, to prevent air or fluid from reentering the pleural space, and to reestablish normal intrapleural and intrapulmonic pressures.

A chest tube is a catheter inserted through the thorax to remove fluid and/or air. There are a variety of chest tubes on the market. In some settings the traditional reusable glass three-bottle systems may still be used. The newest system available is the mobile chest drain. Regardless of the system used, the principles of client management are the same (Carroll, 2002). Chest tubes are commonly used after chest surgery and chest trauma and for pneumothorax or hemothorax to promote lung reexpansion.

A pneumothorax is a collapse of the lung caused by a collection of air in the pleural space. The loss of negative intrapleural pressure causes the lung to collapse. There are a variety of mechanisms for a pneumothorax. It may occur spontaneously or as a result of chest trauma, such as a stabbing or the chest striking the steering wheel in an automobile accident. A pneumothorax may result from the rupture of an emphysematous bleb on the surface of the lung (a large bulla resulting from the destruction caused by emphysema) or from an invasive procedure, such as insertion of a subclavian intravenous (IV) line. A client with a pneumothorax usually feels pain as atmospheric air irritates the parietal pleura. The pain may be sharp and pleuritic. Dyspnea is common and worsens as the size of the pneumothorax increases.

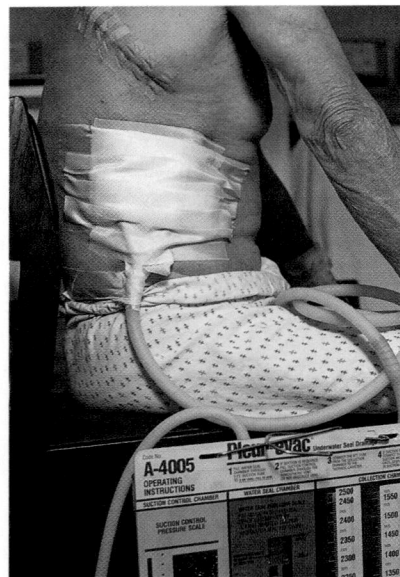

FIGURE **25-2** Pleural chest tube in place following open heart surgery.

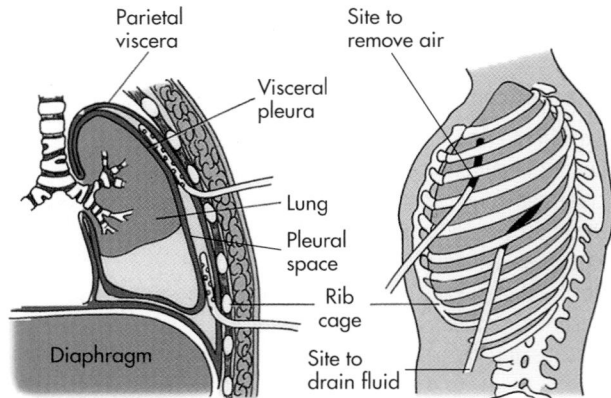

FIGURE **25-3** Diagram of sites for chest tube placement.

A hemothorax is a collapse of the lung caused by an accumulation of blood and fluid in the pleural cavity between the parietal and visceral pleurae, usually as a result of trauma. It produces a counterpressure and prevents the lung from full expansion. A hemothorax can also be caused by rupture of small blood vessels from inflammatory processes, such as pneumonia or tuberculosis. In addition to pain and dyspnea, signs and symptoms of shock can develop if blood loss is severe.

A pleural chest tube (Figure 25-2) is inserted when air or fluid enters the pleural space, compromising oxygenation or ventilation (e.g., chest trauma, open chest surgery, or in the case of a large pleural leak). A closed chest drainage system with or without suction is attached to the chest tube to promote drainage of air and fluid. Lung reexpansion occurs as the fluid or air is removed from the pleural space.

The location of the chest tube indicates the type of drainage expected. Apical (second or third intercostal space) and anterior chest tube placement promotes removal of air, which is necessary in the case of a pneumothorax. Because air rises, these chest tubes are placed high, allowing evacuation of air from the intrapleural space and allowing the lung to reexpand (Figure 25-3). The air is discharged into the atmosphere, and there is little or no drainage in the collection chamber.

Chest tubes are placed low (usually in the fifth or sixth intercostal space) and posterior or lateral to drain fluid (Figure 25-3). Fluid in the intrapleural space is affected by gravity and localizes in the lower portion of the lung cavity when the client is sitting upright. Tubes placed in these positions drain blood and fluid. Frequently applying suction assists this drainage. Fluid drainage is expected after open chest surgery and with some chest trauma.

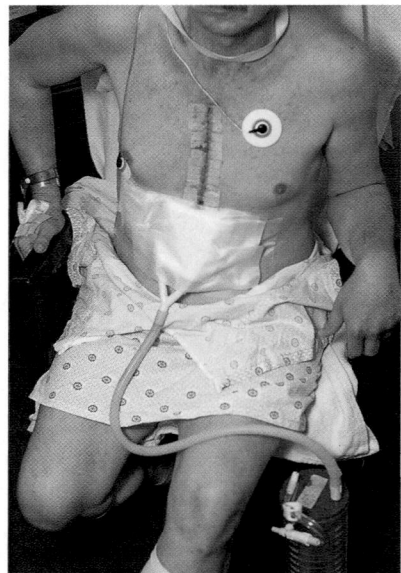

FIGURE **25-4** Mediastinal chest tube.

A mediastinal chest tube is placed in the mediastinum, just below the sternum (Figure 25-4), and is connected to a drainage system. This tube drains blood or fluid, preventing its accumulation around the heart. A mediastinal tube is commonly used after open heart surgery.

The disposable systems, such as a Thora-Sene III or Pleur-evac chest drainage system (Dekental), are one-piece molded plastic units that provide for a single or multiple chamber closed drainage system (Figure 25-5). The disposable units appear to be the system of choice because they are cost-effective and some facilitate autotransfusion, a common practice in open heart surgeries. Knowledge of the basics of chest tube management and troubleshooting maneuvers reduces the client's risk of complications.

Occasionally, in emergency situations and for some small pneumothoraces, a catheter is inserted through the chest wall, and a rubber flutter one-way valve (Heimlich valve) is at-

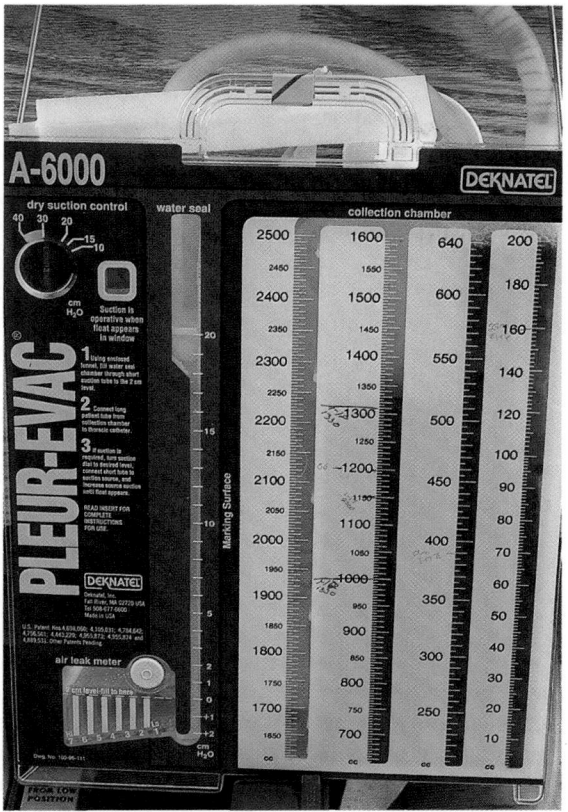

FIGURE 25-5 Disposable chest drainage system.

tached to the catheter (Connor, 1987). The valve opens whenever the pressure is greater than atmospheric pressure and closes when the reverse occurs. As a result, air and fluid exit from the pleural space on expiration, but the valve prevents air from reentering during inspiration (Lewis and others, 2004). No drainage chamber is used with this simple device.

New smaller "pigtail catheters" are also used. These smaller chest tubes are less traumatic than the large bore tubes. In addition, if they occlude, the physician can irrigate them using sterile water. These small chest tubes are not used for trauma or for the drainage of blood (Lewis and others, 2004).

A variety of disposable commercial chest drainage systems are available. A one-bottle system allows air from the pneumothorax to bubble out of the water seal and escape through the air outlet while preventing air from reentering the intrapleural space. This system is not recommended for the evacuation of fluid because drainage would raise the level of the water-seal liquid. An increased height of fluid in the water seal increases the resistance to drainage on expiration and eventually stops the drainage entirely.

A two- or three-chamber system drains both a hemothorax and a pneumothorax effectively (see Figure 25-5). Water-seal or the newer waterless chest drainage systems can be used. Researchers are trying to determine which system is most effective. Marshall and others (2002) compared the two

systems in clients who had lung resection surgery. They concluded that placing chest tubes on water seal for a brief period following surgery decreased the duration of air leak and length of time needed for the chest tube.

The water-seal and waterless systems, which use multiple chambers, are presented in this text. The two-chamber system permits liquid to flow into the collection chamber, and air flows into the water seal chamber. A three-chamber system promotes the drainage of fluid and air with controlled suction. In both systems the first chamber provides a compartment for fluid or blood drainage and a second compartment for either a water seal or a one-way valve. In the three-chamber system, the third compartment is for suction control, which may or may not be used.

Evidence-Based Practice Trends

There has and continues to be controversy as to whether to "strip or milk" the chest tube. Stripping or milking the chest tube is a process used to clear the tube of clots. Milking or stripping is done when the nurse manually compresses the chest tube, and attempts to move the chest tube drainage toward the collection device. This technique should never be routinely done. Careful management of chest tube drainage can prevent the need to milk or strip the chest tube.

Whenever possible, measures should be instituted to maintain tube patency. These interventions include avoiding dependent loops of the drainage tube, or when these loops cannot be avoided, such as when the client is sitting, the nurse should lift and clear the tube every 15 minutes (Schmelz and others, 1999). In addition, it is important to tailor the length of the drainage tube to the client, which can also reduce dependent loops (Allibone, 2003). If the tubing is coiled, looped, or clotted, the drainage is impeded and can result in a tension pneumothorax (Allibone, 2003). A tension pneumothorax is an emergent condition in which there is a rapid accumulation of air in the pleural space, and it may occur when chest drainage is impeded. The end result is a rapidly forming pneumothorax, causing high intrapleural pressure and tension on the heart and major vessels. If left unrecognized and untreated, the affected lung collapses. In addition, the contents within the mediastinum shift to the unaffected side and compress the underlying structures (e.g., vena cava). Cardiac output falls because the pressure from the mediastinal shift compresses the vena cava and venous return is reduced.

When occlusions due to clotting occur, the literature is contradictory regarding interventions. Parkin (2002) noted a wide variety of practices regarding chest tube milking or stripping. Ideally the tube should be changed if a blockage is detected (Allibone, 2003). However, in some select situations, such as with early postoperative chest surgeries, it may be necessary to clear the tube of blood clots. In these situations milking or stripping of the chest tube is done by experienced nurses who are following specific agency guidelines. The danger of stripping or milking the chest tube is a sudden rise in suction pressure, which can in turn cause lung injury or injure the surgical area. However, a nonfunctional chest tube may cause a more severe problem, and milking the chest tube may be the only option (Parkin, 2002).

Skill Performance Guidelines

1. Document client's baseline vital signs, oxygen saturation, lung sounds, and respiratory status. Changes in the vital signs or respiratory status can indicate a malfunction of the chest drainage system.

2. Observe the water seal for intermittent bubbling from its U tube or a rise and fall of fluid that is synchronous with respirations. (For example, in a non–mechanically ventilated client the fluid rises during inspiration, and the fluid level falls during expiration. When a client is on a mechanical ventilator, the opposite occurs.)
   a. Constant bubbling in the water seal or a sudden, unexpected stoppage of water-seal activity is considered abnormal and requires immediate attention.
   b. Unexpected stoppage of activity may indicate a blockage.
      In these situations immediate attention and correction are indicated. After 2 to 3 days, tidaling or bubbling on expiration is expected to stop, indicating that the lung has reexpanded.

3. In the waterless system look for a rise and fall of fluid in the diagnostic air-leak indicator synchronous with respirations. Constant left-to-right bubbling (when facing the indicator) or violent rocking is considered abnormal and may indicate an air leak.

4. Know the amount of expected chest tube drainage.
   a. A sudden decrease in the amount of chest tube drainage can indicate a possible clot or obstruction in the chest tube.
   b. A sudden increase of more than 100 ml of drainage can indicate fresh bleeding from the thorax.
   c. Drainage from a pneumothorax is generally limited. Any fluid buildup is caused by chest tube insertion trauma. The chest tubes drain for a pneumothorax assist in the removal of air from the intrapleural space.

5. Know the expected color of the drainage. Drainage from recent open chest surgery is initially bright red and gradually becomes serous as the postoperative course continues. Pleural effusions usually drain straw-colored fluid. Empyema is a collection of pus in the pleural cavity, and the drainage is pus colored (Coote, 2000).

6. In the water system, observe for constant, gentle bubbling in the suction control chamber when it is connected to suction. In the waterless system, a designated amount of suction is maintained by setting the suction source and dialing the prescribed suction level in the float ball column.

7. Assess both types of systems for air leaks. If an air leak exists, determine whether the air leak is in the client (client-centered air leak) or in the chest tube system (system-centered air leak). Remember that continuous bubbling in the water seal chamber with an absence of bubbles in the suction control chamber indicates that there is a leak in the system (Shuster, 1998). Ensure that all tubing connections are tight.

8. Note the color and amount of chest tube drainage on a regular basis (e.g., every hour initially and then every 4 hours). Make a mark to indicate the fluid level on the side of the drainage collection chamber at the end of the shift. Note the drainage amount as output.

SKILL 25-1   Caring for Clients With Chest Tube Connected to Disposable Drainage Systems

There are two types of commercial drainage systems: the water-seal and the waterless systems.

Water-Seal Systems

Two-Chamber Water-Seal System

On expiration, fluid or air is forced out of the intrapleural space. Gravity pulls air or fluid through the chest tube into the drainage collection chamber. On entering the drainage collection chamber, this fluid or air displaces the air present in the chamber by pushing it through the water seal and out of the system into the atmosphere. The water-seal chamber must be left open to air in order to drain. If the tubing is clamped, there is no mechanism for air to vent. To maintain the water-seal system, the chest tube system must remain upright. When it is tipped or overturned, the water seal is disrupted.

Three-Chamber Water-Seal System

If suction is to be used, the three-chamber water-seal system (see Figure 25-5, p. 857) is set up with the suction control chamber added. A prescribed amount of sterile fluid (e.g., 20 cm of water) is poured into the suction control chamber, which is then attached to a suction source by tubing. The amount of sterile water added depends on the manufacturer's recommendations. The chamber is filled to the set volume for the prescribed amount of suction. Sterile water may need to be added several times a day because of evaporation. As the fluid level decreases, the amount of suction also declines. The wall or portable suction device is turned up until the water in the suction control bottle exhibits a continuous, gentle bubbling. This provides the prescribed amount of suction (negative pressure).

If the suction source delivers more negative pressure than the suction control chamber water level allows, there is no danger because atmospheric air is pulled into the suction control chamber through an inlet, causing the excess suction to dissipate. The extra air pulled into the chamber causes vigorous bubbling. If this occurs, the suction source setting needs to be lowered to reduce noise and evaporation of the fluid. The absence of bubbling indicates that no suction is being exerted into the system. The suction setting should be raised to restore gentle bubbling.

Waterless Systems

Two-Chamber Waterless System

The waterless system's principles are similar to those of the water-seal system except that fluid is not required for setup. Because water is not used, accidentally tipping over the system does not compromise the client's condition.

The water seal is replaced by a one-way valve (Figure 25-6) located near the top of the system. Most of the container serves as the drainage chamber. The suction chamber does not depend on water. Instead, it contains a float ball, which is set by a suction control dial after the suction source is turned on. A diagnostic air-leak indicator is located on the face of the unit. It does require the addition of 15 ml of fluid for visualization. The indicator's function is to identify one of the following:

1. That the lung is expanding normally. This is indicated by a gentle tidaling of the fluid in the diagnostic indicator.
2. That the lung is probably reexpanded if after 2 or 3 days the tidaling has stopped.
3. An air leak is in the system if, while facing the system, the observer sees the fluid bubbling left to right. The source of the air leak must be located and corrected.

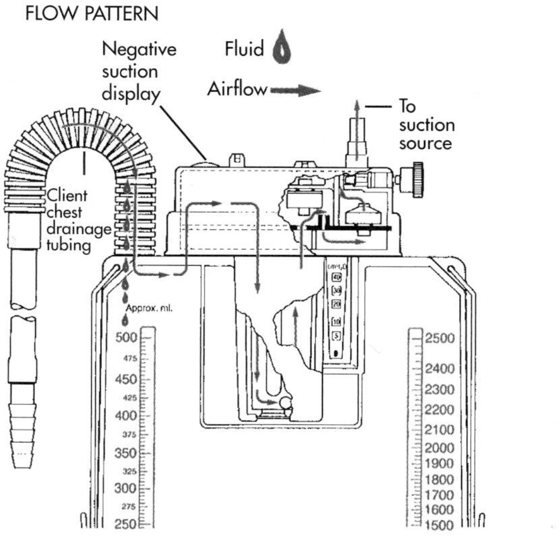

FIGURE **25-6** Disposable waterless chest drainage system with suction.

Three-Chamber Waterless System

If suction is ordered, attach the suction chamber port to the suction source by tubing, turn the suction on, and set the float ball at the prescribed setting. If the float ball will not rise to the prescribed level, increase the suction source setting until it does. The system is now functioning with suction.

There are usually two suction settings: one at either the suction control chamber or the float ball setting and the other at the suction source. The chamber or float ball setting is a safety factor to reduce the possibility that the intrapleural tissues will receive too much suction, causing injury.

DELEGATION CONSIDERATIONS

This skill should not be delegated to assistive personnel. However, assistive personnel may assist with other aspects of the client's care, such as monitoring vital signs. Before delegating aspects of care the nurse should inform assistive personnel about:

- Proper positioning of the client with chest tubes to facilitate chest tube drainage and optimal functioning of the system

- How to ambulate and transfer client with chest drainage
- To inform the nurse of any changes in vital signs, chest pain, or sudden shortness of breath, or excessive bubbling in water-seal chamber
- To notify the nurse immediately if there is disconnection of system, change in type and amount of drainage, sudden bleeding, or sudden cessation of bubbling

EQUIPMENT

❑ Disposable chest drainage system as ordered
❑ Suction source and setup (wall canister or portable)
  • Water suction system add: sterile water or normal saline (NS) solution to cover the lower 2.5 cm (1 inch) of water-seal U tube, sterile water or NS to pour into the suction control chamber if suction is to be used (see manufacturer's directions)
  • Waterless system add vial of 30 ml injectable sodium chloride or water, 20-ml syringe, 21-gauge needle, and antiseptic swab
❑ Nonsterile gloves
❑ Sterile gauze sponges
❑ Local anesthetic, if this is not an emergent procedure

❑ Chest tube tray (all items are sterile): knife handle (1), chest tube clamp, small sponge forceps, needle holder, knife blade No. 10, 3-0 silk sutures, tray liner (sterile field), curved 8-inch Kelly clamps (2), 4 × 4 inch sponges (10), suture scissors, hand towels (3)
❑ Dressings: petrolatum gauze, split chest-tube dressings, several 4 × 4 inch gauze dressings, large gauze dressings (2), and 4-inch tape or elastic bandage (Elastoplast)
❑ Head cover
❑ Face mask/face shield
❑ Sterile gloves
❑ Rubber-tipped hemostats for each chest tube (2)
❑ 1-inch adhesive tape for taping connections

STEP	RATIONALE

ASSESSMENT

STEP	RATIONALE
1. Obtain baseline and serial vital signs, oxygen saturation (SpO$_2$), and level of orientation.	Baseline vital signs are essential for any invasive procedure. Clients requiring chest tube insertion frequently have respiratory distress, and vital signs are taken serially. Changes in level of orientation may indicate decreased levels of oxygen and/or hypoxia.
2. Assess pulmonary status, including: **a.** Respiratory distress, abnormal breath sounds over affected lung area **b.** Signs and symptoms of increased respiratory distress: decreased breath sounds over the affected and nonaffected lungs, marked cyanosis, asymmetrical chest movements **c.** Chest pain on inspiration, hypotension, and tachycardia (Carroll, 2002).	Clients in need of chest tubes have impaired oxygenation and ventilation. The degree of the signs and symptoms associated with respiratory distress is related to the size of the pneumothorax or hemothorax or preexisting illness of the client. Sharp stabbing chest pain with or without decreased blood pressure and increased heart rate may indicate a tension pneumothorax (Woodruff, 1999).
3. If possible, ask client to rate level of comfort on a scale of 0 to 10.	The presence of a pneumothorax or hemothorax is painful, frequently causing a sharp inspiratory pain. In addition, there is also discomfort associated with the presence of a chest tube, not just with the insertion of the tube. As a result of this discomfort clients tend to not cough or change position in an effort to minimize this pain (Owen and Gould, 1997; Puntillo, 2003).
4. Assess client for known allergies. Ask clients if they have had a problem with medications, latex, or anything applied to the skin.	Povidone-iodine is an antiseptic used to cleanse the skin. Lidocaine is a local anesthetic administered to reduce pain. The chest tube will be held in place with tape. Iodine, lidocaine, and tape are common allergens.
5. Review client's medication record for anticoagulant therapy.	Anticoagulation therapy such as aspirin, warfarin, heparin, or platelet aggregation inhibitors such as ticlopidine can increase procedure-related blood loss.
6. For clients who have chest tubes, observe: **a.** Chest tube dressing and site surrounding tube insertion **b.** Tubing for kinks, dependent loops, or clots **c.** Chest drainage system, which should be upright and below level of tube insertion	Ensures that dressing is intact and occlusive seal remains without air or fluid leaks and that area surrounding insertion site is free of drainage or skin irritation (Carroll, 2002). Maintains a patent, freely draining system, preventing fluid accumulation in chest cavity. The presence of kinks, dependent loops, or clotted drainage increases the client's risk for infection, atelectasis, and tension pneumothorax (Allibone, 2003). Facilitates drainage; system must be in this position to function properly.

STEP	RATIONALE

NURSING DIAGNOSES

* Anxiety
* Acute pain
* Impaired gas exchange

Related factors are individualized based on client's condition or needs.

PLANNING

1. Expected outcomes following completion of procedure:
   * Client is oriented and more relaxed.
   * Vital signs are stable.
   * Client reports no chest pain.
   * Breath sounds are auscultated in all lobes. Lung expansion is symmetrical, SpO$_2$ is stable or improved, and respirations are nonlabored.
   * Chest tube remains in place, and chest drainage system remains airtight.
   * Gentle tidaling (fluctuations or rocking) is evident in water seal or diagnostic indicator.
2. Check agency policy, and determine whether informed consent is needed.
3. Review physician's role and responsibilities for chest tube placement (Table 25-1).
4. Explain procedure to client.
5. Perform hand hygiene.
6. Set up the prescribed drainage system. *Open system when physician is ready to insert chest tube.*
   a. Water-seal system (check manufacturer's guidelines)
      (1) Obtain a chest drainage system. Remove wrappers, and prepare to set up the system.

      (2) While maintaining sterility of the drainage tubing, stand the system upright, and add sterile water or NS to the appropriate compartments.
         (a) For a two-chamber system (without suction), add sterile solution to the water-seal chamber (second chamber), bringing fluid to the required level as indicated.
         (b) For a three-chamber system (with suction), add sterile solution to the water-seal chamber (second chamber). Add amount of sterile solution prescribed by physician to the suction control (third chamber), usually 20 cm (8 inches). Connect tubing from suction control chamber to suction source.
      (3) The suction control chamber vent must be without occlusion when suction is used.

Hypoxia relieved.
Decreased hypoxia improves vital sign measure.
Reexpansion of the lung reduces chest pain.
Reexpansion of the lung promotes normal respirations.

Indicates correct placement and patency of the chest tube drainage system.
Indicates system is functioning normally. Reflects changes in intrapleural pressure.
In nonemergent situations most institutions require informed, written permission for chest tube insertion.
Helps differentiate physician and nurse roles so that the nurse can function more effectively.
Reduces anxiety and promotes client cooperation.
Reduces transmission of microorganisms.
Premature opening of the sterile chest drainage system increases risk of contamination of sterile equipment.
Permits displaced air to pass into the atmosphere.
Maintains sterility of the system. The system is packaged in this manner so it can be used under sterile operating room conditions (Carroll, 1991).
Reduces possibility of contamination.

Maintains water seal.

Depth of fluid level dictates the highest amount of negative pressure that can be present within the system (Shuster, 1998). For example, 20 cm of water is approximately −20 cm of water pressure.

Provides a safety factor of releasing excess negative pressure into the atmosphere through the suction control vent. Too little suction prevents lung reexpansion and increases the client risk for infection, atelectasis, and tension pneumothorax. Too much suction damages the lung tissue and perpetuates existing air leaks (Allibone, 2003).

STEP	RATIONALE

TABLE 25-1 PHYSICIAN'S ROLE AND RESPONSIBILITY IN CHEST TUBE PLACEMENT

ROLE	RESPONSIBILITY
Explain purpose, procedure, and possible complications to the client, and have client sign consent form.	Provides informed consent.
Perform hand hygiene. Cleanse chest wall with antiseptic.	Reduces transmission of microorganisms.
Apply mask and gloves.	Maintains surgical asepsis.
Drape area of chest tube insertion with sterile towels.	Maintains surgical asepsis.
Inject local anesthetic, and allow time to take effect.	Decreases pain during procedure.
Use blunt or sharp dissection to create incision in the skin and chest wall.	Opens chest for insertion of chest tube. A trocar is no longer used and increases risk of tissue damage.
Thread a clamped chest tube through the incision. Physician clamps chest tube until system is connected to water seal.	Inserts chest tube into the intrapleural space. Clamping prevents entry of atmospheric air into the chest and worsening of the pneumothorax.
Suture chest tube in place, if suturing is policy or physician preference.	Secures chest tube in place.
Cover the chest insertion site with sterile petrolatum gauze, 4 × 4 inch gauze, and large dressing to form an occlusive dressing supported with an elastic bandage (Elastoplast).	Holds chest tube in place and occludes site around chest tube. Helps stabilize chest tube and holds dressing tightly in place. Helps prevent bacteria entry and air leak.
Water-seal system: Remove connector cover from client's end of chest drainage tubing with sterile technique. Secure drainage tubing to the chest tube and drainage system.	Physician is responsible for making certain that the system is set up properly, the proper amount of water is in the water seal, the dressing is secure, and the chest tube is securely connected to the drainage system.
Water-seal suction: Connect system to suction, or supervise a nurse connecting it to suction, if suction is to be used.	The physician is responsible for determining and checking the amount of fluid that is to be added to the suction control chamber and prescribing the suction setting.
Waterless system: Remove connector cover from client's end of chest drainage tubing with sterile technique. Secure drainage tubing to the chest tube and drainage system.	Physician is responsible for making certain that the system is set up properly and the chest tube is securely connected to the drainage system.
Waterless suction: Turn on suction source. Set float ball level to prescribed setting.	Physician is responsible for prescribing level of float ball and prescribing the suction setting.
The physician or nurse adds sterile water or NS to diagnostic indicator.	Allows quick assurance that the system is functioning properly.
Unclamp the chest tube.	Connects chest tube to drainage.
In both systems the physician orders and reviews chest x-ray studies.	Verifies correct chest tube placement.

b. Waterless system (check manufacturer's guidelines)

(1) Remove sterile wrappers, and prepare to set up equipment.

Maintains sterility of the system. The system is packaged in this manner so it can be used under sterile operating room conditions.

(2) For a two-chamber system (without suction) nothing is added or needs to be done to the system.

The waterless two-chamber system is ready for connecting to the client's chest tube after opening the wrappers.

(3) For a three-chamber waterless system with suction, connect tubing from suction control chamber to the suction source.

The suction source provides additional negative pressure to the system.

STEP	RATIONALE

TABLE 25-2   PROBLEM SOLVING WITH CHEST TUBES

ASSESSMENT	INTERVENTION
Air leak can occur at insertion site, connection between tube and drainage, or within drainage device itself. Continuous bubbling is noted in water-seal chamber and water seal.	Locate leak by clamping tube at different intervals along the tube. Leaks are corrected when constant bubbling stops.
Assess for location of leak by clamping chest tube with two rubber-shod or toothless clamps close to the chest wall. If bubbling stops, air leak is inside client's thorax or at chest insertion site.	Unclamp tube, reinforce chest dressing, and notify physician immediately. Leaving chest tube clamped can cause collapse of lung, mediastinal shift, and eventual collapse of other lung from buildup of air pressure within the pleural cavity.
If bubbling continues with the clamps near the chest wall, gradually move one clamp at a time down drainage tubing away from client and toward suction control chamber. When bubbling stops, leak is in section of tubing or connection between the clamps.	Replace tubing, or secure connection and release clamps.
If bubbling still continues, this indicates the leak is in the drainage system.	Change the drainage system. Make sure chest tubes are patent: remove clamps, eliminate kinks, or eliminate occlusion.
Notify physician immediately, and prepare for another chest tube insertion. Assess for tension pneumothorax; indicated by: • Severe respiratory distress • Low oxygen saturation • Chest pain • Absence of breath sounds on affected side • Tracheal shift to unaffected side • Hypotension and signs of shock • Tachycardia	Obstructed chest tubes trap air in intrapleural space when air leak originates within the thorax. A flutter (Heimlich) valve or large-gauge needle may be used for short-term emergency release of pressure in the intrapleural space. Have emergency equipment, oxygen, and code cart available because condition is life-threatening.
Water seal tube is no longer submerged in sterile fluid due to evaporation.	Add sterile water to water-seal chamber until distal tip is 2 cm under surface level.

(4) Instill 15 ml of sterile water or NS into the diagnostic indicator injection port located on top of the system.

NOTE: This step is not necessary for mediastinal drainage because there will be no tidaling. Also, in an emergency it is not necessary because the system does not require water for setup.

Instillation of water into the injection port enables the nurse to observe for a rise and fall in the diagnostic air-leak window. Constant left-to-right bubbling or rocking is abnormal and may indicate an air leak.

7. Provide two shodded hemostats or approved clamps for each chest tube, attached to top of client's bed with adhesive tape. Chest tubes are only clamped under the following specific circumstances per physician order or nursing policy and procedure:

a. To assess air leak (Table 25-2)

b. To quickly empty or change disposable systems; performed by a nurse who has received education in the procedure

c. To assess if client is ready to have chest tube removed (which is done by physician's order); monitor the client for recurrent pneumothorax

Shodded hemostats have a covering to prevent hemostat from penetrating chest tube once changed. The use of these shodded hemostats or other clamps prevents air from reentering the pleural space (Allibone, 2003).

8. Position the client: During the chest tube insertion, the client will need to be positioned so the client's back or the side in which the tube will be placed is accessible to the physician.

Permits optimal drainage of fluid and/or air.

STEP	RATIONALE

IMPLEMENTATION

1. Perform hand hygiene, and apply gloves.
2. Administer parenteral premedications, such as sedatives or analgesics, as ordered.

Reduces transmission of microorganisms.
Reduces client anxiety and pain during procedure.

- **Critical Decision Point**
  Sedatives and analgesics may alter vital signs depending on the dose and client's tolerance. Monitor closely for changes in blood pressure and respirations.

3. Assist physician in providing psychological support to the client. (See physician's responsibilities in Table 25-1.)
   a. Reinforce preprocedure explanation.

   b. Coach and support client throughout procedure.
4. Show local anesthetic to physician.

5. Hold anesthetic solution bottle upside down with label facing physician. Physician will withdraw solution and inject into client's skin.
   a. Physician places chest tube. (A standard procedure is detailed in Table 25-1.)
6. Help physician attach drainage tube to chest tube.

7. After the chest tube is inserted, tape all connections in a double spiral fashion with 1-inch adhesive tape (Note taping of the chest tube is usually done by the physician at time of tube placement). Then:
   a. Check systems for proper functioning by
      (1) Clamping the drainage tubing that will connect the client to the system
      (2) Connecting tubing from the float ball chamber to the suction source
      (3) Turning on the suction to the prescribed level

Reduces client anxiety and assists in efficient completion of procedure.

Allows physician to read label of drug before administering it to client.
Allows physician to withdraw solution properly while maintaining surgical asepsis.

Connects drainage system and suction (if ordered) to the chest tube.
Secures chest tube to drainage system and reduces risk of air leak causing breaks in airtight system.

Provides a chance to ensure an airtight system before connecting it to the client. Allows correction or replacement of system if it is defective before connecting it to the client. NOTE: Bubbling will be seen at first because there is air in the tubing and system initially. This should stop after a few minutes unless there are other sources of air entering the system.

- **Critical Decision Point**
  If bubbling continues, check connections and locate source of the air leak, as described in Table 25-2.

8. Turn off suction source, and unclamp drainage tubing before connecting client to the system.

Having the client connected to suction when it is being inserted could damage pleural tissues from sudden increase in negative pressure. The suction source is turned on again after the client is connected to the three-chamber system.

9. Check patency of air vents in system:
   a. Water-seal vent must not be occluded.
   b. Suction control chamber vent must not be occluded when suction is used.
   c. Waterless systems have relief valves without caps.

Permits the displaced air to pass into the atmosphere.
Provides safety factor of releasing excess negative pressure into the atmosphere.
Provides safety factor of releasing excess negative pressure.

STEP	**RATIONALE**
10. Coil excess tubing on mattress next to the client. Secure with a rubber band and safety pin or the system's clamp.	Prevents excess tubing from hanging over the edge of the mattress in a dependent loop. Drainage could collect in the loop and occlude the drainage system.
11. Adjust tubing to hang in a straight line from the chest tube to the drainage chamber.	Promotes drainage and prevents fluid or blood from accumulating in the pleural cavity.
12. If the chest tube is draining fluid, indicate the date and time (e.g., 0900) that drainage was begun on the drainage chamber's write-on surface.	Provides a baseline for continuous assessment of the type and quantity of drainage.
13. Strip or milk chest tube only if indicated (this means compressing the tube to encourage clots to press through the tube): *Stripping*—compression along length of the tubing beginning at client and continuing until drainage unit is reached. *Milking*—compressing and releasing the tube sequentially.	Stripping may cause complications because it creates excessive negative intrapleural pressure (over -100 cm H_2O). Milking causes less of a pressure change.

- *Critical Decision Point*

    Check institutional policy before stripping or milking chest tubes. This practice is being discontinued at most institutions because it is believed that stripping the tube greatly increases intrapleural pressure, which could damage the pleural tissue and cause or worsen an existing pneumothorax. However, even though the literature is contradictory, stripping or milking may be done in selected clients (e.g., fresh postoperative thoracic surgery, chest trauma). The rationale for this selective use of stripping or milking is that the presence of clotted tube drainage causes decreased rate of reexpansion and increases risk of tension pneumothorax (Allibone, 2003). In these selected cases the benefits outweigh the risks.

a. Postoperative mediastinal chest tubes are manipulated if nursing assessment indicates an obstruction of drainage resulting from clots or debris in the tubing.	Stripping is controversial and should be performed only if hospital policy permits and there is a physician's order (Phipps and others, 1999). Stripping creates a high degree of negative pressure and has potential of pulling lung tissue or pleura into drainage holes of the chest tube (Carroll, 1991).
14. After the tube is placed, assist client to a comfortable position.	Reduces client anxiety and promotes cooperation.
a. Semi-Fowler's to high-Fowler's position to evacuate air (pneumothorax)	Air rises to the highest point in the chest. Pneumothorax tubes are usually placed on the anterior aspect at the midclavicular line, second or third intercostal space (Woodruff, 1999).
b. High-Fowler's position to drain fluid (hemothorax)	Permits optimal drainage of fluid. Posterior tubes are placed on the midaxillary line, fifth or sixth intercostal space.
15. Remove gloves, and dispose of used soiled equipment.	Prevents accidents involving contaminated equipment.
16. Perform hand hygiene.	Reduces spread of microorganisms.

▎ EVALUATION

1. Monitor vital signs, oxygen saturation, and insertion site every 15 minutes for the first 2 hours.	Provides immediate information about procedure-related complications such as respiratory distress.
2. Monitor chest tube drainage:	
a. Assessment after chest-tube insertion is done every 15 minutes for the first 2 hours. This assessment interval then changes *on the basis of client's status.* Mark the time and level of drainage on the calibrated write-on strip periodically.	Permits timely and efficient account of the amount of drainage from the chest tube. Drainage is marked at specified periods of time and documented on the nurses' notes and intake and output (I&O) sheet. Ensures early detection of complications.
b. *Expected drainage in the adult:* Less than 50 to 200 ml/hr immediately after surgery in a mediastinal chest tube. Approximately 500 ml in the first 24 hours.	Dark-red drainage is expected only during the immediate postoperative period. This drainage turns serous over time.

STEP	RATIONALE
c. *Expected drainage in the adult:* Between 100 and 300 ml of fluid may drain from a pleural tube during the first 3 hours after insertion. The 24-hour rate is 500 to 1000 ml. Drainage is grossly bloody during the first several hours after surgery and then changes to serous. Remember that a sudden gush of drainage may be retained (dark) blood and not active (bright red) bleeding. This increased drainage can result from client position changes.	Reexpansion of the lungs forces drainage into the tube. Coughing can also cause large gushes of drainage or air. Acute bleeding indicates hemorrhage.

• *Critical Decision Point*

If drainage suddenly increases, is bright red, or there is more than 100 ml/hr of bloody drainage (except for the first 3 hours postoperatively), the nurse should notify the physician and remain with the client and assess vital signs and cardiopulmonary status.

3. Assess client for decreased respiratory distress and chest pain, breath sounds over affected lung area, and change in SpO_2.	Increase in respiratory distress and/or chest pain, decrease in breath sounds over the affected and nonaffected lungs, marked cyanosis, asymmetrical chest movements, presence of subcutaneous emphysema around tube insertion site or neck, hypotension, tachycardia, and/or mediastinal shift are critical and indicate a severe change in client status, such as excessive blood loss or tension pneumothorax. Notify physician immediately (Godden, 1998).
4. Ask client to rate level of comfort on a scale of 0 to 10.	Indicates need for analgesia. Client with chest tube discomfort hesitates to take deep breaths and as a result is at risk for pneumonia and atelectasis.
5. Observe: **a.** Chest tube dressing and drainage.	Ensures that dressing is occlusive.

• *Critical Decision Point*

Check the dressing carefully. It can come loose from the skin, although this may not be readily apparent.

b. Tubing should be free of kinks and dependent loops.	Straight and coiled drainage tube positions are optimal for pleural drainage. However, when dependent loop is unavoidable, periodic lifting and draining of the tube will also promote pleural drainage (Schmelz and others, 1999).
c. The chest drainage system should be upright and below level of tube insertion. Note presence of clots or debris in tubing.	System must be in this position to function and to facilitate proper drainage (Gordon and others, 1997).

• *Critical Decision Point*

Monitor the position of the system relative to the chest tube carefully, especially during client transport.

STEP	RATIONALE
d. Water seal for fluctuations with client's inspiration and expiration.	
(1) Waterless system: diagnostic indicator for fluctuations with client's inspirations and expirations.	In the non–mechanically ventilated client, fluid should rise in the water seal or diagnostic indicator with inspiration and fall with expiration. The opposite occurs in the client who is mechanically ventilated. This indicates that the system is functioning properly (Lewis and others, 2000).
(2) Water-seal system: bubbling in the water-seal chamber (see Table 25-2).	When system is initially connected to the client, bubbles are expected from the chamber. These are from air that was present in the system and in the client's intrapleural space. After a short time the bubbling stops. Fluid continues to fluctuate in the water seal on inspiration and expiration until the lung is reexpanded or the system becomes occluded.
(3) Water-seal system: bubbling in the suction control chamber (when suction is being used) (see Table 25-2).	Suction control chamber has constant, gentle bubbling. Tubing to the suction source should be free of obstruction, and the suction source should be turned to the appropriate setting.
e. *Waterless system:* bubbling in diagnostic indicator.	Mechanism to observe for the presence of tidaling.
f. *Type and amount of fluid drainage:* Nurse should note color and amount of drainage, client's vital signs, and skin color. Look at the fluid in the collection tubing, not just the fluid in the collection chamber. Is the drainage bright red, dark red, or pink? Is it opaque, or can you see through it?	Character of drainage indicates if normal or if infection or hemorrhage is developing.
g. *Waterless system:* The suction control (float ball) indicates the amount of suction the client's intrapleural space is receiving.	The suction float ball dictates the amount of suction in the system. The float ball allows no more suction than dictated by its setting. If the suction source is set too low, the suction float ball cannot reach the prescribed setting. In this case the suction must be increased for the float ball to reach the prescribed setting.
6. After first 2 hours, assess client's physical and psychological status at least every 4 hours or according to agency policy.	Detects early signs and symptoms of complications: *Apprehension*—increase in client anxiety, restlessness, and inability to concentrate. *Respiratory distress*—alteration in rate and/or depth of respirations, difficulty breathing, and breath sounds. *Subcutaneous emphysema*—air that is being trapped in the subcutaneous tissue.

Recording and Reporting

- Record level of client comfort, baseline vital signs, including SaO_2. If postoperative client, record vital signs and SpO_2 every 15 minutes for at least 2 hours postoperatively. Record chest drainage output hourly for at least 2 hours, and then record as client status indicates. Document time, type, and amount of drainage. Record integrity of chest suction system (e.g., record the amount of bubbling in the water-seal suction control chamber, level of suction, intactness of system).
- Report client response to chest tube insertion or continuation, noting level of comfort, drainage, and intactness of the system.

Unexpected Outcomes	Related Interventions
1. Air leak unrelated to client's respirations occurs.	• Locate source (see Table 25-2). • Notify physician.
2. There is no chest tube drainage.	• Observe for kink in chest drainage system. • Observe for possible clot in chest drainage system. • Observe for mediastinal shift or respiratory distress (medical emergency). • Notify physician.
3. Chest tube is dislodged.	• Immediately apply pressure over chest tube insertion site. • Have assistant apply gauze dressing and tape three sides. • Notify physician.
4. Substantial increase in bright red drainage occurs.	• Obtain vital signs. • Monitor drainage. • Assess client's cardiopulmonary status. • Notify physician.
5. Continuous bubbling is seen in water-sealed chamber, indicating leak between client and water seal.	• Tighten loose connections. • Check agency policy, and if instructed, cross-clamp chest tube closer to client's chest. If bubbling stops, air leak is inside client's thorax or at chest tube insertion site. • Unclamp chest tube. • Reinforce dressing. • Notify physician.

Teaching Considerations

- Instruct client and family regarding proper functioning of chest tube and drainage system.
- Instruct client to immediately report any changes in chest comfort.

Pediatric Considerations

- If possible, using pictures and special dolls, familiarize child and family with equipment before inserting chest drainage system (Hockenberry and others, 2003).
- Allow child to play with equipment and special dolls before inserting chest drainage system.
- Chest tube drainage greater than 3 ml/kg/hr for more than 2 consecutive hours is excessive and may indicate postoperative hemorrhage (Hockenberry and others, 2003).

Gerontological Considerations

- Fragility of the older adult's skin requires special care and planning for management of chest tube dressing. Frequently assess surrounding skin for signs of skin breakdown (Lueckenotte, 2000).

Home Care Considerations

- Clients with chronic conditions (e.g., uncomplicated pneumothorax, effusions, empyema) that require long-term chest tube may be discharged with smaller mobile drains. These systems do not have a suction control chamber and use a mechanical one-way valve instead of a water-seal chamber (Carroll, 2002).
- Instruct client how to ambulate and remain active with a home chest tube drainage system.
- Provide client and caregiver information as to when to contact health care professionals regarding changes in the drainage system (e.g., chest pain, breathlessness, change in color or amount of drainage).

Actual removal of a chest tube is the function of physicians and advanced practice nurses (APNs). An APN is a nurse with a master's degree in a specialized area of nursing. If nurses are to remove a chest tube, this procedure should be a written component of the agency's policy and procedure standards.

The nurse prepares the client for chest tube removal by (1) assessing the need for preremoval analgesia and obtaining the required medication orders (Houston and Jesurum, 1999) and (2) instructing the client about the process and what will be requested of the client (Mimnaugh and others, 1999). During removal of the chest tube, it is important that the client take a deep breath and hold it until the physician has removed the tube. This maneuver prevents air from being sucked into the chest as the tube is pulled out and before an occlusive dressing is applied.

This skill details for the nurse the actual nursing responsibilities and physician action for chest tube removal.

DELEGATION CONSIDERATIONS

This skill should not be delegated to assistive personnel. The nurse should instruct assistive personnel who care for the client post chest tube removal to:

- Immediately report client sensations of shortness of breath, increased chest pain, dizziness, increased anxiety
- Report any dislodgement or drainage on the dressing

EQUIPMENT

- ❑ Suture set
- ❑ Sterile scissors
- ❑ Sterile forceps
- ❑ Clean gloves
- ❑ Sterile gloves
- ❑ Face mask/face shield
- ❑ Prepared sterile dressing: petrolatum-impregnated gauze, 4 × 4 inch gauze dressings, and large dressings
- ❑ 4-inch adhesive tape or elastic bandage (Elastoplast) cut into strips

STEP	RATIONALE

ASSESSMENT

1. Assess status of client's lung reexpansion:
   a. Provide physician with results of chest x-ray film.

   b. Note trend in water-seal fluctuation over last 24 hours.

   c. Drainage decreases to less than 50 ml/day.
   d. Percuss lung for resonance.
   e. Auscultate lung sounds.
2. Assess client's level of comfort using a 0 to 10 scale, and determine when the last analgesic medication was given.

3. Determines client's understanding of the chest tube removal procedure.
4. Clamp chest tube before removal as ordered by the physician. Assess for changes in vital signs, SpO$_2$, chest pain, and level of apprehension.

Reveals position of lung tissue in chest cavity and whether sufficient lung reexpansion has occurred.
Pleura of the expanded lung seals the holes on the internal tip of the chest tube, halting fluctuation in the water seal. A halt in fluctuation for 24 hours indicates lung is expanded.
Drainage has been removed, allowing the lung to reexpand.
Normal percussion occurs with reexpansion.
Normal breath sounds are heard bilaterally with reexpansion.
Presence of chest tubes is painful, and client frequently requires analgesic medication. It is important to note the last dose of the medication. Chest tube removal is painful, and additional analgesia may be necessary (Houston and Jesurum, 1999; Owen and Gould, 1997).
Assists in determining what the client needs to know about the procedure and assists in reducing anxiety.
Physician orders tube clamping before removal to assess client's tolerance.

- **Critical Decision Point**
   If the client develops respiratory distress when the tube is clamped, assess the client, unclamp the tube, and call the physician.

STEP	RATIONALE

NURSING DIAGNOSES
- Risk for impaired gas exchange
- Acute pain
- Anxiety

Related factors are individualized based on client's condition or needs.

PLANNING

1. Expected outcomes following completion of procedure:
   - Lung reexpansion is maintained.
   - Client does not experience discomfort.
   - Spontaneous healing of chest tube insertion site occurs after removal of tube without infection or other complications.
2. Explain procedure to client.

3. Verify that analgesia will be administered for pain before chest tube removal.

Source of air or fluid loss is sealed or has healed.
Pain management is achieved.
Large nonporous occlusive dressing at puncture site promotes uncomplicated healing.

Reduces anxiety and promotes client cooperation (Mimnaugh and others, 1999).
Anticipatory management of pain related to chest tube removal will reduce client's anxiety and will also assist client in taking the required deep breath (Puntillo, 2003). After procedure, the client will be able to deep breathe and cough more effectively.

IMPLEMENTATION

1. Administer prescribed medication for pain relief about 30 minutes before procedure.

Reduces discomfort and relaxes client. Medication reaches peak effect at time of tube removal. Clients do report sensations ranging from pain to pulling when the chest tube is removed (Houston and Jesurum, 1999; Mimnaugh and others, 1999).

2. Perform hand hygiene, and apply gloves and face shield if needed.

Reduces transmission of microorganisms.

3. Assist client in sitting on edge of bed or lying supine or on the side without chest tubes.

Physician prescribes client's position to facilitate tube removal.

4. Physician or APN prepares an occlusive dressing of petroleum gauze on a pressure dressing and sets it aside on a sterile field and applies sterile gloves.

Essential to prepare in advance for quick application to the wound on tube withdrawal.

5. Support client physically and emotionally while physician or APN removes dressing and clips sutures.

Clients state that when they know the tube is being pulled, they can mentally prepare themselves for the procedure. Support from the health care team reduces anxiety and promotes cooperation (Mimnaugh and others, 1999).

6. Physician or APN asks the client to take a deep breath and hold it or exhale completely and hold it.

Prevents air from being sucked into the chest as the tube is removed.

7. Physician or APN quickly pulls out the chest tube.

Prevents entry of air through the chest wound.

8. Aseptically apply sterile prepared dressing over the wound, and firmly secure it in position with elastic bandage (Elastoplast) or wide tape. Sometimes skin clips or purse-string sutures are used to hold the wound together before dressing is applied.

Keeps wound aseptic. Prevents entry of air into the chest. Wound closure occurs spontaneously. Clips or sutures aid in skin closure.

9. Assist client to a comfortable position.

Assists in client's return to a comfortable status. Clients report that proper positioning and rest following chest tube removal assist in relief of procedure-related sensations of pain and pulling (Mimnaugh and others, 1999).

STEP	RATIONALE
10. Remove used equipment from bedside. Place it in appropriate area for medical waste products.	Prevents spread of microorganisms.
11. Remove gloves, and perform hand hygiene.	Reduces transmission of microorganisms.

EVALUATION

1. Assess lung sounds. Palpate over lung where tube was inserted, and observe client for subcutaneous emphysema. Assess for respiratory distress immediately after tube removal and during the first few hours after removal.	Provides for early notification of physician if adverse symptoms occur. Chest tubes may need reinsertion. Subcutaneous emphysema results from the entrance of air into the subcutaneous space. It is painful, and as a result, clients may not take full lung expansion.
2. Assess client's vital signs, SpO$_2$, pulmonary status, and psychological status.	Detects early signs and symptoms of complications.
3. Review chest x-ray film.	Identifies early signs of incomplete lung expansion.
4. Ask about the client's level of pain or comfort. Observe for nonverbal cues of pain, and assess level of discomfort on a scale of 0 to 10.	Could be signs that wound has not closed well. Determines client's tolerance of procedure.
5. Check chest dressing for drainage and patency. When changing dressing, note wound for signs of healing.	Ensures occlusion and proper healing of chest wound.

Recording and Reporting

- Record removal of tube, amount of drainage in the collection bottle, appearance of wound and dressing, and client's response. Client's response should also include vital signs and respiratory assessment.
- Report client's response to chest tube removal to next shift.

Unexpected Outcomes	Related Interventions
1. Dyspnea, labored respirations	• Potential recurrence of pneumothorax or hemothorax.
	• Notify physician, obtain vital signs and SpO$_2$, and remain with client.
	• Prepare for possible chest tube reinsertion.

Teaching Considerations

- Instruct client and family to immediately report signs of chest pain, shortness of breath, or sensations of chest discomfort.

Pediatric Considerations

- Pediatric clients usually require analgesia (e.g., morphine sulfate 0.1 mg/kg in combination with midazolam [Versed]) before the chest tube removal (Hockenberry and others, 2003).

- EMLA (locally applied anesthetic patch) placed under the occlusive dressing at the chest tube insertion site 1 hour before tube removal reduces pain of procedure. However, child may still feel the "pulling" sensation of tube removal (Hockenberry and others, 2003).

SKILL 25-3 Reinfusion of Chest Tube Drainage

Reinfusion of chest tube drainage into the client's circulatory system has become more widely used since the public has become aware of the risks associated with blood transfusions. When reinfusion is linked with chest drainage, it becomes a relatively risk-free, inexpensive, and easy method of replacing mediastinal blood previously lost during emergencies and open heart or thoracic surgery. Clients requiring this skill must also have an IV line in place (see Chapter 27).

DELEGATION CONSIDERATIONS

This skill should not be delegated to assistive personnel. However, the nurse should notify assistive personnel who may be providing select portions of client care to inform nurse of:
* Changes in client vital signs
* Increased drainage from mediastinal tube
* Decreased drainage from mediastinal tube

EQUIPMENT

❑ Adult/pediatric single-use chest drainage and autotransfusion unit (Figure 25-7)
❑ Replacement bag
❑ Gown, gloves, and mask as needed

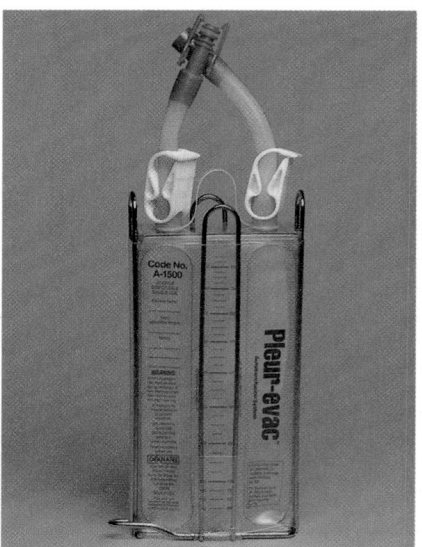

FIGURE **25-7** Example of reinfusion replacement bag.

STEP	RATIONALE

ASSESSMENT

1. See Assessment for Skill 25-1.

2. Determine presence of active bleeding, at least 50 to 100 ml/hr through mediastinal tube. | Indicates the need for possible reinfusion of mediastinal tube drainage.
3. Assess IV site (see Chapter 28). | Determines presence of adequate and patent IV site for the administration of blood products (e.g., 18-gauge angiocatheter).

4. Obtain baseline laboratory data (e.g., hemoglobin and hematocrit). | Provides data to measure the effectiveness of the reinfusion of chest drainage on the client's circulating blood volume.

NURSING DIAGNOSES
* Risk for infection
* Risk for injury

Related factors are individualized based on client's condition or needs.

STEP	RATIONALE

PLANNING

1. Expected outcomes following completion of procedure:
   - Vital signs, hematocrit, and hemoglobin will stabilize.

   - The drainage system will function correctly, and the lung will reexpand in 48 to 72 hours.
   - The IV line will remain patent.

2. Explain procedure to client.

Reinfusion reduces significant blood loss associated with closed chest drainage.
Negative pressure will have been reestablished in the intrapleural space.
A patent IV is necessary for reinfusion of cleansed mediastinal tube drainage.
Reduces anxiety and promotes client cooperation.

IMPLEMENTATION

1. System setup
   a. Set up the autotransfusion system (ATS) according to technique that maintains the sterility of the unit and following the three steps printed on the front of the unit.
   b. Make certain all connections are tight, and all clamps are open.
   c. A 200-μm double-sided mesh filter is located in the ATS bag to filter the drainage.
   d. The ATS collection bag has a capacity of 1000 ml marked in increments of 25 ml and an area for marking times and amounts.

Contamination of the unit provides a ready source of infection to client.

Tight connections ensure an airtight system, and open clamps allow chest drainage to enter the ATS bag.
Filtering the drainage removes extraneous materials and microemboli.
Expected drainage in the adult: Less than 50 to 200 ml/hr immediately after surgery in a mediastinal chest tube. Approximately 500 ml in the first 24 hours. Dark-red drainage is expected only during the immediate postoperative period. This drainage turns serous over time.

2. Perform hand hygiene, and apply gloves.
3. Prepare chest drainage for reinfusion:
   a. Following manufacturer's directions, open a replacement bag, and close the two white clamps.

   b. Use the high-negativity relief valve to reduce excessive negativity.
   c. Bag transfer:
      (1) Close clamp on chest drainage tubing.

      (2) Close the two white clamps on the top of the initial ATS collection bag.
      (3) Connect the chest drainage tube to the new ATS bag with the red connectors.
      (4) Make certain that all connections are tight.
      (5) Open all clamps on chest drainage tube and replacement bag.
   d. Connect the red and blue connectors on top of the initial collection bag, and remove it by lifting it from the side hook and then from the foot hook.
   e. Secure the replacement bag by connecting the foot hook, replacing the metal frame into the side hook of the chest drainage unit, and pushing down to secure the frame onto the hook.
   f. The replacement bag is removed by placing the thumbs on the top of the metal frame and pushing up with the fingers to slide the bag out.

Reduces transmission of microorganisms.

Contamination of the unit provides a ready source of contamination to the client. The closed clamps maintain a closed system during replacement.
This eases the removal of the initial collection bag from the metal support stand.

Prevents air from entering the chest cavity through the tube and collapsing the lung.
Maintains a closed system for the reinfusion, preventing contamination of the blood.
Establishes a new autotransfusion system.

Ensures an airtight system.
Reestablishes an autotransfusion collection system.

Maintains a closed system within the bag and removes it for use in autotransfusion.

Provides safe attachment of the replacement bag to the chest drainage unit.

STEP	RATIONALE
4. Reinfusion:	
a. Use a new microaggregate filter to reinfuse each autotransfusion bag.	Prevents the infusion of microemboli and provides maximal filtration for each bag.
b. Access the bag by inverting it and spiking the bag through the spike port with the microaggregate filter and twisting.	Connects the autotransfusion bag to the transfusion tubing.
c. With the bag upside down, gently squeeze the bag to remove the air, and prime the filter with blood.	Gentle pressure is used to prevent hemolysis.
d. Hang the bag on an IV pole, and continue to prime the tubing until all air is gone. Clamp the tubing, attach it to the client's IV access, and adjust the clamp to deliver the reinfusion at the appropriate rate.	Removes all air from the transfusion tubing. Reinfusion delivered either by gravity, application of a blood cuff (not to exceed 150 mm Hg pressure), or a blood-compatible IV pump (see Chapter 28).
e. If ordered, anticoagulants (citrate phosphate dextrose or heparin) can be added to the reinfusion through the self-sealing port in the autotransfusion connector.	Prevents clotting in the autotransfusion.
5. Discontinuing autotransfusion:	
a. Clamp the chest drainage tube, and connect it directly to the chest drainage unit with the red and blue connectors.	Prevents air from entering the chest cavity through the tube and collapsing the lung.
b. Open the chest drainage tube clamp.	All drainage will be collected directly in the drainage unit and must be appropriately discarded.
6. Discard used supplies, and perform hand hygiene.	Reduces transmission of microorganisms.

EVALUATION

1. Monitor vital signs, hematocrit, and hemoglobin. — Helps determine the effects of the treatment.
2. Monitor chest drainage system and client's lung sounds. — Helps determine the proper functioning of the system and its effectiveness.
3. Assess the IV infusion site for infiltration and phlebitis. — A patent IV infusion site must be maintained.

Recording and Reporting

- Record drainage and reinfusion with times and amounts of each. Describe condition of IV infusion site.
- Report unusual findings and client responses to nurse in charge or physician.

Unexpected Outcomes	Related Interventions
1. Chest tube is displaced.	• Immediately apply pressure over chest tube insertion site. • Have assistant apply sterile petroleum occlusive dressing. • Notify physician.
2. Client has dyspnea, chest pain, and labored respirations.	• Verify that chest tube is patent and draining. • Obtain vital signs. • Notify physician.
3. Client has signs of infection, fever, chills.	• Obtain wound cultures as ordered. • Obtain vital signs.

Teaching Considerations

- Prepare client and family for the procedure so they will understand when the client's blood from the previous mediastinal drainage is reinfused. Client and their families may have had this instruction preoperatively and need reinforcement. Clients who have had emergent thoracic surgery will need more in-depth and frequent information.

FOCUS on CLINICAL PRACTICE

Mr. Robert is in his first postoperative day following open heart surgery. He has a pleural and mediastinal chest tube to drainage. His last vital signs were blood pressure (BP), 110/64 mm Hg; pulse (P), 126 beats per minute; respirations (R) on mechanical ventilator, 16 breaths per minute; SpO_2, 90%; temperature (T), 99.0° F (rectally). The last hourly chest tube drainage was 75 ml from the pleural tube and 100 ml from the mediastinal tube.

1. Why is it important to check vital signs, check for air leaks, and note the amount of chest drainage every 15 to 30 minutes for at least 2 hours after he returns from surgery?
2. Mr. Robert's chest tube drainage has ranged from 75 to 100 ml from both chest tubes over the last 3 hours. What measures do you take to assist in maintaining chest tube patency?

3. It is now 12 hours postoperative, and Mr. Robert is transferred from bed to chair. Immediately following this transfer you note a drainage of 50 ml of dark red fluid. What are your actions?
4. Mr. Robert is discharged to the step-down area. His chest tube is out. Your assessment of this client noted that the dressing over the puncture site was occlusive and without visible drainage. Vital signs were stable, client was free of pain, and sitting in a chair. The assistive personnel tell you he is "breathing funny." You immediately reassess Mr. Robert and find your client is in respiratory distress. His vital signs are BP, 90/60 mm Hg; pulse, 120 beats per minute; respirations, 32 breaths per minute; and SpO_2, 82%. Mr. Robert complains of severe chest pain and is pale. What are your actions?

NCLEX REVIEW QUESTIONS

1. You are caring for a client with a new chest tube. The client is anxious and is fearful of taking pain medications because he knows he needs to be active, take deep breaths, and cough. He feels that taking pain medications will make him sleepy. You actions include:
   1. Telling him that the medication won't make him sleepy
   2. Explaining that by controlling pain he will be able to be active and cough well
   3. Notifying his physician
   4. Giving him the medication anyway
2. Your postoperative thoracotomy client complains of increased sharp chest pain. Your assessment reveals an increased respiratory rate, increased pulse, and increased anxiety. When you assess the chest tube system, you note the water seal chamber of the collection tubing is empty. The client's chest pain is due to:

   1. Improper function of the chest tube system
   2. Improved pneumothorax
   3. Worsening pneumothorax
   4. Incisional pain
3. Clients with chest tubes that assist in the removal of bloody drainage from the chest cavity have many care priorities. Two important priorities related to management of the chest tube system include:
   1. Monitoring chest tube drainage and maintaining chest tube patency
   2. Monitoring chest tube drainage and promoting activity
   3. Promoting airway clearance and maintaining chest tube patency
   4. Promoting activity and airway clearance

Continued

NCLEX REVIEW QUESTIONS

4. Clients who have a pneumothorax have which type of chest tubes?
   1. Pleural tubes placed in the 2-3 intercostal space
   2. Pleural tubes placed in the 5-6 intercostal space
   3. Pleural tubes placed laterally
   4. Pleural tubes placed posteriorly

5. You are caring for a client with a chest tube to treat a pneumothorax. His tube and occlusive dressing become dislodged. Your immediate action is to:
   1. Call for help and take vital signs
   2. Take vital signs and perform a pulmonary assessment
   3. Place an occlusive dressing over chest tube site and take vital signs
   4. Notify the physician and prepare to insert a new chest tube

References

Allibone L: Nursing management of chest drains, *Nurs Stand* 17(22):45, 2003.

Carroll P: A guide to mobile chest drains, *RN* 65(5):56, 2002.

Carroll PF: What's new in chest-tube management, *RN* 54(5):34, 1991.

Connor PA: When and how do you use a Heimlich flutter valve? *Am J Nurs* 87:288,1987.

Godden J: Managing the patient with a chest drain: a review, *Nurs Stand* 12(32):35, 1998.

Gordon PA and others: Positioning of chest tubes: effects on pressure and drainage, *Am J Crit Care* 6:33, 1997.

Hockenberry MJ and others: *Nursing care of infants and children,* ed 7, St. Louis, 2003, Mosby.

Lewis ML and others: *Medical-surgical nursing: assessment and management of clinical problems,* ed 6, St. Louis, 2004, Mosby.

Lueckenotte AG: *Gerontologic nursing,* ed 2, St. Louis, 2000, Mosby.

Phipps WJ and others, editors: *Medical-surgical nursing: concepts and clinical practice,* ed 6, St. Louis, 1999, Mosby.

Shuster PM: Chest tubes: to clamp or not to clamp, *Nurse Educ* 23(3):9, 1998.

Woodruff DW: Pneumothorax, *RN* 62(9):62, 1999.

Research References

Coote N: Surgical versus non-surgical management of pleural empyema (Cochrane Review). *The Cochrane Library,* issue 2, Oxford, UK, 2000, Update Software.

Houston S, Jesurum J: The quick relaxation technique: effect on pain associated with chest tube removal, *Appl Nurs Res* 12(4):196, 1999.

Marshall MB and others. Suction vs. water seal after pulmonary resection: a randomized prospective study, *Chest* 121(3):831, 2002.

Mimnaugh L and others: Sensations experienced during removal of tubes in acute postoperative patients, *Appl Nurs Res* 12(2):78, 1999.

Owen S, Gould D: Underwater seal chest drains: the patient's experience, *J Clin Nurs* 6(3):215, 1997.

Parkin C: A retrospective audit of chest drain practice in a specialist cardiothroacic center and current review of chest drain literature, *Nurs Crit Care* 7(1):30, 2002.

Puntillo K: Pain assessment and management in the critically ill: wizardry or science? *Am J Crit Care* 12(4):10, 2003.

Schmelz JO and others: Effects of position of chest drainage tube on volume drained and pressure, *Am J Crit Care* 8(5):319, 1999.

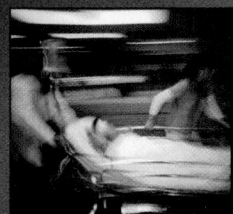

26

Emergency Measures for Life Support

26-1   Inserting an Oropharyngeal Airway

26-2   Use of an Automated External Defibrillator

26-3   Code Management

MEDIA RESOURCES

Evolve Site *evolve*
http://evolve.elsevier.com/Perry/skills
• Weblinks

OBJECTIVES

Mastery of content in this chaper will enable the nurse to:

- Discuss indications for an oral airway.
- Identify indications for automated external defibrillator (AED) application and use.
- State indications for cardiopulmonary resuscitation (CPR).
- Discuss code management organization.
- State the goals for CPR.
- Demonstrate in a laboratory or clinical situation: insertion of an oral airway, use of an AED, and performance of CPR.

KEY TERMS

Advance directive

Automated external
 defibrillator (AED)

Bag-valve-mask (BVM)

Cardiac arrest

Cardiopulmonary arrest

Cardiopulmonary
 resuscitation (CPR)

Diffusion

Dysrhythmia

Endotracheal intubation

Manual defibrillator

Oral airway

Perfusion

Respiratory arrest

Ventilation

The oxygen transport system consists of the respiratory (lungs) and cardiovascular (heart) systems. Adequacy of oxygen delivery depends on the amount of oxygen entering the blood and carbon dioxide leaving the lungs (ventilation), movement of oxygen to the red blood cells at the alveolar level (diffusion), and the blood flow to the lungs and tissues (perfusion). An emergency situation requiring life support occurs when one or more of the above mechanisms fail.

Respiratory and cardiac arrests are emergency situations that the nurse must be prepared to handle at any time. Respiratory arrest, or cessation of ventilation, results in the absence of oxygen delivery to the alveoli. Causes of a respiratory arrest may include airway obstruction, cardiopulmonary illnesses, or ingestion of toxic substances. Early intervention of a respiratory arrest usually prevents a cardiac arrest. Cardiac arrest is the cessation of circulating blood flow that eliminates oxygen transport or perfusion. Many cardiac arrests are caused by an irregular heart rhythm or dysrhythmia. Lethal ventricular dysrhythmias require defibrillation or electrical shock for treatment. Early defibrillation may quickly return the heart to normal, and the client may not progress to a respiratory arrest. The majority of arrests involve the collapse of both the respiratory and cardiovascular systems. This is defined as a cardiopulmonary arrest. Unless otherwise indicated, such as a client having an advance directive for final health care or do not resuscitate (DNR) status, all clients receive cardiopulmonary resuscitation (CPR) in the event of an arrest.

A resuscitation attempt is approached in a systematic and organized fashion to ensure the most expedient care. Within most hospitals this arrest situation is referred to as a "code" (e.g., "code blue," "code 7"). Each institution has a specific code or signal for a cardiac and/or respiratory arrest. The goal is to provide resuscitation in a timely manner and to restore cardiopulmonary function as soon as possible so the likelihood of an adverse outcome is decreased. Most nurses or nursing students are required to be trained in the basic life support measures either through the American Heart Association (AHA) or the American Red Cross. Because of this requirement, the skill of basic CPR is not covered in detail within this chapter. Two specific skills of inserting an oropharyngeal airway and use of an automated external defibrillator (AED) will be covered, as well as the organizational skill of code management.

Evidence-Based Practice Trends

The Committee on Emergency Cardiac Care (AHA, 2000) continues to research cardiac arrest treatment and outcomes and has created guidelines for the initial care of these situations (basic CPR). Specific guidelines for emergency cardiac drugs, manual defibrillation, and supportive measures are included in the advanced cardiac life support (ACLS) guidelines (Cummins, 2001).

The basic life support measures taken by the first responder in the first 2 to 3 minutes of the client's collapse is what appears to have the greatest effect on survival. Early CPR followed by electrical defibrillation of the heart within 3 to 5 minutes (when indicated) can improve the survival of arrest victims to as high as 49%, twice the rate of those previously reported (AHA, 2000). Statistics show that defibrillation within 1 minute can result in a successful rescue as high as 90%; however, statistics drop off rapidly to 50% after 5 minutes, 30% after 7 minutes, and 10% after 9 to 11 minutes (AHA, 2000). Because of these statistics, many hospitals and large public areas are providing the tools needed for the first 2 to 3 minutes of an arrest, including AEDs. AEDs are very user friendly and provide an automated analysis of the heart's rhythm and recommendation for electrical shock. Because of the ease of use and its impact on survival, use of the AED is included in basic CPR training to laypersons and health care professionals. The AHA (2000) has recommended that hospitals be able to provide defibrillation within 3 minutes of the client's collapse. Hospitals must facilitate their code teams to meet this time goal or provide a mechanism to provide early CPR and defibrillation within their facilities.

The delivery of defibrillation is accomplished by sending a jolt of electricity through the heart. In the past the method of electrical delivery was in the form of a monophasic waveform. This waveform provides one unidirectional wave of high energy moving once through the heart. A newer method of electrical delivery using a biphasic waveform has recently been studied and added to most manual defibrillators, as well as AEDs. A biphasic waveform provides bidirectional defibrillation using lower energy delivery through the heart. The lower energy of a biphasic waveform offers some theoretical benefit such as decreased cardiac damage with defibrillation, longer battery life of the defibrillator, and higher conversion rate. The research to date has shown that the lower energy, biphasic waveform is at least equivalent to the monophasic waveform (AHA, 2000). More studies need to be conducted to demonstrate superiority over the monophasic waveforms. In the clinical areas many defibrillators have already been adapted to the biphasic waveform. Clinicians who perform manual defibrillation must adjust to the lower energy levels used with the biphasic waveform.

Practice trends have also been updated in the management of airway and breathing. To provide artificial ventilation, a trained physician, nurse, or therapist may place a plastic tube through the trachea. This is known as endotracheal intubation. It is important to ensure that this tube is placed correctly in the trachea and not in the esophagus to successfully ventilate the lungs. Primary confirmation of the tube placement can be performed by auscultating the breath sounds, but the AHA (2000) now recommends a secondary confirmation of tube placement (i.e., chest x-ray examination, carbon dioxide [CO_2] detectors). Devices to detect CO_2, such as end-tidal CO_2 detectors or color changers, can be attached to end of the endotracheal tube.

Advance directives offer valuable information concerning resuscitation status and individual client decisions regarding resuscitation efforts. Although advance directives may be addressed before or during the client's hospital admission, the nurse can play an important role in encouraging clients to complete the document. Nurses, because of their unique relationship with clients and the associated high level of trust, are the ideal facilitators for the initiation of advance directives. The American Nurses Association (ANA) *Position Statement of Nursing and the Patient Self-Determination Acts* states that it is the nurse's responsibility to facilitate informed decision making for clients making choices about end-of-life care, and they expect providers to initiate these conversations. Though further research is required on the degree of improvement of end-of-life care, there is some evidence that advance directives give clients a means of controlling treatment decisions about the end of their life (Ditto and others, 2001). An advance directive may be used as a tool to minimize disagreements among family members regarding resuscitation status determinations when the client is physically unable to make decisions. Many hospitals have a mechanism to assist the client/family regarding this issue. Health care providers may consult with social services and/or hospital-based ethics committees to assist clients and their families.

Hospitals have begun to allow family members and loved ones to remain in the client's room during actual resuscitative efforts. Evaluations of these programs, pioneered by critical care and emergency nurses, have confirmed a remarkable level of approval and gratitude by participating family members (Emergency Nurses Association, 2001; MacLean and others, 2003). These evaluations, mostly in pediatric cases, have noted significant reduction in posttraumatic stress and self-reports of a greater sense of resolution and fulfillment. In the 2000 pediatric resuscitation guidelines (AHA, 2000), family presence in a resuscitative event has a positive recommendation. Provision must be made for a professional to accompany the family members during these observed attempts, to direct positioning, to answer questions, and to explain procedures. In addition, the accompanying professional can observe for signs of acute discomfort in the family members and can end the observations. There is a lack of sufficient evidence about family presence during adult resuscitations, but this may be due to an absence of research in adults. Although few hospitals have written policies and guidelines to support this practice, most critical care and emergency nurses have allowed family to be present (MacLean and others, 2003).

Cultural Considerations

Whenever a client requires life support measures, the family is a prime nursing responsibility. When caring for clients of diverse cultures and religions, the nurse and health care team members must consider the meaning of life support and resuscitation. For example, Amish families may not see the value of using technological support because it only prolongs the existence of the physical body (Brewer and Bonalumi, 1995). Hmongs believe that there is a pool of blood in the chest that serves as a life force and may misinterpret cardiopulmonary resuscitation as an attempt to kill the client or hasten the client's death (Johnson, 2002). It is also very important to address needs of other clients in the unit or area. Assist clients in their understanding of culturally diverse practices of other clients on the unit. In addition, assure them that their needs, as well as all clients' needs, will be addressed. There are many interventions the nurse can select to assist the family during emergency situations, such as the following:

- Have a staff member available to give support to family members during emergency.
- Use a professional interpreter to explain what is happening to the client.
- Use cultural and religious brokers to facilitate understanding by family members of the events. Accommodate religious and cultural practices of the clients.
- Be prepared to handle large numbers of visitors who would remain at the bedside to provide support for the family and/or pray for the client. Collaborate with the family decision maker and leader in planning rotating visits of family and kin at the bedside. Designate a waiting area to accommodate the group. Assign a contact person from the unit to deal with the client's family and visitors. Promote cultural understanding by staff, and involve them in providing accommodation.
- Consult religious leader and family decision maker regarding measures to be taken during an emergency.

- Discussion about advance directives, DNR, and organ donation should be initiated with the guidance of the religious leader and consent of the family decision maker.
- Autopsy and organ donation may be refused by Muslims who believe that they have to be whole to meet their creator (Meleis, 1996).

Groups may also vary in defining parameters of death. For example, brain death may not be acceptable to those groups that believe in the concept of soul and afterlife. Some African Americans may not readily accept advance directives because of their distrust of the health care system stemming from the Tuskegee experiment (Dupree, 2000). Buddhists and Hindus generally believe that life is determined by one's karma or deeds in previous life. Muslims believe in predestination of life by Allah (Pacquiao, 2001).

Collectivistic groups (e.g., Asians or Hispanics) make decisions together rather than use individual decision making (Doorenbos, 2003). A Sudanese family may generally abide by the decisions of the community elders (Kemp and Rasbridge, 2001).

Skill Performance Guidelines

1. Know the client's baseline vital signs, noting any irregularities in cardiac rhythm. Dysrhythmias can precipitate a cardiopulmonary arrest. Cardiovascular conditions that place the client at risk for dysrhythmias include coronary artery disease, myocardial infarction, open heart surgeries, and fluid/electrolyte imbalances.
2. Know a client's most recent serum electrolyte values. Electrolyte imbalances (e.g., those involving potassium and calcium) can precipitate cardiopulmonary arrest.
3. When an overdose of a chemical or illicit substance is present, know the type and amount of the substance ingested. Certain chemicals, such as alcohol, tranquilizers, and depressants, depress the respiratory center and can result in a respiratory arrest. Overdoses of some drugs, such as heroin, can cause ventricular dysrhythmias and cardiopulmonary arrest.

SKILL 26-1 Inserting an Oropharyngeal Airway

An oropharyngeal airway is a semicircular, minimally flexible, curved piece of hard plastic (Figure 26-1). When inserted, it extends from just outside the lips, over the tongue, and to the pharynx (Figure 26-2). Oral airways enable the nurse to suction through a central core or along the side of the airway, facilitate resuscitation, and maintain airway patency in the unconscious client.

The oral airway is sized for adults and children, varying in length and width. Pediatric sizes are 000, 00, 0, 1, 2, and 3. School-age children are usually size 3 or 4. Adult sizes are 4 through 10 or small, medium, and large. The nurse chooses the size of an oral airway based on the client's age and the width and length of the client's mouth. Size is correct if, when the flange is held parallel to the front teeth with the airway against the client's cheek, the end of the curve reaches the angle of the jaw. General size guidelines for choosing an oral airway for children are provided in Table 26-1.

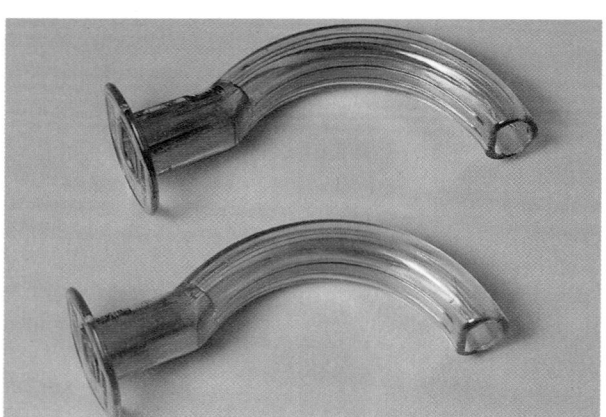

FIGURE **26-1** Oral airways.

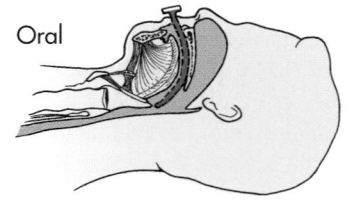

Oral

FIGURE **26-2** Placement of oral airway.

TABLE 26-1   ORAL AIRWAY GUIDELINES FOR SIZE BY AGE

SIZE	AGE
000	Premature neonates
00	Newborn
0	Newborn to 1 yr
1	1 to 2 yr
2	2 to 6 yr
3	6 to 18 yr
4 and larger	18 yr

DELEGATION CONSIDERATIONS

The skill of inserting an oropharyngeal airway should not be delegated to assistive personnel. When assistive personnel care for clients with an oropharyngeal airway, the care provider must be instructed to recognize and report signs of airway distress.

EQUIPMENT

- ❑ Appropriate-size oral airway
- ❑ Nonsterile gloves
- ❑ Tissues or washcloths
- ❑ Suction equipment, if indicated
- ❑ Tape (optional)
- ❑ Face shield, if indicated
- ❑ Tongue blade

STEP	RATIONALE

ASSESSMENT

1. Identify need to insert oral airway. Signs and symptoms include upper airway "gurgling" with respiratory cycle, no gag reflex, increased oral secretions or excretions, excessive drooling, grinding teeth, clenched teeth, biting of oral tracheal or gastric tubes, labored respirations, and increased respiratory rate.

2. Determine factors that normally influence upper airway functioning, such as age (children have a proportionally larger tongue), presence of nasal and oral airway, and drainage tubes (swallowing is more difficult with tubes in place).

3. Assess for presence of gag reflex; gently place tongue blade on back of client's tongue.

These conditions place clients at risk for obstruction of upper airway. This airway is only used with unconscious client because in conscious client the gag reflex causes vomiting or retching when something is placed in pharynx. Oral airways may stimulate vomiting or laryngospasm if inserted in the semiconscious patient.

Allows nurse to accurately assess need for oral airway. Clients at greater risk for upper airway obstruction are infants, children, and adults with cold and flu, loss of consciousness, seizure disorders, neuromuscular diseases, increased oral secretions or excretions, or facial trauma.

Provides guide as to when oral airway can be safely removed in a postoperative client.

- ● *Critical Decision Point*
  Never insert an oropharyngeal airway in a conscious client or a client with recent oral trauma, oral surgery, or loose teeth.

4. Assess client's and family's knowledge of procedure.

Identifies learning needs and facilitates client's cooperation with procedure.

NURSING DIAGNOSES

- ● Ineffective airway clearance
- ● Risk for aspiration
- ● Ineffective breathing pattern

- ● Impaired gas exchange
- ● Risk for infection

Related factors are individualized based on client's condition or needs.

STEP	RATIONALE

PLANNING

1. Expected outcomes following completion of procedure:
   - Client's respiratory status improves, as evidenced by easier respirations with normal rate, easier removal of secretions, and lack of gurgling noise in throat with respirations.

     Airway is cleared of secretions.

   - Client is not able to grind teeth or bite tubes.

     Oral airway prevents tooth contact with other teeth or with tubes.

   - Client's tongue does not relax back into pharynx and obstruct airway.

     Oral airway keeps tongue in correct position to maintain patent airway.

2. Position client; semi-Fowler's position is preferred.

   Promotes client comfort and provides easy access to oral cavity.

IMPLEMENTATION

1. Perform hand hygiene, and apply nonsterile gloves and face shield (when possible).

   Reduces transmission of microorganisms.

2. Whenever possible use padded tongue blade to open client's mouth; if necessary, use thumb and forefinger of nondominant hand to pry jaws and teeth apart.

   Provides access to oral cavity.

3. Insert oral airway:

   When inserting airway, take care not to push client's tongue into pharynx.

   a. Hold oral airway with curved end up, insert distal end until airway reaches back of throat, then turn airway over 180 degrees, and follow natural curve of tongue. Nurse may also hold airway sideways, insert halfway, and then rotate airway 90 degrees while gliding it over natural curvature of tongue. Outer flange should be just outside client's lips.

   Provides patent airway and prevents displacement of client's tongue into posterior oropharynx.

- *Critical Decision Point*

  In some clients it may be possible to depress tongue with tongue blade and insert airway with tip pointing down, sliding it over tongue.

4. Secure with tape if client attempts to push out with tongue.

   Prevents expulsion of airway. Taping an airway in place can limit client's ability to expel vomitus.

5. Suction secretions, as needed.

   Removes secretions; maintains patent airway.

6. Reassess client's respiratory status.

   Directs nurse to initiate intervention.

7. Clean client's face with soft tissue or washcloth.

   Promotes hygiene.

8. Discard tissue into appropriate receptacle, place washcloth in dirty or soiled linen bag, remove gloves and face shield, and discard in appropriate receptacle; perform hand hygiene.

   Reduces transmission of microorganisms.

9. Administer mouth care frequently.

   Increases client comfort and removes debris. It also provides moisture to oral mucosal tissues.

- *Critical Decision Point*

  Do not use lemon glycerin swabs for oral care because they are drying to mucosal tissues and promote bacterial growth. Oral airway may also need to be removed, cleaned, and reinserted in clients with a lot of oral mucous secretions. If secretions are left in place, they could occlude oral airway.

STEP	RATIONALE
EVALUATION	
1. Observe client's respiratory status, and compare respiratory assessments before and after insertion of oral airway.	Identifies client's response to insertion of airway.
2. Assess that airway is patent, that client does not occlude airway by biting tube, and that client's tongue does not obstruct airway.	Ensures oxygen delivery to client.

Recording and Reporting

- Record in nurses' progress notes:
  - Assessment finding while inserting oral airway
  - Size of oral airway
  - Placement
  - Other procedures performed at same time, especially positioning, secretions obtained
  - Client's tolerance of procedure
- Report in addition to material recorded:
  - Respiratory distress
  - Vomiting
  - Pain

Unexpected Outcomes	Related Interventions
1. Client continually coughs and gags when airway is inserted.	• Do not continue inserting airway if client begins to gag. Stimulation of gag reflex can cause vomiting and risk of aspiration. • Remove oral airway, and position client on side. Replace with smaller-size airway. • Assess need for airway.
2. Airway obstruction not relieved.	• Obtain immediate assistance. • Reinsert airway.
3. Client pushes airway out of place or out of mouth.	• Airway may not be properly secured. • Reassess client's need for oral airway.
4. Nurse is unable to insert oral airway in client; client may be combative, or nurse may be unable to pry mouth open.	• Obtain assistance. • Reassess client's need for oral airway.

Teaching Considerations

- Instruct family members in proper cleaning techniques. Observe their technique for adequacy.

Pediatric Considerations

- Oral airways are seldom used in treatment of airway obstruction in children and infants. Due to narrowness of child's airway, oral airways are often more occlusive than beneficial (Hockenberry and others, 2003).
- For infants and children the preferred method for inserting airway is with tip pointing to roof of mouth.

SKILL 26-2 Use of an Automated External Defibrillator

The advantage of the AED is that laypersons or health care providers trained in basic life support, who have less training than ACLS personnel, can defibrillate. AEDs eliminate the training in rhythm interpretation and make early defibrillation practical and achievable. The AED is an automated external defibrillator that incorporates a rhythm analysis system. The device attaches to a client by two adhesive pads and connecting cables. The technology of the AED is available in several different devices. Most AEDs are stand-alone boxes with very simple three-step function (Figure 26-3) and verbal prompts to guide the responder. Some defibrillator manufacturers have incorporated the AED technology into their manual defibrillators. All AEDs offer the automated rhythm analysis whereby the rhythm is compared to thousands of other rhythms stored in the AED's computer software. Upon rhythm identification, some AEDs will automatically provide the electrical shock after a verbal warning (fully automated). Other AEDs will recommend a shock, if needed, and then prompt the responder to press the shock button.

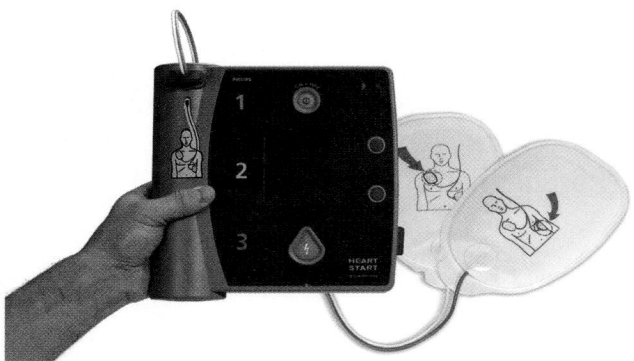

FIGURE 26-3 Automated external defibrillator device. (Courtesy Philips Medical Systems.)

DELEGATION CONSIDERATIONS
Basic life support certification provides hands-on training with an AED for laypersons, assistive personnel, and licensed health care professionals. Most hospitals using AEDs have given the authority to use an AED to all CPR-trained personnel, including assistive personnel. Refer to the specific hospital policies for use of the AED.

EQUIPMENT
❑ Automated external defibrillator
❑ Pair of AED adhesive pads

STEP	RATIONALE

ASSESSMENT
1. Establish loss of consciousness, and call for help.

   This information assists the nurse in determining if the client is unconscious rather than asleep, intoxicated, or hearing impaired.

2. Establish absence of respirations and the lack of circulation: no pulse, no respirations, no movement.

• *Critical Decision Point*
An AED should only be applied to a client who is unconscious, breathless, and pulseless. An AED should NOT be used on children less than 8 years old, unless the AED and AED pads have been specially designed for children less than 8 years old (AHA, 2000).

NURSING DIAGNOSES
• Deceased cardiac output
• Ineffective breathing pattern

• Impaired spontaneous ventilation
• Ineffective tissue perfusion

Related factors are individualized based on client's condition or needs.

STEP	RATIONALE

PLANNING

1. Expected outcomes following completion of procedure:
   - Client's cardiac rhythm is converted back to stable rhythm.
   - Client regains pulse and respirations.
2. Activate the code team in accordance with hospital policy and procedure.
3. Place AED next to the client near the chest or head.

Defibrillation provides the electrical shock to convert a lethal dysrhythmia.

CPR and defibrillation was successful.

First available person to bring the resuscitation cart and AED.

IMPLEMENTATION

1. Start chest compressions until AED arrives and is ready to be attached.

- *Critical Decision Point*

   It is essential that the AED be applied as soon as possible even if chest compressions are interrupted. If the AED is immediately available, attach AED to patient before chest compressions. The faster time to defibrillation, the better the survival rate.

2. Turn on the power (see illustration).

Turning on the power will begin the verbal prompts to guide you through the next steps.

USE THIS AED IF: VICTIM IS UNRESPONSIVE AND NOT BREATHING NORMALLY

TURN ON

FOLLOW PROMPTS

PRESS SHOCK BUTTON IF INSTRUCTED

STEP 2 Power panel with prompts. (Courtesy Philips Medical Systems.)

STEP	**RATIONALE**

3. Attach the device. Stop CPR before attaching the pads. Place the first AED pad on the upper right sternal border directly below the clavicle. Place the second electrode pad lateral to the left nipple with the top of the pad a few inches below the axilla (Figure 26-4). Ensure that the cables are connected to the AED. Do not attach pads to a wet surface, over a medication patch, or over a pacemaker or implanted defibrillator.

Survival rates after ventricular fibrillation arrest decrease approximately 7% to 10% with every minute that defibrillation is delayed (AHA, 2000).

Wet surface, implanted defibrillator, and medication patch may reduce the effectiveness of the defibrillation attempt and result in complications.

4. Allow the AED to analyze the rhythm. Some devices will require that an analysis button be pressed. Clear rescuers and bystanders from the victim, and ensure that no one is touching the victim. The AED will take approximately 5 to 15 seconds to analyze the rhythm.

Each brand of AED is different, so familiarity with the model is important.
Clearing the victim prevents artifact errors, avoids all movement during analysis (Cummins, 2001), and prevents shock from being delivered to bystanders.

5. Deliver the shock in a series of three as indicated by the AED. Before pressing the shock button, announce loudly to clear the victim, and perform a visual check to ensure that no one is in contact with victim. Do not resume CPR until the AED verbal prompts instruct you to do so.

Series of three repeated shocks decreases intrathoracic pressure to the electrical current (AHA, 2000). Clearing the client ensures safety for those involved in rescue efforts.

6. After three shocks, check for signs of circulation: pulse, respirations, movement. If no pulse, resume CPR for 1 minute, then begin the shock sequence again as prompted by the AED.

Most AEDs will analyze the heart rhythm between each shock. If rhythm conversion occurs, the AED will prompt you to check for signs of circulation before the end of the three-shock series.

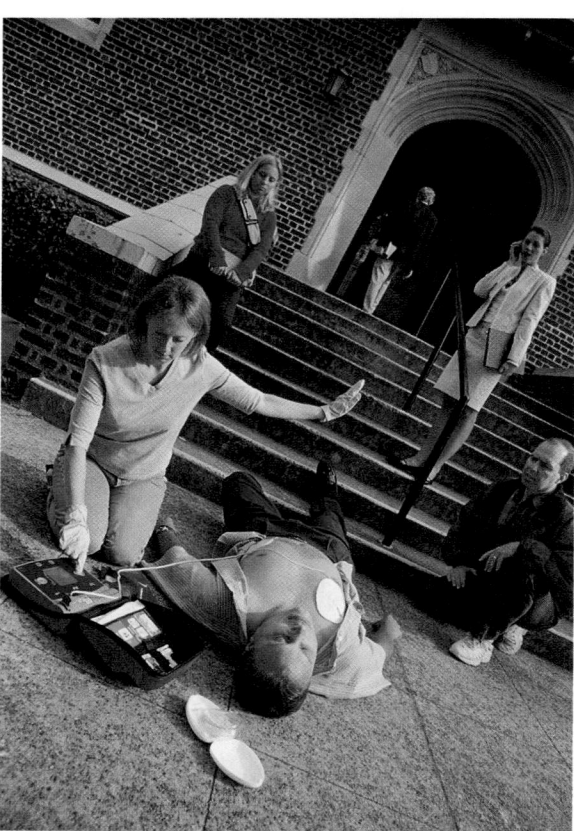

FIGURE **26-4** Placement of AED pads with device next to client. (Courtesy Philips Medical Systems.)

STEP	RATIONALE
EVALUATION	
1. Inspect the pad adhesion to chest wall between series of shocks.	If the pads are not in good contact with chest wall, remove the AED pads, and apply a new set. Attach new set of pads to the AED.
2. Continue resuscitative efforts until the client regains pulse or until the physician determines cessation of efforts.	

Recording and Reporting

- Immediately report arrest, indicating exact location of victim.
- Cardiopulmonary arrest requires precise documentation. Most hospitals use a form designed specifically for in-hospital arrests.
- Record in nurses' notes or on designated CPR worksheet: onset of arrest, time and number of AED shocks (you will not know the exact energy level used by the AED), time and energy level of manual defibrillations, medications given, procedures performed, cardiac rhythm, use of CPR, and the client's response.

Unexpected Outcomes	Related Interventions
1. Client's heart rhythm does not convert into a stable rhythm with pulse after defibrillation.	• Assess pad contact on client's chest wall. • Do not touch client during AED's rhythm analysis. • Avoid placing AED pads over medication patches, pacemaker, or implantable defibrillator generators.
2. Client's skin has burns under AED pads.	• Assess AED pad contact on the chest. • Ensure the chest is dry before applying pads to chest.

Teaching Considerations

- If the client is at risk for cardiopulmonary arrest, the family or caregivers should be instructed and certified in CPR and AED use.
- Client and family should keep emergency numbers taped to phone.

Pediatric Considerations

- Cardiac arrest requiring defibrillation is rare in children. If defibrillation must be considered, lower energy requirements are necessary in the pediatric population. Most AEDs are specifically designed for adult use only and are therefore not recommended for use in children less than 8 years old or less than 25 kg body weight (AHA, 2000). An AED should be used on a pediatric client only if the AED and AED pads have been specially designed for children less than 8 years old. Manual defibrillation performed by health care personnel using lower energy is still the most common method of pediatric defibrillation.

Home Care Considerations

- AEDs and other devices that monitor and defibrillate remotely are available for use in the community and home setting.

SKILL 26-3 Code Management

All who respond to cardiopulmonary arrests should arrive well trained in a simple, easy-to-remember approach. The ACLS Provider Course (AHA, 2000) teaches the primary and secondary survey approach to arrest situations. This memory aid describes two sets of four steps: A-B-C-D. With each step the responder performs an assessment and then, if the assessment so indicates, a management intervention. Initially, a code is managed by the first responder performing the basic skills of CPR, which includes the primary survey of A (airway), B (breathing), C (circulation), D (early defibrillation). This survey must be continued until the code team arrives. The initial process also includes the notification of the hospital's resuscitation team or code team. The team usually includes a physician, critical care nurse, respiratory therapy personnel, anesthesia personnel, and other ancillary support. Most of the code team members have been trained in the ACLS guidelines and the performance of the secondary survey: A (airway intubation), B (confirmation of airway and ventilation), C (rhythm analysis of cardiac rhythm), D (differential diagnosis of the cause). Both surveys must be continually reassessed and managed as appropriate throughout the code situation.

An early primary survey of ABCD is crucial for a favorable client outcome. Without oxygen delivery, brain damage can begin within 4 minutes of arrest; brain damage almost always occurs at 6 minutes, and brain death is certain at 10 minutes (AHA, 2000). The ability of a non–ACLS-trained nurse to initiate resuscitative efforts can prevent lethal dysrhythmias such as ventricular fibrillation from deteriorating to asystole (absence of cardiac electrical activity) and improve the chance of the heart returning to normal rhythm. This improves the ability of the heart and brain to function and improves survivability. Equipment may be readily available at the bedside or in a designated area of the hospital unit. It is the nurse's responsibility to know the location, use of the emergency equipment, and the contents of the resuscitation or crash cart (see Figure 26-5)

As stated earlier in this chapter, CPR certification is required of most nurses and nursing students and will not be covered in detail within this chapter. A few summary points regarding CPR skills have been addressed, including the differences in adult, child, and infant techniques as outlined in Table 26-2.

TABLE 26-2   ADULT, CHILD, AND INFANT CPR TECHNIQUES

TECHNIQUE	ADULT	CHILD (1-8 YEARS OLD)	INFANT
Airway opening	Head-tilt or jaw thrust.	Head-tilt or jaw thrust.	Do not hyperextend the neck.
Mouth-to-mask ventilations	2 slow breaths. $1\frac{1}{2}$-2 sec per breath. 12 breaths/min.	2 slow breaths. 1-$1\frac{1}{2}$ sec per breath. 20 breaths/min.	2 slow breaths. 1-$1\frac{1}{2}$ sec per breath over nose and mouth. 20 breaths/min.
Bag-valve-mask	All ages: Insert oral airway, if available. Slow breaths by squeezing the bag over 1-2 sec. If no oxygen, provide breath over 2 sec.		
Foreign body removal	Abdominal thrusts and blind finger sweeps.	Abdominal thrusts. NO finger sweeps.	Back blows and chest thrusts. Finger sweep only if object visualized.
Chest compressions	Heel of both hands, one atop the other, on lower half of sternum. $1\frac{1}{2}$-2 in. *One-rescuer:* 15 compressions, 2 breaths. *Two-rescuers:* 5 compressions, 1 breath. 80-100 compressions/min.	Heel of one hand on lower half of sternum. Try to maintain open airway with other hand. 1-$1\frac{1}{2}$ in. 5 compressions to 1 breath. 100 compressions/min.	Two fingers one finger width below nipple line. $\frac{1}{2}$-1 in. 5 compressions to 1 breath. >100 compressions/min.

Data from American Heart Association: *Guidelines 2000 for cardiopulmonary resuscitation and emergency cardiovascular care: international consensus on science*, Dallas, 2000, The Association.

DELEGATION CONSIDERATIONS

The basic skills of CPR can be performed by assistive personnel who are certified in basic life support techniques by the American Heart Association or the American Red Cross. Hospitals may differ in how the skill of defibrillation is delegated. In most hospitals, CPR-certified assistive personnel or nurses can use the AED to perform defibrillation. In situations in which the AED is unavailable, a manual defibrillator must be used. Most hospitals reserve the skill of manual defibrillation for licensed personnel who are ACLS trained or have received specialized training to perform manual defibrillation. All others skills required in the code situation will require physician-directed interventions performed by nurses, respiratory therapists, and other physicians.

EQUIPMENT

❑ Crash cart or resuscitation cart (Figure 26-5): Most carts have the following equipment:
  ❑ Gloves, gown, protective eyewear
  ❑ Oxygen source
  ❑ Bag-valve-mask (BVM)
  ❑ Laryngoscope, handle, straight and curved blades
  ❑ Endotracheal tube, various sizes (6 to 8 Fr)
  ❑ Tape
  ❑ Backboard
  ❑ AED and/or manual defibrillator
  ❑ Intravenous (IV) needles (14 to 20 gauge)
  ❑ Central vascular access kit
  ❑ IV tubing and fluids (normal saline and 5% dextrose in water [D_5W])
  ❑ Syringes
  ❑ Laboratory specimen tubes

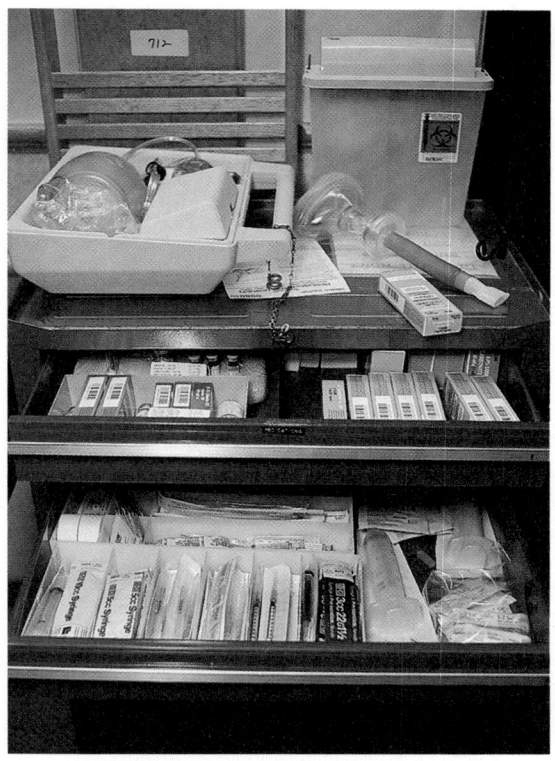

FIGURE 26-5 Emergency resuscitation cart.

❑ Arterial blood gas kit
❑ Code medications
❑ ACLS guidelines or algorithms
❑ Suction source and suction equipment if not with crash cart already

STEP	RATIONALE

PRIMARY SURVEY ABCD

ASSESSMENT

1. Determine if client is unconscious by shaking the client and shouting, "Are you OK?"

Confirms that client is unconscious as opposed to intoxicated, sleeping, or hearing impaired. Unconsciousness can also be caused by substance abuse, hypoglycemia, ketoacidosis, and shock.

● *Critical Decision Point*
  If unconscious person has adequate respirations and pulse, remain until further assistance is present. Place victim in a modified lateral recovery position (see illustration, step 1). Continue to determine presence of respirations and pulse because respiratory or cardiopulmonary arrest is still possible.

STEP	RATIONALE

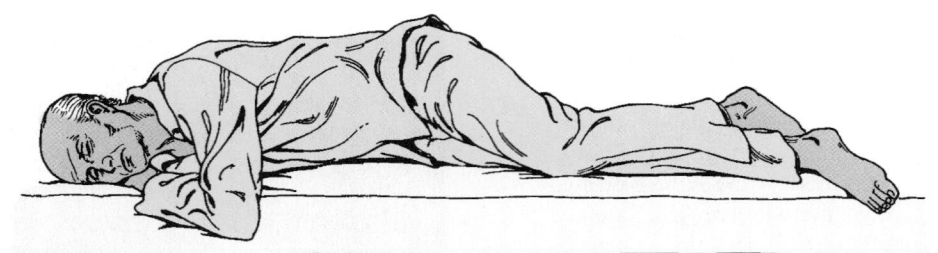

STEP **1** Recovery position.

NURSING DIAGNOSES
- Ineffective breathing pattern
- Ineffective tissue perfusion
- Decreased cardiac output
- Impaired gas exchange
- Impaired spontaneous ventilation

Related factors are individualized based on client's condition or needs.

PLANNING

1. Expected outcomes following completion of procedure:
   - Client regains pulse and respirations.
   - Physician may terminate CPR.

   CPR was successful.
   Decision results when irreversible brain or cardiac damage occurs as expected or there is knowledge of advance directive.

2. Immediately activate the hospital's code team or emergency medical services (EMS). Tell co-workers to bring AED (if available) and crash cart to bedside. For an infant or child, perform CPR for 1 minute before activating EMS.

   Ensures timely application of defibrillation, CPR, and ACLS to the arrest victim.

3. Apply gloves and face shield.

   Reduces transmission of microorganisms.

IMPLEMENTATION
PRIMARY SURVEY: A (AIRWAY)

1. Open airway using:
   a. Head tilt-chin lift (no trauma) *or*
   b. Jaw thrust (trauma is suspected)
   (see illustrations)

   Determine if client has spontaneous respirations. The tongue is the most common cause of blocked airway in an unresponsive client.
   Spinal cord injury should be suspected with any kind of trauma. In these situations a rescuer must use jaw-thrust maneuver. Prevention of head extension and neck movement is very important to prevent paralysis or spinal cord injury. A cervical brace should be applied as soon as possible to maintain cervical-spine stability.

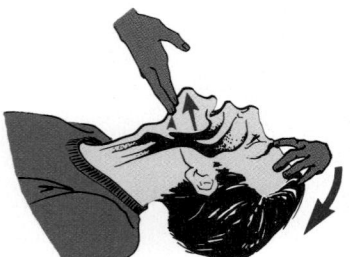

STEP **1a** Head tilt-chin lift.

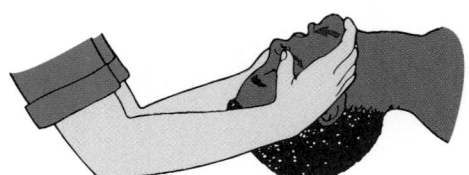

STEP **1b** Jaw thrust without head tilt.

STEP	RATIONALE

PRIMARY SURVEY: B (BREATHING)

2. Attempt to ventilate the client using one of these methods:
   a. Mouth-to-mouth using a barrier device
   b. Mouth-to-mask using a pocket mask (see illustration)
   c. Bag-valve-mask (see illustrations)

Airtight seal is formed, and air is prevented from escaping through nose.

If available, attach BVM or mouth-to-mask device to supplemental oxygen supply.

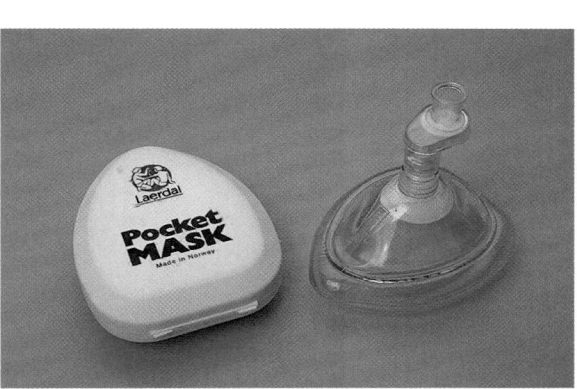

STEP **2b** Pocket mask.

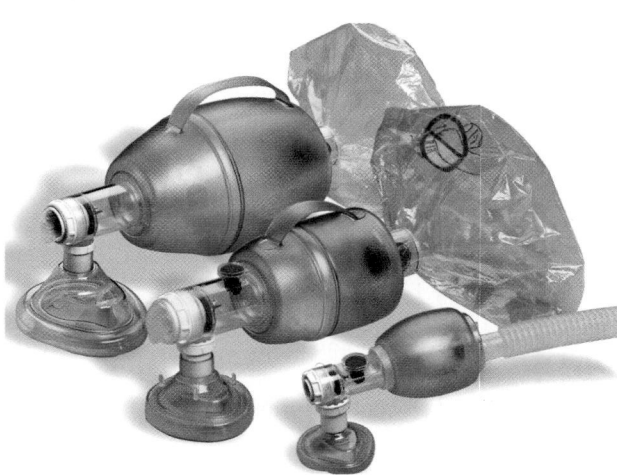

STEP **2c(1)** Bag-valve-mask. (Courtesy AMBU USA.)

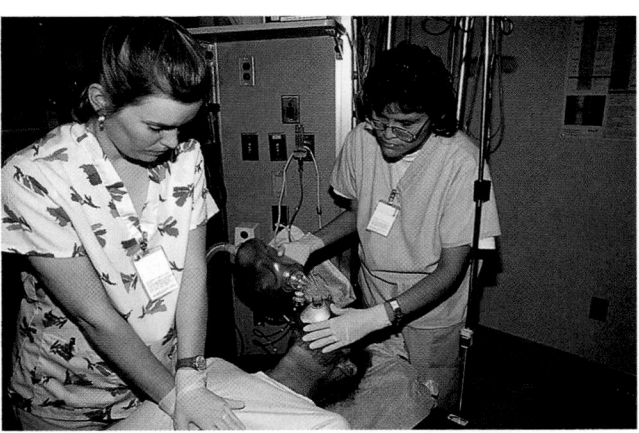

STEP **2c(2)** Two-rescuer breathing with bag-valve-mask.

- *Critical Decision Point*
  Give breaths with only enough force to make the chest rise. Slow breaths deliver air at a low pressure to reduce the risk of gastric distention.

3. If readily available, insert oral airway (see Skill 26-1).

Maintains tongue on anterior floor of mouth and prevents obstruction of posterior airway by tongue.

4. Suction secretions if necessary, or turn victim's head to one side, unless trauma is suspected.

Suctioning prevents airway obstruction. Turning client's head to one side allows gravity to drain secretions.

STEP	**RATIONALE**

PRIMARY SURVEY: C (CIRCULATION)

5. Check carotid pulse on an adult or child.
   Check for brachial pulse in an infant. Feel for 3 to 5 seconds on the side you are on.

6. Place victim on hard surface such as floor, ground, or backboard. Victim must be flat. If necessary, logroll victim to flat, supine position using spine precautions.

7. If pulse is absent and an AED is available, apply AED immediately (see Skill 26-2).

   a. After three shocks, check for signs of circulation: pulse, respirations, movement. If no pulse, resume CPR for 1 minute, then begin the shock sequence again.

8. If pulse is absent and an AED is unavailable, immediately initiate chest compressions:

   a. Assume correct hand position and compression ratio for the client (see illustration).

Carotid pulse is present when other peripheral pulses are not palpable. The neck of an infant is usually short, so the carotid pulse is difficult to locate. Delivering cardiac compressions in the presence of a pulse is contraindicated.

External compression of heart is facilitated. Heart is compressed between sternum and spinal vertebrae, which must be on hard and firm surface.

Survival rates after ventricular fibrillation arrest decrease approximately 7% to 10% with every minute the defibrillation is delayed (AHA, 2000).

ACLS guidelines specify initial three shocks should be followed by chest compressions for 1 minute to provide blood movement and improved perfusion before another set of shocks is delivered (AHA, 2000).

Specific hand position, compression depth, and ratio are different for adult, child, and infant to avoid injury to the heart, lung, or liver.

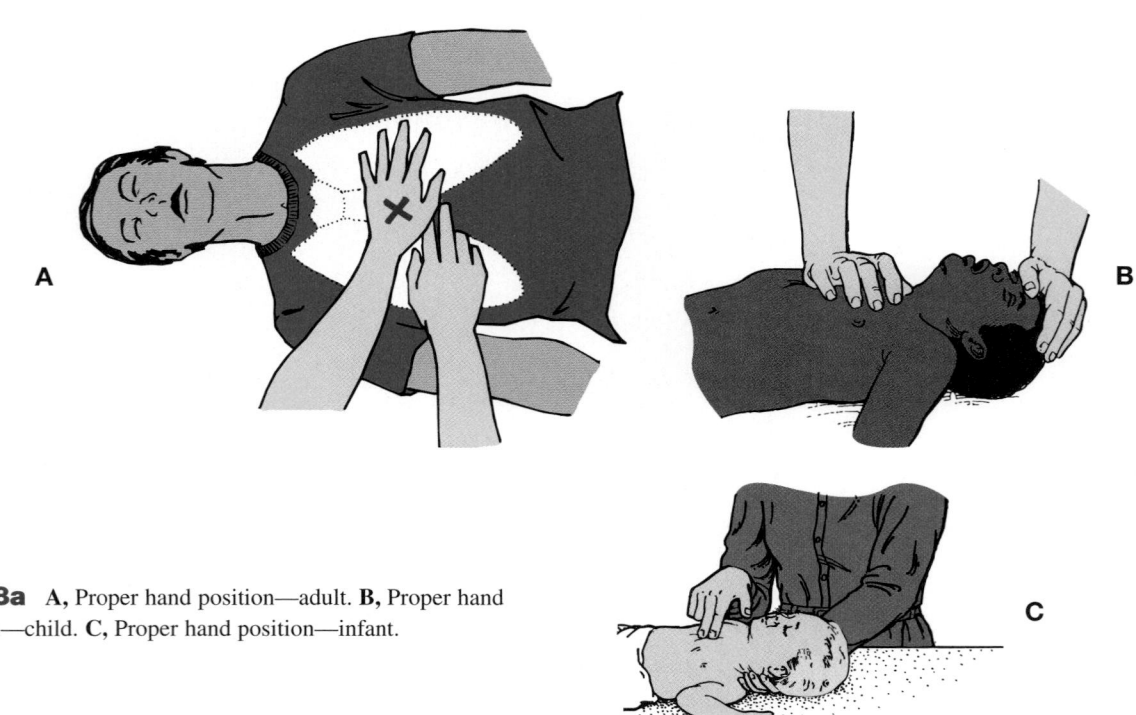

STEP 8a   **A,** Proper hand position—adult. **B,** Proper hand position—child. **C,** Proper hand position—infant.

- *Critical Decision Point*
  Ensure fingers are off the ribs and the lowermost part of the xiphoid process. This minimizes the chance of rib fracture that could result in punctured lung or liver laceration, which can further compromise cardiopulmonary status.

9. Continue chest compressions, ventilations, and AED use (if available).

STEP	RATIONALE

IMPLEMENTATION
SECONDARY SURVEY ABCD

1. Upon arrival of sufficient personnel, delegate tasks as appropriate.

   Assist the victim's roommate or visitors away from the code scene. Assign pastoral care or other nurses to communicate with family. Delegate someone to remove excess furniture or equipment from the room. Have someone bring client's chart to the bedside or be able to refer to the client's electronic chart for latest data and to clarify code status and allergies. Assign a fresh person to perform chest compressions. Assign a nurse as recorder to record/document the events of the code. Another nurse needs to be assigned as the crash cart nurse to get medications from the crash cart to hand them off to code team members. The bedside nurse will be involved with medication administration, vital signs, assisting with procedures, and so on.

   Delegation of duties is essential to meet all the needs of the client and his or her family in a timely matter.

2. Give code leader brief verbal report on events just before code, vital signs, medical diagnosis, and code interventions performed before the code team's arrival.

   This information is critical in the selection of appropriate treatment for the client

SECONDARY SURVEY: A (INTUBATE AIRWAY)

3. If respirations are absent, assist the code team with endotracheal intubation.

   Intubation provides a client airway and increases pulmonary ventilation (Cummins, 2001).

   a. Have available laryngoscope, handle, curved and straight blades, and endotracheal tubes. Ensure that the light source on the laryngoscope is functional.

   Light must be functional on the laryngoscope in order to visualize the vocal cords and provide intubation of the trachea.

SECONDARY SURVEY: B (CONFIRMATION OF AIRWAY AND VENTILATION)

4. Assist in confirmation of endotracheal tube placement by auscultating lungs for bilateral breath sounds and the epigastric area for lack of breath sounds. Secondary confirmation is usually performed by the intubation personnel using a carbon dioxide monitor.

   Tracheal tube placement in the esophagus would not provide ventilation of the lungs.

5. Ventilate using a bag-valve-mask upon intubation.

   BVM will provide a larger volume of air for improved ventilation when attached to an endotracheal tube.

STEP	**RATIONALE**

SECONDARY SURVEY: C (ANALYSIS OF CARDIAC RHYTHM)

6. Attach manual defibrillator/monitor to client using electrocardiogram (ECG) electrodes, Quick-Look paddles, or "hands-off" defibrillation electrodes to visualize heart rhythm.

Quick-Look paddles' placement on the chest can immediately reveal the client's heart rhythm.

7. If cardiac rhythm is shockable, assist code team with manual defibrillation.

Manual defibrillation is performed only by trained personnel.

   a. Turn defibrillator on, and select proper energy level.

Energy is delivered in monophasic waveforms at 200 joules and increased as necessary to 200 to 300 joules, then 360 joules. Some defibrillators deliver energy in biphasic waveforms starting at lower joules.

   b. Apply conductive gel or gel pads to client's chest where defibrillator paddles will be placed. Some defibrillators use "hands-off pads" which are applied to client's chest and directly connected to the manual defibrillator.

Decreases electrical opposition and helps minimize burns to skin (Cummins, 2001).

"Hands-off" pads allow defibrillation without coming into contact directly with the client during shock delivery.

   c. Paddles are charged and placed on the client's chest wall by trained personnel.

Placement ensures appropriate discharge of current.

8. Establish IV access with large-bore needle (14 to 20 gauge), and begin infusion of 0.9% normal saline.

Provides a route for rapid drug administration, access for blood samples, and fluid administration.

Physiological saline is isotonic.

9. Assist with procedures as needed.

Much of the equipment needed for special procedures during a code are found on the crash cart. Knowledge of the crash cart contents is very helpful in the code to provide personnel with the appropriate equipment.

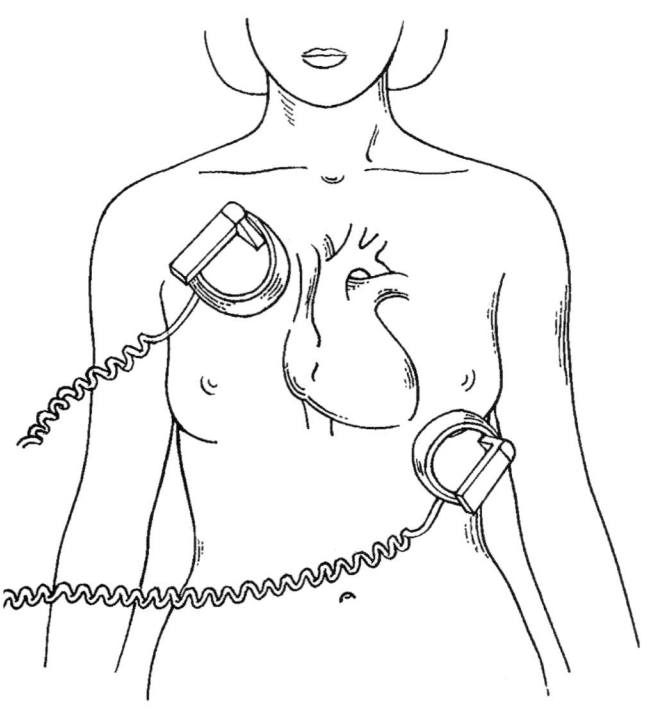

STEP **7b** Electrode placement for defibrillation.

STEP	RATIONALE
10. Continue CPR until relieved, until victim regains spontaneous pulse and respirations, until rescuer is exhausted and unable to perform CPR effectively, or until physician discontinues CPR.	Artificial cardiopulmonary function is maintained. Cardiopulmonary resuscitation is interrupted when changing CPR personnel, during defibrillation, or when transporting victim. During intubation, CPR may be interrupted for more than 5 seconds but should not exceed 30 seconds. Nurse should remind rescue team of number of seconds elapsing during intubation.

SECONDARY SURVEY: D (DIFFERENTIAL DIAGNOSIS)

STEP	RATIONALE
11. Assist physician with differential diagnosis.	Physician may need laboratory or diagnostic information regarding the client to help identify the cause of the arrest.
12. Remove and discard into appropriate receptacle: gloves, face shield, pocket mask, and sharps.	Reduces transmission of microorganisms and needle sticks.

EVALUATION

1. Reassess the primary and secondary survey ABCDs throughout the code event.	This will keep the process organized and address all the needs of the client.
2. Palpate carotid pulse at least every 5 minutes after first minute of CPR.	Documents adequacy of external cardiac compressions.
3. Observe for spontaneous return of respirations or heart rate.	Performance of CPR on client with a pulse is dangerous.
4. Cardiopulmonary resuscitation is not interrupted for more than 5 seconds unless the interruption is for AED application or manual defibrillator use.	Maintains adequacy of oxygenation and circulation.

Recording and Reporting

- Immediately report arrest, indicating exact location of victim.
- In hospital setting, follow hospital policy. In community setting, activate the emergency response system.
- Cardiopulmonary arrest requires precise documentation. Most hospitals use a form designed specifically for in-hospital arrests.
- Record in nurses' notes or on designated CPR worksheet: onset of arrest, time and number of AED shocks (you will not know the exact energy level used by the AED), time and energy level of manual defibrillations, medications given, procedures performed, cardiac rhythm, use of CPR, and the client's response.

Unexpected Outcomes	Related Interventions
1. Client develops skeletal injury, such as fractured ribs or sternum, or internal organ injury, such as lacerated lung or liver.	• Obtain appropriate diagnostic tests to document rib fracture. • Assess client's postarrest breathing for symmetry and pain. • Observe for hemoptysis or gastrointestinal bleeding. • Observe for distending abdomen.
2. Client's CPR is unsuccessful.	• Contact chaplain services. • Contact social worker. • Complete postmortem care on client. • Provide for privacy for client's family to say their goodbyes to client.
3. Rescuer is unassisted, tires, and is unable to continue.	• Obtain assistance.

Teaching Considerations

- If client is at risk for cardiopulmonary arrest, the family or caregivers should be instructed and certified in CPR by certified instructor from institution, American Red Cross, or American Heart Association.
- Client and family should keep emergency numbers taped to the phone or consider programming them into speed dial function on both home and mobile phones. These numbers may include fire department, ambulance, hospital, and physician. Instruct client and family about whom to call. Family may also need to know what to do when client is found unresponsive.
- It is extremely helpful if family has list of medications client is presently taking.

Pediatric Considerations

- All persons involved in administering CPR must understand different breathing/compression ratios, hand (fingers) placement, and depth of compression in children and infants compared with adults.
- Infants and children experience only respiratory arrest much more frequently than full cardiopulmonary arrest.

Gerontological Considerations

- In older adult, compressions often result in rib or cartilage fractures. Cardiopulmonary resuscitation should be continued.

- Loose-fitting dentures should be removed to avoid obstructing the airway. If dentures fit securely, leave them in to ensure a tight seal when providing ventilations.

Home Care Considerations

- In the community and long-term care settings, clients may have implanted defibrillators. For these clients, families should know how to administer CPR. After the first 30 to 60 seconds of an arrest, proceed with CPR as for any other client.
- Soft surface such as mattress, car seat, or grassy surface decreases efficiency of external cardiac compressions.

Long-Term Care Considerations

- It is important for the clients and their families to ensure that the client's code status is clarified upon entering a long-term care environment. Specifics regarding the resuscitative care the client wishes to receive need to be detailed in an advance directive or other legal document. Families must also understand that a copy of the client's advance directive should accompany the client upon transfer to another health care facility if necessary. Families may consider keeping a copy of this document to take with them to the health care facility if their family member is transferred.

FOCUS on CLINICAL PRACTICE

You are the charge nurse for night shift on a general medicine floor. On your rounds you find your client, Ethel Waters, lying unresponsive on the floor of the bathroom. She is 85 years old and was admitted with congestive heart failure. An AED is available down the hall.

1. What should you do first?
   A. Apply AED.
   B. Call for help.
   C. Check for a pulse.
   D. Open airway and provide artificial ventilations.
   Explain your choice:
2. You bend over Mrs. Waters and speak her name loudly, touching her shoulder. She does not respond and is clearly unconscious. You open her airway and deliver two artificial ventilations. Which of the following is NOT an appropriate method to provide artificial ventilations?
   A. Mouth-to-mouth
   B. Mouth-to-mouth with barrier device
   C. Mouth-to-mask
   D. Bag-valve-mask
   Explain your choice.

3. After you successfully ventilate Mrs. Waters, your co-worker arrives with the AED. What is your next step?
   A. Check for a pulse.
   B. Start chest compressions.
   C. Apply the AED.
   Explain your choice.
4. Your co-worker has started chest compressions on Mrs. Waters. Under which of the following circumstances should you interrupt performance of the chest compressions?
   A. Arrival of the code team
   B. AED application and use
   C. Bag-valve-mask use
   D. IV insertion
   Explain your choice.
5. The code team has arrived to continue resuscitation attempts on Mrs. Waters. What activities will be involved in the code team's work? How can you participate?

NCLEX REVIEW QUESTIONS

1. Which of the following is true about an oral airway?
   1. It eliminates the need to position the head of the unconscious client.
   2. It eliminates the possibility of an upper airway obstruction.
   3. It is of no value once an endotracheal tube is inserted.
   4. It may stimulate vomiting or laryngospasm if inserted in the semiconscious client.

2. Which of the following choices lists in correct order the major steps of CPR and AED operations for an unresponsive victim?
   1. Call for help, check for a pulse, attach the AED, open the airway, provide two breaths if needed, then turn on the AED.
   2. Wait for the AED, then open the airway, provide two breaths if needed, check for a pulse, and if no pulse, attach the AED.
   3. Call for help, get the AED, open the airway, provide two breaths if needed, check for a pulse, and if no pulse is present, attach the AED.
   4. Provide two breaths, check for a pulse, call for the AED, provide chest compressions until the AED arrives, attach the AED.

3. Name the preferred technique to open the airway in a known or suspected trauma victim.
   1. Head tilt
   2. Chin lift
   3. Jaw thrust
   4. Lateral lying position

4. Delegation of nurses' roles during a resuscitative event may include which of the following?
   1. Bedside nurse
   2. Crash cart nurse
   3. Recorder
   4. All of the above

5. Which of the following is the time goal from victim collapse to first defibrillation?
   1. 4 minutes
   2. 3 minutes
   3. 6 minutes
   4. 10 minutes

References

American Heart Association: *Guidelines 2000 for cardiopulmonary resuscitation and emergency cardiovascular care: international consensus on science,* Dallas, 2000, The Association.

Brewer JA, Bonalumi NM: Health care beliefs and practices among the Pennsylvania Amish, *J Emerg Nurs* 21(6):494, 1995.

Cummins RO, editor: *ACLS provider manual,* Dallas, 2001, American Heart Association.

Hockenberry MJ and others: *Wong's nursing care of infants and children,* ed 7, St. Louis, 2003, Mosby.

Kemp C, Rasbridge LA: Culture and the end of life: East African cultures. II. Sudanese, *J Hosp Palliat Nurs* 3(3):110, 2001.

Meleis A: Arab Americans. In Lipson J and others, editors: *Culture and nursing care: a pocket guide,* San Francisco, Calif, 1996, UCSF Nursing Press.

Pacquiao DF: Cultural incongruities of advance directives, *Bioethics Forum* 17(1):27, 2001.

Research References

Bernard SA and others: Treatment of comatose survivors of out-of-hospital cardiac arrest with induced hypothermia, *N Engl J Med* 346:557, 2002.

Ditto PH and others: Advance directives as acts of communication: a randomized control trial, *Arch Intern Med* 161(3):421, 2001.

Doorenbos AZ: The use of advance directives in a population of Asian Indian Hindus, *J Transcult Nurs* 14(1):17, 2003.

Dupree CY: The attitudes of black Americans toward advance directives, *J Transcult Nurs* 11(1):12, 2000.

Emergency Nurses Association: *Presenting the option for family presence,* ed 2, Des Plaines, Ill, 2001, ENA.

Hypothermia After Cardiac Arrest Study Group: Mild therapeutic hypothermia to improve the neurological outcome after cardiac arrest, *N Engl J Med* 346:549, 2002.

Johnson SK: Hmong health beliefs and experiences in the Western health care system, *J Transcult Nurs* 13(2):126, 2002.

MacLean S and others: Family presence during cardiopulmonary resuscitation and invasive procedures: practices of critical care and emergency nurses, *Am J Crit Care* 12:246, 2003.

Nolan JP and others: Therapeutic hypothermia after cardiac arrest: an advisory statement by the advanced life support task force of the International Liaison Committee on Resuscitation, *Circulation* 108:118, 2003.

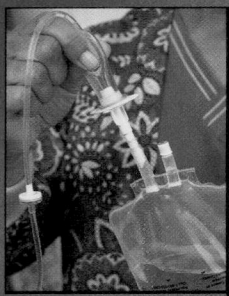

27

Intravenous and Vascular Access Therapy

MEDIA RESOURCES

Evolve Site *evolve*
http://evolve.elsevier.com/Perry/skills
- Weblinks
- Video clips
- Mosby's Nursing Skills Video Exercises

Mosby's Nursing Skills Videos/CD-ROM
- *Administering Intravenous Fluid Therapy Video:* Initiating a peripheral IV, identifying infusion site, promoting venous distention, venipuncture, initiating

MEDIA RESOURCES—cont'd

infusion, and dressing infusion site; troubleshooting intravenous infusions, assessment for potential complications, regular assessments, use of infiltration and phlebitis scales; discontinuing IV therapy, removal of dressing, stabilizing catheter while site is cleansed, removal of catheter, dressing venipuncture site

- *Intravenous Medications Video:* Adding medications to IV fluid containers, use of needleless systems, mixing medication with IV fluid, use of IV flow strip; administering IV piggyback medications, establishing piggyback step-up, reestablishing primary infusion; administering IV medications by mini-infusion pump, filling syringe, securing in pump and re-establishing primary infusion; administering medications by IV bolus, preparing injection lock, rates and techniques for injecting medication, flushing the injection lock after injection
- *Managing Intravenous Fluid Therapy:* Regulating IV infusions, calculating drip rate, using the roller-clamp method and infusion pumps; changing IV tubing and fluids; changing IV dressings, assessment of the infusion site
- *Vascular Access Video:* Dressing care, types of dressings, assessment of the insertion site, maintaining asepsis, documentation; blood draws and fluid administration, scheduling considerations, flushing to check for patency, recapping catheter, connecting to IV fluid; troubleshooting, checking the integrity of vascular access, signs of potential problems

OBJECTIVES

Mastery of content in this chaper will enable the nurse to:

- Discuss conditions requiring intravenous (IV) therapy.
- Explain how to prepare the client and family for IV therapy.
- Discuss factors that increase the risk of complications from IV therapy.
- Identify individualized outcomes for clients requiring IV therapy.
- Explain techniques used to prevent transmission of infection for a client receiving IV therapy.
- Demonstrate initiation of IV therapy, regulation of IV flow rate, changing of IV solutions, changing of IV tubing, changing of IV dressings, and discontinuing a peripheral IV.
- Identify common types of vascular access devices (VADs) and describe their care and maintenance.
- Identify the educational needs of clients with VADs.

KEY TERMS

Cannula	Fluid volume excess (FVE)
Central venous catheter (CVC)	Heparin lock
Drop factor	Hypertonic
Electrolyte	Hypotonic
Electronic infusion device (EID)	Implanted infusion port
Embolus (Emboli)	Infiltration
Exit site	Infusion pump
Fluid volume deficit (FVD)	Injection cap

KEY TERMS-cont'd

Isotonic	Phlebitis
IV plug	Saline lock
Noncoring Huber needle	Sharps container
Over-the-needle catheter (ONC)	Subcutaneous tunnel
Percutaneous	Thrombosis
Peripherally inserted central catheter (PICC)	Vascular access device (VAD)
	Venipuncture

Parenteral Replacement of Fluids

Fluids may be infused directly into the circulating blood volume to supplement or replace body fluids. This form of therapy is common for clients requiring surgery and for clients unable to tolerate oral or enteral nutrition. Parenteral fluid replacement includes intravenous (IV) fluid and electrolyte therapy, blood therapy (see Chapter 28), total parenteral nutrition (TPN), and peripheral parenteral nutrition (PPN) (see Chapter 31). The goal of IV fluid administration is to correct or prevent fluid and electrolyte imbalances, correct or prevent nutritional imbalances, or to provide IV medication therapy. When IV therapy is necessary, the nurse must know the correct solution and equipment needed and how to initiate an infusion, regulate the fluid infusion rate, care for and maintain the system, identify and correct problems, and discontinue the infusion. In addition to knowledge and understanding, IV therapy requires many nursing skills. As with any skill, time, patience, and repetition foster the development of proficiency.

Intravenous Solutions

Prepared IV solutions fall into three general categories: isotonic, hypotonic, and hypertonic (Table 27-1). An isotonic solution has a total electrolyte content of approximately 310 mEq/L. A hypotonic solution has a total electrolyte content of less than 250 mEq/L. A hypertonic solution has a total electrolyte content of 375 mEq/L or greater (Metheny, 2000). All IV fluids should be carefully given, especially hypertonic solutions, because these solutions pull fluid into the vascular space by osmosis, resulting in an increased vascular volume that can result in pulmonary edema, particularly in clients with cardiac or renal diseases. The type and amount of IV solution ordered by the physician are determined by the client's serum electrolyte values and fluid volume balance. The nurse must understand the rationale for IV fluid administration and the type of IV solution ordered. Because the names of IV solutions are often abbreviated or shortened, the nurse must be careful to give the correct solution (Box 27-1).

In addition to the specific IV fluid ordered, the physician often includes additives such as vitamins or electrolytes. Manufactured prepared containers of IV fluids with potassium already added should be used when available to decrease the chance of contamination and error; otherwise, admixture should occur in a pharmacy using a laminar flow

TABLE 27-1 COMPOSITION AND USE OF COMMONLY PRESCRIBED CRYSTALLOID SOLUTIONS

SOLUTION	TONICITY	mOsm/L (mmol/L)	GLUCOSE (g/L)	INDICATIONS AND CONSIDERATIONS
DEXTROSE IN WATER				
5%	Isotonic	278	50	Provides free water necessary for renal excretion of solutes Used to replace water losses and treat hypernatremia Provides 170 calories/L Does not provide any electrolytes
10%	Hypertonic	556	100	Provides free water only, no electrolytes Provides 340 calories/L
SALINE				
0.45%	Hypotonic	154	0	Provides free water in addition to Na^+ and Cl^- Used to replace hypotonic fluid losses Used as maintenance solution although it does not replace daily losses of other electrolytes Provides no calories
0.9%	Isotonic	308	0	Used to expand intravascular volume and replace extracellular fluid losses Only solution that may be administered with blood products Contains Na^+ and Cl^- in excess of plasma levels Does not provide free water, calories, other electrolytes May cause intravascular overload or hyperchloremic acidosis
3.0%-5.0%	Hypertonic	1026	0	Used to treat symptomatic hyponatremia Must be administered slowly and with extreme caution because it may cause dangerous intravascular volume overload and pulmonary edema
DEXTROSE IN SALINE				
5% in 0.225%	Isotonic	355	50	Provides Na^+, Cl^-, and free water Used to replace hypotonic losses and treat hypernatremia Provides 170 calories/L
5% in 0.45%	Hypertonic	432	50	Same as 0.45% NaCl except provides 170 calories/L
5% in 0.9%	Hypertonic	586	50	Same as 0.9% NaCl except provides 170 calories/L
MULTIPLE ELECTROLYTE SOLUTIONS				
Lactated Ringer's solution	Isotonic	309	0	Similar in composition to plasma except that it has excess Cl^-, Mg^{2+}, and no HCO_3^- Does not provide free water or calories Used to expand the intravascular volume and replace extracellular fluid losses
(Hartmann's) solution	Isotonic	274	0	Similar in composition to normal plasma except does not contain Mg^{2+} Used to treat losses from burns and lower gastrointestinal tract May be used to treat mild metabolic acidosis but should not be used to treat lactic acidosis Does not provide free water or calories

Modified from Heitz EU, Horne MM: *Pocket guide to fluid, electrolyte, and acid-base balance,* ed 4, St. Louis, 2001, Mosby.

hood. The body is very sensitive to changes in potassium brought on by lack of intake or increased fluid loss. IV solutions nearly always include added potassium to correct insensitive loss or loss created by the medical condition of the client. The nurse should monitor the client's laboratory values and assess for fluid and electrolyte balance during IV therapy.

Intravenous Catheters

The majority of peripheral venous catheters in the United States are made of polymers, such as polyurethane, silicone, or polyethylene (Thomas, 2002). Metal needles, once the only type of intravenous device, are used infrequently because of the high degree of vein trauma and complication of

IV infiltration and phlebitis. Many companies make a winged catheter with a removable stylet. Despite advancements in catheter products, there is still risk of injury to blood vessel walls. Various cellular processes come into play once an injury to a vein occurs, resulting in clinical signs of redness, edema, infiltration, thrombosis, and pain at a catheter entrance site.

Venous access poses significant risks to clients; however, intravenous therapy is often critical to a client's proper clinical management and recovery. Commonly used over-the-needle catheters (ONCs) comprise a metal stylet, which is used to pierce the skin, and a Teflon, polyurethane, or silicone catheter, which is threaded into a vein and remains there for the instillation of fluid. These flexible catheters do not

BOX 27-1   Common Names for Intravenous Solutions

SOLUTION	COMMON NAMES
0.9% sodium chloride	Normal saline 0.9% NaCl 0.9% NS NS
0.45% sodium chloride	One-half-strength normal saline 0.45% NaCl 0.45% NS $\frac{1}{2}$ NaCl $\frac{1}{2}$ NS
Dextrose 5% in 0.9% sodium chloride	D_5 normal saline D_5 0.9% NaCl D_5 0.9% NS D_5 NS
Dextrose 5% in 0.45% sodium chloride	D_5 One-half-strength normal saline D_5 0.45% NaCl D_5 0.45 NS D_5 $\frac{1}{2}$ NaCl D_5 $\frac{1}{2}$ NS
Lactated Ringer's	LR
Dextrose 5% in lactated Ringer's	D_5 LR

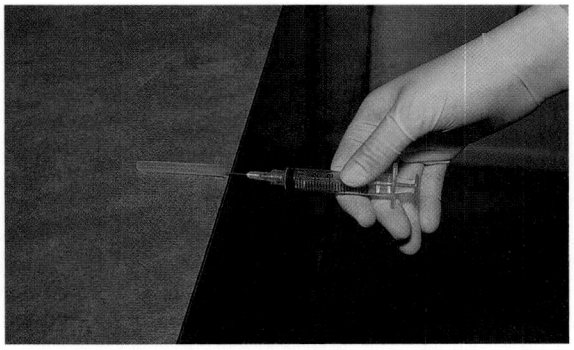

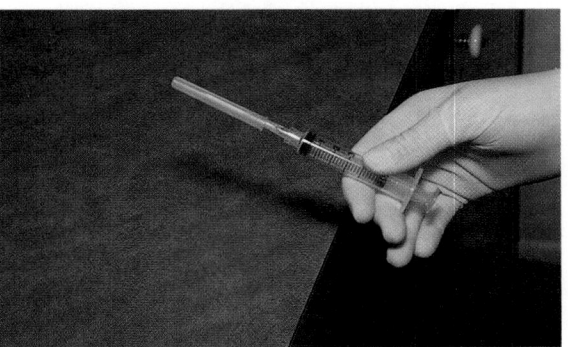

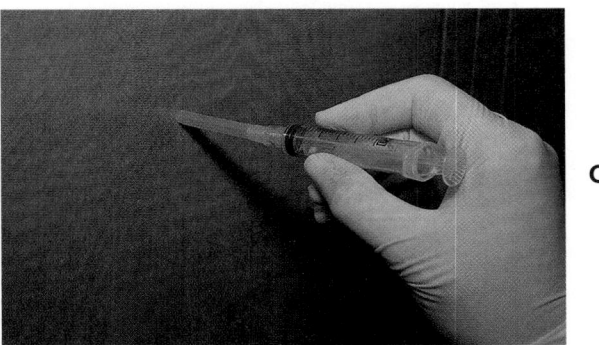

FIGURE **27-1** **A,** Insert contaminated needled into cap using one hand. **B,** Have cap slip fully over needle. **C,** Push cap against firm surface.

dislodge from the vein as easily as stainless steel needles. In addition, large volumes of fluids and medications can be quickly administered through the catheter without a high risk of infiltration. A 20- to 22-gauge flexible catheter is used in most situations for adults, whereas a 22- to 24-gauge catheter can be used for children and older adults or for any other client with small or fragile veins. In general, use the smallest catheter that will deliver the needed fluids at the appropriate rate. If the administration of large volumes of IV fluids or blood or blood products is anticipated, a large size (20- or 18-gauge) catheter is preferred to allow rapid infusion of IV fluids or viscous blood product solutions.

Health care workers are at high risk for accidental needle sticks and sharp injuries. Common causes of accidental needle-stick injuries include recapping incidents, assembling or accessing IV tubing devices with needles attached, disposing of contaminated sharps, using alternative methods to cover used needles on IV assemblies, and intentionally detaching IV lines. IV catheters and winged catheters are devices commonly associated with a high risk for injuries. To help prevent accidental injury, needles should not be recapped, but placed directly in puncture-proof containers, referred to as sharps containers. In emergencies a one-handed "scoop" technique may be used to cover needles (Occupational Safety and Health Administration [OSHA], 2001a) (Figure 27-1). The caregiver places the cap on a flat surface and *with one hand only* slides the needle into the cap. Most health care agencies now use needleless devices that eliminate the use of needles altogether. The needleless devices use protective covers and valvelike systems and come in a variety of needle, catheter, and tubing products.

Evidence-Based Practice Trends

The dwell time for peripheral IV catheters can be up to 96 hours unless a complication arises (Catney and others, 2001; Centers for Disease Control and Prevention [CDC], 2002; White, 2001). Early recognition of complications is paramount and requires immediate discontinuation of a catheter and rotation of the site. Advanced catheter materials such as polyurethane are more biocompatible and are associated with less traumatic insertions, more vascular preservation, and increased cost savings (Mayer and Wong, 2002; OSHA, 2000).

The Needlestick Safety and Prevention Act was enacted to prevent risks related to inadvertent injuries with vascular access devices (VADs) and sharps (Deacon, 2004; OSHA, 2001a, b; Powers, 2002). VADs and ancillary sharps such as Huber access needles are available with safety features, and health care workers should be compliant in their use (Rivers and others, 2003).

BOX 27-2 CDC Guidelines to Decrease Intravascular Infection Related to IV Therapy

- Palpate catheter insertion site for tenderness daily through the intact dressing.
- Visually inspect a catheter site if client develops tenderness at site, fever without obvious source, or symptoms of local or bloodstream infection.
- Perform hand hygiene before and after palpating, inserting, replacing, or dressing any intravascular device.
- Cleanse skin site before venipuncture with an appropriate antiseptic.
- Do not palpate insertion site after skin has been cleansed with antiseptic.
- Use transparent or sterile gauze dressing to cover a catheter site.
- Replace IV tubing, including piggyback tubing and stopcocks, no more frequently than at 72-hour intervals unless clinically indicated.
- Replace tubing used to administer blood, blood products, or lipid emulsions within 24 hours of initiating infusion.
- There are no recommendations for the hang time of IV fluids.
- Replace dressing over peripheral venous catheters when catheter is replaced or when dressing becomes damp, loosened, or soiled.
- Clean injection ports with antiseptic agent before accessing system.
- Do not use in-line filters routinely for infection control.
- Replace short, peripheral venous catheters and rotate sites every 72 to 96 hours or immediately when complications appear.
- Do not routinely apply topical antimicrobial ointment to the insertion site of peripheral venous catheters or central venous catheter insertion sites.
- There is no recommendation for the frequency of replacement of peripherally inserted central catheter (PICC).

Modified from Centers for Disease Control and Prevention: Guidelines for the prevention of catheter-related infections, *MMWR* 51(No. RR-10):1-26, 2002.

BOX 27-3 Standards for Reducing Occupational Exposure to Bloodborne Pathogens

1. Gloves must be worn when there is a reasonable expectation that the employee may contact blood, for example, during venipuncture or while changing IV administration sets.
2. Contaminated needles, needleless devices, and other sharps must be placed in puncture-resistant containers properly labeled as a biohazard; when the containers are full, they are to be sealed and disposed of properly.
3. Contaminated needles should not be bent, sheared, recapped, or removed from the syringe after use.
4. Reports to OSHA of needle-stick injuries are required, and the health care agency must provide medical evaluation and follow-up.
5. Hepatitis B vaccination is to be made available to all employees who have occupational exposure.
6. Training and education must be offered to high-risk workers, such as nurses who initiate IV therapy, concerning precautions for prevention of exposure and use of personal protective equipment.
7. Each facility must have an infection control plan, including methods for reduction of the health care worker's exposure to biohazardous wastes.
8. Facilities must have engineering and work practice controls to eliminate or minimize employee exposure. Controls may include sharps disposal containers and self-sheathing needles.

Occupational Safety and Health Administration: Occupational exposure to bloodborne pathogens; needlestick and other sharps injuries; final rule, *Federal Register* 66(5317-5325), Jan 18, 2001a, http://www.osha-sic.gov/, accessed November 2003.

Skill Performance Guidelines

1. Know the client's normal range of vital signs before instituting intravenous therapy. Fluid or electrolyte imbalances can affect vital signs. Dehydration can produce hypotension and tachycardia. Fluid overload can result in hypertension and a bounding pulse. Disturbances in serum potassium can result in an irregular pulse.

2. Know the client's developmental stage. The proportion of total body water to body mass changes from infancy to the older adult years.

3. Know the client's weight. Body size affects total body water. Fat contains no water; the obese client thus has proportionately less body water.

4. Know the client's medical history and present medications or therapies. Certain drugs such as diuretics or steroids affect fluid and electrolyte balance. Likewise, a client may be on a specific diet, such as a low-sodium diet for water retention. Determine whether the client has previous experience with IV therapy.

5. Beware of prolonged environmental conditions that can affect the client's fluid status. Prolonged exposure to hot, humid weather can lead to fluid and electrolyte imbalances, particularly in the infant, the older adult, and the chronically ill client.

6. Know if the client is right- or left-handed. When possible, place an IV in the nondominant arm.

7. Determine that the present IV system is intact and there are no signs of phlebitis or infiltration. A system in which none of the connections have separated ensures that the sterility of the system has been maintained and that no fluid or medication has been lost. If the nurse suspects that the infusion tubing has separated from the IV cannula, sterility is no longer assumed, and a new system, including sterile tubing, solution, and VAD must be reestablished. Luer-lok connections are recommended.

8. Note when the last IV tubing and dressing change occurred (Box 27-2).

9. Maintain sterility of a patent IV system using the Centers for Disease Control (CDC) recommendations (see Box 27-2).

10. Know the standard precautions for infection control and the Occupational Safety and Health Administration (OSHA) standards for occupational exposure to bloodborne pathogens (Box 27-3).

SKILL 27-1   Initiating Intravenous Therapy

The goal of intravenous (IV) fluid administration is correction or prevention of fluid and electrolyte disturbances in clients who are or may become acutely ill. For example, a client with third-degree burns over 40% of the body is critically ill and has severe fluid and electrolyte imbalances. Fluid therapy must be continuously regulated in a burn client because of continual changes in fluid and electrolyte balance. A client who is NPO (nothing by mouth) after surgery receives IV fluid replacement to prevent fluid and electrolyte imbalances; the infusion is usually discontinued when the client resumes oral intake. Another reason to perform a venipuncture is to provide IV access for intermittent or emergency medication administration. This administration route is often accomplished through the use of a heparin or normal saline lock, which is an IV catheter attached to an injection cap to maintain a closed system. Sometimes a short piece of extension tubing is used. The heparin or saline lock is flushed with a heparin or normal saline solution once a day or after each administration of medication to maintain patency of the IV catheter (see Chapter 21). Peripheral IV access should be used with caution for administration of medications that are irritants; a central venous access is preferred. Vesicants should be administered only through a central venous access site (see Chapter 31).

Concern for the personal safety of nurses who work with IV therapy products is very important because of the possibility of transmission of organisms such as hepatitis B virus (HBV) and human immunodeficiency virus (HIV). The most common cause of exposure of nurses to blood during IV therapy is by needle stick. To prevent this, there are products that decrease the chance of an accidental needle stick. Needleless device products allow for the connection and access of IV tubings without the use of needles. Vascular access devices are available with recessed needles or needle guards to prevent contact with exposed needles.

DELEGATION CONSIDERATIONS

The skill of initiating peripheral intravenous therapy may be within the scope of practice for licensed practical (vocational) nurses in some states. Delegation to assistive personnel is inappropriate.

Other aspects of care may be delegated to assistive personnel. The nurse should instruct assistive personnel to:
- Inform the nurse if client complains of burning, bleeding, swelling, or coolness at catheter insertion site.
- Inform nurse if IV dressing becomes wet.
- Inform nurse if the volume of fluid in the bag is low.

EQUIPMENT
- ❏ Correct IV solution (with time tape attached)
- ❏ Proper IV safety access device for venipuncture (will vary with client's body size and reason for IV fluid administration) (Figure 27-2)
- ❏ IV start kit (available in some agencies): may contain a sterile drape to place under the client's arm, cleansing and antiseptic preparations, dressings, and a small roll of sterile tape

   For IV Fluid Infusion
- ❏ Administration set (choice depends on type of solution and rate of administration; infants and children require microdrip tubing, which provides 60 gtt/ml)
- ❏ 0.22-mm filter (if required by agency policy or if particulate matter is likely)

- ❏ Extension tubing
- ❏ Antiseptic swabs (i.e., chlorhexidine, alcohol, or povidone-iodine)
- ❏ Disposable gloves
- ❏ Tourniquet (can be a source of contamination; use a single-use product)
- ❏ Arm board, if needed (used to maintain wrist or elbow joint position when catheter is placed close to or over a joint [Figure 27-3]; will help prevent infiltration of IV)
- ❏ Nonallergenic tape
- ❏ Towel (to place under client's hand or arm)
- ❏ IV pole, rolling or ceiling mounted
- ❏ Special gown with snaps at shoulder seams (makes removal with IV tubing easier), if available
- ❏ Needle disposal container (also called sharps container)

   For Heparin or Normal Saline Lock
- ❏ Injection cap (also called IV plug, PRN adapter, INT)
- ❏ IV loop or short piece of extension tubing, if necessary
- ❏ 1 to 3 ml of normal saline or heparin flush (10 units/ml as ordered)
- ❏ Syringes and 25-gauge needles

   Transparent Dressing Only
- ❏ Transparent dressing

   Gauze Dressing Only
- ❏ 2 × 2 or 4 × 4 sterile gauze sponge
- ❏ Sterile tape

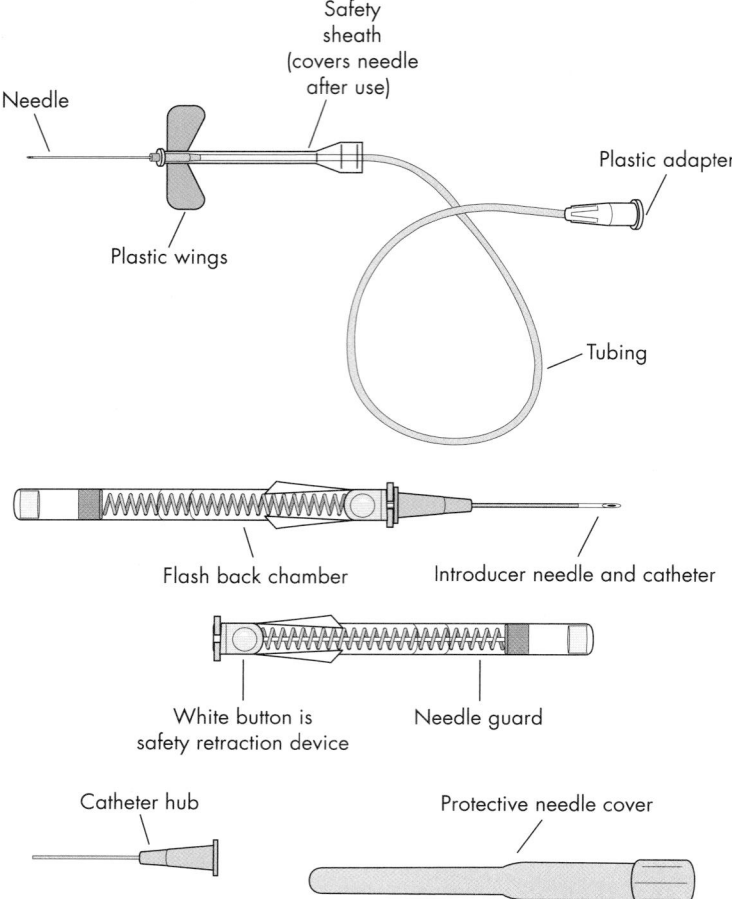

FIGURE 27-2 IV access device options.

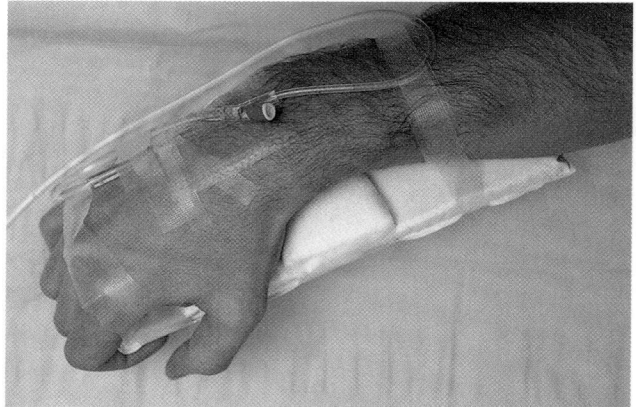

FIGURE 27-3 Arm positioned and taped on arm board.

STEP	RATIONALE

ASSESSMENT

1. Review physician's order for type and amount of IV fluid and rate of fluid administration. Nurse follows six rights of medication administration (see Chapter 19).

An order requesting the initiation of a peripheral IV access and administration of an IV solution must be made by a physician before the initiation of this therapy.

- *Critical Decision Point*

In most medical facilities, physicians do not write an order to "initiate peripheral access" or "perform venipuncture." "Start IV" may be written followed by the exact IV therapy order. The order to perform the venipuncture is implied. If the order is confusing or in question, clarify with the physician before proceeding.

2. Assess for clinical factors/conditions that will respond to or be affected by IV fluid administration:

Provides baseline to determine effect IV fluids have on client's fluid and electrolyte balance.

   a. Peripheral edema—can be rated for severity by assessing pitting over bony prominences. 1+ indicates barely detectable edema to 4+ for deep persistent pitting (see Chapter 18).

   Indicates expanded interstitial volume. This is usually most evident in dependent areas (i.e., feet and ankles). Fluid overload will worsen edema.

   b. Body weight.

   Daily weights document fluid retention or loss. Change in body weight of 1 kg corresponds to 1 L of fluid retention or loss (Heitz and Horne, 2001).

   c. Dry skin and mucous membranes.

   Suggests fluid volume deficit.

   d. Distended neck veins.

   Suggests fluid volume excess.

   e. Blood pressure changes.

   Elevated blood pressure may indicate volume excess due to increase in stroke volume. Decreased blood pressure may indicate fluid volume deficit due to a decrease in stroke volume.

   f. Irregular pulse rhythm; increased pulse rate.

   Rhythm changes may occur with potassium, calcium, and/or magnesium abnormalities; rate change may occur with fluid volume deficit.

   g. Auscultation of crackles or rhonchi in lungs.

   May signal fluid buildup in the lungs due to fluid volume excess.

   h. Inelastic skin turgor (after pinching, fails to return to normal position within 3 seconds).

   With fluid volume deficit, the pinched skin stays elevated for several seconds.

- *Critical Decision Point*

This is a less reliable indicator for older adults because their skin has lost elasticity naturally due to aging.

   i. Anorexia, nausea, and vomiting.

   May occur with acute fluid volume deficit or fluid volume excess.

   j. Thirst.

   Symptomatic of fluid volume deficit.

   k. Decreased urine output.

   During dehydration, kidney attempts to restore fluid balance by reducing urine production. Average daily adult urine output is 1500 ml; urine output of less than 400 ml/24 hr (oliguria) signals the retention of metabolic wastes (Heitz and Horne, 2001).

   l. Behavioral changes (e.g., restlessness, confusion).

   May occur with fluid volume deficit or acid-base imbalance.

   m. Decreased capillary refill.

   Indicates poor tissue perfusion.

3. Assess client's previous or perceived experience with IV therapy and arm placement preference.

   Determines level of emotional support and instruction needed.

STEP	RATIONALE
4. Obtain information from drug reference books or pharmacist about composition of IV fluids, purposes of administration, potential incompatibilities, and side effects to monitor for.	This allows detection of an inadvisable IV fluid order and helps to determine priority assessments.
5. Determine if client is to undergo any planned surgeries or is to receive blood infusion later.	Allows nurse to anticipate and place large-gauge catheter for fluid infusion and avoids placement of catheter in an area that will interfere with medical procedures.
6. Assess for the following risk factors: child or older adult; presence of heart failure or renal failure, skin lesions, infection, low platelet count; or receiving anticoagulants.	Persons at extremes in age develop fluid imbalances more rapidly because they have a proportionately larger extracellular fluid volume; persons with heart failure cannot adapt to sudden increases in vascular volume, and persons with renal failure cannot eliminate excess extracellular fluid. Skin lesions or infection may influence choice of access site. Low platelets or use of anticoagulants increase client's risk for bleeding from IV site and affects venous integrity, increasing the risk of seepage of blood from puncture site during venipuncture attempt.
7. Assess laboratory data and client's history of allergies.	May reveal information that affects insertion of devices, such as fluid volume deficit or allergy to iodine, adhesive, or latex.

NURSING DIAGNOSES

- Risk for imbalanced fluid volume
- Risk for deficient fluid volume
- Risk for infection

- Anxiety
- Deficient knowledge regarding IV therapy

Related factors are individualized based on client's condition or needs.

PLANNING

1. Expected outcomes following completion of procedure:	
• Fluid and electrolyte balance returns to normal; vital signs and other abnormal assessment parameters stabilize and return to normal.	Indicates correction of fluid and electrolyte imbalances and circulatory system's response to fluid and electrolyte replacement.
• IV line is patent.	Ensures instillation of IV fluids without obstruction.
• Infiltration is absent with no swelling and pallor at venipuncture site.	Infiltration results from cannula dislodgement allowing fluid to infuse into subcutaneous space.
• Inflammation is absent.	Inflammation results from irritation of vein by catheter, IV solution, additives, or bacteria.
• Client will understand purpose and risks of IV therapy.	Increases likelihood of client and family adherence to IV treatment modalities.
2. Prepare client and family by explaining the procedure, its purpose, and what is expected of client. Also explain sensations client is to expect.	Cognitive and sensory information decrease anxiety and help to promote cooperation.
3. Assist client to comfortable sitting or supine position. Nurse should be positioned at level position with client. Provide adequate lighting.	Promotes comfort and relaxation to client. Provides proper body mechanics for nurse. Aids in successful vein location.
4. Check client's identification.	Ensures right client receives right intravenous fluid.
5. Perform hand hygiene. Organize equipment on clean, clutter-free bedside stand or table.	Reduces transmission of infection and risk of accidents.

STEP	RATIONALE

IMPLEMENTATION

1. Change client's gown to the more easily removed gown with snaps at the shoulder, if available.

2. Open sterile packages using sterile aseptic technique (see Chapter 9).

3. Prepare IV infusion tubing and solution.

   a. Check IV solution, using six rights of medication administration (see Chapter 19). Make sure prescribed additives, such as potassium and vitamins, have been added. Check solution for color, clarity, and expiration date. Check bag for leaks, which is best if done before reaching the bedside.

   b. Open infusion set, maintaining sterility of both ends of tubing. Many sets allow for priming of tubing without removal of end cap.

   c. Place roller clamp (see illustration) about 2 to 5 cm (1 to 2 inches) below drip chamber, and move roller clamp to "off" position (see illustration).

   d. Remove protective sheath over IV tubing port on plastic IV solution bag (see illustration).

Use of a special IV gown facilitates safe removal of the gown once IV has been inserted.

Maintains sterility of equipment and reduces spread of microorganisms.

IV solutions are medications and should be carefully checked to reduce risk of error. Solutions that are discolored, contain particles, or are expired are not to be used. Leaky bags present an opportunity for infection and must not be used.

Prevents microorganisms from entering infusion equipment and bloodstream.

Close proximity of roller clamp to drip chamber allows more accurate regulation of flow rate. Moving clamp to "off" prevents accidental spillage of IV fluid on client, nurse, bed, or floor.

Provides access for insertion of infusion tubing into solution.

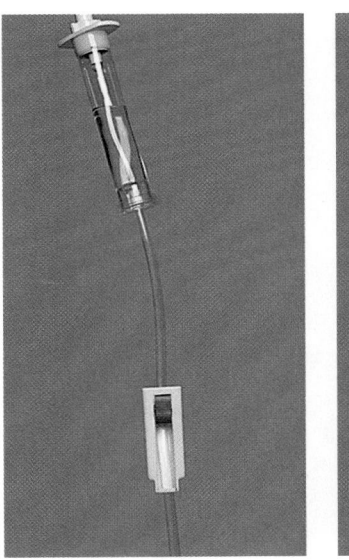
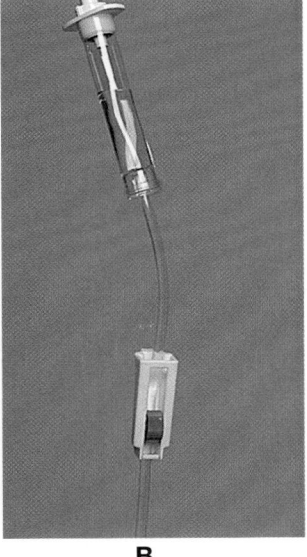

A   **B**

STEP 3c A, Roller clamp in open position. **B,** Roller clamp in closed position.

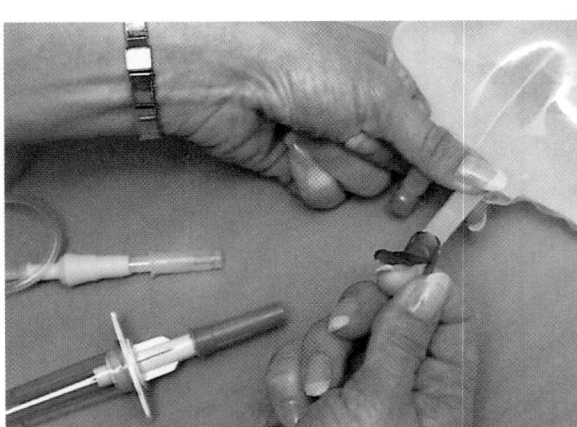

STEP 3d Removing protective sheath from IV bag port.

STEP	**RATIONALE**
e. Insert infusion set into fluid bag or bottle: Remove protector cap from tubing insertion spike, not touching spike, and insert spike into opening of IV bag (see illustration). Cleanse rubber stopper on bottled solution with antiseptic, and insert spike into black rubber stopper of IV bottle.	Flat surface on the top of bottled solution may contain contaminants, whereas opening to plastic bag is recessed. Prevents contamination of bottled solution during insertion of spike.

• *Critical Decision Point*
Do not touch spike because it is sterile. If contamination occurs (e.g., spike is accidentally dropped on the floor), then discard that IV tubing, and obtain a new one.

f. Prime infusion tubing by filling with IV solution: Compress drip chamber and release, allowing it to fill one-third to one-half full (see illustration).	Ensures tubing is cleared of air before connection with IV site. Creates suction effect; fluid enters drip chamber to prevent air from entering tubing.
g. Remove protector cap on end of tubing (some tubing can be primed without removal), and slowly open roller clamp to allow fluid to travel from drip chamber through tubing to needle adapter. Return roller clamp to "off" position after tubing is primed (filled with IV fluid).	Slow fill of tubing decreases turbulence and chance of bubble formation. Removes air from tubing and permits tubing to fill with solution. Closing the clamp prevents accidental loss of fluid.
h. Be certain tubing is clear of air and air bubbles. To remove small air bubbles, firmly tap IV tubing where air bubbles are located. Check entire length of tubing to ensure that all air bubbles are removed (see illustration). If multiple port tubing is used, turn ports upside down, and tap to fill and remove air.	Large air bubbles can act as emboli.

• *Critical Decision Point*
An extension tubing may be added to IV tubing to allow for more length, which will enable client to move more freely while still keeping IV line stable.

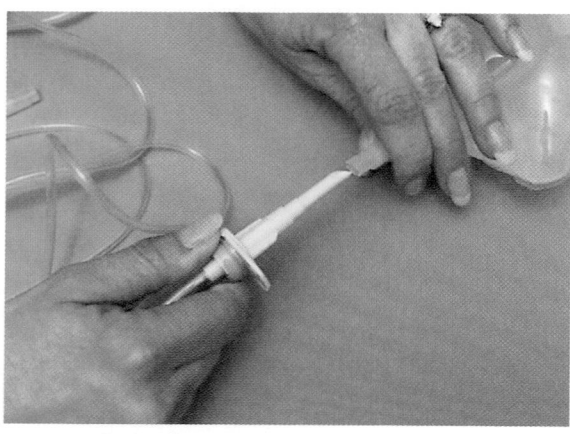

STEP **3e** Inserting spike into IV bag.

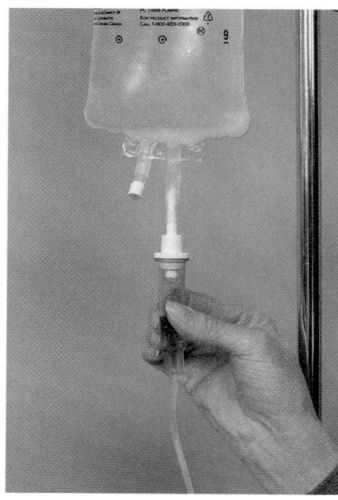

STEP **3f** Squeezing drip chamber to fill with fluid.

STEP	RATIONALE

  i. Replace cap protector on end of infusion tubing.

Maintains system sterility.

4. Prepare heparin or normal saline lock for infusion:

  a. If a loop or short extension tubing is needed because of an awkward IV site placement, use sterile technique to connect the IV plug to the loop or short extension tubing. Inject 1 to 3 ml normal saline through the plug and through the loop or short extension tubing before connecting to IV site.

Removes air to prevent introduction into the vein. Do the same with the saline plug.

5. Apply disposable gloves. Eye protection and mask may be worn (see agency policy) if splash or spray of blood is possible.

Reduces transmission of microorganisms. Decreases exposure to HIV, hepatitis, and other blood-borne organisms (CDC, 2002) and prevents spraying of blood on nurse's mucous membranes.

6. Identify accessible vein for placement of IV cannula. Apply flat tourniquet around arm, above antecubital fossa or 4 to 6 inches (10 to 15 cm) above proposed insertion site (see illustration). Do not apply tourniquet too tightly to avoid injury or bruising to skin. Check for presence of radial pulse. Tourniquet may be applied on top of a thin layer of clothing such as a gown sleeve to protect fragile skin or excess hair. It may become necessary to remove tourniquet and move lower down arm.

Tourniquet impedes venous return but should not occlude arterial flow. If vein cannot be found in antecubital fossa, move down along arm to locate vessel in lower arm or hand.

  Optional: Apply blood pressure cuff instead of tourniquet. Inflate to a level just below client's normal diastolic pressure. Maintain inflation at that pressure until venipuncture is completed.

Use of BP cuff creates less trauma to skin.

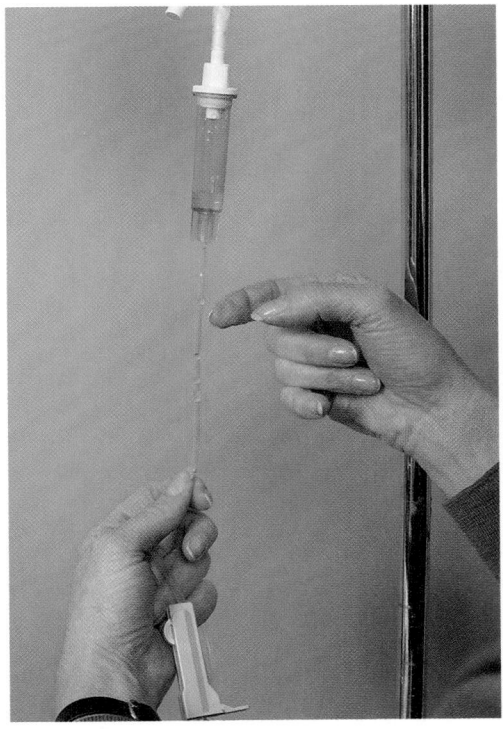

STEP **3h** Removing air bubbles from tubing.

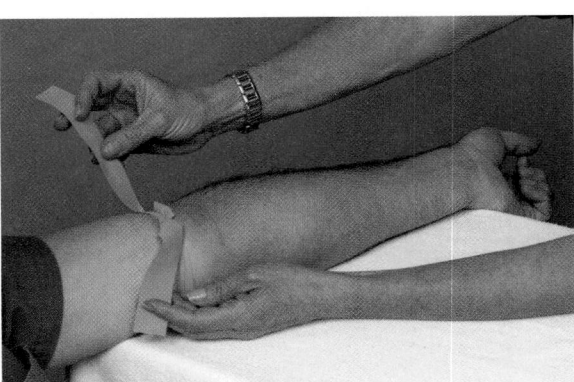

STEP **6** Tourniquet placed on arm for initial vein selection.

STEP	RATIONALE

STEP **7** Cephalic, basilic, and medial cubital veins are best for IV placement in adults.

7. Select the vein for IV insertion (see illustration). The cephalic, basilic, and median cubital are preferred in adults.

   Ensures adequate vein that is easier to puncture with needle and less likely to rupture.

   a. Use the most distal site in the nondominant arm, if possible. Clip arm hair with scissors if necessary.

   Venipuncture should be performed distal to proximal, which increases the availability of other sites for future IV therapy. Hair impedes venipuncture or adherence of dressing.

• *Critical Decision Point*
Do not shave area. Shaving may cause microabrasions and predispose to infection.

   b. Avoid areas that are painful to palpation.

   May indicate inflamed vein.

   c. Select a vein large enough for catheter placement.

   Prevents interruption of venous flow while allowing adequate blood flow around the catheter.

   d. Choose a site that will not interfere with client's activities of daily living (ADLs) or planned procedures.

   Keeps client as mobile as possible.

   e. With the index finger, palpate the vein by pressing downward and noting the resilient, soft, bouncy feeling as the pressure is released.

   Finger tip is more sensitive and is better to assess vein condition.

   f. If possible, place extremity in dependent position.

   Permits venous dilation and visibility.

   g. Select well-dilated vein (see illustration). Other methods to foster venous distention include:

   Increases the volume of blood in the vein at the venipuncture site.

     (1) Stroking the extremity from distal to proximal below the proposed venipuncture site.

   Promotes venous filling.

     (2) Applying warmth to the extremity for several minutes, for example, with a warm washcloth.

   Increases blood supply and fosters venous dilation.

• *Critical Decision Point*
Vigorous friction and multiple tapping of the veins, especially in older adults, may cause hematoma and/or venous constriction.

STEP	RATIONALE

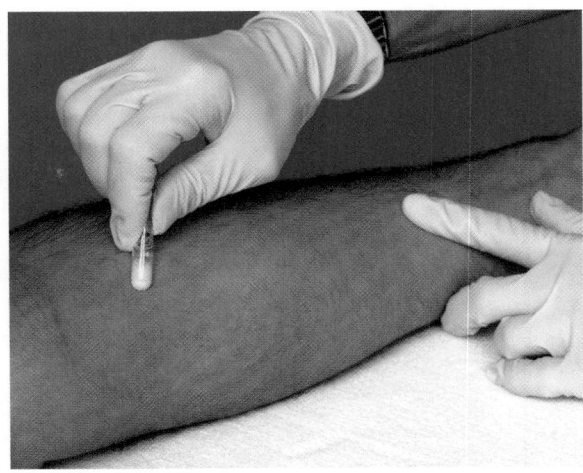

STEP **7g** Palpate vein.   STEP **10** Cleansing site with chlorhexidine.

   h. Avoid sites distal to previous venipuncture site, sclerosed or hardened cordlike veins, infiltrate site or phlebotic vessels, bruised areas, and areas of venous valves or bifurcation.

   i. Avoid fragile dorsal veins in older adult clients and vessels in an extremity with compromised circulation (e.g., in cases of mastectomy, dialysis graft, or paralysis).

8. Release tourniquet temporarily and carefully.

9. Place connection of infusion set or IV plug nearby, maintaining sterility of the system.

10. (If area of insertion appears to need cleansing, use soap and water first.) Use antiseptic swab agent to cleanse insertion site using friction in a horizontal plane, then a vertical plane followed with a circular motion (middle to outward); allow the agent to dry (2 to 3 minutes povidone-iodine, 60 seconds alcohol, 30 seconds chlorhexidine) (see illustration). Refrain from touching the cleansed site unless using sterile technique.

11. Reapply tourniquet 10 to 12 cm (4 to 5 inches) above anticipated insertion site. Check presence of distal pulse.

Such sites can cause infiltration of newly placed IV catheter and excessive vessel damage. Antecubital fossa area is used for blood draws; also limits mobility.

Venous alterations can increase risk of complications (e.g., infiltration, decreased catheter dwell time).

Restores blood flow while preparing for venipuncture.
Permits smooth, quick connection of cannula to IV system.

Mechanical friction in this pattern allows penetration of the antiseptic solution into the cracks and fissures of the epidermal layer of the skin (Crosby and Mares, 2001).

Antiseptic solutions should be allowed to air-dry completely to effectively reduce microbial counts (Intravenous Nurses Society [INS], 2000). If antiseptic agents are used in combination, allow each to air-dry separately. Chlorhexidine 2% preparation is preferred (CDC, 2002).

Touching cleansed area introduces microorganisms from nurse's finger to site. The site would need to be prepped again.

Diminished arterial flow prevents venous filling. The pressure of the tourniquet should cause the vein to dilate.

STEP	RATIONALE
12. Perform venipuncture. Anchor vein by placing thumb over vein and by gently tightening the skin distal to the site $1\frac{1}{2}$ to 2 inches (4 to 5 cm) (see illustration). Warn client of a sharp, quick stick.	Stabilizes vein for needle insertion.
a. *Over-the-needle catheter (ONC):* Insert with bevel up at 10- to 30-degree angle slightly distal to actual site of venipuncture in the direction of the vein.	Places needle at a 10- to 30-degree angle to the vein. When vein is punctured, risk of puncturing posterior vein wall is reduced. Superficial veins require a smaller angle. Deeper veins require a greater angle.
b. *IV catheter safety device:* Insert using same position as for ONC (see illustration).	IV safety device should be available and used.
c. *Winged needle:* Hold needle at 10- to 30-degree angle with bevel up, slightly distal to actual site of venipuncture.	

- ***Critical Decision Point***
  Each cannula should be used only once for each insertion attempt.

13. Observe for blood return through flashback chamber of catheter or tubing of winged cannula, indicating that bevel of needle has entered vein (see illustration). Lower needle until almost flush with skin. *(Advance catheter approximately $\frac{1}{4}$ inch into vein and then on ONC loosen stylet.)* Continue to hold skin taut, and advance catheter into vein until hub rests at venipuncture site. *Do not reinsert the stylet once it is loosened.* Advance the safety device by using push-off tab to thread the catheter (see illustration). Advance winged cannula until hub rests at venipuncture site.	Increased venous pressure from tourniquet increases backflow of blood into catheter or tubing. Allows for full penetration of the vein wall, placement of the catheter in the vein's inner lumen, and advancement of the catheter off the stylet. Reduces risk of introduction of infectious microorganisms along catheter. Reinsertion of stylet can cause catheter shearing in the vein and potential catheter embolization.

- ***Critical Decision Point***
  No more than two attempts at initiating the IV access should be made by a single nurse.

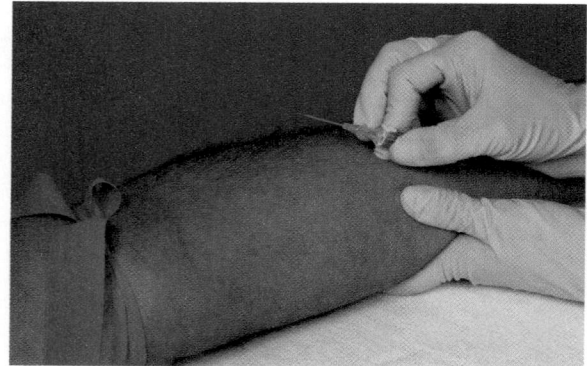

STEP **12** Stabilize vein below insertion site.

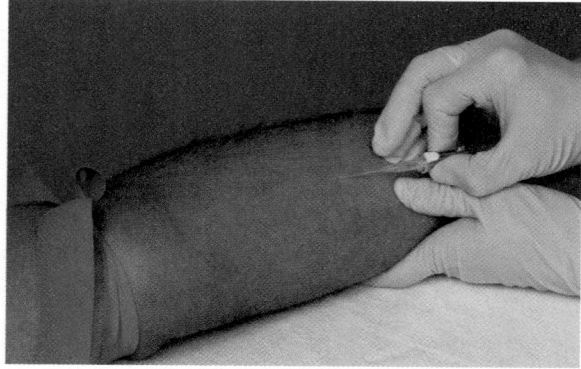

STEP **12b** Puncture skin with catheter at 10- to 30-degree angle.

STEP	**RATIONALE**
14. Stabilize cannula with one hand, and release tourniquet with other. Apply gentle pressure with middle finger of nondominant hand 1¼ inches (3 cm) above the insertion (see illustration). Keep cannula stable with index finger. For a safety device, slide the catheter off the stylet while gliding the protective guard over the stylet, or retract stylet by pushing safety tab (see illustration). A click indicates the device is locked over the stylet. (NOTE: Techniques will vary with each IV device.) Remove the stylet of ONC. Place directly into sharps container.	Permits venous flow, reduces backflow of blood, and allows connection with administration set with minimal blood loss. Prevents transmission of infection.

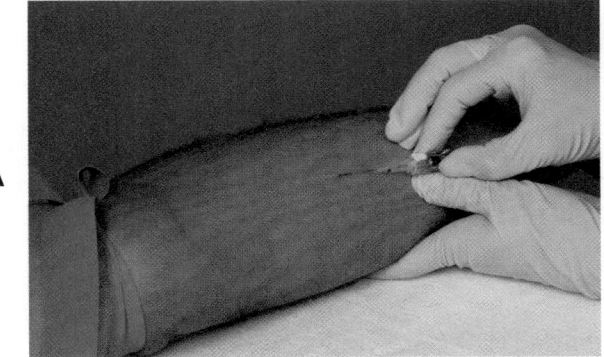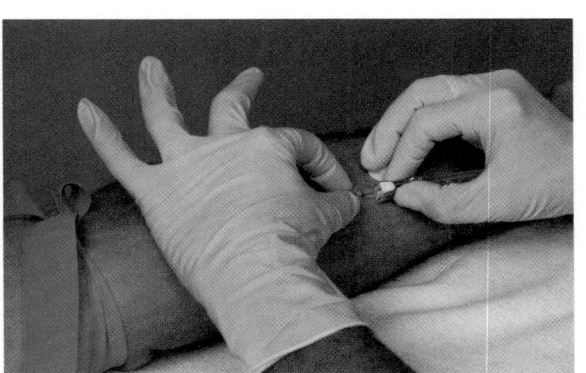

STEP **13 A,** Blood return in flashback chamber. **B,** Advance catheter into vein.

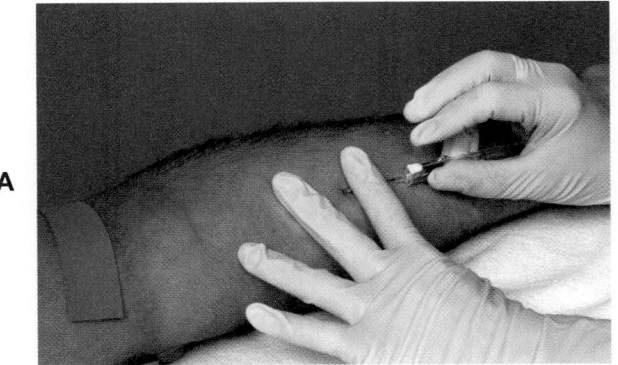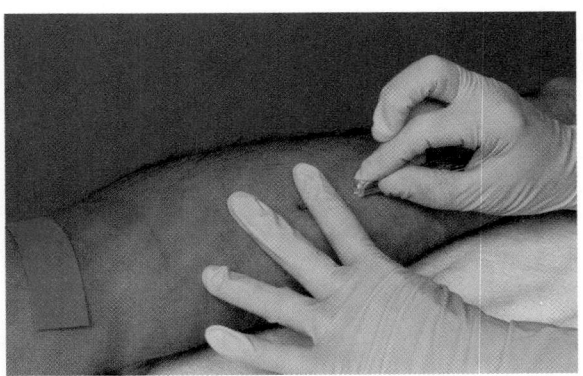

STEP **14 A,** Apply pressure above insertion site. **B,** Retract stylet by pushing safety tab.

STEP	RATIONALE

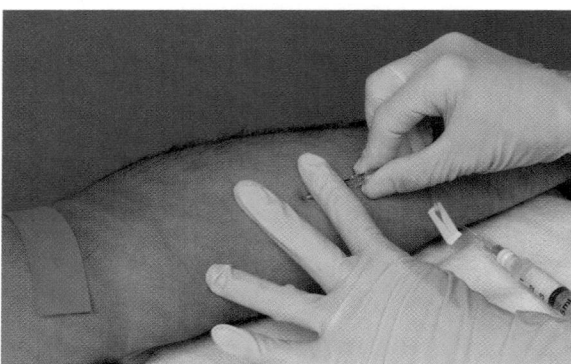

STEP **15** Connecting end of saline lock.

15. Quickly connect end of the prepared saline lock (see illustration) or the infusion tubing set to end of cannula. Do not touch point of entry of connection. Secure connection.

Prompt connection of infusion set maintains patency of vein and prevents risk of exposure to blood. Maintains sterility.

16. *Intermittent infusion:* Hold the heparin/saline lock firmly with nondominant hand, and clean with alcohol. Insert prefilled syringe containing flush solution into injection cap (see illustration). Flush injection cap slowly with flush solution. Use positive flow adapter or withdraw the syringe while still flushing.

"Positive pressure flushing" allows fluid to displace the removed needle, creates positive pressure in the catheter, and prevents reflux of blood during flushing (Phillips, 2001). Stabilizing the cannula prevents accidental withdrawal or dislodgement.

17. *Continuous infusion:* Begin infusion by slowly opening the clamp of the IV tubing.

Initiates flow of fluid through IV catheter, preventing clotting of device.

• **Critical Decision Point**
Be sure to calculate rate so as not to infuse IV solution too rapidly or too slowly.

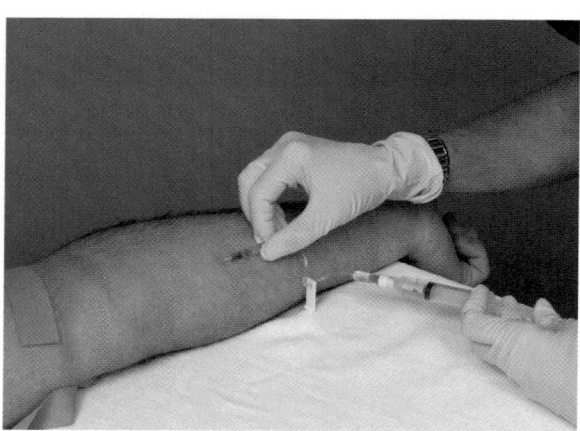

STEP **16** Flush injection cap.

STEP	**RATIONALE**

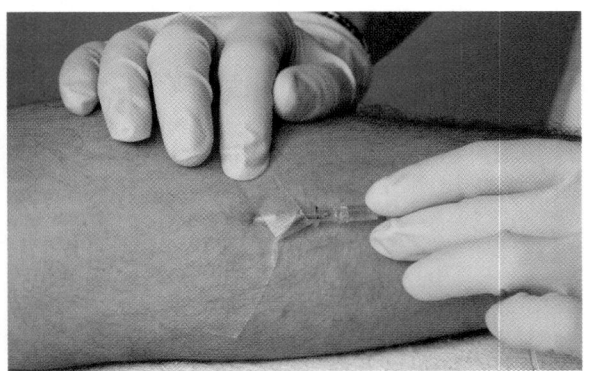

STEP **18b** **A,** Place tape under catheter hub. **B,** Chevron applied before gauze dressing.

18. Secure cannula (procedures can differ; follow agency policy):

    a. Transparent dressing: Secure cannula with nondominant hand while preparing to apply dressing.

Prevents accidental dislodgement of catheter.

    b. Sterile gauze dressing: Place narrow piece (½ inch) of tape under cannula hub with sticky side up, and cross tape over catheter hub to make a chevron (see illustrations). Place tape only on the cannula, *never* over the insertion site. Secure site to allow easy visual inspection. Avoid applying tape around the arm.

Prevents accidental removal of catheter from vein. Prevents back-and-forth motion, which can irritate the vein and introduce microorganisms on the skin into the vein.

19. Apply sterile dressing over site.

    a. Transparent dressing:

        (1) Carefully remove adherent backing. Apply one edge of dressing, and then gently smooth remaining dressing over IV site, leaving connection between IV tubing and catheter hub uncovered (see illustration). Remove outer covering, and smooth dressing gently over site.

Occlusive dressing protects site from bacterial contamination. Connection between administration set and hub needs to be uncovered to facilitate changing the tubing if necessary. CDC (2002) no longer recommends application of antimicrobial ointment to catheter site.

        (2) Take a 1-inch piece of tape, and place it from end of hub of catheter to insertion site, over transparent dressing (see illustration).

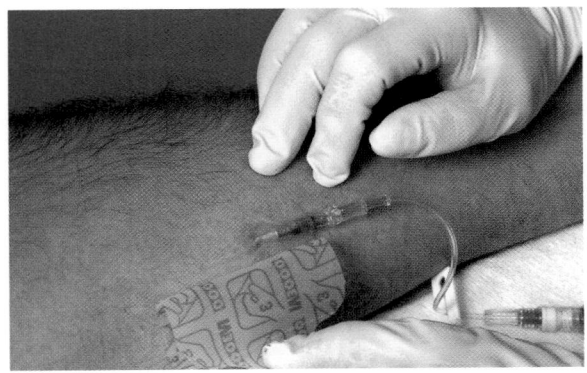

STEP **19a(1)** Applying transparent dressing.

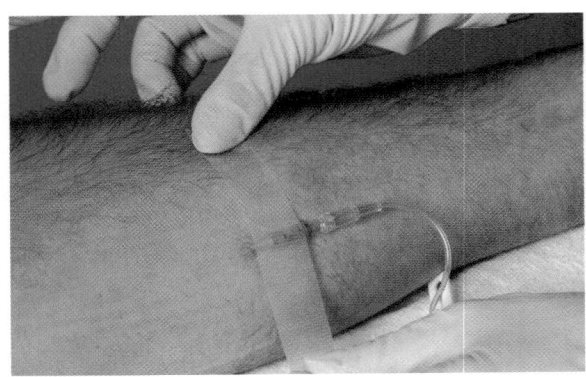

STEP **19a(2)** Place tape over transparent dressing.

STEP	RATIONALE

    (3) Apply chevron, and place only over tape, not the transparent dressing (see illustration).

  b. Sterile gauze dressing:

    (1) Fold a 2 × 2 gauze in half, and cover with a 1 inch–wide tape extending about an inch from each side. Place under the tubing/catheter hub junction (see illustration). Curl a loop of tubing alongside the arm, and place a second piece of tape directly over the tubing and padded 2 × 2, securing tubing in two places

    (2) Place 2 × 2 gauze pad over insertion site and catheter hub. Secure all edges with tape. Do not cover connection between IV tubing and catheter hub (see illustration).

Tape on top of gauze makes it easier to access hub/tubing junction. Gauze pad elevates hub off skin to prevent pressure area. Securing loop of tubing reduces risk of dislodging catheter should the IV tubing get pulled (i.e., the loop would come apart before the catheter dislodges).

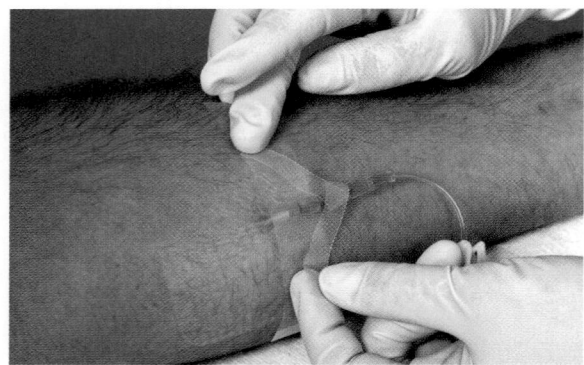

STEP 19a(3) Chevron tape pattern.

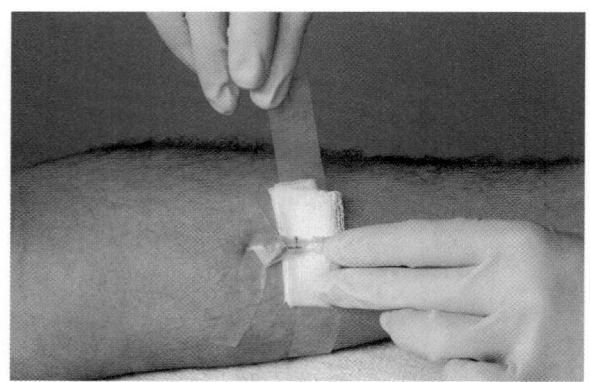

STEP 19b(1) Place folded 2 × 2 gauze under cannula hub.

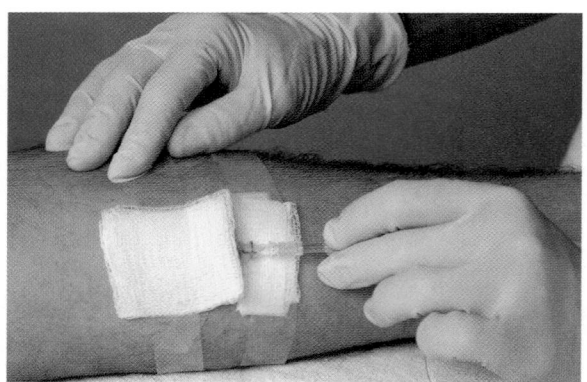

STEP 19b(2) Apply 2 × 2 gauze dressing.

STEP	RATIONALE

20. Loop tubing alongside the arm, and place a second piece of tape directly over the tape covering the transparent dressing (see illustration) or over the padded 2 × 2.

21. For IV fluid administration, recheck flow rate to correct drops per minute (Skill 27-3) and connect to EID as per agency policy.

Manipulation of catheter during dressing application may alter flow rate. Maintains correct rate of flow for IV solution. Flow can fluctuate, so it must be checked at intervals for accuracy.

22. Write date and time of IV placement, cannula gauge size and length, and nurse's initials on dressing (see illustration).

Provides immediate access to data as to when IV was inserted and rotation is needed.

23. Dispose of used stylet or other sharps in appropriate sharps container. Discard supplies. Remove gloves, and perform hand hygiene.

Reduces transmission of microorganisms and protects staff from infection and injury.

24. Instruct client in how to move or turn without pulling on IV catheter.

Prevents accidental dislodgement of catheter.

25. Peripheral IV access should be changed every 72 to 96 hours (CDC, 2002) or per physician orders or more frequently if complications occur.

Incidence of complications may be higher when peripheral IV is allowed to remain in a vein over 72 hours (Catney and others, 2001).

26. When solution has less than 100 ml remaining, next solution should be available at client's bedside.

Subsequent container provides continuation of IVs without interruption and risk of occlusion from empty container.

EVALUATION

1. Observe client every 1 to 2 hours:
   a. Check if correct amount of IV solution has infused by comparing time tape on IV container or electronic infusion device (EID) record.

   Correct administration of fluid volume prevents fluid imbalance.

   b. Count drip rate (if gravity drip), or check rate on infusion pump.

   Accurate monitoring of drip rate further ensures correct volume administration.

   c. Check patency of IV cannula.

   Flow rate will be slowed or stopped.

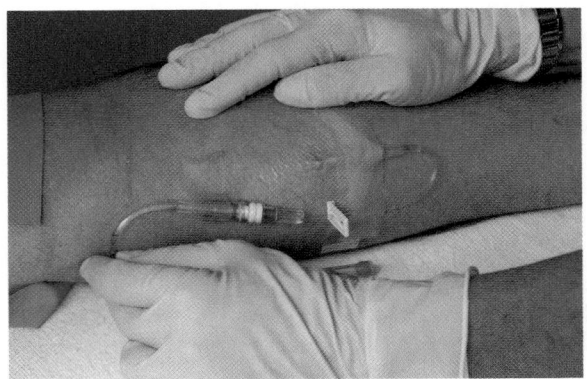

STEP **20** Loop and secure tubing.

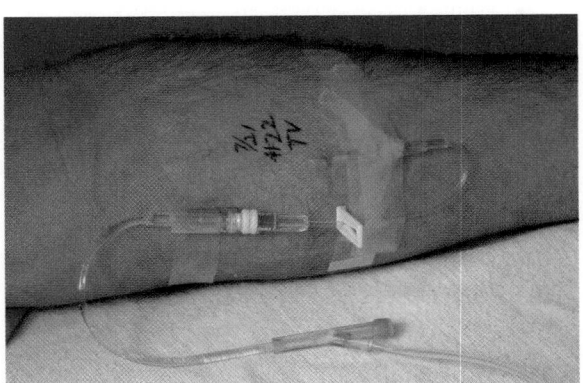

STEP **22** Label IV dressing.

STEP	RATIONALE

- **Critical Decision Point**
  If IV is positional, fluid will run less slowly or stop depending on position of client's arm. Instruct client to position arm to maintain flow; if this continues, IV may have to be restarted.

d. Observe client during palpation of vessel for signs of discomfort.	Tenderness can be early sign of phlebitis.
e. Inspect insertion site, note color (e.g., redness, pallor). Inspect for presence of swelling, infiltration (Table 27-2), and phlebitis (Table 27-3). Palpate temperature of skin above dressing.	Redness or inflammation along with tenderness and warmth indicate vein inflammation or phlebitis. Swelling above insertion site and cool temperature may indicate infiltration of fluid into tissues.
2. Observe client to determine response to therapy (e.g., intake and output [I&O], weights, vital signs, postprocedure assessments).	IV fluids and additives are given to maintain or restore fluid and electrolyte balance. Early recognition of complications leads to prompt treatment.

Recording and Reporting

- Record in nurses' notes number of attempts at insertion, type of infusion, insertion site by vessel, flow rate, size and type of cannula, and when infusion was begun. A special parenteral therapy flow sheet may be used (Figure 27-4).
- If an electronic infusion device is used, document type and rate of infusion.
- Record client's response to IV fluid, amount infused, and integrity and patency of system according to agency policy (usually hourly for vulnerable populations).
- Report to oncoming nursing staff: type of infusion, flow rate, status of venipuncture site, amount of fluid remaining in present solution, expected time to hang subsequent infusion, and any side effects.
- Report to physician adverse reactions such as pulmonary congestion, shock, thrombophlebitis.

Unexpected Outcomes	Related Interventions
1. Fluid volume deficit (FVD) as manifested by decreased urine output, dry mucous membranes, decreased capillary refill, a disparity in central and peripheral pulses, tachycardia, hypotension, shock.	• Notify physician. • May require readjustment of infusion rate.
2. Fluid volume excess (FVE) as manifested by crackles in the lungs, shortness of breath, edema.	• Reduce IV flow rate if symptoms appear. • Notify physician.
3. Electrolyte imbalances as manifested by abnormal serum electrolyte levels, changes in mental status, alterations in neuromuscular function, cardiac arrhythmias, changes in vital signs, and other manifestations.	• Notify physician. • Additives in IV or type of IV fluid may be adjusted.
4. Infiltration at site as indicated by swelling and possible pitting edema, pallor, coolness, pain at insertion site, possible decrease in flow rate (Table 27-2).	• Stop infusion, and discontinue IV (see Skill 27-7). • Elevate affected extremity. • Restart new IV if continued therapy is necessary. • Document degree of infiltration and nursing intervention (see Table 27-2).
5. Phlebitis is indicated by pain, increased skin temperature, erythema along path of vein (Table 27-3).	• Stop infusion, and discontinue IV (see Skill 27-7). • Restart new IV if continued therapy is necessary. • Place moist warm compress over area of phlebitis. • Document degree of phlebitis and nursing interventions per agency policy and procedure (see Table 27-3).

Continued

TABLE 27-2   INFILTRATION SCALE

GRADE	CLINICAL CRITERIA
0	No symptoms
1	Skin blanched
	Edema <1 inch in any direction
	Cool to touch
	With or without pain
2	Skin blanched
	Edema 1–6 inches in any direction
	Cool to touch
	With or without pain
3	Skin blanched, translucent
	Gross edema >6 inches in any direction
	Cool to touch
	Mild-moderate pain
	Possible numbness
4	Skin blanched, translucent
	Skin tight, leaking
	Skin discolored, bruised, swollen
	Gross edema >6 inches in any direction
	Deep pitting tissue edema
	Circulatory impairment
	Moderate to severe pain
	Infiltration of any amount of blood product, irritant, or vesicant

From Intravenous Nurses Society: Infusion nursing standards of practice, *J Intraven Nurs* 23(6S):S57, 2000.

TABLE 27-3   PHLEBITIS SCALE

GRADE	CLINICAL CRITERIA
0	No symptoms
1	Erythema at access site with or without pain
2	Pain at access site with erythema and/or edema
3	Pain at access site with erythema and/or edema
	Streak formation
	Palpable venous cord
4	Pain at access site with erythema and/or edema
	Streak formation
	Palpable venous cord >1 inch in length
	Purulent drainage

From Intravenous Nurses Society: Infusion nursing standards of practice, *J Intraven Nurs* 23(6S):S56, 2000.

Unexpected Outcomes	Related Interventions
6. Bleeding occurs at venipuncture site. Bleeding from vein is usually slow, continuous seepage. Common in clients who have received heparin, have a bleeding disorder, or if the IV site is over a bend in arm/hand.	• If bleeding occurs around venipuncture site and catheter is within vein, gauze dressing may be applied over site. Be aware that if gauze dressing is used, it must be removed to accurately assess insertion site. • Blood on the dressing can result when the administration set becomes disconnected from the catheter's hub. When blood appears on the dressing, verify that the system is intact, and change the dressing.

Teaching Considerations

* Instruct client about signs and symptoms of infiltration, phlebitis, and inflammation. Client can report early onset to nurse.
* Instruct client to inform nurse if flow slows or stops or blood is seen in the tubing or on the dressing.
* Instruct client how to ambulate with IV pole or stand.
* Instruct client to protect IV when performing hygiene activities.

Pediatric Considerations

* Pediatric veins are very fragile. Avoid sites that are easily moved or bumped. Use commercial protective device to cover area.
* In addition to the usual venipuncture sites, the veins in the scalp or the foot are used in infants.

* A rubber band may be used to dilate scalp and small extremities. Aim the cannula toward the heart when using scalp veins (Hankins and others, 2001).
* If clients are older children, allowing them to select IV site may increase cooperation because they have some control over their treatment.
* Most IV infusions in pediatric clients require a 24-gauge catheter, but range is 22 to 26 gauge.
* There is no recommendation for the use of chlorhexidine as a prepping agent in infants less than 2 months of age (CDC, 2002).
* When child is critically ill or long-term IV access is anticipated, a peripherally inserted central catheter (PICC), Broviac catheter, or implanted port may be used to access larger vein.

Continued

ST. JOHN'S HOSPITAL
Springfield, Illinois
I.V. MAINTENANCE RECORD

I.V. FLUID & I.V. MEDICATION

Site Code:
- R.J. or L.J. – Right or Left Jugular
- R.S.V. or L.S.V. – Right or Left Subclavian Vein
- R.L.L. or L.L.L. – Right or Left Lower Leg
- R.H. or L.H. – Right or Left Hand
- R.F.A. or L.F.A. – Right or Left Forearm
- R.U.A. or L.U.A. – Right or Left Upperarm
- R.F. or L.F. – Right or Left Foot
- R.S., L.S. or M.S. – Right, Left or Mid Scalp
- R.F.V. or L.F.V. – Right or Left Femoral Vein
- R.A.C. or L.A.C. – Right or Left Antecubital
- R.W. or L.W. – Right or Left Wrist

- K.V.O. – Keep Vein Open
- H.L. – Heparin Lock
- P.B. – Piggyback
- P. – Push

Triple Lumen Catheter:
- Proximal - 18 gauge (White) Draw blood, Blood Adm, Medications
- Middle - 18 gauge (Blue) TPN Medications
- Distal - 16 gauge (Brown) Blood Adm. Colloids, Viscous Fluids, CVP Monitoring Medications

Allergy:

No. of last I.V. _____ Letter of last expander _____

No. of last Blood/Component _____

Signature:

DATE			
Night Nurse			
Day Nurse			
Evening Nurse			

Order Date	Amount, Solution, Infusing Time or Rate, Medication, Dose, Time	Site(s)	Pump	Time	Time
	One Time I.V Meds.				
No.	I.V. Fluids				

I.V. SITE ASSESSMENT

SITE CODE
- R.J. or L.J. – Right or Left Jugular
- R.S.V. or L.S.V. – Right or Left Subclavian Vein
- R.L.L. or L.L.L. – Right or Left Lower Leg
- R.H. or L.H. – Right or Left Hand
- R.F.A. or L.F.A. – Right or Left Forearm
- R.U.A. or L.U.A. – Right or Left Upperarm
- R.F. or L.F. – Right or Left Foot
- R.S., L.S. or M.S. – Right, Left or Mid Scalp
- R.F.V. or L.F.V. – Right or Left Femoral Vein
- R.A.C. or L.A.C. – Right or Left Antecubital
- R.W. or L.W. – Right or Left Wrist

- K.V.O. – Keep Vein Open
- H.L. – Heparin Lock
- P.B. – Piggyback
- P. – Push
- Cath – Catheter
- NA – Not Applicable

TYPE CODE
- M.C. – Medicut
- A.C. – Angiocath
- S.V. – Scalpvein
- A.S. – Angio-set
- C.D. – Cutdown
- I.C. – Intracath
- I.P. – Infuse A Port
- H.C. – Hickman Catheter
- B.C. – Broviac Catheter
- M.L.C. – Multi-lumen Catheter
- M.L.P. – Multi-lumen Proximal
- M.L.M. – Multi-lumen Middle
- M.L.D. – Multi-lumen Distal
- I. – Introducer

Document on each site once each shift & P.R.N. No space is to be left blank. Place "NA" in spaces which do not apply.

Date	Time	I.V. Site Start	d/c	Site Code	Cath Size	Type Code	Site Day	Cap Change	Dressing Change	I.V. Site: s̄ tenderness redness, edema, drainage	Signature

FIGURE 27-4 IV maintenance record. (Courtesy St. John's Hospital, Springfield, Ill.)

- Choosing age-appropriate activities compatible with the maintenance of the IV infusion is important to maintain normal growth and development.
- Have extra help when starting an IV on a child for safety in positioning. Assistive personnel can help with positioning. Parents may also be allowed to stay with their child to help him or her cope with the procedure.
- Local anesthesia cream LMX4 may be used before preparation of skin and venipuncture to lessen needle-related pain.

Gerontological Considerations

- Gerontological veins are very fragile; there is less subcutaneous support tissue, and there is thinning of the skin (Schelper, 2003). Take more time to select a site. Avoid sites that are easily moved or bumped. Sometimes dorsal metacarpal veins may not be the best choice. Use commercial protective device to protect site (Figure 27-5).
- In older clients, use the smallest gauge possible. For example, a 22-gauge needle is adequate for fluid and medication therapy; a 24-gauge is increasingly more popular in older adults This is less traumatizing to the vein and allows better blood flow to provide increased hemodilution of the IV fluids or medications.
- If possible, avoid the back of the older adult's hand or the dominant arm for venipuncture because these sites greatly interfere with the older adult's independence.

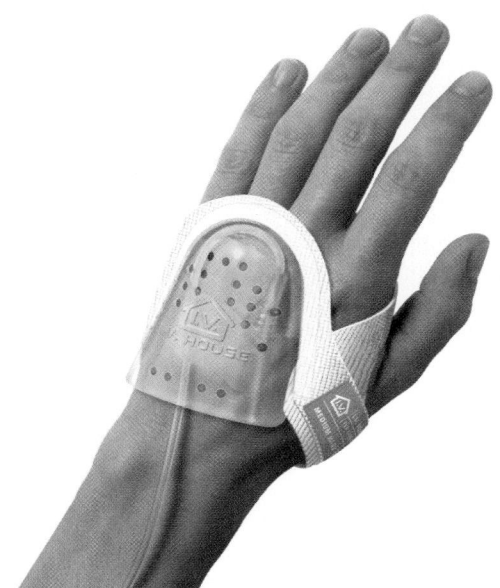

FIGURE 27-5 I.V. House Protective Device. (Courtesy I.V. House.)

- If the older adult has fragile skin and veins, use minimal tourniquet pressure or no tourniquet at all. When a tourniquet is applied, venous pressure goes up sharply, the vein is overstretched, and puncture with even a thin needle can rupture wall of vein (Chukhraev and Grekov, 2000).
- As older adults lose subcutaneous tissue, the veins lose stability and roll away from the needle. To stabilize the vein, apply traction to the skin below the projected insertion point.
- Use a lower angle of approach (e.g., 5 to 15 degrees on insertion) to accommodate more superficial veins (Coulter, 2004).
- Use mesh dressing or securement device on fragile skin (Coulter, 2004).
- Older adults may not complain of pain at the insertion site. A large amount of fluid may infiltrate before a client experiences discomfort. Be vigilant in checking an older adult's IV site.

Home Care Considerations

- Ensure that the client is able and willing to self-administer IV therapy or that there is a reliable caregiver to provide IV therapy care at home.
- Determine the client's ability to obtain help, for example, availability of caregiver, presence of and ability to use telephone.
- Ensure that all sharps and equipment contaminated by blood are disposed of in puncture-resistant containers with lids. Some suppliers will provide sharps containers for needle disposal (see Chapter 41).
- Instruct client and primary caregiver about procedures of IV therapy, including hand hygiene and aseptic technique while manipulating syringes and other supplies.
- Teach client and primary caregiver to protect IV site during hygiene activities by covering IV dressing completely with plastic to avoid getting it wet. If EID used, unplug around water.
- Instruct client to wear clothes that avoid pressure on IV site.
- Teach client about activity restrictions, for example, avoiding strenuous exercise of the arm with the IV.

Long-Term Care Considerations

- If a client is highly active or disturbs IV, an arm board and/or securement device is recommended to prevent dislodgement of the cannula. Ensure that arm board does not restrict client's movement or impair circulation.

SKILL 27-2 Care and Maintenance of a Peripherally Inserted Central Catheter

PICCs provide alternate IV access when the client requires intermediate-length venous access (greater than 7 days to 3 months). PICCs are inserted through the larger cephalic and basilic veins in the upper arm and advanced until the tip enters the central venous system (e.g., subclavian vein). In many states the PICC can be inserted by a registered professional nurse who has received special training and has demonstrated competency in PICC line insertion (refer to state Nurse Practice Act).

The nurse caring for clients with PICCs must understand what they are and be aware of their appropriate care and maintenance. In comparison with centrally placed venous catheters, the PICC has less risk of pneumothorax, hemothorax, or air embolism and is more cost-effective to maintain. Compared with peripheral IV catheters, PICCs have less risk of infiltration and phlebitis. This allows them to be maintained in place longer (more than 72 to 96 hours) because IV fluids and medications are diluted in the greater volume of blood flow present in the larger veins (superior vena cava) where the catheter tip placement should reside. In fact, PICC lines may remain in place as long as there are no signs of problems. Complications associated with PICC use include clotting, leaking, migration, infection, and breaking of the catheter. For successful catheter placement, the client must have a usable cephalic or basilic vein located in the antecubital fossa or upper arm.

PICCs vary in size from 16 to 24 gauge and in length from 40 to 65 cm (16 to 26 inches). The length is chosen based on the distance from the client's proposed insertion site to the desired point of tip placement. Catheters can have a single or double lumen. The catheter is made of soft materials, which cause minimal irritation to the vein. PICCs can be used to infuse IV fluids, parenteral nutrition, blood and blood products, and medications such as antibiotics. The nurse should be aware of product advantages and limitations of each device used.

DELEGATION CONSIDERATIONS

The skill of maintaining a peripherally inserted central catheter should not be delegated to assistive personnel. The nurse provides information and direction, including:

- Instructing assistive personnel involved in caring for clients with PICC lines to report any client complaint regarding the PICC immediately.
- Instructing assistive personnel in how to position and assist clients in moving when PICC lines are in place.

EQUIPMENT

Blood Drawing
- ❑ Antimicrobial swabs (i.e., chlorhexidine, povidone-iodine, alcohol)
- ❑ Four to five syringes (preferably needleless access)
- ❑ Sterile drape
- ❑ Saline flush

- ❑ Heparin flush (100 units/ml)
- ❑ Sterile needleless access
- ❑ Blood tubes, labels, requisitions
- ❑ Gloves, masks

Dressing Change
- ❑ Antimicrobial swabs
- ❑ Gloves, mask, gown
- ❑ Sterile tape
- ❑ Transparent occlusive dressing
- ❑ Gauze dressing: 2 × 2 sterile gauze
- ❑ Steri-Strips or securement device
- ❑ Adhesive remover (if needed)

Heparinization
- ❑ Antimicrobial swabs
- ❑ Access syringe (5 ml or 10 ml—see agency policy)
- ❑ Saline flush
- ❑ Heparin flush (100 units/ml)
- ❑ Sterile needleless access

STEP	RATIONALE

▌ASSESSMENT

1. Assess stage of client's disease and plan of therapy by reviewing medical record.

2. Review physician's order, and assess treatment schedule: times for administration of fluids, drugs, blood products, nutrition, and blood sampling.

Allows nurse to identify client's need for vascular access, evaluate response to therapy, and determine education needs about disease process and plan of therapy using PICC.

Allows nurse to schedule use of PICC for simultaneous administration of products, to educate client about schedule of administration, and to provide for comfort and reduction of anxiety about therapy.

STEP	RATIONALE
3. Assess type of PICC in place. Review manufacturer's directions concerning the catheter and maintenance. Each manufacturer publishes guidelines for its specific catheter.	Care and management depends on type and size of catheter, number of lumens, purpose of therapy.
4. Assess need to use PICC for blood sampling.	Scheduling blood sampling allows nurse to minimize entering PICC system and allows for timely collection of specimens. Risk of infection increases with multiple entries into vascular system, especially in immunocompromised clients.

• *Critical Decision Point*

In most situations, several tests can be run from one blood tube sample. For example, potassium, calcium, and magnesium test results can all be obtained from one full tube of blood versus three separate tubes. Always anticipate the need for a blood test (e.g., blood cultures if a client has developed an elevated temperature). If your next task is to draw blood for electrolyte results, you could eliminate reaccessing the PICC at a later time by asking the physician if blood cultures are to be drawn. Consultation with the laboratory services can provide and confirm specific instructions.

STEP	RATIONALE
5. Assess PICC placement site for skin integrity and signs of infection (i.e., redness, swelling, tenderness, exudate, bleeding).	Clients requiring long-term IV therapy often have conditions placing them at risk for alterations in skin integrity and immune function. PICC site is an insult to skin integrity and provides access for pathogens through the skin as well as pathogens to migrate from the catheter.
6. Assess for proper function of PICC before therapy: integrity of catheter, ability to irrigate or infuse fluid, ability to aspirate blood.	Ensures proper function of PICC with minimal complications.
7. Assess need for irrigation and dressing change by referring to medical record, nurses' notes, agency policies, and manufacturer's recommended guidelines for use.	Provides guidelines for maintaining catheter patency and preventing infection.
8. Assess client's acceptance of PICC and teaching needs related to knowledge of purpose, care, and maintenance. Ask client to discuss steps in care and to perform procedure (e.g., catheter site cleansing or dressing change).	Determines client's level of understanding. Allows nurse to educate client for home care of PICC.

NURSING DIAGNOSES

- Risk for infection
- Impaired skin integrity
- Risk for injury
- Deficient knowledge regarding use of PICC

Related factors are individualized based on client's condition or needs.

PLANNING

1. Expected outcomes following completion of procedure.
   - Site is intact and has no redness or swelling. — Local signs of infection are absent.
   - Systemic signs of infection (fever, malaise, increased white blood cell count [WBC]) are absent. — Catheter system remains free of microbial growth.
   - Fluids, medications, blood products infuse without difficulty. — Patency of catheter is maintained.
   - Blood can be aspirated from catheter. — Indicates patency and placement.
   - Catheter and connecting tube are intact. — Integrity of system is maintained.

STEP	RATIONALE
• Catheter tip is correctly placed, as confirmed by x-ray examination.	Correct placement minimizes chances of malplacement or occlusion.
• Client and family are able to explain the purpose of PICC therapy and perform dressing changes and skin care.	Demonstrates client and family understanding and competency.
2. Position client in semi-Fowler's position. Position level of bed for easy access to client.	Provides access to client.
3. Explain procedure and purpose to client and family. Instruct client to be still during procedure.	Decreases anxiety and promotes cooperation during procedure.

IMPLEMENTATION

STEP	RATIONALE
1. **Administration of Infusion or Sampling of Blood From PICC**	
a. Perform hand hygiene.	Reduces transmission of microorganisms.
b. Apply gloves. Apply gown and goggles (check agency policy) if drawing blood sample.	Prevents transfer of body fluids.
c. Use antimicrobial preparation swabs to cleanse injection cap or catheter hub according to agency policy.	Prevents introduction of microorganisms into catheter.
d. Prepare two syringes with 10 ml normal saline each.	Used to flush catheter.
e. If injection cap will be removed, **clamp catheter.**	Catheter must be clamped if injection cap is removed to prevent entrance of air.
f. If injection cap is in place, insert needleless access syringe containing 10 ml normal saline, and flush. If injection cap is removed, connect syringe tip to catheter hub, release clamp, flush with positive pressure, and reclamp.	Flushing ensures patency of catheter. Catheter must always be clamped during change of syringe or tubing to prevent exposure to air.

• **Critical Decision Point**
If catheter is occluded and resistance is felt, do not force flushing. Vigorous flushing may cause catheter rupture or catheter emboli.

STEP	RATIONALE
g. Connect syringe for blood sampling, and release clamp. Aspirate 5 ml fluid, reclamp, and discard aspirate. (Do not discard if drawn for blood culture.)	Discarding initial 5 ml of aspirate avoids diluting sample.
h. Attach or insert syringe of size equal to volume of blood sample to withdraw to catheter. Release clamp. Withdraw necessary blood for samples, and reclamp.	Samples should be collected at one time to minimize time with open catheter system.
i. Attach or insert syringe filled with 10 ml normal saline to catheter. If clamp is present, release, flush vigorously, and reclamp.	Catheter should be cleared of all blood or medications that may clog catheter lumen or precipitate with additives in IV fluids.
j. If no continuous infusion is indicated, flush catheter with heparin or normal saline (see agency policy). Connect syringe containing 5 ml heparin (100 units/ml) or normal saline flush solution. If clamp is present, release, flush with positive pressure, and reclamp.	A catheter not in use must be flushed to prevent clot formation. This is commonly done with heparin; however, Groshong catheters are flushed with normal saline only.
(1) Attach new cap to end of catheter, and remove clamp.	Maintains sterile seal to catheter.

STEP	RATIONALE
k. If IV fluids will be administered, connect IV tubing to end of catheter, being sure both ends are sterile.	IV system should be closed to maintain sterility.
(1) Regulate IV infusion as ordered.	Maintains ordered fluid intake and keeps catheter patent.
(2) Secure all tubing connections.	Prevents accidental tubing disconnection and catheter displacement. Luer-Lok connections should be used.
l. Dispose of soiled equipment and used supplies. Remove gloves and perform hand hygiene.	Reduces transmission of microorganisms.
2. Dressing Change	
a. Perform hand hygiene and apply clean gloves.	Reduces transmission of microorganisms.
b. Mask self and client, if indicated (check agency policy).	Prevents exposure of catheter exit or placement site to airborne microorganisms.
c. Carefully remove old dressing in the direction the catheter was inserted, noting drainage and appearance of catheter.	Remove tape carefully because clients frequently have alterations in skin integrity. Prevents dislodgement of catheter.
d. Inspect site for signs of redness, swelling, inflammation, tenderness, or exudate.	This is a potential site of infection.
e. Inspect catheter and hub for intactness, and remove clean gloves.	Catheter may become torn, cut, displaced, cracked, or split.
f. Perform hand hygiene, and open dressing kit in a sterile manner. Most agencies have dressing kits that contain all needed dressing change supplies.	Reduces transmission of microorganisms.
g. Apply sterile gloves.	Prevents direct transmission of microorganisms to skin exit site.
h. Clean site with antimicrobial swab, moving first in a horizontal pattern. With a new swab move in a vertical plane, and then use a final swab in a circular pattern, moving outward in concentric circles from insertion site out. Allow to dry.	It is impossible to sterilize skin. Organisms that accumulate must be eliminated by mechanical and chemical means. Mechanical friction in this pattern allows penetration of the antiseptic solution into the cracks and fissures of the epidermal layer of the skin (Crosby and Mares, 2001). Antiseptic solutions should be allowed to air-dry completely to effectively reduce microbial counts (INS, 2000). If antiseptic agents are used in combination, allow each to air-dry separately.
i. Place Steri-Strip (see illustration) or securement device over catheter.	Provides security to prevent catheter dislodgement. PICC lines may be sutured in place, preventing placement of gauze underneath.
j. Redress site using sterile gauze and tape or transparent dressing as indicated (see Skill 27-4).	Prevents entrance of bacteria into exit or placement site.

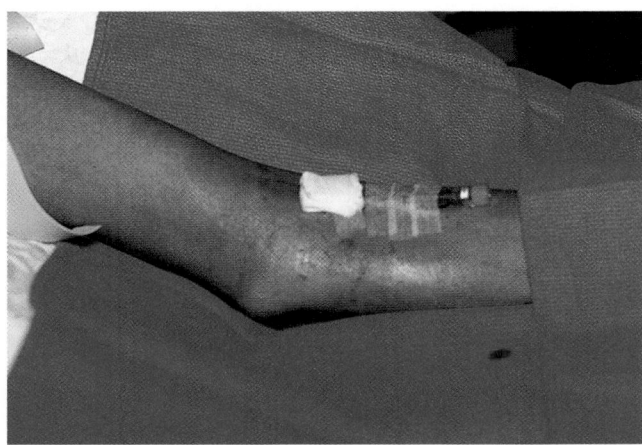

STEP 2i Anchor PICC catheter hub with Steri-Strips.

STEP	RATIONALE
k. Secure connections. Luer-Lok connections are preferred.	Prevents accidental pulling and displacement.
l. Label date, time of dressing change, and size of cannula in place.	Documents dressing change. Provides guideline for time of next change.
m. Dispose of soiled supplies; remove gloves, and perform hand hygiene.	Reduces transmission of microorganisms.

EVALUATION

1. When continuous infusions are administered, observe and calculate drip rate hourly. Note ease with which fluid rate can be increased.	To maintain proper fluid infusion, desired drip rate should be regulated continuously. A gradual slowing in rate or inability to increase rate may indicate catheter occlusion.
2. Routinely assess vital signs of client, noting changes symptomatic of infection.	Catheter-related sepsis can cause fever, chills, flushed skin, tachycardia.
3. Observe site when dressing removed (Table 27-4).	Continual monitoring for signs of inflammation or infection is essential.
4. Observe all catheter connection points periodically.	An intact system prevents accidental blood loss or entrance of air.
5. Inspect condition of catheter and connecting tubing daily for leaks, holes, tears, splits, or cracked hubs.	Break in integrity of system predisposes client to hemorrhage or air embolus.
6. Measure amount of catheter that remains external with each dressing change.	Detects catheter migration.
7. Consult x-ray examination reports for catheter placement.	A routine chest x-ray examination can locate position of catheter tip.
8. Evaluate ability of client and family to provide care and maintain catheter or infusion port through discussion and return demonstrations of dressing changes and skin care. Determine need for restrictions on daily activities.	Measures client's ability to care for self and any additional learning needs.

Recording and Reporting

- Record blood samples obtained, patency of lines, and type of IV fluids administered. Note rate of fluid infusion.
- Report status of PICC, therapy being administered, and development of complications and their treatment.

Unexpected Outcomes	Related Interventions
1. There is blocked or difficult infusion of fluids through catheter, indicating occlusion that is either mechanical, nonthrombotic, or thrombotic.	• Assess tubing for kinks and inspect site to rule out external cause of obstruction. • Tight sutures may need to be removed. • Chest x-ray examination may be ordered to determine internal compression. • Know drug incompatibilities to prevent precipitation of infused solution. • Assess change in ability to aspirate or withdraw from catheter. Look for clots visible in external portion of line. Physician or independent practitioner (IP) or qualified RN may attempt aspiration of clot. • Fibrinolytic therapy may be used (see agency policy).
2. Client experiences pain and erythema at insertion site; blood or fluids leak from PICC insertion site.	• Reinsertion in opposite arm with new sterile catheter may be necessary.

Continued

TABLE 27-4   COMPLICATIONS OF VASCULAR ACCESS DEVICES

COMPLICATION	ASSESSMENT	PREVENTION	INTERVENTION
Catheter damage, Breakage	Observe for pinholes, leaks, tears, every shift. Assess for drainage after flushing.	Follow proper clamping procedure. Avoid sharp objects near the catheter. Use needleless system device.	Use a catheter stylet for temporary repair. Use permanent repair kit. Remove catheter.
Occlusion: thrombus, precipitation, malposition	Assess for blood return. Assess for inability to infuse fluid. Assess equipment. If port, reaccess and verify Huber needle placement. Assess with syringe directly on catheter. Assess for discomfort or pain in shoulder, neck, or arm at insertion site. Assess for neck or shoulder edema. Assess sutures to ensure no restriction or pinching of catheter.	Follow routine flushing with positive pressure and/or use positive pressure valve injection cap. Avoid tugging on CVC. Administer low-dose oral anticoagulant therapy. Avoid using excessive force. Flush between drugs. Flush vigorously after viscous solutions. Avoid mixing incompatible drugs. Avoid kinking catheter.	Reposition client. Have client cough and deep breathe. Raise client's arm. Obtain venogram if ordered. Administer thrombolytics if ordered. Remove catheter (CVC requires order). Obtain x-ray examination as ordered. If precipitate, try hydrochloric acid or ethanol solution per orders. Do not use a 1-ml syringe to instill saline because pressure exceeds 200 psi.
Infection: exit site, tunnel, thrombus, port pocket	Assess exit site for redness, drainage, edema, or tenderness. Assess vital signs. Monitor laboratory findings.	Use aseptic technique. Adhere to dressing change technique. Apply dressing over exit site.	Administer antibiotic therapy as ordered. (Draw blood cultures first when ordered.) Remove catheter (CVC requires order). Administer thrombolytic agent if ordered. Replace catheter. Obtain blood cultures peripheral and from CVC if ordered.
Dislodgement	Assess length of catheter daily. Inform client of possible catheter dislodgement. Identify edema at exit site or drainage. Palpate exit site and tunnel for coiling (catheter can be felt and traced underneath the skin). Assess for distended neck veins.	Loop and tape the catheter securely. Use occlusive dressing. Avoid pulling on CVC. Handle with care. Avoid manipulating catheter by hand. Protect site with soft outer cover.	Insert new catheter. Secure catheter with securement device. Teach client not to manipulate catheter.
Catheter migration, pinch-off syndrome, port separation	Assess for client complaints of gurgling sounds. Assess for change in patency of catheter by evaluating change in flow rate, local irritation, swelling, occlusion, tenderness, pain, inability to aspirate fluid and/or blood. Obtain x-ray examination. Assess edema of arm and hand on side of insertion. Assess for distended neck veins. Assess for inability to infuse fluids. Assess length of catheter daily.	Avoid trauma. Avoid placement near site of local infection, scarring, or skin disorder.	Reposition under fluoroscopy as ordered. Remove catheter as ordered. Stop all fluid administration.

Continued

TABLE 27-4 **COMPLICATIONS OF VASCULAR ACCESS DEVICES—CONT'D**

COMPLICATION	ASSESSMENT	PREVENTION	INTERVENTION
Skin erosion, hematomas, cuff extrusion, scar tissue formation over port	Assess for loss of viable tissue over septum site. Assess for separation of exit site edges. Assess for drainage at exit site. Assess for redness. Assess for edema, contusions. Note if tunneled catheter is exposed.	Maintain nutritional status. Avoid pressure or trauma. Rotate site with each port access.	Remove CVC as ordered. Improve nutrition. Provide appropriate skin care.
Infiltration, extravasation	Assess for erythema. Assess for edema. Assess for spongy feeling. Assess for swelling around the IV site and at the termination of the catheter tip. Assess for labored breathing. Assess for aspiration of fluid and/or blood. Assess for complaints of pain. Assess for no free-flow IV drip.	Stop vesicant administration immediately. Administer antidote or therapeutic medications to maintain tissue integrity according to protocol.	Apply cold/warm compresses according to specific vesicant protocol. Provide emotional support. Obtain x-ray examination if ordered. Use antidotes per protocol. Discontinue IV fluids.
Pneumothorax, hemothorax, air emboli, hydrothorax	Assess for subcutaneous emphysema by inspecting and palpating skin around insertion site and along arm. Inspection may reveal edema where the air is located, and the air may travel if the skin is loose. Palpation reveals a crackling sensation such as popping plastic bubble wrap. Assess for chest pain. Assess for dyspnea, apnea, hypoxia, tachycardia, hypotension, nausea, confusion.	Use injection cap on distal end when not in use. Do not leave catheter open to air.	Administer oxygen as ordered. Elevate feet. Aspirate air, fluid. If air emboli suspected, place client on left side with head elevated slightly. Remove catheter as ordered. Assist with insertion of chest tubes as ordered.
Incorrect placement	Assess for cardiac dysrhythmias. Assess for hypotension. Assess for neck distention. Assess for narrow pulse pressure. Assess for inadequate blood withdrawal. Assess for retrograde flow of blood (the flow of blood back into the tubing usually caused by decreased pressure gradient between the venous system and the access device unit [e.g., IV infusion, heparin lock]).	Obtain x-ray examination after placement. Reposition catheter as warranted.	Stop all fluid administration until placement is confirmed. Discontinue catheter (CVC requires order). Obtain x-ray examination and electrocardiogram (for PICC and CVC). Administer support medications as ordered.

Unexpected Outcomes	Related Interventions
3. Client develops a fever, elevated WBC, and culture of PICC tip is positive, indicating catheter sepsis.	• Remove PICC line as ordered. • Antibiotic therapy may be ordered.
4. Client develops fluid volume deficit, fluid volume excess, or electrolyte imbalances.	• Volume and/or rate of fluid to be infused will be revised by prescriber. • Additions or deletions may be made to additives in IV fluid.
5. Client develops sudden respiratory distress, which may indicate pulmonary embolus.	• Place client in high-Fowler's position. • Notify physician or IP immediately. • Be prepared to obtain chest x-ray examination if ordered.
6. Client develops irregular pulse.	• May indicate malposition of catheter in the right atrium, causing atrial irritation. Catheter may need to be withdrawn several centimeters. • Interventional radiology may be necessary to diagnose and reposition PICC.

Teaching Considerations

- Because PICC insertion and care may be unfamiliar to the client, careful and repeated verbal explanations with written follow-up are important.
- Instruct client and caregiver about signs and symptoms of the most common complications: phlebitis, clotting, leaking at catheter insertion site, or breaking of the catheter. Instruct client in how to respond to each of these complications.
- Because the dressing is the anchor for the PICC, client and caregiver need to notify nurse if dressing becomes loose. Nurse will perform a dressing change.
- If PICC becomes clotted, client should promptly seek care so that declotting measures can be instituted.
- The PICC dressing should not become wet, so bathing must be adapted to keep cannulated arm dry.
- Client should avoid vigorous activities (e.g., weight lifting) because catheter may be damaged.
- Client can move arm freely because there is less chance of infiltration and dislodgement than with a peripheral venipuncture using a short catheter.

Pediatric Considerations

- An advantage of the use of PICCs is the longer duration and stability of use compared with traditional peripheral catheters. PICCs have a reduced risk of infections compared with umbilical venous catheters in neonates.
- In neonates the antecubital veins, long saphenous vein, and superficial temporal vein in the scalp are most commonly used. The external jugular vein, popliteal vein, veins in the ankle, and axillary veins may be used.

Home Care Considerations

- Ensure that client is able and willing to care for PICC line and administer IV therapy or that there is a reliable caregiver or nursing support personnel at home to provide IV therapy care before insertion.
- The catheter can be inserted in the home, or client may have it inserted before discharge from the hospital.
- Common uses for PICCs in the home are long-term antibiotic/antiviral administration, pain control, parenteral nutrition, and hydration.
- Because client in the home setting may be more active, a secure dressing is required.

SKILL 27-3 Regulating Intravenous Flow Rate

After an IV infusion is initiated and the line is patent, the nurse is responsible for regulating the rate of infusion according to the physician's orders. An infusion rate that is too slow can lead to further cardiovascular and circulatory collapse in a client who is dehydrated, in shock, or critically ill. In addition, if an infusion runs too slowly, the chances of a thrombus occluding the cannula are greater. An infusion rate that is too rapid can result in fluid overload, which can result in grave consequences in certain cardiovascular, kidney, and neurological disorders and in the very young and very old.

The nurse calculates the infusion rate to infuse at the prescribed amount. Children, older adults, clients with severe head trauma, and clients susceptible to FVE must be protected from sudden increases in infusion volumes by using an infusion device to regulate flow. Sudden increases can occur accidentally. For example, a restless client may loosen the roller clamp with a sudden movement and thus increase the flow rate, or the flow rate may be accidentally changed with gravity influence. A sudden increase in volume can lead to a critical condition or even to death in some cases. Two types of infusion devices, an electronic infusion device (EID) and an IV volume controller assist the nurse in maintaining correct flow rates, maintaining catheter patency, and preventing runaway bolus IV infusions. Their use also assists the nurse when an IV container volume is complete or when an IV obstruction occurs. Many infusion devices also provide a record for the volume of fluid infused.

An EID is designed to deliver a measured amount of fluid over a period of time, that is, milliliters per hour. An alarm also signals if the pressure in the system increases. For example, when an infiltration of IV fluids forms within the subcutaneous tissue or if the client's arm position obstructs intravenous flow, pressure will build up and the alarm will sound. An infiltration may be extensive before a positive-pressure EID alarm responds. The nurse must frequently inspect and palpate the IV site to ensure timely detection of an infiltration. EIDs have a high degree of accuracy and precision to ensure that the rate of IV fluid therapy is infused precisely.

An IV volume-control device delivers fluid with the aid of gravity. The IV container must be placed approximately 36 inches above the IV site to overcome venous resistance and operate properly. IV volume controllers deliver fluids based on a determination of drops per minute, which is in turn based on milliliters per hour. The nurse must monitor the volume delivered each hour to ensure that the calculated drops per minute deliver the actual volume desired. The actual volume delivered depends on several factors such as the rate of infusion, the IV tubing size, and fluid viscosity. Because IV controllers cannot overcome increased resistance in the IV system, infiltrations can be more quickly detected by an IV controller than by an EID. This sensitivity also increases the frequency of alarm responses that occur when client movement creates a temporary increased resistance to flow. One example of a volume-control device is a calibrated chamber placed between the IV container and the insertion spike and drip chamber of the administration set (Figure 27-6). A small volume of IV fluid is placed in the chamber from the IV fluid container. This smaller volume is then regulated for administration. The advantage of this system is that only the smaller volume of fluid infuses if the rate of the IV is inadvertently increased. Volume-control devices should be used when administering IV fluid to neonates, very young children, and older adults.

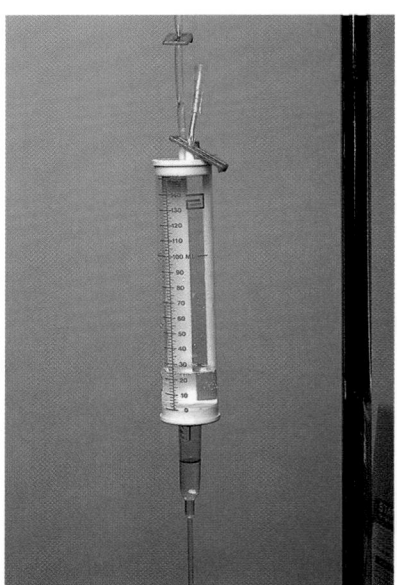

FIGURE 27-6 Volume-control device.

DELEGATION CONSIDERATIONS

The skill of regulating intravenous flow rate should not be delegated to assistive personnel. The nurse provides information and direction including:

- Instructing assistive personnel to inform the nurse when the electronic infusion device alarm signals, the fluid container is almost empty, and the client complains of any discomfort at the IV site

EQUIPMENT

- ❏ Watch with second hand
- ❏ Calculator or pad and pen/pencil
- ❏ Tape
- ❏ Label
- ❏ IV regulating device (EID, volume-control device [optional])

STEP	RATIONALE

ASSESSMENT

1. Check client's medical record for correct solution and additives. Follow six rights of drug administration (see Chapter 19). Usual order includes solution, additives or medications (if included), infusion rate or volume in specified time period. Occasionally, IV order contains only 1 L to keep vein open (KVO). Record also shows time over which each liter is to infuse.

IV fluids are medications. Six rights prevent medication administration error.

2. Perform hand hygiene. Observe for patency of IV line and cannula.

For fluid to infuse at proper rate, IV line and cannula must be free of kinks and thrombi.

3. Assess client's knowledge of how positioning of IV site affects flow rate.

Fosters client participation in maintaining most effective position of arm with IV equipment. Position or setting of control clamp or infusion device rate should be done only by nurse or practitioner.

4. Inspect IV site, and verify with client how venipuncture site feels; for example, determine if there is pain or burning. Palpate site for tenderness.

Pain or burning may be early indication of phlebitis. Includes client in decision making.

NURSING DIAGNOSES

- Deficient fluid volume
- Excess fluid volume
- Risk for imbalanced fluid volume

Related factors are individualized based on client's condition or needs.

PLANNING

1. Expected outcomes following completion of procedure:
   - Serum electrolytes remain within normal limits.
   - Client receives prescribed volume of fluid/medication over desired time interval.
2. Have paper and pencil or calculator to calculate flow rate.
3. Know calibration (drop factor) in drops per milliliter (gtt/ml) of infusion set used by agency:
   Microdrip: 60 gtt/ml
   Macrodrip (Metheny, 2000):
      Abbott: 15 gtt/ml
      Travenol: 10 gtt/ml
      McGaw: 15 gtt/ml

IV fluid assists in maintaining fluid and electrolyte levels.

When infusion rate remains within prescribed range, the therapeutic aim is achieved.

Use mathematical calculations to obtain correct rate.

Microdrip tubing, also called pediatric tubing, universally delivers 60 gtt/ml and is used when small or very precise volumes are to be infused. However, there are different commercial parenteral administration sets for macrodrip tubing. Macrodrip tubing should be used when large quantities or fast rates are necessary.

STEP	RATIONALE

4. Select one of the following formulas to calculate flow rate after determining ml/hr.
 	
     (a) ml/hr/60 min = ml/min
 	
     (b) Drop factor × ml/min = drops/min
 	
        or
 	
     (c) ml/hr × drop factor/60 min = drops/min
	Once hourly rate has been determined (see below), these formulas give correct flow rate.

IMPLEMENTATION

1. Obtain IV fluid/medication and appropriate tubing. Intravenous fluids may be ordered for 24-hour period, indicating how long each liter of fluid should run; for example, IV order for client is:	Use of correct tubing ensures more accurate infusion delivery. Determines volume of fluid that should infuse hourly.

Bottle 1: 1000 ml D_5W with 20 mEq KCl @ 125 ml/hr

Bottle 2: 1000 ml D_5W with 20 mEq KCl @125 ml/hr

Bottle 3: 1000 ml D_5W with 20 mEq KCl @ 125 ml/hr

    Total 24-hour IV intake: 3000 ml

- **Critical Decision Point**

    It is common for physicians to write an abbreviated IV order such as: "D_5W with 20 mEq KCl 125 ml/hr continuous." This order implies that the IV should be maintained at this rate until order has been written for IV to be discontinued.

2. Determine hourly rate by dividing volume by hours, for example:	Provides even infusion of fluid over prescribed hourly rate.

$$ml/hr = \frac{total\ infusion\ (ml)}{hours\ of\ infusion}$$

    1000 ml/8 hr = 125 ml/hr

    or if 3 L is ordered for 24 hours

    3000 ml/24 hr = 125 ml/hr

STEP	RATIONALE

3. Place marked adhesive tape or commercial fluid indicator tape on IV container next to volume markings (see illustration)

Time taping IV bag gives nurse visual cue as to whether fluids are being administered over correct period of time. Time tapes should be used for all IV infusions, including those on therapies infused via EIDs.

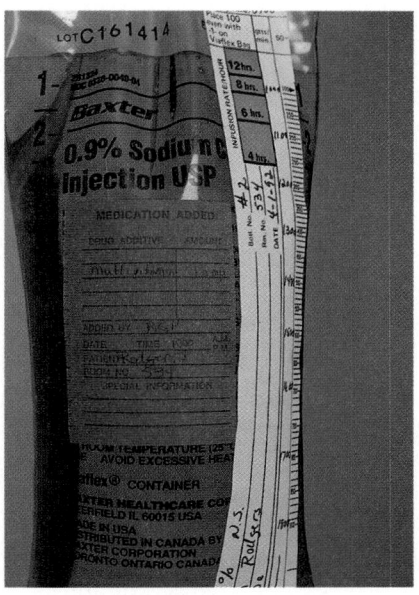

STEP **3** IV fluid bag with time tape.

- *Critical Decision Point*

  On IV bags made of polyvinylchloride (PVC) avoid drawing directly with felt-tip pens or permanent markers because the ink could leech into the solution (Hadaway, 2003).

4. After hourly rate has been determined, calculate minute rate based on drop factor of infusion set. Microdrip infusion set has a drop factor of 60 gtt/ml. Regular drip or macrodrip infusion set used in this example has drop factor of 15 gtt/ml. Using formula (see Planning, step 4), calculate minute flow rate for bottle 1:1000 ml with 20 mEq KCl @ 125 ml/hr.

   Microdrip:

   Allows nurse to calculate minute flow rate for regulation of infusion.

   When using microdrip, ml/hr always equals gtt/min.

   $$125 \text{ ml/hr} \times 60 \text{ gtt/ml} = 7500 \text{ gtt/hr}$$

   $$7500 \text{ gtt} \div 60 \text{ minutes} = 125 \text{ gtt/min}$$

   Macrodrip:

   $$125 \text{ ml/hr} \times 15 \text{ gtt/ml} = 1875 \text{ gtt/hr}$$

   $$1875 \text{ gtt} \div 60 \text{ minutes} = 31\text{-}32 \text{ gtt/min}$$

   Volume is multiplied by drop factor, and the product is divided by time (in minutes).

STEP	RATIONALE
5. Determine flow rate by counting drops in drip chamber for 1 minute by watch, then adjust roller clamp to increase or decrease rate of infusion (see illustration).	Regulate to prescribed rate.
6. Follow this procedure for infusion gravity controller or EID pump:	
a. Consult manufacturer's directions for setup of the infusion. Place electronic eye over drip chamber (see illustration). If a gravity controller is used, ensure that IV container is 36 inches above IV site.	IV controller works by gravity.
b. Insert IV tubing into chamber of control mechanism (see manufacturer's directions) (see illustration).	Most electronic infusion pumps use positive pressure to infuse.

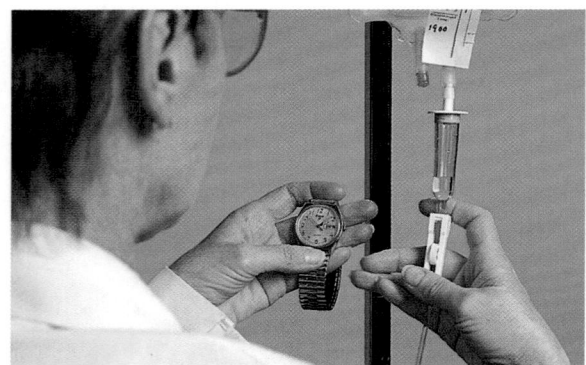

STEP **5** Counting IV drip rate.

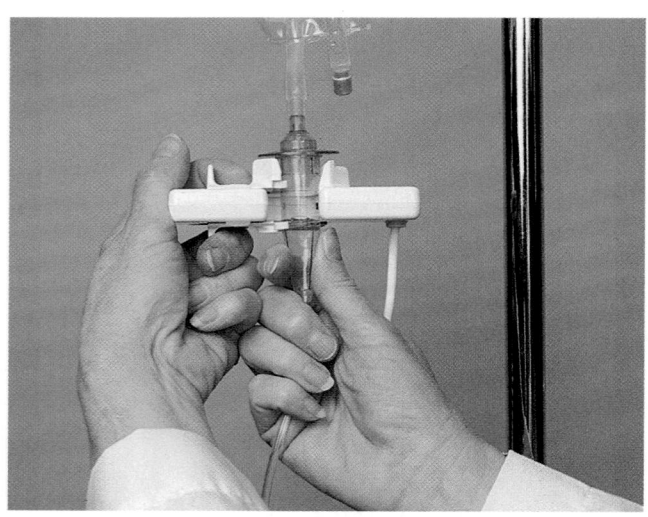

STEP **6a** Electronic eye placed over drip chamber.

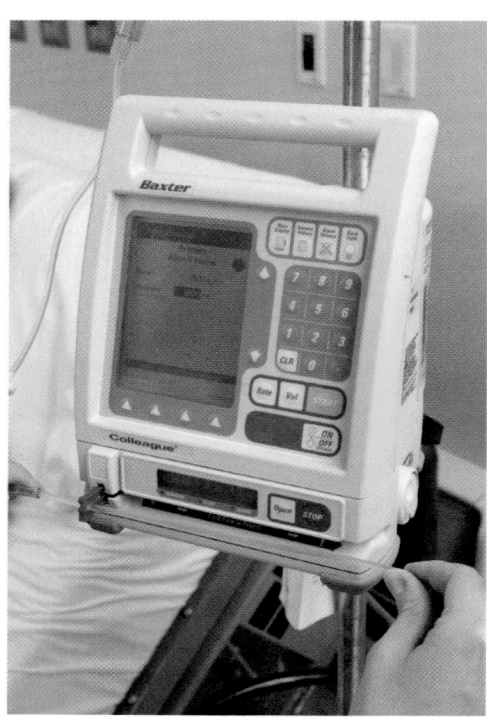

STEP **6b** Insert IV tubing into chamber of control mechanism.

STEP	RATIONALE

    c. Required drops per minute or volume per hour are selected, door to control chamber is closed, power button is turned on, and start button is pressed (see illustrations).

- **Critical Decision Point**
  Special infusion tubing is required for some pumps. Check agency equipment and associated policies.

    d. Open drip regulator completely while EID is in use.   Ensures that pump freely regulates infusion rate.

    e. Monitor infusion rate and IV site for infiltration according to agency policy. Rate of infusion should be checked by comparing volume in the container with the calculated amount that should have been infused even when EID is used.

Infusion controllers or pumps are not infallible and do not replace frequent, accurate nursing evaluation. Infusion pumps may continue to infuse IV fluids after an infiltration has begun.

    f. Assess patency of system when alarm signals.

Alarm on infusion pump can be triggered by empty solution container, tubing obstruction, closed drip regulator, infiltration, thrombus formation, air in the tubing, and/or low battery.

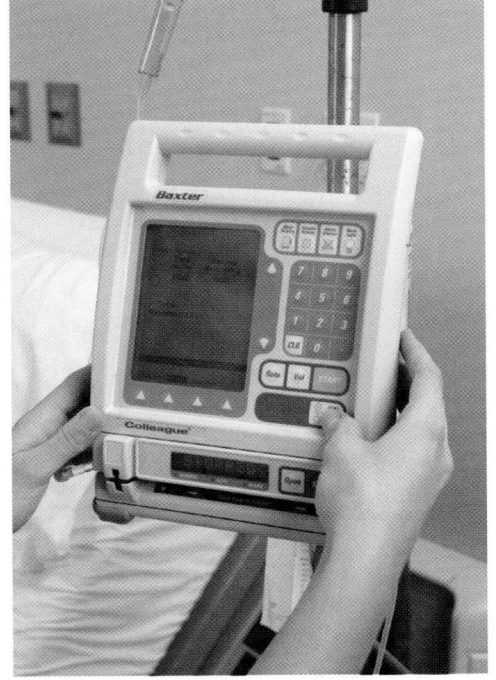 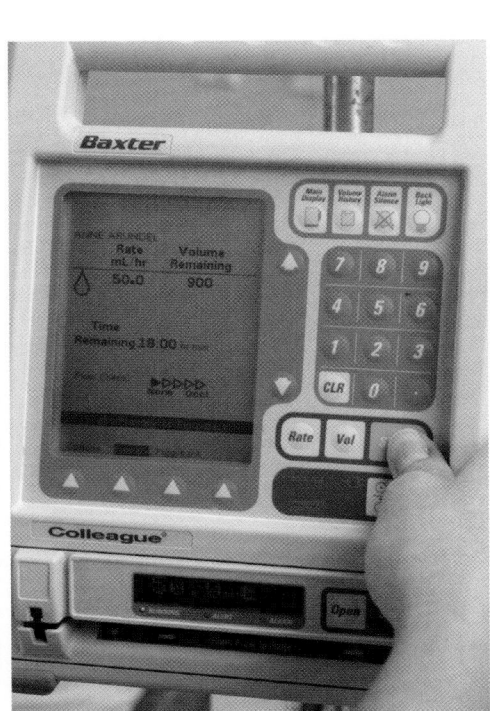

STEP 7c A, Select rate and volume to be infused. **B,** Press start button.

STEP	RATIONALE
7. Follow this procedure for gravity volume-control device:	
a. Place gravity volume-control device between IV container and insertion spike of infusion set using aseptic technique (see Figure 27-6).	Delivers small volume, but must be refilled as it becomes low.
b. Place no more than 2 hours' allotment of fluid into device by opening clamp between IV bag and device.	Allows a safeguard for the nurse if unable to return in exactly 60 minutes. Should infusion rate accidentally increase in rate, allows at most only a 2-hour allotment of fluid to infuse.
c. Assess system at least hourly; add fluid to volume control device. Regulate flow rate.	Maintains patency of system.

EVALUATION

1. Monitor IV infusion at least every hour, noting volume of IV fluid infused and rate.	Ensures correct volume infuses over prescribed time period.
2. Observe client for signs of overhydration or dehydration to determine response to therapy and restoration of fluid and electrolyte balance.	Signs and symptoms of dehydration or overhydration warrant changing rate of fluid infused.
3. Evaluate for signs of infiltration, inflammation at site, clot in catheter, kink or knot in infusion tubing.	Prevents decrease or cessation of flow rate.

Recording and Reporting

- Record rate of infusion, gtt/min, and ml/hr in nurses' notes or parenteral fluid form according to agency policy.
- Immediately record in nurses' notes any ordered change in IV fluid rates.
- Document use of any electronic infusion device or controlling device and number on that device.
- At change of shift or when leaving on break, report rate of infusion and volume left in container to nurse in charge or next nurse assigned to care for client.

Unexpected Outcomes	Related Interventions
1. Sudden infusion of large volume of solution occurs with client having symptoms of dyspnea, crackles in the lung, and increased urine output, indicating fluid overload.	• Slow infusion to KVO rate, and notify physician immediately. • Place client in high-Fowler's position. • New IV orders will be required. • Client may require diuretics.
2. IV fluid container is completed with subsequent loss of IV line patency.	• Discontinue present IV, and restart IV.
3. The IV infusion is slower than ordered.	• Check client for positional change that might affect rate, height of IV container, tubing obstruction. • An infiltration may be developing at IV site. • Check condition of site. • If volume infused is deficient, consult physician/IP for new order to provide necessary fluid volume.

Teaching Considerations

- Instruct client to contact staff if a problem develops.
- If an EID is used, client should know its preset rate and the significance of alarms.
- Teach client about factors affecting flow rate, to protect IV site, and importance of not altering rate control.

Pediatric Considerations

- Children are not small adults. Physiological differences must be remembered, particularly focusing on total body weight (85% to 90% water). Dehydration is a common cause of fluid and electrolyte imbalance; assessment of fluid needs includes meter square weight or caloric method (Phillips, 2001).
- Infusion pumps (especially syringe pumps) are almost always used in pediatrics because they infuse very small amounts of fluids and accurately provide the prescribed volume of IV solution.
- Use only small-volume containers for infusions (250 ml for children younger than 12 months, 500 ml for older children) (Hockenberry and others, 2003). Microdrip tubing is recommended for children.

Geriatric Considerations

- Renal changes in older adults may reduce the kidney's ability to concentrate and dilute urine in response to water or salt excess. Combined with cardiac deficiencies and decreased blood flow to organs, the older client is precariously balanced between dehydration and fluid overload. Use an EID and microdrip. Monitor levels of electrolytes, blood urea nitrogen (BUN), and creatinine, urine output, and daily weight.
- Dextrose infused too rapidly may cause cerebral edema more readily in older clients and those with head injuries. Normal saline, given to an older client with impaired renal function, can cause hypernatremia.

Home Care Considerations

- Ensure that client is able and willing to operate an infusion pump (if applicable) and administer IV therapy. If client is unable to provide self-care, be sure that a reliable caregiver is available in the home.
- Nurse should check proper function of EID before use with client.
- If gravity administration is used, teach client and primary caregiver to time drops per minute using watch with second hand.
- Ensure that client's electrical outlets are properly grounded.

SKILL 27-4   Changing a Peripheral Intravenous Dressing

Peripheral IV cannulas and certain fluid infusions are frequently associated with complications such as local or systemic infections, phlebitis, and infiltration. Dressing applications are done for IV infusion sites at the time when the IV is inserted or when the IV site is changed. The insertion site is the most common source of colonization and infection for IV cannulas. A peripheral IV dressing should be securely applied and must be changed when it becomes, wet, soiled, or loosened/ removed (CDC, 2002). The type of material used for the IV dressing depends on agency policy. A transparent dressing should be changed with cannula site rotation and immediately if integrity of the dressing is compromised. Gauze dressings should be changed routinely every 48 hours and immediately if integrity is compromised. Gauze used underneath a transparent dressing is considered a gauze dressing and should be changed every 48 hours (CDC 2002; INS, 2000).

DELEGATION CONSIDERATIONS

The skill of changing a peripheral intravenous dressing should not be delegated to assistive personnel. The nurse provides information and direction, including:

- Instructing assistive personnel caring for clients with peripheral IVs to report if a client complains of moistness or loosening of an IV dressing.

EQUIPMENT

- ❑ Antiseptic swab
- ❑ Adhesive remover (if needed)
- ❑ Skin protectant swab
- ❑ Disposable gloves, mask, gown
- ❑ Strips of nonallergenic tape
- ❑ Hand or arm board or IV housing device if needed
  For Transparent Dressing
- ❑ Sterile transparent dressing
  For Gauze Dressing
- ❑ Sterile 2 × 2 gauze pad or
- ❑ Sterile 4 × 4 gauze pad

STEP	RATIONALE

ASSESSMENT

1. Determine when dressing was last changed. Many institutions require nurse to write date and time on dressing and date the device was first placed.

2. Observe present dressing for moisture and intactness.

3. Observe IV system for proper functioning or complications: current flow rate, presence of kinks in infusion tubing or IV catheter. Palpate the cannula site through the intact dressing for subjective complaints of pain or burning.

4. Inspect exposed catheter site for inflammation and swelling.

5. Monitor body temperature.
6. Assess client's understanding of the need for continued IV infusion.

Rationale column:

Provides information regarding length of time that present dressing has been in place. In addition, nurse is able to plan for dressing change.

Moisture is medium for bacterial growth and renders dressing contaminated. Nonadhering dressing increases risk of bacterial contamination to venipuncture site or displacement of IV catheter.

Unexplained decrease in flow rate requires nurse to investigate placement and patency of IV cannula. Pain can be associated with both phlebitis and infiltration.

Inflammation indicates phlebitis. Swelling indicates infiltration, with fluid infusing into surrounding tissues. These signs require removal of IV cannula.

Elevated temperature may be related to infection at IV site.
Reveals need for client instruction.

NURSING DIAGNOSES

- Risk for infection
- Pain (acute)

Related factors are individualized based on client's condition or needs.

PLANNING

1. Expected outcomes following completion of procedure:
   - Client will have patent IV as evidenced by absence of infiltration, phlebitis, or thrombus.
   - Client's temperature remains normal.
   - IV insertion site is without pain, redness, swelling, or exudate.
2. Explain procedure and purpose to client and family. Explain that affected extremity must be held still and how long procedure will take.

Rationale column:

Proper care maintains IV infusion as prescribed.

Site remains uninfected.
Site remains uninfected.

Decreases anxiety, promotes cooperation, and gives client time frame around which personal activities can be planned.

IMPLEMENTATION

1. Perform hand hygiene. Apply disposable gloves.

2. Remove tape, gauze, and/or transparent dressing from old dressing one layer at a time by pulling toward the insertion site (see illustration), leaving tape that secures IV cannula intact. Be cautious if cannula tubing becomes tangled between two layers of dressing. When removing transparent dressing, hold cannula hub and tubing with nondominant hand.

Rationale column:

Reduces transmission of microorganisms. Infections related to IV therapy are most often caused by catheter hub contamination, so careful technique must be used throughout the dressing change. Gloves reduce nurse's risk of exposure to HIV, hepatitis, and other blood-borne viruses or bacteria.

Prevents accidental displacement of cannula.

STEP	RATIONALE

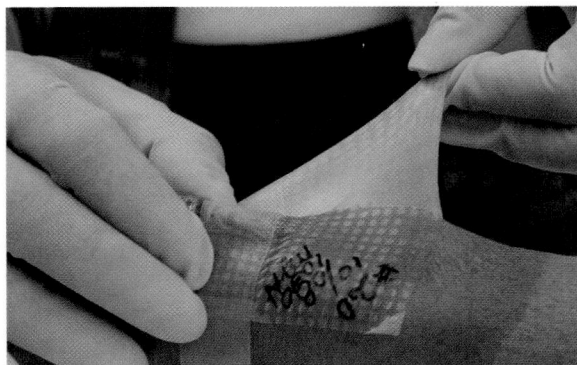

STEP **2** Remove transparent dressing by pulling side laterally.

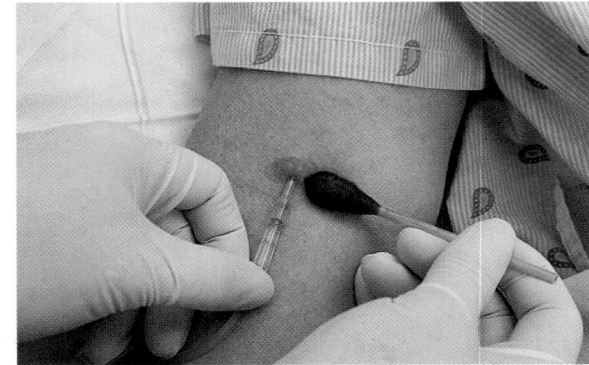

STEP **7** Cleanse peripheral insertion site with antiseptic swab.

3. Observe insertion site for signs and/or symptoms of infection: tenderness, redness, swelling, and exudate.

Presence of infection indicates need to discontinue IV at current site.

4. If complication exists or if ordered by physician, discontinue infusion (see Skill 27-7).

5. If IV is infusing properly, gently remove tape securing cannula. Stabilize cannula with one hand. Use adhesive remover to cleanse skin and remove adhesive residue, if needed.

Exposes venipuncture site. Stabilization prevents accidental displacement of cannula. Adhesive residue decreases ability of new tape to adhere securely to skin.

- **Critical Decision Point**
  Keep one finger over cannula at all times until dressing is applied.

7. Cleanse insertion site with antiseptic swab using friction. Use the first swab in a horizontal plane, cleansing the skin from side to side. Apply the second swab on a vertical plane, up and down. Apply the final swab in a circular pattern moving outward from the insertion site (see illustration). Allow each swab to dry.

Mechanical friction in this pattern allows penetration of the antiseptic solution into the cracks and fissures of the epidermal layer of the skin (Crosby and Mares, 2001).

Antiseptic solutions should be allowed to air-dry completely to effectively reduce microbial counts (INS, 2000). If antiseptic agents are used in combination, allow each to air-dry separately.

8. *Option:* Apply skin protectant solution to the area where the tape or dressing will be applied. Allow to dry.

Coats the skin with protective solution to maintain skin integrity, prevent irritation from the adhesive, and promote adhesion of the dressing.

9. Tape or secure catheter.
   a. Applying transparent dressing: Secure catheter with nondominant hand while preparing to apply dressing.

Prevents catheter dislodgement.

   b. Applying gauze dressing: Place a narrow piece (½ inch) of tape under cannula hub with adhesive side up; cross tape over hub to make a chevron. Place tape only on the cannula, *never over* the insertion site.

Chevron secures cannula. Inspection of the insertion site is essential.

- **Critical Decision Point**
  Do not tape over connection of access tubing or port to IV catheter.

STEP	RATIONALE

10. Apply sterile dressing over site:
    a. Transparent dressing

        (1) Carefully remove adherent backing. Apply one edge of dressing, and then gently smooth remaining dressing over IV site, leaving connection between IV tubing and catheter hub uncovered. Remove outer covering; smooth dressing over site.

Secures catheter and provides tight dressing seal.
Access to cannula hub is needed for access to change tubing and in emergencies.

        (2) Place a 1-inch piece of tape from end of catheter hub to insertion site, over transparent dressing. Apply chevron.

    b. Gauze dressing

        (1) Fold a 2×2 gauze in half, and cover with a 1 inch–wide piece of tape extending about an inch from each side. Place gauze under the tubing/cannula hub junction (see illustration). Curl a loop of tubing alongside the arm, and place a second piece of tape directly over the padded 2×2, securing tubing in two places (see illustration).

Gauze prevents pressure of cannula hub against skin. Securing loop of tubing reduces risk of dislodging catheter from accidental pull.

        (2) Place another 2×2 gauze pad over the venipuncture site and cannula hub. Secure all edges with tape. Do not cover connection between IV tubing and cannula hub.

Gauze dressings must be occlusive to prevent air flow (Hankins and others, 2001).
Access to catheter hub is needed in times of emergency and when changing tubing.

11. Remove and discard gloves.

Prevents transmission of microorganisms.

12. *Option:* Apply hand board or securement device if insertion site or dressing is affected by the motion of the joint.

Reduces the risk of phlebitis and infiltration from mechanical motion.

13. Anchor IV tubing with additional pieces of tape if necessary. When using transparent dressing, avoid placing tape over dressing.

Prevents accidental displacement of IV cannula.

14. Place date and time of dressing change and size and gauge of cannula directly on dressing.

Provides information about dressing change.

15. Discard equipment, and perform hand hygiene.

Reduces transmission of microorganisms.

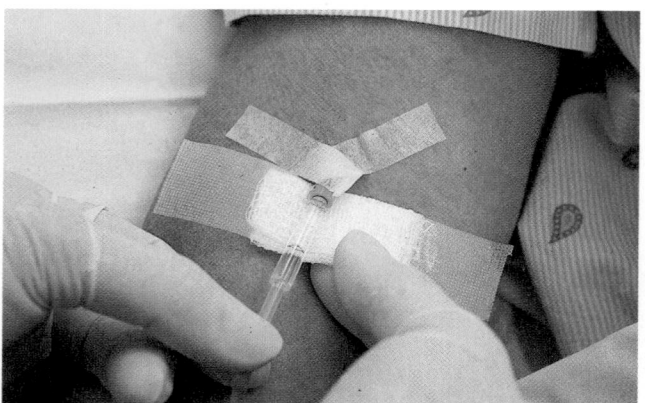
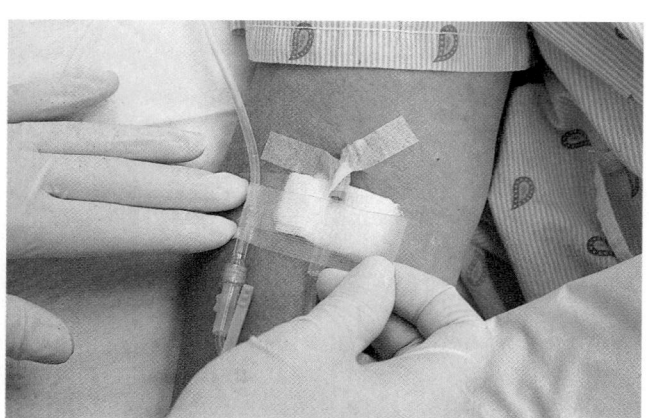

STEP 10b(1) **A,** Place a folded 2×2 under catheter hub. **B,** Secure dressing and loop of IV tubing.

STEP	RATIONALE

■ EVALUATION

1. Ensure flow rate is accurate.

Validates that IV is patent and functioning correctly. Manipulation of cannula and tubing may affect rate of infusion.

2. Inspect condition of IV site, noting color. Palpate for skin temperature, edema, and tenderness.

Complications such as phlebitis and infiltration require discontinuance of IV and location of another site for cannula.

3. Monitor client's body temperature.

Elevated temperature indicates an infection that may be associated with contamination of the venipuncture site.

Recording and Reporting

* Record in nurses' notes time IV dressing was changed and type of dressing used. Include patency of system and description of venipuncture site.
* Report to nurse in charge or oncoming nursing shift that dressing was changed and any significant information about integrity of system.
* Report to physician/IP any complications.

Unexpected Outcomes	Related Interventions
1. IV cannula is infiltrated, as evidenced by decreased flow rate or edema, pallor, or decreased temperature around insertion site.	• Stop infusion, and discontinue IV (see Skill 27-7). • Restart new IV in other extremity if continued therapy is necessary. • Elevate affected extremity.
2. Phlebitis is present, as evidenced by erythema and tenderness along vein pathway.	• Stop infusion, and discontinue IV (see Skill 27-7). • Restart new IV in other extremity if continued therapy is necessary.
3. IV cannula is accidentally removed.	• Restart IV if continued therapy is needed.
4. Client has an elevated temperature.	• Notify physician/IP. IV may be removed and restarted. • Client will be evaluated for source of infection.
5. Insertion site is red and/or edematous and/or painful and/or has presence of exudate, indicating infection at venipuncture site.	• Notify physician/IP. • Culture of the cannula may be ordered. (Confirm before removal of IV.) • Discontinue IV (see Skill 27-7). • Antibiotic therapy may be ordered. (Do not begin until culture is obtained, if ordered.)

Teaching Considerations

* Client should be instructed to notify nurse if skin under dressing or tape becomes reddened, itches, or burns or if dressing becomes compromised.

Pediatric Considerations

* Pediatric clients may not be able to fully understand nurse's explanation. Presence of parent or security toy during procedure can help to decrease fear and increase cooperation. Perform procedure on client's toy or doll first.
* Assistance is required to keep client still and protect IV cannula from dislodgement.

Gerontological Considerations

* In the older adult with fragile skin, prevent skin tears by minimizing the use of tape directly on the skin and applying protectant for adhesive.

Home Care Considerations

* Ensure that there is a reliable caregiver or person at home to provide this IV therapy care.
* Call nurse whenever IV dressing becomes compromised.

SKILL 27-5 Changing Intravenous Solutions

Clients receiving IV therapy may require frequent changing of IV solutions depending upon the rate of infusion and the volume in the container. The nurse must allow adequate time for this procedure and follow proper technique to prevent infection. Fluid containers on ambulatory infusions commonly used with clients in alternate settings may remain longer than 24 hours if aseptic technique is used, the system remains closed without injection ports or add-on tubing, and the medication is stable for the anticipated infusion time (Hankins and others, 2001; INS 2000). The Centers for Disease Control and Prevention (2002) does not have a recommendation for hang time of IV fluids.

DELEGATION CONSIDERATIONS

The skill of changing an intravenous solution should not be delegated to assistive personnel.

- Assistive personnel should inform the nurse when an IV container is near completion.

EQUIPMENT

- ❏ Bottle/bag of IV solution/medication as ordered by physician
- ❏ Time tape

STEP	RATIONALE
ASSESSMENT	
1. Check physician's orders for type of fluid and infusion rate. Follow six rights of medication administration.	Ensures that correct solution will be used. Prevents medication error.
2. If order is written for KVO or to keep open (TKO), note date and time when solution was last changed.	A hang time is no longer recommended by the Centers for Disease Control and Prevention (2002) to ensure sterility of solutions in bag or bottle. Refer to agency policy.
3. Determine the compatibility of all IV fluids and additives by consulting appropriate literature or the pharmacy.	Incompatibilities may lead to precipitate formation and can cause physical, chemical, and therapeutic client changes.
4. Determine client's understanding of the need for continued IV therapy.	Reveals need for client instruction.
5. Determine if current IV access is patent by carefully adjusting the roller clamp to see an increase in flow rate then regulating back to ordered rate. Lowering IV container below level of IV site for presence of blood return (retrograde) is an unreliable indicator. Assess swelling, coolness to touch, or tenderness around IV site, which may indicate infiltration.	If patency is not verified, a new IV access site may be needed. Notify physician. When obstruction is absent, flow rate will increase as roller clamp is adjusted.

- *Critical Decision Point*
  If flow rate does not increase when clamp is adjusted open, systematically check the IV system starting at the IV site up to the IV container for catheter and dressing integrity, tubing kinks, secure connections, inadvertent clamps, tubing puncture, tubing spike communicated with IV container, and distance between IV site and IV container for adequate gravity.

NURSING DIAGNOSES

- Deficient fluid volume
- Risk for infection
- Risk for imbalanced fluid volume
- Deficient knowledge related to purpose for IV therapy

Related factors are individualized based on client's condition or needs.

PLANNING

1. Expected outcomes following completion of procedure:	
• Fluid infusion is correct.	Client receives correct fluid volume.
• IV line remains patent.	Ensures infusion of fluid into intravascular space.

STEP	RATIONALE

2. Have next solution prepared and available at least 1 hour before needed. Check that solution is correct and properly labeled. Check solution expiration date. Observe for precipitate, discoloration, and leakage.

    Adequate planning reduces risk of thrombus formation in vein caused by disruption of flow with empty IV container. Checking prevents medication error.

3. Check client's identification by checking identification band and asking client to state name.

    Ensures correct solution is administered to correct client.

4. Prepare to change solution when less than 25 to 50 ml fluid remains in container.

    Prevents air from entering tubing and vein from clotting from lack of flow. IV containers contain an estimated 5% overfill to compensate for priming of tubing and subsequent container changes.

5. Prepare client and family by explaining the procedure, its purpose, and what is expected of client.

    Decreases anxiety and promotes cooperation.

6. Be sure drip chamber is at least half full.

    Provides fluid to vein while bag is changed.

IMPLEMENTATION

1. Perform hand hygiene.

    Reduces transmission of microorganisms.

2. Prepare new solution for changing. If using plastic bag, remove protective cover from IV tubing port. If using glass bottle, remove metal cap and metal rubber disks.

    Permits quick, smooth, and organized change from old to new solution.

3. Move roller clamp to stop flow rate on existing infusion.

    Prevents solution remaining in drip chamber from emptying while changing solutions.

4. Remove old IV fluid container from IV pole.

    Brings work to nurse's eye level. Prevents fluid from pouring out when spike is removed.

5. Quickly remove spike from old solution container and, without touching tip, insert spike into new container.

    Reduces risk of solution in drip chamber running dry and maintains sterility.

- **Critical Decision Point**
  If spike is contaminated, a new IV tubing set is required. Sterile IV tubing may be used for 72 hours unless compromised.

6. Hang new container of solution.

    Position allows gravity to assist with delivery of fluid into drip chamber.

7. Check for air in tubing. If bubbles form, they can be removed by closing roller clamp, stretching tubing downward, and tapping tubing with finger (bubbles rise in fluid to drip chamber) (see illustration). For a larger amount of air, insert a needleless syringe into a port below the air, and aspirate the air into the syringe. Swab port with alcohol, and allow to dry before inserting syringe into port. Reduce air in tubing by priming slowly instead of allowing a wide-open flow.

    Reduces risk of air embolus. Use of an air-eliminating filter also reduces this risk.

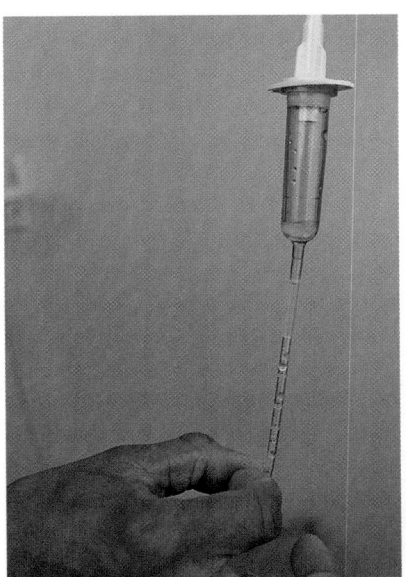

STEP 7 Tap tubing to cause air bubbles to rise up to drip chamber.

STEP	RATIONALE

8. Make sure drip chamber is one-third to one-half full. If the drip chamber is too full, pinch off tubing below drip chamber, invert container, squeeze drip chamber (see illustration), release tubing, and hang bottle.

Reduces risk of air entering tubing. If chamber is completely filled, nurse cannot observe drip rate and rate cannot be accurately regulated.

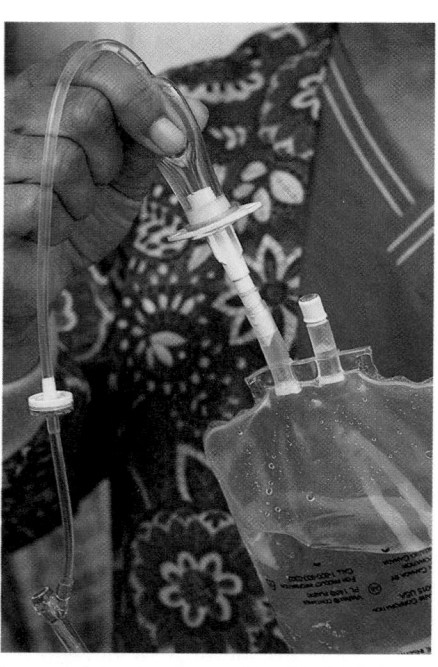

STEP **8** Squeeze drip chamber to fill with fluid. Be sure to leave chamber one-third to one-half full.

9. Regulate flow to prescribed rate.

Maintains measures to restore fluid balance and deliver IV fluid as ordered.

10. Place time label on the side of container, and label with the time hung, the time of completion, and appropriate intervals. If using PVC containers, mark only on the label and not the container.

Provides the nurse with a visual comparison of volume infused compared with prescribed rate of infusion. Ink may leech into PVC containers.

EVAULATION

1. Observe client for signs of overhydration or dehydration to determine response to IV fluid therapy.
2. Periodically check infusion rate.

Provides ongoing evaluation of client's fluid and electrolyte status.
Prevents improper fluid infusion.

Recording and Reporting

- Record amount and type of fluid infused and amount and type of new fluid according to agency policy. A special flow sheet may be used for parenteral fluids.

Unexpected Outcomes	Related Interventions
1. Flow rate is incorrect; client receives too little or too much fluid.	• Readjust infusion rate to ordered rate. • Evaluate client for adverse effects; notify physician. • Determine and correct the cause of the incorrect flow rate. • Use EID when accurate flow rate is critical. • Notify physician if client's anticipated infusion is 100 to 200 ml less than or greater than expected (check agency policy).

Teaching Considerations

* Inform client of new solution, additives, flow rate, and potential side effects.

Home Care Considerations

* Ensure that client is able and willing to self-administer IV therapy (including changing IV solutions) or that there is a reliable caregiver or support person at home to provide this IV therapy care.

* Instruct client and primary caregiver how to perform an IV solution change.
* If medications are delivered to client's home, be sure to instruct client and/or caregiver in proper storage of these IV medications.

SKILL 27-6 Changing Infusion Tubing

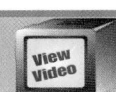

Changing infusion tubing is much simpler and more efficient if changed when hanging a new fluid container. The CDC (2002) recommends changing tubing no more frequently than every 96 hours. The Intravenous Nurses Society (INS) (2000) recommends 72-hour intervals for continuous tubing changes, adding that 48-hour tubing changes may be considered if the rate of catheter-related infection and phlebitis in an institution exceeds 5%. The INS also states that tubing used for inter-mittent infusion through an injection/access port should be changed every 24 hours because both ends of this tubing are manipulated more frequently than tubing used for continuous infusion. If the system has been contaminated, the solution should be changed immediately. Situations arise when the nurse needs to change tubing without hanging a new bag. Such situations include accidental puncture of the tubing or after infusion of blood or a blood product (see Chapter 28).

DELEGATION CONSIDERATIONS

The skill of changing infusion tubing should not be delegated to assistive personnel. The nurse provides information and direction, including:

* Informing assistive personnel to report to the nurse when IV solution container is almost empty.

EQUIPMENT

If a new IV dressing must be applied, assemble additional equipment (see Skill 27-4).

❑ Disposable nonsterile gloves
❑ Label or tape
❑ 2 × 2 gauze (optional)
  Continuous IV Infusion
❑ Infusion tubing
  Intermittent Saline/Heparin Lock
❑ Syringe filled with normal saline or heparin flush solution (check agency policy)
❑ Loop of extension tubing, inspection cap
❑ Antiseptic swab or stick (e.g., chlorhexidene, povidone-iodine, alcohol)

STEP	RATIONALE

ASSESSMENT

1. Determine when new infusion set is needed:
   a. Agency policy will indicate frequency of routine change for IV administration sets and heparin flushes.
   b. Puncture of infusion tubing requires immediate change.
   c. Contamination of tubing requires immediate change.

CDC (2002) and INS (2000) recommend tubing change no more often than 72-hour intervals or whenever tubing has been compromised.

Punctured tubing results in fluid leakage and bacterial contamination.

Contamination of tubing allows entry of pathogens into client's bloodstream.

STEP	RATIONALE
d. Occlusions in tubing requires immediate change. Such occlusions can occur after infusion of packed red cells, whole blood, albumin, other blood components, or administration of incompatible mixtures.	Whole blood or blood component products can occlude or partially occlude tubing because viscous solutions adhere to walls of tubing and decrease size of lumen.
2. Determine client's understanding of the need for continued IV infusions.	Reveals need for client instruction.

NURSING DIAGNOSIS

- Risk for infection

Related factors are individualized based on client's condition or needs.

PLANNING

1. Expected outcomes following completion of procedure:	
• Client's IV site will be free from redness, swelling, pain, or exudate.	Sterile IV tubing prevents microbial growth.
• Client will experience no leakage of solution from tubing.	Intact system decreases risk of microbial contamination.
• Client's IV tubing will be patent.	Brief interruption of IV infusion will not result in thrombus formation.
2. Prepare client and family by explaining the procedure, its purpose, and what is expected of client.	Decreases anxiety, promotes cooperation, and prevents sudden movement of extremity, which could dislodge IV cannula.

IMPLEMENTATION

1. Perform hand hygiene.	Reduces transmission of microorganisms.
2. Open new infusion set, keeping protective coverings over infusion spike and connector and connector site for cannula. Secure all connections.	Provides nurse with ready access to new infusion set and maintains sterility of infusion set.
3. Apply nonsterile, disposable gloves.	Reduces risk of exposure to HIV, hepatitis, and other blood-borne bacteria (CDC, 2002).
4. If cannula hub is not visible, remove IV dressing as directed in Skill 27-4. Do not remove tape securing cannula to skin.	Cannula hub must be accessible to provide smooth transition when removing old and inserting new tubing.
5. For continuous IV infusion:	
a. Move roller clamp on new IV tubing to "off" position.	Prevents spillage of solution after container is spiked.
b. Slow rate of existing infusion by regulating drip rate on old tubing. Be sure rate is at KVO rate.	Prevents complete infusion of solution remaining in tubing. Complete infusion of solution remaining in tubing increases risk of occlusion of IV cannula.
c. Compress drip chamber of old tubing and fill chamber.	Provides surplus of fluid in drip chamber so there is enough fluid to maintain IV patency while changing tubing.
d. Remove existing container from IV pole.	Brings work to nurse's eye level.
e. Invert container and remove old tubing from container; keep spike sterile until new tubing connected. *Option:* Tape old drip chamber to IV pole without contaminating spike.	Allows fluid to continue to flow through IV cannula while nurse is preparing new tubing.
f. Place insertion spike of new tubing into old solution container opening, and hang solution container on IV pole.	Permits flow of fluid from solution into new infusion tubing.

- *Critical Decision Point*
  If spike becomes contaminated, a new IV tubing set is required.

STEP	RATIONALE

g. Compress and release drip chamber on new tubing; slowly fill drip chamber one-third to one-half full (see Skill 27-1).

Allows drip chamber to fill and promotes rapid, smooth flow of solution through new tubing.

h. Slowly open roller clamp, remove protective cap from adapter (if necessary), and flush tubing with solution. Stop infusion. Replace cap. Place end of adapter near client's IV site.

Removes air from tubing and replaces it with fluid. Position equipment for quick smooth connection of new tubing.

i. Turn roller clamp on old tubing to "off" position.

Prevents spillage of fluid as tubing is removed from cannula hub.

6. For Saline/Heparin Lock

a. If a loop or short extension tubing is needed because of an awkward IV site placement, use sterile technique to connect the new injection cap to the loop or tubing.

Prevents transmission of infection.

b. Swab injection cap with antiseptic swab. Insert syringe with 1 to 3 ml saline or heparin flush solution and inject through the injection cap into the loop or short extension tubing.

Removes air to prevent introduction into the vein.

7. *Option:* Place 2 × 2 gauze under cannula hub.

Prevents tubing from accidentally contacting skin and collects blood that may leak from cannula hub.

8. Stabilize cannula hub, and apply pressure over vein just above cannula tip (at least 1½ inches above insertion site). Gently disconnect old tubing from cannula hub, and quickly insert adapter of new tubing into cannula hub (see illustrations).

Allows smooth transition from old to new tubing, minimizing time system open to infection.

A

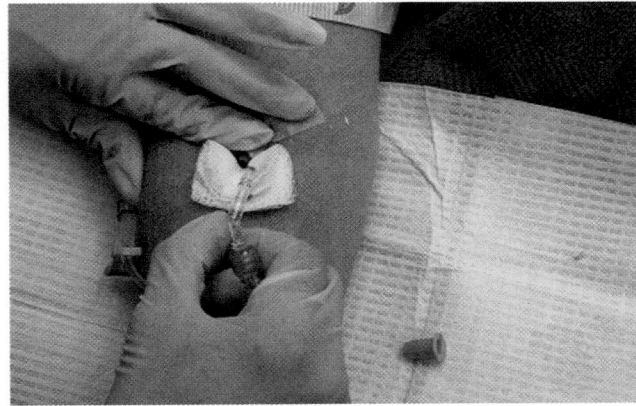

C

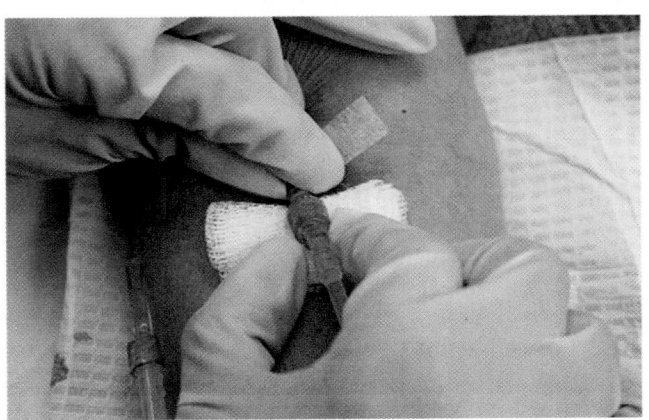

B

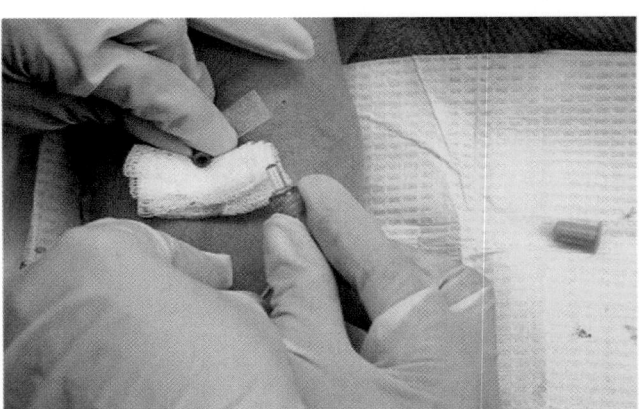

STEP 8k A, Disconnect old tubing. **B,** While compressing vein, attach end of new tubing. **C,** Make sure connection is secure.

STEP	RATIONALE

l. Open roller clamp on new tubing, allowing solution to run rapidly for 30 to 60 seconds, then regulate IV drip according to physician's orders, and monitor rate hourly (see illustration). *Optional:* Connect new tubing to EID and regulate.

Ensures patency of cannula and maintenance of venous access.

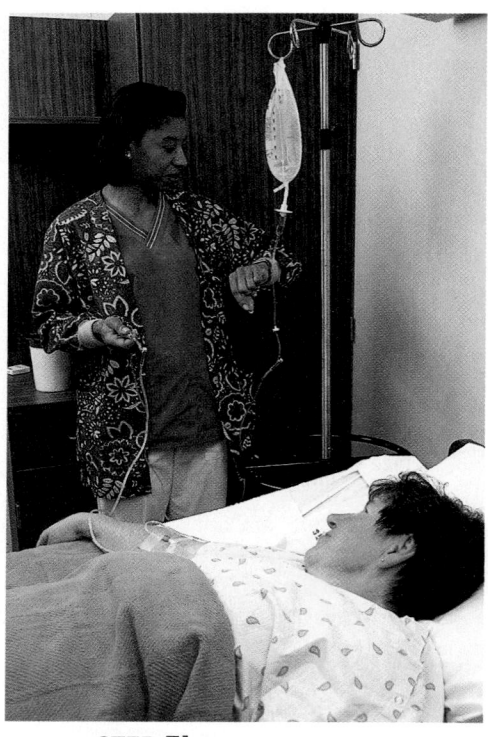

STEP 5l Regulate flow of IV.

m. Attach a piece of tape or a preprinted label with date and time of tubing change onto tubing below the drip chamber.

Provides reference to determine next time for tubing change.

n. Form a loop of tubing, and secure it to client's arm with a strip of tape.

Avoids accidental pulling against site and cannula movement.

o. Remove and discard 2 × 2 gauze (if used) and old IV tubing. If necessary, apply new dressing (see Skill 27-4). Dispose of gloves. Perform hand hygiene.

Reduces transmission of microorganisms.

Recording and Reporting

- Record changing of tubing and solution on client's record. A special parenteral therapy flow sheet may be used.
- Mark a piece of tape or preprinted label with date and time of tubing change, and attach to tubing below the level of drip chamber.

Unexpected Outcomes	Related Interventions
1. Decreased or absent flow of IV fluid is indicated by decreased rate.	• Assess IV infusion system for patency. • Recalibrate drip rate on new tubing. • Assess IV site for infiltration.

Teaching Considerations
- Instruct client to notify nurse if fluid leaks around IV site or from the tubing itself or if tubing separates from cannula.

Home Care Considerations
- Instruct client or primary caregiver in procedure for performing a sterile IV tubing change.

- Ensure that client is able and willing to change infusion tubing and maintain IV access site or that there is a reliable person at home to provide this IV therapy care.

SKILL 27-7   Discontinuing Peripheral Intravenous Access

View Video

The technique for discontinuing a peripheral IV line is relatively simple. The nurse follows infection control guidelines to minimize the chance of the client acquiring an infection. In addition, the nurse takes precautions to not cause discomfort or injury to the client.

DELEGATION CONSIDERATIONS
The skill of discontinuing a peripheral IV should not be delegated to assistive personnel.
- Assistive personnel should be instructed to report any bleeding after the cannula has been removed.

EQUIPMENT
- ❑ Disposable gloves
- ❑ Sterile 2 × 2 or 4 × 4 gauze sponge
- ❑ Antiseptic swab
- ❑ Tape

STEP	RATIONALE
ASSESSMENT	
1. Observe IV site for signs and symptoms of infection, infiltration, or phlebitis.	Findings will determine if therapy is needed following cannula removal.
2. Review physician's orders for discontinuation of IV.	Order required for discontinuation of IV therapy. The order for cannula removal may be implied.
3. Assess client's understanding of the need for IV to be discontinued.	Determines need for instruction.
NURSING DIAGNOSIS	
• Risk for infection	

Related factors are individualized based on client's condition or needs.

STEP	RATIONALE
PLANNING	
1. Expected outcomes following completion of procedure:	
• IV will be removed with minimal trauma to client.	Hemostasis will be maintained.
• IV site will remain free of infection.	Venipuncture wound properly cleansed.
2. Explain procedure to client, describing sensation (burning) to be felt when catheter is removed. Explain that affected extremity must be held still and how long procedure will take (about 5 minutes or less).	Prepares client to cooperate during procedure.
IMPLEMENTATION	
1. Perform hand hygiene. Apply disposable gloves.	Reduces transmission of microorganisms.
2. Turn IV tubing roller clamp to "off" position or turn EID off and then turn roller clamp to "off" position.	Prevents spillage of IV fluid.

STEP	RATIONALE
3. Remove IV site dressing, stabilizing IV device (see Skill 27-4). Then remove tape securing cannula.	Exposes cannula with minimal discomfort.
4. Hold cannula, and clean site with antimicrobial swab.	Removes secretions around skin puncture site.
5. Place clean sterile gauze over venipuncture site, apply light pressure, and remove cannula by pulling straight away from insertion site in a slow, steady motion (see illustration). Keep the cannula parallel to the skin during withdrawal. Inspect catheter for intactness after removal.	Dry pad causes less irritation to the puncture site. Prevents damage to client's vein; determines if catheter tip is intact. Tips of catheter can break off, causing an embolus, and emergency situation. Notify physician/IP immediately if tip is broken.

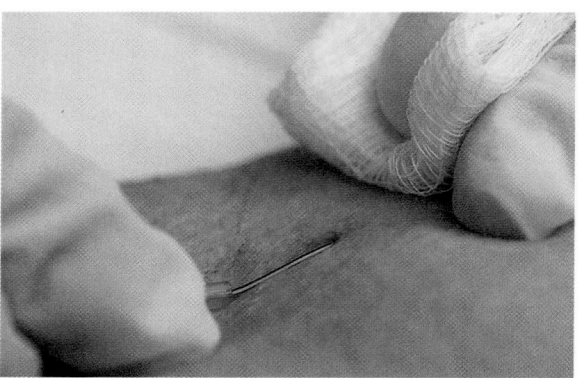

STEP 5 Withdraw IV catheter.

- **Critical Decision Point**
  Do not raise or lift catheter before it is completely out of the vein to avoid trauma or hematoma formation.

6. Keep gauze in place, and apply continuous pressure to site for 2 to 3 minutes.	Controls bleeding and hematoma formation. Contraction is enhanced by pressure to site for at least 2 to 3 minutes (Chukhraev and Grekov, 2000).

- **Critical Decision Point**
  If client has received anticoagulants (e.g., low-dose aspirin, warfarin sodium [Coumadin], heparin), or has a low platelet count, apply steady pressure for 5 to 10 minutes and assess bleeding.

7. Apply clean folded gauze dressing over insertion site, and secure with tape.	Maintains pressure to prevent bleeding and reduces bacterial entry into puncture site.
8. Discard used supplies, remove gloves, and perform hand hygiene.	Reduces transmission of microorganisms.

EVALUATION

1. Observe site for evidence of bleeding through dressing.	Additional pressure may be needed.
2. Observe site for redness, pain, drainage, or swelling.	May indicate infection or phlebitis at old IV site.

Recording and Reporting

- Record in nurses' notes the time peripheral IV was discontinued. Include site assessment information and status of catheter including gauge, length, and catheter tip integrity.
- Report to nurse in charge or oncoming nursing shift that IV was discontinued and any significant complications.

Unexpected Outcomes	Related Interventions
1. Venipuncture site is inflamed and/or has purulent drainage.	• Remove IV. • Notify physician. • Cultures may be ordered. • Cover site with dressing if drainage present. • If area is infected, initiate appropriate wound care protocol (see Chapter 37).
2. Catheter tip is missing upon withdrawal.	• Apply tourniquet high on the extremity to restrict mobility of emboli. • Notify physician immediately.

Teaching Considerations

• Instruct client to notify nurse if bleeding or drainage is noted at insertion site or if pain or tenderness is experienced. Postinfusion phlebitis may occur 48 to 96 hours after catheter removal.

SKILL 27-8 Caring for Central Venous Access Devices

Clients with chronic disease often need long-term IV therapy, which requires safe, repeated access to the venous system for administration of drugs, fluids, nutrition, and blood products. Frequent venipuncture and multiple IV lines pose problems and risks, including infection, pain, and bruising. Clients with chronic disease are generally more susceptible to infection and bleeding. Clients receiving multiple doses of chemotherapeutic drugs experience vein sclerosis or hardening. Eventually no suitable peripheral veins remain for drug administration.

The need for safe and convenient long-term IV therapy has led to the development of catheters and ports designed for long-term access to the venous or arterial systems. These devices generally are placed in the central venous system. The nurse must be able to maintain the integrity of central venous access devices (CVADs) and educate clients about the care and maintenance for the duration of their use.

To manage long-term IV therapy effectively the nurse must be familiar with the various types of CVADs. Knowing the type of CVADs can be confusing because catheters are often referred to by brand name instead of type and placement (e.g., Hickman, Groshong, Raaf, Port-a-Cath). Also, the literature does not indicate universal acceptance of one term to describe a particular catheter. For this skill these CVADs will be divided into three types: tunneled and percutaneous central venous catheters (CVCs) and implanted infusion ports. CVCs are threaded into a large vein, typically the internal or external jugulars or the superior vena cava that leads to the right atrium of the heart. The large vessel lumen minimizes the

risks of vessel irritation, inflammation, or sclerosis that commonly occur when smaller peripheral veins are used. These catheters are used to administer IV fluids, antibiotics, chemotherapy, and parenteral nutrition, to infuse medications and blood products, and to obtain blood samples.

Tunneled CVCs are surgically inserted with the client in the operating room under general or local anesthesia. First a tunnel is made through subcutaneous tissue, usually between the clavicle and nipple (Figure 27-7). The subcutaneous tunnel allows the catheter to remain in place longer because it creates space between the end of the catheter and the actual vein. The risk of infection is lower. Next, the catheter tip is inserted into the subclavian vein and threaded into the superior vena cava (see Figure 27-8). The catheter is held in place with a Dacron cuff that surrounds the catheter located on the chest wall. These catheters have single, double, or triple lumens, which are hollow tubes inside the catheter that allow simultaneous administration of several infusions.

The second type of CVC is the percutaneously placed catheter. The percutaneous catheter is inserted directly through the skin and into a large vein of the neck, usually the internal or external jugular (Figure 27-9), or superior vena cava (see Chapter 31). If not inserted directly into a central vein, a CVC may also be inserted through the cephalic or basilic veins and threaded into the superior vena cava. Various types of percutaneously placed central catheters are available. The length of time catheters are left in place depends on the type and the manufacturer's recommendations, the

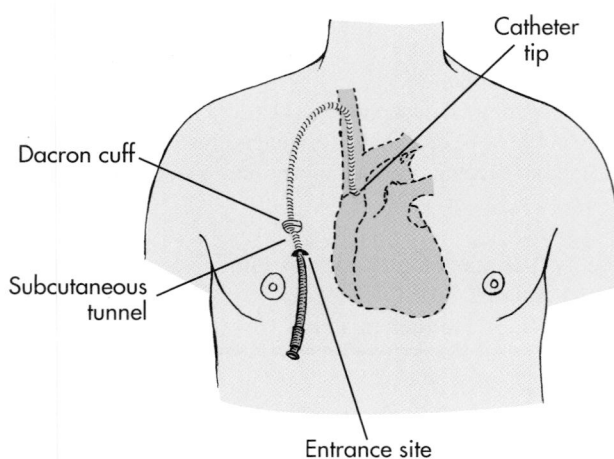

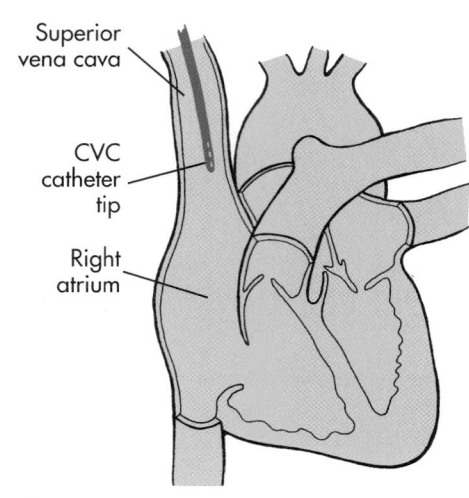

FIGURE **27-7** Small-gauge tunneled catheter is in place, threaded into superior vena cava.

FIGURE **27-8** Catheter tip from CVAD lies in superior vena cava.

length of therapy, and the condition/ functionality of the catheter.

Another type of CVC is the implanted infusion port, which consists of a portal body, a central septum, a reservoir, and a catheter (Figure 27-10, *A*). The port is also available with a double lumen catheter. The physician implants the infusion port under sterile conditions in an operating room with the client under local anesthesia. The infusion port usually rests in a subcutaneous pocket in the infraclavicular fossa, and the catheter is inserted into a large vein and threaded into the superior vena cava (Figure 27-10, *B*). The port can be easily palpated to determine placement. Specially designed non-coring Huber needles (straight or with 90-degree angles) are inserted through the skin to enter the port (Figure 27-10, *C*). Implanted infusion ports are used for administration of injections and for continuous infusions of all types: medications, chemotherapy, parenteral nutrition, and blood products. When not in use, no external catheter is present, and the port manufacturers recommend the port be heparinized every 4 weeks to maintain its patency. No other care is required for a port that is not being used.

Care of CVADs is simple as long as nurses and clients are aware of the purpose and function of the devices and the

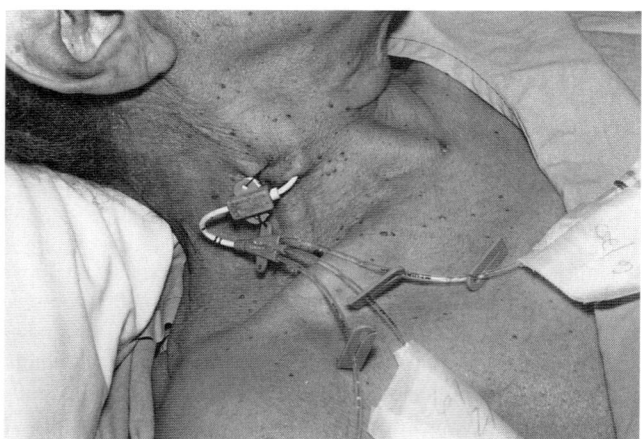

FIGURE **27-9** CVC placed in jugular vein.

two most common complications, infection and cannula occlusion. In the home, most clients learn to use clean technique for dressing changes and catheter care. Clients can learn to initiate infusions, heparinize devices, and discontinue infusions.

DELEGATION CONSIDERATIONS

The skill of caring for a central vascular access device in an acute care setting should not be delegated to assistive personnel. The nurse provides information and direction, including:

* Instructing assistive personnel in the signs and symptoms of CVC complications to report.

EQUIPMENT
Blood Drawing

❑ Antimicrobial swabs (e.g., chlorhexidine, povidone-iodine, alcohol preparation swabs)
❑ Four to five syringes (10 ml)
❑ Sterile drape
❑ Saline flush
❑ Heparin flush (100 units/ml)
❑ Plastic clamp
❑ Sterile Huber injectable (20 to 22 gauge)
❑ Sterile injectable (20 to 22 gauge)

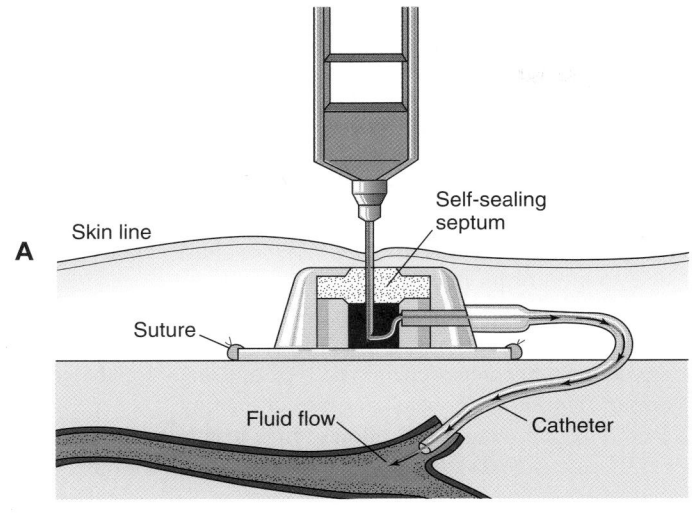

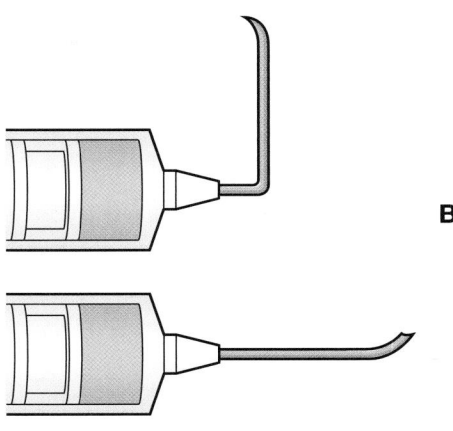

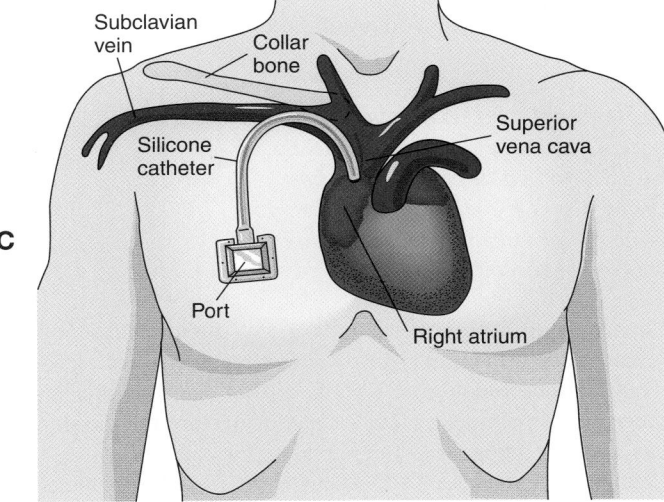

FIGURE **27-10** **A,** Cross section of implantable port showing access of the port with the Huber needle. **B,** Two Huber needles used to enter implanted port. The 90-degree needle is used for top-entry ports for continuous infusion. **C,** Implant port and catheter.

EQUIPMENT, cont'd

Blood Drawing, cont'd
❑ Blood tubes, labels, requisitions
❑ Gloves, gowns, masks

Administration of Drugs, Fluids, Blood Products
❑ Antimicrobial swabs (e.g., chlorhexidine, povidone-iodine, alcohol swabs)
❑ Drug, fluid, blood product to be infused
❑ Sterile IV tubing
❑ IV pole, infusion pump, or blood pump
❑ Sterile drape
❑ Saline flush
❑ Sterile Huber safety needle (infusion port only)
❑ Sterile needleless access
❑ Dressing supplies as indicated
❑ Gloves, gown, masks

Dressing Change
❑ Antimicrobial swabs (e.g., chlorhexidine, povidone-iodine, alcohol swabs)
❑ Gloves (clean and sterile), mask

Dressing Change, cont'd
❑ Tape
❑ Transparent occlusive dressing (transparent dressing)
❑ Sterile gauze 4 × 4 or 2 × 2 sponges (gauze dressing)

Heparinization
❑ Antimicrobial swabs (e.g., chlorhexidine, povidone-iodine, alcohol preparation swabs)
❑ Access syringe (5 ml or 10 ml—see agency policy)
❑ Saline flush
❑ Heparin flush (100 units/ml)
❑ Plastic clamp
❑ Sterile needleless access

Discontinuance of a Percutaneous CVC
❑ Antimicrobial swabs
❑ Petroleum-based or antimicrobial ointment
❑ Gloves and gown, mask, goggles (based on risk)
❑ Sterile gauze 4 × 4 or 2 × 2 sponges
❑ Sterile hypoallergenic tape
❑ Suture removal kit (if sutures are in place)

STEP	RATIONALE

▮ ASSESSMENT

1. Assess stage of client's disease and plan of therapy by review of the medical record.

   Allows nurse to understand need for vascular access in treatment of disease and in evaluation of response to therapy and to determine need to educate client about disease process and plan of therapy using CVAD.

2. Review physician's order, and assess treatment schedule: times for administration of fluids, drugs, blood products, nutrition, and blood sampling.

   Allows nurse to schedule use of CVAD for simultaneous administration of products, to educate client about schedule of administration, and to provide for comfort and reduction of anxiety about therapy.

3. Assess type of CVAD in place.

   Care and management depends on type and size of catheter or port, number of lumens, purpose of therapy.

4. Assess need to use CVAD for blood sampling.

   Scheduling sampling needs allows nurse to minimize number of times CVAD system is entered and allows for timely collection of specimens to evaluate therapy. Risk of infection increases with multiple entries into vascular system, especially in immunocompromised clients.

● *Critical Decision Point*

In most situations, several tests can be run from one blood tube sample. For example, potassium, calcium, and magnesium test results can all be obtained from one full tube of blood versus three separate tubes. Always anticipate the need for a blood test (e.g., blood cultures if a client has developed an elevated temperature). If your next task is to draw blood for electrolyte results, you could eliminate reaccessing the CVAD at a later time by asking the physician if blood cultures are also to be drawn. Consultation with laboratory services can provide specific instructions.

5. Assess CVAD placement site for skin integrity and signs of infection (i.e., redness, swelling, tenderness, exudate, bleeding).

   Clients requiring long-term IV therapy often have conditions placing them at risk for alterations in skin integrity and immune function. CVAD site is an insult to skin integrity and provides access for pathogens through the skin as well as pathogens to migrate from the catheter.

6. Assess for proper function of CVAD before therapy: integrity of catheter, septum port (if used), ability to irrigate or infuse fluid, ability to aspirate blood.

   Ensures proper function of CVAD with minimal complications.

7. Assess need for irrigation and dressing change by referring to medical record, nurses' notes, agency policies, and manufacturer's recommended guidelines for use.

   Provides guidelines for maintaining catheter patency and preventing infection.

8. Assess client's reaction to CVAD and knowledge of purpose, care, and maintenance. In cases where catheter has been in place for a time, ask client to discuss steps in care and to perform procedure (e.g., catheter site cleansing or dressing change).

   Determines client's level of understanding.
   Allows nurse to educate client for home care of CVAD.

9. Assess client's understanding of discontinuance of CVAD.

   Promotes cooperation with procedure.

▮ NURSING DIAGNOSES

- Risk for infection
- Impaired skin integrity

- Risk for injury
- Deficient knowledge regarding use of CVAD

Related factors are individualized based on client's condition or needs.

STEP	RATIONALE

PLANNING

1. Expected outcomes following completion of procedure.
   - Site is intact and has no redness or swelling.
   - Systemic signs of infection (fever, malaise, increased WBC) are absent.
   - Fluids, medications, blood products infuse without difficulty.
   - Blood can be aspirated from catheter.
   - Catheter and connecting tube are intact.
   - Catheter tip is correctly placed, as confirmed by x-ray examination.
   - Client and family are able to explain the purpose of CVAD therapy and perform dressing changes and skin care.
2. Position client in comfortable position with head slightly elevated.
3. Explain procedure and purpose to client and family. Instruct client to be still during procedure.

Local signs of infection are absent.
Catheter system remains free of microbial growth.

Patency of catheter is maintained.

Indicates patency and placement.
Integrity of system is maintained.
Correct placement minimizes chances of malplacement or occlusion.
Demonstrates that client and family have an understanding and competency for caring for CVAD.

Provides access to client. Infusion port requires palpation.

Decreases anxiety and promotes cooperation.

IMPLEMENTATION

1. **Administration of Infusions or Sampling of Blood From Implanted Infusion Port**
   a. Perform hand hygiene. Mask self and client. Not all institutions require masking of the client. The client may, instead, be asked to turn head away from port site. Refer to agency policy.
   b. Prepare sterile field (see Chapter 9), and open sterile supplies. Prepare 10-ml syringe filled with saline.
   c. Using antimicrobial swab, prepare client's skin overlying port septum, moving first in a horizontal pattern, secondly with a vertical plane, and the final swab in a circular pattern moving outward in concentric circles from insertion site out. Allow to dry.
   d. Apply sterile gloves.
   e. Apply sterile drape to port site (may be optional in some agencies).
   f. Attach one end of sterile extension tubing to syringe, and attach appropriate-size Huber needle to other end. Fill tubing with saline solution.
   g. Palpate port septum with nondominant hand, observing aseptic technique (see illustration). The dominant hand remains sterile for safety Huber needle insertion.

Reduces transfer of microorganisms, prevents spread of airborne microorganisms while access to system is exposed.

Provides work space for use of sterile items.

Rigorous skin preparation is necessary to prevent introducing microbes into system. This pattern allows penetration of the antiseptic solutions into the cracks and fissures of the epidermal layer of the skin (Crosby and Mares, 2001).

Prevents transmission of microorganisms by nurse's hands.
Provides sterile work area.

Removes all air from tubing, reducing risk of air embolus.

Septum port must be located to ensure proper Huber safety needle entry.

STEP	RATIONALE

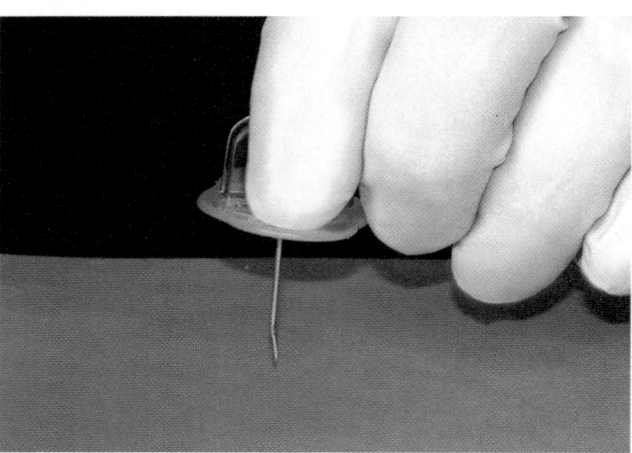

A

B

STEP **1g A,** Palpate port septum before inserting Huber needle. **B,** Close-up of insertion of Huber needle. (**B** Courtesy B. Braun Medical, Inc.)

h. While holding wings or needle hub, insert Huber safety needle through skin at a 90-degree angle, and push firmly down until needle penetrates silicone septum and is in portal chamber.

Do not push too hard. If tip of the needle bends, septum can be damaged upon removal of needle.
Safety needle device should be used.

i. Check for proper placement by aspirating blood return with the attached syringe (see illustration).

j. If a good blood return is present, flush tubing with remaining saline in syringe. If a blood return is not obtained, fill another syringe, and attempt to flush port with 10 ml normal saline.

If blood is unable to be aspirated, it may signal presence of clots in the catheter lumen and/or at catheter tip. Forceful irrigation against resistance may propel clotted blood into the client's vascular system.

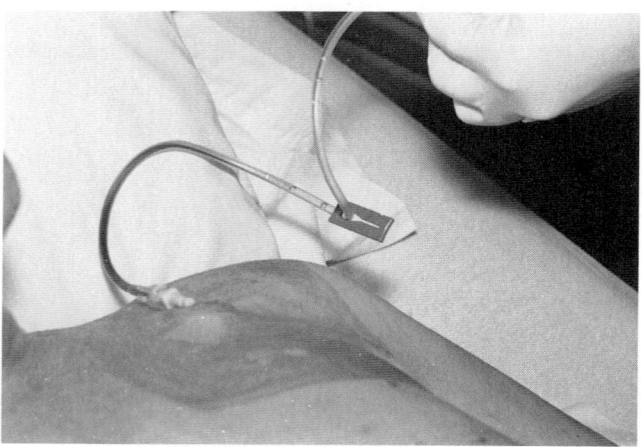

STEP **1i** Aspirate blood return from port.

STEP	RATIONALE

- *Critical Decision Point*
  Do not irrigate forcefully if resistance is felt. If unable to flush, reposition needle without completely withdrawing it from the skin. If Huber needle is withdrawn, prepare skin for new insertion with a sterile Huber needle. Never use a syringe less than 10 ml because the pounds per square inch (psi) pressure is too high.

k. Observe for swelling. If swelling occurs around needle insertion site, stop procedure, and notify physician.

This may indicate that needle is not in port, but in surrounding subcutaneous tissue, or that there is a tear in the catheter.

l. To draw blood samples, first aspirate and discard 5 ml of serous fluid.

Avoids dilution of sample.

m. Withdraw necessary blood for each sample, using two 10-ml syringes equal to total volume withdrawn.

Eliminates repeated need to puncture infusion port for sampling.

n. Flush port with 10 ml normal saline. (Refer to agency policy.)

Any fluid other than normal saline has potential for clotting blood or precipitating in catheter.

o. If continuous infusion is not indicated, heparinize port by flushing with 3 ml heparin (100 units/ml) flush solution or amount and solution per agency policy using positive pressure or injection cap valve.

Prevents clot formation.

p. If IV fluid will be continuously administered, secure Huber needle with Steri-Strips (see illustration) or commercial securement device. Cover the Huber needle and insertion site with a transparent dressing. If Huber needle does not sit flush on skin, place folded 2 × 2 gauze under hub, and then cover with dressing.

Prevents accidental dislodging of needle at insertion site.
Gauze underneath transparent dressing is considered a gauze dressing and should be changed every 48 hours.

q. Connect IV infusion tubing with sterile tubing connected to Huber needle.

IV infusion system should be closed to maintain sterility.

r. Regulate IV infusion as ordered.

Maintains desired fluid intake and patency of catheter.

s. If infusion is intermittent, turn off infusion, and deaccess port by withdrawing needle (see illustration). Discard needle in appropriate safety container.

Avoids needle-stick injury.
Reduces transmission of microorganisms.

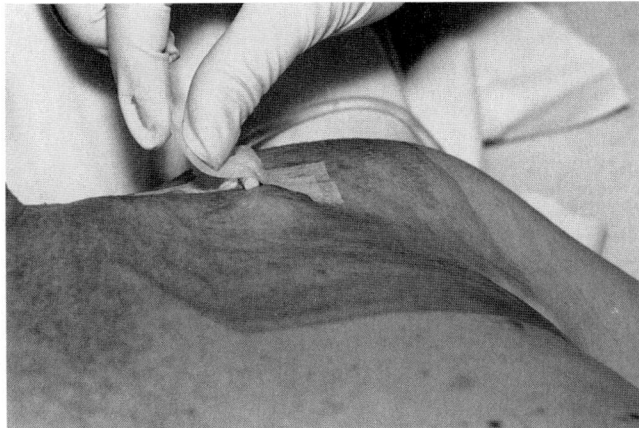

STEP **1p** Secure Huber needle with Steri-Strips.

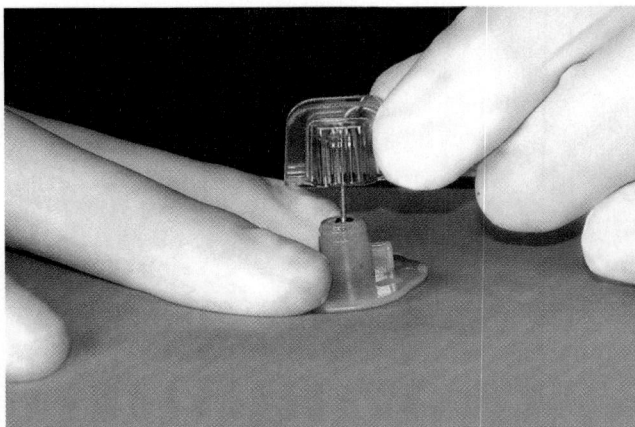

STEP **1s** Demonstration of how to deaccess port; first stabilize base, and then withdraw needle. The safety clip will automatically activate. (Courtesy B. Braun Medical, Inc.)

STEP	RATIONALE
t. Dispose of all soiled supplies and used equipment. Send labeled specimens to laboratory. Remove gloves, and perform hand hygiene.	Reduces spread of microorganisms.
2. Administration of Infusion or Sampling of Blood From Central Venous Catheter	
a. Perform hand hygiene.	Reduces transmission of microorganisms.
b. Apply gloves. Apply gown and goggles (check agency policy) if blood sampling.	Prevents transfer of body fluids.
c. Use antimicrobial preparation swabs to cleanse injection cap or catheter hub according to agency policy.	Prevents introduction of microorganisms into catheter.
d. Prepare two syringes with 10 ml normal saline each.	Used to flush catheter.
e. If injection cap will be removed, clamp catheter.	Catheter must be clamped if injection cap is removed to prevent entrance of air.
f. If injection cap is in place, insert needleless access of syringe containing 10 ml normal saline, aspirate for blood return and if present, flush. If injection cap is removed, connect syringe tip to catheter hub, release clamp, aspirate for blood return and if present, flush with positive pressure, and reclamp.	Aspiration of blood return indicates catheter placement in venous system. Flushing ensures patency of catheter. Catheter must always be clamped during change of syringe or tubing to prevent exposure to air.

• *Critical Decision Point*

If catheter is occluded and resistance is felt, do not force flushing. Vigorous flushing may cause catheter rupture or catheter emboli.

STEP	RATIONALE
g. Connect syringe for blood sampling, and release clamp. Aspirate 5 ml fluid, reclamp, and discard aspirate.	Avoids diluting sample.
h. Attach or insert syringe of size equal to volume of blood sample to withdraw to catheter. Release clamp. Withdraw necessary blood for samples, and reclamp.	Samples should be collected at one time to minimize time with open catheter system.
i. Attach or insert syringe filled with 10 ml normal saline to catheter. If clamp is present, release, flush vigorously, and reclamp.	Catheter should be cleared of all blood or medications that may clog catheter lumen or precipitate with additives in IV fluids.
j. If no continuous infusion is indicated, flush catheter with heparin or normal saline as appropriate. Connect syringe containing 5 ml heparin (100 units/ml) or normal saline flush solution. If clamp is present, release, flush with positive pressure, and reclamp.	A catheter not in use must be flushed to prevent clot formation. This is commonly done with heparin; however, Groshong catheters are flushed with normal saline only.

STEP	RATIONALE
k. Attach new cap to end of catheter, and remove clamp.	Maintains sterile seal to catheter.
l. If IV fluids will be administered, connect IV tubing to end of catheter, being sure both ends are sterile.	IV system should be closed to maintain sterility.
m. Regulate IV infusion as ordered.	Maintains ordered fluid intake and keeps catheter patent.
n. Secure all tubing connections.	Prevents accidental tubing disconnection and catheter displacement. Luer-lok connections should be used.
o. Dispose of soiled equipment and used supplies. Remove gloves, and perform hand hygiene.	Reduces transmission of microorganisms.
3. Dressing Change	
a. Perform hand hygiene, and apply clean gloves.	Reduces transmission of microorganisms.
b. Mask self and client, if indicated (check agency policy).	Prevents exposure of catheter exit or placement site to airborne microorganisms.
c. Carefully remove old dressing in the direction the catheter was inserted.	Remove tape carefully because clients frequently have alterations in skin integrity.
d. Inspect placement or exit site for signs of redness, swelling, inflammation, tenderness, or exudate.	This is a potential site of infection. Drainage or inflammation indicates catheter site infection.
e. If catheter is tunneled, palpate Dacron cuff in subcutaneous tunnel.	Documenting position of cuff verifies proper placement.
f. Inspect catheter and hub for intactness, and remove clean gloves.	Catheter may become torn, cut, displaced, cracked, or split.
g. Perform hand hygiene, and open dressing kit in a sterile manner (see Chapter 9). Most agencies have dressing kits that contain all needed dressing change supplies.	
h. Apply sterile gloves.	Prevents direct transmission of microorganisms to skin exit site.
i. Clean placement or exit site with antimicrobial swab, moving first in a horizontal pattern, secondly with a vertical plane, and the final swab in a circular pattern moving outward in concentric circles from insertion site out. Allow to dry (see illustration).	It is impossible to sterilize skin. Organisms that accumulate must be eliminated by mechanical and chemical means. Mechanical friction in this pattern allows penetration of the antiseptic solution into the cracks and fissures of the epidermal layer of the skin (Crosby and Mares, 2001).
	Antiseptic solutions should be allowed to air-dry completely to effectively reduce microbial counts (INS, 2000). If antiseptic agents are used in combination, allow each to air-dry separately.

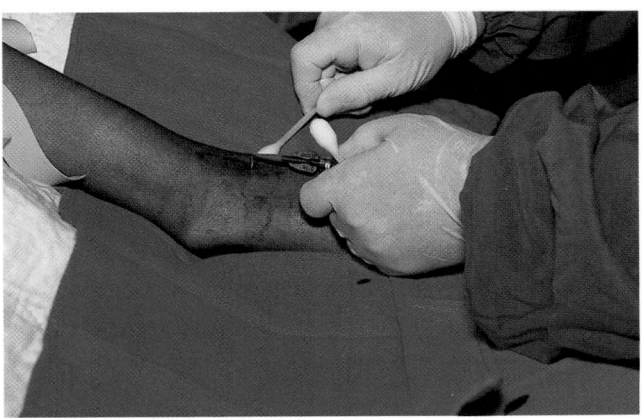

STEP **3i** Cleanse central venous access device site.

STEP	RATIONALE
j. Redress site using sterile gauze and tape or transparent dressing as indicated (see Skill 27-4).	Prevents entrance of bacteria into exit or placement site.
k. Secure connections.	Prevents accidental pulling and displacement. Luer-lok connections should be used.
l. Label date, time of dressing change, and size of cannula in place.	Documents dressing change. Provides guideline for time of next change.
m. Dispose of soiled supplies; remove gloves, and perform hand hygiene.	Reduces transmission of microorganisms.
4. Discontinuance of a Percutaneous CVC	
a. Confirm physician orders.	CVCs require physician orders for removal.
b. Gather supplies, and place on designated area. Clamp catheter, or turn off infusion.	Ensures that all supplies needed are available in area.
c. Position client in supine position. If client has difficulty tolerating supine position, may delay positioning until actual withdrawal.	Reduces gravitational release of venous fluid at exit site.
d. Don gloves and personal protective equipment.	Standard precautions are necessary when blood exposure is possible.
e. Remove dressing, being careful not to remove CVC.	Dressing removal exposes CVC site and provides unobstructed access.
f. Apply antimicrobial swabs starting at CVC site and working outward.	Cleanses CVC site to avoid introduction of microorganisms.
g. If sutures are present, use sterile scissors to remove. Dispose of scissors in sharps container.	Sutures must be removed before removal of CVC. Immediate sharps disposal reduces risk of injury.
h. Place 2 × 2 gauze sponge with petroleum-based or antimicrobial ointment on CVC site.	Provides protected covering when CVC is removed to absorb blood and serous fluid (INS, 2000).
i. Have client perform Valsalva maneuver as you slowly and steadily remove CVC.	Promotes negative intrathoracic pressure thus reducing the risk of introduction of air into the venous system.
j. When CVC completely removed, apply firm pressure on IV site.	Pressure on IV site assists in clot formation. Clients who have been on anticoagulant therapy may require 5 minutes of pressure.
k. Position sterile gauze (4 × 4 or 2 × 2) over site and secure with sterile hypoallergenic tape.	Protects insertion site from microorganisms.
l. Inspect integrity of catheter tip.	CVCs may fracture or shear.
m. Dispose of CVC and other IV equipment in appropriate manner.	Reduces transmission of blood.

STEP	RATIONALE

EVALUATION

1. When continuous infusions are administered, observe and calculate drip rate hourly. Note ease with which fluid rate can be increased.

2. Routinely assess vital signs of client, noting changes symptomatic of infection.

3. Observe catheter or port exit or placement site when sites are exposed (see Table 19-4).

4. Observe all catheter connection points periodically.

5. Inspect condition of catheter and connection tubing daily for leaks, holes, tears, splits, or cracked hubs.

6. Consult x-ray examination reports for catheter placement.

7. Evaluate ability of client and family to provide care and maintain catheter or infusion port through discussion and return demonstrations of dressing changes and skin care. Determine need for restrictions on daily activities.

To maintain proper fluid infusion, desired drip rate should be regulated continuously. A gradual slowing in rate or inability to increase rate may indicate catheter occlusion.

Catheter-related sepsis can cause fever, chills, flushed skin, tachycardia.

Continual monitoring for signs of inflammation or infection is essential.

An intact system prevents accidental blood loss or entrance of air.

Break in integrity of system predisposes client to hemorrhage or air embolus.

A routine chest x-ray examination can locate position of catheter tip.

Measures client's ability to care for self and any additional learning needs.

Recording and Reporting

- Chart date and time of medications, blood products, parenteral fluids given, and blood samples obtained on medical record.
- Chart condition of exit site or port insertion site, including skin integrity, signs of infection, placement, integrity, and functionality of catheter.
- Chart dressing change procedure, label date, time, type, and size of Huber needle in port.
- Chart patency of catheter, ability to draw blood, and difficulty with infusions.
- Chart measures taken to educate client in self-care and response to education.
- Chart date, time, and condition of CVC when discontinued, description of site and how site was dressed.
- In emergency situations (damage to catheter, loss of patency, blood loss, air embolus, septic episode, local signs of infection), notify nursing or medical personnel immediately. Instruct client and family when to contact medical personnel.

Unexpected Outcomes	Related Interventions
1. For catheter complications see Table 27-4.	
2. Client or family member is unable to explain or perform CVAD care.	• May indicate need for home care referral or additional instruction.

Teaching Considerations

- Discuss and provide written emergency measures and telephone numbers of health care personnel to be used in case of catheter damage, displacement, swelling, redness, or leakage at insertion site; occlusion of port or catheter; temperature above 100° F; and shaking chills.
- Provide written instruction for dressing changes, inspection of insertion site, irrigations, and tubing changes.
- Arrange for instruction and return demonstration of skills by client or caregiver.
- Have client or caregiver maintain a list of caregivers and telephone numbers (e.g., physician, nurse, social worker, pharmacist, dietitian).

Pediatric Considerations

- Chlorhexidine as a skin disinfectant is not recommended in neonates less than 7 days or gestational age less than 26 weeks (CDC, 2002).
- Amount and dosage of flush solution (heparin/saline) varies with age and size.

Geriatric Considerations

- Skin protectants promote adhesion and skin protection.
- Pathological atrophy of the veins may lead to hidden lethal bleeding into the chest cavity when the central venous structures are injured by trauma (Schelper, 2003).

Home Care Considerations

- Initiate early referral for discharge planning to social service, counselor, or home care coordinator for assessment of resources.
- Determine client and caregiver's acceptance of client's altered body image.
- Provide client with written list of providers for supplies and equipment.
- Assess willingness and ability of primary caregiver to assist in home management of device. Acceptance of altered body image influences primary caregiver's readiness to assist with care.
- Instruct client and caregiver in adaptations of hospital procedures that can be made at home (e.g., good hand hygiene instead of sterile gloves).
- Discuss troubleshooting and emergency care routines with caregiver in home.
- Assess home environment, and determine suitable area for dressing changes, avoiding areas where contaminants are potential hazards.
- Determine ability of client to meet expenses of equipment involved in caring for CVCs.

FOCUS *on* CLINICAL PRACTICE

Eleanor Rodriguez is scheduled for a colonoscopy in the outpatient clinic. She is a 52-year-old, Hispanic woman who has been referred by her general practitioner to undergo her initial diagnostic screening evaluation. The physician has ordered 1000 ml D_5 ½ NS to be started in the right hand upon admission to run at 60 ml/hr. She has had previous IVs when she was hospitalized with the birth of her children, which was in another country. She has been admitted and is waiting in the treatment room by herself.

SAMPLE DOCUMENTATION

1. Using a microdrip tubing, what would be the correct drip rate for this IV?

2. When you obtain the IV fluids for Ms. Rodriguez, what steps are necessary before you initiate the IV?
3. If the first attempt to insert a cannula for the IV was unsuccessful, what nursing measures should the nurse take before another attempt is made?
4. The IV has been started and is infusing by gravity drip. What teaching considerations should the nurse share with the client?

NCLEX REVIEW QUESTIONS

1. At what drop rate per minute should a liter of D_5 RL ordered at 12 hours with a drop factor of 15 gtt/ml be set?
   1. 10
   2. 21
   3. 33
   4. 83

2. Mr. Rogers had his IV catheter inserted 48 hours ago to receive antibiotic therapy. On assessment of his IV site, the nurse observes redness and tenderness upon palpation. The nurse documents that the IV was discontinued and restarted due to:
   1. Complaints from the client.
   2. Infiltration
   3. Phlebitis
   4. Termination of therapy.

3. Where should the termination site of the PICC tip be located?
   1. Antecubital fossa
   2. Basilic vein
   3. Cephalic vein
   4. Superior vena cava

4. An implanted infusion port should be accessed with:
   1. A Huber needle
   2. A PICC
   3. An extension tubing
   4. The smallest gauge catheter available

5. Which of the following nursing measures MOST promotes positive outcome in a client with a central venous catheter?
   1. Change the administration set with every new IV container.
   2. Use aseptic technique in related procedures.
   3. Refrain from using catheters for blood draws.
   4. Rotate the site every 7 days.

6. Jeremy, a 7-month-old infant, is admitted with a diagnosis of gastroenteritis. Which of the following IV cannulas is MOST appropriate for receiving IV fluids and possible medications for 2 days?
   1. 24-gauge catheter
   2. 20-gauge catheter
   3. 16-gauge catheter
   4. Peripherally inserted central catheter

7. Which of the following measures is MOST appropriate for a nurse to assist in infusing the IV fluid at the prescribed delivery?
   1. Use a permanent marker to indicate the hourly volume on the bag.
   2. Instruct the client to keep the arm with the IV very still.
   3. Use an electronic infusion device.
   4. Set the rate at KVO.

8. The physician discontinued Mr. Wong's heparin IV therapy. What nursing intervention is MOST appropriate when the nurse terminates his IV catheter?
   1. Apply pressure to the IV site for 5 minutes.
   2. Convert the catheter to an intermittent heparin lock for 24 hours.
   3. Encourage Mr. Wong to ambulate.
   4. Use sterile technique to clean the site.

References

Centers for Disease Control and Prevention: Guidelines for the prevention of intravascular catheter-related infections, *MMWR Morb Mort l Wkly Rep* 51(No. RR-10):1-26, 2002.

Coulte K: Older adult patient. In Macklin D, Chernecky C: *Real wo d nursing survival guide IV therapy,* St. Louis, 2004, Saunders.

Crosby TC, Mares AK: Skin antisepsis past, present, and future, *JVAD* 6(2), 2001.

Hadaway LC: ON the road to successful IV starts, *Nursing* 33(S1):S1, 2003.

Hankins J and others: *Infusion therapy in clinical practice,* Philadelphia, 2001, Saunders.

Heitz UE, Horne MM: *Pocket guide to fluid, electrolyte, and acid-base balance,* ed 4, St. Louis, 2001, Mosby.

Hockenberry MJ and others: *Wong's nursing care of infants and children,* ed 7, St. Louis, 2003, Mosby.

Intravenous Nurses Society: Infusion nursing standards of practice, *J Intraven Nurs* 23(6S):556, 2000.

Metheny N: *Fluid and electrolyte balance: nursing considerations,* ed 4, Philadelphia, 2000, Lippincott.

Occupational Safety and Health Administration: Needlestick safety and prevention act (HR 5178), 2000.

Occupational Safety and Health Administration: Occupational exposure to bloodborne pathogens; needlestick and other sharps injuries; final rule, *Federal Register* 66(5317-5325), Jan 18, 2001a, http://www.osha.gov/FedReg_osha_pdf/FED200101118A.pdf, accessed November 2003.

Occupational Safety and Health Administration: *Revision to OSHA's bloodborne pathogen standard,* April 2001b, http://www.osha-sic.gov/needlesticks/needlefact.html.

Phillips D: *Manual of IV therapeutics,* ed 3, Philadelphia, 2001, FA Davis.

Powers F: Effectively evaluating and converting your organization to the use of infusion safety products, *J Infus Nurs* 25(6S):S10, 2002.

Schelper R: The aging venous system, *JVAD* 8(3):8, 2003.

Thomas JR: The use of polymers in IV catheters: structure, properties, and future developments, *JVAD* 7(1):25, 2002.

Chukhraev AM, Grekov IG: Local complications of nursing interventions on peripheral veins, *J Infus Nurs* 23(3):167, 2000.

Deacon VL: The Safe Medical Device Act and its impact on clinical practice, *J Infus Nurs* 27(1):31, 2004.

Mayer T, Wong DG: The use of polyurethane PICCs and alternative to other catheter materials, *JVAD* 7(2):26, 2002.

Rivers D and others: Predictors of nurses' acceptance or an intravenous catheter safety device, *Nurs Res* 52(4):249, 2003.

White SA: Peripheral intravenous therapy-related phlebitis rates in an adult population, *J Infus Nurs* 24(1):19, 2001.

Research References

Catney MR and others: Relationship between peripheral intravenous catheter dwell time and the development of phlebitis and infiltration, *J Infus Nurs* 24(5):332, 2001.

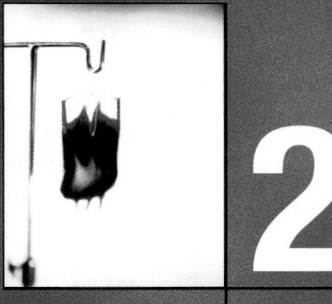

28

Blood Therapy

28-1   Initiating Blood Therapy

28-2   Monitoring for Adverse Reactions
to Transfusion

MEDIA RESOURCES

Evolve Site *evolve*
http://evolve.elsevier.com/Perry/skills
• Weblinks

OBJECTIVES

Mastery of content in this chaper will enable the nurse to:

- Discuss indications for blood therapy.
- Describe various transfusion reactions.
- Demonstrate the following skills on selected clients: initiating blood therapy, implementing autotransfusion, and monitoring for adverse reactions to transfusion.

KEY TERMS

Agglutinate	Blood type
Allogeneic	Hemolysis
Anemia	Neutropenic
Autologous transfusion	Reinfusion device
Autotransfusion	Thrombocytopenia
Blood group	Transfusion reaction
Blood transfusion	

Transfusion therapy is the intravenous (IV) administration of whole blood or blood components for therapeutic purposes. Most transfusions involve administration of allogenic units, units donated by an unknown compatible donor. Transfusions are used to restore intravascular volume with whole blood or albumin, to restore the oxygen-carrying capacity of blood by replacing red blood cells (RBCs), to replace clotting factors and/or platelets to reverse coagulopathy, or to replace white blood cells in neutropenic clients. Transfusion of components separated from whole blood may be pooled, transferred into one transfusion container, to facilitate infusion.

Transfused blood may be allogenic, donated by another person, or autologous, donated in advance by the client. Autologous transfusion, or autotransfusion, is the collection and reinfusion of a client's own blood. The blood for an autologous transfusion is commonly obtained by preoperative donation. Blood for an autologous transfusion can also be salvaged perioperatively (during a surgical procedure), using a machine that washes and filters the blood to remove anticoagulants and activated clotting factors before reinfusion into the client's circulation (American Association of Blood Banks [AABB], 2002).

A client's blood can also be salvaged postoperatively. The client's blood is removed through tubes from the site of bleeding and filtered before reinfusion. An anticoagulant such as heparin, acid citrate dextrose, or citrate phosphate dextrose (CPD) may be used to prevent clotting (AABB, 2002). Salvaged blood must be reinfused within 6 hours of the beginning of collection. If more than 50% of the client's total blood volume is reinfused, replacement of clotting factors is necessary.

There are several advantages to autologous transfusions. They generally are safer for the client because they reduce the risk of incompatibility reactions. However, clerical errors and infectious disease contamination still are potential risks. When preoperative donation is used, the need to carefully identify the blood unit and the client is as important as it is for an allogeneic transfusion, or the advantages are negated. The reinfused blood from perioperative blood salvage contains more viable red blood cells than does stored blood, its pH is normal, and there is a higher level of 2,3-diphosphoglycerate (2,3-DPG, a chemical that increases the oxygen-carrying capacity of hemoglobin). Another advantage of autologous transfusion is the conservation of the blood supply, especially if the client has a rare blood type (Vernon and Pfeifer, 2003).

Despite precautions, blood component therapy is not without risk. Clerical errors (e.g., improper labeling or completion of requisition), either in the collection or distribution of blood, may lead to the administration of incompatible units of blood. In addition, unforeseeable incompatibility and/or disease transmission remain a remote possibility, and careful testing has reduced these occurrences considerably. To decrease some of the risks of transfusion, a client scheduled for major surgery in which a large volume of blood loss is anticipated (e.g., open heart surgery, some orthopedic surgeries) may choose to preoperatively donate 1 to 5 units of his or her own blood for an autologous transfusion, for perioperative or postoperative reinfusion (Goodnough, 2003). It is recommended that the client's donations cease more than 72 hours before surgery to ensure the client's hemodynamic stability. Like allogeneic blood, autologous units are tested for disease and virus transmissions. A unit of RBCs can be stored for 5 to 6 weeks, or if frozen, for several years (AABB, 2002).

Another method used by clients as an alternative to anonymous allogeneic transfusion is the directed donation: a friend or relative donates blood specifically for a particular client's use. These donations must meet the same standards as any blood donation. Disadvantages include overt and covert pressure placed on the potential donor to donate blood. Directed donations are no safer than other allogeneic donations because potential donors may engage in behaviors that place them at high risk for hepatitis or human immunodeficiency virus (HIV) infection that they may be reluctant to admit. Questions to screen potential donors at blood donation centers help eliminate this risk.

Although the decision to transfuse is made by a physician, the nurse assesses the client before, during, and after a transfusion. The nurse must understand the rationale for transfusion of any component to be given, the expected outcomes, and any possible unanticipated outcomes so that the nurse may immediately identify any adverse effects of the therapy.

ABO System

Blood type in the ABO system is determined by the presence or absence of specific antigens on the surface of red blood cells. When the type A antigen is present, the blood group is called type A. When the type B antigen is present, the blood group is type B. When both A and B antigens are present, the blood group is type AB, and when neither A nor B antigens are present, the blood group is type O (Table 28-1).

TABLE 28-1   ABO System

CLIENT'S BLOOD TYPE	RED BLOOD CELLS ANTIGEN	TRANSFUSION WITH TYPE A	TRANSFUSION WITH TYPE B	TRANSFUSION WITH TYPE AB	TRANSFUSION WITH TYPE O	TRANSFUSION OPTIONS
A	A	Yes	No	No	Yes	A, O
B	B	No	Yes	No	Yes	B, O
AB	AB	Yes	Yes	Yes	Yes	A, B, AB, O Universal recipient
O	None	No	No	No	Yes	O Universal donor

Antibodies that react against the A and B antigens are naturally present in the plasma of people whose red blood cells do not carry the antigen. These antibodies (agglutinins) react against the foreign antigens (agglutinogens). Incompatible red blood cells agglutinate (clump together) and result in a life-threatening hemolytic transfusion reaction. People with type A blood have anti-B antibodies; people with type B blood have anti-A antibodies. People with type AB blood have neither antibody and therefore can receive all blood types, and people with type O blood have both A and B antibodies, and therefore can receive only type O blood.

Rh System

Although six common types of Rh antigen may be present on the surface of red blood cells, the type D antigen is widely prevalent and is most likely to incite an immune response. It is the presence or absence of the D antigen that determines a person's Rh type. A person with the D antigen is considered Rh positive, and a person without the D antigen is considered Rh negative. Unlike the ABO antigens, there are no naturally occurring antibodies to the Rh (D) antigen. A person with Rh-negative blood must first be exposed to Rh-positive blood before any Rh antibodies are formed. A person with Rh-negative blood who is exposed to a large amount (200 ml or more) of Rh-positive blood will develop enough antibodies to mount a severe transfusion reaction with repeat exposure. These antibodies take up to 2 weeks to form. Therefore, in the case of massive transfusion as used in trauma situations, Rh-positive blood may be used for a person with Rh-negative blood without adverse effect, provided that the person has not been exposed to Rh-positive blood in the past.

An Rh-negative mother previously exposed to Rh antigen can transfer her Rh antibodies across the placenta to an Rh-positive fetus. This can result in severe fetal hemolysis, the breakdown of red blood cells, with resultant anemia and jaundice, and can be fatal to the infant.

Evidence-Based Trends

Safety and risk management are key factors in transfusion therapy. ABO incompatibility is one of the most serious errors and often has fatal outcomes. ABO incompatibility is estimated to occur with 1 of every 14,000 units administered in the United States (Goodnough, 2003). Systems designed to improve identification processes, such as barcode tech-

nology, have demonstrated improved practice and the need for further development (Turner and others, 2003). Almost all fatal hemolytic transfusion reactions occur as a result of human error. A barcode system incorporates technology as an additional safeguard in the identification process between the client and the compatible blood unit. The development of laboratory screening procedures is another method of ensuring safe transfusion; new viruses such as the West Nile virus emerge and threaten transmission infection. Blood alternative therapies with pharmacological developments such as colloids, crystalloids, and erythropoietin are used to reduce the risks associated with transfusing human blood (Rudnicke, 2003). Conservation of the blood supply through transfusion-free surgery and medical decisions is another trend gaining support. Blood conservation requires excellent nursing care and anticipation of complications and relevant interventions (Vernon and Pfeifer, 2003).

Cultural Considerations

When administering blood products, it is essential that the nurse consider a client's cultural beliefs and his or her acceptance of blood therapy. There are religions that do not allow blood transfusions. For example, members of Jehovah's Witness do not allow blood transfusions or organ donation if it involves blood exchange (Andrews and Hanson, 2003). It may prove helpful to consult a religious leader when caring for clients in need of blood therapy. Be aware of organizational policies and procedures to follow when clients refuse blood transfusion. Inform the physician of a client's decision.

SKILL PERFORMANCE GUIDELINES

1. Review hospital or agency policy and procedure regarding administration of blood or blood products. These are designed to ensure safe administration of blood products.
2. Know the client's normal range of vital signs and medical history, including allergies. Administration of blood products increases intravascular volume and may elevate a client's blood pressure. This may be one of the desired effects of therapy. However, some clients cannot tolerate the volume load of a blood transfusion and may develop fluid volume excess, leading to markedly elevated blood pressure, tachycardia, pulmonary edema, or cardiac failure.
3. Monitor and document the client's temperature and vital signs immediately before initiation of therapy and

closely during blood therapy as well. Policies differ between institutions regarding timing of vital sign monitoring during blood transfusions. An elevation in temperature or heart rate may be one of the first signs that a person is having an adverse reaction to a transfusion. A client may also experience marked hypotension if a severe reaction occurs (Table 28-2).

4. Understand the indications for and the goal of the transfusion therapy. This will allow the nurse to assist the physician in evaluating the outcome and assessing the need for any further therapy.

5. Assess the client's most recent serum electrolyte values. When blood is stored, there is continual destruction of

RBCs, which releases potassium from the cells into the plasma. If blood is transfused rapidly, there may be transient hyperkalemia before the potassium is reabsorbed. Blood that is preserved with CPD contains a high concentration of citrate ions. The excess citrate may combine with the ionized calcium in the recipient's blood, resulting in transient low ionized calcium levels. Although ionized calcium deficiency resulting from blood transfusions is rare, it is more likely to occur in young children, older adults, or clients with osteoporosis.

6. Verify the client's understanding of the procedure and its rationale. This may help to alleviate any anxiety the client may have over receiving blood products.

TABLE 28-2 ADVERSE REACTIONS TO BLOOD TRANSFUSIONS

REACTION	MECHANISM	ONSET	SIGNS AND SYMPTOMS	PREVENTION	MANAGEMENT
Acute hemolytic transfusion reaction	ABO, Rh incompatibility; causes intravascular destruction of transfused RBCs as antibodies in recipient's plasma attach to antigens on donor RBCs	Within 5-15 minutes of initiation of transfusion	Characteristically begins with increased temperature, increased heart rate; sensation of heat and pain along vein receiving blood; chills, low back pain, headache, nausea, chest or back pain, chest tightness, dyspnea, bronchospasm, anxiety, hypotension, vascular collapse, hemoglobinemia, hemoglobinuria (Hgb molecules from hemolysis of RBCs are released into the plasma; this free Hgb, when filtered by the kidneys, may obstruct the renal tubules, leading to renal failure), disseminated intravascular coagulation, possibly death	Carefully identify client and the blood sample obtained for blood typing and compatibility screening. When blood released from blood bank, match with client information. Follow organization's verification procedures at bedside before transfusion.	Stop transfusion. Maintain IV access. Notify physician. Monitor vital signs at least every 15 minutes. Correct arterial blood pressure, correct coagulopathy if present. Monitor intake and ouput hourly. (Attempts may be made to alkalinize the urine and initiate diuresis because this may prevent precipitation of hemoglobin within the renal tubules.) Dialysis may be required. Obtain blood and urine samples and send to laboratory with unused portion of unit of blood. Document reaction according to agency policy.
Delayed hemolytic transfusion reaction	Immune response mounted by recipient against non-ABO donor antigens; usually the result of destruction of transfused RBCs by alloantibodies not detected during the crossmatch	2-14 days	Unexplained fever, unexplained decrease in Hgb/Hct, increased bilirubin levels, jaundice	Careful crossmatching of donor and recipient blood. Potential to be missed because it may occur several days after transfusion.	Monitor laboratory values for anemia. (Recognition is important because subsequent transfusions may cause an acute hemolytic reaction.) If detected, notify physician and blood bank. Most delayed hemolytic reactions require no treatment.
Febrile, nonhemolytic	Accompanies <1% of transfusions; possible sensitivity of recipient to the leukocytes or platelets in donor's blood	30 minutes after initiation to 6 hours after completion of transfusion	Fever >1° C above baseline, flushing, chills, headache, muscle pain; occurs most frequently in immunosuppressed clients	Use leukocyte-reduced blood products in clients who have experienced febrile nonhemolytic reactions in the past.	Stop transfusion. Administer antipyretics as ordered. Monitor temperature every 4 hours.

Data from Otto SE: *Mosby's pocket guide to intravenous therapy,* ed 4, St. Louis, 2001, Mosby; American Association of Blood Banks: *Technical manual,* ed 4, Bethesda, Md, 2002, The Association.
Hct, Hematocrit; *Hgb,* hemoglobin; *PRBCs,* packed red blood cells; *RBC,* red blood cells.

TABLE 28-2 **ADVERSE REACTIONS TO BLOOD TRANSFUSIONS — CONT'D**

REACTION	MECHANISM	ONSET	SIGNS AND SYMPTOMS	PREVENTION	MANAGEMENT
Allergic reaction (mild to moderate)	Caused by recipient allergy to a plasma protein in donor's blood	During transfusion to 1 hour after transfusion	Local erythema, hives and urticaria, itching or pruritus	May administer antihistamines before transfusion if prescribed.	Stop transfusion. Notify physician and blood bank. Administer antihistamines as ordered. Monitor and document vital signs every 15 minutes. Transfusion may be restarted if fever, dyspnea, and wheezing are not present.
Allergic reaction (severe)	Caused by recipient allergy to a donor antigen (usually IgA) Agglutination of RBCs obstructing capillaries and blocking blood flow, causing symptoms to all major organ systems	Within 5-15 minutes of initiation of transfusion	Coughing, nausea, vomiting, respiratory distress, wheezing, hypotension, loss of consciousness, possible cardiac arrest	Transfusion of saline-washed or leukocyte-depleted RBCs.	This is a life-threatening reaction. Stop transfusion. Maintain IV access. Notify physician and blood bank. Administer antihistamines, corticosteroids, epinephrine, and antipyretics as ordered. Measure and document vital signs every 5-15 minutes. Initiate cardiopulmonary resuscitation if necessary.
Graft-versus-host disease	Reproduction of donor lymphocytes, usually in an immunocompromised recipient, which attack recipient's RBCs as if they were foreign proteins	Days to weeks	Skin rash, fever, jaundice due to liver dysfunction, bone marrow suppression	Administer irradiated blood products as prescribed.	Administer methotrexate, corticosteroids as ordered.
Circulatory overload	Occurs with transfusion of excessive volume or excessively rapid rate; can lead to pulmonary edema	Any time during or within 1-2 hours after transfusion	Dyspnea, cough, crackles at lung bases, tachypnea, headache, hypertension, tachycardia, increased central venous pressure, distended neck veins	Administer blood or component at prescribed rate, usually no greater than 2-4 ml/kg/hr; pay particular attention to rate and volume in older adults, young children, and clients with cardiac and renal disorders. Administer PRBCs instead of whole blood. Minimize amount of saline infused with transfusion.	Slow or stop transfusions as ordered. Elevate client's head. Notify physician.
Bacterial sepsis	Bacterial contamination of infused product	During transfusion to 2 hours after transfusion	High fever, chills, abdominal cramping, vomiting, diarrhea, profound hypotension	Proper care of blood or blood product from time of procurement through end of administration. Complete transfusion within 4 hours.	Stop transfusion. Maintain IV access. Notify physician. Monitor and document vital signs. Obtain samples for blood culture and Gram's stain from recipient. Administer IV fluids, broad-spectrum antimicrobials, vasopressors, and steroids as ordered.

SKILL 28-1 Initiating Blood Therapy

The physician determines which blood component is needed to treat a client's medical condition. Clinical indications differ among blood products (Table 28-3). The nurse is responsible for understanding which components are appropriate in various situations. Before requesting a blood component for a client, the nurse must first ensure that a sample of the client's blood has been sent to the laboratory within the past 72 hours for blood typing and general compatibility screening. When sending a sample of a client's blood to the blood bank for crossmatching, the nurse must be meticulous in verifying the client's identifying information on the sample.

If a client is bleeding severely and requires massive replacement of blood products, special infusion tubing may be obtained and hung through a pump that allows for rapid transfusion. Using a blood warmer warms the tubing and thus the infused product. Blood is refrigerated in the blood bank for storage. Rapid transfusion of cold blood is discouraged because it is likely to cause dysrhythmias and a reduction of core temperature. Heating a unit of blood in a microwave or under hot water can destroy blood cells.

DELEGATION CONSIDERATIONS

This skill may not be delegated to assistive personnel. Depending upon the agency's policy, assistive personnel may:
- Obtain blood components from the blood bank
- Assist in the verification procedure before the initiation of blood therapy; many inpatient facilities require two licensed professionals to verify blood units

After the transfusion has been started and the client is stable, assistive personnel can monitor the client's vital signs. Assistive personnel should be taught the signs and symptoms of a transfusion reaction and the importance of immediately reporting if any signs or symptoms occur. Monitoring of a client by assistive personnel does not relieve the nurse of the responsibility and accountability to continue to assess the client during the transfusion.

EQUIPMENT
- ❏ Blood administration set
- ❏ 0.9% NaCl (normal saline) IV solution
- ❏ Alcohol wipes
- ❏ Disposable clean gloves
- ❏ Tape
- ❏ Blood pressure cuff and stethoscope
- ❏ Thermometer
- ❏ Signed transfusion consent form

  If Needed
- ❏ Rapid infusion pump
- ❏ Leukocyte-depleting filter
- ❏ Blood warmer
- ❏ Pressure bag
- ❏ Pulse oximeter

  For Perioperative Blood Salvage
- ❏ Cell saver or continuous collection container and appropriate tubing

  For Postoperative Salvage via Drainage Tubes
- ❏ Drainage collection and reinfusion device
- ❏ 0.9% normal saline IV solution
- ❏ Anticoagulant, if needed
- ❏ Transfer bag and tubing
- ❏ Label
- ❏ Disposable gloves

STEP	RATIONALE

ASSSSMENT

1. Verify that IV cannula is patent and without complications such as infiltration or phlebitis. In emergency situations that require rapid transfusions, a 16- or 18-gauge cannula is preferred; however, transfusions for therapeutic indications may be infused with cannulas ranging from 20 to 24 gauge.

Patent IV ensures that transfusion will be initiated and infused within established time guidelines. The gauge of the IV cannula should be appropriate for accommodating the infusion of blood and/or blood components (Infusion Nursing Standards of Practice, 2000). Large cannulas, such as 18 gauge, promote optimal flow of blood components. Use of a smaller cannula such as 22 to 24 gauge may require blood bank to divide the unit so that each half can be infused within the allotted time or may require pressure-assisted devices. Infiltration or signs of infection at IV site contraindicate use of that line.

TABLE 28-3   BLOOD AND BLOOD COMPONENT PRODUCTS*

BLOOD PRODUCT AND SOURCE	VOLUME AND INFUSION TIME	ABLE TO TRANSMIT HIV/HBV†	ABO/RH TESTING NEEDED	ACTIONS/USES
Whole blood—single donor: allogeneic or autologous	300-550 ml <4 hr	Yes	Yes—Must be ABO identical Rh—Yes	Replaces red cell mass and plasma volume; expected to raise hemoglobin 1 g/100 ml and hematocrit by 3% in nonhemorrhaging adult.
Packed RBCs—single donor: allogeneic or autologous	300-350 ml <4 hr	Yes	Yes/Yes	Preferred method of replacing red blood cell mass; expected to raise Hgb/Hct level same as whole blood.
Leukocyte-poor RBCs†— single donor: allogeneic or directed	200-250 ml <4 hr	Yes	Yes/Yes	Replaces RBCs while preventing febrile, non-hemolytic transfusion reactions; reduces risk of CMV† transmission.
Irradiated RBCs—single donor: allogeneic or directed	250-350 ml <4 hr	Yes	Yes/Yes	Replaces RBCs while preventing transfusion-associated graft-versus-host disease; used in immunodeficient clients (any blood component can be irradiated).
Fresh frozen plasma— single donor	200-250 ml <4 hr	Yes	Yes/No	Replaces plasma without RBCs or platelets; contains most coagulation factors and complement; used in the control of bleeding where replacement of coagulation factors is needed (e.g., DIC, TTP).
Cryoprecipitate—multiple donors, pooled	5-20 ml/unit; 1 unit/10 kg body weight 1-2 ml/min	Yes	No/No	Replaces factors VIII, XIII, von Willebrand's factor, and fibrinogen.
Platelets—multiple/random donor, pooled	40-70 ml/unit; 1 unit/10 kg body weight <4 hr	Yes	Yes/Yes	Used in clients with thrombocytopenia. Certain microaggregate filters are not to be used with platelets—check manufacturer's instructions.
Platelets—single donor	200-500 ml <4 hr	Yes	Yes/Yes	Single-donor platelets are most useful in immunologically refractory clients when given as HLA matched with recipient. Each unit expected to raise platelet count by 5000-10,000/ml in a 70-kg client.
Colloid components— albumin 5% pooled	250-500 ml 1-10 ml/min	No	No/No	Oncotically equivalent to plasma, used to treat hypoproteinemia in burns and hypoalbuminemia in shock and ARDs; used to support blood pressure in dialysis and acute liver failure.
Colloid components— albumin 25% pooled	50-100 ml 0.2-0.4 ml/min	No	No/No	Increased circulating blood volume by increasing intravascular oncotic pressure.

Data from http://www.redcross.org/services/biomed/profess/pgbtscreen.pdf, accessed Dec 14, 2003; McKenry L, Salerno E: *Mosby's pharmacology in nursing*, ed 21, St. Louis, 2003, Mosby.
*Other less commonly used blood components include factors VIII and IX concentrates, granulocytes, immunoglobulin, and saline-washed RBCs.
ARD, Acute respiratory disease; *CMV*, cytomegalovirus; *DIC*, disseminated intravascular coagulation; *HBV*, hepatitis B virus, *Hct*, hematocrit; *Hgb*, hemoglobin; *HIV*, human immunodeficiency virus; *HLA*, human leukocyte antigen; *RBC*, red blood cell; *TTP*, thrombotic thrombocytopenic purpura.

STEP	RATIONALE
2. Obtain client's transfusion history.	Identifies client's prior response(s) to transfusion of blood components. If client has experienced a reaction in the past, anticipate a similar reaction, and be prepared to rapidly intervene.
3. Review physician's order for blood component transfusion. Check that transfusion consent has been properly completed and signed by client.	A physician's order must be present before transfusing a blood product. Verifying order helps to ensure that appropriate blood component will be administered. Most agencies require clients to sign consent forms before receiving blood component therapy because of the inherent risks.
4. Know indication for blood product to be transfused (e.g., packed red blood cells [PRBCs] for a client with a low hematocrit level from gastrointestinal bleeding or surgery blood loss).	Knowing rationale for product to be transfused facilitates evaluation of outcome of therapy.
5. Obtain and record vital signs, including temperature, immediately before initiation of transfusion.	Change from baseline vital signs during infusion will alert nurse to a potential transfusion reaction or adverse effect of therapy.
6. Assess client's level of comfort.	Pain increases oxygen demand. When RBCs are depleted, the body's ability to meet that demand is reduced. Client may need to be medicated for comfort to decrease metabolic demand. Also, if IV medications are necessary during transfusion, a second IV site is necessary because the blood line may not be used because of incompatibilities and the increased risk of contamination.
7. Assess client's understanding of procedure and rationale.	Clarifying client's need for and associated benefits of therapy may alleviate some of the anxiety client may have.

NURSING DIAGNOSES

- Activity intolerance
- Ineffective peripheral tissue perfusion
- Decreased cardiac output

- Deficient fluid volume/excess fluid volume
- Deficient knowledge regarding purpose and risks of blood transfusions

Related factors are individualized based on client's condition or needs.

PLANNING

1. Expected outcomes following completion of the procedure:	
• Client will verbalize understanding of rationale for therapy.	Indicates learning has occurred.
• Client experiences improved activity tolerance.	Oxygenation is improved.
• Mucous membranes are pink, and client has brisk capillary refill.	Tissue perfusion is improved.
• Client's cardiac output returns to baseline.	Intravascular volume is restored.
• Client's systolic blood pressure improves, and urine output is 0.5 to 1 ml/kg/hr.	Parameters reflect optimal fluid status and adequate renal blood flow.
• Laboratory values will reflect improvement in targeted areas (hematocrit, coagulation values).	Components in blood are reflected in improved targeted laboratory values such as complete blood count [CBC], RBC, hemoglobin [Hgb], hematocrit [Hct], and/or coagulation values.
2. Explain procedure to client and family.	Promotes client's cooperation and ability to report complications.

STEP	RATIONALE

IMPLEMENTATION

1. Preadministration

   a. Obtain blood component from blood bank following agency protocol.

Timely acquisition ensures product is safe to administer. Agency protocol usually encompasses safeguards to ensure quality control throughout transfusion process.

   b. Correctly verify product and identify client with a person considered qualified by your agency (e.g., RN, licensed practical nurse [LPN], client care technician).

Strict adherence to verification procedures before administration of blood or blood components reduces risk of administering the wrong blood to client. Most hemolytic transfusion reactions are caused by clerical errors (AABB, 2002).

      (1) Check client's first and last names by having client state name, if able. Also check client's identification number and date of birth on arm band and client record.

When a discrepancy is noted during verification procedure, do not administer the product. Notify blood bank and appropriate personnel as indicated by agency policy.

      (2) Verify that component received from blood bank is component ordered by physician.

Ensures client receives correct therapy.

      (3) Check that client's blood type and Rh type are compatible with donor blood type and Rh type. Be sure that transfusion is not discolored, clotted, or leaking and does not have bubbles present.

Verifies accurate donor blood type. Air bubbles, clots, or discoloration may indicate bacterial contamination or inadequate anticoagulation of the stored component and would be contraindications for transfusion of that product.

      (4) Check that unit number on unit of blood and on form from blood bank match.

Prevents accidental administration of wrong component.

      (5) Check expiration date and time on unit of blood.

Expired blood should never be used, because the cell components deteriorate and may contain excess citrate ions.

      (6) Record verification process as directed by agency policy.

Documentation on legal medical record.

      (7) Check appearance of blood product for leaks, bubbles, clots, or purplish color.

Do not transfuse blood if integrity is compromised. Blood serves as a medium for bacterial growth.

   c. Empty urine drainage collection container, or have client void.

If a transfusion reaction occurs, a urine specimen containing urine produced after initiation of the transfusion will be sent to the laboratory.

2. Administration

   a. Perform hand hygiene, and apply clean disposable gloves and appropriate attire.

Using standard precautions reduces risk for transmission of microorganisms.

   b. Autologous transfusion only:

      (1) Connect drainage tubes to collection container or cell-processing system.

Allows collection of client's blood for reinfusion, storage (no longer than 6 hours), or washing and spinning.

      (2) Minimize air bubbles by establishing secure connections. Follow agency and manufacturer's procedure for setup and maintenance of system.

STEP	**RATIONALE**
c. Open Y tubing blood administration set.	Y tubing is used to facilitate maintenance of IV access in case a client will need more than 1 unit of blood. Both a unit of blood and a container of normal saline are connected to the system. With Y tubing, normal saline can be easily infused at a keep vein open (KVO) rate (10 to 12 gtt/min) to maintain venous patency while obtaining the next transfusion unit following each transfusion (follow manufacturer's guidelines regarding the number of units that can be given before tubing must be changed).
	If the client is to receive only 1 unit of blood, a piggyback infusion of 0.9% saline IV solution should be connected with the blood administration set, using a stopcock or needleless valve. Saline should be readily available in case of a transfusion reaction.
d. Set roller clamp(s) to "off" position.	Moving roller clamps to "off" position prevents accidental spilling and wasting of product.
e. Spike 0.9% normal saline IV bag with one of Y tubing spikes (see illustration). Invert filter, open roller clamps of IV bag and component side of Y, keeping the common tubing clamp below the filter closed. Set IV bag on table, and gently press down to squeeze IV bag to fill both sides of Y tubing. Close tubing clamp of component side of Y, and open common tubing clamp below the filter. Continue to press down on IV saline bag to completely fill filter and half of drip chamber. Close both tubing clamps. All three tubing clamps should be closed.	Primes tubing with fluid to eliminate air on both sides of Y. Inverting the filter to fill from top to bottom reduces the formation of air pockets. Closing the roller clamp prevents spillage and waste of fluid.

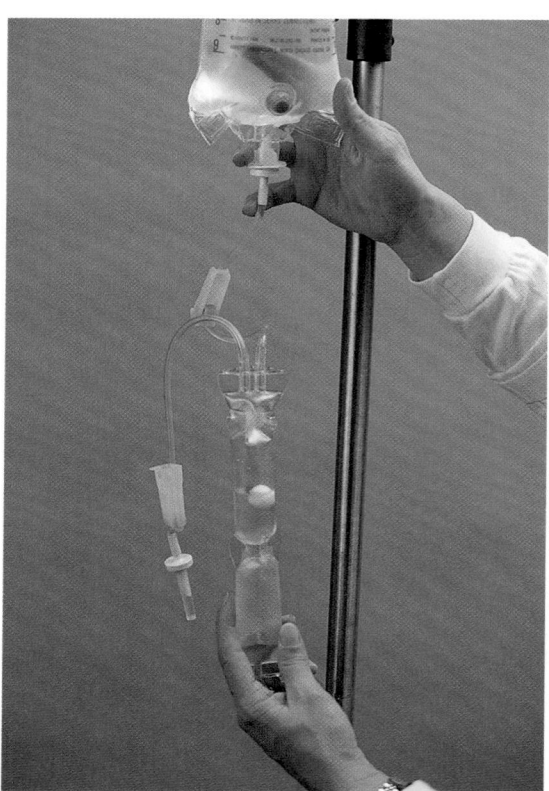

STEP 2e Blood administration set primed with normal saline.

STEP	RATIONALE

f. Hang on IV pole. Open common tubing clamp to finish priming the tubing to the distal end of tubing connector. Close tubing clamp when tubing is filled with saline. Maintain protective sterile cap on tubing connector

This will completely prime the tubing with saline, and the IV line is ready to be connected to the client's vascular access device (VAD).

g. Prepare blood component for administration. Remove protective covering from access port. Spike blood component unit with other Y connection (see illustration). Hang on IV pole. Open clamp of Y connected to blood unit, and open common tubing clamp to prime tubing with blood. Allow saline in tubing to flow into receptacle, being careful to ensure any blood spillage is contained in blood precaution container.

A protective barrier drape may be used to catch any potential blood spillage. The tubing is primed with the blood unit and ready for transfusion into the client.

- **Critical Decision Point**

Normal saline is compatible with blood products, unlike solutions that contain dextrose, which causes coagulation of donor blood.

h. Maintaining asepsis, attach primed tubing to client's VAD. Open common tubing clamp.

This initiates infusion of blood product into client's vein.

i. Remain with client during the first 5 to 15 minutes of a transfusion. Initial flow rate during this time should be 2 ml/min, or 20 gtt/min.

Most transfusion reactions occur within the first 5 to 15 minutes of a transfusion (Doughty, 2000). Infusing a small amount of blood component initially minimizes the volume of blood to which the client is exposed, thereby minimizing the severity of a reaction.

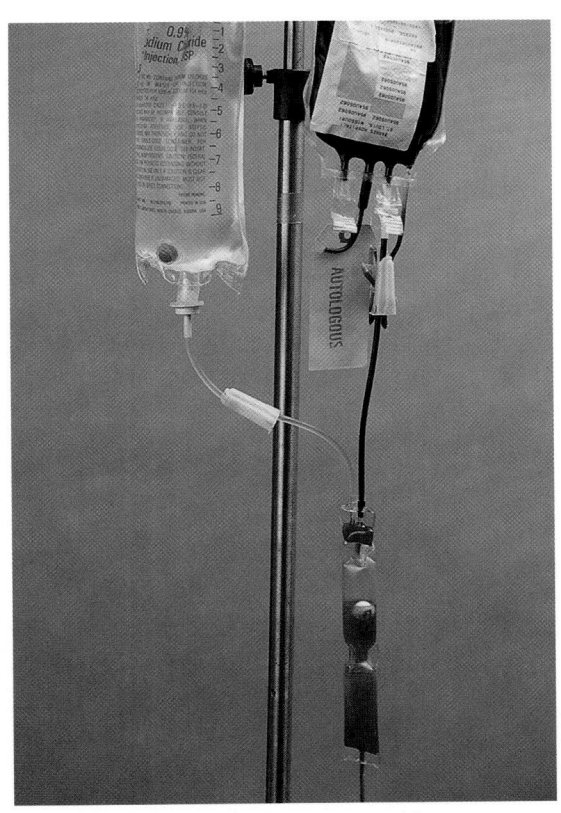

STEP 2g Unit of blood connected to Y tubing setup.

STEP	RATIONALE

- **Critical Decision Point**
  If signs of a transfusion reaction occur, stop the transfusion, start normal saline with new primed tubing directly to the VAD at KVO, and notify the physician immediately. (Refer to Skill 28-2 for signs and symptoms of a transfusion reaction.)

j.	Monitor client's vital signs 5 minutes after the blood product has begun infusing and per agency policy after that.	Frequent monitoring of vital signs will help to quickly alert nurse to a transfusion reaction.
k.	Regulate rate of transfusion according to physician's orders. (Drop factor for blood tubing is 10 gtt/ml.)	Maintaining the prescribed rate of flow decreases risk of fluid volume excess while restoring vascular volume.

- **Critical Decision Point**
  A unit of blood should not hang for more than 4 hours because of the danger of bacterial growth.

- **Critical Decision Point**
  Medication should never be injected into the same IV line with a blood component because of the risk of contaminating the blood product with pathogens and the possibility of incompatibility. A separate IV line must be maintained if the client requires IV infusion (total parenteral nutrition [TPN], pain control) during the transfusion.

l.	After blood has infused, clear IV line with 0.9% normal saline, and discard blood bag according to agency policy.	Infusing IV saline solution infuses remainder of blood in IV tubing and keeps IV line patent for supportive measures in case of a transfusion reaction (Hanna and Raad, 2001).
m.	Appropriately dispose of all supplies. Remove gloves, and perform hand hygiene.	Standard precautions during a transfusion reduce transmission of microorganisms.

EVALUATION

1. Monitor IV site and status of infusion each time vital signs are taken.

   Detects presence of infiltration or phlebitis and verifies continuous and safe infusion of blood product.

2. Observe for any changes in vital signs and for chills, flushing, itching, dyspnea, rash, or other signs of transfusion reaction.

   These may be early signs of a transfusion reaction (see Table 28-2).

3. Observe client and assess laboratory values to determine response to administration of blood component.

   This aids in determining whether goals of therapy have been reached or if further blood component therapy will be required.

Recording and Reporting

- Record type of blood component and amount administered, along with client's response to therapy. This may be documented on transfusion record itself, in nurses' notes, medication administration record, and/or intake and output sheet, depending on agency policy.
- Report signs and symptoms of a transfusion reaction immediately.
- Record amount of blood received by autotransfusion and client's response to therapy.
- Report to physician any deterioration in cardiac status.

Unexpected Outcomes	Related Interventions
1. Client displays signs and symptoms of a transfusion reaction, which occurs when donor blood is incompatible with recipient's blood or when recipient has a sensitivity to a plasma protein in the transfused (donor's) blood.	• Stop transfusion. • Normal saline should be connected at VAD hub to prevent any subsequent blood from infusing from tubing. Disconnect blood tubing at VAD hub, and cap distal end with sterile connector to maintain sterile system. Keep vein open with slow infusion of normal saline at 10 to 12 gtt/min to ensure venous patency and maintain venous access for medication or to resume transfusion. It is important to regulate flow rate to minimize administration of excess IV fluid, especially in clients who are prone to fluid overload such as clients with cardiac and renal disorders, pediatric clients, and older adults. Notify physician. • See Table 28-2 for interventions.
2. Client develops infiltration or phlebitis at venipuncture site.	• Remove IV and insert new VAD in different site. The product may be restarted if remainder can be infused within 4 hours of initiation of transfusion. • Institute nursing measures to reduce discomfort at infiltrated or infected site.
3. Rate of infusion slows in the absence of infiltration.	• Gently flush IV line with normal saline, or use a pressure bag to increase rate of flow of product.
4. Fluid overload occurs, and/or client exhibits difficulty breathing or has crackles upon auscultation.	• Slow or stop transfusion, elevate head of bed, and inform physician of physical findings. • Administer diuretics, morphine, and/or oxygen as ordered by physician. • Continue frequent assessments, and closely monitor vital signs, intake and output
5. Client displays signs and symptoms associated with decreased cardiac output: hypotension, tachycardia, cold skin, decreased urine output.	• Ensure that transfusion is infusing at ordered rate, so that rate of volume replacement is sufficient. • If blood loss is too rapid, allogenic transfusion may be necessary.

Teaching Considerations

- Instruct client regarding rationale for transfusion and anticipated amount of time for completion of transfusion.
- Discuss with client and family the rationale for frequent vital sign monitoring throughout transfusion.
- Inform client and family to notify nurse in case of itching, swelling, dizziness, dyspnea, low back pain, or chest pain, because these may be indicative of a transfusion reaction.
- Instruct client to inform nurse if pain, swelling, or redness occurs at IV site, because these are indicative of infiltration.

Pediatric Considerations

- The first 50 ml or 20% of volume (whichever is smaller) of a blood transfusion should be run very slowly in a pediatric client, and nurse should stay with child for that time.

- Smaller aliquots of blood are often available for use with pediatric clients (AABB, 2002).
- Twenty-seven gauge cannulas can be used to infuse packed red cells without significant hemolysis (Hankins and others, 2001). The use of a small-gauge cannula will require positive pressure through an infusion pump because the blood will not infuse by gravity alone.
- Blood replacement is recommended when a child's blood loss totals 5% to 7% of total blood volume.

Gerontological Considerations

- Older adults may have decreased cardiac function, thus requiring a slower infusion time. Half units may be obtained if a client is unable to tolerate the volume in a whole unit of blood or blood component.

Home Care Considerations

- Clients who have had prior transfusion reactions, acute angina, or congestive heart failure are not considered good candidates for home transfusion.
- The transfusion must be initiated as soon as possible after component is obtained from blood bank. It should be transported in an insulated container with ice. Blood bank will determine appropriate temperature.
- The nurse must plan for client to have nursing personnel present during the entire transfusion process and for 30 to 60 minutes after transfusion.

- When blood sample is obtained for blood typing and crossmatching, identity band should be attached to client, with full name and identification number used by laboratory. This provides clear identification of client when blood component transfusion is initiated.
- Client and caregiver should be instructed regarding signs and symptoms of a delayed hemolytic transfusion reaction (unexplained fever, decrease in hemoglobin and hematocrit levels 2 to 14 days after transfusion) so that they can report them and receive treatment if necessary

SKILL 28-2 Monitoring for Adverse Reactions to Transfusion

During the transfusion of blood products, a client is at risk for adverse reactions, particularly during the first 15 minutes. The nurse should remain with the client for that period to assess vital signs and the client's physiological response. Selected transfusion reactions are described in Table 28-2.

A transfusion reaction is a systemic response to the administration of a blood product that is either incompatible with that of the recipient, contains allergens to which the recipient is sensitive or allergic, or is contaminated with pathogens. Some clients with sensitivities to blood products as a result of frequent transfusions may require premedication with diphenhydramine.

Several types of adverse reactions may result from a blood transfusion. General adverse reactions (see Table 28-2) may have symptoms ranging from fever, chills, and skin rash to hypotension and cardiac arrest. A client may also experience a delayed transfusion reaction, which will not manifest itself for days or weeks. The primary risk for transfusion-associated death is the erroneous transfusion of ABO-incompatible allogeneic units (Goodnough, 2003). Fatalities that occur as the result of a transfusion reaction must be reported to the Food and Drug Administration by the agency.

Other possible adverse outcomes that may result from transfusion therapy include circulatory overload and transmission of diseases such as hepatitis, cytomegalovirus, or HIV. Currently all units of blood undergo extensive serological testing, thereby minimizing the risk of clients acquiring a blood-borne disease.

DELEGATION CONSIDERATIONS

Assistive personnel should be instructed regarding the signs and symptoms of a transfusion reaction and should immediately report if any of these occur; however, the nurse is responsible and accountable for assessing, monitoring, and evaluating the client.

STEP	RATIONALE

ASSESSMENT

1. Observe for fever with or without chills.

Fever may be indicative of onset of an acute hemolytic reaction, febrile nonhemolytic reaction, or bacterial sepsis.

2. Assess client for tachycardia and/or tachypnea and dyspnea.

May indicate acute hemolytic reaction or circulatory overload. These symptoms may be accompanied by a cough in the case of circulatory overload.

3. Observe client for hives or skin rash.

These may be early indications of an allergic reaction, anaphylaxis, or graft-versus-host disease, which occurs after transfusion.

STEP	RATIONALE
4. Observe client for flushing.	Flushing may be present in an acute hemolytic reaction or a febrile nonhemolytic reaction. Localized flushing may be present with an allergic reaction.
5. Observe client for gastrointestinal symptoms.	Nausea and vomiting may be present in acute hemolytic transfusion reactions, anaphylactic reactions, or sepsis. Diarrhea may be present in graft-versus-host disease or sepsis.
6. Observe client for a fall in blood pressure.	Hypotension may be indicative of an acute hemolytic reaction, anaphylaxis, or sepsis.

- **Critical Decision Point**
  Sepsis and other infections due to blood transfusion should be reported to the blood bank and your agency's infection control department, which will then communicate that information to the state health department and the Centers for Disease Control and Prevention.

7. Observe the client for wheezing, chest pain, and possible cardiac arrest.	These are all indications of an anaphylactic reaction.
8. Be alert to client complaints of headache or muscle pain in the presence of a fever.	Both may be indicative of a febrile nonhemolytic reaction.
9. Monitor client for disseminated intravascular coagulation, renal failure, and hemoglobinemia/hemoglobinuria by reviewing laboratory test results.	All are late signs of an acute hemolytic reaction.
10. Auscultate client's lungs, and monitor central venous pressure, if possible.	Crackles in bases of lungs and a rising central venous pressure (CVP) are indications of circulatory overload.
11. Observe client for jaundice and increased liver enzymes, indicating liver damage, and decreased red blood cells, white blood cells, and platelets, indicating bone marrow suppression.	These are indicative of graft-versus-host disease and would occur following transfusion.
12. Monitor client's laboratory values (e.g., CBC, Hgb, Hct) for anemia refractory to transfusion therapy.	This could signify a delayed hemolytic reaction.
13. In clients receiving massive transfusions, observe client for mild hypothermia, cardiac dysrhythmias, hypotension, and hypocalcemia.	Cold blood products can affect the cardiac conduction system, resulting in ventricular dysrhythmias. Other cardiac dysrhythmias, hypotension, and tingling may indicate hypocalcemia, which occurs when citrate (used as a preservative for some blood products) combines with client's calcium.

NURSING DIAGNOSES

- Anxiety
- Decreased cardiac output
- Excess fluid volume
- Hyperthermia

- Hypothermia
- Impaired gas exchange
- Pain (acute)

Related factors are individualized based on client's condition or needs.

PLANNING

1. Expected outcomes following completion of the procedure:
   - Client will have pink mucous membranes and brisk capillary refill.
   - Client's cardiac output will return to baseline.
   - Client will maintain core body temperature of 97° to 99° F.

Tissue perfusion is improved.

Intravascular volume is restored.
Helps to confirm absence of transfusion reaction.

STEP	RATIONALE
• Client will have urine output of 0.5 to 1 ml/kg/hr.	Reflects optimal fluid status.
• Client will maintain stable blood pressure.	Intravascular volume is restored. Absence of transfusion reaction.
• Client will maintain oxygen saturation of greater than 95%.	Improved tissue perfusion.
• Client will be comfortable and calm.	Absence of transfusion reaction. Appropriate nursing measures applied to keep client at ease.
2. Explain treatment of a reaction to client and family.	Allays anxiety and helps client/family anticipate nurse's actions.

IMPLEMENTATION

IN THE EVENT OF TRANSFUSION REACTION

1. Stop the transfusion.	Severity of reaction is related to amount of component infused.
2. Remove tubing containing blood product, and replace it with new tubing (see Chapter 27), except as noted below, in the case of mild allergic reaction.	Prevents additional blood in tubing from being infused.
3. Maintain patent IV line using 0.9% normal saline.	Normal saline tubing should be connected at the cannula hub to prevent additional blood from being infused. Medications and fluids will need to be administered for certain reactions.
4. Notify physician.	Transfusion reactions require immediate medical intervention. In the event of a mild allergic reaction, transfusion should be stopped and antihistamine administered per physician's order. Transfusion may then be restarted per physician's order.
5. Notify blood bank.	Blood bank will have a procedure to follow when notified of a transfusion reaction.
6. Obtain blood samples (if needed) from arm opposite transfusion. Check agency policy regarding number and type of tubes to be used.	Typically, one tube of blood will be crossmatched to pretransfusion sample to ensure that correct blood was given to recipient, and the blood will be checked for antibodies to determine the type of reaction. A second blood sample will be checked for free hemoglobin in the serum, indicating hemolysis, and a bilirubin level should be obtained.
7. Return remainder of blood component and attached blood tubing to the blood bank according to agency policy. (Blood will not usually need to be returned in the case of circulatory overload.)	A sample of this blood will be crossmatched to client's pretransfusion and posttransfusion samples to determine if error in crossmatching occurred.
8. Monitor and document client's vital signs every 15 minutes or more frequently if needed.	Maintains ongoing assessment of client's cardiopulmonary status.
9. Administer prescribed medications according to type and severity of transfusion reaction.	
a. Epinephrine	Stimulates sympathetic nervous system to relieve respiratory distress and combat vasodilation in anaphylaxis.
b. Antihistamine	Parenteral antihistamine diminishes some aspects of allergic response by blocking histamine receptors. May also be ordered before transfusion in some cases.
c. Antibiotics	Administered when bacterial contamination/sepsis is suspected.
d. Antipyretics/analgesics	Administered to relieve fever and discomfort in acute hemolytic reactions, febrile nonhemolytic reactions, graft-versus-host disease, and bacterial sepsis.

STEP	RATIONALE
e. Diuretics/morphine	May be administered in circulatory overload to reduce intravascular volume and decrease vascular tone.
f. Corticosteroids	Stabilizes cell membranes, decreasing histamine release. Administered in severe allergic reactions.
10. IV fluids.	Rapid administration of IV fluids may help to counteract some of symptoms of anaphylactic shock.
11. In the event of cardiac arrest, initiate cardiopulmonary resuscitation (see Chapter 26).	Anaphylaxis can quickly lead to cardiopulmonary arrest. Prompt resuscitation may prevent further complications.
12. Obtain first voided urine sample and send to laboratory. A catheter may need to be inserted to obtain the urine (see Chapter 32).	Hemoglobinuria occurs with acute hemolytic reactions. Degree of damage to kidneys is influenced by pH of urine and rate of urinary excretion. Attempts will be made to initiate diuresis and alkalinize the urine. If kidney damage is severe, dialysis may be required.

EVALUATION

1. Observe client, and conduct necessary nursing measures to determine response to discontinuing transfusion or instituting measures to reduce transfusion reaction.	Provides continued monitoring of client's cardiopulmonary status and physiological response.

Recording and Reporting

- Document client's response to transfusion in nurse's notes/transfusion form/appropriate operative form.
- Immediately report presence of transfusion reaction and client's physical assessment findings to nurse in charge and physician.
- Record exact time of transfusion reaction, assessment findings, and nursing and medical actions taken.

Unexpected Outcomes	Related Interventions
1. Client's physiological status worsens.	• Appropriate interventions will be dictated by nature of crisis. Table 28-2 provides general guidelines.

Teaching Considerations

- Clients and caregivers should be taught signs and symptoms of transfusion reactions and steps to be taken should they occur.

Pediatric Considerations

- Irradiated red blood cells and platelets are preferable in children under 6 years of age because of their immature immune systems and to avoid graft-versus-host disease.

Gerontological Considerations

- Administer blood components cautiously to older adults, considering both rate and amount of infusion, because they are more likely to develop circulatory overload than younger clients.

Home Care Considerations

- Certain adverse outcomes (development of hepatitis) or transfusion reactions (delayed hemolysis) occur days to weeks after client has received transfusion and may become evident in the home setting. It is important that client, family, and home care workers are aware of signs and symptoms of these adverse occurrences and steps to be taken should they occur.

FOCUS on CLINICAL PRACTICE

You are assigned to care for Mr. Jack Norris, a 45-year-old African-American who is admitted with sickle cell anemia. He has shortness of breath and acute pain. The physician has ordered 2 units of packed red blood cells to be transfused when ready.

1. What assessments are necessary before initiating the transfusion?
2. Mr. Norris has an IV infusing in his left cephalic vein that was started in the emergency department. The blood bank has notified the nurse that the packed red blood cells are ready. What should the nurse do before bringing the unit of PRBCs to the nursing unit?
3. Once the PRBCs are started, at what rate should they infuse? What is the nurse's responsibility during the transfusion?
4. Within 10 minutes of the transfusion, Mr. Norris gets restless and spikes a temperature of 101.2° F. His pretransfusion temperature was 99.4° F. What should the nurse suspect, and what actions should be taken?

NCLEX REVIEW QUESTIONS

1. Which of the following solutions should the nurse set up as a piggyback infusion when initiating a blood transfusion?
   1. 0.45% sodium chloride (½ NS)
   2. Dextrose 5% in 0.45% sodium chloride (D_5 ½ NS)
   3. 0.9% sodium chloride (normal saline)
   4. Dextrose 5% in 0.9% sodium chloride (D_5 NS)
2. Which of the following types of blood is appropriate for a client who is A+?
   1. ABO
   2. A
   3. B
   4. AB
3. Which of the following clients is a candidate for autologous transfusion?
   1. 7-year-old scheduled for hernia repair
   2. 36-year-old scheduled for colon resection
   3. 54-year-old scheduled for cholecystectomy
   4. 72-year-old scheduled for total hip replacement
4. Which of the following actions has the greatest impact on reducing a potential transfusion reaction?
   1. Administering an antihistamine 15 minutes before the transfusion
   2. Comparing the client's identification bracelet with the blood bag label number
   3. Ensuring that the client knows what his or her blood type is
   4. Obtaining client's previous transfusion history

References

American Association of Blood Banks: *Technical manual,* ed 14, Bethesda, Md, 2002, The Association.

Andrews M, Hanson P: Religion, culture, and nursing. In Andrews M, Boyle J: *Transcultural concepts in nursing care,* Philadelphia, 2003, Lippincott.

Doughty RR: Observation and documentation of bedside blood transfusion, *Br J Nurs* 9(16):1054, 2000.

Goodnough LT: Risks of blood transfusion, *Crit Care Med* 31(12S):S678, 2003.

Hankins J and others: *Infusion therapy in clinical practice,* Philadelphia, 2001, WB Saunders.

Infusion nursing standards of practice, *J Intraven Nurs* 23(6S):S1, 2000.

McKenry L, Salerno E: *Mosby's pharmacology in nursing,* ed 21, St. Louis, 2003, Mosby.

Otto SE: *Mosby's pocket guide to intravenous therapy,* ed 4, St. Louis, 2001, Mosby.

Rudnicke C: Transfusion alternatives, *J Infus Nurs* 26(1):27, 2003.

Vernon S, Pfeifer GM: Blood management strategies for critical care patients, *Crit Care Nurse* 23(6):34, 2003.

Research References

Hanna H, Raad I: Blood products: a significant risk factor for long-term CRBSI in cancer patients, *Infect Control Hosp Epidemiol* 22(3):165, 2001.

Turner CL, Casbard AC, Murphy MF: Barcode technology: its role in increasing the safety of blood transfusion, *Transfusion* 43(9):1200, 2003.

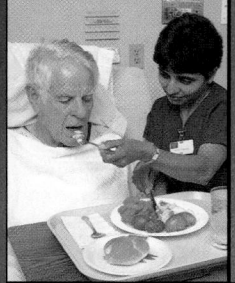

29

Oral Nutrition

MEDIA RESOURCES

Evolve Site *evolve*

http://evolve.elsevier.com/Perry/skills
- Weblinks
- Video clips
- Mosby's Nursing Skills Video Exercises

Mosby's Nursing Skills Videos/CD-ROM

- *Nutrition and Fluids Video:* Preparing for meals; serving meal trays, use of the "clock" technique for a visually impaired person; feeding the dependent person, positioning and observations for a person with dysphagia, signs of aspiration, and difficulty swallowing and "pocketing" of food

OBJECTIVES

Mastery of content in this chaper will enable the nurse to:

- Perform accurate nutritional screening.
- Identify and refer clients appropriate for nutritional assessment to a registered dietitian.
- Assess client's ability to swallow.
- Identify the client at risk for aspiration related to dysphagia.
- Evaluate the client's tolerance of oral nutrition.
- Prepare the client to receive appropriate meals.
- Demonstrate how to properly feed the client who cannot self-feed.
- Provide mouth care after feeding a client.

KEY TERMS

Albumin	Gag reflex
Anthropometrics	Malnutrition
Aspiration	National Dysphagia Diet
Basal energy expenditure (BEE)	Nutritional risk
Body mass index (BMI)	Nutritional screening
Bolus	Prealbumin
Dysphagia	Registered dietitian

BOX 29-1   Factors Related to Nutritional Risk in Adults

The presence of one of more of the following factors denotes potential nutrition risk:

- Involuntary weight change of $\geq$5% in $\leq$3 months
- Decreased appetite
- Nausea and vomiting
- Drug-nutrient interactions
- Compromised dentition
- Change in bowel habits for more than 3 days
- Inappropriate use of dietary supplements
- Chronic disease
- Increased energy and nutrient requirements (major surgery, trauma)
- Inadequate nutrition intake, including not receiving food or nutrition products for <7 days

From Shopbell J and others: Nutrition screening and assessment. In *The science and practice of nutrition support*, Dubuque, Iowa, 2001, American Society for Parenteral and Enteral Nutrition.

Nutritional status reflects general health and can affect rate of recovery from procedures, surgery, or illness. When a client is unable to obtain adequate oral nutrition, nutritional status can be compromised. A nurse's role includes performing nutritional screening to determine the client's risk status for malnutrition, assessing and assisting an adult client with feeding issues, and identifying clients at risk for aspiration during oral feeding.

Screening for Nutritional Risk

Malnutrition is present in up to 50% of all hospitalized adult clients (Hall, 1999). Nutritional screening is the process of identifying client characteristics associated with nutritional problems and risk factors (ASPEN Board of Directors, 1997; Hammond, 2003; Shopbell and others, 2001). It is the first step in the nutritional assessment process. The purpose of a nutritional screening is to quickly identify individuals who are malnourished or at risk of malnutrition (ASPEN Board of Directors, 1997; Hammond and others, 2003; Shopbell and others, 2001). Nutritional risk is the potential to become malnourished because of factors that are primary, such as inadequate intake, or secondary, such as disease. Box 29-1 provides a list of factors related to nutritional risk (Shopbell and others, 2001). An effective nutritional screen is simple, uses readily available data or data that is easy to obtain, includes data relevant to nutritional status, leads to an intervention, and is cost effective. Box 29-2 provides an example of a nutritional screening tool used by nurses in an urban teaching hospital (Brody, 2002).

Health care professionals can work with the registered dietitian (RD) to complete a nutritional assessment. No single biochemical test, such as serum albumin, can accurately indicate poor nutritional status, but collectively biochemical tests, measurements of height and weight, and a thorough diet and nutritional history can reflect the client's nutritional status. A registered dietitian is a food and nutrition expert who has met the minimum academic and professional requirements to qualify for the credential RD (American Dietetic Association, 2003).

The continuing decrease in length of stay in acute care facilities makes nutritional screening and assessment an essential component of care. Once the RN or other responsible professional completes nutritional screening, clients at nutritional risk are referred to the RD for formal nutritional assessment. Clients may be assessed for a variety of reasons, including diagnoses associated with nutritional risk (such as gastrointestinal [GI] problems, trauma, burns, sepsis, or malabsorption), recent rapid weight loss, or history of poor dietary intake. The Joint Commission on Accreditation of Healthcare Organizations (JCAHO) (2003) standards require the identification of clients who are nutritionally at risk by means of an initial screening mechanism. This screening must be completed within 24 hours of admission to a hospital, within 14 days of admission to a long-term care facility, or within a facility-defined period of time in ambulatory care and home care settings (JCAHO, 2003). Clients who are identified to be at risk should have a nutritional assessment completed by an RD. A multidisciplinary nutritional plan of care should be designed, implemented, and periodically reevaluated based on individual client needs. JCAHO also re-

BOX 29-2   Nutritional Screening Tool

All clients are screened by a Registered Nurse within 8 hours of admission date for the presence of "nutritional risk triggers."
Nutritional risk triggers include:

Adults:
- New-onset diabetes, new-onset insulin therapy, or diabetic ketoacidosis
- Presence of pressure ulcers (stage 2 or greater), Braden Scale score 13-14 (moderate risk) or <12 (high risk), or specialty bed required
- Swallowing problems
- Alternative route of feeding: total parenteral nutrition (TPN), peripheral parenteral nutrition (PPN) or enteral nutrition (tube feeding)
- Recent unintentional weight loss (> 5 lb in 2 months)
- Client with renal dialysis dependence
- Immunocompromised status
- Eating disorder (Anorexia nervosa or bulimia)
- Severe liver disease or pancreatitis
- Uncontrolled blood sugar

Maternity:
- Adolescent pregnancy (<18 years of age)
- Antepartum
- Multigestation (twins or greater)
- Substance abuse in pregnancy
- Lactating women
- Diabetes in pregnancy

Pediatrics:
- HIV
- Cancer
- Lead poisoning
- Prematurity <2 years old
- Chewing/Swallowing difficulty
- Feeding Tube
- Weight Loss

Nursing notifies the Department of Food and Nutrition Services within 24 hours of admission date via computer system if one or more "nutritional risk triggers" are present.

The Registered Dietitian performs a nutritional assessment within 24 hours of notification of the trigger.

Reprinted with permission from *Newark Beth Israel Medical Center nutrition screening, assessment, and reassessment policy.*

quires education and training of clients related to nutritional intervention, modified diets, and oral health.

Nutrition Screening Initiative

The aging of America has led to increased prevalence of age-related chronic disease. Disease-specific nutritional screening and intervention are fundamental to the management of many of these chronic diseases. The Nutrition Screening Initiative (NSI) (1997) was a multidisciplinary endeavor led by the American Academy of Family Physicians and the American Dietetic Association from 1990 to 2003. Although funding for the program has ended, the materials and processes established still exist and are in use. Disciplines represented include nutrition, dentistry,

pharmacology, mental health, managed care, home care, and community social services. The NSI's goal is to accelerate the incorporation of nutritional screening and intervention into the nation's health care delivery system for older Americans (American Academy of Family Physicians, 2003). One tool designed to identify individuals at nutritional risk as a result of the NSI is the DETERMINE Your Nutritional Health Checklist (Figure 29-1). This 10-item questionnaire is intended to be completed by the client and brought to the physician's office. Based on the outcomes of each individual client's form, referral(s) to an appropriate health care professional are made (NSI, 1997). The NSI also designed two screening tools for use by health care professionals. The Level I Screen (Figure 29-2) was designed for administration by nonphysician health care providers and does not include laboratory assessment. The Level II Screen was designed for administration by physicians or other individuals whose scope of practice includes ordering laboratory tests and administering cognitive tests (White and others, 2002).

Global Assessment

Subjective Global Assessment (SGA) and Mini Nutritional Assessment (MNA) are two tools, based on client history and a simple physical status, used by RDs and physicians to assess nutritional status (Persson and others, 1996). These tools were designed to allow practitioners to assess nutritional status without using objective measures (Edel and others, 2000).

SGA (Figure 29-3) is an overall evaluation of a client that includes assessment of five components of the medical history: weight and weight change, dietary intake, gastrointestinal symptoms, disease state, and the client's functional status. It also includes a physical examination for changes in body composition such as loss of subcutaneous fat in the triceps and chest, muscle wasting in the quadriceps and deltoids, and signs of ankle or sacral edema or ascites (Detsky and others, 1987; McCann, 1996; Shopbell and others, 2001). Following evaluation, the clinician categorizes the client as well nourished, mildly to moderately malnourished, or severely malnourished based on the information obtained (Detsky and others, 1987; McCann, 1996).

The MNA (Figure 29-4), developed by Guigoz with Nestle Nutritional Corporation, is an assessment tool that can be used to identify geriatric clients (over 65 years of age) at risk of malnutrition. It is an 18-item tool in which questions are divided into one of two main components, screening or assessment. The screening includes questions related to change in oral intake, weight loss, mobility, stress, and body mass index (BMI). A score of less than 11 in the screening component suggests malnutrition and the need to complete the remainder of the form. The assessment component includes arm and calf circumference, specific questions related to eating habits, and questions related to medical history. A total score is calculated (0 to 30 points) to provide a subjective judgment of protein energy malnutrition (PEM). A total

Text continued on p. 991

The Warning Signs of poor nutritional health are often overlooked. Use this checklist to find out if you or someone you know is at nutritional risk.

Read the statements below. Circle the number in the yes column for those that apply to you or someone you know. For each yes answer, score the number in the box. Total your nutritional score.

DETERMINE YOUR NUTRITIONAL HEALTH

	YES
I have an illness or condition that made me change the kind and/or amount of food I eat.	2
I eat fewer than 2 meals per day.	3
I eat few fruits or vegetables, or milk products.	2
I have 3 or more drinks of beer, liquor or wine almost every day.	2
I have tooth or mouth problems that make it hard for me to eat.	2
I don't always have enough money to buy the food I need.	4
I eat alone most of the time.	1
I take 3 or more different prescribed or over-the-counter drugs a day.	1
Without wanting to, I have lost or gained 10 pounds in the last 6 months.	2
I am not always physically able to shop, cook and/or feed myself.	2
TOTAL	

Total Your Nutritional Score. If it's —

0-2   **Good!** Recheck your nutritional score in 6 months.

3-5   **You are at moderate nutritional risk.** See what can be done to improve your eating habits and lifestyle. Your office on aging, senior nutrition program, senior citizens center or health department can help. Recheck your nutritional score in 3 months.

6 or more   **You are at high nutritional risk.** Bring this checklist the next time you see your doctor, dietitian or other qualified health or social service professional. Talk with them about any problems you may have. Ask for help to improve your nutritional health.

These materials developed and distributed by the Nutrition Screening Initiative, a project of:

 AMERICAN ACADEMY OF FAMILY PHYSICIANS

 THE AMERICAN DIETETIC ASSOCIATION

 NATIONAL COUNCIL ON THE AGING

Remember that warning signs suggest risk, but do not represent diagnosis of any condition. Turn the page to learn more about the Warning Signs of poor nutritional health.

FIGURE **29-1** Tool for nutritional screening of older adults.

The Nutrition Checklist is based on the Warning Signs described below. Use the word <u>DETERMINE</u> to remind you of the Warning Signs.

DISEASE

Any disease, illness or chronic condition which causes you to change the way you eat, or makes it hard for you to eat, puts your nutritional health at risk. Four out of five adults have chronic diseases that are affected by diet. Confusion or memory loss that keeps getting worse is estimated to affect one out of five or more of older adults. This can make it hard to remember what, when or if you've eaten. Feeling sad or depressed, which happens to about one in eight older adults, can cause big changes in appetite, digestion, energy level, weight and well-being.

EATING POORLY

Eating too little and eating too much both lead to poor health. Eating the same foods day after day or not eating fruit, vegetables, and milk products daily will also cause poor nutritional health. One in five adults skip meals daily. Only 13% of adults eat the minimum amount of fruit and vegetables needed. One in four older adults drink too much alcohol. Many health problems become worse if you drink more than one or two alcoholic beverages per day.

TOOTH LOSS/ MOUTH PAIN

A healthy mouth, teeth and gums are needed to eat. Missing, loose or rotten teeth or dentures which don't fit well or cause mouth sores make it hard to eat.

ECONOMIC HARDSHIP

As many as 40% of older Americans have incomes of less than $6,000 per year. Having less--or choosing to spend less--than $25-30 per week for food makes it very hard to get the foods you need to stay healthy.

REDUCED SOCIAL CONTACT

One-third of all older people live alone. Being with people daily has a positive effect on morale, well-being and eating.

MULTIPLE MEDICINES

Many older Americans must take medicines for health problems. Almost half of older Americans take multiple medicines daily. Growing old may change the way we respond to drugs. The more medicines you take, the greater the chance for side effects such as increased or decreased appetite, change in taste, constipation, weakness, drowsiness, diarrhea, nausea, and others. Vitamins or minerals when taken in large doses act like drugs and can cause harm. Alert your doctor to everything you take.

INVOLUNTARY WEIGHT LOSS/GAIN

Losing or gaining a lot of weight when you are not trying to do so is an important warning sign that must not be ignored. Being overweight or underweight also increases your chance of poor health.

NEEDS ASSISTANCE IN SELF CARE

Although most older people are able to eat, one of every five have trouble walking, shopping, and buying and cooking food, especially as they get older.

ELDER YEARS ABOVE AGE 80

Most older people lead full and productive lives. But as age increases, risk of frailty and health problems increase. Checking your nutritional health regularly makes good sense.

The Nutrition Screening Initiative, 2626 Pennsylvania Avenue, NW, Suite 301, Washington, DC 20037

© The Nutrition Screening Initiative is funded in part by a grant from Ross Laboratories, a division of Abbott Laboratories.

A5944(1.00)/DECEMBER 1995

FIGURE **29-1, cont'd**

Level I Screen

Body Weight

Measure height to the nearest inch and weight to the nearest pound. Record the values below and mark them on the Body Mass Index (BMI) scale to the right. Then use a straight edge (ruler) to connect the two points and circle the spot where this straight line crosses the center line (body mass index). Record the number below.

Healthy older adults should have a BMI between 22 and 27.

Height (in): _____
Weight (lb): _____
Body Mass Index: _____
(number from center column)

Check any boxes that are true for the individual:

❑ Has lost or gained 10 lb (or more) in the past 6 mo

❑ Body mass index <22

❑ Body mass index >27

For the remaining sections, please ask the individual which of the statements (if any) is true for him or her and place a check by each that applies.

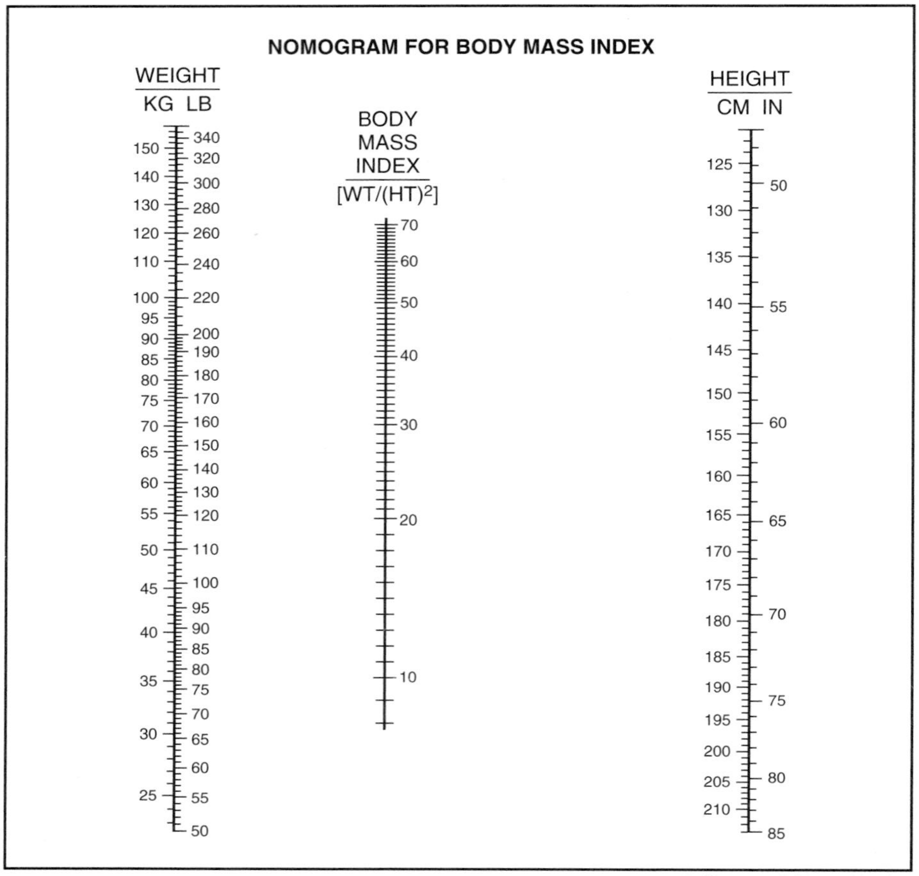

NOMOGRAM FOR BODY MASS INDEX

WEIGHT
KG LB

BODY
MASS
INDEX
[WT/(HT)^2]

HEIGHT
CM IN

© George A Bray 1978

Eating Habits

❑ Does not have enough food to eat each day

❑ Usually eats alone

❑ Does not eat anything on one or more days each month

❑ Has poor appetite

❑ Is on a special diet

❑ Eats vegetables two or fewer times daily

❑ Eats milk or milk products once or not at all daily

❑ Eats fruit or drinks fruit juice once or not at all daily

❑ Eats breads, cereals, pasta, rice, or other grains five or fewer times daily

❑ Has difficulty chewing or swallowing

❑ Has more than one alcoholic drink per day (if woman); more than two drinks per day (if man)

❑ Has pain in mouth, teeth, or gums

Level Screen

Name:

Date:

FIGURE 29-2 NSI Level I Screen.

MEDICAL HISTORY

	SGA Rating		
	A	B	C
1. Weight Change Clothing Size _____ No Change _____ Change Overall loss in past month: _____ _____ 6 months _____ 1 year			
% Loss of usual weight _____ <5% _____ 5–10% _____ >10%			
Change in past 2 weeks _____ Increase (gain) _____ No change (stabilization) _____ Decrease (continued loss)			
2. Dietary Intake Reduction _____ Unintentional _____ Intentional Overall Change _____ No Change _____ Change Increase or Decrease			
Duration _____ Weeks _____ Months			
Diet Change _____ Suboptimal solids (i.e., 75%, 50%, 25% intake) _____ Full liquid diet _____ Hypocaloric fluids _____ NPO (starvation)			
3. Gastrointestinal Symptoms (persisting daily for >2 weeks) _____ None _____ Diarrhea _____ Dysphagia/Odynaphagia _____ Nausea _____ Vomiting _____ Anorexia			
4. Functional Impairment Overall impairment _____ None _____ Mild _____ Severe			
Duration _____ Days _____ Weeks _____ Months			
Type _____ Ambulatory (Walking or Wheelchair) _____ Bedridden			

PHYSICAL EXAMINATION

	SGA Rating		
	Well (A)	Mild/Mod (B)	Severe (C)
5. Muscle Wasting _____ Bicep _____ Tricep _____ Quadricep _____ Deltoid _____ Temple			
6. Subcutaneous Fat Loss _____ Tricep _____ Chest _____ Eyes _____ Perioral _____ Interosseous _____ Palmar			
7. Edema _____ Hands _____ Sacral _____ Lower extremity			

(A) Well Nourished _____ **(B) Mild/Moderate Undernutrition** _____ **(C) Severe Undernutrition** _____

Reference:
Journal of the American College of Nutrition: 2000 Oct:19(5): 570-7

Use of Subjective Global Assessment to Identify Nutrition-Associated Complications and Death in Geriatric Long-Term Care Facility Residents

Gordon S. Sacks, PharmD, Kaye Dearman, PharmD, William H. Replogle, PhD, Virginia L. Cora, DSN, RNCS, Mark Meeks, MD and Todd Canada, PharmD

Department of Clinical Pharmacy (G.S.S., K.D.), The University of Mississippi Jackson, Mississippi
Department of Family Medicine (W.H.R.), The University of Mississippi Jackson, Mississippi
Department of Medicine (V.L.C., M.M.), The University of Mississippi Jackson, Mississippi
Department of Pharmacy Services (T.C.), Parkland Memorial Hospital, Dallas, Texas

FIGURE **29-3** Subjective Global Assessment tool to evaluate components of medical history.

Mini Nutritional Assessment
MNA®

Last name: _____ First name: _____ Sex: _____ Date: _____

Age: _____ Weight, kg: _____ Height, cm: _____ I.D. Number: _____

Complete the screen by filling in the boxes with the appropriate numbers.
Add the numbers for the screen. If score is 11 or less, continue with the assessment to gain a Malnutrition Indicator Score.

Screening

A Has food intake declined over the past 3 months due to loss of appetite, digestive problems, chewing or swallowing difficulties?
0 = severe loss of appetite
1 = moderate loss of appetite
2 = no loss of appetite ☐

B Weight loss during the last 3 months
0 = weight loss greater than 3 kg (6.6 lbs)
1 = does not know
2 = weight loss between 1 and 3 kg (2.2 and 6.6 lbs)
3 = no weight loss ☐

C Mobility
0 = bed or chair bound
1 = able to get out of bed/chair but does not go out
2 = goes out ☐

D Has suffered psychological stress or acute disease in the past 3 months
0 = yes   2 = no ☐

E Neuropsychological problems
0 = severe dementia or depression
1 = mild dementia
2 = no psychological problems ☐

F Body Mass Index (BMI) (weight in kg)/(height in m)^2
0 = BMI less than 19
1 = BMI 19 to less than 21
2 = BMI 21 to less than 23
3 = BMI 23 or greater ☐

Screening score (subtotal max. 14 points) ☐ ☐

12 points or greater Normal–not at risk–no need to complete assessment
11 points or below   Possible malnutrition–continue assessment

Assessment

G Lives independently (not in a nursing home or hospital)
0 = no   1 = yes ☐

H Takes more than 3 prescription drugs per day
0 = yes   1 = no ☐

I Pressure sores or skin ulcers
0 = yes   1 = no ☐

J How many full meals does the patient eat daily?
0 = 1 meal
1 = 2 meals
2 = 3 meals ☐

K Selected consumption markers for protein intake
• At least one serving of dairy products (milk, cheese, yogurt) per day?   yes ☐   no ☐
• Two or more servings of legumes or eggs per week?   yes ☐   no ☐
• Meat, fish or poultry every day   yes ☐   no ☐
0.0 = if 0 or 1 yes
0.5 = if 2 yes
1.0 = if 3 yes ☐.☐

L Consumes two or more servings of fruits or vegetables per day?
0 = no   1 = yes ☐

M How much fluid (water, juice, coffee, tea, milk...) is consumed per day?
0.0 = less than 3 cups
0.5 = 3 to 5 cups
1.0 = more than 5 cups ☐.☐

N Mode of feeding
0 = unable to eat without assistance
1 = self-fed with some difficulty
2 = self-fed without any problem ☐

O Self view of nutritional status
0 = views self as being malnourished
1 = is uncertain of nutritional state
2 = views self as having no nutritional problem ☐

P In comparison with other people of the same age, how does the patient consider his/her health status?
0.0 = not as good
0.5 = does not know
1.0 = as good
2.0 = better ☐.☐

Q Mid-arm circumference (MAC) in cm
0.0 = MAC less than 21
0.5 = MAC 21 to 22
1.0 = MAC 22 or greater ☐.☐

R Calf circumference (CC) in cm
0 = CC less than 31   1 = CC 31 or greater ☐

Assessment (max. 16 points) ☐☐.☐

Screening score ☐☐

Total Assessment (max. 30 points) ☐☐.☐

Malnutrition Indicator Score
17 to 23.5 points   at risk of malnutrition ☐
Less than 17 points   malnourished ☐

Ref.: Guigoz Y, Vellas B and Garry PJ. 1994. Mini Nutritional Assessment: A practical assessment tool for grading the nutritional state of elderly patients. *Facts and Research in Gerontology*. Supplement #2:15–59.
Rubenstein LZ, Harker J, Guigoz Y and Vellas B. Comprehensive Geriatric Assessment (CGA) and the MNA: An Overview of CGA, Nutritional Assessment, and Development of a Shortened Version of the MNA. In: "Mini Nutritional Assessment (MNA): Research and Practice in the Elderly". Vellas B, Garry PJ and Guigoz Y, editors. Nestlé Nutrition Workshop Series. Clinical & Performance Programme, vol. 1. Karger Bale, in press.

FIGURE 29-4 The Nestle Mini Nutritional Assessment tool is particularly useful in assessing the nutrition status of geriatric clients.

score of less than 17 points denotes malnutrition; a score of 17 to 23.5 indicates risk for malnutrition (Nestle Clinical Nutrition, 2003; Persson and others, 1996).

Nutritional Assessment by the Registered Dietitian

The nutritional care provided by a registered dietitian is often termed medical nutrition therapy (MNT). MNT is defined by the 2001 Medicare MNT benefit legislation as "nutritional diagnostic, therapy, and counseling services for the purpose of disease management which are furnished by a registered dietitian or nutrition professional" (Lacey and Pritchett, 2003). In 2003 the American Dietetic Association published the Nutrition Care Process (NCP) and model. The process provides structure to the provision of nutritional care to all clients and provides a framework by which the registered dietitian can think critically and make decisions regarding medical nutrition therapy (Lacey and Pritchett, 2003). There are four steps to the process: nutrition assessment, nutrition diagnosis, nutrition intervention, and nutrition monitoring and evaluation (Lacey and Pritchett 2003). The nutritional assessment is a comprehensive evaluation of a client's nutritional status, performed by a registered dietitian. Components of the assessment include medical, social, nutritional, and medication history, physical examination, anthropometric measurements, and laboratory data. The nutritional assessment builds on information collected from the nutritional screening (Hammond and others, 2003). The goal of the assessment is to develop an effective nutritional plan of care that addresses issues identified from the assessment and screening (Shopbell and others, 2001). From assessment a decision on nutritional diagnosis is made. A nutritional diagnosis is a label that describes "an actual occurrence, risk of, or potential for developing a nutritional problem that dietetics professionals are responsible for treating independently" (Lacey and Pritchett, 2003). The nutritional intervention is the activity intended to address that problem. The effects of this intervention are then monitored and evaluated with changes made as necessary.

Malnutrition and Its Consequences

Malnutrition is defined as "a pathologic state resulting from a relative or an absolute deficiency or excess of one or more of the essential nutrients" (Shopbell, and others, 2001). Human nutritional reserves are depleted as a result of the inadequacy of nutrient intake to meet nutrient requirements. This inadequacy can result from a disorder in food ingestion, digestion, or absorption. It can occur from inability to ingest adequate nutrients, inability to digest nutrients, or inability to absorb nutrients (Hammond and others, 2003) or increased losses. Consequences of malnutrition include increased length of hospital stay, compromised immune function, delayed wound healing, increased complication rate, and increased mortality. Early identification of malnutrition or the risk of malnutrition can decrease the incidence of these side effects (Shopbell and others, 2001). In order to effectively identify nutrition-related problems, nutritional

screening and assessment strategies have been implemented in hospitals, ambulatory care centers, and long-term care institutions.

Evidence-Based Practice Trends

Throughout this chapter, evidence-based practice is integrated into the various sections. Studies by Brody and others (2000) and Huhmann and others (2003) provide evidence in support of dysphagia screening. Similar evidence-based approaches and outcomes are integrated in nutritional screening and assessment.

Dysphagia screening is recommended as part of the multidisciplinary approach to dysphagia management. The dietary intake of clients with dysphagia may be affected for long periods of time, and the malnutrition that occurs in these individuals is secondary to insufficient protein, calorie, and micronutrient intake (Elmstahl and others, 1999; Perry and Love, 2001). Registered nurses, registered dietitians, physicians, or speech language pathologists can perform these screenings in clients (Daniels and others, 2000; Davies, 1999; DePippo and others, 1994). Early screening and treatment of dysphagia leads to more cost-effective treatment and improved quality of care and ensures optimal outcomes (Elmstahl and others, 1999; Hinds and Wiles, 1998).

Skill Performance Guidelines

1. Know the normal ranges of laboratory values and physical assessment characteristics. Identify which characteristics are abnormal in the client. Weight is a valuable indicator of changes in nutritional status.

2. Be aware of signs and symptoms associated with malnutrition (see Table 29-1). Identify those clients who are at risk for malnutrition and other nutritional abnormalities, such as iron deficiency anemias.

3. Use a systematic and organized approach when obtaining a nutritional assessment.

4. Be aware of clients' social history, cultural preferences, and economic factors. Clients may be interested in healthy nutritional practices but may be unable to implement them (e.g., no refrigeration at home, lack of money to buy food or infant formula). The nurse needs to be aware of limitations and work with the client toward realistic goals. Each of these factors alone and in combination impact a client's nutritional status and his or her ability to adhere to therapeutic diets.

5. Review the client's medical history. Certain diseases, medications, and medical problems can influence nutritional status. Clients with some medical problems or nonfunctioning GI tracts cannot be treated with oral nutrition. Parenteral therapies may be necessary (American Society for Parenteral and Enteral Nutrition [ASPEN], 1997).

6. Verify that the type of feeding ordered is what has been provided to the client at the proper temperature. Knowledge of the different types of oral diets (e.g., di-

abetic diet, lactose intolerant diet) helps the nurse properly plan and recommend changes to meet client needs.

7. Promote factors that improve the client's appetite, such as encouraging the client to select foods; providing small, frequent meals; and arranging pleasant and comfortable surroundings.

8. An organized approach when feeding a client of any age helps the client feel more at ease, and appetite may increase in an unhurried atmosphere.

9. Be aware of the psychological impact on the adult client who cannot self-feed. Feeding in a timely, well-paced, and understanding manner that allows maximal client independence can lessen the negative aspects of being fed by someone else. Instruct family members to provide a relaxed, social atmosphere when feeding the client and to allow the client to be as independent in feeding as possible. Assistive devices may enable the client to perform self-care.

10. Encourage clients and family members to keep menus from the hospital meal tray to use as a guide for preparing meals at home.

Cultural Considerations

It is important to assess the meaning of food to the client and family. Foods are generally associated with caring and love, especially in collectivistic cultures. Food is also associated with health promotion, maintenance, and restoration. For example:

- For Asians a balance between yin and yang is achieved through dietary practices (Purnell and Kim, 2003; Sharts-Hopko, 2003; Wang, 2003).
- Among Koreans, seaweed soup is given to mothers post-partum to cleanse the blood, promote lactation, and restore yang because postpartum is a predominantly yin state.
- Many cultures, including Asians, Hispanics, Eastern Europeans, and Africans, believe in the heat and cold theory of health and illness. Foods are classified as cold or hot based on their characteristics, independent of the temperature at which they are served. There is no universal agreement across cultures on which foods are hot or cold.
- Early infant feeding and use of additives in the baby's formula have been associated with the low-income Puerto Rican belief that a rotund (gordito/a) baby is healthy (Higgins, 2000).

Determine the nutritional practices of the client and family. Collect information on the types of foods and beverages that are generally given for different types of conditions. For example, some pregnant Hispanics and African-American women are known to have specific cravings to eat starch or red clay that need to be satisfied to promote the baby's health (Glanville, 2003; Purnell, 2003). Some African-Americans

also believe that certain foods build blood, thereby preventing anemia (Glanville, 2003). When providing nutritional care to clients of diverse cultures and religions:

- Avoid making value judgments about their practices.
- Understand the practice, and collaborate to develop healthy alternatives.
- Recognize and assess differences in food preparation practices. For example, determine types of spices and condiments indigenous to the culture. For example, Indians use strong spices such as cumin, coriander, cardamom, pepper, ginger, garlic, onions, chilies, and saffron in their cooking (Jambunathan, 2003). Koreans eat fermented cabbage (kimchee) with each meal (Purnell and Kim, 2003). Japanese eat fresh, uncooked seafood such as seaweed and tuna (Sharts-Hopko, 2003).
- Assess religious and cultural influences on nutritional practices.
  - Buddhists and Hindus are generally vegetarians because of their respect for life and belief in transmigration of the soul.
  - Hindus generally avoid eating beef, but some may eat chicken and lamb (Jambunathan, 2003).
  - Muslims eat *Halal* foods and avoid those that are classified as *Haram* (pork, alcohol) (Lawrence and Rozmus, 2001).
  - Orthodox Jews generally eat kosher foods and avoid serving meat and dairy at the same time, eat fish with fins and scales, and eat animals that chew their cud and nonpredatory birds.
  - Muslims fast all day during the month of Ramadan, including food and water. They eat before dawn and during evenings (Rassoul, 2000).
  - Some Hindus fast to obtain blessing from their gods.
- Accommodate food patterns of the culture.
  - Assess which ingredient or food content needs to be reduced. For example, a Chinese client on a low-sodium diet should use low-sodium soy sauce and avoid shrimp paste and oyster sauce (Wang, 2003).
  - A diabetic Puerto Rican should be counseled how to use exchanges within the cultural dietary pattern (Adams, 2003). Rice, beans, corn, potatoes, and plantains all belong to the same carbohydrate food group (Juarbe, 2003).
  - Note that most Southeast Asians, Jews, and Africans are lactose intolerant.
  - Allow family members to prepare food for the client by teaching them how to accommodate the prescribed modification. Note that some groups may not be able to read food labels.
  - Use an interpreter to provide culture-specific teaching. Instruct family members in how to store and heat the food they bring for the client.

SKILL 29-1   Performing Nutritional Screening

There are four basic components of nutritional screening: (1) client history (medical, psychological, and social); (2) physical examination and anthropometric measurements; (3) biochemical parameters; and (4) dietary history (Grodner and others, 2000; Lacey and Pritchett, 2003). Elements of the client history, such as appetite, psychosocial factors affecting intake, economics, and cultural issues, give background to factors influencing current nutritional status. The medical history indicates medications, surgery, and co-existing medical conditions compromising nutrition. Depression or abnormal psychiatric behavior leading to decreased food intake can be identified in the psychological history. A social history can give important insight into beliefs, the financial ability to obtain food, and food customs influencing nutritional education. Assessment of dietary intake by eating habits can indicate food practices or avoidance of food groups that may impair nutritional status. A physical examination can reveal signs of impaired nutrition. Finally, biochemical parameters offer information on the status of circulating proteins.

Physical Examination

Physical examination is an important component of a thorough nutritional screening. Malnutrition has both internal and external effects. Table 29-1 lists some of the external manifestations of malnutrition.

Anthropometrics

Height and weight are useful in determining the nutritional status of both children and adults. The height and weight of children are plotted on growth charts and evaluated against standards based on the normal U.S. population. This information is essential to track children's' growth over time, which reflects nutritional adequacy. Height can be measured directly or indirectly. The direct measurement of height involves a measuring rod, or statiometer, and the individual must be able to stand or lie flat. This is sometimes impossible due to the client's condition, so indirect methods such as recumbent length, arm span, or knee height are used to estimate height.

Weight information can also be gathered in several ways, including usual body weight (UBW), ideal body weight (IBW), actual body weight (ABW), and BMI. A thorough nutritional assessment usually requires the collection of all of these measures of weight. The change in a client's weight over time is an inexpensive and relatively accurate method of predicting nutritional status. Box 29-3 illustrates two ways of categorizing the severity of weight loss and malnutrition according to amount of weight lost (Hammond and others, 2003). BMI provides a definition for adiposity and can be calculated or obtained from a BMI chart (see Figure 29-5). Box 21-4 lists BMI by degree of adiposity. BMI alone is not a perfect predictor of overweight or obesity. Clinical judgment must be used when evaluating muscular clients such as body builders or those clients with large amounts of edema or ascites because these physiological states may lead to false overestimation of the degree of fatness (Expert Panel on the Identification, 2000).

Biochemical Indices

Biochemical indices further assist in the classification of nutritional status. Table 29-2 lists select biochemical parameters important to the determination of nutritional risk status. It is important to remember that disease state and therapy can affect laboratory data and thus the value may be misleading (Hammond and others, 2003). No single test is a marker of malnutrition. Test results, along with other parameters, help determine the presence and degree of malnutrition.

The liver manufactures serum albumin and prealbumin; therefore values are decreased in the presence of liver disease. Many other disease states such as inflammation, acute phase response, and kidney disease can also decrease serum protein markers of nutritional status (Shopbell and others, 2001). It is important not to look at a single value, but instead to look at a series of values in conjunction with client history and physical examination to evaluate trends over time.

TABLE 29-1 COMPONENTS OF PHYSICAL EXAMINATION FOR NUTRITIONAL SCREENING

BODY AREA	NUTRITIONAL RISK SYMPTOMS	NUTRITION IMPLICATIONS
Hair	Dull, shedding, easily pluckable	Generalized protein calorie malnutrition
Face	Malar pigmentation (dark skin over cheeks and under eyes)	Niacin, B vitamins
	Bitemporal wasting	Malnutrition
	Nasolabial seborrhea	Niacin, riboflavin, B_6 deficiency
	Edematous	Protein deficiency
	Moon face	Corticosteroid impact
	Pallor	Inadequate Fe^{++}, undernutrition
Eyes	Pale eye membranes	Inadequate Fe^{++}
Lips	Cheilosis (red/swelling)	Inadequate niacin, B_6, riboflavin, Fe^{++}
	Angular fissures	
Gingiva	Spongy, bleeding, abnormal redness	Inadequate vitamin C
Tongue	Glossitis (red, raw, fissured)	Inadequate folate, niacin, riboflavin, Fe^{++}, B_6, B_{12}
	Pale, atrophic, smooth/slick (filiform papillary atrophy)	Inadequate Fe^{++}, B_{12}, niacin, folate
	Magenta	Inadequate riboflavin
Nails	Spoon shaped, brittle, ridged	Inadequate Fe^{++}
Back	Bony prominences along shoulder girdle	Malnutrition

BOX 29-3 **Categories of Weight Loss and Malnutrition**

SIGNIFICANT WEIGHT LOSS

5% loss in 1-3 months
7.5% loss in 3-6 months
10% loss in 6 or more months

SEVERE WEIGHT LOSS

>5% loss in 1 month
>7.5% loss in 3 months
>10% loss in 6 months

DEGREE OF MALNUTRITION

Mild: 85%-90% usual body weight
Moderate: 75%-84% usual body weight
Severe: <74% usual body weight

Blackburn G, Bistrian B: Nutritional and metabolic assessment of the hospitalized patient, *JPEN J Parenter Enteral Nutr* 1(1):11, 1977.

BOX 29-4   Body Mass Index

$$BMI = Weight\ (kg)/Height\ (m)^2$$

OR

$$BMI = \frac{Weight\ (lbs)}{(Height\ (inches) \times Height\ (inches))} \times 703$$

CLASSIFICATION OF BMI IN ADULTS

Degree of Adiposity	BMI
Underweight	$<18.5\ kg/m^2$
Normal Weight	$18.5\text{-}24.9\ kg/m^2$
Overweight	$25\text{-}29.9\ kg/m^2$
Obesity (Class 1)	$30\text{-}34.9\ kg/m^2$
Obesity (Class 2)	$35\text{-}39.9\ kg/m^2$
Extreme Obesity (Class 3)	$\geq 40\ kg/m^2$

Body Mass Index (BMI)

BMI	Weight in pounds													
Height	120	130	140	150	160	170	180	190	200	210	220	230	240	250
4'6	29	31	34	36	39	41	43	46	48	52	43	46	48	60
4'8	27	29	31	34	36	38	40	43	45	47	49	52	54	56
4'10	25	27	29	31	34	36	38	40	42	44	46	48	50	52
5'0	23	25	27	29	31	33	35	37	39	41	43	45	47	49
5'2	22	24	26	27	29	31	33	35	37	38	40	42	44	46
5'4	21	22	24	26	28	29	31	33	34	36	38	40	41	43
5'6	19	21	23	24	26	27	29	31	32	34	36	37	39	40
5'8	18	20	21	23	24	26	27	29	30	32	34	35	37	38
5'10	17	19	20	22	23	24	26	27	29	30	32	33	35	36
6'0	16	18	19	20	22	23	24	26	27	28	30	31	33	34
6'2	15	17	18	19	21	22	23	24	26	27	28	30	31	32
6'4	15	16	17	18	20	21	22	23	24	26	27	28	29	30
6'6	14	15	16	17	19	20	21	22	23	24	25	27	28	29
6'8	13	14	15	17	18	19	20	21	22	23	24	25	26	28

KEY

	Obese (30+)
	Overweight (25–29)
	Healthy weight (Below 25)

FIGURE **29-5** Body Mass Index Grid.

From Expert Panel on the Identification, Evaluation, and Treatment of Overweight and Obesity in Adults: *The practical guide identification, evaluation, and treatment of overweight and obesity in adults,* Bethesda, Md, 2000, National Institutes of Health.

TABLE 29-2 SELECTED BIOCHEMICAL TESTS FOR NUTRITIONAL SCREENING

BIOCHEMICAL PARAMETER	LABORATORY TEST	NORMAL RANGE	FUNCTION
Visceral protein status	Serum albumin	3.5-5.0 mg/100 ml	Maintains oncotic pressure; carrier protein; changes slowly; half-life 14-20 days
	Prealbumin	15-36 mg/100 ml	Transport protein for thyroxine; carrier for retinol binding protein; useful in measuring short-term changes; half-life 2-3 days
Lipid status	Cholesterol	<200 mg/100 ml	Blood lipid required for production of steroids, hormones, and cell membranes; levels decrease with malnutrition
Hematological status	Hemoglobin	Male 14-18 g/100 ml Female 12-16 g/100 ml	Measure of the total amount of hemoglobin reflecting the number of red blood cells; levels decrease with dietary deficiency
	Hematocrit	Male 42%-52% Female 37%-47%	Percentage of total blood volume made up of red blood cells; levels decrease with dietary deficiency

Data from *The science and practice of nutrition support*, Dubuque, Iowa, 2001, Kendall; Pagana K, Pagana T: *Mosby's diagnostic and laboratory test reference*, New York, 1999, Mosby.

DELEGATION CONSIDERATIONS

The interpretation of data collected during a nutritional screening is the responsibility of the nurse and should not be delegated to assistive personnel. Certain steps, such as obtaining the client's height and weight, may be delegated. However, when delegating other aspects of care to assistive personnel, it is important that the nurse instruct assistive personnel to:

• Report any signs of coughing, gagging, or choking during meals or when drinking fluids
• Report to the nurse when client does not complete meal or refused to eat

EQUIPMENT

❑ Tongue blade, stethoscope, penlight
❑ Scale
❑ Assessment sheet and pen

STEP	RATIONALE

ASSESSMENT

1. Assess client for usual body weight, noting recent changes in the last 6 months (see Chapter 18).

2. Review results of relevant laboratory tests (see Table 29-2).

3. Determine what medications and other dietary supplements client is taking (over-the-counter and prescribed).

4. Determine client's ability to manipulate eating utensils and self-feed.

Sudden change in body weight unrelated to diet changes can indicate illness (Hernandez and others, 2003).

These biochemical parameters (tests ordered by physician) measure visceral and circulating protein status, lipid status, and hematological status. Albumin, prealbumin, hemoglobin, hematocrit, and cholesterol levels can assist in providing a clue about nutritional status.

Certain medications can inhibit or potentiate action of other medications. Also, medications and nutrients may interact to either decrease medication function (e.g., foods rich in vitamin K, such as dark green vegetables, and coumarin anticoagulants) or impair nutrient use (mineral oil laxatives). Nurses are expected to be aware of drug-drug and drug-nutrient interactions that may impair client care.

Difficulty in self-feeding creates significant risk for malnutrition (Schmid and others, 2003).

STEP	RATIONALE

NURSING DIAGNOSES

- Feeding self-care deficit
- Risk for aspiration
- Risk for deficient fluid volume

- Deficient knowledge regarding nutritional intake
- Imbalanced nutrition: less than body requirement
- Imbalanced nutrition: more than body requirements

Related factors are individualized based on client's condition or needs.

PLANNING

1. Expected outcomes following completion of procedure:
   - Client denies any swallowing or chewing problems or food intolerances.

   - Physical and clinical assessment and laboratory data are consistent with adequate nutritional status.
2. Explain to client purpose for nutritional screening.
3. Prepare environment: quiet, undistracting.

Indicates lack of food intolerance or oral problems interfering with ingestion.
Indicates that client is not at nutritional risk.

Ensures client's participation in care.
Helps nurse to better obtain information.

IMPLEMENTATION

1. Obtain complete and thorough nursing history, including appetite, social, economic, and psychological information.

2. Perform physical assessment.

3. Help client to standing position, and be sure client is free of restrictive clothing.
4. Have client stand on scale, or if client is unable to stand, use chair, bed, or sling type of scale. Record weight.

5. Measure client's height. If client is unable to stand, measure from heel to top of head while client is lying flat on bed, and record.
6. Calculate, or determine via standard height and weight chart, IBW with a range for normal of 10% above and 10% below IBW.
   Calculation of IBW can be accomplished using the following formula:
   Male: 106 pounds (48.1 kg) for the first 5 feet, then add 6 pounds per additional inch (2.7 kg per 2.5 cm).
   Female: 100 pounds (45.4 kg) for the first 5 feet, then add 5 pounds per additional inch (2.25 kg per 2.5 cm).
7. Calculate BMI: Wt (kg)/Ht (m)^2
8. Calculate percent usual body weight using individual's current body weight and the individual's stable weight.
   % Usual body weight = [(usual body weight − current body weight) = usual body weight] × 100
9. Discuss client's diet history, including current diet and explanations for any restrictions, food allergies, food intolerances.
10. Explain to client that nutritional screening is complete.
11. Report diet restrictions and preferences to food and nutrition department.

Allows nurse to identify those clients who are at nutritional risk or are at risk of developing nutrient deficiencies; is of significant importance in the care of acute and chronically ill clients (Correia, 1999).
Through use of physical assessment, nurse will be able to detect signs and symptoms of malnutrition (see Table 29-1).
Clients must be standing for anthropometric measurements.

Weight is a useful index of client's nutritional well-being. Ideally, client should be weighed with same scale at same time of day with same amount of clothing for comparison of weight changes over time.
Correct height measurement assists in calculating ideal body weight.

Allows for assessment against national standards.
Allows for assessment using the client as his or her own standard.

Allows for assessment of factors affecting diet adequacy and appetite.

Allows time for client to ask questions about assessment.
Ensures an inpatient or resident will receive appropriate diet.

STEP	RATIONALE

▌ EVALUATION

1. Review history and physical findings. Note abnormal findings or areas of concern.

   Completeness of data obtained from history and physical findings permits prompt identification of risk, malnutrition, and need for nutritional interventions.

2. Compare client's weight for height with ideal and usual weight.

   Significant weight fluctuations or weight outside of normal range may indicate nutritional risk.

3. Compare anthropometric data with normal measurements.

   Abnormal measurements indicate nutritional risk.

4. Compare biochemical test levels with client's levels.

   Abnormal values, when considered with other nutritional parameters, may indicate malnutrition. Albumin is major protein produced by liver. It is a useful indicator for chronically malnourished clients. In an acute care client, a greater number of factors influence albumin (e.g., stress, hydration, surgery). Transferrin is a more specific indicator of protein and calorie malnutrition than albumin.

Recording and Reporting

- Record results on nutritional screening form, making referral to the RD and documenting any significant differences from the norm.

Unexpected Outcomes	Related Interventions

1. Body weight is below or above usual body weight.	• Check weight weekly, and assess for change. Report significant changes to RD or physician.
	• Document significant changes in intake, especially if client is at risk of malnutrition.
	• If client has experienced an unintentional weight loss, consult the RD for medical nutrition therapy.
	• Registered dietitian will:
	  · Conduct a nutritional assessment.
	  · Calculate caloric needs. Most commonly used formulas include Harris-Benedict equation for basal energy expenditure (BEE), and calculation of calories per kilogram.
	  · Determine amount of protein client requires.
	  · Determine route of nutrition (enteral [oral or tube] or parenteral). For parenteral nutrition (PN) the physician and dietitian will choose either peripheral or central PN and determine whether fat is needed (see Chapter 31).

2. Laboratory test results are not within normal limits.	• Inform physician. • Obtain serial laboratory parameters as ordered by physician or dietitian.

Pediatric Considerations

- Anthropometric data include measurement of length, weight, and head circumference in young children. These measurements are compared with standard growth charts to determine percentiles. The height and weight of children age 2 to 18 years is compared with standard growth charts for interpretation (Hockenberry, 2004).
- Head circumference is measured in children up to 36 months of age and in any child whose head size is questionable. The head circumference is compared with standard growth charts for interpretation (Hockenberry, 2004).

Gerontological Considerations

- The "normal" anthropometric standards were developed based on a healthy middle-age population and may not accurately reflect muscle wasting, decreased subcutaneous fat, or decreased skin elasticity in the older adult (Lueckenotte, 2000).
- Tools available for anthropometric measures for the older adult population have been published (*Nutritional Assessment of the Elderly Through Anthropometry*, 1988).
- Tools available in the Nutrition Screening Initiative (1997) have been designed specifically for nutritional screening of older adults (see Figure 29-2).

SKILL 29-2   Assisting the Adult Client With Oral Nutrition

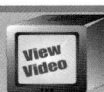

Assisting the adult with oral nutrition requires time, patience, knowledge, and understanding. Most people eat without assistance. However, with illness, trauma, or compromised oral integrity, the client may be physically unable to eat without assistance. Physical impairments that limit self-feeding, compromised dentition, improper fitting dentures, oral lesions or infections, or diseases with resulting impaired digestion may limit the types and consistencies of foods tolerated. Hemiplegia, fractured arm, quadriplegia, debilitating illness, or generalized weakness may also limit self-feeding ability and subsequently appetite. The presence of intravenous (IV) catheters or tubings, dressings, and bandages can also limit self-feeding. In addition, some older adults tire quickly and may need to be assisted even though they can eat independently. The adult who needs help to eat needs compassion and understanding. Merely feeding the adult can be accomplished with common sense, but providing a socially meaningful mealtime requires education and experience on the part of the nurse.

DELEGATION CONSIDERATIONS

The skill of assisting the client with oral nutrition can be delegated to assistive personnel. Such individuals, however, require training not only in "how to feed" but also in strategies to turn a meal into an enjoyable eating experience for the client. The nurse should instruct assistive personnel:

- About any specific swallowing strategies/techniques unique to the client
- To report incidences of coughing, gagging, or difficulty swallowing immediately to the nurse

EQUIPMENT

- ❏ Two-handled cup with lid
- ❏ Plate with plate guard
- ❏ Utensils with splints
- ❏ Utensils with enlarged handles
- ❏ Towels

STEP	RATIONALE

ASSESSMENT

1. Assess that GI tract is functional, and determine what type of diet client can tolerate.
2. Assess client's ability to swallow. In clients with neurological condition, assess cranial nerves V, VII, IX, X, and gag reflex.

Nurse's awareness of specific diet order ensures client gets an appropriate meal tray.

Some clients (those who have neurological diseases or are handicapped) may be at risk for dysphagia and aspiration and may not be able to tolerate a regular diet. Change in consistency of diet (thickened liquids, pureed, soft), swallow training, or alternative means of nutrition may be needed.

STEP	RATIONALE
3. Place a tongue blade on the back of client's tongue.	Clients who do not gag are at risk for aspiration (see Skill 29-3).
4. Determine to what extent client is able to self-feed. Assess physical motor skills, level of consciousness, visual acuity and peripheral vision, and mood.	Clients with any level of independence should not be totally fed by hospital staff. Thorough understanding of client's physical and cognitive limitations alerts the nurse to client's needs.
5. Assess client's appetite, tolerance of foods, cultural and religious preferences, and food likes and dislikes.	Awareness of client's needs before meals prevents misunderstanding and frustration for both nurse and client.

NURSING DIAGNOSES

- Risk for aspiration
- Risk for deficient fluid volume
- Feeding self-care deficit

- Disturbed sensory perception (gustatory)
- Impaired swallowing

Related factors are individualized based on client's condition or needs.

PLANNING

1. Expected outcomes following completion of procedure:	
• Client denies any biting, chewing, or swallowing problem or food intolerances.	Indicates absence of gastric disturbance or food intolerance.
• Client's weight is maintained or changes according to the nutritional care plan.	Nutritional intake meets daily needs.
• Client completes meal.	Prescribed dietary intake consumed.
• Client is able to participate in independent feeding	Enables client to be as independent as possible; provide assistive devices as needed to promote independence; involve family in mealtime if possible.
2. Prepare client's room for mealtime: **a.** Clear over-bed table. **b.** Set up chair for client and for nurse. Place bed in upright back position if client is unable to be up in the chair. Certain conditions, such as pressure ulcer, traction, or spinal surgery, may prevent positioning with head elevated.	Upright position assists client with keeping food toward front of mouth before swallowing, reducing aspiration.
3. Prepare client for meal: **a.** Assist client with elimination needs.	Increases client's comfort and enjoyment of meal, and as a result client's nutritional intake may increase.
b. Help client perform hand hygiene.	Reduces spread of microorganisms.
c. Assist client with mouth care. Clients with dysphagia or dry mouth may benefit from clear water rinsing or swabbing.	Oral hygiene improves taste and increases appetite.
d. Clients with stomatitis (inflammation of oral mucosa) may benefit from rinsing with a solution containing hydrogen peroxide, warm saline, sodium bicarbonate, or a combination of all agents. Consult with physician regarding an oral analgesic (e.g., lidocaine 2% viscous) (Ignatavicius and Workman, 2002).	Clients may avoid foods because of pain from oral infections or lesions.
e. Help client to put in dentures and put on eyeglasses or insert contact lenses if used. Check that dentures fit properly.	Enhances client's ability to bite, chew, and swallow as well as see food. Ill-fitting dentures inhibit normal masticatory function and pose a safety risk.
f. Help client to comfortable sitting position. If client is unable to sit, turn client on side with the head of the bed elevated.	Minimizes risk of aspiration.

STEP	RATIONALE

g. Obtain special devices and needed supplies to facilitate feeding (two-handled cup with lid, plate with plate guard, utensils with splints, utensils with enlarged handles, towels) before meal (see illustration).

Ensures organized, unhurried atmosphere.

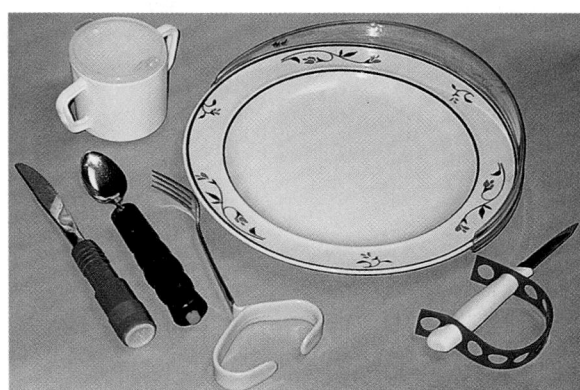

STEP **3g** Mealtime equipment. *Clockwise from upper left:* two-handled cup with lid, plate with plate guard, utensils with splints, and utensils with enlarged handles.

IMPLEMENTATION

1. Perform hand hygiene before preparing client's tray.
2. Assess tray for completeness and correct diet.
3. Prepare tray to meet client's needs: open cartons, remove lids, cut food, and season food after asking client's preferences.
4. If client is able to eat independently, stop here. Return after 10 to 20 minutes.
5. For client who cannot eat independently, begin offering assistance.
   a. Put yourself in a comfortable position.
   b. Ask client about any religious or cultural preferences before beginning feeding.
   c. Ask in what order client would like to eat, and cut food into bite-size pieces.
   d. It may be helpful for disoriented, visually impaired, or easily fatigued clients to have food identified by location on plate as if the plate were a clock (see illustration).

Reduces spread of microorganisms.
Prevents ingestion of incorrect or incomplete meal.
Clients with cognitive or physical impairments may not have the fine motor coordination needed to prepare tray for eating.
Determines how well client is tolerating diet.

Sitting or standing close to client during feeding promotes psychologically comforting and caring environment, which may increase appetite. It is important that the caregiver be comfortable when feeding client, so as not to rush him or her through the meal.
Allows client more independence and control. Small pieces are easier to chew and minimize risk of aspiration.
Assists in client's ability to locate food items.

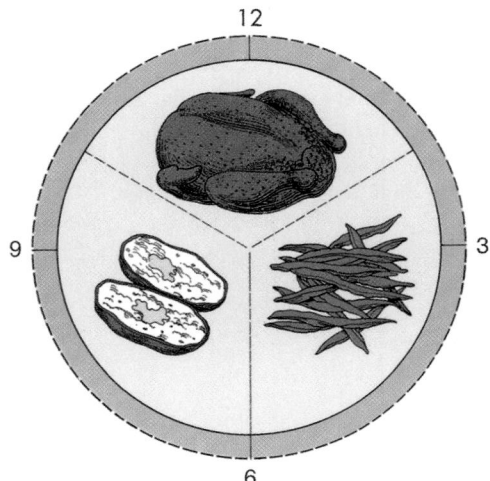

STEP **6a** For the visually impaired client: "The potatoes are at 9 o'clock."

STEP	RATIONALE

6. Feed client in a manner that facilitates chewing and swallowing.

   a. *Older adult:* Feed small amounts at a time, assessing biting, chewing, swallowing, and fatigue.

Decreased saliva production can impair swallowing in the older adult. Aspiration can result because of a decreased or absent gag reflex and relaxation of the lower esophageal sphincter (Williams and Hooper, 1999). Chewing and sitting up for feeding may accelerate onset of fatigue. Frequent rests may be helpful (White and others, 1991; Whitehouse, 1992).

   b. *Neurologically impaired client:* Feed small amounts at a time, and assess for ability to chew, manipulate tongue to form a bolus, and swallow. Give small amounts of thin liquids (soup, beverages), and assess for swallowing.

Clients with limited tongue strength and control may be unable to move bolus to back of mouth for swallowing. Checking for "pocketed" food in mouth prevents aspiration.

- **Critical Decision Point**
  Clients with dysphagia who aspirate thin liquids may benefit from liquids thickened with commercial thickening products or from change in consistency of diet.

   c. *Client with cancer:* Check for food aversions before and during the meal.

May have strong, abnormal sense of taste and smell because of medications.

7. Provide fluids as requested. Do not allow client to drink all liquids at beginning of meal.

Assists with swallowing. Prevents client from filling up on liquids.

8. Talk with client during meal.

Meal should be a pleasant event. Conversation promotes socialization. Involve family if possible.

9. Use meal as an opportunity to educate client (e.g., topics related to nutrition, postoperative exercises, discharge plans).

Education can occur whenever nurse and client are together.

10. Assist client with hand washing and performing mouth care.

Mouth care after meals helps prevent dental caries.

11. Help client to resting position.

Client may feel tired after full meal. If client is prone to aspiration, leave head elevated 45 degrees for 30 minutes after meal.

12. Return client's tray to appropriate place, and perform hand hygiene.

Reduces spread of microorganisms.

EVALUATION

1. Observe client's ability to swallow.

Determines if client develops dysphagia and becomes prone to aspiration.

2. Weigh client daily (if nutrition has been inadequate).

Gradual weight gain reflects improved nutritional status.

3. Determine client's tolerance to diet.

Overfeeding may cause nausea and vomiting. Underfeeding may leave client feeling hungry.

4. Monitor client's fluid and food intake.

Helps to determine whether client's nutritional and fluid needs are being met.

5. Observe client's ability to feed self.

Determines if client is gaining independence in feeding.

Recording and Reporting

- Document in client's chart: client's tolerance of diet, amount eaten, and intake and output.
- If client is on calorie counts, record caloric intake on appropriate form; if intake and output are being evaluated, record fluid intake on appropriate form.
- If client is receiving oral nutritional supplements (special foods or oral supplements such as Ensure, Boost, and Resource), record the amount taken and communicate client tolerance (likes or dislikes, supplements to fill or replace meals) to the health care team to evaluate supplement effectiveness.
- Report any swallowing difficulties, food dislikes, refusal to eat to nurse in charge.

Unexpected Outcomes	Related Interventions
1. Client is unable to complete meal.	• Determine why client is unable to finish meal (e.g., inadequate personnel for feeding assistance, ingestion of large volume of liquids immediately before meal, food preferences). • Determine if client's food preferences are met. • Determine if client is in pain or uncomfortable. • Assess for constipation. • Perform oral assessment.
2. Client chokes on food.	• Suction food and secretions from mouth and airway. • If choking occurs often, contact physician. • Make appropriate referrals (e.g., speech therapy).

Teaching Considerations

- Reinforce diet guidelines with client and family.
- Instruct client and family to maintain a balanced diet and to monitor intake of fluids and percent or amount of meals and snacks consumed. If intake falls below 75% for any length of time, the client should be referred to an RD for medical nutrition therapy.
- Teach family members to assist client in feeding self. Help client do as much as possible in feeding self.
- Instruct client and primary caregiver in importance of providing frequent mouth care.

Pediatric Considerations

- Infant feeding includes bottle or breast-feeding and the introduction of semisolid foods such as cereals at around 6 months; strained vegetables, meats, and fruits at around 8 months; and bite-size table foods at around 1 year. Cup feeding and finger foods are introduced as the child's fine motor skills develop (Hockenberry, 2004).

Gerontological Considerations

- Older adult clients may have diminished appetite because of loss of taste and smell and decreased number of taste buds.
- Interactions between nutrients and medications may affect taste of foods or metabolism, absorption, digestion, or excretion of drugs (Lueckenotte, 2000).

Home Care Considerations

- Assess familiarity of client and primary caregiver with proper nutritional standards.
- Assess financial resources of client and family to determine if they are able to purchase proper foods for client.
- Assess priority given by client and family to provision of a balanced nutritional plan.
- Help client, family, and primary caregiver to make eating an enjoyable experience.

Long-Term Care Considerations

- Meals are part of the resident's social interaction with other residents and staff, and, as a result, residents rarely eat meals in their rooms.
- Meals in long-term care settings may be in a social dining program, where residents eat in a dining room and food is served as in a restaurant; family dining, in which residents serve themselves from a common serving bowl; or in an assistive dining program, in which residents can receive assistance with meals (Sorrentino and Gorek, 1999).

SKILL 29-3 Aspiration Precautions

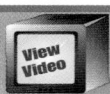

Aspiration in the adult client usually occurs as a result of difficulties in swallowing (dysphagia). Swallowing dysfunction, better known as dysphagia, is associated with multiple neurogenic, myogenic, and obstructive causes (Box 29-5). Dysphagia can produce numerous complications, including increased mortality, increased length of stay, aspiration of food, chest infection, compromised nutritional status, and overall disability (Elmstahl and others, 1999; Perry and Love, 2001; Smithard and others, 1996). Characteristics of dysphagia include cough and/or voice change after swallow; abnormal lip closure and tongue movement; lingual discoordination; hoarse voice; slow, weak, imprecise, or uncoordinated speech; abnormal gag; abnormal volitional cough; de-

layed oral and pharyngeal transit; incomplete oral clearance; regurgitation; pharyngeal pooling; delayed or absent trigger of swallow; and inability to speak consistently (Box 29-6) (Groher, 1997).

The two primary types of dysphagia are oropharyngeal and esophageal dysphagia. Oropharyngeal dysphagia relates to problems with the oral, or voluntary, phase of swallowing and the pharyngeal phase. It can be related to neurogenic disorders, decreased salivation, oropharyngeal lesions, weakness of lips, decreased oral sensitivity, Sjögren's syndrome (dry mouth), or cognitive disorders. Esophageal dysphagia, or involuntary phase, can be related to obstructive disorders, motility disorders, or motor dysfunction (Spieker, 2000).

Complications of dysphagia include increased length of stay, chest infections, disability/decreased functional status, decreased nutritional status, increased likelihood of discharge to institutionalized care, and increased mortality (Elmstahl and others, 1999; Odderson and others, 1995; Smithard and others, 1996). The "silent aspiration," or aspiration that occurs without a cough, is a serious concern with dysphagic individuals and is often the cause of complications (Hammond and others, 2001). Silent aspiration accounts for 40% to 70% of aspiration in clients with dysphagia. (Daniels and others, 2000).

Nutritional Implications of Dysphagia

Dysphagia usually causes a decrease in food intake, which subsequently results in malnutrition. Nutritional status changes as indicated by changes in skinfold thickness and albumin level are apparent in clients who exhibit dysphagia (Smithard and others, 1996). In most instances this is due to difficulty in consuming an adequate volume of solids or liquids. Dietary intake may be affected for long periods of time, and the malnutrition that occurs is secondary to insufficient protein, calorie, and micronutrient intake (Elmstahl

---

BOX 29-5 Causes of Dysphagia

NEUROGENIC

Stroke
Cerebral palsy
Guillain Barré syndrome
Multiple sclerosis
Amyotrophic lateral sclerosis
 (Lou Gehrig disease)
Diabetic neuropathy
Parkinson's disease

MYOGENIC

Myasthenia gravis
Aging
Muscular dystrophy
Polymyositis
Dermatomyositis

OBSTRUCTIVE

Benign peptic stricture
Lower esophageal ring
Candidiasis
Head and neck cancer
Inflammatory masses
Trauma/surgical resection
Zenker's diverticulum
Esophageal webs
Extrinsic structural lesions
Anterior mediastinal masses
Cervical spondylosis

OTHER

Gastrointestinal or esophageal
 resection
Rheumatologic disorders
Connective tissue disorders
Vagotomy

BOX 29-6 Criteria for Dysphagia Referral

Before referral:
If the answer is yes to either of the following two questions, the referral at this time is not appropriate.
- Is the client unconscious or drowsy?
- Is the client unable to sit in an upright position for a reasonable length of time?

Please consider the next two questions before making the referral:
- Is the client near end of life?
- Does the client have an esophageal problem that will require surgical intervention?

When observing the client or giving mouth care, look for:
- Open mouth (weak lip closure)
- Drooling liquids or solids
- Poor oral hygiene/thrush

- Facial weakness
- Tongue weakness
- Difficulty with secretions
- Slurred, indistinct speech
- Change in voice quality
- Poor posture or head control
- Weak involuntary cough
- Delayed cough (up to 2 minutes after swallow)
- General frailty
- Confusion/dementia
- No spontaneous swallowing movements

If any of the above are present, the client may have swallowing problems and may need referral to speech language pathologist.

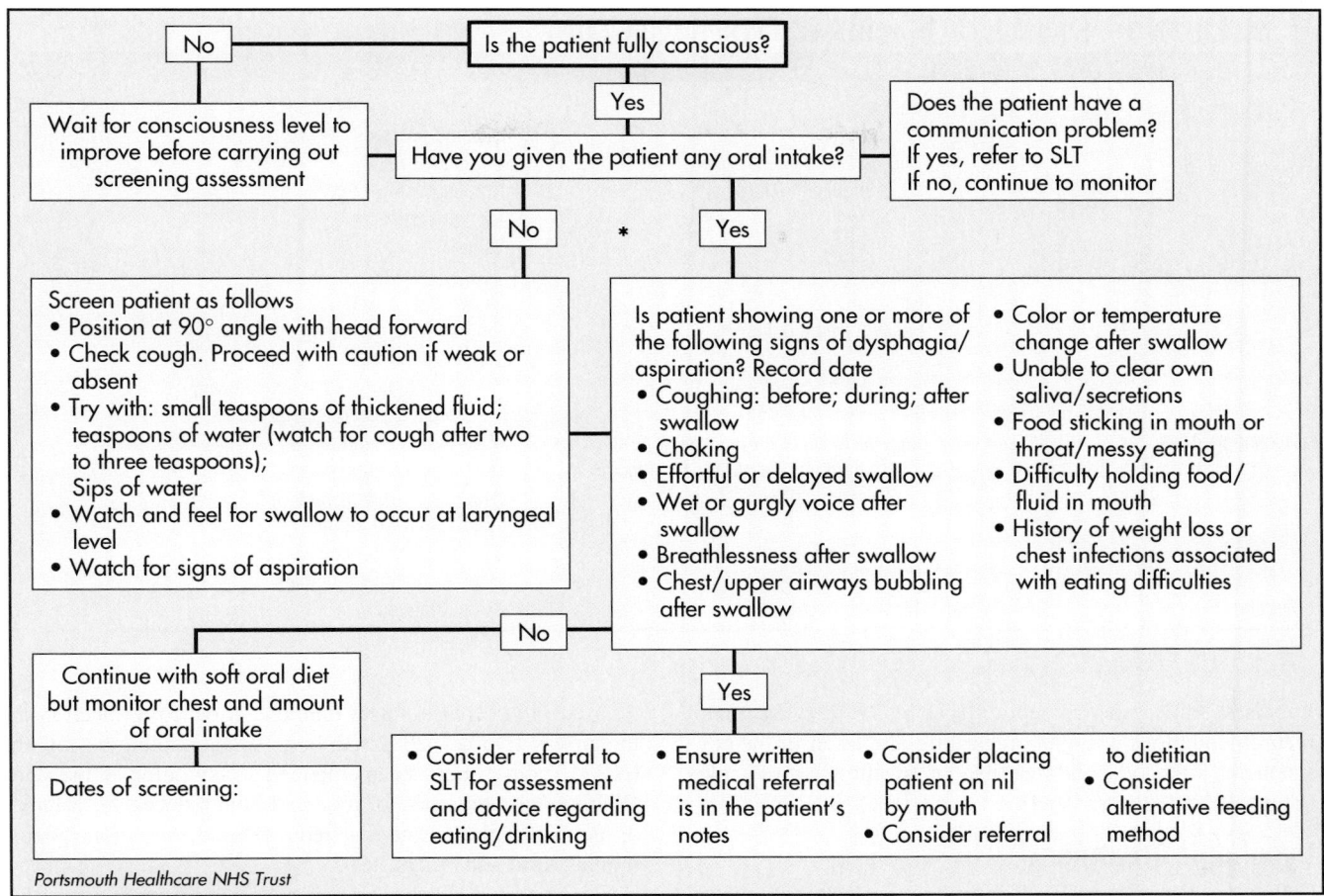

FIGURE 29-6 Screening assessment for dysphagic clients. (From Dangerfield L, Sullivan R: Screening for and managing dysphagia after stroke, *Nurs Times* 95[19]:44, 1999.)

and others, 1999; Perry and Love, 2001). This can significantly impede the recovery process (Bending, 2001).

Dysphagia Screening

Dysphagia screening is defined as "a procedure designed to detect any clinical indication of potential neurological deglutition dysfunction" (Perry and Love 2001). There are many dysphagia screening tools, and they all have similar characteristics (Figure 29-6). The Registered Dietitian (RD) Dysphagia Screening Tool, designed by Brody and others, uses medical record review, client questioning, and observation of a meal. This screening tool includes observation of a client at a meal for change in voice quality, posture and head control, percentage of meal consumed, eating time, drooling of liquids and solids, cough during/after a swallow, facial or tongue weakness, difficulty with secretions, pocketing, and presence of voluntary and dry cough (Brody and others, 2000). Other screening methods for dysphagia include the Burke Dysphagia Screening Test, the Standardized Swallowing Assessment, Hinds and Wiles timed test, and the Smithard Bedside Swallowing Assessment (Perry and Love, 2001). All of these tools assess holding food in mouth, leakage from mouth, cough-

ing, choking, breathlessness, and quality of voice after swallowing (Perry, 2001a; Perry, 2001b; Wood and Emick-Herring, 1997). Registered nurses, registered dietitians, physicians, or speech language pathologists can screen clients (DePippo and others, 1992; Ellul and Barer, 1996; Wood and Emick-Herring, 1997). Early screening and treatment of dysphagia leads to more cost-effective treatment, improved quality of care, and ensures optimal outcomes (Elmstahl and others, 1999; Hinds and Wiles, 1998).

Dysphagia Assessment

Bedside dysphagia assessments identify clients at risk for dysphagia and provide recommendations for dysphagia therapy (Smithard and others, 1996). The assessment includes observation of a range of textures and consistencies, resulting in a comprehensive description of the phases of swallowing, usually accompanied by judgment of degree of dysfunction and aspiration risk (Perry and Love, 2001). A certified speech language pathologist (SLP) must perform the assessment. Clinical assessment focuses on oral-motor and oral-sensory function, protective reflexes, and respiratory status. Observations are made on level of arousal, cognitive-

TABLE 29-3 STAGES OF NATIONAL DYSPHAGIA DIET

STAGE	DESCRIPTION	EXAMPLES
Dysphagia Puree	Uniform Pureed Cohesive "Puddinglike" texture	Smooth hot cereals cooked to a "pudding" consistency Mashed potatoes Pureed meat Pureed pasta or rice Pureed vegetable Yogurt
Dysphagia Mechanically Altered	Moist Soft textured Easily forms a bolus	Cooked cereals Dry cereals moistened with milk Canned fruit (excluding pineapple) Moist ground meat Well cooked noodles in sauce/gravy Well-cooked, diced vegetables
Dysphagia Advanced	Regular foods (with the exception of very hard, sticky, or crunchy foods)	Moist breads (with butter, jelly, etc.) Well-moistened cereals Peeled soft fruits (peach, plum, kiwi) Tender, thin-sliced meats Baked potato (without skin) Tender, cooked vegetables
Regular	All foods	No restrictions

linguistic status, and perception (Davies, 1999). Treatment recommendations are made regarding alteration in the consistencies of foods and the use of swallowing therapies (Elmstahl and others, 1999).

Dysphagia Treatment

Following the diagnosis of dysphagia, treatment should commence. The plan of care for treatment may include the promotion of good nutritional status, weight maintenance, reducing of the risk of aspiration, promotion of eating independence, and enjoyment of mealtime (Dorner, 2002). Treatment typically includes oral motor exercises, swallowing techniques, positioning during feeding, and diet modification. Elmstahl and others (1999) found that the combination of these techniques reduced the degree of oral and pharyngeal dysfunction, which led to improved nutritional status (Elmstahl and others, 1999).

Diet Management

There are social, cultural, and emotional aspects in eating and drinking in all societies (Negus, 1994; Shaw and Power, 1999). A priority for dysphagic clients is the initiation of safe oral nutrition and hydration (Wood and Emick-Herring, 1997). Changes in food and/or liquid consistencies, elimination of oral intake and initiation of tube feeding are common diet modifications. Liquid or pureed foods are sometimes the only consistency tolerated by clients with mechanical disorders that cause dysphagia but may not be the most appropriate choice for individuals with oropharyngeal dysphagia. Clients with oropharyngeal dysphagia have more success with semisolid consistencies that are easy to chew (Groher, 1997). Liquids often have to be thickened with a commercial thickener to decrease transit time and allow for protection of the airway (Dorner, 2002; Groher, 1997). Nothing by mouth (NPO) status should be maintained if aspiration is present. Withholding oral intake of food and fluid reduces the volume of material aspirated and may reduce the severity of the pneumonia (Kidd and others, 1995).

In October 2002 the American Dietetic Association published the National Dysphagia Diet Task Force's (NDDTF's) National Dysphagia Diet (National Dysphagia Diet Task Force, 2002). The diet comprises four levels: Dysphagia Puree, Dysphagia Mechanically Altered, Dysphagia Advanced, and Regular. There are also four levels of liquid consistencies: thin liquids (low viscosity), nectarlike liquids (medium viscosity), honeylike liquids (viscosity of honey), and spoon-thick liquids (viscosity of pudding) (National Dysphagia Diet Task Force, 2002) (Table 29-3).

Compliance with the puree diet can be a problem with clients who previously consumed whole foods. Clients often find pureed foods unappetizing, especially if they are coming from a baby food jar (Dorner, 2002; Groher, 1997; Shaw and Power, 1999). Several food service companies now provide individualized and bulk varieties of pureed foods for the hospitality industry. Unfortunately these items are often very expensive, preventing their widespread use.

Client Positioning

Client positioning is also a very important part of feeding a client with dysphagia. The client must be sitting upright and should be supervised. Correct anatomical alignment is necessary for the passage of food through the pharynx and esophagus. Clients should be well supported whether in a chair or in a bed (Davies, 1999).

DELEGATION CONSIDERATIONS

The assessment of client's risk for aspiration and determination of positioning should not be delegated to assistive personnel. However, assistive personnel may feed clients after receiving instruction on aspiration precautions. The nurse must instruct assistive personnel to:

- Report to the nurse in charge, as soon as possible, any onset of coughing, gagging, or pocketing of food

EQUIPMENT

- ❏ Chair or electric bed (to allow client to sit upright)
- ❏ Thickening agents as needed (rice, cereal, yogurt, gelatin, commercial thickening agent)
- ❏ Tongue blade
- ❏ Penlight

STEP	RATIONALE

ASSESSMENT

1. Perform nutritional screening (see Skill 29-2).

   Clients with aspiration from dysphagia may alter their eating patterns or choose foods that do not provide adequate nutrition (Perry and McLaren, 2003).

2. Assess clients who are at increased risk of aspiration for signs and symptoms of dysphagia (see Box 29-6).

   Client may exhibit symptoms or demonstrate poor lip and tongue control. Clients at risk include those who have neurological or neuromuscular diseases and those who have had trauma to or surgical procedures of the oral cavity or throat (Dangerfield and Sullivan, 1999).

3. Observe chest during mealtime for signs of dysphagia, and allow client to attempt to feed self. Note at end of meal if client fatigues.

   Can detect abnormal eating patterns such as frequent clearing of throat or prolonged eating time. Fatigue increases risk of aspiration.

4. Ask client about any difficulties with chewing or swallowing various textures of food.

   Be alert for symptoms such as coughing, dyspnea, or drooling that suggest difficulty handling food, especially thin liquids.

5. Report signs and symptoms of dysphagia to the physician.

   Client may need to have an evaluation performed by a radiologist or speech language pathologist (Perry, 2001a).

6. Place an identification on client's chart or Kardex indicating that dysphagia is present.

   Identifying client as dysphagic reduces risk of his or her receiving oral nutrients without supervision (Dangerfield and Sullivan, 1999).

NURSING DIAGNOSES

- Risk for aspiration
- Disturbed sensory perception (gustatory)
- Impaired swallowing

Related factors are individualized based on client's condition or needs.

PLANNING

1. Expected outcome following completion of procedure:
   - Client will not exhibit signs or symptoms that suggest aspiration is occurring.

   Interventions for preventing aspiration are successful.

IMPLEMENTATION

1. Perform hand hygiene.
2. Using penlight and tongue blade, gently inspect mouth for pockets of food.

   Pockets of food in the mouth can indicate difficulty swallowing.

3. Elevate head of client's bed so that hips are flexed at a 90-degree angle and head is flexed slightly forward, or help client to same position in a chair.

   Reduces risk of aspiration.

4. Observe client consume various consistencies of foods and liquids.

   Difficulty managing foods may indicate dysphagia. Referral to a dietitian is appropriate if a client has difficulty with a particular consistency.

STEP	RATIONALE
5. Ask client to remain sitting upright for at least 30 minutes after the meal.	Reduces the risk of gastroesophageal reflux, which can cause aspiration.
6. Help client to perform hand hygiene and perform mouth care.	Mouth care after meals helps prevent dental caries.
7. Return client's tray to appropriate place, and perform hand hygiene.	Reduces spread of microorganisms.

EVALUATION

1. Observe client's ability to ingest foods of various textures and thicknesses.	Indicates whether aspiration risk is increased with thin liquids.
2. Monitor client's food and fluid intake.	Client may avoid certain types and textures of food that are difficult to swallow.
3. Weigh client weekly.	Determines if weight is stable and reflects adequate caloric level.
4. Observe client's oral cavity after meal to detect pockets of food.	Determines presence of pockets of food when meal has included foods of various textures.

Recording and Reporting

- Document the following in client's chart: client's tolerance of various food textures, amount of assistance required, position during meal, absence or presence of any symptoms of dysphagia, and amount eaten.
- Report any coughing, gagging, choking, or swallowing difficulties to nurse in charge or physician.

Unexpected Outcomes	Related Interventions
1. Client coughs, gags, complains of food "stuck in throat," or has pockets of food in mouth.	• Client may require a swallowing evaluation (Box 29-6) (see Figure 29-6). • Consider consultation with a speech therapist for swallowing exercises and techniques to improve swallowing and reduce risk of aspiration. • Notify physician of any symptoms that occurred during meal and which foods caused the symptoms.
2. Client avoids certain textures of food.	• Change consistency and texture of food (see Table 29-3).
3. Client experiences weight loss.	• Discuss findings with physician and/or dietitian.

Teaching Considerations
- Instruct caregivers regarding signs of aspiration and dysphagia.
- Instruct caregivers regarding specifics for foods and client positioning to reduce risk of aspiration.
- Teach family to use oral suction as needed.

Gerontological Considerations
- Older adults who have had a stroke or have Parkinson's disease are at risk for aspiration.
- If dysphagia is severe, an enteral feeding tube may be necessary (Lueckenotte, 2000) (see Chapter 30).

FOCUS on CLINICAL PRACTICE

Mrs. Simon is an active 89-year-old woman involved in many charity and community activities. She presents at the emergency department with slurred speech and right-sided facial droop. She is subsequently admitted to the neurological unit.

1. What are your initial concerns related to her nutritional risk, and what other information would you like to have about this client?

2. Mrs. Simon is diagnosed with an acute stroke. What further testing (e.g., biochemical, radiological) would assist you in your evaluation of the client's nutritional risk?
3. The physician has written an order for a regular diet for Mrs. Simon. What precautions would you implement?
4. Mrs. Simon is experiencing much difficulty with eating and feeding herself at mealtime. What referrals would you suggest that the physician make for Mrs. Simon?

NCLEX REVIEW QUESTIONS

1. Factors related to nutritional risk in adults include:
   1. Drug nutrient interactions
   2. Compromised dentition
   3. Anorexia, nausea, vomiting
   4. Poor knowledge of nutrient sources
2. The Nutrition Screening Initiative was:
   1. A federally funded program aimed at identifying older adults at nutritional risk
   2. A federally funded program aimed at identifying children at nutritional risk
   3. A nutritional screening program aimed at early intervention for those lacking food
   4. A federally funded program aimed at early identification of nutritional risk in high-risk populations
3. Ms. Jones is a 60-year-old vegetarian admitted to rule out (r/o) stroke. In doing your physical assessment you note a beefy red, fissured tongue. Which of the following may be the problem?
   1. She has glossitis and a possible vitamin B_{12} deficiency.
   2. She has filiform papillary atrophy and an iron deficiency.
   3. She has a vitamin C deficiency.
   4. She has protein calorie malnutrition.

4. Ms. Jones's biochemical profile now shows she has an albumin level of 2.7 mg/100 ml and a prealbumin level of 12 mg/100 ml. These two parameters indicate:
   1. A micronutrient deficiency
   2. Protein malnutrition because albumin has a long half-life and prealbumin a short half-life
   3. The need for further testing because they are not valid nutrition parameters
   4. Liver disease
5. Mrs. Smith is admitted with the diagnosis of r/o stroke. Upon doing her cranial nerve examination you notice she has no gag reflex. She is at risk for:
   1. Trigeminal neuralgia
   2. Aspiration
   3. Dehydration
   4. Facial palsy
6. You are admitting a new adult client. You will calculate the BMI because body mass index:
   1. Measures subcutaneous fat and muscle
   2. Is based on electron currents
   3. Is a measure of body weight in proportion to height
   4. Determines body frame size

References

American Academy of Family Physicians: *About the Nutrition Screening Initiative (website),* 2003, American Academy of Family Physicians, http://www.aafp.org/x16082.xml, accessed December 30, 2003.

American Dietetic Association: *RD fact sheet,* 2003, http://www.eatright.org/Public/index_13056.cfm.

American Society for Parenteral and Enteral Nutrition (ASPEN) Board of Directors: Standards for nutrition support for adult residents of long term care facilities, *Nutr Clin Pract* 12:284, 1997.

American Society for Parenteral and Enteral Nutrition (ASPEN) *The science and practice of nutrition support: a case-based core curriculum,* Dubuque, Iowa, 2001, Kendall Hunt.

Bending A: Meeting the challenges of managing dysphagia, *Community Nurse* 7(1):13, 2001.

Brody R: *Newark Beth Israel Medical Center nutrition screening, and re-assessment policy and procedure,* Newark, NJ, 2002, Newark Beth Israel Medical Center.

Correia MI: Assessing the nutritional assessment, *Nutr Clin Pract* 14:142,1999.

Dangerfield L, Sullivan R: Screening for and managing dysphagia after stroke, *Nurs Times* 95(19):44,1999.

Davies S: Dysphagia in acute strokes, *Nurs Stand* 13(30):49, 1999.

Dorner B: Tough to swallow, *Today's Dietitian,* p 28, Aug 2002.

Edel J and others: Nutritional assessment of adults. In *Manual of clinical dietetics,* Chicago, 2000, American Dietetic Association.

Expert Panel on the Identification, Evaluation, and Treatment of Overweight and Obesity in Adults: *The practical guide to identification, evaluation, and treatment of overweight and obesity in adults,* Bethesda, Md, 2000, National Institutes of Health.

Glanville CL: People of African American heritage. In Purnell L, Paulanka B: *Transcultural healthcare,* Philadelphia, 2003, FA Davis.

Grodner M and others: *Foundations and clinical applications of nutrition: a nursing approach,* ed 2, St. Louis, 2000, Mosby.

Groher M: *Dysphagia: diagnosis and management,* Boston, 1997, Butterworth-Heinemann.

Hall J: Choosing nutrition support: how and when to initiate, *Nurs Case Manag* 4(5):212,1999.

Hammond K and others: Dietary and clinical assessment. In *Krause's food nutrition and diet therapy,* Philadelphia, 2003, Saunders, http://www.aafp.org/PreBuilt/ NSI_DETERMINE.pdf.

Hockenberry M: *Wong's clinical manual of pediatric nursing,* St. Louis, 2004, Mosby.

Ignatavicious D, Workman ML: *Medical surgical nursing,* ed 4, St. Louis, 2002, Mosby.

Jambunathan J: People of Hindu heritage. In Purnell L, Paulanka B: *Transcultural healthcare* (CD-ROM), Philadelphia, 2003, FA Davis.

Joint Commission on Accreditation of Healthcare Organizations: *Crosswalk of 2003 standards for hospitals to 2004 provision of care, treatment, and service standards for hospitals,* 2003, The Commission, http://www.jcaho.org/accredited+organizations/ hospitals/standards/new+standards/pc_xwalk_hap.pdf, accessed December 31, 2003.

Juarbe TC: People of Puerto Rican heritage. In Purnell L, Paulanka B: *Transcultural healthcare,* Philadelphia, 2003, FA Davis.

Kidd D and others: The natural history and clinical consequences of aspiration in acute stroke, *QJM* 88(6):409, 1995.

Lacey K, Pritchett E: Nutrition care process and model: ADA adopts road map to quality care and outcomes management, *J Am Diet Assoc* 103(8):1061, 2003.

Lueckenotte AG: *Gerontologic nursing,* ed 2, St. Louis, 2000, Mosby.

National Dysphagia Diet Task Force: *National dysphagia diet: standardization for optimal care,* Chicago, 2002, American Dietetic Association.

Negus E: Stroke induced dysphagia in the hospital: The nutritional perspective, *Br J Nurs* 3(6):263, 1994.

Nestle Clinical Nutrition: *MNA—mini nutritional assessment,* 2003, Nestle Nutrition, http://www.mna-elderly.com/, accessed December 31, 2003.

Nutrition Screening Initiative: DETERMINE your nutritional health questionnaire, Washington, DC, 1997, American Academy of Family Physicians.

Nutritional assessment of the elderly through anthropometry, Columbus, Ohio, 1988, Ross Laboratories.

Pagana K, Pagana T: *Mosby's diagnostic and laboratory test reference,* St. Louis, 2005, Mosby.

Perry L: Screening swallowing function of patients with acute stroke. I. Identification, implementation, and initial evaluation of a screening tool for use by nurses, *J Clin Nurs* 10:463, 2001a.

Perry L: Screening swallowing function of patients with acute stroke. II. Detailed evaluation of the tool used by nurses, *J Clin Nurs* 10:474, 2001b.

Perry L, Love C: Screening for dysphagia and aspiration in acute stroke: a systematic review, *Dysphagia* 16:7, 2001.

Purnell L: People of Cuban heritage. In Purnell L, Paulanka B: *Transcultural healthcare,* Philadelphia, 2003, FA Davis.

Purnell L, Kim S: People of Korean heritage. In Purnell L, Paulanka B: *Transcultural healthcare,* Philadelphia, 2003, FA Davis.

Rassoul JH: The crescent of Islam: healing, nursing and the spiritual dimension, *J Adv Nurs* 32(6):1476, 2000.

Sharts-Hopko N: People of Puerto Rican heritage. In Purnell L, Paulanka B: *Transcultural healthcare,* Philadelphia, 2003, FA Davis.

Shopbell J and others: Nutrition screening and assessment. In *The science and practice of nutrition support,* Dubuque, Iowa, 2001, American Society for Parenteral and Enteral Nutrition.

Smithard D and others: Complications and outcome after acute stroke: does dysphagia matter? *Stroke* 27(7):1200, 1996.

Sorrentino SA, Gorek B: *Long-term care assistants,* ed 3, St. Louis, 1999, Mosby.

Spieker M: Evaluating dysphagia, *Am Fam Physician* 61:3639, 2000.

Wang Y: People of Chinese heritage. In Purnell L, Paulanka B: *Transcultural healthcare,* Philadelphia, 2003, FA Davis.

White J and others: Misconceptions on using NSI screens, *J Am Diet Assoc* 102(10):1398, 2002.

White JV and others: Consensus of the Nutrition Screening Initiative: risk factors and indications of poor nutritional status in older Americans, *J Am Diet Assoc* 91(7):783, 1991.

Whitehouse MJ: Nursing assessment of the elderly patient, *J Intraven Nurs* 15:S14, 1992.

Williams LS, Hooper PD: *Understanding medical-surgical nursing,* Philadelphia, 1999.

Wood P, Emick-Herring B: Dysphagia: a screening tool for stroke patients, *J Neurosci Nurs* 29(5):325, 1997.

Research References

Adams CR: Lessons learned from urban Latinas with Type 2 diabetes mellitus, *J Transcult Nurs* 14(3):255, 2003.

Blackburn G, Bistrian B: Nutritional and metabolic assessment of the hospitalized patient, *JPEN J Parenter Enteral Nutr* 1(1):11, 1977.

Brody R and others: Role of registered dietitians in dysphagia screening, *J Am Diet Assoc* 100(9):1029, 2000.

Daniels S and others: Clinical predictors of dysphagia and aspiration risk: outcome measures in acute stroke patients, *Arch Phys Med Rehabil* 81:1030, 2000.

DePippo K and others: Validation of the 3-oz water swallow test for aspiration following stroke, *Arch Neurol* 49:1259, 1992.

DePippo K and others: The Burke dysphagia screening test: validation of its use in patients with stroke, *Arch Phys Med Rehab* 75:1284, 1994.

Detsky A and others: What is subjective global assessment? *J Parenter Enteral Nutr* 11(1):8, 1987.

Ellul J, Barer D: Intraobserver reliability of a standardized bedside swallowing assessment, *Cerebrovasc Dis* 6(suppl 2):152, 1996.

Elmstahl S and others: Treatment of dysphagia improves nutritional conditions in stroke patients, *Dysphagia* 14:61, 1999.

Hammond C and others: Assessment of aspiration risk in stroke patients with quantification of voluntary cough, *Neurology* 56:502, 2001.

Hernandez JL and others: Clinical evaluation for cancer in patients with involuntary weight loss without specific symptoms, *Am J Med* 114(8):631, 2003.

Higgins B: Puerto Rican cultural beliefs: influence on infant feeding practices in western New York, *J Transcult Nurs* 11(1):12, 2000.

Hinds N, Wiles C: Assessment of swallowing and referral to speech and language therapists in acute stroke, *QJM* 919(12): 829, 1998.

Huhmann M and others: Dysphagia screening by a registered dietitian in acute stroke patients, *J Am Diet Assoc* 103:(9) suppl, 2003.

Lawrence P, Rozmus C: Culturally sensitive care of the Muslim patient, *J Transcult Nurs* 12(3):228, 2001.

McCann L: Subjective global assessment as it pertains to the nutritional status of dialysis patients, *Dial Transplant* 24(4):190, 1996.

Odderson I and others: Swallow management in patients on an acute stroke pathway: quality is cost effective, *Arch Phys Med Rehabil* 76:1130, 1995.

Perry L, McLaren S: Eating difficulties after stroke, *J Adv Nurs* 43(4):360, 2003.

Persson M and others: Nutritional status using mini nutritional assessment and subjective global assessment predict mortality in geriatric patients, *J Am Geriatr Soc* 50(12):1532, 1996.

Schmid A and others: Recording the nutrient intake of nursing home residents by food weighing method and measuring the physical activity, *J Nutr Health Aging* 7(5):294, 2003.

Shaw C, Power J: Nutritional management of patients with dysphagia, *Br J Community Nurs* 4(7):338, 1999.

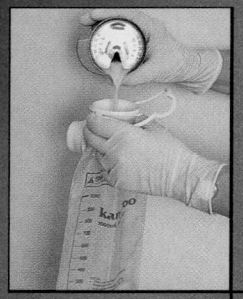

30

Enteral Nutrition

MEDIA RESOURCES

Evolve Site *evolve*

http://evolve.elsevier.com/Perry/skills
- Weblinks
- Video clips
- Mosby's Nursing Skills Video Exercises

Mosby's Nursing Skills Videos/CD-ROM
- ***Enteral Nutrition Video:*** Feeding tube insertion using the nasogastric route, confirmation of tube placement; enteral feedings; feeding tube irrigation; feeding tube removal

OBJECTIVES

Mastery of content in this chaper will enable the nurse to:

- Assess the client who is to receive enteral tube feedings.
- Determine the appropriate route of intubation for the client.
- Demonstrate ability to correctly insert a small-bore feeding tube.
- Discuss the rationale for measuring pH to determine feeding tube placement.
- Identify the typical color of nasogastric (NG) and nasointestinal (NI) tube aspirate.
- Demonstrate the appropriate technique for irrigating a feeding tube.
- Demonstrate the appropriate technique for administering syringe tube feedings.
- Demonstrate the appropriate technique for administering continuous tube feedings.
- Discuss the risk of aspiration for a client receiving gastric versus intestinal tube feeding.
- Evaluate the client's tolerance of enteral feeding.

KEY TERMS

Enteral nutrition
Enteral tube feeding
Gastrostomy feeding tube
Jejunostomy feeding tube
Nasogastric (NG) feeding tube
Nasointestinal (NI) feeding tube

Residual volume
Thrombosis
Vascular access device (VAD)
Venipuncture

Enteral nutrition is the administration of nutrients directly into the gastrointestinal (GI) tract. The most desirable and appropriate method of providing nutrition is the oral route; unfortunately, this is not always possible. When oral feedings are not possible, yet the stomach or intestine is able to digest nutrients, enteral tube feeding is an alternative. Enteral feeding is preferred over parenteral nutrition because it improves utilization of nutrients, is generally safer for clients, maintains structure and function of the gut, and is less expensive (ASPEN, 2002). A variety of enteral feeding formulas are available in whole protein or partially digested form. Special enteral formulas for renal disease, hepatic disease, pulmonary disease, or diabetes are also available. Adult and pediatric formulas can be chosen. The skills presented in this chapter focus on the administration of nutritional feedings directly into the gastrointestinal tract with the goal of restoring the client's nutritional status.

Evidence-Based Practice Trends

Indications for enteral nutrition generally fall into one of three categories: impaired swallowing or gag reflex (which is usually related to a neurological problem); nutritional deficit due to reduced food ingestion or hypermetabolic state even when the client is able to eat; or an inability to eat related to surgery, injury, or disease process. This last category is often associated with altered or decreased level of consciousness. According to a recent investigation, complications associated with enteral nutrition include displacement of the tube, electrolyte alterations, hyperglycemia, constipation, diarrhea, clogging of the tube, vomiting, and pulmonary aspiration (Pancorbo-Hidalgo and others, 2001). Complications of prolonged intubation may also include nasal erosion, nasopharyngeal ulcers, sinusitis, otitis, esophagitis, and vocal cord paralysis (ASPEN, 2002).

One of the most dreaded complications associated with tube feedings is pulmonary aspiration, potentially leading to pneumonia. Two traditional bedside methods used to assess for pulmonary aspiration of enteral feeding into the respiratory tract included the glucose method and the dye method. The premise of the glucose method was that normal tracheal secretions contain minimal levels of glucose. Therefore, if glucose-rich enteral formula were aspirated into the airway, glucose levels of tracheal secretions would increase. However, researchers have shown that the glucose levels of tracheal secretions vary widely (Metheny and others, 1998b).

Another common practice was the addition of food coloring to enteral tube feeding. The supposition was that food coloring, typically blue, added to enteral feeding would cause suctioned tracheal secretions to turn blue if the client aspirated the tube feeding into the respiratory tract. However, the dye may be systemically absorbed, interfere with hemoccult testing of stool, and has questionable safety (Maloney and Metheny, 2002; McClave and others, 2002; Metheny and others, 2002b). There may even be an association between death and the use of dye in enteral feedings (Maloney and Metheny, 2002). The most recent recommendations from members of the North American Summit on Aspiration in the Critically Ill Client indicate that the dye method and the glucose method of testing for aspiration should no longer be used (McClave and others, 2002).

Researchers are currently trying to develop new bedside methods for assessing for pulmonary aspiration, such as assessing for the presence of pepsin, a substance produced in the stomach, in tracheal secretions (Metheny and others, 2002a). Possibly the most important nursing intervention to decrease the risk of aspiration is to keep the head of the bed elevated at least 30 degrees (APEN, 2002; Metheny and others, 2002a). If the client must have the bed in a flat position (e.g., because of spinal precautions), it is possible to keep the bed flat yet elevate the head by placing the bed in reverse Trendelenburg position (Metheny and others, 2002a).

Routine assessment for placement of feeding tubes is primarily a nursing responsibility. Traditionally, the auscultatory method of assessing placement was used. Since the late 1980s there have been several studies showing that the auscultatory method to detect gastric or intestinal feeding tube placement is unreliable. This method cannot detect when a feeding tube has inadvertently been placed into the respiratory tract (Dobranowski and others, 1992; Roubenoff and Ravich, 1989) and cannot distinguish between placement in the stomach versus the intestine (Metheny and others, 1990). Methods to assess tube placement with greater reliability are discussed in Skill 30-2, verification of feeding tube placement.

Lastly, as with all invasive hospital procedures, nasogastric (NG) and nasointestinal (NI) tubes are associated with an increased risk for infection. Besides the risks for infection related to pulmonary aspiration, feeding tubes have recently been demonstrated to be reservoirs for nosocomial pathogens (Mehall and others, 2002). The most important intervention for decreasing colonization of NG and NI tubes is appropriate hand hygiene.

Cultural Considerations

When clients need enteral feedings, it is difficult if not impossible to include culturally specific food preferences. However, it is important to incorporate other cultural practices into the client's care during enteral nutrition. If family caregivers are allowed to be present during feeding, family communications can often be enhanced, because food is generally associated with caring and love in most cultures. Encouraging family participation in feeding the client may also be helpful in some situations.

Be sure to integrate religious and cultural beliefs and practices in feeding. If possible, avoid enteral nutrition sub-strates that are prohibited by the religion or the culture; for example, some Asians may have slight lactose intolerance. Provide privacy when feeding through a gastrostomy or jejunostomy, particularly for Muslims, Hindus, Middle Eastern, and Orthodox Jewish females.

Skill Performance Guidelines

1. Be aware of the purpose for the feeding and which clients are appropriate candidates.
2. Be aware of the psychological implications associated with the insertion of a feeding tube. The client may become frightened and will need reassurance and encouragement throughout the insertion procedure.
3. Be aware of safety measures to prevent dislodgement of the feeding tube and aspiration of gastric contents by the client.
4. Consider the client's medications and their route of delivery. Certain medications should not be administered via a feeding tube (see Chapter 20).
5. Know the client's activity pattern. Clients requiring physical or occupational therapy should have tube feedings completed at least 1 hour before activity to decrease the risk of vomiting or abdominal discomfort.

SKILL 30-1   Intubating the Client With a Nasogastric or Nasointestinal Feeding Tube

Throughout this chapter, feeding tubes are referred to as being nasally placed because that is the most frequent route used, primarily because the nose provides a natural stability for tubes. However, in the event of trauma to the nose, or in the event an endotracheal tube is already placed in the mouth, feeding tubes may also be placed orally. Large-bore NG tubes should be avoided for primary use as a feeding tube because they carry an increased risk of aspiration and are more irritating to the nasopharyngeal and esophageal mucosa (ASPEN, 2002). Occasionally, large-bore tubes that were inserted for gastric decompression will be used to initiate enteral feeding because they are already in place. If the feeding continues for more than a few days, or if the client is at high risk for aspiration, the nurse should consult with the physician about placement of a small-bore feeding tube (Figure 30-1).

Small-bore feeding tubes are available in weighted (tungsten) or nonweighted designs. Weighted tubes were thought to pass more easily into the duodenum or jejunum via peristalsis; however, research has not demonstrated an advantage of the weight in promoting intestinal passage (Lord and others, 1993). Nonetheless, weighted tubes are used more frequently than nonweighted tubes for nasoduodenal and nasojejunal feedings because they are believed to remain in correct position longer than nonweighted tubes. Aside from the weighted tip, small-bore tubes are made of a softer material than large-bore tubes. Hence small-bore tubes can be left in place for an extended period with less irritation to the nasopharyngeal, esophageal, and gastric mucosa. Because the tubes are flexible, a guide wire or stylet is used to pro-

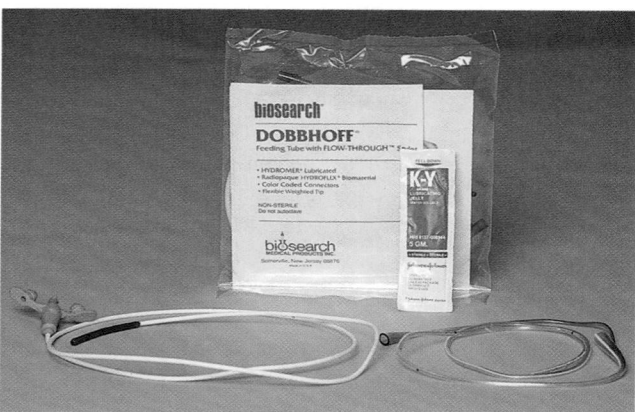

FIGURE 30-1 Small-bore feeding tube.

vide rigidity to facilitate insertion and positioning and then removed once correct placement is verified. Placing an NG or NI feeding tube requires a physician's order.

A rare yet potentially fatal complication associated with the insertion of a feeding tube is inadvertent placement into another part of the body. Placement into the respiratory tract reportedly occurs in approximately 5% of the cases in intensive care settings (Harris and Huseby, 1989). To avoid this problem, initial placement of a feeding tube should be checked with an x-ray examination before the instillation of any substance into the tube (Bankier and others, 1997; Welch and others, 1994). On rare occasions, displacement has also been known to occur into the brain (Metheny, 2002). To avoid this problem, a client who has had a serious injury (e.g., facial fractures) or surgical procedure (e.g., craniofacial surgery) at the site of tube entry, or anywhere along the route the tube is being placed, should not have an NG or NI tube placed by a nurse.

DELEGATION CONSIDERATIONS

This skill should not be delegated to assistive personnel. However, assistive personnel may assist with client positioning during tube insertion.

EQUIPMENT

- ❏ NG or NI tube (8 to 12 Fr) with guide wire or stylet
- ❏ 60-ml or larger Luer-Lok or catheter-tip syringe
- ❏ Stethoscope
- ❏ Hypoallergenic tape and tincture of benzoin or tube fixation device
- ❏ pH indicator strip (scale 0.0 to 14.0)
- ❏ Glass of water and straw for clients able to swallow
- ❏ Emesis basin
- ❏ Towel
- ❏ Facial tissues
- ❏ Clean gloves
- ❏ Suction equipment in case of aspiration
- ❏ Penlight to check placement in nasopharynx
- ❏ Tongue blade

STEP	RATIONALE
ASSESSMENT	
1. Verify client's need for enteral tube feedings and intubation. Also assess client's weight for height, hydration status, electrolyte balance, and organ function.	Identify clients who need tube feedings before they become nutritionally depleted. It is reported that up to 40% of hospitalized clients are malnourished (Pearce and Duncan, 2002).
2. Determine patency of nares. Have client close each nostril alternately and breathe. Examine each naris for patency and skin breakdown.	Nares may be obstructed or irritated, or septal defect or facial fractures may be present.
3. Review client's medical history: nosebleeds, facial trauma, nasal surgery, deviated septum, anticoagulant therapy, coagulopathy.	History of these problems may require nurse to seek physician's order to change route of nutritional support.
4. Assess client for gag reflex. Place tongue blade in client's mouth, touching uvula.	Assists nurse in identifying client's ability to swallow and determines if a greater risk of aspiration exists.
5. Assess client's mental status.	Alert client is better able to cooperate with procedure. If vomiting should occur, an alert client can usually expectorate vomitus, which can help to reduce the risk of aspiration.
6. Auscultate for bowel sounds.	Absence of bowel sounds may indicate decreased or absent peristalsis and increased risk of aspiration. Reassess frequently after initiation of tube feedings. Monitor residual volume.
7. Determine if the physician wants a prokinetic agent administered before the placement of an NI tube.	Prokinetic agents, such as metoclopramide, given BEFORE NI tube placement have been shown to help advance the tube into the intestine (Kittinger and others, 1987).
8. Verify physician's order.	A physician's order is needed to intubate a client with a feeding tube.

STEP	RATIONALE

NURSING DIAGNOSES

- Imbalanced nutrition: less than body requirements
- Readiness for enhanced nutrition
- Impaired swallowing

- Risk for aspiration
- Impaired gas exchange

Related factors are individualized based on client's condition or needs.

PLANNING

1. Expected outcomes following completion of procedure:	
• Verification that tube is in stomach or intestine.	Correct placement (Neumann and others, 1995).
• Feeding tube will remain patent.	Proper irrigation is achieved.
• Client has no respiratory distress (e.g., increased respiratory rate, coughing, poor color), or signs of discomfort or nasal trauma.	Tube correctly placed causes no interference with airway; and tube correctly secured minimizes irritation to nares.
2. Explain procedure to client.	Increases client's cooperation with intubation procedure.
3. Explain to client how to communicate during intubation by raising index finger to indicate gagging or discomfort.	It is important for client to have a way of communicating to alleviate stress. Nurse may pause insertion procedure to decrease gagging.

- *Critical Decision Point*

  NG or NI feeding tubes may be inserted in clients with altered or decreased level of consciousness, but risk of inadvertent respiratory placement is increased if there is an impaired gag reflex (Wendell and others, 1991).

4. Position client sitting with head of bed elevated at least 30 degrees or high-Fowler's position. If client is comatose, place in semi-Fowler's position with head propped forward using a pillow. An assistant may be necessary to help with positioning of confused or comatose clients. If client is forced to lie supine, place in reverse Trendelenburg position.	Reduces risk of pulmonary aspiration in event client should vomit. Head propped assists with closure of airway and passage of the tube into the esophagus. The natural response to an object being inserted into the nose is to tip the head backward; this should be avoided because it opens the airway.
5. Examine feeding tube for flaws: rough or sharp edges on distal end and closed or clogged outlet holes.	Flaws in feeding tube hamper tube intubation and can injure client. Clogged outlets do not allow passage of feeding.
6. Determine length of tube to be inserted, and mark with tape or indelible ink (see illustration).	Being aware of proper length to intubate determines approximate depth of insertion.

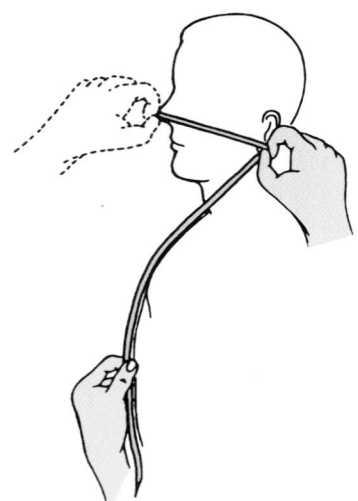

STEP **6** Determine length of tube to be inserted.

STEP	**RATIONALE**

- *Critical Decision Point*
  Tip of tube must reach stomach. Measure distance from tip of nose to earlobe to xyphoid process of sternum (see illustration). Add additional 20 to 30 cm (8 to 12 inches) for NI tube (Hanson, 1979; Lord and others, 1993; Welch, 1996).

7. Prepare NG or NI tube for intubation:
   a. Perform hand hygiene. — Reduces spread of microorganisms.
   b. Inject 10 ml of water from 60-ml Luer-Lok or catheter-tip syringe into the tube. — Aids in guide wire or stylet insertion.
   c. Make certain that guide wire is securely positioned against weighted tip and that both Luer-Lok connections are snugly fitted together. — Promotes smooth passage of tube into GI tract. Improperly positioned stylet can induce serious trauma.
8. Cut adhesive tape 10 cm (4 inches) long, or prepare tube fixation device.

IMPLEMENTATION

1. Put on clean gloves. — Reduces transmission of microorganisms.
2. Dip tube with surface lubricant into glass of room temperature water, or apply water-soluble lubricant. Plastic tubes should *not* be placed in cold water or ice water. — Activates lubricant to facilitate passage of tube into naris and GI tract. Tubes will become stiff and inflexible, causing trauma to mucous membranes.
3. Hand the alert client a glass of water with straw or glass with crushed ice (if able to swallow). — Client will be asked to swallow water to facilitate tube passage.
4. Gently insert tube through nostril to back of throat (posterior nasopharynx). May cause client to gag. Aim back and down toward ear (see illustration). — Natural contours facilitate passage of tube into GI tract.
5. Have client flex head toward chest after tube has passed through nasopharynx. — Closes off glottis and reduces risk of tube entering trachea.

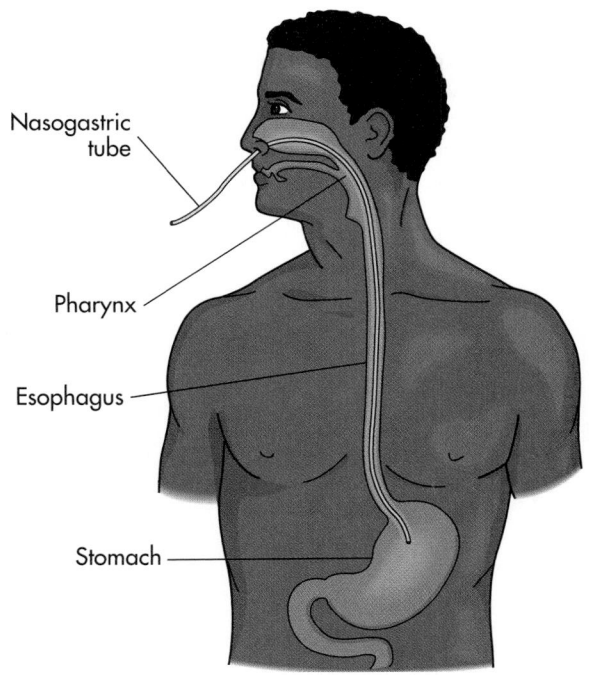

STEP **4** NG tube inserted through nose and esophagus into stomach.

STEP	RATIONALE

- **Critical Decision Point**
  Encourage client to swallow by giving small sips of water or ice chips. Advance tube as client swallows. Rotate tube 180 degrees while inserting. Swallowing facilitates passage of tube past oropharynx. Rotating tube decreases friction.

6. Emphasize need to mouth breathe and swallow during the procedure.	Helps facilitate passage of tube and alleviates client's fears during the procedure.
7. When the tube is inserted to the tip of the carina (approximately 25 cm [10 inches] in the adult), stop and listen for air exchange from the distal portion of the tube.	If air can be heard, tube could be in respiratory tract; remove tube, and start over (Metheny and Titler, 2001).
8. Advance tube each time client swallows until desired length has been passed.	Reduces discomfort and trauma to client.

- **Critical Decision Point**
  Do not force tube. If resistance is met or client starts to cough, choke, or become cyanotic, stop advancing the tube, and pull tube back and start over.

9. Check for position of tube in back of throat with penlight and tongue blade.	Tube may be coiled, kinked, or entering trachea.
10. Temporarily anchor tube to the nose with a small piece of tape, and check placement of tube (see Skill 30-2).	Movement of the tube stimulates gagging. Assesses general position before anchoring tube more securely.
11. Check placement of tube (see Skill 30-2)	Proper tube position is essential before initiating feeding.
12. After gastric aspirates are obtained, anchor tube to nose, and avoid pressure on nares. Mark exit site with indelible ink. Use one of following options for anchoring:	A properly secured tube allows the client more mobility and prevents trauma to nasal mucosa.
a. Apply tape:	
(1) Apply tincture of benzoin or other skin adhesive on tip of client's nose, and allow it to become "tacky."	Helps tape adhere better. Protects skin.
(2) Split one end of the adhesive tape strip lengthwise 5 cm (2 inches).	
(3) Wrap each of the 5-cm strips in opposite directions around tube as it exits nose (see illustration).	

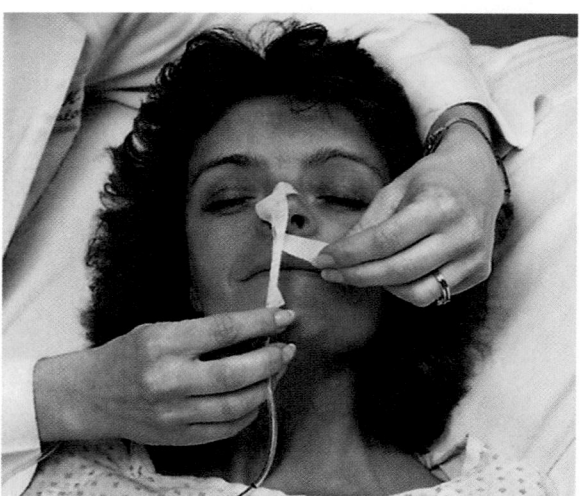

STEP 12a(3) Wrapping tape to anchor nasoenteral tube.

STEP	RATIONALE

   b. **Apply tube fixation device** using shaped adhesive
      patch:
      (1) Apply wide end of patch to bridge of nose
          (see illustration).
      (2) Slip connector around feeding tube as it exits
          nose (see illustration).

13. Fasten end of NG tube to client's gown using a piece of tape. Do not use safety pins to pin the tube to the client's gown.	Reduces traction on the naris if tube moves. Safety pins can become unfastened and cause injury to the client.
14. Assist client to a comfortable position. NOTE: Positioning the client on right side does not facilitate intestinal placement.	Make the patient comfortable. Researchers indicate that placing the patient on the right side does not promotes passage of the tube into the small intestine (Kittinger and others, 1987).

• Critical Decision Point
Leave guide wire or stylet in place until correct position is ensured by x-ray film. Never attempt to reinsert a partially or fully removed guide wire or stylet while feeding tube is in place. This can cause perforation of the tube and injure the client.

15. Obtain x-ray film of chest/abdomen.	X-ray examination is currently the most accurate method to determine feeding tube placement.
16. Apply gloves, and administer oral hygiene (see Chapter 14). Cleanse tubing at nostril with washcloth dampened in mild soap and water.	Promotes client comfort and integrity of oral mucous membranes.
17. Remove gloves, dispose of equipment, and perform hand hygiene.	Reduces transmission of microorganisms.

EVALUATION

1. Observe client to determine response to NG or NI tube intubation. Have the client speak. Check vital signs and oxygen saturation.	A client who is comfortable, able to speak without difficulty, and has normal oxygen saturation is likely to have a correctly placed tube.
2. Confirm x-ray results.	Proper position is essential before initiating feedings.
3. Remove the guide wire or stylet after x-ray verification of correct placement.	
4. Routinely assess location of external exit site marking on the tube, as well as color and pH of fluid withdrawn from the NG or NI tube.	Can reveal if end of tube has changed position. However, it is possible that the tube can change position inside the gastrointestinal tract with no external evidence of the change.

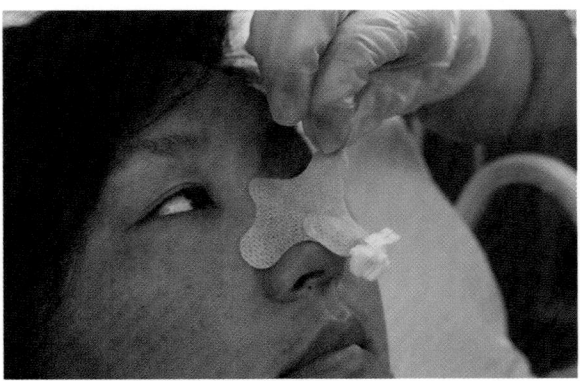

STEP **12b(1)** Applying patch to bridge of nose.

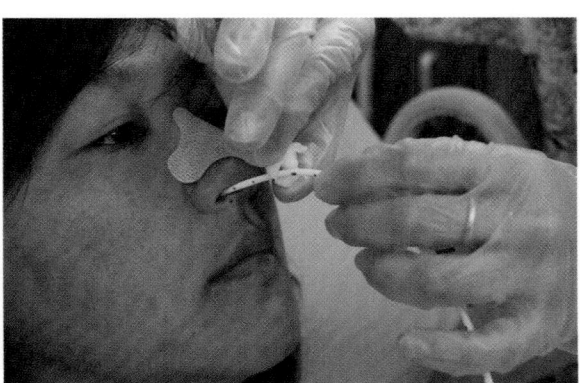

STEP **12b(2)** Slip connector around feeding tube.

Recording and Reporting

- Record and report type and size of tube placed, location of distal tip of tube, client's tolerance of procedure, and confirmation of tube position by x-ray examination. Documentation of nonrespiratory placement by x-ray examination is standard practice when a small-bore tube is initially inserted. Record and report any type of unexpected outcome and the interventions performed.

Unexpected Outcomes	Related Interventions
1. Placement of the tube into the respiratory tract. This may not be discovered until the x-ray report. A small-bore or large-bore tube can enter the airway without causing obvious respiratory symptoms, particularly in a semiconscious or unconscious client.	• Remove the tube, and report the incident to the physician; obtain order for reinsertion.
2. Aspiration of stomach contents into respiratory tract (immediate response) in the alert client, evidenced by coughing, dyspnea, cyanosis, or decreases in oxygen saturation values during the procedure.	• Position the client on side to protect the airway. • Suction the client nasotracheally or orotracheally to try to remove aspirated substance. • Report the event immediately to the physician.
3. Aspiration of stomach contents into respiratory tract (delayed response or small-volume aspiration), evidenced by auscultation of crackles or wheezes, dyspnea, or fever.	• Report change in client condition to the physician; if there has not been a recent chest x-ray film, suggest one be ordered. • Prepare for possible initiation of antibiotics.
4. Displacement of feeding tube to another site (see Skill 30-2).	
5. Clogging of feeding tube.	• Irrigate tube (see Skill 30-3).
6. Nasal mucosa becomes inflamed, tender, and/or eroded.	• Retape the tube in a different position to relieve pressure on mucosa. • If the tube has been in the same site for an extended period, consider reinsertion of the tube in the opposite naris (physician's order required).

Teaching Considerations

- Instruct client or family caregiver to offer oral hygiene frequently and to keep client's lips lubricated.
- Teach client or family caregiver to report tension on feeding tube or displacement of tape or fixation device; instruct client or caregiver to stabilize the tube while help is called.

Pediatric Considerations

- Premature infant and neonate: Measure from the nose or mouth to the earlobe then to the xiphoid process (Hockenberry and others, 2003).
- Older child: Use one of the following techniques; either (1) measure from the nose to the bottom of the earlobe then to the lower end of the xiphoid process or (2) measure from the nose to the earlobe then to a point midway between the xiphoid process and the umbilicus (Hockenberry and others, 2003).

- In infant, observe for vagal stimulation during insertion of feeding tube, resulting in decreased heart rate.

Gerontological Considerations

- Ensure adequate lubrication of tube to decrease discomfort for the older adult, because of the potential for decreased oral or nasopharyngeal secretions in older adults.

Home Care Considerations

- Assess the client or primary caregiver's ability to maintain tube and feeding program.
- Assess the environmental safety and sanitation of client's home to determine potential for infection or injury.
- Teach client or primary caregiver how to assess tube placement (see Skill 30-2).
- Teach the family caregiver correct method for securing feeding tube to nares to eliminate pressure on nares and face and to allow enough tubing for movement.

SKILL 30-2 Verifying Feeding Tube Placement

Nasally or orally placed small-bore feeding tubes can be inserted into the stomach for either intermittent or continuous feedings; they can also be inserted into the small intestine (duodenum or proximal jejunum) for continuous feedings. Large-bore tubes are not suitable for small bowel feedings. Intermittent feedings are boluses administered over a short time period; therefore they are only given into the stomach because it is a natural reservoir for fluid (ASPEN, 2002).

It is possible for an NG or NI enteral feeding tube to move into a different location (from the stomach to the intestine or from the intestine into the stomach) without any external evidence that the tube has moved. The risk for aspiration of regurgitated gastric contents into the respiratory tract is increased when the tip of an NI tube accidentally dislocates upward into the stomach or when the tip of either an NG or NI tube dislocates upward into the esophagus.

Following initial x-ray verification that a tube is positioned in the desired site (either the stomach or small intestine), the nurse is responsible for ensuring that the tube has remained in the intended position before administering formula or medications through the tube. Therefore tube position must be verified every 4 to 12 hours and as needed. Because it is not feasible to do radiographic checks at this frequency, other methods of determining placement have been investigated. Certain characteristics of fluid aspirated from feeding tubes are helpful in assessing placement of the tube. Color may differentiate gastric from intestinal placement. Because most intestinal aspirates are stained by bile to a distinct yellow color, and most gastric aspirates are not, the difference can often distinguish the sites (Metheny and others, 1998a). The pH of an aspirate offers valuable data as well in assessing placement of a feeding tube (Gharpure and others, 2000; Metheny and others, 1999). Bedside testing of pH using pH paper covering a range from 0 to 14 is sufficient for this purpose (Metheny and others, 1994) and should be standard protocol to aid in the assessment of feeding tube placement. More recently, a tool assessing the bilirubin level of aspirated fluid has been tested (Metheny and Titler, 2001). When used in conjunction with pH levels and color, this tool can assess placement of feeding tubes at a high level of accuracy in many cases without the need for obtaining an x-ray film (Metheny and others, 1999; Metheny and Titler, 2001). The algorithm using these assessments could decrease the need for an x-ray examination to exclude respiratory placement to less than 30% of clients with newly inserted feeding tubes (Metheny and others, 1999). This same algorithm was used to accurately predict gastric placement 98% of the time and intestinal placement 92% of the time (Metheny and others, 1999).

Studies have been conducted on the efficacy of testing for pepsin (an enzyme found in gastric juice) and trypsin (an enzyme present in duodenal and jejunal secretions) to assess tube placement. These enzymes, used in conjunction with the appearance, pH, and bilirubin content of feeding tube aspirates, are helpful in assessing feeding tube placement (Metheny and Stewart, 2002) and in the future may eliminate the need for an initial x-ray film to assess placement. They may also lead to near 100% accuracy of routine assessment of feeding tube placement.

DELEGATION CONSIDERATIONS

The verification of tube placement is the responsibility of the nurse and should not be delegated to assistive personnel. However, assistive personnel may take responsibility for other aspects of care. The nurse must instruct assistive personnel to immediately inform nurse:

- If client's respirations change or client complains of shortness of breath, coughing, or choking
- If the client vomits or the assistive personnel notices vomitus in client's mouth during oral hygiene.
- If nasal skin irritation is present
- If displacement of the feeding tube occurs

EQUIPMENT

- ❑ 60-ml Luer-Lok or catheter-tip syringe
- ❑ Stethoscope
- ❑ Clean gloves
- ❑ pH indicator strip (scale of 0.0 to 14.0)

STEP	RATIONALE

ASSESSMENT

1. Be aware of policy and procedures for frequency and method of checking tube placement in your facility.

   Maintains quality of client care. Some facilities allow the auscultation method; regardless of the method, make sure x-ray confirmation was obtained at the time of placement.

2. Identify signs and symptoms of inadvertent respiratory migration of feeding tube: coughing, choking, or cyanosis.

   Signs and symptoms indicate accidental migration of feeding tube into the airway. However, their absence does not ensure that respiratory migration has not occurred, especially in the client with altered level of consciousness and/or altered gag and cough reflexes.

3. Identify conditions that increase the risk for spontaneous tube dislocation from the intended position (e.g., stomach to esophagus, intestine to stomach):
   a. Retching/vomiting
   b. Nasotracheal suctioning
   c. Severe bouts of coughing

   Feeding tubes may become dislocated by increases in intra-abdominal pressure or coughing.

4. Observe the external portion of the tube for movement of the ink mark away from the mouth or naris (see Skill 30-1).

   Increased external length of a tube may indicate that the distal tip is no longer in the correct position.

5. Review client's medication record: Is client receiving a gastric acid inhibitor (e.g., cimetidine, ranitidine, famotidine, nizatidine) or a proton pump inhibitor (e.g., omeprazole)?

   H_2 receptor antagonists reduce volume of gastric acid secretion and the acid content of secretions, thus causing the pH value to be higher, that is, more basic (Metheny and Stewart, 2002).

6. Review client's record for history of prior tube displacement.

   Clients who have a history of tube displacement are at increased risk.

NURSING DIAGNOSES

- Risk for aspiration
- Impaired gas exchange

Related factors are individualized based on client's condition or needs.

PLANNING

1. Expected outcomes following completion of procedure:
   - Color, pH, and appearance of aspirate is consistent with the initial tube placement according to x-ray results.

   Indicates that the tube has likely remained in the correct location initially confirmed by x-ray film (Metheny and others, 1998a).

2. Explain procedure to client.

   Client has a right to be informed regarding all procedures done.

IMPLEMENTATION

1. Perform hand hygiene, and apply gloves.

   Reduces transmission of microorganisms.

2. Measures to verify placement of tube should be conducted at the following times:
   a. For intermittently tube-fed clients, test placement immediately before each feeding and before medications.
   b. For continuously tube-fed clients, test placement every 4 to 12 hours and before medication administration.
   c. Wait at least 1 hour after medication administration by tube or mouth.

   Premature aspiration of contents will remove unabsorbed medication, reducing dose delivered to client. Medication can also interfere with pH testing and appearance of aspirate (Metheny and others, 1994).

STEP	RATIONALE
3. Draw up 30 ml of air into a 60-ml syringe, then attach to end of feeding tube. Flush tube with 30 ml of air before attempting to aspirate fluid. Repositioning the client from side to side may be helpful. More than one bolus of air through the tube may be needed in some cases.	Burst of air aids in aspirating fluid more easily (Metheny and others, 1993). Smaller syringes generate unnecessarily high pressures inside the tube.
	It may be more difficult to aspirate fluid from the small intestine than from the stomach.
4. Draw back on syringe slowly, and obtain 5 to 10 ml of gastric aspirate (see illustration). Observe appearance of aspirate to help assess the position of the tube.	Drawing back quickly, or with a smaller syringe, increases intratubular pressure and may cause the tube to collapse.
	Quantity is sufficient for pH testing. Aspirates from NG tubes of continuously tube-fed clients often have appearance of curdled enteral formula. Aspirates from NI tubes are often stained yellow from bile. Gastric aspirates from intermittently tube-fed clients are not typically bile stained (unless intestinal fluid has refluxed into the stomach).
5. Gently mix aspirate in syringe. Measure pH of aspirated GI contents by dipping the pH strip into the fluid or by applying a few drops of the fluid to the strip (see illustration). Compare the color of the strip with the color on the chart provided by the manufacturer (see illustration) (Metheny and others, 1998a).	Mixing ensures equal distribution of contents for testing. pH paper covering a minimal range of range from 0 to 14 provides most accurate readings of gastric pH levels (Metheny and others, 1994).
a. Gastric fluid from client who has fasted for at least 4 hours usually has pH range of 1 to 4.	Range of 1 to 4 is a reliable indicator of stomach placement, especially when a gastric acid inhibitor is *not* being used.
b. Fluid from NI tube of fasting client usually has pH greater than 6.	Intestinal contents are more basic than stomach contents (Metheny and others, 1999).
c. Client with continuous tube feeding may have pH of 5 or higher.	Formulas contain solutions that are basic.
d. pH of pleural fluid from the tracheobronchial tree is generally greater than 6.	The pH of pleural fluid makes it difficult to differentiate between respiratory and intestinal placement (Metheny and others, 1999). The bilirubin test would help discriminate between intestinal and respiratory placement.

- ***Critical Decision Point***
  Auscultation of an air bolus is no longer considered a reliable or safe method for verification of tube position. (See discussion of evidence-based practice trends.)

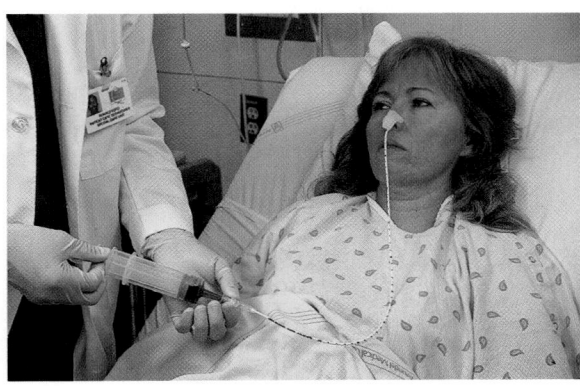

STEP **4** Obtaining gastric aspirate.

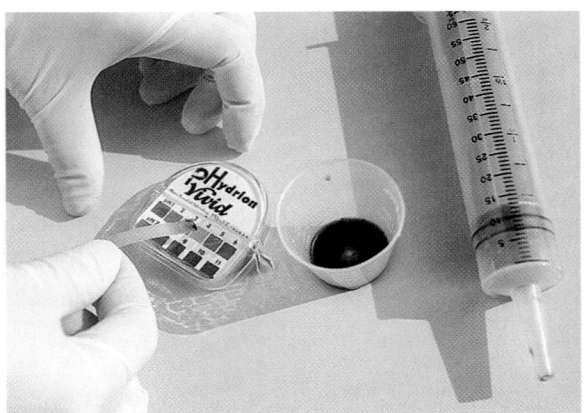

STEP **5** Compare color on test strip with color on pH chart.

STEP	RATIONALE
6. If after repeated attempts it is not possible to aspirate fluid from a tube that was originally established by x-ray examination to be in desired position, and if (a) there are no risk factors for tube dislocation, (b) tube has remained in original taped position, and (c) client is not experiencing respiratory distress, assume tube is correctly placed (Metheny and others, 1993).	It is reasonable to assume tube is correctly placed. When abdominal x-ray films are obtained for clinical reasons, the nurse can take advantage of reports to monitor tube location.
7. Irrigate tube (see Skill 30-3).	Keeps tube patent.
8. Remove and dispose of gloves. Perform hand hygiene.	Reduces transmission of microorganisms.

EVALUATION

1. Observe client for respiratory distress:
   a. Persistent gagging
   b. Paroxysms of coughing
   c. Respiratory patterns (e.g., rate and depth) that are inconsistent with baseline measures.
	Feeding enters airways.

2. Verify that color, pH, and appearance of aspirate are consistent with the initial tube placement according to x-ray results.	Indicates that the tip of the tube is likely to be positioned in the same place as it was following x-ray confirmation.

Recording and Reporting

- Record and report pH and appearance of aspirate.

Unexpected Outcomes	Related Interventions
1. Red or brown coloring (coffee grounds in appearance) of fluid aspirated from a feeding tube is an indicator of new blood or old blood, respectively, in the gastrointestinal tract.	• If the color is not related to medications recently administered, notify the physician.
2. Client develops severe respiratory distress (e.g., dyspnea, decreased oxygen saturation, increased pulse rate), which could result from aspiration of enteral feedings or displacement of feeding tube into the lung.	• Notify physician. • Stop any enteral feedings. • Obtain chest x-ray as ordered.
3. Abdomen becomes distended, which may occur if feeding tube is displaced into esophagus.	• Notify physician. • Stop any enteral feedings.

Teaching Considerations

- Instruct client to not pull or alter position of nasoenteral tube.

Pediatric Considerations

- Decrease the amount of air insufflated according to the size of the client (e.g., an infant may only need 1 ml of air, a small child 5 ml) before aspiration of gastric secretions.

Home Care Considerations

- Instruct client or primary caregiver not to proceed with feedings or medication administration via the tube if there is any doubt as to proper placement of tube.

SKILL 30-3 Irrigating a Feeding Tube

The skill of irrigating a feeding tube maintains patency of the tube. All types of feeding tubes require routine irrigation. Patency of a tube may be questioned when air or fluid cannot be instilled through the tube. Adequacy of nutritional support is essential in client care, and for this reason tubes must remain patent. Unless effort is made to monitor and irrigate feeding tubes routinely, the amount of feeding a client receives is likely 15% to 20% below the amount ordered and 25% to 30% less than the goal (McClave and others, 1999).

There are other types of feeding tubes besides those inserted by nurses at the bedside. When clients cannot tolerate nasally or orally placed tubes, there are options. See Skill 30-5 for descriptions of gastrostomy and jejunostomy tubes. Both of these tubes require routine irrigation.

DELEGATION CONSIDERATIONS
The skill of irrigating a feeding tube should not be delegated to assistive personnel. Assistive personnel should be instructed to report whenever a continuous tube feeding stops infusing.

EQUIPMENT
- ❏ 60-ml catheter-tip syringe
- ❏ Normal saline or tap water
- ❏ Towel
- ❏ Disposable gloves

STEP	RATIONALE

ASSESSMENT

1. Inspect the volume, color, and character of gastric aspirates (if obtainable).

2. Note ease with which tube feeding infuses through tubing.

3. Monitor volume of tube-feeding formula administered during a shift, and compare with ordered amount.
4. Refer to agency policies regarding routine irrigation (usually every 4 to 12 hours).
5. Assess sodium levels.

Thick secretions and a reduced volume of secretions may indicate need to irrigate tube. Excess volume of secretions (more than 200 ml) may indicate delayed gastric emptying.
Failure of formula to infuse as desired may indicate developing obstruction.
Indicates whether sufficient volume of feeding is infusing.

Determines frequency of irrigations. (See discussion of evidence-based practice trends.)
To determine if there is a particular need to choose either normal saline or tap water for irrigation. Obtain physician order for irrigant.

NURSING DIAGNOSES
- Imbalanced nutrition: less than body requirements
- Deficient fluid volume
- Excess fluid volume

Related factors are individualized based on client's condition or needs.

PLANNING

1. Expected outcomes following completion of procedure:
   - Feeding tube remains patent.

   - Client receives prescribed caloric intake.
2. Explain procedure to client.
3. Position client in high-Fowler's (if tolerated) or semi-Fowler's position.

Irrigation fluid clears inner lumen of feeding tube of accumulated solids and secretions.
Feeding infuses without interruption.
Decreases client anxiety.
Reduces risk of aspiration during irrigation.

STEP	RATIONALE

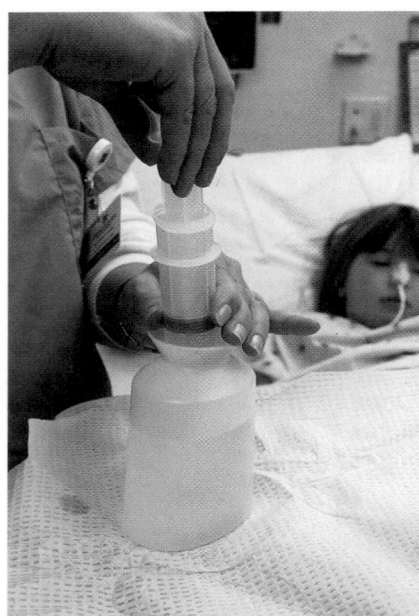

STEP **4** Draw up 30 ml normal saline into syringe.

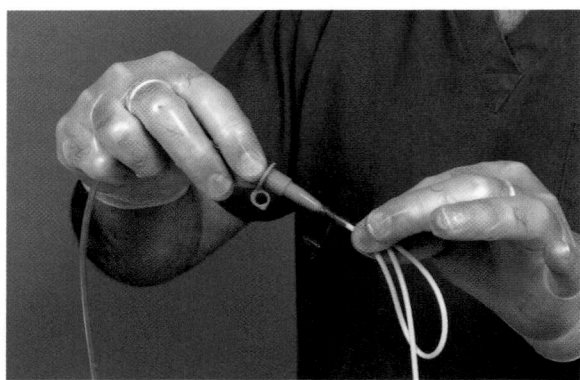

STEP **5** Kink tubing while unplugging feeding tube.

IMPLEMENTATION

1. Perform hand hygiene.

   Reduces transmission of microorganisms.

2. Prepare equipment at client's bedside, and apply gloves.
3. Verify tube placement (see Skill 30-2) if fluid can be aspirated.

   With tip of tube correctly placed in stomach, irrigation will not create risk of aspiration.

4. Draw up 30 ml of normal saline or tap water in syringe (see illustration).

   This amount of solution will flush length of tube. Irrigation fluids should not be used from multidose bottles that are used on other clients. The client should have his or her own bottle of irrigation solution, and bottles should be changed every 24 hours to reduce the risk of contamination.

5. Kink feeding tube while disconnecting it from feeding-bag tubing or while removing plug at end of tube (see illustration). Place end of feeding-bag tubing on towel.

   Prevents leakage of gastric secretions.

6. Insert tip of catheter into end of feeding tube. Release kink, and slowly instill irrigating solution (see illustration).

   Infusion of fluid clears tubing.

7. If unable to instill fluid, reposition client on left side, and try again.

   Tip of tube may be against stomach wall. Changing client's position may move tip away from stomach wall.

STEP	RATIONALE

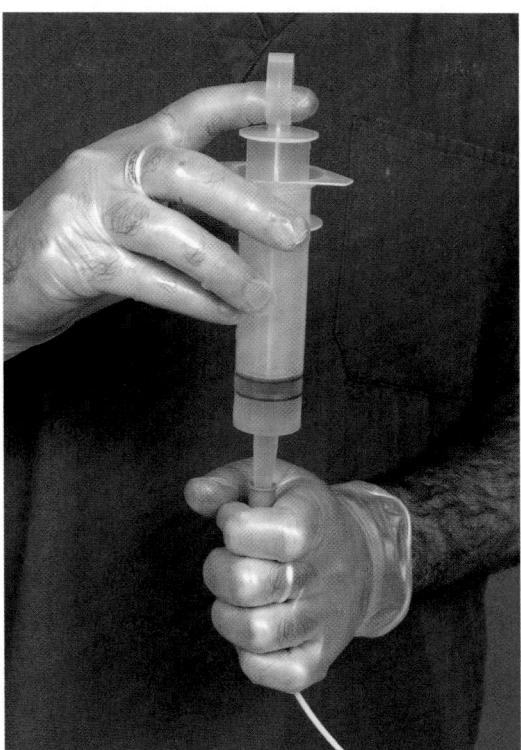

STEP **6** Irrigate feeding tube.

8. When saline or tap water has been instilled, remove syringe. Reinstitute tube feeding, or administer medication as ordered. Irrigate before medications, between different medications, and after the final medication (before feedings are reinstituted).

Tubing is clear and patent.
Certain tube-feeding formulas have properties that predispose to tube clogging (Simon and Fink, 1999). Irrigation prevents mixing of medications in the tube, which may cause clogging. Flushes medications completely through the tube so medications do not mix with enteral nutrition inside the tube and clog.

9. Remove and discard gloves; dispose of supplies. Perform hand hygiene.

Reduces transmission of microorganisms.

EVALUATION

1. Observe ease with which tube feeding instills through tubing.

A successfully irrigated tube is patent, allowing for free flow of tube-feeding solution.

Recording and Reporting

- Record time of irrigation, amount and type of fluid instilled.

Unexpected Outcomes	Related Interventions
1. Tube cannot be irrigated and remains obstructed.	• Reattempt irrigation; if unsuccessful, notify the physician. Tube may need to be removed and a new tube placed.
2. Fluid and electrolyte imbalances occur. Irrigation with excessive amounts of water can cause sodium levels to drop; excessive saline can cause increased sodium levels. Insufficient irrigation can cause water deficiency; excessive irrigations can cause fluid volume excess.	• Notify the physician of abnormal electrolyte levels or imbalanced intake and output.

Pediatric Considerations

- Irrigation of a tube requires a smaller volume of solution in children: 1 or 2 ml for small tubes to 5 to 15 ml or more for large ones (Hockenberry and others, 2003).

SKILL 30-4 Administering Enteral Nutrition via a Nasogastric Feeding Tube

The general indications for enteral feeding were described in the section on evidence-based research trends. Some specific examples of these indications include the following:

1. Clients who cannot eat because of surgery, injury, or disease process (e.g., comatose clients; clients receiving mechanical ventilation; clients recovering from oral, head, and neck surgeries; clients with pancreatitis or inflammatory bowel disease)
2. Nutritional deficit due to reduced food ingestion or hypermetabolic state, even when they are physically capable of eating (e.g., confused clients; clients with eating disorders; clients with cancer, sepsis, burns, trauma, or head injury)
3. Clients with impaired swallowing or gag reflex (e.g., clients who have had a stroke)

Gastric feedings are the most common type of enteral nutrition, allowing tube-feeding formulas to enter the stomach and then pass more gradually through the intestinal tract to ensure absorption. However, gastric ileus (decreased or absent peristalsis affecting the stomach but not the intestines), delayed gastric emptying, or gastric resections contraindicate gastric feedings. Intestinal tubes allow for feeding into the small intestine beyond the pyloric sphincter of the stomach (Kudsk and others, 1992). The advantage of intestinal feedings is decreased gastric volume, which reduces the risk of aspiration, provided that feedings do not reflux back into the stomach.

Tube feeding has been associated with the inadequate delivery of nutrients, potentially leading to malnutrition or electrolyte disturbances, because of interruptions in feeding (McClave and others, 1992). Previously, beginning administration of enteral nutrition was often delayed until bowel sounds were auscultated in the client. However, research has suggested that when compared to total parenteral nutrition (intravenous nutrition), initiation of enteral nutrition within the first 24 hours in critically ill clients helps to lower infection rates and decrease length of intensive care unit admission (Kudsk and others, 1992; Moore and others, 1989). In addition, early enteral nutrition helps to maintain bowel mucosal integrity, improve wound healing, and reduce rates of septic morbidity (Heyland and Mandell, 1992). Furthermore, it is not necessary to wait for the presence of bowel sounds to begin tube feeding. Heyland and others (1995) found that even critically ill clients tolerated enteral feedings to some degree regardless of whether bowel sounds were present. Nevertheless, early enteral feedings are not without risk; therefore care should be taken to balance the benefits and risks by assessing for client tolerance of the feeding (Gottschlich and others, 2002).

DELEGATION CONSIDERATIONS

Administration of nasoenteral tube feeding is a procedure that can be delegated to assistive personnel. However, a nurse must first verify tube placement and patency. The nurse should instruct assistive personnel:

- About the prescribed rate to infuse the feeding
- About any positioning restrictions for a specific client
- To report any difficulty infusing the feeding or any discomfort voiced by the client
- To report any gagging, paroxysms of coughing, or choking

EQUIPMENT

- ❑ Disposable feeding bag and tubing or ready-to-hang system
- ❑ 60-ml Luer-Lok or catheter-tip syringe
- ❑ Stethoscope
- ❑ Infusion pump (required for continuous or intestinal feedings): Use pump designed for tube feedings
- ❑ pH indicator strip (see Skill 30-2)
- ❑ Prescribed enteral feeding
- ❑ Gloves
- ❑ Equipment to obtain blood glucose by finger stick

STEP	RATIONALE

■ ASSESSMENT

1. Assess client's need for enteral tube feedings (clients who are unable to eat, have a nutrition deficit, or have impaired swallowing).

2. Assess client for food allergies.

3. Auscultate for bowel sounds.

4. Obtain baseline weight and laboratory values. Assess client for fluid volume excess or deficit, electrolyte abnormalities, and metabolic abnormalities such as hyperglycemia.

5. Verify physician's order for formula, rate, route, and frequency.

Identify clients who need tube feedings before they become nutritionally depleted.

Prevents client from developing localized or systemic allergic responses.

Absent bowel sounds may indicate decreased ability of GI tract to digest or absorb nutrients.

Enteral feedings are to restore or maintain a client's nutritional status. Provides objective data to measure effectiveness of feedings. Laboratory data (e.g., electrolytes and capillary blood-glucose measurement) are ordered by physician.

Ensures correct formula will be administered in appropriate volume.

■ NURSING DIAGNOSES

- Imbalanced nutrition: less than body requirements
- Readiness for enhanced nutrition

- Impaired swallowing
- Risk for aspiration

Related factors are individualized based on client's condition or needs.

■ PLANNING

1. Expected outcomes following completion of procedure:
   - Nutritional status is improved, as evidenced by increasing weight, improving laboratory values, and improved intake and output.
   - Client has no signs of respiratory distress.

2. Explain procedure to client.
3. Perform hand hygiene.

Indicates that client's nutritional needs are being met.

Entry of feeding tube into airways or aspiration of feeding may cause respiratory distress.

Decreases client anxiety.

Reduces transmission of microorganisms.

STEP	RATIONALE

4. Prepare feeding container to administer formula continuously:
   a. Check expiration date on formula and integrity of container.
   b. Have tube feeding at room temperature.

   c. Connect tubing to container, or prepare ready-to-hang container. Use aseptic technique, and avoid handling the feeding system. If you need to handle the system, perform hand hygiene and wear gloves.
   d. Shake formula container well, and fill container with formula (see illustration). Open stopcock on tubing, and fill tubing with formula to remove air (prime tubing). Hang on pole.
5. For intermittent feeding have syringe ready and be sure formula is at room temperature.
6. Place client in high-Fowler's position, or elevate head of bed at least 30 degrees. For client forced to remain supine, place in reverse Trendelenburg position.

Ensures GI tolerance of formula. Prevents leakage of tube feeding.

Cold formula may cause gastric cramping and discomfort because the liquid is not warmed by mouth and esophagus.

The feeding system, including the bag, connections, and tubing, must be free of contamination to prevent bacterial growth (Padula and others, 2004).

Filling the tubing with formula prevents excess air from entering gastrointestinal tract once infusion begins.

Cold formula causes gastric cramping.

Elevated head helps prevent aspiration.

IMPLEMENTATION

1. Apply gloves.
2. Determine tube placement (see Skill 30-2). Observe aspirate's appearance and note pH measure (see illustration).

Reduces transmission of microorganisms.

Feedings instilled into a misplaced tube may cause serious injury or death. On occasion, color alone may differentiate gastric from intestinal placement because most intestinal aspirates are stained by bile to a distinct yellow color, and most gastric aspirates are not (Metheny and others, 1999) (see illustration).

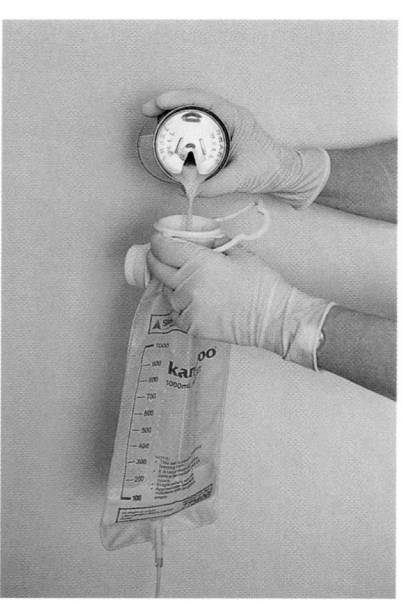

STEP **4d** Pour formula into feeding container.

STEP	**RATIONALE**

3. Check gastric residual volume (see illustration). Residual volume should be assessed before each feeding for intermittent feedings. Researcher recommendations for continuous feeding ranges from every 4 to 12 hours.
   a. Connect syringe to end of feeding tube, pull back slowly, and aspirate the total amount of gastric contents that may possibly be aspirated.
   b. Return aspirated contents to stomach unless volume is excessive (greater than 100 ml). Verify with agency policy.
4. Irrigate tube (see Skill 30-3).

For adults, a volume in excess of 200 ml for NG tubes should raise concern about intolerance; however, feedings may continue while further examinations are conducted (ASPEN, 2002; McClave and others, 1992; McClave and others, 1999; Murphy and Bickford, 1999). Fluids aspirated from the stomach contain electrolytes that, if withheld, may cause electrolyte imbalances. Notify the physician if residual volume is excessive, and request an order regarding whether or not the residual fluid should be returned to the client.

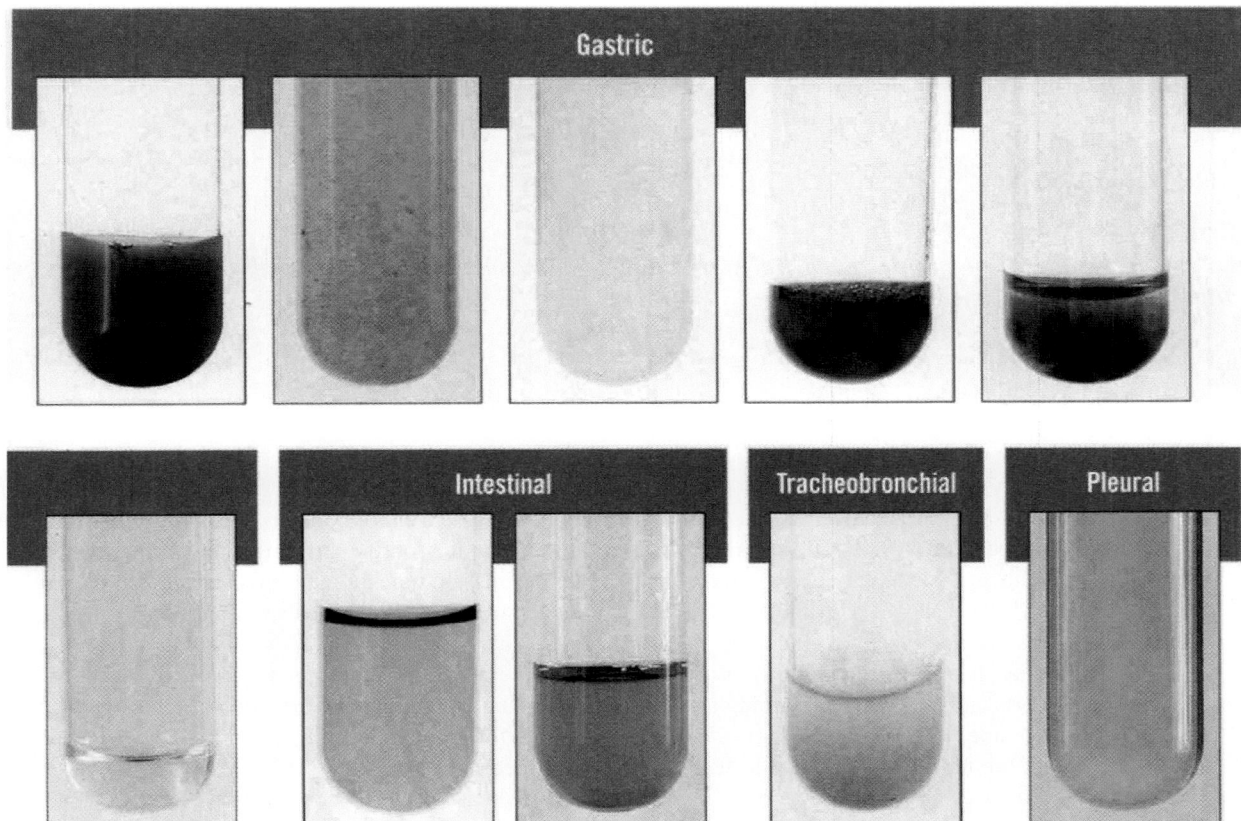

STEP 2 Typical color of aspirates from stomach, intestine, and airway. (Used with permission from Metheny NA and others: pH, color, and feeding tubes, *RN* 61:25, 1998.)

STEP	RATIONALE

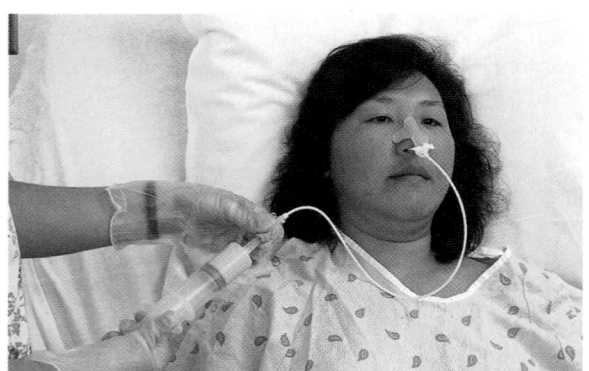

STEP **3** Check for gastric residual volume (small-bore tube).

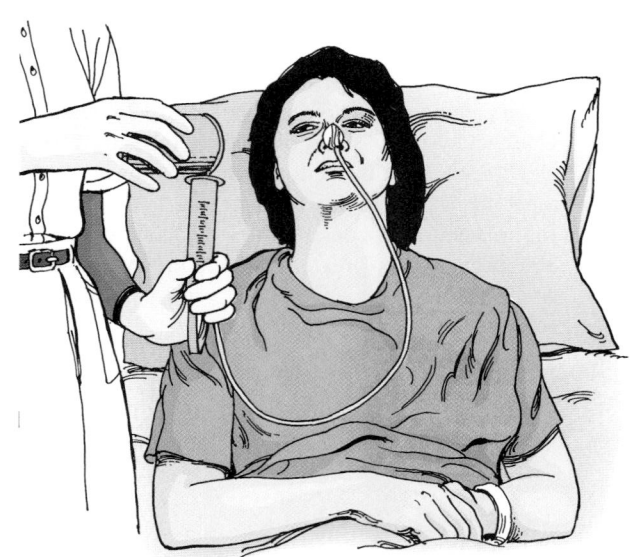

STEP **5a(3)** Fill syringe with formula.

5. Initiate feeding:

• *Critical Decision Point*
Do not add food coloring or dye to enteral nutrition. (See discussion of evidence-based practice trends.)

a.   Syringe or intermittent feeding
   (1)   Pinch proximal end of feeding tube.
   (2)   Remove plunger from syringe, and attach barrel of syringe to end of tube.
   (3)   Fill syringe with measured amount of formula (see illustration). Release tube, and elevate syringe to no more than 18 inches (45 cm) above insertion site, and allow it to empty gradually by gravity. Repeat steps 1 to 3 until prescribed amount has been delivered to client.
   (4)   If a feeding bag (see illustration) is used, prime tubing, and attach gavage tubing to end of feeding tube. Set rate by adjusting roller clamp on tubing or placing on a feeding pump. Allow bag to empty gradually over 30 to 60 minutes. Label bag with tube-feeding type, strength, and amount. Include date, time, and initials. Change bag every 24 hours.
b.   Continuous-drip method
   (1)   Prime and hang feeding bag and tubing on feeding-pump pole.
   (2)   Connect distal end of tubing to proximal end of feeding tube.

Prevents air from entering client's stomach.
Barrel receives formula for instillation.

Height of syringe allows for safe, slow, gravity drainage of formula. Total delivery of bolus feedings may take several minutes, depending on the amount of the bolus. Administering the feeding too quickly may cause abdominal discomfort to the client or increase the risk for aspiration.

Gradual emptying of tube feeding by gravity from syringe or feeding bag reduces risk of abdominal discomfort, vomiting, or diarrhea induced by bolus or too-rapid infusion of tube feedings.
Helps decrease bacterial colonization.

Continuous feeding method is designed to deliver prescribed hourly rate of feeding. This method reduces risk of abdominal discomfort.

| STEP | RATIONALE |

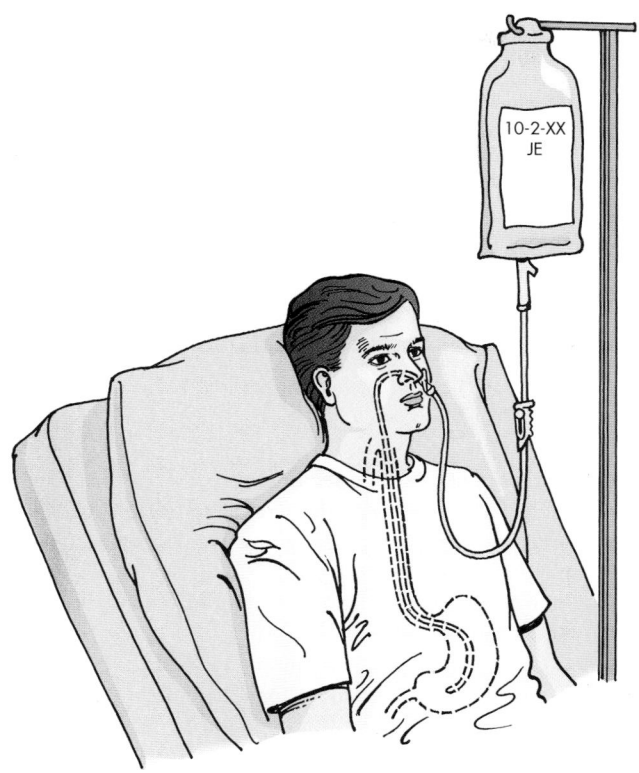

STEP **5a(4)** Administer feeding.

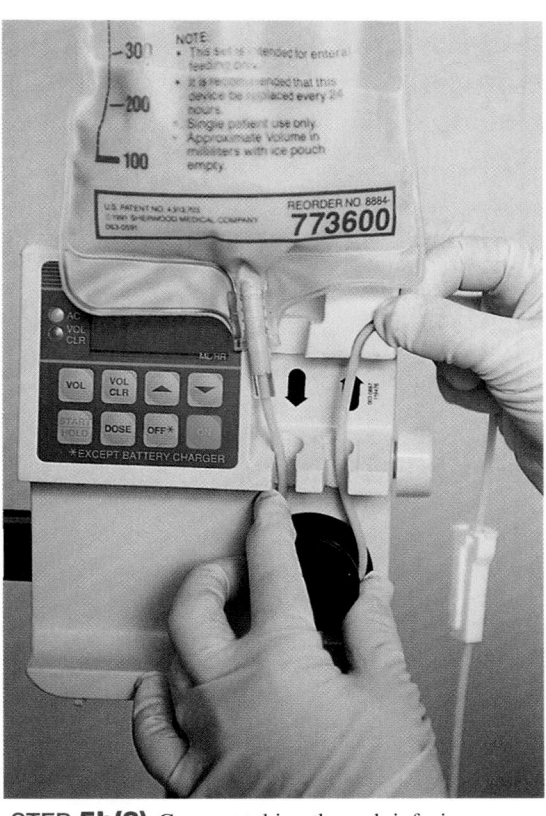

STEP **5b(3)** Connect tubing through infusion pump.

(3) Connect tubing through infusion pump, and set rate (see illustration).

Delivers continuous feeding at a steady rate and pressure. Feeding pump alarms for increased resistance.

- **Critical Decision Point**
  Maximum hang time for formula is 8 hours in an open system, 24 hours in closed, ready-to-hang system (if it remains closed). Refer to manufacturer's guidelines.

6. Advance rate of concentration of tube feeding gradually (Box 30-1).

Helps to prevent diarrhea and gastric intolerance to formula.

7. Following intermittent infusion or at end of infusion irrigate nasogastric feeding tube per hospital policy (see Skill 30-3).

Provides client with source of water to help maintain fluid and electrolyte balance. Clears tubing of formula.

8. When tube feedings are not being administered, cap or clamp the proximal end of the feeding tube.

Prevents air from entering stomach between feedings.

9. Rinse bag and tubing with warm water whenever feedings are interrupted. Use a new administration set every 24 hours.

Rinsing bag and tubing with warm water clears old tube feedings and reduces bacterial growth.

10. Dispose of supplies, and perform hand hygiene.

Reduces transmission of microorganisms.

STEP	RATIONALE

BOX 30-1 Advancing the Rate of Tube Feeding

INTERMITTENT

1. Start formula at full strength for isotonic formulas (300 to 400 mOsm) or at ordered concentration.
2. Infuse formula over at least 20 to 30 minutes via syringe or feeding container.
3. Begin feedings with no more than 150 to 250 ml at one time. Increase by 50 ml per feeding per day to achieve needed volume and calories in six to eight feedings. (NOTE: Concentrated formulas at full strength may be infused at slower rate until tolerance is achieved.)

CONTINUOUS

1. Start formula at full strength for isotonic formulas (300 to 400 mOsm) or at ordered concentration. Usually hypertonic formulas are also started at full strength but at a slower rate.
2. Begin infusion rate at designated rate.
3. Advance rate slowly (e.g., 10 to 20 ml/hr) per day to target rate if tolerated (tolerance indicated by absence of nausea and diarrhea, and low gastric residuals).

EVALUATION

1. Measure residual volume per policy.
2. Monitor finger-stick blood glucose (usually at least every 6 hours until maximum administration rate is reached and maintained for 24 hours).
3. Monitor intake and output at least every 8 hours (Edwards and Metheny, 2000).
4. Weigh client daily until maximum administration rate is reached and maintained for 24 hours, then weigh client 3 times per week.
5. Monitor laboratory values.

6. Observe client's respiratory status.

7. Observe client's level of comfort.
8. Auscultate bowel sounds.

Evaluates tolerance of tube feeding.
Requires a physician order. Alerts nurse to client's tolerance of enteral nutrition. May require physician to revise type of formula administered.
Intake and output are indications of fluid balance or fluid volume excess or deficit.
Weight gain is indicator of improved nutritional status; however, sudden gain of more than 2 pounds in 24 hours usually indicates fluid retention.
Laboratory values (e.g., albumin, transferrin, and prealbumin) are indicators of client nutritional status.
Change in respiratory status can indicate aspiration of tube feeding.
Reduced gastric emptying can lead to abdominal discomfort.
Evaluates status of gastric peristalsis.

Recording and Reporting

- Record amount and type of feeding, client's response to tube feeding, patency of tube.
- Record volume of formula and any additional water on intake and output form.
- Report type of feeding, status of feeding tube, client's tolerance, and adverse effects.

Unexpected Outcomes	Related Interventions
1. The feeding tube becomes clogged. Frequent aspiration of gastric or intestinal contents (Powell and others, 1993) and frequent administration of medications via the tube have been associated with increased clogging of feeding tubes (Pancorbo-Hidalgo and others, 2001; Seifert and others, 2002).	• To avoid this problem, flush the tube with water after checking the residual volume (Edwards and Metheny, 2000). Cranberry juice should not be used to unclog feeding tubes; water works better than cranberry juice (Metheny and others, 1988).
2. Gastric residual volume is excessive.	• Notify physician to determine if feedings need to be held. If feedings are held, reassess residual volume 1 hour after the feeding is stopped to determine if volume has lessened or increased. If it has increased, make sure the physician is aware.
	• Maintain client in semi-Fowler's position; have head of bed elevated at least 30 degrees.

Unexpected Outcomes	Related Interventions
3. Client aspirates formula.	• (See interventions following Skill 30-1.)
4. The client develops diarrhea 3 times or more in 24 hours; may indicate intolerance.	• Notify physician, and confer with dietitian to determine need to modify type of formula, concentration, or rate of infusion. • Consider other causes (e.g., bacterial contamination of the feeding, client infection) (Eisenberg, 2002). • Determine if client is receiving antibiotics or medications (e.g., those containing sorbitol) that can induce diarrhea (Benya and others, 1991; Guenter and others, 1991).
5. Client develops nausea and vomiting.	• May indicate gastric ileus. Withhold tube feeding, and notify physician. • Be sure tubing is patent; aspirate for residual.
6. Aspirated fluid has foul odor or unusual appearance.	• Notify the physician, and document the findings. Do not return aspirated material of unusual odor or appearance without first consulting physician.

Teaching Considerations

- Teach client and family caregiver that, if tolerated, client should remain upright for 1 hour after feedings.
- Instruct client or family caregiver that client may express feelings of fullness, increased gas, belching, or diarrhea.

Pediatric Considerations

- Intermittent feeding is preferred in infants because of possible perforation of the stomach, nasal airway obstruction, ulceration, and irritation to mucous membranes with continuous feedings. When giving intermittent feedings to a small child, administration should take approximately 20 to 30 minutes, or as long as it would take to bottle-feed the child. Hold the infant, and offer a pacifier during the feeding to simulate a more natural bottle-feeding experience (Hockenberry and others, 2003).
- Temporary small-bore NG tubes are often placed in infants just before each feeding and removed afterward.
- For a neonate, an excessive residual volume is more than 20% of the ordered amount. For an older child, an excessive residual volume is greater than 50% of the ordered amount.

- For pediatric clients receiving continuous feedings, assess the residual volume with routine vitals signs, at minimum at least every 4 hours (Hockenberry and others, 2003).

Gerontological Considerations

- Older adult clients may be more susceptible to hyperglycemia related to the glucose concentration in enteral formulas.
- Older adults may have decreased gastric transit time so that formula remains in the stomach longer than for younger clients. Gastric residual checks are of special importance to decrease the risk of vomiting and aspiration during gastric feeding.

Home Care Considerations

- Instruct primary caregiver and/or client to monitor intake and output using household measuring devices.
- Ask client or care provider about any symptoms or discomfort during enteral feedings. Reinforce instruction to contact nurse if symptoms of discomfort occur.
- If enteral feeding is to be used at home for longer than 1 to 2 weeks, discuss potential for gastrostomy placement with physician.

SKILL 30-5 Administering Enteral Nutrition via a Gastrostomy or Jejunostomy Tube

When clients cannot tolerate nasoenteral feeding tubes, require permanent enteral feeding, or when nasoenteral feeding tubes interfere with rehabilitation, other options may be selected. One such option is a gastric feeding. Gastric feedings permit the delivery of partially digested nutrients to the stomach or intestine at a normal physiological rate. Gastric feedings via a gastrostomy feeding tube are relatively safe to administer, provided the client has normal gastric emptying and there is not excessive residual volume. A gastrostomy tube is inserted in the operating room or endoscopy area by a surgeon or gastroenterologist. A large tube is surgically placed in the stomach and exits through an incision in the upper left quadrant of the abdomen, where it is sutured in place. A more current practice is a PEG tube, which is inserted with endoscopic visualization of the stomach. This tube also exits through a puncture wound in the upper left quadrant of the abdomen, but it is held securely in place by virtue of its designs (see Figure 30-2).

When clients have gastric ileus (decreased or absent peristalsis that affects the stomach but not the intestines), delayed gastric emptying, gastric resections, or neurological impairments that place them at greater risk of aspiration, enteral nutrition may be delivered via a jejunostomy tube. Jejunostomy tubes, like gastrostomy tubes, can be inserted during surgery or endoscopy. Endoscopic insertion of a jejunostomy tube is done through a PEG tube. After insertion of the large-bore PEG tube, the PEJ tube is passed through the PEG and advanced into the jejunum (see Figure 30-3). A Y connector attached to the jejunostomy tube caps the PEG tube and closes the system. This Y connector labels the gastrostomy tube and designates the jejunostomy tube for feeding. The nurse must know which tube is gastric and which tube is jejunal.

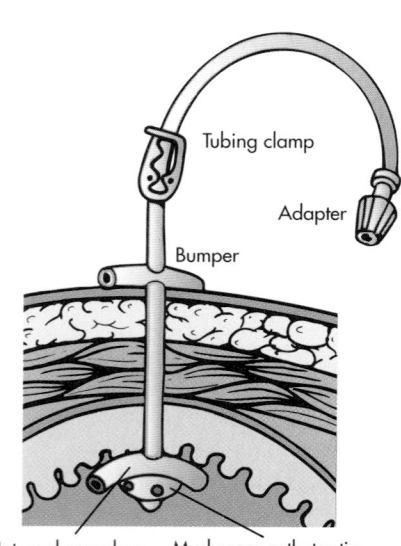

FIGURE **30-2** Placement of PEG tube into stomach.

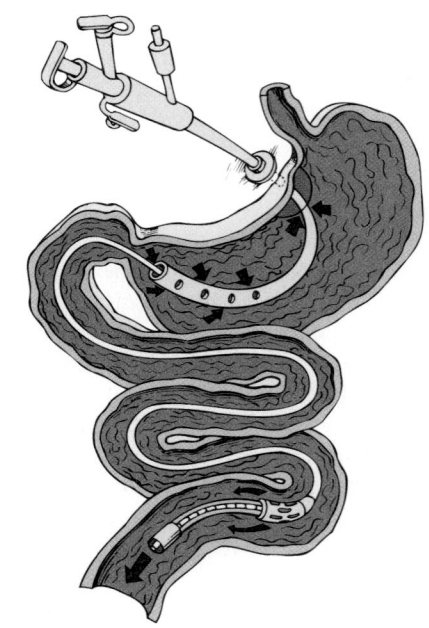

FIGURE **30-3** Endoscopic insertion of jejunostomy tube.

DELEGATION CONSIDERATIONS

Administration of gastrostomy or jejunostomy tube feeding is a procedure that can be delegated to assistive personnel. However, a nurse must first verify tube placement and patency. The nurse should instruct assistive personnel:
- About the prescribed rate to infuse the feeding
- To report any difficulty infusing the feeding or any discomfort voiced by the client
- To report any gagging, paroxysms of coughing, or choking

EQUIPMENT

- ❑ Disposable feeding bag and tubing or ready-to-hang system
- ❑ 30-ml or larger Luer-Lok or catheter-tip syringe
- ❑ Stethoscope
- ❑ Infusion pump (required for continuous or intestinal feedings): Use pump designed for tube feedings
- ❑ pH indicator strip (see Skill 30-2)
- ❑ Prescribed enteral feeding
- ❑ Gloves
- ❑ Equipment to obtain blood glucose by finger stick

STEP	RATIONALE

ASSESSMENT

1. Assess client's need for enteral tube feedings (clients who are unable to eat, have a nutrition deficit, or have impaired swallowing).

   Identify clients who need tube feedings before they become nutritionally depleted.

2. Assess client for food allergies.

   Prevents client from developing localized or systemic allergic responses.

3. Auscultate for bowel sounds. Consult physician if bowel sounds are absent.

   Absent bowel sounds may indicate decreased ability of GI tract to digest or absorb nutrients.

4. Obtain baseline weight and laboratory values. Assess client for fluid volume excess or deficit, electrolyte abnormalities, and metabolic abnormalities such as hyperglycemia.

   Enteral feedings are to restore or maintain a client's nutritional status. Provides objective data to measure effectiveness of feedings. Laboratory data (e.g., electrolytes and capillary blood-glucose measurement) are ordered by physician.

5. Verify physician's order for formula, rate, route, and frequency.

   Ensures correct formula will be administered in appropriate volume.

6. Assess gastrostomy/jejunostomy stoma site for breakdown, irritation, or drainage.

   Infection, pressure from gastrostomy tube, or drainage of gastric secretions can cause skin breakdown.

NURSING DIAGNOSES

- Imbalanced nutrition: less than body requirements
- Readiness for enhanced nutrition
- Impaired swallowing
- Risk for aspiration

Related factors are individualized based on client's condition or needs.

PLANNING

1. Expected outcomes following completion of procedure:
   - Nutritional status is improved, as evidenced by increasing weight, improving laboratory values, and improved intake and output.

     Indicates that client's nutritional needs are being met.

   - Client has no signs of respiratory distress.

     Entry of feeding tube into airways or aspiration of feeding may cause respiratory distress.

   - Skin surrounding stoma site is dry, intact, and without signs of infection.

     Skin breakdown around stoma occurs from pressure of feeding tube or seepage of gastric contents and secretions around the feeding tube.

2. Explain procedure to client.

   Decreases client anxiety.

3. Perform hand hygiene.

   Reduces transmission of microorganisms.

4. Prepare feeding container to administer formula continuously:
   a. Check expiration date on formula and integrity of container.

      Ensures GI tolerance of formula. Prevents leakage of tube feeding.

   b. Have tube feeding at room temperature.

      Cold formula may cause gastric cramping and discomfort because the liquid is not warmed by mouth and esophagus.

   c. Connect tubing to container, or prepare ready-to-hang container. Use aseptic technique, and avoid handling the feeding system. If you need to handle the system, perform hand hygiene and wear gloves.

      The feeding system, including the bag, connections, and tubing, must be free of contamination to prevent bacterial growth (Padula and others, 2004).

STEP	RATIONALE
d. Shake formula container well, and fill container with formula. Open stopcock on tubing, and fill tubing with formula to remove air (prime tubing). Hang on pole.	Filling the tubing with formula prevents excess air from entering gastrointestinal tract once infusion begins.
5. For intermittent feeding have syringe ready and be sure formula is at room temperature.	Cold formula causes gastric cramping.
6. Place client in high-Fowler's position, or elevate head of bed at least 30 degrees.	Elevated head helps prevent aspiration.

IMPLEMENTATION

STEP	RATIONALE
1. Apply gloves.	Reduces transmission of microorganisms.
2. Determine tube placement (see Skill 30-2). Observe aspirate's appearance and note the pH measurement.	Feedings instilled into a misplaced tube may cause serious injury or death. On occasion, color alone may differentiate gastric from intestinal placement because most intestinal aspirates are stained by bile to a distinct yellow color, and most gastric aspirates are not (Metheny and others, 1999) (see Skill 30-4, step 2).
3. Check gastric residual volume. **a.** *Gastrostomy tube:* Attach syringe, and aspirate gastric secretions. Return aspirated contents to stomach unless the volume exceeds 100 ml. If the volume is greater than 100 ml on several occasions, hold feeding and notify physician (McClave and others, 1992). **b.** *Jejunostomy tube:* Aspirate intestinal secretions, observe volume and return contents as above.	For adults, a volume in excess of 100 ml for gastrostomy tubes should raise concern about intolerance; however, feedings may continue while further examinations are conducted (ASPEN, 2002; McClave and others, 1992; McClave and others, 1999; Murphy and Bickford, 1999). Fluids aspirated from the stomach contain electrolytes that, if withheld, may cause electrolyte imbalances. Notify the physician if residual volume is excessive, and request an order regarding whether or not the residual fluid should be returned to the client.

STEP	RATIONALE
4. Irrigate tube with 30 ml water (see Skill 30-3).	Maintains patency following removal of aspirate.
5. Initiate feeding:	

- ### Critical Decision Point
  Do not add food coloring or dye to enteral nutrition. (See discussion of evidence-based practice trends.)

a. Syringe or intermittent feeding	
(1) Pinch proximal end of gastrostomy/jejunostomy tube feeding tube.	Prevents air from entering client's stomach.
(2) Remove plunger from syringe, and attach barrel of syringe to end of tube.	Barrel receives formula for instillation.
(3) Fill syringe with measured amount of formula (see illustration). Release tube, elevate syringe to no more than 18 inches (45 cm) above insertion site, and allow it to empty gradually by gravity. Repeat steps 1 to 3 until prescribed amount has been delivered to client.	Height of syringe allows for safe, slow, gravity drainage of formula. Total delivery of bolus feedings may take several minutes, depending on the amount of the bolus. Administering the feeding too quickly may cause abdominal discomfort to the client or increase the risk for aspiration.
(4) If a feeding bag is used, prime tubing, and attach gavage tubing to end of feeding tube. Set rate by adjusting roller clamp on tubing or placing on a feeding pump. Allow bag to empty gradually over 30 to 60 minutes (see Skill 30-4). Label bag with tube-feeding type, strength, and amount. Include date, time, and initials.	Gradual emptying of tube feeding by gravity from syringe or feeding bag reduces risk of abdominal discomfort, vomiting, or diarrhea induced by bolus or too-rapid infusion of tube feedings.
Change bag every 24 hours.	Helps decrease bacterial colonization.

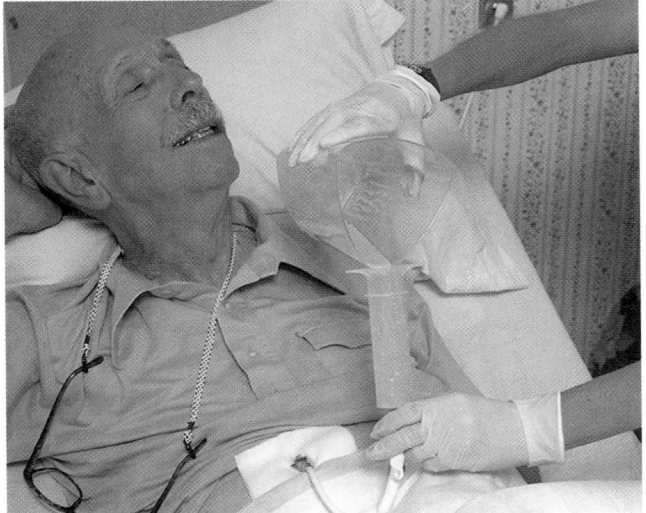

STEP **5a(3)** Syringe method for gastrostomy feeding.

STEP	RATIONALE

b. Continuous-drip method

    (1) Connect distal end of tubing to proximal end of feeding tube.

    (2) Connect tubing through infusion pump, and set rate (see Skill 30-4).

> Delivers continuous feeding at a steady rate and pressure. Alarms for increased resistance. This method reduces risk of abdominal discomfort.

6. Advance rate of concentration of tube feeding gradually (see Box 30-1).

> Helps to prevent diarrhea and gastric intolerance to formula.

7. Administer water via feeding tube as ordered or between feedings.

> Provides client with source of water to help maintain fluid and electrolyte balance. Clears tubing of formula.

8. Flush tube with 30 ml of water every 4 to 6 hours around-the-clock and before and after administering medications via the tube.

> Maintains tube patency.

9. When tube feedings are not being administered, cap or clamp the proximal end of the feeding tube.

> Prevents air from entering stomach between feedings.

10. Rinse bag and tubing with warm water whenever feedings are interrupted. Use a new administration set every 24 hours.

> Rinsing bag and tubing with warm water clears old tube feedings and reduces bacterial growth.

11. The gastrostomy/jejunostomy exit site of the tube is usually left open to air. However, if a dressing is needed because of drainage, change dressing daily or as needed.

> Leaking or gastric drainage may cause irritation and excoriation to the skin. Skin around the feeding tube should be cleansed daily with warm water and mild soap. The area must be dried completely before applying the dressing.

12. Dispose of supplies, and perform hand hygiene.

> Reduces transmission of microorganisms.

EVALUATION

1. Measure residual volume per policy.

> Evaluates tolerance of tube feeding.

2. Monitor finger-stick blood glucose (usually at least every 6 hours until maximum administration rate is reached and maintained for 24 hours).

> Requires a physician order. Alerts nurse to client's tolerance of enteral nutrition. May require physician to revise type of formula administered.

3. Monitor intake and output at least every 8 hours (Metheny, 2000).

> Intake and output are indications of fluid balance or fluid volume excess or deficit.

4. Weigh client daily until maximum administration rate is reached and maintained for 24 hours, then weigh client 3 times per week.

> Weight gain is indicator of improved nutritional status; however, sudden gain of more than 2 pounds in 24 hours usually indicates fluid retention.

5. Monitor laboratory values.

> Laboratory values (e.g., albumin, transferrin, prealbumin) are indicators of client's nutritional status.

6. Observe stoma site for skin integrity.

> Gastric or intestinal secretions can cause injury and necrosis at stoma site.

7. Observe client's level of comfort.

> Reduced gastric emptying can lead to abdominal discomfort.

8. Auscultate bowel sounds.

> Assess gastric peristalsis.

Recording and Reporting

- Record amount and type of feeding, client's response to tube feeding, patency of tube.
- Record volume of formula and any additional water on intake and output form.
- Report type of feeding, status of feeding tube, client's tolerance, and adverse effects.

Unexpected Outcomes	Related Interventions
1. The feeding tube becomes clogged. Frequent aspiration of gastric or intestinal contents (Powell and others, 1993) and frequent administration of medications via the tube have been associated with increased clogging of feeding tubes (Pancorbo-Hidalgo and others, 2001; Seifert and others, 2002).	• To avoid this problem, flush the tube with water after checking the residual volume (Edwards and Metheny, 2000). Cranberry juice should not be used to unclog feeding tubes; water works better than cranberry juice (Metheny and others, 1988).
2. Excessive gastric residual volume.	• Notify physician to determine if feedings need to be held. If feedings are held, reassess residual volume 1 hour after the feeding is stopped to determine if volume has lessened or increased. If it has increased, make sure the physician is aware. • Maintain client in high-Fowler's position or have head of bed elevated at least 30 degrees.
3. Client aspirates formula.	• (See interventions following skill 30-1.)
4. The client develops diarrhea 3 or more times in 24 hours; may indicate intolerance.	• Notify physician, and confer with dietitian to determine need to modify type of formula, concentration, or rate of infusion. • Consider other causes (e.g., bacterial contamination of the feeding, client infection) (Eisenberg, 2002). • Determine if client is receiving antibiotics or medications (e.g., those containing sorbitol) that can induce diarrhea (Benya and others, 1991; Guenter and others, 1991).
5. Drainage (signs of hemorrhage, infection, or obstruction) from the abdominal insertion site of a gastrostomy or jejunostomy (ASPEN, 2002).	• Notify the physician; describe and document the type of drainage. • For purulent drainage anticipate the need for cultures. • Place a dry drain gauze around the site, and change every shift and as needed (prn).

Teaching Considerations

- Teach client and family caregiver that, if tolerated, client should remain upright for 1 hour after feedings.
- Instruct client or family caregiver that client may express feelings of fullness, increased gas, belching, or diarrhea.
- For tubes inserted in the abdominal wall, teach client or primary caregiver to clean around tube with warm water and mild soap.
- For tubes inserted in the abdominal wall, half-strength hydrogen peroxide diluted with water (50:50) can be used for the first few days after insertion of the tube to remove any crusting around exit site. A dressing is usually not necessary or recommended.

Pediatric Considerations

- When giving intermittent feedings to a small child, administration should take approximately 20 to 30 minutes, or as long as it would take to bottle-feed the child. Hold the infant, and offer a pacifier during the feeding to simulate a more natural bottle-feeding experience (Hockenberry and others, 2003).
- A low-profile gastrostomy tube (gastrostomy button) may be used for pediatric clients to decrease the chance of child pulling out or dislodging tube and for increased comfort. Low-profile tube has an adapter to allow syringe feeding or connection to a feeding container.

Gerontological Considerations

- Older adult clients may be more susceptible to hyperglycemia related to the glucose concentration in enteral formulas.
- Older adults may have decreased gastric transit time so that formula remains in the stomach longer than for younger clients. Gastric residual checks are of special importance to decrease the risk of vomiting and aspiration during gastric feeding.

Home Care Considerations

- Instruct primary caregiver and/or client to monitor intake and output using household measuring devices.
- Ask client or care provider about any symptoms or discomfort during enteral feedings. Reinforce instruction to contact nurse if symptoms of discomfort occur.

FOCUS on CLINICAL PRACTICE

At the beginning of your night shift you are told that you will be receiving a new admission any moment. You receive report from the operating room. Your patient is a 33-year-old woman, Mrs. Lake. She was in a motor vehicle accident earlier in the day. She sustained fractures to her left arm and both legs. She did not see a traffic light and rear-ended a stopped vehicle; she was going approximately 35 to 40 mph and was not wearing her seat belt. There was no airbag in her car. The length of the surgical procedure was 2 hours.

1. She arrives at the intensive care unit. In performing the abdominal assessment for this client, what do you particularly want to assess?
2. The physician orders an NG tube to be placed for gastric decompression. In carrying out this order, what should the nurse be particularly careful to do?

3. The NG tube is successfully placed without incident. However, during your shift Mrs. L. has a few more abnormal heartbeats, so the physician chooses to continue mechanical ventilation and cardiac monitoring. Two days later, Mrs. L. has developed pneumonia and is therefore still on the mechanical ventilator. Her NG tube has been clamped. What type of measures are performed to maintain a feeding tube that is clamped?
4. The physician orders tube feeding to begin via the NG tube. What should be assessed before beginning tube feeding via the NG tube?
5. If the client is still mechanically ventilated and receiving feedings via the NG tube 3 days later, what should the nurse recommend to the physician?

NCLEX REVIEW QUESTIONS

1. What is the most important fact that should be documented on any nasally or orally placed feeding tube before the instillation of any type of substance?
   1. Radiographic confirmation of nonrespiratory placement
   2. Confirmation that the tube is in the stomach
   3. Confirmation that the tube is in the intestine
   4. The type and location of the feeding tube placement

2. A new order for enteral nutrition has been written. The client has not yet received any feeding. The nurse checks placement of the small-bore nasally placed feeding tube. The following results were obtained: 10 ml of yellow-stained fluid, pH of 6. Based on these findings, where is the tip of the tube most likely positioned?
   1. Respiratory tract
   2. Stomach
   3. Intestine
   4. Esophagus

NCLEX REVIEW QUESTIONS

3. A new order for enteral nutrition has been written. The client has not yet received any feeding. The nurse checks placement of the small-bore nasally placed feeding tube. The following results were obtained: 20 ml of clear fluid, pH of 4. Based on these findings, where is the tip of the tube most likely positioned?
   1. Respiratory tract
   2. Stomach
   3. Intestine
   4. Esophagus

4. The client has been receiving enteral nutrition for the last 48 hours and is also receiving an H_2 blocker. The nurse checks placement of the small-bore nasally placed feeding tube. The following results were obtained: 80 ml of cream-colored fluid that is curdled in appearance, pH of 6. Based on these findings, where is the tip of the tube most likely positioned?
   1. Respiratory tract
   2. Stomach
   3. Intestine
   4. Esophagus

5. As a result of a motor vehicle accident, the client has had multiple facial fractures and suffered a stroke. Based on these facts, what route should the nurse recognize as the safest and most likely route for feeding tube placement?
   1. NI
   2. G-tube
   3. J-tube
   4. PEG
   5. PEJ

6. What particular electrolyte value should be assessed before choosing the type of feeding tube irrigate?
   1. Magnesium
   2. Sodium
   3. Potassium
   4. Chloride

7. Mr. D is a 74-year-old, semicomatose client who is receiving tube feedings via an NI tube. Based on this information, what is his greatest risk for death?
   1. Respiratory failure
   2. Cardiac failure
   3. Aspiration pneumonia
   4. Malnutrition

8. What is the most important intervention a nurse can do to prevent nosocomial infections associated with enteral nutrition?
   1. Inserting NG tubes sterilely
   2. Performing hand hygiene
   3. Wearing sterile gloves when handling the feeding system
   4. Boiling the tube feedings and allowing them to cool before administration

References

ASPEN: American Society for Parenteral and Enteral Nutrition: Guidelines for the use of parenteral and enteral nutrition in adult and pediatric patients, *JPEN J Parenter Enteral Nutr* 26:1SA, 2002.

Edwards SJ, Metheny NA: Measurement of gastric residual volume: state of the science, *Medsurg Nurs* 9:25, 2000.

Eisenberg P: An overview of diarrhea in the patient receiving enteral nutrition, *Gastroenterol Nurs* 25:95, 2002.

Heyland D, Mandell LA: Gastric colonization by gram-negative bacilli and nosocomial pneumonia in the intensive care unit patient: evidence for causation, *Chest* 101:187, 1992.

Hockenberry MJ and others: *Wong's nursing care of infants and children*, ed 7, St. Louis, 2003, Mosby.

Maloney J, Metheny N: Controversy in using blue dye in enteral tube feeding as a method of detecting pulmonary aspiration, *Crit Care Nurse* 22:84, 2002.

McClave SA and others: North American Summit on Aspiration in the Critically Ill Patient: consensus statement, *JPEN J Parenter Enteral Nutr* 26:S80, 2002.

Metheny NA: Inadvertent intracranial nasogastric tube placement, *Am J Nurs* 102:25, 2002.

Metheny NA, Titler MG: Assessing placement of feeding tubes, *Am J Nurs* 101:36, 2001.

Padula CA and others: Enteral feedings: what the evidence says, *Am J Nurs* 104:62, 2004.

Pearce CB, Duncan HD: Enteral feeding: nasogastric, nasojejunal, percutaneous endoscopic gastrostomy, or jejunostomy—its indications and limitations, *Postgrad Med J* 78:198, 2002.

Roubenoff R, Ravich WJ: Pneumothorax due to nasogastric feeding tubes: report of four cases, review of the literature, and recommendations for prevention, *Arch Intern Med* 149:184, 1989.

Seifert CF and others: Drug administration through enteral feeding catheters, *Am J Health Syst Pharm* 59:378, 2002.

Simon T, Fink AS: Current management of endoscopic feeding tube dysfunction, *Surg Endosc* 13:403, 1999.

Wendell GD and others: Pneumothorax complicating small-bore feeding tube placement, *Arch Intern Med* 151:599, 1991.

Research References

Bankier AA and others: Radiographic detection of intrabronchial malpositions of nasogastric tubes and subsequent complications in intensive care unit patients, *Intensive Care Med* 23(4):406, 1997.

Benya R and others: Diarrhea associated with tube feeding: the importance of using objective criteria, *J Clin Gastroenterol* 13:167, 1991.

Dobranowski J and others: Incorrect positioning of nasogastric feeding tubes and the development of pneumothorax, *Can Assoc Radiol J* 43:35, 1992.

Gharpure V and others: Indicators of postpyloric feeding tube placement in children, *Crit Care Med* 28:2962, 2000.

Gottschlich MM and others: The 2002 Clinical Research Award: an evaluation of the safety of early vs. delayed enteral support and effects on clinical, nutritional, and endocrine outcomes after severe burns, *J Burn Care Rehabil* 23:401, 2002.

Guenter PA and others: Tube feeding-related diarrhea in acutely ill patients, *JPEN J Parenter Enteral Nutr* 15:277, 1991.

Hanson RL: Predictive criteria for length of nasogastric tube insertion for tube feeding, *JPEN J Parenter Enteral Nutr* 3:160, 1979.

Harris MR, Huseby JS: Pulmonary complications from nasoenteral feeding tube insertion in an intensive care unit: incidence and prevention, *Crit Care Med* 17:917, 1989.

Heyland D and others: Enteral nutrition in the critically ill patient: a prospective survey, *Crit Care Med* 23:1055, 1995.

Kittinger JW and others: Efficacy of metoclopramide as an adjunct to duodenal placement of small-bore feeding tubes: a randomized, placebo-controlled, double-blind study, *JPEN J Parenter Enteral Nutr* 11:33, 1987.

Kudsk KA and others: Enteral versus parenteral feeding: effects on septic morbidity after blunt and penetrating abdominal trauma, *Ann Surg* 215:503, 1992.

Lord LM and others: Comparison of weighted vs. unweighted enteral feeding tubes for efficacy of transpyloric intubation, *JPEN J Parenter Enteral Nutr* 17:271, 1993.

McClave SA and others: Enteral tube feeding in the intensive care unit: factors impeding adequate delivery, *Crit Care Med* 27:1252, 1999.

McClave SA and others: Use of residual volume as a marker for enteral feeding intolerance: prospective blinded comparison with physical examination and radiographic findings, *JPEN J Parenter Enteral Nutr* 16:99, 1992.

Mehall JR and others: Enteral feeding tubes are a reservoir for nosocomial antibiotic-resistant pathogens, *J Pediatr Surg* 37:1011, 2002.

Metheny N and others: Effect of feeding tube properties and three irrigants on clogging rates, *Nurs Res* 37:165, 1988.

Metheny N and others: Effectiveness of the auscultatory method in predicting feeding tube location, *Nurs Res* 39:262, 1990.

Metheny N and others: Effectiveness of pH measurements in predicting feeding tube placement: an update, *Nurs Res* 42:324, 1993.

Metheny NA and others: pH testing of feeding-tube aspirates to determine placement, *Nutr Clin Pract* 9:185, 1994.

Metheny NA and others: pH, color, and feeding tubes, *RN* 61:25, 1998a.

Metheny NA and others: Measurement of glucose in tracheobronchial secretions to detect aspiration of enteral feedings, *Heart Lung* 27:285, 1998b.

Metheny NA and others: pH and concentration of bilirubin in feeding tube aspirates as predictors of tube placement, *Nurs Res* 48:189, 1999.

Metheny NA, Stewart BJ: Testing feeding tube placement during continuous tube feedings, *Appl Nurs Res* 15:254, 2002.

Metheny NA and others: Pepsin as a marker for pulmonary aspiration, *Am J Crit Care* 11:150, 2002a.

Metheny NA and others: Efficacy of dye-stained enteral formula in detecting pulmonary aspiration, *Chest* 122:276, 2002b.

Moore FA and others: TEN versus TPN following major abdominal trauma—reduced septic morbidity, *J Trauma* 29:916, 1989.

Murphy LM, Bickford V: (1999) Gastric residuals in tube feeding: how much is too much? *Nutr Clin Pract* 14:304, 1999.

Neumann MJ and others: Hold that x-ray: aspirate pH and auscultation prove enteral tube placement, *J Clin Gastroenterol* 20:293, 1995.

Pancorbo-Hidalgo PL, Garcia-Fernandez FP, Ramirez-Perez C: Complications associated with enteral nutrition by nasogastric tube in an internal medicine unit, *J Clin Nurs* 10:482, 2001.

Powell KS and others: Aspirating gastric residuals causes occlusion of small-bore feeding tubes, *JPEN J Parenter Enteral Nutr* 17:243, 1993.

Welch SK: Certification of staff nurses to insert enteral feeding tubes using a research-based procedure, *Nutr Clin Pract* 11:21, 1996.

Welch SK and others: Comparison of four bedside indicators used to predict duodenal feeding tube placement with radiography, *JPEN J Parenter Enteral Nutr* 18:525, 1994.

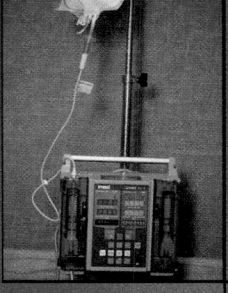

31

Parenteral Nutrition

MEDIA RESOURCES

Evolve Site *evolve*

http://evolve.elsevier.com/Perry/skills

- Weblinks
- Video clips
- Mosby's Nursing Skills Video Exercises

Mosby's Nursing Skills Videos/CD-ROM

- *Vascular Access Video:* Fluid administration, scheduling considerations, flushing to check for patency, re-capping catheter, or connecting to IV fluid; troubleshooting, including checking the integrity of vascular access and signs of potential problems

OBJECTIVES

Mastery of content in this chaper will enable the nurse to:

- Identify clients who are candidates for parenteral nutrition.
- Describe factors influencing selection of appropriate sites for administering parenteral nutrition.
- Identify measures used to prevent complications of central parenteral nutrition.
- Demonstrate appropriate nursing care of the client receiving parenteral nutrition.
- Assist the physician with placement of a central vein catheter.
- Demonstrate a central line dressing change application.

KEY TERMS

Amino acid
Bacteremia
Lipid emulsion
Nutritional support nursing
Parenteral nutrition (PN)

Peripherally inserted central catheter (PICC)
Trendelenburgs position
Valsalva maneuver

BOX 31-1   Indications for Parenteral Nutrition

NONFUNCTIONAL GI TRACT

Massive small bowel resection/GI surgery
Paralytic ileus
Intestinal obstruction
Trauma to abdomen, head, or neck
Severe malabsorption
Intolerance to enteral feeding
Chemotherapy, radiation therapy, bone marrow transplantation

EXTENDED BOWEL REST

Enterocutaneous fistula
Inflammatory bowel disease exacerbation
Severe diarrhea
Moderate to severe pancreatitis

PREOPERATIVE TPN

Preoperative bowel rest
Treatment for comorbid severe malnutrition in clients with nonfunctional GI tracts
Severely catabolic clients when GI tract nonusable for more than 4 to 5 days

Parenteral nutrition (PN) is a form of specialized nutrition support in which nutrients, including amino acids (protein/nitrogen), dextrose (carbohydrate/glucose), fat emulsions (fatty acids), vitamins, electrolytes, minerals, and trace elements are given intravenously (IV). Clients who are unable to digest or absorb enteral nutrition benefit from PN (Box 31-1). When a client's gastrointestinal (GI) tract is functional, enteral nutrition (see Chapter 30) is generally used before initiating parenteral nutrition. Clinical and laboratory monitoring of a client is required throughout PN therapy. The ultimate goal is to resume use of the GI tract through enteral or oral feedings as soon as possible (American Society for Parenteral and Enteral Nutrition [ASPEN], 2002).

Clients with short-term nutritional needs often receive intravenous solutions of less than 10% dextrose via a peripheral vein in combination with amino acids and lipids. Peripheral solutions are not as calorically dense as PN solutions and therefore are used temporarily when clients have high caloric needs. Parenteral nutrition with greater than 10% dextrose requires a central venous catheter (CVC) that is placed into a high-flow central vein such as the superior vena cava. A physician inserts a central venous catheter under sterile conditions (Figure 31-1). Another option for PN infusions is a peripherally inserted central catheter (PICC). Nurses with specialized training insert PICCs that are started in a vein of the forearm and threaded into the subclavian or superior vena cava vein (Figure 31-2) (see Chapter 27). Surgically implanted subcutaneous ports (Figure 31-3) may also be used for PN infusion. PN solutions are usually hyperosmolar and thus must be administered into a large-diameter vein to pre-

vent sclerosis of vein tissue. This chapter discusses the administration of PN using central venous access catheters. The ideal device used for PN is durable, reliable, and user friendly, because many clients receiving PN will continue to receive the nutritional therapy in the home or long-term care setting.

The nurse plays an important role in assessing and identifying a client's need for parenteral nutrition. The first sign of a developing problem may be a pattern of a decline in oral food intake and reduced appetite. Frequently the nurse will be the first to identify risk factors, such as progressive weight loss, restricted or limited fluid intake, intolerance to enteral feedings, increased energy need (burns, sepsis, and trauma), or being NPO (nothing by mouth) for 3 or more days. The nurse's assessment provides information for ultimately consulting with a dietitian and physician in an effort to initiate appropriate parenteral nutrition. The nurse also plays a role in the selection of the best vascular access site for PN administration (Table 31-1). Selection of an ideal vascular access device depends on several factors: client factors, device characteristics, therapeutic issues, and duration of therapy (Orr, 1999). For example, implanted ports and PICCs require the highest level of manual dexterity for home care clients to manage dressing changes and tubing manipulation.

Lipid emulsions provide supplemental kilocalories and prevent essential fatty acid deficiencies. These emulsions can be administered through a separate peripheral line, through the central line by a Y connector tubing (see Chapter 27), or as an admixture to the PN solution. The addition of lipid emulsion to the PN solution is called a three-

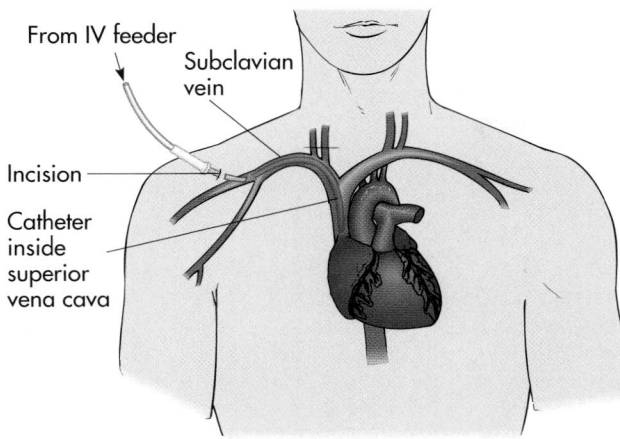

FIGURE 31-1 Placement of central venous catheter inserted into subclavian vein. (Courtesy Rolin Graphics.)

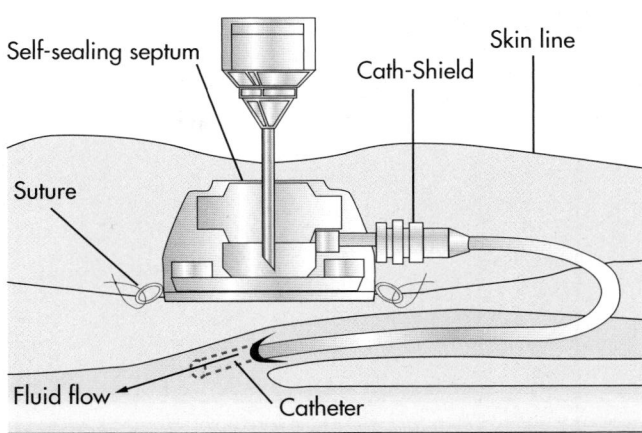

FIGURE 31-3 Cross section of implantable port displaying access of the port with a Huber needle. (Courtesy SIMS Deltec, Inc, St. Paul, Minn.)

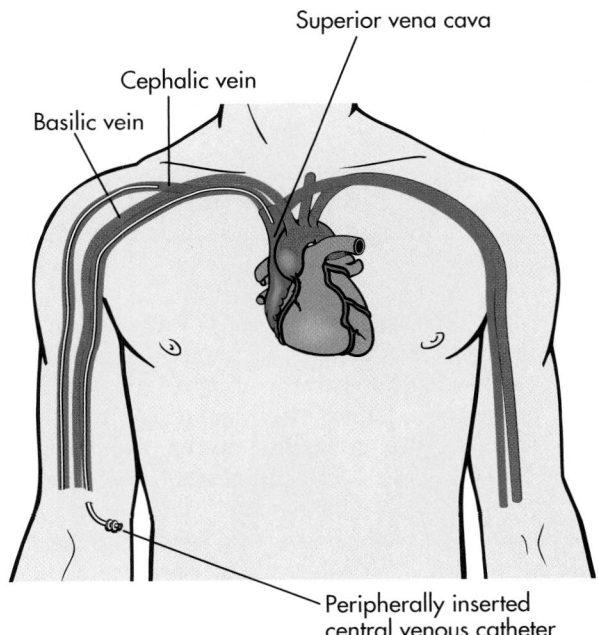

FIGURE 31-2 Placement of peripherally inserted central catheter (PICC) through antecubital fossa. (Modified from *Lewis SM and others:* Medical-surgical nursing: assessment and management of clinical problems, ed 5, St. Louis, 2000, Mosby.)

in-one admixture and is given over a 24-hour period to provide nutritionally complete PN. The essential fatty acid present in lipid emulsion is linoleic acid. This acid cannot be made from other fats in human metabolism and therefore must be supplied. Linoleic acid is an omega-6 fatty acid. A client who is deficient in linoleic acid will be immunosuppressed and thus at risk for infection. A nutritional regimen that does not provide adequate fatty acids can lead to essen-

tial fatty acid deficiency (EFAD). Signs and symptoms of EFAD include dry scaly skin, sparse hair growth, impaired wound healing, decreased resistance to stress, increased susceptibility to respiratory tract infections, anemia, thrombocytopenia, and liver function abnormalities. EFAD is prevented by administering a minimum of 500 ml of 10% lipid emulsion 2 times per week.

Fat emulsion is a soybean or safflower oil base that is isotonic and may be infused with an amino acid and dextrose solution through a central or peripheral vein. When administering fat (lipid) emulsions via piggyback infusion, the solution must be added below the infusion filter and inserted in the port nearest to the venipuncture site. This is because the fat particles are large and cannot pass through the infusion filter without breaking down. Not all clients should receive fat emulsion. Individuals for whom fat emulsions are contraindicated include those who have a disturbance of normal fat metabolism, such as pathological hyperlipemia.

Parenteral nutrition has significant physiological and psychological implications. Clients who are unable to eat may become socially isolated, have food cravings, or even hallucinate about food. A majority of social events focus around food, thereby excluding the client from complete participation. The nurse promotes the client's psychological well-being by discussing possible feelings and sensations; describing possible alternatives to satisfy oral cravings, such as chewing gum or sucking on hard candies (if allowed); and offering activities that can help distract a client from hunger cravings and promote participation in social interactions. Many clients who receive parenteral nutrition are capable of some oral intake. Client and family education helps to alleviate many of the client's and family's fears and concerns.

The nursing committee of the American Society of Parenteral and Enteral Nutrition (ASPEN) has defined nutritional support nursing practice, the scope of nutritional support nursing, and the goals of nutritional support (ASPEN,

TABLE 31-1 FACTORS IN DETERMINING VASCULAR ACCESS DEVICE SELECTION FOR PARENTERAL NUTRITION

CLIENT FACTORS	DEVICE CHARACTERISTICS	THERAPEUTIC FACTORS	DURATION OF THERAPY
PHYSIOLOGICAL Condition of veins Hypercoagulability state Diabetes Skin disorders Previous surgery involving thorax or vascular system Known allergies to catheter materials **FUNCTIONAL** Poor vision Altered dexterity Developmental disabilities Frailty **PSYCHOLOGICAL** Needle phobia Body image impairment Previous experience with vascular access device **SOCIAL SUPPORT** Care provider availability Financial resources	Design of device Low risk for infection (e.g., antibacterial coatings) Numbers of lumens Durability	Characteristics of solutions or emulsions Dextrose concentration >10% requires central vein access Solution with osmolarity >600 mOsm/L requires central vein access Type of disease or condition being treated (e.g., long-term metastatic disease vs. short-term bowel inflammation)	PICCs can be placed for duration of 1 year. Implanted ports may remain in place for life of need or until portal head does not hold needle. Manufacturers recommend 1500 needle sticks with 20-gauge needle. Hickman or Broviac catheter remains in place for life of need unless catheter becomes clotted, infected, or there is breakdown of catheter material. Triple-lumen subclavian catheters used only for duration of acute care.

2001): Nutritional support nursing practice is the care of individuals with potential or known nutrition alterations. The goal of nutritional support nursing is to assist individuals in restoring and maintaining optimal nutritional health.

Cultural Considerations

Parenteral nutrition is obviously a form of nutrition and thus can pose problems for members of ethnic groups who restrict intake of certain types of foods. Consider the following guidelines:

- Accommodate religious and cultural beliefs of clients by making sure that prohibited substances are not added to the parental solution. For example, animal-based products should be avoided for strict vegetarian Hindus and Buddhists.
- Consult religious leaders about continuous feedings during fasting periods such as Ramadan. Although the sick are generally exempted, many devout Muslims will insist on fasting during Ramadan.

Evidence-Based Practice

There is substantial scientific data for the prevention of complications of central venous catheterization. The use of full sterile-barrier precautions during central venous catheter insertion reduces the incidence of catheter-related infections (O'Grady and others, 2002; Raad and others, 1994). Although the efficacy of such precautions has not been studied for PICC insertion, the use of full sterile-barrier precautions is probably applicable to PICCs (O'Grady, 2002). The use of antimicrobial-impregnated catheters lowers the rate of catheter-related bloodstream infections (McGee and Gould, 2003). The most common catheters used are those impregnated with chlorhexidine and silver sulfadiazine or minocycline and rifampin.

Povidone-iodine is widely used for skin preparation before CVC insertion. Recently chlorhexidine has been shown to reduce the risk of catheter colonization and thus may be preferable (McGee and Gould, 2003). More institutions are moving to the use of chlorhexidine. Further study is necessary.

A common nursing practice at one time was to apply antibiotic ointments to catheter-insertion sites during insertion and dressing changes. This practice is no longer recommended because the use of such ointments increases the rate of catheter colonization by fungi, promotes the emergence of antibiotic-resistant bacteria, and has not been shown to lower the rate of catheter-related bloodstream infections (McGee and Gould, 2003).

Guidelines adopted by the Centers for Disease Control and Prevention (CDC) and the Infusion Nurses Society (INS) for CVC insertion and maintenance have been incorporated into Skill 31-1 of this chapter.

Skill Performance Guidelines

1. Know when peripheral vein access can be used instead of central vein access. Clients who require short-term nutrition support, for whom central access placement is contraindicated or not feasible, who have adequate peripheral access, and who can tolerate larger volumes of fluid are candidates for peripheral parenteral nutrition.

2. Be aware of complications associated with PN, including metabolic disturbances, fluid imbalance, technical management of catheter system, and infections.

3. Monitor the client's vital signs, electrolyte levels, triglyceride levels, weight, and fluid status and compare baseline with treatment values. Clients who receive PN may have rapid changes in these values.

4. Know the client's recent temperature range. Clients with peripheral or central IV lines are susceptible to septicemia; an elevated temperature can be an early indicator of a bacterial process.

5. Use strict aseptic technique in the care and maintenance of central venous catheters and PICC devices

---

SKILL 31-1   Caring for the Client Receiving Central Venous Placement for Central Parenteral Nutrition

Central parenteral nutrition (CPN) is a form of nutritional support administered through central vein cannulation. A catheter is usually placed in the subclavian vein through an infraclavicular venipuncture (see Figure 31-1). The subclavian site is preferred because it provides a flat, relatively immobile area on the chest and blood flows at a high rate, decreasing the risk of phlebitis or displacement. The use of the jugular site poses a greater risk for infection (O'Grady and others, 2002).

The nurse has an important role when assisting the physician in placing a CPN line. Attention to asepsis and positioning, being available to reassure the client during the procedure, and ensuring that the right equipment is available are critical to the success of the procedure. Because CPN is associated with numerous complications (Table 31-2), it is vital that the nurse carefully monitor the CPN site and notify the physician of any symptoms or developing problems (Krzywda and others, 1999). Clients receiving CPN are at high risk for catheter-related bloodstream infections (CR-BSI).

DELEGATION CONSIDERATIONS

The skill of caring for a client receiving central venous placement for PN should not be delegated to assistive personnel. Instruct assistive personnel to report the following immediately:

- Client's dressing becomes damp or soiled.
- Catheter line appears to be pulled out farther than original insertion position.
- Intravenous line becomes disconnected.
- Client has a fever.
- Client complains of pain at the site.

EQUIPMENT

Insertion and Dressing Care
- ❏ Hair clippers
- ❏ Subclavian insertion tray *or* the following:
- ❏ Caps
- ❏ Sterile gowns
- ❏ Sterile drapes
- ❏ Masks and protective eyewear
- ❏ Nonsterile gloves
- ❏ Sterile gloves (powder free)
- ❏ Gauze pads
- ❏ Surgical towels
- ❏ Antimicrobial solutions: 2% chlorhexidine-based preparation; alternatively, tincture of iodine, an iodophor, and 70% alcohol as single agents or in combination
- ❏ 1% lidocaine (Xylocaine)
- ❏ Central line catheter kit
- ❏ Sterile drapes
- ❏ 5-ml syringe
- ❏ Bath blanket or towel and protective pad
- ❏ 500-ml bottle of 5% dextrose in water
- ❏ Transparent dressing or gauze dressing for catheter insertion site
- ❏ Tape
- ❏ Intravenous infusion pump
- ❏ Tincture of benzoin (optional)

Discontinuation of CVC
- ❏ Central venous catheter dressing change kit
- ❏ Tape
- ❏ Antimicrobial solutions: 70% alcohol, 2% chlorhexidine-based preparation, or iodophor
- ❏ Sterile scissors and forceps (basic set)
- ❏ Goggles, gown, mask, and clean gloves

TABLE 31-2 COMPLICATIONS OF CENTRAL PARENTERAL NUTRITION

PROBLEM	CAUSE	SYMPTOMS	IMMEDIATE ACTION	PREVENTION
Air embolism	IV tubing disconnected; part of catheter system open or removed without being clamped	Sudden respiratory distress; decreased SpO$_2$ levels, shortness of breath, coughing, chest pain, decreased blood pressure	Clamp catheter; position client in left Trendelenburg position; call physician; administer oxygen as needed.	Make sure all catheter connections are secure; clamp catheter when not in use. Never use a stopcock with a CVC.
Localized infection (exit site or tunnel)	Poor aseptic technique in removal of skin flora during site preparation and dressing care	Exit site: erythema, tenderness, induration or purulence within 2 cm of skin at exit site. Tunnel: same as above but extends beyond 2 cm from exit site	Call physician. Exit: warm compress, daily site care, oral antibiotics. Tunnel: remove catheter.	Use proper aseptic technique. Change transparent dressings every 7 days, gauze dressings every 48 hours. Change dressing if damp, loosened, or soiled. Cleanse site during any dressing change with chlorhexidine or povidone-iodine a minimum of 3 to 5 min. Routine use of antibiotic ointment not recommended.
Systemic infection (catheter sepsis or bacteremia)	Catheter hub contamination; contamination of infusate; spread of bacteria through bloodstream from distant site	Systemic: isolation of same microorganism from blood culture and catheter segment, with client showing fever, chills, malaise, elevated white blood cell count	Systemic: antibiotics intravenously, remove catheter.	Use full sterile-barrier precautions during catheter insertion and dressing change. Use antibiotic-impregnated catheters. Do not disconnect tubing unnecessarily.
Hyperglycemia	Client receiving CPN too quickly; too little insulin in solution; infection	Excessive thirst, urination, blood glucose >160 mg/100 ml, confusion	Call physician; may need to slow infusion rate (physician order).	Review medical history for glucose intolerance or diabetes; keep rate as ordered, never increase CPN to "catch up." Use aseptic technique and routine blood glucose monitoring.
Hypoglycemia	CPN abruptly discontinued; too much insulin	Client is shaky, dizzy, nervous, anxious, senses hunger, blood glucose level <80 mg/100 ml	Call physician; if CPN discontinued abruptly, may need to restart D$_{10}$ NS at previous CPN rate. If client has oral intake, give ½ cup fruit juice. Perform blood glucose monitoring; retest in 15 to 30 min.	Decrease CPN, "tapering" gradually until discontinued; blood glucose monitoring is used to ensure adequate insulin.

Data from Hickey MS: *Handbook of enteral, parenteral, and ARC/AIDS nutritional therapy*, St. Louis, 1992, Mosby; Krzywda EA and others: Catheter infections: diagnosis, etiology, treatment, and prevention, *Nutr Clin Pract* 14:178, 1999; O'Grady and others: Guidelines for the prevention of intravascular catheter-related infections, *MMWR Morbid Mortal Wkly Rep* 51(RR10):1, 2002.

STEP	RATIONALE

ASSESSMENT

1. Assess need for CPN, and determine client's current nutritional status and energy needs. Consult with physician and dietitian.

   a. Weight loss of 10% or more of usual body weight

   b. Reduction in values for prealbumin, serum albumin, and total lymphocyte count, total iron-binding capacity

   c. Prolonged alteration in gastrointestinal function (malabsorption, recent gastrointestinal surgery, or paralytic ileus)

   d. Reduced intake of calories

   e. Intolerance to food/enteral feedings

2. Check physician's order for initiation of CPN and insertion of central vein catheter for size and type of catheter. Be prepared to witness when physician obtains written informed consent from client.

3. Assess client's hydration status: skin turgor, texture, and fluid intake and output.

4. Assess client for any surgical procedures of the upper chest or anatomical irregularities.

5. Consider catheter material to be used, (e.g., silicone, polymers, antibiotic impregnation), and determine if client has allergy to material.

6. Inspect condition of skin overlying supraclavicular and infraclavicular area.

7. Assess client for allergy to iodine, lidocaine, or latex.

8. Assess client's knowledge of purpose of procedure and any previous experience with a CVC insertion/discontinuation.

9. In some institutions initiate a consult with the nutritional support service before insertion.

Rationale column:

Provides baseline to compare changes after CPN is started.

Indicates malnutrition, a criteria for parenteral nutrition when GI function is altered.

Serve as markers for nutritional risk but do not provide clinical measure for efficacy of parenteral nutrition (Bozzetti and others, 2000).

Rules out use of enteral nutrition to restore weight loss.

May result from factors such as loss of appetite, problems with chewing/swallowing, debilitating conditions causing fatigue or shortness of breath.

Rules out use of enteral nutrition as a therapy.

Parenteral nutrition and insertion of central catheter requires informed consent (INS, 2000). Physician may request a certain type or size of catheter.

Dehydration depletes fluid volume and may make insertion of a central vein catheter more difficult.

Previous surgical procedures or central vein catheterizations may indicate that a particular site should not be used. Scoliosis or other spine deformities may make positioning difficult.

Prevents onset of hypersensitivity or allergic reaction from use of catheter.

Certain skin conditions where skin integrity is broken may contraindicate catheter insertion.

Solutions used during catheter insertion and use of gloves could cause serious allergic response.

Helps to allay anxiety and determines level of client teaching required.

Team of experts is best prepared to recommend PN solution and catheter placement.

NURSING DIAGNOSES

- Imbalanced nutrition: less than body requirements
- Risk for infection
- Deficient knowledge regarding catheter insertion

- Deficient fluid volume
- Excess fluid volume

Related factors are individualized based on client's condition or needs.

PLANNING

1. Expected outcomes following completion of procedure:
   - Insertion occurs without complication.
   - Insertion site is free of inflammation or breakdown.

Placement of a central vein catheter carries risks.

Denotes absence of infection and skin changes at central venous site.

STEP	RATIONALE

2. Explain to client steps for central line placement, use of the Valsalva maneuver, the need for CPN, and follow-up care. Provide time for client to ask questions.

Allows client to anticipate steps of procedure to minimize anxiety and to ensure client participation as needed.

3. Verify that consent was signed.

Consent document is required, because central line placement is considered an invasive procedure.

IMPLEMENTATION

1. Catheter Insertion

   a. Physician, with assistance of nurse, positions client flat in bed, lying supine. Place rolled towel or bath blanket between client's scapulas, and place protective pad under shoulder area.

Opens angle between clavicle and first rib; dilates veins to facilitate eventual catheter insertion.

   b. If necessary, use electric clippers to remove any hair around insertion site.

Transient microorganisms reside in body hair. Clippers do not cause microabrasions, which harbor microorganisms (INS, 2000).

   c. Physician applies cap, mask, and eyewear. Performs surgical hand scrub. Applies surgical gown and sterile gloves.

Maximum barrier precautions needed when inserting central venous catheter (INS, 2000).

   d. Nurse puts on cap (optional), mask, and eyewear. Performs hand hygiene. (Check agency policy because more stringent precautions may be required.)

Appropriate barrier precautions necessary for nurse to assist in positioning and comforting client, obtaining additional supplies as needed, regulating IV flow rate once line is inserted.

   e. Physician opens central vein kit and adds any sterile equipment to kit for use during insertion (see Chapter 9).

Maintains sterile field.

   f. Nurse saturates 4 × 4 gauze pads with alcohol, and physician scrubs area using circular motion from shoulder to ear to chin to nipple for approximately 1 minute.

Alcohol cleans and defats skin.

   g. Physician cleans same area for 1 minute using antimicrobial swabs (chlorhexidine or iodophor).

Removes surface skin bacteria.

   h. Allow antimicrobial solution to air-dry completely.

Ensures maximum antimicrobial effect.

   i. Physician removes sterile gloves and applies new pair of sterile gloves.

Gloves become contaminated from surface bacteria picked up in solution.

   j. Physician uses large sterile drape and sterile towels to create a sterile field. Physician finds anatomical landmarks and places fenestrated drape appropriately.

Provides sterile work space for catheter insertion. Clients whose catheters were placed using a mask, cap, sterile gloves, gown, and large drape had lower colonization rate of bacteria than clients where sterile gloves and a small drape were used (Raad and others, 1994).

   k. Physician arranges equipment in kit in preparation for catheter insertion.

Ensures smooth, orderly procedure.

   l. Nurse sets up IV bag, fills tubing, and covers end of tubing with a sterile cap (see Chapter 27).

IV tubing is ready to be connected to IV catheter.

   m. Nurse places client in Trendelenburgs position and turns client's head away from site of insertion (see illustration).

With head down, below heart, position promotes maximal filling and distention of subclavicular vein.

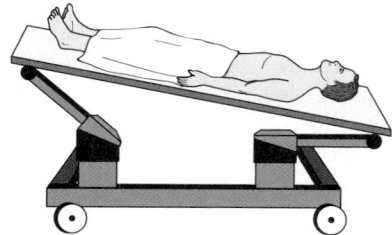

STEP 1m Client positioned in Trendelenburgs position in preparation for central venous catheter insertion.

STEP	RATIONALE

- *Critical Decision Point*

Trendelenburgs position is contraindicated in clients with head injuries, increased intracranial pressure, and spinal cord injuries.

n. Nurse wipes off top of 1% lidocaine bottle with alcohol swabs and holds bottle upside down. Option: Topical transdermal anesthetic agents can be applied before insertion.	Removes surface bacteria; allows physician to withdraw lidocaine while maintaining asepsis. Lidocaine has the potential for creating allergic reaction and tissue damage.
o. Physician injects needle into bottle and withdraws approximately 3 to 4 ml lidocaine. Physician injects needle into site for subclavian puncture and anesthetizes venipuncture site, waiting 1 to 2 minutes for effect to take place.	Minimizes discomfort client feels during venipuncture.

- *Critical Decision Point*

At time of insertion, nurse asks client to hold breath and strain. This is a Valsalva maneuver, which increases intrathoracic pressure and prevents entry of air into the catheter. Maneuver is also performed whenever the catheter will be open to air. If client is unable to perform Valsalva maneuver, nurse compresses client's abdomen gently.

p. Physician inserts IV catheter into subclavian vein. Usually this is done by locating the vein with a large-bore cannula, removing the needle from the cannula, threading a wire into the cannula and vein, removing the cannula over the wire, and threading the central vein catheter over the wire to the appropriate location (Seldinger technique) (Nussbaum and Fischer, 1994).	Large vein is selected because it is less irritated by PN solution.
q. Physician determines patency of line by withdrawing blood with 5-ml syringe. When blood return is evident and catheter placement is judged appropriate, physician connects IV tubing to intravenous catheter.	Connecting IV solution prevents air from entering venous system.
r. Nurse initially runs the IV fluid in at a rapid rate (macrodrip 20 to 30 gtt/min, microdrip 60 gtt/min) for 5 to 10 minutes.	Assesses whether fluid is infusing easily through newly inserted line.

- *Critical Decision Point*

Nurse must remain vigilant and be sure to connect functional line to IV pump or slow rate so that excess fluid is not infused. In addition, excess fluid should not be infused until chest x-ray confirms catheter placement.

s. Nurse adjusts IV infusion to 30 to 40 ml/hr and connects to electronic infusion pump until chest x-ray study is obtained.	Central line cannulations increase risk of pneumothorax (entrance of air into pleural space). Chest x-ray examination verifies absence of pneumothorax and confirms location of intravenous catheter before fluids are administered at a rapid flow.
t. Physician sutures central venous catheter in place. *Option:* Catheter securement device may be used, which avoids the need for a local anesthetic.	Suturing catheter to skin at insertion site or applying a securement device assists in preventing accidental dislodgement.
u. Physician removes sterile drapes and completes procedure.	Occurs only if physician is not applying occlusive dressing to IV site.
v. Physician orders chest film.	X-ray examination is the only method to confirm location of catheter tip.

STEP	RATIONALE
2. Applying Occlusive Dressing	
a. Nurse performs hand hygiene and applies sterile gloves.	Maintains surgical asepsis.
b. With alcohol swab, start at catheter exit site and cleanse skin, working in concentric circles outward approximately 2 to 3 inches. (Repeat with different swab 3 times.) Allow to dry.	Removes blood and defats skin. Drying ensures antimicrobial action.
c. Cleanse insertion site with antiseptic swab using friction. Use the first swab in a horizontal plane, cleansing the skin from side to side. Apply the second swab on a vertical plane, up and down. Apply the final swab in a circular pattern moving outward from the insertion site. Allow each swab to dry.	Mechanical friction in this pattern allows penetration of the antiseptic solution into the cracks and fissures of the epidermal layer of the skin (Crosby and Mares, 2001).

• *Critical Decision Point*
It is no longer recommended to routinely apply antimicrobial ointment to catheter insertion site at time of insertion or during routine dressing changes (McGee and Gould, 2003).

STEP	RATIONALE
d. Change sterile gloves.	Ensures that microorganisms removed during prep are not introduced to catheter site.
e. Apply occlusive transparent or occlusive gauze dressing over site (see Chapter 38).	Reduces transmission of microorganisms to venipuncture site. Transparent dressings reliably secure the device, permit visual inspection of catheter site, require less frequent changes than standard gauze and tape, and can be worn an extended time. However, there is no clinical difference in the incidence of catheter site colonization of bacteria with gauze compared with transparent dressings (O'Grady and others, 2002).
f. Remove and dispose of gloves. Loop and tape tubing securely to client's shoulder. Do not kink tubing or apply tape over transparent dressing. Label dressing with date of insertion and catheter size.	Helps to reduce chance of accidentally pulling on catheter and causing dislodgement. Label provides reference for dressing change schedule.
g. Assist with chest x-ray examination.	Documents line position or presence of pneumothorax or other complications.
h. Reposition client.	Maintains comfort.
i. When position of central vein catheter is confirmed, prepare parenteral nutrition solution obtained from pharmacy for infusion via infusion pump (see Skill 31-2).	Infusion pump will ensure regular infusion of prescribed volume of PN.
j. Dispose of supplies and perform hand hygiene.	Reduces transmission of microorganisms.
3. Discontinuing CVC	
a. Verify physician's order to discontinue line. Check agency policy because most require physician to discontinue CVC. In some settings critical care nurses receive training for competency in removal of line.	Verifies appropriateness of procedure. CVC should be removed only by competent health care professional.
b. If IV fluids and or medications are to continue, ensure that the fluids/medications are converted to a peripheral IV before central line discontinuation (see Chapter 27).	Prevents interruption of IV medication/fluid therapy.
c. Perform hand hygiene.	Prevents transmission of microorganisms.
d. Turn off the IV fluids infusing through the central line.	Prevents fluid loss during CVC removal.

STEP	RATIONALE
e. Apply gown, mask, goggles, and clean gloves.	Prevents transmission of microorganisms and nurse's exposure to blood-borne pathogens.
f. Gently remove the CVC dressing and discard it in appropriate biohazard container.	Prevents skin tears.
g. Remove gloves, wash hands and apply new pair of clean gloves.	Prevents transfer of organisms on soiled dressing to catheter insertion site.
h. Prep CVC insertion site with alcohol, starting at the insertion site and moving outward in concentric circles. Allow to dry.	Removes microorganisms from insertion site. Drying ensures maximal antimicrobial effect.
i. Repeat prep with antiseptic swab (chlorhexidine or povidone-iodine). Allow to dry.	
j. Remove the sutures using sterile scissors.	Reduces transmission of microorganisms.
k. Position client in Trendelenburgs position or with head of bed as low as client can tolerate.	Position promotes venous filling and prevents air embolus during catheter removal.
l. Instruct client to take a deep breath and hold it. Place a sterile 4 × 4 gauze dressing just above site, and withdraw catheter smoothly. Note any resistance while removing the catheter. Inspect the catheter for intactness, especially along tip.	Valsalva maneuver stabilizes intrathoracic pressure and prevents air from entering venous system. Catheter tip can potentially break off to cause an embolus and must be identified immediately.
m. Immediately apply firm pressure to exit site with sterile 4 × 4s for 5 minutes or until bleeding stops.	Prevents hemorrhage from central vein site.

- **Critical Decision Point**
  It may be necessary to apply pressure longer if client is receiving anticoagulation.

STEP	RATIONALE
n. Inspect site after 5 minutes of holding pressure. If there is no bleeding or hematoma, apply a sterile occlusive dressing to the site.	Prevents entrance of microorganisms into old insertion site.
o. Return client to comfortable position. Be sure IV is infusing at correct rate.	Maintains IV fluid therapy.
p. Discard supplies; remove gloves and personal protective equipment. Perform hand hygiene.	Prevents transmission of microorganisms.

EVALUATION

1. Observe client for shortness of breath, pain in the chest or shoulder after CVC insertion.	Symptoms indicate complication of pneumothorax.
2. Observe client for bleeding or swelling at the insertion site and occlusiveness of the dressing.	Symptoms may indicate infiltration of intravenous fluids into subcutaneous tissues or damage to vessel lumen. Dressing must remain occlusive to effectively protect against entrance of microorganisms.
3. Observe insertion site over time for erythema, warmth, tenderness, edema, or drainage.	Symptoms may indicate infection at line insertion site.
4. Measure client's body temperature every 4 hours for 24 hours and then as ordered. Review any diagnostic reports (e.g., white blood cell count, catheter site cultures).	Fever can be early warning sign of systemic infection resulting from entrance of microorganisms into bloodstream. Absence of a confirmed source of infection should raise concern of a catheter-related infection.
5. After discontinuation of CVC observe for possible complications of air embolism, pneumothorax, hematoma at puncture site.	Complications may develop within minutes or hours of line discontinuation.

Recording and Reporting

- Record in nurses notes condition of client before, during, and after procedure.
- Document size, type, and location of central catheter, presence or absence of blood return after placement of central vein catheter, type of dressing, and type and rate of PN infused.
- Document confirmation of appropriate position of central vein catheter following x-ray examination.
- Document discontinuation of line by noting client's tolerance of procedure, presence or absence of complications, condition of skin at insertion site, and application of sterile dressing.

Unexpected Outcomes	Related Interventions
1. Client develops fever and signs of catheter-related infection.	• Obtain two samples of blood for culture from peripheral site to evaluate possibility of bacteremia.
2. Displacement of the central vein catheter into veins of the neck or chest occurs.	• Physician will withdraw catheter and insert new catheter into different site.
3. Pneumothorax results from insertion of catheter into pleural space.	• Call physician immediately. Chest x-ray film will be obtained to confirm diagnosis. • Prepare for removal of catheter and insertion of chest tube (see Chapter 25).
4. Purulence and erythema develop at catheter exit site.	• Call physician for removal of catheter. • Systemic antibiotic therapy may be initiated.
5. Bleeding occurs at the insertion site or into the pleural cavity.	• Call physician. • Prepare for removal of catheter.

Teaching Considerations

- Instruct client to report discomfort around the site; in either arm, shoulder, or side of the neck; or any shortness of breath.

Pediatric Considerations

- Central vein catheters that are of a smaller diameter and shorter length are available for children and infants.
- Care must be taken to secure infant catheters in a manner that does not allow them to twist. The twisting of these fragile small-diameter catheters can cause them to tear.
- Parents must fully understand benefits and risks of central venous placement. Use of pictures can be very helpful.

Gerontological Considerations

- Older adults may have difficulty with lying flat in bed, and a modification of the totally supine position during insertion may be necessary.

Home Care Considerations

- Clients or family members may need to learn to perform catheter site care and dressing changes for long-term central venous catheters.

SKILL 31-2   Caring for the Client Receiving Central Parenteral Nutrition

CPN involves the delivery of parenteral nutrition nutrients via a central vein access. CPN can be delivered through an IV access inserted directly into the subclavian vein or a PICC threaded into the subclavian vein. Caring for clients receiving CPN requires the use of strict aseptic technique and the nurse's application of critical thinking. Because of the composition of CPN fluids, clients can experience metabolic and fluid balance changes quickly. In addition, the clinical condition of clients receiving CPN is usually poor, especially when clients have alterations in host defenses, severe underlying illnesses, and extremes of age. The nurse must be prepared to anticipate changes in the client's condition that may signal developing complications. Similarly, the nurse must use good judgment to maintain the IV system and to ensure it is in proper working order.

Intravenous catheters used to provide parenteral nutrition are at an increased risk for infection compared with catheters used for other therapies such as antibiotics or chemotherapy (Krzywda and others, 1999). At one time it was assumed that the high concentration of dextrose supported bacterial growth. Dextrose, however, is highly acidic and not a good growth medium for many common bacteria and fungi (Orr, 1999). Instead, it is likely that the increased risk of infection is associated with long-term central catheter placement and the numerous factors (e.g. dressing selection and site care) that can lead to catheter-related sepsis. Preventing infection is a nursing priority when preparing and administering fluids and monitoring the infusion system.

DELEGATION CONSIDERATIONS
Caring for clients receiving CPN should not be delegated to assistive personnel. Assistive personnel should be instructed to report the following immediately:
- The CPN infusion pump alarm sounds.
- Client complains of a moist or leaking dressing/tubing.

EQUIPMENT
- ❏ IV infusion tubing
- ❏ CPN solution (IV)
- ❏ IV filter (*optional*—0.22 μm for dextrose/amino acids, 1.2 μm for three-in-one solutions)
- ❏ Intravenous infusion pump
- ❏ Disposable gloves

STEP	RATIONALE

ASSESSMENT

1. Assess client's nutritional status (see Skill 31-1): measure caloric intake and weight. In some institutions a consultation with the nutritional support service is required.

2. Inspect condition of central vein access or PICC access for presence of inflammation, edema, tenderness at site, and whether tubing is patent and not kinked.

3. Assess client's blood glucose level (finger stick—see Chapter 43).

4. Assess factors influencing CPN administration: electrolyte levels, elevated blood glucose level, renal and hepatic function.

5. Assess vital signs, and auscultate client's lung sounds.

Nurse needs to be aware of client's nutritional parameters to monitor and judge response to therapy. Nutritional support clinicians are best prepared to assess indications for CPN.

Nurse monitors site to identify early signs of infection, infiltration, or disruption in system integrity. Development of complication may contraindicate infusion of fluids and may indicate need to establish new IV site.

Provides baseline for measuring tolerance to high concentration of glucose infusion.

Clients may require their CPN therapy to be adapted by composition or volume (requires physician order).

Provides baseline for monitoring client's response to fluid infusion. Crackles in lungs are early indication of fluid volume excess.

STEP	**RATIONALE**
6. Verify physician's order for nutrients, minerals, vitamins, trace elements, and electrolytes, as well as flow rate. TPN is usually ordered in a three-in-one solution (amino acids, carbohydrates, and fats).	CPN must be ordered by physician and is often ordered daily in the hospital setting after review of laboratory values. In the home setting, orders may be obtained less frequently (e.g., weekly)

NURSING DIAGNOSES

* Imbalanced nutrition: less than body requirements
* Excess fluid volume
* Risk for infection

Related factors are individualized based on client's condition or needs.

PLANNING

1. Expected outcomes following completion of procedure:	
• Client's ideal weight gain is usually between 1 and 2 lb/week.	Weight is an indicator of how well the client is doing nutritionally and determines fluid volume. Weight gain greater than 1 lb/day indicates fluid retention.
• Serum glucose levels are less than 200 mg/100 ml.	A serum glucose level less than 200 mg/100 ml will reflect a metabolic tolerance to the concentrated glucose solution in PN.
• Central access catheter or PICC device is patent, and site is free of pain, swelling, redness, or inflammation. PICC site is free of phlebitis.	Ensures that CPN is infusing into the vein rather than into surrounding tissues and that there are no signs of an access device infection.
2. Explain purposes of CPN.	Promotes understanding and reduces anxiety.

IMPLEMENTATION

1. Perform hand hygiene, and apply gloves.	Reduces transmission of microorganisms.
2. Check that ordered PN solution is correct with correct additives and properly labeled. Check solution expiration date. Also check client's name.	Prevents medication error.
3. Inspect PN solution for particulate matter or, if it is a three-in-one solution, inspect emulsion for a cream layer or separation of the fat into a layer. If there is a thin layer of aggregated fat droplets about 1 to 2 cm in thickness, agitate bag (Driscoll and Baron, 2000).	Deterioration of a three-in-one solution results in breakdown of the emulsion.

• *Critical Decision Point*

Do not use PN solution if it has coalesced (thick, dense layer of fat droplets at surface, appearing 10 cm in thickness) or oiled out (fat droplets separate from solution and appear as a clear layer at surface). Notify the pharmacy, and request a new solution (Driscoll and Baron, 2000).

STEP	**RATIONALE**
4. Check client's identification band, and ask client to state name.	Ensures correct client receives correct intravenous solution.
5. Connect PN solution to appropriate intravenous tubing with filter. Prime tubing, being sure no air bubbles remain, and turn off flow with roller clamp. Connect end of tubing to central or peripheral catheter line, and open roller clamp to rate that maintains patency of line.	Air introduced into central circulation can result in an air embolus, a fatal complication. PN solutions need to be connected to new, sterile intravenous tubing every 24 hours (when lipids are infused), or every 48 hours (when lipids not infused).
6. Place IV tubing into an intravenous infusion pump, open roller clamp completely, and regulate flow rate on pump as ordered (see Chapter 27) (see illustration). In some institutions the infusion rate is immediately set at the ordered rate. In other institutions an initial rate of 40 to 60 ml/hr is established, and the rate is gradually increased until client's complete nutritional needs are supplied.	CPN flow rates are ordered to meet client's metabolic and electrolyte needs. Rate must be maintained to prevent electrolyte imbalances. The rate may be advanced each day toward the target rate to provide adequate calories and protein.

• *Critical Decision Point*

Rate of infusion may be increased gradually to prevent metabolic and electrolyte abnormalities (ASPEN, 2001). CPN is hyperosmolar and is usually tolerated when increased in stepwise fashion. Do not abruptly discontinue CPN, because this may lead to hypoglycemia. If discontinued suddenly, hang infusion of 5% dextrose in water at same infusion rate (ASPEN, 2001).

7. Infuse all IV medications through an alternate intravenous line. Do not obtain blood samples or CVP readings through same lumen or port used for CPN infusion.	Prevents drug incompatibility. Prevents occlusion of central line and reduces risk of transmission of infection.

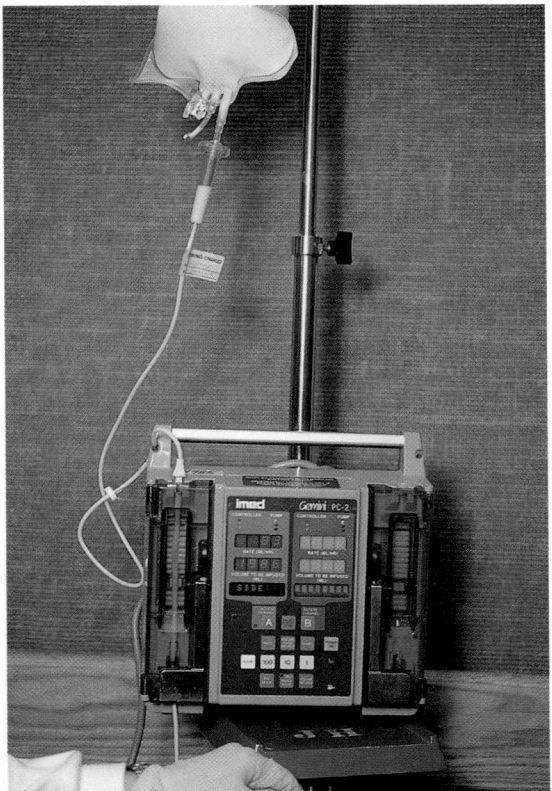

STEP **6** Parenteral nutrition solution infusing via infusion pump.

STEP	RATIONALE
8. Do not interrupt TPN infusion (e.g., showers, transport to procedure, blood transfusion).	Maintains continuous infusion of nutrients, prevents hypoglycemic reaction.
9. Change infusing tubing and filter using strict aseptic technique every 24 hours.	Prevents development of catheter-related bacteremia.
10. Discard used supplies, and perform hand hygiene.	Reduces transmission of infection.

EVALUATION

1. Monitor flow rate routinely, at least hourly.	Too rapid or too slow infusion could result in metabolic disturbances.
2. Monitor fluid intake every 8 hours.	Prevents fluid imbalance from too slow or too rapid infusion.
3. Obtain daily weights or weights as ordered.	Over time, routine measurement of weights will reflect weight gain/loss resulting either from caloric intake or fluid retention.
4. Assess for fluid retention.	Weight gain in excess of 1 lb/day, dependent edema, lung crackles, and intake greater than output per each 24-hour period indicate fluid retention.
5. Monitor client's glucose level and laboratory parameters to determine response to CPN.	Adequate tolerance is demonstrated by maintenance of normal electrolyte levels, satisfactory fluid balance, acceptable serum glucose levels, gradual increase in weight, and improvement in serum proteins.
6. Inspect central venous access site.	Determines IV patency and absence of infection, infiltration, or phlebitis.

Recording and Reporting

- Record condition of central venous access device, rate and type of infusion, lumen used for infusion, intake and output every 8 hours, vital signs, and weights.
- If signs of infection, occlusion, fluid retention, or infiltration occur, notify the physician.

Unexpected Outcomes	Related Interventions
1. There is redness, swelling, and tenderness around the venous access site, indicating possible exit site infection.	• Notify physician. • Apply warm compress, and initiate daily site care as ordered. Systemic antibiotic therapy may begin.
2. Client develops fever, malaise, and chills, indicating systemic infection.	• Check exit site for signs of infection. • Notify physician, and consult about the need to obtain cultures of exit site or blood. Systemic antibiotic therapy may begin.
3. Infusion stops flowing or flows at a rate slower than ordered.	• Venous access device may have become occluded with fibrin or particulate matter. Report the occlusion to the physician. • If the device is a surgically placed device or PICC (see Chapter 27), a thrombolytic agent may be ordered.
4. Client experiences weight gain greater than 1 lb/day. Taut skin turgor may also be present. Crackles auscultated over lung fields.	• Notify physician. • Anticipate need to reduce IV infusion rate.

Unexpected Outcomes	Related Interventions
5. Serum glucose is greater than 200 mg/100 ml. Indicates client's intolerance to glucose load in the CPN solution.	• May document need for addition of insulin to the CPN, modification of CPN solution, or sliding-scale insulin coverage.
6. Serum electrolytes are out of normal range.	• May indicate movement of electrolytes in response to infusion of fluids and glucose. The electrolyte levels in the solution may need to be adjusted.

Teaching Considerations
- Instruct client and family about the purpose and goals of CPN. Keep them informed about daily care of central line.

Pediatric Considerations
- Indications for parenteral nutrition for infants include gastroschisis, congenital anomalies of the gastrointestinal system, short-bowel syndrome, extensive burns, children receiving chemotherapy and/or radiation who are not tolerating oral feedings, and children who are NPO for extended periods.
- CPN can cause hepatobiliary dysfunction in infants.
- With children requiring long-term parenteral nutrition it may be possible to change them to a cycle when they have stabilized. This will allow them to receive the parenteral nutrition at a time when they may be less active, thus allowing more normalcy in the family during the time the child is not receiving the solution (Hockenberry and others, 2003).

Gerontological Considerations
- Older adults may have impaired ability to manage higher fluid volumes or may be at risk for an increased incidence of hyperglycemia.

Home Care Considerations
- Clients requiring long-term PN will benefit from a referral to a home nutrition therapy team.
- Clients or family members may need to learn to perform catheter site care, dressing changes for long-term central venous catheters, and techniques for adding and removing parenteral nutrition solutions.
- Teach client and primary caregiver to monitor client's weight, calorie count, intake and output, and serum glucose level.
- Teach client and primary caregiver about actions to take in case of emergency or unexpected outcomes.
- Observe client and primary caregiver perform procedure in hospital before discharge (see Chapter 42).

SKILL 31-3 Caring for the Client Receiving Peripheral Parenteral Nutrition With Lipid (Fat) Emulsion

The administration of parenteral nutrition via peripheral veins requires the use of lower concentrations of dextrose and amino acids to lower tonicity and lessen the risk of vein damage (Table 31-3). For example, 2 L of peripheral parenteral nutrition (PPN) consisting of 10% dextrose and 10% amino acids supplemented by 500 ml of 1% IV fat emulsion provide 2000 kcal/day. PPN is usually administered in conjunction with fat emulsion. Unfortunately, PPN is often difficult to maintain because of frequent episodes of phlebitis in superficial arm veins and infiltrations of solutions into subcutaneous tissue. Therefore the final dextrose concentration must be no greater than 10%, because the peripheral vein will sclerose at higher concentrations. However, solutions of lower concentration make it difficult to supply adequate calories and amino acids through a peripheral vein.

This problem, in addition to the scarcity of adequate access sites, is the reason many experts recommend PPN for only short periods of time. Nutrients given through central veins may be very concentrated (e.g., 1800 mOsm). However, concentrations this great are not tolerated in peripheral veins because of their relatively low blood flow. Indications for PPN include the following:

1. Short-term need for parenteral nutrition: NPO for more than 5 days but anticipation that the client will tolerate enteral or oral nutrition within 7 to 10 days.
2. History of problems with central vein access or inability to establish central vein access. Clients with a history of multiple central venous catheter infections or occlusions have increased risks associated with catheter

TABLE 31-3 COMPARISON OF CENTRAL PARENTERAL NUTRITION (CPN) AND PERIPHERAL PARENTERAL NUTRITION (PPN)

	CPN	PPN
Osmolality	1800 to 2000 mOsm	600 to 700 mOsm
Route of administration	Central venous catheter	Small peripheral vein
Usual daily caloric intake	2000 to 4000	700 to 2000
Fat emulsion	Minor caloric source; provides essential fatty acid	Major caloric source; provides essential fatty acid
Objectives	Weight maintenance; weight gain	Weight maintenance
Duration of therapy	6 days or longer	3 to 7 days

placement. Multiple catheter placements may deplete access sites.

3. Adequate peripheral access. Despite its lower osmolality, PPN tends to cause phlebitis and may require frequent changes in the access location.

4. Ability to tolerate larger volumes of fluid. Because of the lower concentration of dextrose in PPN, a larger volume of fluid is required to attain adequate calories. Clients with impaired renal or cardiac function may not tolerate PPN.

5. Ability to tolerate lipid emulsions. Lipid is the most calorically dense nutrient, and PPN without lipid would not provide adequate calories unless very large volumes of fluid were provided. One liter of 10% dextrose provides only 340 kcal. Five hundred milliliters of 10% lipid provides 550 kcal.

DELEGATION CONSIDERATIONS

The skill of caring for a client receiving peripheral parenteral nutrition with lipid emulsion should not be delegated to assistive personnel. However, assistive personnel should be instructed to report the following:

- Infusion pump alarm sounds.
- Client complains of burning or pain at insertion site.
- IV dressing becomes moist.

EQUIPMENT

- ❏ PPN solution
- ❏ Lipid emulsion
- ❏ Two sets of IV tubing (filter optional—0.22 μm for amino acid/dextrose solution)
- ❏ Needle (19 gauge), Y connector, or stopcock
- ❏ Alcohol swab
- ❏ Infusion pump
- ❏ Disposable gloves

STEP	RATIONALE

ASSESSMENT

1. Assess client for potential lipid intolerance. Assess serum triglyceride level. Serum triglyceride should be drawn before initiation of fat therapy (baseline) and 6 hours after fat has infused.

Determines client's ability to metabolize lipid.

2. Select or initiate appropriate functional IV site (18-gauge catheter) to administer PPN and lipid emulsion. Assess its patency and function (see Chapter 27).

Large-gauge catheter ensures more efficient flow of infusion.

3. Check physician's order for volume of fat emulsion and PPN solution.

Fat emulsions and PPN must be ordered by physician.

4. Check administration time for fat emulsion.

Fat emulsions may cause adverse symptoms if infused too rapidly as a separate infusion. The infusion time should be at least 4 hours. Fat emulsions should hang no longer than 10 hours as a separate infusion. When admixed with the PPN, fats are administered over 31 hours.

5. Use care in locating fat emulsion from supply area. Read label of solution.

Lipid emulsions are white and opaque; thus care should be taken to avoid confusing enteral formula with parenteral lipids.

STEP	RATIONALE

NURSING DIAGNOSES

- Imbalanced nutrition: less than body requirements
- Risk for infection

Related factors are individualized based on client's condition or needs.

PLANNING

1. Expected outcomes following completion of procedure:
   - Triglyceride level is stable.
   - Venipuncture site is free of phlebitis, pain, swelling, redness, and inflammation.
   - Client does not show signs of systemic infection (e.g., elevated temperature).
2. Explain purposes of PPN.
3. Place client in a comfortable position for IV insertion or initiation of infusion.
4. Check that ordered PN solution is correct with correct additives and properly labeled. Check solution expiration date. Also check client's name. Inspect bottle for opacity and consistency in texture and color.
5. Warm solution to room temperature if refrigerated.

Rationale (Planning):

Indicates physical tolerance to fat.
Ensures proper administration of PPN with lipids.

Temperature is an indication of possible systemic infection related to parenteral nutrition.
Promotes understanding and reduces anxiety.
When clients are comfortable, they tolerate procedures more readily.
Prevents medication error.

Prevents change in body temperature from instillation of cold solution.

IMPLEMENTATION

1. Perform hand hygiene, and apply gloves.
2. Check client's identification band, and ask client to state name.
3. Connect IV tubing to PPN solution, run fat emulsion into IV tubing, and remove excess air. Turn roller clamp to off position.
4. Clean peripheral line tubing injection port of primary IV with alcohol swab. (*Optional:* Use Y connector.)
5. Insert end of fat emulsion infusion tubing into injection port of main IV, proximal to the venipuncture site, below the infusion filter on the main parenteral nutrition line.
6. Open roller clamp completely on fat emulsion infusion, and then set flow rate on infusion pump.

7. Begin PPN at ordered rate—10% fat emulsions are infused over at least 4 hours, and 20% fats are infused over at least 6 hours. All lipids can hang for 12 hours; admixing lipids with parenteral nutrition can hang for 24 hours.
8. Discard supplies, and perform hand hygiene.

Rationale (Implementation):

Reduces transmission of microorganisms.
Ensures correct client receives correct intravenous solution.

To prevent air from entering vascular system, all tubing must be purged.

Removes surface organisms at injection site and prevents organisms from entering blood system.
Fat emulsions cannot infuse through a 0.22-μm IV filter—the emulsion would separate.

Up to 2.5 g fat per kilogram per day may be infused, but fat emulsion should not exceed 60% of total calories. Recommended daily fat percentage is 30% or less of total calories.
The rate of PPN administration does not need to be gradually increased. The lower concentration of dextrose allows most clients to tolerate the full administration rate without difficulty.

Reduces transmission of infection.

EVALUATION

1. Measure vital signs and client's general comfort level every 10 minutes for first 30 minutes.
2. Measure client's laboratory values (e.g., triglycerides) daily.

Rationale (Evaluation):

Monitors client for fat emulsion intolerance.

Provides objective data to measure the response to therapy.

STEP	RATIONALE
3. Monitor temperature every 4 hours, and regularly inspect venipuncture site for signs of phlebitis or infiltration.	Determines onset of fever, a complication of intolerance to fat emulsion or sepsis. Determines integrity of IV system. Weight gain, I&O imbalance, peripheral edema, and crackles in lungs can indicate fluid retention.
4. Assess client's weight, intake and output (I&O), condition of peripheral extremities (for edema), and breath sounds.	

Recording and Reporting

- Record intake and output every 8 hours on flow sheet.
- Record temperature every 4 hours.
- Record condition of IV site, type of PPN, and rate and status of infusion.
- Report development of fever or symptoms of fat intolerance to physician.

Unexpected Outcomes	Related Interventions
1. There is intolerance to fat emulsion, as evidenced by increased triglyceride levels, increased temperature (3° to 4° F), chills, headache, nausea and vomiting, muscle ache, backache, chest pain.	• Confer with physician, and determine if fat emulsion should be discontinued.
2. See Unexpected Outcomes and Related Interventions for Skill 31-2.	

Teaching Considerations

- Teach client and primary caregiver to monitor client's weight, calorie count, intake and output, and IV site.

Pediatric Considerations

- See Skill 31-2.

Gerontological Considerations

- Older adults may have lipid intolerance.

Home Care Considerations

- See Skill 31-2.
- Observe client and primary caregiver perform procedure in hospital before discharge (see Chapter 42).

FOCUS *on* CLINICAL PRACTICE

Mr. Giles is a 43-year-old client admitted to the hospital with a severe exacerbation of Crohn's disease. He has lost 10 pounds in the last 3 weeks and has suffered recurrent abdominal pain, cramping, and loose stools. He is unable to tolerate food orally, becoming easily nauseated. The client is to receive bowel rest and nutritional support with TPN. The physician plans to insert a central line for parenteral nutrition therapy.

1. Identify four physical parameters that can change quickly and should thus be part of the nurse's baseline assessment before initiating TPN.
2. Explain why a client receiving TPN will have an initial blood glucose measurement.
3. Identify the three components of a 3:1 TPN solution.
4. In preparing Mr. Giles for a central line insertion, the nurse explains a Valsalva maneuver as follows, "Mr. Giles, when the physician begins to insert the catheter in your shoulder I will want you to take a deep breath and hold it." Is the nurse's explanation of a Valsalva maneuver correct? What is a Valsalva maneuver?
5. Approximately 48 hours after Mr. Giles's TPN infusion begins, the client develops excessive thirst, confusion, and an increase in urine output. These symptoms may indicate:
   A. Infection
   B. Pulmonary embolus
   C. Hyperlipidemia
   D. Hyperglycemia
6. Two days after TPN infusion has begun, Mr. Giles has experienced a 5-pound weight gain. He comments, "This stuff is great—I am gaining back some of the weight I lost." What would be your response? What would you include in a nursing assessment?

NCLEX REVIEW QUESTIONS

1. A solution of TPN should be administered into a large-diameter vein like the subclavian because the solution is typically:
   1. Acidic
   2. Opaque
   3. Hyperosmolar
   4. Isotonic
2. Which intervention has been proven to reduce the incidence of catheter-related infection from a central line insertion?
   1. Use of full sterile-barrier precautions during insertion
   2. Use of a transparent dressing following catheter insertion
   3. Application of an antibiotic ointment daily to the catheter insertion site
   4. Changing of IV infusion tubing every 48 hours
3. The correct position for preparing a client for a central line insertion is:
   1. Prone
   2. Sims' or side-lying
   3. Trendelenburg
   4. Supine with pillow under shoulder
4. Following the insertion of a central venous catheter into the subclavian vein, a physician will order an x-ray examination to:
   1. Determine presence of pulmonary edema
   2. Determine position of catheter tip
   3. Rule out a pulmonary emboli
   4. Rule out a hemothorax
5. Parenteral nutrition given via a peripheral vein can never have a dextrose concentration greater than:
   1. 2.5%
   2. 5.0%
   3. 7.5%
   4. 10.0%
6. Signs and symptoms of lipid intolerance include the following:
   1. Increased temperature, chills, headache, nausea and vomiting, and chest pain
   2. Respiratory distress, shortness of breath, chest pain, and decreased blood pressure
   3. Increased temperature, chills, malaise, elevated white blood cell count
   4. Bleeding and swelling at insertion site

References

American Society for Parenteral and Enteral Nutrition: Standards of practice: nutrition support nurses, *Nutr Clin Pract* 16(1):56, 2001.

American Society for Parenteral and Enteral Nutrition: Guidelines for the use of parenteral and enteral nutrition in adult and pediatric patients, *JPEN* 26(1):1SA, 2002.

Bozzetti F and others: Perioperative total parenteral nutrition in malnourished gastrointestinal cancer patients: a randomized clinical trial, *JPEN* 24(1):7, 2000.

CDC NNIS System: National Nosocomial Infections Surveillance (NNIS) report, data summary from October, 1986-April 1997, issued May 1997, *Am J Infect Control* 25:477, 1997.

Crosby TC, Mares AK: Skin antisepsis past, present, and future, *JVAD* 6(2), 2001.

Driscoll DF, Baron MN: Physiochemical stability of two types of intravenous lipid emulsions as total nutrient admixture, *JPEN* 24(1):15, 2000.

Hickey MS: *Handbook of enteral, parenteral, and ARC/AIDS nutritional therapy,* St. Louis, 1992, Mosby.

Hockenberry MJ and others: *Wong's nursing care of infants and children,* ed 7, St. Louis, 2003, Mosby.

Infusion Nurses Society: Infusion Nursing Standards of Practice, *J Intraven Nurs* 31(6S):S1, 2000.

Krzywda EA and others: Catheter infections: diagnosis, etiology, treatment, and prevention, *Nutr Clin Pract* 14:178, 1999.

Nussbaum MS, Fischer JE: Parenteral nutrition. In Zaloga GP, editor: *Nutrition in critical care,* St. Louis, 1994, Mosby.

Orr ME: Vascular access device selection for parenteral nutrition, *Nutr Clin Pract* 14:172, 1999.

Research References

McGee DC, Gould MK: Current concepts: preventing complications of central venous catheterization, *N Engl J Med* 348(12): 1131, 2003.

O'Grady NP and others: Guidelines for the prevention of intravascular catheter-related infections, *MMWR Morb Mortal Wkly Rep* 51(RR-10):1, 2002.

Raad II and others: Prevention of central venous catheter-related infections by using maximal sterile barrier precautions during insertion, *Infect Control Hosp Epidemiol* 15:311, 1994.

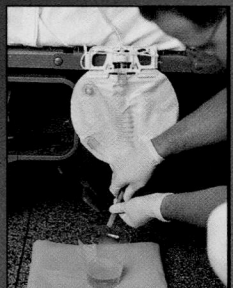

32

Urinary Elimination

MEDIA RESOURCES

Evolve Site *evolve*

http://evolve.elsevier.com/Perry/skills
- Weblinks
- Video clips
- Mosby's Nursing Skills Video Exercises

Mosby's Nursing Skills Videos/CD-ROM
- *Normal Elimination Video:* Assisting with a urinal; assisting with a bedpan, including standard and fracture bedpans; providing catheter care; applying a condom catheter
- *Urinary Catheter Management Video:* Urinary catheter insertion, including indwelling catheter for female patients and the straight catheter for male patients

Urinary elimination is a natural and private process individuals take for granted until it is altered by some uncontrollable physiological factor. Clients needing assistance with urinary elimination may require physiological and psychological assistance from the nurse. Physiological support may require use of an invasive procedure such as the insertion of a catheter into the bladder. Psychological assistance may be needed to help the client adjust to an alteration in urinary elimination. Therefore the nurse must be competent in performing technical skills and sensitive to a client's psychological needs.

Certain disease processes, medications, and stages of growth and development influence fluid and electrolyte status. Physical assessment findings can indicate that a fluid or electrolyte imbalance exists. The nurse must know the factors influencing fluid and electrolyte balance and the signs and symptoms of fluid imbalances. A client's hydration status is an important physiological indicator that is closely monitored, especially when the urinary system is altered. When clients have altered or impaired elimination, their intake (fluids ingested) and output (fluids excreted) (I&O) are often measured to help monitor fluid and electrolyte balance (see Chapter 18).

Cultural Considerations

Provision of care for urinary elimination needs cannot be done compassionately and competently without considering a client's cultural heritage. The potential exposure of perineal structures during elimination care has significant implications for members of those cultures who hold specific beliefs about female modesty and gender-appropriate care. Use the following guidelines when caring for clients with culturally diverse needs:

- Accommodate need for gender-congruent care among cultures emphasizing separate gender roles and female modesty such as African, Hispanic, Asian, Islamic, Arabic, Hindu, Jewish Orthodox, and Amish cultures.
  - Explain the procedure to be done, and ask the client how he or she wants it performed.
  - Allow presence of a family member at the bedside if requested by the client.
  - Provide privacy through adequate draping and use of bedside screens.
  - Prevent entrance of the opposite sex into the client's room during the procedure.
  - Avoid prolonged exposure of the client.
- Control verbal and nonverbal communication when performing catheterization of a female who was circumcised.
  - Avoid judgmental comments, and assess for landmarks in a professional manner.
  - Use a smaller Foley catheter when the area is constricted from scarring.
- Promote clients' understanding of procedure to be done.
  - Use an interpreter if needed.
  - Repeat explanations because client's anxiety about the loss of privacy can pose distraction.
  - Explain measures to protect client's privacy.
- Meticulous hygiene is observed by certain cultures such as Hindus and Muslims that designate the left hand to perform unclean procedures such as catheterization.
  - Wash your hands before touching the client, and use your right hand.
  - Use the left hand to handle the urinal and/or urinary secretions.
  - Do not place the urinal or soiled bed linens on top of the bedside table or surface used for praying or eating.
  - Provide the client with the equipment and supplies for cleansing after elimination (Lawrence and Rozmus, 2001).

Evidence-Based Practice Trends

There is consistent evidence that a significant number of nosocomial infections are related to urinary catheterization. The risk of infection is associated with the method and duration of catheterization, the quality of catheter care, and host susceptibility. (Guidelines for Preventing Infections, 2004). Suprapubic catheterization is becoming increasingly popular because it offers some potential advantages to urethral catheterization, including reduction in urinary infection rates (Addison and Mould, 2000). Continuous ambulatory peritoneal dialysis (CAPD) is a treatment for end-stage renal disease. Because CAPD involves the instillation of fluid into the peritoneal space, peritonitis, or inflammation of the peritoneal lining, is a complication. The onset of peritonitis is the major reason CAPD clients transfer to hemodialysis therapy (Lancaster, 2001). Research has demonstrated that the use of double bag or Y set systems reduces the incidence of peritonitis in clients on CAPD (Ellis, 2002).

Skill Performance Guidelines

1. Know the client's usual fluid intake pattern, including the types and amounts of fluids and when they are ingested, and assess the client's fluid preferences regarding types, temperature, and amount of fluids preferred at one time.

2. Know the client's normal range of vital signs. Abnormal fluid and electrolyte balances can affect the amount of circulating blood volume (see Table 32-1).

3. Know the client's medical history, including diseases and any therapies the client is receiving that may affect kidney and/or bladder function. Clients with injuries from burns or trauma or cardiopulmonary or renal disease frequently have fluid imbalances. Medications may affect fluid and electrolyte balance. For example, diuretics are successfully used to regulate fluid balance; however, side effects can further potentiate fluid and electrolyte imbalances. Steroids are frequently used to treat severe inflammatory conditions, but they may cause the retention of sodium and water and increase excretion of potassium.

4. Be aware of environmental conditions that can affect fluid balance. Prolonged exposure to extreme environmental temperatures can cause increased loss of body fluids.

5. Know the signs of dehydration and fluid overload (see Table 32-1).

6. Institute measurement of I&O when there is an anticipated or suspicious change in fluid balance. The nurse is responsible for the maintenance of accurate records. Measurements are kept throughout the day and totaled every 8 hours, but the nurse may determine that more frequent measurements are required (see Chapter 18).

7. Know the average output range for a client. Adult urinary output averages 1000 to 2400 ml in 24 hours. Minimum average hourly output is 30 ml; output is frequently monitored in acutely ill clients on an hourly or bihourly schedule.

8. It may be necessary to weigh the client to help assess fluid status. Obtain weights with the same scale, same time of day, and with comparable articles of clothing, including bed linen if bed weights are necessary.

9. Consider the client's age when assessing micturition habits. Toilet training and enuresis are concerns that arise in the toddler and preschooler. In the adult, increasing age may bring disease and physiological changes that predispose to incontinence, or the inability to control urination.

10. Encouraging fluids is a nursing responsibility. Any client not restricted in total fluid intake should be assessed; if oral intake is not minimally 1500 ml/day, a plan of care should be developed with the client to increase fluids. Clients with urinary problems may be hesitant to take fluids in fear of incontinence and/or increased urinary frequency. Education on the importance of fluid intake in maintaining urinary and overall health is vital.

11. Know the client's most recent serum electrolyte measurements. Abnormal electrolyte values can affect fluid balance and, if uncorrected, can lead to deterioration of the client's health status or even death.

12. Provide for the client's comfort. A client uncomfortable physically or psychologically may be unable to relax the external urethral sphincter (voluntary muscle at the neck of the bladder) and therefore not be able to

---

TABLE 32-1   SIGNS OF FLUID VOLUME DEFICIT (FVD) AND FLUID VOLUME EXCESS (FVE)

Eyes	*FVD:* Sunken eyes, dry conjunctivae, decreased or absence of tearing
	FVE: Periorbital edema, blurred vision, papilledema
Mouth	*FVD:* Sticky, dry mucous membrane; dry, cracked lips; decreased saliva; increased viscosity of saliva; furrowed, shrunken tongue
	FVE: Excessive salivation
Skin	*FVD:* Increased skin temperature; dry, scaly skin; poor turgor
	FVE: Edema, anasarca
Cardiovascular	*FVD:* Increased pulse rate, weak pulse, hypotension, decreased pulse volume/pressure, decreased capillary filling, increased hematocrit
	FVE: Bounding pulse rate, blood pressure normal with or without orthostatic changes, third heart sound (S_3), distended neck veins
Gastrointestinal	*FVD:* Sunken abdomen
	FVD or FVE: Vomiting, diarrhea, abdominal cramps
Renal	*FVD:* Oliguria or anuria, urine specific gravity increased (normal, 1.010 to 1.030)
	FVE: Decreased urine specific gravity, diuresis (if kidneys are normal)

urinate (void) or completely empty the bladder. The nurse can promote comfort measures by providing privacy, offering the client a warm bedpan, assisting the client into a normal voiding position (standing for a man, squatting for a woman), or reducing pain by administering a prescribed analgesic before helping the client walk to the bathroom. Distraction measures, such as turning on a sink faucet so the client can hear water running, may help the client to void.

13. Identify conditions that weaken abdominal or pelvic muscles such as multiple abdominal or gynecological surgeries or pregnancies. Clients with weak abdominal or pelvic floor muscles can be taught exercises to strengthen these muscles and increase the ability of the bladder to contract and promote better control of the external urethral sphincter.

14. Know the client's normal pattern of urination/micturition. The client should be taught not to ignore the urge to void. The nurse can assist by responding readily to the client's request to use a bedpan, urinal, bathroom, or commode. The nurse can also offer the client the opportunity to void after meals, at regular intervals throughout the day, and before bedtime. Clients taking diuretic medications should receive them early in the morning so they do not need to void during the night.

15. Consider the client's functional status. Mobility and sensory problems may influence access to toileting facilities. Assessments that should be made include use of walking aids, distance to the toilet, ability to remove clothing or to get in and out of the bathroom, and lighting.

SKILL 32-1 Assisting a Client in Using a Urinal

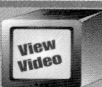

The client's ability to void depends on feeling the urge to urinate and on being able to control the urethral sphincter. One factor that can interfere with urination/micturition is bed rest or immobility, which does not allow the client to assume the normal position for emptying the bladder. The female client is accustomed to squatting, which promotes contraction of the pelvic and abdominal muscles that assist in sphincter control and bladder contraction. The nurse assists the bedridden woman in using a bedpan for voiding (see Chapter 33). A man voids more easily in the standing position. If a man cannot walk to the toilet facilities, he may stand at the bedside and void into a urinal (a plastic or metal receptacle for urine). If he is unable to stand at the bedside, the nurse needs to assist him in using the urinal in bed.

DELEGATION CONSIDERATIONS

This skill may be delegated to assistive personnel. The nurse provides assistive personnel with information, assistance, and direction, including:

- Caution assistive personnel to be sensitive to the privacy needs of the client.
- Instruct assistive personnel to report information about urine such as changes in color, amount, or odor and the presence of incontinence.
- Inform assistive personnel about the amount of assistance the client requires to use the urinal and if standing is permitted.
- Remind assistive personnel to teach the client and family about the procedure, so they can more fully understand and participate in care.

EQUIPMENT

- ❏ Urinal (Figure 32-1)
- ❏ Disposable gloves
- ❏ Graduated cylinder (used for measuring volume if urinal is not marked)
- ❏ Supplies for diagnostic urine tests and specimen collection (see Chapter 43)

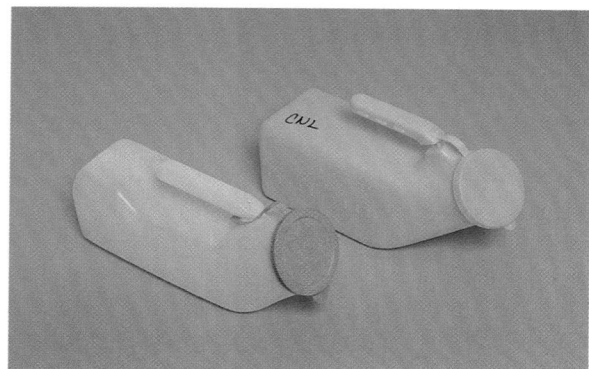

FIGURE **32-1** Types of male urinals.

STEP	RATIONALE

ASSESSMENT

1. Assess client's normal urinary elimination habits.

   Identifies normal pattern of urination; helps nurse to recognize when client may require use of urinal.
2. Assess for periods of incontinence.

   May assist in planning when to offer urinal.
3. Palpate for distended bladder.

   Indicates if bladder is full and client needs to void.
4. Assess client's cognitive and physical status.

   Provides nurse with information about how much assistance is required to use urinal.
5. Assess client's knowledge regarding urinal use.

   Reveals need for client instruction.

NURSING DIAGNOSES

* Deficient knowledge regarding use of urinal
* Impaired urinary elimination

* Impaired physical mobility
* Toileting self-care deficit

Related factors are individualized based on client's condition or needs.

PLANNING

1. Expected outcomes following completion of procedure:
   * Client is able to assist self with urinal.

     Promotes self-care for toileting needs, decreases incontinence and its complications.
   * Client remains continent.

     Urinal offered in timely manner.

IMPLEMENTATION

1. Perform hand hygiene, and apply gloves.

   Reduces transmission of microorganisms.
2. Provide privacy by closing bedside curtain or room door.

   Provides privacy and reduces embarrassment to client, thus promoting relaxation.
3. Assist client into appropriate position: on side, back, or sitting with head of bed elevated, or assist to standing position.

   Men find it easier to void and empty bladder while standing.

* ### Critical Decision Point
  Always determine mobility status before having a client stand to void.

4. If possible, client should hold urinal and position penis in urinal. If client needs assistance, position penis completely within urinal and hold urinal in place or assist client with holding urinal.

   Penis is placed completely within urinal to avoid urine spills.
5. Once client has finished voiding, remove urinal, and wash and dry penis.

   Prevents growth of microorganisms. Prevents skin breakdown.
6. Observe urine, empty and cleanse urinal, and return it to client for future use.

   Avoids spilling and reduces odors.
7. Allow client to perform hand hygiene after voiding.

   Reduces spread of microorganisms.
8. Remove and dispose of gloves; perform hand hygiene.

   Reduces spread of microorganisms.

EVALUATION

1. Observe client's ability to use urinal.

   Determines level of assistance required by client.
2. Monitor for periods of incontinence.

   Determines frequency needed to assist client with using urinal.

Recording and Reporting

* Record and report client's ability to use urinal and characteristics of urinary output in nurses' notes.
* If I&O measurement is being monitored in client, include output data on flow sheet (see Chapter 18).
* Record client's voiding patterns, and report problems with voiding to physician.

Unexpected Outcomes	Related Interventions
1. Client is incontinent.	• Increase frequency of prompted voidings. • Ensure client can reach urinal. • Monitor skin integrity. • Determine type of incontinence.
2. Client unable to void using a urinal.	• Attempt to place client in standing position and provide privacy (see Skill Performance Guidelines).
3. Client experiences persistent urge, stress, or overflow incontinence.	• Refer for urological evaluation.

Teaching Considerations

- Clients should be taught not to ignore the urge to void. Poor habits may contribute to urinary retention (incomplete emptying of the bladder) problems.
- Hand hygiene is the best method for preventing infection. Clients may need this basic hygienic tip reinforced.
- Clients who are having difficulty with incontinence at night should be instructed to avoid tea, coffee, and other caffeine drinks during the evening hours.

Pediatric Considerations

- Children who have been continent may become incontinent as a result of the stress from being ill but also if they are receiving intravenous (IV) fluids through the night. Attempts should be made to offer the urinal at appropriate times during the night such as with vital signs to prevent the embarrassment caused by the unexpected lack of control.
- Privacy norms will vary from household to household and with child's age. If child prefers privacy, nurse tries to prevent interruptions as child voids.
- Physiologically children can control their sphincters between the ages of 18 and 24 months (Hockenberry and others, 2003).

Gerontological Considerations

- Aging process may impair micturition; older men may require urinal use more frequently to avoid urinary incontinence.
- The older man who is accustomed to standing to void may empty his bladder more readily if allowed to stand when using the urinal.
- Nocturia is common in older adults; use of urinal at night may help to prevent falls in an unfamiliar setting such as a hospital (Lueckenotte, 2000).

Home Care Considerations

- Assess level of assistance required by client to determine if additional medical equipment (e.g., over-bed trapeze, bedside commode) is necessary for the client to maintain continence.
- Before hospital discharge consider referral to home care agency to follow up and reinforce teaching concepts.

Long-Term Care Considerations

- Urinary incontinence is a frequent problem in long-term care. All residents should have a baseline assessment of any urinary problem. Assessment for individuals with urinary incontinence should include a history and physical examination, a voiding diary, a urinalysis, and postvoid residual urine determination (Gray and Haas, 2000).

SKILL 32-2 Inserting a Straight or an Indwelling Catheter

Catheterization of the bladder involves introducing a rubber or plastic tube through the urethra and into the bladder. The catheter provides for a continuous flow of urine in clients unable to control micturition or in those with obstruction to urine outflow. Because bladder catheterization carries the risk of the development of urinary tract infection (UTI), it is preferable to rely on less invasive measures to promote bladder emptying.

An indwelling or Foley catheter may remain in place for an extended period especially with critically ill clients. It may be necessary to change indwelling catheters periodi-

cally; however, typically every attempt is made to remove a catheter as soon as a client can void independently. The nurse uses sterile asepsis when inserting an indwelling or straight catheter to reduce the risk of bladder infections. Intermittent catheterization involves insertion of a catheter for a one-time bladder emptying. When a straight catheter is used, the procedure can be repeated as necessary. Intermittent catheterization has been shown to lower UTI rates and eliminate many of the complications associated with indwelling catheters in clients with spinal cord lesions undergoing rehabilitation (Biering-Sorensen and others, 2001).

DELEGATION CONSIDERATIONS

The use of assistive personnel for inserting urinary catheters may occur in some settings (see agency policy). Otherwise, assistive personnel may assist with positioning the client, focusing lighting for the procedure, and aiding in the client's comfort during the procedure by measures such as holding the client's hand or keeping the client warm.

EQUIPMENT

- ❏ Catheterization kit (Figure 32-2) containing the following sterile items: gloves (extra pair optional); drapes, one fenestrated; lubricant antiseptic cleansing solution; cotton balls; forceps; prefilled syringe with sterile water to inflate balloon of indwelling catheter; catheter of correct size and type for procedure (i.e., intermittent or indwelling); sterile drainage tubing with collection bag and multipurpose tube holder or tape, safety pin, and elastic band for securing tubing to bed if client is bedridden (for indwelling catheter); receptacle or basin (usually at the bottom of the catheterization tray); and specimen container
- ❏ Option: Double or triple lumen indwelling catheter if client is to receive catheter irrigation (see Skill 32-5).
- ❏ Blanket

- ❏ Waterproof absorbent pad
- ❏ Disposable gloves, basin with warm water, soap, washcloth, and towel
- ❏ Flashlight or other appropriate additional light as needed

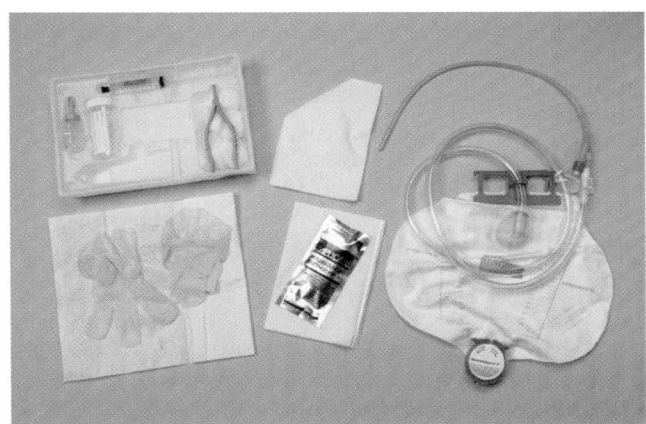

FIGURE **32-2** Kit of indwelling catheterization kit (includes drainage device, specimen cup, sterile drapes, sterile gloves, indwelling catheter, cleansing solution, sterile saline, sterile cotton balls, forceps, and lubricant).

STEP	RATIONALE

■ ASSESSMENT

1. Review client's medical record, including physician's order and nurses' notes.

Determines purpose of inserting catheter: preparation for surgery, urinary irrigations, collection of sterile urine specimen, or measurement of residual urine. Assess for previous catheterization, including catheter size, response of client, and time of last catheterization. Catheters may range in size from 5 Fr to 30 Fr.

STEP	RATIONALE
2. Assess status of client:	
a. Ask client when was time of last urination. Check I&O flow sheet.	Determines time of last voiding and indicates likelihood of bladder fullness.
b. Level of awareness or developmental stage	Reveals client's ability to cooperate during procedure and level of explanation needed.
c. Mobility and physical limitations of client	Affect way that nurse positions client. Nurse can request additional nursing personnel to assist with this procedure if necessary.
d. Client's gender and age	Determines catheter size: 5 to 6 Fr is generally used for an infant; 8 to 10 Fr with 3-ml balloon is generally used for children; 14 to 16 Fr is indicated for adult women; 12 Fr may be considered for young girls; 16 to 18 Fr is used for male clients. Larger sizes may be ordered by physician.
3. Determine if client has distended bladder (bladder palpable above symphysis pubis). When bladder is full, palpation causes urge.	Palpation causes pain. Full bladder with inability to void may indicate need to insert catheter.
4. Assess for perineal anatomical landmarks, erythema, drainage, and odor.	Determines condition of perineum.
5. Identify any pathological condition that may impair passage of catheter (e.g., enlarged prostate gland in men).	Obstruction prevents passage of catheter through urethra into bladder.

• *Critical Decision Point*

Determine allergy to antiseptic, tape, latex, and lubricant. Betadine allergies are common; if the client is unaware of allergy, ask if allergic to shellfish.

6. Assess client's knowledge of the purpose for catheterization and whether client has had catheter placed previously.	Reveals need for client instruction and/or support.

NURSING DIAGNOSES

- Anxiety
- Acute pain
- Urinary retention

- Deficient knowledge regarding need for catheterization
- Risk for infection

Related factors are individualized based on client's condition or needs.

PLANNING

1. Expected outcomes following completion of procedure:	
• Bladder is not palpable.	Removal of urine from bladder relieves sensation of fullness.
• Client will verbalize relief of discomfort in bladder.	Patent catheter system keeps bladder empty and client comfortable.
• Minimum of 30 ml of urine is present in urinary collection bag every hour (see Chapter 18).	Verifies presence of catheter in bladder, catheter patency, and adequate perfusion to kidneys.
• Client verbalizes minimal pain during procedure.	Correct insertion technique minimizes localized trauma to urethra.
• Client verbalizes the purpose and expectations about the procedure.	Promotes cooperation.

IMPLEMENTATION

1. Perform hand hygiene.	Reduces transmission of microorganisms. Infection is common after catheterization. Foley catheter systems are often colonized with bacteria within 48 hours of catheterization (Suchinski and others, 1999).
2. Close curtain or door.	Provides privacy and reduces embarrassment to client, thus promoting relaxation.

STEP	**RATIONALE**

3. Raise bed to appropriate working height.

Promotes use of proper body mechanics by nurse.

4. Facing client, stand on left side of bed if right-handed (on right side if left-handed). Clear bedside table, and arrange equipment.

Successful catheter insertion requires nurse to assume comfortable position with all equipment easily accessible.

5. If side rails in use, raise side rail on opposite side of bed, and lower side rail on working side.

Promotes client safety.

6. Place waterproof pad under client.

Prevents soiling of bed linen.

• *Critical Decision Point*
   Get assistance to position and to support weak or frail clients.

7. Position client:

Provides good visualization of perineal structures.

   a. Female client:

      (1) Assist to dorsal recumbent position (supine with knees flexed). Ask client to relax thighs so the hip joints can be externally rotated.

Legs may be supported with pillows to reduce muscle tension and promote comfort.

      (2) Position female client in side-lying (Sims) position with upper leg flexed at knee and hip if unable to be supine. If this position is used, nurse must take extra precautions to cover rectal area with drape during procedure to reduce chance of cross contamination.

This alternate position is used if client cannot abduct leg at hip joint (e.g., if client has arthritic joints). Also, this position may be more comfortable for client. Support client with pillows if necessary to maintain position.

   b. Male client:

      (1) Assist to supine position with thighs slightly abducted.

Comfortable position for client that aids in visualization of penis.

8. Drape client:

Avoids unnecessary exposure of body parts and maintains client's comfort.

   a. Female client:

      (1) Drape with bath blanket. Place blanket diamond fashion over client, with one corner at client's neck, side corners over each arm and side, and last corner over perineum.

   b. Male client:

      (1) Drape upper trunk with bath blanket, and cover lower extremities with bed sheet, exposing only genitalia.

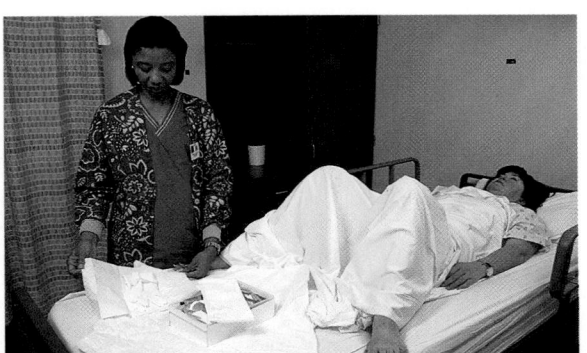

STEP **8a(1)** Position dorsal recumbent with client draped and supplies ready for use.

STEP	RATIONALE
9. Wearing disposable gloves, wash perineal area with soap and water as needed; dry (see Chapter 14).	Reduces microorganisms near urethral meatus (Haberstich, 2002).
10. Position lamp to illuminate perineal area. (When using flashlight, have assistant hold it.)	Permits accurate identification and good visualization of urethral meatus.
11. Perform hand hygiene.	Reduces transmission of microorganisms.
12. Open package containing drainage system; place drainage bag over edge of bottom bed frame, and bring drainage tube up between side rail and mattress.	Prepares bag for attachment to catheter.

• *Critical Decision Point*

This step is necessary only if indwelling catheter is to be inserted and drainage system is not part of the catheterization kit.

STEP	RATIONALE
13. Open catheterization kit according to directions, keeping bottom of container sterile.	Prevents transmission of microorganisms from table or work area to sterile supplies. The materials in the kit are arranged in sequence of use.
14. Place plastic bag that contains kit within reach of work area	Use as waterproof bag to dispose of used supplies.
15. Apply sterile gloves (see Chapter 9).	Allows nurse to handle sterile supplies without contamination.

• *Critical Decision Point*

If underpad is first item in kit, place the pad plastic side down under the client, touching only the edges so as to maintain sterility. Then apply sterile gloves (see Chapter 9 sterile fields).

STEP	RATIONALE
16. Organize supplies on sterile field. Open inner sterile package containing catheter. Pour sterile antiseptic solution into correct compartment containing sterile cotton balls (see illustration). Open packet containing lubricant. Remove specimen container (lid should be loosely placed on top) and prefilled syringe from collection compartment of tray, and set them aside on sterile field if needed.	Maintains principles of surgical asepsis and organizes work area.
17. Before inserting indwelling catheter, a common practice is to test balloon by injecting fluid from prefilled syringe into balloon port (see illustrations).	Checks integrity of balloon. Do not use the catheter if the balloon does not inflate or leaks. This is a controversial step. Follow manufacturer's recommendations. Checking the balloon in this way may stretch the balloon and cause increased trauma on insertion.

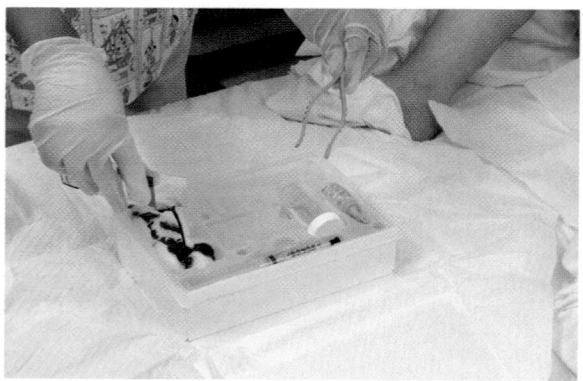

STEP **16** Pouring antiseptic solution over cotton balls.

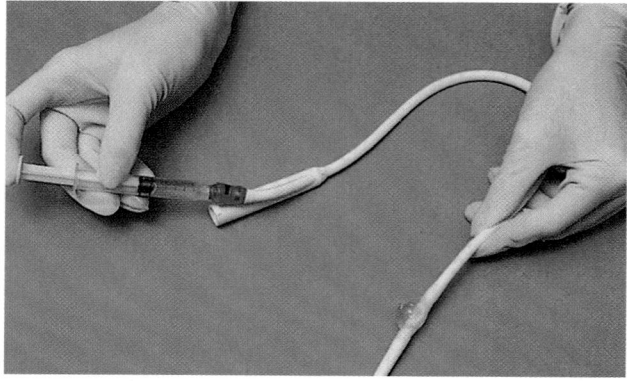

STEP **17** Balloon inflation.

STEP	**RATIONALE**
18. Lubricate catheter 2.5 to 5 cm (1 to 2 inches) for women and 12.5 to 17.5 cm (5 to 7 inches) for men (see illustration). NOTE: Some catheter kits will have a plastic sheath over the catheter that must be removed before lubrication. (*Optional:* Physician may order use of lubricant containing local anesthetic.)	Prevents urethral trauma. Inflamed tissue is more susceptible to infection (Haberstich, 2002).
19. Apply sterile drape, keeping gloves sterile:	
a. Female client:	
(1) Allow top edge of drape to form cuff over both hands. Place drape down on bed between client's thighs. Slip cuffed edge just under buttocks, taking care not to touch contaminated surface with gloves.	Outer surface of drape covering hands remains sterile. Sterile drape against sterile gloves is sterile.
(2) Pick up fenestrated sterile drape, and allow it to unfold without touching an unsterile object. Apply drape over perineum, exposing labia and being sure not to touch contaminated surface (see illustration).	Maintains sterility of work surface.
b. Male client: Two methods are used for draping, depending on preference.	Maintains sterility of work surface.
(1) *First method:* Apply drape over thighs and below penis without completely opening fenestrated drape.	
(2) *Second method:* Apply drape over thighs just below penis. Pick up fenestrated sterile drape, allow it to unfold, and drape it over penis with fenestrated slit resting over penis (see illustration).	
20. Place sterile tray and contents on sterile drape between legs. Open specimen container. NOTE: Client's size and positioning will dictate exact placement. This method works best with flexible, average-size clients.	Provides easy access to supplies during catheter insertion. Maintains aseptic technique during procedure.

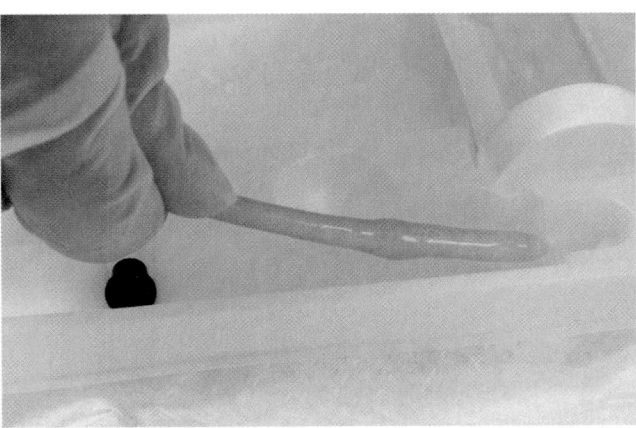

STEP **18** Lubricating catheter.

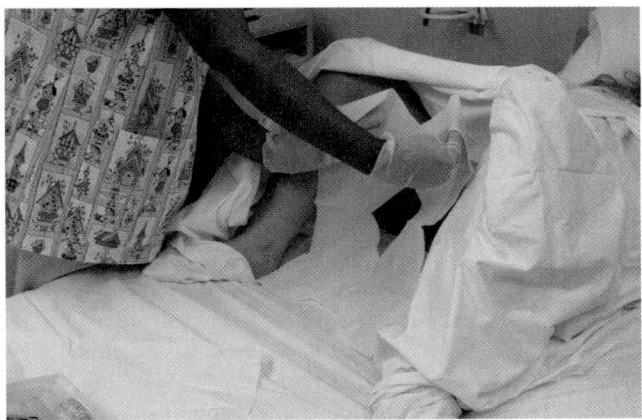

STEP **19a(2)** Place sterile fenestrated drape (with opening in center) over perineum with labia exposed.

STEP	RATIONALE

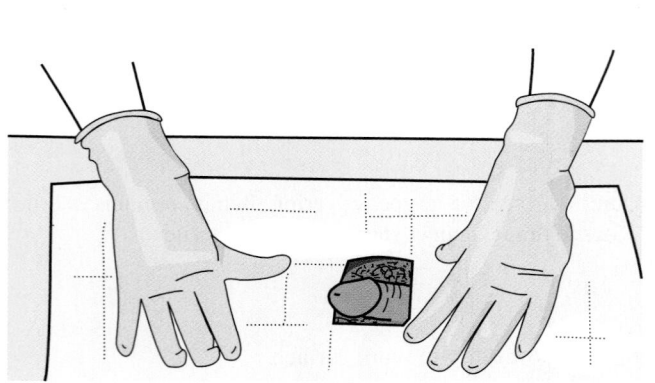

STEP **19b(2)** Draping male with fenestrated drape.

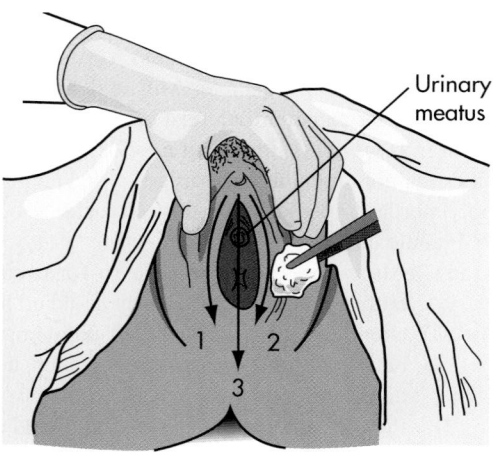

Urinary meatus

STEP **21a(2)** Cleansing female perineum.

21. Cleanse urethral meatus.

    a. Female client:

        (1) With nondominant hand, carefully retract labia to fully expose urethral meatus. Maintain position of nondominant hand throughout procedure.

Full visualization of urethral meatus is provided. Full retraction prevents contamination of urethral meatus during cleansing.

• Critical Decision Point

Closure of labia during cleansing requires that the procedure be repeated because the area has become contaminated.

        (2) Using forceps in sterile dominant hand, pick up cotton ball saturated with antiseptic solution, and clean perineal area, wiping front to back from clitoris toward anus. Using a new cotton ball for each area, wipe along the far labial fold, near labial fold, and directly over center of urethral meatus (see illustration).

Cleansing reduces number of microorganisms at urethral meatus. Cleansing moves from area of least contamination to that of most contamination. Dominant hand remains sterile.

    b. Male client:

        (1) If client is not circumcised, retract foreskin with nondominant hand. Grasp penis at shaft just below glans. Retract urethral meatus between thumb and forefinger. Maintain nondominant hand in this position throughout procedure.

Retraction exposes meatus for catheter insertion. Accidental release of foreskin or dropping of penis during cleansing requires process to be repeated because area has become contaminated.

• Critical Decision Point

If the foreskin does not remain retracted during insertion, then the cleansing procedure must be repeated because the area has become contaminated.

        (2) With dominant hand, pick up cotton ball with forceps, and clean penis. Move cotton ball in circular motion from urethral meatus down to base of glans. Repeat cleansing three more times, using clean cotton ball each time (see illustration).

Reduces number of microorganisms at urethral meatus and moves from areas of least to most contamination. Dominant hand remains sterile.

STEP	RATIONALE

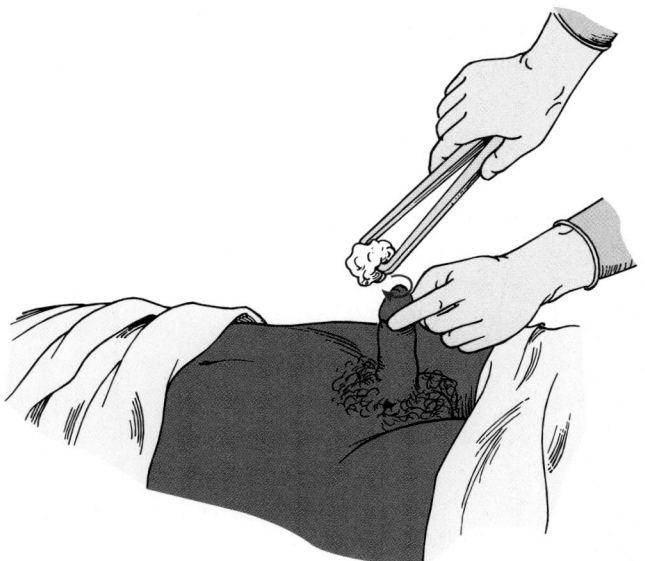

STEP **21b(2)** Cleansing male urinary meatus.

22. Pick up catheter with gloved dominant hand 7.5 to 10 cm (3 to 4 inches) from catheter tip. Hold end of catheter loosely coiled in palm of dominant hand. (*Optional:* May grasp catheter with forceps.) Place distal end of catheter in urine tray receptacle if straight catheterization is being done.

- **Critical Decision Point**
  Hold catheter near tip because it allows easier manipulation during insertion into urethral meatus and prevents distal end from striking contaminated surface.

23. Insert catheter:
    a. Female client:
       (1) Ask client to bear down gently as if to void, and slowly insert catheter through urethral meatus (see illustration).
       (2) Advance catheter a total of 5 to 7.5 cm (2 to 3 inches) in adult **or until urine flows out catheter's end.** As soon as urine appears, advance catheter another 2.5 to 5 cm (1 to 2 inches). Do not force against resistance. Place end of catheter in urine tray receptacle.

Relaxation of external sphincter aids in insertion of catheter.

Female urethra is short. Appearance of urine indicates that catheter tip is in bladder or lower urethra. Advancement of catheter ensures bladder placement.

- **Critical Decision Point**
  If no urine appears, check if catheter is in vagina. If misplaced, leave catheter in vagina as landmark indicating where not to insert, and insert another.

       (3) Release labia, and hold catheter securely with nondominant hand.

Bladder or sphincter contraction may cause accidental expulsion of catheter.

STEP	RATIONALE

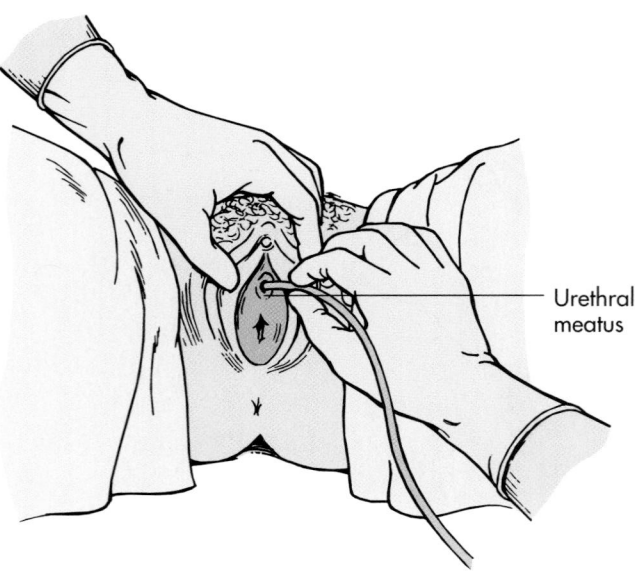

STEP **23a(1)** Inserting the catheter.

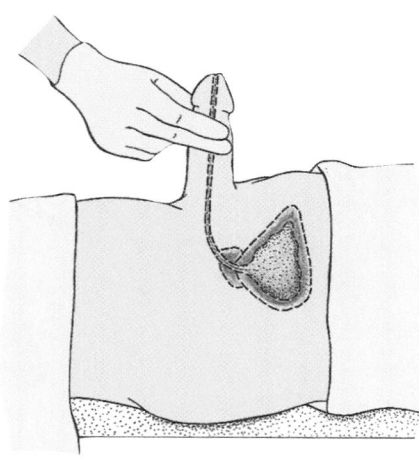

STEP **23b(1)** Position penis perpendicular to body for catheter insertion.

b. Male client:

(1) Lift penis to position perpendicular to client's body, and apply light traction (see illustration).

Straightens urethral canal to ease catheter insertion.

(2) Ask client to bear down as if to void, and slowly insert catheter through urethral meatus.

Relaxation of external sphincter aids in insertion of catheter.

(3) Advance catheter 17 to 22.5 cm (7 to 9 inches) in adult or **until urine flows out catheter's end.** If resistance is felt, withdraw catheter; do not force it through urethra. When urine appears, advance catheter to the bifurcation of the drainage and balloon inflation port (see illustration). **Do not use force to insert a catheter.**

The adult male urethra is long. It is normal to meet resistance at the prostatic sphincter. When resistance is met, nurse should hold catheter firmly against sphincter without forcing catheter. After few seconds, sphincter relaxes and catheter is advanced. Appearance of urine indicates catheter tip is in bladder or urethra. Further advancement of catheter to the bifurcation of the drainage and balloon inflation port ensures proper placement (Daneshgari and others, 2002).

(4) Lower penis, and hold catheter securely in nondominant hand. Place end of catheter in urine tray receptacle.

Catheter may be accidentally expelled by bladder or urethral contraction. Collection of urine prevents soiling and provides output measurement.

(5) Reduce (or reposition) the foreskin.

Paraphimosis (retraction and constriction of the foreskin behind the glans penis) secondary to catheterization may occur if foreskin is not reduced.

24. Collect urine specimen as needed. Fill specimen cup or jar to desired level (20 to 30 ml) by holding end of catheter in dominant hand over cup.

Allows sterile specimen to be obtained for culture analysis.

25. Allow bladder to empty fully unless institution policy restricts maximal volume of urine drained with each catheterization (about 800 to 1000 ml).

Retained urine may serve as reservoir for growth of microorganisms.

• Critical Decision Point

If a straight, single-use catheter was inserted, withdraw catheter slowly but smoothly until removed.

STEP	RATIONALE

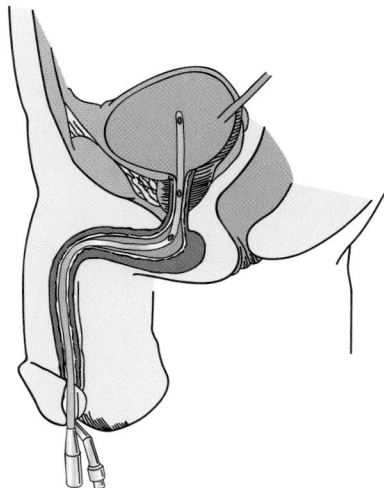

STEP **23b(3)** Male anatomy with correct catheter insertion to the bifurcation of the drainage and balloon inflation port.

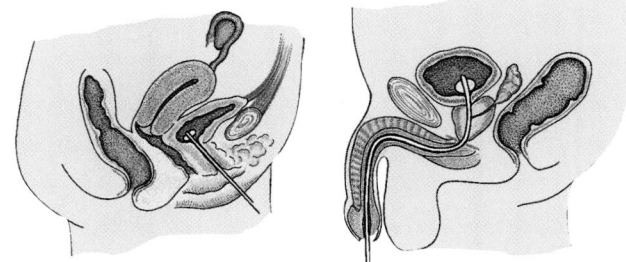

STEP **26** Placement of inflated balloon in bladder.

26. Inflate balloon fully with amount of fluid recommended by manufacturer.

    a. While holding catheter with nondominant hand at urethral meatus, take end of catheter and place it between first two fingers of nondominant hand.

    b. With free dominant hand, attach syringe to injection port at end of catheter.

    c. Slowly inject total amount of solution. If client complains of sudden pain, aspirate solution, and advance catheter further.

    d. After advancing catheter and/or inflating balloon, release catheter, and pull gently to feel resistance. Then move catheter slightly back into bladder.

Inflation of balloon anchors catheter tip in place above bladder outlet to prevent removal of catheter (see illustrations). Note the size of balloon on the catheter. Most commonly a 5-ml balloon is used, but a 30-ml balloon may be ordered. A prefilled syringe may be included with the kit; use only the amount included. Do not overinflate or underinflate the balloon.

• *Critical Decision Point*

    If resistance is noted to inflation or the client complains of pain, the balloon may not be entirely within the bladder. Stop inflation; aspirate any fluid injected into the balloon, and advance the catheter a little more before reattempting to inflate.

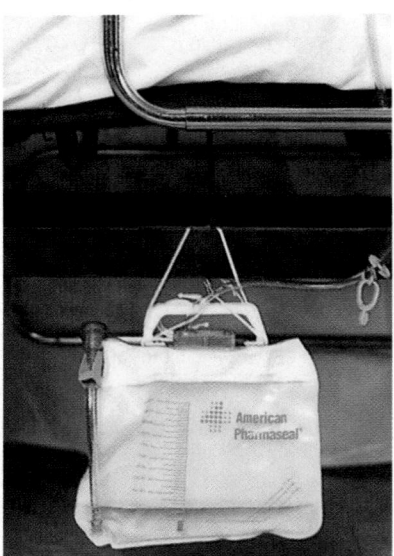

STEP **27** Drainage bag below level of bladder.

27. Attach end of catheter to collecting tube of drainage system. Drainage bag must be below level of bladder (see illustration); do not place bag on side rails of bed.

Establishes closed system for urine drainage. Placement on side rails could result in bag being raised above bladder.

28. Anchor catheter:
   a. Female client:
      (1) Secure catheter tubing to inner thigh with strip of nonallergenic tape (commercial multipurpose tube holders with a Velcro strap are also available). Allow for slack so movement of thigh does not create tension on catheter (see illustration). Clip drainage tubing to edge of mattress.

Anchoring catheter to inner thigh reduces pressure on urethra, thus reducing possibility of tissue injury in this area (Evans, 1999).

   b. Male client:
      (1) Secure catheter tubing to top of thigh or lower abdomen (with penis directed toward chest). Allow slack in catheter so movement does not create tension on catheter (see illustration). Clip drainage tubing to edge of mattress.

Anchoring catheter to lower abdomen reduces pressure on urethra at junction of penis and scrotum, thus reducing possibility of tissue injury in this area.

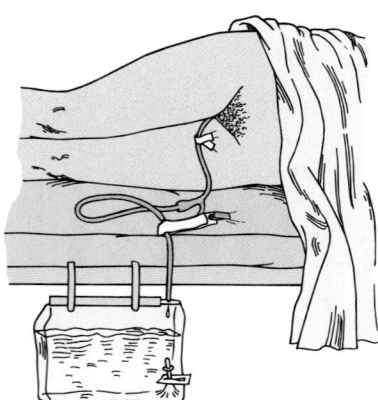

STEP **28a(1)** Securing the female indwelling catheter.

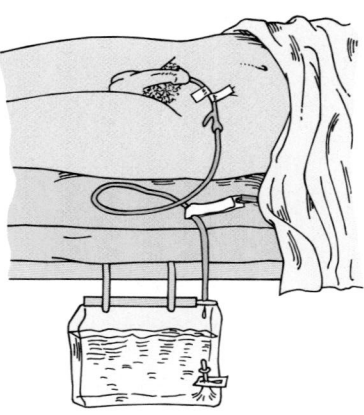

STEP **28b(1)** Securing the male indwelling catheter.

STEP	RATIONALE

- **Critical Decision Point**
  Be sure there are no obstructions in tubing. Coil excess tubing on bed and fasten it to bottom sheet with clip from kit or with rubber band and safety pin.

29. Assist client to comfortable position. Wash and dry perineal area as needed.	Maintains comfort and security.
30. Remove gloves, and dispose of equipment, drapes, and urine in proper receptacles.	Reduces transmission of microorganisms.
31. Perform hand hygiene.	Reduces spread of microorganisms.

EVALUATION

1. Palpate bladder.	Determines if distention is relieved.
2. Ask about client's comfort.	Determines if client's sensation of discomfort or fullness has been relieved.
3. Observe character and amount of urine in drainage system.	Determines if urine is flowing adequately.
4. Determine that there is no urine leaking from catheter or tubing connections.	Prevents injury to client's skin and ensures a closed sterile system.

Recording and Reporting

- Report and record type and size of catheter inserted, amount of fluid used to inflate balloon, characteristics of urine, amount of urine, reasons for catheterization, specimen collection, and, if appropriate, client's response to procedure and teaching topics.
- Empty drainage bag, and record amounts at least every 8 hours. Initiate I&O records (see Chapter 18).

Unexpected Outcomes	Related Interventions
1. No urine is present.	• *Female:* Catheter may be in vaginal opening. • *Male:* Catheter may not be advanced far enough through prostatic urethra. • Urine should drain freely. If not, nurse must further assess catheter placement and client's hydration status. • Assess the client for discomfort, and check intake record. If catheter is in the bladder and no urine is produced within 1 hour, absence of urine should immediately be reported to physician.
2. Catheter cannot be advanced.	• Retry unless client is experiencing discomfort. • If catheter cannot be advanced, notify physician.
3. Bladder discomfort persists despite catheter patency.	• This may indicate urethral spasm or bladder spasm. Notify physician.
4. Leakage of urine from around catheter.	• Indicates improper catheter placement, possible balloon deflation, or too small a catheter. Reinflate balloon, or replace catheter.

Continued

Unexpected Outcomes	Related Interventions
5. More than 500 to 1000 ml of urine drains from the catheter.	• Check institution policy before beginning catheterization; some agencies restrict maximal amount of urine that can be drained at one time. This amount may vary from 500 to 1000 ml.
6. Client with a spinal cord transection experiences the following symptoms: blood pressure (BP) elevated to 200 mm Hg systolic, bradycardia, headache, flushing and sweating above the spinal level of the injury. Spinal cord–injured (SCI) clients run the risk of autonomic dysreflexia (hyperreflexia) when exposed to a noxious stimulus such as a full bladder. Hyperreflexia is an autonomic response of the sympathetic system that results in dangerously high blood pressure. SCI clients who require intermittent catheterization are especially susceptible to dysreflexia.	• Immediately elevate head of bed. • Empty a full bladder by unkinking tubing or removing any blockage in the catheter tubing. • Notify physician (Lombardo and Hartwig, 2003).

Teaching Considerations

- Explain how the client can cooperate during the procedure.
- Explain to client that a burning and/or pressure sensation may be experienced during catheter insertion.
- Instruct client in ways to lie in bed with catheter. In the side-lying position facing the catheter, the tubing should drape over the thigh. In the side-lying position facing away from the catheter, the tubing should extend between the legs.
- Caution client against lying on tubing and against raising catheter bag and tubing above hips.
- Explain what is involved in the care of the catheter and drainage system.

Pediatric Considerations

- For an infant or young child, nurse must explain procedures to parent. Describe procedure to child at level he or she is able to understand (Hockenberry and others, 2003).
- Children and adolescents will experience some discomfort during catheterization. Assistance and gentle holding may be necessary, especially in younger child. Most children prefer to have the parents remain with them during procedure. Ask adolescents if they would like a parent to remain with them.
- Catheterization in infants and children can be made easier by use of an adequate amount of lubricant that contains 2% lidocaine (Hockenberry and others, 2003).
- Never force the catheter. If resistance is met, pause for approximately 20 seconds until sphincter relaxes, and continue to attempt insertion.

Gerontological Considerations

- A client with a catheter is especially vulnerable to UTI. The frail older adult client who is physically compromised runs the additional risk of developing septicemia, an infection that has spread to the blood; therefore indwelling catheters should be used only in select circumstances (Lueckenotte, 2000).
- Ensuring adequate oral fluid intake of 2000 ml/day and assisting the older adult with toileting on a regular timed basis will help bladder retraining and minimize the need for excessive catheterization.
- Attached equipment such as a catheter may make it more likely that the older adult will not be fully ambulatory, thereby increasing the risks associated with decreased mobility. When catheters are required, they should be removed as soon as the client's condition allows.

Home Care Considerations

- Clients who are at home may use a leg bag during the day and switch to a large-volume bag at night so that sleep can remain uninterrupted.
- Clients may catheterize themselves at home on an intermittent basis using clean technique. Self-catheterization may be successful in maintaining continence and can result in fewer infections than the use of indwelling catheters (Biering-Sorensen and others, 2001).

Long-Term Care Considerations

- Appropriate use of indwelling catheters may include incontinent residents who have wounds that are contaminated by urine and in clients who are terminally ill (Doherty, 2001).

SKILL 32-3 Care and Removal of the Indwelling Catheter

Clients with indwelling catheters require specific perineal hygiene care to reduce the risk of UTI. Any secretions or encrustation at the catheter insertion site must be completely removed (see Chapter 14). Perineal care and the cleansing of the first 4 inches of the exposed catheter every 8 hours is minimally expected. This is often referred to as catheter care. The use of powders or lotions on the perineum is contraindicated because of the risk of growth of microorganisms, which may ascend the urinary tract.

Removal of a retention catheter is a skill requiring clean technique. When removing a retention catheter, the nurse must prevent trauma to the urethra. If the retention catheter balloon is not fully deflated, its removal can result in trauma and subsequent swelling of the urethral meatus, and urinary retention can occur.

If the catheter was in place for more than several days, the client may experience dysuria resulting from inflammation of the urethral canal. Because of decreased bladder muscle tone, the client may urinate frequently.

DELEGATION CONSIDERATIONS

The skill of performing routine catheter care and removing a catheter can be delegated to assistive personnel. The nurse provides assistive personnel with information, assistance, and direction, including:

- Instruct assistive personnel to report catheter drainage (color, odor, amount).
- Instruct assistive personnel to report condition of catheter tubing (leaks, discharge, encrustation) and condition of perineum (color, discharge, contamination from fecal incontinence).
- Remind assistive personnel to check size of balloon and size of syringe needed to deflate balloon and to report if balloon does not deflate and/or if there is excessive burning or bleeding.
- Instruct assistive personnel to measure first voiding and to report time and amount to nurse.

EQUIPMENT

- ❑ Disposable gloves (needed for care and removal)
- ❑ Bed protector
- ❑ Bath blanket
  For Catheter Care
- ❑ Soap, washcloth, basin, and water (to cleanse perineum before catheter care)
- ❑ Graduated cylinder (used if urine collection bag will be emptied)
  For Removing a Catheter
- ❑ Syringe (same size as volume of solution used to inflate balloon) (information on balloon size can be obtained directly from balloon inflation valve on catheter)
- ❑ Waterproof pad
- ❑ Correctly labeled sterile specimen container, alcohol or other disinfectant swab, and 25-gauge $\frac{1}{2}$-inch needle (if culture and sensitivity are to be obtained before catheter removal)

STEP	RATIONALE
ASSESSMENT	
1. Determine how long catheter has been in place. Check agency policy to determine how often indwelling catheter must be changed.	Catheters in place for more than a few days are more likely to cause urethral irritation and buildup of encrustation.
2. Observe any discharge or encrustation around urethral meatus.	May indicate inflammatory process and may harbor bacteria.
3. Assess for complaints of pain or discomfort; determine location and type of pain client is experiencing; assess for presence of allergies (e.g., to antiseptic solution).	Indicates potential UTI.
4. Monitor client's temperature.	Increased temperature may be a symptom of UTI.
5. Determine client's fluid intake.	Lack of fluid intake reduces natural flushing of urinary system and increases chance of bacterial growth.
6. Assess urine color, clarity, odor, and amount.	Cloudy urine and urine with a strong odor may indicate UTI; possible indicator of client's volume status.
7. Assess client's knowledge of catheter care or removal procedure.	Reveals need for client instruction.

STEP	RATIONALE
8. Assess need or order for catheter removal.	Indwelling catheters are a primary risk factor for UTIs and should be used only when necessary and discontinued when they are no longer clinically indicated (Haberstich, 2002).

NURSING DIAGNOSES

- Risk for infection
- Impaired urinary elimination
- Deficient knowledge regarding perineal care

- Acute pain
- Toileting self-care deficit

Related factors are individualized based on client's condition or needs.

PLANNING

1. Expected outcomes following completion of procedure:	
• Urethral meatus is free of secretions and encrustation.	Indicates absence of irritation.
• Urine is clear, and volume is sufficient.	Indicates absence of UTI and adequate output.
• Client is afebrile.	Indicates absence of infection.
• Skin under tape site is intact and not abraded, open, or reddened.	
• Client will verbalize feeling of comfort after procedure is completed.	Cleansing relieves local discomfort.
• After catheter is removed, the client voids without discomfort and voids a minimum of 250 ml of urine with each voiding within 6 to 8 hours of catheter removal.	Indicates return of voluntary bladder function without urinary retention.

IMPLEMENTATION

1. Perform hand hygiene, and apply gloves.	Reduces transmission of microorganisms.
2. Close curtain, or close door.	Provides privacy and reduces embarrassment to client, thus promoting relaxation.
3. Raise bed to appropriate working height. If side rails are raised, lower side rail on working side.	Promotes nurse's use of proper body mechanics.
4. Organize equipment for perineal care or removal of catheter.	Increases efficiency of procedure.

- *Critical Decision Point*

  Get assistance for positioning the weak or frail client as necessary.

5. Position client, and cover with bath blanket, exposing only perineal area.
   a. Female in dorsal recumbent position.
   b. Male in supine position.
	Reduces client's embarrassment. Ensures easy access to perineal tissues.

6. **Catheter Care** a. Don gloves and place waterproof pad under client.	Protects bed from soiling.
b. Provide routine perineal care as outlined in Chapter 14.	
c. Assess urethral meatus and surrounding tissues for inflammation, swelling, and discharge, and ask client if burning or discomfort is felt.	Determines local infection and status of hygiene.
d. Using a clean washcloth, wipe in circular motion along length of catheter for about 10 cm (4 inches).	Reduces presence of secretions or drainage on outside catheter surface.

- *Critical Decision Point*

  Note the presence of any encrustation, and clean thoroughly.

STEP	RATIONALE
e. Replace as necessary the adhesive tape or multi-purpose tube holder that anchors catheter to client's leg or abdomen. Remove adhesive residue from skin.	Secures catheter, thus reducing risk of catheter being pulled and exposing portion of catheter that was in urethra. Also prevents drag on catheter and avoids creating pressure from balloon on bladder floor.
f. Avoid placing tension on the catheter.	Tension causes urethral trauma.
g. Replace tubing and collection bag as necessary and/or according to agency policy, adhering to principles of surgical asepsis.	Urinary tubing and collection bag should be changed if there are signs of leakage, odor, or sediment buildup. The catheterization system, including the catheter, may need to be replaced if leaking or blockage occurs.
h. Check drainage tubing and bag to ensure that:	
(1) Tubing is not looped or positioned above level of bladder.	Prevents pooling of urine and reflux of urine into bladder.
(2) Tubing is coiled and secured onto bed linen.	Prevents looping of tubing and subsequent pooling of urine.
(3) Tube is not kinked or clamped.	Prevents stasis of urine in bladder. Also ensures that client is not lying on tubing, causing pressure on skin and increasing risk of pressure ulcer.
(4) Collection bag is positioned appropriately on the bed frame.	Ensures appropriate drainage of urine.
i. Collection bag should be emptied as necessary but at least every 8 hours.	Urine in collection bag is excellent medium for growth of microorganisms.
7. Catheter Removal	
Refer to Steps 1 through 5 as necessary.	
a. Don gloves and place waterproof pad:	Prevents soiling of bed linen. Provides wrapper to cover contaminated catheter after removal, thus eliminating possibility of urine contaminating nurse's gloved hand.
(1) Between female's thighs (if in supine position)	
(2) Over male's thighs	
b. Obtain sterile urine specimen if required (see Chapter 43).	Determines if bacteria are present in urine.
c. Remove adhesive tape or Velcro tube holder used to secure and anchor catheter.	Allows for positioning of catheter for removal.
d. Insert hub of syringe into inflation valve (balloon port). Aspirate entire amount of fluid used to inflate balloon (see illustration).	Deflates balloon to allow for removal. If solution is not completely aspirated, partially inflated balloon causes trauma to urethral wall as catheter is removed.

- *Critical Decision Point*

    Do not use force to make the syringe fit into the valve.

| **e.** Pull catheter out smoothly and slowly. | Prevents trauma to urethral mucosa. |

- *Critical Decision Point*

    Stop pulling catheter if resistance is met; balloon is probably still inflated. Aspirate again to ensure all fluid has been removed. If still meet resistance, notify physician.

f. Wrap contaminated catheter in waterproof pad. Unhook collection bag and drainage tubing from bed.	Prevents contamination of nurse's hands.
8. When catheter care and/or removal is completed:	
a. Reposition client as necessary. Cleanse perineum, and remove any adhesive residue from skin. Lower level of bed, and position side rails accordingly.	Promotes client comfort and safety.
b. Measure and empty contents of collection bag.	Provides accurate recording of urinary output.
c. Dispose of all contaminated supplies correctly, remove gloves, and perform hand hygiene.	Reduces spread of microorganisms.

STEP	**RATIONALE**

EVALUATION

1. Inspect the condition of the urethra and surrounding tissue, and ask client about discomfort.
2. Note character and amount of urine.

3. Observe time and amount of first voided specimen.

Determines if area is cleansed properly and/or if client has any irritation.
Helps indicate if infection is present and output is adequate before and after catheter removed.
Indicates return of bladder function.

Recording and Reporting

- Ensure that times for catheter care are set in the care plan. Clients with indwelling catheters should receive perineal and catheter care every 8 hours and after bowel movements.
- Record in nurses' notes when catheter care was given, removal of catheter and condition of urethral meatus, and character of urine.

Unexpected Outcomes	**Related Interventions**
1. Urethral or perineal irritation is present.	• Observe for leaking, and replace catheter if necessary. • If catheter is present, ensure that indwelling catheter is anchored as outlined in Skill 32-2. • If securing catheter does not help, or if catheter has been removed, notify physician of urethral irritation.
2. Client has fever and/or odor is present, or client experiences small, frequent voidings or any burning or bleeding.	• Monitor vital signs and urine, but report findings to physician because any of these symptoms/signs may indicate a UTI.
3. Client experiences urinary retention and is unable to void after catheter removal	• Ensure adequate intake and privacy, and facilitate urination by relaxation (see Skill Performance Guidelines). • If client unable to void within 6 to 8 hours of catheter removal, notify physician.

Teaching Considerations

- Unless contraindicated, clients with a catheter should drink at least 2000 ml of fluid per day to promote continuous flushing of the bladder, preventing sediment from collecting in the catheter tubing.
- Instruct client to hold collection bag below the level of the bladder when ambulating.
- Instruct client to keep the collection bag off the floor, where microorganisms are abundant.
- Instruct client not to disconnect the catheter from the collection tubing and bag.

Pediatric Considerations

- Do not force catheter out of bladder if resistance is met. When excessive tubing has been inserted in bladder, there have been occurrences of knotting of the tube (Hockenberry and others, 2003).

Gerontological Considerations

- The older adult client may exhibit atypical signs and symptoms of UTI. Although the usual symptoms of dysuria, urgency, frequency, odor, and hematuria should be assessed, they may not be present. The assessment must also include assessing for less specific signs such as fever and/or mental status changes including agitation, lethargy, and confusion.

Home Care Considerations

- Assess client and primary caregiver for ability and motivation to participate in routine catheter care.
- Silicone catheters may be a better choice for client in the home or in long-term care facilities, where catheterization for longer periods of time may be done, because the silicone is less likely to become encrusted. Encrustation harbors microorganisms and increases irritation.

SKILL 32-4 Obtaining Catheterized Specimens for Residual Urine

Residual urine is the volume of urine in the bladder after a normal voiding. Clients suspected of retaining urine are assessed for residual urine. Urinary retention is the inability of the bladder to fully empty.

Clients at risk for large residual volumes include those receiving bladder training exercises, such as those with spinal cord injuries, those who have suffered a cerebrovascular accident, and those who have had bladder surgery.

DELEGATION CONSIDERATIONS

The skill of obtaining catheterized specimens for residual urine should not be delegated to assistive personnel. Assistive personnel may assist with positioning clients, adjusting lighting, or comforting client during procedure.

EQUIPMENT

❑ Equipment listed in Skill 32-3
❑ Straight catheter

STEP	RATIONALE
ASSESSMENT	
1. Review prior I&O record.	Identifies usual amount of urine client voids during each voiding.
2. Determine if client experiences pain or discomfort when voiding.	Pain may be associated with bladder spasms.
3. Review physician's order to determine how often residual urine must be checked.	Order must be obtained from physician before nurse can catheterize client. Physician's order indicates when this procedure is no longer necessary (e.g., check residual urine twice a day until amount obtained is less than 100 ml).
4. Check time of last voiding before catheterization.	Residual urine determinations should be performed immediately after voiding to obtain accurate information about amount of urine remaining in bladder.
5. Assess client's knowledge regarding urinary retention and previous experience with catheterization.	Reveals need for client education and support.

NURSING DIAGNOSES

- Anxiety
- Deficient knowledge regarding residual urine
- Impaired urinary elimination

- Risk for infection
- Urinary retention

Related factors are individualized based on client's condition or needs.

PLANNING

1. Expected outcomes following completion of procedure:	
• Successive catheterizations result in decreasing amount of residual urine.	Client gains improved bladder control.
• Urine remains clear and dilute, without foul odor.	Removal of retained urine reduces medium for bacterial growth.
• The client explains the purpose of the procedure and what is expected.	Helps to minimize anxiety.

STEP	RATIONALE

IMPLEMENTATION

1. Ask client to void completely, and measure volume of urine. | Determines how much client is able to void compared to how much urine remains in bladder, which will be measured by catheterization.

• **Critical Decision Point**
Remind ambulatory clients not to dispose of urine and that it must be measured.

2. Perform hand hygiene.	Reduces transmission of infection.
3. Proceed as for inserting straight catheter (see Skill 32-2).	Insertion of straight catheter drains residual urine.
4. Accurately measure urine obtained.	Allows amount retained (catheterized amount) to be compared to amount voided.
5. Remove catheter by pulling it out smoothly and slowly.	Prevents urethral trauma.
6. Dispose of contaminated supplies, remove gloves, and perform hand hygiene.	Reduces transmission of microorganisms.

EVALUATION

1. Compare amount of urine voided and amount obtained on catheterization.	Difference indicates whether procedure should be repeated. Volume should be less than 100 ml.
2. Urine is clear, dilute, and odor free.	Indicates absence of infection.

Recording and Reporting

• Report and record amount of urine voided, amount obtained from catheterization, and client's response.
• Report presence of unexpected outcomes to physician and other team members as appropriate.
• Initiate a voiding diary if frequency or incontinence persist.

Unexpected Outcomes	Related Interventions
1. Residual volume is greater than 100 ml of urine.	• Indicates inadequate bladder emptying; physician should be notified.
2. Urinary incontinence of small amount of urine occurs.	• Results from overflow incontinence from bladder distension. Physician should be notified.
3. Client has signs and symptoms associated with bladder infection.	• Monitor vital signs, and notify physician.

Teaching Considerations

- Although straight catheters are normally used to drain residual urine, the physician may order an indwelling Foley catheter insertion if residual urine volumes exceed a certain volume. This provides the option of keeping the catheter inserted if residual volume is high. If physician's order is written in such a manner, nurse may elect to perform residual catheterization with Foley catheter. This procedure will need to be clarified and explained to the client, who may be anxious about urinary problems.
- Clients need to be informed about symptoms of UTI. Infections can increase bladder spasms and lead to worsening of urine retention.
- Urine retention predisposes the client to UTI and urinary calculi. Signs and symptoms of UTI are a change in urinary elimination such as frequency or nocturia; pain in back or on urination (dysuria); changes in urine including odor, blood, or sediment in urine and color changes to dark yellow or pink; and systemic symptoms as fever and chills. The major symptom of urinary calculi is pain that is described as dull and aching to intense, and the pain can be localized in the flank, back, lower abdomen, or groin. In addition, the client may present with fever, chills, nausea, and vomiting.

Pediatric Considerations

- For infant or child, nurse must explain procedures to parent. Describe procedure to child at the level he or she is able to understand.
- Technique may be used when use of urine bags for obtaining specimens has not been successful.

Gerontological Considerations

- Urine retention is not considered a normal part of aging and therefore should not be dismissed.
- UTI that occurs as a result of residual urine can be devastating to the frail older adult. Septicemia, an infection that spreads into the circulation, may be life threatening.

SKILL 32-5 Performing Catheter Irrigation

Catheter irrigations are performed on an intermittent or continuous basis to maintain catheter patency. There are two types of irrigation systems: closed bladder irrigation systems and open irrigation systems. A closed bladder irrigation system provides intermittent or continuous irrigation of the system without disrupting the sterile alignment of the catheter and drainage system (Figure 32-3), thus decreasing the risk of bacteria entering the urinary tract. The closed system is used most frequently in clients who have had genitourinary surgery. These clients are at risk for occlusion of the Foley catheter by small blood clots and mucous fragments; they are also at risk for UTI.

The open irrigation system is also used to maintain catheter patency (Figure 32-4). However, this system is used when bladder irrigations are required less frequently (e.g., every 8 hours) and there are no blood clots or large mucous shreds in the urinary drainage. This type of irrigation requires the nurse to aseptically break the closed drainage system and maintain surgical asepsis throughout the procedure. Both systems can be used to irrigate the bladder with a medication to treat an infection or local bladder irritation.

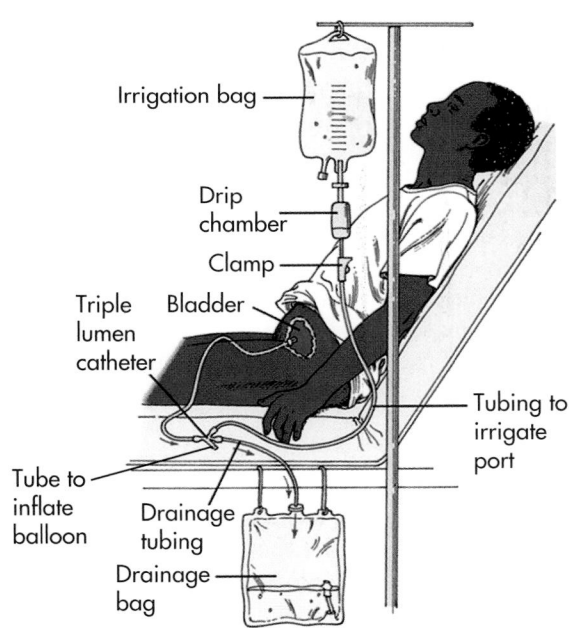

FIGURE **32-3** Closed continuous irrigation.

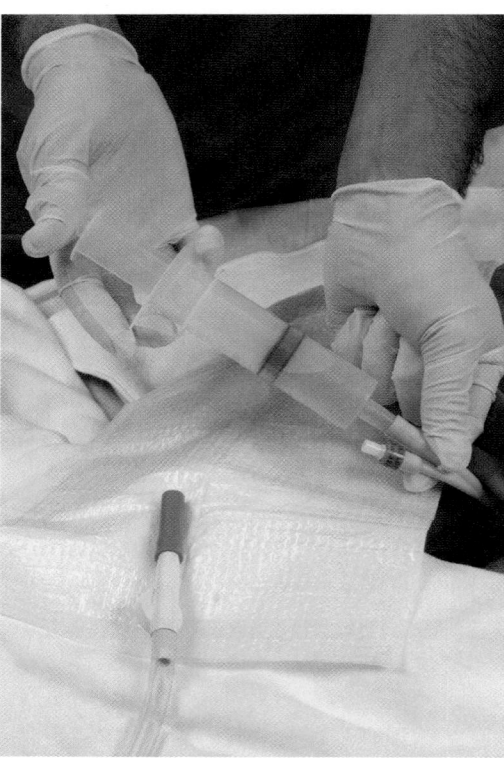

FIGURE **32-4** Aspirating fluid to deflate balloon.

DELEGATION CONSIDERATIONS

The skill of catheter irrigation should not be delegated to assistive personnel.

The nurse provides assistive personnel with the following directions:

- Instruct assistive personnel to inform nurse about complaints of pain, discomfort, or fever.
- Instruct assistive personnel to inform nurse about presence of blood clots in the drainage or a change in color of the drainage.
- Instruct assistive personnel to inform nurse about any decrease in drainage amount.

EQUIPMENT

Closed Continuous Method

- ❏ Sterile irrigating solution (unless otherwise specified in order) at room temperature
- ❏ Irrigation tubing with clamp (with or without Y connector) (clamp regulates irrigation flow rate; Y connector allows IV bags to be connected to tubing)
- ❏ IV pole
- ❏ Y connector (optional) (used to connect irrigation tubing to double-lumen catheter)

Closed Intermittent Method

- ❏ Sterile irrigating solution at room temperature
- ❏ Sterile graduate container
- ❏ Sterile 30- to 50-ml irrigation or cone syringe (used to instill irrigant into catheter)
- ❏ Sterile 19- to 22-gauge 1-inch needle
- ❏ Antiseptic swab
- ❏ Screw clamp (used to temporarily occlude catheter as irrigant is instilled)

Open Intermittent Method

- ❏ Sterile irrigating solution at room temperature (normal saline is most commonly used)
- ❏ Disposable sterile irrigation tray and set
- ❏ Bulb syringe or 60-ml piston type of syringe
- ❏ Sterile collection basin
- ❏ Waterproof drape
- ❏ Sterile solution container
- ❏ Antiseptic swabs
- ❏ Gloves
- ❏ Tape

STEP	RATIONALE

ASSESSMENT

1. Check client's record to determine:

   a. Purpose of bladder irrigation.

   Allows nurse to anticipate observations to make (e.g., blood or mucus in urine).

   b. Physician's order for type and amount of irrigant (e.g., saline).

   Order required to initiate therapy. Ensures that correct medication or solution and amount will be administered. Amount of solution used to flush system may be a nurse judgment or indicated by physician or institutional policy. Frequency of irrigation is based on need of client (e.g., client who has just had prostate gland surgery may require continuous irrigations for 24 hours).

   c. Type of irrigation: continuous or intermittent.

   Allows nurse to select proper equipment. In continuous irrigation, clamp regulates slow, steady flow into bladder. Because outflow should correspond to regulated irrigation drip, patency of catheter must be checked frequently to prevent distention of bladder. For intermittent irrigation, flow from irrigating solution is clamped for specified time and then opened, and designated amount of irrigating solution is allowed to flush into bladder. Intermittent irrigation requires close observation of catheter patency between irrigations.

   d. Type of catheter used (NOTE: Appropriate catheter should be inserted at time of original catheterization):

   Indicates if it is necessary to break system for irrigation.

      (1) Single lumen—used primarily with open irrigation.

      (2) Double lumen (one lumen to inflate balloon, one to allow outflow of urine).

      (3) Triple lumen (one lumen to inflate balloon, one to instill irrigant solution, and one to allow outflow of urine) (see Figure 32-3).

2. Assess the following:

   a. Color of urine and presence of mucus, clots, or sediment.

   Indicates if client is bleeding or sloughing tissue and determines necessity for increasing irrigation rates with continuous irrigations or increasing irrigation frequency with intermittent irrigations.

   b. Palpate bladder.

   Determines if urine is draining freely from bladder.

   c. Existing closed irrigation system:

   Determines presence of bladder distention.

      (1) Note if fluid entering bladder and fluid draining from bladder are in appropriate proportions.

      (2) Determine that drainage tubing is not kinked, clamped off incorrectly, or looped below bladder level.

   Determines if system is obstructed. One would expect more output than fluid instilled because of urine production.

      (3) Note amount of fluid remaining in existing irrigating solution container.

   Allows nurse to anticipate hanging of new irrigation bag.

STEP	RATIONALE

- **Critical Decision Point**
  If fluid cannot enter, or if fluid draining is less than amounts going in, stop the irrigation, assess, and notify the physician.

STEP	RATIONALE
3. Review I&O record.	Determines baseline for prior output measures. All clients with continuous bladder irrigations should have I&O measurements (see Chapter 18).
4. Assess client for presence of bladder spasms and discomfort.	Reveals need for bladder irrigation.
5. Assess client's knowledge regarding purpose of performing catheter irrigation.	Reveals need for client instruction.

NURSING DIAGNOSES

- Acute pain
- Impaired urinary elimination
- Risk for infection

- Deficient knowledge regarding the need for bladder irrigation

Related factors are individualized based on client's condition or needs.

PLANNING

1. Expected outcomes following completion of this procedure:
   - Output is greater than volume of irrigating solution used.

   - Absence of pain or discomfort.
   - Absence of fever; urine is not concentrated or foul smelling.
   - Client can explain purpose of procedure and what to expect.

   Indicates patency of drainage system. Patency promotes drainage of clots and mucus, which if trapped cause bladder spasms.
   Bladder empties, avoiding irritation and spasm.
   Indicates infection not likely present.

   Helps client relax and promotes cooperation.

IMPLEMENTATION

1. Perform hand hygiene.
2. Provide privacy: Pull curtains around bed, and fold back covers so catheter is exposed at junction where it connects to drainage tubing. Cover client's chest with bath blanket.
3. Position client in supine position, and remove tape or Velcro tube holder that is anchoring catheter to client. Be careful not to pull on catheter.
4. Organize appropriate supplies according to type of irrigation being performed.

   Reduces transmission of microorganisms.
   Promotes client's self-esteem; shows respect for client while exposing only area nurse must see.

   Allows for client comfort. Removing tape enables nurse to manipulate catheter.

STEP	RATIONALE
5. **Closed Intermittent Irrigation**	
a. Pour prescribed room-temperature sterile irrigating solution in sterile container. Be sure solution is not cold.	Cold solution may cause bladder spasm.
b. Clamp indwelling retention catheter below soft injection port or on drainage tubing.	Occlusion of catheter provides resistance against which irrigant can be forcefully instilled into catheter.
c. Draw sterile solution into syringe using aseptic technique. Keep tip of syringe sterile.	Ensures sterility of irrigating fluid.
d. Apply gloves.	Reduces risk of exposure to body fluids.
e. Cleanse catheter injection port with antiseptic swab (this same port is used for specimen collections).	Reduces transmission of infection.
f. Insert needle of syringe through port at 30-degree angle. (See manufacturer's instructions for possible variation.)	Ensures needle tip enters lumen of catheter and that needle does not puncture tubing.
g. Inject fluid into catheter and bladder.	The injection dislodges clots and sediment.

• *Critical Decision Point*

If catheter does not irrigate, tip may incorrectly be lodged in the urethra and not in the bladder. Use slow, even pressure when injecting fluid. Too much pressure may traumatize the bladder wall.

STEP	RATIONALE
h. Withdraw syringe, and remove clamp; allow solution to drain into urinary drainage bag. (Tubing is clamped temporarily to allow instilled fluid to remain in bladder, especially if irrigant is medicated.)	Allows drainage to flow via gravity.
6. **Closed Continuous Irrigation**	
NOTE: Supplies for closed irrigation system may be kept at bedside. Irrigating solution should be at room temperature. This practice is similar to that when bag of IV fluid is added to IV infusion. Using principles of medication safety, check that solution, volume, client, route, and time are correct. Discard any sterile solution not used within 24 hours of opening. Check institutional policy. When irrigant is opened, it should be marked with the date and time.	
a. Apply gloves, and using aseptic technique, insert (spike) tip of sterile irrigation tubing into bag containing irrigation solution.	Reduces transmission of microorganisms.
b. Close clamp on tubing, and hang bag of solution on IV pole.	Prevents loss of irrigating solution.
c. Open clamp, and allow solution to flow through tubing, keeping end of tubing sterile; close clamp, and recap end of tubing.	Removes air from tubing.
d. Use aseptic technique to connect tubing to drainage port of Y connector on double/triple lumen catheter.	

• *Critical Decision Point*

Be sure drainage bag and tubing are securely connected to drainage port of Y connector.

STEP	RATIONALE
e. For continuous irrigation, calculate drip rate, and adjust clamp on irrigation tubing accordingly to begin flow of solution into bladder; be sure clamp on drainage tubing is open, and check volume of drainage in drainage bag.	Ensures continuous, even irrigation of catheter system. Prevents accumulation of solution in bladder, which may cause bladder distention and possible injury.
f. For intermittent flow, clamp tubing on drainage system, open clamp on irrigation tubing, and allow prescribed amount of fluid to enter bladder (100 ml is normal for adult); close irrigation tubing clamp, and then open drainage tubing clamp.	Fluid is instilled through catheter in a bolus into bladder, flushing system. Fluid drains out after irrigation is complete.

- **Critical Decision Point**
  Do not leave a clamped drainage bag unattended. Check frequently, at least every hour.

7. **Open Irrigation**

STEP	RATIONALE
a. Apply gloves.	Reduces transmission of infection. Irrigation is a sterile procedure, but only parts of the system coming in contact with the inside of the catheter must remain sterile. The tip of the syringe, end of the catheter, end of the catheter tubing, and irrigant must remain sterile. Therefore the use of sterile gloves is optional.
b. Open sterile irrigation tray; establish sterile field, and pour required amount of sterile solution into sterile solution container. Replace cap on large container of solution.	Adheres to principles of surgical asepsis.
c. Position waterproof drape under catheter.	Prevents soiling of bed linen.
d. Aspirate 30 ml of solution into irrigating syringe. Place syringe in sterile solution container until ready to use.	Prepares irrigant for instillation into catheter. Maintains sterility of irrigating syringe.
e. Move sterile collection basin close to client's thigh.	Prevents soiling of bed linen and prohibits reaching over sterile area.
f. Wipe connection point between catheter and tubing with antiseptic wipe before disconnecting.	Reduces transmission of microorganisms.
g. Disconnect catheter from drainage tubing, allowing urine to flow into sterile collection basin; cover open end of drainage tubing with sterile protective cap, and position tubing so it stays coiled on top of bed.	Maintains sterility of inner aspect of catheter lumen and drainage tubing; reduces potential of introducing pathogens into bladder.
h. Insert tip of syringe into lumen of catheter, and gently instill solution.	Reduces incidence of bladder spasm but clears catheter of obstruction.

- **Critical Decision Point**
  If strong resistance is noted, do not force the irrigation.

STEP	RATIONALE
i. Withdraw syringe, lower catheter, and allow solution to drain into basin. Repeat, instilling solution and draining several times until drainage is clear of clots and sediment.	Allows drainage to flow by gravity. Provides for adequate flushing of catheter.
j. If solution does not return, have client turn onto side facing nurse; if changing position does not help, reinsert syringe and gently aspirate solution.	Change in position may move tip of catheter in bladder, increasing likelihood that fluid instilled will flow out.

STEP	RATIONALE
k. After irrigation is complete, remove protector cap from urinary drainage tubing adapter, cleanse adapter with alcohol swab, and reinsert adapter into lumen of catheter.	Reestablishes closed urinary drainage system.
8. Anchor catheter to client's leg or thigh with tape or Velcro multipurpose tube holder (see Skill 32-2).	Prevents trauma to urethral tissue.
9. Assist client into comfortable position.	Promotes relaxation and rest.
10. Lower bed to lowest position, and position side rails accordingly.	Promotes client safety.
11. Dispose of contaminated supplies, remove gloves, and perform hand hygiene.	Reduces spread of microorganisms.

EVALUATION

1. Calculate fluid used to irrigate bladder and catheter, and subtract from volume drained.	Determines accurate urinary output.
2. Assess characteristics of output: viscosity, color, and presence of clots.	Data serve as baseline to judge response to therapy.
3. Observe for catheter patency.	Ensures bladder emptying freely.
4. Observe client for signs of pain and fever.	Evaluates for presence of infection.
5. Observe urine to determine clarity, concentration, and odor.	Determines presence of bacteria in urine.

Recording and Reporting

- Record amount of solution used as irrigant, amount returned as drainage, characteristics of output, and urine output of drainage in nurses' notes and I&O sheet.
- Report catheter occlusion, sudden bleeding, infection, or increased pain to physician.

Unexpected Outcomes	Related Interventions
1. Irrigating solution is not returned or is not flowing at prescribed rate, which indicates possible occlusion of Foley catheter.	• Examine tubing for clots, sediment, and kinks. • Notify physician if irrigant is retained, client complains of pain, or bladder is distended.
2. Signs of fever or cloudy, foul urine are present.	• May indicate infection; physician should be notified. • Monitor vital signs and character of urine.
3. Increase in bladder spasms occurs. May indicate occlusion of catheter with foreign object (e.g., blood clot).	• Notify physician if large clots or sediment is returned or if spasms increase or are unrelieved. May need to change from intermittent to continuous irrigation.

Teaching Considerations

- Instruct client and primary caregiver to observe urine daily for changes in color, presence of mucus or blood, and changes in consistency and odor.
- Clients should be taught that bleeding is common after transurethral prostatectomy and that bright red–tinged urine during first 48 hours postoperatively followed by pink-tinged to clear urine by fifth postoperative day is expected.
- Instruct client to maintain adequate oral intake of 2 L/day (unless contraindicated).

Gerontological Considerations

- Benign prostatic hypertrophy is common as men age, and surgical intervention on the prostate gland may be required. After surgery, continuous and rapid irrigation of the bladder with a three-way Foley catheter is often necessary to prevent clotting and obstruction of the catheter. Often irrigant is adjusted to keep urine pink rather than a set rate.

Home Care Considerations

- Assess the client and primary caregiver for ability and motivation to perform catheter irrigation.
- Assess client's environment for appropriate storage space for materials needed for procedure.
- Observe client and primary caregiver while they perform procedure.

SKILL 32-6 Applying a Condom Catheter

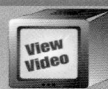

The external application of a urinary drainage device is a convenient, safe method of draining urine in male clients. The condom catheter is suitable for incontinent or comatose clients who still have complete and spontaneous bladder emptying. The condom is a soft, pliable rubber sheath that slips over the penis and is kept in place with the use of an elastic adhesive strip (Figure 32-5). The catheter may be attached to a leg drainage bag or a standard urinary drainage bag. Often this is a nursing-instituted procedure, but check policies to determine if a physician's order is required.

The often advised frequency for changing a condom catheter is every 24 hours. However, close monitoring every 4 hours to detect potential problems is necessary. With each catheter change, the nurse cleanses the urethral meatus and penis thoroughly and looks for signs of skin irritation.

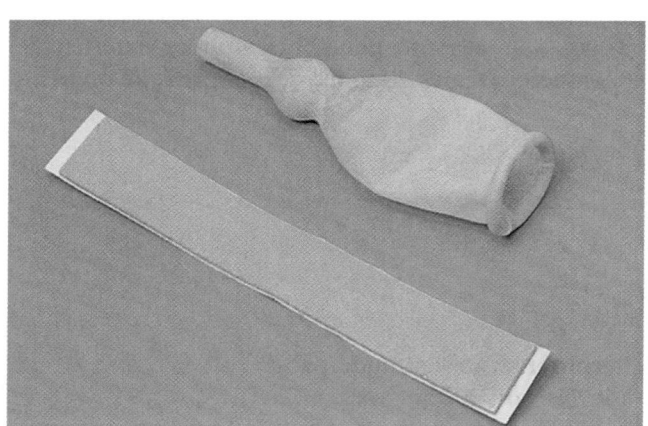

FIGURE **32-5** Condom catheter.

DELEGATION CONSIDERATIONS

The skill of applying a condom catheter can be delegated to assistive personnel. Consult policy, because delegation may vary with agencies. Before delegation the nurse assesses the skin of the client's penile shaft, making sure it is intact and free from swelling, redness, or open lesions. The nurse provides assistive personnel with information, assistance, and direction, including:

- Instruct assistive personnel to ask whether the client has a latex allergy.
- Instruct assistive personnel to follow manufacturer's directions on how to apply the adhesive strip that secures the condom catheter because methods for applying the catheter differ from manufacturer to manufacturer.

EQUIPMENT

- ❑ Condom catheter kit (rubber condom sheath of appropriate size, strip of elastic adhesive, skin preparation)
- ❑ Urinary collection bag with drainage tubing or leg bag and straps
- ❑ Basin with warm water and soap
- ❑ Towels and washcloth(s)
- ❑ Bath blanket
- ❑ Nonsterile disposable gloves
- ❑ Scissors and/or safety razor

STEP	RATIONALE

ASSESSMENT

1. Assess urinary elimination pattern, client's ability to voluntarily urinate, and continence.

2. Assess mental status of client so appropriate teaching related to condom catheter can be implemented.

Clients who are incontinent are at risk for skin breakdown and thus candidates for a condom catheter.

Some male clients may be incontinent only at night. Teaching can be implemented to instruct client on self-application.

STEP	RATIONALE
3. Assess condition of penis.	Provides baseline to compare changes in condition of skin after condom catheter application.
4. Assess client's knowledge of the purpose of a condom catheter.	Reveals need for client instruction.

NURSING DIAGNOSES

- Toileting self-care deficit
- Risk for impaired skin integrity
- Total urinary incontinence

     • Deficient knowledge regarding application of condom catheter

Related factors are individualized based on client's condition or needs.

PLANNING

1. Expected outcomes following completion of procedure:
   - Client is continent with condom catheter intact.   Catheter is secure; normal voiding occurs.
   - Penile shaft is free of skin irritation or breakdown.   Indicates absence of irritation.
   - Client can explain the purpose of the procedure and what to expect.   Reduces anxiety and promotes cooperation.

IMPLEMENTATION

1. Perform hand hygiene.	Reduces transmission of microorganisms.
2. Provide privacy by closing room door or bedside curtain.	Reduces embarrassment to client, thus promoting relaxation.
3. Raise bed to appropriate working height. If side rails raised, lower side rail on working side.	Promotes nurse's use of good body mechanics.
4. Assist client into supine position. Place bath blanket over upper torso. Fold sheets so lower extremities are covered; only genitalia should be exposed.	Promotes comfort; draping prevents unnecessary exposure of body parts.
5. Prepare urinary drainage collection bag and tubing. Clamp off drainage bag port. Secure collection bag to bed frame; bring drainage tubing up through side rails onto bed. *Optional:* Prepare leg bag for connection to condom.	Provides easy access to drainage equipment after condom catheter is in place.
6. Apply disposable gloves. Provide perineal care (see Chapter 14), and dry thoroughly.	Removes irritating secretions. Rubber sheath of condom rolls onto dry skin more easily.

- **Critical Decision Point**

   Clip hair at base of penis. In some cases shaving the hair at the base of the penis may be necessary. Hair adheres to condom and is pulled during condom removal or may get caught in rubber as condom catheter is applied.

7. Apply skin preparation to penis, and allow to dry. If client is uncircumcised, return foreskin to normal position.	Skin preparation has an alcohol base. Evaporation is necessary to prevent irritation.

STEP	RATIONALE

8. With nondominant hand, grasp penis along shaft. With dominant hand, hold condom sheath at tip of penis and smoothly roll sheath onto penis.

Prepares penis for easy condom placement.

- **Critical Decision Point**
  Allow 2.5 to 5 cm (1 to 2 inches) of space between tip of glans penis and end of condom catheter (see illustration step 8).

9. Apply adhesive.
    a. Spiral wrap penile shaft with strip of elastic adhesive. Strip should be spiral wrapped and not overlap itself (see illustration). Do not use any tape except that provided by the manufacturer. Other tapes will not provide the flexibility needed for spiral wrap and may impair circulation to the penis.
    b. For newer catheters that are self-adhesive, apply catheter as in steps 7 and 8, then apply gentle pressure on penile shaft for 10 to 15 seconds to secure catheter.

Condom must be secured firmly so it is snug and stays on but not tight enough to cause constriction of blood flow. With some brands of catheters the adhesive strip is applied before the condom is applied.

- **Critical Decision Point**
  Never use adhesive tape in the application of the condom catheter because it may impede circulation.

10. Connect drainage tubing to end of condom catheter. Be sure condom is not twisted. Catheter can be connected to large-volume bag or leg bag (see illustration).

Allows urine to be collected and measured. Keeps client dry. Twisted condom obstructs urine flow.

11. Place excess coiling of tubing on bed, and secure to bottom sheet.

Prevents looping of tubing and promotes free drainage of urine.

12. Place client in safe, comfortable position. Lower bed, and place side rails accordingly.

Promotes safety and comfort.

13. Dispose of contaminated supplies, and perform hand hygiene.

Reduces spread of microorganisms.

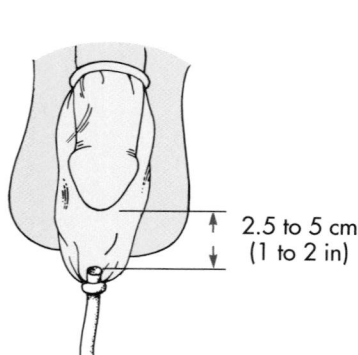

STEP 8 Distance between end of penis and tip of condom.

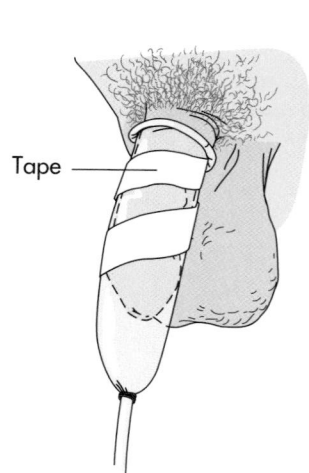

STEP 9a Tape applied in spiral fashion.

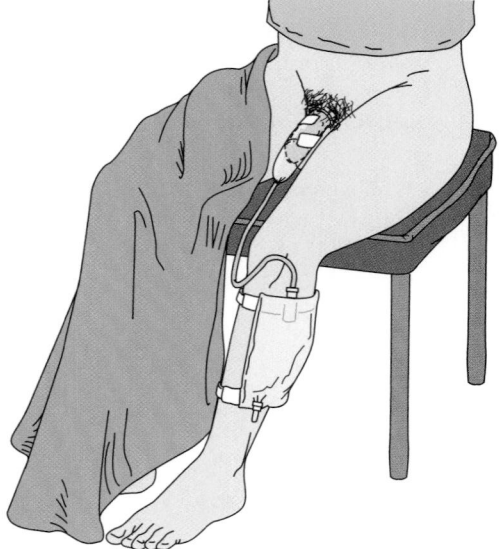

STEP 10 Leg bag.

STEP	RATIONALE

EVALUATION

1. Observe urinary drainage.
2. Inspect penis with condom catheter in place within 30 minutes after application. Look for swelling and discoloration, and ask client if there is any discomfort.
3. Remove and change condom, and inspect skin on penile shaft for signs of breakdown or irritation at least daily when hygiene is performed and when condom is reapplied.

Determines if normal voiding is occurring.
Determines if catheter has been applied incorrectly.

Indicates if condom or urine is causing irritation or if adhesive is too restrictive. Frequent assessment of circulation of glans penis is important to determine if condom has been applied too tightly.

Recording and Reporting

- Report and record pertinent information: condom application, condition of penis, skin, and scrotum, and voiding pattern.
- Monitor I&O as indicated.

Unexpected Outcomes	Related Interventions
1. Skin around penis is reddened and excoriated. Results from pressure of adhesive or contact with urine.	• Check for allergy. • Remove condom, and notify physician. • Do not reapply until penis and surrounding tissue are free from irritation. • Some institutions apply a thin layer of plasticized skin spray to skin of penile shaft to protect skin from ulceration and irritation caused by rubber condom and adhesive holding it in place.
2. Urination is reduced in amount and frequency.	• Assess for kink in tubing. • Assess condom application 30 minutes after applying, and inspect every 4 hours to determine if the penis circulation is adequate. • Observe whether urine is pooling at tip of condom, bathing the penis in urine; reapply.
3. Penile swelling or discoloration occurs.	• Catheter has been improperly applied, or adhesive has been applied too snugly, resulting in impaired circulation. Remove catheter. Notify physician.
4. Condom does not stay on.	• Reapply as necessary. Reassess current condom size. See manufacturer's size chart.
5. Venous circulation in leg impaired from leg bag strap.	• Assess leg every 8 hours for circulatory impairment. • Apply a large Foley bag at night or continuously for a bedridden client

Teaching Considerations

- Teach client to keep condom and catheter kink free and positioned below the level of the bladder.
- Teach client with leg bag to periodically assess leg straps for tightness and to report pain in leg.
- Teach client a collection bag that fills completely may put unnecessary tension on the catheter and contribute to problems keeping the catheter intact. Client should have bag emptied regularly.

Pediatric Considerations

- Condom catheters are rarely used in pediatrics. When used in adolescents, take precautions to minimize child's embarrassment.

Gerontological Considerations

- Condom catheters are not recommended in clients with chronic urinary obstruction such as benign prostatic hypertrophy.
- Clients with neuropathy should be carefully evaluated before application of the condom catheter.

Home Care Considerations

- Caregivers should be taught assessments to be made and what to report.
- Teach client to switch from leg bag to drainage bag at night.
- Modifications may need to be made in clothing to promote optimal drainage.

SKILL 32-7   Care of a Suprapubic Catheter

Suprapubic catheters are inserted surgically into the bladder through the lower abdomen above the symphysis pubis (Figure 32-6). There are advantages to the suprapubic catheter; the client may void naturally when the catheter is clamped, and it is more comfortable than the indwelling catheter. The procedure can be performed at the bedside with the client under local anesthesia, or it may be performed in surgery.

The nurse is responsible for maintaining the catheter while the client is in the nursing home or hospital and for teaching the client or caregiver about routine care. Daily care will depend on the institution's policy, but the cleaning and dressing of the catheter site is similar to that for any surgical drain.

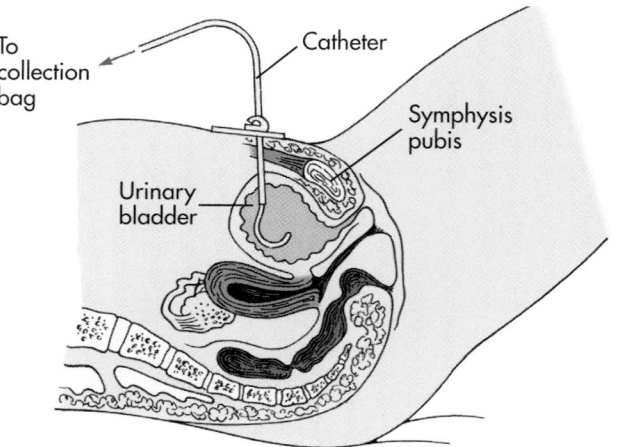

FIGURE 32-6 Suprapubic catheter in place.

DELEGATION CONSIDERATIONS

The skill of caring for a newly established suprapubic catheter should not be delegated to assistive personnel. However, assistive personnel may care for established suprapubic catheters.

- Instruct assistive personnel to report any change in client's comfort from tube, appearance of foul-smelling or discolored urine, or fever.

EQUIPMENT

- ❑ Gloves, sterile and clean
- ❑ Cleansing agent
- ❑ Sterile gauze for cleaning
- ❑ Sterile drain sponge (split gauze)
- ❑ Tape
- ❑ Dressing bag

STEP	RATIONALE

ASSESSMENT

1. Assess urine in bag for amount, clarity, color, odor, and sediment.

Abnormal findings may indicate potential complications such as UTI, decreased urinary output, and blockage.

2. Observe dressing for drainage and intactness.

Drainage indicates potential complication such as infection. Dressing coming off may be caused by tape choice or client picking at dressing.

3. Assess catheter insertion site for signs of inflammation such as redness, swelling, and discharge. Ask client if there is any pain at site.

If insertion is new, slight inflammation may be expected as part of wound healing. May indicate potential infection.

4. Assess how catheter is held in place.

The catheter may be sutured or may be retained by a manufactured seal or a water-filled balloon (much like an indwelling catheter in this latter example).

5. Observe tape site for signs of irritation.

Taping over the same area over a prolonged period may lead to skin irritation and breakdown.

6. Assess for fever.

An increased temperature may indicate infection.

7. Check for allergies.

Client may be sensitive to tape, latex, or antiseptic solution.

8. Assess client's knowledge of purpose of catheter and its care.

Determines level of instruction required.

NURSING DIAGNOSES

- Acute pain
- Impaired urinary elimination
- Impaired skin integrity

- Risk for infection
- Deficient knowledge regarding care of suprapubic catheter

Related factors are individualized based on client's condition or needs.

PLANNING

1. Expected outcomes following completion of procedure:
   - Client will verbalize no pain or discomfort at insertion site.

Patent catheter system keeps bladder empty and client comfortable and without signs of infection.

   - Minimum of 30 ml of urine is present in urinary collection bag every hour.

Verifies that there is adequate perfusion to kidneys and that catheter is not blocked.

   - Urine remains clear and dilute without foul odor.

Removal of retained urine reduces medium for bacterial growth.

   - Site remains dry, clean, and intact.

No indication of infection or skin breakdown develops.

   - Client remains afebrile.

Indicates that no infection is developing.

   - Client can explain the purpose and expected outcome.

Helps to minimize anxiety.

IMPLEMENTATION

1. Perform hand hygiene.

Reduces transmission of infection.

2. Close curtain or room door.

Provides privacy and reduces embarrassment to client, thus promoting relaxation.

3. Prepare supplies and cleansing agent as for applying a dry dressing (see Chapter 38).

The catheter site is surgically made and therefore is treated similarly to other incisions. Once the suprapubic catheter is established and healed, dressings are not advocated unless there is an infection/discharge (Sanders, 2001).

STEP	RATIONALE
4. Use nondominant sterile gloved hand to hold catheter erect while cleaning. Use gauze moistened with cleansing agent to clean site by swabbing in circular motion starting closest to the drain and continuing in outward widening circles for approximately 2 inches (5 cm) (see illustration).	Follows principle of sterile technique to move from area of least contamination to most. Cleanses microorganisms that could migrate to site.

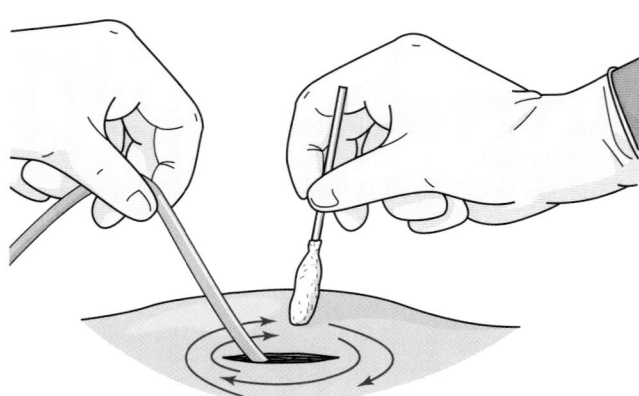

STEP 4 Clean in a circular pattern.

STEP	RATIONALE
5. Use a new piece of moistened gauze to gently clean the base of the catheter, moving up and away from site of insertion. Do not pull catheter.	Removes microorganisms that reside on any drainage that adheres to tubing.
6. With dominant sterile gloved hand, apply split gauze around catheter and tape in place.	Serves to collect secretions.
7. Secure catheter to abdomen with tape or Velcro multi-purpose tube holder to reduce tension on insertion site.	This technique is similar to that used for indwelling urinary catheter. Secures catheter and reduces risk of excessive tension on suture and/or body seal.
8. Check bag and tubing placement.	

● ***Critical Decision Point***
Be sure there are no obstructions in tubing. Coil excess tubing on bed, and fasten it to bottom sheet with clip from kit or with rubber band and safety pin.

EVALUATION

1. Ask client whether there is any pain or discomfort from suprapubic catheter.	Determines if bladder is draining and client is free of infection.
2. Observe client's urine for sediment, odor, or discoloration.	Possible signs of infection when present.
3. Inspect dressing at least every shift.	Drainage may indicate infection.
4. Monitor for signs of infection: elevated white blood cell count (WBC), positive urine culture, or elevated temperature.	Indicates systemic infection from UTI.

Recording and Reporting

- Report and record dressing replacement, including assessments of wound and tolerance of client to dressing.
- Clients may have both an indwelling and a suprapubic catheter after gynecological or bladder surgery. Urine must be assessed in both drainage systems. (Most urine will be found in the suprapubic drainage system.) Record both outputs.
- Residual urine can be assessed by having client void while suprapubic drainage tubing is clamped; the residual urine is then measured by releasing the clamp. Residual urine amounts of less than 50 ml may indicate that bladder function has returned postoperatively.

Unexpected Outcomes	Related Interventions
1. Catheter becomes obstructed.	• Catheter is blocked by clots, accumulation of sediment, or position of catheter in bladder. The suprapubic catheter is often small bore and is easily blocked. Encourage client to drink at least 2000 ml of fluids per day if no restrictions. • Notify physician if blockage is persistent.
2. Site continues to bleed after removal of old dressing.	• Notify physician. • Monitor site, and assess vital signs.
3. Client develops a UTI.	• Encourage fluids, and notify physician. • Observe urine for color, consistency. • Monitor I&O.
4. Leakage of urine at site and skin breakdown.	• Inspection and dressing changes are important in monitoring for these problems. • Notify physician.

Teaching Considerations

- Encourage clients to consume a minimum of 2000 ml of fluids daily if not contraindicated.
- Clients should be taught to keep the drainage bag lower than the bladder and to keep tubing free of kinks.
- Clients should be informed that they may experience bladder spasms. The diameter of the suprapubic catheter is small and is easily occluded with clots, mucus, or sediment. Occlusion can lead to bladder irritation and spasms.
- Clients with both suprapubic and indwelling catheters should be informed that they will have the indwelling urinary catheter removed first, usually between the second and fourth postoperative day.

Home Care Considerations

- With shortened hospital stays it is common for the post-surgery client to go home with a suprapubic catheter.
- Client or caregiver needs to be taught how to clean and dress the suprapubic site and assess signs of infection at the site.
- Client or caregiver needs to be taught how to empty a catheter bag and assess urine for color, odor, clarity, and amount.

SKILL 32-8 Peritoneal Dialysis and Continuous Ambulatory Peritoneal Dialysis

The kidneys are organs that filter and excrete excess fluid and solute wastes. When the kidneys fail, little to no urine is produced, electrolyte imbalances occur, and toxins accumulate in the blood. If excess fluid and toxins are not removed, death results.

Dialysis is a process that removes fluid and solute wastes from the blood or lymph. There are two major types of dialysis: hemodialysis and peritoneal dialysis. Hemodialysis nursing is a specialty practice that involves the shunting of the client's blood through a machine. Peritoneal dialysis is a procedure that infuses a hypertonic solution into the peritoneal cavity. The solution is left for a specified period of time and then drained. The semipermeable peritoneal membrane serves as a filter to remove excess water, electrolytes, and toxins from the blood. Peritoneal dialysis has three steps, each of which varies in length: (1) infusing the dialysate into the cavity, (2) allowing the fluid to dwell in the cavity, and (3) draining the dialysate from the cavity. These are sometimes referred to as "fill, dwell, and drain times."

Peritoneal dialysis can be performed for the acutely ill client or for the client with chronic renal failure. Acute intermittent peritoneal dialysis (IPD) is used within the hospital setting and involves the surgical insertion of a temporary catheter into the peritoneal cavity (Figure 32-7). An exchange or dialysis cycle in acute peritoneal dialysis ranges from $\frac{1}{2}$ hour to 2 hours.

A second form of peritoneal dialysis is used with clients who need ongoing dialysis. Clients who require dialysis because of a chronic condition have long-term peritoneal catheters inserted and, based on need, may receive their dialysis in a variety of settings, including their homes. Therapy can be intermittent or continuous depending on the need.

CAPD is a type of therapy that has made home peritoneal dialysis feasible for the client with end-stage renal disease. With this type of dialysis, a permanent catheter is surgically implanted into the peritoneal cavity, and the processes of osmosis and diffusion remove fluid, excess electrolytes, and toxins from the blood. CAPD has the same three phases as acute peritoneal dialysis; however, the time cycle differs. Exchanges during the day are 3 to 6 hours long, and night-

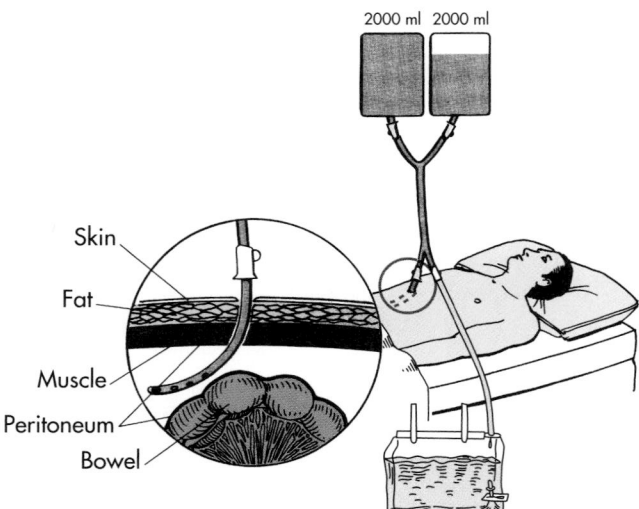

FIGURE 32-7 Patient receiving peritoneal dialysis. Dialysis fluid is being inserted into peritoneal cavity. (From Phipps WJ and others: *Medical-surgical nursing,* ed 6, St. Louis, 1999, Mosby.)

time exchanges last 8 to 12 hours. During the "dwell time" an empty bag and drainage tubing are folded and concealed under the client's clothes (unless a bagless system is used). Afterward the client drains the abdominal cavity, which is followed by reinstillation of fresh dialysate into the peritoneal cavity. The dialysate must be changed 3 to 5 times a day. One major advantage of CAPD is that it allows the client to be out of the hospital, maintain the system at home, and continue with daily activities.

A variation of the CAPD is continuous cyclic peritoneal dialysis (CCPD), which uses a cycler that automates the infusion of the dialysate. CCPD is often used to automate nighttime exchanges for clients in the home, or it may be used by hospital staff to automate the cycling process. When used for the client at night in the home, this process is referred to as nightly intermittent peritoneal dialysis.

DELEGATION CONSIDERATIONS

The skills of peritoneal and continuous ambulatory dialysis should not be delegated to assistive personnel.

EQUIPMENT

- ❑ Ordered bag of dialysate solution at 37° C (98.6° F)
- ❑ Sterile on-off pack containing titanium or plastic adapter and catheter cap
- ❑ Hydrogen peroxide
- ❑ Antimicrobial solution
- ❑ Mask, sterile gloves, goggles, and gown.
- ❑ IV pole
- ❑ Connector tubing (CAPD clients may not need)
- ❑ Sterile drainage bag
- ❑ IV bag label (IPD only)
- ❑ Peritoneal dialysis flow sheet (see Figure 32-8, p. 1112)

STEP	RATIONALE

ASSESSMENT

STEP	RATIONALE
1. Obtain client's weight.	Provides baseline information about weight attributed to fluid retention. A daily weight gain of 1 kg is equivalent to 1 L of fluid.
2. Obtain vital signs.	Fluid volume changes associated with dialysis increase risk for hemodynamic blood pressure changes. In clients undergoing IPD, increased abdominal pressure may lead to bradycardia subsequent to vagal nerve stimulation.
3. Assess respiratory rate, and auscultate lungs.	Pressure from fluid that is cycled into the peritoneal cavity may cause difficulty with breathing. Fluid volume changes may lead to fluid volume overload.
4. Measure abdominal girth.	Mark midpoint of client's abdomen. Keep mark as reference for future measurements. Provides baseline data regarding amount of fluid in peritoneal cavity.
5. Monitor for fluid and electrolyte balance.	Clients may experience hypervolemia or hypovolemia. Signs of hypervolemia include increased blood pressure, difficulty breathing, edema, and neck vein distention. Signs of hypovolemia include tachycardia, hypotension, poor skin turgor, and dry mucous membranes. With potassium imbalance, either hypokalemia or hyperkalemia may occur. Laboratory work must be performed to monitor for a potassium level alteration.
6. Inspect catheter site for erythema, tenderness, drainage, and swelling.	Indicates infection at catheter entry site, which increases risk for peritonitis.
7. Measure body temperature.	Provides baseline data about client's febrile status.
8. Review hospital or dialysis unit's procedure for IPD or CAPD.	There may be institutional variations regarding ordering of supplies; fill, dwell, and drain times; catheter care; and discharge teaching plan.

STEP	RATIONALE
9. Review physician's orders:	
a. Verify dialysis solution and any medications added to solution.	IPD and CAPD require specific orders individualized to client's fluid needs and disease process.
b. Verify number of exchanges and infusion, dwell and drain times.	
10. Obtain laboratory data as ordered:	Establishes baseline of fluid and electrolyte status for monitoring changes that occur from IPD or CAPD.
a. IPD: every 12 to 24 hours.	
b. CAPD: can vary depending on individual needs.	
11. Assess client's and family members' knowledge regarding the purpose of dialysis.	Reveals need for client instruction.

NURSING DIAGNOSES

- Deficient fluid volume
- Risk for deficient fluid volume
- Excess fluid volume
- Impaired home maintenance

- Deficient knowledge regarding peritoneal dialysis
- Acute pain
- Risk for infection

Related factors are individualized based on client's condition or needs.

PLANNING

1. Expected outcomes following completion of procedure:

• Client experiences decreased weight.	Indicates that excess fluid was removed. Indicates that more fluid was removed than was instilled.
• Vital signs are stable.	Indicates that there are no adverse hemodynamic responses.
• Client experiences decreased abdominal girth with IPD.	Indicates that no fluid was retained in peritoneal cavity.
• No erythema, tenderness, or drainage is present at catheter site.	Indicates absence of local inflammation at catheter site.
• No fever is present.	Indicates that no systemic infection is present.
• Dialysate return is clear or slightly light yellow.	Expected color of returned fluid; indicates absence of blood or bacteria in peritoneal cavity.
• Client is able to discuss principles of asepsis and peritoneal dialysis.	Discussing principles allows nurse to document cognitive learning.
• Client or caregiver will perform CAPD.	Demonstration is an effective measure to evaluate psychomotor learning.

IMPLEMENTATION

1. Perform hand hygiene, and apply mask.	Reduces transmission of microorganisms.

- *Critical Decision Point*

  When client is performing peritoneal dialysis in the home, client must wear mask.

2. Place client in semi-Fowler's or high-Fowler's position.	Instilling fluid into peritoneal cavity decreases diaphragmatic excursion. The semi-Fowler's or high-Fowler's position promotes optimal lung expansion.

STEP	RATIONALE
3. Add medications to dialysate bag using six rights of medication administration (see Chapter 19). Use aseptic technique to add medications immediately before beginning instillation of dialysate. This involves disinfecting multiple-dose vials and injection ports of plastic bags. Label and record all medications added (Lancaster, 2001).	Reduces transmission of microorganisms into dialysate.

• **Critical Decision Point**
Maintain strict asepsis when adding medications to dialysate.

a. Heparin	Reduces accumulation of fibrin around catheter tip.
b. Prophylactic antibiotics	Reduce risk of peritonitis.
c. Insulin	Regular insulin is added to control serum glucose (Lancaster, 2001).
4. Attach two warmed dialysate bags to inflow tubing, and attach to IV pole. Bags are spiked exactly as IV solution bags (see Chapter 21) or with special spiking devices.	Dialysate is warmed by dry heat through the use of warming pad, incubator, or microwave warming device. Hanging two bags promotes timely, organized follow-up exchanges. Standard IPD usually includes 24 exchanges in 24 hours. CAPD clients are instructed to hang only one bag because these clients have three to five exchanges daily.

• **Critical Decision Point**
Immersing dialysate in warm water is not recommended because of the chance of contamination (Lancaster, 2001). Dialysate that is too cold results in intolerance, cramps, and hypothermia.

5. Apply sterile gloves.	
6. Disinfect catheter cap and end of catheter with antimicrobial solution; remove cap and disinfect adapter. Connect tubing, maintaining sepsis.	Reduces transmission of microorganisms.
7. With the CAPD system a Y connector that attaches on one side to the dialysate and on the other side to the drainage bag may be used. The Y connector is attached aseptically.	This connection allows for flushing about 100 ml of dialysate into the drainage bag and then draining dialysate from the peritoneum. Research has shown this procedure, called the "flush before fill," to be effective in reducing the incidence of peritonitis (Lancaster, 2001).
8. Open clamp on first dialysate bag, and clamp on client line. Infuse solution over prescribed time (usually 2 L/ 10-15 min).	Permits instillation of dialysate into peritoneal cavity.
9. Clamp inflow tubing for prescribed dwell time. **a.** IPD: usually 30 minutes. **b.** CAPD: 3 to 5 hours. (CAPD client folds tubing and infusion bag on abdomen, which is concealed by clothing, and uses same bag and tubing for drain cycle.)	Prevents air from entering peritoneal cavity. Dwell time permits peritoneal membrane to exchange fluid, electrolytes, and toxins from blood.

STEP	RATIONALE

- **Critical Decision Point**

  Monitor infusion and dwell time carefully. A timer may be used to signal the scheduled interval for each phase.

STEP	RATIONALE
10. Remove first dialysate bag from IV pole. Place third warmed bag on pole.	Promotes organized procedure. When multiple exchanges are ordered, nurse should have two dialysate bags on IV pole.
11. Unclamp outflow tubing and drain (usually for 20 minutes). Evaluate drainage for clarity and color.	Permits drainage of dialysate and wastes from peritoneal cavity. During first two or three exchanges, it is common for dialysate to remain in cavity; excess should drain with later exchanges. The used dialysate should be clear (Scott, 1999).
12. Clamp outflow tubing.	Prevents untimed drain during subsequent exchange.
13. Apply gloves, mask, eye protection, and/or gown, and empty and measure fluid in drainage bag.	Protective equipment chosen to protect nurse from accidental splashes of fluid. Provides assessment of fluid balance of dialysate solution. If volume of fluid infused is more than amount drained, balance is positive (e.g., if 2000 ml of dialysate was infused and 1800 ml was drained, balance is positive 200 ml [+200 ml], meaning the client is retaining the fluid).

- **Critical Decision Point**

  Wear gloves, mask, eye protection (or face shield), and gown when emptying because splashes may occur.

STEP	RATIONALE
14. Remove contaminated items. Perform hand hygiene.	Prevents transmission of microorganisms.
15. Repeat steps until all exchanges are complete.	
16. During first exchanges, monitor client's vital signs every 15 minutes.	Promotes timely documentation of hemodynamic effects of IPD.
17. When all exchanges are complete: a. Acute-use catheter (short-term use): Disinfect, disconnect connections, and discard tubing. Disinfect catheter rim, and securely place sterile cap on end.	Keeps sterile catheter secure and closed to entrance of microorganisms.
b. Chronic-use catheter (long-term use): See guidelines made specifically for catheter.	Maintains patency of catheter insertion site.
18. Inspect catheter site; if dressing is reapplied, apply a clear transparent occlusive dressing (see Chapter 38).	Intact, dry dressing reduces risk of infection. If encrustations have developed, clean gently. Removal of crusts may cause further injury and may increase chance of infection (Scott, 1999).
19. Perform hand hygiene, and dispose of contaminated supplies according to agency policy.	Reduces transmission of microorganisms and blood-borne pathogens.

STEP	RATIONALE

▌EVALUATION

1. Obtain weight.

2. Obtain dialysis fluid balance measurements. Fluid balance measurements will demonstrate presence or absence of retained fluid in peritoneal cavity.

3. Obtain vital signs.
4. Obtain body temperature.
5. Measure abdominal girth.

6. Inspect catheter site for erythema, tenderness, drainage, and swelling.
7. Auscultate lungs for crackles.

8. Inspect returned dialysate solution.

9. Observe client performing CAPD.
10. Assess client's comfort level.

11. Monitor laboratory work.

RATIONALE

Decrease indicates removal of excess fluid; increase indicates retention of fluid.
Determines adequacy of fluid removal.

Documents tolerance to IPD.
Denotes presence or absence of infection.
Provides an indirect measurement of fluid retention in peritoneal cavity.
Determines if symptoms of infection are present.

Provides a measurement of fluid overload. As intravascular fluid increases, crackles are auscultated in bases of lungs.
Note blood, purulent discharge, fecal contents, or urine that may indicate infection, perforation, or fistula development.
Documents learning of skill.
Clients may have incisional pain after access insertion. Clients undergoing peritoneal dialysis may also describe a feeling of fullness following instillation of a large volume of dialysate in the abdominal cavity.
Imbalances in potassium may occur. A relative increase or decrease in hematocrit may indicate hypovolemia or hypervolemia, respectively.

Recording and Reporting

- Document client's weight, abdominal girth, and dialysis fluid balance before and after IPD.
- Document client's vital signs, respiratory status, temperature, and status of catheter site.
- Record presence of pain or discomfort, including location, quality, and duration of pain.
- Record color of dialysate drainage, condition of catheter dressing, and whether new dressing is applied.
- Note any unexpected outcomes and actions taken by nurse and physician.
- Individual hospitals have individual flow sheets to record IPD fluids (Figure 32-8).
- When charting, it is important to note that if client is losing fluid weight, a negative balance is achieved. A positive balance means client is retaining instilled fluid.
- Report pain that is severe or unexpected.

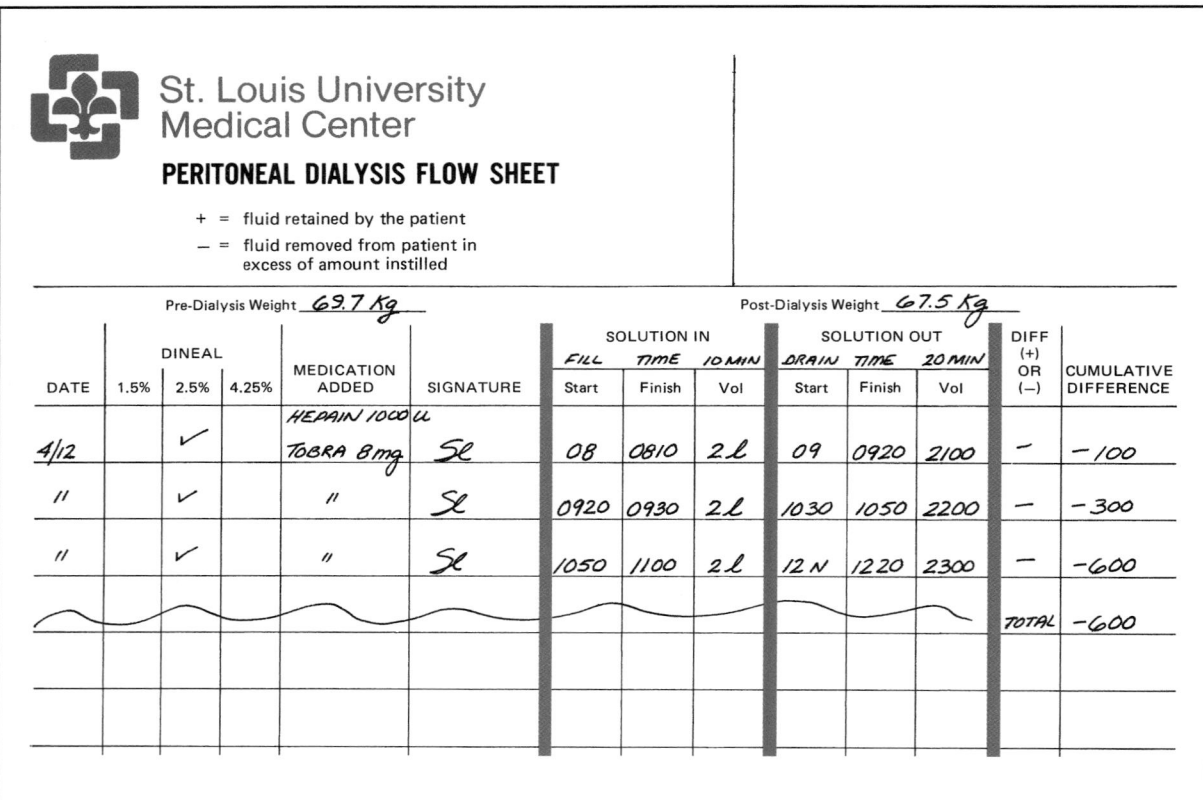

FIGURE **32-8** Peritoneal dialysis flow sheet. (Courtesy Saint Louis University Medical Center, St. Louis.)

Unexpected Outcomes	Related Interventions
1. Client experiences increased weight or no weight change. Indicates fluid retained in peritoneal cavity.	• Report to physician.
2. Fluid balance is positive. Indicates excess fluid retained.	• Report to physician.
3. Client experiences decreased blood pressure and tachycardia. Client unable to tolerate fluid volume, or catheter may have perforated bowel.	• Report to physician. • Monitor client frequently.
4. Client experiences increased abdominal girth. Indicates retained fluid.	• Report to physician. • Assess for kinking in dialysis tubing.
5. Erythema, tenderness, and drainage are present at catheter site. Indicates local inflammatory response.	• Report to physician.
6. Fever is present. Indicates systemic infection.	• Report to physician.
7. Dialysate drainage is abnormal.	• Report to physician.
8. Client experiences cramps. Indicates that dialysate is too cold, infusion is too rapid, volume is too much for client to tolerate, or electrolyte imbalances have occurred.	• Check temperature of dialysate, check electrolyte levels, and compare volume to previous records. • Report to physician.

Unexpected Outcomes	Related Interventions
9. Client experiences sudden respiratory distress. Indicates that volume is too excessive for client to tolerate.	• Raise head of bed. • Report to physician.
10. Instillation flow is poor, or drainage is poor.	• Check for kink in inflow/outflow tubing or catheter.
11. Dialysate is leaking from peritoneum.	• Look for edema in abdominal wall, perineum, or penis (Lancaster, 2001). • Notify physician.
12. Leak at catheter site occurs. Indicates catheter displacement toward abdominal surface.	• Notify physician.

Teaching Considerations

- Teach IPD clients what to expect during and after procedure.
- Teach scrub and exchange procedures to CAPD clients and/or caregivers according to policy, and ask client to correctly demonstrate scrub and exchange procedure.
- Instruct client and/or caregivers in the common symptoms of fluid excess and deficit, and instruct client to weigh self correctly.
- Review teaching plan with client before discharge and during each clinic visit.
- Periodically review potential complications and signs and symptoms, including common symptoms associated with peritonitis.
- Review medications and dietary and fluid restrictions.
- Instruct client when and whom to contact in emergency.
- Instruct client and/or caregivers how to take blood pressure correctly.
- Client receiving IPD should be encouraged to move around in bed. However, movements should avoid stressing catheter or tubing. CAPD clients who are ambulatory should be encouraged to ambulate in between exchanges.
- Teach the client to check labels carefully. Peritoneal dialysis solutions are available in four dextrose concentrations (1.5%, 2.5%, 3.5%, and 4.25%), each with increasing osmolality to enhance fluid removal by osmosis (Scott, 1999).

Pediatric Considerations

- Parents of young children learn to manage CAPD. Older children and adolescents are able to perform the procedure themselves, thus providing them with some control and less dependency.

Gerontological Considerations

- A major risk factor for death with CAPD is age greater than 65 years (Lancaster, 2001).
- The older adult client may be at risk for malnutrition related to loss of protein during dialysis, dietary restrictions, and loss of appetite.
- Clients on dialysis often suffer many complications; older adults are no exception. However, older adult clients may be taking medications for other chronic health problems. Monitoring and assessment of medication therapy are ongoing.

Home Care Considerations

- CAPD clients must do the following correctly to complete CAPD exchanges:
  - Demonstrate CAPD scrub and aseptic exchange procedure.
  - State signs of infection.
  - Adhere to fluid, dietary, and medication therapies.
  - Perform activities of daily living. CAPD is designed so client can maintain normal daily activities.
- The training interval for client undergoing CAPD is individualized to the client and family.
- Properly dispose of any used dialysate fluid.

FOCUS *on* CLINICAL PRACTICE

You are assigned to care for a 69-year-old woman admitted to the clinical unit for urinary retention. The physician writes an order to catheterize the client for residual urine The only history available is that she has arthritic joints.

1. What other assessment data would be pertinent to obtain about this client?
2. Explain what teaching you should implement before the procedure.
3. Based on the client's gender and age, what catheter size would you use for this client?
   A. 8 Fr
   B. 10 Fr
   C. 12 Fr
   D. 16 Fr

4. Explain what type of catheter you would obtain and why.
5. Based on the client's history, you would anticipate that the client may need to assume which position for the procedure?
   A. Sims
   B. Dorsal recumbent
   C. Supine
   D. Prone
   Explain your choice.

NCLEX REVIEW QUESTIONS

1. What is the most important action when caring for a client with a condom catheter?
   1. Provide perineal hygiene every 8 hours.
   2. Use sterile technique.
   3. Place glans penis at the end of condom catheter.
   4. Ensure the elastic adhesive is not tight.
2. When changing a condom catheter on an uncircumcised client, the nurse will:
   1. Replace foreskin over the glans penis
   2. Cleanse the urethral meatus in a circular motion
   3. Use adhesive tape to secure condom
   4. Lubricate condom for easier application
3. When caring for the client with an indwelling catheter, the nurse should:
   1. Routinely irrigate the catheter to maintain patency
   2. Secure catheter tubing to the thigh
   3. Check for bladder distention every shift
   4. Assess intake and output every 4 hours
4. What is the most important action to ensure an accurate measure of urine residual?
   1. Use a sterile specimen container.
   2. Collect the urine from the catheter port.
   3. Have the client void before obtaining the specimen.
   4. Ask the client when he or she last voided.
5. Which statement is true regarding catheterization of a female client with an indwelling catheter?
   1. The catheter must be inserted 1 to 2 inches after urine flows.
   2. The catheter will be inserted a total of $1\frac{1}{2}$ to 2 inches.

3. Clean technique is used for this procedure.
   4. The catheter can be removed after the bladder is emptied.
6. The female client asks why the indwelling catheter is taped to her inner thigh. The nurse explains it is important to prevent:
   1. Urine leakage around the catheter
   2. Slippage of the catheter from the bladder
   3. Possible urethral trauma
   4. Accidental removal
7. The most important action to prevent client injury before removing an indwelling catheter is to:
   1. Put on sterile gloves
   2. Place a water proof pan under the client
   3. Empty the collection bag
   4. Deflate the balloon
8. When cleansing female genitalia immediately before catheterization, the proper technique includes:
   1. Using warm water and soap
   2. Cleansing in a circular motion
   3. Wiping from back to front using sterile cotton balls and solution
   4. Using a single sterile cotton ball for each wipe
9. When performing a catheterization, sterile gloves are applied:
   1. Before draping the client
   2. After cleansing the client's perineal area with antiseptic solution
   3. Before lubricating the catheter
   4. After applying the drape over the perineal area

NCLEX REVIEW QUESTIONS

10. When placing an indwelling catheter in a male, the balloon can be inflated after:
    1. Urine returns in the tubing
    2. Emptying the bladder
    3. Inserting the catheter to the bifurcation of the catheter ports
    4. Advancing the catheter a total of 1 to 2 inches
11. When inserting an indwelling catheter, the nurse sees urine flowing in the tubing. The nurse should hold the catheter with his or her nondominant hand until the:
    1. Balloon is inflated
    2. Urine stops flowing in the tubing
    3. Collection bag is full
    4. Catheter is anchored appropriately
12. Which statement is true regarding the open method of catheter irrigation?
    1. Always use sterile gloves for the procedure.
    2. Use maximal pressure when inserting the fluid.
    3. Clamp the catheter below soft injection port or drainage tubing.
    4. If strong resistance is noted, do not force the irrigation.
13. To minimize blockage of the suprapubic catheter, the nurse teaches the client to:
    1. Irrigate the catheter every 4 hours
    2. Maintain fluid intake of at least 2000 ml

3. Keep the drainage bag lower than the bladder
4. Observe the urine for color and consistency
14. When cleansing the suprapubic insertion site, the nurse:
    1. Starts close to the drain site and cleans in a circular motion outward
    2. Starts furthest from the drain site and cleans in a circular motion inward
    3. Cleanses in any pattern as long as the site is not contaminated
    4. Uses principles of medical asepsis
15. With peritoneal dialysis, a negative balance means:
    1. The client is losing fluid weight
    2. The client is retaining fluid
    3. There is poor instillation flow or poor drainage
    4. There is no weight change
16. Which of the following should be implemented to prevent infection in the patient receiving CAPD?
    1. Use strict aseptic technique.
    2. Increase fluid intake to at least 1500 ml/day.
    3. Add heparin to the dialysate.
    4. Change an intact, dry dressing every shift.

References

Addison R, Mould C: Risk assessment in suprapubic catheterization, *Nurs Stand* 14(36): 43, 2000.

Biering-Sorensen F and others: Urinary tract infection in patients with spinal cord lesions, *Drugs* 61(9):1275, 2001.

Doherty W: Promoting planned care for patients with indwelling catheters, *Br J Community Nurs* 6(1):11, 2001.

Evans E: Indwelling catheter care: dispelling the misconceptions, *Geriatr Nurs* 20(5):85, 1999.

Gray M, Haas J: Assessment of the patient with urinary incontinence. In Doughty D: *Urinary and fecal incontinence*, ed 2, St. Louis, 2000, Mosby.

Guidelines for preventing infections associated with insertion and maintenance of short-term indwelling urethral catheters, htpp://www.doh.gov.uk/HAI, retrieved Jan 4, 2004.

Haberstich N: Protecting catheterized patients from infection, *Nurs Residential Care* 4(10):482, 2002.

Hockenberry MJ and others: *Wong's nursing care of infants and children*, ed 7, St. Louis, 2003, Mosby.

Lancaster L: *ANNA: curriculum for nephrology nursing*, ed 4, Pitman, NJ, 2001, Anthony J. Janetti.

Lawrence P, Rozmus C: Culturally sensitive care of the Muslim patient. *J Transcult Nurs* 12(3):228, 2001.

Lombardo M, Hartwig M: Central nervous system injury. In Price S, Wilson L: *Pathophysiology: clinical concepts of disease,* ed 6, St. Louis, 2003, Mosby.

Lueckenotte A: *Gerontological nursing*, ed 2, St. Louis, 2000, Mosby.

Phipps WJ and others: *Medical-Surgical nursing*, ed 6, St. Louis, 1999, Mosby.

Sanders C: Suprapubic catheterization: risk management, *Pediatr Nurs* 13(10):14, 2001.

Scott M: Caring for the orthopaedic patient receiving continuous ambulatory peritoneal dialysis, *Orthop Nurs* 18(4):59, 1999.

Suchinski G and others: Treating urinary infections in the elderly, *Dimens Crit Care Nurs* 18(1):21, 1999.

Research References

Ellis PA: Review: double bag or Y set systems reduce peritonitis in patients on continuous ambulatory dialysis, *Evid Based Nurs* (5): 14, 2002.

Daneshgari F and others: Evidence based multidisciplinary practice: improving the safety and standards of male bladder catheterization, *Medsurg Nurs* 11(5):236, 2002.

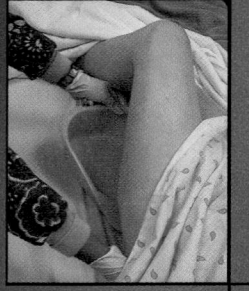

33

Bowel Elimination and Gastric Intubation

MEDIA RESOURCES

Evolve Site *evolve*

http://evolve.elsevier.com/Perry/skills
- Weblinks
- Video clips
- Mosby's Nursing Skills Video Exercises

Mosby's Nursing Skills Videos/CD-ROM
- *Normal Elimination Video:* Assisting with a bedpan, standard and fracture bedpans, administering a cleansing enema

OBJECTIVES

Mastery of content in this chaper will enable the nurse to:

- Describe factors that promote and impede normal bowel elimination.
- Discuss methods to relieve constipation or impaction.
- Describe precautions to follow in administering an enema.
- Describe approaches for managing a client's comfort during nasogastric tube insertion.
- Implement the following skills: assisting client in using a bedpan, digital removal of stool, enema administration, and insertion of a nasogastric tube.

KEY TERMS

Cathartic	Fracture pan
Cleansing enema	Hemorrhoids
Colon	Impaction
Constipation	Medicated enema
Decompression	Obstipation
Defecation	Occult blood
Enema	Oil-retention enema

BOX 33-1   Common Causes of Constipation

- Irregular bowel habits and ignoring the urge to defecate.
- Chronic illnesses (e.g., Parkinson's disease, multiple sclerosis, rheumatoid arthritis, chronic bowel diseases, depression, eating disorders) (Annells and Koch, 2002; Richmond, 2003).
- Low-fiber diet high in animal fats (e.g., meats, dairy products, eggs) and refined sugars (rich desserts). Also, low fluid intake slows peristalsis (Bliss and others, 2001).
- Situational stress (e.g., illness of a family member, death of a loved one, divorce) (Dosh, 2002).
- Lengthy bed rest or lack of regular exercise.
- Secondary effects of medications (e.g., antacids, antidepressants, iron, narcotics, anticholinergics).
- Heavy laxative use causes loss of normal defecation reflex. In addition, the lower colon is completely emptied, requiring time to refill with bulk (Annells and Koch, 2002).
- Older adults experience slowed peristalsis, loss of abdominal muscle elasticity, and reduced intestinal mucus secretion. Older adults often eat low-fiber foods.
- Neurological conditions that block nerve impulses to the colon (e.g., spinal cord injury, tumor).
- Organic illnesses such as hypothyroidism, hypocalcemia, or hypokalemia (Richmond, 2003).

Regular elimination of bowel waste products is essential for normal body functioning. Because bowel function depends on the balance of several factors, physical and psychological, elimination patterns and habits vary among individuals. When clients' functional status changes or they become ill at home or in a health care setting, they may not be able to maintain normal elimination habits and require assistance, such as the use of a bed pan or enema administration. It is important for the nurse to always show respect for a client's privacy, provide necessary comfort measures, and attend to the client's emotional needs when performing required skills.

To manage clients' elimination problems, the nurse must understand normal elimination and factors that promote, impede, or cause alterations in elimination, such as constipation, diarrhea, and fecal incontinence. Supportive nursing care respects the client's privacy and emotional needs. In addition, interventions designed to promote normal bowel elimination should be performed in a way that minimizes discomfort.

The nurse must be able to assist immobilized clients with the elimination process by helping them on and off bedpans. Often a nurse may be responsible for collecting stool specimens and ensuring that they are properly handled (see Chapter 43). If a client is constipated, the nurse may be expected to competently administer enemas or to digitally remove impacted stool. When clients undergo surgery or experience an alteration in gastrointestinal peristalsis, the insertion of a nasogastric tube may become necessary.

Evidenced-Based Practice Trends

Constipation is a symptom, its cause is multifaceted, and it is not a disease (Box 33-1). The signs of constipation vary among clients, but they usually include infrequent bowel movements fewer than 2 times per week, difficulty in evacuating feces, inability to defecate at will, and hard fecal material (Dosh, 2002). Constipation is a significant health hazard; it is more common in women, in nonwhites, in children than in adults, and older adults than in younger adults (Lembo and Camilleri, 2003).

Straining to evacuate a hardened feces causes problems to the client with recent abdominal, gynecological, or rectal surgery because the act of straining may cause the sutures to separate, reopening the wound. In addition, clients with history of cardiovascular diseases, glaucoma, and increased intracranial pressure should avoid straining.

There are interventions for the control of constipation. Initially lifestyle changes of increased dietary fiber, increased fluids, moderate exercise, and elimination of laxative use should be tried (Hinrichs and Huseboe, 2001; Lembo and Camilleri, 2003). If these measures are unsuccessful, then stepwise levels of interventions should be tried. Bulk-forming laxatives (e.g., psyllium [Metamucil] or methylcellulose [Citrucel]) are safe and add bulk to the fecal material. These laxatives can then be followed by or used in combination with a saline laxative (e.g., magnesium hydroxide [Milk of Magnesia]) or osmotic laxative (e.g., lactulose [Chronulac]). If the constipation continues, stimulant laxatives (e.g., bisacodyl [Dulcolax] or senna [Senokot]) may provide relief. Emollient laxative, such as mineral oil, is avoided because it has been associated with lipoid aspiration pneumonia (Dosh, 2002).

Fecal incontinence is the client's inability to control the passage of feces and gas. Management of fecal incontinence requires a complete understanding of the causes. The presence of diarrhea is frequently associated with the incontinence episodes. This diarrhea may be due to diet or antibiotic use, which alters the normal flora in the gastrointestinal tract (Bartlett, 2002). In addition, these clients have little or no warning before the incontinence episode of loose, watery diarrhea, and the diarrhea may be present without a positive stool culture (Bliss and others, 2000). Management strategies for fecal incontinence are diverse. Whenever possible the diarrhea should be controlled; supplementing with dietary fiber slows intestinal transit time and increases the bulk of the fecal contents (Bliss and others, 2001). Agents to control the diarrhea will encourage the stool to become more formed, and thus the frequency of incontinence declines. However, when a client has organism-related diarrhea (e.g., *Clostridium difficile*), treatments to slow intestinal transit should be avoided (Bliss and others, 2000).

Cultural Considerations

When caring for clients from other cultural and ethnic groups, modifications of care are frequently needed. The modifications go beyond language and communication issues; for example, there may be specific hygiene practices or dietary needs. In meeting the elimination needs of clients from other cultures it is important to consider the following aspects:

- Accommodate the need for gender-congruent care among cultures emphasizing separate gender roles and female modesty such as African, Hispanic, Asian, Islamic, Arabic, Hindu, Jewish Orthodox, and Amish cultures.
- Provide for hygiene needs of clients.
  - Distinct hygienic practices are observed by certain cultures, such as Hindus and Muslims, that designate the left hand to perform unclean procedures such as bowel elimination.
  - Wash your hands before touching the client, and use your right hand to first touch the client.
  - Use the left hand to handle the bedpan and to assist the client in cleansing after bowel movement (Lawrence and Rozmus, 2001).

- Promote client's understanding of the procedure.
  - Use an interpreter if needed.
  - Repeat explanations because client's anxiety about the loss of privacy can pose distraction.
  - Explain measures to protect client's privacy.

Skill Performance Guidelines

1. Determine a client's normal pattern of bowel elimination, and try to accommodate that pattern while the client is in a health care setting. Determine the time the client normally has a bowel movement and the amount of assistance needed.
2. Provide privacy, and try to reduce the client's embarrassment. If possible, the client should be encouraged to use the bathroom. However, if the nature of the illness limits physical activity, ensure as much privacy as possible during use of the bedpan or bedside commode.
3. Be aware of foods that promote normal peristaltic movement, including high-fiber foods such as raw fruit, whole grains, and green leafy vegetables, that are consistent with the client's prescribed diet. Immobilized clients should receive foods that promote peristalsis but not those that adversely affect bowel routine.
4. Unless contraindicated, encourage adequate hydration. Normally a person should drink 6 to 8 glasses of water per day. Warm fluids are especially effective in increasing peristalsis.
5. Encourage clients to be as active as physically possible. Physical activity promotes peristalsis, whereas immobilization decreases it.
6. Promote client comfort. The procedures designed to promote normal elimination or bowel decompression can create discomfort if not performed correctly.
7. Be aware of the side effects of medications the client receives. Some drugs may impair the normal elimination pattern by causing constipation or diarrhea. Also, general anesthetic agents used during surgery cause temporary cessation of peristalsis, which can affect the normal elimination pattern after surgery and increase the risk for constipation.
8. Consider the developmental changes that affect bowel functioning throughout the life span. For example, an older adult might become less active, muscle tone might be decreased, and eating patterns might change. These factors could result in constipation.
9. When handling or coming in contact with fecal matter, always use standard precautions.

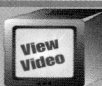

SKILL 33-1 Assisting the Client in Using a Bedpan

A client restricted to bed must use a bedpan for defecation. Women use bedpans to pass urine and feces, whereas men use bedpans only for defecation. Sitting on a bedpan can be extremely uncomfortable. The nurse should help the client assume a position similar to the natural squatting position.

Two types of bedpans are available (Figure 33-1). The regular bedpan, made of metal or hard plastic, has a curved, smooth upper end and a tapered lower end. The pan is approximately 5 cm (2 inches) deep. A fracture pan, designed for clients with body or leg casts or clients restricted from raising their hips (e.g., following total joint replacement), has a shallow upper end approximately 1.3 cm ($\frac{1}{2}$ inch) deep that slips easily under a client. The upper end of either pan fits under the client's buttocks toward the sacrum, with the lower end just under the upper thighs.

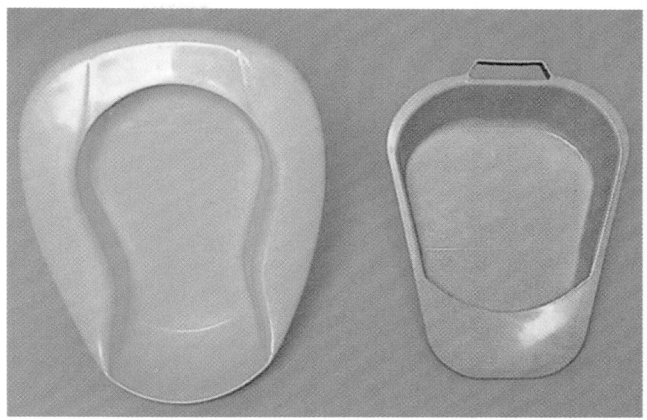

FIGURE **33-1** Types of bedpans. *Left,* Regular bedpan. *Right,* Fracture bedpan.

DELEGATION CONSIDERATIONS

The skill of assisting a client onto a bedpan can be delegated to assistive personnel. The nurse provides information, assistance, and direction, including:

* Inform and assist assistive personnel in proper way to position clients who have mobility restrictions.
* Instruct assistive personnel regarding positioning of clients with therapeutic equipment present, such as drains, intravenous catheters, or traction.

EQUIPMENT

❑ Disposable gloves
❑ Appropriate type of clean bedpan
❑ Bedpan cover
❑ Toilet tissue
❑ Specimen container (if necessary), plastic bag, clearly labeled with date, client's name, and identification number
❑ Washbasin, washcloths, towels, and soap
❑ Waterproof, absorbent pads
❑ Clean drawsheet (optional)

STEP	RATIONALE

⬛ ASSESSMENT

1. Assess client's normal bowel elimination habits: routine pattern, effect of certain foods/fluids and eating habits on bowel elimination, effect of stress and level of activity on normal bowel elimination patterns, current medications, normal fluid intake.

Managing a client's elimination problems depends on a thorough understanding of normal elimination and factors that may create alterations. Mass peristalsis is strongest during the hour after first meal of the day. Nurse should anticipate when to offer bedpan.

2. Auscultate abdomen for bowel sounds, and palpate for abdominal distention.

Normal bowel sounds occur irregularly at the rate of 5 to 35 per minute (Seidel and others, 2003). A fecal-filled colon is palpated as a firm rounded mass. A distended bladder can be palpated as a smooth, round mass above the symphysis pubis.

3. Assess client to determine level of mobility and amount of assistance required.

Determines if client can assist in positioning on bedpan or if totally dependent on nurse's help. Older adults, obese clients who have had hip or knee surgery, and debilitated clients may require assistance of two or more nurses to help them onto or off of the bedpan (Ebersole and others, 2004). Assistance from additional personnel promotes safety for client and nurses.

    a. Assess if client is allowed to sit up or must lie flat when using bedpan.

Determines most appropriate type of bedpan.

STEP	RATIONALE
4. Assess client's level of comfort. Especially note presence of rectal or abdominal pain or presence of hemorrhoids or irritation of skin surrounding anus.	Pain can limit client's ability to assist with positioning. Rectal or abdominal pain can reduce client's ability to bear down during defecation.
5. Determine if a stool specimen is needed.	Provides ample opportunity to obtain specimen container before placing the client on the bedpan.

NURSING DIAGNOSES

- Bowel incontinence
- Risk for constipation
- Diarrhea

- Acute, chronic pain
- Impaired physical mobility

Related factors are individualized based on a client's condition or needs.

PLANNING

1. Expected outcomes following completion of procedure:	
• Client is able to successfully defecate in bedpan.	Indicates normal elimination.
• Perianal skin is clear and intact.	No irritation has occurred; perianal skin is cleaned appropriately.
• Client eliminates without pain.	Client is positioned comfortably on bedpan.
2. Explain procedure to client, including self-help tips, such as how to use a trapeze, how to move hips, etc.	Information promotes client's independence, reduces anxiety, and helps client to better assist nurse during procedure.
3. Obtain assistance from additional nursing personnel as warranted.	Adequate personnel resources minimize muscle strain for client and nurse. Reduces client's discomfort.

IMPLEMENTATION

1. Perform hand hygiene, and apply gloves.	Reduces transmission of microorganisms.
2. Provide privacy by closing curtains around bed or door of room.	Reduces embarrassment and promotes bowel elimination.
3. Place bedpan under warm, running water for few seconds, then dry. Be careful that pan is not too hot.	Metal bedpans are very cold. Warm pan helps client to relax anal sphincter. Although plastic bedpans may not be as cold to touch as metal, warming them before use is still wise.
4. Put side rail up on opposite side of bed.	Protects client from falling out of bed. Client can use side rail to grasp onto and assist self to move about in bed and onto the bedpan.
5. Raise bed horizontally according to nurse's height.	Promotes use of good body mechanics and minimizes muscle strain for nurse and client.
6. Have client assume supine position.	Position eases eventual pan placement.

- **Critical Decision Point**
  Observe for the presence of drains, dressings, intravenous fluids, and traction. These devices may impede a client from assisting with the procedure and may also necessitate more personnel to assist in placing the client on a bedpan.

7. Place client who is mobile in bed and can assist with procedure on bedpan.	
a. Raise client's head 30 to 60 degrees.	Prevents hyperextension of back and provides support to upper torso when client raises hips. Sitting position promotes defecation.
b. Remove upper bed linens just enough so they are out of the way, but do not unduly expose client.	Prevents embarrassment to client; demonstrates respect for client's sense of dignity.

STEP	**RATIONALE**

c. Remove bedpan cover, and place in accessible location.

d. Instruct client in how to flex knees and lift hips upward.

Little effort should be required of client, whose body weight is supported by lower legs and feet and upper torso and arms.

e. Place, hand palm up, closest to the client's head, under client's sacrum, to assist lifting. As the client raises the hips, use other hand to slip bedpan under client (see illustration). Be sure open rim of bedpan is facing toward foot of bed. **Do not shove pan under client's hips.** (*Optional:* Have client use overhead trapeze frame to raise hips.)

Nurse must ensure that bedpan is placed high enough under buttocks so feces enters pan. Incorrect placement of bedpan can cause discomfort for client and spillage of contents. Raise knee gatch (unless contraindicated) or ask client to bend the knees. Shoving the bedpan under the client increases the risk of friction injury to the underlying skin and tissues.

f. *Optional:* If using a fracture pan, simply slip it under the client as the hips are raised (see illustration).

Requires less maneuvering by client.

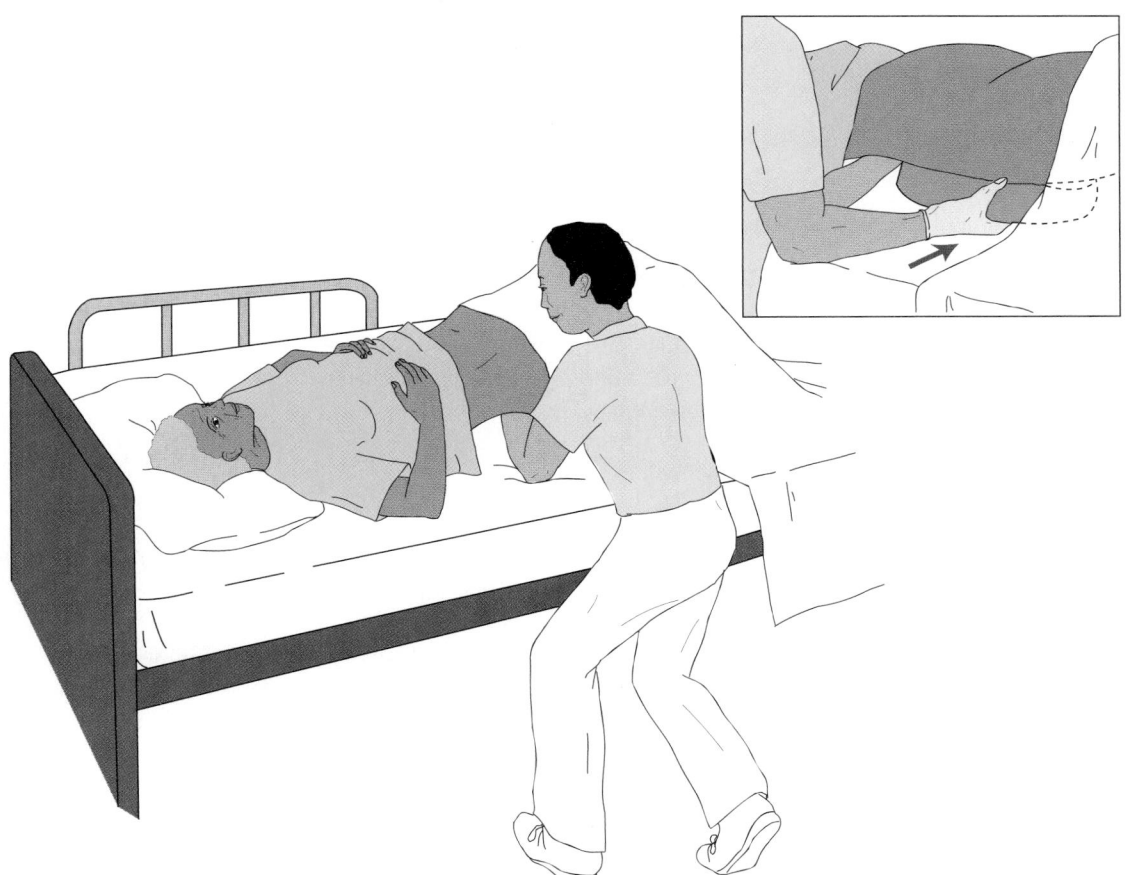

STEP 7e The client raises the hips and buttocks off the bed as the bedpan is slid underneath. (From Sorrentino SA: *Mosby's textbook for nursing assistants,* ed 5, St. Louis, 2000, Mosby.)

STEP	RATIONALE

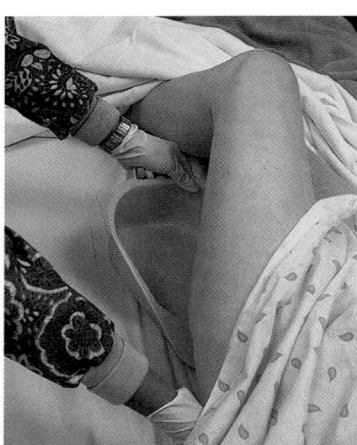

STEP **7f** Client lifts hips as fracture pan is positioned.

8. Place client who is immobile or has restrictions in mobility on bedpan.

    a. Lower the head of the bed flat (if tolerated by medical condition).

        Assists client for whom it is unsafe to exert effort when lifting hips, who must remain flat, or who is unable to lift hips to roll onto bedpan.

    b. Remove top linens as necessary to turn client while minimizing exposure.

        Prevents embarrassment to client; demonstrates respect for client's sense of dignity.

    c. Remove bedpan cover, and place in accessible location.

    d. Assist the client with rolling onto one side, backside toward you, or turn client into side-lying position. Place bedpan firmly against client's buttocks and down into mattress. Be sure that open rim of bedpan is facing toward foot of bed (see illustrations).

        Incorrect placement can cause discomfort to client and spillage of contents.

- **Critical Decision Point**

    If client has had total hip replacement, the abduction pillow placed between the legs to prevent dislocation of the new joint must remain in place. Use a fracture pan.

    e. Keeping one hand against the bedpan, place the other around the client's far hip. Ask the client to roll back onto the bedpan, flat in bed. **Do not shove the pan under the client.**

        Positions client squarely on pan with minimal exertion. Shoving the bedpan under the client increases the risk of friction injury to the underlying skin and tissues.

    f. Raise client's head 30 degrees to a comfortable level, unless contraindicated.

        Client can assume sitting position unless the condition necessitates maintaining flat position. Sitting position promotes defecation.

    g. Raise knee gatch (unless contraindicated), or ask client to bend the knees.

        Relieves stress on back.

9. Ensure that client is comfortable; cover client for warmth. Place small pillow or rolled towel under lumbar curve of back.

    Provides added comfort. Pain reduces or eliminates urge to defecate, which can result in bowel elimination problems.

10. Ensure that call bell and toilet tissue are within easy reach for client.

    Promotes safety by preventing client from reaching over edge of bed for objects out of reach.

STEP	**RATIONALE**

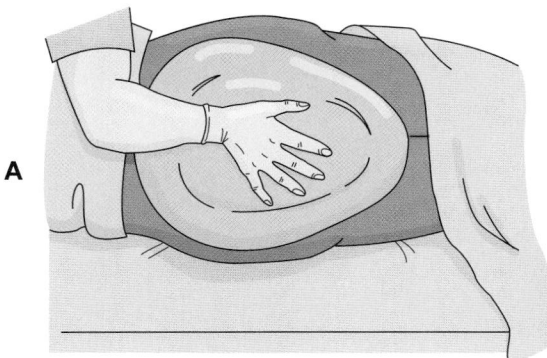

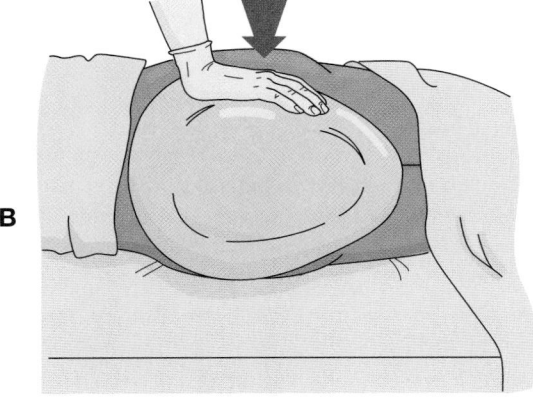

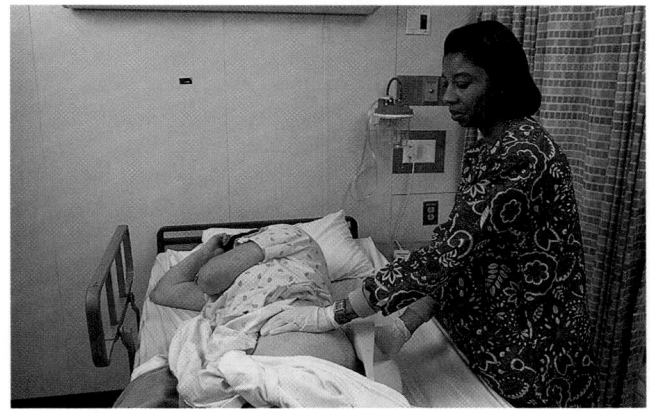

STEP 8d A, Position the client on one side, and place the bedpan firmly against the buttocks. **B,** Push down on the bedpan and toward the client. **C,** Nurse places bedpan in position. (**A** and **B** from Sorrentino SA: *Mosby's textbook for nursing assistants,* ed 5, St. Louis, Mosby.)

11. Ensure that bed is in lowest position and upper side rails are up.	Promotes client safety and enables the client to reposition the pan as needed.
12. Remove gloves, and perform hand hygiene.	Reduces transmission of microorganisms.
13. Allow client to be alone, but monitor status and respond promptly to call signal.	Reassures client that nurse has not forgotten. Client may not be able to call nurse; the nurse is responsible for assessing client's status while on bedpan.
14. Apply new pair of gloves.	Reduces transmission of microorganisms.
15. Position client's bedside chair close to working side of bed.	Provides area to place bedpan and contents on chair after removal from client. Prevents spillage that could occur if full bedpan placed on bed surface.
16. Collect basin of warm water.	Allows client to perform hand hygiene after wiping perineal area (if appropriate); also allows nurse, wearing gloves, to use water to wash client's perineal area if client is unable to wipe thoroughly.
17. Move aside upper linens, keep client covered with towel.	Prevents undue embarrassment; maintains privacy.
18. Determine if client is able to wipe own perineal area.	Determines client's need for assistance in hygiene following use of bedpan.

STEP	RATIONALE
19. Remove bedpan of mobile client.	
a. Ask client to flex knees, placing body weight on lower legs, feet, and upper torso; lift buttocks up from bedpan. At same time, place hand farthest from client on side of bedpan to support it (prevent spillage) and place other hand (closest to client) under sacrum to assist in lifting. After client is completely lifted off bedpan, remove pan and place it on bedside chair.	Nurse should avoid pulling or shoving pan from under hips because this action can pull skin and cause tissue injury.
b. Offer client opportunity to perform hand hygiene after having wiped perineal area (if appropriate).	Reduces spread of microorganisms.
20. Remove bedpan of immobile client.	
a. Lower head of bed.	Facilitates turning of client.
b. Assist client with rolling onto side and off bedpan. Hold bedpan flat and steady while client is rolling off it; otherwise spillage will occur. Place bedpan and contents on bedside chair.	
c. Wipe client's anal area using several layers of toilet tissue or perineal wipes, wipe from mons pubis toward rectal area (for female client only); deposit contaminated tissue in bedpan. If necessary, wash perineal area with warm, soapy water, drying area thoroughly.	Cleansing from area of lesser contamination to greater contamination reduces spread of microorganisms. Prevents excoriation and skin breakdown. Promotes personal hygiene. This is an excellent time to perform perineal hygiene (see Chapter 14).
21. Cover bedpan and contents with bedpan cover as soon as possible.	Reduces spread of offensive odors.
22. Return client to comfortable position, ensuring that bottom linens are clean and as wrinkle-free as possible. Soiled linens must be changed.	Reduces chance of skin breakdown when bedridden client lies on dry, wrinkle-free linens.
23. Position bed in its lowest position. Ensure that call bell, phone, drinking water, and desired personal items (e.g., books) are within easy access.	Promotes comfort and reduces risk of injury to client.
24. If stool specimen is to be obtained, this is appropriate time to collect it. Wearing gloves, empty contents of bedpan into toilet or in special receptacle in appropriate utility room. Spray faucet attached to most institution toilets allows bedpan to be rinsed thoroughly. Use disinfectant if required by institution.	This should be done as soon as possible to prevent spread of offensive odor. Client uses same bedpan each time. (If it becomes very soiled, it could be replaced with clean one and soiled one sent for resterilization).
25. Replace all used equipment in appropriate location for subsequent use when required. Dispose of soiled linens correctly.	
26. Remove gloves, and perform hand hygiene.	Reduces transmission of microorganisms.

EVALUATION

1. Assess characteristics of stool. Note color, odor, consistency, frequency, amount, shape, and constituents. Also assess characteristics of urine, if client voided in bedpan.	Identifies significant changes or findings.
2. Evaluate client's ability to use bedpan.	Provides continual assessment of ability to use bedpan.
3. Inspect client's perianal area and surrounding skin while removing bedpan.	Liquid stool predisposes client to skin breakdown.
4. Evaluate client's overall activity tolerance and comfort.	Defecation and use of the bedpan can be energy consuming.

Recording and Reporting

• Record and report character and amount of stool in nurses' notes. Record urine output if client also voids.
• Complete laboratory requisition if stool or urine specimen was collected, and send to laboratory.

Unexpected Outcomes	Related Interventions
1. Client is unable to use bedpan.	• If client's mobility allows, obtain order for use of a bedside commode.
2. Client is incontinent of stool, resulting from client's embarrassment in using bedpan or nursing staff's delay in offering bedpan.	• Establish a regular schedule of offering bedpan, or improve responsiveness when client calls for assistance. • Discuss with staff the need to answer the client's request for toileting assistance promptly.
3. Client becomes constipated, resulting from pain of defecation, immobility, or unnatural position for defecation.	• Consult with physician regarding administration of a stool softener. • Try offering dietary foods high in fiber. • Increase fluid intake if appropriate for client's medical condition.
4. Client develops irritation and breakdown of skin around perianal area.	• Administer regular perineal care (see Chapter 14).
5. Blood in stool or black stool.	• This diagnostic finding requires fecal occult blood testing (FOBT) (see Chapter 43).

Teaching Considerations

• Some bedridden clients have overhead trapeze frame connected to bed to help lift them on and off bedpan. Teaching this activity can help to maintain strength of client's arms.
• Teach female clients to cleanse from area of lesser contamination to greater contamination (i.e., wiping from front to back). This reduces transmission of anal bacteria to urinary meatus and reduces risk of urinary tract infections.

Pediatric Considerations

• Constipation in early childhood results from environmental changes, such as being hospitalized and needing to use a bedpan.
• Repeated stool withholding leads to stretching or dilating of the rectum and decreases the sensation or "urge" to defecate (Hockenberry and others, 2003; Lembo and Camilleri, 2003).

Gerontological Considerations

• Older adults have some loss of sphincter control and often will require a quick response in providing a bedpan.
• Older adults may have limited movement in hips, requiring modification in pan placement (Ebersole and others, 2004).

• Incidence of constipation is greater because there is impaired rectal sensation to defecate. As a result the older adult does not perceive the need to defecate (Ebersole and others, 2004).
• Reinforce with older adult clients that as long as the consistency of the stool remains normal and that the bowel movements occur with regularity there is no need to have a bowel movement daily. Therefore clients should not place themselves on laxatives to avoid constipation (Ebersole and others, 2004; Lueckenotte, 2000).
• With increased age, transit time through the bowel increases, causing a normal lengthening of the time between bowel movements (Lueckenotte, 2000).

Home Care Considerations

• Assess client's home environment, routines, and activity of family members. When a bedpan must be used, determine availability of privacy and adequate time to use bedpan.

SKILL 33-2 Removing Fecal Impaction Digitally

Constipation is a relatively common health problem for many adults who believe that a regular bowel habit requires having a daily bowel movement or a bowel movement at the same time each day (or both) (Prather and Ortiz-Camacho, 1998). Constipation is usually defined medically as infrequent stools. However, a consensus definition of functional constipation includes two or more of the following factors noted for at least 3 months: (1) straining with defecation at least one fourth of the time, (2) lumpy or hard stools (or both) at least one fourth of the time, (3) sensation of incomplete evacuation at least one fourth of the time, or (4) two or fewer bowel movements in a week (Dosh, 2002; Lembo and Camilleri, 2003). There are a variety of interventions that can successfully relieve constipation. However, there are clients who develop obstipation, the absolute inability to pass stool.

Fecal impaction, the inability to pass a hard collection of stool, occurs in all age-groups. Physically and mentally incapacitated persons and institutionalized older adult clients are at greatest risk (Prather and Ortiz-Camacho, 1998). Symptoms of fecal impaction include constipation, rectal discomfort, anorexia, nausea, vomiting, abdominal pain, diarrhea (around the impacted stool), and urinary frequency. The treatment for fecal impaction is prevention, but once it occurs digital removal of stool is the only alternative (Lembo and Camilleri, 2003). This procedure can be very uncomfortable and embarrassing for the client. Excessive rectal manipulation may cause irritation to the mucosa, bleeding, and stimulation of the vagus nerve, which can cause a reflex slowing of the heart rate.

DELEGATION CONSIDERATIONS

This skill should not be delegated to assistive personnel. In some institutions only physicians perform this procedure. When delegating care to a client who has undergone digital removal of stool, the nurse provides information, direction, and assistance, including:

- Instruct assistive personnel to provide perineal care following each bowel movement.
- Instruct assistive personnel to observe any evacuated stool for color and consistency.
- Instruct assistive personnel to immediately report any signs of blood or bloody mucous discharge to the nurse for further assessment.

EQUIPMENT
- ❏ Disposable gloves
- ❏ Water-soluble local anesthetic lubricant (NOTE: Some institutions require use of water-soluble lubricant without anesthetic when nurse performs procedure.)
- ❏ Waterproof, absorbent pads
- ❏ Bedpan
- ❏ Bedpan cover
- ❏ Bath blanket
- ❏ Washbasin, washcloths, towels, and soap

STEP	RATIONALE

ASSESSMENT

1. Assess client to determine:
   a. Medical history of fecal impaction.

   b. Last bowel movement.

   c. Consistency of stool, seepage of liquid stool. This situation may occur particularly in immobilized client. Client seems to continually or frequently be incontinent of liquid stool.

   d. Expression of desire to defecate but inability to do so.
   e. Complaints of pain when trying to defecate.

Can be a recurrent problem for institutionalized or disabled clients (Prather and Ortiz-Camacho, 1998).

Infrequent defecation increases chances of hard stool forming in rectum. Constipation is defined as two or fewer stools per week (Dosh, 2002).

Symptomatic of an impaction high in colon. Client may be able to pass small pieces of hard stool or have episodes of passing small amounts of liquid stool (Prather and Ortiz-Camacho, 1998).

Large fecal mass causes rectal distention and increases perception of urge to evacuate the rectum (Dosh, 2002).

Pain often suppresses urge to defecate and compounds problem.

STEP	RATIONALE
f. Normal bowel patterns; eating habits; exercise pattern or level of mobility; medications, especially narcotic analgesics.	Nurse must determine if these are contributing factors and attempt to include nursing actions in care plan that may help to prevent situation from recurring.
g. Obtain baseline vital signs.	Provides baseline measure. The sacral branch of the vagus nerve is stimulated during digital stimulation; this stimulation may result in reflex slowing of heart rate (Seidel and others, 2003).

• *Critical Decision Point*
Because of the potential to stimulate the sacral branch of the vagus nerve, clients with a history of dysrhythmia or heart disease have a greater risk of changes in heart rhythm. Be sure to monitor client's pulse before and during procedure. This procedure may be contraindicated in cardiac clients; if in doubt, verify with physician.

STEP	RATIONALE
h. Bowel sounds and abdominal distention.	Indicates presence of peristalsis but does not conclusively confirm gastrointestinal patency. Distention can contribute to constipation.
2. Check client's record to determine if physician's order exists to remove stool manually.	Because this procedure may involve excessive stimulation of vagus nerve, physician's order must be written in client's record before nurse can perform procedure.

NURSING DIAGNOSES
- Constipation
- Diarrhea
- Acute pain

Related factors are individualized based on client's condition or needs.

PLANNING

1. Expected outcomes following completion of procedure:	
• Impacted stool is successfully removed.	Indicates rectum is clear of stool.
• Client is free of abdominal or rectal discomfort.	Fecal impaction causes direct pain to rectum and indirect abdominal discomfort through abdominal distention.
• Vital signs remain within client's baseline.	Indicates absence of vagal stimulation.
2. Explain procedure to client.	Information reduces anxiety and encourages client participation in a therapeutic elimination protocol.

IMPLEMENTATION

1. Perform hand hygiene, and apply gloves.	Prevents transmission of microorganisms.
2. Obtain assistance to help change client's position, if necessary. Raise bed horizontally to comfortable working height.	Promotes client safety and use of good body mechanics by nurse.
3. Keeping the far side rail raised, assist client to left side-lying position with knees flexed and back toward nurse.	Promotes client safety. Provides access to rectum.
4. Pull curtains around bed, or close door to room. With near side rail lowered, drape the client's trunk and lower extremities with bath blanket, and place a waterproof pad under the client's buttocks.	Maintains client's sense of privacy and prevents unnecessary exposure of body parts.
5. Place bedpan next to client.	Bedpan is receptacle for stool.
6. Don disposable gloves. Lubricate gloved index finger and middle finger of dominant hand with anesthetic lubricant.	Permits smooth insertion of finger into anus and rectum.

STEP	**RATIONALE**

- *Critical Decision Point*
  Observe for the presence of perianal skin irritation. Presence of such indicates the need for postprocedure skin care to the perianal region to reduce pain during subsequent bowel elimination.

7. Instruct client to take slow deep breaths, and gradually and gently insert gloved index finger, and feel the anus relax around the finger. Then insert the middle finger (Prather and Ortiz-Camacho, 1998).	Slow deep breaths may help to relax the client. Gradual insertion of index finger helps to dilate the anal sphincter.
8. Gradually advance fingers slowly along rectal wall toward umbilicus.	Allows nurse to reach impacted stool high in rectum.
9. Gently loosen fecal mass by moving fingers in a scissors motion to fragment the fecal mass (Prather and Ortiz-Camacho, 1998). Work fingers into hardened mass.	Loosening and penetrating mass allows nurse to remove it in small pieces, resulting in less discomfort to client.
10. Work stool downward toward end of rectum. Remove small sections of feces and discard into the bedpan.	Prevents need to force finger up into rectum and minimizes trauma to mucosa.
11. Periodically assess heart rate, and look for signs of fatigue.	Vagal stimulation slows heart rate and may cause dysrhythmia. Procedure may exhaust client.

- *Critical Decision Point*
  Stop procedure if heart rate drops or rhythm changes from the client's baseline.

12. Continue to clear rectum of feces, and allow client to rest at intervals.	Rest improves client's tolerance of procedure, allowing heart rate to slow.
13. After removal of impaction, provide washcloth and towel to wash buttocks and anal area.	Promotes client's sense of comfort and cleanliness.
14. Remove bedpan, and inspect feces for color and consistency. Dispose of feces. Remove gloves by turning inside out and discarding in proper receptacle.	Reduces transmission of microorganisms.
15. Assist client to toilet or clean bedpan. (Procedure may be followed by enema or cathartic.)	Disimpaction may stimulate defecation reflex.
16. Perform hand hygiene.	Reduces transmission of microorganisms.

EVALUATION

1. Perform rectal examination for stool, and observe anal and perianal area for irritation or skin breakdown.	Determines if rectum is clear.
2. Reassess vital signs, and compare to baseline values. Continue to monitor the client for 1 hour for bradycardia.	Determines extent of vagal stimulation.
3. Assess bowel sounds.	Determines presence of peristaltic activity.
4. Palpate abdomen to determine if it is soft and nontender.	Discomfort is relieved.

Recording and Reporting

- Record client's tolerance to procedure, amount and consistency of stool removed, and adverse effects.
- Report any adverse effects to nurse in charge or physician.

Unexpected Outcomes	Related Interventions
1. Client experiences bleeding from rectum.	• Assess anal and perianal region for source of bleeding. • Stop if bleeding is excessive.
2. Changes from baseline vital signs occur.	• Stop procedure, and retake vital signs. • Notify prescriber if vital signs remain altered.
3. Diarrheal stool is present.	• Assess client for continuing impaction. • Administer suppositories or enemas as ordered. • Increase client's fluid intake and dietary fiber.

Teaching Considerations

* If constipation and subsequent impaction are diet related, teach client about high-fiber nutritional products to increase bulk and the need for adequate fluid intake.
* If necessary, teach family caregivers about the effects of immobility, hydration, and nutrition on normal bowel elimination.

Pediatric Considerations

* Digital removal of stool is not recommended in pediatrics due to the risk of anal fissures and pain that may trigger stool withholding (Hockenberry and others, 2003).

Gerontological Considerations

* Many older adult clients are especially prone to dysrhythmia and other problems related to vagal stimulation; monitor heart rate and rhythm closely.
* At least 28% of older adult clients are constipated as a result of insufficient dietary bulk, inadequate fluid intake, laxative abuse, diminished muscle tone and motor function, decreased defecation reflex, mental or physical illness, and presence of tumors (Ebersole and others, 2004).
* For older adults, instituting a diet adequate in dietary fiber (6 to 10 g per day) adds bulk, weight, and form to stool and improves defecation (Ebersole and others, 2004).
* Consider development of a regular toileting routine that includes responding to the urge to defecate (Lueckenotte, 2000).

SKILL 33-3 Administering an Enema

An enema is the instillation of a solution into the rectum and sigmoid colon. The instillation of an enema solution promotes defecation by stimulating peristalsis. The volume or type of fluid breaks up the fecal mass, stretches the rectal wall, and initiates the defecation reflex.

Typically an enema is given to treat constipation or to empty the bowel before diagnostic procedures or certain types of abdominal surgery. Mosimann and Cornu (1998) suggest that clients who do not receive an enema before noncolonic abdominal operations have a return of peristalsis before those clients who have had enemas. Nevertheless, preoperative enemas are still very common for a number of surgeries.

Cleansing enemas promote complete evacuation of feces from the colon. They act by stimulating peristalsis through infusion of large volumes of solution. Oil-retention enemas act by lubricating the rectum and colon. Feces absorb oil and become softer and easier to pass. Medicated enemas contain pharmacological therapeutic agents and may be prescribed to reduce dangerously high serum potassium levels, as with use of a sodium polystyrene sulfonate (Kayexalate) enema, or to reduce bacteria in the colon before bowel surgery, as with use of a neomycin enema. Types of enemas include the following:

Tap water (hypotonic) enema should not be repeated after first installation because water toxicity or circulatory overload can develop.

Physiological normal saline is safest. Infants and children can tolerate only this type because of their predisposition to fluid imbalance. If solution is prepared at home, mix 500 ml (1 pint) of tap water with 1 teaspoon table salt.

Hypertonic solution is useful for clients who cannot tolerate large volumes of fluid. Only 120 to 180 ml (4 to 6 ounces) is usually effective (e.g., commercially prepared Fleet enema).

Harris Flush enema is a return flow enema that helps to expel intestinal gas. Fluid alternately is flowed into and out of the large intestine. This stimulates peristalsis in the large intestine and assists in expelling gas.

Soapsuds solution is pure castile soap added to either tap water or normal saline, depending on client's condition and frequency of administration. Use *only* castile pure soap. Recommended ratio of pure soap to solution is 5 ml (1 teaspoon) to 1000 ml (1 quart) warm water or saline. Soap should be added to enema bag after water is in place.

Oil-retention enema uses an oil-based solution. Permits administration of a small volume, which is absorbed by the stool. The absorption of the oil softens stool for easier evacuation.

Carminative solution provides relief from gaseous distention. An example is MGW solution, which contains 30 ml of magnesium, 60 ml of glycerin, and 90 ml of water.

DELEGATION CONSIDERATIONS

The skill of administering an enema can be delegated to assistive personnel. However, before delegating this skill, the nurse provides information, assistance, and direction, including:

- Inform and assist assistive personnel in proper way to position clients who have mobility restrictions.
- Instruct assistive personnel regarding positioning of clients with therapeutic equipment present, such as drains, intravenous catheters, or traction.
- Instruct assistive personnel regarding signs and symptoms of client not tolerating the procedure, and when it enema must be stopped. These signs and symptoms may include abdominal pain more than a pressure sensation, abdominal cramping, abdominal distention, or rectal bleeding.
- Explain to assistive personnel the expected outcome of the enema and to immediately inform the nurse about the presence of blood in the stool or around the rectal area, any change in client vital signs, or new symptoms so the nurse can further evaluate the client.

EQUIPMENT

- ❑ Disposable gloves
- ❑ Water-soluble lubricant
- ❑ Waterproof, absorbent pads
- ❑ Toilet tissue
- ❑ Bedpan, bedside commode, or access to toilet
- ❑ Washbasin, washcloths, towel, and soap
- ❑ Intravenous (IV) pole
  Enema Bag Administration
- ❑ Disposable gloves
- ❑ Enema container (Figure 33-2)
- ❑ Tubing and clamp (if not already attached to container)
- ❑ Appropriate-size rectal tube (adult: 22 to 30 Fr; child: 12 to 18 Fr)
- ❑ Correct volume of warmed solution (adult: 750 to 1000 ml; adolescent: 500 to 700 ml; school-age child: 300 to 500 ml; toddler: 250-350 ml; infant: 150 to 250 ml)
  Prepackaged Enema
- ❑ Prepackaged enema container with rectal tip (Figure 33-3)

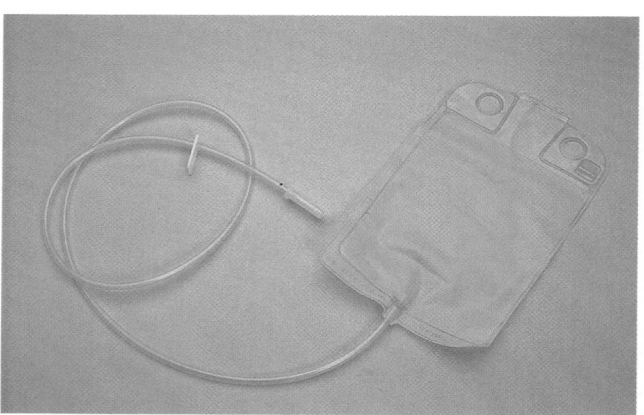

FIGURE **33-2** High-volume enema bag with tubing.

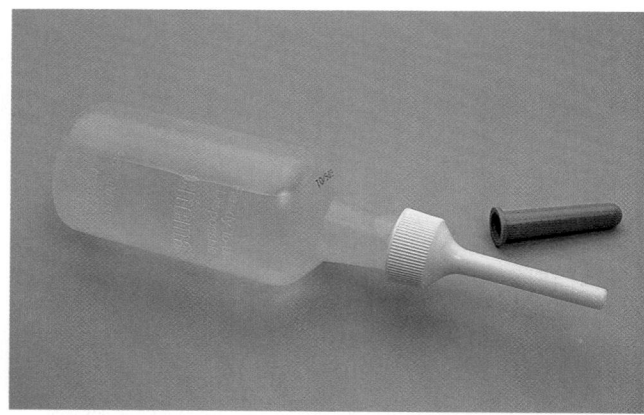

FIGURE **33-3** Prepackaged enema container with rectal tip.

STEP	RATIONALE

ASSESSMENT

1. Assess status of client: last bowel movement, normal versus most recent bowel pattern, presence of hemorrhoids, mobility, bowel sounds, presence of abdominal pain.

2. Assess medical record for presence of increased intracranial pressure, glaucoma, or recent rectal or prostate surgery.

Determines factors indicating need for enema and influencing the type of enema used. Also establishes baseline for bowel function.

Conditions contraindicate use of enemas.

STEP	RATIONALE
3. Inspect abdomen for presence of distention.	Establishes a baseline for determining effectiveness of enema.
4. Determine client's level of understanding of purpose of enema.	Allows nurse to plan for appropriate teaching measures.
5. Check client's medical record to clarify rationale for enema.	Determines purpose of enema administration: preparation for special procedure or relief of constipation.
6. Review physician's order for enema.	Order by physician is usually required for hospitalized client. Used to determine how many enemas client will require, type of enema to be given.

- **Critical Decision Point**
  "Enemas until clear" order means that enemas are repeated until client passes fluid that is clear of fecal matter. Check agency policy, but usually client should receive only three consecutive enemas to avoid disruption of fluid and electrolyte balance.

NURSING DIAGNOSES
- Constipation
- Risk for constipation
- Acute pain

Related factors are individualized based on client's condition or needs.

PLANNING

1. Expected outcomes following completion of procedure:	
• Stool is evacuated.	Solution clears rectum and lower colon of stool.
• Enema return is clear.	All feces in colon have passed.
• Abdomen is flat, nontender, with no distention.	Gas and feces have been expelled.
2. Collect appropriate equipment, and arrange at bedside.	Ensures smooth procedure.
3. Correctly identify client, and explain procedure.	Information promotes client cooperation and reduces anxiety.

IMPLEMENTATION

1. Perform hand hygiene, and apply gloves.	Reduces transmission of microorganisms.
2. Provide privacy by closing curtains around bed or closing door.	Reduces embarrassment for client.
3. Raise bed to appropriate working height for nurse; raise side rail on client's left side.	Promotes good body mechanics and client safety.
4. Assist client into left side-lying (Sims') position with right knee flexed. Children may also be placed in dorsal recumbent position.	Allows enema solution to flow downward by gravity along natural curve of sigmoid colon and rectum, thus improving retention of solution.

- **Critical Decision Point**
  If client is suspected of having poor sphincter control, position the client on the bedpan in comfortable dorsal recumbent position. Clients with poor sphincter control cannot retain all of enema solution. Administering enema with client sitting on toilet is unsafe because curved rectal tubing can abrade rectal wall.

5. Place waterproof pad under hips and buttocks.	Prevents soiling of linen.
6. Cover client with bath blanket, exposing only rectal area, clearly visualizing anus.	Provides warmth, reduces exposure of body parts, allows client to feel more relaxed and comfortable.
7. Separate buttocks, and examine perianal region for abnormalities, including hemorrhoids, anal fissure, rectal prolapse (Moppett, 1999).	Findings will influence nurse's approach to insertion of enema tip. Prolapse contraindicates enema.

STEP	RATIONALE
8. Place bedpan or commode in easily accessible position. If client will be expelling contents in toilet, ensure that toilet is free. (If client will be getting up to bathroom to expel enema, place client's slippers and bathrobe in easily accessible position.)	Used in case client is unable to retain enema solution.
9. Administer enema	
a. Administer prepackaged disposable commercial Fleet enema.	
(1) Remove plastic cap from tip of container. Tip of nozzle is already lubricated, but more water-soluble jelly can be applied as needed.	Lubrication provides for smooth insertion of rectal tube without causing rectal irritation or trauma.
(2) Gently separate buttocks, and locate rectum. Instruct client to relax by breathing out slowly through mouth.	Breathing out promotes relaxation of external rectal sphincter.
(3) Expel any air from the enema container.	Introducing air into colon can cause further distention and discomfort (Moppett, 1999).
(4) Insert nozzle of container gently into anal canal, angling towards the umbilicus. *Adult:* 7.5 to 10 cm (3 to 4 inches) (see illustration) *Adolescent:* 7.5 cm to 10 cm (3 to 4 inches) *Child:* 5 to 7.5 cm (2 to 3 inches) *Infant:* 2.5 to 3.75 cm (1 to 1½ inches)	Gentle insertion prevents trauma to rectal mucosa (Saltzstein and others, 1988).

- **Critical Decision Point**
  If pain occurs or resistance is felt at any time during procedure, stop and confer with physician.

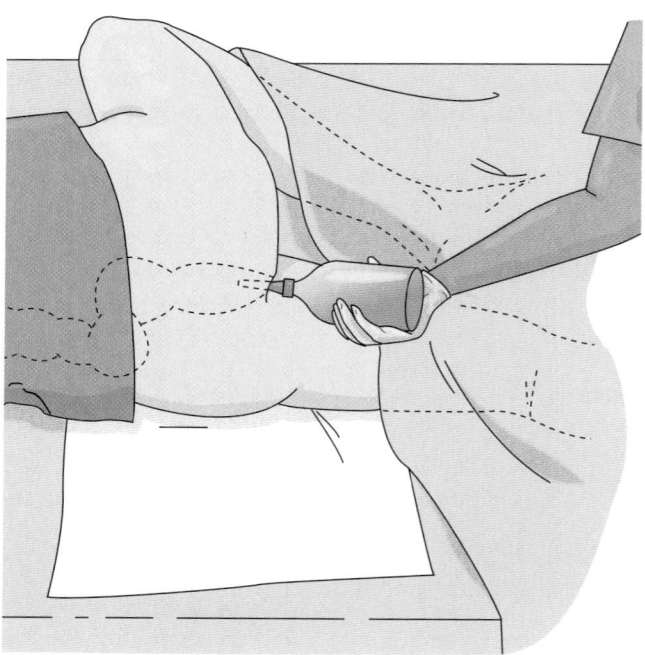

STEP **9a(4)** The tip of the commercial enema is inserted into the rectum. (From Sorrentino SA: *Mosby's textbook for nursing assistants,* ed 5, St. Louis, 2000, Mosby.)

STEP	**RATIONALE**

(5) Squeeze bottle until all of solution has entered rectum and colon. Instruct client to retain solution until the urge to defecate occurs, usually 2 to 5 minutes.

Hypertonic solutions require only small volumes to stimulate defecation.

b. Administer enema using enema bag.

(1) Add warmed solution to enema bag: warm tap water as it flows from faucet, place saline container in basin of hot water before adding saline to enema bag, and check temperature of solution by pouring small amount of solution over inner wrist.

Hot water can burn intestinal mucosa. Cold water can cause abdominal cramping and is difficult to retain.

(2) Raise container, release clamp, and allow solution to flow long enough to fill tubing.

Removes air from tubing.

(3) Reclamp tubing.

Prevents further loss of solution.

(4) Lubricate 6 to 8 cm (2½ to 3 inches) of tip of rectal tube with lubricating jelly.

Allows smooth insertion of rectal tube without risk of irritation or trauma to mucosa.

(5) Gently separate buttocks, and locate anus. Instruct client to relax by breathing out slowly through mouth.

Breathing out promotes relaxation of external anal sphincter.

(6) Insert tip of rectal tube slowly by pointing tip in direction of client's umbilicus (see illustration). Length of insertion varies:
Adult: 7.5 to 10 cm (3 to 4 inches)
Adolescent: 7.5 cm to 10 cm (3 to 4 inches)
Child: 5 to 7.5 cm (2 to 3 inches)
Infant: 2.5 to 3.75 cm (1 to 1½ inches)

Careful insertion prevents trauma to rectal mucosa from accidental lodging of tube against rectal wall. Insertion beyond proper limit can cause bowel perforation.

- *Critical Decision Point*
  If tube does not pass easily, do not force. Consider allowing a small amount of fluid to infuse, and then try to slowly reinsert the tube. The instillation of fluid may relax the sphincter and provide additional lubrication.

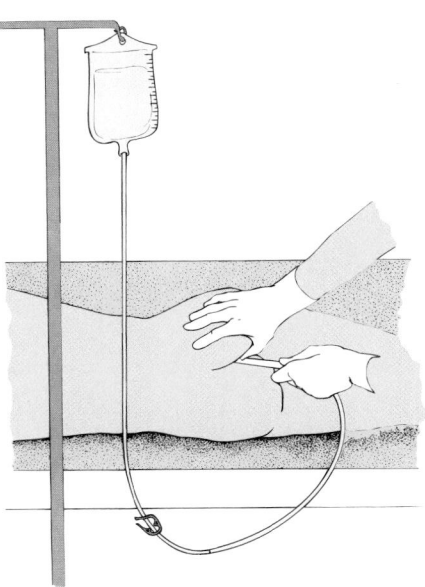

STEP **9b(6)** Insertion of rectal tube into rectum.

STEP	**RATIONALE**
(7) Hold tubing in rectum constantly until end of fluid instillation.	Bowel contraction can cause expulsion of rectal tube.
(8) Open regulating clamp, and allow solution to enter slowly with container at client's hip level.	Rapid instillation can stimulate evacuation of rectal tube.
(9) Raise height of enema container slowly to appropriate level above anus: 30 to 45 cm (12 to 18 inches) for high enema, 30 cm (12 inches) for regular enema, 7.5 cm (3 inches) for low enema. Instillation time varies with volume of solution administered (e.g., 1 L/10 min) (see illustration).	Allows for continuous, slow instillation of solution; raising container too high causes rapid instillation and possible painful distention of colon. High pressure can cause rupture of bowel in infant.
(10) Lower container or clamp tubing if client complains of cramping or if fluid escapes around rectal tube.	Temporary cessation of instillation prevents cramping, which may prevent client from retaining all fluid, altering effectiveness of enema.
(11) Clamp tubing after all solution is instilled.	Prevents entrance of air into rectum.
10. Place layers of toilet tissue around tube at anus and gently withdraw rectal tube and tip.	Provides for client's comfort and cleanliness.
11. Explain to client that feeling of distention is normal, as well as some abdominal cramping. Ask client to retain solution as long as possible while lying quietly in bed. (For infant or young child, gently hold buttocks together for few minutes.)	Solution distends bowel. Length of retention varies with type of enema and client's ability to contract rectal sphincter. Longer retention promotes more effective stimulation of peristalsis and defecation.

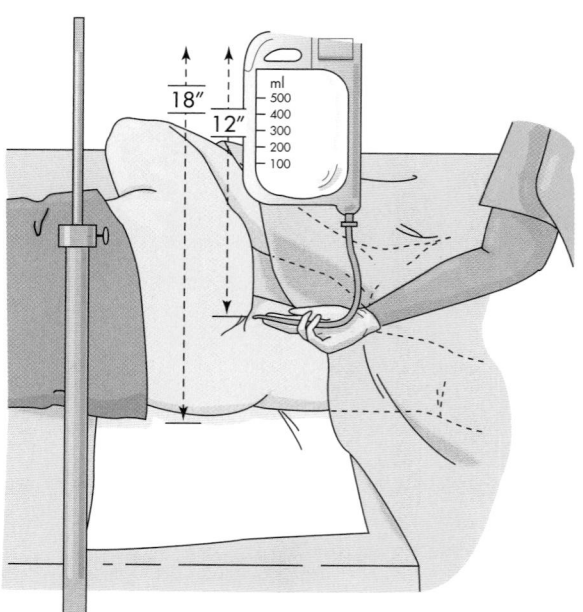

STEP 9b(9) An enema is given in the Sims' position. The IV pole is positioned so that the enema bag is 12 inches above the anus and approximately 18 inches above the mattress (depending on the client's size). (From Sorrentino SA: *Mosby's textbook for nursing assistants,* ed 5, St. Louis, 2000, Mosby.)

STEP	RATIONALE
12. Discard enema container and tubing in proper receptacle, or rinse out thoroughly with warm soap and water if container is to be reused.	Reduces transmission and growth of microorganisms.
13. Assist client to bathroom, or help to position client on bedpan.	Normal squatting position promotes defecation.
14. Observe character of feces and solution (caution client against flushing toilet before inspection).	

• **Critical Decision Point**
When enemas are ordered "until clear," it is essential to observe contents of solution passed. The enema return is considered "clear" when no solid fecal material exists, but the solution may be colored.

STEP	RATIONALE
15. Assist client as needed with washing anal area with warm soap and water (if nurse administers perineal care, use gloves). If client is using a toilet, caution against flushing toilet before inspection of enema return.	Fecal contents can irritate skin. Hygiene promotes client's comfort.
16. Remove and discard gloves, and perform hand hygiene.	Reduces transmission of microorganisms.

EVALUATION

1. Inspect color, consistency, and amount of stool, odor, and fluid passed.	Determines if stool is evacuated or fluid is retained. Note abnormalities such as presence of blood or mucus.
2. Assess condition of abdomen.	Determines if distention is relieved.

Recording and Reporting

• Record type and volume of enema given, time administered, and characteristics of results.
• Report failure of client to defecate and any adverse effects to physician.

Unexpected Outcomes	Related Interventions
1. Abdomen becomes rigid and distended.	• Stop enema. • Obtain vital signs. • Notify prescriber.
2. Abdominal cramping or pain develops.	• Slow the rate of instillation.
3. Bleeding occurs.	• Stop the enema. • Notify prescriber. • Obtain vital signs, and assess abdomen and rectum.

Teaching Considerations

• Client should be instructed that enemas should not be given to treat cause of constipation.
• For self-administration, client should be instructed to lie in dorsal recumbent position with knees and hips flexed toward chest.

Pediatric Considerations

• The use of oral stool softeners is the initial recommended treatment of constipation in children.

• Children and infants usually do not receive prepackaged hypertonic enemas because hypertonic solutions can cause rapid fluid shift (Hockenberry and others, 2003).

Gerontological Considerations

• Caution is needed when enemas are ordered "until clear" in the older adult population. Older adults may become fatigued, are at risk for fluid and electrolyte imbalances, and may experience changes in vital signs.

- Instruct older adults and their caregivers in how to modify diet to avoid constipation.
- Older adult may have difficulty retaining fluid. The nurse may gently hold buttocks together to assist.

Home Care Considerations

- Assess client's and primary caregiver's ability and motivation to administer enema, and provide instruction as needed.

- Assess client's ability to manipulate equipment and self-administer enema.
- Assess client's environment to identify location where enema may be administered with privacy.

SKILL 33-4 Inserting and Maintaining a Nasogastric Tube for Gastric Decompression

There are times following major surgery or as a result of conditions affecting the gastrointestinal tract when normal peristalsis temporarily becomes altered. Because peristalsis is slowed or absent, a client cannot eat or drink fluids without causing abdominal distention. The temporary insertion of a nasogastric tube into the stomach serves to decompress the stomach, keeping it empty until normal peristalsis returns.

A nasogastric (NG) tube is a pliable tube that is inserted through the client's nasopharynx into the stomach. The tube has a hollow lumen that allows the removal of gastric secretions and the introduction of solutions into the stomach. There are times when a nasogastric tube can be used for enteral feedings, but a softer small-bore feeding tube is preferred for feeding purposes (see Chapter 30). The Levin and Salem sump tubes are the most common for stomach decompression. The Levin tube is a single lumen tube with holes near the tip. It may be connected to a drainage bag or an intermittent suction device to drain stomach secretions. The Salem sump tube is preferable for stomach decompres-

sion. The tube has two lumina: one for removal of gastric contents and one to provide an air vent. A blue "pigtail" is the air vent that connects with the second lumen. When the sump tube's main lumen is connected to suction, the air vent permits free, continuous drainage of secretions. *The air vent should never be clamped off, connected to suction, or used for irrigation.*

Nasogastric tube insertion does not require sterile technique. Clean technique is adequate. The procedure is uncomfortable, with clients experiencing a burning sensation as the tube passes through the sensitive nasal mucosa. One of the greatest nursing care challenges is keeping the client comfortable because the tube is a constant irritation to mucosa. The nurse routinely assesses the condition of the nares and mucosa for inflammation and excoriation. Supportive care includes changing soiled tape or fixation devices when they become soiled, keeping the nares lubricated and clean, and providing frequent mouth care to minimize the dehydration from mouth breathing.

DELEGATION CONSIDERATIONS

The skill of inserting and maintaining an NG tube should not be delegated to assistive personnel. The nurse is responsible for the proper function and drainage of the nasogastric tube, all relevant assessments, and determining the client's level of comfort. The nurse instead directs assistive personnel to:

- Measure and record the drainage from an NG tube
- Provide oral and nasal hygiene measures
- Perform selected comfort measures, such as positioning, offering ice chips if allowed
- Anchor the tube to the client's gown during routine care to prevent accidental displacement

EQUIPMENT

- ❑ 14 or 16 Fr NG tube (smaller-lumen catheters are not used for decompression in adults because they must be able to remove thick secretions)
- ❑ Water-soluble lubricating jelly
- ❑ pH test strips (measure gastric aspirate acidity)
- ❑ Tongue blade
- ❑ Flashlight
- ❑ Emesis basin
- ❑ Asepto bulb or catheter-tipped syringe
- ❑ 1-inch (2.5-cm) wide hypoallergenic tape or commercial fixation device

EQUIPMENT—cont'd

❑ Safety pin and rubber band
❑ Clamp, drainage bag, or suction machine or pressure gauge if wall suction is to be used
❑ Towel
❑ Glass of water with straw

❑ Facial tissues
❑ Normal saline
❑ Tincture of benzoin (optional)
❑ Suction equipment
❑ Disposable gloves

STEP	RATIONALE

ASSESSMENT

1. Inspect condition of client's nasal and oral cavity.

Baseline condition of nasal and oral cavity determines need for special nursing hygiene measures after tube placement.

2. Ask if client has had history of nasal surgery, and note if deviated nasal septum is present.

Nurse should insert tube into ***uninvolved*** nasal passage. Procedure may be contraindicated if surgery is recent.

3. Palpate client's abdomen for distention, pain, and rigidity. Auscultate for bowel sounds.

Baseline determination of level of abdominal distention and function later serves as comparison once tube is inserted. Decreased bowel sounds occur with peritonitis and paralytic ileus. In the presence of diminished or absent bowel sounds the abdomen should be auscultated for 5 minutes in all four quadrants to make sure that no sounds are missed and to localize specific sounds (Seidel and others, 2003).

4. Assess client's level of consciousness and ability to follow instructions.

Determines client's ability to assist in procedure.

• *Critical Decision Point*
If client is confused, disoriented, or unable to follow commands, obtain assistance from another staff member to insert the tube.

5. Determine if client has had an NG tube insertion in the past and which naris was used.

Procedure is uncomfortable and requires thorough explanation. Client's previous experience will complement any explanations.

6. Check medical record for physician's order, type of NG tube to be placed, and whether tube is to be attached to suction or drainage bag.

Procedure requires physician's order. Adequate decompression depends on NG suction.

NURSING DIAGNOSES

• Deficient knowledge regarding purpose of gastric decompression
• Impaired oral mucous membrane

• Risk for impaired skin integrity
• Acute pain

Related factors are individualized based on client's condition or needs.

PLANNING

1. Expected outcomes following completion of procedure:
   • Stomach will remain soft, nontender, and without distention.

NG tube is positioned in stomach, remains patent, and drains gastric secretions.

   • Client nares and surface of nose remain clear, without abrasions or excoriation.

Absence of irritation from NG tube.

   • Client's nasal mucosa will remain moist and intact.

Reduces risk of erosion developing.

2. Prepare equipment at the bedside. Have a 4-inch (10-cm) piece of tape ready with one end split in half.

Ensures well-organized procedure. Tape will be used to initially hold tube in place after insertion.

3. Identify client, and explain procedure. Let client know there will be a burning sensation in nasopharynx as tube is passed.

Identification prevents error of placing tube in wrong client. Explanation gains client's cooperation and ability to anticipate nurse's action.

STEP	RATIONALE

IMPLEMENTATION

1. Perform hand hygiene, and apply disposable gloves.

   Reduces transmission of microorganisms.

2. Position client in high-Fowler's position with pillows behind head and shoulders. Raise bed to a horizontal level comfortable for the nurse.

   Promotes client's ability to swallow during procedure. Good body mechanics prevents injury to nurse or client.

3. Place bath towel over client's chest; give facial tissues to client. Place emesis basin within reach.

   Prevents soiling of client's gown. Tube insertion through nasal passages may cause tearing and coughing with increased salivation.

4. Pull curtain around the bed, or close room door.

   Provides privacy.

5. Stand on client's right side if right-handed, left side if left-handed.

   Allows easiest manipulation of tubing.

6. Instruct client to relax and breathe normally while occluding one naris. Then repeat this action for other naris. Select nostril with greater airflow.

   Tube passes more easily through naris that is more patent.

7. Measure distance to insert tube:

   a. *Traditional method:* Measure distance from tip of nose to earlobe to xiphoid process (see illustration).

      Tube should extend from nares to stomach; distance varies with each client.

   b. *Hanson method:* First mark 50-cm point on tube, then do traditional measurement. Tube insertion should be to midway point between 50 cm (20 inches) and traditional mark.

8. Mark length of tube to be inserted with small piece of tape placed around tube so it can be easily removed.

   Marks amount of tube to be inserted from naris to stomach.

9. Curve 10 to 15 cm (4 to 6 inches) of end of tube tightly around index finger, then release.

   Curving tube tip aids insertion and decreases stiffness of tube.

10. Lubricate 7.5 to 10 cm (3 to 4 inches) of end of tube with water-soluble lubricating gel.

    Minimizes friction against nasal mucosa and aids insertion of tube. Water-soluble lubricant is less toxic than oil-soluble if aspirated.

11. Alert client that procedure is to begin.

    Decreases client anxiety and increases client cooperation.

12. Initially instruct client to extend neck back against pillow; insert tube slowly through naris with curved end pointing downward (see illustration).

    Facilitates initial passage of tube through naris and maintains clear airway for open naris.

13. Continue to pass tube along floor of nasal passage, aiming down toward ear. When resistance is felt, apply gentle downward pressure to advance tube (do not force past resistance).

    Minimizes discomfort of tube rubbing against upper nasal turbinates. Resistance is caused by posterior nasopharynx. Downward pressure helps tube curl around corner of nasopharynx.

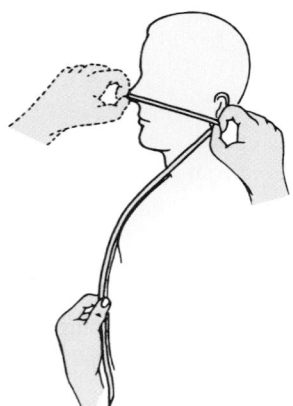

STEP **7a** Technique for measuring distance to insert NG tube.

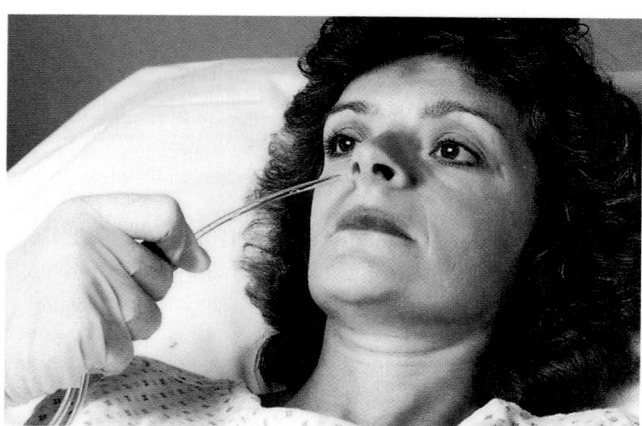

STEP **12** Insert NG tube with curved end pointing downward.

STEP	RATIONALE
14. If resistance is met, try to rotate the tube, and see if it advances. If still resistant, withdraw tube, allow client to rest, relubricate tube, and insert into other naris.	Forcing against resistance can cause trauma to mucosa. Helps relieve client's anxiety.

• **Critical Decision Point**
If unable to insert tube in either naris, stop procedure and notify physician.

STEP	RATIONALE
15. Continue insertion of tube until just past nasopharynx by gently rotating tube toward opposite naris.	
a. Once past nasopharynx, stop tube advancement, allow client to relax, and provide tissues.	Relieves client's anxiety; tearing is natural response to mucosal irritation, and excessive salivation may occur because of oral stimulation.
b. Explain to client that next step requires that client swallow. Give client glass of water unless contraindicated.	Sipping of water aids passage of NG tube into esophagus.
16. With tube just above oropharynx, instruct client to flex head forward, take a small sip of water, and swallow. Advance tube 2.5 to 5 cm (1 to 2 inches) with each swallow of water. If client is not allowed fluids, instruct to dry swallow or suck air through straw. Advance tube with each swallow.	Flexed position closes off upper airway to trachea and opens esophagus. Swallowing closes epiglottis over trachea and helps move the tube into the esophagus. Swallowing water reduces gagging or choking. Water can be removed later from stomach by suction.
17. If client begins to cough, gag, or choke, withdraw slightly and stop tube advancement. Instruct client to breathe easily and take sips of water.	Tubing may accidentally enter larynx and initiate cough reflex, and withdrawal of the tube reduces risk of laryngeal entry. Gagging is eased by swallowing water, which must be given cautiously to reduce the risk of aspiration.

• **Critical Decision Point**
If vomiting occurs, assist client in clearing airway; oral suctioning may be needed. Do not proceed until airway is cleared.

STEP	RATIONALE
18. If client continues to cough during insertion, pull tube back slightly.	Tube may enter larynx and obstruct airway.
19. If client continues to gag and cough or complains that the tube feels as though it is coiling in the back of the throat, check back of oropharynx using flashlight and tongue blade. If tube is coiled, withdraw it until the tip is back in the oropharynx. Then reinsert with the client swallowing.	Tube may coil around itself in back of throat and stimulate gag reflex.
20. After client relaxes, continue to advance tube with swallowing until tape or mark on tube is reached, which signifies the tube is in the desired distance. Temporarily anchor tube to client's cheek with a piece of tape until tube placement is verified.	Tip of tube should be within stomach to decompress properly. Anchoring of tube prevents accidental displacement while the tube placement is verified.
21. Verify tube placement: Check agency policy for preferred methods for checking tube placement.	
a. Ask client to talk.	Client is unable to talk if NG tube has passed through vocal cords.
b. Inspect posterior pharynx for presence of coiled tube.	Tube is pliable and can coil up in back of pharynx instead of advancing into esophagus.

STEP	RATIONALE
c. Aspirate gently back on syringe to obtain gastric contents, observing color (see illustration).	Gastric contents are usually cloudy and green, but may be off-white, tan, bloody, or brown in color. Aspiration of contents provides means to measure fluid pH and thus determine tube tip placement in gastrointestinal tract.
	Other common aspirate colors include the following: duodenal placement (yellow or bile stained), esophagus (may or may not have saliva-appearing aspirate).
d. Measure pH of aspirate with color-coded pH paper with range of whole numbers from 1 to 14 (see illustration).	Gastric aspirates have decidedly acidic pH values, preferably 4 or less, compared with intestinal aspirates, which are usually greater than 4, or respiratory secretions, which are usually greater than 5.5 (Metheny and others, 1993, 1994, 1998; Metheny and Titler, 2001).

- **Critical Decision Point**
  Be sure to use gastric (Gastrocult) pH test and not Hemoccult test.

e. Have ordered x-ray examination performed of chest/abdomen.	X-ray film verifies initial placement of the tube (Metheny and Titler, 2001).
f. If tube is not in stomach, advance another 2.5 to 5 cm (1 to 2 inches), and repeat steps 21a to d to check tube position.	Tube must be in stomach to provide decompression.

22. Anchoring tube:

a. After tube is properly inserted and positioned, either clamp end or connect it to drainage bag or suction machine.	Drainage bag is used for gravity drainage. Intermittent suction is most effective for decompression. Client going to the operating room often has tube clamped.
b. Tape tube to nose; avoid putting pressure on nares. Cut tape about 5 inches (10 cm), and split down the middle, halfway.	Prevents tissue necrosis. Tape anchors tube securely.
(1) Before taping tube to nose, apply small amount of tincture of benzoin to lower end of nose, and allow to dry *(optional)*. Apply tape to nose, leaving the split end free. Be sure top end of tape over nose is secure.	Benzoin prevents loosening of tape if client perspires.

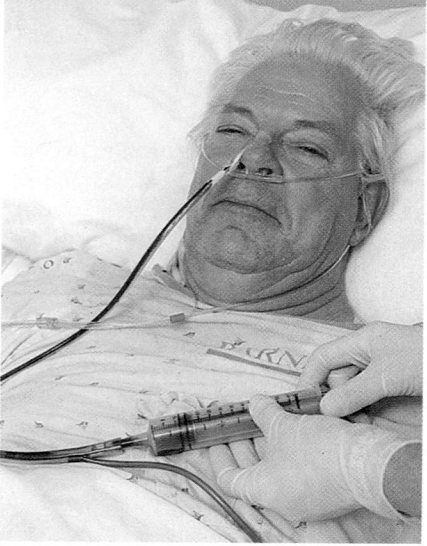

STEP **21c** Aspiration of gastric contents.

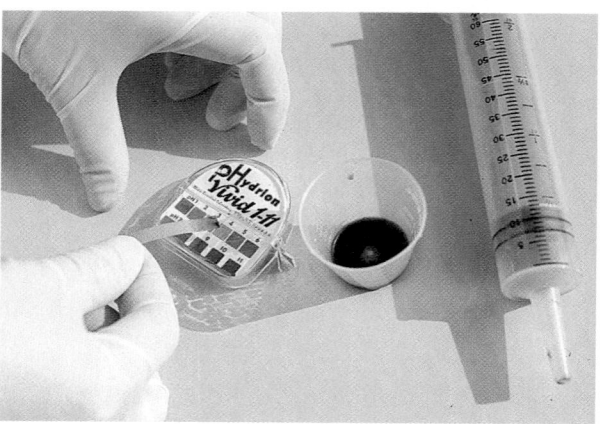

STEP **21d** Checking pH of gastric aspirate.

STEP	RATIONALE

(2) Carefully wrap two split ends of tape around tube (see illustration).

(3) Alternative: Apply tube fixation device using shaped adhesive patch (see illustration).

c. Fasten end of NG tube to client's gown by looping rubber band around tube in slipknot. Pin rubber band to gown (provides slack for movement).

Reduces pressure on nares if tube moves.

d. Unless physician orders otherwise, head of bed should be elevated 30 degrees.

Helps prevent esophageal reflux and minimizes irritation of tube against posterior pharynx.

e. Explain to client that sensation of tube should decrease somewhat with time.

Adaptation to continued sensory stimulus.

f. Remove gloves, and perform hand hygiene.

Reduces transmission of microorganisms.

23. Once placement is confirmed:

a. Place a mark, either a red mark or tape, on the tube to indicate where the tube exits the nose.

The mark or tube length is to be used as a guide to indicate whether displacement may have occurred.

b. Measure the tube length from nares to connector as an alternate method.

c. Document the tube length in the client record.

Information assists in determining tube placement.

24. Tube irrigation:

a. Perform hand hygiene, and apply gloves.

Reduces transmission of microorganisms.

b. Check for tube placement in stomach (see step 21). Reconnect NG tube to connecting tube.

Prevents accidental entrance of irrigating solution into lungs.

c. Draw up 30 ml of normal saline into Asepto or catheter-tip syringe.

Use of saline minimizes loss of electrolytes from stomach fluids.

d. Clamp NG tube. Disconnect from connecting tubing, and lay end of connection tubing on towel.

Reduces soiling of client's gown and bed linen.

e. Insert tip of irrigating syringe into end of NG tube. Remove clamp. Hold syringe with tip pointed at floor, and inject saline slowly and evenly. Do not force solution.

Position of syringe prevents introduction of air into vent tubing, which could cause gastric distention. Solution introduced under pressure can cause gastric trauma.

- **Critical Decision Point**

  Do not introduce saline through blue "pigtail" air vent of Salem sump tube.

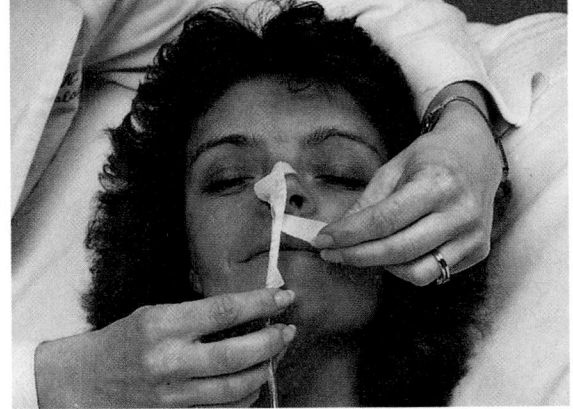

STEP **22b(2)** Tape is crossed over and around NG tube.

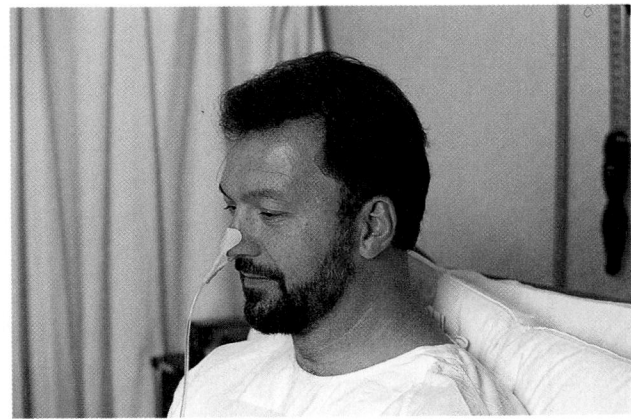

STEP **22b(3)** Client with tube fixation device.

STEP	RATIONALE
f. If resistance occurs, check for kinks in tubing. Turn client onto left side. Repeated resistance should be reported to surgeon.	Tip of tube may lie against stomach lining. Repositioning on left side may dislodge tube away from the stomach lining. Buildup of secretions will cause distention.
g. After instilling saline, immediately aspirate, or pull back slowly on syringe to withdraw fluid. If amount aspirated is greater than amount instilled, record the difference as output. If amount aspirated is less than amount instilled, record the difference as intake.	Irrigation clears tubing, so stomach should remain empty. Fluid remaining in stomach is measured as intake.
h. Reconnect NG tube to drainage or suction. (If solution does not return, repeat irrigation.)	Reestablishes drainage collection; may repeat irrigation or repositioning of tube until NG tube drains properly.
i. Remove gloves, and perform hand hygiene.	Reduces transmission of microorganisms.
25. Discontinuation of NG tube:	
a. Verify order to discontinue NG tube.	Physician's order required for procedure.
b. Explain procedure to client, and reassure that removal is less distressing than insertion.	Minimizes anxiety and increases cooperation. Tube passes out smoothly.
c. Perform hand hygiene, and apply disposable gloves.	Reduces transmission of microorganisms.
d. Turn off suction, and disconnect NG tube from drainage bag or suction. Remove tape or fixation device from bridge of nose, and unpin tube from gown.	Have tube free of connections before removal.
e. Stand on client's right side if right-handed, left side if left-handed.	Allows easiest manipulation of tube.
f. Hand the client facial tissue; place clean towel across chest. Instruct client to take and hold a deep breath.	Client may wish to blow nose after tube is removed. Towel may keep gown from getting soiled. Airway will be temporarily obstructed during tube removal.
g. Clamp or kink tubing securely and then pull tube out steadily and smoothly into towel held in other hand while client holds breath.	Clamping prevents tube contents from draining into oropharynx. Reduces trauma to mucosa and minimizes client's discomfort. Towel covers tube, which can be an unpleasant sight. Holding breath helps to prevent aspiration.
h. Measure amount of drainage, and note character of content. Dispose of tube and drainage equipment into proper container.	Provides accurate measure of fluid output. Reduces transfer of microorganisms.
i. Clean nares, and provide mouth care.	Promotes comfort.
j. Position client comfortably, and explain procedure for drinking fluids, if not contraindicated.	Depends on physician's order. Sometimes clients are allowed nothing by mouth (NPO) for up to 24 hours. When fluids are allowed, the order usually begins with a small amount of ice chips each hour and increases as client is able to tolerate more.
26. Clean equipment, and return to proper place. Place soiled linen in utility room or proper receptacle.	Proper disposal of equipment prevents spread of microorganisms and ensures proper exchange procedures.
27. Remove gloves, and perform hand hygiene.	Reduces transmission of microorganisms.

EVALUATION

1. Observe amount and character of contents draining from NG tube. Ask if client feels nauseated.	Determines if tube is decompressing stomach of contents.
2. Palpate client's abdomen periodically, noting any distention, pain, and rigidity, and auscultate for the presence of bowel sounds. Turn off suction while auscultating.	Determines success of abdominal decompression and the return of peristalsis. The sound of the suction apparatus may be transmitted to abdomen and be misinterpreted as bowel sounds.

STEP	RATIONALE
3. Inspect condition of nares and nose.	Evaluates onset of skin and tissue irritation.
4. Observe position of tubing.	Determines if tension is being applied to nasal structures.
5. Ask if client feels sore throat or irritation in pharynx.	Evaluates level of client's discomfort.

Recording and Reporting

- Record length, size, and type of gastric tube inserted and through which nostril it was inserted, client's tolerance of procedure, confirmation of tube placement, character of gastric contents, pH value, whether the tube is clamped or connected to drainage or to suction, and the amount of suction supplied.
- Record difference between amount of normal saline instilled and amount of gastric aspirate removed on intake and output (I&O) sheet. Record in nurses' notes or flow sheet amount and character of contents draining from NG tube every shift.

Unexpected Outcomes	Related Interventions
1. Client's abdomen is distended and painful.	• Assess patency of the tube. • Irrigate tube. • Verify that suction is on as ordered.
2. Client complains of sore throat from dry, irritated mucous membranes.	• Perform oral hygiene more frequently. • Ask physician whether client can suck on ice chips or throat lozenges.
3 Client develops irritation or erosion of skin around naris.	• Provide frequent skin care to area. • Retape tube to avoid pressure on naris. • Consider switching tube to other naris.
4. Client develops signs and symptoms of pulmonary aspiration: fever, shortness of breath, or pulmonary congestion.	• Perform complete respiratory assessment. • Notify physician. • Obtain chest x-ray examination as ordered.

Gerontological Considerations

- Check for ill-fitting dentures, and remove them for the client's safety and comfort during the insertion.
- Oral and nasal mucosal drying may be present. Be sure that the tube is adequately lubricated for insertion.

FOCUS *on* CLINICAL PRACTICE

Mrs. Feld is a 78-year-old woman with a history of diabetes mellitus who is hospitalized following a fall in her home during which she fractured her right hip. The hip was surgically repaired 3 days ago. At present she is in bed and is not allowed to bear any weight on her right leg. Mrs. Feld's last bowel movement was the day before she fell, so that she has gone 4 days without a bowel movement. For the last 2 days she has been on a 1200-cal diabetic diet.

Her abdomen is nontender, slightly distended. Her bowel sounds are active and within normal range in all 4 quadrants. She attempted a bowel movement with a great deal of straining and expelled small, hard brown stool. You have talked to her doctor, and he provided orders for a Fleet enema.

1. You have explained the enema procedure to Mrs. Feld and have prepared your supplies. You need to provide a bedpan or commode for Mrs. Feld to expel the fecal material following the enema. Please make your selection and provide a rationale.
2. A Fleet enema was given to Mrs. Feld; an assistive personnel is also providing care to Mrs. Feld. What is the expected outcome of Mrs. Feld's enema? What if any instructions will you give to the assistive personnel?

3. The assistive personnel just reported to you that Mrs. Feld is complaining of stomach pain. From the following select and prioritize the correct actions:
   A. Notify the doctor.
   B. Instruct the assistive personnel to palpate Mrs. Feld's abdomen.
   C. Give postoperative pain medication as ordered.
   D. Perform an abdominal assessment.
   E. Obtain vital signs, and instruct assistive personnel to obtain vital signs every 15 to 30 minutes thereafter.
4. Mr. Dale has pancreatitis and is NPO. To reduce the pain from pancreatitis it is important that his stomach remain empty and decompressed; as a result he has a Salem sump nasogastric tube set to low suction. When you assessed Mr. Dale at the beginning of your shift, his abdomen was soft and nontender, the NG tube was draining dark green secretions, and he was not nauseated. Two hours later, the assistive personnel reports that he is nauseated and vomited dark green material. You go to his bedside and inspect the vomitus and assess the client. He is diaphoretic; temperature, 99° F; pulse, 110 beats per minute; blood pressure, 140/88 mm Hg. His abdomen is distended, slightly tender, and there is no drainage from the NG tube. What are your actions?

NCLEX REVIEW QUESTIONS

1. Which assessment finding is not associated with constipation/impaction?
   1. Diarrhea
   2. Abdominal distention
   3. Hard, small stools
   4. Absent bowel sounds
2. When selecting interventions to reduces the risk of constipation, which is the appropriate stepwise order?
   1. Lifestyle changes, bulk-forming laxatives, saline or osmotic laxatives, stimulating laxatives
   2. Bulk-forming laxatives, lifestyle changes, saline or osmotic laxatives, stimulating laxatives
   3. Lifestyle changes, stimulating laxatives, bulk-forming laxatives, saline or osmotic laxatives
   4. Bulk-forming laxatives, stimulating laxatives, lifestyle changes, saline or osmotic laxatives

3. Fecal incontinence can be managed by dietary fiber. The rationale for this intervention is:
   1. Dietary fiber increases intestinal transit time and increases bulk of fecal contents.
   2. Dietary fiber decreases intestinal transit time and increases bulk of fecal contents.
   3. Dietary fiber increases intestinal transit time and decreases water reabsorption into the fecal contents.
   4. Dietary fiber decreases intestinal transit time and decreases water reabsorption into the fecal contents.
4. The normal frequency for bowel sounds is:
   1. 5 to 10 per minute
   2. 10 to 30 per minute
   3. 5 to 35 per minute
   4. 10 to 30 per minute

NCLEX REVIEW QUESTIONS

5. Absent bowel sounds occur with:
   1. Intestinal viruses and bacteria
   2. Constipation and impaction
   3. Overuse of laxatives
   4. Peritonitis and paralytic ileus
6. One risk associated with digital removal of impacted stool is stimulation of the vagus nerve. When this nerve is stimulated, what can occur?
   1. Reflex vomiting
   2. Reflex tachycardia

3. Reflex bradycardia
4. Reflex urination

7. Verification of placement of a nasogastric tube is an important nursing assessment. To adequately verify tube placement before each NG irrigation, the nurse must:
   1. Auscultate bowel sounds
   2. Aspirate gastric contents
   3. Determine pH of gastric contents
   4. Auscultate abdomen for insufflations of air

References

Ebersole P and others: *Toward a healthy aging: human needs and nursing response,* ed 6, St. Louis, 2004, Mosby.

Hockenberry MJ and others: *Wong's nursing care of infants and children,* ed 7, St. Louis, 2003, Mosby.

Lawrence P, Rozmus C: Culturally sensitive care of the Muslim patient, *J Transcult Nurs* 12(3):228, 2001.

Lueckenotte AG: *Gerontolgic nursing,* ed 2, St. Louis, 2000, Mosby.

Moppett S: Administration of an enema, *Nurs Times* 95:insert 2p, 1999.

Richmond J: Prevention of constipation through risk management, *Nurs Stand* 17(16):39, 2003.

Saltzstein R and others: Anorectal injuries incident to enema administration: a recurring avoidable problem, *Am J Phys Med Rehabil* 67:186, 1988.

Seidel HM and others: *Mosby's guide to physical examination,* ed 5, St. Louis, 2003, Mosby.

Sorrentino SA: *Mosby's textbook for nursing assistants,* ed 5, St. Louis, 2000, Mosby.

Research References

Annells M, Koch T: Older people seeking solutions to constipation; the laxative mire, *J Clin Nurs* 11(5):603, 2002.

Bartlett JG: Antibiotic-associated diarrhea, *N Engl J Med* 346(5):334, 2002.

Bliss DZ and others: Fecal incontinence in hospitalized patients who are acutely ill, *Nurs Res* 49(2):101, 2000.

Bliss DZ an others: Supplementation with dietary fiber improves fecal incontinence, *Nurs Res* 50(4):203, 2001.

Dosh SA: Evaluation and treatment of constipation, *J Fam Pract* 51(6):555, 2002.

Hinrichs M, Huseboe J: *Evidenced-based protocol: management of constipation,* The University of Iowa, Iowa City, Iowa, Gerontological Nursing Interventions Research Center, Research Dissemination Core, reviewed March 2001.

Lembo A, Camilleri M: Current concepts: chronic constipation, *N Engl J Med* 349(14):1360, 2003.

Metheny N, Titler M: Assessing placement of feeding tubes, *Am J Nurs* 101(5):36, 2001.

Metheny N and others: Effectiveness of pH measurements in predicting feeding tube placement: an update, *Nurs Res* 42(6):324, 1993.

Metheny N and others: Visual characteristics of aspirates from feeding tubes as a method for predicting tube location, *Nurs Res* 43:282, 1994.

Metheny N and others: pH, color, and feeding tubes, *RN* 61(1):277, 1998.

Mosimann F, Cornu P: Are enemas given before abdominal operations useful? A prospective randomized trial, *Eur J Surg* 164(7):527, 1998.

Prather CM, Ortiz-Camacho CP: Evaluation and treatment of constipation and fecal impaction in adults, *Mayo Clin Proc* 73(9): 881, 1998.

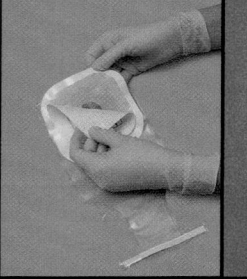

34

Ostomy Care

MEDIA RESOURCES

Evolve Site *evolve*

http://evolve.elsevier.com/Perry/skills

- Weblinks
- Video clips
- Mosby's Nursing Skills Video Exercises

Mosby's Nursing Skills Videos/CD-ROM

- *Ostomy Care Video:* Pouching a colostomy; pouching a ureterostomy

OBJECTIVES

Mastery of content in this chaper will enable the nurse to:

- Identify types of bowel and bladder diversions.
- Explain differences in color and consistency of drainage based on the location of an ostomy.
- Discuss factors influencing enterostomy drainage.
- Describe methods used to maintain skin integrity during pouching of ostomies.
- Pouch an incontinent urinary diversion.
- Catheterize a urinary diversion.

KEY TERMS

Colon conduit	Maculopapular
Colostomy	Nosocomial infection
Continent ostomy or diversion	Ostomy
Cystectomy	Peristalsis
Effluent	Peristomal
Enterostomy	Skin barrier
Ileal conduit	Stent
Ileostomy	Stoma
Incontinent diversion	Ureterostomy
Intubation	Urinary diversion
Maceration	Urostomy

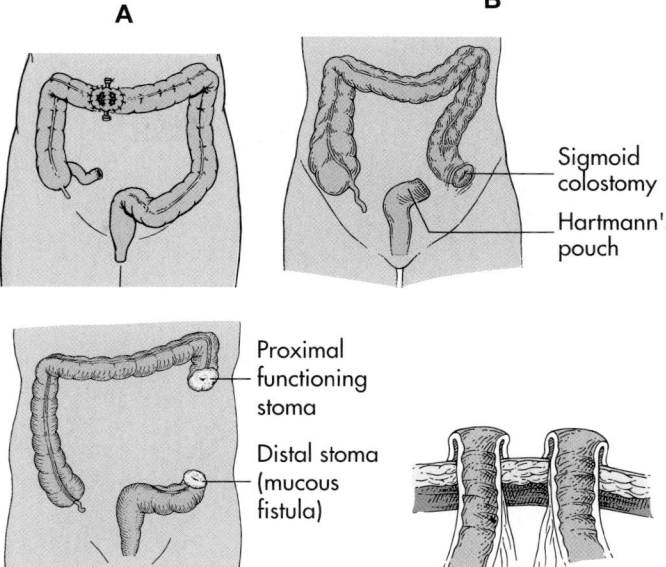

FIGURE 34-1 Types of enterostomies. **A,** Abdominal view of loop colostomy in transverse colon. **B,** Sigmoid colostomy. Distal bowel is oversewn and left in place to create a Hartmann's pouch. **C,** Double-barrel colostomy in the descending colon. **D,** Cross-sectional view of double-barrel stoma. (From Hampton BG, Bryant RA: *Ostomies and continent diversions: nursing management*, St. Louis, 1992, Mosby.)

Certain diseases or conditions require surgical intervention to create an opening into the abdominal wall for fecal or urinary elimination. For example, colon cancer, bladder cancer, or trauma may require a permanent ostomy for elimination. An enterostomy is any surgical procedure that produces an artificial stoma in a portion of intestine through the abdominal wall. The drainage from the stoma is often called effluent. A temporary ostomy may be created for elimination when healing needs to take place in the case of diverticulitis or trauma, such as a gunshot wound of the colon. That type of colostomy is often termed a "loop" or "double-barrel" colostomy with the proximal stoma producing effluent and the distal portion allowed to heal. After healing, the ends are reconnected to allow normal bowel elimination (Thompson, 2000). A portion of intestinal mucosa or segment of ureter is brought out to the abdominal wall, and a stoma, or opening, is formed to allow feces or urine to drain. This opening is called an ostomy. The piece of intestine that is brought out onto the client's abdomen is called a stoma.

The forms of bowel enterostomy are ileostomy, which involves the ileum of the small intestine, and colostomy, which can involve various segments of the colon (Figure 34-1). Ostomies can be temporary or permanent and continent or incontinent. An example of a continent ileostomy is the Kock

reservoir. In addition, the three-loop S and the two-loop J ileoanal pouches provide continence using the client's anal sphincter (Figure 34-2).

The location of the ostomy in the bowel determines the consistency of stool or effluent passed. An ileostomy bypasses the entire large intestine; thus stools are liquid and frequent, contain digestive enzymes, and must be pouched at all times. The same fecal characteristics hold true for a colostomy of the ascending colon. A colostomy of the transverse colon generally results in a thicker, semiformed stool. The sigmoid colostomy emits stool almost identical to that normally passed through the rectum.

For the urinary system the surgical procedures (Figure 34-3) involved in creating a stoma for urinary drainage are called urinary diversions, which may be either continent or incontinent. Clients who have an incontinent diversion cannot control when the urine exits from their stoma and therefore must wear an external urinary ostomy pouch at all times. Examples of incontinent urinary diversions are an ileal conduit and other forms of ureterostomies (Figure 34-3). Continent urinary diversion surgery creates an internal pouch where urine is stored. Clients who have continent diversions, such as the Kock or Indiana pouch, do not need to wear an external ostomy pouch over their urinary stoma.

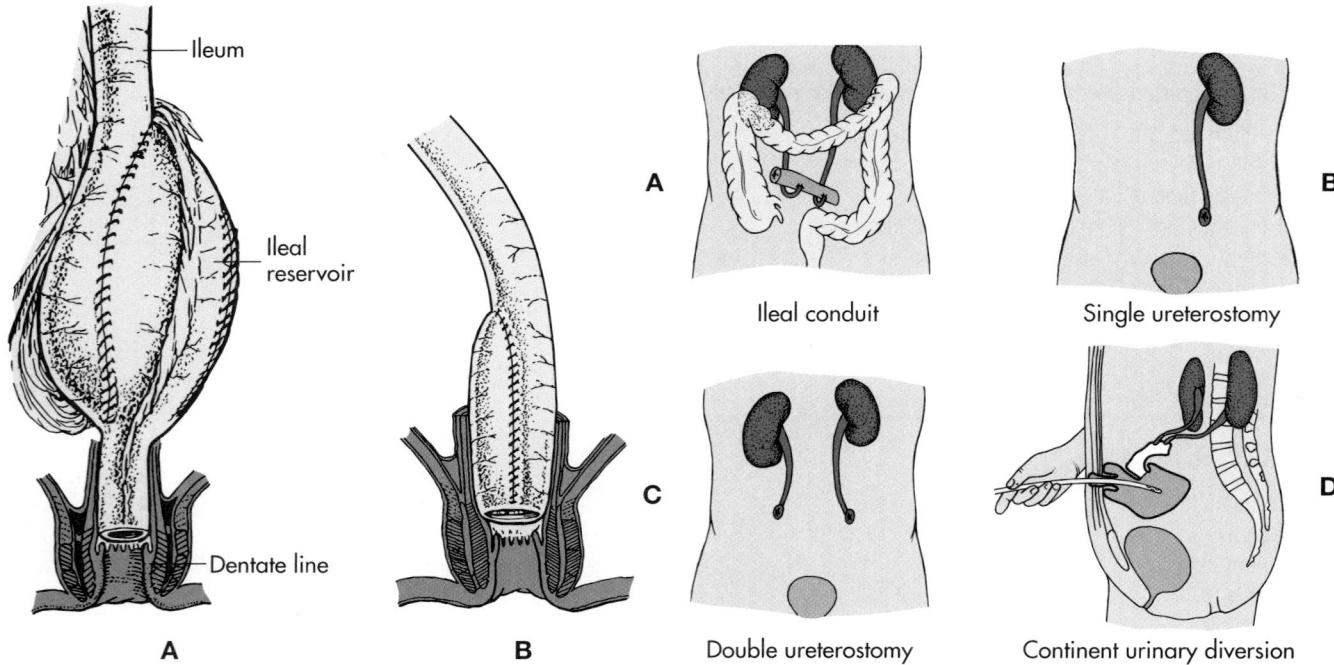

FIGURE 34-2 Ileoanal reservoirs (IARs). **A,** S-shaped configuration. **B,** J-shaped configuration. (From Hampton BG, Bryant RA: *Ostomies and continent diversions: nursing management*, St. Louis, 1992, Mosby.)

FIGURE 34-3 Types of incontinent ureterostomies. **A,** Ileal loop. **B,** Single ureterostomy. **C,** Double ureterostomy. **D,** Continent urinary diversion (Indiana pouch).

Instead, these clients are taught to insert a catheter into their stoma to drain out the urine periodically throughout the day (see Skill 34-4).

The surgical procedure for a utreterstomy may or may not involve cystectomy (removal of the bladder). For an ileal conduit, usually 6 to 8 inches of ileum are separated from the bowel. One end is used to create an external stoma, usually in the lower right quadrant, and the other end is sutured closed. The ureters are internally implanted into this piece of bowel. The client must wear an external ostomy pouch or appliance at all times to collect the urine. The rest of the bowel is sutured together so the client has normal bowel movements as before surgery.

An ureterostomy involves bringing the end of one or both ureters directly to the abdominal surface. An ureterostomy is small, difficult to pouch, or may become occluded in certain body positions. Irritation of the skin from leakage of urine is a common problem. Continent urinary diversions include the Kock urinary reservoir/pouch, Indiana pouch (see Figure 34-3, *D*), and the neobladder procedures, such as the Camay procedure, which use the client's existing urinary sphincter (Beitz and Zuzelo, 2003).

Regardless of the type of ostomy, peristomal skin care is vital to prevent irritation from fecal or urinary irritants. Most ostomy stomas will need to be pouched at all times. Because of its anatomical location, a sigmoid colostomy can often evacuate formed stool with some regularity so that the client

need wear only a protective pad or cap over the stoma for much of the day.

Clients with ostomies face a threat to body image (Erwin-Toth, 2001; Thompson, 2000). Clients with ostomies have concerns about leakage and odor, body image changes, social support, self-care, health and life expectations, and surgical complication management. Some other concerns clients may have are fears of mutilation, rejection by friends or family, and even a loss of normal sexual function (Smith, 2000; Thompson, 2000). Foul-smelling odors, spillage or leakage of liquid stools or urine, and the inability to regulate elimination give clients a sense of powerlessness and loss of self-esteem (Secord and others, 2001). Clients who have other conditions, such as spinal cord injuries, have additional care concerns that must be addressed (Thomason, 2000).

Education and counseling of clients with ostomies is a major intervention for the nurse (Ball, 2000; Secord and others, 2001). To assist clients in self-care, instruction for clients should begin on admission during the preoperative period and resume early postoperatively as the client's physical condition permits. A variety of teaching strategies must be used for each client based on his or her physical ability, learning style, and emotional readiness to learn (O'Shea, 2001). A clinical pathway for a client with an ostomy in the home care setting allows assistance in returning the client to independence (Figure 34-4). The nurse must

OSTOMY CLINICAL PATH

PATIENT _____ **ID #** _____ **DATE** _____

Medical diagnosis _____ **ICD-9 code** _____

SOC: _____ **Discharge date:** _____ **Care Coordinator:** _____

GOALS:

PHYSIOLOGIC – Patient will achieve optimal bowel function without complications. Patient's wound will heal with no sign of infection.

PSYCHOLOGIC – Patient will demonstrate a level of acceptance of modified lifestyle.

COGNITIVE – Patient/Primary care person will demonstrate independence with ostomy care.

Outcome Achieved

Y/N DATE VC

Problem: **ALTERATION IN BOWEL FUNCTIONS**
    1. optimal bowel function without complications   1. _____

Problem: **POTENTIAL/ACTUAL SKIN IMPAIRMENT**
                R/T SURGICAL INCISION/OSTOMY EFFLUENT
    1. verbalizes/demonstrates wound care   1. _____
    2. verbalizes s/s of infection   2. _____
    3. verbalizes/demonstrates stoma/peristomal skin care   3. _____
    4. achieves/maintains intact skin   4. _____

Problem: **KNOWLEDGE DEFICIT R/T OSTOMY**
    1. verbalizes A & P of bowel   1. _____
    2. verbalizes/demonstrates appliance removal   2. _____
    3. verbalizes/demonstrates wafer preparation   3. _____
    4. verbalizes/demonstrates wafer application   4. _____
    5. verbalizes pouch application   5. _____
    6. verbalizes/demonstrates clip use   6. _____
    7. verbalizes/demonstrates pouch care   7. _____
    8. verbalizes odor control/flatus release   8. _____
    9. verbalizes potential complications   9. _____
    10. verbalizes frequency of change   10. _____
    11. verbalizes balanced diet   11. _____
    12. verbalizes supply sources   12. _____
    13. verbalizes activity levels   13. _____
    14. achieves independence with ostomy care   14. _____

Problem: **ALTERATION IN BODY IMAGE**
    1. verbalizes fears/demonstrates appropriate coping mechanisms   1. _____
    2. demonstrates adjustment to ostomy by active participation in care as able   2. _____
    3. discusses activities resumed   3. _____
    4. demonstrates ability to cope with illness   4. _____

Problem: **KNOWLEDGE DEFICIT R/T MEDICATIONS/SAFETY**
    1. verbalizes/demonstrates knowledge and compliance with medications   1. _____
    2. verbalizes/demonstrates safety measures   2. _____

Code: Outcome Achieved
    Y = yes
    N = no
    VC = variance code 1, 2, or 3

_____
Patient signature

1. patient   2. environment   3. agency

_____
Case manager signature

FIGURE 34-4 Ostomy care clinical pathway. (From Mitchel JV: A clinical pathway for ostomy care in the home: process and development, *J Wound Ostomy Continence Nurs* 25(4):200, 1998.)

help the client to understand that a normal lifestyle is possible with an ostomy.

Evidence-Based Practice Trends

The primary changes in ostomy care since the early 1990s are related to improvements in surgical techniques for both bowel and urinary diversions. One simple though profound change has been preoperative stoma site assessment and marking for most ostomy surgeries (Banks and Razor, 2003). Many ostomy leakage problems are traceable to a poorly sited stoma that is difficult to pouch effectively (Erwin-Toth, 2000). Preoperative planning of stoma locations has resulted in stomas that are easier to maintain with fewer complications (Thompson, 2000).

The development of continent ileostomy and urostomy reservoirs has progressed to the development of a variety of ileoanal reservoirs for bowel and urinary effluent that are controlled using the client's anal or urinary sphincter or a surgically created nipple valve (Ball, 2000; Beitz and Zuzelo, 2003). Care of pouched stomas (incontinent colostomy, ileostomies, and urostomies) has improved as drainage devices have improved. These improvements include a wider variety of sizes, specialty shapes (convex skin flange, oval flanges), and better skin barriers (Smith, 2000; Thompson, 2000). An improved array of products for neonatal and pediatric use has been shown to enhance the care of that population (Rogers, 2003).

Fecal or urinary diversions are frequently recommended for a variety of conditions, such as trauma, cancer, or congenital abnormalities (Colwell and others, 2001). Adjustment in the client's body image, activities of daily living, and self-care that result from these diversions or ostomies can be eased by a wound, ostomy, and continence (WOC) nurse. Not only does the ostomy nurse assist the client with managing the ostomy, but WOC nurses are influential in defining best practices for ostomy management (Colwell and others, 2001; Mowdy, 1998).

One major issue is how ostomy surgery affects a person's life. The Montreux study used the Stoma Care Quality of Life Index to determine the effect of an ostomy (Marquis and others, 2003). Approximately 4700 clients with ostomies completed the survey immediately postoperatively and at 3, 6, 9, and 12 months after surgery. Quality-of-life (QOL) scores improved steadily, but the greatest change occurred between the immediate postoperative measurement and the one 3 months after surgery. Clients who perceived solid and accurate teaching from the WOC nurse rated their QOL scores higher. In addition, clients who felt that they had continued access to the nurse specialist immediately following hospital discharge rated their scores higher as well (Marquis and others, 2003). This study demonstrated the effect of individualized discharge teaching and continued fol-

low-up on a group of clients who had surgeries that affected both their body image and quality of life.

Cultural Considerations

In any culture the presence and care of an ostomy presents unique challenges. New ostomies require monitoring and observation, and clients from other cultures may find this more invasive and embarrassing. Most cultures consider bowel and urinary secretions as not fit for public display. However, exposure of the lower torso, which is needed for ostomy care, is generally avoided among Asians, Africans, Hispanics, Hindus, Muslims, Arabic, Orthodox Jewish, and Amish groups. When caring for clients with ostomies from these cultures, it is helpful to assign gender-congruent caregivers if possible and to allow presence of a family member if requested by the client.

It is important to avoid communication during the procedure that may be interpreted as disrespectful by the client. As always, prepare adequately for the procedure, seek necessary assistance, and maintain a calm, professional demeanor.

Skill Performance Guidelines

1. Know how to assess your client's stoma (Box 34-1).
2. Know what type of effluent is expected from the ostomy. Some ostomies, such as an ileostomy, normally have liquid drainage. Due to normal enzymes in the small bowel, ileostomy drainage is most damaging to skin. Copious output may result in dehydration and electrolyte imbalance. An ileal conduit, though draining urine, normally has mucus because the bowel still produces mucus.
3. Know if the ostomy is continent or incontinent. This information indicates to the nurse whether the lack of spontaneous drainage signals a problem (i.e., incontinent ostomy) or whether it requires insertion of a catheter to drain the effluent (i.e., continent ostomy). Just because a client has a stoma does not mean there will be spontaneous drainage. Clients who have continent ostomies (Kock or Indiana pouches) need to self-catheterize periodically during the day to drain the fecal or urine contents (see Skill 34-4).
4. Know the client's usual elimination pattern so the client can return to or maintain a usual schedule while receiving nursing care.
5. Know the client's routine for self-care of the ostomy. A client who has independently cared for an ostomy should be encouraged to resume self-care as soon as possible.
6. Know the equipment options available. Various types of equipment are used for different types of stomas, ostomy drainage, and skin irritations.

BOX 34-1   ABCDs of Stoma Assessment and Pouching

A IS FOR ASSESSMENT

Number of stoma(s)
How many stomas does your client have? (Single or double)

Stoma location
Where on the abdomen is your client's stoma?
What part of the bowel is the stoma?
Is the stoma near structures that will affect care?

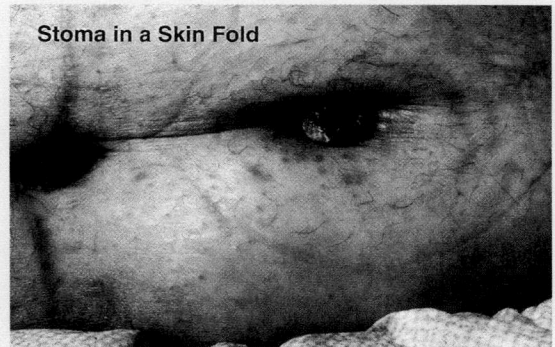

Stoma in or near a skinfold. (Courtesy ConvaTec, Princeton, NJ.)

Stoma type
Is this a matured stoma?
What is the length or protrusion of the stoma?
  Bud, flush, or spout

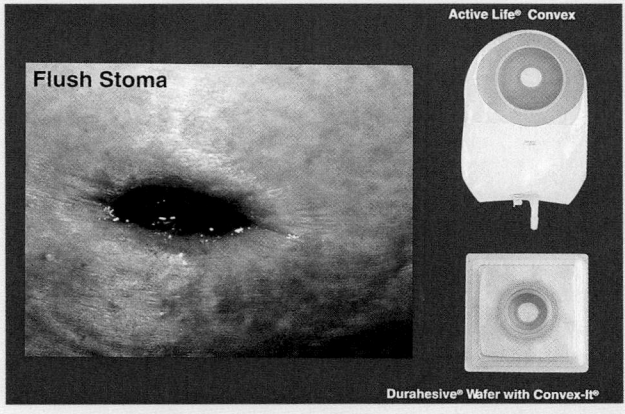

Normal flush stoma. (Courtesy ConvaTec, Princeton, NJ.)

Stoma shape
What shape is the client's stoma?
  Round, oval, regular/irregular

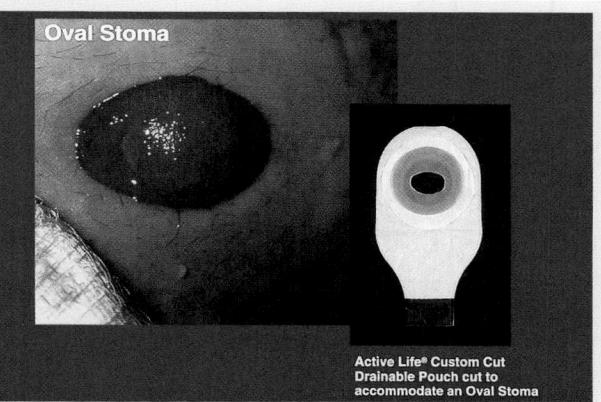

Oval stoma. (Courtesy ConvaTec, Princeton, NJ.)

Stoma viability
How do you monitor stoma viability?
  Color, tissue turgor, bleeding
Stoma construction
How is stoma made?
  End, loop, double barrel
What is the direction of the stoma lumen?

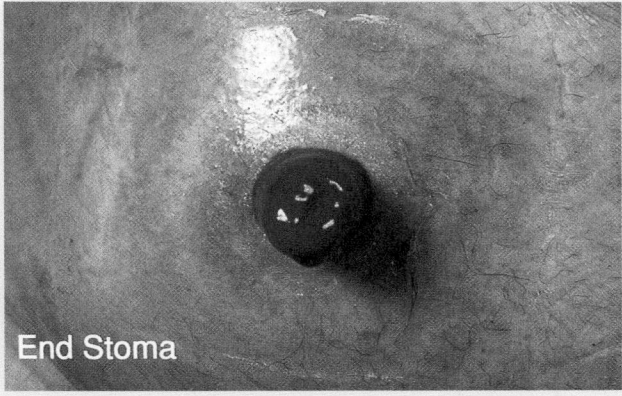

End stoma (bud type). (Courtesy ConvaTec, Princeton, NJ.)

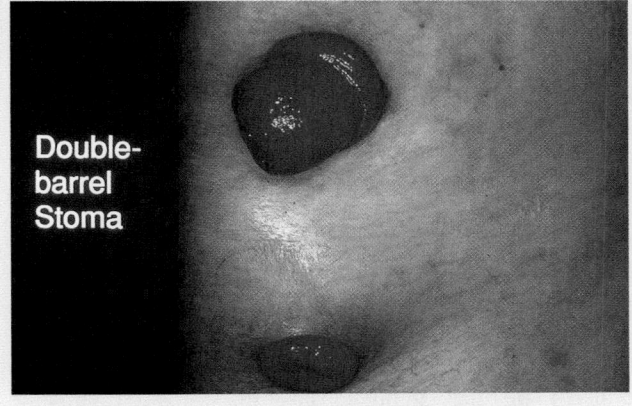

Double-barrel stoma. (Courtesy ConvaTec, Princeton, NJ.)

From Ayello E: The ABCD's of stoma assessment and pouching (Personal correspondence, 2000).

Continued

BOX 34-1   ABCDs of Stoma Assessment and Pouching—cont'd

A IS FOR ASSESSMENT—cont'd

Stoma drainage
Is this a continent or incontinent stoma?
What is the normal amount and consistency of stoma output?

Stoma size
What size is the stoma?
How do I measure it?

B IS FOR CERTIFICATION BOARDS

Wound, Ostomy, Continence Nurses (WOCN)
1550 S Coast Highway, Suite 201
Laguna Beach, CA 92651
(888) 224-9626
Fax (714) 376-3456
www.wocn.org

C IS FOR COMPLICATIONS

Bleeding
Necrosis
Prolapse
Hernia
Laceration
Irritation
Retraction
Stenosis

D IS FOR DIFFERENT AND DETERMINING POUCHING SYSTEMS

Differences in pouching systems
Fecal versus urinary
Adhesive versus nonadhesive
One piece versus two piece
Precut versus cut to fit
Disposable versus reusable
Drainable (open ended) versus closed end (nondrainable)

Determining pouching systems
Is the correct skin barrier and pouch being used?
Does the skin barrier and pouch fit correctly?
How do you measure the stoma and determine the correct pouching system sizing for each product?
Is the skin barrier intact?
Are there any peristomal skin problems or abdominal contours that will alter the pouching system needed?
How often does this pouching system need to routinely be changed?
When should the pouch be emptied?

From Ayello E: The ABCD's of stoma assessment and pouching (Personal correspondence, 2000).

SKILL 34-1   Pouching an Enterostomy

Immediately after surgical diversion or removal of a portion of bowel, it is necessary to place a pouch over the newly created stoma because in some incontinent ostomies effluent may begin immediately. The pouch collects all effluent and protects the skin from irritating drainage. A pouch with its skin barrier should fit comfortably, cover the skin surface around the stoma, and create a good seal. The postoperative pouch should allow visibility of the stoma.

The technique of pouching a newly formed stoma differs from techniques used to pouch a stoma several days or weeks old. The new stoma is edematous during the postoperative healing process for up to 6 weeks. An incision line from the bowel resection may lie close to or around the stoma.

The stoma itself often has a series of small stitches around its perimeter. A pouch and its skin barrier must be applied so that they do not constrict the stoma or traumatize healing tissues. Initially the pouch over a postoperative colostomy may not need to be emptied frequently because drainage is diminished or lacking. Several days may pass be-fore a client's normal elimination pattern returns. In the case of an ileostomy, the client will have frequent liquid stools when peristalsis returns (Erwin-Toth, 2001).

Many types of pouches and skin barriers are available (Schiff, 2000). Some pouches have skin barriers directly preattached and are called one-piece pouching systems. Some of these one-piece pouches already are precut to size by the manufacturer, whereas others must be custom cut to size for the client's stoma measurement. Other systems are two separate pieces. The pouch can be applied to the skin barrier by attaching it to the flange (a plastic ring) on the barrier. Often the skin barrier needs to be custom cut to the client's specific stoma size. For two-piece systems the skin barrier with flange must be used with the corresponding size pouch that fits that flange *from the same manufacturer* to use the system correctly without leakage. Nurses should understand how to use each of these different pouching systems (Figure 34-5). Modifications for preventing complications related to leakage of feces or urine are essential (Erwin-Toth, 2001; Thompson, 2000).

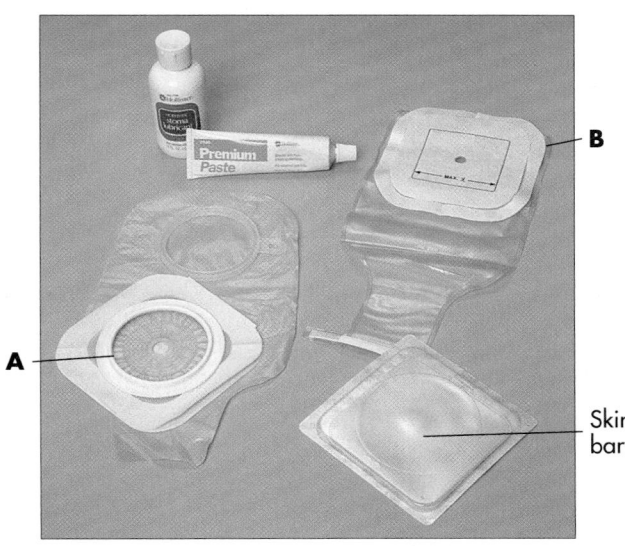

FIGURE **34-5** Examples of pouching systems. **A,** Two-piece detachable system. (NOTE: The skin barrier would need to be custom cut by the client according to self-stoma size obtained by measurement.) The pouch opening is already precut by the manufacturer to fit the size of the flange on the skin barrier. **B,** One-piece pouch with skin barrier attached.

DELEGATION CONSIDERATIONS

This skill should not be delegated to assistive personnel. The one exception in some agencies is that care of an enterostomy (6 weeks postoperative plus) may be delegated to assistive personnel. When delegating this skill, the nurse must inform assistive personnel about:

- The expected amount, color, and consistency of drainage from the enterostomy
- The expected appearance of the stoma
- Special equipment needed to complete procedure
- When to report changes in the client's stoma and surrounding skin integrity

EQUIPMENT

❑ Pouch, clear drainable colostomy/ileostomy/urostomy in correct size for two-piece system (see Figure 34-5, *A*) or custom cut-to-fit, one-piece type with attached skin barrier (see Figure 34-5, *B*)
❑ Pouch closure device, such as a clamp or pouch valve
❑ Adhesive remover (optional)
❑ Clean disposable gloves
❑ Ostomy deodorant, if needed
❑ Gauze pads or washcloth
❑ Towel or disposable waterproof barrier
❑ Basin with warm tap water
❑ Scissors
❑ Skin barrier such as sealant wipes or wafer
❑ Ostomy belt (optional)
❑ Stethoscope

STEP	RATIONALE

ASSESSMENT

1. Perform hand hygiene, and put on disposable gloves.

   Reduces transmission of microorganisms.

2. Auscultate for bowel sounds.

   Documents presence of peristalsis.

3. Observe existing skin barrier and pouch for leakage and length of time in place. Depending upon type of pouching system used (such as opaque pouch), nurse may have to remove pouch to fully observe stoma. Clear pouches permit viewing of stoma without their removal.

   Determines likelihood of pouch loosening from stoma and failing to collect effluent. Routine observation allows for early detection of potential problems (Thompson, 2000). Leaking may indicate need for different pouch or sealant.

- *Critical Decision Point*

   Intact skin barriers with no evidence of leakage do not need to be changed daily and can remain in place for 3 to 5 days (Erwin-Toth, 2001).

4. Observe stoma for color, swelling, trauma, and healing; stoma should be moist and reddish pink. Assess type of stoma. Stomas can be almost flush with the skin or be a budlike protrusion on the abdomen. (An example of a normal bud stoma can be found in Box 34-1.)

   Stoma characteristics should be one of the factors to consider when selecting an appropriate pouching system.

STEP	RATIONALE

- **Critical Decision Point**
  Stoma should be measured with each pouching system change to determine correct size of equipment needed. Follow each ostomy pouch manufacturer's directions and measuring guide as to which size ostomy pouch to use based on client's actual stoma measurement size (Erwin-Toth, 2000).

5. Observe effluent from stoma and record of intake and output. Ask client about skin tenderness.

   Plan on routine changing of skin barrier pouch at times of less effluent output. Generally avoid changing after meals, when gastrocolic reflux increases chance of fecal effluent output.

- **Critical Decision Point**
  Because of stomal and abdominal characteristics, some clients may need convexity in their ostomy pouching system to avoid leakage (Thompson, 2000).

6. To minimize skin irritation, avoid unnecessary changing of entire pouching system. A one-piece pouch with attached skin barriers or the skin barrier of a two-piece pouching system should be changed every 3 to 5 days, *not* daily.

   Pouches should be emptied when one-third to one-half full because weight of contents may dislodge skin seal, and ostomy drainage is irritating to the skin. Also, pouches collect flatus (gas), which needs to be expelled because it can disrupt skin seal.

- **Critical Decision Point**
  Do not put holes in pouch for flatus to escape because effluent may also leak. Instead, encourage client to empty pouch of flatus.

7. Assess abdomen for best type of pouching system to use. Consider:
   a. Contour and peristomal plane

   Determines pouching system selection and need for other equipment.
   A firm/flat and round/hard abdomen usually needs a flexible or soft pouching system, whereas a flabby or soft abdomen usually needs a firmer system (see illustration). Convexity may be needed for stomas that are retracted or in skinfolds, and different pouching systems are needed to prevent leaking.

   b. Presence of scars, incisions
   c. Location and type of stoma
8. Discard gloves.

- **Critical Decision Point**
  Pouching system options include the following:
  - *Adhesive and nonadhesive systems, which are also available for both urinary and fecal drainage.*
  - *One-piece pouch with skin barrier already attached; precut pouch and skin barrier; or two-piece pouch system, which consists of pouch that can detach from skin barrier, which remains around client's stoma for several days. Bottom of ostomy pouch is either open ended, which is closed with a clip, valve, rubber band, or some other type of closure device between emptying, or closed ended, in which end of pouch is sealed closed. One-piece pouches should be open-ended pouches that can be opened periodically to empty effluent without removing pouch from around stoma.*
  - *Two-piece pouches give client choice of using either an open-ended or closed-ended pouch. This is because client can remove pouch from skin barrier to empty effluent. For some clients accessory products, such as karaya paste or careful use of a pouch belt, will enhance the seal and prevent leakage (Erwin-Toth, 2001).*

STEP	RATIONALE

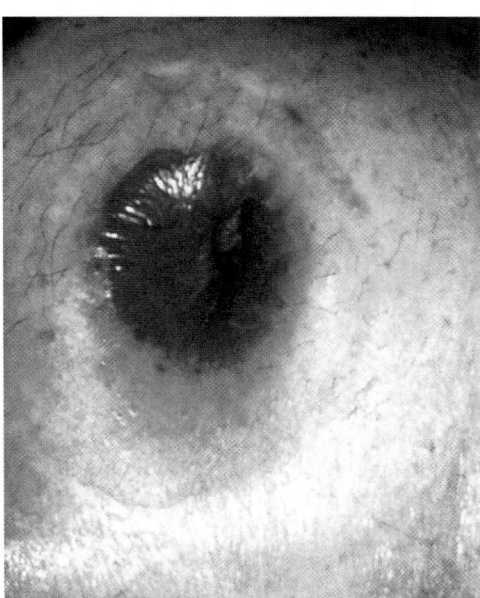

STEP 7 Irregular stoma (flush on right side, raised on left with skin irritation).

9. Assess the client's condition as to the best type of pouching system to use. Assess vision, dexterity or mobility, and cognitive function.

Clients with poor vision may benefit by using yellow-tinted sunglasses to reduce glare and improve contrast and by using magnification mirrors (Jeffries and MacKay, 1997). Clients who also have mobility problems or spinal cord injuries may benefit by using equipment that has a longer pouch, which is easier to empty independently when sitting (Erwin-Toth, 2003; Thomason, 2000). Clients who have difficulty using their hands or who have limited vision may find a one-piece system or a precut pouch and skin barrier more desirable to use; others prefer being able to keep the skin barrier in place for several days, changing just the pouch, and therefore prefer the two-piece system.

10. Remove existing pouch if any, by gently pushing skin from adhesive barrier; properly dispose of soiled pouch (save clamp if attached to pouch). After skin barrier and pouch removal, assess skin around stoma, noting scars, folds, skin breakdown, and peristomal suture line if present.

Prevents skin irritation and controls odor. Determines need for barrier paste to increase adherence of pouch to skin or to fill in irregularities. Many enterostomal pouch systems have a flexible adhesive, a pectin, karaya, or synthetic wafer flange that assists in leak prevention. Karaya is a natural gum product that softens with body heat and conforms to the contours around the stoma. A deeper skin crease will need a paste to fill in the defect and prevent leakage (Erwin-Toth, 2000).

11. Determine client's and family's emotional response and knowledge and understanding of an ostomy and its care.

Assists in determining extent to which client is able to participate in care and need for teaching and information clarification (O'Shea, 2001; Secord and others, 2001).

STEP	RATIONALE

NURSING DIAGNOSES

- Disturbed body image
- Constipation
- Ineffective coping
- Diarrhea

- Deficient knowledge regarding ostomy self-care
- Acute pain
- Risk for impaired skin integrity

Related factors are individualized based on client's condition or needs.

PLANNING

1. Expected outcomes following completion of procedure:
   - Client denies discomfort.
   - Stoma is moist and reddish pink. Skin is intact and free of irritation; sutures are intact.

   - Stoma drains moderate amount of liquid or soft stool and flatus in pouch.
   - Flatus is noted by bulging of pouch in absence of drainage; flatus initially indicates return of peristalsis after surgery.
   - Client observes stoma and steps of procedure carefully.

   - Client asks questions about procedure and may attempt to assist with pouch change.
2. Explain procedure to client; encourage client's interaction and questions.
3. Assemble equipment, and close room curtains or door.

Stoma and surrounding skin intact.
Normal findings in client with postoperative enterostomy that is healing. Stoma initially is edematous and shrinks over next 6 to 8 weeks.
Stoma functioning normally. Skin is free of irritation.

Snug seal around stoma has been attained.

Reveals acknowledgment of body alteration and interest in self-care.
Asking to assist indicates readiness to learn and to begin self-care (O'Shea, 2001).
Lessens client's anxiety and promotes client's participation.

Optimizes use of time; conserves client's and nurse's energy. Provides privacy.

IMPLEMENTATION

1. Position client either standing or supine, and drape. If seated, position client either on or in front of toilet.

2. Perform hand hygiene, and apply new pair of disposable gloves.
3. Place towel or disposable waterproof barrier under client.
4. Remove used pouch and skin barrier gently by pushing skin away from barrier. An adhesive remover may be used to facilitate removal of skin barrier.
5. Cleanse peristomal skin gently with warm tap water using gauze pads or clean washcloth; do not scrub skin; dry completely by patting skin with gauze or towel.

When client is supine, there are fewer skin wrinkles, which allows for ease of application of pouching system; maintains client's dignity.
Reduces transmission of microorganisms.

Protects bed linen.
Reduces skin trauma. Improper removal of pouch and barrier can irritate client's skin and can cause skin tears.

Avoid use of soap because it leaves a residue on skin that interferes with pouch adhesion to skin (Thompson, 2000). Skin must be dry as skin barrier; pouch does not adhere to wet skin. If blood appears on gauze pad, do not be alarmed. If rubbed, stoma may ooze some blood as a result of cleaning process. Stoma's surface is highly vascular mucous membrane. Bleeding into pouch is abnormal. Do not use adhesive remover on open skin of any client or peristomal skin of neonates if they contain alcohol because they will cause discomfort and skin damage (Rogers, 2003).

STEP	**RATIONALE**
6. Measure stoma for correct size of pouching system needed, using the manufacturer's measuring guide (see illustration).	Ensures accuracy in determining correct pouch size needed. Stoma shrinks and does not reach usual size for 6 to 8 weeks (Thompson, 2000).
7. Select appropriate pouch for client based on client assessment. With a custom cut-to-fit pouch, use an ostomy guide to cut opening on the pouch $\frac{1}{16}$ to $\frac{1}{8}$ inch larger than stoma before removing backing. Prepare pouch by removing backing from barrier and adhesive. With ileostomy, apply thin circle of barrier paste around opening in pouch; allow to dry (see illustrations).	Size of pouch opening keeps drainage off skin and lessens risk of damage to stoma during peristalsis or activity. Pouch and skin barrier are changed whenever leaking. Change when client is comfortable; before a meal is better because this avoids increased peristalsis and chance of evacuation during pouch change. Can also be changed before or after tub bath or shower. Paste facilitates seal and protects skin. Stool is alkaline and contains enzymes, and this irritates skin; fecal bacteria can colonize on skin and increase risk of infection.

● *Critical Decision Point*

If client has large amount of liquid stool from an ileostomy, consider using a "high-output" pouch that will contain this effluent and reduce frequency of pouch emptying.

8. Apply skin barrier and pouch. If creases next to stoma occur, use barrier paste to fill in; let dry 1 to 2 minutes.	

● *Critical Decision Point*

When applying skin barrier to stoma that is close to client's abdominal incision, skin barrier may have to be trimmed to fit.

a. For one-piece pouching system:	
(1) Use skin sealant wipes on skin directly under adhesive skin barrier or pouch; allow to dry. Press adhesive backing of pouch and/or skin barrier smoothly against skin, starting from the bottom and working up and around sides.	Ensure smooth, wrinkle-free seal. Be aware of any irritated or open areas because the skin sealant wipes often contain alcohol.
(2) Hold pouch by barrier, center over stoma, and press down gently on barrier; bottom of pouch should point toward client's knees when sitting (see illustration).	A different positioning of the pouch may be necessary to allow better gravity flow. For example, a client confined to bed may need to have pouch positioned horizontally over the side of the abdomen (Thomason, 2000).
(3) Maintain gentle finger pressure around barrier for 1 to 2 minutes.	Gentle pressure and body heat assist in adhesion.

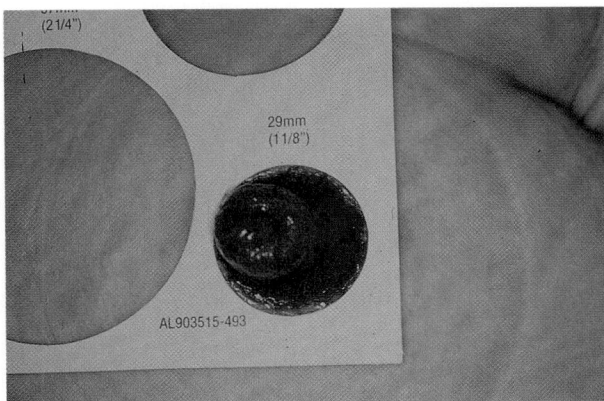

STEP **6** Measuring an ostomy.

STEP	RATIONALE

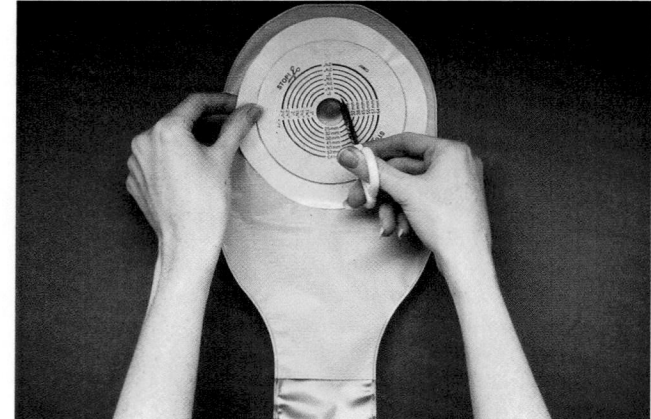

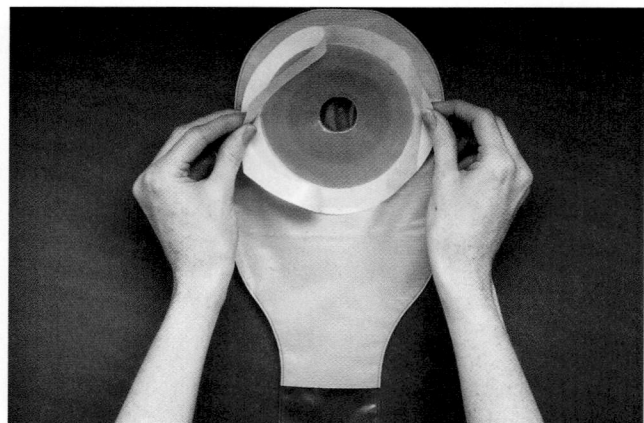

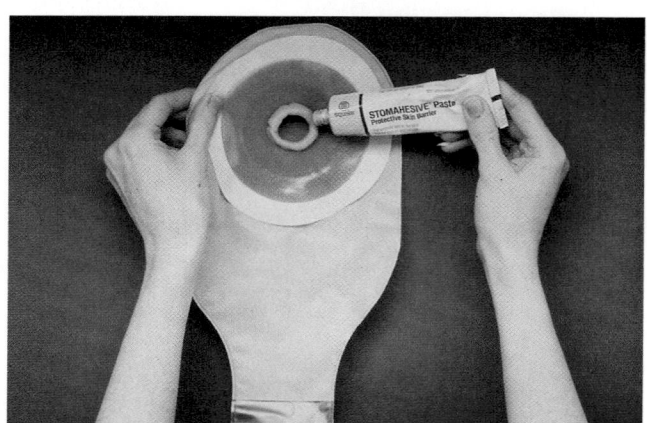

STEP **7 A,** Cut-to-fit, one-piece drainable ostomy pouch.
B, Removing the backing paper for the barrier on a one-piece
pouch. **C,** Applying barrier paste to a one-piece ostomy pouch.
(Courtesy ConvaTec, Princeton, NJ.)

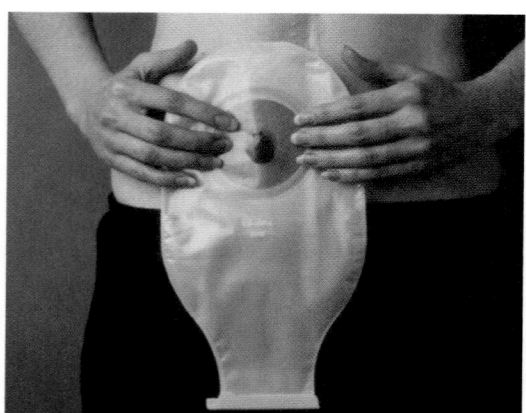

STEP **8a(2)** Applying a one-piece pouch. (Courtesy ConvaTec,
Princeton, NJ.)

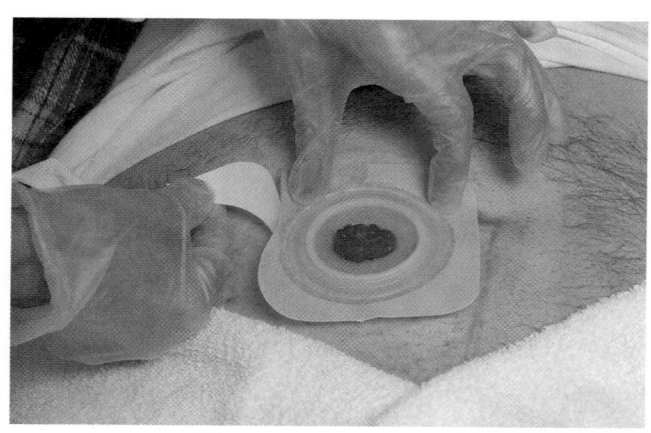

STEP **8b(1)** Application of barrier-paste flange.

STEP	RATIONALE

b. If using two-piece pouching system:
  (1) Apply barrier-paste flange (barrier with adhesive) as in steps above for one-piece system. Then snap on pouch, and maintain finger pressure (see illustration).

Creates wrinkle-free, secure seal; decreases irritation from adhesive on skin. Some two-piece pouching systems may have a snapping or clicking sound that occurs when attaching pouch to skin barrier.

c. For both pouching systems gently tug on pouch in a downward direction.

Determines that pouch is securely attached.

9. Gently press on the pectin or karaya flange to facilitate adhesion.

A pectin, karaya, or synthetic skin barrier keeps pouch system attached securely (Erwin-Toth, 2001). Some clients may prefer a belt attached to the pouch for extra security.

• *Critical Decision Point*
Make sure client who chooses to wear an ostomy belt does not have the belt too tight. To check for appropriate tightness, two fingers placed between belt and client's skin should fit comfortably.

10. Although many ostomy pouches are odor-proof, some nurses and clients like to add a small amount of ostomy deodorant into pouch. Do not use "home remedies," which can harm stoma, to control ostomy odor. Do not make hole in pouch to release flatus.

Causes damage to pouch and defeats purpose of odor-proof pouch. A hole for flatus may also allow effluent to leak.

• *Critical Decision Point*
Aspirin should never be added to ostomy pouch. It can cause stomal bleeding.

11. Fold bottom of drainable open-ended pouches up once, and close using a closure device such as a clamp (or follow manufacturer's instructions for closure).

Maintains secure seal to prevent leaking.

12. Properly dispose of old pouch and soiled equipment. Client may also request spraying of room air freshener in room if needed.

Lessens odors in room.

13. Remove gloves, and perform hand hygiene.

Reduces transmission of microorganisms.

14. Change one- or two-piece pouch every 3 to 5 days or longer unless leaking; pouch can remain in place for tub bath or shower; after bath, pat the pouch and underlying skin dry.

Avoids unnecessary trauma to skin from too-frequent changes. If pouch is removed for bathing or shower, have client use a mild soap without oils or deodorants. Make sure all soap residue is rinsed off. Drying ensures adhesion of pouch and prevention of skin irritation under pouch (Erwin-Toth, 2001).

• *Critical Decision Point*
Sometimes pouch needs to be reapplied after showering or bathing because adhesion is decreased.

EVALUATION

1. Ask if client feels discomfort around stoma.

Determines presence of skin irritation.

2. Note appearance of stoma around skin and existing incision (if present) while pouch is removed and skin is cleansed. Reinspect condition of skin barrier and adhesive. Inspect edges of pouch for "tracking" of effluent under edges. This may signal a potential leak due to skinfold or wrinkle.

Determines condition of tissues and progress of healing. Determines presence of leaks or potential problems.

Determines return of peristalsis and bowel elimination.

STEP	RATIONALE
3. Auscultate bowel sounds, and observe characteristics of stool.	
4. Observe client's nonverbal behaviors as pouch is applied. Ask if client has any questions about pouching.	May indicate emotional response to stoma and readiness for teaching. Determines level of understanding of procedure (O'Shea, 2001).

Recording and Reporting

- Chart type of pouch and skin barrier applied.
- Record amount and appearance of stool or drainage in pouch, size of stoma, color and texture of stool, condition of peristomal skin, and sutures.
- Document abdominal distention and excessive tenderness, nature and location of bowel sounds.
- Record client's level of participation and need for teaching.
- Report any of the following to nurse in charge and/or physician: Abnormal appearance of stoma, suture line, peristomal skin, or character of output and absence of bowel sounds. No flatus in 24 to 36 hours and no stool by third day.

Unexpected Outcomes	Related Interventions
1. Skin around stoma is irritated, has burning sensation.	• Assess stoma as mucosal layer of stoma separates from skin. • May be caused by undermining of pouch seal by fecal contents. • May indicate an allergic reaction, which can be manifested by erythema and blistering, usually confined to one area immediately under allergen (Erwin-Toth, 2000). • Remove pouch more slowly. • Obtain referral for enterostomal therapy (ET/WOC) nurse.
2. Necrotic stoma is manifested by purple or black color, dry instead of moist texture, failure to bleed when washed gently, or presence of tissue sloughing.	• Assess circulation to stoma. • Determine presence of excessive edema or excessive tension on bowel suture line.
3. Client complains of irritation and burning around stoma.	• Assess skin for breaks in integrity, skin inflammation, maceration, or infection.
4. Client refuses to view stoma or participate in care.	• Obtain information about ostomy support groups in community. • Refer client and family to other volunteer clients with an ostomy in community for individual support. • Knowledge and acceptance by staff facilitate understanding and adjustment.

Teaching Considerations

- Include family members or significant other in teaching because this may facilitate client's readiness to learn (Secord and others, 2001).
- Client's readiness to learn may be judged, for example, by willingness to look at stoma and asking questions. If client is apprehensive about touching or looking at stoma, have client hold gauze pad over stoma and clean around stoma (O'Shea, 2001; Thompson, 2000).

- Some clients acknowledge stoma with minimal emotional difficulty; some may never completely adjust to it. Individualize care according to client's situation and circumstances (Thompson, 2000).
- Teach client to avoid diarrhea or constipation by eating a balanced diet and having adequate fluids (Thompson, 2000).
- Client should be given a teaching manual with steps clearly stated, or audiotaped instructions. With client

who has learning disability, a "picture book" of the steps may be more appropriate.

- Adult clients may wear usual clothes because abdominal peristalsis pushes stool out of stoma, and snug clothes do not interfere with effluent emptying into external pouch. Tight girdles and undergarments, however, should not be worn without consent of surgeon. For babies, one-piece garments are preferred because they can help keep baby from pulling off ostomy pouch (Rogers, 2003).

Pediatric Considerations

- Because most ostomy surgery done on neonates is for emergency situations, often no time is available for pre-operative selection of stoma site. Most stomas, however, are temporary with stoma being "taken down" (removed or closed) when baby is about 1 year old. Colostomies are the most frequent type of stomas in neonates. They are usually done because baby has necrotizing enterocol-itis (NEC), Hirschsprung's disease, or imperforate anus (Colwell, 2003; Rogers, 2003).
- Although normal stoma color is red, a temporary change in stoma color to white or purple may occur when baby is crying (Colwell, 2003).
- Neonates often have multiple stomas on their tiny ab-domens that may be the result of corrective bowel surg-eries. Select a cut-to-fit pouch that allows multiple stoma openings in skin barrier, yet still fits on neonate's tiny ab-domen (Colwell, 2003).
- Because babies swallow large amounts of air while suck-ing, it is normal to expect considerable amounts of flatus. Make sure pouch can accommodate increased amount of flatus, or be prepared to release flatus frequently (Rogers, 2003).
- Use equipment that is designed by manufacturers for use with pediatric clients (Colwell, 2003).
- If caring for a preterm infant, be aware that the peri-stomal skin is not fully developed and as a result skin sealants and adhesive removers should not be used be-cause they will damage the epithelium (Rogers, 2003).
- Usually a baby triples its birth weight in the first year. A stoma does not delay baby's growth. As baby grows in size, so too does the stoma. Therefore stoma should be measured frequently, and appropriate adjustments in pouching and skin barrier size made accordingly.

- Rogers (2003) has stated that the one characteristic of pouch skin barriers for preterm infants that is most im-portant is flexibility to cover the infant's rounded abdom-inal contour. Otherwise, the same considerations that are important for adults with ostomies need to be addressed (size and shape of the stoma, consistency of effluent, vol-ume of stool and flatus, and peristomal skin integrity).
- Whenever possible, adolescents requiring an ostomy benefit from presurgical contact with other adolescents who have an ostomy (Erwin-Toth, 1999).

Gerontological Considerations

- Evaluate older adult's cognitive status for understanding ostomy self-care instructions.
- Evaluate older adult's motor and visual ability to prepare ostomy equipment. For clients who are unable to custom cut the size of their skin barriers, consider having barri-ers precut by ostomy equipment supplier or using a pre-cut two-piece system (Erwin-Toth, 2001).
- Older clients need teaching about change in number of eliminations (from an incontinent ostomy) that would be normal on a daily basis. Older clients may have some physical limitations, but most are able to learn self-care if given enough time (O'Shea, 2001).
- Financial concerns about cost of ostomy supplies and re-imbursement may be an important issue for some clients on fixed income.

Home Care Considerations

- Client should understand that although the nurse may have used sterile gauze to clean stoma, it is not necessary to use sterile gauze. In fact, gauze is not needed at all; a washcloth or any soft material can be used.
- Evaluate client's home toileting facilities. This includes:
  - Presence of adequate toileting facilities in client's home
  - Privacy
  - Flushing toilet facilities
  - Number and location of toileting facilities
  - Number of other people living with client who must share toileting facilities

SKILL 34-2 Pouching an Incontinent Urinary Diversion

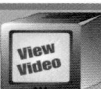

Because urine flows continuously from an incontinent urinary diversion, a urinary pouch is usually placed over the opening immediately after surgery. Placement of the pouch may be more challenging than the enterostomy because urine flow keeps the skin moist and in the immediate postoperative period urinary stents may be in place in the stoma.

The stoma of a urinary diversion is normally reddish. It is made from a portion of the gastrointestinal tract, either the ileum or the colon, and has the same mucosal surface. Ideally the stoma should protrude ½ to ¾ inch above the skin. An ileal conduit is usually located in the right lower quadrant; a colon conduit is usually located in the left lower quadrant. Ureterostomies are usually performed in infants, and a conduit is performed when the child approaches school age (see Figure 34-3).

DELEGATION CONSIDERATIONS

The skill of pouching a new incontinent urinary diversion should not be delegated to assistive personnel. Care of an established incontinent urinary diversion can be delegated. When delegating this skill, the nurse must inform assistive personnel about:

- The baseline assessment findings of the client's ostomy and when to report changes
- Expected amount and character of the output, and when to report changes
- Special equipment needed to complete procedure

EQUIPMENT

- ❑ Pouch, urinary (with antireflux flap) and skin barrier (Figure 34-6)

NOTE: Use two-piece system (pouch and flange) if stents are present (see Figure 34-6); use measuring guide to measure the stoma to determine the correct size of pouch and skin barrier

- ❑ Bedside urinary drainage bag
- ❑ Clean disposable gloves (sterile gloves optional)
- ❑ Hand-held hair dryer
- ❑ Sterile gauze pads
- ❑ Towel or disposable waterproof barrier
- ❑ Basin with warm tap water
- ❑ Scissors
- ❑ Skin-sealant wipes
- ❑ Sterile forceps (if stents present)
- ❑ Vinegar

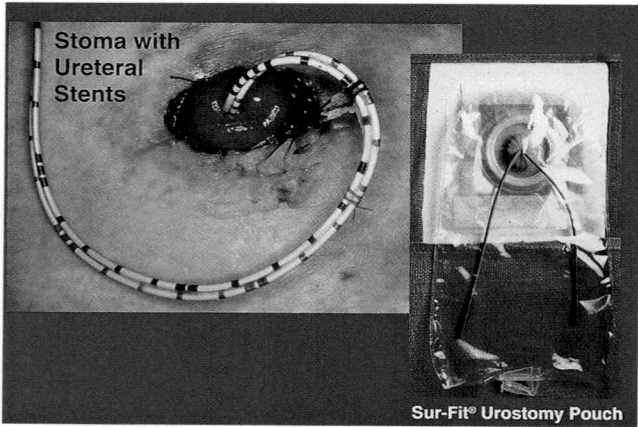

Stoma with Ureteral Stents

Sur-Fit® Urostomy Pouch

FIGURE 34-6 Viable ileal conduit stoma with stents present and normal peristomal skin and pouch. (Courtesy Hollister, Inc, Libertyville, Ill.)

STEP	RATIONALE

ASSESSMENT

1. Perform hand hygiene and apply disposable gloves. Check pouch for leakage, length of time in place; ask client about skin tenderness or discomfort. Check stoma for color, healing. Check abdominal incision (if present) for relationship to stoma for proper placement of pouch. To prevent skin irritation, one-piece pouch or skin barrier from two-piece system should be changed, if not leaking, every 3 to 7 days, or when checking for skin irritation. Stoma should be moist and reddish pink; immediately after surgery it is edematous and usually has urinary stents in place (see Figure 34-6).

   Pouches should be emptied when one-third to one-half full because weight of urine in pouch may weaken or dislodge skin seal (Thompson, 2000).

2. Observe output from stoma. Immediately after surgery, ureteral stents are in place and remain for up to 10 to 14 days. The physician then removes the stents.

   Urinary output must be monitored on all postoperative clients with urinary diversions to monitor renal status and patency of stents and whether volume of output is within acceptable limits (minimum of 30 ml/hr). Stents (an internal support device) are used to maintain patency of ureters at surgical anastomoses. These stents are sutured in place with dissolvable sutures.

3. Assess abdomen for best type of pouch to use. After pouch is off, assess skin around stoma, observing scars, folds, skin breakdown; also check peristomal suture line if present. Discard gloves.

   Maximizes secure fit and minimizes chance of leakage. Pouch and skin barrier are changed with any leakage. Determines need for barrier paste and additional intervention.

4. Determine client's emotional response, knowledge, and understanding of ostomy. Determine client's family and other significant support.

   Helps determine extent client is able to participate in care and need for teaching (O'Shea, 2001). Helps anticipate discharge needs.

NURSING DIAGNOSES

- Disturbed body image
- Deficient knowledge regarding ostomy self-care
- Risk for impaired skin integrity

Related factors are individualized based on client's condition or needs.

PLANNING

1. Expected outcomes following completion of procedure:
   - Stoma is moist, reddish pink, oozes blood only slightly if rubbed. Peristomal skin is free of irritation and is intact. Sutures are intact, and incision is well approximated.

     Normal findings for postoperative urinary diversion.

   - Urine drains freely from stents or stoma. Urine is yellowish with mucous shreds and is without foul odor. Volume of output is within acceptable limits (30 ml/hr).

     These are normal findings in postoperative phase. The mucosal surface of the stoma is easily traumatized. Mucous shreds are normal when bowel is used as urinary diversion. Urine should flow freely if unobstructed.

   - Client denies discomfort.

     Reflects ongoing healing without complications.

   - Client, family member, or significant other is willing to view stoma and asks questions about procedural steps.

     Shows adjustment to body image change and willingness to learn self-care (O'Shea, 2001).

2. Assemble equipment.

   Optimizes use of time; conserves client's and nurse's energy.

3. Close room curtains or door.

   Provides privacy.

4. Explain procedure to client; encourage client's participation and questions.

   Lessens anxiety and promotes client's participation.

STEP	RATIONALE

IMPLEMENTATION

1. Position client standing or supine, and drape. Some clients may prefer to do pouch change while sitting because this may make it easier for them to see stoma. However, when skin barrier and pouch are applied in sitting position, skin may have folds and wrinkles. Because of this, skin barriers and pouches applied with client in sitting position may leak.

   When client is supine, fewer wrinkles occur, allowing for ease of pouch application; maintains client's dignity.

2. Prepare pouch by removing backing from barrier and adhesive; if using cut-to-fit, cut opening ¹⁄₁₆ to ⅛ inch larger than stoma before removing backing. Some urinary pouches have special skin barrier that melts and forms secure seal around base of stoma. This is referred as a "turtleneck" effect and will not harm stoma.

   Barrier facilitates seal and protects skin; size of opening keeps urine off skin and lessens risk of maceration with skin irritation; avoids risk of damage to stoma. Stoma shrinks and does not reach optimal size for 6 to 8 weeks (Thompson, 2000). Pouch and skin barrier are changed whenever leaking. Change when client is comfortable; better time is in morning on arising because urinary output is reduced.

3. Perform hand hygiene, and apply gloves.

   Reduces transmission of microorganisms.

4. Place towel or disposable waterproof barrier under client. Tightly roll several gauze pads separately (should resemble tampon). (*Optional:* If gauze pads [called "wicks"] are to come in contact with stents, roll with sterile gloves on. Place wicks on sterile barrier [can use the inside of gauze wrapper].)

   Protects bed linen. Rolled gauze pads used to absorb urine during pouch change.

5. Remove used pouch carefully and gently by pushing skin away from barrier. If stents are present, *do not pull on them*. Immediately place a wick or sterile gauze pad over stomal opening. If stents are present, place sterile gauze pad underneath tips.

   Reduces risk of trauma to skin and risk of injury to ureters if stents are present; jerking irritates skin and can cause skin tears. Keeps urine from leaking onto skin. Immediately after surgery copious mucus exists over stoma because bowel has not adjusted to presence of urine.

6. Cleanse peristomal skin gently with warm tap water using gauze pads; do not scrub skin. Dry skin.

   Avoid soap. It leaves residue on skin, which interferes with pouch adhesion (Thompson, 2000). Pouch does not adhere to wet skin. Stents are sutured in place to decrease risk of damage. Do not be alarmed if a small amount of blood appears on stoma because stomal surface may ooze blood if rubbed. Bleeding into pouch is abnormal. Using a vinegar soak will remove uric acid crystals that may be deposited on peristomal skin.

- *Critical Decision Point*

  If uric acid crystals are present on skin, apply washcloth with a vinegar soak (one-third vinegar and two-thirds warm water) to peristomal skin. Rinse with warm tap water, and dry completely by patting skin with dry gauze or towel. Can use hand-held dryer set on cool. If copious mucus is on surface of stoma, carefully remove while stabilizing stents with sterile forceps.

7. Wick stoma continuously during pouch measurement and change. Place tip of gauze at stomal opening. Measure stoma.

   Using a wick at stoma tip prevents peristomal skin from becoming wet with urine during pouching-change procedure.

   a. If creases form next to stoma, use barrier paste or seal to fill in; let dry 1 to 2 minutes.

   Flattening of creases with paste or seal creates smooth surface for pouch placement (Thompson, 2000).

- *Critical Decision Point*

  For some clients, a pouch system with convexity may be needed to get a good seal and prevent leaks (Thompson, 2000).

STEP	**RATIONALE**
b. Apply skin sealant in circular area around base of stoma to any skin not protected by barrier; let dry. Hold pouch by barrier, center over stoma and stents, and press down gently on barrier. Bottom of pouch should be angled slightly to attach to bedside urinary drainage bag. Use another skin sealant on skin coming in contact with adhesive; allow to dry. Press adhesive backing smoothly against skin, starting from the bottom and working up and around sides. Never use a karaya skin barrier with a urinary diversion.	Urine renders karaya in skin barrier ineffective and results in leakage.
c. Maintain gentle finger pressure around barrier for 1 to 2 minutes.	Helps to ensure molding and adherence of skin barrier.
d. If using two-piece pouch, apply flange (barrier with adhesive) as above, then snap on pouch. If the client is mostly out of bed and ambulatory, apply pouch vertically.	Urine drains almost continuously. Flange waterproofs any skin that may contact urine. Creates wrinkle-free secure seal. Angling pouch avoids uneven twisting, which can disrupt seal. Prevents trauma to skin.
8. During the night, open drain spout, attach specific manufacturer adapter piece to end of pouch, and then attach this to bedside urinary bag. Place bag at a point close to foot of bed.	Constant flow of urine results in frequent emptying; overfilling of pouch may break skin seal. Placing night bag at foot of bed maximizes straight drainage that avoids urine accumulation in pouch.

- **Critical Decision Point**
  Know the specific urinary equipment that is being used. Many urinary pouches need an adapter piece that is specific to their brand to attach urinary pouch to bedside urinary drainage bag. Even within some manufacturers, adapter piece varies with different types of urinary pouches available.

9. Properly dispose of used pouch and soiled equipment.	Avoids odor in room.

- **Critical Decision Point**
  Do not throw used pouch and skin barrier into toilet. Most pouching equipment clogs toilet.

10. Remove gloves; perform hand hygiene.	Reduces transmission of microorganisms.
11. Change skin barrier and pouch every 3 to 7 days unless leaking; pouch can remain in place for tub bath or shower; after bath pat adhesive dry, or use hand-held dryer set on cool.	Avoids unnecessary trauma to skin from too-frequent changes. Drying ensures adhesion of pouch.

EVALUATION

1. Observe appearance of stoma, peristomal skin, and suture line during pouch change.	Determines condition of stoma and peristomal skin and progress of wound healing.
2. Evaluate character and volume of urinary drainage.	Determines if stoma and/or stents are patent. Character of urine can reveal degree of concentration and alterations in renal function.

- **Critical Decision Point**
  Mucus is a normal finding in urine from an ileal conduit or colon conduit. Other sediment in urine needs to be evaluated.

3. Ask if client notes discomfort around stoma.	Evaluates presence of skin irritation.
4. Observe client's, family member's, or significant other's willingness to view stoma and ask questions about procedure.	Determines level of adjustment and understanding of stoma care and pouch application.

Recording and Reporting

- Record type of pouch, time of change, condition and appearance of stoma and peristomal skin, and character of urine.
- Record urinary output.
- Document client's, family's, or significant other's reaction to stoma, and level of participation.
- Report abnormalities in stoma or peristomal structures and absence of urinary output to nurse in charge or physician.

Unexpected Outcomes	Related Interventions
1. Peristomal skin is irritated, reddened, tender, or has overgrowth.	• Keep peristomal skin dry. • Determine if client has an allergy to barrier and adhesive or infection. • Remeasure stoma before each change to ensure best fit of pouch. Change size of pouch opening as needed to protect skin (Erwin-Toth, 2003). • Culture any drainage.
2. No urinary output for several hours or output is less than 30 ml/hr. Urine has foul odor.	• Determine patency of stents or stoma. • Obtain urine specimen for culture and sensitivity to test for possible infection (see Chapter 43). • Notify physician.
3. Client reports burning sensation around base of stoma.	• Assess for presence of yeast infection around stoma, which causes itching, burning; appears as reddened area with maculopapular rash (Erwin-Toth, 2000). • Notify physician. • Apply medicated cream if ordered.
4. Client, family member, or significant other is unable to observe stoma, ask questions, or participate in care.	• Adjustment takes time, and process of grieving is individualized. • Further client education may be needed.

Teaching Considerations

- Use opportunity to teach whenever doing pouch change even if client does not appear interested. Do not force client to look at stoma; allow time for adjustment.
- Teach clients significance and importance of drinking at least 2 quarts of water daily and of helping to prevent urinary infections through intake of fluids and foods such as cranberry juice and blueberries (Gray, 2002).
- Teach clients that some mucus in urine is expected, but they should report any blood in their urine, excessively cloudy urine, chills, fever (101° F or higher), and back pain to their physician.
- Client should be given a teaching manual with steps clearly stated, or audiotaped instruction.
- Clients should be given a list of equipment and name, address, and phone number of a supplier in their community.

Pediatric Considerations

- In neonates, urinary diversions are less common than fecal ostomies.
- The type of urostomy done in neonates is usually a ureterostomy. Because these stomas are *very* tiny, are flush to the skin, and are often in skin creases in the flank area, they are very difficult to pouch and maintain a good intact seal with skin barrier and pouch. Sometimes parents may decide not to use an ostomy pouching system. Because urine is less erosive to the skin than fecal effluent, some parents may opt to use diapers with good skin care to manage their baby's urostomy (Boarini, 1989).

Gerontological Considerations

- Some older clients feel that they can cope with continuous flow of urine from stoma by decreasing amount of fluid they drink so they will have less output. This can be very dangerous to client's health. Client needs appropriate teaching to change this misconception.
- Limitations in physical and visual ability may require adjustments in self-care routine.

Home Care Considerations

- At home, pouch spout should be opened and connected to straight drainage at night. Make sure client understands that using wrong adapter piece causes leakage.
- Many different types of pouching systems are available. Some are one-piece and others two-piece. All disposable pouches are odor-proof, and most have an antireflux valve. Clients should be encouraged to find a pouch that they can apply easily and that satisfies them (Erwin-Toth, 2001).
- Clients should avoid placing pouches in extremely hot or cold locations because temperature may affect barrier and adhesive materials.
- Advise clients when they travel to always keep spare ostomy supplies with them in case luggage gets lost.
- While swimming, clients may find that applying waterproof tape to skin barrier and/or wearing an ostomy belt prevents pouch and skin barrier from becoming dislodged.
- See also Home Care Considerations given for Skill 34-1.

SKILL 34-3   Catheterizing a Urinary Diversion

Catheterization of a urinary diversion is the only way to obtain an accurate culture and sensitivity specimen for screening of infection (see Chapter 43). When necessary to obtain a specimen from a urinary diversion, the best method is to insert a sterile double-tip catheter into the stoma. Obtaining a specimen from urine in the pouch does not provide an accurate finding. If a specimen is needed from a client with a continent urinary diversion, it is important to have client or nurse perform a clean catheterization first to empty the diversion of stagnant urine and then perform a sterile procedure to obtain the specimen for culture.

With the use of strict aseptic technique, catheterization is relatively safe and easy. To prevent trauma of tissues, the nurse should understand how the stoma and implanted ureters are constructed.

Reflux of urine into the ureters can cause infection. Incorrect pouch placement, large volumes of urine in the pouch or a urinary pouch without an antireflux valve may promote reflux. The risk of reflux may be reduced by attaching the urinary pouch to straight drainage when high urinary output is expected. A client must understand the importance of draining the pouch frequently and using clean technique during stomal and skin care.

DELEGATION CONSIDERATIONS

This skill should not be delegated to assistive personnel. Instead, the nurse must instruct assistive personnel to:

- Inform nurse if client complains of peristomal pain or back pain
- Inform nurse if there is a change in color or amount of urinary drainage or if there is mucus or blood in the urinary drainage

EQUIPMENT

- ❑ Urinary catheterization supplies (may be contained in prepackaged sterile catheter kit or may need to be gathered separately). All items must be sterile.
- ❑ 14 to 16 Fr red rubber catheter (most use a double-tip catheter)
- ❑ Water-soluble lubricant
- ❑ Antiseptic swab (e.g., povidone-iodine or chlorhexidine)
- ❑ Sterile disposable gloves
- ❑ Sterile specimen container
- ❑ Gauze pads
- ❑ Bed protection barrier
- ❑ Towels
- ❑ Urinary diversion pouch (if client is using one-piece system; if using two-piece system, pouch can be snapped off for procedure)
- ❑ Nonsterile disposable gloves

STEP	RATIONALE

ASSESSMENT

1. Determine need to perform catheterization to obtain a sterile specimen from urinary diversion; note signs and symptoms of urinary tract infection (UTI) such as elevated temperature, chills, foul-smelling urine, elevated white blood cell (WBC) count.

   Urinary diversion may pose risk for reflux of urine back to kidneys, resulting in infection (Lewis and others, 2004).

2. Obtain physician's order for catheterization.

   Invasive procedure requires physician's order.

3. Assess client's understanding of need for procedure and how procedure is done.

   Determines willingness to cooperate and indicates extent of explanation nurse should provide.

NURSING DIAGNOSES

- Risk for infection
- Deficient knowledge regarding urinary diversion catheterization

Related factors are individualized based on client's condition or needs.

PLANNING

1. Expected outcomes following completion of procedure:
   - No bacteria are present in urine.   *No infection is present.*
   - Skin and stoma are intact, without signs of irritation.   *Urinary pouch is intact.*
   - Client describes risks of infection and techniques to prevent infection.   *Demonstrates client's learning.*
2. Assemble equipment.   *Optimizes use of time; conserves client's and nurse's energy.*
3. Close room curtains or door.   *Provides privacy.*
4. Explain procedure to client; if possible; attempt to obtain specimen when client is due to change pouch if using one-piece system.

   Lessens anxiety and promotes client's cooperation. Changing pouch too frequently can result in skin breakdown (Thompson, 2000).

IMPLEMENTATION

1. Position client sitting, if possible, and drape towel across pelvic area.

   Gravity facilitates flow of urine. Maintains client's dignity. Towel absorbs urine.

2. Perform hand hygiene and apply disposable gloves.

   Reduces transmission of microorganisms; wicks absorb urine from stomal opening of an incontinent urinary diversion.

3. Remove used pouch according to Skill 34-2, Implementation, step 5.

4. Remove and discard gloves. Open sterile catheterization set according to instructions, or open needed equipment and place on sterile barrier. Apply fresh sterile gloves and prepare several sterile gauze wicks. Place on barrier inside of sterile gauze wrapper. If not using catheterization kit, place gauze pad on sterile field, and squeeze small amount of lubricant onto gauze.

   Protects skin from trauma.

   Avoids contamination.
   An incontinent ostomy will continue to dribble urine.

5. If needed, have client wick stoma while waiting by placing a sterile gauze over stoma.

6. Cleanse "face" of stoma with antiseptic swabs using circular motion from center outward. Using new swab each time, repeat twice.

   Removes surface bacteria.

7. Allow some urine to flow out of stoma of incontinent ostomy. For continent ostomy flush stoma with sterile saline.

   Flushes antiseptic off face of stoma. Iodine in specimen alters results.

8. Lubricate tip of catheter with water-soluble lubricant.

   Lubricant facilitates passage of catheter through stoma.

STEP	RATIONALE
9. Remove lid from specimen container. Place distal end of catheter into specimen container. Hold catheter in container with nondominant hand.	Only a few drops of urine are obtained; care should be used to direct all into container.
10. With dominant hand, gently insert catheter 2 to 2½ inches (5 to 6.5 cm) into stoma. If using a double-tip catheter, insert the catheter into the stoma first, then gently advance the inner catheter. Do not force catheter, redirect course as needed. Use gentle but firm pressure similar to regular catheterization of urethra. Have client cough or turn slightly to facilitate passage of catheter.	Care must be taken to avoid perforation. Some resistance is common at muscle level in conduit or at "nipple" level of continent ostomy. Allow catheter to enter slowly. Have client breathe slowly and deeply with mouth open; may relax abdominal muscles.
11. Maintain container below level of stoma. Have client cough as needed. Urine may flow around and through catheter. This is acceptable, but only urine from catheter is desired. Normally, wait 5 minutes; if no urine is in container, pinch catheter and remove; direct urine "trapped" in catheter into cup.	Facilitates drainage of urine. Only 3 to 5 ml of urine is needed for culture and sensitivity studies.
12. After withdrawing catheter, place gauze pad over stoma.	Keeps skin dry.
13. Apply lid to specimen container. Remove gloves, and label specimen with required information.	Prevents accidental spillage. Labeling ensures acceptance of specimen by laboratory and processing.
14. Reapply new pouch (see Skill 34-1).	Pouch is necessary to contain urine; proper technique is important to avoid skin and stoma irritation (Thompson, 2000).
15. Remove used pouch and equipment, and dispose of properly.	Avoids unpleasant odor in room and eliminates source of bacterial colonization.
16. Perform hand hygiene, and send specimen to laboratory at once.	Avoids transmission of infection. Allowing urine to sit for long periods at room temperature affects laboratory results (Lewis and others, 2004).

EVALUATION

1. Refer to laboratory report, and compare results of culture and sensitivity with normal expected findings. Remember that mucus is a normal finding in the urine of a client with an ileal or colon conduit.

Determines presence of infection. If contamination appears likely, second specimen will need to be sent.

2. Observe stoma and peristomal area for skin breakdown.

Exposure of skin to urine increases the risk of skin breakdown.

3. Check that urinary pouch and skin barrier are intact with no leakage.

A properly applied pouch and skin barrier that are the correct size minimize chance of leakage (Erwin-Toth, 2003).

4. Ask client about signs and symptoms of UTI.

An informed client will seek attention for a problem earlier if aware of signs and symptoms (O'Shea, 2001).

Recording and Reporting

- Record time specimen collected, client's tolerance of procedure, and appearance of urine, skin, and stoma.
- Report results of laboratory test to nurse in charge or physician.

Unexpected Outcomes	Related Interventions
1. Culture reveals evidence of bacteria in urine.	• Notify physician. • Initiate prescribed medications. • Encourage fluids.
2. Skin or stoma reveals complications.	• Provide additional skin care. • Culture any drainage. • Consult with stoma specialist.

Teaching Considerations

- Explain common symptoms of UTI: flank pain, dark or bloody urine, foul-smelling urine, fever (101° F or higher), cloudy urine (not mucus), and nausea.
- Encourage client to maintain fluid intake, and notify physician if symptoms of infection develop.

- Instruct client or primary caregiver about clean technique during pouch application.
- Reinforce importance of fluid intake (2 L/day).

SKILL 34-4 Maintaining a Continent Diversion

Continent diversions can be done to contain either urine or stool. These newer surgical procedures provide clients with the option of having an ostomy that does not spontaneously drain effluent, but rather must be drained from the internal pouch by the client. Figure 34-7 shows an example of an internal pouch created for a continent stool diversion. The pouch is emptied when the client inserts a catheter or tube into the external stoma to drain the stool. Because the ostomy is continent, the client does not have to wear an external ostomy pouch over the external stoma.

A continent urinary diversion is a reservoir or pouch that collects urine. Urine is evacuated only when a catheter is inserted into the stoma to empty the urine. This is unlike a conventional urinary diversion such as an ileal conduit, which serves only as a passageway for urine to flow to the outside of the abdomen. Many techniques are available for construction of a continent urinary diversion using various portions of the small and/or large bowel (see Figure 34-3). Depending on the surgical technique used, the continent urinary diversion may be a Kock pouch, an Indiana continent urinary diversion, or some other type (Colwell and others, 2001). Because this reservoir is continent, the client does not have to wear an external pouch. The reservoir is intubated (or catheterized) at scheduled times to drain urine. The opening (called a stoma) into the reservoir generally is placed in the right lower quadrant of the abdomen below where an ileal conduit would be. The stoma is flush with the skin or slightly budded and is reddish pink.

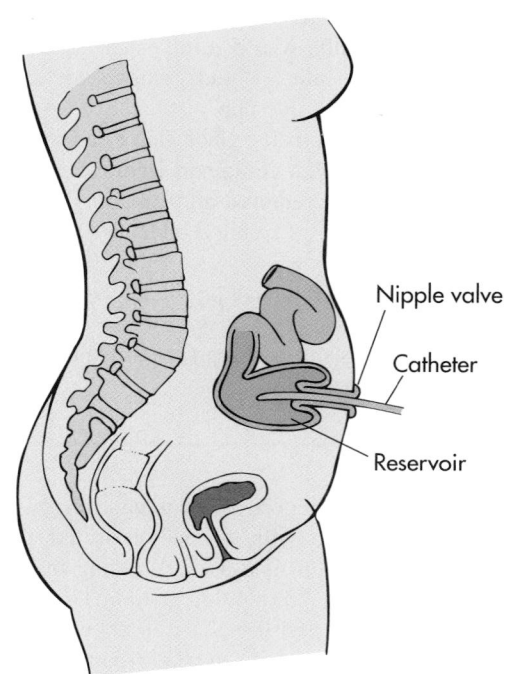

FIGURE 34-7 Continent ileal reservoir showing placement of catheter at surgery to maintain drainage during healing. After healing, catheter inserted intermittently for drainage. (Modified from Hull TL, Erwin-Toth P: The pelvic pouch procedure and continent ostomies: overview and controversies, *J Wound Ostomy Continence Nurs* 23(3):156, 1996.)

DELEGATION CONSIDERATIONS

The skill of maintaining a continent diversion should not be delegated to assistive personnel. The nurse should inform assistive personnel to:

- Immediately report any leaks of urine or feces seeping around the stoma
- Report any changes in client's level of comfort

EQUIPMENT

Varies with recovery phase.
Postoperative Care to 3 Weeks
- Sterile normal saline (NS)
- Sterile catheter tip irrigating syringe
- Sterile gauze pads
- Sterile gloves
- Antiseptic swab (e.g., povidone-iodine or chlorhexidine)
- Sterile specimen cup
- Sterile water
- Towels

EQUIPMENT—cont'd

Postoperative Care 4 to 6 Weeks
- ❑ Sterile NS
- ❑ Sterile catheter tip irrigating syringe
- ❑ Sterile gauze pads
- ❑ Sterile gloves
- ❑ Antiseptic swab (e.g., povidone-iodine or chlorhexidine)

- ❑ Sterile basin
- ❑ Sterile 14 to 16 Fr red rubber catheter
- ❑ Water-soluble lubricant
- ❑ Stoma cover (commercial or adhesive strip or nonstick dressing)
- ❑ Liquid antimicrobial soap
- ❑ Towels

STEP	RATIONALE

ASSESSMENT

1. Observe all tubes for intactness and patency, nature of drainage, and connection to appropriate collection system. Label all collecting bags with origin of urine or drainage contained in them. Keep intake and output record.

Clients return immediately after surgery with a catheter in stoma. Avoids errors in input and output record. Minimal acceptable urine output is 30 ml/hr from all sites.

• *Critical Decision Point*

If client had a continent urinary diversion, then ureteral stents that exit through stoma or another site on abdomen will also be present; stents are connected to a separate drainage system. If a continent ileostomy, usually a single large tube will direct effluent out of internal pouch.

2. Observe stoma for color, peristomal skin for maceration, and condition of all external suture lines.

Determines potential circulatory problems and reflects healing progress. Stoma should be red or pink, glistening with a mucous coating. A dusky or bluish stoma has compromised circulation (Lewis and others, 2004).

3. Assess bowel sounds and lung sounds. Assess serum values of chloride and creatinine.

Manipulation of large portions of bowel may lead to an ileus. Underventilation by client after surgery may lead to respiratory complications. Immediately after surgery, intestinal segment used for reservoir may absorb chloride and hydrogen ions. Creatinine measures effectiveness of kidney function (Pagana and Pagana, 2004).

4. Palpate lightly around stoma, noting any localized tenderness or guarding.

May be sign of infection along internal suture lines.

5. Determine client's emotional response, knowledge, and understanding of continent reservoir or pouch; determine family and other significant support.

Helps determine extent client is able to participate in care and need for teaching. Assists in anticipating discharge needs (O'Shea, 2001).

NURSING DIAGNOSES

- Disturbed body image
- Risk for infection

- Deficient knowledge regarding ostomy self-care
- Risk for impaired skin integrity

Related factors are individualized based on client's condition or needs.

PLANNING

1. Expected outcomes following completion of procedure:
   - Stoma is moist, reddish pink, and oozes blood only slightly if rubbed. Peristomal skin is free of irritation and intact. Sutures are intact, and incision is well approximated. Client denies discomfort.

These are normal findings in postoperative phase. Reflects ongoing healing without complications.

STEP	RATIONALE

- Effluent is normal depending on type of continent diversion:
  - Urine drains freely from stents, stomal catheter, or intubation catheter. Urine is clear yellowish with mucous shreds and is without foul odor. Volume of output is within acceptable limits.

  Character of urine and consistency of stool will depend on many factors, for example, location and hydration status. Urine should flow freely if unobstructed.

  - Effluent is brown, may be semiformed or semiliquid.

  Mucous shreds are normal when bowel is used as reservoir.

- Client has no pain at stoma or peristomal skin.

  Pain might be an indicator of infection.

- Client, family member, or significant other is willing to view stoma and asks questions about procedural steps.

  Shows adjustment to body image change and willingness to learn self-care (O'Shea, 2001).

- Client is able to intubate and irrigate bowel pouch before discharge.

  Reflects comprehensive teaching. Continent diversion requires a knowledgeable client to maintain optimal functioning. If unable to care for self, client is at risk for complications.

2. Assemble equipment.

   Optimizes use of time; conserves client's and nurse's energy.

3. Close room curtains or door.

   Provides privacy.

4. Explain procedure to client; encourage client's interaction and questions.

   Lessens anxiety and promotes client's participation.

IMPLEMENTATION

POSTOPERATIVE CARE TO 3 WEEKS

1. Position client supine or sitting, and drape with towels.

   Facilitates instilling NS into reservoir; sitting is a better position for drainage. Maintains client's dignity.

2. Perform hand hygiene, and open sterile equipment. Remove lid from sterile specimen cup, and place lid with open side up. Pour 20 to 30 ml sterile NS into sterile specimen cup. Open sterile syringe and antiseptic swabs, and position them for use.

   Reduces transmission of microorganisms.

3. Put on sterile gloves, and draw 20 to 30 ml sterile NS into syringe. Cleanse connection point of indwelling stomal catheter and drainage tubing with antiseptic swabs using a circular motion; use each swab once; wait 30 seconds.

   Reduces risk of nosocomial infection.

4. Disconnect catheter and tubing, and gently irrigate stomal catheter by infusing saline; do not contaminate tip of drainage tubing. If a new urinary diversion, gently irrigate to avoid forcing solution and retained urine into implanted ureters.

   Large numbers of internal surgical sites require strict asepsis during postoperative phase. Reflux into ureters may cause infection (Lewis and others, 2004).

- *Critical Decision Point*
  Do not aspirate because this increases risk of damage to internal suture lines. Irrigation maintains patency of stomal catheter because large amount of mucus is secreted initially by reservoir.

5. Reconnect drainage system. Record volume used for irrigation. For urinary diversions, subtract this from total urine output at end of each shift. Follow agency protocol for changing bedside urinary drainage bags.

   Keeps accurate urinary output record. Reduces risk of colonization of microorganisms.

STEP	**RATIONALE**
6. Using remaining antiseptic swabs, cleanse "face" of stoma around catheter. Use another swab, and cleanse skin around base of stoma; allow to dry 30 seconds, and gently remove antiseptic with a gauze pad moistened with sterile water.	Mucus accumulates on face of stoma and seeps onto skin. Maintains skin integrity and reduces risk of infection. Some clients are allergic to iodine, so assess for allergy to iodine or shellfish before this step (Lewis and others, 2004).
7. Discard soiled equipment; remove gloves. Maintain sterile specimen cup and sterile NS and water containers for next irrigation. Label these with date, time, and nurse's initials. NOTE: Hospital protocols vary; generally, immediately after surgery continent diversions are gently irrigated every 2 to 4 hours to maintain patency of stomal catheter, allowing urine to drain freely.	Reduces transmission of microorganisms. Maintains sterility of cup so it can be used for 8 hours. Some supplies can stay at bedside for 8 hours if strict aseptic technique is followed; this helps contain costs.

POSTOPERATIVE CARE 4 TO 6 WEEKS

STEP	**RATIONALE**
1. Follow steps 1 and 2 in preceding section. Omit setting up sterile specimen cup.	Generally stoma catheter is removed the third postoperative week.
2. Open sterile basin, and maintain inside of wrapper as sterile field. Pour 30 to 60 ml of sterile NS into basin. Open gauze pads onto sterile wrapper; squeeze small amount of water-soluble lubricant onto gauze pad. Open wrapper of sterile red catheter for use, or place catheter onto sterile basin wrapper.	Maintains strict aseptic technique to reduce risk of nosocomial infection during recovery phase.
3. Apply sterile gloves, and draw 30 to 60 ml of sterile NS into syringe. Cleanse "face" of stoma with antiseptic swab starting from center and using circular movements to outer edge; wait 30 seconds.	Reduces risk of nosocomial infection; removes any accumulation of mucus.
4. Lubricate tip of catheter well. Insert into stoma by gently rotating during insertion; insert until urine starts to drain.	Reduces trauma to continence mechanism (valve) during insertion; some resistance to insertion is normal as catheter passes through layer of abdominal fascia. Client may need to change position to facilitate insertion. Taking slow, deep breaths also helps by relaxing abdominal muscles.
5. If no effluent starts to drain, problem solving is needed. The illustration can be used to help solve problem of inadequate effluent from pouch. For example, try moving catheter in and out slightly, have client move side to side, or ask patient to cough. If these actions do not cause drainage then gently irrigate the catheter with 30 to 60 ml of sterile saline.	Mucus may plug the catheter. Catheter may need to be irrigated to establish flow.

STEP	**RATIONALE**

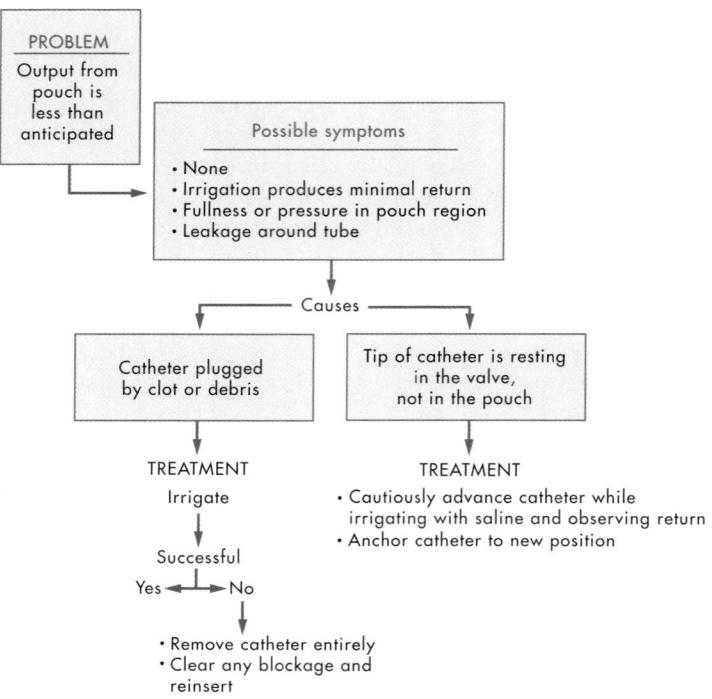

PROBLEM
Output from pouch is less than anticipated

Possible symptoms
• None
• Irrigation produces minimal return
• Fullness or pressure in pouch region
• Leakage around tube

Causes

Catheter plugged by clot or debris

Tip of catheter is resting in the valve, not in the pouch

TREATMENT
Irrigate

Successful
Yes ◄──┴──► No

TREATMENT
• Cautiously advance catheter while irrigating with saline and observing return
• Anchor catheter to new position

• Remove catheter entirely
• Clear any blockage and reinsert

STEP 5 Problem solving when output from the pouch is lower than anticipated. (Modified from Hull TL, Erwin-Toth P: The pelvic pouch procedure and continent ostomies: overview and controversies, *J Wound Ostomy Continence Nurs* 23(3):156, 1996)

6. Before withdrawing catheter, have client cough three or four times, then slowly remove.

Positive pressure inside abdomen clears residual urine or stool from pouch and continence valve; clears mucus from catheter.

7. Gently cleanse peristomal skin with gauze pads and liquid antimicrobial soap; rinse; pat dry.

Reduces bacterial colonization and removes any dried mucus to maintain skin integrity.

8. Cover stoma with stomal covering.

Some leakage of effluent occurs until full recovery from surgery; mucus will always be produced.

9. Discard soiled equipment; remove gloves. Maintain sterile NS; label with date, time, and nurse's initials.

Reduces transmission of microorganisms. Some equipment can stay at bedside for 8 hours if strict aseptic technique is followed; this helps reduce costs.

10. Record output and amount used for irrigation.

Keeps accurate output record.

NOTE: *Postoperative week 3:* Stoma is intubated every 2 to 3 hours and once at night to drain urine; it is irrigated every 4 hours. Schedule should be known to client and to all caregivers. A time card at bedside facilitates this. *Weeks 4 through 6:* Intubate every 4 hours and as needed (prn) at night; irrigate twice a day (bid) and prn. Fully recovered client with continent urinary diversion must intubate (or be intubated if unable to do) every 4 hours and prn at night; irrigate bid and prn. Physician's protocols may vary somewhat.

The scheduled intubation times allow for gradual expansion of the pouch. Pouches or reservoirs vary as to maximum amount of urine they can hold after complete recovery; may range from 150 to 600 ml. Reservoirs constructed from bowel always secrete mucus and must be routinely irrigated.

STEP	RATIONALE

▮ EVALUATION

1. Note appearance of stoma, peristomal skin, and abdominal suture lines.

Determines condition of stoma and peristomal skin and progress of wound healing.

2. Evaluate character and volume of output.

Determines if stomal catheter, stents, and residual catheter (e.g., cecostomy tube) are patent. Alerts nurse for need to irrigate stomal catheter. Minimal urinary output is 30 ml/hr.

3. Palpate for discomfort over pouch site and over peristomal skin.

May indicate large amount of residual urine, residual stool, or infection. Determines if any skin irritation is present.

4. Observe client's, family member's, or significant other's willingness to participate in care.

Determines level of adjustment, need for teaching, and risk for complications.

Recording and Reporting

- Record time of irrigation and/or intubation, size of catheter used, ease of intubation, amount of NS used, amount and character of output, and client's tolerance.
- Document client's and family's responses and their level of participation in care.
- Report abnormalities of stoma and peristomal skin.

Unexpected Outcomes	Related Interventions
1. Continence valve leaks excessively and continuously after stomal catheter is removed.	• Replace valve. • Empty reservoir more often to avoid overdistention.
2. Catheter cannot be inserted.	• Remove catheter, and start again. • Pouch may be overdistended; empty pouch more frequently.
3. Stool is especially thick.	• Encourage client not to take a laxative but rather to increase daily fluid intake, including intake of prune juice.
4. See also Unexpected Outcomes and Related Interventions for Skill 34-1.	

Teaching Considerations

- Give instruction according to client's level of understanding and ability and readiness.
- Use the opportunity to teach whenever doing pouch irrigation or intubation even if client does not appear interested. Do not force client to look at stoma; allow time for adjustment (O'Shea, 2001; Secord and others, 2001).
- Include family member or significant other in teaching if possible.
- Client should be given a teaching manual with steps clearly stated, or audiotaped instructions. For someone with a learning disability, a "picture book" of steps may be more appropriate.
- Client should be given a list of equipment and name, address, and phone number of a supplier in the community.
- Teach clients that some mucus in urine is expected; they should report any blood in urine, excessively cloudy urine, chills, fever (101° F or higher), and back pain to physician immediately.

- Teach clients to *not* use petroleum-based products for lubricating the catheter because this increases risk of infection; client may use plain warm tap water or water-soluble lubricant (preferred). May use plain warm tap water to irrigate after week 6 (this may vary with physician's protocol).

Gerontological Considerations

- Clients should be carefully assessed preoperatively for their suitability for having a continent diversion. Clients must have physical, visual, and mental ability to intubate stoma and drain internal pouch on prescribed schedule.

Home Care Considerations

- Teach clients proper care of intubation catheters: After use, rinse inside to clear any mucus, and wash with warm, soapy water; rinse well inside and out; suspend catheter so that it hangs to dry. Dry completely, and keep in a clean plastic bag or toothbrush holder container.
- Clients must always carry their catheter with them.

FOCUS *on* CLINICAL PRACTICE

You are assigned to care for Janeé Bell, a 28-year-old customer service representative. She has been admitted for elective colon removal secondary to a 10-year history of ulcerative colitis. She is scheduled for a Kock procedure for a continent ileostomy.

1. What other information will you need to adequately care for her both preoperatively and postoperatively?
2. As you review preoperative teaching with Janeé, you realize that she has a good understanding when she states:
   A. "I will need to drain the pouch with a catheter regularly."
   B. "The stoma surface should be pink and dry."
   C. "The drainage will be formed."
   D. "I will wear a drainage bag all the time."
   Explain your choice.

3. After Janeé returns from surgery you assess the stoma. You should expect the stoma to (choose all that apply):
   A. Have a mucous coating
   B. Be even with the skin level
   C. Appear red and shiny
   D. Have a catheter placed into the pouch
   E. Be pink and dry
   Explain your choices.
4. When teaching Janeé about care at home, you explain that:
   A. All equipment must be sterile
   B. Petroleum jelly is used as a lubricant
   C. The catheter may be washed and dried between uses
   D. After a few weeks she will insert the catheter only once a day
   Explain your choice.

NCLEX REVIEW QUESTIONS

1. A client with a continent ileostomy pouch (fecal) has inserted the catheter, but only a small amount of effluent has drained. What should he do first?
   1. Remove the catheter
   2. Gently insert catheter a little more
   3. Massage the abdomen
   4. Irrigate catheter with ½ to 1 ounce of tap water
2. A client has a new ileal conduit (loop) urostomy secondary to bladder cancer. Which of the following behaviors by the client suggests the most acceptance of this body image change? Client:
   1. Watches the nurse empty the pouch
   2. Looks at the site
   3. Reads the product literature
   4. Holds the gauze wick on stoma during a pouch change
3. The nurse recognizes the main disadvantage of an ileal conduit (loop) is that:
   1. Constipation may occur
   2. Stool remains liquid
   3. Urine drains continuously
   4. Nutrients are lost
4. The nurse will teach the client to protect the peristomal skin around most ostomies by:
   1. Cleansing with alcohol
   2. Lubricating skin with mineral oil
   3. Using karaya barrier
   4. Applying benzoin patches

5. The nurse caring for a client with a permanent colostomy should emphasize which dietary instruction?
   1. As normal a diet as possible
   2. Limiting liquids to prevent diarrhea
   3. A low-residue diet to decrease amount of stool
   4. Avoiding spices and gas-producing foods
6. A client about to have an ileostomy to cure his ulcerative colitis asks the nurse, "Will I really be able to have a normal life with this procedure?" What should the nurse do?
   1. Notify the physician to talk to the client
   2. Call in a clergy person for the client
   3. Tell client not to worry about it now
   4. Invite a person with an ostomy to speak with client
7. A client with a continent Kock pouch for stool will be taught that the following solution may be used to irrigate the pouch, if necessary, after complete healing has taken place:
   1. 10 to 20 ml of sterile saline
   2. 30 to 60 ml of warm tap water
   3. 50 to 60 ml of sterile saline
   4. 120 ml of sterile water

References

Ball EM: Ostomy guide. II. A teaching guide for continent ileostomy, *RN* 63(12):35, 2000.

Boarini JH: Principles of stoma care for infants, *J Enterostom Ther* 16(1):21, 1989.

Erwin-Toth P: The effect of ostomy surgery between the ages of 6 and 12 years on psychological development during childhood, adolescence, and young adulthood, *J Wound Ostomy Continence Nurs* 23(1):77, 1999.

Erwin-Toth P: Ostomies and fistulas: prevention and management of peristomal skin complications, *Adv Skin Wound Care* 13(4):175, 2000.

Erwin-Toth P: Caring for a stoma is more than skin deep, *Nursing* 31(5):36, 2001.

Erwin-Toth P: Ostomy pearls, *Adv Skin Wound Care* 16(3):146, 2003.

Gray M: Are cranberry or cranberry products effective in the prevention or management of urinary tract infection? *J Wound Ostomy Continence Nurs* 29(3):122, 2002.

Hampton BG, Bryant RA: *Ostomies and continent diversions: nursing management*, St. Louis, 1992, Mosby.

Hull TL, Erwin-Toth P: The pelvic pouch procedure and continent ostomies: overview and controversies, *J Wound Ostomy Continence Nurs* 23(3):156, 1996.

Jeffries C, MacKay AT: Improving stoma management in the low-vision patient, *J Wound Ostomy Continence Nurs* 24(6):302, 1997.

Lewis SM and others: *Medical-surgical nursing: assessment and management of clinical problems*, ed 6, St. Louis, 2004, Mosby.

Mitchel JV: A clinical pathway for ostomy care in the home: process and development, *J Wound Ostomy Continence Nurs* 25(4):200, 1998.

Mowdy S: The role of the WOC nurse in an ostomy support group, *J Wound Ostomy Continence Nurs* 25:51, 1998.

O'Shea HS: Teaching the adult ostomy patient, *J Wound Ostomy Continence Nurs* 28(1):47, 2001.

Pagana KD, Pagana TJ: *Mosby's diagnostic and laboratory test reference,* ed 6, St. Louis, 2004, Mosby.

Rogers VE: Ostomy care: managing preemie stomas—more than just the pouch, *J Wound Ostomy Continence Nurs* 30(2):100, 2003.

Schiff L: Ostomy products, *RN* 63(11):71, 2000.

Secord C and others: Adjusting to life with an ostomy, *Can Nurse* 97(1):29, 2001.

Smith D: Tackling the issue of patient sexuality after stoma surgery, *Community Nurse* 6(1):18, 2000.

Thompson J: A practical ostomy guide, part I, *RN* 63(11):61, 2000.

Research References

Banks N, Razor B: Preoperative stoma site assessment and marking, *Am J Nurs* 103(3):64A (Hospital Extra), 2003.

Beitz JM, Zuzelo PR: The lived experience of having a neobladder, *West J Nurs Res* 25(3): 294, 2003.

Colwell JC and others: The state of the standard diversion, *J Wound Ostomy Continence Nurs* 28(1):6, 2001.

Marquis P and others: Quality of life in patients with stomas: the Montreux study, *Ostomy Wound Manage* 49(2):48, 2003.

Thomason SS: Promoting outcomes for patients with spinal cord impairments and ostomies, *Medsurg Nurs* 9(2):77, 2000.

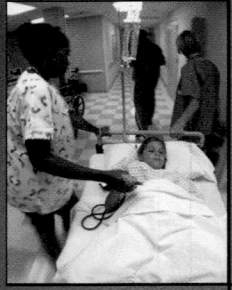

35

Preoperative and Postoperative Care

MEDIA RESOURCES

Evolve Site *evolve*
http://evolve.elsevier.com/Perry/skills
- Weblinks
- Video clips
- Mosby's Nursing Skills Video Exercises

Mosby's Nursing Skills Videos/CD-ROM
- ***Preoperatvie Nursing Care Video:*** Preoperative assessment, nursing history, informed consent, risk factors, physical assessment parameters, and review of laboratory and diagnostic test results; family support and participation, assessment of postdischarge needs; postoperative exercises and pain management, diaphragmatic breathing, incentive spirometry, controlled coughing, PCA, and nonpharmacological methods of pain relief; surgical preparation, preoperative checklist, and surgical consent
- ***Postoperative Nursing Care Video:*** Postanesthesia recovery room transfer; pain management, use of PCA; promoting postoperative recovery, breathing and coughing exercises, splinting, pneumatic compression stockings, wound care, and NG tube management

OBJECTIVES

Mastery of content in this chaper will enable the nurse to:

- Describe the activities needed to prepare a client for surgery.
- Explain the rationale for preoperative procedures.
- Discuss cultural differences that might affect the implementation of preoperative and postoperative procedures.
- Adequately prepare a client for surgery.
- Describe the benefits of structured preoperative teaching.
- Explain the rationale for each of the four postoperative exercises.
- Successfully instruct a client in performing postoperative exercises.
- Discuss the differences in nursing assessment during the immediate postoperative period and the convalescent phase of recovery.
- Conduct an assessment of a postoperative client.

KEY TERMS

Analgesia	Jackson-Pratt drain
Anesthesia	Malignant hyperthermia
Aspiration	Paralytic ileus
Atelectasis	Penrose drain
Coagulopathies	Phlebothrombosis
Decompression	Postanesthesia care unit (PACU)
Dehiscence	Postoperative
Ecchymosis	Postural hypotension
Evisceration	Preoperative
Hemostasis	Preoperative checklist
Hemovac drain	Procedural sedation
Homans' sign	Thrombophlebitis
Hypovolemic shock	Urinary retention
Incentive spirometer	Venous thrombosis
Informed consent	

BOX 35-1   JCAHO Client and Family Education Standards

The client's learning needs, abilities, preferences, and readiness to learn are assessed. The assessment considers cultural and religious practices, emotional barriers, desire and motivation to learn, physical and cognitive limitations, and language barriers. When called for by the age of the client and the length of stay, the hospital assesses and provides for client's academic education needs. Clients are educated about:

- The plan for care, treatment, and services (i.e., postoperative monitoring)
- Basic health practices and safety (i.e., out of bed [OOB] only with assistance)
- The safe and effective use of medication, according to their needs (i.e., the patient is only one allowed to press patient-controlled analgesia [PCA])
- Nutrition interventions, modified diets, or oral health (i.e., progression of diet postoperatively)
- The safe and effective use of medical equipment (i.e., incentive spirometer)
- Pain—understanding pain, the risk for pain, the importance of effective pain management, the pain assessment process, and methods for pain management (i.e., reporting of pain, frequency of medications, nonmedication pain relief techniques)
- Rehabilitation techniques to help them reach maximum independence possible (i.e., early ambulation)

Modified from Joint Commission on Accreditation of Healthcare Organizations: *Accreditation manual for hospitals*, Chicago, 2004, The Commission.

Any form of surgery is a stressful event, whether it is a major surgical procedure occurring in a large medical center or a minor procedure occurring in an outpatient center. The client must frequently make the decision to undergo a procedure that is associated with pain, possible disfigurement, dependence, or even the threat of death. Psychologically, the experience of surgery can cause considerable fear and anxiety. Physiologically, the more complex the surgery, the more likely a client will undergo changes in most major body systems.

The nurse uses a variety of skills to help the surgical client adequately prepare for the physiological and psychological stressors of surgery. During the preoperative phase the nurse performs a thorough assessment of the client's physical and emotional status. Coordination of a variety of diagnostic tests ensures that the surgeon and the anesthesia care provider have the information needed to determine the client's risks

during surgery and the postoperative period. In preparation for surgery, the nurse instructs the client and family concerning postoperative care in compliance with the Joint Commission on Accreditation of Health Care Organizations (JCAHO) client and family education standards (Box 35-1). The instructional topics enable the client and family to actively participate in the recovery process. Certain procedures, such as surgical skin preparation, the insertion of an indwelling catheter (see Chapter 32) or nasogastric (NG) tube (see Chapter 33), may be performed to protect the client from risks associated with surgery.

It is imperative that the nurse inquire about cultural practices and religious beliefs that may alter the client's and/or family's acceptance of perioperative teaching and procedures. The nurse remains nonjudgmental and adapts the client's care to encompass these practices and beliefs whenever possible. Each client's plan of care is individualized to provide an improved state of wellness and to maximize the client's ultimate level of independence. The nurse also communicates pertinent information to all members of the health care team so that the client receives comprehensive and holistic care.

A potential complication from surgery is that of surgical site infection. To decrease this risk the client's skin overlying the proposed surgical site is thoroughly cleansed to minimize skin contamination and the risk of postoperative wound infection. Preparation of the incisional area sometimes begins the evening before surgery and involves washing the skin (Centers for Disease Control and Prevention [CDC], 1999). For same-day surgery, clients may be asked to do this at home.

The skin is cleansed by scrubbing with an antimicrobial soap (e.g., chlorhexidine) two or more times. The client may perform the scrubbing during either a bath or shower. If an enema is given in preparation for surgery, the final shower or bath should be given after the enema. The client also may be required to shampoo hair if surgery involves the head, neck, or even the upper chest.

According to the Centers for Disease Control and Prevention (CDC) (1999), the Association of PeriOperative Registered Nurses (AORN) (2002b), and other agencies, hair is best left at the surgical site. If it is necessary for hair to be removed, the preferred method is by clipping outside of the operating room (OR) shortly before the incision is made (CDC, 1999; AORN, 2002b). Shaving the surgical site removes hair that serves as a reservoir for bacterial growth. However, evidence shows that infection can form in small cuts made by a razor. Wound infection occurs more often in clients who are shaved preoperatively than clients who are not shaved.

If the client is to be admitted for same-day surgery, the preoperative assessment and teaching of postoperative exercises may be done several days before surgery. This may be done by the surgeon's office nurse or, more typically, by the preoperative nurse in the outpatient department. The nurse ensures the completion of operative permits, blood work, testing (e.g., electrocardiogram [ECG]), and any other ordered procedures before the start of the procedure.

During the postoperative phase, when the client returns from the OR, the nurse is initially responsible for assessing the client's physical status to monitor any changes during the recovery process. Once the client's condition stabilizes, the nurse focuses efforts on returning the client to a functional level of wellness as soon as possible within the limitations created by surgery. The speed of a client's recovery depends on how effectively the nurse can anticipate potential complications, initiate necessary supportive and preventive therapies, and actively involve the client and family in the recovery process.

Evidence-Based Practice Trends

The health care industry is in a continuous state of technological advancement. These constant changes are responsible for the development of new diagnostic and interventional devices (e.g., endoscopic examination and laser surgery) that have contributed to a shortened surgical length of stay and changes in roles for care providers. A majority of clients now undergo surgery in an ambulatory care setting. Most surgical clients who must be hospitalized are not admitted until the day of surgery. Although preoperative education has been shown to improve client outcomes postoperatively (Oetker-Black and others, 2003), this shift in the provision of surgical services poses special challenges to health care professionals to meet their clients' educational needs in a reduced time frame. It is essential that ambulatory care clients receive adequate information to ensure the client

and/or family members can manage postoperative care activities in the home setting.

It has been reported that among surgical clients, surgical site infections (SSI) are the most common nosocomial infections, accounting for 38% of all such infections (Mangram and others, 1999). The sound judgment and proper technique of the surgical team and general overall health state of the client are among the most critical factors in the prevention of postoperative infections (Nichols, 2001). In 1999 the CDC Health Care Infection Control Practices Advisory Committee published revised guidelines for the prevention of infections. Some of the guidelines include the following recommendations:

- Do not remove hair unless it will interfere with the operation.
- If hair is to be removed, it is preferably done just before the operation with electric clippers.
- Require clients to shower or bathe with an antiseptic agent at least the night before surgery.
- Identify and treat all remote infections before elective operation.
- Keep hospital stay as short as possible.

Strict guidelines for use of antibiotics were recommended as well. In general, it is recommended that prophylactic antibiotics be given as close to the time of incision as possible (within 30 to 60 minutes) and not be given for longer than 24 hours postoperatively. In fact, it has been found that antibiotic usage after incision closure does not reduce infection rate, and when the antibiotics are continued, infections are more likely to be caused by a resistant organism (CDC, 2003).

Cultural Considerations

To provide culturally competent care to the surgical client, the nurse begins by assessing the family hierarchy to determine who needs to be involved in the client's decisions regarding surgery. Collectivist groups such as Africans, Asians, and Hispanics make decisions as a group. When providing preoperative teaching, the nurse includes family members. Use of professional interpreters may prove beneficial.

Preoperatively it is important to accommodate a client's religious and cultural needs. For example, the nurse allows religious articles to be worn until just before surgery. It is important to request information from the client, family, or religious leader about how these articles can be removed if absolutely necessary. Similarly, these same articles should be returned promptly after surgery. A Mormon who has received full sacraments will likely request to wear an undergarment. A male Sikh may request to wear a turban, keep his long hair and beard, metal bracelet, and symbolic sword (Singh, 2000). An East Indian woman may wish to wear her wedding necklace.

Preoperatively it can be helpful to assess client preferences for pain medication. Certain groups such as Filipinos believe that pain medications may lead to addiction. Buddhists and Hindus may prefer to endure the pain without medication (Pacquiao, 2003). Cultures (Latinos and Muslims) that value men being in control of their emotions may prevent members from verbalizing pain.

Skill Performance Guidelines

1. Know the type and nature of any previous surgery. Anatomical and physiological alterations may affect the client's health care needs.
2. Identify the factors and conditions that may increase a client's risks during surgery. Preoperative preparation and postoperative care depend upon the knowledge of these risk factors.
3. Know the rationale for and extent of impending surgery. Each type of surgical procedure requires a different type of nursing care.
4. Administer pain relief therapies according to the client's needs perioperatively. Pain can slow the surgical client's recovery.
5. Encourage the client's independence as soon as possible during the postoperative period. This minimizes the occurrence of postoperative complications.
6. Anticipate how surgery will affect the client's ability to return home to a functional lifestyle. Early discharge planning, client education, referral to community resources, and rehabilitation measures are needed to prepare the client to return home.
7. Identify cultural and religious beliefs and practices that may affect clients' and/or family members' reactions to the surgical experience, such as who can give consent, blood transfusions, and disposal of body parts, including hair.

SKILL 35-1   Preparing the Client for Surgery

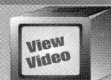

Preparing the client for surgery involves activities and procedures that help to decrease anxiety, ensure client safety, and decrease the risks of complications. A thorough nursing assessment is needed to document baseline data for future comparisons to determine the effect of instruction and to monitor clients at risk for complications during the perioperative experience.

Anxiety can interfere with the effectiveness of anesthesia and the ability of clients to actively participate in their care. The nurse provides information to clients about what will occur during the perioperative experience, as well as what sensations the client can expect to feel. Demonstration of a caring attitude toward the client, family members, and significant others can increase feelings of trust and reduce anxiety (Figure 35-1).

Client safety is ensured through a number of interventions and activities. Informed consent is required by law to help protect clients' rights, their autonomy, and their privacy. The client should be given information by the surgeon about the extent and type of surgery, alternative therapies, usual risks and benefits, and consequences of not having surgery in a nonthreatening manner as outlined in *The Patient Care Partnership* developed by the American Hospital Association (2003) (Table 35-1). The client or the client's legal guardian must sign a surgical consent form that includes this information. If the client's cultural practices include male dominance, as in many Asian and Middle Eastern cultures (D'avanzo Geissler, 1998), the husband, father, or oldest brother of a female client may also need to sign the consent form. The consent must also be signed by a witness to verify that the person who signed the consent is the client so named or the client's legal guardian. It is the nurse's ethical (not legal) responsibility, acting as the client's advocate, to ensure

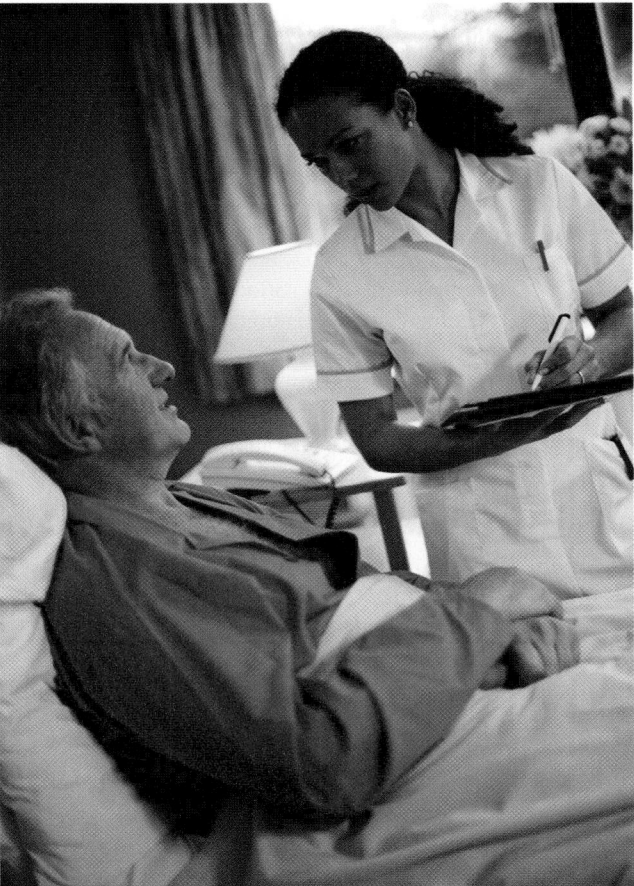

FIGURE 35-1 Nurse establishes a trusting relationship with client.

TABLE 35-1 INFORMATION NEEDED FOR INFORMED CONSENT

PARAMETERS	EXAMPLES
Name of procedure/surgery	Abdominal hysterectomy under general anesthesia.
Description of procedure/surgery	Removal of uterus only through an incision in the abdominal wall at the top of the pubic hairline done while unconscious.
Person performing the procedure/surgery	Doctor Richard Jones assisted by Doctor William Smith.
Benefits of procedure/surgery	To remove uterus with fibroids and stop excessive bleeding. Abdominal route is necessary due to anticipated adhesions from prior abdominal surgery.
Potential risks and adverse effects of procedure/surgery	Risks of hemorrhage and infection from surgery, risks of excessive sedation and allergic reaction to drugs used with general anesthesia, accidental damage to bladder, intestines, and/or nerves controlling these organs.
Approximate length of time for procedure/surgery	About 1 hour; 1 to 2 hours in recovery room.
Approximate length of time needed for recovery	3 to 4 days on surgical unit; 4 to 6 weeks before resuming physically stressful work.
Alternative treatments	Removal of uterus vaginally, radiation to shrink fibroids.
Consequences of refusing treatment	Continuation of pain and vaginal bleeding, risk of developing anemia. After menopause, fibroids should regress.

that the client understands the information and that the form has been signed and witnessed before the client receives preoperative medication.

Some clients with "do not resuscitate" (DNR) orders may require surgery for palliative care. DNR orders should not routinely be upheld nor should they be routinely suspended during anesthesia and surgery. The client's physicians are responsible for discussing and documenting issues with the client and/or family to determine whether the DNR order is to be maintained or whether it is to be partially or completely suspended during surgery. This discussion should describe potential resuscitation efforts that may be required during surgery and whether withholding resuscitation initiatives would alter the client's goals for having the surgery. Considerations that should be included in the discussion are the goals of the surgical treatment, the possibility of resuscitative measures, a description of what these measures include, and possible outcomes with and without resuscitation. If the client has opted to alter the DNR order during the intraoperative period, clear documentation should be in the medical record indicating when the DNR order is to be reinstated (AORN, 2003c).

Another aspect of maintaining safety is to minimize risk of client injury due to falls. Client activity is typically restricted after administration of preoperative sedatives. The preoperative checklist (Figure 35-2) must be completed to ensure that all procedures have been carried out and all necessary information and documentation for safe delivery of care is in the client's chart.

The risks for postoperative complications are decreased in a number of ways, some of which are specific to the type of procedure. For example, any client with a surgical incision of the thorax or abdomen will be expected to have pain postoperatively, and this reduces lung expansion. The client will be encouraged to learn how to use an incentive spirometer to reduce the incidence of atelectasis postoperatively. Skin preparation and deep breathing and coughing

exercises are examples of other procedures used to reduce complications.

Food and fluids are routinely withheld for a period of time preoperatively. However, in 1999, the American Society of Anesthesiologists (ASA) revised its practice guidelines for preoperative fasting in healthy clients undergoing elective procedures. These more liberal guidelines allow for the consumption of clear liquids up to 2 hours before elective surgery, a light breakfast (e.g., tea and toast) 6 hours before the procedure, and a heavier meal 8 hours beforehand (American Society of Anesthesiologists, 1999). These are merely guidelines. Each client should have orders written by anesthesia personnel outlining preoperative fasting requirements. In general, food and fluids are withheld for 4 to 8 hours before surgery requiring general anesthesia to minimize the risk of aspiration. The client may need to be allowed nothing by mouth (NPO) even when spinal or epidural anesthesia is administered. Hypotension due to autonomic nervous system blockade can induce nausea and vomiting (Lewis and others, 2004). Clients who are dehydrated or are at risk for hypovolemia will have intravenous fluids ordered. Medications may be given to decrease respiratory and gastrointestinal (GI) secretions, as an adjunct to anesthesia, and to decrease the risk of infection and development of stress ulcers.

The type of surgery dictates the preparation required preoperatively; for example, low-residue and clear liquid diets, enemas, cathartics, and oral antibiotics are ordered for clients before they undergo bowel surgery. Povidone-iodine douches may be used before many gynecological procedures.

Clients who smoke should be encouraged to stop the use of all tobacco products for at least 30 days before surgery. Nicotine delays wound healing and increases the risk of wound infection by constricting blood flow (CDC, 1999). Clients whose blood work indicates a low hemoglobin level and/or abnormal electrolyte levels or coagulopathies may require inpatient therapy before surgery.

A-1c4 NURSE'S DETAILED PERIOPERATIVE NOTE

1. Place initials in the space preceding the appropriate response (YES/NO, MET/NOT MET, NOT APPLICABLE)
2. Explain any "NO" or "NOT MET" in the space provided adjacent to the item or in the comment section provided, except for * items.
3. Record additional information in the comment section.
4. Record initials immediately following narrative entry.

DATE

HOSP. #

NAME

BIRTH DATE

ADDRESS

SS#

IF NOT IMPRINTED, PLEASE PRINT DATE, HOSP. #, NAME AND LOCATION

PERIOPERATIVE TRANSPORT BY:	METHOD:	PREOPERATIVE UNIT/AREA:
TIME RECEIVED IN PRESURGICAL CARE UNIT:	TIME RECEIVED IN OR:	

PATIENT ASSESSMENT/PREPARATION	YES	NO	COMMENT
PATIENT IDENTIFIED			ID Band Location
BLOOD BAND PRESENT*			#/Location
ALLERGIES* (If yes, please list)			
LATEX PRECAUTIONS INDICATED*			
CONSENT			
NPO			
HEALTH CHANGED SINCE LAST APPT			If Yes, Specify: Physician Notified:
INFECTIONS, PROBLEMS WITH HEART OR LUNGS			If Yes, Specify: Physician Notified:
TAKING ANY NEW MEDICATIONS			If Yes, Specify: Physician Notified:
PREOPERATIVE ORDERS COMPLETED			
SKIN ASSESSMENT COMPLETED			
VITALS OBTAINED DAY OF SURGERY			
HISTORY AND PHYSICAL PRESENT			
LAB VALUES REVIEWED			
LEVEL OF CONSCIOUSNESS—Answers questions/responds appropriately for age			
IMPLANTS/PROSTHESIS* (If yes, please list)			

Preoperative pain score (0–10) _____
Surgical site verified and marked with patient ☐ _____
Patient voided @ _____ Belongings: _____
Nursing comments _____

NURSING DIAGNOSIS	NURSING ORDERS/INTERVENTIONS	EXPECTED PATIENT OUTCOMES
ANXIETY—Risk of, Related to Surgical Intervention and Outcomes	1. Psychologic & physiologic comfort measures are provided. ___ Yes ___ No	The patient reports and/or demonstrates a reduction in anxiety. ___ MET ___ NOT MET
KNOWLEDGE DEFICIT—Risk of, Related to Surgical Intervention	1. The patient's understanding is assessed and questions/concerns are addressed by the appropriate individuals. ___ Yes ___ No	The patient's (guardian's) description of surgery corresponds with the Operative Consent (G-2d). ___ MET ___ NOT MET
INJURY—Risk for, Related to Tubes, Catheters, Lines ___ Not Applicable	1. Integrity of tubes, catheters, and lines is maintained. ___ Yes ___ No Catheters/Tubes/Drains/Lines: _____	The patient's risk for injury related to care and management of tubes, catheters, and lines is minimized. ___ MET ___ NOT MET

Initials	Standards Implemented By:	Initials	Standards Implemented By:

26304/9-01/MH05859   **UNIVERSITY OF IOWA HOSPITALS AND CLINICS**

Tab labels (right margin): A -1c4 / B CLIN. NOTES / C LABORATORY / D X-RAY EXAM / E CONSULTATION / F SPEC. EXAM / G THERAPY / H PATHOLOGY / I PT. QUES.

FIGURE 35-2 Preoperative assessment form. (Courtesy University of Iowa Hospitals and Clinics.)

Because many clients are admitted on the day of surgery, much of the preoperative preparation is often the responsibility of the client or the primary caregiver. It is important therefore that the hospital preadmission nurse or a nurse in the surgeon's practice be designated to provide adequate instructions. Client teaching should include any food and fluid restrictions, which medications, if any, are permitted on the morning of surgery, and the need for surgical site preparation the evening before surgery. It is also important to include action to be taken if any of these instructions are mistakenly omitted. Written instructions are a useful adjunct to teaching because the client and/or family can refer to them for any points that are unclear or forgotten. Videos and pamphlets are also useful adjuncts in preparing clients and their families.

To ensure client safety, the correct person, procedure, and surgical site are verified at the time of scheduling the procedure; upon admission or entry into the facility; and each time the responsibility for care of the client is transferred to another caregiver. A final verification check occurs immediately before the start of the procedure involving the entire surgical team. If the case involves laterality (right versus left), multiple structures (e.g., fingers, toes, lesions) or multiple levels (e.g., spine), then the final verification should include a site marking by the person performing the procedure. Clients should be involved in this process when they are awake and aware if possible. Immediately before starting the procedure (in the location where the procedure will be done) a "time out" is called. The entire operative team, using active communication verifies the correct client identity, correct side and site, agreement on the procedure to be done, correct client position, and availability of correct implants and any special equipment or special requirements. This final verification process should be documented (JCAHO, 2004).

DELEGATION CONSIDERATIONS

The skills of assessment and teaching should not be delegated to assistive personnel. Assistive personnel may administer an enema or a douche, obtain vital signs, apply antithrombotic stockings, and assist clients in removing clothing, jewelry, and prostheses. Before delegating these skills, the nurse must:

- Instruct assistive personnel in any precautions needed for the assigned client

EQUIPMENT

- ❏ Stethoscope
- ❏ Informed consent form
- ❏ Preoperative checklist
- ❏ Enema set and prescribed solution (if ordered—see Chapter 33)
- ❏ Douche set and prescribed solution (if ordered)
- ❏ Intravenous (IV) solutions and equipment (if ordered—see Chapter 27)
- ❏ Indwelling catheter set (if ordered—see Chapter 32)
- ❏ Antiembolism stockings (if ordered—see Skill 11-3)
- ❏ Medications (if ordered—see Chapter 20)

STEP	RATIONALE

ASSESSMENT

1. Correctly identify client by having client state (if able) name and a second client identifier (verify agency policy regarding identifiers to use such as date of birth or client registration number). Verify correct information on identification band.

Ensures correct client. Two distinct identifiers are to be used to verify correct client identification (JCAHO, 2004).

2. Determine ability of client to answer questions regarding health history and pending surgery.

Identifies reliability of client and need to supplement with information from family members or significant others. May indicate need for further information for informed consent.

3. Perform physical examination (Table 35-2 and Chapter 18). Focus on body systems likely to be affected by surgery.

Provides baseline data for future assessments and interventions. Also confirms or disputes information from history and may uncover new information.

• Critical Decision Point

If client is having emergency surgery, nurse focuses on assessment of primary body system affected.

4. Collect nursing history, and identify risk factors (see Table 35-2).

Allows for anticipation of possible complications and planning for interventions to reduce risks. Allergies, particularly to latex, can be life threatening.

STEP	RATIONALE

TABLE 35-2   ASSESSMENT OF THE SURGICAL CLIENT

ASSESSMENT CATEGORY	KEY CRITERIA
Nursing history	Previous personal/family experience with surgery and anesthesia (malignant hyperthermia)
Physical examination	General system review:
	• Head and neck
	• Integument
	• Thorax and lungs
	• Heart and vascular
	• Abdomen
	• Neurological status
	• Age
	• Nutrition
	• Radiotherapy, chemotherapy, medications that depress immune system
	• Fluid and electrolyte balance
	• Preexisting infection
	• Chronic respiratory disease (emphysema, bronchitis, asthma)
	• Immunological disorders (leukemia, acquired immunodeficiency syndrome
	• Allergies/sensitivities (including medications, food, latex, and environmental)
Risk factors	Medication history (prescription, over-the-counter [OTC], and herbal remedies)
	Physical or mental impairments
	Mobility limitations
	Prostheses (including hearing aids)
	Smoking habits
	Alcohol ingestion
	Family support and coping mechanisms
	Occupation
	Emotional health
	Temperature, blood pressure, pulse and respiratory rates
	Height and weight
	Oxygen saturations
	Electrocardiogram
	Laboratory values (e.g., Hgb, K$^+$, glucose, coagulation studies)
	Radiology and diagnostic test findings

STEP	RATIONALE
5. Apply allergy/sensitivity band if applicable.	Alerts health care providers to client's allergies and sensitivities.
6. Ask about client's and family members' expectations of surgery and care to be provided. Include questions concerning fears, cultural practices, and religious beliefs if applicable.	Allows nurse to anticipate client's/family's priorities and to adapt plan so that appropriate instruction and support can be given.
7. Review client's preoperative orders.	Identifies specific procedures and diagnostic tests to be done and medications to be given.
8. If client is same-day admit or ambulatory client, validate that preoperative preparations were completed as ordered. Specific preparations to review include NPO status, administration of medications, skin preparation, and bowel preparation if applicable.	Failure to complete preparation could lead to perioperative or postoperative complications and may necessitate the postponement or cancellation of surgery.
9. Ask if client has an advance directive. If so, place it in client's record.	Document conveys client's wishes if life support measures are necessary.

STEP	RATIONALE

NURSING DIAGNOSES

- Ineffective airway clearance
- Anxiety
- Risk for aspiration
- Risk for disturbed body image
- Ineffective breathing pattern
- Fear
- Impaired gas exchange
- Risk for infection

- Risk for perioperative-positioning injury
- Deficient knowledge regarding the surgical experience
- Impaired oral mucous membrane
- Acute pain
- Impaired physical mobility
- Risk for impaired skin integrity
- Ineffective tissue perfusion

Related factors are individualized based on client's condition or needs.

PLANNING

1. Expected outcomes following completion of procedure:
   - Client can state what surgical procedure is being performed and risks and benefits of surgery.
   - Client participates in preoperative and postoperative care.
   - Client states anxiety is decreased.

2. Prepare client's chart using preoperative checklist, and assemble equipment as needed.
3. Explain procedures, and allow client, family members, and significant others to ask questions and express concerns.

Identifies readiness to sign informed consent.

Preoperative preparations are effective.

Anxiety may interfere with effectiveness of teaching and of anesthesia.

Ensures that all preoperative procedures will be completed.

Decreases anxiety and increases cooperation.

IMPLEMENTATION

1. Orient client to room or presurgical (holding) area.
2. Physician obtains informed consent. Act as client advocate as needed; include considering any culturally sensitive issues. Witness form if allowed by agency.

Decreases anxiety and promotes feelings of control.
Surgery cannot be legally performed without client receiving information about need and extent of the surgery, alternatives, risks, and benefits. Client and/or family may be afraid to ask questions or express concerns regarding diverse practices.

• Critical Decision Point
Clients who are illiterate can sign with a mark if properly witnessed. Minors, unless married or declared emancipated, or individual considered incompetent cannot legally sign a consent form. Parent or legal guardian must provide consent. Some cultures do not allow female members to give consent.

3. Check medical record, and review or complete preoperative checklist (see Figure 35-2).

4. Provide preoperative teaching, including explanation of postoperative exercises (see Skill 35-2), skin preparation, pain-control measures (see Chapter 6), and postoperative care in recovery room and nursing division (see Skill 35-3).
5. Instruct client on need and rationale for NPO for period specified before surgery.

Ensures that pertinent laboratory and diagnostic test results are available and that all preoperative preparations are completed.
Decreases anxiety and promotes cooperation in care.

GI tract should be empty to decrease risk of vomiting and aspiration.

STEP	RATIONALE

- **Critical Decision Point**

  Client may brush teeth but should not swallow water. Client may take oral medications with sips of water (30 ml) if they are specially ordered to be taken preoperatively (e.g., antiarrhythmic or seizure medications). All other oral medications are withheld. The nurse must later check postoperative orders to ensure that scheduled medications unrelated to surgery are not forgotten.

6. Assess that any preoperative orders for enemas, douches, and skin preparations have been followed. Insert IV and/or indwelling catheter if ordered.	May delay or postpone surgery if not completed. IV and/or indwelling catheter may be inserted in holding or preanesthesia area.
7. Provide for hygiene measures, ensuring client privacy. Instruct client to remove all clothing, including undergarments, and to apply disposable cap and hospital gown with opening in back.	Prevents client's hair from contaminating sterile surfaces and provides easy access to client's body in OR.
8. Instruct client to remove hairpins, clips, wigs, hairpieces, jewelry, including rings used in body piercing, and makeup (including nail polish and acrylic nails). Religious medals may be pinned to gown if agency policy permits. In some institutions, acrylic nails or nail polish may be removed from only one finger if a pulse oximeter is used. Check institution's policy.	Hair appliances and jewelry anywhere on the body may become dislodged and cause injury during positioning and intubation (Armstrong, 1998). Rings may decrease circulation in fingers. Makeup, nail polish and false nails impede assessment of skin and oxygenation. In addition, acrylic nails may harbor pathogenic organisms (AORN, 2002a).

- **Critical Decision Point**

  Wedding rings that cannot be removed may be taped in place. Be careful not to create tourniquet effect with tape around finger.

9. Assist client in removing prostheses, including dentures and oral appliances, glasses and contact lenses, artificial limbs and eyes, artificial eyelashes, and hearing aids. Inventory items, and give to family members or have security lock them up. Document list of items and their location in preoperative checklist and/or nurses' notes per agency policy.	Prostheses can be lost or damaged during surgery and could cause injury. Oral appliances may occlude airway.

- **Critical Decision Point**

  If client will be required to follow instructions in the OR, hearing aid may be left in place. Decision may be made to leave wig or dentures in place until entering OR suite if removal will cause embarrassment. Check agency policy.

10. Secure all valuables, or give to family member or significant other. Have release form signed if required by agency.	Valuables left in client's room may be lost or stolen.
11. Apply antiembolism stockings as ordered (see Chapter 4).	Promotes venous return and reduces risk of thrombus formation.
12. Assess vital signs immediately before going to OR.	Abnormal vital signs may indicate conditions that increase risk for surgery.

- **Critical Decision Point**

  Vital signs not within normal range or client's baseline must be reported to physician and may require surgery to be postponed. Document abnormal vital signs and any action taken in nurses' notes and/or preoperative checklist according to agency policy.

STEP	RATIONALE
13. If client does not have an indwelling catheter, assist him or her in voiding before receiving preoperative medication.	Prevents incontinence and bladder distention during surgery and urinary retention with overflow postoperatively. Preoperative medication may cause drowsiness and decreased voiding sensation.
14. Administer preoperative medications as ordered. (These medications may be given in preoperative or holding area. Check preoperative orders.)	Reduces pain, anxiety, respiratory secretions, and amount of anesthesia required. Promotes relaxation. Antibiotics may be ordered prophylactically but are given within 30 to 60 minutes of incision.

• *Critical Decision Point*

Check that informed consent is signed before giving preoperative medications. Times on consent form and on medication administration record (MAR) must attest to this. Preoperative medications may alter level of consciousness and make the consent invalid.

15. Client is placed on bed rest with call light within reach and is told not to get out of bed without assistance.	There is an increased chance of injury in attempting to ambulate to void when client is sedated and unattended.

EVALUATION

1. Have client describe surgical procedure and its benefits and risks.	Confirms level of knowledge needed to sign informed consent.
2. Compare all assessment data with client's baseline and expected normals.	Evaluates client's risk for complications and possible need to postpone surgery.
3. Have client repeat preoperative instructions and demonstrate postoperative exercises.	Provides evidence that client understands preoperative instructions and can perform exercises.
4. Monitor client for signs and symptoms of anxiety, and ask how client and family are feeling.	Increased heart rate and blood pressure, dilated pupils, dry mouth, increased sweating, and muscle rigidity or shaking are responses to stress and anxiety. Asking client about feelings gives permission to express concerns, which can be further explored.

Recording and Reporting

- Document all preoperative preparations in nurses' notes and/or checklist.
- Document client's condition on transfer to OR in nurses' notes and/or on flow sheet.
- Document presence of any allergies/sensitivities on arm band, medical record, and medication administration record.
- Record disposition of client valuables/belongings (i.e., whether locked up according to agency policy or sent with family).
- Report and record any abnormal assessment findings, lack of signed and witnessed consent form, or failure of client to maintain NPO status and action taken.
- Report and record client's cultural practices and/or religious beliefs that affect perioperative care and any modification of care planned.

Unexpected Outcomes	Related Interventions
1. Client is unable to give consent, and family member is unavailable.	• In emergency situations, telephone consent from next of kin may be obtained. Two persons must witness oral consent.
	• Documentation must include explanation of situation and fact that oral consent was obtained and so witnessed.
	• At the earliest opportunity, person giving oral consent must sign a written consent. Signed telegram or signed fax may also be considered oral consent. Follow agency policy.

Unexpected Outcomes	Related Interventions
2. Vital signs are above or below client's baseline or expected range.	• This may indicate infection, anxiety, pain, or cardiovascular dysfunction, which increases surgical risk. • Clients who are dehydrated or malnourished may require hydration with IV solutions (see Chapter 27), parenteral nutrition (see Chapter 31), or antibiotic therapy before surgery.
3. Informed consent has not been signed and witnessed. Physician did not provide information and/or ensure that consent form was signed.	• Client is not ready for surgery. Client must sign consent before administration of preoperative medications or any medication that alters central nervous system.
4. Client did not remain NPO, which may indicate that the client did not understand instructions or forgot.	• Notify surgeon and anesthesiologist. Surgery may be postponed or cancelled.
5. Client is unable to state instructions or demonstrate postoperative exercises.	• Assessment of client's level of understanding or method of instruction was insufficient. Revision of instruction and reteaching is necessary.
6. Client did not void before receiving preoperative medication.	• Perhaps client did not need to void or was unable to void. Assess for bladder distention. If distended, client can use urinal or bedpan or may need order to be catheterized (see Chapter 32).

Teaching Considerations

- JCAHO client and family education standards are guidelines that should ensure that client, family member, and/or primary caregiver be taught about surgical procedure, healing process, sutures, dressing, drains, feeding tubes, pain control, and diet with rationale for each. Adults learn best when they understand the purpose or meaning of what is being taught (JCAHO, 2004).

Pediatric Considerations

- Parents should be involved in preoperative preparation to decrease children's anxiety. Preadmission programs to prepare parents and children for same-day surgery have been shown to decrease anxiety in both parents and children. Part of preoperative teaching should include giving children the opportunity to handle equipment they will see such as an anesthesia mask or drainage tube.
- Hospital programs that involve well-prepared parents during anesthesia induction in OR "virtually eliminated the need for heavy preoperative sedation—and shortened the child's post-op recovery period" (Fennell, 1999).
- Preoperative preparation should take into consideration developmental level of child; for example, toys and games may be used to demonstrate preoperative procedures (Hockenberry, 2005).
- Allow parents to accompany their child to the holding area.

Gerontological Considerations

- Physiological changes that occur with aging may require admission to hospital before surgery for additional diagnostic tests and stabilization of condition (Table 35-3).
- Focus on wellness and the person's strength.
- Teach when client is alert and rested. Keep teaching sessions short.
- Age-related changes such as decreased vision, hearing, and short-term memory may require presence of family members or primary caregiver during preoperative preparation.

Home Care Considerations

- Clients admitted on day of surgery must be instructed about NPO status, skin preparation, and procedures such as enemas and douches before admission. Often enemas or douches are done at home.
- Clients having surgery performed in ambulatory surgery centers must be accompanied by a family member or friend to allow for discharge after the procedure (Box 35-2).

TABLE 35-3 PHYSIOLOGICAL FACTORS THAT PLACE OLDER ADULT CLIENTS AT RISK FOR SURGERY

ALTERATIONS	SURGERY RISKS	NURSING IMPLICATIONS
CARDIOVASCULAR		
Degenerative change in myocardium and valves	Reduced cardiac reserve.	Assess baseline vital signs.
Rigidity of arterial walls and reduction in sympathetic and parasympatheticinnervation to heart	Predisposes client to postoperative hemorrhage and rise in systolic and diastolic blood pressure.	Maintain adequate fluid balance to minimize stress to the heart. Ensure blood pressure is adequate to meet circulatory demands.
Increase in calcium and cholesterol deposits within small arteries; arterial walls thickened	Predisposes client to clot formation in lower extremities.	Instruct client on techniques for performing leg exercises and proper turning. Apply antiembolism stockings, sequential compression devices (SCDs).
INTEGUMENTARY SYSTEM		
Decreased subcutaneous tissue and decreased fragility of skin	Prone to pressure ulcers and skin tears.	Assess skin every 4 hours; pad all bony prominences during surgery. Turn or reposition.
PULMONARY		
Rib cage stiffens and enlarges	Reduced vital capacity.	Instruct client in proper technique for coughing and deep breathing exercises, and use of spirometer.
Reduced diaphragm excursion	Greater residual capacity or volume of air left in lung after normal breath increases, reducing amount of new air brought into lungs with each inspiration.	Encourage deep breathing. Use incentive spirometer to enhance exhalation.
Lung tissue less distensible; alveoli enlarged	Reduced blood oxygenation.	Assess oxygen saturation via oximetry (SpO_2).
RENAL		
Reduced blood flow to kidneys	Blood loss causes a decrease in circulation to the kidney.	Monitor urinary output and laboratory data (i.e., BUN, creatinine).
Reduced glomerular filtration rate and excretory times	Limits ability to remove drugs or toxic substances.	Assess for adverse effects of medications.
Reduced bladder capacity	Voiding frequency increases, and larger amount of urine stays in the bladder after voiding. Sensation of need to void may not occur until bladder is filled.	Instruct client to notify nurse immediately when sensation of bladder fullness develops. Keep call light or bedpan within easy reach.
NEUROLOGICAL		
Sensory losses, including reduced tactile sense, increased pain tolerance	Client less able to respond to early warning signs of surgical complications.	Inspect bony prominences for signs of pressure. Orient client to surrounding environment. Observe for nonverbal signs of pain.
Decreased reaction time	Client becomes confused easily after anesthesia.	Reorient as needed. Maintain safe environment. Institute fall precautions.
METABOLIC		
Lower basal metabolic rate	Reduced total oxygen consumption and nutritional needs.	Ensure adequate nutritional intake once diet is resumed.
Reduced number of red blood cells and hemoglobin levels	Reduces ability to carry adequate oxygen to tissues.	Administer necessary blood products. Assess for adequacy of oxygenation, fatigue, and infection.
Change in total amounts of body potassium and water volume	Greater risk for fluid or electrolyte imbalance.	Monitor electrolyte levels.

BOX 35-2 Postanesthesia and Ambulatory Surgery Discharge Criteria

POSTANESTHESIA DISCHARGE CRITERIA

Client awake (or baseline)
Vital signs stable
No excess bleeding or drainage
No respiratory depression
Oxygen saturation >90%
Report given

AMBULATORY SURGERY DISCHARGE CRITERIA

All postanesthesia care unit (PACU) discharge criteria met
No intravenous (IV) narcotics for last 30 minutes
Minimal nausea and vomiting
Voided (if appropriate to surgical procedure/orders)
Able to ambulate if age-appropriate and not contraindicated
Responsible adult present to accompany client
Discharge instructions given and understood

SKILL 35-2 Demonstrating Postoperative Exercises

Structured preoperative teaching has a positive influence on a surgical client's recovery (Shuldham, 1999). The nurse provides information and teaches skills that help clients understand the surgical experience and participate actively in the recovery process. The skills of coughing, deep breathing, turning, and use of an incentive spirometer are important in preventing circulatory and respiratory postoperative complications.

In the past, teaching occurred the evening before surgery when clients were most anxious. But due to cost reduction efforts, many clients are admitted to the hospital or ambulatory surgery center on the day of surgery. Preoperative teaching done at this time may not be highly effective because of the client's high anxiety level.

Some clients undergoing surgery in ambulatory care settings prefer the inclusion of discharge information with preadmission teaching (Bernier and others, 2003). Many health care institutions have developed comprehensive outpatient client education programs to better enable clients to receive the knowledge and skills needed to participate in their own care before coming to the hospital or ambulatory care center. Teaching booklets and videotapes are often available to supplement any instruction a nurse provides.

Postoperative exercises include diaphragmatic breathing and effective coughing, turning, and leg exercises. The use of incentive spirometry to encourage voluntary deep breathing through an apparatus that provides visual feedback may also be included. The physician may order incentive spirometry for clients especially at risk for atelectasis or pneumonia (e.g., chronic smokers or clients on prolonged bed rest). During the discussion of these exercises, the nurse explains the relationship between the exercises and the physiological principles that make them important. Through specific explanations and guided practice the nurse helps develop client commitment to the recovery process. The nurse demonstrates the exercises and then continues to coach the client through several return practice sessions. Commitment to the exercise regimen is evidenced by the client's independent practice.

Whenever possible the nurse includes family members or other significant persons in the practice sessions. Frequently these individuals are with the client during the postoperative period and can thus serve as coaches. The nurse also provides clients with information about the sensations typically experienced after surgery, such as incisional pain, nausea, tightness of dressings, and what can be done to alleviate them. The information helps clients interpret realistically the events that occur in the postoperative period. As a result, clients are able to decrease anxiety, conserve their energies, and attend to performing the exercises that assist in their recovery.

A potential postoperative complication is deep vein thrombosis (DVT). One of the simplest ways to prevent the formation of DVT is to encourage and assist the client in early ambulation and leg exercises. When this is not possible or the client's age, past history, or surgical procedure place him or her at an increased risk, additional devices may be used to help prevent the formation of DVT. Compression stockings are frequently applied before surgery and remain on clients until they are fully ambulatory. Intermittent pneumatic compression devices are also frequently used on the surgical client (see Chapter 11). These devices compress the leg and increase venous flow thereby decreasing venous pooling and stasis. Another device used in the prevention of DVT is the venous plexus foot pump (Figure 35-3). This pump mimics the natural action of walking by intermittently compressing the sole of the foot and then relaxing it, so the venous plexus can fill with blood. Neither the intermittent pneumatic compression device nor the venous plexus foot pump should be used on clients with an acute DVT, significant peripheral vascular ischemia, large open wounds or skin grafts, or cancer of the extremity (Day, 2003). None of these devices should replace the need for early and frequent ambulation.

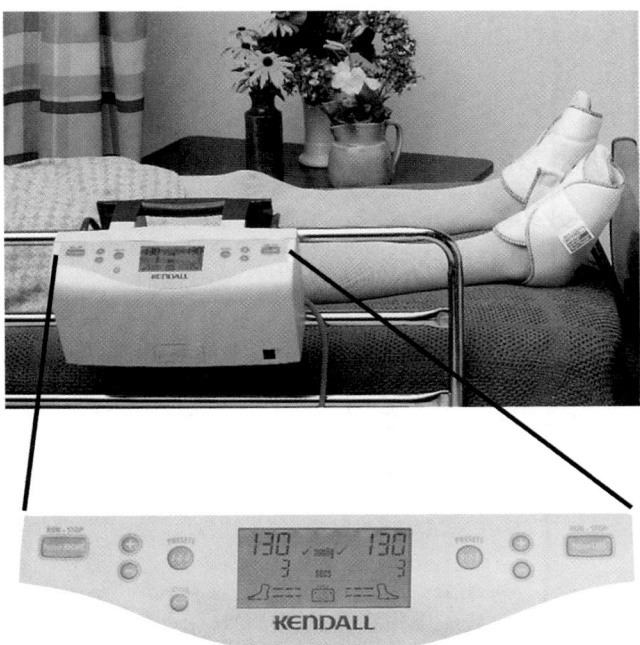

FIGURE **35-3** Venous plexus foot pump with bedside controls. (Courtesy Tyco Healthcare Group LP.)

DELEGATION CONSIDERATIONS

The teaching of postoperative exercises should not be delegated to assistive personnel. Assistive personnel can reinforce and assist clients in performing postoperative exercises. The nurse should instruct assistive personnel about:

* Any precautions unique to a particular client
* When to report if the client is unable or unwilling to perform the exercises correctly

EQUIPMENT

❑ Pillow (optional; used to splint the incision when coughing to reduce discomfort)
❑ Incentive spirometer

STEP	RATIONALE

ASSESSMENT

1. Assess client's risk for postoperative respiratory complications: identify presence of chronic pulmonary condition (e.g., emphysema, chronic bronchitis, asthma); any condition that affects chest wall movement, such as obesity, advanced pregnancy, thoracic or abdominal surgery; history of smoking; and presence of reduced hemoglobin level.

General anesthesia predisposes client to respiratory problems because lungs are not fully inflated during surgery, cough reflex is suppressed, and mucus collects within airway passages. Postoperatively, inadequate lung expansion can lead to atelectasis and pneumonia. Chronic lung conditions create greater risk for developing respiratory complications. Smoking damages ciliary clearance and increases mucus secretion. A reduced hemoglobin level can lead to reduced oxygen delivery.

* **Critical Decision Point**

Assess and report to physician and/or anesthesiologist if client has had a cold or upper respiratory infection within past week.

2. Auscultate lungs.
3. Assess client's ability to deep breathe and cough by placing hand on client's abdomen, having client take a deep breath, and observing movement of shoulders, chest wall, and abdomen. Observe chest excursion during a deep breath. Ask client to cough into tissue after taking a deep breath.

Establishes baseline for postoperative comparison.
Reveals maximum potential for chest expansion and ability to cough forcefully; serves as baseline to measure client's ability to perform exercises postoperatively. Diaphragmatic breathing allows for complete lung expansion and improved ventilation and increases blood oxygenation. Deep breathing also allows air to pass by partially obstructing mucous plugs, thus increasing force with which to expel mucous plug. Coughing loosens secretions and helps to remove them from pulmonary alveoli and bronchi.

4. Assess client's risk for postoperative thrombus formation (older adults, immobilized clients, clients with personal or family history of clots, and women over 35 who smoke and are taking birth control pills are most at risk). Observe the calves for redness, warmth, and tenderness. Palpate pedal pulses. Check for a Homans' sign, calf pain on dorsiflexion of the foot (which may or may not be present) (see Skill 18-5). Calf pain is usually unilateral. Compare legs for bilateral equality.

Following general anesthesia, circulation is slowed, causing a greater tendency for clot formation. Immobilization results in decreased muscular contraction in lower extremities, which promotes venous stasis. The physical stress of surgery creates a hypercoagulable state in most individuals. Manipulation and positioning during surgery may inadvertently cause trauma to leg veins.

* **Critical Decision Point**

A Homans' sign is not always present when a deep vein thrombosis exists (Maher and others, 2002). Checking for Homans' sign may be contraindicated in a suspected DVT because some researchers think that vigorous dorsiflexion may dislodge a thrombus. If a thrombus is suspected, notify physician and refrain from manipulating extremity any further. Surgery will usually be postponed. Antiembolism stockings or pneumatic compression cuffs may be ordered for clients at risk for thrombus formation (see Chapter 11).

STEP	RATIONALE
5. Assess client's ability to move independently while in bed.	Clients confined to bed rest, even for limited periods, will need to turn regularly. Determines existence of any mobility restrictions.
6. Assess client's willingness and capability to learn exercises; note factors such as attention span, anxiety level, level of consciousness, language skills, and level of pain, if any.	Capacity to learn depends on readiness, ability, and learning environment.

• *Critical Decision Point*
Highly anxious clients or those in severe pain have difficulty learning and performing postoperative exercises.

STEP	RATIONALE
7. Assess family members' or significant others' willingness to learn and to support client postoperatively.	Family's or significant other's presence postoperatively can be potential motivating factor for client's recovery; family member or significant other can coach clients on exercise performance.
8. Assess client's medical orders preoperatively and postoperatively.	May require adaptations in way exercises are performed.

NURSING DIAGNOSES

- Ineffective airway clearance
- Ineffective breathing pattern
- Impaired gas exchange
- Risk for infection
- Impaired memory

- Impaired physical mobility
- Acute pain
- Risk for impaired skin integrity
- Ineffective tissue perfusion

Related factors are individualized based on client's condition or needs.

PLANNING

1. Expected outcomes following completion of procedure:	
• Client is able to correctly deep breathe, use incentive spirometer, cough, turn, and perform leg exercises throughout postoperative period.	Client's ability to perform exercises should reduce risk of postoperative complications.
• Postoperatively, chest excursion meets or exceeds preoperative level.	Turning, deep breathing, and coughing exercises help client maintain full lung expansion and clear airways postoperatively.
• Lungs are clear to auscultation preoperatively and postoperatively.	Absence of secretions reduces risk for postoperative pneumonia.
• No redness, warmth, or tenderness in lower extremities, pedal pulses palpable.	Leg exercises prevent circulatory and mobility problems postoperatively.
• Client initiates exercises spontaneously.	Client values importance of exercises to recovery.
2. Prepare equipment as needed.	
3. Prepare room for teaching.	Quiet, private area free from distractions enhances client's ability to learn.

IMPLEMENTATION

1. **Teach Diaphragmatic Breathing**	
a. Assist client to comfortable semi-Fowler's or high-Fowler's position with knees flexed. If client chooses to sit, assist to side of bed or to upright position in chair. If client is sitting in a chair, knees should be at or higher than hips. Use stool if necessary.	Upright position facilitates diaphragmatic excursion by using gravity to keep abdominal contents away from diaphragm. Prevents tension on abdominal muscles, which allows for greater diaphragmatic excursion.

STEP	RATIONALE

• *Critical Decision Point*
Postoperatively client can usually be positioned upright with head of bed elevated. If client must remain flat in bed, stress that exercises can still be performed.

b. Stand or sit facing client.

Client will be able to observe breathing exercises performed by nurse.

c. Instruct client to place palms of hands across from each other along lower borders of anterior rib cage; place tips of third finger lightly together. Demonstrate for client (see illustration).

Position of hands allows client to feel movement of chest and abdomen as diaphragm descends and lungs inside chest wall expand.

d. Have client take slow, deep breaths, inhaling through nose, and pushing abdomen against hands. Tell client to feel middle fingers separate as client inhales. Explain that client will feel normal downward movement of diaphragm during inspiration. Explain that abdominal organs descend as chest wall expands. Demonstrate for client.

Slow, deep breath allows for more complete lung expansion than is ordinarily done and prevents panting or hyperventilation. Inhaling through nose warms, humidifies, and filters air. Explanation and demonstration focus on normal ventilatory movement of chest and abdominal wall. Client learns to understand how diaphragmatic breathing feels.

e. Avoid using chest and shoulder muscles while inhaling, and instruct client in same manner.

Using auxiliary chest and shoulder muscles during breathing increases unecessary energy expenditures and does not promote full lung expansion.

f. Take a slow, deep breath and hold for count of 3, and then slowly exhale through mouth as if blowing out a candle (pursed lips). Explain that client will feel middle fingertips touch as chest wall contracts (see illustration).

Allows for gradual, controlled expulsion of air.

g. Repeat breathing exercise three to five times.

Allows client to observe slow, rhythmic breathing pattern.

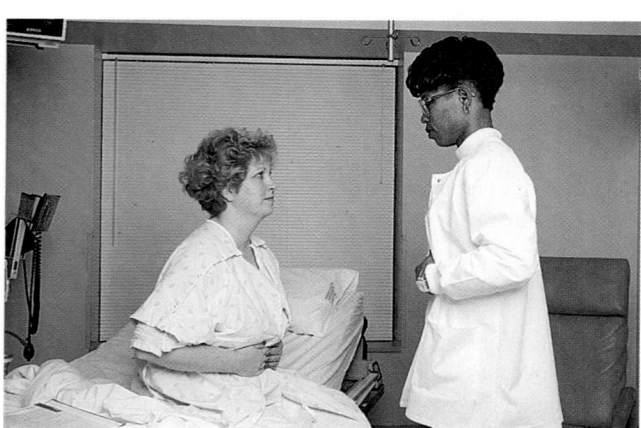

STEP 1c Client and nurse practice deep breathing.

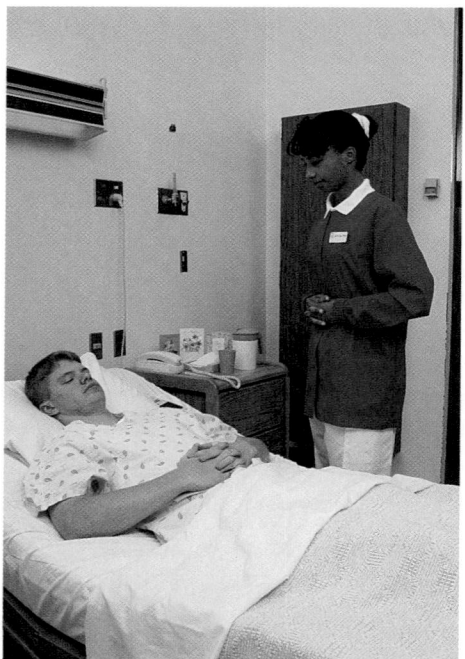

STEP 1f Deep breathing exercise—placement of hands on upper abdomen during inhalation. (From *Mosby's medical, nursing, and allied health dictionary,* ed 5, St. Louis, 1998, Mosby.)

STEP	RATIONALE

h. Have client practice exercise. Client is instructed to take 10 slow, deep breaths every 2 hours while awake during postoperative period until mobile. Another option is to have client use incentive spirometry (see illustration).

Repetition of exercise reinforces learning. Regular deep breathing will prevent or minimize postoperative respiratory complications. Incentive spirometer gives a visual incentive to breathe as deeply as possible.

2. **Teach Controlled Coughing**

a. Explain importance of maintaining an upright position.

Position facilitates diaphragm excursion and enhances thorax and abdominal expansion.

b. Demonstrate coughing. Take two slow, deep breaths, inhaling through nose and exhaling through pursed lips.

Deep breaths expand lungs fully so that air moves behind mucus and facilitates effective coughing.

c. Inhale deeply a third time, and hold breath to count of 3. Cough fully for two to three consecutive coughs without inhaling between coughs. (Tell client to push all air out of lungs.)

Consecutive coughs help remove mucus more effectively and completely than one forceful cough.

• *Critical Decision Point*
Coughing may be contraindicated after brain, spinal, or eye surgery due to an increase in intracranial pressure.

d. Caution client against just clearing throat instead of coughing deeply.

Clearing throat does not remove mucus from deeper airways.

e. If surgical incision is to be either thoracic or abdominal, teach client to place either hands or a pillow over incisional area and place hands over pillow to splint incision (see illustration). During breathing and coughing exercises, press gently against incisional area for splinting and support (see illustration).

Surgical incision cuts through muscles, tissues, and nerve endings. Deep breathing and coughing exercises place additional stress on suture line and cause discomfort. Splinting incision with hands or pillow provides firm support and reduces incisional pulling and pain.

f. Client continues to practice coughing exercises, splinting imaginary incision. The client is instructed to cough two to three times every 2 hours while awake.

Value of deep coughing with splinting is stressed to effectively expectorate mucus with minimal discomfort.

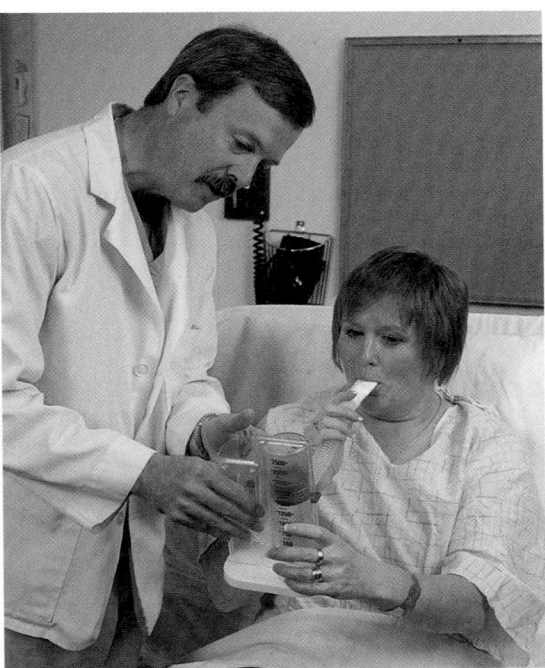

STEP **1h** Client demonstrates incentive spirometry.

STEP	RATIONALE

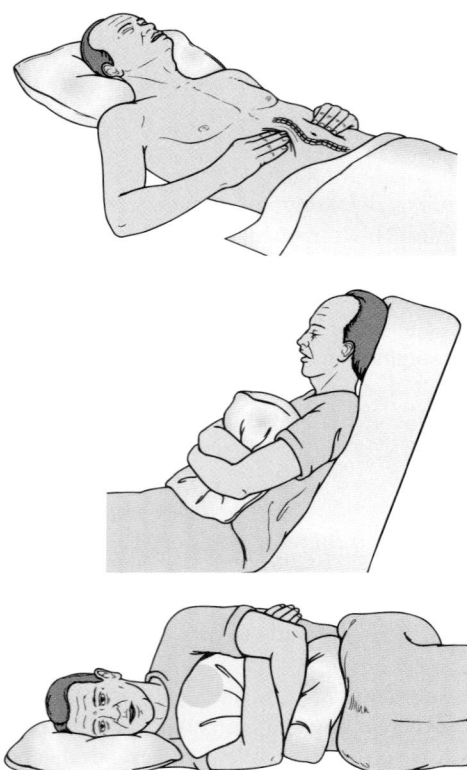

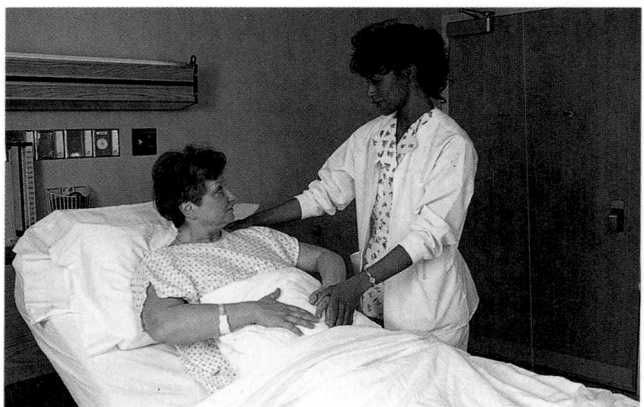

STEP **2e(2)** Client splinting abdomen with pillow.

STEP **2e(1)** Techniques for splinting incision when coughing or moving. (From Lewis S and others: *Medical-surgical nursing: assessment and management of clinical problems,* ed 6, St. Louis, 2004, Mosby.)

g. Instruct client to examine sputum for consistency, odor, amount, and color changes and to notify nurse if any changes are noted.

Sputum consistency, odor, amount, and color changes may indicate the presence of a pulmonary complication such as pneumonia.

• *Critical Decision Point*
For clients with preexisting pulmonary disease, know usual character of mucus to determine if change has occurred.

3. **Teach Turning** (*Example:* turning on right side)
    a. Instruct client to assume supine position and move toward left side of the bed. This is easily accomplished by bending knees and pressing heels against mattress to raise buttocks (see illustration).
    b. Have client place the right hand or a pillow over incisional area to splint it
    c. Instruct client to keep right leg straight and flex left knee up (see illustration).

Positioning begins in this example on left side of bed so that turning to right side will not cause client to roll off bed's edge. Buttocks lift prevents shearing force from body moving against sheets.

Splinting incision supports and minimizes pulling on suture line during turning.

Straight leg stabilizes the client's position. Flexed left leg shifts weight for easier turning.

STEP	**RATIONALE**

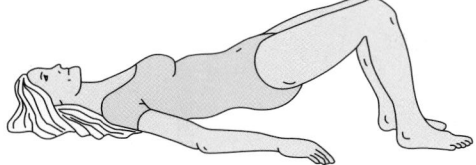

STEP **3a** Buttocks lift. (From Lowdermilk D and others: *Maternity nursing,* ed 5, St. Louis, 1999, Mosby.)

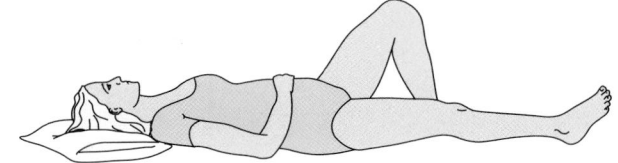

STEP **3c** Leg position when turning to the right. (From Lowdermilk D and others: *Maternity nursing,* ed 5, St. Louis, 1999, Mosby.)

• **Critical Decision Point**

Some clients, such as those who have had back surgery or vascular repair, may be restricted from flexing their legs postoperatively. Client may be restricted from turning or may need assistance for positioning (see Chapter 10).

d. Have client grab right side rail with left hand, pull toward right, and roll onto right side.	Pulling toward side rail reduces effort needed for turning.
e. Instruct client to turn every 2 hours from side to back to other side, while awake. If client is unable to perform above maneuver, note in chart that staff or primary caregiver must turn client every 2 hours. May need to place pillows behind client to help maintain side-lying position.	Reduces risk of vascular complications by contraction of leg muscles around veins to improve venous return. Also reduces pulmonary complications by shifting mucus to prevent consolidation.
4. Teach Leg Exercises	
a. Have client assume supine position in bed. Demonstrate leg exercises by performing passive range-of-motion exercises and simultaneously explaining exercise.	Provides for normal anatomical position of lower extremities and normal joint motion of each joint of lower extremities.

• **Critical Decision Point**

If client's surgery involves one or both lower extremities, surgeon must order leg exercises in postoperative period. Leg unaffected by surgery can be safely exercised unless client has preexisting phlebothrombosis (blood clot formation) or thrombophlebitis (inflammation of vein wall).

b. Rotate each ankle in complete circle. Instruct client to draw imaginary circles with big toe (see illustration). Repeat five times.	Ankle circle exercises maintain joint mobility and promote venous return.
c. Alternate dorsiflexion and plantar flexion by moving both feet, pointing toes up toward head and then down toward end of mattress. Direct client to feel calf muscles contract and relax alternately (see illustration). Repeat five times.	Calf pumping stretches and contracts gastrocnemius muscles, which enhances venous return.
d. Perform quadriceps setting by tightening thigh and bringing knee down toward mattress, then relaxing (see illustration). Repeat five times.	Quadriceps setting exercises contract muscles of upper legs and maintain knee mobility and improve venous return to the heart.
e. Client alternately raises each leg from bed surface; client begins by keeping leg straight and then bends leg at hip and knee (see illustration). Repeat five times.	Leg raise promotes contraction and relaxation of quadriceps muscles and promotes hip and knee movements by keeping leg straight and bending hip and knee joints.

STEP	RATIONALE

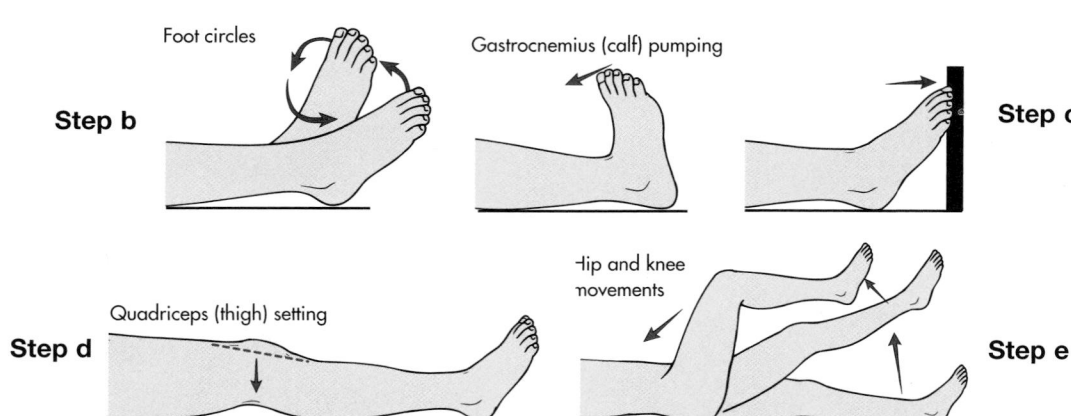

Step 4b-e Leg exercises. (From Lewis S and others: *Medical-surgical nursing: assessment and management of clinical problems,* ed 5, St. Louis, 2000, Mosby.)

• *Critical Decision Point*

If client is unable to perform exercises, note on Kardex that staff or primary caregiver must do passive range of motion to lower extremities every 2 hours while awake. Alternatively, notify surgeon, and request an order for pneumatic compression cuffs (see Chapter 11).

f. Have client continue to practice exercises at least every 2 hours while awake. Client is instructed to coordinate turning and leg exercises with diaphragmatic breathing, incentive spirometry, and coughing exercises.

Repetition of exercise sequence reinforces learning. Establishes routine for exercises that develops habit for performance. Sequence of exercises should be leg exercises, turning, deep breathing, and coughing. Exercises before coughing should enhance ability to move secretions so that they may be expectorated.

EVALUATION

1. Observe client performing all four exercises independently.
2. Observe family members' or significant other's ability to coach client.
3. Evaluate client's chest excursion.
4. Auscultate client's lungs.
5. Check calves for redness, warmth, and tenderness. Assess pedal pulses.

Provides opportunity for practice and return demonstration of exercises. Ensures client has learned correct technique.

Family member or significant other can assist positively or interfere with correct technique.

Determines extent of lung expansion.

Breath sounds reveal if airways are clear.

Absent signs and normal pulses usually indicate that no venous thrombosis is present.

Recording and Reporting

• Record physical assessment findings in nurses' notes or flow sheet.
• Report and record any assessed complications and action taken.
• Record in nurses' notes which exercises have been demonstrated to client and whether or not client can perform exercises independently.
• Report any problem client has in practicing exercises to nurse assigned to client on next shift.

Unexpected Outcomes	Related Interventions
1. Client is unwilling to perform exercises due to incisional pain of thorax or abdomen (deep breathing and coughing, turning) or due to surgery in lower abdomen, groin, buttocks, or legs (leg exercises).	• Instruct client to ask for pain medication 30 minutes before performing postoperative exercises or use patient-controlled analgesia (PCA) immediately before exercising.
2. Client is unable to perform exercises correctly. Anxiety, and fatigue alter client's performance.	• Additional instruction is needed. • Client may benefit from stress reduction techniques.
3. Client develops pulmonary complications such as atelectasis postoperatively. Breaths are shallow; cough is ineffective.	• Notify physician. • Start oxygen as ordered, and increase frequency of coughing exercises.
4. Client develops circulatory complications such as venous stasis or thrombophlebitis postoperatively. Leg exercises are inadequate.	• Notify physician. • Place client on bed rest with affected leg elevated as ordered. • Continue to have client do exercises with unaffected leg.

Teaching Considerations

- Clients do better with combination of procedural explanations, skills teaching, and psychosocial support (Shuldham, 1999).
- Explain postoperative exercises to client and primary caregiver, including their importance to recovery and physiological benefits. Adults learn best when they understand how they will benefit from activity.

Pediatric Considerations

- Parents should encourage and allow children to move within limits posed by surgery.
- Adolescents should receive same preoperative instructions and teaching as adults to support their developmental stage. Adolescents are searching for identity, and treating them with respect will enhance their self-esteem and independence and should increase compliance.
- Young children's normal responses of crying and moving extremities will maintain lung expansion and peripheral circulation. Therefore teaching coughing, deep breathing, and leg exercises is not usually necessary for young children.
- Children need family members and/or nursing staff to assume coach's role of reminding and encouraging.

Gerontological Considerations

- Changes related to aging such as decreased vision, hearing, and short-term memory may affect teaching effectiveness. Shorter sessions with frequent reinforcement and use of teaching aids with large print may be necessary. Including family members or primary caregiver in teaching sessions is strongly encouraged. Take time to instruct client properly.
- Aging process decreases ventilatory capacity and increases risk for respiratory complications.
- Aging process decreases muscle mass, thus decreasing energy level and increasing risk of venous stasis.

Home Care Considerations

- Review coughing, deep breathing, abdominal splinting, relaxation, and leg exercises before admission to hospital or surgical clinic and after discharge.

SKILL 35-3 Performing Postoperative Care of the Surgical Client

Nursing care of the postoperative surgical client is divided into two phases: immediate recovery and postoperative convalescence. During both phases the nurse must make comprehensive and detailed assessments of the client's condition. The effects of anesthesia and the physiological stressors imposed by surgery can place the client at risk for a variety of physiological alterations. It is also important for the nurse to facilitate communication among all members of the health care team, the client, and the client's family or significant other.

The first phase of postoperative care takes place during the immediate recovery period. For hospitalized clients this extends from the time the client leaves the OR to the time the client has stabilized in the recovery room (RR), postanesthesia room (PAR), or postanesthesia care unit (PACU) and has been transferred to the nursing division. For an ambulatory surgical client, the first phase of recovery normally lasts 1 to 2 hours before discharge home. The first phase is the most critical postoperative phase for assessing aftereffects of anesthesia, airway clearance, cardiovascular complications, temperature control, and neurological function. The client's condition can change rapidly. The nurse in the recovery area must make timely, intelligent, and accurate assessments to select the most appropriate measures of care for the client.

Each hospital has its own policies for directing the process for recovering clients during the immediate postoperative period. Frequently, for example, clients undergoing cardiac or central vascular repair transfer from the OR to an intensive care unit (ICU). In this situation the client is not sent to the RR/PACU area. The conditions of these clients are potentially so unstable as to require the monitoring available only in an ICU.

The second phase of recovery is the postoperative convalescent period. This period extends from the time the client is discharged from the RR or PACU to the time the client is discharged from the hospital for inpatient clients. Outpatient surgical clients undergo convalescence at home. All clients who have undergone surgical procedures have similar postoperative needs. However, nursing care becomes very individualized and depends on the nature of the client's surgery, preexisting medical conditions, the onset of complications, and the speed of recovery. Not all surgical clients recover at the same rate. During the convalescent period the nurse begins preparation for discharge and actively includes client, family, and significant others in the process. The nurse promotes the client's independence, educates the client and/or family about any limitations imposed by surgery, and provides resources needed for the client to assume an improved state of wellness.

DELEGATION CONSIDERATIONS

The skill of initiating and managing postoperative care of the client should not be delegated to assistive personnel. Assistive personnel may obtain vital signs and provide comfort and hygiene measures. Before delegating these measures the nurse must:

- Instruct assistive personnel to report specific changes in client's vital signs, behavior, or level of consciousness

EQUIPMENT

Phase 1: Immediate Recovery Period

❑ Stethoscope, sphygmomanometer, or automatic blood pressure machine
❑ Thermometer
❑ Pulse oximeter and monitor
❑ IV fluid poles/infusion pump(s) and IV fluids ordered
❑ Emesis basin
❑ Oxygen equipment such as mask, nasal cannula, tubing, and oxygen regulator
❑ Continuous suction equipment (to suction airway)
❑ Intermittent suction (for nasogastric [NG] tube suction if ordered) and irrigation supplies (irrigation set up, normal saline, pH paper)

❑ Dressing supplies
❑ Warmed blankets
❑ Graduated container for measuring output
❑ Additional equipment for physical assessment as ordered

Phase 2: Postoperative Convalescent Period

❑ Stethoscope, sphygmomanometer, thermometer
❑ IV fluid poles and IV fluids ordered
❑ Intermittent external pneumatic compression equipment (if ordered)
❑ Emesis basin
❑ Washcloth and towel
❑ Waterproof pads
❑ Equipment for oral hygiene
❑ Pillows
❑ Facial tissue
❑ Oxygen equipment (if ordered)
❑ Continuous suction equipment (for airway suction and wound drainage systems if ordered)
❑ Intermittent suction (for NG suction if ordered) and irrigation supplies (irrigation set up, normal saline, pH paper)
❑ Dressing supplies
❑ Orthopedic appliances (if skeletal traction ordered)
❑ Graduated containers for measuring output

STEP	RATIONALE

ASSESSMENT

PHASE 1: IMMEDIATE RECOVERY PERIOD

1. Receive report from circulating nurse, including procedure performed, range of vital signs, any complications, estimated blood loss (EBL), other fluid loss, fluid replacement, type of anesthesia, medications given, type of airway and size, extent of surgical wound, and any preoperative medical and/or nursing diagnoses.

Determines client's general status and allows nurse to anticipate need for special equipment, nursing care, and activities in RR/PACU.

• *Critical Decision Point*

Client's usual first complaint is of pain. Know how much sedative and/or analgesic have already been given and how long ago.

2. Upon client's arrival in RR/PACU, obtain report from surgeon and anesthesia provider.

Review provides detailed analysis of client's physiological status, allowing nurse to make appropriate observations and interventions. Provides baseline data to determine any change in condition.

3. Consider type of surgery client underwent, restrictions to movement, and type of anesthesia used.

Influences type of assessments nurse initiates, type of complications to observe for, and specific nursing interventions needed.

4. After receiving report, perform a thorough client assessment, including vital signs, pulse oximetry, and respiratory, cardiac, neurological, GI, genitourinary (GU), and fluid status. Monitor client's temperature, surgical site and drains, skin integrity, comfort, safety, and anxiety level.

Provides baseline for further postoperative evaluations. Identifies priority nursing interventions.

• *Critical Decision Point*

Be sure to turn client on side (when possible) to observe underlying skin and accumulation of blood or serous drainage not visible otherwise.

PHASE 2: CONVALESCENT PERIOD

1. Obtain phone report from nurse in RR/PACU.

Preliminary report allows nurse to prepare hospital room with necessary supplies and equipment for client's special needs.

2. Upon client's arrival at division, collect more detailed report from nurse accompanying client.

Detailed report helps nurse plan appropriate assessment and nursing care measures. Data provide baseline to detect any change in client's condition.

3. Review client's chart for information pertaining to type of surgery, complications, medications administered, preoperative medical risks, baseline vital signs, and client's usual medications given/not given preoperatively.

Nature of surgery, intraoperative complications, and presence of medical risks dictate complications for which to observe. Vital signs provide means to measure postoperative changes. List of client's usual medications may necessitate a call to physician for orders concerning timing and dose of drugs not given preoperatively.

4. Review postoperative orders.

Offers additional guidelines for type of care to provide.

5. Assess client's knowledge and expectations of surgical recovery.

Client will be better prepared to participate in care.

STEP	RATIONALE

■ NURSING DIAGNOSES

- Ineffective airway clearance
- Risk for aspiration
- Disturbed body image
- Ineffective breathing pattern
- Impaired verbal communication
- Acute confusion
- Deficient fluid volume
- Excess fluid volume
- Impaired gas exchange
- Deficient knowledge regarding postoperative care

- Impaired physical mobility
- Acute pain
- Ineffective protection
- Disturbed sensory perception: visual, auditory
- Impaired skin integrity
- Impaired swallowing
- Ineffective thermoregulation
- Ineffective tissue perfusion
- Urinary retention
- Impaired spontaneous ventilation

Related factors are individualized based on client's condition or needs.

■ PLANNING

1. Expected outcomes following completion of procedure:

   - Client's vital signs, including oxygen saturation, remain within previous baseline or normal expected range.

     No occurrence of cardiovascular, pulmonary, or thermoregulatory changes except those expected from effects of anesthetic or analgesic.

   - Client reports relief of discomfort after analgesic or other pain relief measures.

     Pain relief measures effectively alter client's reception or perception of pain.

   - Surgical wound remains intact without redness, edema, ecchymosis, or discharge. If opaque dressing covers incision, dressing remains dry and intact.

     Indicates wound healing without signs of bleeding or infection.

   - Breath sounds remain clear to auscultation; mucus is clear.

     Postoperative exercises and activity promote lung expansion and alveolar stability.

   - Normal bowel sounds present within 48 to 72 hours after bowel or abdominal surgery and/or general anesthetic. Normal bowel sounds are heard within 24 hours in cases of minor surgery.

     Indicates return of intestinal peristalsis.

   - Intake and output remain relatively in balance.

     Adequate urinary elimination maintained. Fluid intake (IV and/or by mouth [PO]) adequately maintained.

   - Legs remain without signs and symptoms of thrombophlebitis.

     Postoperative leg exercises and early ambulation minimize venous stasis and clot formation.

   - Client is able to discuss recovery and discharge plans. Verbalizes no specific physical complaints.

     Client coping with physical and psychological stress of surgery.

2. Prepare the equipment as necessary at bedside, and test equipment for function.

   Prepared for use if needed.

3. Explain to client all procedures you are to perform and rationale for each. On nursing division include family members and/or significant other in explanations. In ambulatory surgery centers, families are allowed at the bedside during recovery period.

   Involves client in plan of care and minimizes anxiety. As recovery progresses, client is able to make more choices regarding how procedures should be performed. Family can serve as coach and can help client remember explanations given.

■ IMPLEMENTATION

PHASE 1: IMMEDIATE RECOVERY PERIOD

1. Perform hand hygiene.

   Reduces transmission of microorganisms.

2. Check equipment setup in cubicle of RR/PACU.

   All equipment must be operational and ready to use on client's arrival.

STEP	**RATIONALE**
3. As client enters RR/PACU on stretcher, immediately attach oxygen tubing to regulator, hang IV fluids, check IV flow rates, and attach pulse oximeter (see Skill 17-6). Connect any drainage tubes to gravity drainage, continuous or intermittent suction as ordered. Attach cardiac monitor. Ensure indwelling catheter and bag are in drainage position and patent.	Maintaining oxygenation and circulation are two priorities. Inhaled oxygen improves percentage delivered to alveoli. Pulse oximeter provides information on arterial oxygen saturation. IV fluids maintain circulatory volume and provide route for emergency drugs. Drainage tubes must remain patent and in proper position to allow fluid to drain.
4. Conduct complete assessment of all vital signs. Compare findings with client's normal baseline. Continue assessing vital signs at least every 15 minutes until client stabilizes. Provide warm blankets as needed for client comfort.	Vital signs can reveal onset of postoperative complications, for example, respiratory depression, hypothermia or hyperthermia, pulse irregularity, or hypotension. Respiratory depression can result from anesthetics. Hypotension can result from anesthetics or acute blood loss. Acute blood loss may lead to hypovolemic shock with signs of reduced blood pressure, elevated heart and respiratory rates, pale skin, and restlessness. General anesthetic may affect temperature-regulating center, and lower metabolic rate causes hypothermia. Malignant hyperthermia is a rare inherited condition that develops after receiving an anesthetic and is a medical emergency (AORN, 2003a).

• *Critical Decision Point*

If client underwent a short procedure under procedural sedation, check agency policy for sedation recovery guidelines. The RN monitoring a client who receives procedural sedation/ analgesia should have no other responsibilities that would compromise continuous client monitoring (AORN, 2003b). Oxygenation should be monitored periodically until clients are no longer at risk for hypoxemia. Ventilation and circulation should be monitored at regular intervals until clients are suitable for discharge. Discharge criteria should be designed to minimize the risk of central nervous system or cardiorespiratory depression following discharge from observation by trained personnel (American Society of Anesthesiologists, 2002).

5. Maintain patent airway:	
a. Position client on side with head facing down and neck slightly extended (see illustration). Never position client with hands over chest (reduces chest expansion).	Extension prevents occlusion of airway at pharynx. Downward position of head moves tongue forward, and mucus or vomitus can drain out of mouth, preventing aspiration.
b. Place small folded towel under client's head. If client is restricted to supine position, elevate head of bed approximately 10 to 15 degrees, extend neck, and turn head to side. Have emesis basin available if client becomes nauseated.	Supports head in extended position. Prevents aspiration if client should vomit.
c. Clients with spinal anesthetic should be positioned supine, without elevation of head, for up to 24 hours. Fluids should be encouraged.	To prevent spinal headache from loss of cerebrospinal fluid. Increased IV or PO fluids aids body in replacing cerebrospinal fluid.

• *Critical Decision Point*

If client is not able to hyperextend neck, turn head to side if possible; suction oropharynx (see Chapter 24) frequently.

d. Encourage client to deep breathe and cough on awakening.	Promotes lung expansion and expectoration of mucous secretions
e. Suction artificial airway and oral cavity as secretions accumulate.	Clears airway of secretions.

STEP	RATIONALE

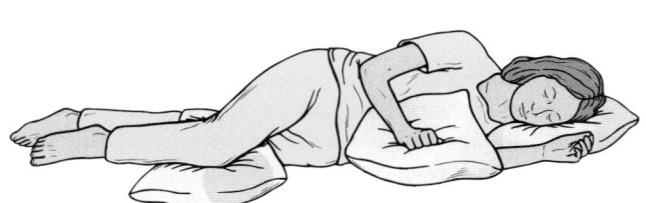

STEP **5a** Position of client during recovery from general anesthesia. (From Lewis S and others: *Medical-surgical nursing: assessment and management of clinical problems,* ed 6, St. Louis, 2004, Mosby.)

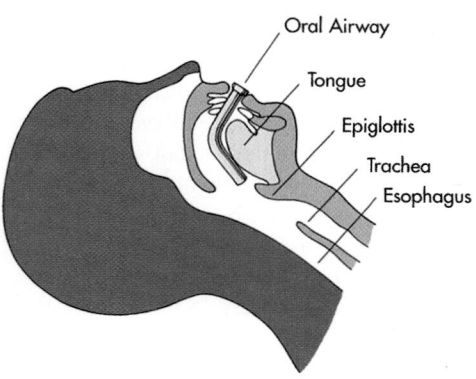

Oral Airway
Tongue
Epiglottis
Trachea
Esophagus

STEP **5f** Oral airway position before removal.

f. Once gag reflex returns, client spits out oral airway (see illustration). Do not tape oral airway.

Indicates client can clear airway independently. If airway is taped, client will gag and may obstruct airway.

• Critical Decision Point
Due to shorter half-life of drugs used today, many clients have oral airway removed before leaving OR. PACU nurse must assess that respiratory effort is adequate; otherwise airway may need to be replaced, and client may need a ventilator.

6. Call client by name in moderate tone of voice. If there is no response, attempt to arouse client by touching or gently moving a body part. Explain that client is in RR/PACU.

Determines client's level of consciousness and ability to follow commands.

7. Assess circulatory perfusion by inspecting color of nail beds, mucous membranes, and skin. Palpate for skin temperature. Test for capillary refill.

Pink or normal color of skin, nail beds, and mucous membranes and brisk (less than or equal to 3 seconds) capillary refill indicate adequate perfusion. Warm extremities reveal adequate circulation.

8. Observe condition of dressing and drains for any evidence of bright red blood. Also look underneath client for any pooling of bloody drainage.

Hemorrhage from surgical wound usually occurs within first few hours, indicating that a blood vessel was incompletely tied or cauterized during surgery. When dressing becomes saturated, blood oozes down client's side and collects underneath client.

9. Inspect surgical area for swelling or discoloration. Note condition of surgical dressing, including amount, color, odor, and consistency of drainage. Mark dressing with circle around drainage using a black pen. Place time of marking and check area every 10 to 15 minutes, marking any changes and noting vital signs.

A progressive increase in or changes in characteristics of drainage warrants call to surgeon because it could indicate hemorrhage (Academy of Medical-Surgical Nurses, 2004). Determines extent of fluid loss and condition of underlying wound. Size, location, and depth of wound influence amount of drainage (see Chapter 38).

10. Reinforce pressure dressing, or change simple dressing as ordered and needed. Make observations of condition of incision, surrounding tissue, and amount and color of any drainage if incision is exposed or covered with transparent dressing.

Pressure dressing should not be removed because it helps to maintain hemostasis (termination of bleeding) and to absorb drainage. Changing dressings immediately postoperatively can disrupt wound edges and aggravate drainage. First dressing changes most often occur 24 hours postoperatively and are usually done by physician. Minor surgical wounds may not have dressings but simply skin closure or wounds may be covered with transparent dressing, which allows for observation of incision and surrounding tissue (Academy of Medical-Surgical Nurses, 2004).

STEP	RATIONALE

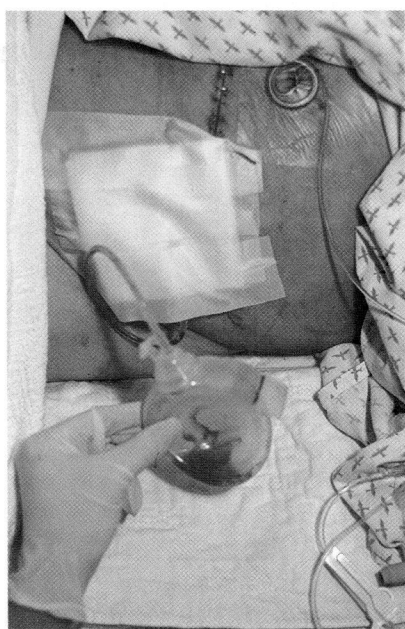

STEP 11 Jackson-Pratt drain charged (collapsed) and client's wound.

STEP	RATIONALE
11. Inspect condition and contents of any drainage tubes and collecting devices. Note character and volume of drainage (see illustration). See Chapter 37 for other types of drains and collection devices.	Determines drainage tube patency and extent and character of wound drainage.
12. Observe patency and intactness of urinary catheter system (if present). Note volume and character of urine.	Patent drainage system prevents bladder distention. Urine volume monitors renal function and perfusion. Decreased output (less than 30 ml/hour in an adult) is an early sign of hypovolemic shock.
13. If NG tube is present, validate correct placement, and irrigate periodically (see Chapter 33) with normal saline, if ordered.	Maintains patency of tube to ensure gastric decompression (removal of pressure caused by gas or liquid). Normal saline is isotonic and will not increase loss of fluid and electrolytes from stomach.
14. Continue monitoring of IV fluid rates. Observe IV site for signs of infiltration, such as swelling, edema, redness, warmth, discomfort, and leakage of IV fluid.	Continuous regular infusion of IV fluids maintains client's fluid intake to maintain adequate hydration and circulatory function.
15. As client awakens, provide mouth care by placing moistened washcloth to lips, swabbing oral mucosa with dampened swab, or applying petrolatum to lips. Sips of tap water and ice chips may also be ordered.	Client remains at risk for aspiration and should not be given fluids to rinse mouth. Moist cloth, swab, or sips of water and/or ice chips can be soothing to dry mucosa.
16. Assess level of pain as client awakens. Provide pain medication as ordered and when vital signs have stabilized (JCAHO, 2004).	Pain can increase the stress response and interfere with postoperative exercises. Pain medication can further depress vital signs if effect of anesthetic is still present. Client with spinal anesthesia is unable to feel sensation below level of spinal cord. Client will need pain medication as regional anesthetic wears off.

STEP	RATIONALE
17. Encourage client to practice ankle circles and calf-pumping exercises.	These leg exercises encourage venous return. If spinal or epidural anesthetic was used, leg exercises help effects of regional anesthetic to wear off once drug has been substantially metabolized by liver.
18. Explain to client how he or she is progressing and that plans for transfer to a nursing division are being made.	Helps client remain oriented to surroundings and recovery activities.
19. Once all physiological signs have stabilized, contact physician for order to release client to nursing division. Measure all intake and output (I&O) before transferring client to nursing division.	Physician is responsible for dictating level of observation and care required by client. Intake and output while in PACU is important baseline information to include in report to nurse in nursing division.

- **Critical Decision Point**
  If client is to be discharged to home, ensure that client has someone to drive him or her home and to observe client for signs and symptoms of complications. Review with client and driver reportable signs and symptoms and emergency care needed.

PHASE 2: CONVALESCENT PERIOD

1. Make final check of equipment setup in client's room, including emesis basin and waterproof pads. Be sure bed is placed in high horizontal position and to side so that stretcher can easily be moved beside bed.	During transfer, client's status may change, necessitating quick interventions upon arrival. Availability of equipment ensures smooth transfer process.
2. Upon arrival at client's room assist RR/PACU staff, and use three-person carry or slide board to transfer client to bed (see Chapter 10).	Technique avoids strain on nurses' back muscles and maintains client's safety.
3. Once client is transferred to bed, immediately attach any existing oxygen tubing, hang IV fluids, check IV flow rate, attach NG tube to suction, and place indwelling catheter in drainage position.	Maintains client's oxygenation, circulation, and elimination functions. Allows for frequent monitoring of I&O. Provides for client's comfort. Prevents potentially contaminated urine backflow into sterile bladder, thus decreasing incidence of bladder infections.
4. Conduct complete assessment of all vital signs. Compare findings with vital signs in recovery area and client's baseline values. Continue monitoring as ordered and as condition warrants (e.g., a typical order might read: VS q 15 min × 4, q 30 min × 2, q 1 hr × 4). A nurse should not assume that further monitoring is unnecessary if the client appears normal during the initial assessment.	Client should be stabilized once transferred to nursing division. Change in vital signs can reveal early onset of postoperative complications.

- **Critical Decision Point**
  Report to the anesthesiologist and/or physician any findings deviating from previous assessment.

5. Maintain client's airway:	
a. Position client on side (if allowed); if client remains sleepy or lethargic, keep head extended.	Positioning minimizes chances of aspiration.
b. Encourage deep breathing and coughing using pillow as an incisional splint every 1 to 2 hours.	Promotes lung expansion and expectoration of mucus.
6. Be sure any drainage tubes are connected to proper suction or drainage device. If NG tube is present, validate correct placement, and irrigate as ordered and connect to proper drainage device (see Chapter 33).	Maintains drainage tube patency so that wound beds remain dry for healing. Occlusion of NG tube can lead to abdominal distention, vomiting, and aspiration.

STEP	RATIONALE
7. Assess client's surgical dressing for intactness and presence and character of drainage. Reinforce as ordered. If no dressing present, inspect condition of wound (see Chapter 37).	Wound can hemorrhage quickly during early postoperative period. Observations of wound and dressings provide data to measure progress of wound healing.

• Critical Decision Point

If unable to change dressing, mark area of drainage, and label with time, date, and initials. Record frequency of reinforcement. Never use felt tip marker to mark dressing because ink can bleed into gauze, contaminating incision site.

8. Assess for bladder distention if client does not have indwelling catheter. Offer bedpan if client senses urge to void (see Chapter 32).	Anesthetics and analgesics depress sensation of bladder fullness. Client may still have no sensations below level of spinal or epidural anesthetic.

• Critical Decision Point

Initiate measures to stimulate voiding within 4 hours of surgery or removal of indwelling catheter to prevent urinary retention with overflow.

9. Measure and record all sources of fluid intake and output (IV, irrigation fluids, ice chips, PO fluids; Foley/ voided urine, NG drainage, wound drainage, and excessive perspiration) (see Chapter 18).	Assists in monitoring fluid and electrolyte balance.
10. Position client for comfort, maintaining airway and correct body alignment. Avoid positioning on surgical wound site or with pressure on popliteal space.	Good positioning reduces stress on suture line and decreases risks of aspiration and impaired circulation. Comfortable position helps client relax.
11. Encourage client to continue with leg exercises every 1 to 2 hours. If client is unable or unwilling to do them, nurse should do passive range of motion (see Chapter 11).	Leg exercises increase venous return, which decreases risk of thrombophlebitis. Range-of-motion exercises maintain joint mobility.
12. If ordered, apply elastic stockings or pneumatic compression cuffs to lower extremities, and attach to compressor (see Skill 11-3). Explain to client that compression cuffs will inflate and deflate intermittently.	Increases venous return. Explanation decreases anxiety and fosters cooperation.
13. Explain to client that you have completed all observations and that you will ask family members or significant other to enter room. Place bed in lowest position and call light within reach, and raise side rails.	Promotes client's orientation and sense of well-being. Lowest position minimizes injury should client become confused and try to get out of bed. Call light and side rail positioning ensure client's safety as effects of anesthetic continue to diminish.
14. Explain client's general status to family and/or significant other, describe purpose of any equipment in room, and explain reason for frequent observations and procedures.	Family and significant others are normally anxious to learn about client's status. Unfamiliar sights (equipment and client's appearance) can be anxiety provoking. Family's and significant other's understanding can promote their participation in client's care.

• Critical Decision Point

It can be helpful to give family simple tasks to perform, such as wiping client's face with washcloth and coaching postoperative exercises.

15. Refer to recovery record to determine if pain medication was administered. Always ask client to rate the severity of pain on an analog scale and to indicate the amount of analgesic he or she wants (JCAHO, 2004). Administer analgesic if vital signs remain stable, or initiate patient-controlled analgesia (PCA), if ordered (see Skill 6-2).	Pain relief is essential for client to be able to begin postoperative exercises. Client is best judge of his or her pain. Pain scale provides an objective measure for nurse to interpret client's progress.

STEP	RATIONALE
16. Provide oral hygiene, and repeat as needed.	Maintenance of moist mucous membranes facilitates expectoration of secretions and promotes comfort.
17. As client stabilizes over the next hours or days, perform the following measures:	
a. Have client participate in postoperative exercises.	Promotes pulmonary and circulatory function to minimize onset of postoperative complications.
b. Encourage use of incentive spirometer if ordered. Watch client use spirometer first few times to judge efficacy of breathing pattern. Chart level that client can achieve.	Promotes lung expansion. Can monitor progress and encourage client to inhale more deeply.
c. Begin activity orders. Assess vital signs first time client sits or stands to judge tolerance.	Early ambulation promotes circulation, lung expansion, and peristalsis. Sudden positional changes can cause postural hypotension.
d. Monitor bowel sounds every 4 to 8 hours. Must wait to have at least hypoactive bowel sounds before advancing diet beyond ice chips. Begin dietary orders slowly according to client's tolerance. Medicate with antiemetic if client is nauseated. Give analgesic with antiemetic until client is eating well.	Promotes normal fluid and electrolyte balance, restores nutritional intake, and promotes normal GI function and wound healing. Analgesics often cause nausea on an empty stomach.
e. Assist client in assuming normal urinary voiding pattern (see Chapter 32). Male clients may need assistance to stand to void. Female clients may need to sit on bedpan in bed or chair so legs can be bent and dangling or helped to bathroom.	Promotes normal urinary elimination and prevents bladder distention and urinary retention with overflow. A more natural position may help client to void.

• Critical Decision Point
If client does not void within 8 hours after surgery or bladder becomes distended, notify physician. Urinary catheter may have to be inserted.

f. Closely monitor progress of wound healing, and change dressings as ordered.	Wound infection occurs most often within 3 to 6 days postoperatively. Wound dehiscence occurs most often 3 to 11 days postoperatively.

• Critical Decision Point
Delayed wound healing may result in wound dehiscence or evisceration. This occurs most frequently after coughing, sneezing, vomiting, or getting up from a sitting position. Caution should be observed when client performs these activities. Remind client to use pillow to splint incision during these activities. Evisceration is a medical emergency (see Chapter 38).

g. Monitor and maintain wound drainage devices, such as Jackson-Pratt, Hemovac, or Penrose drains. Jackson-Pratt and Hemovac drainage systems must be emptied whenever they are half full of drainage or air and be recharged (compressed to discharge air) (see illustration).	Wound drainage devices promote healing from inside to outside and relieve pressure on suture line. Compressing a flexible closed container and then plugging drainage hole creates negative suction pressure.
h. Monitor drainage for color, consistency, and amount every 4 to 8 hours. Compare to previous assessment.	Drainage should progress from sanguineous to serosanguineous to serous in color, become more watery, and decrease in amount as wound heals.
18. Gradually increase client's involvement in decision making and in any explanations about surgery and related implications.	Promotes client's sense of control and independence. Encourages feeling of self-esteem.

STEP	**RATIONALE**

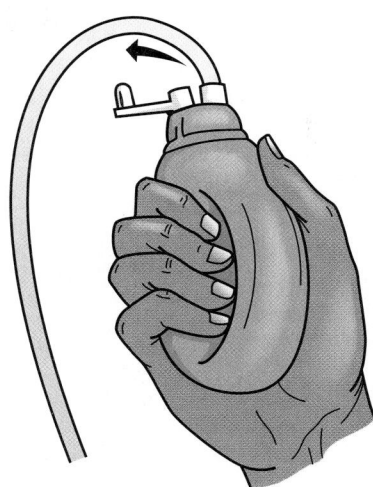

STEP **17g** Charging a Jackson-Pratt drainage system.

19. Teach client and family signs and symptoms of complications such as infection, dehiscence, excessive bleeding, and need for nutrition for wound healing and techniques of wound care if needed.	Early discharge necessitates client and family involvement because complications often occur after client goes home.
20. Discuss with client and family or significant other plans for discharge.	Allows nurse to anticipate client's needs in home setting and discuss any problems that might arise.
21. Prepare to make referral for home care or convalescent care as client's condition dictates. Get order from physician.	If client continues to need nursing care or rehabilitation after discharge, physician's order is necessary. Referral provides continuity of care.

EVALUATION

1. Compare all vital sign assessment measurements with client's baseline and expected normals.	Allows nurse to evaluate client's respiratory, cardiovascular, and thermoregulatory status throughout recovery.
2. Evaluate effects of pain-relief measures, such as positioning, and use of analgesics.	Determines level of comfort achieved and effectiveness of pain-relief measures.
3. Monitor changes in surgical wound at least every shift.	Provides data for nurse to measure progress of wound healing.
4. Monitor lung sounds following postoperative exercises.	Determines status of airways.
5. Auscultate bowel sounds at least each shift.	Allows nurse to evaluate return of peristalsis and diet tolerance.
6. Monitor intake and output balance for each shift.	Can indicate onset of fluid imbalances.
7. Discuss with client general level of comfort and progress toward recovery.	Gives client sense of participation in care. Client's perceptions can also be helpful in noting onset of complications. Reveals readiness to learn about discharge.
8. Conduct physical assessments appropriate for client's unique type of surgery.	Allows nurse to monitor course of recovery.

Recording and Reporting

- Document client's arrival in RR/PACU or nursing division; record vital signs, assessment findings, and all nursing measures initiated in nurses' notes. Continue documentation every 15 minutes until stable, then every 30 minutes times 2, every hour times 4, then every 4 to 8 hours as condition warrants.
- Record vital signs and I&O on appropriate flow sheets.
- Report any abnormal assessment findings and signs of complications to nurse in charge and/or physician.

Unexpected Outcomes	Related Interventions
1. Vital signs are above or below client's baseline or expected range.	• Alterations may result from anesthetic effects. Ensure client is fully awake from anesthesia before giving large doses of narcotics. Ensure client's family does not medicate client with PCA. Monitor geriatric client closely for opiate sensitivity—client may require use of opiate antagonist such as Narcan in presence of bradypnea. • Medicate for pain as indicated; titrate analgesics to maximize pain relief; assess client's use of and understanding of PCA device. • Notify physician for symptoms of internal bleeding or shock such as hypotension or tachycardia.
2. Client continues to experience incisional pain. Analgesic dosage may be insufficient.	• Initiate different nonpharmacologic relief measures. • Call physician for additional analgesic orders.
3. Abnormal or absent breath sounds are auscultated. This may be due to bronchial constriction or mucus secretions in large airways immediately postoperatively or result of atelectasis a day or more later.	• Notify physician, and request order for incentive spirometer, if not already ordered. • Encourage client to turn, deep breathe, and cough more often. • Investigate history of asthma or allergic response to medication when wheezing or stridor is auscultated.
4. Client complains of calf tenderness and warmth; may exhibit positive Homans' sign, redness, and edema in lower extremity.	• These are signs and symptoms of venous thrombosis or thrombophlebitis. Notify physician, and anticipate orders for bed rest, leg elevation, and initiation of anticoagulation (e.g., heparin intravenous drip). • Do not massage affected leg. • Continue to have client do leg exercises with unaffected leg.
5. Bowel sounds are absent or decreased.	• Paralytic ileus can develop as common complication after bowel or abdominal surgery. Intestinal motility may return slowly depending on anesthetic effects. • Keep IV in place. • Encourage turning and ambulation. • Assess for bowel sounds and flatus every 4 hours. • Report findings to physician.
6. Client develops fever, tenderness, and pain at wound site; increased white blood cell count or purulent drainage is present.	• These are signs and symptoms of wound infection. Notify physician, and anticipate orders for culture of wound drainage and IV antibiotics.

Unexpected Outcomes	Related Interventions
7. Client reports feeling something in wound "give way." Increased serosanguineous drainage is noted.	• May indicate wound dehiscence or evisceration. Report wound dehiscence and/or evisceration to surgeon immediately because it could be life threatening. • If evisceration has occurred, cover abdominal contents with sterile gauze saturated with sterile normal saline, and prepare client for emergency surgery.
8. Intake and output measurements reflect imbalance.	• Indicates possible fluid volume excess or deficit. Continue to monitor strict I&O, and contact physician if 24-hour totals continue to reflect imbalance.
9. Client is unable to discuss discharge plans or has negative view of recovery.	• May indicate client is coping poorly with stress of surgery. Discuss discharge plans and instructions with significant family member or friend. • Encourage client to express fears and concerns. • Refer client to support group if appropriate. • Notify physician, and request referral for counseling if necessary.

Teaching Considerations

- If client had spinal or epidural anesthetic, remind family or significant other that loss of extremity movement is normal for several hours.
- Reinforce preoperative teaching regarding coughing, deep breathing, and leg exercises and information concerning ambulation and pain control.
- Instruct client and primary caregiver to identify signs and symptoms and appropriate actions to take for infection, respiratory, circulatory, or GI difficulties and wound disruptions.
- Provide important phone numbers to client and primary caregiver for use in event of emergency and for follow-up care on discharge.
- Teach client about appropriate wound care, diet recommendations, and activity restrictions.
  Client Teaching for Ambulatory Surgical Clients
- Physician's office telephone number (24-hour answer)
- Surgery center's telephone number
- Follow-up appointment, date, time
- Review of prescribed medications
- Guidelines related to specific surgery
- Dressing and wound care
- Activity restrictions
- Guidelines related to anesthesia
- Dietary restrictions
- Activity restrictions
- Warning signs of complications

Pediatric Considerations

- Parent-child separation should be kept to minimum time possible. When a parent cannot be present, it is important to leave a favorite possession with child.

- Nurse must be alert for allergic responses and signs and symptoms of malignant hyperthermia in children who have not been exposed to drugs or anesthetic agents. Family history of allergies makes child at high risk for experiencing similar reactions.
- Vomiting is a major concern in young children due to increased risk of fluid and electrolyte imbalances and risk of aspiration. Vomiting is also more likely because surgery in children is often necessitated by accidental injuries without benefit of NPO status.
- Mandatory fluid intake guidelines are not usually necessary because of aggressive fluid replacement in children.
- Voiding before discharge from ambulatory surgery is not usually required for young children.
- Undermedicating young children may be based on myth that narcotics are more dangerous for infants. The fact is that "by 3-6 months of age, healthy infants can metabolize opioids similarly to older children" (Hockenberry, 2005). Observing the normalizing of vital signs and behavior after administration of analgesics is a valuable clue that pain really existed before treatment (Hockenberry, 2005).

Gerontological Considerations

- The ability of older adults to tolerate surgery depends on extent of physiological changes that have occurred with aging, presence of any chronic diseases, and duration of surgical procedure.
- Undermedicating older adults is common. Asking clients to rate their pain before and after administration of analgesics and asking what numerical rating is acceptable to them are better methods of individualizing care.

Home Care Considerations

- Teach primary caregiver about any postoperative exercises, home modifications, or activity limitations.
- If client is discharged with dressing changes, bedroom or bathroom is usually an ideal location for procedure. Have primary caregiver perform return demonstration of dressing change.

FOCUS on CLINICAL PRACTICE

You are assigned to care for Mrs. Edmonds, an obese 42-year-old attorney. She is a same-day surgery admit and is to undergo an abdominal hysterectomy for fibroid tumors and a bladder neck suspension. Her past medical history includes 2-packs-per-day cigarette smoking and birth control pills for 20 years.

1. What constitutes informed consent? Who may obtain informed consent?

2. When should Mrs. Edmonds receive her preoperative antibiotic prophylaxis?
3. What topics should be included in Mrs. Edmonds' preoperative teaching?
4. What postoperative complication is Mrs. Edmonds at risk for developing? Give rationale.
5. Before performing postoperative exercises, what should the client be instructed to do?

NCLEX REVIEW QUESTIONS

1. Informed consent must include which of the following?
   1. An explanation of the risks of having the procedure
   2. The exact time needed to perform procedure
   3. The names of the scrub and circulating nurses
   4. A written advance directive
2. Which of the following is true regarding "do not resuscitate" (DNR) orders?
   1. DNR orders should remain in effect throughout all stages of surgical procedures.
   2. DNR orders should automatically be suspended during and immediately following surgical procedures.
   3. Physicians should discuss and document issues with the client and/or family to determine whether DNR orders are to be maintained or modified during surgical procedures.
   4. Clients with DNR orders typically are not candidates for surgical procedures.
3. Prophylactic antibiotics should be administered:
   1. Within 30 minutes of incision
   2. Within 90 minutes of incision

   3. Within 2 hours of incision
   4. Within 4 hours of incision
4. Which intervention is used to prevent DVT?
   1. Maintaining bed rest for 8 to 12 hours after surgery
   2. Turning from side to side every 4 hours
   3. Applying an intermittent pneumatic compression device
   4. Performing a Homans' assessment every 8 hours
5. Which client condition contributes least risk for postoperative respiratory complications?
   1. Asthma
   2. Crohn's disease
   3. Advanced pregnancy
   4. Decreased hemoglobin level
6. Which symptom might support a suspicion of deep vein thrombosis?
   1. Positive Homans' sign
   2. Bilateral edema to lower extremities
   3. Absence of pedal pulse to the affected leg
   4. Lack of hair growth to lower extremities

NCLEX REVIEW QUESTIONS

7. A 67-year-old woman was admitted from the PACU to the medical/surgical unit status post colectomy. Upon initial examination, a dime-sized amount of shadowing is noted on her dressing. Which intervention should be implemented next?
   1. Do nothing because this is an expected outcome for the postoperative client.
   2. Using a black pen, mark the dressing with a circle around the drainage.
   3. Remove the dressing to determine the exact amount of bleeding.
   4. Immediately notify the physician.

8. Immediately postoperatively, the postcolectomy client states she is thirsty. Which describes the best intervention?
   1. Explain to the client that she may not have anything to eat or drink until the return of peristalsis.
   2. Provide the client with mouth care only by swabbing oral mucosa with a dampened swab.
   3. Provide the client with a small cup of a clear liquid beverage.
   4. Increase her IV fluids to satisfy her thirst.

9. Which medical equipment would the nurse prepare for a postcolectomy client upon admission to the PACU?
   1. Ventilator
   2. Arterial line transducer
   3. Cardiac-respiratory monitor
   4. Cooling blanket

References

Academy of Medical-Surgical Nurses: *Core curriculum for medical-surgical nursing,* ed 3, Pitman NJ, 2004, The Academy.

American Hospital Association: *The patient care partnership,* Chicago, 2003, The Association.

American Society of Anesthesiologists: Practice guidelines for preoperative fasting and the use of pharmacologic agents to reduce the risk of pulmonary aspiration: application to health clients undergoing elective procedures: a report by the American Society of Anesthesiologists Task Force on Preoperative Fasting, *Anesthesiology* 90(3):896, 1999.

American Society of Anesthesiologists: practice guidelines for sedation and analgesia by non-anesthesiologists: an updated report by the American Society of Anesthesiologists Task Force on Sedation and Analgesia by Non-anesthesiologists, 2002, The Society.

Armstrong M: A clinical look at body piercing, *RN* 61(9):26, 1998.

Association of Operating Room Nurses: *Standards, Recommended practices and guidelines,* Denver, 2002a, The Association.

Association of Operating Room Nurses: recommended practices for skin preparation of patients, *AORN J* 75(1):184, 2002b.

Association of Operating Room Nurses: *Standards and recommended practices for perioperative nursing: malignant hyperthermia guideline,* Denver, 2003a, The Association.

Associate of Operating Room Nurses: *Standards and recommended practices for perioperative nursing: managing the patient receiving moderate sedation/analgesia,* Denver, 2003b, The Association.

Association of Operating Room Nurses: *Standards and recommended practices for perioperative nursing: perioperative care of patients with do-not-resuscitate (DNR) orders,* Denver, 2003c, The Association.

Centers for Disease Control and Prevention: *Guidelines for prevention of surgical site infections,* Atlanta, 1999, Hospital Infection Control Programs, US Department of Health and Human Services.

D'Avanzo C, Geissler E: *Pocket guide to cultural assessment,* ed 3, St. Louis, 2003, Mosby.

Day M: Recognizing and managing deep vein thrombosis, *Nursing* 33(5):36, 2003.

Dunn D: Preoperative assessment criteria and patient teaching for ambulatory surgery patients, *J Perianesth Nurs* 13(5):274, 1998.

Fennell MD: Parents in, you bet! *RN* 62(12):38, 1999.

Hockenberry M: *Wong's essentials of pediatric nursing,* ed 7, St. Louis, 2005.

Joint Commission on Accreditation of Healthcare Organizations: *Accreditation manual for hospitals,* Chicago, 2004, The Commission.

Lewis S and others: *Medical-surgical nursing, assessment and management of clinical problems,* ed 6, St. Louis, 2004, Mosby.

Lowdermilk D, Perry S: *Maternity nursing,* ed 6, St. Louis, 2003, Mosby.

Maher A and others: *Orthopaedic nursing,* ed 3, Philadelphia, 2002, Saunders.

Mosby's medical, nursing, and allied health dictionary, ed 5, St. Louis, 2002, Mosby.

Nichols R: Preventing surgical site infections: a surgeon's perspective, *Emerg Infect Dis* 7(2):2001.

Pacquiao DF: Cultural competence in ethical decision-making. In Andrews B, Boyle J: *Transcultural concepts in nursing care,* Philadelphia, 2003, Lippincott.

Singh P: *The Sikhs,* New York, 2000, Random House.

Research References

Bernier M and others: Preoperative teaching received and valued in a day surgery setting, *AORN J* 77(3):563, 2003.

Centers for Disease Control and Prevention: *National surgical infection prevention: Medicare quality improvement project—evidence base for duration of antimicrobial prophylaxis*, Aug 12, Atlanta, 2003, Centers for Disease Prevention and Control.

Hathaway D: Effect of preoperative instruction on postoperative outcomes: a meta-analysis, *Nurs Res* 35(5):269, 1986.

Mangram A and others: Guideline for prevention of surgical site infection, 1999, *Infect Control Hosp Epidemiol* 20(4):247, 1999.

Oetker-Black SL and others: Preoperative teaching and hysterectomy outcomes, *AORN J* 77(6):1215, 2003.

Shuldham C: A review of the impact of pre-operative education on recovery from surgery, *Int J Nurs Stud* 36:171, 1999.

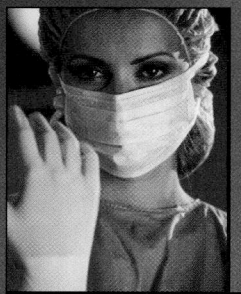

36

Intraoperative Care

MEDIA RESOURCES

Evolve Site *evolve*

http://evolve.elsevier.com/Perry/skills
- Weblinks
- Video clips
- Mosby's Nursing Skills Video Exercises

Mosby's Nursing Skills Videos/CD-ROM
- *Wound Care Video:* Sterile gloving, latex precautions

OBJECTIVES

Mastery of content in this chaper will enable the nurse to:

- Describe the meaning of a sterile conscience.
- Describe the roles of a registered nurse in the operating room.
- Identify guidelines for use of sterile technique in the operating room.
- Correctly perform surgical hand antisepsis.
- Correctly don a sterile surgical gown.
- Correctly apply sterile gloves using the closed technique.

KEY TERMS

Asepsis	Scrub nurse
Aseptic technique	Sponge
Circulating nurse	Sterile
Contamination	Sterile conscience
Perioperative	Sterile field
Registered nurse first assistant (RNFA)	Strike through
	Surgical scrub

The perioperative role of the nurse practicing in the operating room (OR) suite encompasses the client's surgical experience from the preoperative throughout the intraoperative period and into the postoperative phase (see Chapter 35). The standards of clinical practice that registered nurses follow within the OR are designed to provide an optimal level of care that ensures the client's safety and comfort (Association of Perioperative Registered Nurses [AORN, 2003b]). In addition, the nurse exercises judgment, critical thinking, and interpersonal communication skills in applying the nursing process to ensure clients receive appropriate nursing care during the perioperative experience.

Members of the surgical team may include the surgeon, registered nurse first assistant (RNFA), certified registered nurse anesthetist (CRNA) and/or anesthesiologist, circulating nurse and scrub nurse, or surgical technologist. The intraoperative phase begins when the client enters the OR suite and ends with admission to the postanesthesia care unit (PACU). During the intraoperative phase, the registered nurse assumes the role of either first assistant to the surgeon, scrub nurse, or circulating nurse. The RNFA is a nurse with advanced education (including a clinical practicum or internship) who assists the surgeon with the surgical procedure, performing a combination of nursing and medical functions and/or skills (Box 36-1). The scrub nurse (Box 36-2) provides the surgeon with instruments and supplies, disposes of soiled sponges, and accounts for sponges, needles, and instruments on the surgical field. Registered nurses, licensed practical nurses, or surgical technologists may assume the

BOX 36-1 Role and Responsibilities of a Registered Nurse First Assistant

The RNFA role is an expansion of the traditional perioperative nursing role and areas of responsibility will overlap. Responsibilities specific to the practice of first assisting include:
- Providing surgical exposure (assists in retraction of tissues and suctioning of surgical field)
- Providing hemostasis (control of bleeding)
- Handling tissue safely
- Using surgical instruments and suturing
- Performing wound closure
- Applying human anatomical and physiological considerations in practice; recognizes structure, function and location of tissues and organs; manipulates tissues accordingly to avoid injury

From Association of Operating Rooms Nurses: Revised AORN official statement of RN first assistants. In *AORN standards and recommended practices for perioperative nursing*, Denver, 2003, The Association.

BOX 36-2 Role of the Scrub Nurse

- Assists circulating nurse in preparing OR, opening supplies
- Performs surgical hand scrub and dons sterile gown and gloves
- Prepares sterile field with procedure-appropriate supplies and instruments, verifying all are in working order
- Performs sponge, sharp, and instrument counts with circulating nurse before incision is made, at the beginning of wound closure, and at the end of the surgical procedure
- Gowns and gloves surgeons and assistants as they enter the OR
- Assists surgeons with sterile draping of client
- Keeps sterile field orderly and monitors progress of procedure and any breaks in aseptic technique
- Passes sterile instruments and supplies to surgeons and assistants
- Handles surgical specimens per institutional policy
- Constantly monitors location of all sponges and sharps in the sterile field

scrub nurse role. The circulating nurse (Box 36-3) is always a registered nurse and is considered to be the charge nurse in the room (AORN, 2003a). The circulating nurse assumes responsibility and accountability for maintaining client safety and continuity of quality care. This includes supervising the conduct of the nonprofessional staff. The circulating nurse is also an assistant to the first assistant, scrub nurse, and surgeon.

It is essential that perioperative nurses fully understand and follow the principles of aseptic technique. The overall goal of asepsis is to minimize contamination of the surgical wound. Before the client reaches the OR, supplies, instruments, and equipment must be thoroughly sterilized to remove all microorganisms. Members of the surgical team follow specific guidelines for performing a surgical scrub and donning surgical attire before handling sterile items. The

BOX 36-3 Role of the Circulating Nurse

- Organizes and prepares OR before start of surgical procedure; checks to see that equipment works properly
- Gathers supplies for surgical procedure and opens sterile supplies for scrub nurse
- Counts sponges, sharps, and instruments with scrub nurse before incision is made, at the beginning of wound closure, and at the end of the surgical procedure
- Sends for client at appropriate time
- Conducts preoperative client assessment, including the following:
  - Explains role and identifies client
  - Reviews medical record and verifies procedure and consents
  - Confirms dentures and prostheses removed
  - Confirms client's allergies, nothing by mouth (NPO) status, laboratory values, electrocardiogram (ECG), x-ray studies, skin condition, circulatory and pulmonary status
- Safely assists client to operating table and positions client according to surgeon preference and procedure type, using safety precautions (e.g., safety belt, securing arms, padding bony prominences)
- Applies conductive pad to client if electrocautery used; may prepare client's skin; may apply ECG electrodes
- Explains briefly to client what the circulating nurse and the scrub nurse are doing
- Assists surgical team by tying gowns and arranging equipment
- Assists anesthesia personnel during induction and extubation
- Continuously monitors procedure for any breaks in aseptic technique and anticipates needs of the team; opens additional sterile supplies for scrub nurse
- Handles surgical specimens per institutional policy
- Documents on perioperative nurses' notes
- Communicates to family and PACU personnel during the surgical procedure

special preparation of the client's skin before application of sterile drapes helps reduce the numbers of microorganisms around the surgical incision. The scrub nurse and surgeons create a sterile field around the surgical wound and maintain it throughout the procedure in accordance with strict aseptic principles. The surgical procedure itself finally ends with sterile application of dressings.

All OR personnel must develop a sterile conscience, a personal commitment to safe, quality client care. A sterile conscience means a nurse must know what is sterile, what is unsterile, and how to keep sterile and unsterile items apart. The practice of strict aseptic technique requires discipline, integrity, honesty, and assertiveness concerning any short-comings in aseptic practice. For example, the scrub nurse, who accidentally touches the faucet with one hand while rinsing, rescrubs the hands; the circulating nurse, who accidentally touches a sterile item, has it removed from the sterile field; the surgeon, who contaminates a sterile glove, has the affected glove changed. These are all examples of following one's sterile conscience.

During the postoperative phase, the registered nurse assists in transferring the client to the recovery room or PACU. The OR nurse is an important resource in planning the client's postoperative care.

Evidence-Based Practice Trends

The practice of surgical scrubbing in perioperative settings is changing. In recent years, manufacturers have begun to introduce new hand scrub products that are replacing traditional lengthy scrub routines that use water, brushes, and nonalcohol antiseptic solutions. Recent research demonstrates that hand scrub preparations containing 50% to 90% alcohol combined with chlorhexidine gluconate are just as effective as the traditional scrubbing method in preventing surgical site infections (Parienti and others, 2002). The benefits of using a brushless, alcohol-based surgical hand product (with added emollients) include fast and easy application, limited or decreased damage to the user's skin, improved compliance with hand antisepsis protocols, simplified application technique, and reduced material waste (i.e., water, brushes, packaging) (Conner, 2003).

Skill Performance Guidelines

1. All items used within a sterile field must be sterile.
2. Gowns used by scrub persons must be sterile before donning. Once in place, gowns are considered sterile from the front chest and shoulders to table level and on the sleeves to 2 inches (5 cm) above the elbow.
3. Sterile persons must keep their hands in view, above waist level and below neckline, to avoid contamination.
4. When wearing a sterile gown, arms should not be folded with hands tucked in the axillary region. This area is not considered sterile once the gown is donned. Perspiration can lead to strike through, or contamination that occurs when moisture permeates a sterile barrier.
5. Sterile draped tables should be considered sterile only at table level. Sides of the drape extending below table level are unsterile.
6. All personnel moving around or within a sterile field must do so in a manner consistent with maintaining the sterility of that field. Scrubbed persons move from sterile areas to other sterile areas, contacting a sterile field only with sterile gowns and gloves. Unscrubbed persons should always stay at least 1 foot away from the sterile field while keeping it in constant view and should contact only unsterile areas.
7. All sterile supplies and equipment should be grouped around the sterile-draped client.
8. Unsterile persons must avoid reaching over the sterile field.
9. Scrubbed persons should remain close to the sterile field. When changing position, they should turn face to face or back to back.

SKILL 36-1 Surgical Hand Antisepsis

In the operating room setting it is imperative that hand hygiene or surgical hand antisepsis be achieved through effective surgical scrub or antiseptic hand rub (Boyce and Pittet, 2002). To reduce the risk that clients may acquire postoperative infections, use of an antimicrobial preparation for hand antisepsis is an integral part of the presurgical scrubbing procedure for operating room personnel. Although the skin cannot be sterilized, the number of microorganisms can be greatly reduced by chemical, physical, and mechanical means.

The surgical hand scrub has been the traditional method for surgical asepsis. Through the use of an antimicrobial agent and sterile brushes, the surgical hand scrub removes debris and transient microorganisms from the nails, hands, and forearms; reduces the resident microbial count to a minimum; and inhibits rapid/ rebound growth of microorganisms (AORN, 2003d). New evidence suggests that a brushless technique, with or without water, containing at least 60% alcohol, is an alternative to the traditional hand scrub with a brush with the same microbial efficacy (Gruendemann and Bjerke, 2001).

Both hand antiseptic methods are currently used in operating room settings. This skill will address both techniques.

Surgical attire (i.e., scrubs) is worn in the operating room to reduce the chance for contamination from surgical personnel to clients, and vice versa. Fingernails should be short, clean, and healthy. If polish is worn, it should not be chipped or worn more than 4 days. Artificial nails should not be worn (AORN, 2003d). All rings, watches, and bracelets are removed before the surgical scrub.

The Association of Perioperative Registered Nurses (AORN) recommends a 3- to 4-minute hand and arm scrub with an approved antimicrobial agent for all surgical procedures. The institution should standardize the surgical hand scrub procedure for all staff using either the anatomical timed scrub or the counted stroke method (AORN, 2003d) (see agency policy). Some procedures, described as clean procedures, require performing hand hygiene but not necessarily a surgical scrub. Some examples of clean procedures are laryngoscopy, esophagoscopy, and proctoscopy.

DELEGATION CONSIDERATIONS

Surgical hand antisepsis is performed by a scrub nurse or RNFA. The role of the scrub nurse can be delegated to a surgical technologist or licensed practical nurse. Nonlicensed personnel can assist the RN in the circulating role by:
- Setting up gown and glove supplies
- Opening sterile supplies
- Setting up sterile fields
- Running errands under the direction of the RN

EQUIPMENT

- ❑ Deep sink with foot or knee controls for dispensing water and soap
- ❑ Antimicrobial agent approved by agency
- ❑ Surgical scrub brush with plastic nail file
- ❑ Paper face mask, cap or hood, surgical shoe covers
- ❑ Sterile towel
- ❑ Sterile pack containing sterile gown
- ❑ Protective eyewear (glasses or goggles)

STEP	RATIONALE

▌ASSESSMENT

1. Determine type and length of time for hand hygiene per agency policy.

2. Remove bracelets, rings, and watches.

3. Inspect fingernails, which must be short, clean, and healthy. Artificial nails should not be worn.

Guidelines vary regarding ideal time needed for surgical scrub.

Jewelry may harbor or protect microorganisms from removal. Allergic skin reactions may occur as a result of scrub agent or glove powder accumulating under jewelry.

Long nails and chipped or old polish increase number of bacteria residing on nails. Long fingernails can puncture gloves, causing contamination. Artificial nails may harbor gram-negative microorganisms and fungus (AORN, 2003d).

- **Critical Decision Point**
  Nail polish should be removed if chipped or worn longer than 4 days because there is a tendency after that time for the nails to harbor greater numbers of bacteria (AORN, 2003d).

STEP	RATIONALE

4. Inspect condition of cuticles, hands, and forearms for presence of abrasions, cuts, or open lesions.

Cuts, abrasions, exudative lesions, and hangnails tend to ooze serum, which may contain pathogens. Broken skin permits microorganisms to enter various layers of the skin, providing deeper microbial breeding grounds (AORN, 2003d).

NURSING DIAGNOSES
- Risk for infection
- Risk for injury

Related factors are individualized based on client's condition or needs.

PLANNING
1. Expected outcomes following completion of procedure:
   - Client will not develop signs of surgical wound infection.

Indicates microorganisms are not transferred to the client and sterile field.

IMPLEMENTATION
1. Don surgical shoe covers, cap or hood, face mask, and protective eyewear.

Protective eyewear is mandated to prevent exposure to blood or body fluids splashing from the sterile field, causing the risk of infection (e.g., human immunodeficiency viirus [HIV], hepatitis B virus [HBV]). Laser surgery requires special protective eyewear to prevent eye damage from stray laser energy.

2. Turn water on using foot or knee control, and adjust to comfortable temperature.

Knee or foot controls prevent contamination of hands after scrub.

3. Prescrub wash/rinse: Wet hands and arms under running lukewarm water, and lather with antimicrobial agent up to 2 inches above elbows.

A short prescrub wash/rinse removes gross debris and superficial microorganisms and is an essential step before surgical antisepsis.

4. Keep hands elevated above elbows. Rinse hands and arms thoroughly under running water.

Water runs from fingertips to elbows by gravity; hands are maintained as the cleanest part of the upper extremity.

5. Under running water, clean under nails of both hands with file (see illustration); discard file.

Removes dirt and organic materials that harbor microorganisms.

6. Surgical hand scrub (with brush):
   a. Wet brush, and apply antimicrobial agent. Visualize each finger, hand, and arm as having four sides. Wash all four sides effectively. Scrub the nails of one hand with 15 strokes. Scrub the palm, each side of thumb and fingers, and the posterior side of the hand with 10 strokes each (see illustration).

Ensures removal of resident microorganisms on all surfaces of hands and arms.

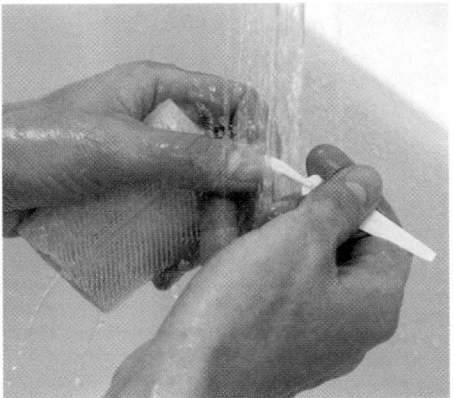

STEP **5** Cleaning under fingernails.

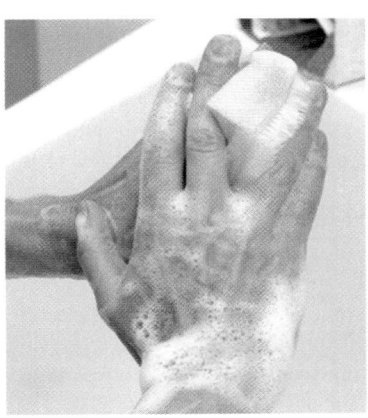

STEP **6a** Scrubbing side of fingers.

STEP	RATIONALE

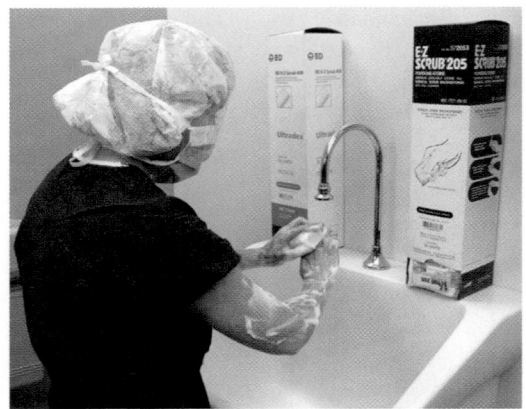

STEP **6b** Scrubbing forearms.

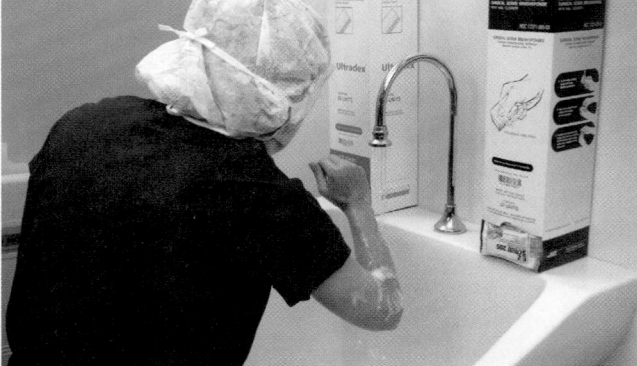

STEP **6c** Rinsing arms.

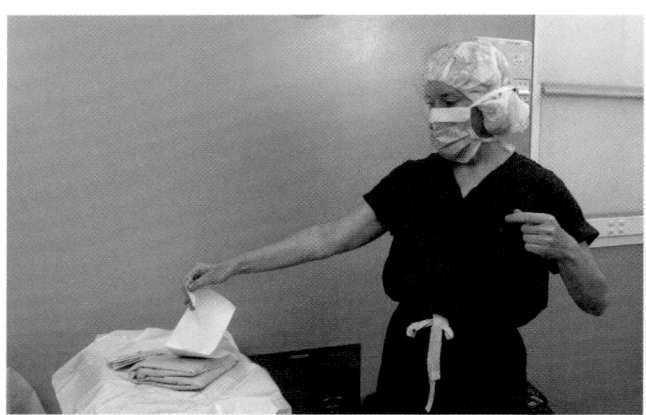

STEP **6e** Grasping sterile towel.

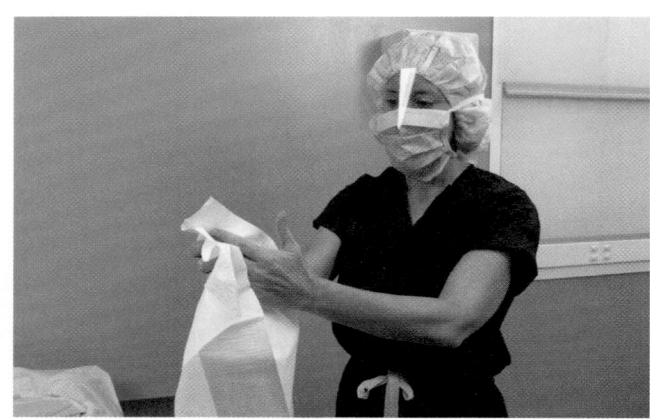

STEP **6f** Drying sequence.

STEP	RATIONALE
b. Divide the arm mentally into thirds; scrub each third 10 times (see illustration) (AORN, 2003d). Some agency policies requrire scrub by time rather than 10 strokes. Rinse brush, and repeat the sequence for the other arm. A two-brush method may be substituted. Check agency policy.	Eliminates transient microorganims and reduces resident hand flora.
c. Discard brush; flex arms, and rinse from fingertips to elbows in one continuous motion, allowing water to run off at elbow (see illustration).	Hands remain cleanest part of upper extremities.
d. Turn off water with foot or knee control, with hands elevated in front of and away from body. Enter OR suite by backing into room.	Keeps hands free of microorganisms.
e. Approach sterile setup, and grasp sterile towel, taking care not to drip water on the sterile field (see illustration).	Water would contaminate field.
f. Bending slightly at the waist, keeping hands and arms above the waist and outstretched, grasp one end of the sterile towel to dry one hand thoroughly, moving from fingers to elbow in a rotating motion (see illustration).	Avoids sterile towel from contacting unsterile scrub attire and transferring contamination to hands. Dry skin from cleanest (hands) to least clean (elbows).

| STEP | RATIONALE |

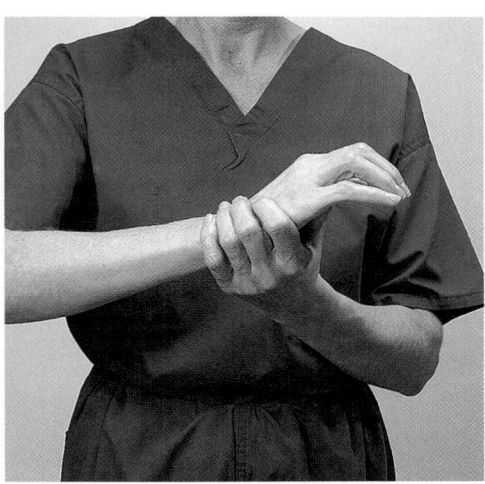

STEP **7b** Application of antimicrobial agent for brushless hand scrub. (Courtesy 3M Health Care.)

   g. Use the opposite end of the towel to dry the other hand.

   h. Drop towel into linen hamper or into circulating nurse's hand.

7. *Optional:* Brushless antiseptic hand rub

   a. After prescrub wash, dry hands and forearms thoroughly with a paper towel.

   b. Dispense 2 ml of antimicrobial agent hand preparation into the palm of one hand (see illustration). Dip the fingertips of the opposite hand into the hand preparation, and work it under the nails. Spread the remaining hand prep over the hand and up to just above the elbow covering all surfaces (see illustration).

   c. Using another 2 ml of hand preparation, repeat above procedure with the other hand.

* **Critical Decision Point**
   This is an example of one particular brushless product. Please see manufacturer's instructions for application. There are many new products on the market, and strict adherence to their guidelines is essential to achieving surgical asepsis.

   d. Dispense another 2 ml of hand preparation into either hand, and reapply to all aspects of both hands up to the wrist. Allow to dry before donning gloves.

Avoids transfer of microorganisms from elbow to opposite hand.

Promotes reduction in microorganisms on all surfaces of hands and arms.

EVALUATION

1. Observe the client for signs of localized wound infection (usually occurs 2 to 3 days postoperatively).

Signs of infection include redness, heat, swelling, pain, and purulent drainage.

Recording and Reporting

* No recording is required for surgical hand antisepsis. Record area and description of surgical site postoperatively to provide baseline for monitoring wound.

Unexpected Outcomes	Related Interventions
1. Redness, heat, swelling, pain, or purulent drainage may develop at surgical site as a result of infection.	• Institute appropriate wound care (see Chapter 37). In the event a pattern of surgical wound infections occurs, the hospital infection control team will monitor trends from the operating rooms in an effort to trace the origin. This may include cultures of nails and hands of staff, soap dispensers, and so on.

Teaching Considerations
• Instruct client and family or significant other to observe surgical site for signs of infection.

SKILL 36-2 Donning Sterile Gown and Closed Gloving

Immediately following a surgical scrub, a sterile gown should be applied, followed by application of sterile gloves. All members of the surgical team must prepare in this manner before entering the sterile field. Once applied, the surgical gown is considered sterile in the front from chest to waist or table level. The sleeves are considered sterile from 5 cm (2 inches) above the elbow to fingertips. The back of the gown is not considered sterile when worn.

Surgical gowns should cover all garments worn underneath. All sterile gowns that are free of tears, punctures, strain, and abrasion provide an effective barrier against microorganisms passing between unsterile and sterile areas (AORN, 2003c).

The scrub nurse should use the closed-glove method when initially entering the sterile field. If a glove becomes contaminated during the surgery, the circulating nurse, wearing protective unsterile gloves, grasps the outside of the glove and pulls off the glove inside out, leaving the stockinette cuff of the gown in place. Another sterile team member assists in regloving, or the open-glove method can be used. If both the scrub nurse's gloves become contaminated, it is recommended to regown and reglove using the closed-glove method (Elkin and others, 2004).

DELEGATION CONSIDERATIONS
Application of a sterile gown and gloves is usually performed by a scrub nurse or RNFA. The role of a scrub nurse can be delegated to a surgical technologist or licensed practical nurse. Nonlicensed personnel can assist the RN by:
• Setting up sterile gown and glove packages

EQUIPMENT
❑ Package of proper-size sterile gloves (latex-free if nurse or client has sensitivity or allergy)
❑ Sterile pack containing sterile gown
❑ Clean, flat, dry surface (table or Mayo stand) on which to open gown and gloves
❑ Paper face masks, cap or hood, surgical shoe covers
❑ Protective eyewear/face shield

STEP	RATIONALE

ASSESSMENT
1. Select proper size and type of sterile gloves. Latex-free gloves should be selected if latex sensitivity of client or any surgical personnel in the room is suspected.

Proper fit ensures ease of handling instruments and supplies. Prevents latex allergic response.

2. Select proper size and type of sterile surgical gown.

Ill-fitting gown may impede movement of nurse's extremities.

STEP	RATIONALE

NURSING DIAGNOSIS

- Risk for infection

Related factors are individualized based on client's condition or needs.

PLANNING

1. Expected outcomes following completion of procedure:
   - No break in surgical technique will occur. Client is not exposed to microorganisms.

Nurse maintains aseptic practice and does not contaminate gown or gloves.

IMPLEMENTATION

1. Open sterile gown and glove package on a clean, dry, flat surface. This can be done by the scrub nurse (before scrubbing hands) or circulating nurse.

Preferably on a small table separate from the sterile field containing the sterile instruments and supplies.

2. Perform surgical hand antisepsis (see Skill 36-1).

3. After drying hands, pick up gown (folded inside out) from sterile package, grasping the inside surface of gown at the collar.

The hands are not completely sterile. The inside surface of the gown will contact the skin's surface and is thus considered contaminated.

4. Lift folded gown directly upward and step back, away from the table.

Prevents gown from touching unsterile object.

5. Locate neckband; with both hands, grasp the inside front of gown just below neckband.

Clean hands may touch inside of gown without contaminating outer surface.

6. Keeping at arm's length away from body, allow gown to unfold with the inside of gown toward body. Do not touch outside of gown or allow it to touch the floor.

Outside of gown remains sterile.

7. With hands at shoulder level, slip both arms into armholes simultaneously (see illustration). Do not allow hands to move through cuff opening. Have circulating nurse pull gown over shoulders by reaching inside arm seams. Gown is pulled on, leaving sleeves covering hands.

Careful application prevents contamination. Gown covers hands to prepare for closed gloving.

8. Have circulating nurse tie gown at neck and waist (see illustration). If gown is wraparound style, sterile front flap is not touched until the scrub nurse has gloved.

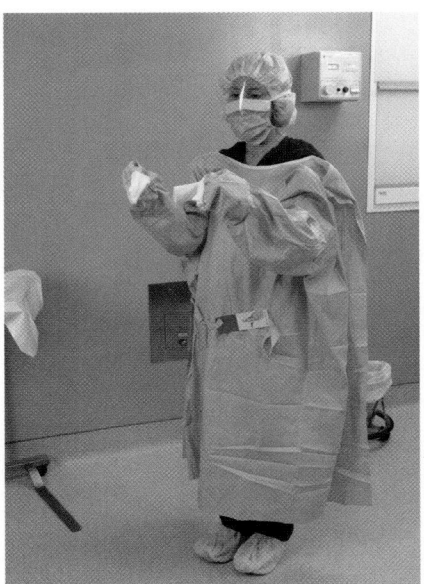

STEP **7** Placing arms in sleeves.

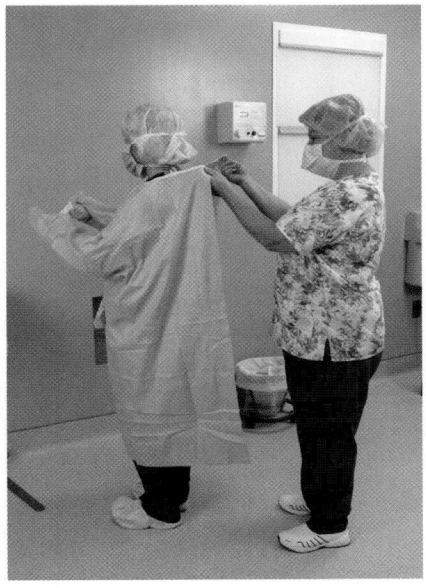

STEP **8** Circulating nurse ties scrub gown.

STEP	RATIONALE

9. Apply gloves using the closed-glove method:
   a. With hands covered by gown cuffs and sleeves, open inner sterile glove package (see illustration).

   Sterile gown cuff will touch sterile glove surface.

   b. Grasp folded cuff of glove for dominant hand with the nondominant hand.

   Sterile gown touches sterile glove.

   c. Extend dominant forearm forward with palm up, and place palm of glove against palm of dominant hand. Gloved fingers point toward elbow.

   Positions glove for application over cuffed hand, keeping glove sterile.

   d. While holding glove cuff through gown with dominant hand on which it was placed, grasp back of glove cuff with nondominant hand and turn glove cuff over end of dominant hand and gown cuff (see illustration).

   Positions glove over gown for hand insertion.

   e. Grasp top of glove and underlying gown sleeve with covered nondominant hand. Carefully extend fingers into glove, being sure glove's cuff covers gown's cuff.

   f. Glove nondominant hand in same manner with gloved, dominant hand (see illustration). Keep hand inside sleeve. Be sure fingers are fully extended into both gloves (see illustration).

   Gloves remain sterile.

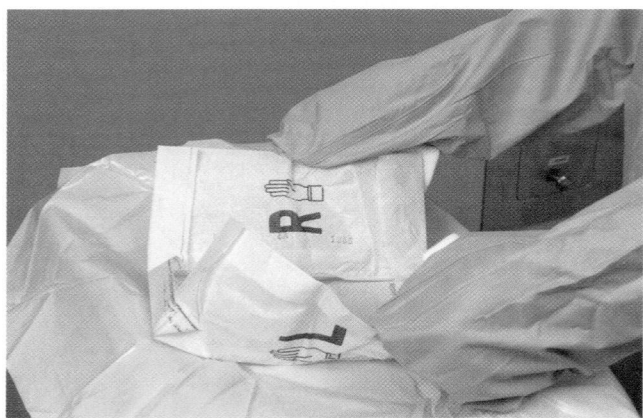

STEP **9a** Scrub nurse opens glove package.

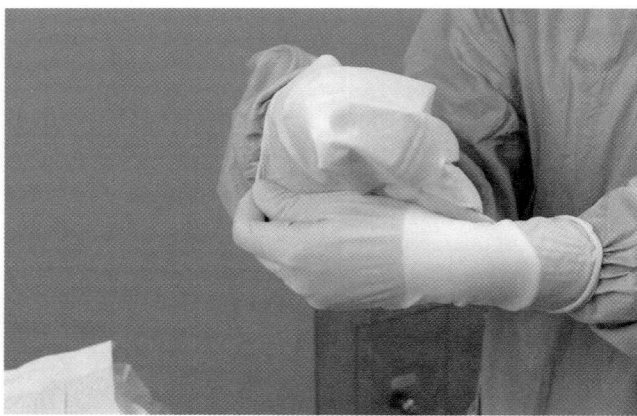

STEP **9f(1)** Second glove applied.

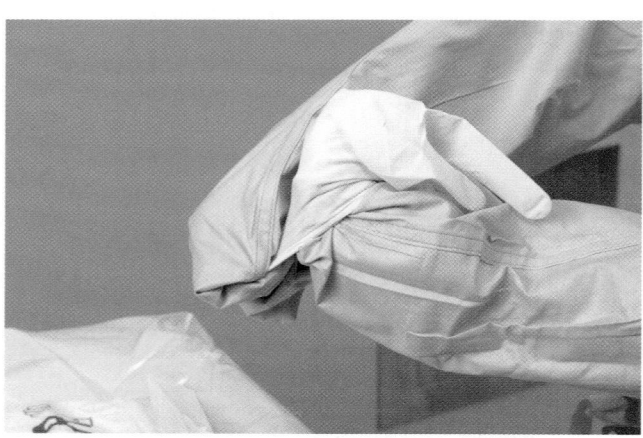

STEP **9d** Glove applied as hands remain inside cuff.

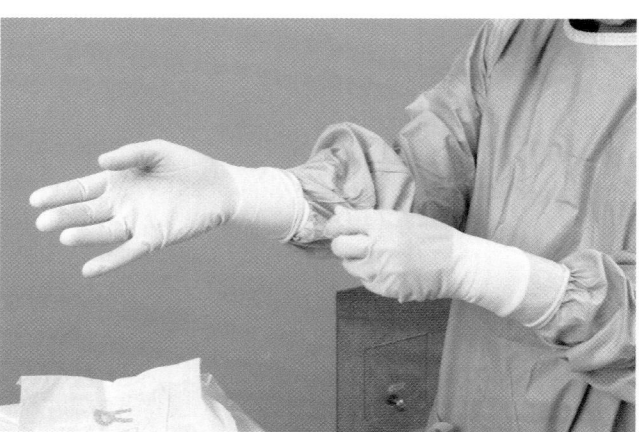

STEP **9f(2)** Gloved fingers extended.

STEP	RATIONALE

10. For wraparound gown:

   a. Grasp sterile front flap/waist tie with gloved hands, and untie.

   Front of gown is sterile.

   b. Pass tie to circulating nurse, who stands still as scrub nurse turns. This may also be held by another team member with sterile gloves. Keep gown tie in left hand.

   c. Allowing margin of safety, turn to the left one-half turn, covering back with extended gown flap. Retrieve tie only from team member, and secure both ties in place.

   Maneuver covers entire body with gown.

   NOTE: On disposable sterile gowns, there is often a paper tab attached to the tie that can be passed to a nonsterile team member for turning, and then is pulled off and discarded (see illustration).

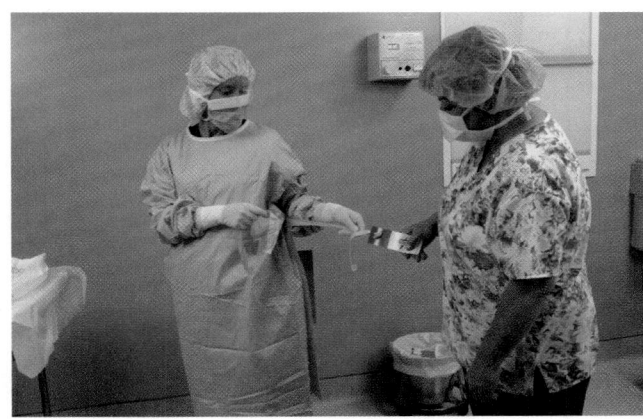

STEP **10c** Disposable paper gown with paper tab.

EVALUATION

1. Observe the client for signs of localized wound infection (usually occurs 2 to 3 days postoperatively).

Signs of infection include redness, heat, swelling, pain, and purulent drainage.

Recording and Reporting

- No recording is required for sterile gowning and gloving. Record area and description of surgical site postoperatively to provide baseline for monitoring wound.

Unexpected Outcomes	Related Interventions
1. Redness, heat, swelling, pain, or purulent drainage may develop at surgical site as a result of infection.	• Institute appropriate wound care (see Chapter 37). In the event a pattern of surgical wound infections occurs, the hospital infection control team will monitor trends from the operating rooms in an effort to trace the origin. This may include cultures of nails and hands of staff, soap dispensers, etc.

Teaching Considerations

- Instruct client and family or significant other to observe surgical site for signs of infection.

FOCUS on CLINICAL PRACTICE

You are assigned to be the circulating nurse for Mr. James's total hip replacement. He is a 68-year-old retired engineer with no significant medical history except for severe arthritis in his left hip. The surgical team includes Dr. R. Jones, orthopedic surgeon; B. Best, RNFA; Sarah Williams, ST (surgical technologist), and Dr. L. O'Brien, anesthesiologist. Sarah is a new scrub nurse on the orthopedic team. She has only been scrubbing by herself for 1 week (without a preceptor).

1. Sarah is running late because of the staff meeting this morning. While she is at the sink performing a surgical hand scrub with a brush, you notice her scrubbed hand hits the faucet. You tell her what you observed, but she states she did not feel it. What should Sarah do in this situation?
   A. Scrub that hand 1 minute longer
   B. Switch to use of antiseptic rub
   C. Start the surgical hand scrub over
   D. Nothing because she is about to apply sterile gloves
   Explain your choice.
2. Sarah just had artificial nails applied last night because she is in a wedding tonight. They are polished with no signs of chipping. Is it okay for Sarah to scrub for Mr. James's total hip replacement today?

A. Yes, because the polish was applied just last night
B. Yes, because the polish is not chipped
C. No, artificial nails may not be worn
Explain your choice.
3. Dr. Jones performs a brushless antiseptic hand rub before gowning and gloving. Does he need to perform a prescrub wash/rinse?
   A. Yes
   B. No
   Explain your choice.
4. While Sarah is gowning and gloving Dr. Jones, you notice the sleeve of his gown touches an intravenous pole. Sarah and Dr. Jones do not seem to notice. He starts to raise his voice at Sarah to hurry up and pass him the sterile drapes. What should you do?
   A. Do not say anything, Dr. Jones is already mad and in a hurry.
   B. Wait until the patient is draped and all equipment/tables are in place before you tell Sarah.
   C. Immediately tell Dr. Jones his gown is contaminated.
   Explain your choice.

NCLEX REVIEW QUESTIONS

1. The role of the circulating nurse includes:
   1. Performing surgical hand scrub and donning sterile gown and gloves
   2. Providing surgical exposure (assisting in retraction of tissues and suction of surgical field)
   3. Conducting perioperative assessment, reviewing medical record, verifying consent forms
   4. Gowning and gloving surgeons and assistants as they enter the OR
2. The traditional method for surgical asepsis is:
   1. The surgical hand scrub
   2. Alcohol foam rub
   3. Brushless scrub
   4. Waterless scrub

3. Before beginning surgical asepsis, the scrub nurse should:
   1. Remove nail polish even if it is not chipped
   2. Inspect fingernails, cuticles, hands, and forearms for presence of abrasions, cuts, or open lesions
   3. Count all instruments, sponges, and sharps with circulating nurse
   4. Remove rings and bracelets; watches may be left on
4. To apply gloves using the closed-glove method:
   1. Both hands should be covered with the cuffs of the gown
   2. Both hands should be through the cuffs of the gown
   3. Dominant hand should be covered with the cuff of the gown
   4. Nondominant hand should be covered with the cuff of the gown

NCLEX REVIEW QUESTIONS

5. An example of not following one's sterile conscience is:
   1. Scrub nurse who accidentally touches the faucet with one hand while scrubbing rescrubs the hands
   2. Circulating nurse accidentally touched a sterile item, removes it from the sterile field
   3. Surgeon who contaminates sterile glove has the affected glove changed
   4. Before scrub nurse dries hands with a towel, she drips water on the sterile gown she is about to put on but does not replace the gown

References

Association of Operating Room Nurses: AORN Official Statement on unlicensed assistive personnel. In *AORN standards, recommended practices, and guidelines*, Denver, 2003a, The Association.

Association of Operating Room Nurses: Position statement—statement on mandate for the registered professional nurse in the perioperative practice setting. In *AORN standards, recommended practices, and guidelines*, Denver, 2003b, The Association.

Association of Operating Room Nurses: Recommended practices for selection and use of surgical gowns and drapes. In *AORN standards and recommended practices for perioperative nursing*, Denver, 2003c, The Association.

Association of Operating Room Nurses: Recommended practices for surgical hand scrubs. In *AORN standards and recommended practices for perioperative nursing*, Denver, 2003d, The Association.

Association of Operating Room Nurses: Revised AORN official statement on RN first assistants. In *AORN standards and recommended practices for perioperative nursing*, Denver, 2003e, The Association.

Conner R: Clinical issues: fire blankets; alcohol-based hand scrubs; peel pouch indicators; aseptic technique definitions; shaving, *AORN J* 78(3):484, 2003.

Elkin M, Perry A, Potter P: *Nursing interventions and clinical skills*, ed 3, St. Louis, 2004, Mosby.

Research References

Boyce JM, Pittet D: Guidelines for hand hygiene in health care settings, *Am J Infect Control* 30(8):S1, 2002.

Gruendemann BJ, Bjerke NB: Is it time for brushless scrubbing with an alcohol-based agent? *AORN J* 74(6):859, 2001.

Parienti JJ and others: Hand-rubbing with an aqueous alcoholic solution vs. traditional surgical hand-scrubbing and 30-day surgical site infection rates: a randomized equivalence study, *JAMA* 288(6):722, 2002.

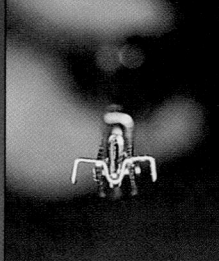

37

Wound Care and Irrigations

37-1 Performing Wound Irrigation

37-2 Performing Suture and Staple Removal

37-3 Managing Drainage Evacuation

MEDIA RESOURCES

Evolve Site *evolve*

http://evolve.elsevier.com/Perry/skills
- Weblinks
- Video clips
- Mosby's Nursing Skills Video Exercises

Mosby's Nursing Skills Videos/CD-ROM

- *Wound Care Video:* Sterile gloving, latex precautions; wound assessments, indirect and direct assessments, wound drainage systems, and types of wound drainage

OBJECTIVES

Mastery of content in this chaper will enable the nurse to:

- Discuss the body's response during each stage of the wound-healing process.
- Differentiate between primary and secondary intention.
- Explain factors that impair or promote normal wound healing.
- Perform a wound irrigation.
- Remove sutures or staples.
- Demonstrate care of a wound-drainage system.

KEY TERMS

Dehiscence

Eschar

Evisceration

Granulation tissue

Healing ridge

Hemostasis

Hemovac drain

Irrigation

Jackson-Pratt (JP) drain

Keloid

Penrose drain

Primary intention

Secondary intention

Staples

Tertiary intention

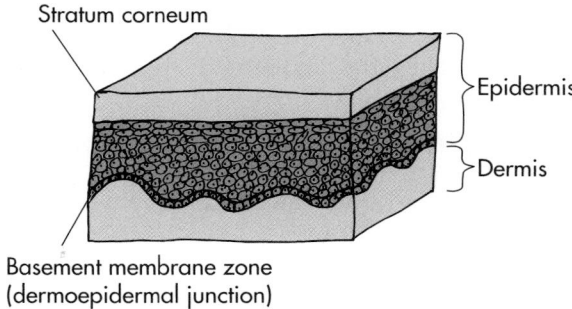

FIGURE **37-1** Layers of the integument.

Proper wound care is necessary to promote healing that results in an intact skin layer. An intact skin is the body's first line of defense against invasion by infectious microorganisms. The skin defends the body in other ways by serving as a sensory organ for pain, touch, and temperature, and it has an acid pH, which is often called the "acid mantle."

The skin or integument, the largest external organ, has two layers: the epidermis and the dermis (Figure 37-1). The outer layer, the epidermis, has five layers. The outermost layer, the stratum corneum, consists of flattened dead keratinized cells. The thin layer of the stratum corneum prevents dehydration of underlying cells and is a physical barrier to the entry of certain chemicals. The barrier is selective; it does allow absorption of topical medications in paste, ointment, and dermal patch forms. The next layers in the epidermis are the stratum lucidum, stratum granulosum, and stratum spinosum. The innermost layer of the epidermis, the stratum germinativum, is sometimes called the basal layer. It is from this single layer of keratinocytes that cells migrate up toward the stratum corneum. Important features of the stratum germinativum are the epidermal protrusions, or "peaks and valleys," that point downward into the dermis. These provide resiliency and integrity to the skin structure. Also found in this layer are the melanocytes, which are the cells that give the skin its color. The area that separates the epidermis from the dermis is called the dermoepidermal junction or the basement membrane zone.

Beneath the epidermis is the dermis. The dermis contains no skin cells. Collagen (a tough fibrous protein layer), blood vessels, and nerves compose the dermal layer. Collagen composes about 70% of the dermis and is therefore extremely important in wound healing. The dermis restores the physical properties of the skin and its structural integrity. Restoration of both the epidermal and dermal layers is necessary to promote healing. Risk of local or systemic infection, impaired circulation, and breakdown of tissue directly impair the wound-healing ability of the skin layers (Waldrop and Doughty, 2000).

Physiologically, wound healing occurs in the same way for all clients, with skin cells and some tissues (including the vascular tissues) regenerating quickly and others regenerating slowly or not at all. The latter group includes cells of the liver, renal tubules, and central nervous system neurons.

Wound healing in the adult skin is complex and involves a series of physiological processes among cells and tissues (Box 37-1). These processes can be affected by the location, severity, and extent of the injury and the tissue layer or layers involved (Waldrop and Doughty, 2000). In addition, there are underlying factors that inhibit the ability of cells and tissues to regenerate, return to normal structure, or resume normal functioning (Box 37-2).

The color of an open wound represents the balance between nonviable tissue called eschar or slough and new healthy granulation tissue (Davidson, 2002). A wound that is healing well is red or pink in color (Table 37-1). Necrotic wounds are without proper circulation and provide an excellent medium for bacterial growth, resulting in wound infections.

Collagen deposition begins in the inflammatory phase and peaks during the proliferative phase. It is important for nurses to assess for the accumulation of this new tissue (Cooper, 2000). This "healing ridge" is composed of newly formed collagen and can be felt along a healing wound (Waldrop and Doughty, 2000) (Figure 37-2). It is usually present directly under the suture line between days 5 and 9 (Cooper, 2000). Absence of the healing ridge may indicate a wound at risk for dehiscence or infection (Waldrop and Doughty, 2000) (Figure 37-3).

Types of healing are primary intention, secondary intention, and tertiary intention (Figure 37-4). Healing by primary intention is expected when the edges of a clean surgi-

BOX 37-1 Stages of Wound Healing (Full-Thickness Wounds)

INFLAMMATORY STAGE

Starts when skin integrity is impaired and continues in a clean wound for 3 days.

- Hemostasis—Blood vessels constrict, gathering of platelets stops bleeding. Clots form a fibrin matrix. Scab forms, preventing entry of infectious organisms.
- Inflammatory response—Increases blood flow to wound and vascular permeability to plasma, resulting in localized redness and edema.
- White blood cells arrive at wound.
    Neutrophils ingest bacteria and small debris, then die in a few days and leave enzyme exudate, which either attacks bacteria or interferes with tissue repair.
    Monocytes become macrophages.
    Macrophages clean cell of debris by phagocytosis; aid in wound repair by recycling normal amino acids and sugars.
- Epithelial cells move from wound margins to base of clot or scab (for period of approximately 48 hours).

PROLIFERATIVE STAGE

Follows inflammatory stage and continues for 2 to 3 weeks.

- Neoangiogenesis—Vascular integrity restored as production of new capillaries occurs.
- Fibroblasts—Function with help of vitamins B and C; oxygen and amino acids synthesize collagen.
- Collagen—Provides strength and structural integrity to the wound.
- Contraction—Occurs only in open wounds and greatly reduces healing time because it reduces the amount of matrix that must be produced to fill the wound.
- Epithelial cells—Differentiate to duplicate damaged cells (e.g., intestinal mucosal cells acquire their columnar appearance).

REMODELING PHASE

The final phase in full-thickness wound healing and may continue for 1 year or more.

Data from Waldrop J, Doughty DB: Wound healing physiology. In Bryant RA, editor: *Acute and chronic wounds: nursing management*, ed 2, St. Louis, 2000, Mosby.

BOX 37-2 Systemic Factors Affecting Wound Healing

- Tissue perfusion and oxygenation
- Nutritional status
- Infection
- Diabetes mellitus
- Corticosteroid therapy or hypercortisolemia
- Chemotherapy and radiation
- Age
- Stress—both psychological and physiological
- Immunosuppression
- Systemic conditions that affect health status such as renal or hepatic disease, sepsis, cancer
- Hematopoietic disorders

From Waldrop J, Doughty DB: Wound healing physiology. In Bryant RA, editor: *Acute and chronic wounds: nursing management*, ed 2, St. Louis, 2000, Mosby.

cal incision remain close together. The wound heals quickly, and tissue loss is minimal or absent (Waldrop and Doughty, 2000). The skin cells quickly regenerate, and capillary walls stretch across under the suture line to form a smooth surface as they join.

Wounds that are left open and allowed to heal by scar formation are classified as healing by secondary intention (Waldrop and Doughty, 2000). There is tissue loss and open, jagged wound edges. Granulation tissue gradually fills in the area of the defect with scar tissue (Figure 37-5). This process is typical of severe laceration or massive surgical intervention with skin loss. In secondary intention there is some gap between the edges. A thin fibrinous exudate covers the edges of the wound, prevents bacterial invasion, and coagulates surface bleeding. New capillaries are supported by connective tissue. This form of healing results in a thicker surface closure. The slowness of this process places the client at greater risk for infection and collection of body fluids that must be drained to permit healing. Some clients who heal by secondary intention may develop an excessive amount of connective tissue in the scar surface. This tissue is known as keloid. Other developments may include the formation of a fistula in response to the presence of bacteria in the wound.

Healing by tertiary intention is sometimes called delayed primary intention or closure. It occurs when surgical wounds are not closed immediately but left open for 3 to 5 days to allow edema or infection to diminish. Then the wound edges are sutured or stapled closed. Scarring is usually minimal (Waldrop and Doughty, 2000). During the healing process a wound may have some type of dressing covering it.

An initial surgical dressing is not removed for direct wound inspection until a physician writes a medical order to remove it. Certain situations and some institutional policies govern who changes the dressing the first time. Special attention is paid to maintaining the position of drains during dressing changes (Waldrop and Doughty, 2000). To promote client comfort, an analgesic, as ordered, should be administered 30 to 45 minutes before changing the dressing. However, the nurse's assessment determines the best time for analgesic administration before wound care. Skin cleansing in the area of the suture line or drain site is indicated when an excessive amount of drainage occurs. The presence of wound exudate is an expected stage of epithelial cell growth.

Recently a new method, vacuum-assisted closure (VAC), for wound healing has been used to treat difficult-to-heal wounds. VAC uses controlled negative pressure on wounds. Negative pressure stretches and distorts the cells within the wound, pulling them close together. It is believed that this

TABLE 37-1	**WOUND COLOR**
Black wounds	Black eschar represents full-thickness tissue destruction. Black is used to describe necrotic tissue or desiccated tissue like tendon. It is also common with stage III and IV pressure ulcers and the gangrenous lesions secondary to peripheral vascular disease.
	Moisture-retentive dressings or synthetic dressings are contraindicated. These wounds are usually treated conservatively. As long as the wound is noninfected and eschar is dry and intact, the wound may be left alone.
	If the client is ambulatory, chemical enzymes may be used as an alternative to debridement. However, this treatment may not be as effective as debridement in some clients.
Yellow wounds	Yellow represents death of subcutaneous fat tissue and muscle degeneration. It can be yellow, cream-colored, or gray necrotic slough, which is usually accompanied by purulent drainage.
	For clients with a low infection risk, the use of moisture-retentive dressings enhances debridement. These moisture-retentive dressings may include wet-to-dry dressings, as well as hydrocolloids, hydrogels, or alginates.
Red wounds	Red wounds occur when the yellow slough is removed. The red color is the result of an increasing amount of red or pink granulation tissue.
	The goal in red wound management is to select a dressing that maintains a clean and slightly moist wound environment and minimizes damage to healing tissue.

Data from Beitz JM, Bates-Jensen B: Algorithms, critical pathways, and computer software for wound care: contemporary status and future potential, *Ostomy Wound Manage* 47(4):33, 2001; Cooper DM: Assessment, measurement, and evaluation: their pivotal roles in wound healing. In Bryant RA: *Acute and chronic wounds: nursing management,* ed 2, St. Louis, 2000, Mosby.

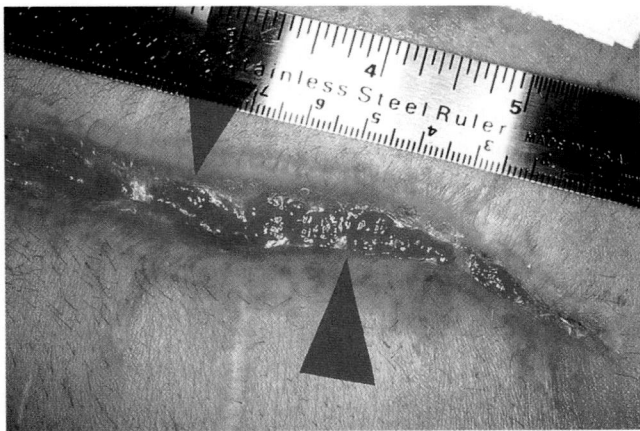

FIGURE **37-2** Surgical wound with epithelialization occurring: epithelial healing ridge apparent. (From Bryant RA, editor: *Acute and chronic wounds,* ed 2, St. Louis, 2000, Mosby.)

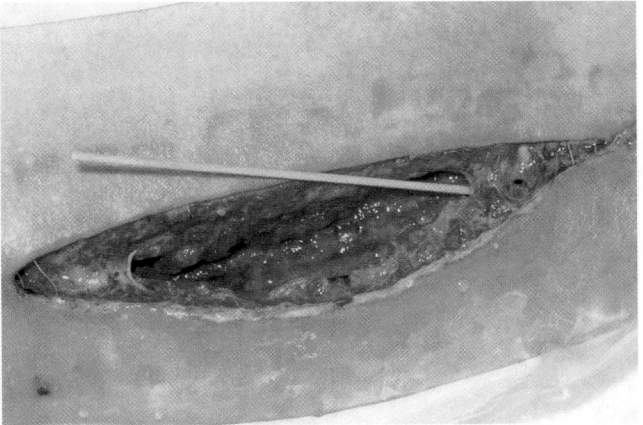

FIGURE **37-3** Surgical wound lacking evidence of healing epithelial ridge. (From Bryant RA, editor: *Acute and chronic wounds,* ed 2, St. Louis, 2000, Mosby.)

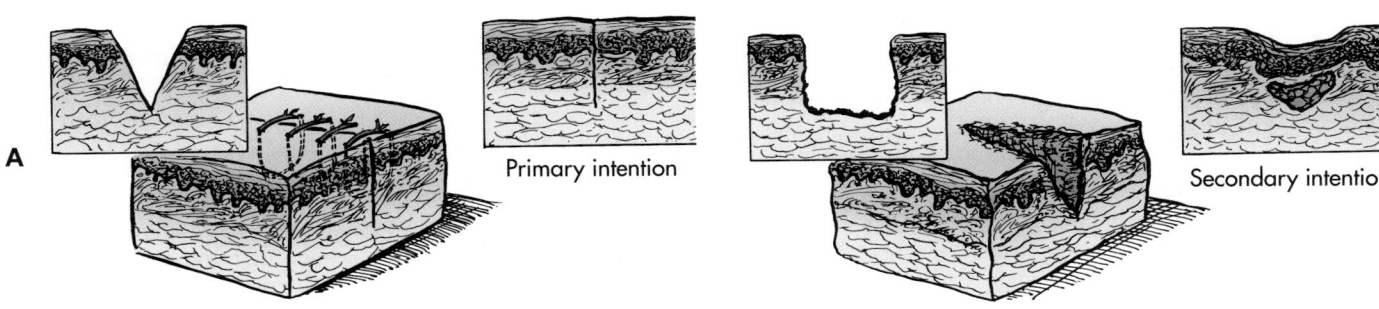

A, Primary intention

B, Secondary intention

FIGURE **37-4** **A,** Wound healing by primary intention, such as with a surgical incision. Wound healing edges are pulled together and approximated with sutures, staples, or adhesive tapes, and healing occurs by connective tissue deposition. **B,** Wound healing by secondary intention. Wound edges are not approximated, and healing occurs by granulation tissue formation and contraction of the wound edges (Used with permission: Bryant RA, editor: *Acute and chronic wounds: nursing management,* ed 2, St. Louis, 2000 Mosby.)

TABLE 37-2 WOUND CLEANSING PROTOCOL

	MECHANICAL FORCE	
PHASE OF HEALING	HIGH PRESSURE INFLAMMATORY	LOW PRESSURE PROLIFERATIVE
Wound base characteristics	• Presence of necrotic tissue (eschar, fibrin slough), debris, or other particulate matter • Significant bacterial burden • Moderate/large amount of exudate • Residue from wound care products	• Presence of granulation tissue or new epithelial cells • Non/minimum serous or serosanguineous exudate • Residue from wound care products
Clinical outcome(s)	• Loosen, soften, and remove devitalized tissue from wound • Separate eschar from fibrotic tissue/fibrotic tissue from granulating base • Remove wound care product residue	• Prevent trauma to viable wound tissue • Remove wound care product residue
Solutions: Wound cleansers	• Normal saline • Volume of solution depends on size of wound	• Normal saline • Volume of solution depends on size of wound
Delivery systems*	• 35-ml syringe/19-gauge angiocatheter • Irrijet® DS • Pleurovac	• Pouring saline directly from bottle • Bulb syringe • Piston syringe

From Barr JE: Principles of wound cleansing, *Ostomy Wound Manage* 7A(suppl 41):15S, 1995.

*This is not an all-inclusive list of delivery systems available. Inclusion does not imply endorsement.

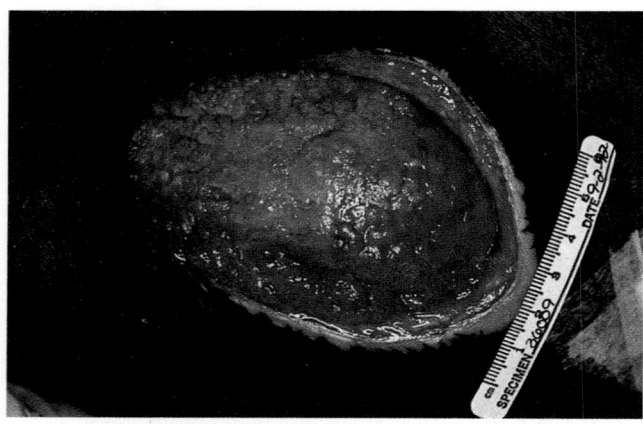

FIGURE **37-5** Open wound with a granulating base.

distortion causes the epithelial cells to multiply rapidly and form granulation tissue (Mendez-Eastman, 2001). The negative pressure of VAC also removes third-space fluid in the open wound, allowing increased blood flow to the wound. The VAC dressing keeps the wound bed moist (Mendez-Eastman, 2001). There have been good results with VAC on chronic wounds such as stasis ulcers and stage III and IV pressure ulcers. This technique appears to decrease the time it takes to heal stubborn, chronic wounds (Mendez-Eastman, 2001). Changing the dressing of a VAC is discussed in Chapter 38.

Meticulous hand hygiene and proper infection control procedures before and after removing soiled dressings, coupled with proper wound-cleansing procedures, limit the risk of nosocomial infection. Using clean gloves prevents exposure to body fluids, exudate, or bloody drainage from a wound. Wound cleansing delivers a fluid or cleansing solution to the wound surface by means of a specific mechanical force and assists with the separation and removal of necrotic debris, particulate matter, bacteria, and residue of wound care products (Barr, 1995). Effective wound cleansing can be accomplished by using an appropriate cleansing solution that does not harm the tissue and is delivered by adequate mechanical cleansing action of soaking, scrubbing, or irrigation (Barr, 1995). Irrigation is the method of wound cleansing most used by nurses.

Irrigation uses the mechanical force (either high or low) of a stream of solution to remove particulate matter, debris, bacteria, and necrotic tissue from a wound. A pressure needed to irrigate wounds is between 4 and 15 psi. In addition to cleansing via irrigation (Table 37-2), prescribed medications may be introduced in the wound irrigant. Principles of basic wound irrigation include the following:

1. Cleanse in a direction from the least contaminated area to the most contaminated.
2. When irrigating, all the solution flows from the least contaminated to the most contaminated area.

When irrigating a wound, be sure that the flow of irrigation moves from the area being cleansed to an area that is both distal to it and lower. In wound care the area being cleansed is considered "clean" and the surrounding skin surfaces are considered "contaminated" without respect to whether the wound is infected. Within the wound the irrigation flow is directed from healthy tissue toward infected tissue. Irrigating solutions are sterile. In the event that the irri-

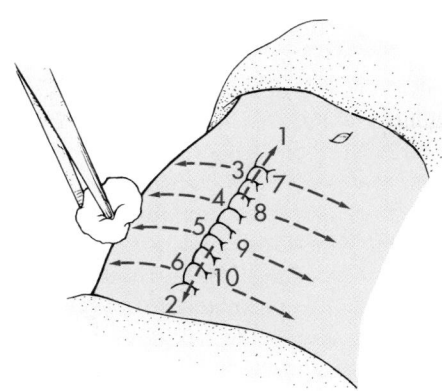

FIGURE **37-6** Method of cleansing the suture line area.

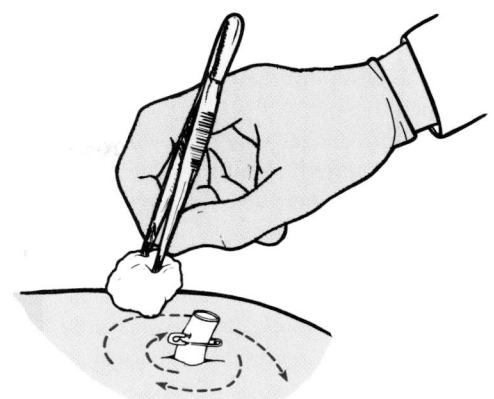

FIGURE **37-7** Cleansing a drain site.

gant has caustic or irritating properties, protect the skin with a skin protectant product and place the collection basin close to the area of the exiting fluid.

The suture line is the "least contaminated" area and is always cleansed first (Figure 37-6). The center is the most important part of the suture line; therefore, using a new sterile swab or gauze, clean the suture line by starting at the center of the suture line and working toward one end. With another sterile swab or gauze, start at the center of the incision and work toward the other end. All other cleansing involves moving from one end to the other on each side of the incision. Work in straight lines, moving away from the suture line with each successive stroke.

The drain site is cleansed using a circular stroke starting with the area immediately next to the drain (Figure 37-7). With each new swab start immediately next to drain and attempt to cleanse a little further out from the drain.

Evidence-Based Practice Trends

Guidelines for the nursing care of wounds are written in an effort to improve client outcomes and decrease costs related to chronic wound management (Beitz and Bates-Jensen, 2001). The Agency for Health Care Policy and Research (AHCPR) guidelines for pressure ulcers in adults, (1994) are valid for nursing today (Shekelle and others, 2001). The Association for the Advancement of Wound Care has developed "The Wound Patient's Bill of Rights" (Bryant, 2000). These rights make the client an active participant in the management of his or her wounds. The Wound, Ostomy and Continence Nurses Society (WOCN) provides a website with resources for nurses related to wound care. The website is found at www.wocn.org (Bryant, 2000).

A wound care team is an effective strategy to improve client outcomes for chronic wounds and to decrease costs of supplies and nursing visits related to wound care (Bedell and others, 2003). The wound care team provides early identification of client needs, facilitates continuity of client care,

and acts as a resource for evidence-based practice related to wound care.

Research has shown that wound cleansing and debridement are effective methods to prevent wound infection (Campany and others, 2000). Irrigation of wounds by nurses is a technique used for wound cleansing. Effective wound irrigation is best achieved through the use of a 35-ml syringe with a 19-gauge needle or angiocatheter with irrigation pressures delivered between 4 and 15 psi (Campany and others, 2000). When irrigation pressures exceed 15 psi, additional harm can occur to the tissues (AHCPR, 1994). There is an increased risk of wound infection because the high pressures can drive bacteria into the wound. Professional nurses need to be knowledgeable about correct wound irrigation techniques and be able to achieve effective irrigation pressures in practice (Campany and others, 2000).

Hydrodebridement with pulsed lavage, a type of irrigation using a handheld device, has been found to be an effective wound-cleansing option for clients receiving nursing care at home for chronic wounds (Morgan and Hoelscher, 2000). It allows the nurse to deliver site-specific wound care that avoids cross contamination of the wound. This type of therapy is less expensive than whirlpool therapy. Clients receiving wound cleansing with pulsed lavage experienced no pain with the treatment (Morgan and Hoelscher, 2000).

Cultural Considerations

- Assess the cultural meaning of blood and secretions.
  - Blood may be perceived as dirty (Muslims and Hindus), and stained bed linens and gowns should be changed promptly.
  - Some Asians believe that blood is the life force; hence presence of bloodstained secretion and drainage should be explained thoroughly.
  - Showing negative reactions toward the client's bloody secretions may be perceived as disrespectful by some Africans.

- Provide for privacy needs of clients from cultures that emphasize gender-congruent care and separate gender roles.
  - Prevent exposure of the client by proper draping and using bed screens.
  - Assign same-gender caregiver when giving care requiring exposure of client's private parts.
- Include family members when giving explanations about the nursing care regimen.
  - In collectivistic cultures, presence of family members at the bedside is to be expected.
  - Among Arabic families, at least one family member, usually a female, stays at the bedside all the time (Miller and Petro-Nustas, 2002).

Skill Performance Guidelines

1. Know the client's age. With age, vascular changes occur, collagen tissue is less pliable, and scar tissue is tighter. Because the epidermodermal junction becomes flatter in older adults, their skin tears more easily from mechanical trauma such as tape removal.
2. Know the client's nutritional status. Tissue repair and infection resistance are directly related to adequate nutrition, including proteins, carbohydrates, lipids, vitamins, and minerals. Clients who are malnourished are at increased risk of wound infections and wound infection-related sepsis (Rudolph, 2002).
3. Understand the risks of obesity. Inadequate vascularization decreases delivery of nutrients and cellular elements required for healing. The client is at greater risk for wound infection and dehiscence or evisceration (Mathison, 2003).
4. Identify factors that decrease oxygenation, such as decreased hemoglobin level, smoking, and underlying cardiopulmonary conditions. Adequate oxygenation at the tissue level is essential for white blood cell (WBC) activity and phagocytosis, for fibroblast proliferation and collagen synthesis, and for reepithelialization (Waldrop and Doughty, 2000). Tissue repair is negatively influenced by a hematocrit value below 33% and a hemoglobin value below 10 g/100 ml. Hemoglobin level is reduced and oxygen release to tissues is reduced in smokers.
5. Know the types of medications prescribed. Steroids reduce inflammatory response and slow collagen synthesis. Cortisone depresses fibroblast activity and capillary growth. Chemotherapy depresses bone marrow production of white blood cells and impairs immune function.
6. Identify the presence of chronic diseases or chronic trauma, such as diabetes or radiation. Decreased tissue perfusion and failure to release oxygen to tissues result from diabetes. In radiation therapy, wound healing is most effective when surgery is performed within 4 to 6 weeks of irradiation before the anticipated vascular scarring and fibrosis.
7. Unwounded skin is always stronger than healed skin that has been wounded.

SKILL 37-1 Performing Wound Irrigation

Wound cleansing and irrigation is accomplished using sterile technique for surgical wounds or clean technique for some chronic wounds. The cleansing solution is introduced directly into the wound with a syringe, syringe and catheter, shower, or whirlpool. When a syringe is used, the tip should remain 2.5 cm (1 inch) above the wound. If the client has a deep wound with a narrow opening, a soft catheter is attached to the syringe to permit the fluid to enter the wound. Irrigation should not cause tissue injury or discomfort. Fluid retention is avoided by positioning the client on the side to encourage the flow of the irrigant away from the wound. With small wounds, it is often helpful to use a 35-ml syringe with a 19-gauge needle attached to facilitate optimal pressure for cleansing with minimal risk of tissue injury (Campany and others, 2000). Ambulatory clients may benefit from the use of a handheld shower for wound cleansing, holding the shower spray approximately 12 inches (30 cm) from the wound. If the force applies too much pressure for the client's comfort, a clean washcloth may be tied around the showerhead to disperse the force. An alternative is the shower table, frequently used in burn and trauma wound care, which allows cleansing in the acute care area. For clients who require mechanical debridement and cleansing but cannot tolerate the above methods, a whirlpool bath is a useful method. The whirlpool procedure is frequently performed by or with the assistance of physical therapists, who then help to apply dressings.

There are two types of wound irrigation: high-pressure and pulsatile high-pressure lavage. High-pressure irrigation is the cleansing of a necrotic wound with irrigating fluid delivered at 4 to 15 psi, with a 35-ml syringe and a 19-gauge angiocatheter. This procedure provides force to remove wound debris without damaging healthy tissue. Pulsatile high-pressure lavage is an alternative to high-pressure irrigation. It is the use of a machine to deliver intermittent high-pressure irrigation, combined with suction to remove the irrigant and wound debris (Ramundo and Wells, 2000). A whirlpool is also commonly used to remove bacteria and debris from the surface of large wounds. In addition, a whirlpool will soften and loosen adherent necrotic tissue and cleanse and remove wound exudate.

Wound irrigations promote wound healing through removing debris from a wound surface, decreasing bacterial counts, and loosening and removing eschar. Eschar is "thick, leathery, necrotic, devitalized tissue" (AHCPR, 1994). Solutions used for irrigations include normal saline, warm water, or mild wound cleansers such as Cara Klenz, Saf Clens, and Biolex. Skin cleansers are not the same as wound cleansers and should not be indiscriminately substituted for them.

DELEGATION CONSIDERATIONS

Check institutional policy and the state's Nurse Practice Act regarding which wound care interventions can be delegated to assistive personnel. The skill of wound irrigation should not be delegated to assistive personnel. However, cleansing of chronic wounds using clean technique can be delegated. It is the nurse's responsibility to assess and document wound characteristics. Before delegating the skill the nurse must:

- Discuss modifications of the skill such as increased frequency of wound cleansing other than once a shift
- Instruct assistive personnel what to report when a wound is cleansed (e.g., wound color, presence of bleeding, drainage)
- Instruct assistive personnel to report client pain

EQUIPMENT

- ❑ Irrigant/cleansing solution (volume 1.2 to 2 times the estimated wound volume)
- ❑ Irrigation delivery system, depending on amount of pressure desired: sterile irrigation 35-ml syringe with sterile soft angiocatheter or 19-gauge needle (AHCPR, 1994) or handheld shower or whirlpool
- ❑ Clean or sterile gloves
- ❑ Waterproof underpad, if needed
- ❑ Dressing supplies (Table 37-3)
- ❑ Disposable waterproof biohazard bag
- ❑ Gown
- ❑ Goggles
- ❑ Extra towels and padding (to use to protect bed)

STEP	RATIONALE

ASSESSMENT

1. Review physician's order for irrigation of open wound and type of solution to be used.

2. Assess recent recording of signs and symptoms related to client's open wound:

   a. Extent of impairment of skin integrity, including size of wound (measure length, width, and depth). Wounds should be measured in centimeters and in the following order: length, width, and depth (Cooper, 2000).

   b. Elevation of body temperature.

   c. Drainage from wound (amount and color). Amount can be measured by part of dressing saturated or in terms of quantity (e.g., scant, moderate, copious).

   d. Odor. Must state whether or not there is odor. More frequent cleansing is needed if wound has a foul odor (AHCPR, 1994).

   e. Wound color (see Table 37-1).

   f. Consistency of drainage.

   g. Culture reports.

   h. Stage of healing of the client's wound.

Open wound irrigation requires medical order including type of solution(s) to use (Waldrop and Doughty, 2000).

This assesses volume of irrigation solution needed. Data also used as baseline to indicate change in condition of wound.

May indicate response to infection (Rudolph, 2002).
Expect amount to decrease as healing takes place. Serous drainage is clear like plasma; sanguineous or bright red drainage indicates fresh bleeding; serosanguineous drainage is pink; purulent drainage is thick and yellow, pale green, or white.
Strong odor indicates infectious process.

Color represents a balance between necrotic tissue and new scar tissue. Proper selection of wound products, based on the color of the wound, facilitates removal of necrotic tissue and promotes new tissue growth (Rolstad and others, 2000).
Type and color of drainage is dependent on moisture of the wound and type of organisms present (Cooper, 2000).
Chronic wounds heal by secondary intention, and they are often colonized with bacteria.
Client's wound characteristics determine type and amount of pressure to use during irrigation.

TABLE 37-3 COMMON WOUND DRESSING CATEGORIES

CATEGORY	DESCRIPTION	INDICATIONS	SIDE EFFECTS	EXAMPLES
Absorptive fillers	• Variety of product types including absorptive powders, pastes, and beads • Highly absorptive • Oxygen permeable • Moisture retentive • Requires secondary cover dressing	• Absorption in full-thickness wounds with moderate to heavy exudate • Autolytic debridement of yellow slough in deep wounds with uneven wound beds • Odor control • Hydrophilic cleansing action and reduction of surface bacteria	• Will desiccate wound and cause further damage if exudate is minimal • Some products may be difficult to remove if wound is deep with tunneling	Bard Absorption Dressing Chronicure Comfeel Powder DuoDERM Paste HydraGran Multidex Iodosorb Gel
Alginates	• Nonwoven mass of calcium-sodium alginate fibers that form moisture-retentive gel on contact with wound fluid • Moisture retentive • Nonocclusive • Varying levels of absorbency • Nonadhesive • Available in pads and ropes for packing • Requires secondary cover dressing to secure	• Absorption of heavy to moderate wound exudate in superficial and deep wounds • Autolytic debridement of yellow slough • Infected wounds (after appropriate intervention and with close monitoring of wound progress) • "Filler" for deep or tunneling wounds (rope form) • Hemostasis	• May contribute to wound desiccation if wound exudate is minimal and gel dries (saturate with saline to soften) • Contraindicated for use on third-degree burns • Limited hemostatic properties	CURASORB Kaltostat Sorbsan
Foams	• Semipermeable polyurethane foam dressings that have varying barrier properties • Moisture retentive • Conformable • Available in pads and pillows for filling wound cavities • Available in adhesive and nonadhesive forms • Some products require tape or secondary cover dressing to secure	• Absorption of moderate to heavy exudate in superficial and deep wounds • Protection of friable peri-wound skin (nonadhesive pads) • Infected wounds (after appropriate intervention and with close monitoring of wound progress) • Autolytic debridement of yellow slough • Padding of tracheostomy sites • Padding and protection of high-trauma areas (pretibial area, forearms, etc.)	• May promote wound dehydration and desiccation if exudate is minimal • Contraindicated for sinus tracts	Allevyn CURAFOAM Flexzan LyoFoam MitraFlex
Gauze (woven)	• Absorbent • Woven gauze is 100% meshed cotton fabric woven into squares, rolls, and packing strips • Nonwoven gauze is made of synthetic fibers pressed together to look like woven fabric • Available in sterile and nonsterile packing	• Absorption of moderate to heavy exudate in superficial and deep wounds • Protection of surgical wounds • Mechanical debridement of yellow slough (wet-to-dry gauze) • Autolytic debridement (saline-moistened gauze) • Absorption of minimal to heavy exudate in superficial and deep wounds • "Filler" for packing dead space in large, deep wound cavities • Infected wounds (moistened or impregnated with topical antimicrobials)	• May adhere to healthy tissue and cause injury on removal • Some products may shed, leaving lint in wound	Curity Gauze Sponges KERLIX Super Sponge KLING gauze rolls NUGAUZE packing strips
Hydrocolloids	• Conformable material made of gelatin, pectin and carboxymethylcellulose particles suspended in adhesive base • Moisture retentive • Highly occlusive • Wafers are available in regular and extra-thin forms and in variety of shapes	• Autolytic debridement of minimal to moderate amount of yellow slough • Protection of high-friction areas • Protection from exogenous contamination (excellent barrier function) • Absorption of minimal to moderate exudate in superficial and shallow full-thickness wounds • Fibrinolytic activity (venous leg ulcers)	• Occlusive properties can promote infection in high-risk patients (especially anaerobic infection) • Contraindicated for third-degree burns • May promote hypertrophic granulation tissue • Some products leave residue in wound on removal • Some products have an unpleasant odor on dressing removal	Comfeel Cutinova DuoDERM Restore Tegasorb

Data from Cuzzell J: Wound assessment and evaluation of wound dressings—confusion or choice? *Dermatol Nurs* 14(3):187, 2002; Hess CT: How to use gauze dressings, *Nursing* 30(9):88, 2000.

STEP	RATIONALE
i. Dressing: dry and clean; evidence of bleeding, profuse drainage.	Provides an initial assessment of present wound drainage.
3. Assess comfort level or pain on a scale of 0 to 10, and identify symptoms of anxiety.	Discomfort may be related directly to wound or indirectly to muscle tension or immobility. Anxiety results from multiple factors (e.g., surgery, diagnosis, awaiting pathology reports) and anticipation of unknown nursing interventions (e.g., first wound irrigation).
4. Assess client for history of allergies to antiseptics, tapes, or dressing material.	Known allergies suggest application of a sample of prescribed antiseptic as skin test before flushing wound with large volume of solution or selection of different tape or dressing material.

NURSING DIAGNOSES

- Risk for injury
- Pain (acute, chronic)

- Impaired skin integrity
- Impaired tissue integrity

Related factors are individualized based on client's condition or needs.

PLANNING

1. Expected outcomes following completion of procedure:
   - Client states acceptable level of comfort on 0 to 10 scale after wound irrigation.
   - Wound begins to heal; dressing is clean and dry; wound is free of drainage and inflammation, or drainage is decreased in amount or type (e.g., less bloody or serous as opposed to serosanguineous).
   - Skin integrity is maintained; no redness, edema, or inflammation noted in surrounding tissue.
2. Explain procedure of wound irrigation and cleansing.
3. Administer prescribed analgesic 30 to 45 minutes before starting wound irrigation procedure.

4. Position client.
   - Position comfortably to permit gravitational flow of irrigating solution through wound and into collection receptacle (see illustration).

   - Position client so that wound is vertical to collection basin. Place container of irrigant/cleansing solution in basin of hot water to warm solution to body temperature.
   - Place padding or extra towel in the bed.
   - Expose wound only.

Premedication, gently administered irrigation, application of clean dressing, and repositioning client ensure comfort.
Healing progresses in absence of debris and presence of protective covering.

No further skin and tissue damage has resulted from wound irrigation.
Information will reduce client's anxiety.
Promotes pain control and permits client to move more easily and be positioned to facilitate wound irrigation (Dochterman and Bulechek, 2004).

Directing solution from top to bottom of wound and from clean to contaminated area prevents further infection. Position client during planning stage keeping in mind the bed surfaces needed for later preparation of equipment.
Warmed solution increases comfort and reduces vascular constriction response in tissues.

Protects bedding.
Prevents chilling of client.

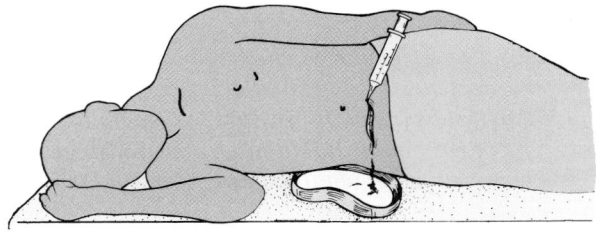

STEP 4 Client position for wound irrigation.

STEP	RATIONALE

IMPLEMENTATION

1. Perform hand hygiene.
2. Form cuff on waterproof biohazard bag, and place it near bed.

3. Close room door or bed curtains.
4. Apply gown and goggles.

5. Apply clean gloves, and remove soiled dressing and discard in waterproof bag. Discard gloves.
6. Prepare equipment; open sterile supplies.
7. Apply sterile gloves.
8. To irrigate wound with wide opening:
   a. Fill 35-ml syringe with irrigation solution.

   b. Attach 19-gauge angiocatheter.

   c. Hold syringe tip 2.5 cm (1 inch) above upper end of wound and over area being cleansed.
   d. Using continuous pressure, flush wound; repeat steps a, b, and c until solution draining into basin is clear.
9. To irrigate deep wound with very small opening:
   a. Attach soft angiocatheter to filled irrigating syringe.

   b. Lubricate tip of catheter with irrigating solution; then gently insert tip of catheter, and pull out about 1 cm (½ inch).

Rationale column:

Reduces transmission of microorganisms.

Cuffing helps to maintain large opening, thereby permitting placement of contaminated dressing without touching refuse bag itself.

Maintains privacy.

Protects nurse from splashes or sprays of blood and body fluids (Centers for Disease Control and Prevention [CDC], 1997).

Reduces transmission of microorganisms.

Prevents transfer of microorganisms to wound surface.

Flushing wound helps remove debris and facilitates healing by secondary intention.

Catheter lumen delivers ideal pressure for cleansing and removal of debris (Ramundo and Wells, 2000).

Prevents syringe contamination. Careful placement of the syringe prevents unsafe pressure of the flowing solution.

Clear solution indicates all debris has been removed.

Catheter permits direct flow of irrigant into wound. Expect wound to take longer to empty when opening is small.

Removes tip from fragile inner wall of wound.

• *Critical Decision Point*
Do not force catheter into the wound because this could cause tissue damage.

   c. Using slow, continuous pressure, flush wound.

Use of slow mechanical force of a stream of solution loosens particulate matter on the wound surface and promotes healing (Ramundo and Wells, 2000).

• *Critical Decision Point*
CAUTION: Splashing may occur during this step.

   d. Pinch off catheter just below syringe while keeping catheter in place.
   e. Remove and refill syringe. Reconnect to catheter, and repeat until solution draining into basin is clear.

Prevents aspiration of solution into syringe and contamination of sterile solution (Dochterman and Bulechek, 2004).

• *Critical Decision Point*
Pulsatile high-pressure lavage may be the irrigation of choice for necrotic wounds. The amount of irrigant is wound-size dependent. Pressure settings on the device should remain between 4 and 15 psi. The nurse should not use pulsatile high-pressure lavage on exposed blood vessels, muscle, tendon, and bone. This type of irrigation should not be used with graft sites and should be used with caution in clients receiving anticoagulant therapy (Ramundo and Wells, 2000).

STEP	RATIONALE
10. To cleanse wound with handheld shower:	
a. With client seated comfortably in shower chair, adjust spray to gentle flow; water temperature should be warm.	Useful for clients able to shower with assistance or independently. May be accomplished at home. A shower table is helpful for bed-bound or acutely ill clients.
b. Cover showerhead with clean washcloth if needed.	Reduces pressure released at shower head.
c. Shower for 5 to 10 minutes with shower head 12 inches (30 cm) from wound.	Ensures wound is thoroughly cleansed.
11. To cleanse wound with whirlpool:	
a. Adjust water level and temperature; add prescribed cleansing agent.	Wound is hypersensitive to hot temperature.

- *Critical Decision Point*
  To avoid tissue damage, position client so that water jets are not directly over clean granulating wound tissue.

b. Assist client into whirlpool, or place extremity into whirlpool.	
c. Allow client to remain in whirlpool for prescribed interval.	Ensures thorough wound cleansing.

- *Critical Decision Point*
  Clients who are confused, have poor activity tolerance, or have impaired mobility should never be left alone in the whirlpool.

12. When indicated, obtain cultures (see Chapter 43) after cleansing with nonbacteriostatic saline.	Routine culturing of open wounds is not recommended by AHCPR (1994). AHCPR (1994) recommends using quantitative bacterial cultures (tissue biopsy or wound fluid by needle aspiration) rather than swab cultures, which often detect only surface bacterial contaminants.

- *Critical Decision Point*
  Consider culturing a wound if it has a foul, purulent odor; inflammation surrounds the wound; a nondraining wound begins to drain; or client is febrile.

13. Dry wound edges with gauze; dry client if shower or whirlpool is used.	Prevents maceration of surrounding tissue from excess moisture.
14. Apply appropriate dressing (see Chapter 38).	Maintains protective barrier and healing environment for wound.
15. Remove gloves, mask, goggles, and gown.	Prevents transfer of microorganisms.
16. Assist client to comfortable position.	
17. Dispose of equipment and soiled supplies, and perform hand hygiene.	Reduces transmission of microorganisms.

▌ EVALUATION

1. Assess type of tissue in wound bed.	Identifies wound healing progress and determines type of wound cleansing and dressing needed.
2. Inspect dressing periodically.	Determines client's response to wound irrigation and need to modify plan of care.
3. Evaluate skin integrity.	Determines if extension of wound has occurred.
4. Observe client for signs of discomfort.	Client's pain should not increase as a result of wound irrigation.
5. Observe for presence of retained irrigant.	Retained irrigant is a medium for bacterial growth and subsequent infection.

Recording and Reporting

- Chart in the nurses' notes wound assessment before and after irrigation; amount, color, and odor of drainage on dressing removed; amount and type of solution used; irrigation device used; client's tolerance of the procedure; type of dressing applied after irrigation.
- Immediately report to attending physician any evidence of fresh bleeding, sharp increase in pain, retention of irrigant, or signs of shock.

Unexpected Outcomes	Related Interventions
1. Bleeding or serosanguineous drainage appears.	• Flush wound during next irrigation using less pressure. • Notify physician of bleeding.
2. Retained fluid and debris appear.	• Increase amount of fluid used during irrigation. • Increase amount of pressure when flushing wound. • Make sure wound is clear of retained fluid and debris before applying dressing.
3. Increased pain or discomfort occurs.	• Decrease force of pressure during wound irrigation. • Assess client for need for additional analgesia before wound care. • Assess client for need for additional analgesia if discomfort increases.
4. Suture line opening extends.	• Notify physician. • Reevaluate amount of pressure to use for next wound irrigation.

Teaching Considerations

- Instruct and provide written handouts to client and primary caregiver to observe wound care, and provide time for return demonstrations.
- Explain the need for specialized supplies such as irrigating solutions and dressings and the need to maintain asepsis when performing care.
- Instruct client and caregiver where and how additional supplies are obtained.
- Instruct client and primary caregiver about signs of improper wound healing and wound infection.
- Stress aseptic technique.
- Assess client's and primary caregiver's understanding of need for and methods of wound care.
- Teach client and caregiver how to make normal saline, especially if cost is an issue. Normal saline can be made by using 2 teaspoons of salt in 1 L (1 quart) of boiling water (Barr, 1995).
- Provide written instruction on dressing change.
- Client may need to receive wound care management in a free-standing wound care clinic. Be sure client has directions to clinic and knows where to park and where to obtain dressing supplies.

Pediatric Considerations

- Pediatric clients may be very frightened. They might verbally and physically try to prevent nurse from cleaning wound. Having child active in parts of procedure or working out child's feelings about wound irrigation using play therapy on a doll with a wound may help child to be more cooperative with procedure.
- Skin on neonates is immature and can easily be damaged from pressure and wound care products. Check that products are approved for use with this population. Remember that in neonates the skin readily absorbs products.
- Topical anesthetic solutions (e.g., lidocaine, adrenaline, and tetracycline [LAT] and tetracycline-phenylephrine [tetraphen]) applied to wounds supply short-term (10 to 15 minutes) anesthesia (Hockenberry and others, 2003).
- Assess need for pain management. Provide pain management before performing wound irrigation (Hockenberry and others, 2003).

Gerontological Considerations

- Wound irrigations can be traumatic, frightening, and painful to some older clients. Nurse should assess client's cooperation before doing wound irrigation. Nurse should be mindful of client's cognitive level of understanding when performing wound irrigation.

- Older adult's skin has increased potential for irritation from products used and increased risk for infection (Myer, 2000).
- Older skin loses many of its normal characteristics; therefore it is more easily damaged from trauma due to the cleaning process (Lueckenotte, 2000).

Home Care Considerations

- Assess client's home environment to determine adequacy of facilities for performing wound care; check especially for adequate lighting, running water, and storage of supplies.

- Tell client and caregiver that because normal saline has no preservatives, the bottle should be labeled with day and time, and it should be thrown out 24 to 48 hours after it is first opened or made (Barr, 1995).
- Wound care is planned in conjunction with client's total rehabilitation goals. The objective of wound care management in a subacute care setting is to return the client to his or her home environment (Beshara and others, 2000).
- Provide support for the client and caregiver during the wound healing process. Chronic wounds can take months to years to heal (Thomas and Kamel, 2000).

SKILL 37-2 Performing Suture and Staple Removal

Institutional policy determines whether *only* the physician or the physician *and* nurse may remove sutures and staples. The physician's written order is always obtained before implementing either skill. The time of removal is based on the stage of incision healing and the extent of surgery.

Sutures and staples are generally removed within 7 to 10 days after surgery if healing is adequate. Retention sutures usually remain in place 14 to 21 days. Timing the removal of sutures and staples is important. They must remain in place long enough to ensure initial wound closure with enough strength to support internal tissues and organs. Leaving the sutures in too long increases the risk of infection at the puncture sites. Sutures left in longer than 14 days generally leave scar marks (Autio and Olson, 2002). The physician determines and orders removal of all sutures or staples at one time or removal of every other suture or staple as the first phase, with the remainder removed in the second phase.

Sutures are threads of wire or other materials used to sew body tissues together. Sutures come in different sizes and are absorbent or nonabsorbent. Sutures are placed within tissue layers in deep wounds and superficially as the final

means for wound closure. The deeper sutures are usually an absorbable material that disappears in several days. Superficial sutures repair the skin using nonabsorbent sutures (Autio and Olson, 2002).

Staples are stainless steel wire. Their use is restricted by the location of the incision, because there must be adequate distance between the skin and structures that lie below the skin, including bone and vascular structures. The cosmetic result may not be as desirable as that obtained with finer suture material. Staples do provide ample strength. Removal requires a sterile staple extractor and aseptic technique.

The client's history of wound healing, site of wound, tissues involved, and the purpose of the sutures determine the suture material selected. For example, a client with repeated abdominal surgeries might require wire sutures for greater strength to promote wound closure.

The physician and/or nurse judge whether to remove all sutures if any sign of suture line separation is evident during the process of suture or staple removal. It is not uncommon to remove every other suture initially, removing the balance several days to a week later.

DELEGATION CONSIDERATIONS

This skill should not be delegated to assistive personnel. The nurse must:

- Instruct assistive personnel to report drainage, bleeding, swelling at the site or an elevation in the client's temperature to the nurse
- Instruct assistive personnel to report client's complaints of pain to the nurse
- Inform assistive personnel about any special hygiene practices following suture removal

EQUIPMENT

- ❑ Disposable waterproof bag
- ❑ Sterile suture removal set (forceps and scissors) or sterile staple extractor
- ❑ Sterile applicators or antiseptic swabs
- ❑ Steri-Strips or butterfly adhesive strips
- ❑ Clean gloves
- ❑ Sterile disposable gloves

STEP	RATIONALE

ASSESSMENT

1. Identify client with need for suture or staple removal:
   a. Check physician's order.　　Removal of sutures or staples is a dependent intervention.
   b. Review specific directions related to suture or staple removal.　　Indicates specifically which sutures are to be removed (e.g., every other suture).
   c. Determine history of conditions that may pose risk for impaired wound healing: advanced age, cardiovascular disease, diabetes, immunosuppression, radiation, obesity, smoking, poor cellular nutrition, very deep wounds, and infection.　　Preexisting health disorders affect speed of healing and may result in dehiscence.

2. Assess client for history of allergies.　　Determines if client is sensitive to antiseptic.
3. Assess client's comfort level or pain on a scale of 0 to 10.　　Provides baseline of client's comfort level to determine response to therapy.
4. Assess healing ridge and skin integrity of suture line for uniform closure of wound edges, normal color, and absence of drainage and inflammation.　　Indicates adequate wound healing for support of internal structures without continued need for sutures or staples.

- *Critical Decision Point*
  If wound edges are separated or signs of infection are present, wound has not healed properly. Notify physician because sutures or staples may need to remain in place and/or other wound care initiated.

NURSING DIAGNOSES

- Risk for infection
- Impaired skin integrity
- Risk for impaired skin integrity

Related factors are individualized based on client's condition or needs.

PLANNING

1. Expected outcomes following completion of procedure:
   - All suture material or staples are removed.　　Removes source of infection or irritation from retained sutures.
   - Suture line is intact.　　Wound is healing and does not require protective dressings.
   - Client states acceptable level of comfort on 0 to 10 scale following removal of sutures or staples.　　Client may require premedication with pain medicine before suture or staple removal.
2. Explain to client that suture removal is usually not a painful procedure but client may feel pulling or tugging of the skin.　　Gains client cooperation and reduces anxiety.

IMPLEMENTATION

1. Close curtains or room door.　　Provides privacy.
2. Position client comfortably, while exposing suture line.　　Prepares area for staple or suture removal.

- *Critical Decision Point*
  For client who is highly anxious or who has an extensive wound, consider need to administer analgesic 30 minutes before suture removal.

STEP	RATIONALE
3. Ensure direct lighting is on suture line.	Aids visibility and correct placement of forceps or extractor during removal process, ultimately reducing soft tissue injury.
4. Perform hand hygiene.	Reduces risk of infection.
5. Place cuffed refuse disposal bag within easy reach.	Provides for easy disposal of contaminated dressings and prevents passing items over sterile work area.
6. Prepare sterile field with dressing change supplies: **a.** Open sterile suture removal tray or staple extract tray, and slide contents onto prepared field, maintaining sterility of inside surface of wrapper or tray (see Chapter 9). **b.** Open sterile antiseptic swabs, and place on inside surface of tray. **c.** Open sterile glove package, exposing cuffed ends.	Allows nurse to freely handle sterile supplies.
7. Apply clean gloves. Carefully remove dressing, and discard dressing and clean gloves in prepared refuse disposal bag.	Reduces transmission of infection.
8. Inspect wound (see illustration).	Determines adequacy of wound healing.
9. Apply sterile gloves, if required by policy.	Allows nurse to handle sterile supplies.
10. Cleanse sutures or staples and healed incision with antiseptic swabs.	Removes surface bacteria from incision and sutures or staples.
11. Remove staples: **a.** Place lower tips of staple extractor under first staple. As you close handles, upper tip of extractor depresses center of staple, causing both ends of staple to be bent upward and simultaneously exit their insertion sites in the dermal layer (see illustration).	Avoids excess pressure to suture line and secures smooth removal of each staple.
b. Carefully control staple extractor.	Avoids suture-line pressure and pain.

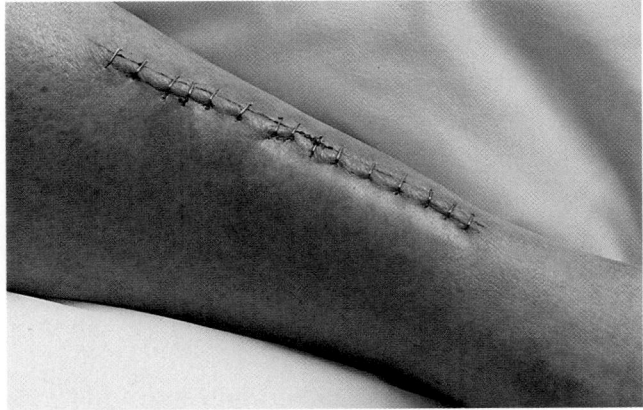

STEP 8 Suture line secured with staples.

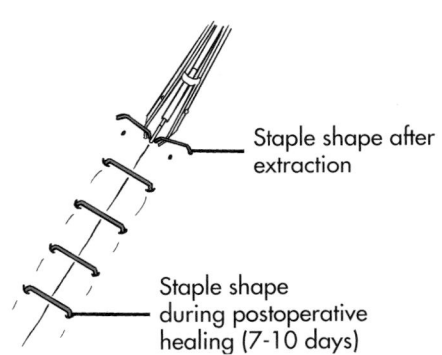

STEP 11a Staple extractor placed under staple.

Staple shape after extraction

Staple shape during postoperative healing (7-10 days)

STEP	RATIONALE

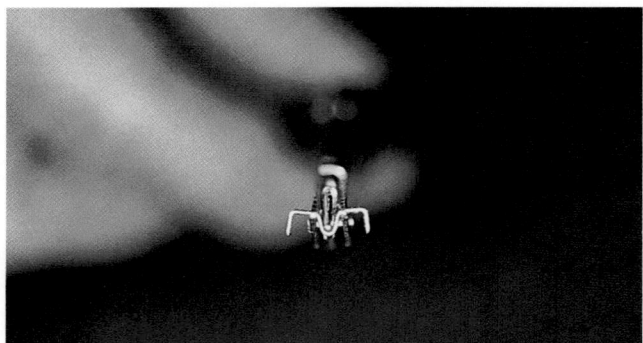

STEP **11c** Metal staple removed by extractor.

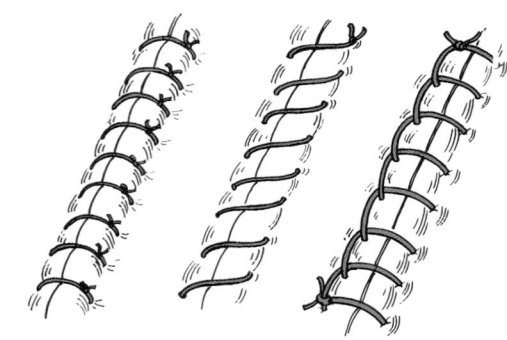

STEP **12** Types of sutures: *Left,* Intermittent; *middle,* continuous; *right,* blanket.

   c. As soon as both ends of staple are visible, move it away from skin surface, and continue on until staple is over refuse bag (see illustration).

   d. Release handles of staple extractor, allowing staple to drop into refuse bag.

   e. Repeat steps a through d until all staples are removed.

12. Remove intermittent sutures (see illustration):

   a. Place gauze a few inches from suture line. Grasp scissors in dominant hand and forceps in nondominant hand.

Prevents scratching tender skin surface with sharp pointed ends of staple for comfort and infection control.

Avoids contaminating sterile field with used staples.

Gauze serves as receptacle for removed sutures. Placement of scissors and forceps allows for efficient suture removal.

• *Critical Decision Point*
Placement of scissors and forceps is very important. Avoid pinching the skin around the wound when lifting up the suture. Likewise, avoid cutting the skin around the wound by accident when snipping the suture.

   b. Grasp knot of suture with forceps, and gently pull up knot while slipping tip of scissors under suture near skin (see illustration).

   c. Snip suture as close to the skin as possible.

Releases suture.

• *Critical Decision Point*
Never snip both ends of suture; there will be no way to remove the part of the suture situated below the surface.

   d. Grasp knotted end with forceps, and in one continuous smooth action pull the suture through from the other side (see illustration). Place removed suture on gauze.

Smoothly removes suture without additional tension to suture line.

• *Critical Decision Point*
Never pull exposed surface of any suture into tissue below epidermis. The exposed surface of any suture is considered contaminated.

STEP	**RATIONALE**

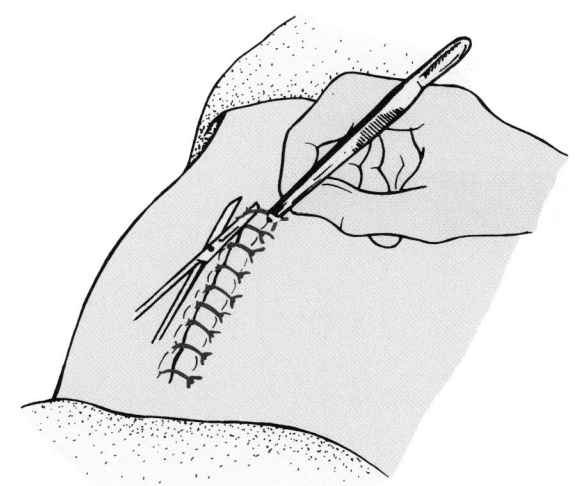

STEP **12b** Removal of intermittent suture. Nurse cuts suture as close to skin as possible, away from the knot.

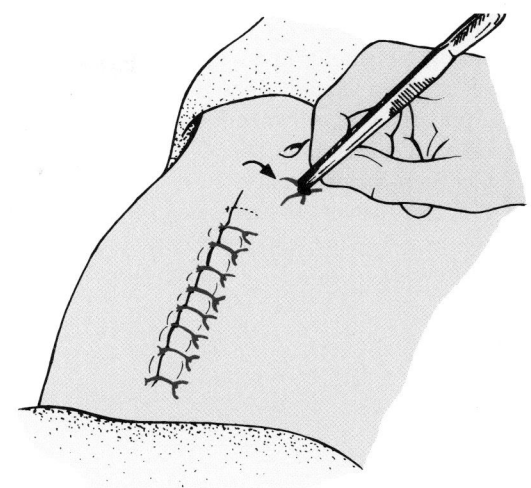

STEP **12d** Nurse removes suture and never pulls the contaminated stitch through tissues.

e. Repeat steps a through d until every other suture has been removed.	
f. Observe healing level. Based on observations of wound response to suture removal and physician's original order, determine whether remaining sutures will be removed at this time. If so, repeat steps a through d until all sutures have been removed.	Determines status of wound healing and if suture line will remain closed after all sutures are removed.
g. If any doubt, stop and notify physician.	
13. Remove continuous sutures, including blanket stitch sutures:	
a. Place sterile gauze a few inches from suture line. Grasp scissors in dominant hand and forceps in nondominant hand.	Gauze serves as receptacle for removed sutures. Placement of scissors and forceps allows for efficient suture removal.
b. Snip first suture close to skin surface at end distal to knot.	Releases suture.
c. Snip second suture on same side.	Releases interrupted sutures from knot.
d. Grasp knotted end, and gently pull with continuous smooth action, removing suture from beneath the skin. Place suture on gauze compress.	Smoothly removes sutures without additional tension to suture line. Prevents pulling of contaminated portion of suture through the skin.
e. Repeat steps a through d in consecutive order until the entire line has been removed.	
14. Inspect incision site to make sure all sutures are removed and to identify any trouble areas. Gently wipe suture line with antiseptic swab to remove debris and cleanse wound.	Reduces risk of further incision line separation.

- ***Critical Decision Point***
  Make sure that the entire suture has been removed and that no part of it has been retained in the client's wound.

STEP	**RATIONALE**

15. Apply Steri-Strips if *any* separation greater than two stitches or two staples in width is apparent to maintain contact between wound edges.
    a. Apply tincture of benzoin or Skin Prep to the skin on each side of the suture line. Allow to dry.
    b. Cut Steri-Strips to allow strips to extend 4 to 5 cm (1½ to 2 inches) on each side of the incision.
    c. Remove backing, and apply across incision (see illustration).

Supports the wound by distributing tension across the wound and eliminates closure technique scarring (Autio and Olson, 2002).
Promotes increased adherence of the Steri-Strips.

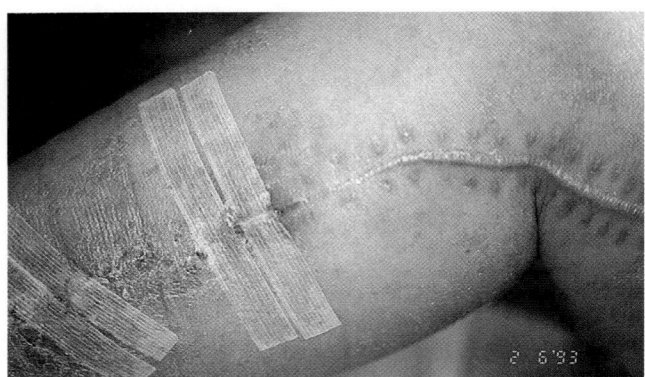

STEP 15c Steri-Strips over incision.

    d. Inform client to take showers rather than soak in bathtub according to physician's preference.
16. Apply light dressing, or expose to air if no clothing will come in contact with suture line. Instruct client about applying own dressing if it will be needed at home.
17. Discard all contaminated materials, and remove and dispose of gloves.
18. Route reusable items such as staple extractor for resterilization, and perform hand hygiene.

Steri-Strips are not removed and are allowed to fall off gradually.
Healing by primary intention eliminates need for dressing.

Reduces transmission of infection.

Reduces transmission of infection.

▌ EVALUATION

1. Assess site where sutures or staples were removed; inspect condition of soft tissues, including skin. Look for any pieces of removed suture that were left behind.
2. Determine if client has pain along incision.

Sources of infection have been removed.

Determines comfort level. Can indicate if suture material remains in skin.

Recording and Reporting

- Chart on the nurses' notes the time the sutures or staples were removed; the number of sutures or staples removed; cleansing of the suture line; appearance of the wound; level of healing of the wound; type of dressing applied if one is used; and client's response to suture or staple removal.
- Immediately notify physician of suture line separation, dehiscence, evisceration, bleeding, or purulent drainage.

Unexpected Outcomes	Related Interventions
1. Retained suture is present.	• Assess suture line closely to determine if any suture material remains. • Notify physician. • Instruct client to notify physician if signs of suture line infection develop following discharge from agency.
2. Client experiences wound separation or drainage secondary to healing problems.	• Leave remaining sutures or staples in place. • Place supportive butterfly closures across suture line. • Notify physician.

Teaching Considerations

* Crusting from around sutures can be removed with half-strength hydrogen peroxide or normal saline as long as skin is intact.
* Teach client to observe for any sign of separation of wound edges before removing remaining sutures.
* Have client apply own dressing and inspect suture line for continued healing.
* Continue instruction on resumption of bathing and showering activities, prevention of abdominal strain during defecation, and provision of adequate nutrition and ambulation.
* Explain gradual suture line skin color changes (e.g., in light-tone clients from red to natural color).
* Teach client not to put additional stress on suture line from such activities as lifting or bending (Dochterman and Bulechek, 2004). Client with abdominal surgery or injury must avoid lifting heavy packages or equipment for several weeks.
* Instruct primary caregiver and client to maintain clean technique when treating suture line and changing dressings.

* Instruct client that sometimes there may be a small amount of drainage from wound immediately after suture removal.
* Instruct client to avoid exposing wounds to the sun because this can increase scarring (Autio and Olson, 2002).

Pediatric Considerations

* Assistance may be needed to keep babies from moving during the suture removal procedure.
* Topical anesthetic solutions (e.g., lidocaine, adrenaline, and tetracycline [LAT] and tetracycline-phenylephrine [tetraphen]) applied to wounds supply short-term (10 to 15 minutes) anesthesia (Hockenberry and others, 2003).

Gerontological Considerations

* Older adults may need reassurance about suture removal procedure. Depending on their mental status, they may not understand procedure.
* Older skin may be at higher risk for dehiscence after sutures are removed.

SKILL 37-3 Managing Drainage Evacuation

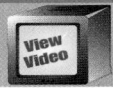

If drainage accumulates in the wound bed, wound healing is delayed. Removal of even small amounts of drainage is accomplished by either a closed or open drain system. The drain may be inserted directly through the suture line into the wound or through a small stab wound near the suture line into the wound.

An open drain system (e.g., a Penrose drain [Figure 37-8]) removes drainage from the wound and deposits it onto the skin surface. A sterile safety pin is inserted through this drain, outside the skin, to prevent the tubing from moving into the wound.

To remove the Penrose drain the physician advances the tubing in stages as the wound heals from the bottom up. Nursing interventions include caution to prevent accidental removal of the drain during dressing changes and to protect skin surfaces in direct contact with the irritating drainage. Because of the danger of accidental dislodgement and the need to assess the drain placement accurately, Penrose drains that are covered with gauze pads are managed by the nurse and are not delegated to assistive personnel. Some Penrose drains are contained within wound pouches due to the high volume of drainage from the wound.

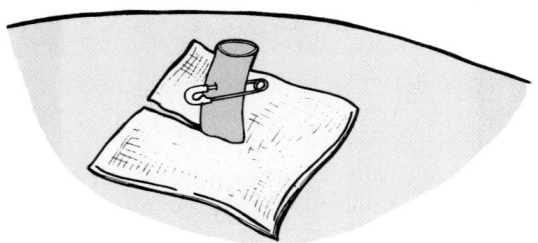

FIGURE **37-8** Penrose drain with a drain-split gauze.

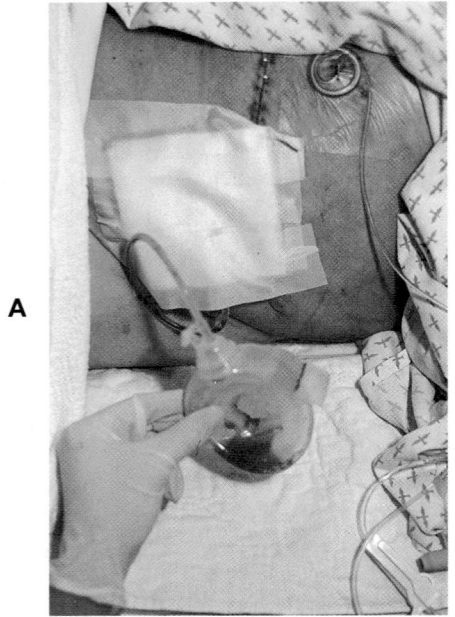

A

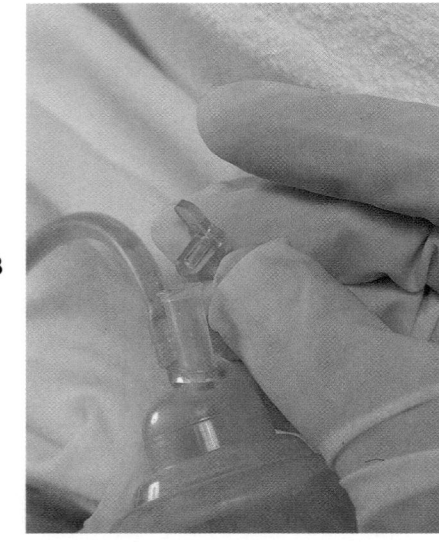

B

FIGURE **37-9** **A,** Jackson-Pratt wound drainage system.
B, Emptying Jackson-Pratt device.

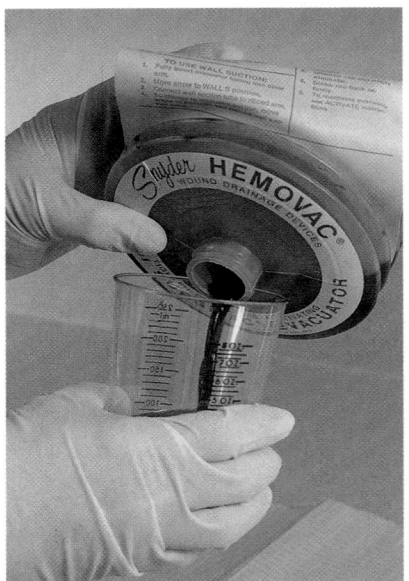

FIGURE **37-10** Hemovac contents drained into sterile measuring container.

BOX 37-3 Attaching Wound Suction Devices to Wall Suction

HEMOVAC

- Connect graduated adapter to emptying port and then to wall suction tubing.
- Set suction level as prescribed or on *low* if suction level not specified.

JACKSON-PRATT

- Attach connecting adapter to suction tubing.
- Set suction level as prescribed or on *low* if suction level not specified.
- Attach tubing with graduated connector to open port, and secure with tape.

A closed drain system (e.g., the Jackson-Pratt [JP] drain [Figure 37-9]), Hemovac drain (Figure 37-10), VacuDrain, or Constavac) relies on the presence of a vacuum to withdraw accumulated drainage from a wound bed. The drain system is connected to a clear plastic drain with multiple perforations. Drainage collects in a closed reservoir, suction bladder, or bag (Box 37-3). The closed system ensures dry skin but operates only if the tubing is patent and a vacuum exists. Drainage is emptied periodically from the reservoir, and the vacuum is reestablished.

DELEGATION CONSIDERATIONS

Assessment of wound drainage and maintenance of drains and the drainage system should not be delegated to assistive personnel. However, emptying a closed drainage container or pouch, measuring the amount of drainage, and reporting the amount on the client's intake and output (I&O) record may be delegated to assistive personnel. Before delegating this aspect of the skill the nurse must:

- Discuss with assistive personnel any modification of the skill such as increased frequency of emptying the drain other than once a shift
- Instruct assistive personnel to report any change in amount, color, or odor of drainage
- Review the intake and output procedure with assistive personnel

EQUIPMENT

- ❑ Graduated measuring cylinder
- ❑ Alcohol sponge
- ❑ Gauze sponges
- ❑ Goggles if needed
- ❑ Sterile specimen container, if culture is needed
- ❑ Sterile dressings or pouch, if drain is needed
- ❑ Clean disposable gloves
- ❑ Safety pin(s)

STEP	RATIONALE

ASSESSMENT

1. Identify presence, location, and purpose of closed wound drain and drainage system as client returns from surgery. Assess drainage present on client's dressing.

   Drainage tubing may be placed within wound or through small surgical incision near major wound.

2. Identify *number* of wound drain tubes and what drainage each one ought to be draining. Label each drain tube with a number or label.

   Assigning a labeling system to each drain helps with consistent documentation when client has multiple drainage tubes.

3. Assess if drain tube needs self-suction, wall suction, or no suction by checking physician's orders.

   Some drain tubes such as Hemovacs can be used with self-suction or wall suction.

4. Inspect system to determine presence of one straight tube or Y-tube arrangement with two-tube insertion sites.

   Allows nurse to plan skin care and identifies quantity of sterile dressing supplies needed.

5. Inspect system to ensure proper functioning. A complete systematic inspection should include the insertion site, drainage moving through tubing in direction of reservoir (tubing patent), airtight connection sites, and presence of any leaks or kinks in the system.

   Properly functioning system maintains suction until reservoir is filled; drainage is no longer being produced or accumulated. Tension on drainage tubing increases injury to skin and underlying muscle.

6. Assess client's comfort level or pain on a scale of 0 to 10.

   Provides baseline of client's comfort level to determine response to therapy.

- *Critical Decision Point*

  Attach drainage tubing with tape and a safety pin to client's gown so that it does not pull on insertion site.

7. Be sure Penrose drain has a sterile safety pin in place. Penrose drains may be covered with a gauze dressing or a wound pouch. Use caution and do not accidentally pull on drain while positioning gauze.

   Pin prevents drain from being pulled below the skin's surface.

8. Identify type of drainage container client has.

   Determines frequency for emptying drainage.

NURSING DIAGNOSES

- Risk for injury
- Risk for infection
- Impaired skin integrity

Related factors are individualized based on client's condition or needs.

STEP	RATIONALE

PLANNING

1. Expected outcomes following completion of procedure:
   - Wound healing continues.

   Client will be comfortable, and epithelialization will continue in the absence of infectious pathogens or accumulated debris.

   - Vacuum is reestablished.
   Suction system is intact.
   - Client states acceptable level of comfort on 0 to 10 scale following removal of sutures or staples.
   Client may require pain medication due to discomfort caused by wound drain.
   - Tubing is patent.
   Fluid is draining away from wound.
2. Explain procedure to client.
   Promotes client's cooperation.

IMPLEMENTATION

1. Close room door or bedside curtains.
   Provides privacy.
2. Perform hand hygiene, and apply gloves.
   Reduces transmission of microorganisms.
3. Place open specimen container or measuring graduate on bed between you and client.
   Permits measuring and discarding of wound drainage.
4. When emptying evacuator, maintain asepsis while opening port:
   Avoids entry of pathogens.
   a. Hemovac (see Figure 37-10):
       (1) Open plug on port indicated for emptying drainage reservoir.
   Vacuum will be broken, and reservoir will pull air in until chamber is fully expanded.
       (2) Tilt evacuator in direction of plug.
   Drains fluid toward plug.
       (3) Slowly squeeze two flat surfaces together while draining into sterile laboratory specimen container if culture is ordered, then drain remainder into graduated cylinder. Cover specimen container.
   Prevents splashing of contaminated drainage.
       (4) Hold uncovered alcohol sponge in dominant hand; place evacuator on flat surface with open outlet facing upward; continue pressing downward until bottom and top are in contact; hold surfaces together with one hand, quickly cleanse opening and plug with other hand, and immediately replace plug; secure evacuator on client's bed.
   Compression of surface of Hemovac creates vacuum. Cleansing of plug reduces transmission of microorganisms into drainage evacuation.
       (5) Check evacuator for reestablishment of vacuum, patency of drainage tubing, and absence of stress on tubing.
   Facilitates wound drainage and prevents tension on drainage tubing.
   b. Jackson-Pratt evacuator (see Figure 37-9, A):
       (1) Open emptying cap on side of bulb-shaped reservoir (see Figure 37-9, B).
   Breaks vacuum for drain.
       (2) Tilt drain toward direction of plug, and drain toward opening. Empty drainage from evacuator.
       (3) Compress bulb over drainage container. Cleanse ends of emptying port with alcohol sponge while continuing to compress container. Replace cap immediately. Secure evacuator below wound site with safety pin through indicated perforation to client's gown.
   Reestablishes vacuum. Reduces transmission of microorganisms into drainage evacuator and prevents tension on drainage tubing.

STEP	**RATIONALE**
5. Place and secure drainage reservoirs to prevent any pull on tubing insertion sites.	Pinning drainage tubing to client's gown will prevent tension or pulling on tubing and insertion site (Dochterman and Bulechek, 2004).

• *Critical Decision Point*
  Be sure there is slack in tubing from reservoir to wound.

6. Send labeled specimen to laboratory if ordered by physician or if purulence is noted.	Allows for culture testing to reveal infection.
7. Discard soiled supplies, remove gloves, and perform hand hygiene.	Reduces transmission of microorganisms.
8. Apply new sterile gloves, and proceed with dressing change (see Chapter 38) around drain site and inspection of skin if indicated or ordered. Split-drain sponge dressings are often used around drain tubes (see illustrations) and then covered with gauze. Penrose drains are either covered with gauze dressings or a wound pouch.	Prevents entrance of bacteria into surgical wound.
9. Discard contaminated materials, and perform hand hygiene.	Reduces transmission of microorganisms.

EVALUATION

1. Observe for drainage in drainage evacuator.	Indicates presence of vacuum, patency of tubing, and functioning of drainage evacuator.

• *Critical Decision Point*
  Clots or large collections of debris may prohibit drainage flow. An area especially prone to clogging from drainage is the Y site in the drainage tubing.

2. Inspect wound for drainage or collection of drainage fluid under the skin, causing a seroma.	Drainage should not be significant under suture line. Indicates inadequate functioning of drainage evacuator. New wound drainage appears very red at first and later changes to lighter color.

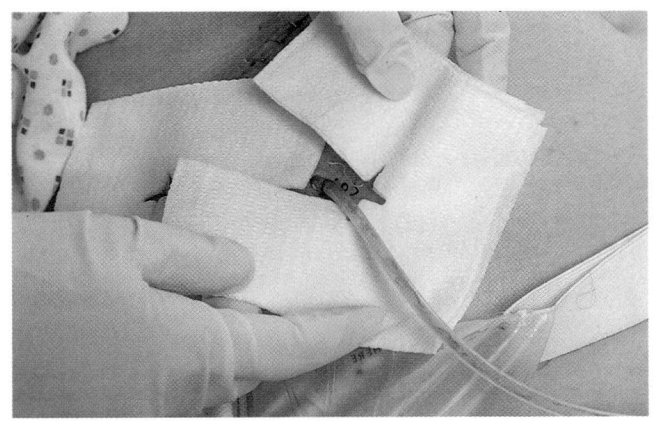 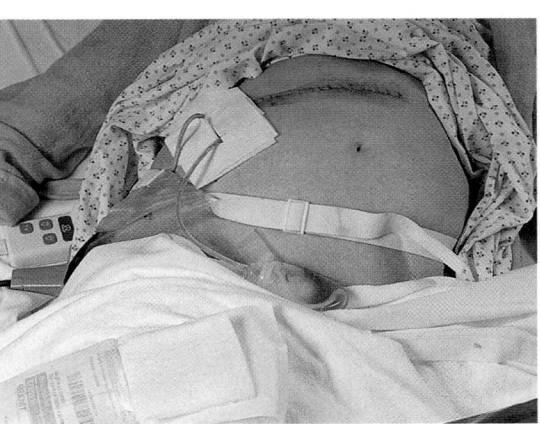

STEP 8 A, Jackson-Pratt (JP) split gauze dressing. Applying split dressing around a JP drain tube. **B,** Split dressing in place around a JP drain tube.

STEP	RATIONALE
3. Empty drainage system, and measure drainage.	Drainage collection reservoir is emptied every 8 to 12 hours and as needed for large drainage volume. The nurse collects diagnostic specimen in the presence of unexpected purulence or pungent odor, reports findings to physician, and records in progress note.
4. Assess client's level of comfort using the 0 to 10 scale.	Procedure should not increase client's pain.

Recording and Reporting

- Chart in the nurses' notes emptying of the drainage evacuator; reestablishment of vacuum in evacuator; amount, color, odor of drainage; dressing change to drain site; and appearance of drain insertion site.
- Record amount of drainage on intake and output record.
- Immediately report to the physician a sudden change in amount of drainage, either output or absence of drainage flow; pungent odor of drainage or new evidence of purulence; severe pain; or dislodgement of the drainage tube.
- Report presence of functioning drainage evacuator and emptying frequency at a change-of-shift report to nurse.

Unexpected Outcomes	Related Interventions
1. Wound becomes infected.	• Notify physician about the presence of signs of infection: purulent drainage, odor, reddened site, increased WBC count, and temperature elevation. • Use aseptic technique when changing dressings.
2. Bleeding appears.	• Determine amount of bleeding, and notify physician if excessive. • Assess for tension on client's drainage tubing. • Secure tubing to prevent pulling and pain.
3. Client experiences pain.	• Assess client's level of pain. • Medicate client. • Stabilize drainage tubing to reduce tension and pulling against incision. • Notify physician if signs of wound infection are present.
4. Drainage evacuator system is not accumulating drainage.	• Assess drainage tubing for clots. • Assess drainage system for air leaks or kinks. • Notify physician.

Teaching Considerations

- Instruct client about anticipated postoperative drainage, expected progress of wound healing and drainage volume, and estimated date of removal of drain as volume diminishes.
- Instruct client or caregiver in how to empty and record amount of drainage.
- Unexplained dark red drainage is major concern to any client. Being aware of what to expect reduces anxiety.
- Instruct primary caregiver and client in how to change dressings located around drain site.
- Instruct client to wear loose-fitting clothes.
- Instruct client to keep drain lower than waist level when ambulating, sitting, or lying down.
- Instruct client not to pull or tug on tubing; secure drain with safety pin.

Pediatric Considerations

- Have parents help to prevent pediatric clients from dislodging drainage tubes.

Gerontological Considerations

- Be aware that older adult clients with large amounts of drainage will need additional fluid intake because they are more apt to become dehydrated.
- Measures may need to be taken to prevent a confused client from pulling out drain collector.

Home Care Considerations

- Dispose of drainage in toilet.
- Wear clean gloves, and perform hand hygiene before and after procedure.
- Provide written instructions on drain care.
- Arrange for home care nurse if needed.

FOCUS *on* CLINICAL PRACTICE

You are assigned to care for Mrs. Tobias, who was readmitted to the hospital with wound dehiscence and infection following a colon resection.

1. Which factors in Mrs. Tobias's history contributed to her poor wound healing? Check all that apply. Explain your choices.
   A. Takes Prednisone daily for respiratory disease
   B. Has type 2 diabetes mellitus
   C. Takes aspirin daily due to myocardial infarction (MI) 6 years earlier
   D. Eats six small high-protein meals a day
   E. Is 74 years old
   F. Drinks 2 L of water daily
2. The physician orders Mrs. Tobias's wound to be irrigated once a shift. Mrs. Tobias asks why she has to have this done. How would you respond to Mrs. Tobias?
3. As you prepare to do the wound irrigation, how should you position Mrs. Tobias? Explain your choice.
   A. Supine with irrigation basin vertical to wound
   B. High-Fowler's with basin at base of wound
   C. Lying on her side with basin vertical to wound
   D. Low-Fowler's with basin at base of wound
4. Which intervention will help to reduce the risk of infection during wound irrigation? Check all that apply.
   A. Use sterile technique.
   B. Direct the flow of solution from healthy tissue to infected tissue.
   C. Warm irrigation solution to body temperature.
   D. Clean suture line after doing wound irrigation.
   E. Irrigate with a continuous pressure of 3 psi.
5. You note that during the wound irrigation the wound surfaces begin to bleed. What action should you take? Explain your answer.
   A. Increase amount of fluid used to irrigate wound.
   B. Assess the client's need for analgesics before irrigation.
   C. Apply a pressure dressing to wound after irrigation.
   D. Decrease pressure used to irrigate wound.

NCLEX REVIEW QUESTIONS

1. Which statement made by the client indicates a need for further teaching related to irrigating a wound after discharge?
   1. "I'll lie so the wound is vertical to the basin during the irrigation."
   2. "I'll use slow continuous pressure while irrigating my wound."
   3. "I'll warm the irrigation solution to body temperature before using."
   4. "I'll irrigate the wound starting at the bottom and move to the top."
2. The nurse assesses the color of a wound with increasing granulation tissue as:
   1. Black
   2. Red
   3. Yellow
   4. Tan
3. The nurse selects which instrument as being appropriate to irrigate a wound that has a wide opening?
   1. 10-ml syringe with 14-gauge angiocatheter
   2. 20-ml syringe with 25-gauge angiocatheter
   3. 35-ml syringe with 19-gauge angiocatheter
   4. 60-ml syringe with 23-gauge angiocatheter

Continued

NCLEX REVIEW QUESTIONS

4. Which action does the nurse take first when performing suture removal?
   1. Assemble needed equipment.
   2. Obtain the physician's order for removal.
   3. Perform hand hygiene.
   4. Instruct the client on steps in the removal.
5. Which behavior by a newly graduated nurse removing intermittent sutures needs to be corrected?
   1. Snips suture at end proximal to knot
   2. Clips suture close to skin surface
   3. Removes suture in smooth continuous manner
   4. Holds scissors in dominant hand
6. Which action should the nurse take when removing staples from an extensive abdominal wound?
   1. Position the patient in a semi-Fowler's position.
   2. Place upper tip of staple remover under staple to ease removal.
   3. Administer an analgesic 30 minutes before staple removal.
   4. Lift up on the staple when depressing the extractor handles.
7. The client asks the nurse why he has a drain in the abdomen after his surgery. What is the nurse's best response?
   1. To remove abdominal fluids to reduce stress on the suture line

2. To decrease swelling of the suture line by allowing fluid to be removed
3. To allow antibiotics to be instilled into the suture line to prevent wound infection
4. To remove drainage from the wound area to promote healing
8. Which nursing intervention should be included on the care plan for a client who has a Jackson-Pratt drain?
   1. Empty the drain every 24 hours.
   2. Pin the drainage tubing to the client's gown.
   3. Place Vaseline gauze around the tube insertion site.
   4. Secure the evacuator above the level of the wound.
9. In the first 3 hours after surgery, the 60 ml of drainage in the Jackson-Pratt drain appears very red. Which action should the nurse take?
   1. Continue to monitor the color and amount of drainage.
   2. Notify the physician immediately of the color and amount.
   3. Irrigate the drain until the drainage is pink.
   4. Increase the client's fluid intake.

References

Agency for Health Care Policy and Research: *Treatment of pressure ulcers*, Clinical practice guideline No. 15, AHCPR Pub No. 95-0653, Rockville, Md, 1994, U.S. Department of Health and Human Services, Public Health Service.

Autio L, Olson KK: The four S's of wound management: staples, sutures, Steri-strips, and sticky stuff, *Holist Nurs Pract* 16(2):80, 2002.

Barr JE: Principles of wound cleansing, *Ostomy Wound Manage* 7A(suppl 41):15S, 1995.

Beitz JM, Bates-Jensen B: Algorithms, critical pathways, and computer software for wound care: contemporary status and future potential, *Ostomy Wound Manage* 47(4): 33, 2001.

Beshara M, Jameson G, Barr B: Practice development in acute and long-term care settings. In Bryant RA, editor: *Acute and chronic wounds: nursing management,* ed 2, St. Louis, 2000, Mosby.

Bryant RA, editor: *Acute and chronic wounds,* ed 2, St. Louis, 2000, Mosby.

Centers for Disease Control and Prevention: *Part II:* Recommendations for isolation precautions in hospitals, *1997, http://wonder. cdc.gov/wonder/prevguid/p000049/p0000419.asp.*

Cooper DM: Assessment, measurement, and evaluation: their pivotal roles in wound healing. In Bryant RA, editor: *Acute and chronic wounds,* ed 2, St. Louis, 2000, Mosby.

Cuzzell J: Wound assessment and evaluation of wound dressings—confusion or choice? *Dermatol Nurs* 14(3):187, 2002.

Davidson M: Sharpen your wound assessment skills, *Nursing* 32(10):32, 2002.

Dochterman JC, Bulechek GM: *Nursing interventions classification (NIC),* ed 4, St. Louis, 2004, Mosby.

Hess CT: How to use gauze dressings, *Nursing* 30(9):88, 2000.

Hockenberry MJ and others: *Wong's nursing care of infants and children,* ed 7, St. Louis, 2003, Mosby.

Lueckenotte AG: *Gerontologic nursing,* ed 2, St. Louis, 2000, Mosby.

Mathison CJ: Skin and wound care challenges in the hospitalized morbidly obese patient, *J Wound Ostomy Continence Nurs* 30:78, 2003.

Mendez-Eastman S: Guidelines for using negative pressure wound therapy, *Adv Skin Wound Care* 14(6):314, 2001.

Myer AH: The effects of aging on wound healing, *Top Geriatr Rehabil* 16(2):1, 2000.

Ramundo J, Wells J: Wound debridement. In Bryant RA, editor: *Acute and chronic wounds: nursing management,* ed 2, St. Louis, 2000, Mosby.

Rolstad BS and others: Principles of wound management. In Bryant RA, editor: *Acute and chronic wounds: nursing management,* ed 2, St. Louis, 2000, Mosby.

Rudolph DM: Why won't this wound heal? Understand the causes of and interventions for chronic wounds, *Am J Nurs* 102(2): 24, 2002.

Thomas DR, Kamel HK: Wound management in postacute care, *Clin Geriatr Med* 16(4):783, 2000.

Waldrop J, Doughty DB: Wound healing physiology. In Bryant RA, editor: *Acute and chronic wounds: nursing management,* ed 2, St. Louis, 2000, Mosby.

Research References

Bedell B and others: How a wound resource team saved expenses and improved outcomes, *Home Healthc Nurse* 21(6):397, 2003.

Campany E and others: Nurses' knowledge of wound irrigation and pressures generated during simulated wound irrigation, *J Wound Ostomy Continence Nurs* 27:296, 2000.

Miller J, Petro-Nustas W: Context for care of Jordanian women, *J Transcult Nurs* 13(3):228, 2002.

Morgan D, Hoeslscher J: Pulsed lavage: promoting comfort and healing in home care, *Ostomy Wound Manage* 46(4):44, 2000.

Shekelle PG and others: Validity of the Agency for Healthcare Research and Quality clinical practice guidelines: how quickly do guidelines become outdated, *JAMA* 286(12):1461, 2001.

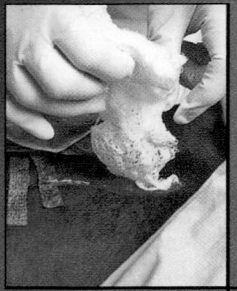

38

Dressings

MEDIA RESOURCES

Evolve Site *evolve*

http://evolve.elsevier.com/Perry/skills
- Weblinks
- Video clips
- Mosby's Nursing Skills Video Exercises

Mosby's Nursing Skills Videos/CD-ROM
- *Wound Care Video:* Dressing changes, wet-to-dry dressings and use of wound V.A.C. system

OBJECTIVES

Mastery of content in this chaper will enable the nurse to:

- Properly assess a wound.
- Choose the correct dressing for a wound.
- Understand the technique of a dressing application.
- State advantages and disadvantages of the types of dressings used.
- Correctly apply dry, wet-to-dry, pressure, and synthetic dressings.
- Correctly change a Wound Vacuum Assisted Closure dressing.

KEY TERMS

Dead space	Hydrogel
Debridement	Macerated
Dehiscence	Neovascularization
Epithelialization	Occlusive dressing
Erythema	Pressure dressing
Evisceration	Primary dressing
Excoriated	Secondary dressing
Exudate	Wound Vacuum Assisted
Granulation	Closure
Hydrocolloid	

Wound characteristics identified during assessment, along with treatment goals, determine the type of dressing needed (Agency for Health Care Policy and Research [AHCPR], 1994)). Wounds heal best in a moist environment. The concept of moist wound healing revolutionized wound management and served as a catalyst for the development of many moisture-retentive dressings (see Skills 38-3 through 38-5). This was especially true for treatment of pressure ulcers (Box 38-1). Dressings are two types. A primary dressing comes in direct contact with the wound bed. Secondary dressings are used to cover or hold primary dressings in place.

Dressings serve several functions, including maintenance of a moist environment (Ovington, 2001b), protection from outside contaminants, protection from further injury, prevention of the spread of microorganisms, increased client comfort, and control of bleeding. The ideal dressing is based on the purpose of the dressing. For example, to control bleeding, a dressing must be applied with pressure. When wound drainage is present, the dressing must be highly absorbent. An alginate, foam, or hydrocolloid dressing is used in a non-infected wound that is draining a moderate to large amount of exudate (Nelson and Dilloway, 2002) (see Chapter 37).

Another factor to consider when choosing a dressing is ease of application. The dressing should conform to body contours and should be durable but flexible, cost-effective, able to absorb or contain exudate, easily removed without damage to the healing surface, and acceptable in appearance (Ovington, 2001b).

BOX 38-1   AHCPR 1994 Dressing Recommendations

- Use a dressing that keeps the ulcer bed continuously moist. Wet-to-dry dressings should be used only for debridement and are not considered continuously moist saline dressings.
- Use clinical judgment to select a type of moist wound dressing suitable for the ulcer. Studies of different types of moist wound dressings showed no differences in pressure ulcer healing outcomes.
- Choose a dressing that keeps the surrounding (periulcer) intact skin dry while keeping the ulcer bed moist.
- Choose a dressing that controls exudate but does not desiccate the ulcer bed.
- Consider caregiver time when selecting a dressing.
- Eliminate wound dead space by loosely filling all cavities with dressing material. Avoid overpacking the wound.
- Monitor dressings applied near the anus, because they are difficult to keep intact.

When changing a dressing the nurse must be knowledgeable about wound healing to differentiate a normal or expected appearance from abnormal changes. Assessment of the exudates absorbed by the dressing provides valuable diagnostic information.

Primary healing takes place when tissue is cleanly cut and the margins are reapproximated. Repair should occur without complication. New capillary circulation bridges the wound quickly in 3 to 4 days, and once normal tissue oxygenation is achieved, the wound is considered to be healed. A wound closed for primary healing is most susceptible to infection during the first 4 days.

Healing by secondary intention occurs when a wound is left open. Healing results in the formation of granulation tissue from the bottom of the wound and eventual epithelialization from the sides of the wound to close the defect made by the wound. During the process of epithelialization, epithelial cells migrate and proliferate from the wound edges to cover the wound surface. Burns, infected wounds, and deep pressure ulcers heal in this manner (Waldrop and Doughty, 2000).

The type of dressing used depends on the wound characteristics and the goal of wound management, which can be wound debridement or wound healing. Various types of dressings can be applied to wounds (Cuzzell, 2002b; Milne and Houle, 2002; Ovington, 2001b, 2002). Given the many types of dressings that are now available, the nurse may find it difficult to decide which dressing is best to use on a particular wound. Some nurses may find the flow sheet in Figure 38-1 helpful in selecting the appropriate dressing to care for a particular wound (Maklebust and Palleschi, 1996).

Woven gauze dressings, the oldest and most common type, do not interact with wound tissues and thus cause little wound irritation (Hess, 2000). Gauze comes in a variety of sizes and shapes. The nurse applies gauze either moist or dry, depending on whether the wound needs debridement, a moist healing environment, or a covering to prevent trauma.

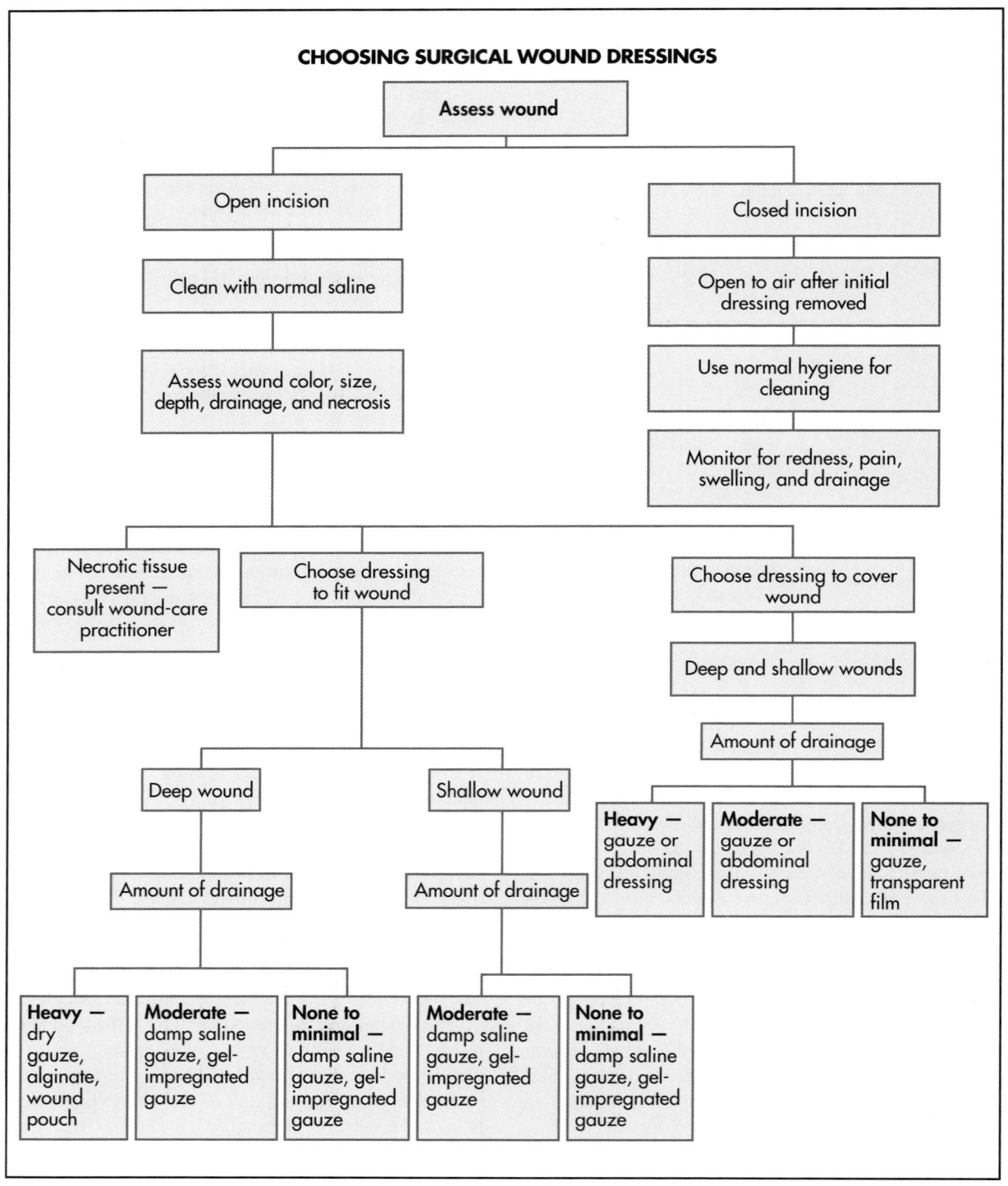

FIGURE **38-1** Flow chart for dressing selection.

Wet-to-dry (also called moist-to-dry) dressings are used for wounds requiring debridement (see Skill 38-1). The nurse moistens the gauze layer that touches the wound surface (primary dressing). *This dressing should not be so moist that it will never dry out.* The moistened gauze increases the absorptive ability of the dressing to collect exudate and wound debris. This then is covered with a secondary dressing layer that is dry. When the inner moistened gauze dressing is dried, it is then removed from the wound. As the gauze is pulled from the wound, the wound tissue that has adhered to the gauze is removed, thus effectively debriding the wound. Wet-to-dry dressings are an example of mechanical nonselective debridement (Capasso and Munro, 2003). For example, to maintain the moist environment needed for wound healing, wet-to-wet (damp-to-damp or moist-to-moist) dressings rather than dry dressings should be used in a clean granulating wound.

Telfa gauze dressings contain a shiny, nonadherent surface on one side. When used as a contact layer, the Telfa gauze usually does not stick to incisions or wound openings. Drainage passes through the nonadherent (shiny) surface to the softened gauze above.

Dressings are also available as thin, self-adhesive elastic films (e.g., Op-Site, Bioclusive, Blisterfilm, Acu-derm, Tegaderm, PRO-CLUDE, Polyskin) (see Skill 38-3). The dressing is a synthetic permeable membrane that acts as a temporary second skin. This type of dressing has several advantages: (1) it adheres to undamaged skin to contain exudate and minimize wound contamination, (2) it serves as a barrier to external fluids and bacteria but allows the wound surface to "breathe," (3) it promotes a moist environment that speeds epithelial cell growth, and (4) it can be removed without damaging underlying tissues (Cuzzell, 2002b; Nelson and Dilloway, 2002). Other advantages are that it allows the client to shower and it permits direct observation of the wound. A disadvantage of such a dressing is that it cannot debride an infected wound. The film is ideal for small, superficial wounds. This type of dressing can be used to autolytically debride a necrotic wound. It is also useful as a dressing over an intravenous catheter site. The transparent film allows the nurse to assess the wound without removing the dressing.

The hydrocolloid dressings (DuoDERM, Comfeel, Restore, Tegasorb, and others) represent a category of hydroactive dressings (see Skill 38-4). These dressings provide a moist environment for wound healing while facilitating the softening and subsequent removal of wound debris. The dressing promotes wound healing by providing an occlusive protective barrier that absorbs drainage from the wound into the dressing. In addition, the dressing stays in place through an adhesive backing, reduces local pain, and may be used with wound exudate absorbers (e.g., DuoDERM granules) to increase time between dressing changes (Cuzzell, 2002b).

Hydrogel dressings (e.g., Vigilon, Biolex, Nu-Gel, IntraSite Gel, Carrington-Gel) have a high moisture content (95%), causing them to swell and retain fluid (see Skill 38-4). They are useful over clean, moist, or macerated tissues. The dressing provides a nonadherent, protective barrier with the ability to absorb wound drainage (Cuzzell, 2002b). These dressings are very soothing and cooling, thus making them especially useful for painful burn wounds. A secondary dressing is needed to hold these dressings in place.

Foam dressings (e.g., Allevyn, LyoFoam, Epi-Lock, BIOPATCH, CURAFORM) absorb light-to-heavy amounts of exudate, are conformable, and can easily be made to fit a wound (see Skill 38-4). These properties make them especially useful for treating leg ulcers.

Evidence-Based Practice Trends

The type of wound care and dressing change required will determine whether clean or sterile technique should be used (Wooten and Hawkins, 2001). Currently there is not sufficient research evidence in nursing to demonstrate whether using clean or sterile technique is more effective at decreasing wound infection rates and promoting wound healing (Gray and Doughty, 2001). Current practice recommends using sterile gloves for postoperative dressing changes in the first 24 to 48 hours after surgery (St. Clair and Larrabee, 2002). The use of clean technique does reduce the cost of supplies for wound care (Gray and Doughty, 2001). Nurses should follow the guidelines established at their health care institution related to use of clean or sterile technique for dressing changes (Gray and Doughty, 2001; St. Clair and Larrabee, 2002).

Different types of dressings demonstrate comparable healing outcomes for wounds but vary in cost (Capasso and Munro, 2003; Graumlich and others, 2003). Hydrocolloid and collagen dressings were shown to be equally effective in healing pressure ulcers. However, the collagen dressings were more expensive (Graumlich and others, 2003). A comparison of wet-to-dry normal saline gauze dressings and hydrogel dressings showed equivalent healing rates in the treatment of arterial and diabetic wounds. The use of hydrogel dressings resulted in a lower cost (Capasso and Munro, 2003).

A new technique called woundoscopy is available to assess nonhealing wounds (Kehoe and Elmore, 2002). The technique uses a sterilized endoscope to view deep sinus tracts in wounds without the client's having to go to surgery. The benefits of woundoscopy include improved ability to assess sinus tracts, detection and removal of foreign bodies in the wound, and avoidance of surgery for clients (Kehoe and Elmore, 2002).

A "Wound Burden" Scale has been developed to describe the severity of wounds and estimate the cost of wound care (Pompeo, 2001). The scale has been found to be an effective measure in estimating wound care costs in a long-term care setting. Clients who had higher wound burden had significantly higher wound care costs (Pompeo, 2001).

Cultural Considerations

Different cultures and religious practices attribute different meanings to wounds and trauma. It is important to assess and try to understand the different meaning about blood and wounds and how it may affect clients and their families. Some cultures, such as those from East Asia, may interpret loss of blood and secretions as loss of one's spiritual and vital life energy. Orthodox Jewish clients consider blood and secretions of the individual as part of his spiritual being that should be treated with care and respect. Other cultures, such as Muslims and Hindus, may perceive blood as dirty; hence soiled dressings and linens must be disposed of promptly.

Dressing changes always require a respect for the client's privacy. However, clients from other cultures may have additional privacy needs such as the need for gender-congruent caregivers, especially if dressings are located in areas considered private. If possible, drape the client and prevent entrance of the opposite sex into the room with the client uncovered. In addition, the client may find it helpful if a family member is present during the procedure.

Dressing changes are at times painful. Take time to understand cultural differences in expressions of pain and beliefs toward pain medications. For some cultural groups (Hindus, Russians, Asians), the nurse may offer the pain medication even if the client does not complain of pain. Some clients (Koreans) may express somatic symptoms such as improved sleep and appetite (Park and others, 2001). When possible and appropriate, be sure to accommodate cultural care modalities such as heat and cold when performing wound irrigations. If permitted, use warm or room temperature solutions when the condition is categorized as cold to achieve balance and healing. Most Asians believe that clients in cold conditions (febrile conditions, postpartum) are considered vulnerable to the cold and wind (Andrews, 2003; Nowak, 2003).

Skill Performance Guidelines

1. Determine the goals of wound management. For example, certain dressings can be used to debride wounds, whereas others can be used to maintain a moist wound

---

BOX 38-2 Types of Wound Exudate

- *Serous,* which is a clear, watery plasma
- *Sanguineous,* which indicates fresh bleeding
- *Serosanguineous,* which is a pale, more watery drainage than sanguineous drainage
- *Purulent,* which is a thick, yellow, green, or brown drainage

---

environment necessary for granulation tissue to fill wound defects in a clean wound.

2. Know the cause or type of wound. Wounds caused by vascular insufficiency, diabetes, pressure, trauma, and surgery are all very different and must have an individualized treatment plan (Cuzzell, 2002a). Not knowing the cause of the wound can have serious negative effects if the nurse uses treatments that are contraindicated for certain types of wounds.

3. Know the expected amount and type (Box 38-2) of wound exudate or drainage. Wounds that have large amounts of drainage require more frequent dressing changes or need dressings that are capable of absorbing large amounts of drainage. Such wounds include fresh postoperative sites, open wounds, and fistulae.

4. Know the type of dressing ordered. Wet-to-dry dressings require more equipment than do dry dressings. Pressure dressings require elastic bandages to maintain the pressure.

5. Determine if wound drainage tubes are present. This prevents their accidental dislocation when the old dressing is removed (see Skill 37-3).

6. Determine the presence of any further break in skin integrity adjacent to the wound. Breaks in skin integrity further increase the client's risk for infection.

7. The location of the wound, the care setting that the client is in, and the client's level of activity influence the decision of what dressing to use.

SKILL 38-1 Applying a Dressing (Dry or Wet-to-Dry)

A dry dressing may be chosen for wound healing by primary intention with little drainage. The dressing protects the wound from injury, prevents introduction of bacteria, reduces discomfort, and speeds healing.

Dry dressings are most commonly used for abrasions and nondraining postoperative (primary intention healing) incisions. The dry dressing does not debride the wound and should not be selected for wounds requiring debridement. In addition, a dry dressing is not appropriate for an open

wound that is healing by secondary intention. If a dry dressing adheres to a wound, the nurse should moisten the dressing with sterile normal saline or water before removing the woven gauze. Moistening the dressing in this manner decreases the adherence of the dressing to the wound and reduces the risk of further trauma to the wound.

Wet-to-dry dressings are gauze moistened with an appropriate solution. For this reason, wet-to-dry dressings are sometimes called moist-to-dry or damp-to-dry dressings be-

TABLE 38-1	PROBLEMS ASSOCIATED WITH WOUNDS REQUIRING DEBRIDEMENT
PROBLEM	**NURSING ACTIVITIES**
Solutions used may be irritating to healthy skin around wound.	Protect healthy skin with protective barrier, such as Stomahesive, or apply topical ointments, such as zinc oxide. If zinc oxide is used, it should be removed with mineral oil. Avoid scrubbing of the skin because the scrubbing can cause harm to the epithelial layer.
Wound becomes excessively dry.	Continually moist dressing (with a physician's order) might be tried. Eliminate fine mesh gauze, and lightly pack wound with fluffy gauze dampened with prescribed solution.
Wound is deep, and retention of dressing in cavity is suspected.	Irrigate wound copiously with prescribed solution to loosen dressing for removal. Use continuous "ribbon" or strip of gauze to dress deep wounds.
Wound drainage is damaging healthy tissue.	Protect healthy tissue with skin barrier, such as a hydrocolloid. Wounds with large amounts of drainage may benefit from occlusive drainage collection device.
Client's skin is irritated by tape.	Use hydrocolloid under tape, use Montgomery ties as needed, use fabric tape that has multidirectional stretch, secure dressing with binder, or wrap with roll gauze if on extremity.

cause this terminology more accurately describes what the dressing should be. In clinical practice these terms (wet-to-dry, moist-to-dry, and damp-to-dry) are considered synonymous.

The primary purpose of wet-to-dry dressings is to mechanically debride a wound. The moistened contact layer of the dressing (primary dressing) increases the absorptive ability of the dressing to collect exudate and wound debris (Ovington, 2001a). As the dressing dries, it adheres to the wound and debrides the wound of the tissue when the dressing is removed. One must *take care not to apply a dressing so wet that it remains wet continuously* (Table 38-1). A dressing that is too wet may cause tissue maceration and bacterial growth. It also does not dry out and therefore does not remove the necrotic tissue when being removed from the wound. The moistened gauze must be covered with a secondary dressing layer that is dry. Disadvantages to wet-to-dry dressings are that the dressing needs to be changed every 4 to 6 hours and the removal of the dry dressing is likely to cause pain to the client (Nelson and Dilloway, 2002).

Woven gauze should be used to pack wounds (Hess, 2000). Principles for correctly packing a wound can be found in Box 38-3. Commonly used wetting agents include normal saline and lactated Ringer's solution, which are isotonic solutions that aid in mechanical debridement. Acetic acid is effective against *Pseudomonas aeruginosa* but is toxic to fibroblasts in standard dilutions.

Povidone-iodine, usually one-quarter to one-half strength, is a rapid-acting antimicrobial agent for cleansing *intact* skin. It should never be used on a healthy granulating wound bed. This agent should be used only in select situations for short-

> **BOX 38-3   Principles for Packing a Wound**
>
> - Use the wound characteristics to decide what type of packing is appropriate.
> - Make sure the packing material can be safely used to pack a wound.
> - Moisten the packing material with a noncytotoxic solution such as normal saline. Never use cytotoxic solutions (e.g., povidone-iodine) to pack a wound.
> - If using woven gauze, fluff it before packing it into the wound.
> - Loosely pack the wound.
> - Do not let the packing material drag or touch the surrounding wound tissue before you put it into the wound.
> - Fill all the wound dead space with the packing material.
> - Pack the wound until you reach the wound surface; never pack the wound higher than the wound surface.

term use. In open wounds this solution is toxic to fibroblasts (AHCPR, 1994). No well-controlled research studies document that bacteria levels decrease in chronic open wounds when povidone-iodine was applied (Milne and Houle, 2002). Other antibiotic solutions may be ordered, although their use is controversial. See Chapter 37 for a more detailed discussion of appropriate solutions to use to clean wounds. Because they can harbor microorganism growth, solutions should be discarded 24 to 48 hours after opening and replaced with fresh solutions. All solution bottles must be clearly labeled with date and time of opening.

DELEGATION CONSIDERATIONS

The care of acute new wounds and those that require sterile technique or a wet-to-dry dressing for dressing change should not be delegated to assistive personnel. The skill of applying a dry dressing or changing the top dressing may be delegated to assistive personnel. The assessment of the wound must be done by the RN and is not delegated to assistive personnel. If the dressing change is delegated to assistive personnel, the nurse must still assess the wound. Before delegating this aspect of skill, the nurse must:

- Discuss with assistive personnel any unique modifications of the skill, such as the need for use of special tape or taping techniques to secure the dressing
- Instruct assistive personnel about the signs of infection and poor wound healing and to immediately report the findings for further assessment

EQUIPMENT

- ❑ Clean disposable gloves
- ❑ Sterile gloves
- ❑ Sterile dressing set (scissors, forceps) (may be optional, check institution policy)
- ❑ Sterile drape (optional)
- ❑ Dressings: Fine mesh gauze, sterile dressings, abdominal (ABD) pads
- ❑ Sterile basin (optional)
- ❑ Antiseptic ointment (as prescribed)
- ❑ Cleansing solution as prescribed
- ❑ Sterile normal saline or prescribed solution
- ❑ Tape, ties, or bandage as needed (include nonallergic tape if necessary)
- ❑ Protective waterproof underpad
- ❑ Waterproof bag
- ❑ Adhesive remover (optional)
- ❑ Measurement device (optional): tape measure, camera (optional)
- ❑ Protective gown, mask, goggles used when spray from wound is a risk
- ❑ Additional lighting if needed (e.g., flashlight, treatment light)

STEP	RATIONALE

ASSESSMENT

1. Assess size of wound to be dressed (see Chapters 15 and 37).	Assists nurse in planning for proper type and amount of supplies needed.
2. Assess location of wound.	Wound location alerts nurse to dressing type needed and if assistance is needed to hold dressings in place.
3. Ask client to rate pain using a scale of 0 to 10.	Removal of dressing can be painful; client may require pain medication before dressing change to allow drug's peak effect during procedure.
4. Assess client's knowledge of purpose of dressing change.	Determines level of support and explanation required by client.
5. Assess need and readiness for client or family member to participate in dressing wound.	Prepares client or family member if dressing must be changed at home.
6. Review medical orders for dressing change procedure.	Indicates type of dressing or applications to use.
7. Identify clients with risk factors for wound-healing problems, including:	Physiological changes due to aging, chronic illness, poor nutrition, medications, and cancer treatments have the potential to affect wound healing (Wysocki, 2002).
a. Aging	Physiological changes of aging alter the immune system, resulting in decreased resistance to pathogens (Myer, 2000).
b. Prematurity	The skin of premature babies is not mature and does not have the immune functions of normal skin.
c. Obesity	Subcutaneous tissue has diminished vascularity.
d. Diabetes	Vascular changes associated with diabetes reduce blood flow to peripheral tissues; also leukocyte malfunction occurs secondary to hyperglycemia.
e. Compromised circulation	Results in inadequate supply of nutrients, blood cells, and oxygen to wound.
f. Poor nutritional state	Impairs stages of inflammation and collagen formation states.
g. Immunosuppressive drugs	Decreases inflammatory response and decreases collagen synthesis.

STEP	RATIONALE
h. Irradiation in area of wound	Decreases blood supply to tissues.
i. High levels of stress	Increased cortisol levels reduce number of lymphocytes and decrease inflammatory response.
j. Steroids	Slows rate of epithelialization and neovascularization and inhibits contraction.

NURSING DIAGNOSES

- Risk for infection
- Deficient knowledge regarding dressing application
- Acute pain
- Impaired skin integrity

Related factors are individualized based on client's condition or needs.

PLANNING

1. Expected outcomes following completion of procedure:	
• Client's wound is free of infection; drainage begins to diminish in amount, and wound closure is progressing.	Indicates wound is healing appropriately.
• Client reports minimal discomfort.	Indicates dressing procedure and choice are appropriate.
• Client or family explains method of dressing application.	Indicates learning has occurred.
2. Explain procedure to client.	Decreases client's anxiety.
3. Position client to allow access to area to be dressed.	Facilitates application of dressing.
4. Plan dressing change to occur 30 minutes following administration of analgesic.	Dressing change is better tolerated by client if pain medication has been administered at least 30 minutes before dressing change.

IMPLEMENTATION

1. Close room or cubicle curtains. Perform hand hygiene. Apply gown, goggles, and mask if risk of spray exists.	Provides for privacy and reduces transmission of microorganisms.
2. Position client comfortably, and drape to expose only wound site. Instruct client not to touch wound or sterile supplies.	Draping provides access to the wound yet minimizes unnecessary exposure.
3. Place disposable bag within reach of work area. Fold top of bag to make cuff. Put on clean disposable gloves.	Ensures easy disposal of soiled dressings. Prevents contamination of bag's outer surface. Prevents transmission of infectious organisms.
4. Remove tape: pull parallel to skin, toward dressing, and hold down uninjured skin. If over hairy areas, remove in the direction of hair growth. Remove remaining adhesive from skin.	Pulling tape toward dressing reduces stress on suture line or wound edges and reduces irritation and discomfort (Nelson and Dilloway, 2002).
5. With clean gloved hand or forceps remove dressings. Carefully remove outer secondary dressing first, and then remove inner primary dressing that is in contact with the wound bed. If drains are present, slowly and carefully remove dressings one layer at a time. Keep soiled undersurface from client's sight.	The purpose of the primary dressing is to remove necrotic tissue and exudate. Appearance of drainage may be upsetting to client. Avoids accidental removal of drain.

- **Critical Decision Point**

  In wet-to-dry dressing, the inner primary dressing if applied properly will have dried and will adhere to underlying tissues; do not moisten it. It is incorrect technique and a common error by some clinicians to moisten the dried gauze before removing it. This defeats the purpose of using this type of dressing and reduces the amount of debris the dressing will remove (Ramundo and Wells, 2000).

STEP	RATIONALE
6. Inspect wound for color, edema, drains, exudate, and integrity (see illustration). Observe appearance of drainage on dressing. Assess for odor. Gently palpate the wound edges for drainage, bogginess, or client report of increased pain. Measure wound size (length, width, and depth [if indicated]) (see Chapters 15 and 37).	Provides assessment of drainage and of wound's condition. Indicates status of healing. Presence of bleeding during this type of dressing change is an indication that healthy tissue is being injured (Capasso and Munro, 2003).

• **Critical Decision Point**
Dressings that are heavily saturated with exudate indicate a need to add more absorbent gauze dressing to the wound. Assess the wound for any changes in color, drainage, odor, or edema.

STEP	RATIONALE
7. Describe the appearance of the wound and any indicators of wound healing to the client.	Wounds may appear unsettling and frightening to clients; it is helpful for the client to know that the wound appearance is as expected and what healing is taking place.
8. Dispose of soiled dressings in disposable bag. Remove gloves by pulling them inside out. Dispose of gloves in bag. Perform hand hygiene.	Reduces transmission of microorganisms to other persons.
9. Open sterile dressing tray or individually wrapped sterile supplies. Place on bedside table (see illustration).	Sterile dressings remain sterile while on or within sterile surface. Preparation of all supplies prevents break in technique during dressing change.
10. Open prescribed cleansing solution, and pour over sterile gauze.	Keeps supplies sterile. Solution may be packaged to spray/pour directly on wound.

• **Critical Decision Point**
If sterile drape or gauze packages become wet from solution, this causes contamination; repeat preparation of supplies.

STEP	RATIONALE
11. Put on gloves, clean or sterile depending on institution policy.	Sterile gloves allow handling of sterile supplies without contamination. Follow the guidelines of the health care institution related to clean versus sterile gloves. There is insufficient research to support either sterile or clean gloves as being more effective in decreasing infection and improving wound healing (Gray and Doughty, 2001).

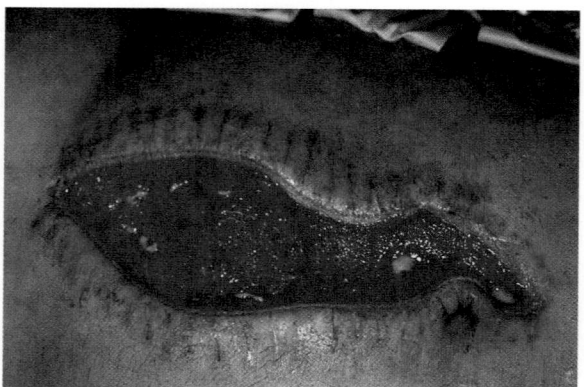

STEP 6 Abdominal wound with beefy red granulation tissue present and attached wound edges. (From Bryant RA: *Acute and chronic wounds: nursing management,* ed 2, St. Louis, 2000, Mosby.)

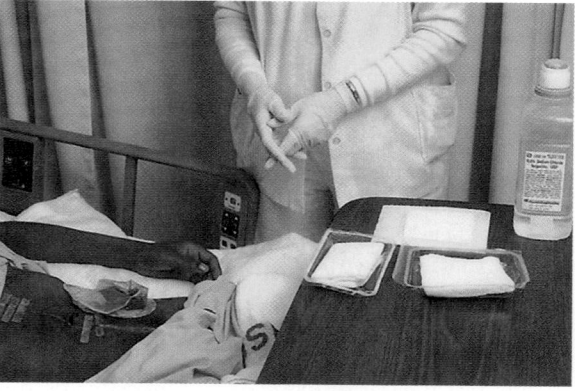

STEP 9 Sterile dressing supplies.

STEP	RATIONALE
12. Cleanse wound (see Chapter 37):	
a. Use separate swab for each cleansing stroke, or spray wound surface.	Prevents contaminating previously cleaned area.
b. Clean from least contaminated area to most contaminated.	Cleansing in this direction prevents introduction of organisms into wound.
c. Cleanse around the drain (if present), using circular stroke starting near drain and moving outward and away from the insertion site.	Correct aseptic technique in cleansing to prevent contamination.
13. Use dry gauze to blot in same manner as in step 12 to dry wound.	Drying reduces excess moisture, which could eventually harbor microorganisms.
14. Apply antiseptic ointment if ordered, using same technique as for cleansing.	Helps reduce growth of microorganisms.
15. Apply dressings to incision or wound site:	A dressing over a wound can help clients gradually adjust to changes in body image (West and Gimbel, 2000).
a. Dry dressing	
(1) Apply loose woven gauze as contact layer.	Promotes proper absorption of drainage.
(2) Cut 4 × 4 gauze flat to fit around drain if present or use precut split-drain flat.	Secures drain and promotes drainage absorption at site (see Skill 37-3).
(3) Apply additional layers of gauze as needed.	Layering ensures proper coverage and optimal absorption.
(4) Apply thicker woven pad (e.g., Surgipad, abdominal dressing).	This type of dressing is often used for postoperative wounds. Soft dressings over wounds protect the wound from irritation and provide support (West and Gimbel, 2000).
b. Wet-to-dry dressing	
(1) Place fine mesh gauze in container of sterile solution.	

● *Critical Decision Point*

Open or "fluff" the woven gauze that will be placed directly against the wound bed. Sometimes "packing strip" may be used to pack the wound (see Figure 38-2). When using packing strip, with sterile scissors cut the amount of dressing that is anticipated to be used to pack the wound. Do not let the packing strip touch the side of the bottle. Pour prescribed solution over the packing gauze or strip to moisten it. Contact layer must be totally moistened to increase dressing's absorptive abilities (Ramundo and Wells, 2000).

(2) Wring out excess fluid, and apply moist, fluffed woven-mesh gauze or packing strip directly onto wound surface without having the gauze touch the surrounding skin (see illustration A).	Moist gauze absorbs drainage and adheres to debris (Hess, 2000). The inner gauze should be moist but not dripping wet. The moist gauze must be able to dry in the wound. Having the inner gauze too wet so it does not dry is a common error in technique for this type of dressing.

● *Critical Decision Point*

If wound is deep, gently lay moistened woven gauze over wound surface with forceps until all surfaces are in contact with moist gauze and the wound is loosely filled. Fill the wound, but avoid packing the wound too tightly or having the gauze extend beyond the top of the wound (see illustration step 15b[2], B).

STEP	**RATIONALE**

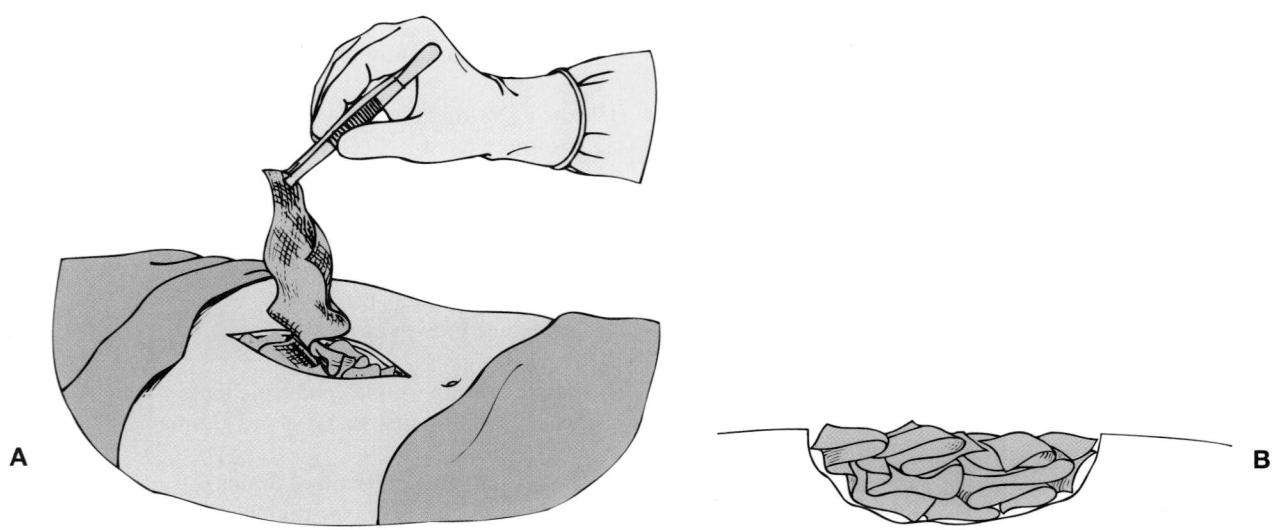

STEP **15b(2)** **A,** Packing wound. **B,** Wound packed loosely,

(3) Make sure any dead space from sinus tracts, undermining, or tunneling is loosely packed with gauze.

(4) Apply dry sterile gauze over wet gauze.

(5) Cover the packed wound with a secondary dressing such as an ABD pad, Surgipad, or gauze (see illustration).

Do not overpack the wound too tightly; it can cause wound trauma when the dressing is removed (Ramundo and Wells, 2000).

Dry layer pulls moisture from wound.

Protects wound from entrance of microorganisms.

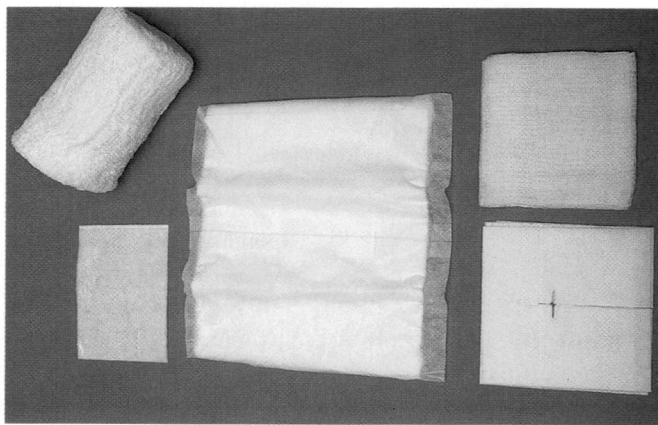

STEP **15b(5)** Secondary wound dressings.

STEP	**RATIONALE**

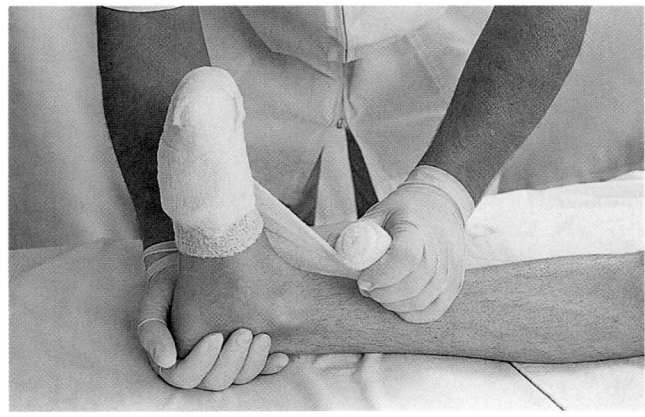

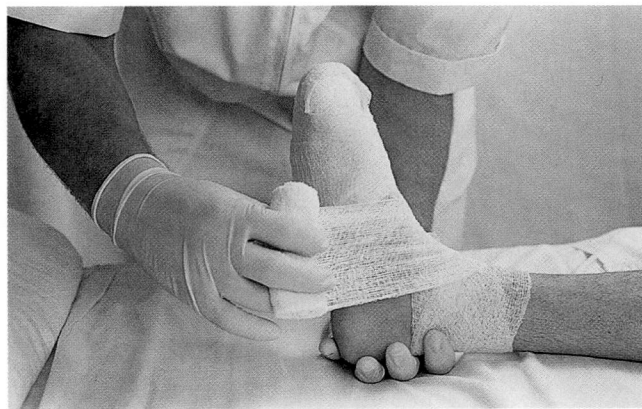

STEP **16(1)** Application of roll gauze.

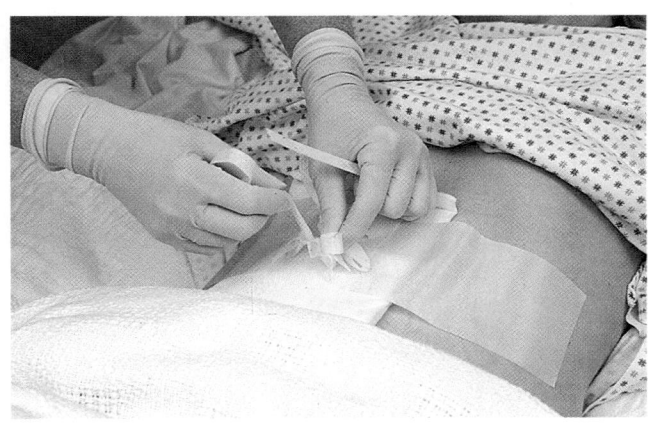

STEP **16(2)** Securing Montgomery ties.

16. Secure dressing with roll gauze (for circumferential dressings) (see illustrations), tape, Montgomery ties or straps (which are applied perpendicular to the wound) (see illustration), or binder.

Supports wound and ensures placement and stability of dressing.

- *Critical Decision Point*
  If areas of redness appear from tape, paper tape or alternatives, such as elastic bandage, Kerlix, or a binder may be used to secure dressing. Sometimes strips of a hydrocolloid dressing are placed on the skin under the Montgomery ties to further protect the skin.

17. Remove gloves, gown if worn, and dispose of them in bag. Dispose of all supplies. Remove goggles if worn.

Reduces transmission of microorganisms. Clean environment enhances client comfort.

18. Assist client to comfortable position.

Promotes client's sense of well-being.

19. Perform hand hygiene.

Reduces transmission of microorganisms.

STEP	RATIONALE

▌ EVALUATION

1. Inspect condition of wound and presence of any drainage.

Determines rate of healing.

2. Ask if client has pain during procedure.

Pain may be early indication of wound complication or result of dressing pulling tissue.

3. Inspect condition of dressing at least every shift.

Determines status of wound drainage.

4. Ask client to describe steps and techniques of dressing change.

Evaluates client's learning.

Recording and Reporting

- Chart in the nurses' notes appearance of wound, color, presence and characteristics of exudate, change in wound characteristics, especially drainage amount, type and amount of dressings applied, and tolerance of client to dressing change.
- Report to physician unexpected appearance of wound drainage or accidental removal of drain, bright red bleeding, or evidence of wound dehiscence or evisceration.
- Record frequency of dressing change and supplies needed on care plan.
- Write nurse's initials, date, and time of dressing change on a piece of tape in ink (not marker), and place on dressing.

Unexpected Outcomes	Related Interventions
1. Wound drainage increases.	• Increase frequency of dressing changes. • Notify physician, who may consider drain placement or alternate dressing method.
2. Wound bleeds during dressing change.	• Assess patient medication history and history of bleeding disorder. • If excessive, may need to apply pressure. • Observe color and amount of drainage. • Notify physician.
3. Client reports sensation that "something has given way under the dressing."	• Remove dressing, and inspect wound for dehiscence or evisceration. • Protect wound. Cover with sterile moist dressing. • Instruct client to lie still. • Remain with client to monitor vital signs. • Notify physician.
4. Before discharge, client is unable to describe proper application of dressing.	• Provide additional teaching or support. • Include caregiver in teaching plan. • Obtain services of home care agency if needed.
5. Skin around wound margins becomes red, macerated, or excoriated.	• The outer layer of the wet-to-dry dressing is too moist. • Securing method for dressing is causing irritation. Change to paper tape.

Teaching Considerations
* Explain risks of improper wound care.
* Wounds out of client's reach and vision require assistance from another caregiver.
* Anxiety or fear can decrease the client's learning capacity. Include family member or caregiver in teaching.
* Explain expected wound appearance, what should be reported, and risks of improper wound care. Provide client with a written list of what should be reported.
* After demonstrating wound care, allow client or caregiver to perform dressing change with and without supervision.

Pediatric Considerations
* Check that dressing products are safe to use on pediatric clients, especially on premature infants.
* Pediatric clients may be fearful of dressing changes. Obtaining client's cooperation and/or having another person available to keep child from moving during dressing change procedure may be needed (Hockenberry and others, 2003).
* Older child may need something to do during dressing changes. Listening to music or watching video helps to relieve some of the boredom or stress during procedure (Hockenberry and others, 2003).

Gerontological Considerations
* Dressing change procedure may be a source of pain and misunderstanding for a confused or disoriented client.

* Normal aging results in loss of thickness, elasticity, vascularity, and strength of skin tissue. As a result, there is an increased risk for skin tear when removing adhesive from older adult's skin (Lueckenotte, 2000).
* Normal aging changes of skin tissue may also delay wound-healing process (Lueckenotte, 2000).

Home Care Considerations
* Ability of caregiver and amount of time needed to change a particular dressing should be considered when selecting a dressing procedure in the home care setting. "In the home care setting, caregivers may choose more expensive dressing materials to reduce the frequency of dressing changes" (AHCPR, 1994).
* Assess extent of wound or incision in relation to client's level of activity to determine type of dressing that will achieve desired purpose.
* Assess area where procedure will be performed for adequate lighting. Determine if a table or cabinet is available on which sterile supplies may be placed with reasonable security.

Long-Term Care Considerations
* Centers with subacute care units often provide specialized wound care. Clients are admitted to center for continued wound care management (Thomas and Kamel, 2000).
* Be sure dressing is secure so that client can actively participate in physical therapy and other activities that increase independence.

SKILL 38-2   Applying a Pressure Bandage

A pressure bandage is a temporary treatment for the control of excessive bleeding. The bleeding is usually sudden and not anticipated. It may follow surgical intervention, or it may be a life-threatening occurrence related to accidental trauma, stabbing, suicide attempt, or other injury. Following application of the pressure dressing itself, sandbags are placed adjacent to the dressing to augment pressure.

An adult weighing 154 pounds (70 kg) has a total volume of 5 L of circulating blood. All nursing actions must be rapidly and effectively executed when excessive blood loss occurs. Once pressure has been applied, it must continue until definitive actions can be executed by the health care team. Surgical repair is most often the option of choice.

DELEGATION CONSIDERATIONS
The skill of applying a pressure dressing should not be delegated to assistive personnel. The *assessment* of the wound, condition of the pressure dressing, and the circulation status distal to the pressure dressing is the nurse's responsibility. Instruct assistive personnel to:
* Observe the pressure dressing to make sure that it remains in place and that there is no visible bleeding from the site
* Observe under the client for bleeding

EQUIPMENT
* ❑ Sterile gauze
* ❑ Gauze roll bandage
* ❑ Adhesive tape
* ❑ Gloves
* ❑ Sandbags
* ❑ Protective gown, mask, goggles (used when spray from wound is a risk)

STEP	RATIONALE

ASSESSMENT

1. Identify clients at risk for unexpected bleeding:

   a. Traumatic injury
   b. Donor graft site
   c. Arterial puncture sites
   d. Postoperative wounds
   e. Wounds after surgical debridement
   f. History of bleeding disorder

Nurse should be familiar with conditions associated with unexpected bleeding to rapidly respond to bleeding.

Nurse should review the client's history for potential problems.

PHASE I: IMMEDIATE ACTION—FIRST NURSE

1. Identify client with sudden hemorrhage:
   a. Locate external bleeding site.

   Maintaining asepsis and privacy are considered only if time and severity of blood loss permit inclusion of these activities. NOTE: Wounds to the groin area can result in large amounts of blood loss, which is not always visible.

   b. Apply direct pressure immediately.

   Hemostasis maintained as supplies are prepared.

2. Seek assistance.

   Bandage must be quickly secured.

PHASE II: APPLYING PRESSURE BANDAGE—SECOND NURSE

1. Quickly observe location of bleeding.

   Bleeding source determines method and supplies needed for applying pressure bandage. Arterial bleeding is bright red and gushes forth in waves, related to heart rhythm; if vessel is very deep, flow will be steady. Venous bleeding is dark red and flows smoothly. Capillary bleeding is oozing of dark red blood; self-sealing controls this bleeding. Hemorrhage is loss of a large amount of blood either externally or internally in short period of time.

2. Quickly observe area underneath client for blood.

   Blood will flow with gravity to the lowest point. Frequently a large volume of blood may be underneath client and not initially visible.

3. Quickly assess client's pulse, blood pressure, skin color, anxiety/restlessness, and changes in level of consciousness. Reassess every 5 to 15 minutes until client is stabilized.

   Findings of tachycardia, hypotension, diaphoresis, restlessness, and diminished urinary output indicate impending hypovolemic shock.

NURSING DIAGNOSES

- Decreased cardiac output
- Deficient fluid volume

- Impaired skin integrity
- Ineffective peripheral tissue perfusion

Related factors are individualized based on client's condition or needs.

PLANNING

1. Expected outcomes following completion of procedure:
   - Bleeding is temporarily controlled.
   - Circulation to distal parts is adequate.
   - Fluid loss is minimal.
   - Client's blood pressure and pulse remain within normal range.

   Source of bleeding is controlled with pressure.
   Blood flow to periphery is maintained.
   Loss of blood is controlled.

STEP	RATIONALE

IMPLEMENTATION

1. Apply clean gloves. *If client's condition permits,* perform hand hygiene, apply clean gloves, and provide privacy.

Maintaining asepsis and privacy are considered only if time and severity of blood loss permit inclusion of these activities.

2. First person presses on site of bleeding. Second person unwraps roller bandage and places within easy access.

Hemostasis maintained as supplies are prepared. Pressure dressing provides interim control of bleeding.

3. Second person quickly cuts three to five lengths of adhesive tape and places them within easy reach.

Bandage must be quickly secured.

4. In *simultaneous coordinated actions:*

   a. Rapidly cover bleeding area with many thicknesses of gauze compresses. First person slips fingers out as other nurse exerts adequate pressure to continue controlling bleeding.

   Gauze is absorbent. Layers provide bulk against which local pressure can be applied to bleeding site.

• *Critical Decision Point*

   As soon as possible elevate extremity or area of bleeding. Elevation assists in decreasing the rate of blood loss.

   b. Adhesive strips are placed 7 to 10 cm (3 to 4 inches) beyond width of dressing with even pressure on both sides of nurse's fingers as close as possible to central bleeding source. Secure tape on distal end, pull tape across dressing, and maintain firm pressure as proximate end of tape is secured.

   Tape exerts downward pressure, promoting hemostasis.

   To ensure blood flow to distal tissues and prevent tourniquet effect, adhesive tape must not be continued around entire extremity.

• *Critical Decision Point*

   Do not tape around circumference.

   c. Remove fingers temporarily, and quickly cover center of area with third strip of tape.

   Provides pressure to source of bleeding.

   d. Continue reinforcing area with tape as each successive strip is overlapped on alternating sides of center strip. Also continue applying pressure.

   Prevents tape from loosening.

   e. When pressure bandage is on extremity, apply roller gauze: apply two circular turns tautly on both sides of fingers that are pressing gauze. Compress over bleeding site. Simultaneously remove finger pressure and apply roller gauze pressure over center. Continue with figure-eight turns. Secure end with two circular turns and strip of adhesive (see Skill 38-1).

   Roller gauze acts as pressure bandage, exerting more even pressure over extremity.

• *Critical Decision Point*

   Start pressure bandage from distal to proximal working toward the heart.

5. Remove gloves, and perform hand hygiene.

Reduces the spread of microorganisms.

STEP	RATIONALE
■ EVALUATION	
1. Immediately evaluate client to determine response to pressure dressing.	
a. Observe for control of bleeding	Effective pressure bandage controls bleeding without blocking distal circulation.
b. Evaluate adequacy of circulation (distal pulse, skin characteristics)	Determines level of perfusion to distal body parts.
c. Estimate volume of blood loss (e.g., count number of dressings used, weigh saturated dressing)	Determines blood and fluid replacement needs.
d. Measure vital signs	Identifies client's adaptation to blood loss and early stages of hypovolemic shock.

Recording and Reporting

- Report immediately to physician present status of client's bleeding control, time bleeding was discovered, estimated blood loss, nursing interventions (including effectiveness of applied pressure bandage), apical and distal pulses, blood pressure, sensorium level, signs of restlessness, and need for physician to administer to client without delay.
- Record and implement physician's verbal orders in response to above reporting. (NOTE: Institutional policy on telephone/verbal orders varies.)
- Chart in nurses' notes status of client's bleeding control, time bleeding was discovered, estimated blood loss, nursing interventions (including effectiveness of applied pressure bandage), vital signs, distal pulses, consciousness level, signs of restlessness, and notification of physician.
- Shift-change report includes emergency situation, intervention and evaluation as reported to physician, and need for continuous bedside monitoring of bleeding control, distal pulse, vital signs, intravenous (IV) therapy, consciousness level, oxygenation or hypoxia, and anxiety level.

Unexpected Outcomes	Related Interventions
1. Excessive pressure is exerted that results in pain, weak or absent pulses, edema of distal body part, or tissue necrosis.	• Release pressure slightly, and monitor distal circulation every 5 to 10 minutes.
2. Uncontrolled hemorrhaging progresses to fluid and electrolyte imbalance, tissue hypoxia, confusion, hypovolemic shock, cardiac arrest, and death.	• Initiate IV therapy (physician's order is required) for fluid replacement. • Initiate nothing-by-mouth (NPO) order because surgical intervention may be needed. • Apply pressure to pressure point as needed; place client in Trendelenburg's position; provide warmth. • Monitor vital signs every 5 to 15 minutes (apical, distal rate, blood pressure). • Monitor dressing for signs of bleeding. • Reinforce dressing with tape as needed to prevent seepage. If dressing is saturated, replace only top layers so as not to disturb any clot formation at the wound site.

Teaching Considerations

- Explain purpose of pressure bandage.
- Explain need to monitor vital signs.
- Explain need for client to remain quiet and stay in position to reduce bleeding.

Pediatric Considerations

- Child will calm down if care providers and family remain calm.

Gerontological Considerations

- Due to the normal changes of aging, the older adult has an increased risk for vascular and tissue changes distal to the pressure dressing. Therefore assess skin and pulse distal to the pressure bandage frequently.

Home Care Considerations

- At home client may apply pressure with clean towels or linen.
- Emergency system (911) should be activated.
- Client should be positioned to promote elevation of affected body part (if extremity) and promote relaxation.
- If a puncture wound occurs from a penetrating object (e.g., knife, toy, building materials), do not remove the object. Removal of object will cause more rapid blood loss and may damage underlying structures.

SKILL 38-3   Applying a Transparent Dressing

A film dressing is a "clear, adherent, nonabsorptive, polymer-based dressing that is permeable to oxygen and water vapor but not to water" (AHCPR, 1994) (Figure 38-2). Polyurethane moisture and vapor-permeable film dressing were developed to manage superficial wounds. They are often used following laparoscopic surgery. Film dressings can also be used prophylactically on high-risk intact skin (Rolstad and others, 2000).

Transparent dressings can also be used for autolytic debridement of small wounds with little or no exudate (Rolstad and others, 2000). Pain and discomfort are diminished with the use of a transparent dressing, and the film conforms well to different body contours. Therefore bodily movement is less restricted. Transparent dressings may be with or without adhesives. If without adhesives, secure with hypoallergenic tapes.

With the use of a transparent dressing, a moist exudate forms over the wound surface, which prevents tissue dehydration and allows for rapid, effective healing by speeding epithelial cell growth. Because these dressings are clear, the wound can be visualized without removing the dressing. For best results these dressings should be used on clean, de-

brided wounds that are not actively bleeding. The film should be applied wrinkle free but not stretched over the skin. Should the fluid accumulation take on a white, opaque appearance with erythema of the surrounding tissue, one must assume an infectious process is under way, and the dressing should be removed and a wound culture obtained.

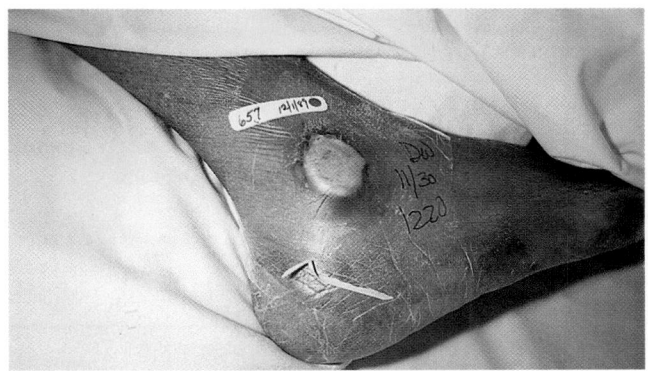

FIGURE **38-2** Transparent dressing.

DELEGATION CONSIDERATIONS

The skill of applying a transparent dressing may be delegated to assistive personnel. However, the care of acute new wounds and those that require sterile technique for dressing change generally remain within the domain of professional nursing. The assessment of the wound should not be delegated to assistive personnel even if the dressing change is delegated. The nurse should assess the wound after the dressing is removed by assistive personnel. Before delegating this skill the nurse must:

- Discuss with assistive personnel any unique modification of the skill such as removal or special taping needed
- Instruct assistive personnel about the signs of infection or poor wound healing to report

EQUIPMENT

- ❑ Sterile gloves (optional)
- ❑ Dressing set (optional)
- ❑ Sterile saline or other agent (as ordered)
- ❑ Clean disposable gloves
- ❑ Cotton swabs
- ❑ Waterproof bag for disposal
- ❑ Mineral oil (optional)
- ❑ Transparent dressing (size as needed)
- ❑ Sterile gauze pads (4 × 4 inches)
- ❑ Skin preparation materials (optional)
- ❑ Protective gown, mask, goggles (used when spray from wound is a risk)

STEP	RATIONALE

ASSESSMENT

1. Assess location and size of wound to be dressed (see Chapter 37). | Allows nurse to determine supplies and assistance needed.
2. Review physician's orders for frequency and type of dressing change. | Physician orders frequency of dressing changes and special instructions.
3. Assess client's level of comfort. | Client who is comfortable during procedure is less likely to move suddenly, causing wound or supply contamination. Dressing change procedure can be painful, and client may need pain management.
4. Assess client's knowledge of purpose of dressing. | Identifies client's learning needs.
5. Assess risk for impaired wound healing (see Chapter 37). | Physiological changes due to aging, chronic illness, poor nutrition, medications, and cancer treatments have the potential to affect wound healing (Wysocki, 2002).

NURSING DIAGNOSES

- Risk for infection
- Acute pain
- Impaired skin integrity

Related factors are individualized based on client's condition or needs.

PLANNING

1. Expected outcome following completion of procedure:
   - Wound heals rapidly with little pain and mobility restriction for client. | Dressing effective in preventing infection and promoting healing.
2. Explain procedure to client. | Relieves anxiety and promotes understanding of healing process.
3. Position client to allow access to dressing site. | Facilitates application of dressing.

IMPLEMENTATION

1. Close door or cubicle curtains; keep sheet or gown draped over body parts not requiring exposure. | Provides privacy and decreases transfer of microorganisms.
2. Cuff top of disposable waterproof bag, and place within reach of work area. | Cuff prevents accidental contamination of tip of outer bag.
3. Perform hand hygiene, and put on clean disposable gloves. Moisture-proof gown, mask, and eye goggles are worn when risk of spray exists. | Reduces transmission of infectious organisms from soiled dressings to nurse's hands (Nelson and Dilloway, 2002).

STEP	**RATIONALE**
4. Remove old dressing. For easier removal, ease off using cotton swab soaked in mineral oil, or secure piece of tape to corner of dressing and pull back slowly in a direction parallel to the wound rather than upward.	Reduces excoriation or irritation of skin following dressing removal. The stretching action breaks the seal to increase ease of removal (Rolstad and others, 2000).
5. Dispose of soiled dressings in waterproof bag, remove disposable gloves by pulling them inside out, dispose of them in waterproof bag, and perform hand hygiene.	Reduces transmission of microorganisms.
6. Prepare sterile dressing supplies.	Reduces risk of break in sterile technique.
7. Pour saline or prescribed solution over 4 × 4 sterile gauze pads.	Maintains sterility of dressing.
8. Apply clean or sterile gloves (check institution policy).	Allows nurse to handle dressings.
9. Cleanse area gently with moist 4 × 4 sterile gauze pads, or spray with wound cleanser. Cleanse from least contaminated to most contaminated area (see Chapter 37).	Reduces introduction of organisms into wound.
10. Pat dry skin around wound thoroughly with dry 4 × 4 sterile gauze pads.	Transparent dressing with adhesive backing does not adhere to damp surface (Rolstad and others, 2000).
11. Inspect wound for tissue type, color, odor, and drainage; measure if indicated.	Appearance indicates state of wound healing.

- *Critical Decision Point*
  If wound has a large amount of drainage, choose another dressing that can absorb this amount of wound drainage rather than transparent film dressing, which can absorb only light to moderate amounts of drainage.

12. Apply transparent dressing according to manufacturer's directions (see Figure 38-2). *Film should not be stretched during application.* Avoid wrinkles in film.	Wrinkles would provide tunnel for exudate drainage.

- *Critical Decision Point*
  Know specific characteristics of the brand of film dressing you are applying. Some film dressings can be removed during application process and reapplied to correct application errors such as being applied too tight or too loose with wrinkles.

13. Remove gown and goggles. Remove gloves by pulling inside out, and discard in prepared bag.	Reduces risk of microorganism transfer.
14. Assist client to comfortable position.	Enhances client comfort and relaxation.
15. Discard soiled dressing change materials properly, and perform hand hygiene.	Reduces transmission of microorganisms.

EVALUATION

1. Inspect condition of wound on ongoing basis.	Determines status of wound healing. Wound can be easily viewed.
2. Evaluate client's level of comfort.	Determines if pain resulted from procedure.

Recording and Reporting

- Report signs and symptoms of infection and poor wound healing to the physician.
- Chart in the nurses' notes the characteristics of wound: color, odor, viscosity, and amount of drainage; application of dressing; what was reported to physician and completion of physician orders received.
- Write date and time on a sticker, and place on peripheral aspect of dressing.

Unexpected Outcomes	Related Interventions
1. Wound becomes infected.	• Dressing changes may need to be done more frequently. • Different type of dressing may be required. • Obtain wound culture per agency policy.
2. Dressing does not stay in place.	• Evaluate size of dressing used for adequate wound margin (1 to 1½ inches [2.5 to 3.75 cm]). • Client's skin may be too dry or too moist.
3. Skin tears can occur with this type of dressing.	• Adhesive backing may be too strong for fragile skin. • Consider other dressing type.

Teaching Considerations
* Explain wound-healing process with film dressing.
* Explain need to change dressing should edges loosen.
* Explain to client and family that collection of wound fluid under dressing is not "pus," but normal interaction of body fluids with dressing.
* Allow client or caregiver to demonstrate dressing change should self-care need be identified.

Pediatric Considerations
* Adhesive backing may cause skin tears on premature babies' immature skin (Hockenberry and others, 2003).
* To remove: raise one edge of dressing, and pull parallel to skin to loosen adhesive.
* Children may find this procedure more tolerable if they know that the longer the dressing is left on, the easier it is to remove (Hockenberry and others, 2003).

Gerontological Considerations
* Adhesive backing may be too strong for the skin of older adults. Do not use a film dressing that has an adhesive backing that has a stronger bond to the epidermis than the epidermis has to the dermis (Lueckenotte, 2000).

Home Care Considerations
* Wound may be cleansed in shower, if approved by physician.
* Client may shower or bathe with dressing in place.
* Many types of transparent dressings exist. Explore types with client, and recommend type client finds easy to work with and has access to.
* Make sure client has a source of dressing supplies for purchase after discharge.

SKILL 38-4 Applying Hydrocolloid, Hydrogel, Foam, or Absorption Dressings

Hydrocolloid dressings can be used for a variety of reasons. These include (1) maintaining a moist wound environment for healing of clean, shallow to moderately deep wounds, (2) autolytic debriding of necrotic wounds, (3) protecting high-friction areas on intact skin, (4) protecting from contamination, and (5) providing absorption of minimal amount of exudates in superficial and shallow wounds (Cuzzell, 2002b). A hydrocolloid dressing may be applied beneath Montgomery ties or on bony prominences to reduce injury to the subcutaneous tissues (see Chapter 15). Pain and discomfort are diminished with the use of hydrocolloid dressings. Their "cushioning" effect provides protection to the wound and skin beneath bony prominences. These adhesive-backed dressings conform well to different body contours. Hydrocolloids come in the form of granules, paste, or wafer dressings. Wound exudate is absorbed into the dressing, forming a jellylike substance next to the wound surface.

The dressing maintains a moist, insulated environment that promotes rapid, effective healing.

A hydrogel dressing is a semipermeable "water-based nonadherent, polymer based dressing that has some absorptive properties" (AHCPR, 1994). Hydrogel dressings serve the same functions as a hydrocolloid dressing (Cuzzell, 2002b). These dressings are available in several forms, including a "sheet," amorphous gels, and impregnated gauze that can be placed in the wound. These dressings facilitate wound debridement by rehydration. They absorb exudate and encourage healing by maintaining a moist wound-healing environment (Figure 38-3). The gel dressings are nonadherent and must be covered with a secondary dressing to hold them in place.

The hydrocolloid or hydrogel dressings are used frequently over venous stasis ulcers, arterial ulcers, and pressure ulcers. Hydrocolloid dressings are one of the most fre-

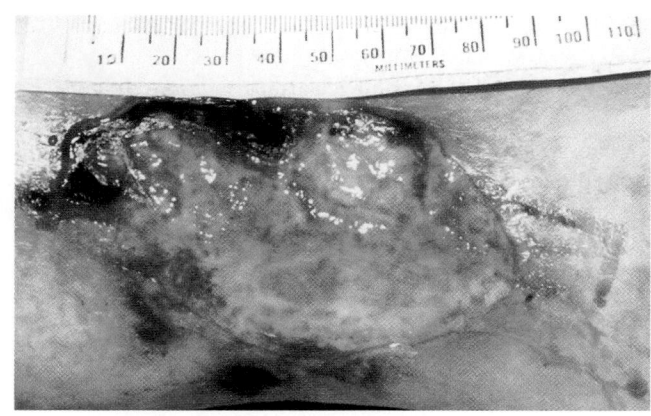 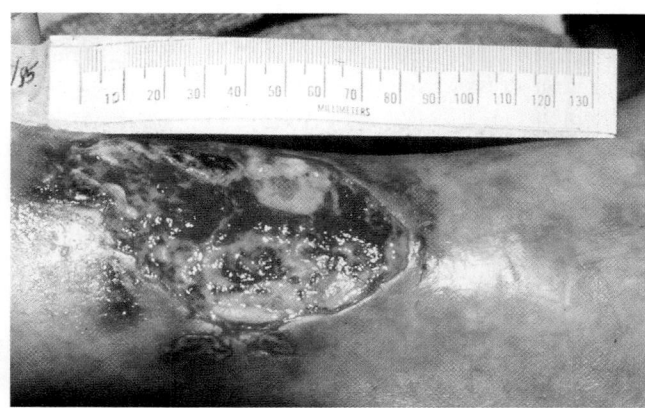

A

B

FIGURE **38-3** **A,** Highly exudative venous ulcer with slough present in wound bed and eschar present along superior aspect. **B,** One week after treatment with hydrocolloids and compression therapy, venous ulcer has granulation tissue present. The amount of slough and eschar is reduced. (From Bryant RA: *Acute and chronic wounds: nursing management,* ed 2, St. Louis, 2000, Mosby.)

quently used dressings for pressure ulcers in home and long-term care settings (Meehan and others, 1999). Because of their "cooling" and soothing properties, hydrogel dressings are used with burns and to protect the skin from radiation. When used in combination with wound exudate absorbers, these dressings are useful over stage III pressure ulcers (see Chapter 15). Hydrogel dressings do not stick to the wound and can be easily removed.

A foam dressing is "a sponge-like polymer dressing that may or may not be adherent; it may be impregnated or coated with other materials and has some absorptive properties" (AHCPR, 1994). These hydrophilic dressings are used in full-thickness wounds with minimal to moderate amounts of drainage. Foam dressings absorb moderate to heavy exudates in superficial or deep wounds, protect friable periwound skin, provide autolytic debridement, pad and protect high-trauma areas (e.g., pretibial area, forearms), and can be used with infected wounds following appropriate intervention and close monitoring of wound healing (Cuzzell, 2002b). More heavily draining wounds may be covered with foam dressings when absorptive wound fillers are also used. These dressings require a secondary dressing to secure the foam in place, or they may be secured with tape or a sheet of flexible tape.

The foam dressings protect the wound surface while maintaining a moist, insulated environment. The result is a well-hydrated wound bed that can heal rapidly with little discomfort to the client. Application directions for the different brands of foam dressings vary. The nurse should read and follow the specific directions for the particular brand of foam dressings that is being used.

Absorption dressings can contain large amounts of wound exudate. They may take the form of pastes, granules, sheeting, or rope. This group of dressings include calcium alginate materials, which are manufactured from natural material (seaweed) and are known for their absorptive properties, forming a gel over the wound surface as exudate is contained. The exudate absorbers are nonadhesive, nonocclusive dressings that can be used in combination with other dressings. These dressings are appropriate for full-thickness wounds with moderate to high amounts of drainage. Deep tracking wounds can safely be packed with calcium-sodium alginate preparation, which allows easy removal with little risk of retained dressing deep in the wound cavity. Calcium-sodium alginate dressings may be further useful in control of wound odor, achieving hemostasis, and control of pain (Cuzzell, 2002b). Generally absorption and alginate dressings require a secondary dressing, and that dressing can be changed as needed (Cuzzell, 2002b). The typical frequency of dressing changes is daily to once or twice a week.

DELEGATION CONSIDERATIONS

The skill of applying a hydrocolloid, hydrogel, foam, or absorption dressing should not be delegated to assistive personnel.

EQUIPMENT

❏ Sterile gloves (optional)
❏ Dressing set (optional)
❏ Sterile saline or other cleansing solution (as ordered)

❏ Clean disposable gloves
❏ Waterproof bag for disposal
❏ Wound measurement devices (tape measure, tracing paper, camera)
❏ Dressing (size as needed) as prescribed (hydrocolloid, hydrogel, foam, absorption)
❏ Sterile gauze pads (4 × 4 inches)
❏ Secondary dressing of choice (if needed)
❏ Protective gown, mask, goggles (used when spray from wound is a risk)

STEP	RATIONALE

ASSESSMENT

1. Assess wound location and size of wound to be dressed (see Skill 38-1, Assessment, and Chapter 37).

   Allows nurse to determine supplies and assistance needed.

2. Determine the type of dressing. Do not use alginate or absorption dressings on nonexuding wounds. Most of these dressings are designed to absorb moderate to large amounts of wound drainage and therefore should not be used in wounds with minimal or no drainage (Cuzzell, 2002b).

   Dressing selection is based on type of wound, location of wound, amount and type of exudate (Nelson and Dilloway, 2002).

- *Critical Decision Point*

  Some brands of hydrocolloid dressings are available in custom shapes and sizes to better fit certain difficult body parts such as the sacrum, heels, or elbows. The variety of shapes aids in flexibility of dressing selection and better dressing adherence.

3. Review physician's orders for frequency and type of dressing change.

   Physician orders mode of therapy.

4. Assess client's level of comfort on a scale of 0 to 10.

   Client who is comfortable during procedure is less likely to move suddenly, causing wound or supply contamination. Client may require pain medication before dressing change to allow drug's peak effect during procedure.

5. Assess client's knowledge of purpose of dressing.

   Identifies client's learning needs.

NURSING DIAGNOSES

- Risk for infection
- Deficient knowledge regarding wound care

- Acute pain
- Impaired skin integrity

Related factors are individualized based on client's condition or needs.

PLANNING

1. Expected outcomes following completion of procedure:
   - Wound heals rapidly with little pain and mobility restriction for client.

     Dressing effective in preventing infection and promoting healing.
   - Wound exudate is adequately absorbed.

     Dressing effective in exudate management for draining wounds.
   - Wound drainage is contained, and skin surrounding wound remains intact.

     Dressing effective in controlling wound exudate.
   - Client explains procedure correctly.

     Indicates learning has occurred.

2. Explain procedure to client.

   Relieves anxiety and promotes understanding of healing process.

3. Position client to allow access to dressing site.

   Facilitates application of dressing.

STEP	RATIONALE

■ IMPLEMENTATION

1. Close room door or cubicle curtains.

   Provides for client privacy and reduces transfer of microorganisms.

2. Expose wound site, and cover client.

   Draping provides access to wound while minimizing client exposure.

3. Cuff top of disposable waterproof bag, and place within reach of work area.

   Cuff prevents accidental contamination of top of outer bag. Nurse should not reach across sterile field.

4. Perform hand hygiene and put on clean disposable gloves. Moisture-proof gown, mask, and goggles are worn when risk of spray exists.

   Reduces transmission of infectious organisms.

5. Remove old dressing. For easier removal, pull back slowly across dressing in direction of hair growth.

   Reduces irritation and possible injury to skin (Nelson and Dilloway, 2002).

● *Critical Decision Point*
Check removal directions for specific brand of dressing that is being used. Some brands need to have old dressing soaked or moistened for removal. With some types of dressings, adhesive remover may be used to ease off dressing. Use caution to avoid contact of adhesive remover with the wound.

6. Dispose of soiled dressings in waterproof bag. Remove disposable gloves by pulling them inside out, and dispose of them in waterproof bag. Avoid having client see old dressing because the sight of wound drainage may be upsetting to the client.

   Reduces transmission of microorganisms.

● *Critical Decision Point*
Hydrocolloid dressings interact with wound fluids and form a soft whitish-yellowish gel, which is hard to remove and may have a faint odor. Normal discoloration may occur with some brands of foam dressings. A residual gel substance occurs in wound beds with some brands of absorption dressings (Cuzzell, 2002b). These are normal occurrences and should not be confused with pus or purulent exudate, wound infection, or deterioration of the wound.

8. Prepare sterile dressing supplies.

   Reduces risk of break in sterile technique.

9. Pour saline or prescribed solution over 4 × 4 sterile gauze pads, or open spray wound cleanser.

   Maintains sterility of dressing.

10. Put on gloves, sterile if required by policy.

    Allows nurse to handle dressings.

11. Cleanse area gently with moist 4 × 4 sterile gauze pads, swabbing exudate away from wound, or spray with wound cleanser (see Chapter 37).

    Reduces introduction of organisms into wound. Cleansing effectively removes any residual dressing gel without injuring newly formed delicate granulation tissue formed in the healing wound bed.

12. Thoroughly pat wound surface dry with dry 4 × 4 sterile gauze pads. Dry intact skin around the wound.

    Dressing will not adhere to damp surface. Periwound skin should be kept dry to prevent breakdown.

13. Inspect wound for tissue type, color, odor, and drainage. Measure wound size and depth (see Chapter 37).

    Appearance and measurement indicates state of wound healing.

14. Apply dressing according to manufacturer's directions.
    a. Hydrocolloid dressings

    Ensures proper application of dressing. Different brands of dressings require different application techniques.

● *Critical Decision Point*
For some brands of hydrocolloid wafers, size of dressing used should be larger than wound size by a 1- to 1½-inch margin beyond wound edges.

STEP	RATIONALE
(1) Apply hydrocolloid granules or paste before wafer dressing in deeper wounds.	Dressing should not be stretched during application. Avoid wrinkles that would provide tunnel for exudate drainage. Hydrocolloid granules assist in absorbing drainage to increase wearing time of dressing (Rolstad and others, 2000).

• *Critical Decision Point*
  Edges may be notched to help mold around wound. Consider using custom shapes to better conform to certain parts of the body such as heels, elbows, and sacrum.

STEP	RATIONALE
(2) Apply amorphous gels approximately ¼- to ½-inch thick across wound surface, or put hydrogel sheet over wound bed. Cover with secondary dressing such as gauze, hydrocolloid, or foam.	Fluid gels take form of cavity type of wounds. A secondary dressing must be used with a hydrogel to hold it in place; it has no adhesive.
(3) If necessary, apply tape around the edges of the hydrocolloid dressing to assist in keeping the dressing in place.	
b. Foam dressings	
(1) Know removal and application characteristics of specific brand of foam dressing you are using.	Most foam dressings should be applied smoothly; avoid wrinkles. May be used with absorptive dressings to accommodate more highly draining wounds.
(2) Make sure you know which side of foam dressing should be placed toward wound bed and which side should be facing away from wound bed.	Ensures proper absorption.
(3) With some brands, dressings can be trimmed to fit wound size, whereas other brands of dressings cannot be cut.	Dressing should not overlap wound so as to avoid maceration of healthy skin.
(4) Check with manufacturer as to which types of secondary dressings to avoid when covering foam dressing that could reduce effectiveness of foam dressing.	
(5) Some brands of foam dressings need slight tension on the dressing while being applied. Some brands of foam dressings need to be covered with a secondary dressing (Rolstad and others, 2000).	
c. Absorption or alginate dressings	
(1) Fill wound cavity, but fill one-half to two-thirds full to allow for expansion with absorption.	
(2) Allows for expansion with absorption. For most brands of alginate dressings, dressing can be cut or folded to fit wound. For others, it is important not to completely fill wound bed with dressing but rather to allow space for alginate dressing to expand to fill wound bed. For some brands the alginate dressing should be applied moist, and for others it should be dry. Some brands need a secondary dressing that extends at least 1¼ inches beyond wound edges.	
(3) Apply secondary dressing, if needed (check manufacturer's directions).	Some secondary dressings may reduce effectiveness of alginate or absorption dressing (Cuzzell, 2002b).

STEP	RATIONALE
15. Remove sterile gloves by pulling them inside out, and discard in prepared bag.	Reduces transfer of microorganisms.
16. Assist client to comfortable position.	Enhances client comfort and relaxation.
17. Discard soiled dressing change materials properly. Perform hand hygiene.	Reduces transmission of microorganisms.

EVALUATION

1. Inspect condition of wound on ongoing basis. Note drainage and odor.	Determines status of wound healing.
2. Evaluate client's level of comfort.	Determines if pain resulted from procedure.
3. Ask client to explain wound care method.	Evaluates client's level of learning.

Recording and Reporting

- Report unusual observations immediately, then chart what was reported and when.
- Chart in nurses' notes the characteristics of wound tissue type: color, odor, viscosity, and amount of drainage; application of dressing; and client's tolerance to dressing change.
- Graph wound surface area or volume if wound is chronic wound.
- Write date, time, and nurse's initials in ink (not marker) on the dressing.

Unexpected Outcomes	Related Interventions
1. Wound becomes infected.	• Dressing changes may need to be done more frequently. • Different type of dressing may be required. • Discontinue use of dressing.
2. Dressing does not stay in place.	• Evaluate size of dressing used for adequate margin (1 to 1½ inches [2.5 to 3.75 cm]), or dry skin more thoroughly before reapplication. • Consider custom shapes for difficult body parts. "Picture frame" the edges of the hydrocolloid dressing using tape. • Dressing may be secured with roll gauze, tape, transparent dressing, or dressing sheet.
3. Wound develops more necrotic tissue and increases in size.	• In rare instances, wounds do not tolerate hypoxia induced by hydrocolloid dressings. In these clients use should be discontinued. • Evaluate appropriateness of wound care protocol. • Evaluate client for other impediments to wound healing.
4. Wound drainage is more than dressing can absorb.	• Change type of dressing to one that can absorb amount of wound drainage. • Foam dressings may be used over wound exudate absorbers.
5. Absorption wound dressing is dry and adherent when removed.	• Wound drainage has diminished, and an alternative dressing should be considered.
6. Client is unable to describe proper application of dressing.	• Provide additional teaching or support. • Obtain services of home care agency if needed.

Teaching Considerations

- Instruct client and caregiver to observe wound for signs and symptoms of infection.
- Instruct client and family regarding proper handling of dressing to avoid contamination of sterile adhesive surface.
- Explain expected wound appearance, fluid or gel accumulation in wound bed, and possible odor with use of specific dressing.
- Explain frequency of dressing changes required. Often the dressing is not changed daily.
- Because application technique can vary with different brands, tell client and caregiver not to purchase a brand different from the one for which nurse gave them instructions. If a different brand must be used, client and caregiver should check with nurse for any additional instructions or modifications in application and removal techniques.

Pediatric Considerations

- See Pediatric Considerations for Skills 38-1, 38-2, and 38-3.

Gerontological Considerations

- See also Gerontological Considerations for Skills 38-1, 38-2, and 38-3.
- Avoid early and frequent removal of a hydrocolloid dressing to reduce injury to surrounding intact skin.

Home Care Considerations

- Dressing is easily applied and readily adaptable for home use.
- Dressing may not be available at every pharmacy. Client may need assistance locating dressing.

SKILL 38-5 Wound Vacuum Assisted Closure

Wound Vacuum Assisted Closure (Wound V.A.C.) is a type of therapy that speeds wound healing by applying localized negative pressure to draw the edges of a wound together (Figures 38-4 and 38-5). Wound V.A.C. accelerates wound healing by promoting the formation of granulation tissue, collagen, fibroblasts, and inflammatory cells to completely close or improve the health of a wound. Often the treatment prepares a wound for a skin graft. The use of negative pressure removes fluid from the area surrounding the wound, thus reducing local peripheral edema and improving circulation to the area (Chua and others, 2000) (Figure 38-6). In addition, Wound V.A.C. reduces bacterial counts in wounds, which improves healing because the body can focus on healing rather than fighting infection (Mendez-Eastman, 2001).

Wound V.A.C. may be used to treat acute and chronic wounds, including surgical wounds that have dehisced and pressure ulcers. To use Wound V.A.C., necrotic tissue, malignancy, and fistula to body organs in the wound need to be absent (Mendez-Eastman, 2002).

The cycle and amount of negative pressure to the wound are ordered by the physician or wound care specialist (Mendez-Eastman, 2002). The target negative pressures for wound healing range from 50 mm Hg to 125 mm Hg. The negative pressure can be continuous or intermittent depending on the stage

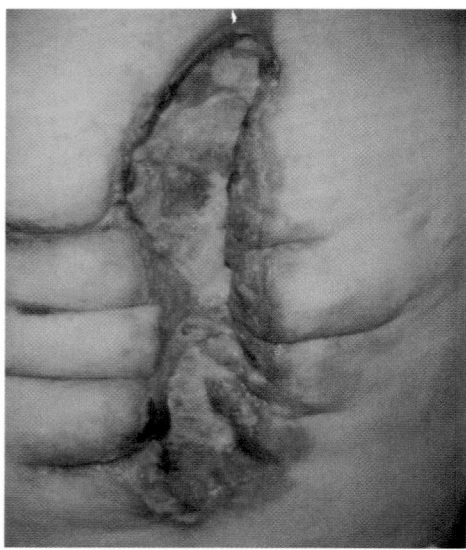

FIGURE **38-4** Dehisced wound before Wound V.A.C. therapy. (Courtesy Kinetic Concepts, Inc. [KCI], San Antonio, Tex.)

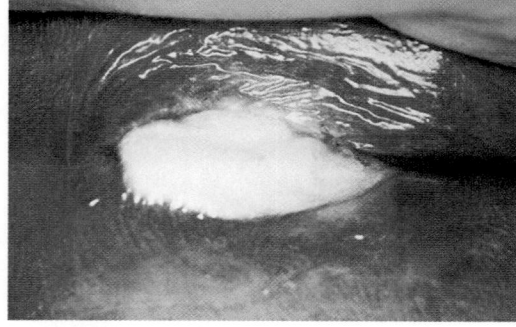

FIGURE **38-5** Dehisced wound after Wound V.A.C. therapy. (Courtesy Kinetic Concepts, Inc. [KCI], San Antonio, Tex.)

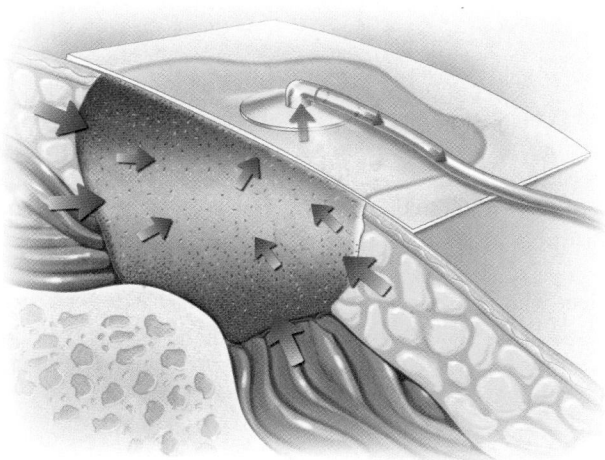

FIGURE **38-6** Wound V.A.C. system using negative pressure to remove fluid from area surrounding the wound, reducing edema, and improving circulation to area. (Courtesy Kinetic Concepts, Inc. [KCI], San Antonio, Tex.)

of wound healing. To optimize wound healing, negative pressure should be maintained 22 out of 24 hours per day (KCI, 2003). As the wound heals, the settings may change.

The schedule for changing Wound V.A.C. dressings varies. An infected wound may need a dressing change every 24 hours, whereas a clean wound can be changed 3 times a week (Chua and others, 2000; Mendez-Eastman, 2002). As the wound heals, the wound base becomes redder as perfusion increases. Granulation tissue will line the surface of the wound, and new epithelial growth is seen along the wound edges. Last, the surface area of the wound should show a steady decrease as healing occurs (KCI, 2003).

DELEGATION CONSIDERATIONS

The skill of Wound Vacuum Assisted Closure should not be delegated to assistive personnel.

* Instruct assistive personnel to use caution in positioning or turning client to avoid tubing displacement.

EQUIPMENT

❏ Wound V.A.C. unit (requires physician order [Figure 38-7])
❏ Wound V.A.C. foam dressing
❏ Tubing for connection between V.A.C. unit and V.A.C. dressing
❏ Gloves, clean and sterile
❏ Scissors, sterile
❏ Waterproof bag for disposal
❏ Skin preparation/skin barrier
❏ Moist washcloth
❏ Linen bag
❏ Protection gown, mask, goggles (used when spray from wound is a risk)

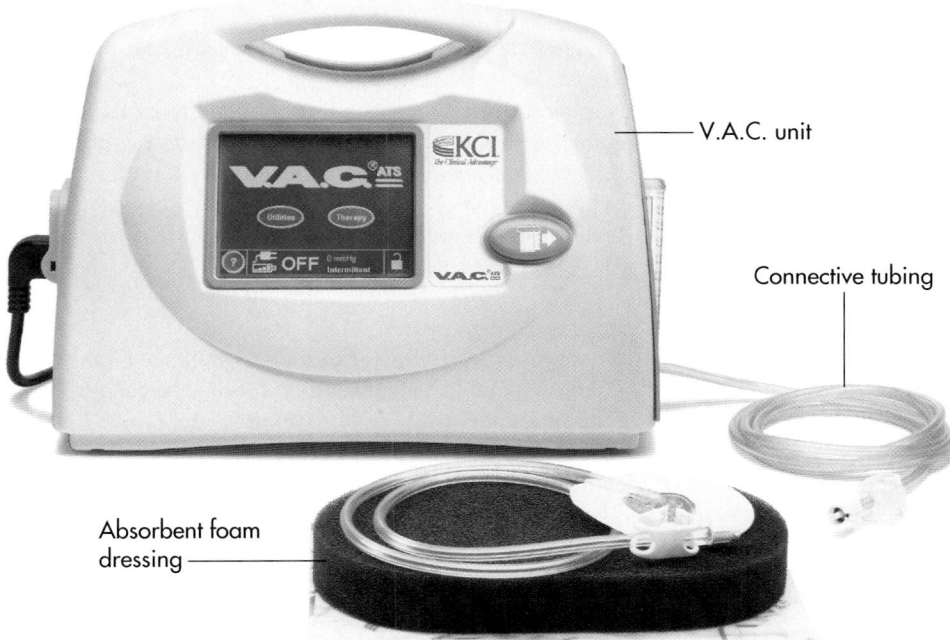

V.A.C. unit

Connective tubing

Absorbent foam dressing

FIGURE **38-7** Wound V.A.C. unit. *Top to bottom*: V.A.C. unit itself, connective tubing to go between V.A.C. unit and V.A.C. dressing, absorbent foam. (Courtesy Kinetic Concepts, Inc. [KCI], San Antonio, Tex.)

STEP	RATIONALE
ASSESSMENT	
1. Assess location, appearance, and size of wound to be dressed (see Chapter 37).	Allows nurse to gather information regarding status of wound healing, presence of complication, and type of supplies and assistance needed to apply Wound V.A.C. dressing.
2. Review physician's orders for frequency of dressing change, type of foam to use, and amount of negative pressure to be used.	Physician orders frequency of dressing changes and special instructions.
3. Assess client's level of comfort using a scale of 0 to 10.	Client who is comfortable during procedure is less likely to move suddenly, causing wound or supply contamination.
4. Assess client's and family member's knowledge of purpose of dressing.	Identifies client's learning needs. Prepares client and family if dressing will need to be changed at home.

NURSING DIAGNOSES

- Risk for infection
- Deficient knowledge regarding wound care
- Acute pain
- Impaired skin integrity

Related factors are individualized based on client's condition or needs.

STEP	RATIONALE
PLANNING	
1. Expected outcomes following completion of procedure:	
• Client's wound shows evidence of healing by smaller size and less drainage, redness, or swelling.	Dressing effective in promoting healing and preventing infection.
• Client reports pain less than previously assessed level during and after dressing changes.	Analgesic and comfort measures effective in controlling client pain.
• Dressing remains intact with airtight seal and prescribed negative pressure.	Dressing effective in maintaining negative pressure and promoting healing.
• Client or family member demonstrates correct method of dressing changes.	Indicates client and family learning has occurred.
2. Explain procedure to client.	Relieves anxiety and promotes understanding of healing process.
3. Position client to allow access to dressing site.	Facilitates application of dressing.

STEP	RATIONALE
IMPLEMENTATION	
1. Close room door or cubicle curtains.	Provides for client privacy and reduces transmission of organisms.
2. Position client, expose wound site, and cover client.	Draping provides access to wound while minimizing exposure. Positioning ensures client comfort during procedure.
3. Cuff top of disposable waterproof bag, and place within reach of work area.	Cuff prevents accidental contamination of top of outer bag.
4. Perform hand hygiene, and put on clean disposable gloves. If risk of spray exists, apply protective gown, goggles, and mask.	Reduces transmission of infectious organisms from soiled dressings to nurse's hands.
5. Push therapy on/off button on Wound V.A.C.	Deactivates therapy.
6. Raise the tubing connectors above the level of the Wound V.A.C. unit, and disconnect tubes from each other to drain fluids into canister. Before lowering, tighten clamp on canister tube.	Allows for proper drainage of fluid in drainage tubing (KCI, 2003). Wound V.A.C. canister unit should be changed when full or at least once a week to control odor (KCI, 2003).
7. With dressing tube unclamped, introduce 10 to 30 ml of normal saline, if ordered, into tubing to soak underneath foam. Let set for 15 to 30 minutes.	Facilitates loosening of foam when tissue adheres to foam (KCI, 2003; Krasner, 2002).
8. Gently stretch transparent film horizontally, and slowly pull up from the skin.	Reduces stress on suture line or wound edges and reduces irritation and discomfort.

STEP	**RATIONALE**
9. Remove old Wound V.A.C. dressing, observing appearance and drainage on dressing. Use caution to remove dressing around drains. Dispose of soiled dressings in waterproof bag. Remove gloves by pulling them inside, out, and dispose of them in waterproof bag. Avoid having client see old dressing because the sight of wound drainage may be upsetting to the client. Perform hand hygiene.	Determines dressings needed for replacement. Avoids accidental removal of drains. Reduces transmission of microorganisms.
10. Apply sterile or clean gloves. Irrigate the wound with normal saline or other solution ordered by the physician. Gently blot to dry (see Skill 37-1).	Irrigation removes wound debris and cleanses wound bed.
11. Measure wound as ordered: at baseline, first dressing change, weekly, and discharge from therapy. Remove and discard gloves. Perform hand hygiene.	Provides objective measure of wound healing progress in response to negative pressure therapy (KCI, 2003).

- **Critical Decision Point**

  Wound cultures may be ordered on a routine basis. Wound cultures should be obtained during the dressing change when drainage looks purulent, there is change in amount or color, or drainage has a foul odor (Chua and others, 2000).

12. Depending on the type of wound, apply sterile or new clean gloves.	Fresh sterile wounds require sterile gloves. Chronic wounds may require clean technique. Do not use the same gloves worn to clean wound, because cross contamination may occur.
13. Select appropriate foam dressing depending on wound type and stage of healing. Use sterile scissors to cut foam to exact wound size, making sure to fit the size and shape of the wound, including tunnels and undermined areas.	Black polyurethane (PU) foam has larger pores and is most effective in stimulating granulation tissue and wound contraction. White polyvinyl alcohol (PVA) soft foam is denser with smaller pores and is used when the growth of granulation tissue needs to be restricted (KCI, 2003; Mendez-Eastman, 2002).

- **Critical Decision Point**

  Use of black foam may cause clients to experience more pain because of excessive wound contraction. Clients may need to be switched to the PVA soft foam.

14. Gently place foam in wound, being sure that the foam is in contact with entire wound base, margins, and tunneled and undermined areas.	Maintains negative pressure to entire wound. Edges of the foam dressing must be in direct contact with the client's skin (Mendez-Eastman, 2002).
15. Apply tubing to foam in the wound (see illustration).	Connects the negative pressure from the Wound V.A.C. unit to the wound foam.

- **Critical Decision Point**

  For deep wounds regularly reposition tubing to minimize pressure on wound edges. Clients with restricted mobility or sensation must be repositioned frequently so that they do not lie on the tubing and cause skin damage (KCI, 2003).

16. Apply skin protectant, such as skin preparation or Stomahesive wafer, to skin around the wound.	Protects periwound skin from injury that may result from the occlusive dressing and will help decrease pain associated with wound margins (Krasner, 2002).

STEP	RATIONALE

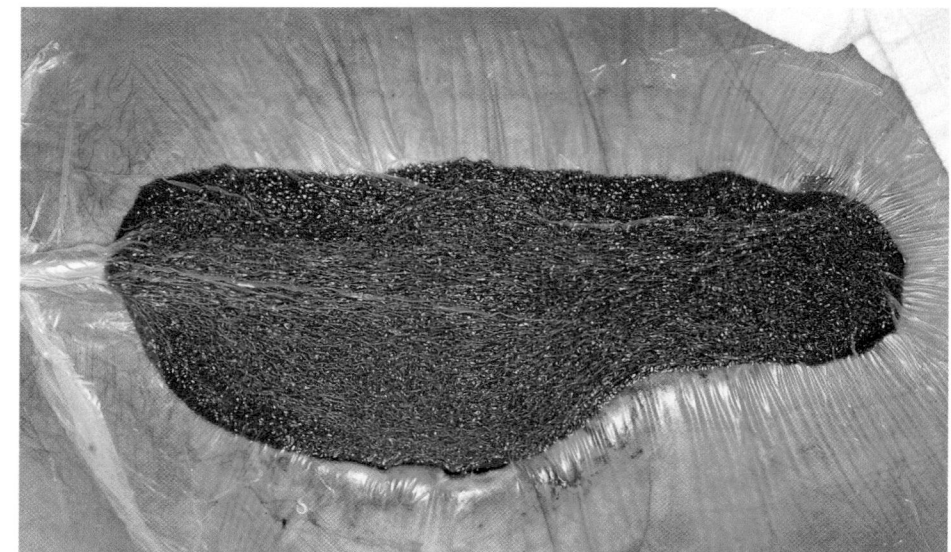

STEP 15 Dressing application. **A,** Properly sized foam to cover wound. **B,** Wrinkle-free transparent dressing applied over foam. **C,** Secure tubing to the foam and transparent dressing unit (step 17). (Courtesy Kinetic Concepts, Inc. [KCI], San Antonio, Tex.)

STEP 17 Foam dressing, transparent dressing, and Wound V.A.C. tubing secured over existing wound. (Courtesy Kinetic Concepts, Inc. [KCI], San Antonio, Tex.)

17. Apply Wound V.A.C. transparent dressing, covering the Wound V.A.C. foam and 3 to 5 cm of surrounding healthy tissue. Make sure transparent dressing is wrinkle-free. Secure tubing to transparent film, aligning drainage hole to ensure an occlusive seal (see illustration). Make sure not to apply tension to drape and tubing.

Ensure that the wound is properly covered and a negative pressure seal can be achieved (Box 38-4). Excessive tension may compress foam dressing, impede wound healing, and produce a shear force on periwound area (KCI, 2003).

STEP	RATIONALE

> **BOX 38-4   Maintaining an Airtight Seal**
>
> Once Wound V.A.C. therapy is initiated, the wound must stay sealed to avoid wound desiccation. Wounds around joints and near the sacrum are problem areas to seal. The following points may assist in maintaining an airtight seal:
> - Shave hair around wound.
> - Cut transparent film to extend 3 to 5 cm beyond wound perimeter.
> - Avoid wrinkles in transparent film.
> - Patch leaks with transparent film.
> - Use multiple small strips of transparent film to hold dressing in place before covering dressing with large piece of transparent film.
> - Avoid adhesive remover because it leaves a residue that hinders film adherence.
>
> From Chua PC and others: Vacuum-assisted wound closure, *Am J Nurs* 100(12):46, 2000.

18. Secure tubing several centimeters away from the dressing.

    Prevents pull on the primary dressing, which can cause leaks in the negative pressure system (Chua and others, 2000; KCI, 2003).

19. After the wound is completely covered, connect the tubing from the dressing to the tubing from the canister and Wound V.A.C. unit.

    Intermittent or continuous negative pressure can be administered at 50 mm Hg to 175 mm Hg, according to physician orders and client comfort. The average is 125 mm Hg (Chua and others, 2000; KCI, 2003).

    a. Remove canister from sterile packaging and push into Wound V.A.C. unit until a click is heard. **An alarm will sound if the canister is not properly engaged.**

    b. Connect the dressing tubing to the canister tubing. Make sure both clamps are open.

    c. Place Wound V.A.C. unit on a level surface, or hang from the foot of the bed. The Wound V.A.C. unit will alarm and deactivate therapy if the unit is tilted beyond 45 degrees.

    d. Press in green-lit power button, and set pressure as ordered.

    Activates negative pressure.

20. Discard soiled dressing change materials properly. Perform hand hygiene.

    Reduces transmission of organisms.

21. Inspect Wound V.A.C. system to verify that negative pressure is achieved.

    Negative pressure is achieved when an airtight seal is achieved (see Box 38-4).

    a. Verify that display screen reads THERAPY ON.
    b. Be sure clamps are open and tubing is patent.
    c. Identify air leaks by listening with stethoscope or by moving hand around edges of wound while applying light pressure.
    d. If a leak is present, use strips of transparent film to patch areas around the edges of the wound.

22. Assist client to a comfortable position.

    Enhances client comfort and relaxation.

STEP	RATIONALE

■ EVALUATION

1. Inspect condition of wound on ongoing basis; note drainage and odor.

Determines status of wound healing.

2. Ask client to rate pain using a scale of 0 to 10.

Determines client's level of comfort following the procedure.

3. Verify airtight dressing seal and correct negative pressure setting.

Determines effective negative pressure being applied.

4. Observe client or family member's ability to perform dressing change.

Indicates client and family learning has occurred.

Recording and Reporting

- Chart in the nurses' notes the appearance of wound, color, characteristics of any drainage, presence of wound healing augmentation, such as Wound V.A.C, dressing change, and client response to dressing change.
- Record date and time of dressing change on new dressing.
- Report brisk, bright red bleeding, evidence of poor wound healing, evisceration or dehiscence, and possible wound infection to physician.

Unexpected Outcomes	Related Interventions
1. Wound appears inflamed and tender, drainage has increased, and an odor is present.	• Notify the physician. • Obtain wound culture. • Increase frequency of dressing changes.
2. Client reports increase in pain.	• Client may need more analgesia when V.A.C. is initiated or changed. • If using black foam, switch to the PVA foam. • Negative pressure may need to be reduced and gradually titrated upward.
3. Negative pressure seal has broken.	• Take preventive measures (see Box 38-4). • Shave surrounding skin.
4. Client or caregiver is unable to perform dressing change.	• Provide additional teaching and support. • Obtain services of home care agency.

Teaching Considerations

- Instruct client and caregiver to observe wound for signs and symptoms of infection.
- Explain expected wound appearance with use of dressing. Instruct client and caregiver in appearance of foam dressings.
- Instruct client and family in points to follow to maintain negative pressure seal.
- Explain frequency of dressing changes required. Often the dressing is not changed daily.
- Explain need to change Wound V.A.C. canister when full or at least once a week to help to control odor (KCI, 2003).

Pediatric Considerations

- Wound V.A.C. therapy is not appropriate for fragile neonatal skin.
- Parents need to actively participate in Wound V.A.C. treatment.

Gerontological Considerations

- Use skin care practices to protect periwound tissue. Transparent film may be irritating to fragile skin. Skin protectant is one method to reduce the risk of tissue injury.
- May need to start with lower negative pressures such as 75 mm Hg and slowly titrate up to 125 mm Hg (KCI, 2003).
- Visual impairment may prevent self-care and require home care services.

Home Care Considerations

- Client and family may benefit from visits with home care agency to monitor initial treatments.
- Provide information to family and caregiver regarding proper disposal of contaminated product.

FOCUS on CLINICAL PRACTICE

You are caring for a 65-year-old client who has been admitted for treatment of a nonhealing venous leg ulcer. The physician has ordered a hydrocolloid dressing as wound therapy for the ulcer.

1. The client tells you, "I just cover the ulcer with a piece of gauze at home, and it has been healing fine." The client asks you why you are putting that wafer material on the wound. What will you tell the client?
2. What advantage do hydrocolloid dressings have over wet-to-dry dressings? Explain your answer.
   1. Are less time consuming for the nurse to apply
   2. Produce increased debridement of the wound edges
   3. Decrease pain and discomfort for the client during removal
   4. Provide increased leg mobility for the client
3. The client says to you that she does not know why the physician just doesn't "stitch up" the leg ulcer. You understand that the healing in wounds such as venous ulcers occurs due to the formulation of granulation tissue and epithelialization. This type of wound healing is called:
   1. Primary intention
   2. Secondary intention
   3. Direct intention
   4. Indirect intention
4. Which intervention is appropriate when changing the venous leg ulcer dressing? Explain your choice.
   1. Clean the wound with prescribed wound cleanser, and dry thoroughly.

2. Remove soiled dressing using sterile gloves.
3. Soak hydrocolloid dressing in saline before packing wound.
4. Stretch hydrocolloid dressing to cover all wound edges.
5. When changing the dressing you assess all the following. Which need to be reported to the physician? Explain your answers.
   1. Pink wound bed
   2. Strong unpleasant odor
   3. Whitish-yellowish gel in wound bed
   4. Moist wound bed
   5. Brisk bleeding in the wound bed
   6. Thick creamy yellow drainage on dressing
   7. Dry and black wound edges
6. You are preparing the client for discharge and are teaching her how to change the dressing on a venous ulcer. Which statement made by the client indicates the need for further teaching? Explain your answer.
   1. "I'll call the doctor if there is a strong odor when I change the dressing."
   2. "I'll pull the old dressing off in the direction that the hair is growing."
   3. "I'll expect to see a whitish-yellowish gel under the wound dressing."
   4. "I'll wet the dressing with normal saline before I remove it."

NCLEX REVIEW QUESTIONS

1. The nurse explains to the client that the purpose of the wet-to-dry dressing is to:
   1. Keep the wound bed moist
   2. Remove unhealthy or dead tissue from the wound
   3. Prevent bacteria from entering the wound
   4. Prevent heat loss from the open wound

2. Which is the appropriate intervention used by the nurse to remove a wet-to-dry dressing from a wound?
   1. Remove all layers of the dressing together.
   2. Apply saline to dressing to loosen from wound.
   3. Administer an analgesic at the beginning of the dressing change.
   4. Pull off tape parallel to skin toward the dressing.

3. Which finding assessed by the nurse during the dressing change is indicative of wound infection?
   1. Wound packing is saturated with serosanguineous drainage.
   2. Waterlike translucent exudate is pooled in the wound bed.
   3. Packing removed from wound has strong foul odor.
   4. Wound surface bleeds when dressing is removed.

4. Which action should the nurse take first when the client has a sudden hemorrhage from a wound site?
   1. Notify the physician.
   2. Take the client's vital signs.
   3. Apply direct pressure.
   4. Increase the IV flow rate.

5. Which taping technique for a pressure dressing to a lower leg wound observed by the nurse requires intervention?
   1. Tape is wrapped around the leg to secure the dressing.
   2. Each tape strip is overlapped for reinforcement.
   3. Tape is secured on distal end first then secured on proximal end.
   4. Strip of tape is placed down center of dressing.

6. Which nursing action will assist in decreasing the rate of blood loss?
   1. Initiate intravenous therapy.
   2. Apply ice to the bleeding wound.

3. Monitor distal circulation every 5 to 10 minutes.
4. Elevate the area of bleeding.

7. The nurse understands that a transparent film dressing is most appropriate for which type of wound?
   1. Surgical incision with large amount of drainage
   2. Small wound with no exudate
   3. Stage IV pressure ulcer
   4. Third-degree burn of the hand

8. Which intervention is appropriate as the nurse changes a transparent film dressing?
   1. Stretch the film over the wound during application.
   2. Pull film dressing upward to break seal to remove.
   3. Press out wrinkles by applying outward strokes.
   4. Apply lubricant on wound edges to protect skin.

9. The nurse is changing a Wound V.A.C. dressing, and the dressing sponge is adhered to the wound. Which is the best action for the nurse to take?
   1. Instill 10 to 30 ml of saline into the foam, and remove dressing in 15 minutes.
   2. Pull back on the sponge horizontally starting at the top.
   3. Lift the sponge by pulling up from the middle of the dressing.
   4. Gently cut the sponge away from the wound using sterile scissors.

10. During Wound V.A.C. therapy, which nursing intervention will help maintain an airtight seal?
    1. Use adhesive remover to clear away old adhesive.
    2. Cut film to extend 1 to 2 cm beyond wound edges.
    3. Shave hair around wound edges.
    4. Use adhesive tape to anchor dressing in place.

11. Which assessment finding in a client with Wound V.A.C. therapy alerts the nurse to a possible wound infection?
    1. Bleeding and tenderness of wound
    2. Pain and serosanguineous drainage
    3. Stinging sensation and increased redness
    4. Increased drainage and odor

References

Andrews M: The influence of cultural and health belief systems on health care practices. In Andrews M, Boyle J: *Transcultural concepts in nursing care,* Philadelphia, 2003, Lippincott.

Agency for Health Care Policy and Research: *Treatment of pressure ulcers,* Clinical practice guideline No. 15, Rockville, Md, 1994, U.S. Department of Health and Human Services, Public Health Service.

Chua PC and others: Vacuum-assisted wound closure, *Am J Nurs* 100(12):45, 2000.

Cuzzell J: Wound assessment and evaluation: characteristics of common problem wounds, *Dermatol Nurs* 14(2):129, 2002a.

Cuzzell J: Wound assessment and evaluation wound dressings—confusion or choice? *Dermatol Nurs* 14(3):187, 2002b.

Hess CT: How to use gauze dressings, *Nursing* 30(9):88, 2000.

Hockenberry MJ and others: *Wong's nursing care of infants and children*, ed 7, St. Louis, 2003, Mosby.

KCI USA: *The V.A.C.: Vacuum Assisted Closure: V.A.C. therapy clinical guidelines*, product information, San Antonio, Tex, 2003.

Kehoe A, Elmore MF: Woundoscopy: a new technique for examining deep, nonhealing wounds, *Ostomy Wound Manage* 48(4):30, 2002.

Krasner DL: Managing wound pain in patients with vacuum-assisted closure devices, *Ostomy Wound Manage* 48(5):38, 2002.

Lueckenotte AG: *Gerontologic nursing*, ed 2, St. Louis, 2000, Mosby.

Maklebust J, Palleschi M: Promoting surgical wound healing, *Nursing* 26(6):24c, 1996.

Mendez-Eastman S: Guideline for using negative pressure wound therapy, *Adv Skin Wound Care* 14(6):314, 2001.

Mendez-Eastman S: Wound therapy, *Nursing* 32(5):59, 2002.

Milne C, Houle T: Current trends in wound care management, *Orthop Nurs* 21(6):11, 2002.

Myer AH: The effects of aging on wound healing, *Top Geriatr Rehabil* 19(2):1, 2000.

Nelson DB, Dilloway MA: Principles, products, and practical aspects of wound care, *Crit Care Nurs Q* 25(1):33, 2002.

Nowak T: People of Vietnamese heritage. In Purnell L, Paulanka B: *Transcultural healthcare,* Philadelphia, 2003, FA Davis.

Ovington LG: Hanging wet-to-dry dressings out to dry, *Home Healthc Nurse* 19(8):477, 2001a.

Ovington LG: Wound care products: how to choose, *Home Healthc Nurse* 19(4):224, 2001b.

Ovington LG: Dealing with drainage: the what, why and how of wound exudate, *Home Healthc Nurse* 20(6):368, 2002.

Ramundo J, Wells J: Wound debridement. In Bryant RA: *Acute and chronic wounds: nursing management*, St. Louis, 2000, Mosby.

Rolstad B and others: Wound care product formulary. In Bryant RA: *Acute and chronic wounds: nursing management*, St. Louis, 2000, Mosby.

Waldrop J, Doughty D: Wound-healing physiology. In Bryant RA: *Acute and chronic wounds: nursing management*, St. Louis, 2000, Mosby.

West JM, Gimbel M: Acute surgical and traumatic wound healing. In Bryant RA: *Acute and chronic wounds: nursing management*, St. Louis, 2000, Mosby.

Wysocki AB: Evaluating and managing open skin wounds: colonization versus infection, *AACN Clin Issues* 13(3):382, 2002.

Research References

Capasso V, Munro BH: The cost and efficacy of two wound treatments, *AORN J* 77(5):984, 2003.

Graumlich JF and others: Healing pressure ulcers with collagen or hydrocolloid: a randomized controlled trial, *J Am Geriatr Soc* 51(2):147, 2003.

Gray M, Doughty DB: Clean versus sterile technique when changing wound dressings, *J Wound Ostomy Continence Nurs* 28(3):125, 2001.

Meehan M and others: Report on the prevalence of skin ulcers in a home health agency population, *Adv Wound Care* 12(9):459, 1999.

Park Y-J and others: A survey of Hwa-Byung in middle-age Korean women, *J Transcult Nurs* 12(2):115, 2001.

Pompeo MG: The role of "wound burden" in determining the costs associated with wound care, *Ostomy Wound Manage* 47(3):65, 2001.

St. Clair KL, Larrabee J: Clean versus sterile gloves: which to use for postoperative dressing changes? *Outcomes Manag* 6(1):17, 2002.

Thomas DR, Kamel HK: Subacute care for seniors: wound management in post acute care, *Clin Geriatr Med* 16(4):783, 2000.

Wooten MK, Hawkins K: Clean versus sterile: management of chronic wounds (position statement), *J Wound Ostomy Continence Nurs* 28(5):24a, 2001.

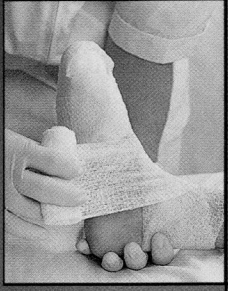

39

Binders and Bandages

MEDIA RESOURCES

Evolve Site *evolve*
http://evolve.elsevier.com/Perry/skills
• Weblinks

OBJECTIVES

Mastery of content in this chaper will enable the nurse to:

- Discuss the purposes of binders and bandages.
- Describe the precautions for use of binders and bandages.
- Demonstrate correct technique for applying turned bandages.
- Demonstrate correct application of binders.
- Describe the elements to document when applying binders and bandages

⬤ **KEY TERMS**

Binder
Chronic venous insufficiency
Elastic bandage
Excoriation
Maceration

Binders and elastic bandages applied over dressings can provide extra protection and therapeutic benefits by:

1. Creating pressure over a body part (e.g., a compression bandage applied over venous leg ulcers)
2. Immobilizing a body part (e.g., an elastic bandage applied around a sprained ankle)
3. Supporting a wound (e.g., an abdominal binder applied over a large abdominal incision and dressing)
4. Reducing or preventing edema (e.g., a breast binder used to minimize swelling between skin and tissue layers after a mastectomy)
5. Securing a splint (e.g., a bandage applied around hand splints for correction of deformities)
6. Securing dressings (e.g., elastic webbing applied around leg dressings after a vein stripping)
7. Maintaining the position of special equipment for applying traction (e.g., Buck's extension) (see Chapter 12)
8. Enabling the client to participate in effective respiratory functions of deep breathing, coughing, and clearing of airway sections (e.g., an abdominal binder used to support local incisions, reducing the pain from respiratory maneuvers)

Elasticized bandages are available in rolls of various widths and materials, including gauze, elasticized knit, elastic webbing, flannel, and muslin. Gauze bandages are lightweight and inexpensive, mold easily around contours of the body, and permit air circulation to prevent skin maceration, which is softening and breakdown of the skin due to fluid. (See Chapter 15 on pressure ulcer formation.) Flannel and muslin bandages are thicker than gauze and thus stronger for supporting or applying pressure. A flannel bandage also insulates to provide warmth. Elastic bandages conform well to body parts but can also be used to exert pressure over a body

part. Elastic compression bandages are categorized as either long-stretch or short-stretch (Kunimoto, 2001).

Long-stretch bandages provide sustained compression regardless of a client's activities. Short-stretch bandages provide compression only when a client activates his or her calf muscle pump, as in walking. Gauze and elastic bandages are used to secure dressings on extremities, amputation stumps, and the hand (Table 39-1). In addition, elastic bandages are used for compression therapy on lower extremities to promote the return of blood from the peripheral veins to the central circulation.

Binders are bandages made of large pieces of material specially designed to fit a specific body part. Most binders are made of elastic, cotton, muslin, or flannel. The most common type of binder is the abdominal binder. Breast binders continue to be used in limited circumstances.

An abdominal binder supports large abdominal incisions that are vulnerable to tension or stress as the client moves or coughs (Figure 39-1). A breast binder looks like a tight-fitting sleeveless vest. Although used less often because of changes in surgical techniques, the breast binder helps to reduce swelling of tissues following major breast surgery. The binder conforms to the shape of the chest wall and is available in different sizes. Breast binders can provide support after breast surgery or exert pressure to reduce lactation in a woman after childbirth. The nurse secures a binder with Velcro strips, metal fasteners, or safety pins.

Evidence-Based Practice Trends

Compression therapy using elastic compression bandages is one of the primary treatments for venous ulcers. The use of compression therapy corrects the problem of venous insufficiency, allowing the ulcer to heal (Kunimoto, 2001). Pressures of 30 to 40 mm Hg at the ankle reducing to pressures of 15 to 20 mm Hg at the thigh have been shown to be most effective in reducing venous insufficiency (Lorimer and others, 2003). Elevation of the legs above the level of the heart 3 to 4 times daily for 30 minutes and at night can decrease swelling and improve venous circulation in clients who cannot or will not tolerate compression therapy (deAraujo and others, 2003; Kunimoto, 2001).

Elastic compression bandages have advantages over the nonelastic, rigid bandages. Elastic bandages are easier to use, conform better to the leg, require less frequent dressing changes, and will sustain needed pressures (deAraujo and others, 2003). Long-stretch bandages such as the four-layer bandage are used most frequently because they maintain constant pressure for several days, thus reducing the need for frequent dressing changes (Kunimoto, 2001). Four-layer dressings are more expensive than single-layer dressings, but they promote more rapid healing of the ulcer; therefore they seem to be less expensive (deAraujo and others, 2003).

Correct application of the graduated compression bandage by a trained practitioner is the single most effective therapy in managing venous ulcers (Lorimer and others, 2003). Compression dressings for treatment of venous ulcers

TABLE 39-1	TYPES OF BANDAGE TURNS	
TYPE	**DESCRIPTION**	**PURPOSE OR USE**
Circular Circular turns.	Bandage turn overlapping previous turn completely	Anchors bandage at the first and final turn; covers small part (finger, toe)
Spiral Spiral turns.	Bandage ascending body part with each turn overlapping previous one by one-half or two-thirds width of bandage	Covers cylindrical body parts such as wrist or upper arm
Spiral-reverse Spiral-reverse turns.	Turn requiring twist (reversal) of bandage halfway through each turn	Covers cone-shaped body parts such as the forearm, thigh, or calf; useful with non-stretching bandages such as gauze or flannel
Figure eight Figure-eight turns.	Oblique overlapping turns alternately ascending and descending over bandaged part; each turn crossing previous one to form figure eight	Covers joints, applies low-grade pressure for venous return; snug fit provides excellent immobilization
Recurrent Recurrent turns.	Bandage first secured with two circular turns around proximal end of body part; half turn made perpendicular up from bandage edge; body of bandage brought over distal end of body part to be covered with each turn folded back over on itself	Covers uneven body parts such as head or stump

need to be used cautiously in persons with arterial insufficiency of the legs and cardiac insufficiency (deAraujo and others, 2003; Kunimoto, 2001). In clients with lower extremity arterial insufficiency, compression dressings can decrease the arterial blood flow to the legs, causing ischemia. Indicators of arterial circulation such as peripheral pulses, color, temperature, and capillary refill need to be assessed frequently. Decision trees are available to assist nurses in assessment and treatment of venous ulcers (Cuzzell, 2002).

Breast binders or support bras have been used following childbirth as mechanical methods to suppress lactation. No difference has been found between the two products in producing symptoms of breast engorgement, but breast binding was found to cause greater breast tenderness and milk leakage than did using a support bra (Swift and Janke, 2003).

Cultural Considerations

- Assess cultural practices relevant to use of binders and bandages.
  - Among Pacific Islanders abdominal binders may be applied tightly immediately postpartum to promote abdominal firmness and uterine healing.
  - Some Filipinos and Mexicans apply abdominal binders (fajitas) to the infant to prevent gas and hernia (Berry, 1999; Pacquiao, 2003).
  - Bandages on certain body parts such as the face and the head may be perceived as disfiguring.
- Consider ethnocultural differences when teaching signs and symptoms of decreased circulation resulting from increased pressure from binders or bandages (see Chapter 15).

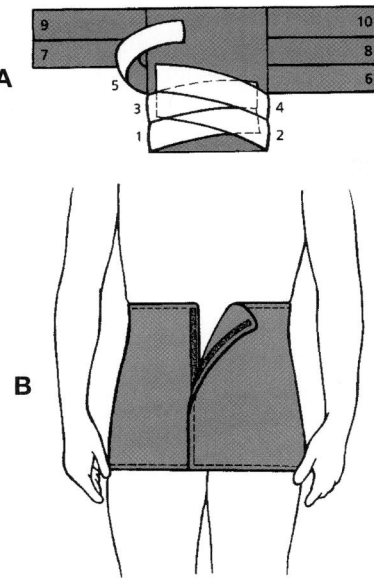

FIGURE **39-1** Abdominal binders. **A,** Scultetus binder with crossover strap closures. **B,** Straight binder with Velcro closure.

Skill Performance Guidelines

1. The nurse who applies a bandage or binder can loosen or readjust it as necessary. The nurse should have a physician's order before loosening or removing a bandage or binder applied by a physician.
2. Assess the status of circulation frequently below a site where a bandage has been applied.
3. Assess the status of ventilation frequently when an abdominal binder or breast binder has been applied.
4. Correctly applied binders or bandages should not cause injury to underlying and nearby body parts and should not create discomfort or reduce ventilatory expansion.

SKILL 39-1   Applying Gauze and Elastic Bandages

Both gauze and elastic bandages are used to hold dressings securely in hard-to-cover areas. For example, a dressing covering the length of a client's lower leg will be held in place more firmly when the dressing is surrounded by a well-secured gauze bandage. An elastic bandage is also used to apply compression to an area. Elastic compression is used most often on the lower extremities to prevent edema and to support varicosities. Many clients use elastic bandages to reduce dependent edema in the extremities.

Continuous compression therapy, the treatment of choice for chronic venous insufficiency, has multiple therapeutic benefits (Box 39-1). The principle of compression therapy is consistent with Laplace's law of physics. Following the natural shape of the lower leg, gradient compression therapy delivers higher pressures at the ankle (smaller radius) with a decline in pressure at the knee (larger radius). This provides for normal venous flow (Kunimoto, 2001). Continuous compression therapy typically involves the application of four layers of bandages to remain in place without slipping, designed to apply 30 to 40 mm Hg of pressure at the ankle reducing to 15 to 20 mm Hg of pressure at the thigh (Lorimer and others, 2003). Nurses require advanced training to apply continuous compression bandages, which is beyond the scope of this text.

Other uses of elastic bandages include support of the knee, ankle, elbow, and wrist in conditions such as strains and sprains (Phipps and others, 2003). When fully stretched, an elastic bandage extends to 3 yards (270 cm). Shorter lengths of 1½ yards (135 cm) are available for bandaging the wrist or a child's foot or knee. Gauze bandages likewise come in a va-

> **BOX 39-1   Therapeutic Benefits of Continuous Compression Therapy**
>
> - Alleviation of venous hypertension
> - Increased return of venous blood to the central circulation and heart
> - Stimulation of fibrinolysis
> - Removal of sodium from subcutaneous tissue
> - Reduction of local edema
> - Increased local oxygenation
> - Promotion of an environment favorable for wound healing
>
> Modified from Kunimoto BT: Management and prevention of venous leg ulcers: a literature-guided approach, *Ostomy Wound Manage* 47(6):36, 2001.

riety of lengths. Gauze and elastic bandages are available in widths ranging from 2 inches (5 cm) to 8 inches (20 cm).

When gauze or elastic bandages are selected to secure a dressing, the type of bandage turn and selected width are determined by the size and shape of the body part to be bandaged. For example, 3- and 4-inch bandages are most commonly used for the adult leg. A smaller 2-inch bandage would be used for the wrist.

Gauze and elastic bandages come supplied in a roll with an inner and outer surface. In preparation for bandaging, the outer surface is placed next to the skin and then rolled around the surface to be covered. Even tension is applied during application. When an elastic bandage is applied to an extremity, the bandage is started at the site farthest from the heart (distal) and proceeds toward the heart (proximal).

DELEGATION CONSIDERATIONS

The skill of applying an elastic bandage for compression should not be delegated to assistive personnel. The nurse is responsible for assessment of the wound or injury and evaluation of the response to the elastic bandage. The skill of applying bandages to secure nonsterile dressings can be delegated following assessment. Before delegating this skill the nurse must:

- Discuss with assistive personnel any unique modification of the skill such as special taping

- Instruct assistive personnel to report client's complaint of pain, numbness, or tingling after a bandage has been applied or any changes in client's skin color or temperature

EQUIPMENT

- ❑ Correct width and number of gauze or highly elastic bandages
- ❑ Clips or adhesive tape
- ❑ Disposable gloves, if wound drainage is present

STEP	RATIONALE
ASSESSMENT	
1. Review client's medical record and nursing prescriptions for specific orders related to application of elastic bandage. Note area to be covered, type of bandage required, frequency of change, and previous response to treatment.	Specific prescription may direct procedure, including such factors as extent of application (e.g., toe to knee, toe to groin) or duration of treatment.
2. Inspect skin of area to be bandaged for alterations in integrity as indicated by presence of abrasion, discoloration, or chafing. Pay close attention to areas over bony prominences.	Altered skin integrity may contraindicate use of elastic bandage to be applied directly to the skin because of applied pressure. May require a dressing before bandage is applied (Kunimoto, 2001).
3. Inspect any surgical dressing.	Surgical dressing replacement or reinforcement precedes application of any bandage.

- **Critical Decision Point**

  If incision/wound is to be covered by a bandage, it should be covered with a dressing to avoid soiling of bandage and irritation of wound.

STEP	RATIONALE
4. Observe adequacy of circulation by noting surface temperature, skin color, pulses (distal to area to be bandaged), presence of edema, and sensation and movement of body parts to be wrapped.	Comparison of area before and after application of bandage is necessary to ensure continued adequate circulation. Impairment of circulation may result in pain, coolness to touch when compared with opposite side of body, cyanosis or pallor of skin, diminished or absent pulses, edema or localized pooling, and numbness and/or tingling of body part.
5. Assess client's comfort level using visual analog scale of 0 to 10 (see Chapter 6), and note any other objective signs of discomfort.	Provides baseline to determine effects of therapy and client's response.
6. Assess for size of bandage.	
a. *Gauze or basic elastic bandage to secure a dressing:* Assess size of area to be covered. Each successive role of gauze/elastic should overlap previous layer. Smaller widths are used for upper extremities, larger widths for lower extremities.	Proper size bandage avoids bulkiness and ensures adequate coverage.
b. *Elastic bandage to provide simple compression:* Assess circumference of lower extremity before or shortly after client gets out of bed in the morning or after client has been in bed for at least 15 minutes. Select width that will cover and overlap without bulkiness.	Assures clinician that dependent edema is at a minimum, so true leg circumference can be estimated (Reichardt, 1999). Compression bandages not applied correctly may produce pressures that are either too low or too high to promote venous return (Lorimer and others, 2003).
7. Identify client's and primary caregiver's present knowledge level of skill if bandaging will be continued at home.	Ensures that planning and teaching are individualized.

STEP	RATIONALE

NURSING DIAGNOSES

- Deficient knowledge regarding bandage application
- Pain (acute, chronic)

- Impaired physical mobility
- Impaired tissue integrity

Related factors are individualized based on client's condition or needs.

PLANNING

1. Expected outcomes following completion of procedure:
   - Client states pain or discomfort is decreased or absent on a scale of 0 to 10.

     Indicates proper application of elastic bandage without excess pressure or compression that could impair local blood flow.

   - No tingling or numbness is noted by client.

     Bandage is not causing pressure on peripheral nerves or arterial circulation.

   - Distal parts (toes, fingers) feel warm (symmetrically) to touch, pulse is present, no cyanosis or blanching is present, and motion is not unnecessarily impaired.

     Indicates adequate circulation to distal regions.

   - Localized edema is reduced.

     Elastic bandage promotes venous return.

   - Client applies bandage correctly.

     Demonstrates learning and ensures continuity of care after discharge.

2. Explain procedure to client. Reinforce during teaching that smooth, even pressure will be applied to improve venous circulation, prevent clot formation, reduce or prevent swelling, immobilize body part, secure surgical dressings, and provide pressure.

   Increased knowledge needed to promote cooperation, reduce anxiety, and ensure correct technique for self-application.

3. Teach skill to client or significant other when bandage will be applied in the home.

   Reduces anxiety and ensures continuity of care.

IMPLEMENTATION

1. Close room door or curtains.

   Maintains client's comfort and dignity.

2. Assist client to assume comfortable, anatomically correct position, lying in bed.

   Maintains alignment. Facilitates application of bandage in anatomical position.

3. Perform hand hygiene, and apply gloves if drainage is present.

   Reduces transmission of microorganisms.

- **Critical Decision Point**

  With client in bed, elevation of dependent extremities for 15 minutes before elastic bandage application will enhance venous return.

4. Apply bandage
   a. Gauze or elastic bandage to secure dressing:
      (1) Hold roll of bandage in dominant hand, and use other hand to lightly hold beginning layer of bandage at distal body part. While rolling bandage around body part, continue transferring roll to dominant hand as bandage is wrapped (see illustration).

      Maintains appropriate and consistent bandage tension.

STEP	RATIONALE

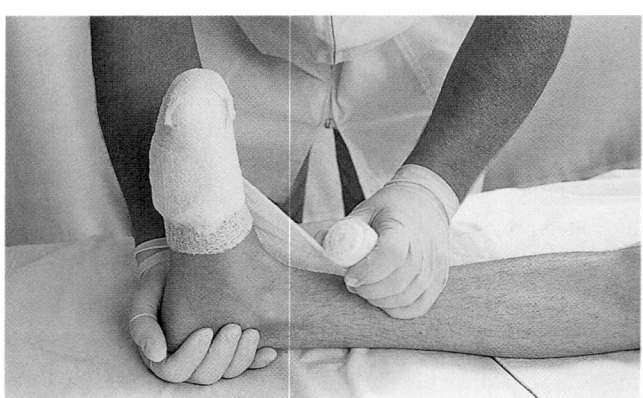

STEP **4a(1)** Nurse applies roller gauze to foot.

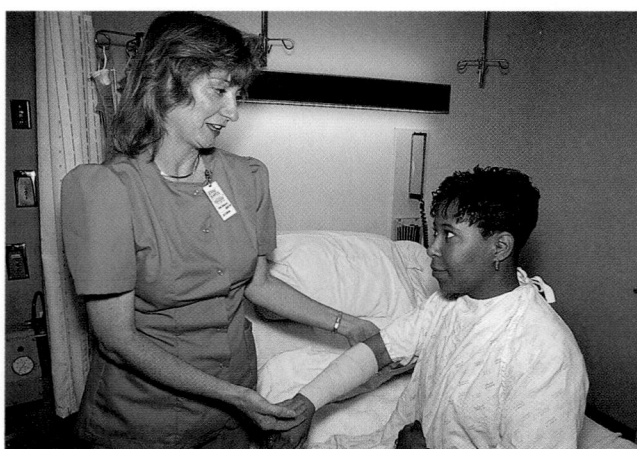

STEP **4a(1a)** Nurse checks temperature of skin below site of bandage application.

- ## Critical Decision Point
  Except in cases where toes or fingers are treated because of wounds, toes or fingertips should remain uncovered and visible for follow-up circulatory assessment.

(2) Apply bandage from distal point toward proximal boundary using variety of turns to cover various shapes of body parts (see Table 39-1). (For bandaging of amputation stump, see illustration.)

Bandage is applied in manner that conforms evenly to body part and promotes venous return.

(3) While unrolling elastic bandage, stretch bandage slightly.

Maintains uniform bandage tension.

- ## Critical Decision Point
  Avoid wrapping bandage too tightly because this may cause numbness and tingling from impaired circulation and/or pressure on peripheral nerves.

(4) Overlap turns by one-half to two-thirds width of bandage roll.

Prevents uneven bandage tension and circulatory impairment.

(5) Secure first bandage with clip or tape before applying additional rolls.

Maintains a smooth bandage surface.

(6) Apply additional rolls without leaving any uncovered skin surface. Secure last bandage applied.

Prevents wrinkling or loose ends.

b. Elastic bandage for simple intermittent compression:

(1) Have client lie in bed with leg slightly elevated.

Promotes venous return during application.

(2) Hold roll of bandage in dominant hand, and use other hand to lightly hold beginning layer of bandage at distal body part. While rolling bandage around body part, continue transferring roll to dominant hand as bandage is wrapped.

Maintains appropriate and consistent bandage tension.

STEP	RATIONALE

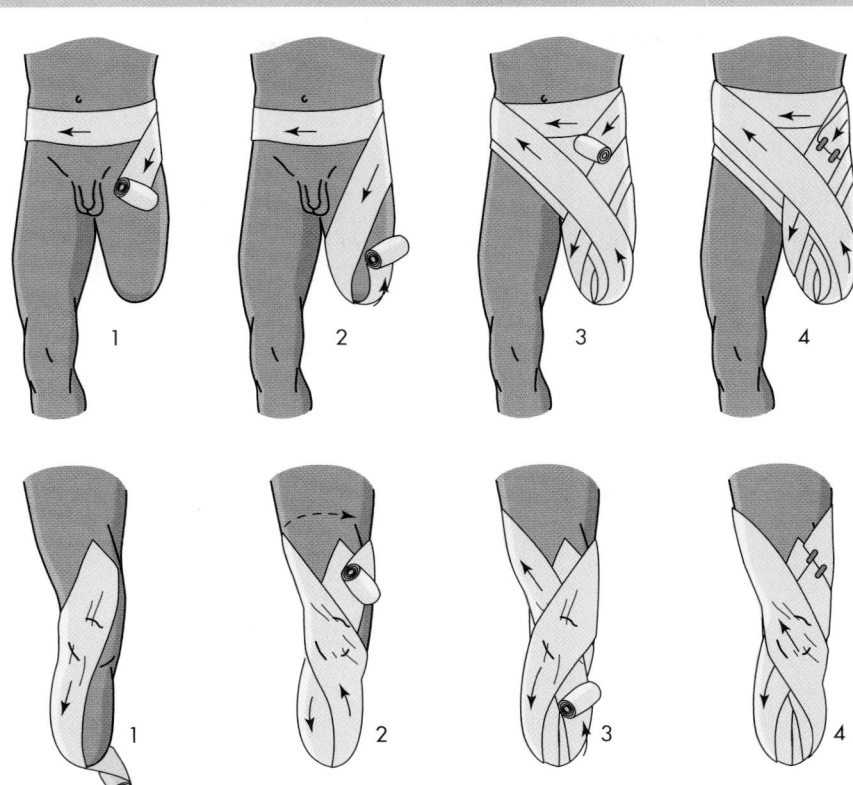

STEP 4a(2) *Top,* Correct method for bandaging midthigh amputation stump. Note that bandage must be anchored around patient's waist. *Bottom,* Correct method for bandaging midcalf amputation stump. Note that bandage need not be anchored around the waist. (From Phipps J and others: *Medical-surgical nursing: health and illness perspectives,* ed 7, St. Louis, 2003, Mosby.)

(3) Apply the highly elastic conformable bandage using a figure-eight turn. Apply from distal (just above toes) to most proximal boundary.	Applies higher compression pressure at the ankle while reducing at the thigh to promote venous return (Kunimoto, 2001; Lorimer and others, 2003).
(4) Stretch bandage slightly while applying.	Maintains uniform tension.
(5) After applying only one layer of bandage, secure with tape or clips.	Prevents excess pressure over limb. Continuous pressure bandage using multiple layers requires trained clinician to apply.
5. Remove gloves if worn, and perform hand hygiene.	Reduces transmission of microorganisms.
6. Remove and reapply elastic bandage once every 8 hours unless otherwise directed by physician.	Single layer bandage can slip easily, causing excess pressure where bandage rests.

EVALUATION

1. Evaluate distal circulation when bandage application is complete and at least twice during 8-hour period.	Measurements determine if bandage is applied too tightly, compromising circulation or movement.
a. Observe skin color for pallor or cyanosis.	Determines if circulation is compromised.
b. Palpate skin for warmth.	
c. Palpate pulses, and compare bilaterally.	Early detection and management of circulatory impairment ensures healthy neurovascular status.
d. Ask if client is aware of pain, numbness, tingling, or other discomfort.	Neurovascular changes indicate impaired venous return.
e. Observe mobility of extremity.	Determines if bandage is too tight, which restricts movement, or if intended therapeutic joint immobility is attained.

STEP	RATIONALE
2. Evaluate as needed for wrinkles, looseness, or tightness; client discomfort or itchiness; and changes, including drainage.	Slippage of bandage can cause pressure on underlying tissue, leading to impaired circulation or pressure on nerves.
3. Have client demonstrate bandage application.	Return demonstration validates client's learning.

Recording and Reporting

- Chart in nurses' notes condition of wound, integrity of dressing, application of bandage, type of bandage applied, circumference of lower extremity, circulation, and client's comfort level before and after bandage application.
- Report any changes in neurological or circulatory status to nurse in charge or physician.

Unexpected Outcomes	Related Interventions
1. Circumferential ridging develops with deep indentations into skin; client may note tingling, numbness, or pain.	• Bandage is too tight, causing impaired circulation. • Remove, and wait 30 minutes before reapplying.
2. Extremity distal to wrap is cool, cyanotic, or blanched.	• Remove bandage. • Notify physician.
3. Dressing is loose, slipping, or improperly wrapped, providing improper support.	• Remove dressing. • Reapply using correct technique.
4. Extremity has decreased range of joint motion.	• Notify physician. • Check dressing for correct application.

Teaching Considerations

- Applying elastic bandage to oneself is difficult. Teach significant other if treatment will continue after hospitalization.
- Unless total immobilization is prescribed for client, instruct on proper range-of-motion exercises. Encourage client to practice regularly.

Pediatric Considerations

- Use adhesive tape rather than loose clips or safety pins to fasten bandage on small child or infant.

Gerontological Considerations

- As clients age, skin becomes more fragile, which increases their susceptibility to skin breakdown. Once skin/tissue injury occurs, wound healing is delayed. Assess these clients more frequently for evidence of skin breakdown or decrease in circulation over the areas covered by and distal to the bandage (Ebersole and others, 2004).

Home Care Considerations

- Advise client on best resources for obtaining bandage supplies. Consult with home care nurse as needed.
- Assess client's and primary caregiver's ability, motivation, and availability to participate in bandaging procedure.
- Assess client's understanding of bandaging and willingness to leave bandage in place.
- Assess client's environment to determine potential for permitting bandaged area to remain free from contaminants.
- The elastic bandage is washable and is placed in large folds over a line to dry. Do not use an electric dryer because bandage can shrink.

SKILL 39-2 Applying an Abdominal Binder and a Breast Binder

Binders are indicated for the support of underlying muscles and large incisions. The muscles and viscera surrounding an operative site may require support during the postoperative period to reduce trauma and edema. This promotes healing and permits a client to move more freely without additional discomfort. The basic shape of an abdominal binder is a rectangle that is wide enough to extend from the groin to the waistline and long enough to encircle the abdomen with an overlap for closure. Breast binders are made in the form of tight-fitting vests.

DELEGATION CONSIDERATIONS

The skill of applying a binder can be delegated to assistive personnel. The assessment of the client is the nurse's responsibility and should be conducted before binder application. Before delegating this skill the nurse must:

- Discuss with assistive personnel any unique modification of the skill such as special wrapping or manner of securing the binder
- Instruct assistive personnel to report client's complaint of pain, numbness, or tingling, difficulty breathing after an abdominal or breast binder has been applied, or any changes in client's skin color or temperature.

EQUIPMENT

❑ Gloves, if wound drainage present
  Abdominal Binder
❑ Correct size cloth/elastic straight binder
❑ Safety pins (6 to 8) unless Velcro closure or metal fasteners are attached
  Breast Binder
❑ Correct size binder
❑ Safety pins (approximately 12) unless Velcro closure is attached

STEP	RATIONALE

ASSESSMENT

1. For client who needs support of abdomen, observe ability to breathe deeply, cough effectively, and turn or move independently.

2. Determine if client has allergy to adhesive tape.

3. Inspect skin for actual or potential alterations in integrity. Observe for irritation, abrasion, skin surfaces that rub against each other, and allergic response to adhesive tape used to secure dressing.

4. Inspect any surgical dressing for intactness, presence of drainage, and coverage of incision. Change any soiled dressing before applying binder.

5. Assess client's comfort level, using visual analog scale of 0 to 10 (see Chapter 6) and note any other objective signs and symptoms.

6. Gather necessary data regarding size of client and appropriate binder to use (see manufacturer's guidelines).

Baseline assessment determines client's ability to breathe and cough. Impaired ventilation of lung can lead to alveolar atelectasis and inadequate arterial oxygenation.

Contraindicates use of tape to secure binder.

Actual impairments in skin integrity can be worsened with application of a binder. Binder can cause pressure and excoriation.

Dressing replacement or reinforcement precedes application of any binder. If left uncovered, a wound can be damaged from rubbing of binder.

Data will provide baseline to later determine effectiveness of binder placement.

Ensures proper fit of binder.

NURSING DIAGNOSES

- Ineffective breathing pattern
- Deficient knowledge regarding binder application
- Impaired physical mobility

- Acute pain
- Impaired skin integrity
- Impaired tissue integrity

Related factors are individualized based on client's condition or needs.

PLANNING

1. Expected outcomes following completion of procedure:
   - Client's respirations are unrestricted. Coughing is effective, and secretions are expectorated.

Ability to fully expand lungs and cough must continue after application of binder to enhance oxygenation and avoid pulmonary complications.

STEP	**RATIONALE**
• Client is able to move within prescribed limits and states pain is absent or reduced.	Support to incision from binder promotes comfort during turning, ambulation, or deep breathing.
• Client's suture line is intact, with no drainage or separation.	Binder decreases tension on suture line to promote healing. Snug support helps maintain intact suture line.
2. Explain procedure to client.	Promotes client's understanding and cooperation.
3. Teach skill to client or significant other.	Reduces anxiety and ensures continuity of care after discharge.

IMPLEMENTATION

1. Close curtains or room door.	Maintains client's comfort and dignity.
2. Perform hand hygiene, and apply gloves (if likely to contact wound drainage).	Reduces transmission of microorganisms.
3. Apply abdominal binder:	
a. Position client in supine position with head slightly elevated and knees slightly flexed.	Minimizes muscular tension on abdominal organs.
b. Assist client in rolling on side away from nurse toward raised side rail while firmly supporting abdominal incision and dressing with hands.	Reduces pain and discomfort.
c. Place binder flat on bed, right side up. Fanfold far side of binder toward midline of binder. (For a scultetus binder, be sure tails are smoothly placed against client's side as far side is fanfolded.)	Gathers binder together so client can roll over with minimal effort.
d. Place fanfolded ends of binder under client.	Permits placement and centering of binder with minimal discomfort.
e. Instruct or assist client in rolling over folded binder.	Positions client over binder.
f. Unfold and stretch ends out smoothly on far side of bed. Then stretch out ends on near side of bed.	Smooth, even binder maintains skin integrity and comfort.
g. Instruct client to roll back into supine position.	Facilitates an even application of binder over abdomen.
h. Adjust binder so that supine client is centered over binder, using symphysis pubis and costal margins as lower and upper landmarks.	Centers support from binder over abdominal structures, which reduces incidence of decreased lung expansion while ensuring adequate wound support.
i. If client is very thin, pad iliac prominences with gauze bandage.	Reduces pressure on prominences.
j. Close binder. Pull one end of binder over center of client's abdomen. While maintaining tension on that end of binder, pull opposite end of binder over center and secure with Velcro closure tabs, metal fasteners, or horizontally placed safety pins.	Provides continuous wound support and comfort.

• ***Critical Decision Point***
Recheck client's ability to breathe deeply and cough effectively. Shallow respirations, continuing after a tight binder has been loosened, may indicate beginning of serious respiratory problems, including alveolar atelectasis and pulmonary embolus, among others.

k. Assess client's comfort level.	Helps determine effectiveness of binder placement.
l. Adjust binder as necessary.	Promotes comfort and chest expansion.
4. Apply breast binder:	
a. Have client lie supine with head elevated 45 degrees.	Facilitates normal anatomical position of breasts and eases application of binder.
b. Thoroughly wash and dry under pendulous breasts before applying a breast binder.	Reduces risk of growth of microorganisms.
c. Assist client in placing arms through binder's armholes.	Eases binder placement process.

STEP	RATIONALE

   d. Lightly pad area under breasts with 4 × 4 gauze dressing if necessary.

Prevents skin contact with undersurface.

   e. Using Velcro closure tabs or horizontally placed safety pins, secure binder at nipple level first. Continue closure process above and then below nipple line until entire binder is closed (see illustration).

Horizontal placement of pins may reduce risk of uneven pressure or localized irritation. Applying support at nipple line ensures even alignment of breasts.

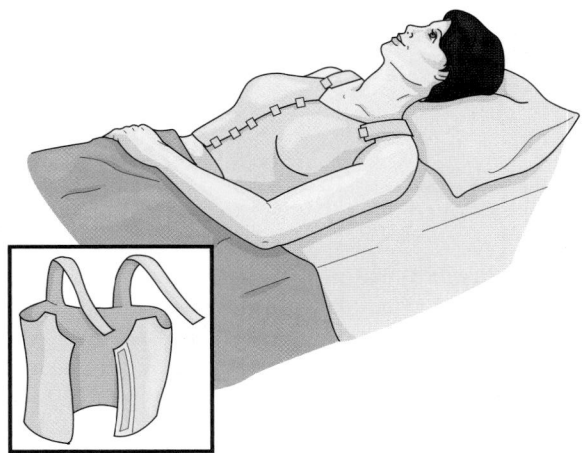

STEP **4e** Client with breast binder applied. (From Sorrentino SA: *Mosby's textbook for nursing assistants*, ed 5, St. Louis, 2000, Mosby.)

   f. Make appropriate adjustments, including individualizing fit of shoulder straps and pinning waistline darts to reduce binder size.

Maintains support to client's breasts.

   g. Instruct and observe skill development in self-care related to reapplying breast binder.

Self-care is integral aspect of discharge planning. Skin-integrity and comfort-level goals are ensured.

5. Remove gloves, and perform hand hygiene.

Prevents cross infections.

EVALUATION

1. Observe site for skin integrity, circulation, and characteristics of the wound. Remove binder and surgical dressing to assess wound characteristics at least every 8 hours.

Determines that binder has not resulted in complications (e.g., rubbing or abrasion of skin, disruption of wound).

2. Evaluate comfort level of client, using visual analog scale of 0 to 10, and note any other objective signs and symptoms.

Binders should not increase discomfort.

3. Evaluate client's ability to ventilate properly, including deep breathing and coughing, every 4 hours.

Identifies any impaired ventilation and potential pulmonary complications.

4. Identify client's need for assistance with activities such as hair combing, dressing, and ambulating.

Mobility of upper extremities may be limited, depending on severity and location of incision.

Recording and Reporting

- Record type and application of binder, condition of skin, circulation, integrity of underlying dressing, and client's comfort level.
- Report any complications (e.g., pain, skin irritation, impaired ventilation) to nurse in charge.
- Report reduced lung expansion to physician immediately.

Unexpected Outcomes	Related Interventions
1. Impaired breathing as evidenced by shallow, rapid respirations leads to ineffective oxygenation.	• Remove binder. • Reapply binder using correct technique.
2. Tight binder impairs circulation to tissues.	• Remove binder. • Consult with physician, and reapply if appropriate.
3. Skin integrity is impaired, resulting from uneven pressure and irritation.	• Remove binder. • Administer skin care according to agency policy. • Consult with physician, and reapply if appropriate.
4. Pain and discomfort are increased.	• Binder or dressing support may be applied incorrectly. • Remove binder. • Reapply using correct technique.

Teaching Considerations

• Instruct client that a properly fitting brassiere that extends to lower rib cage and has front closure may be substituted for breast binder.
• Consider client's dexterity in reapplying binder to self, opportunities to practice skill, and need to teach significant other.

Pediatric Considerations

• Use adhesive tape rather than loose clips or pins to fasten binder on small child or infant.

Gerontological Considerations

• As clients age, skin becomes more fragile, which increases their susceptibility to skin breakdown. Once skin/tissue injury occurs, healing is delayed. Assess these clients more frequently for evidence of skin breakdown over area covered by binder (Ebersole and others, 2004).

Home Care Considerations

• Assess primary caregiver's understanding, ability, and motivation to participate in application of binder.
• Assess client's understanding of purpose of binder and willingness to permit binder to remain in place.
• Abdominal and breast binders are washable and are placed over a line to dry.

FOCUS on CLINICAL PRACTICE

You are assigned to care for Mr. Dodson after surgery to repair his ventral hernia. Mr. Dodson is 6 feet tall and weighs 260 pounds. The physician orders an abdominal binder for Mr. Dodson.

1. What assessment data should you gather in preparation for applying the binder on Mr. Dodson?
2. Mr. Dodson asks you why the physician ordered an abdominal binder for him. What explanation should you give Mr. Dodson?
3. Which of the following should be used in evaluating Mr. Dodson's response after applying the abdominal binder? Check all that apply.
   A. Remove the binder at least every 8 hours to assess the wound integrity, circulation, and characteristics.
   B. Assess Mr. Dodson's appetite level.
   C. Assess Mr. Dodson's hourly urine output.
   D. Assess Mr. Dodson's comfort level.
   E. Monitor Mr. Dodson's apical pulse every 4 hours.
   F. Assess Mr. Dodson's ability to deep breathe and cough and ventilate every 4 hours.
   G. Assess Mr. Dodson's need for assistance with hair combing, ambulation, bathing, and dressing.
4. Provide appropriate documentation for application of Mr. Dodson's abdominal binder.
5. An hour after having the binder put on, Mr. Dodson tells you he cannot seem to get comfortable and rates his pain as 8/10. His previous pain rating was 4/10. You note that his respiratory rate is 24 breaths per minute and shallow. What action should you take? Explain your answer.

NCLEX REVIEW QUESTIONS

1. The nurse recognizes that a primary reason for applying a compression bandage is to:
   1. Prevent wound infection
   2. Reduce wound inflammation
   3. Decrease pain perception
   4. Promote venous return.

2. The nurse should evaluate distal circulation to an extremity after bandage application at least every:
   1. 4 hours
   2. 8 hours
   3. 12 hours
   4. 24 hours

3. Which of the following may contraindicate the use of an elastic bandage applied to the skin of the lower extremity?
   1. Edema of the lower leg
   2. Abraded chafed skin on the lower leg
   3. Varicose veins of the leg
   4. A sprain of the ankle

4. The nurse teaches the client that the reason for the abdominal binder following surgery is to:
   1. Decrease abdominal edema
   2. Stimulate granulation healing of the incision
   3. Support the abdominal muscles
   4. Absorb drainage from the wound

5. Which action is most appropriate for the nurse to take if after applying an abdominal binder, the client experiences shallow, rapid respirations?
   1. Notify the physician.
   2. Elevate the head of the client's bed.
   3. Encourage the client to deep breathe and cough.
   4. Remove the binder, and reapply it.

6. The nurse should place the client in which position to apply an abdominal binder?
   1. Upright in a chair
   2. Supine
   3. Semi-Fowler's
   4. Reverse Trendelenburg's

References

Berry A: Mexican American women's expressions of the meaning of culturally congruent prenatal care, *J Transcult Nurs* 10(3):203, 1999.

Cuzzell J: Wound assessment and evaluation: venous ulcer decision tree, *Dermatol Nurs* 14(5):346, 2002.

Ebersole P and others: *Toward healthy aging: human needs and nursing response*, ed 6, St. Louis, 2004, Mosby.

Phipps J and others: *Medical-surgical nursing: health and illness perspectives*, ed 7, St. Louis, 2003, Mosby.

Reichardt LE: Venous ulceration: compression as the mainstay of therapy, *J Wound Ostomy Continence Nurs* 26(1):39, 1999.

Sorrentino SA: *Mosby's textbook for nursing students,* ed 5, St. Louis, 2000, Mosby.

Research References

deAraujo T and others: Managing the patient with venous ulcers. *Ann Intern Med* 138(4):326, 2003.

Kunimoto BT: Management and prevention of venous leg ulcers: a literature guided approach, *Ostomy Wound Manage* 47(6):36, 2001.

Lorimer KR and others: Venous leg ulcer care: how evidence-based is nursing practice? *J Wound Ostomy Continence Nurs* 30(30): 132, 2003.

Pacquiao DF: People of Filipino heritage. In Purnell L, Paulanka B: *Transcultural health care,* Philadelphia, 2003, FA Davis.

Swift K, Janke F: Breast binding . . . is it all that it's wrapped up to be? *J Obstet Gynecol Neonatal Nurs* 32(3):332, 2003.

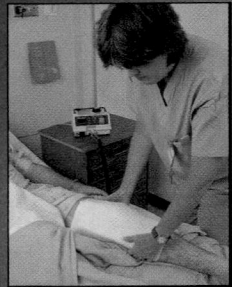

40

Warm and Cold Therapy

MEDIA RESOURCES

Evolve Site *evolve*
http://evolve.elsevier.com/Perry/skills
• Weblinks

OBJECTIVES

Mastery of content in this chaper will enable the nurse to:

- Identify the effects of heat and cold on the client.
- Differentiate the types of injuries or conditions that benefit from warm and cold applications.
- Identify the risks to clients related to warm and cold applications.
- Explain common guidelines used to protect clients who receive warm and cold applications.
- Correctly apply warm and cold applications.

KEY TERMS

Compress	Piloerection
Conduction	Pyrogen
Cryotherapy	Sitz bath
Evaporation	Vasoconstriction
Insulator	Vasodilation
Neuropathy	

The local application of heat and cold to body parts can have a beneficial effect. To use warm and cold therapies safely, the nurse must understand how the body normally responds to temperature variations and the risks connected with these applications.

Exposure to heat or cold causes both systemic and local responses. The hypothalamus acts as the thermostat of the body to maintain body temperature at approximately 37° C, or 98.6° F. Systemically, when the skin is exposed to warm or hot temperatures, vasodilation and perspiration occur to promote heat loss. As perspiration evaporates from the skin, cooling occurs. In cryotherapy, when the skin is exposed to cool or cold temperatures, the systemic response includes vasoconstriction and piloerection to conserve heat. Shivering occurs in response to cooler temperatures, producing heat through muscular contraction.

The local response to heat and cold results from changes in blood vessel size, which affects blood flow to the exposed area. This physiological response explains the effectiveness of warm and cold therapies (Table 40-1).

When receptors for heat or cold are stimulated, sensory impulses travel via somatic afferent fibers to the hypothalamus and cerebral cortex. The cerebral cortex makes a person aware of temperature sensations. The person can then adapt as necessary to maintain normal body temperature; if cold, the person can put on additional clothing, or if warm, the person can cool down by bathing the face with a tepid damp cloth. The hypothalamus simultaneously controls physiological reflexes needed to regulate normal body temperature. The body also has a protective reflex response for exposure to temperature extremes. Exposure to an extremely hot or cold stimulus sends impulses traveling to the spinal cord, synapsing at the spinal cord, and returning by way of motor nerves to cause withdrawal from the stimulus. The person becomes aware of the discomfort as withdrawal occurs.

Sensory adaptation to local temperature extremes can occur quickly within the body. Although a person may initially feel a temperature extreme, once the sensory receptors adapt, the person may become unaware of any temperature variation. Eventually excessive heat causes a burning sensation; excessive cold causes a numbing sensation before pain

TABLE 40-1 THERAPEUTIC EFFECTS OF WARM AND COLD APPLICATIONS

THERAPY	PHYSIOLOGICAL RESPONSES	THERAPEUTIC BENEFIT	EXAMPLES OF CONDITIONS TREATED
Warm application	Vasodilation	Improves blood flow to injured body part, promotes delivery of nutrients and removal of wastes, decreases venous congestion in injured tissues	Inflamed or edematous body part; new surgical wound; infected wound; arthritis, degenerative joint disease; localized joint pain, muscle strains; low back pain, menstrual cramping; hemorrhoidal, perianal, and vaginal inflammation; local abscesses
	Reduced blood viscosity	Improves delivery of leukocytes and antibodies to wound site	
	Reduced muscle tension	Promotes muscle relaxation and reduces pain from spasm or stiffness	
	Increased tissue metabolism	Increases blood flow; provides local warmth	
	Increased capillary permeability	Promotes movement of waste products and nutrients	
Cold application	Vasoconstriction	Reduces blood flow to injured body part, prevents edema formation, reduces inflammation	Immediately after direct trauma such as sprains, strains, fractures, muscle spasms, after superficial lacerations or puncture wound; after minor burns; when malignancy is suspected in area of injury or pain; after injections; for arthritis, joint trauma
	Local anesthesia	Reduces localized pain by slowing or blocking peripheral nerve conduction	
	Reduced cell metabolism	Reduces enzyme function and oxygen needs of tissues	
	Increased blood viscosity	Promotes blood coagulation at injury site	
	Decreased muscle tension	Prevents muscle spasm by decreasing spasticity/tone and relieves pain	

Data from Stitik T, Nadler S: I. When—and how—to use cold most effectively, *Consultant* 38(12):2881, 1998; Stitik T, Nadler S: II. When—and how—to apply the heat, *Consultant* 39(1):144, 1999.

TABLE 40-2 CONDITIONS THAT INCREASE RISK OF INJURY FROM WARM AND COLD APPLICATION

CONDITION	RISK FACTORS
Areas with little body fat	Thinner layers in children increase risk of burns; older adults have reduced sensitivity to painful stimuli.
Open wounds, broken skin, stomas	Subcutaneous and visceral tissue are more sensitive to temperature variations; also contain no temperature receptors and fewer pain receptors than normal skin.
Areas of edema or immature scar tissue	Reduced sensation to temperature stimuli because of thickening of skin layers from fluid buildup or scar formation.
Peripheral vascular disease (e.g., diabetes, arteriosclerosis)	Body's extremities are less sensitive to temperature and pain stimuli because of circulatory impairment and local tissue injury; cold applications would further compromise blood flow.
Confusion or unconsciousness	Reduced perception of sensory or painful stimuli.
Spinal cord injury	Alteration in nerve pathway preventing reception of sensory or painful stimuli.
Abscessed tooth or appendix	Infection highly localized; application of heat may cause rupture with systemic spread of microorganisms.

Data from Stitik T, Nadler S: I. When—and how—to use cold most effectively, *Consultant* 38(12):2881, 1998; Stitik T, Nadler S: II. When—and how—to apply the heat, *Consultant* 39(1):144, 1999.

TABLE 40-3 TEMPERATURE RANGES FOR WARM AND COLD APPLICATIONS

TEMPERATURE	CENTIGRADE RANGE (DEGREES)	FAHRENHEIT RANGE (DEGREES)
Hot	37-41	98-106
Warm	34-37	93-98
Tepid	26-34	79-93
Cool	18-26	65-80
Cold	10-18	50-65

is sensed. Because of this physiological phenomenon, the risk of tissue injury from heat and cold applications is great. Certain clients are more at risk than others for injury from warm and cold applications (Table 40-2). The nurse plays an important role in maintaining the client's safety in the application of heat and cold. The nurse must always have an order for a heat or cold application, and the order should include the duration of the treatment and the desired temperature to be used when settings can be controlled (Table 40-3). In health care agencies, central supply departments typically set temperature settings on heat and cold devices. Because many of these therapies can be used at home, the nurse must instruct clients and their families in the proper use of these therapies.

When using heat or cold therapies, the nurse can use either dry or moist applications. The selection of dry or moist application is determined by the nature of temperature conduction and the result desired from therapy. Temperature travels from an external source such as a compress or water pad to the skin's surface. A substance that conducts temperatures poorly is a good insulator and thus a protector for skin and tissues. For example, cloth placed over a heating pad insulates the skin from hot temperature extremes. Plastic, which is the external covering for most commercial heating pads, and the fluid in moist compresses both conduct heat well, thus placing the client at risk for injury during heat applications. However, there are distinct advantages to using both dry and moist applications (Table 40-4). The nurse should be familiar with the effects of each application type.

Evidence-Based Practice Trends

Heat is used primarily for acute muscular strain injuries and can selectively affect either superficial or deep tissue (Stitik and Nadler, 1999). If deep muscle penetration is desired, moist heat is the preferred application method. When areas are prone to muscle spasm in response to an acute injury, heat can be applied for 20 to 30 minutes every 2 hours. Due to the analgesic effects of moist heat, clients will usually be more compliant with treatment.

The application of cold is a popular and established method for treating soft tissue injuries. The use of cryotherapy for various injuries has shown a positive effect on pain relief (Weiner, 2003) and has been shown to be effective in the postoperative period after reconstructive surgery of the joints (Airaksinen and others, 2003). Cold is also used to reduce recovery time as part of the rehabilitation program for the treatment of both acute and chronic injuries (Airaksinen and others, 2003; Poddar, 2003). This is thought to be due to the positive physiological effects, such as pain relief, decrease of nerve conduction, and decrease in edema by constriction of blood vessels (Poddar, 2003; Wilke and Weiner, 2003).

Very little information is written comparing the effects of heat to the effects of cryotherapy. In ankle sprains, the early application of ice (within 36 hours) decreased time to recovery (Poddar, 2003). The application of ice—but not heat—also reduced edema. Heat may increase swelling and subsequently slow recovery.

The hypothermia-hyperthermia blanket raises, lowers, or maintains body temperature through conductive heat or cold transfer between the blanket and the client. There is little re-

TABLE 40-4	**CHOICE OF DRY OR MOIST WARM APPLICATION**	
TYPE	**ADVANTAGES**	**DISADVANTAGES**
Moist application	Reduces drying of skin and softens wound exudate	Can cause maceration of the skin with prolonged exposure
	Conforms well to body area being treated	Cools rapidly because of moisture evaporation
	Penetrates deeply into tissue layers	Creates greater risk for burns to skin because moisture conducts heat
	Lessens sweating and insensible fluid loss	
Dry application	Less likely to burn skin	Increases body fluid loss through sweating
	Does not cause skin maceration	Does not penetrate deep into tissue
	Retains temperature longer because not influenced by evaporation	Causes increased drying of skin

search to support using physical cooling methods to treat fevers, and in fact these methods could actually harm the client (Nicoll, 2002). Febrile responses occur in three phases: chill phase, plateau phase, and defervescence phase. During the chill phase of a febrile response, the increasing gradient between the body temperature and the set point of the hypothalamus stimulates a warming response. Shivering and vasoconstriction occur to elevate the body temperature to a new set point. The hypothalamus maintains the body temperature at the new set point during the plateau phase, until the pyrogen becomes inactive, and the set point drops to its normal level. When the defervescence phase occurs, the hypothalamus initiates a cooling response with chills, shivering, and diaphoresis signaling a break in the fever and a return to normal body temperature. Cooling a client using a hypothermia blanket during the chill phase is counterproductive and could stimulate further warming response (Nicoll, 2002).

In the treatment of hypothermia a variety of methods are used to gain normothermia (Ruffolo, 2002). The methods are divided into three groups: passive external/surface rewarming (i.e., placing warm blankets on top of the client), active external/surface rewarming and active internal/core rewarming (i.e., infusing warmed intravenous fluids) (Nicoll, 2002; Ruffolo, 2002; Sicoutris, 2001). Hyperthermia blankets fall into the second method—active external or surface rewarming. As the body surface is rewarmed, the peripheral blood vessels will dilate, transporting colder peripheral blood to the warmer core, causing a decrease in core temperature (Sicoutris, 2001). In addition, rewarming shock has been documented when peripheral vasodilation occurs in the presence of volume depletion (Nicoll, 2002; Sicoutris, 2001). Hyperthermia blankets, which make contact with only 20% to 30% of the body surface area, are somewhat inefficient and should be placed on top of the client to prevent tissue necrosis and further heat loss (Ruffolo, 2002).

Cultural Considerations

When explaining the use of warm and cold therapy to clients, the meaning and significance of the therapy can take on very different interpretations based on a client's culture.

It is therefore important to assess the culture-specific applications of warm and cold principles from the client and family members.

- Assess how warm and cold are used normally in the care of the client.
  - Many cultures such as Hispanics, Arabic culture, Asians, Africans, Caribbeans, and Eastern Europeans believe in the holistic concept of hot and cold to promote balance and wellness (Andrews and Boyle, 2003; Levy Miller, 2000).
  - Heat and cold applications are reflected in dietary, environmental, herbal, and medicinal use.
  - The goal of hot and cold principles is restoring balance by giving the opposite of the cause or problem.
- In oriental therapy, hot and cold concepts are subsumed under the broad umbrella of yin and yang that integrates the concept of balance and holistic health.
- Accommodate generic beliefs and practices of the client.
  - In general, water (bathing), cold (air-conditioned rooms), and ice (ice in beverages) are avoided when the client's condition is classified as cold, as well as in a hot condition when the client is considered vulnerable to environmental conditions.
- Use cultural brokers such as family members, physicians, and religious leaders to increase acceptance of critical therapies such as hypothermia or ice packs that contradict the client's/family's beliefs and practices.
- Accommodate client's need for privacy.
  - Clients may refuse being exposed to reduce body temperature.

Skill Performance Guidelines

1. Protect damaged skin. Exposed layers of skin are more sensitive to temperature variations than intact skin.
2. Time all applications carefully. A person tolerates temperature extremes better when the duration of exposure is short (10 to 20 minutes). Prolonged exposure can injure tissues and eliminate the benefits of therapy (Stitik and Nadler, 1998). Keep a timer or clock close by so that the client can help the nurse time applications.

3. Know the temperature of the application being used. Many devices, such as heating pads or water flow pads (e.g., Aqua-K pads), have thermostats to regulate temperature. Always check the temperature of moist compresses applied directly to the skin.

4. Certain body parts, such as the extremities or perineum, are more sensitive than others to temperature extremes. The nurse can modify the intensity of heat and cold when sensitive skin areas are being treated.

5. Check the client frequently during a warm or cold application. The condition of the skin indicates whether tissue injury is occurring. Be observant for signs of excessive redness, maceration, or blistering.

6. Know the client's risk for injury from heat or cold. Certain clients are more predisposed to injury than others (see Table 40-2).

7. Do not allow the client to adjust temperature settings. It is common for the client to adapt to a temperature extreme and then think that the temperature should be adjusted.

8. Never position the client so that the client cannot move away from the temperature source. This avoids the risk of injuries from temperature exposure. The hospitalized client should always have a call light within reach.

9. Do not leave the client unattended if the person is unable to sense temperature changes or move away from the temperature source. The nurse is responsible for the client's safety.

10. Discourage the client from moving an application. This may cause injury to an unprotected area of the body and decrease the effectiveness of therapy.

SKILL 40-1 Application of Moist Heat (Compress and Sitz Bath)

Warm compresses and commercial heat packs are examples of moist heat applications. A warm compress is a section of sterile or clean gauze moistened with a prescribed heated solution (i.e., normal saline, sterile water) and applied directly to an open wound or the skin's surface. A sterile compress is necessary only when there is a break in skin integrity.

Commercially packaged sterile, premoistened compresses are available in some agencies (Figure 40-1). They require the use of a special infrared lamp to heat. Plain sterile or clean gauze can be heated by adding the gauze to a container of warmed solution. Often the nurse applies an aquathermia heating pad over a compress to deliver a continuous, con-

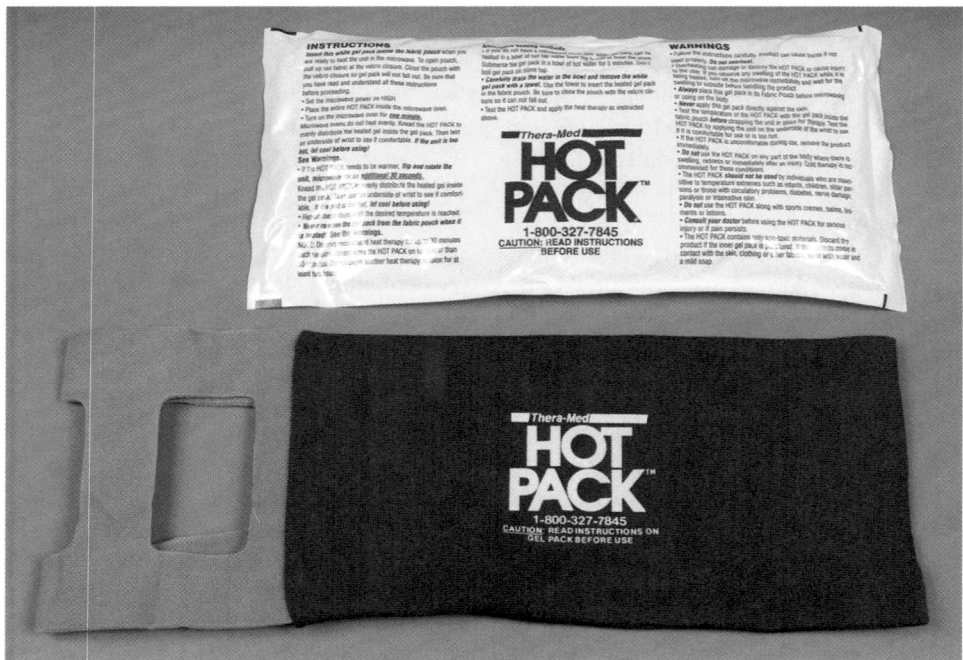

FIGURE **40-1** Commercial moist heat pack.

trolled source of heat to improve the application's therapeutic effects (see Skill 40-2). Moist warm compresses are used to improve circulation, relieve edema, promote consolidation of exudate in a wound, and promote comfort.

Moist heat application also includes the use of warm baths, soaks, and sitz baths. A warm bath or soak usually involves immersion of a body part into a warmed solution. Warm soaks and sitz baths are used to promote circulation, reduce edema and inflammation, promote muscle relaxation, debride wounds, and apply medicated solutions. If a body part is too large to immerse, a soak can be accomplished by wrapping the affected body part in a dressing saturated with the prepared, warmed solution.

A sitz bath is given by use of a special tub or chair basin that allows a client to sit in water without immersing the legs, feet, and upper trunk (Figure 40-2). Sitz basins are disposable and especially easy to use in the home. Portable baths fit easily on top of toilets. Clients who have undergone perineal or rectal surgery, who have had an episiotomy during childbirth, or who have painful hemorrhoids or perineal inflammation may benefit from a sitz bath.

When preparing a soak or bath, the nurse should remember that the heated solution is in direct contact with the

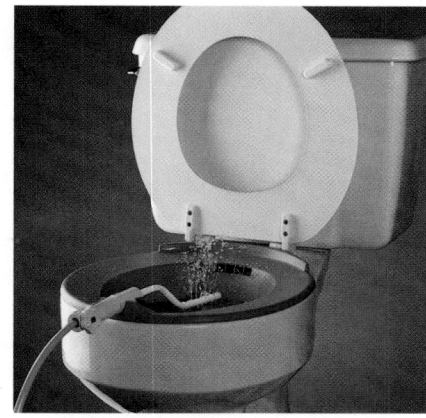

FIGURE **40-2** Disposable sitz bath.

client's skin. It is very important to check water temperature frequently and carefully to prevent burns. It is also desirable to keep the solution temperature constant to enhance the moist heat's therapeutic effects. Whenever heated solution is added to a soak basin or bath, the client's body part should be removed and then reimmersed once the solution has mixed.

DELEGATION CONSIDERATIONS

When the client is assessed by the nurse to be stable, and there are no risks or complications, the skill of applying moist heat can be delegated to assistive personnel. The nurse provides assistive personnel with information, assistance, and direction, including:

- Discuss with assistive personnel the need to maintain proper temperature of the application throughout the treatment and to keep the application in place for only the required length of time.
- Caution assistive personnel to inform the nurse if any discomfort develops, requiring termination of the treatment.
- Caution assistive personnel to inform the nurse if the client complains of dizziness or light-headedness.
- Instruct assistive personnel to report when treatment is complete so that an evaluation of the client's response can be made.

EQUIPMENT

- ❑ Clean basin, tub, or sitz bath (basin may need to be sterile if body part to be soaked has an open wound)
- ❑ Prescribed solution warmed to appropriate temperature (tap water is commonly used for sitz baths)
- ❑ Absorbent gauze dressing, cloth rolls, or commercially prepared compresses
- ❑ Prescribed medication (if ordered)
- ❑ Dry bath towel
- ❑ Disposable gloves
- ❑ Sterile gloves
- ❑ Waterproof pad
- ❑ Ties or tape
- ❑ Aquathermia or electric heating pad (optional)
- ❑ Bath blanket

STEP	RATIONALE

▌ ASSESSMENT

1. Refer to physician's order for type of moist heat application, location and duration of application, desired temperature, and institutional policies regarding temperature.

2. Assess skin around area to be treated for sensitivity to temperature and pain by measuring light touch, pinprick, and temperature sensation (see Chapter 18).

Ensures safe and correct application.

Certain conditions alter conduction of sensory impulses that transmit temperature and pain Clients insensitive to heat or cold sensations must be monitored closely during treatment.

STEP	RATIONALE

- *Critical Decision Point*

  Clients with diabetes, victims of stroke or spinal cord injury, and clients with peripheral neuropathy are particularly at risk for thermal injury (Stitik and Nadler, 1999).

| 3. Refer to medical record to identify any systemic contraindications to moist heat application. Clients with history of myocardial infarction, angina pectoris, or hypotension and those using nitroglycerin transdermal patch or ointment and smoking cessation patches are at risk. | Certain cardiovascular conditions and side effects of certain medications place clients at risk for sudden changes in blood pressure and blood flow caused by vasodilation. Heat causes vasodilation, which aggravates active bleeding. Heat applied to localized area of acute inflammation or tumor may cause rupture or activate cell growth (Stitik and Nadler, 1999). |

- *Critical Decision Point*

  Use caution when there is an area of active bleeding or inflammation.

4. Assess client's blood pressure and pulse.	Establishes a baseline for comparison.
5. Assess client's ability to position self for soak application or to position self in bath.	Determines level of assistance needed to place client in position for treatment.
6. Assess client's level of comfort using an appropriate pain scale (0 to 10).	Provides baseline for client's comfort level. Soak or bath may soothe inflamed or injured body parts (Stitik and Nadler, 1999).
7. Assess client's understanding of application and its purpose.	Determines need for health teaching.

NURSING DIAGNOSES

- Risk for injury
- Deficient knowledge regarding moist heat applications
- Impaired physical mobility
- Pain (acute, chronic)

- Disturbed sensory perception (tactile)
- Impaired skin integrity
- Ineffective (peripheral) tissue perfusion

Related factors are individualized based on client's condition or needs.

PLANNING

1. Expected outcomes following completion of procedure:	
• Affected area is pink and warm to touch immediately after application.	Vasodilation increases blood flow to site.
• After multiple applications, wound shows signs of healing (e.g., granulation; reduced edema, inflammation, drainage).	Moist heat increases blood flow, enhances white blood cell infiltration, and removes waste products from cells (Stitik and Nadler, 1999).
• Client denies burning sensation.	Indicates appropriate temperature applied.
• Client will relate a measurable decrease in pain.	Moist heat reduces edema/inflammation and relaxes stiff and strained muscles. Heat applications cause pain signals to be overridden as they enter dorsal horn of spinal column and decreases pain perception in cerebral cortex (Stitik and Nadler, 1999).
• Blood pressure and pulse are within client's normal range.	No systemic vascular changes occur. The goal of therapy is to achieve a localized vascular response.
• Client able to safely apply therapy.	Measures level of learning.
2. Assemble and prepare equipment and supplies.	Organization of supplies prevents unnecessary delays in procedure.

STEP	**RATIONALE**
3. Explain steps of procedure and purpose to client. Describe sensations to be felt, such as decreasing warmth and wetness. Explain precautions to prevent burning.	Minimizes client's anxiety and promotes cooperation during procedure.

IMPLEMENTATION

STEP	**RATIONALE**
1. Close door if in private room, and/or close bedside curtains.	Decreases drafts, thus decreasing the transmission of microorganisms. Provides for client privacy.
2. Perform hand hygiene.	Reduce transmission of microorganisms.
3. Apply moist sterile compress.	
a. Assist client in assuming comfortable position in proper body alignment, and place waterproof pad under area to be treated.	Compress remains in place for several minutes. Limited mobility in uncomfortable position causes muscular stress. Pad prevents soiling of bed linen.
b. Expose body part to be covered with compress, and drape client with bath blanket.	Prevents unnecessary cooling and exposure of body part.
c. Prepare compress.	
(1) Pour solution into sterile container.	
(2) If using portable heating source, warm solution. Commercially prepared compresses may remain under infrared lamp until just before use.	When using gauze compress, open sterile packages, and drop gauze into container to become immersed in solution.

- **Critical Decision Point**

  To avoid injury to client, test temperature of sterile solution by applying drop to nurse's forearm (without contaminating solution).

STEP	**RATIONALE**
d. Prepare aquathermia pad (if needed) (see Skill 40-2)	
e. Apply disposable gloves. Remove any existing dressing covering wound. Dispose of gloves and dressings in proper receptacle.	Reduces transmission of microorganisms.
f. Assess condition of wound and surrounding skin. Inflamed wound appears reddened, but surrounding skin is less red in color.	Provides baseline to determine response to moist heat.

- **Critical Decision Point**

  If skin surrounding wound is reddened, application may be contraindicated.

STEP	**RATIONALE**
g. Apply sterile gloves.	Allows nurse to manipulate sterile dressing and touch open wound.
h. Pick up one layer of immersed gauze, wring out any excess solution, and apply it lightly to open wound and avoid surrounding skin.	Excess moisture macerates skin and increases risk of burns and infection. Skin is sensitive to sudden change in temperature.
i. In few seconds, lift edge of gauze to assess for redness.	Increased redness indicates burn.
j. If client tolerates compress, pack gauze snugly against wound. Be sure all wound surfaces are covered by warm compress.	Packing of compress prevents rapid cooling from underlying air currents.
k. Cover moist compress with dry sterile dressing and bath towel. If necessary, pin or tie in place. Remove sterile gloves.	Dry sterile dressing will prevent transfer of microorganisms to wound via capillary action caused by moist compress. Towel insulates compress to prevent heat loss.
l. Apply aquathermia or waterproof heating pad over the towel *(optional)* (see Skill 40-2). Keep it in place for desired duration of application.	Provides constant temperature to compress.

STEP	RATIONALE

- *Critical Decision Point*

Removing warm compress after 20 minutes and then reapplying in 15 minutes, if desired, maintains vasodilation and positive therapeutic effects. Local application of heat for more than 20 minutes may result in reflex vasoconstriction (Stitik and Nadler, 1999).

STEP	RATIONALE
m. If an aquathermia pad is *not* used to maintain temperature of application, change warm compress using sterile technique every 5 to 10 minutes or as ordered during duration of therapy.	Prevents cooling and maintains therapeutic benefit of compress.
n. After prescribed time, apply disposable gloves, and remove pad, towel, and compress. Reassess wound and condition of skin, and replace dry sterile dressing as ordered.	Continued exposure to moisture will macerate skin. Prevents entrance of microorganisms into wound site.
o. Assist client to preferred comfortable position.	Maintains client's comfort.
p. Dispose of equipment and soiled compress. Perform hand hygiene.	Reduces transmission of microorganisms.
4. Provide sitz bath or soak to intact open skin.	
a. Apply disposable gloves. Remove any existing dressing covering wound. Dispose of gloves and dressings in proper receptacle.	Reduces transmission of microorganisms.
b. Assess condition of wound and surrounding skin. Pay particular attention to suture line.	Provides baseline to determine response to warm soak.
c. Fill basin or tub with warmed solution. Check temperature.	Checking for correct temperature reduces risk of burns.

- *Critical Decision Point*

Test temperature of solution by applying small amount to forearm.

STEP	RATIONALE
d. Assist client to immerse body part in tub or basin.	Prevents falls.
e. Cover client with bath blanket or towel as desired.	Prevents chilling and enhances client's ability to relax.
f. Maintain constant temperature throughout 15-to-20-minute soak:	Ensures proper therapeutic effect.
(1) Keep large sheet or blanket over container or basin.	Prevents heat loss through evaporation. Therapeutic effects of soak can be obtained only from constant temperature.
(2) After 10 minutes, remove body part from soak, check to see that skin is not burned, empty cooled solution, add newly heated solution, and reimmerse body part.	Presence of burn contraindicates completing the soak. Adding warmed solution to basin with body part immersed can cause burn.
g. After 15 to 20 minutes, remove client from soak or bath; dry body parts thoroughly. (Clean gloves are required if drainage is present.)	Avoids chilling. Enhances client's comfort.
h. Drain solution from basin or tub. Clean and place in proper storage area. Dispose of soiled linen and gloves (if used); perform hand hygiene.	Reduces transmission of microorganisms.

▌EVALUATION

STEP	RATIONALE
1. Inspect condition of body part or wound treated for redness, burns, and pain.	Evaluates effectiveness of treatment and risk for potential injury.
2. Question client regarding presence of burning sensation, severity of pain, and general response to therapy.	Determines if client was exposed to temperature extreme, resulting in burn. Evaluates client's subjective response to therapy.

STEP	RATIONALE
3. Assess vital signs if client complains of dizziness or light-headedness.	Determines if vascular response to vasodilation has occurred.
4. Have client demonstrate application of therapy and explain its purpose.	Measures level of learning and ability to perform application.

Recording and Reporting

- Record procedure, noting type, location, and duration of application, as well as solution and temperature in nurses' notes.
- Record condition of body part, wound, and skin before and after treatment and client's response to therapy.
- Record preprocedure and postprocedure vital signs (as indicated).
- Record any instructions given and client's ability to explain and perform procedure.
- Report all client complaints and any unusual findings to nurse in charge or physician.

Unexpected Outcomes	Related Interventions
1. Client's skin is reddened and sensitive to touch. Extreme warmth caused burning of skin layer.	• Discontinue moist application immediately. • Notify physician.
2. Client complains of burning and discomfort. Individuals vary in their tolerance to heat and pain.	• Extreme temperature for client to tolerate—reduce temperature. • Assess for skin breakdown. • Notify physician.
3. Client unable to explain purpose of application or performs it incorrectly.	• Reinstruction or clarification needed.

Teaching Considerations

- If heat applications are to be continued after discharge, have client or family member give a return demonstration before discharge.
- Teach client to gently pack wound, when using sterile compresses, to avoid discomfort.
- Caregivers and clients need to be taught that careful assessment is needed for clients with reduced sensation to determine if temperature of compress is too hot.

Pediatric Considerations

- The skin of infants and children is thin and fragile and therefore easily damaged. Use special caution in this population (Hockenberry and others, 2003). Remain with children during procedure for safety and effectiveness.
- It is often helpful to incorporate play into the time the child is required to soak. Placing items in the basin for the child to interact with is helpful. Boats or other similar water toys may be placed in the bath with the child who requires a bath soak. Adult supervision is necessary.

Gerontological Considerations

- The older adult client who is receiving long-term steroid therapy or is malnourished can develop thin, fragile skin, which is more easily damaged.
- The older adult may have impaired circulation to a given skin region or impaired sensation for pain/or temperature (Lueckenotte, 2000).
- Older adult clients, whose aging process has resulted in loss of subcutaneous tissue and fat and consequently the insulating effect of these substances, may experience alterations in thermoregulation (Lueckenotte, 2000).
- In some clients, such as frail, older clients with cardiac conditions, it may be necessary to monitor vital signs throughout procedure.

Home Care Considerations

- When necessary, assess availability of primary caregiver to assist client in application of moist heat, caregiver's understanding of purpose of procedure, and willingness of caregiver to comply with procedure and not leave client.
- Assess physical environment to determine adequacy of facilities for use by client. Medical equipment companies may be contacted for assistance in determining best product for client.

SKILL 40-2   Applying Aquathermia and Heating Pads

Aquathermia and heating pads are common forms of dry heat therapy used in health care settings and in the home (Figure 40-3). Both are covered and applied directly to the skin's surface, and for this reason extra precautions are needed to prevent burns. The aquathermia pad (water flow pad) consists of a waterproof rubber or plastic pad connected by two hoses to an electrical control unit that has a heating element and motor. Distilled water circulates through hollowed channels in the pad to the control unit where water is heated (or cooled). The nurse can adjust the temperature setting by inserting a plastic key into the control unit. In most health care institutions, the central supply department sets the temperature regulators to the recommended temperature, approximately 40.5° to 43° C (105° to 109.4° F). Because of the constant temperature control, aquathermia pads tend to be safer than heating pads. If distilled water in the unit runs low, the nurse simply adds more distilled water to the reservoir at the top of the control unit. Rubber and plastic conduct heat, so the pad should be encased in a towel or pillowcase to avoid direct exposure to the skin.

The conventional heating pad, used mostly in the home care setting, consists of an electric coil enclosed in a water-

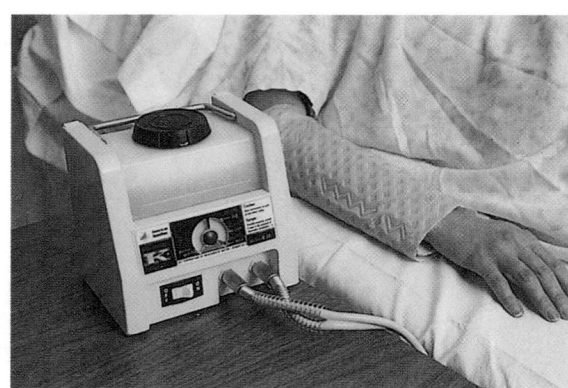

FIGURE **40-3** Aquathermia pad.

proof cover. A cotton or flannel cloth covers the outer pad. The pad connects to an electrical cord that has a temperature-regulating unit for high, medium, or low settings. Because it is so easy to readjust temperature settings on heating pads, clients should be instructed not to turn the setting higher once they have adapted to the temperature. It is wise to avoid ever using the highest setting.

DELEGATION CONSIDERATIONS
The skill of applying an aquathermia or heating pad may be delegated to assistive personnel. The nurse should assess the condition of the area to be treated and explain the purpose of the treatment. If there are no risks or complications, this skill can be delegated. The nurse provides assistive personnel with information, assistance, and direction, including:
- Caution assistive personnel to maintain proper temperature of the application throughout the treatment and to keep the application in place for only the length of time specified based on physician order or hospital policy.
- Caution assistive personnel to check client's skin for excessive redness and pain during application and to report any changes to the nurse.

- Instruct the assistive personnel to report when treatment is complete so that an evaluation of the client's response can be made.

EQUIPMENT
- ❑ Aquathermia (acute care) or heating pad (home care)
- ❑ Electrical control unit
- ❑ Distilled water (for aquathermia pad)
- ❑ Bath towel or pillowcase
- ❑ Tape, ties, or gauze roll

STEP	RATIONALE

ASSESSMENT
1. Refer to physician's order for location of application and duration of therapy. Institutional policy usually sets recommended temperature for aquathermia pad.

2. Assess condition of skin over which pad is to be applied.

3. Assess level of discomfort and range of motion if client is being treated for muscle sprain.

4. Assess area to be treated for sensitivity to temperature, light touch, and pain (see Chapter 18).

Order required to help ensure client's safety.

Provides baseline to determine change in skin condition after heat application.

Provides baseline to determine if pain relief is achieved.

Determines if client is insensitive to heat extremes.

STEP	RATIONALE
5. Check electrical plugs and cords for obvious fraying or cracking.	Prevents injury from accidental electrical shock.
6. Determine client's or family members' knowledge of procedure, including steps for application and safety precautions.	Heating pads are frequently used in home. Assessment determines extent of health teaching required.

NURSING DIAGNOSES

- Risk for injury
- Deficient knowledge regarding moist heat applications
- Impaired physical mobility
- Pain (acute, chronic)

- Disturbed sensory perception (tactile)
- Impaired skin integrity
- Ineffective peripheral tissue perfusion

Related factors are individualized based on client's condition or needs.

PLANNING

1. Expected outcomes following completion of procedure:	
• Skin is pink and warm to touch after application.	Vasodilation from heat exposure increases blood flow to affected part.
• Client reports less discomfort of inflamed tissues or strained muscles.	Heat applications lower pain perception by stimulating large-diameter sensory nerve fibers and blocking pain impulses of smaller nerve fibers (Stitik and Nadler, 1999).
• Client may be able to move strained muscles more freely.	Heat reduces stiffness and improves range of motion (Stitik and Nadler, 1999).
• Client correctly applies pad.	Documents learning.
2. Prepare equipment and supplies.	Organization of supplies prevents unnecessary delays in procedure.
3. Explain procedure and precautions.	Improves likelihood of client's compliance with therapy.

IMPLEMENTATION

1. Close door if in private room, and/or close bedside curtains.	Provides for client's privacy.
2. Perform hand hygiene, and position client comfortably so area to be treated may be exposed.	Reduces transfer of microorganisms. Client must be able to assume position for several minutes during application.
3. For aquathermia or uncovered heating pad, cover or wrap affected area with bath towel, or enclose pad with pillowcase.	Prevents heated surface from touching client's skin directly and increasing risk for injury to client's skin.

- **Critical Decision Point**
  Do not pin the wrap to pad because this may cause a leak in device.

4. Place pad over affected area (see Figure 40-3), and secure with tape, tie, or gauze as needed.	Pad delivers dry warm heat to injured tissues. Pad should not slip onto different body part.

- **Critical Decision Point**
  Never position client so that client is lying directly on pad. This position prevents dissipation of heat and increases risk of burns.

5. Turn heating pad on to low or medium setting. Check temperature of aquathermia pad.	Prevents exposure of client to temperature extremes.
6. Monitor condition of skin every 5 minutes during application, and question client regarding sensation of burning.	Determines if heat exposure is resulting in burn.

STEP	RATIONALE
7. After 20 to 30 minutes (or time ordered by physician), remove pad and store.	Continued exposure will result in burns. Some clients should not have access to pad without supervision.
8. Assist client in returning to preferred comfortable position, dispose of soiled linen, and perform hand hygiene.	Promotes relaxing environment. Reduces spread of microorganisms.

EVALUATION

1. Inspect condition of skin exposed to heat.	Evaluates response of skin to heat exposure.
2. Ask client if strained muscle or inflamed area continues to be painful. Evaluate pain severity.	Heat reduces edema and relieves pain from muscle stiffness and spasm (Stitik and Nadler, 1999).
3. Note if client is able to move strained muscle with less discomfort.	Heat relaxes strained muscle.

- *Critical Decision Point*
  Do not have client actively exercise muscle to evaluate results of therapy. Active exercise can aggravate muscle strain.

4. Observe client apply pad.	Measures level of learning.

Recording and Reporting

- Record site of application, duration of therapy, and client's response.
- Describe any instruction given and client's success in demonstrating procedure.
- Report changes in skin integrity such as burns.

Unexpected Outcomes	Related Interventions
1. Skin is reddened and sensitive to touch. Symptoms indicate first-degree burn.	• Remove the pad, and reassess in 5 to 10 minutes. • If symptoms continue, notify nurse in charge, or contact physician.
2. Edema and inflammation are increased. Applying heat too soon after an injury can increase edema through vasodilation.	• Notify nurse in charge, or contact physician.
3. Body part is painful to move. Movement stretches burn-sensitive nerve fibers in skin.	• Discontinue aquathermia or heating pad use. Wait for swelling to resolve before attempting to reapply. • Notify nurse in charge, or contact physician.
4. Client applies heat incorrectly or is unable to relate precautions.	• Reinstruct client as necessary.

Teaching Considerations
- Highlight safety precautions as they are followed during application.

Pediatric Considerations
- Due to the risk of injury from heating pads, this treatment is used infrequently in children.
- The skin of infants and children is thin and fragile and therefore easily damaged. Use special caution in this population. Remain with children during procedure for safety and effectiveness.
- Assess body temperature gain and loss, which occurs more readily in pediatric clients.

Gerontological Considerations
- Older adults are more at risk for burns because of loss of heat sensation. Check site frequently during all treatments.
- Older clients have thin, more fragile skin that is susceptible to burns.

Home Care Considerations

- Assess client and primary caregiver as to their understanding, ability, and motivation to comply with procedure.
- Assess home environment for facilities (e.g., condition of electrical outlets) to comply with implementation of procedure.

SKILL 40-3 Applying Cold Applications

Application of cold, or cryotherapy, can be accomplished through many therapeutic modalities, such as moist cold compresses, chemical or cold packs, electromechanical or compression devices, or immersion of a body part into a cold soak. Cold therapy is used to treat localized inflammatory responses that lead to edema, hemorrhage, muscle spasm, or pain (see Table 40-1). Cold can exert a profound physiological effect on the body, reducing inflammation caused by injuries to the musculoskeletal system (Airaksinen and others, 2003; Poddar, 2003; Stitik and Nadler, 1998). Because reduction of inflammation is the primary goal, cryotherapy is the treatment of choice for the first 24 to 48 hours after an injury.

Vasoconstriction resulting from cold application reduces blood flow to the injured part and thus reduces fluid accumulation and slows bleeding and hematoma formation associated with trauma. The lower temperature also suppresses muscle spasm and produces a local anesthetic response. When used appropriately, cold applications can significantly lessen pain and immobility by reducing swelling of injured tissues (Airaksinen and others, 2003; Poddar, 2003; Stitik and Nadler, 1998). This is an important point for nurses to know when deciding on the choice of heat or cold for the treatment of acute injuries. Cold is also indicated as an adjunct analgesic for chronic pain and spasticity control. It can also be used as an analgesic after arthroscopic surgical procedures (Airaksinen and others, 2003).

A cold compress usually consists of a commercial cold pack, a gauze dressing, or a washcloth that has been immersed in iced or chilled solution to achieve the desired temperature. The compress may be sterile or clean; however, a clean compress is most commonly used. Any open wounds require sterile applications. A variety of sizes or thicknesses of gauze can be used, depending on the site of injury. For example, a cold compress to the eye requires thicker gauze that fits a small area to maintain a cold temperature. Thin gauze works more effectively for larger areas such as the face.

Ice bags and cold packs come in a variety of sizes to fit different body parts (Figure 40-4). When a commercial ice bag or cold pack is unavailable, the client can use a plastic bag or glove filled halfway with crushed ice. The bag or glove should be squeezed to expel air, which hampers cold conduction. In the home setting, a bag of frozen vegetables can be substituted for an ice bag. All of these items should be wrapped in a towel or cloth before application.

There are electrically controlled cooling devices that work much like an aquathermia pad. The cooling pad has the advantage of delivering a constant cool temperature. This type of machine can be recommended as an alternative aid to postoperative pain management in clients undergoing certain orthopedic surgeries (Wilke and Weiner, 2003). Cold modalities that simultaneously provide compression are extremely effective in treating acute musculoskeletal injuries that are associated with soft-tissue swelling (Arnold and Shelbourne, 2000; Kannus, 2000). Elevating the extremity during treatment further augments venous return. A person who undergoes treatment with one of these devices is simultaneously receiving all four components of the rest, ice, compression, and elevation (RICE) method for managing this type of injury.

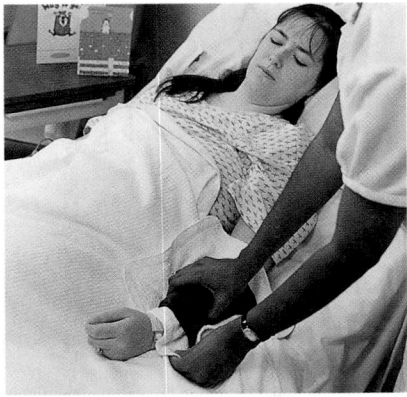

FIGURE **40-4** Placement of ice pack (or bag) on extremity.

DELEGATION CONSIDERATIONS

The skill of applying cold applications may be delegated to assistive personnel in special situations. The client should be assessed and the purpose of the treatment explained. If there are no risks or complications, this skill may be delegated. The nurse provides assistive personnel with information, assistance, and direction, including:

- Caution assistive personnel to maintain proper temperature of the application throughout the treatment and to keep the application in place for only the length of time specified in the physician's order.
- Caution assistive personnel to check client's skin for excessive redness or pain and to report immediately to the nurse if any adverse reactions occur.
- Instruct assistive personnel to report when treatment is complete so that an evaluation of the client's response can be made.

EQUIPMENT

- ❑ Cold compress
- ❑ Absorbent gauze (clean or sterile) folded to desired size
- ❑ Clean or sterile basin with ice and water at desired temperature
- ❑ Bath towel or absorbent pad
- ❑ Two pairs of disposable or sterile gloves (according to agency policy)
- ❑ Cool water flow pad
- ❑ Cooling pad and electrical pump
- ❑ Compression device with appropriate extremity attachments
- ❑ Tapes, ties, gauze roll, or elastic wrap bandage
- ❑ Ice bag or collar with water
- ❑ Ice pack
- ❑ Towel or pillowcase
- ❑ Cloth ties or tape
- ❑ Disposable gloves (if blood or body fluids are present)

STEP	RATIONALE

ASSESSMENT

1. Refer to physician's order for location and duration of application.

   Physician's order is required for all cold applications.

2. Inspect condition of injured or affected part. Gently palpate area.

   Provides baseline for determining change in condition of injured tissues.

- **Critical Decision Point**

  Keep injured part immobilized and in alignment. Movement can cause further injury to strains, sprains, or fractures.

3. Consider time in which injury occurred.

   Cold should be applied quickly after an injury to prevent edema. Application of cold is most effective if started within 24 hours of injury.

4. Ask client to describe severity and character of pain on a scale of 0 to 10.

   Provides baseline for determining pain relief with therapy.

5. Assess area to be treated for sensitivity to temperature, light touch, and pain and for adequate circulation (see Chapter 18).

   Determines if client is insensitive to cold extremes.

6. Assess client's understanding of procedure.

   Determines need for health teaching.

NURSING DIAGNOSES

- Risk for injury
- Deficient knowledge regarding moist cold applications
- Impaired physical mobility

- Pain (acute, chronic)
- Impaired skin integrity
- Ineffective peripheral tissue perfusion

Related factors are individualized based on client's condition or needs.

PLANNING

1. Expected outcomes following completion of procedure:
   - Affected area is slightly pale and cool to touch.
   - Extent of edema is decreased.

   - Client relates measurable decrease in pain.

   Result of vasoconstriction.
   Cold reduces blood flow to affected part, reducing edema formation (Airaksinen and others, 2003; Stitik and Nadler, 1998).
   Cold creates local anesthetic effect (Airaksinen and others, 2003; Poddar, 2003).

STEP	RATIONALE
• Client correctly states how to apply cold compress and provides demonstration.	Documents learning.
2. Prepare equipment and supplies.	Organization prevents unnecessary delays.
3. Explain procedure and precautions.	Improves likelihood of client's compliance with therapy.

IMPLEMENTATION

1. Close room door and bedside curtain.	Provides privacy for client.
2. Perform hand hygiene.	Reduces spread of microorganisms.
3. Position client carefully, keeping body part in proper alignment and exposing only area to be treated.	Prevents further injury to body part. Avoids unnecessary exposure of body parts, maintaining client's comfort and privacy.

• *Critical Decision Point*
In cases of strains, sprains, or fractures, extremity or body part should remain aligned to prevent further injury.

4. Place towel or absorbent pad under area to be treated.	Prevents soiling of bed linen.
5. Apply disposable gloves.	Reduces spread of infection.
6. Cold compress:	
a. Check temperature of solution, and submerge gauze into filled basin at bedside; wring out excess moisture.	Extreme temperature can cause tissue damage. Dripping gauze is uncomfortable to client.
b. Apply compress to affected area, molding it gently over site.	Ensures that cold is directed over site of injury.
7. Electrically controlled cooling device:	
a. Wrap cool water flow pad around body part (see illustration).	Ensures even application of cold temperature.
b. Be sure correct temperature is set.	Ensures effective therapy.
c. Secure with elastic wrap bandage, gauze roll, or ties.	
8. Prepare ice bag or collar:	
a. Fill bag with water, secure cap, and invert.	Checks for leaks.
b. Empty water, and then fill bag two-thirds full with small ice chips.	Bag can be more easily molded over body part.

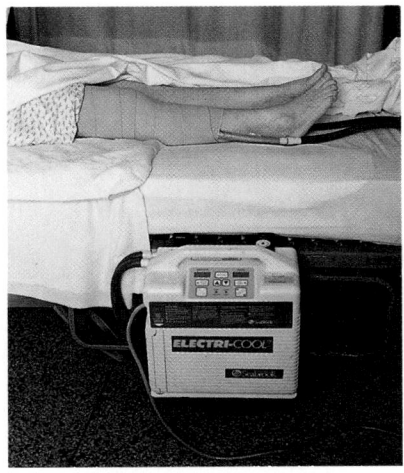

STEP **7a** Cooling device.

STEP	RATIONALE
c. Release excess air from bag by squeezing its sides before securing cap.	Excess air interferes with cold conduction (Ruffolo, 2002).
d. Wipe bag dry.	Prevents skin maceration.
e. Apply snugly over area. Secure with tape as needed.	Cold should be directly over injury to maximize therapeutic effect.
9. Prepare ice pack:	
a. Commercial packs are squeezed or kneaded.	Releases alcohol-based solution to create cold temperature.

• Critical Decision Point
Moisture may form on outside of bag if room temperature is warm. This does not indicate a leak.

b. Apply pack directly over area. Wrap prepared bag or pack with towel or pillowcase.	Cold should be applied directly over injury. Protects client's tissue and absorbs condensation. Prevents direct exposure of cold against client's skin.

• Critical Decision Point
Do not reapply ice pack to red or bluish areas; continual use of ice pack makes ischemia worse.

10. Remove gloves, and dispose of in proper container.	Reduces transfer of microorganisms.
11. Check condition of skin every 5 minutes for duration of application.	Determines if there are adverse reactions to cold. These include mottling, redness, burning, blistering, and numbness (Stitik and Nadler, 1998).
a. If area is edematous, sensation may be reduced, and extra caution must be used during cold therapy.	
b. Numbness and tingling are common sensations with cold applications and indicate adverse reactions only when severe and coupled with other symptoms. Stop when client complains of burning sensation or skin begins to feel numb.	When applying cold, skin will initially feel cold, followed by relief of pain. As cryotherapy continues, client will feel a burning sensation, then pain in the skin, and finally numbness (Stitik and Nadler, 1998).
12. After 15 to 20 minutes (or as ordered by the physician), apply clean gloves, remove compress or pad, and gently dry off any moisture.	Drying prevents maceration of skin. Prolonged application of cold can result in diminished blood flow and tissue ischemia or compensatory vasodilation to provide warmth to area being treated (Stitik and Nadler, 1998).

• Critical Decision Point
Areas with little body fat (such as knee, ankle, and elbow) do not tolerate cold as well as fatty areas (such as thigh and buttocks). For bony areas, decrease time of cold application to lower range.

13. Assist client to comfortable position.	Maintains relaxing environment.
14. Remove and dispose of supplies. Empty basin, if used, and dry. Dispose of soiled linen and gloves. Perform hand hygiene.	Reduces transfer of microorganisms.

EVALUATION

1. Inspect affected area for changes in condition of skin.	Determines reaction to cold application.
2. Palpate affected area gently.	Determines level of edema.
3. Question client about level of comfort.	Determines if pain has been relieved.
4. Ask client to apply cold application and explain risks of treatment.	Measures level of learning.

Recording and Reporting

- Record procedure, including type, location, duration of application, and client's response, in nurses' notes.
- Describe any instruction given and client's success in demonstrating procedure.
- Report undesirable changes in condition of skin to nurse in charge or physician.

Unexpected Outcomes	Related Interventions
1. Skin takes on mottled, reddened, or bluish purple appearance as a result of prolonged exposure.	• Stop the treatment. • Notify nurse in charge or physician. • Injury from prolonged exposure requires different therapy.
2. Client complains of burning type of pain and numbness.	• Stop the treatment because these are signs of ischemia. • Notify nurse in charge or physician.
3. Client is unable to describe application or use compress correctly.	• Reinstruction and clarification are necessary.

Teaching Considerations

- Injuries requiring this type of therapy usually occur away from health care settings. Clients active in sports should know steps to take to minimize extent of injury.

Pediatric Considerations

- A greater metabolic rate and larger trunk in relation to rest of body make children more prone to hypothermia (Nicoll, 2002). Exercise caution with young clients.
- Infants have an unstable temperature control mechanism, so mottling of extremities is common and may not indicate an adverse reaction if this symptom is seen alone (Nicoll, 2002).
- Cool soaks may also be used to decrease itching with some skin lesions. The same precautions and use of play should be used as with warm soaks.

Gerontological Considerations

- Older adults are more at risk for tissue damage due to loss of cold sensation (Nicoll, 2002). Check site frequently during all treatments.

Home Care Considerations

- Clean cloth can be used in home setting as long as there is no open wound.
- Assess client and primary caregiver as to understanding, ability, and motivation to comply with procedure.
- Assess client's home environment for adequacy of facilities with which to implement procedure.
- An ice pack can be improvised by placing ice cubes in a zippered plastic bag or by using a bag of frozen peas or corn. Place a thin towel between bag and skin.

SKILL 40-4　Caring for Clients Requiring Hypothermia or Hyperthermia Blankets

The hypothermia-hyperthermia blanket raises, lowers, or maintains body temperature through conductive heat or cold transfer between the blanket and the client. When operated manually, the unit maintains a set temperature regardless of the client's temperature. Because the client's temperature is assessed using conventional thermometers, the unit's temperature is manually adjusted to reach a different temperature setting.

When operating in the automatic setting, the unit continually monitors the client's temperature using a thermistor probe (rectal, skin, or esophageal). Temperature heating and cooling cycles alternate to achieve and maintain the desired temperature.

Clients can have high, prolonged fevers from infectious and neurological diseases and as side effects from anesthesia. When the client presents with hyperthermia caused by injury to the anterior hypothalamus or as side effect of anesthesia, the application of a hypothermia (cooling) blanket is recommended (Nicoll, 2002). Hypothermia blankets are fluid-filled rubberized blankets that circulate cooled solution (usually distilled water) through the blanket. When placed on top of the client, the cooling blanket helps to reduce the client's body temperature (Figure 40-5). The application of a hypothermia (cooling) blanket is not recommended in caring for the client with a diagnosis of fever (Nicoll, 2002).

Conversely, clients whose body temperature is abnormally low due to extreme exposure to cold or due to hypothermia induced for neurological or cardiac surgery require a hyperthermia (warming) blanket to assist the body in returning to near-normal temperature (Nicoll, 2002; Sicoutris, 2001). In the case of hyperthermia or rewarming therapy, a warmed solution is circulated through the blanket to help return the client's body temperature to normal.

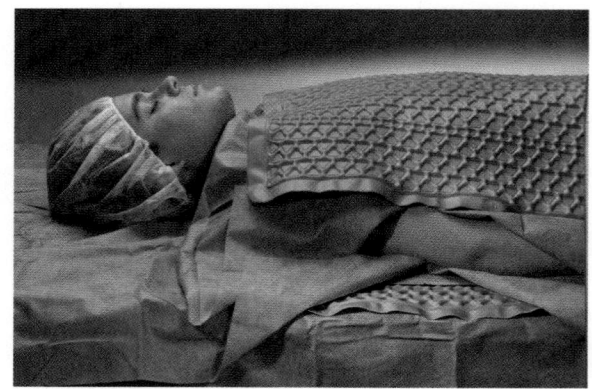

FIGURE 40-5 Hypothermia cooling blanket before sheet applied to bed. (Courtesy Cincinnati Sub-Zero Maxi-Therm Hyper-Hypothermia Blanket.)

DELEGATION CONSIDERATIONS

This skill may be delegated to assistive personnel. The nurse should initially assess the client and explain the purpose of the treatment. If there are no risks or complications, this skill can be delegated. The nurse provides assistive personnel with information, assistance, and direction, including:

- Caution assistive personnel to maintain proper temperature of the application throughout the treatment and to discontinue the application as specified in the physician's order.
- Caution assistive personnel to inform the nurse of any unexpected outcomes such as shivering or redness to the skin.
- Instruct assistive personnel to report when treatment is complete so that an evaluation of the client's response can be made.

EQUIPMENT

- ❑ Hypothermia or hyperthermia blanket with control panel and rectal probe
- ❑ Sheet or thin bath blanket
- ❑ Distilled water to fill the units if necessary
- ❑ Disposable gloves
- ❑ Rectal thermometer

STEP	RATIONALE

ASSESSMENT

1. Refer to physician's order, and double-check that client's current body temperature requires use of hypothermia or hyperthermia blanket.

Institution of therapy requires physician's order.

2. Assess vital signs, neurological status, mental status, and peripheral circulation.

Establishes baseline data to use for comparison during therapy.

3. Verify that other, less intensive measures cannot return client's body temperature to normal.

Use of hypothermia and hyperthermia blanket is not without risk and should be instituted only when other measures are not effective (Nicoll, 2002).

- *Critical Decision Point*

    Antipyretic therapy should be attempted for fever. Physiological manifestations of fever include increased oxygen consumption, increased heart rate, increased cardiac output, and elevated levels of catecholamines, which can be detrimental to seriously or critically ill clients (Nicoll, 2002).

STEP	RATIONALE

4. Assess client's skin on chest and extremities, paying close attention to bony prominences such as hands and feet.

These areas are more exposed to blanket and consequently are at greater risk for injury. Baseline data enable nurse to quickly determine if injury to skin is result of therapy.

NURSING DIAGNOSES

- Fever
- Risk for injury
- Deficient knowledge regarding implications of hypothermia or hyperthermia blanket
- Impaired physical mobility

- Pain (acute, chronic)
- Disturbed sensory perception (tactile)
- Impaired skin integrity
- Ineffective peripheral tissue perfusion

Related factors are individualized based on client's condition or needs.

PLANNING

1. Expected outcomes following completion of procedure:
   - Temperature is within normal range.
   - Absence of shivering with hypothermia blanket.

   Indicates that therapy is effective.
   Shivering increases metabolic rate and heat production but also increases oxygen consumption. This mechanism contributes to body temperature elevation and can cause client's body temperature to rise (Nicoll, 2002). In addition, shivering causes vasoconstriction, which can injure skin of distal body regions (Nicoll, 2002).

   - Skin clear without signs of injury or burns.

   Distal regions of client's skin are at greatest risk for injury from blanket. Indicates that treatment is causing no adverse effects.

2. Explain procedure to client.
   Increases cooperation and reduces anxiety.
3. Position client comfortably.
4. Prepare blanket according to agency policy and manufacturer's instructions.

   Agencies have specific policies as to who should maintain equipment in functional order. Each type of blanket varies from one manufacturer to another. Manufacturer's instructions are located on machine. Read before using.

IMPLEMENTATION

1. Perform hand hygiene, and apply gloves.
   Reduces transmission of microorganisms.
2. Measure temperature, pulse, respirations, and blood pressure.
   Provides baseline for determining response to therapy.
3. Apply lanolin or mixture of lanolin and cold cream to client's skin where it will touch blanket.
   Helps protect skin from heat and cold sensations.
4. Turn on blanket, and observe that cool or warm light is on. Precool or prewarm blanket, setting pad temperature to desired level.
   Verifies that blanket is correctly set to assist in reducing (cool) or increasing (warm) client's body temperature. Prepares blanket for prescribed therapy.
5. Verify that pad temperature limits are set at desired safety ranges.
   Safety ranges prevent excessive cooling or warming. The blanket automatically shuts off when preset body temperature is achieved.
6. Cover the hypothermia or hyperthermia blanket with a thin sheet or bath blanket.
   Protects client's skin from direct contact with blanket, thus reducing risk of injury to skin. Sheet or blanket covers plastic and provides insulation between client and appliance.

STEP	**RATIONALE**
7. Position hypothermia or hyperthermia blanket on top of client.	Provides wide distribution of blanket against client's skin.

- **Critical Decision Point**
  When using a blanket for hypothermia, the client has the potential to develop pressure ulcers because of decreased blood flow in the skin.

STEP	**RATIONALE**
a. Wrap client's hands and feet in gauze.	Reduces risk of thermal injury to body's distal areas.
b. Wrap scrotum with towels.	Protects sensitive tissue from direct contact with cold.
8. Lubricate rectal probe and insert into client's rectum.	When using hypothermia or hyperthermia blanket, it is imperative that nurse continuously monitor client's core interior (rectal) temperature.
9. Turn and position client regularly to protect from pressure ulcer development and impaired body alignment (see Chapter 10). Keep linens free of perspiration and condensation.	Client has an increased risk of pressure ulcer development because of skin moisture created by blanket and client's body temperature.
10. Double-check fluid thermometer on control panel of blanket before leaving room.	Verifies that pad temperature is maintained at desired level.
11. Remove gloves, and perform hand hygiene.	Reduces transmission of microorganisms.

EVALUATION

STEP	**RATIONALE**
1. Monitor client's temperature and vital signs every 15 minutes during first hour, and every 30 minutes of therapy thereafter.	Provides continuous evaluation of response of client's body temperature to therapy during initial and continual therapy.
2. Evaluate automatic temperature control every 30 minutes visually and every 4 hours by taking client's rectal temperature.	Ensures removal of hypothermia or hyperthermia blanket when client's temperature returns to desired level. Decreases risk of subnormal body temperature. Verifies accuracy of rectal probe and automatic temperature control device.

- **Critical Decision Point**
  It is generally accepted to discontinue hypothermia treatment when the client's core temperature is 1° F above desired temperature.

STEP	**RATIONALE**
3. Observe skin for indications of burns, change in color, and other signs of injury.	Hypothermia and hyperthermia blankets have the potential to cause skin injuries.
4. Observe client for signs of shivering.	Early signs of shivering, which may harm client, include electrocardiographic changes, facial muscle twitching, or hyperventilation.
5. Determine client's level of comfort.	Therapy has the potential to cause discomfort. Prompt assessment reduces risk for severe injuries.

Recording and Reporting

- Record baseline data: vital signs, neurological and mental status, status of peripheral circulation and skin integrity when therapy was initiated.
- Note type of hyperthermia-hypothermia unit used; control settings (manual or automatic, and temperature settings); date, time, duration, and client's tolerance of treatment.
- Chart on temperature graphic repeated measurements of vital signs to document response to therapy.
- Report any unexpected outcome to physician. Further treatment may be needed.

Unexpected Outcomes	Related Interventions
1. Client's core body temperature decreases or rises rapidly. This indicates that temperature is too extreme and might produce injury to client.	• Adjust blanket temperature no more than 1° F every 15 minutes to avoid complications.
2. Client's core temperature remains unchanged.	• Client may need hypothermic or hyperthermic treatment of additional sites, such as axilla, groin, and neck, in addition to those covered by blanket. • Discuss use of an antipyretic with physician.
3. Client begins to shiver. Shivering increases metabolic rate and heat production, causing client's core body temperature to rise, and increases oxygen consumption.	• Adjust the temperature to a more comfortable range, and assess if shivering decreases. • If shivering continues, stop treatment and notify physician.
4. Skin breaks down, indicating that client's skin may have received thermal injury (frostbite or burn) from blanket.	• Stop treatment. • Notify physician.

Teaching Considerations
• Clients and their families need to be instructed not to move client off blanket.

Pediatric Considerations
• A greater metabolic rate and larger trunk in relation to rest of body make children more prone to hypothermia (Nicoll, 2002). Exercise caution with young clients.

• Infants have an unstable temperature control mechanism, so mottling of extremities is common and may not indicate an adverse reaction.

Gerontological Considerations
• Older adults are more at risk for tissue damage because of loss of cold sensation. Check client frequently during all treatments.

FOCUS *on* CLINICAL PRACTICE

You are assigned to care for an 82-year-old client with a complaint of right ankle pain after slipping on a wet spot on the floor. The client is currently unable to bear weight on the extremity. It appears to be bruised and swollen.

1. What other information would you like to have about this client?
2. The emergency department (ED) attending physician has been in to examine your client and orders a cold compress to the right foot and ankle. What do you need to do to begin an application? Check all that apply. Explain your choice(s).
   A. Notify the charge nurse of the need for a cold application.
   B. Refer to physician's order for location and duration of the application.
   C. Explain the procedure and precautions to avoid injury to the skin.
   D. Assess condition of injured or affected body part.
3. List information to include in an explanation to the client about the cold application treatment.
4. Your client has been diagnosed with a severe muscle strain of the right shoulder, and the physician has ordered heat applications to the shoulder for 24 hours. The therapeutic benefits of heat application include:
   A. Local anesthesia
   B. Vasodilation
   C. Increased muscle tension
   D. Vasoconstriction

NCLEX REVIEW QUESTIONS

1. A client has been diagnosed with severe muscle strain of the lower back, and the physician has ordered heat applications to the lower back for 48 hours. The main advantage of using moist heat application instead of dry heat in treating this client is:
   1. Moist heat is less likely to burn the skin.
   2. Moist heat penetrates deeper into tissue layers.
   3. Moist heat causes skin maceration.
   4. Moist heat cools rapidly due to moisture evaporation.

2. Conditions that increase the risk of injury from heat applications include:
   1. Areas with a lot of body fat
   2. Anxiety
   3. Peripheral vascular disease
   4. Dehydration

3. When applying dry heat using a heating pad, what would be a reason for discontinuing the application?
   1. Skin is pink and warm to touch.
   2. Skin is reddened and sensitive to touch.
   3. Client reports less discomfort of inflamed tissue or muscle strain.
   4. Client can move strained muscle more freely.

4. Which of the following interventions will prevent burns when using an aquathermia pad on an older client?
   1. Place the client on top of the aquathermia pad.
   2. Turn the aquathermia pad to the highest setting.
   3. Wrap the uncovered aquathermia pad around the injured body part.
   4. Monitor the condition of the skin every 5 minutes during the application.

5. You have just completed a cold application to your client's knee. Which of the following is an expected outcome?
   1. Affected area is slightly pale and cool to touch.
   2. Extent of edema had increased.
   3. Client relates measurable increase in pain.
   4. Affected area is mottled, reddened, or bluish purple.

6. Cold applications affect the injured body part by:
   1. Causing vasodilation, which increases blood flow
   2. Causing vasoconstriction, which decreases blood flow
   3. Increasing pain and immobility
   4. Increasing muscle spasms

7. When applying a cold application to a bony prominence, such as an ankle or elbow, you should:
   1. Decrease the time of the cold application
   2. Increase the time of the cold application
   3. Keep the time length of the cold application the same as when the application is over a fatty area
   4. Leave the cold application in place until it naturally cools to allow for deeper penetration

8. Shivering during the application of a hypothermia (cooling) blanket decreases the effectiveness of treatment by:
   1. Decreasing the metabolic rate and heat loss
   2. Decreasing oxygen consumption
   3. Increasing metabolic rate and heat production
   4. Causing vasodilation

References

Andrews M, Boyle J: *Transcultural concepts in nursing care,* Philadelphia, 2003, Lippincott.

Hockenberry and others: *Nursing care of infants and children,* ed 7, St. Louis, 2003, Mosby.

Levy Miller N: Haitian ethnomedical systems and biomedical practitioners: directions for clinicians, *J Transcult Nurs* 11(3):204, 2000.

Lueckenotte AG: *Gerontologic nursing,* ed 2, St. Louis, 2000, Mosby.

MacAuley DC: Ice therapy: how good is the evidence, *Int J Sports Med* 22(5):379, 2001.

Nicoll L: Heat in motion: evaluating and managing temperature, *Nursing* 32(5):s1, 2002.

Ruffolo D: Hypothermia in trauma, *RN* 65(2):46, 2002.

Stitik T, Nadler S: I. When—and how—to use cold most effectively, *Consultant* 38(12):2881, 1998.

Stitik T, Nadler S: II. When—and how—to apply the heat, *Consultant* 39(1):144, 1999.

Wilke B, Weiner RD: Postoperative cryotherapy: risks versus benefits of continuous-flow cryotherapy units, *Clin Podiatr Med Surg* 20(2):307, 2003.

Research References

Airaksinen O and others: Efficacy of cold gel for soft tissue injuries, *Am J Sports Med* 31(5), 680, 2003.

Poddar S: Heat or ice for acute ankle sprain, *J Fam Pract* 52(8): 642, 2003.

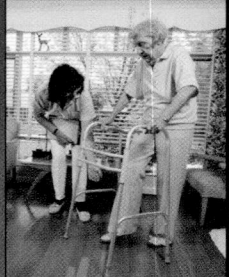

41

Home Care Safety

MEDIA RESOURCES

Evolve Site *evolve*

http://evolve.elsevier.com/Perry/skills
• Weblinks

Mastery of content in this chaper will enable the nurse to:

- Identify clients at risk for safety problems and possible accidents.
- Promote self-care of clients in the home.
- Describe factors within a home environment that create risks for injury for clients.
- Perform a home safety risk assessment.
- Identify interventions that will modify the home environment for physical safety.
- Identify interventions to reduce safety risks for clients with sensory, cognitive, and mental status alterations.
- Recommend strategies to ensure safe drug administration within the home.

/ **KEY TERMS**

Alzheimer's disease
Dementia
Polypharmacy
Reminiscing
Respite care
Wandering

Safety has been described as being in an environment where people feel secure in their surroundings. In Maslow's hierarchy of needs, safety includes security, stability, protection, and freedom from fear and anxiety (Maslow, 1954). Thus safety has both a physical and an emotional component. For example, if a wheelchair-bound client has removed door frames to allow for better bathroom access, the physical improvements will enhance the client's confidence to maneuver within the home. When a person's environment is safe, the potential to provide self-care is maximized. In addition, the client will emotionally feel less anxious about trying to move about and to interact within the environment.

Accidents are a common health problem in the United States, Canada, and other nations. Billions of dollars are spent annually as a result of accidents in the home. Accidents often occur as a result of environmental barriers coupled with the presence of intrinsic risks (e.g., neurological or visual disabilities, postural hypotension, and gait disturbances). Accident prevention often begins with making timely and adequate home repairs. However, many clients do not have the resources needed to maintain a safe home environment. The nurse plays an important role in improving a client's safety. The nurse collaborates with clients, family members, and other health care providers in the community in finding the best approaches for meeting a client's safety needs. The ultimate goal is to create an environment in which the client and family can provide self-care safely and effectively.

Nurses care for clients who develop serious physical and emotional limitations and who are unable to fully recover before having to return home. In many cases it may take clients weeks, months, or years to recover from traumatic injuries. For example, the nurse faces basic questions such as can clients reach the things they need if they are bed- or chair-bound? Is the immediate environment safe for other family members? What care requirements does the client have that cannot be easily accomplished in the home environment? Anticipation of the client's needs is essential so that clients and families can adapt the home environment as necessary. Home care nurses must continually be alert for safety factors that place clients at risk for injury. Family caregiving is on the rise as more people are providing ongoing support to family members and friends in the home. The home care nurse becomes very adept at partnering closely with clients and family members so that the client's nursing care needs can be met within the home without disrupting normal lifestyles unnecessarily. Finally, nurses in any setting must assess for patterns of health care problems (e.g., falls, burns, or medication errors) that may point to safety problems in the home.

Home care clients include the chronically ill, disabled children with physical and mental impairment, victims of acute medical illness and traumatic accidents, and the terminally ill. One group of clients that has significant risk for threats to safety within the home is older adults, because of the physiological changes that accompany aging. Because of older adults' vulnerability, it becomes the nurse's responsibility to restore pattern, order, and environmental predictability to a client's personal life space as possible (Ebersole and Hess, 2003). Despite older adults' risks, they learn how to negotiate their environments relatively well and are usually more aware of potential dangers. Thus, older adults may often be more cautious than younger persons and are amenable to changes that bring a sense of security and safety. However, the onset of an acute illness can change this and may require special effort to restore the older adult's sense of security.

A common misconception about aging is that cognitive impairments are widespread among older adults. However, when an older adult does begin to experience disorientation, loss of language skills, loss of the ability to calculate, and poor judgment, investigation of the underlying cause is indicated. Dementia is a generalized impairment of intellectual functioning, with the most common form being Alzheimer's disease. As Alzheimer's disease progresses, safety becomes a key concern. The older adult suffers memory loss, confusion, poor orientation, and a reduced attention span. Care providers are challenged with the choice of maintaining a person's autonomy versus taking steps to prevent accidents or injuries that ensure the person's physical safety and protection (Lueckenotte, 2000).

Clients of all ages have safety risks when they experience alterations that impair their mobility, sensory function, or cognitive thought processes. If a loss or reduction in a person's ability to function within the environment occurs suddenly, the person may resist environmental changes, attempting to deny any limitations. In this case, the client may try to initiate self-care actions without needed guidance or modification to the environment. For the client whose functional loss has been gradual, the accommodation may require only minimal revision. However, for the client whose alteration has been gradual and unnoticed by the client, such as with Alzheimer's disease, more aggressive revisions may be needed from the client, family, and/or nurse.

Lueckenotte (2000) defines preventive safety as the interruption of a sequence of events that could result in an accident. To successfully prevent or reduce the number of accidents in the home, it is necessary to consider what predisposes a person to an accident and how the environment can be modified to minimize the risk. The skills within this chapter are focused on helping clients retain their independence while implementing preventive safety measures within the home

Evidence-Based Practice Trends

An important source of evidence-based practice guidelines for patient safety is in the area of fall prevention. The rate of falling and the prevalence of risk factors for falling increase steeply after the age of 70 years (Tinetti, 2003). Strategies that have proven effective among older adults deemed at risk for falling include professionally supervised balance and gait training, muscle-strengthening exercise, gradual discontinuation of psychotropic medications, and modification of hazards in the home after discharge (Campbell and others, 1997; Gillespie and others, 2001; Robertson and others, 2001). Exercise programs found to be effective have been short term, usually lasting 1 year or less (Tinetti, 2003). Most of the benefits of exercise are maintained only as long as a client maintains the exercise regimen.

Health professionals are able to recommend any number of modifications to the home. Generally these recommendations can be effective in reducing trip and slip hazards, which are more commonly linked to falls (Gill and others, 2000). The most commonly recommended modifications in a study that saw a 20% reduction in the risk of falling included removal of throw rugs, change to safer footwear, use of nonslip bathmats, use of lighting at night, and the addition of stair rails (Cummings and others, 1999). Changes in the environment alone are not enough to prevent falls. Recent research shows that controlling and reducing intrinsic risk factors (e.g., hypotension, visual limitations, and heart palpitations) are critical to fall prevention.

Cultural Considerations

A client's culture influences his or her lifestyle and manner in which the home environment is structured and maintained. It is important for the nurse who is attempting to promote safety within the client's home to consider the following:

- Collaborate with the client in assessing the home environment. Assess cultural practices that may pose risks such as burning incense (Asians) and lighting candles (Jewish, Asians) when a client is on oxygen therapy.
- Assess availability of home care equipment. Amish families, for example, do not have electricity in the home to support operation of equipment such as apnea monitors, nebulizers, or refrigeration of medical supplies (Brewer and Bonalumi, 1995).
- When assessing the availability of family caregivers in the home, recognize that many collectivistic cultures (e.g., Jewish, Hispanic, Arabic, and Asians) value an active presence and caring for ill family members.
- Facilitate client access to necessary support services. Family obligation is a burden for many Asian families whose support system is decreased markedly by immigration. Seeking outside help in caring for elder parents may not be accepted by other family members. Clients with limited English language proficiency may not be able to access support services on their own.

Skill Performance Guidelines

1. When changing a client's home environment, retain as much of the client's independence and ability to provide self-care as possible.
2. Reinforce with family or friends who assume the role of caregiver the importance of preserving client autonomy as much as possible.
3. Any modifications to the home environment should be made after considering clients' physical strengths, remaining functional abilities, and resources for making change.

SKILL 41-1   Modifying Safety Risks in the Home Environment

The home environment should be a place where individuals feel healthy, comfortable, and safe. People want to be able to move about freely within their homes, regardless of the home's size, and to have a sense of control over daily living routines. This requires maintenance of personal space and a sense of privacy. All persons seek to create a personal space in their homes with which they can identify and maneuver about without having to think about every action or movement.

Clients requiring home care often experience physical alterations that require changes to be made in their home environment. In the case of older adults, the progressive physical changes of aging can create the same type of need. The changes should complement the client's remaining strengths. For example, if a client has poor balance but good upper arm strength, modifications should be made so that the client can safely walk or move throughout the house, ascend and descend stairs, and enter and exit a bathtub or shower. Side rails along hallways and stairwells and grab bars in the bathroom are good solutions. A nurse who cares for a client who re-

quires changes in the home environment must respect the concept of personal space. Making changes too rapidly without the client's consent may cause more problems than benefits. The nurse must appreciate the arrangement of the client's space within the home and not move things or suggest modifications without permission. Knowing the rooms the client most frequently uses can help in making the adjustments that will most likely create a safe environment.

An important part of making changes in the home environment is conducting a safety assessment. The home safety assessment covers all major living areas and helps to identify which changes are of greater priority than others. Frequently the nurse consults with physical and occupational therapists on the type of adjustments necessary. Independence can be enhanced to secure a better quality of life for clients and family members. When older adults were asked to identify the skills most important for remaining independent, they selected balance, being able to see, being able to lock/unlock doors, using a toilet, and managing medications (Mastrian, 2001).

DELEGATION CONSIDERATIONS

The skill of conducting an initial home safety assessment should not be delegated to assistive personnel. An RN is best qualified to determine what alterations or revisions are preferred based on a client's physical and/or cognitive limitations. However, principles involved in changing the home environment are both practical and commonsense in approach.

- Assistive personnel should inform the RN when they make suggestions for ways to make the home safer.

EQUIPMENT

❑ Home safety checklist

STEP	RATIONALE
ASSESSMENT	
1. Review previous physical findings, or assess the client's vision, hearing, musculoskeletal, and neurological function (see Chapter 18).	May reveal sensory alterations or problems with strength, coordination, or balance that predispose client to injury.
2. Determine if client has had a history of falls or other injuries within the home. Be specific in your assessment. Use the mnemonic, SPLATT: *S*ymptoms at time of fall *P*revious fall *L*ocation of fall *A*ctivity at time of fall *T*ime of fall *T*rauma postfall (Lueckenotte, 2000)	Key symptoms can be helpful in identifying cause for fall. Onset, location, and activity associated with fall provide further details on causative factors and how future falls might be prevented.
3. Have client who has had near fall or actual fall maintain a fall diary (Box 41-1).	Information in fall diary is very helpful in determining antecedents and consequences of falling (Lueckenotte, 2000).

STEP	RATIONALE

BOX 41-1 Fall/Near Fall Diary

- Maintain a notebook with 8½ × 11 inch paper. Across the longest edge of the paper, write the headings: "Date," "Time of Fall," "Activity at Time of Fall," "Symptoms," and "Injury."
- As soon as possible after a fall has occurred, complete information under each heading.
- If a family member witnesses the fall, have him or her record on a separate page what was observed.
- Have listed in the fall diary an emergency contact number for clients to call in case a fall results in a serious injury.
- Have client who has experienced a fall bring diary to the health care provider's office at the next scheduled visit or give to visiting nurse on next home visit.

Modified from Lueckenotte A: *Gerontologic nursing*, ed 2, St. Louis, 2000, Mosby.

4. Conduct a screening, using the "Get Up and Go" test. The test requires the examiner to look for unsteadiness as a client gets up from a chair without using the arms, walks a few feet, and returns.

Simple screening examination is very useful in detecting difficulties with balance or gait (Tinetti, 2003).

5. Review risk factors that predispose clients to accidents within the home:

   a. Known visual impairment

   Reduced visual function may alter client's balance, depth perception, or adaptation to the dark or glaring light.

   b. Hearing impairment

   Prevents client from hearing normal environmental sounds clearly as a source of orientation. Also prevents clear perception of any home-installed alarms (e.g., smoke alarm).

   c. Neuromuscular dysfunction (e.g., lower extremity weakness, unsteady gait, impaired balance, poor ankle dorsiflexion)

   Factors predispose clients to fall. Recurrent falls are associated with difficulty standing up from a chair. Poor ankle dorsiflexion impairs reflex to right oneself during phases of a fall (Tideiksaar, 1998).

   d. Reduced energy or fatigue

   Predisposes to falls.

   e. Incontinence

   Frequent trips to bathroom often cause client with other deficits to accidentally trip or fall over barriers.

   f. History of stroke, parkinsonism, arthritis, and drug related hypotension

   Factors found to be predominant causes for falls in long-term care facilities (Gill and others, 2000; Lipsitz and others, 1991).

   g. Postural hypotension, palpitations, difficulty breathing, or shortness of breath

   Dizziness or light-headedness predisposes to falls.

   h. Medication usage and history, including polypharmacy and use of sedatives, antihypertensives, antidepressants, and diuretics

   Multiple use of medications has been associated with falls. Medications that alter sensorium can affect balance and judgment. Diuretics cause increased trips to bathroom.

6. Determine if client has a fear of falling. Possible indicators include apprehension during ambulation (observed in facial expressions), sweating or trembling while ambulating, clutching persons or objects while ambulating, reluctance to change position or ambulate, and new onset of wobbly, reduced mobility after a fall (Gray-Micelli, 1997).

Fear of falling occurs variably in older adult population (Arfken and others, 1994; Gray-Micelli, 1997). Clinicians believe that fear of falling causes individual to take unnatural precautions that may predispose client to fall.

- **Critical Decision Point**
  Use family as a resource in assessment. Family may witness accident trends or patterns.

STEP	RATIONALE
7. Partner with client and family and conduct home safety assessment:	Provides comprehensive review of all areas within home that may pose hazardous situations.
a. Front and back entrances	
(1) Are walkways to the front/back door even and free from holes or cracks?	Entrances may pose barriers in surfaces over which client must walk.
(2) Are home entrances well lighted, including walkways?	Poorly lit areas prevent individuals from seeing variations in walking surface.
(3) Does client have nonskid strips/safety treads or bright-colored paint on outdoor steps? What colors are most easily seen by client? Are these colors used?	Nonskid surfaces cause fewer slips on stairs. Color on steps permits individual to see edges, accommodating for any reduced depth perception.
(4) Are doormats in good repair with nonskid backing and tapered edge?	
(5) Are doors in good repair and open and close easily? Can client open and close all doors easily?	Act of opening and closing door can cause a fall.
(6) Is there a sturdy handrail on both sides of stairs leading to entrance?	Handrails provide greater support while ascending and descending stairs.
(7) Are steps in good condition with even, flat surfaces?	Uneven surfaces predispose to tripping.
b. Kitchen	Kitchen is one of the most hazard-oriented rooms in a home and poses serious hazards for fire.
(1) Does client wear clothing with short or close-fitting sleeves when cooking?	Short or close fitting sleeves are less likely to accidentally catch on fire when a person works at a stove.
(2) Does client always stay in kitchen when cooking?	Lack of attention when using fire can pose a risk.
(3) Does client have a loud timer to signal when food is cooked?	Prevents burning of food and risk of fire.
(4) Does client keep stove top and oven clean and grease free?	Grease is highly flammable.
(5) Are stove control dials easy to see and use?	Client may accidentally use higher flame than is needed for cooking safely.
(6) Is a charged, easy-to-use fire extinguisher close at hand?	Extinguisher should be ready for use at all times.

• *Critical Decision Point*

Have client demonstrate steps of how to use extinguisher.

(7) Are there emergency numbers for police, fire, and poison control posted on or near telephone?	Emergency phone numbers and extinguisher ensure quick response should fire break out.
(8) Can items in kitchen cabinets and shelves be reached without climbing on a stool or chair? Is step stool sturdy and in good repair?	Climbing on step stools or chairs poses risks for falls.
(9) Is there adequate lighting over sink, stove, and work areas?	Poor lighting may make it difficult to see control knobs or dials or provides inadequate illumination when using sharp knives or utensils.
(10) Are kitchen throw rugs and mats slip resistant?	Rugs or mats not slip resistant can easily slide on tile or wood floors.
c. Bathrooms	
(1) Can bathroom door lock be unlocked from both sides of door?	Functional locks prevent person from being trapped in bathroom.
(2) Is tub or shower equipped with nonskid mats, abrasive strips, or surfaces that are not slippery?	Bathrooms are hazardous rooms. Wet floors and tub or shower bottoms can be very slippery, creating risk of falls.

STEP	RATIONALE
(3) Does bathroom floor have nonslip surface or rug with nonskid backing?	Slippery tile predisposes to falls.
(4) Does client avoid using slippery bath oils when bathing?	Use of bath oils can make tub surface slippery and increase risk of falls.
(5) Do bathtub and shower have at least one grab bar that is different color than that of the wall?	Grab bars provide extra support while maneuvering into and out of tubs or showers.
(6) Is client careful not to place towels on grab bars?	Client may accidentally grab towel instead of bar when needing support. Towel can slip off bar.
(7) Does shower have stable stool or chair and hand-held sprayer?	Shower stool allows client to sit while showering.
(8) Are cold and hot water faucets clearly marked, and is temperature on water heater 120° F or lower?	Accidental burns can occur from exposure to hot water.
d. Bedroom	
(1) Is a night-light placed in bedroom and/or bath?	Older adults have poor night vision.
(2) Is a working smoke detector just outside bedroom door?	Alarm situated just outside bedroom can awaken person early enough to escape fire.
(3) Can client turn on light without having to get out of bed in the dark? .	Getting out of bed, without proper lighting or ability to adjust to light changes, and reaching for necessary objects can predispose client to fall
(4) Is furniture arranged to provide clear path from bed to bathroom?	Obstructed path creates barrier that can cause tripping and falls.
(5) Is phone with emergency numbers within easy reach of bed?	Clients may develop physical symptoms while in bed, requiring easy access to phone.
(6) Are other alarm systems available? Push buttons that call for help? Nursery listening devices for invalid clients?	Alarm systems placed in readily accessible location can alert family/caregivers when person requires immediate assistance.
e. Living room/family room	
(1) Are electrical or extension cords removed from under furniture and carpeting? Kept out of the way of traffic?	Clients can easily trip or fall over electrical cords.
(2) Can client turn on light without having to walk into dark room?	Darkened room can disorient and prevent client from seeing uneven surfaces.
(3) Are hallways and walkways free from objects and clutter?	The common walkway through the living room should be barrier and clutter free.
(4) Are loose area rugs securely attached to floor and not placed over carpeting? (For best safety, consider removal of throw rugs.)	Loose edges of rugs are easy for persons to trip over.
(5) Is furniture arranged in each room so that client can walk around easily?	Furniture can create obstacles to walking in a room.
(6) Is all furniture steady and without sharp edges?	Clients often use edge of furniture for support when standing.
f. Around the house	
(1) Are all living areas and stairways well lighted?	Adequate lighting helps persons to see any barriers or uneven walking surfaces.
(2) Is flooring or carpeting throughout house in good repair?	Frayed carpet or irregular surfaces can cause tripping and result in a fall.
(3) Are all thresholds level with floor or no more than ½ inch in height?	

STEP	RATIONALE
(4) Is there a light switch at both top and bottom of stairs?	Prevents individual from having to walk a portion of stairs in dark.
(5) Does lighting produce glare or shadows on stairs?	Older adults are sensitive to glare.
(6) Do handrails run continuously from top to bottom of flights of stairs?	
(7) Are step coverings in good condition? Stairs free of clutter?	
g. General fire safety	
(1) Does client have properly working smoke detectors with good batteries?	Smoke alarms properly located, well functioning, and with batteries replaced twice a year can provide timely alert for fire.

• *Critical Decision Point*
Check to see when battery was last changed; it should be changed every 6 months.

(2) Does client have several emergency exit plans in case of fire?	Exit plan helps persons to anticipate route of escape when fire does occur. Exit should be route that is not barred by difficult-to-open locks or any physical barriers.
(3) Has family determined a meeting place in event of emergency, such as at mailbox in front of home?	Use of a common emergency meeting location is an efficient method for determining that all family members are safely out of the house.
(4) Does client use portable space heaters? Are they kept 3 feet away from flammable items?	Heaters, furnaces, and chimneys pose risks for fire.
(5) Is furnace area free of things that can catch on fire?	
(6) Does a qualified professional check furnace and chimney annually?	
(7) Does client who smokes report smoking in bed?	The leading cause of fire deaths is careless smoking, with most fire deaths occurring between 10 PM and 6 AM (National Fire Protection Association [NFPA], 2001).
h. General electrical safety	
(1) Are electrical cords in good condition, not frayed, spliced, or cracked?	Damaged cords can short-circuit and lead to fire.
(2) Are electrical cords kept away from water?	Use of any appliance or device that is exposed to water creates risk for electrical shock.
(3) Does client use extension cord/outlet extenders with built-in circuit breaker or fuse?	Prevents overloading of circuit that can lead to fire.
(4) Do all wall outlets and switches have cover plates?	Prevents physical contact with wiring.
(5) Does client use lightbulbs of correct wattage for each fixture?	Use of excessive wattage can lead to fire.
(6) Is main electrical fuse box for home easily accessible and clearly labeled?	In event of emergency, fuse box should be easy to access so that proper circuit can be cut off.
i. Carbon monoxide prevention	
(1) Are furnace flues checked regularly for patency?	Common cause of carbon monoxide toxicity (Droscher and others, 1999).
(2) Is there a carbon monoxide detector in home?	
8. Assess client's financial resources; determine monthly income used for ongoing expenses.	Determines potential for making repairs to home. May reveal need for low-cost community service support.

STEP	RATIONALE

9. Assess client's and family member's willingness to make changes. Has client accepted limitations that pose risk for injury? Determine how important functional independence is for client.

Attempts to improve safety within home can be perceived as intrusive. If it can be shown that necessary revisions to home environment will preserve independence, client may participate more willingly.

NURSING DIAGNOSES

- Anxiety
- Ineffective health maintenance
- Health-seeking behaviors regarding home safety
- Impaired home maintenance
- Risk for injury

- Deficient knowledge regarding home safety risks
- Impaired memory
- Impaired physical mobility
- Disturbed sensory perception (visual, auditory, and/or tactile)

Related factors are individualized based on client's condition or needs.

PLANNING

1. Expected outcomes following completion of procedure:
   - Client and/or family will describe potential environmental risks within home that may predispose to accidents.
   - Client and/or family will initiate actions to correct environmental risks, making home safer.
   - Client will remain free of injury.

2. Prioritize with client and family environmental barriers that pose greatest risk.

3. Recommend calling in reliable contractor if major home repairs are necessary.

During home safety assessment nurse instructs client on those risks that are of greatest concern.

Client sees value in altering living environment.

Environmental barriers are reduced or removed to minimize injuries.
Client's own physical and/or cognitive deficits will make certain environmental risks more hazardous. Prioritization helps client make best choices.
Ensures repairs are made safely and correctly.

IMPLEMENTATION

1. Recommend taking steps to reduce physical hazards that can predispose to falls:
   a. Paint edges of concrete stairs bright yellow, orange, or white.
   b. Install treads with uniform depth of 9 inches (22.5 cm) and 9-inch risers (vertical face of steps)
   c. Rearrange furniture to open up space through hallways and major rooms.
   d. Reduce clutter within living areas (e.g., footstools, flower pots, extension cords, children's toys).
   e. Secure all carpeting, mats, and tile; place nonskid backing under small rugs and doormats.
   f. Pad floor, and use specialized tile that absorbs impact of falls.
   g. Use low-rise beds, or use futon beds or a mattress on the floor.
   h. Have enough electrical outlets installed to be able to plug light or electronic device (e.g., TV, video) into nearby outlet. Secure electrical cords against baseboards.
   i. Install nonskid strips on surface of bathtub and/or shower stall.

This highlights visual target for client to see edge of stairs more clearly.
If stairs are of uniform size, client does not have to continually adjust vision or stride.
Creates unobstructed pathway for ambulation.

Reduces chance of client's slipping when stepping on rug surface.
Cushions person's fall.

Lowers distance to floor surface.

Prevents need to run extension cords across walkways.

Reduces chances of slipping on tub/shower stall surface.

STEP	**RATIONALE**

    j. Have grab bar installed in studs at tub, toilet, and/or shower (see illustration). Have client select vertical or horizontal placement if choice available. Be sure bar is different color than that of wall

Bar provides stability for maneuvering in bathroom. Should be easily visible.

    k. Have handrails installed along the side of any stairway (see illustration). Be sure stairways are well lighted, with switches at top and bottom of steps.

Older adults have difficulty seeing edges of stairs.

    l. Install appropriate broad-beam lighting for outside walkways.

    m. Keep a lighted phone easily accessible, next to the client's bed.

Prevents client from having to get up out of bed, often in the dark.

2. Have client use padding or types of clothing that will cushion bony prominences, especially high-risk bony prominences (e.g., hips). Specially designed hip protectors are available.

Helps to absorb impact of falling body.

3. Make modifications to promote safe practice of activities of daily living (ADLs):

    a. Provide direct light source in areas where client reads, cooks, uses tools, or conducts hobby work. High-intensity light on object or surface that is involved works best.

Older adults require three times as much light to see objects as they did when they were in their twenties (Ebersole and Hess, 2003).

- **Critical Decision Point**

  Avoid fluorescent lighting because it can create excessive glare.

    b. Consider satin and nongloss finishes for walls, cabinets, and countertops in kitchen. Have sheer curtains or adjustable shades in other living areas.

Reduces glare, to which older adults are very sensitive.

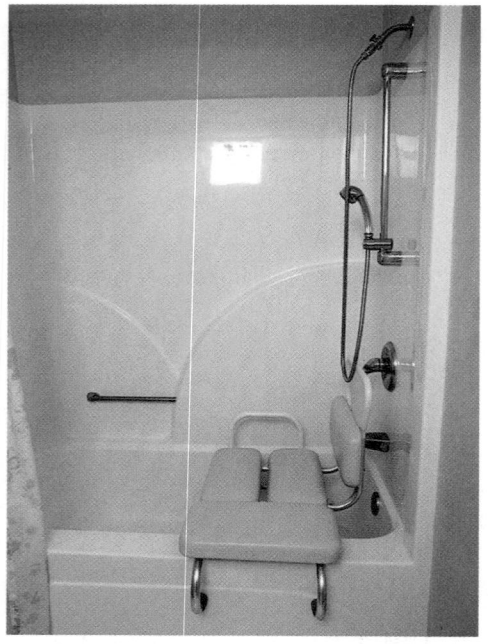

STEP 1J Grab bars and safety seat installed in a shower.

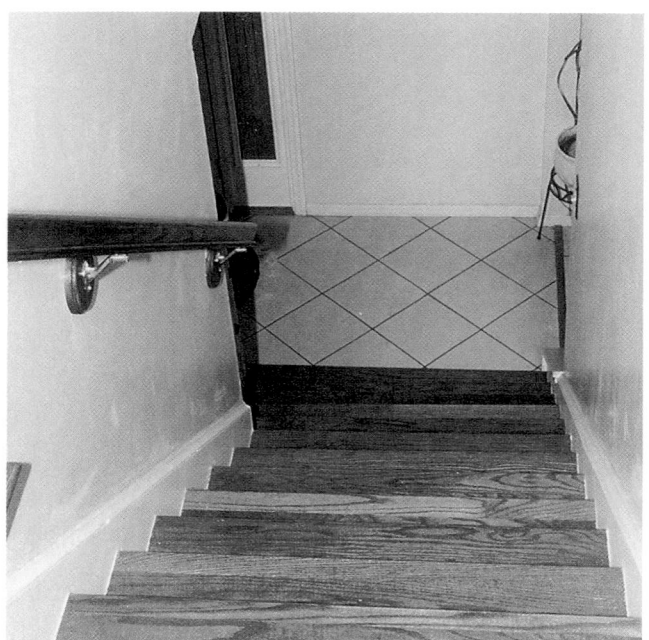

STEP 1k Handrails installed along stairways provide security for clients with visual, balance, and coordination problems.

STEP	RATIONALE
c. Apply colored tape or paint to color code controls of stove, oven, dryer, toaster, and other appliances.	Clients with reduced visual acuity may adjust appliance to wrong setting, creating potential risk of fire or burning.
d. Consider installing lazy Susans and pull-out drawers with glide mechanisms in kitchen cabinets. Also install C-ring handles in lower cabinets.	Makes access to food and kitchen supplies easier.
4. Take steps to eliminate fire hazards:	
a. Have smoke detectors installed near each bedroom, kitchen, and in basement of home. Be sure detector is on each floor of home.	Fires most frequently start in basement near furnace, dryer, or electrical wiring; kitchen; or in living areas where extensive wiring can be found. Alarm should be close by to alert client and family when sleeping.
b. Have client select fire extinguisher that is easy to handle and manipulate (see illustration). Ask client to read instructions and demonstrate its proper use.	Older adult or client with disability may have difficulty gripping mechanisms on certain extinguishers.
c. Have area around furnace cleared of any flammable items.	Reduces risk for fire.
d. Instruct client to never place portable space heater within 3 feet of flammable items. Have client buy model that turns off automatically as soon as change in position occurs (Lueckenotte, 2000).	Intense heat can ignite flammable items easily. Safety device can shut off heater and prevent ignition of fire.
e. Have client make appointments for maintenance of furnace and chimney cleaning in appropriate season.	Furnace maintenance prevents short circuits and fires. Accumulation of creosote on chimney walls can lead to fire.
f. Have client check lightbulb wattage in all fixtures.	Ensures proper wattage being used.
g. Have client establish routine during cooking that keeps client in kitchen. Be sure cooking range is kept clean and items such as potholders and towels are kept away from burners.	Food cooking on stove can easily boil over or begin to burn when unattended.
h. If client is a smoker, review need to keep ashtrays clean and emptied. Placing a small amount of water or sand in bottom of ashtray is useful if client is visually impaired.	Client with reduced vision may be unable to tell if cigarette, cigar, or match has extinguished.

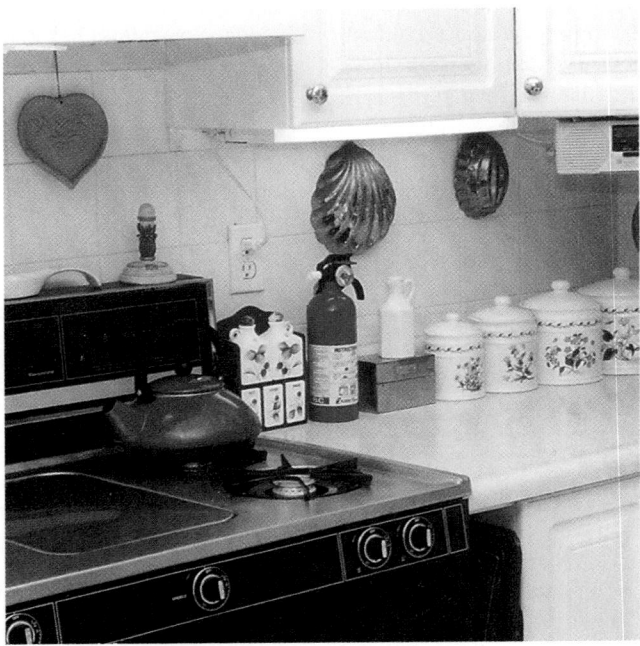

STEP 4b Fire extinguisher accessible in kitchen.

STEP	RATIONALE

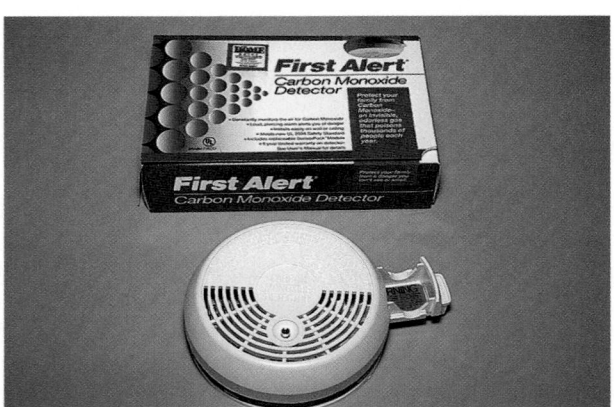

STEP **6c** Carbon monoxide detector.

i. Strongly discourage smoking in bed, smoking in a chair when there is a possibility of falling asleep, and smoking after taking a medication that diminishes alertness.

Risks factors for burns, as well as fire.

j. Recommend client install power strips or surge protectors for plugging in multiple appliances/devices.

Prevents risk of electrical short, which can cause a fire.

5. Take steps to reduce chances of injury from burns:

a. Have setting on hot water heater adjusted to 120° F or lower. To check water temperature, let water run until steam is noted, fill container, and check temperature with a meat thermometer.

Scalds are typically caused from bathing and showering when hot water tank temperatures are in excess of 140° F or 60° C (Harper and Dickson, 1995).

b. Instruct client to always turn cold water on first.

Prevents direct exposure to hot water.

c. Install touch pads on lamps.

Light can be easily turned on without risk of touching hot lightbulb.

d. Use color codes of red for hot and blue for cold on water faucets. (If client cannot distinguish colors, choose two that are easily distinguished.)

Prevents accidental burning from turning on wrong faucet.

6. Take steps to prevent carbon monoxide exposure in the home:

a. Have condition of furnace venting checked annually just before time of season when furnace is turned on.

Improper venting prevents escape of carbon monoxide, a poisonous gas. Carbon monoxide combines irreversibly with hemoglobin, preventing formation of oxyhemoglobin and reducing oxygen supply to tissues.

b. Caution clients against using a gas stove or barbecue grill for heating inside of home.

Both are sources of carbon monoxide.

c. Have carbon monoxide detector installed in home (see illustration).

Detector alarms when carbon monoxide reaches unsafe levels.

EVALUATION

1. Have client and family member(s) identify safety risks revealed in home safety assessment.

Demonstrates what client recognizes as a risk and its relative importance for changing.

2. During follow-up visit or call to home ask client to discuss plans for making any modifications, and observe what changes have been implemented.

Evaluates extent to which client sees risks as potentially harmful and complies with suggested changes.

STEP	**RATIONALE**
3. During follow-up visits or calls ask if client has experienced any falls or other injuries within home.	May reveal if risks have been eliminated, depending on client's previous history of injury.

Recording and Reporting

- Retain copy of home safety assessment in client's home care record.
- Record any instruction provided, client's response, and changes made within environment in progress notes.

Unexpected Outcomes	**Related Interventions**
1. Client and family do not acknowledge risks identified from home safety assessment.	• Determine if reluctance to make changes is due to limited resources, disbelief concerning need to make changes, fear of loss of autonomy, or other reasons. • Review implications of risks to client's safety and welfare.
2. Client fails to make changes agreed on in previous plan.	• Determine reason for failure to make changes. • Help prioritize greatest risks.
3. Client suffers fall or burn within home.	• Conduct an assessment of contributing factors and conditions in environment at time of injury. • Make revisions based upon assessment findings.

Teaching Considerations

- Family caregivers may benefit from learning how to safely assist client in ambulating or transferring from bed to chair or wheelchair to chair, depending on client's mobility limitations.
- Instruct client and caregiver in what to do in case client falls, including access to emergency assistance and how to prevent further injury. Many communities have a service available that is designed for persons who live alone. The service company provides a small device that client wears around the neck and a special monitor connected to client's telephone. Clients summon help by pressing button on device if phone is inaccessible. When alarm is received by company, a call is initiated to client to determine the problem. If there is no answer, the company will contact family members, friends, or a rescue squad to check on client. This service is a valuable option to frail older adults who live alone or are left at home alone for periods of time.

Pediatric Considerations

- Caution parents when working in the kitchen to never pour hot liquids when an infant or young child is close by.
- Remove all crib toys that are strung across crib or playpen when child begins to push up on hand or knees (4 to 7 months).
- Keep faucets out of reach of children.

Gerontological Considerations

- If client is wheelchair-bound, lower light switches and other control devices within easy reach. Similarly, kitchen cabinets and other storage closets can be redesigned for access. A high-rise toilet with vertically hinged arm support allows client to transfer sideways from wheelchair to toilet seat (Shamberg and Shamberg, 1995). Another option is placing a bedside commode (with bedpan removed) over a conventional toilet seat. Commode level is usually higher than toilet. Then commode can also be moved near the bed for nighttime use.

Long-Term Care Considerations

- Staff should maintain close supervision of confused clients.

SKILL 41-2 Adapting the Home Setting for Clients With Cognitive Deficits

An important aspect of safety is a person's ability to perform routine ADLs and to make correct decisions about home management activities. Home management includes use of the telephone, cleaning, shopping, money management, meal preparation, and taking medication. A person who is unable to perform these activities or who requires assistance from another may have physical disabilities and/or cognitive limitations. When the limitations are cognitive, a person's autonomy is clearly threatened. Family members often misunderstand certain behaviors associated with cognitive changes and become concerned as to whether the individual can function safely within the home. The nurse may enter into situations where decisions must be made as to whether a client is competent to perform self-care.

Two of the most common cognitive conditions affecting clients in the home are dementia and depression. Dementia is a chronic generalized impairment of intellectual functioning that leads to a decline in the ability to perform basic and instrumental activities of daily living. Dementia is characterized by a gradual, progressive, irreversible cerebral dysfunction. Alzheimer's disease is the most common form of dementia. It has the characteristic progressive symptoms of loss of memory (amnesia), loss of the ability to recognize objects and persons (agnosia), loss of the ability to perform familiar tasks (apraxia), and loss of language skills (aphasia). As Alzheimer's disease progresses, older adults become more dependent on caregivers for assistance.

Individuals who are in the early to middle stage of dementia are at risk for wandering. Wandering is defined by the North American Nursing Diagnosis Association (2003) as meandering, aimless, or repetitive locomotion that exposes the individual to harm and is frequently incongruent with boundaries, limits, or obstacles. For example, a wandering client may walk around the house trying repeatedly, but ineffectively, to carry out a task independently. Another example of wandering is when the client may try to leave his or her place of residence but is stopped by family caregivers. Wandering can be managed by modifying the environment, using physical and psychosocial interventions, and installing technological devices (e.g., motion detectors and portable alarms) (Futrell and Melillo, 2002). This skill will focus on environmental modifications.

Depression is a chronic, insidious emotional disorder characterized by feelings of sadness, melancholy, dejection, and worthlessness that are inappropriate and out of proportion to reality. It can occur alone or in combination with cognitive disorders such as dementia. Depression can also occur secondarily to isolation when the older adult is homebound and has few social visitors.

Making accurate assessments of older adults' mental status and cognitive function takes practice. Mental status is an overlap between affective and cognitive function. A person may have certain mental processes intact (e.g., orientation to name, time, and place), while at the same time other processes are diminished or compromised (e.g., short-term memory of life events). Assessment of a client's level of orientation alone is not an accurate indicator of cognitive functioning (Ebersole and Hess, 2003).

This skill does not cover the complexity of assessing the full range of cognitive dysfunction in older adults. Instead it attempts to give the nurse guidelines for how to help clients who have varying degrees of cognitive dysfunction make adaptations to preserve their ability to function safely within the home. Similarly the skill addresses techniques for the family to use in assisting the older adult.

DELEGATION CONSIDERATIONS

Aspects of the skill of adapting the home environment for clients with cognitive deficits can be delegated to assistive personnel. However, assessment of cognitive function should not be delegated to assistive personnel. Assistive personnel can make helpful suggestions in regard to how to help clients adapt approaches to performing daily activities.

* Have assistive personnel inform nurse when there is a change in client's mood, memory, and ability to maintain home.

EQUIPMENT

❑ Mini-Mental State Examination (MMSE)
❑ Short Geriatric Depression Scale (SGDS)
❑ Calendar
❑ Paper for making lists
❑ Medication organizer (optional)
❑ Bulletin board or poster board (optional)
❑ Motion detector (optional)

STEP	RATIONALE

ASSESSMENT

1. Assess client over a short period of time, and be sensitive to client's sensory needs or disabilities.

   Improves likelihood of gathering relevant data (Ebersole and Hess, 2003).

2. Be sure the room in which you meet with client and family is well lit with minimal outside noises or interruptions. Speak clearly and in normal tone of voice.

   An optimal environment for the assessment of the client's cognitive and mental status will provide a more valid assessment.

3. Ask client to describe own level of health and have him or her describe how it affects the ability to perform self-care skills (e.g., bathing, dressing, eating, toileting).

   Question will require client to attend to one topic. Allows nurse to assess attention and concentration. Also determines if client is fully perceptive of physical capabilities.

- *Critical Decision Point*

  Family members may be used to confirm description. Do not create situation in which client feels you are not listening to his or her views. The additional person supplements answers with the client's consent, but the client remains the focus of the interview.

4. Ask how the client is doing with home management responsibilities: "Tell me what bills you pay each month. Can you tell what each one is for? Can you tell me about your normal day—when do you get up, eat meals, dress? Do you have problems dressing or bathing?"

   Provides good comparison of client and family perceptions. Interaction will help to measure short-term memory, judgment, and problem solving.

5. Assess client's medications. Review number and type of medications, purpose as prescribed, time of day taken, and dosages. Give special attention to pain medications, anticonvulsants, antihypertensives (especially beta-adrenergic blockers), diuretics, digoxin, aspirin, and anticoagulants.

   Older adults frequently suffer drug interactions from polypharmacy, the concurrent prescribing of multiple medications. Select drugs and/or combinations of drugs can place client at risk for side effects that may increase chances of injury as a result of physical or cognitive changes.

6. Determine if client has family member or friend who assists with self-care or home management responsibilities. What level of support is provided by caregiver? How frequent is the caregiver available? Does client perceive satisfaction in caregiver's support? What level of satisfaction does caregiver perceive? Does caregiver take advantage of respite care?

   The relationship between a family caregiver and a client help define how difficult it is to provide caregiving support. The role of family caregiver can be stressful, particularly if the individual has other responsibilities such as parenting, work, or school. Determines availability of resource to client and quality of that support.

7. During discussion, observe client's dress, nonverbal expressions, appearance, and cleanliness.

   Conditions such as depression and dementia can result in client's inability to attend to personal appearance.

- *Critical Decision Point*

  Do not confuse behavioral changes with lack of available resources to maintain hygiene. Also be aware of signs and symptoms of abuse or neglect (see Chapter 18). Report suspected abuse to appropriate social service agency.

8. Observe immediate home environment. Is it well kept and orderly?

   Behavioral changes associated with cognitive dysfunction may be first detected in disorderly home and inappropriate placement of objects (e.g., carton of orange juice placed inside kitchen cabinet instead of in refrigerator).

9. If you suspect a cognitive or mental status change:
   a. Complete a Mini-Mental State Examination (e.g., Folstein's examination) for dementia.
   b. Complete Short Geriatric Depression Scale for depression.

   Mini-Mental State Examination screens orientation, attention and calculation, recall, language, and intelligence.

   SGDS is a 15-item screening tool for depression in older adults.

STEP	RATIONALE
10. If wandering is suspected, observe for the following behaviors (family caregivers might provide information as well): • Repeated shadowing or seeking whereabouts of caregiver • Revisiting one destination many times • Inability to locate landmarks or getting lost in a familiar setting • Going into unauthorized or private places • Searching for "missing" people or places • Walking with no apparent destination or purpose • Haphazard or continuous moving, walking, or pacing • Walking that cannot easily be redirected	Persons prone to wandering exhibit these behaviors and might be prone to wander away from their home (Futrell and Melillo, 2002).
11. Assess what current environmental strategies are being used by family caregivers in dealing with wandering (e.g., latches and alarms on doors, visual cues such as STOP signs, constant supervision).	Assists in determining level of intervention necessary.

NURSING DIAGNOSES

* Caregiver role strain
* Acute confusion
* Ineffective health maintenance
* Impaired home maintenance
* Risk for injury
* Impaired memory

* Ineffective role performance
* Self-care deficit (feeding, toileting, bathing/hygiene, dressing/grooming)
* Disturbed thought processes
* Wandering

Related factors are individualized based on client's condition or needs.

PLANNING

1. Expected outcomes following completion of procedure:
   * Client is able to complete home management responsibilities within existing limitations.
   * Client receives appropriate combination of medications for diagnosed conditions.
   * Caregiver describes techniques to use in helping client perform self-care and home management activities.
   * Caregiver uses techniques that help client complete self-care and home management activities.
   * Family caregivers will describe steps to take in minimizing wandering.
   * Client will experience less problem wandering.
2. If client has difficulty with self-care skills, refer family to occupational therapy, homemaker services, or respite care as appropriate.

Modifications are made that help client apply remaining cognitive functions.
Assistive devices enable client to follow prescribed medication regimen.
Instruction will prepare caregiver with variety of caregiving techniques.
Caregiver preserves client's autonomy and maximizes client's functionality.
Instruction will prepare caregivers with wandering management strategies.
Wandering management strategies will be effective.
Occupational therapists can provide assistive devices and recommend self-care adaptations. Homemaker services provide added resource for meal preparation and home cleaning. Respite care provides family caregiver temporary rest away from continuous responsibilities.

STEP	RATIONALE

3. If client has physical disability affecting fine motor skills, consult with physical and/or occupational therapist.

Can offer assistive devices to make bathing, dressing, writing, and feeding easier (see illustration).

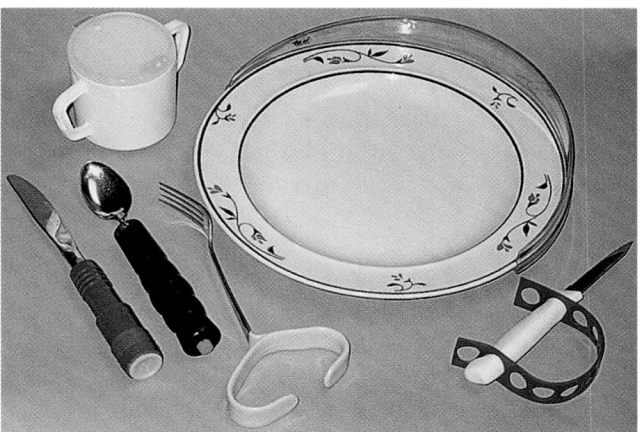

STEP 3 Assistive feeding devices.

4. Consider client's level of cognitive impairment before implementing strategies that will require changes in living environment. Some clients may require only minor adaptations, and others will depend more on assistance of caregivers.

Retention of client's independence and autonomy is ultimate goal.

5. Determine best time of day for approaches that result in desired response.

Client may be more alert and responsive in morning versus afternoon or vice versa.

IMPLEMENTATION

1. If client has difficulty remembering when to perform tasks (e.g., paying bills, taking medicines), help to create a list, or post reminder notes in a conspicuous location (e.g., bulletin board, front of refrigerator), provide a medication container organized by days of week, recommend a wristwatch with alarm to signal medication administration times.

Memory function in older adults tends to be preserved for relevant, well-learned material (Lueckenotte, 2000). Lists and organizers will help client cope with memory loss and still safely perform activities.

2. When client has difficulty completing tasks such as writing checks for bills or bringing groceries into home to store, reduce steps it takes to complete task. Find ways to consolidate steps or simplify task.

Prevents frustration in completing task and/or forgetting step that leads to task being unfinished.

3. Help client and caregiver determine routine schedule for daily activities such as eating, bathing, daily exercise, home management activities, and napping. Have large calendar posted in conspicuous area to write in appointments or special planned events.

Consistency creates sense of security and keeps client more easily oriented to daily activities. Routines are important in providing security, but client must also have option of making changes as necessary.

4. Instruct caregiver to focus on client's abilities rather than disabilities. Use abilities in modifying approaches to daily activity performance. For example, if client has limited use of right hand, develop approaches that maximizes use of left hand.

Retains client's autonomy and sense of self-worth.

STEP	RATIONALE
5. Have caregiver assist with setting-up activities so that client can complete task (e.g., chopping up vegetables before actual cooking, placing wash basin on table in bedroom for sponge bath, placing clothes to wear for the day on bed, unpacking groceries on countertop for eventual storage, arranging food on plate with items in clockwise orientation—vegetables at 9, salad at 3, meat at 6).	Helps client master task even though unable either physically or cognitively to perform all steps.
6. Discuss with client, caregiver, and primary care provider options for scheduling multiple medications:	Drugs may cause physiological changes that create risk for injury.
a. Medications that are likely to cause confusion should be administered at bedtime.	Reduces risk of confusion during waking hours contributing to disorientation and risk for falling.

- **Critical Decision Point**
  Do not recommend this if client has nocturia.

STEP	RATIONALE
b. Space antihypertensives and antiarrhythmics at different times to minimize side effects.	These drugs may cause blood pressure changes and dizziness, thus increasing risk of falls.
c. Reduce number of pain medications used when possible.	
d. Have diuretics taken early in day and not at night.	Diuretic effect occurs during the day while client is awake.
7. Instruct caregiver in how to use simple and direct communication:	Relays care and support through therapeutic communications techniques.
a. Sit or stand in front of client in full view.	Promotes reception of verbal and nonverbal messages.
b. Face the client with a hearing impairment while speaking; do not cover the mouth.	Client can see speaker's lips. Prevents voice distortion.
c. Use a calm and relaxed approach.	
d. Use eye contact and touch.	Helps to reinforce messages.
e. Speak in simple words and short sentences.	Enhances understanding of messages.
f. Use nonverbal gestures that complement verbal messages.	
8. Keep clocks, calendars, and personal mementos (e.g., pictures, scrapbooks) situated throughout rooms within the home. Enhance the environment with addition of tactile boards or three-dimensional art.	Reinforces reality orientation when client's memory is failing. Increasing visual appeal of environment helps to reduce wandering (Futrell and Melillo, 2002).
9. Have caregiver routinely orient client to who caregiver is and what activities they are going to complete.	This strategy is useful in clients with progressive dementia. This improves their productivity and responses (Lueckenotte, 2000).
10. Be sure client has regular naps or rest periods during the day.	Fatigue can add to any mental status changes. Provides client energy to perform planned activities.
11. Have caregiver encourage and support frequent visits by family and friends. Instruct caregiver in how to use humor and reminiscing of favorite stories to promote social interaction.	Participation in social activities prevents boredom and restlessness.
12. Provide a safe place for a person to wander (e.g., large family room or fenced yard).	May reduce risk of injury and leaving residence.
13. Provide clues, such as pictures and signs, to guide the client to a desired location (e.g., sign for the bathroom or bedroom) (Futrell and Melillo, 2002).	Reduces aimless wandering.
14. Recommend family of wandering client install multiple and different kinds of locks (e.g., deadbolt plus a chain lock placed low or high on door) (Futrell and Melillo, 2002).	Reduces client's ability to exit residence.

STEP	RATIONALE
15. Disguise a door that leads to a dangerous area (e.g., a stairwell) with a mural that looks like a bookshelf or set of pantry shelves (Futrell and Melillo, 2002).	Prevents falls. Murals are available on the Web at www.alzstore.com.
16. Address the cause of wandering (e.g., feed a person who is hungry, provide regular exercise). Eliminate stressors (e.g., changes in daily routines, excess stimulation) (Futrell and Melillo, 2002).	Reduces stimuli that prompt wandering.
17. Install a motion detector near an exit site, with a portable alarm that can accompany caregiver.	Alerts caregiver to client's attempt to exit residence.

EVALUATION

1. During follow-up visits ask client to review the home management activities completed the morning of that day, as well as the previous day.	Determines client's ability to recall events and evaluates if planned activities were completed.
2. Review with client and caregiver revised schedule for medication administration.	Evaluates understanding of regimen.
3. Have caregiver keep track of doses client takes over a 1-week period.	Tracking doses will confirm if client is adherent to regimen.
4. Ask caregiver to describe ways that will increase client's success in completing home management and self-care activities.	Measures learning.
5. Have caregiver show schedules of daily routines and review specific approaches used. Observe environment for presence of reality orientation cues.	Determines caregiver's success in applying information and making environmental changes.
6. Have family caregivers describe options for minimizing wandering.	Measures learning.
7. Have family caregivers report number of occurrences of wandering.	Determines if reduction in wandering has occurred.

Recording and Reporting

- Record assessment of client's cognitive and mental status, recommended interventions, and client's and caregiver's response in progress notes.
- Report to physician any change in client's behavior that might reflect a decline in cognitive or mental status.

Unexpected Outcomes	Related Interventions
1. Client is unable to complete daily activities as planned.	• Further modifications may be needed. Reassess what occurred when a task was not completed. Caregiver and client conflict could have played a role rather than client being unable cognitively to complete task.
2. Client experiences drug interaction from multiple medications.	• Have physician evaluate client's medication regimen. • Recommend feasibility of pharmacy consult.
3. Caregiver is unable to describe/implement techniques that will improve client's orientation and ability to complete activities.	• Reinstruction and discussion are necessary. • Support for caregiver may be necessary before caregiver can learn how to support someone else. • Consider that caregiver may not be able to provide necessary support; other options may need to be analyzed.

Continued

Unexpected Outcomes	Related Interventions
4. Caregiver is unable to describe/implement strategies to decrease wandering.	• Reinstruction and discussion are necessary. • Caregiver may not have resources available to adapt environment.
5. Client's wandering increases.	• Reconsider strategies used. Reassess factors prompting wandering.

Teaching Considerations

• Instruct caregiver in signs and symptoms of dementia and depression. If client's functionality continues to decline, caregiver may choose to learn more ADL support skills (e.g., how to assist with hygiene, dressing, transfer and turning, toileting).

Pediatric Considerations

• Children with cognitive impairment are often not aware of inherent dangers during play and other activities. Parental supervision is critical.

Gerontological Considerations

• Stress created for caregiver by older adult demonstrating problematic behaviors may be reduced if awareness of meaning of behaviors and methods of managing these is encouraged (Lueckenotte, 2000).

SKILL 41-3 Medication and Medical Device Safety

Clients frequently must manage the administration of medications and the use of medical devices such as syringes, blood glucose monitoring equipment, dressing supplies, and even intravenous devices. This includes administration, storage, and disposal. Safety is critical in ensuring that medications are administered correctly, devices are used properly, and equipment is cleaned and/or removed as waste. Infection control is just one principle the client and/or caregiver must learn to ensure a safe environment within the home.

One of the nurse's responsibilities within the home environment is to assist the client with sensory, mobility, or cognitive deficits. Clients who require special consideration include those with acute sensory or neurological impairment, clients with chronic illness such as diabetes or arthritis, and older adults who frequently have physical limitations that make manipulation of medical devices and dispensing of medications difficult. For example, clients with arthritic hands are sometimes unable to open medication containers because of the lack of strength in the hands and the pain created by pressure on the joints. This skill reviews steps to take to ensure safe use of medications and medical devices. Chapter 42 addresses how to instruct clients in medication use.

DELEGATION CONSIDERATIONS

Assessment of the client's risks in using medical devices and in administering medication should not be delegated to assistive personnel. Identification of the adaptations needed within the home based on the client's limitations should not be delegated. However, assistive personnel, such as home health aides, will frequently be in situations enabling them to see how clients use adaptations. Assistive personnel can make suggestions that further ensure client safety regarding the use of basic infection control practices and how to dispose of sharps, needles, and contaminated supplies.

EQUIPMENT

❑ Colored marking pens
❑ Labels
❑ Puncture-resistant sharps container or 2-L soda bottle with cap
❑ Duct or adhesive tape
❑ Assistive devices (e.g., syringe magnifier)

STEP	RATIONALE

ASSESSMENT

1. Assess client's sensory, musculoskeletal, and neurological function (see Chapter 18).

   Helps to reveal any deficits that may affect preparation and use of medications or medical devices.

2. If family caregiver provides routine assistance, assess his or her function as above.

   Determines level of assistance caregivers can provide.

3. Assess client's medication regimen and length of time client has been receiving each drug.

   Determines complexity of medication regimen and extent to which client should be familiar with regimen.

4. Ask client to show you where medications are stored in home. Look at each container.

   Determines condition and labeling of containers.

• *Critical Decision Point*

   Note temperature of storage area. Medications should not be stored in extreme heat. Insulin should be kept in a cool place.

5. Have client describe daily schedule for drug administration and whether there are any problems in following that schedule.

   Helps to reveal client's adherence to or misunderstanding of instructions (see Chapter 42).

6. If client self-administers injections, ask to see where those supplies are stored and what is used to dispose of used syringes and needles.

   Determines sterility of equipment and whether method of disposal creates risk to client or family for needle-stick injuries.

7. If client uses a glucose-monitoring device, ask to see where monitor, lancets, and glucose strips are stored. Also ask about how client disposes of lancets.

   Allows nurse to examine cleanliness of equipment, sterility of lancets, and condition of glucose strips. Sharps should be disposed of in puncture-proof container.

8. If client applies dressings to a wound, ask to see where dressings are stored and determine how client disposes of soiled dressings.

   Determines if dressings supplies are kept clean and are properly discarded.

NURSING DIAGNOSES

• Ineffective health maintenance
• Health-seeking behaviors regarding medication safety
• Risk for infection
• Risk for injury

• Deficient knowledge regarding medication and medical device safety
• Noncompliance (sharps disposal)

Related factors are individualized based on client's condition or needs.

PLANNING

1. Expected outcomes following completion of procedure:
   • Client and caregiver will discuss principles of medication safety.

   Nurse provides knowledge base for safe medication administration.

   • Client and caregiver will be able to prepare medications independently.

   Adaptations are made to accommodate client's and/or caregiver's deficits in handling and manipulating equipment.

   • Client and caregiver will identify correct conditions for storing medications, medical devices, and supplies.

   Instruction focuses on infection control measures.

   • Client and caregiver will dispose of used medical equipment and supplies correctly.

   Appropriate receptacles and methods for disposal are made available.

IMPLEMENTATION

1. Instruct client and caregiver in principles to ensure medications are safe to use:

   a. Never take a medicine prescribed for another member of household.

   Medications must be of full strength and used for the appropriate pharmacological reason to have therapeutic benefit.

   b. Do not take any medicine more than a year old or past expiration date on container.

   Expired medication may be toxic or no longer effective.

STEP	RATIONALE
c. Do not place different medicines in same container.	Prevents accidental "mix-up" of medications and medication error.
d. Always finish a prescribed medication; do not save for a future illness.	Prevents underdosing or inappropriate dosing.
2. Recommend approaches to facilitate preparation of medications:	
a. For clients with weakened grasp or pain of hands and fingers, have local pharmacist place medications in a screw-top container.	Tops of childproof containers are difficult to remove, especially if hand and finger grasp are weakened.

• *Critical Decision Point*

If client has children or grandchildren who have easy access to medication storage area or client's purse, be sure medications are stored in secure place.

b. For clients with visual alterations, have pharmacy type larger labels on all medication containers.	Ensures client is able to read drug name and dosage schedule clearly.
c. For clients who are legally blind, have braille labels placed on medication containers.	Labels embossed with drug name, strength, and prescription numbers can be easily read by client trained in use of braille.
d. For clients taking multiple medications, introduce a color-coding system. Colors could be used for drugs that are to be taken at the same time. Tops of bottle caps can be marked with a colored marking pen.	Technique may help to ensure correct drugs and doses are taken at correct times of day.
e. Provide specially designed syringes with large numerals or syringe magnifier for clients with visual alterations (see illustration).	Ensures accurate dose of drug is prepared in syringe.
f. For clients who have difficulty manipulating syringes, offer a spring-loaded needle insertion aid.	Delivers injection safely without manipulation of plunger.

• *Critical Decision Point*

Family caregivers should be instructed to know what to do following a needle-stick injury: wash the affected area thoroughly with soap and water, then dry. If client has acquired immunodeficiency syndrome (AIDS), hepatitis, or other communicable disease, caregivers should pursue appropriate laboratory testing.

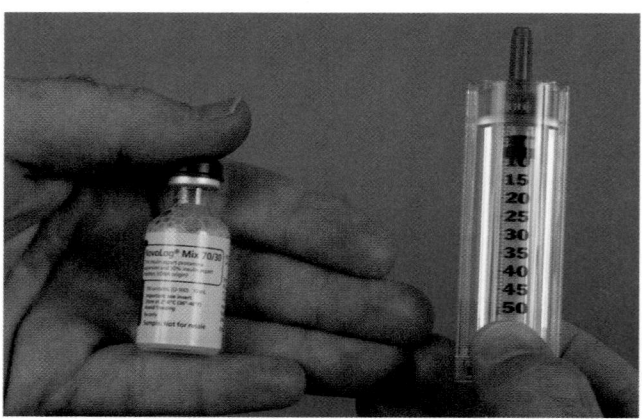

STEP 2e Syringe with magnifier.

STEP	RATIONALE

g. Instruct caregivers in how to properly draw up prescribed volume of medication into syringe. When necessary, have caregiver prepare extra prefilled syringes for client's use when caregiver is absent.

Ensures caregiver knows proper preparation techniques. Ensures client has access to injections.

● *Critical Decision Point*

Refer to medication insert or pharmacist as to whether doses can be stored in syringe over several hours or days. Keep all prefilled insulin syringes refrigerated, and use within 21 days (Rice, 2000).

3. Recommend approaches for medication and supply storage:

   a. Store medications in a safe place, preferably in the kitchen.

Moisture in bathroom may cause medications to decompose.

   b. Keep liquid medications and parenteral drugs, especially insulin, in a cool place.

Prevents decomposition of drug.

● *Critical Decision Point*

Insulin may be stored in refrigerator, but it is not necessary. The vial in use can be stored at room temperature for up to 30 days without losing potency (Rice, 2000). Otherwise, store in refrigerator. If it is stored in refrigerator, be sure drug is kept in a bin or container, away from food.

   c. Keep medical supplies such as syringes, dressing supplies, and glucose meter in airtight container (e.g., plastic storage bin) and stored in cool place, such as bedroom closet.

Ensures supplies are not exposed to moisture or other contaminants.

4. Review for client and caregiver the proper techniques for disposal of medications, "sharps," and disposable medical supplies:

   a. Discard unused portions of drugs or outdated drugs in sink or toilet.

Ensures that no one in household uses drug not prescribed for their use or drugs that will be ineffective pharmacologically.

   b. Obtain sharps container from medical supply store or intravenous (IV) equipment supplier. (If finances are limited, have client use a small-neck plastic bottle, such as a soda bottle.) Dispose of all needles and lancets in container (see illustration).

Puncture-proof container prevents exposure to contaminated needle stick. Small-neck container makes it difficult for anyone to easily retrieve a used needle or sharp.

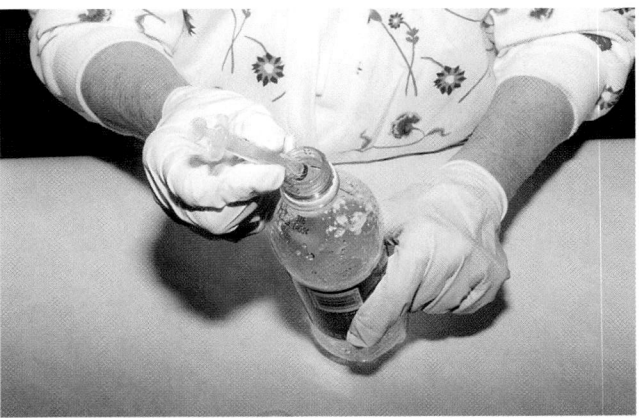

STEP 4b Disposing of syringe in hard plastic soda bottle.

STEP	RATIONALE
c. Caution against filling container to a point where needles protrude out opening. Discard when three-fourths full, securing top with duct tape or adhesive tape.	Prevents needle sticks.
d. Store sharps container in an area inaccessible to children.	Prevents injury to child.
e. Dispose of soiled dressings, used glucose testing reagent strips, and IV tubing in a separate, sealed, plastic garbage bag. Then place in second plastic bag (double bagged), and discard appropriately as trash.	Prevents contamination with other items in home. Minimizes chances of caregiver being exposed to infectious waste.
f. Consult local public health department or community authorities regarding proper way to dispose of waste.	Most communities have strict guidelines for waste disposal.

EVALUATION

1. Have client and/or caregiver describe steps to take to ensure medications are safe to use.	Demonstrates learning.
2. Observe client and/or caregiver prepare and administer a medication dose.	Evaluates ability to physically manipulate medications and necessary equipment.
3. Observe home setting for location of medications and supplies.	Evaluates client's and/or caregiver's adherence to recommendations.
4. Have client describe how sharps or medical equipment is discarded.	Demonstrates learning.
5. Do pill counts (pills remaining in containers) at successive intervals, such as twice a week for 2 weeks.	Verifies client takes correct number of medications over a period of time.

Recording and Reporting

- Record instructions and recommendations to client and caregiver and results of return demonstrations in progress notes.

Unexpected Outcomes	Related Interventions
1. Client and/or caregiver is unable to recall principles for safe use of drugs.	• Reinstruction necessary, or client and caregiver may need chance to ask more questions regarding benefit of precautions. • Offer written, simple, and clear instructions.
2. Client and/or caregiver has difficulty or is unable to prepare and self-administer a medication.	• Offer further assistance in setting up equipment. Offer assistive aids. • Reinstruct in steps used to prepare medication.
3. Medications and medical devices are not stored in a secure or appropriate location.	• Client may choose to store items conveniently rather than safely or may have limited resources. • Reinstruction and discussion are necessary.
4. Sharps and disposable medical equipment are not disposed of properly.	• Reinstruction is required. • Arrange to provide appropriate containers.
5. Excess or insufficient number of pills found during pill count.	• Incorrect dosage is being taken. Review with client daily drug prescribed. Reevaluate use of dosage reminders.

Teaching Considerations

- Instruct clients in care of linen. Use of lancets or application of dressings may cause soiling of client's linen supply. Infected or soiled linen should be kept in a separate, leakproof plastic bag. Contaminated items should be washed separately from household laundry in hot water with 1 cup of bleach and detergent for *two* regular wash cycles.

Pediatric Considerations

- It is vital to keep medications and other equipment out of the reach of small children. If teaching self-management skills, this needs to initially occur with adult supervision and input. Never refer to medications as candy.

FOCUS on CLINICAL PRACTICE

Mrs. Gleason is a 78-year-old woman who lives in her own two-bedroom home. She has a history of arthritis, hypertension, and glaucoma. She takes four different oral medications and eye drops. Her daughter checks on her mother every evening after work. The daughter assists with giving Mrs. Gleason a complete bath once a week. Mrs. Gleason cooks her own meals and performs routine ADLs. She also has been managing her own instrumental activities, but her daughter periodically reviews her mother's bill schedule and checkbook for accuracy.

1. Based upon her medical history, offer two reasons why Mrs. Gleason is at risk for falls.
2. To assess the client's adherence to her medication regimen:
   A. Ask client to show you where medications are stored in home.
   B. Have client describe daily schedule for drug administration.
   C. Determine caregiver's knowledge of medication schedule.
   D. Examine the condition of storage area for medications.
3. Mrs. Gleason's daughter tells you she is concerned about her mother's safety, "I worry that she will fall. I tried to reorganize things in her house, but that just made her angry." What advice might you give the daughter?

4. For each of the interventions listed below, provide a rationale for why the intervention is effective in reducing falls.
   A. Install treads with uniform depth of 9 inches (22.5 cm) and 9-inch risers (vertical face of steps).
   B. Rearrange furniture to open up space through hallways and major rooms.
   C. Apply colored tape or paint to color the control knobs on stove.
   D. Have grab bar installed in studs at tub, toilet, and/or shower.
   E. Have handrails installed along the side of any stairway.
5. Mrs. Gleason's arthritis affects fine motor movement of her hands. List two aspects of medication administration that might be affected by Mrs. Gleason's disability.
6. Mrs. Gleason's daughter expresses a concern that her mother is not taking her medications regularly. What action might the daughter take to determine her mother's medication compliance?

NCLEX REVIEW QUESTIONS

1. A client with the Alzheimer's form of dementia exhibits all of the following except:
   1. Progressive loss of memory
   2. Loss of the ability to recognize objects and persons
   3. Loss of the ability to perform familiar tasks
   4. Feelings of dejection
2. Exercise programs found to be most effective in reducing the incidence of falls are best described as:
   1. Long-term regimens incorporating client's activity patterns
   2. Short-term regimens lasting 1 year or less
   3. Programs focused on maintaining range of motion
   4. Long-term endurance exercise
3. A simple screening examination useful in detecting difficulties with balance or gait is the:
   1. Mini-Mental State Examination
   2. "Get Up and Go" test
   3. SPLATT screening tool
   4. Fall diary
4. A client at home is changing a dressing daily on a foot ulcer. The old dressing should be discarded in a:
   1. Wide-mouth plastic bottle
   2. Plastic storage bin
   3. Standard garbage pail
   4. Plastic garbage bag placed into a second plastic bag

References

Arfken C and others: The prevalence and correlates of fear of falling in elderly persons living in the community, *Am J Pub Health* 84(4):565, 1994.

Brewer JA, Bonalumi NM: Health care beliefs and practices among the Pennsylvania Amish, *J Emerg Nurs* 21(6):494, 1995.

Droscher MJ and others: Heating oil company responses to inquiries concerning carbon monoxide toxicity, *Ann Emerg Med* 33(4):406, 1999.

Ebersole P, Hess P: *Toward healthy aging,* ed 6, St. Louis, 2003, Mosby.

Gray-Micelli D: Falling among older individuals: exploring psychological issues, *Adv Nurse Pract* 5:7, 1997.

Harper RD, Dickson WA: Reducing the burn risk to elderly persons living in residential care, *Burns* 21(3):205, 1995.

Lueckenotte A: *Gerontologic nursing,* ed 2, St. Louis, 2000, Mosby.

National Fire Protection Association: *Fact sheets: home fires,* Quincy, Mass, 2001, http://www.nfpa.org/research/nfpafactsheets.

Maslow A: *Motivation and personality,* ed 2, New York, 1954, Harper and Row.

North American Nursing Diagnosis Association: *Nursing diagnoses: definitions and classification 2003-2004,* Philadelphia, 2003, The Association.

Rice R: *Home health nursing practice,* ed 3, St. Louis, 2000, Mosby.

Shamberg S, Shamberg A: Reentry begins at home, *Rehab Manag* 8(5):24, 1995.

Tideiksaar R: *Falls in older persons: prevention and management,* ed 2, Baltimore, 1998, Health Professions Press.

Research References

Campbell AJ and others: Randomised controlled trial of a general practice programme of home based exercises to prevent falls in elderly women, *Br Med J* 315:1065, 1997.

Cummings RG and others; Home visits by an occupational therapist for assessment and modification of environmental hazards: a randomized trial of falls prevention. *J Am Geriatric Soc* 47:1417, 1999.

Futrell M, Melillo KD: *Evidence-based protocol: wandering,* The University of Iowa Gerontological Nursing Interventions Research Center, Research Dissemination Core, Iowa City, Iowa, 2002, University of Iowa.

Gill T and others: Environmental hazards and the risk of nonsyncopal falls in the homes of community-living older persons, *Med Care* 38(12):1174, 2000.

Gillespie LD and others: Interventions for preventing falls in elderly people, *Cochrane Database Syst Rev* 3:CD000340, 2001.

Lipsitz L and others: Causes and correlates of recurrent falls in ambulatory frail elderly, *J Gerontol* 46(4):114, 1991.

Mastrian K: Differing perceptions in defining safe independent living for elders, *Nurs Outlook* 49:213, 2001.

Robertson MC and others: Effectiveness and economic evaluation of a nurse delivered home exercise programme to prevent falls. I. Randomised controlled trial, *Br Med J* 322:697, 2001.

Tinetti M.E.: Preventing falls in elderly persons, *N Engl J Med* 348(1):42, 2003.

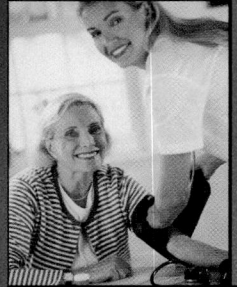

42

Home Care Teaching

MEDIA RESOURCES

Evolve Site *evolve*

http://evolve.elsevier.com/Perry/skills
• Weblinks

OBJECTIVES

Mastery of content in this chaper will enable the nurse to:

- Identify factors that influence clients' learning and skill performance of home care.
- Discuss the collaborative nature of home care teaching.
- Assess safety factors that may impair or prohibit the client's skill performance in the home setting.
- Discuss situations and conditions that require client and/or family to learn skills that support and achieve health maintenance.
- Understand variances in teaching strategies in the home setting.
- Implement and evaluate appropriate learning strategies that support positive client outcomes.

KEY TERMS

Antipyretic
Clean technique
Dementia
Febrile
Gastrostomy feeding tube
High-Fowler's position
Infusion pump
Intake and output (I&O) record

Nasal cannula
Nasogastric feeding tube
Over-the-counter drug
Oxygen therapy
Piloerection
prn
Transtracheal oxygen catheter

Changes in the health care delivery system in recent times have shifted the site of care delivery from the acute inpatient setting to the home care arena. Although acute- and long-term care settings continue to provide inpatient services, many clients recover from or are treated for illnesses in the home environment. The psychosocial, emotional, and financial issues surrounding the ongoing needs of individuals and families dealing with chronic or episodic illnesses are often best managed in the home setting.

The home care nurse is faced with a diverse client population with varying acuity levels. Treatments that historically were provided strictly in an inpatient setting are now commonplace in home care. In addition, clients are expected to assume greater responsibility for managing their care at home, resulting in a greater demand on home care nurses to provide client education on a variety of complex topics (Falvo, 2004).

Client teaching is an essential part of home care nursing practice. Evidence-based practice guidelines, which define the standard of practice based on current best knowledge, are now widely used in health care settings to improve the quality of care. Client education is often included in these guidelines (Redman, 2001). For example, the American Diabetes Association's standards (2004) indicate that intensive client education about self-management principles is integral to successful diabetes management plans. According to these standards, interdisciplinary teams that include nurses, physicians, advanced practice nurses, dietitians, pharmacists, and mental health professionals provide diabetes self-management education about topics such as blood sugar control, dietary choices, and prevention of long-term and short-term complications of diabetes.

All nurses, including home care nurses, have an ethical responsibility to teach their clients. In *Patient Care Partnership*, the American Hospital Association (2003) indicates that clients have the right to make informed decisions about their care. Information must be relevant, current, and clearly presented. The home care nurse often clarifies information provided to the client by other health care professionals and may become the client's primary source of information.

An additional challenge facing home care nurses today is illiteracy. In the United States, illiteracy may affect the client's ability to read, write, and speak English and to compute and solve problems related to self-care (Falvo, 2004). To overcome challenges presented by illiteracy, home care nurses assess the client's ability to learn and understand information in different ways before, during, and after client education is provided (Dreger and Trembeck, 2002). For example, nurses assess clients' reading abilities and understanding levels by asking clients to review printed information and answer open-ended questions, such as, "After reading this medication teaching sheet, tell me how this medication will help you" (Osborne, 2001). To assess math skills, home care nurses ask clients to calculate dosages of prescribed medications. To assess the ability to problem solve, nurses pose pertinent problems and ask clients to solve the problem. For example, if a nurse is helping an obese client with a weight management program, the nurse may give the client a menu from a restaurant and ask the client to identify healthy food choices.

To enhance learning of all clients, the nurse provides printed client education information and videotapes or audiotapes to reinforce learning when possible. Effective supplemental client education material is presented at a level that matches the client's ability to read and understand information. In addition, the home care nurse presents information in an organized manner and presents only essential information on a topic, allowing adequate time for the client to learn. For example, to teach a woman how to feed her husband who has a feeding tube, the nurse first teaches the wife how to measure the tube feeding and how to manipulate the equipment. Once this is accomplished, the process of administering the feeding occurs. The nurse provides the wife with written materials that outline the steps required for administering the tube feeding and watches the wife perform a return demonstration of the tube feeding to assess learning.

Home care nurses must be creative and adapt to each client's unique physical, psychosocial, and cultural needs. Home care nurses assess their clients' health status, and identify, coordinate, and intervene with various interdisciplinary services and resources that are required to support their clients' successful health maintenance. Nurses involved in home care collaborate with the client, family, or designated caregivers, as well as interdisciplinary teams that may include the prescribing physician, pharmacists, physical therapists, occupational therapists, and organizations that provide and maintain medical equipment. Many times a variety of other social services and/or health-related organizations are also involved in making clients' home care plans successful. For collaboration to be successful, the nurse identifies who is involved in the client's care and the contributions and abilities of each person. The nurse establishes mutual trust and respect for each person's abilities and contributions through open and honest communication.

Home care nurses design interventions to help their clients overcome barriers that affect the ability to comply with recommended health care, such as lack of transportation or inadequate funds for medication, food, and equipment. Clients' cultural beliefs or values must be considered in the design of interventions and in the manner in which other family members are involved. It is very important for the client to become an active partner in the plan of care.

Client education is an essential component of home care and a major factor in clients' compliance with therapies (Falvo, 2004). Home care nurses must assess intrinsic and extrinsic factors that affect clients' abilities and willingness to manage self-care. If a person does not want to learn, it is unlikely that learning will occur. However, many clients can be motivated to return to a previous level of health or function. For example, a client who has recently experienced a below-the-knee amputation may be motivated to learn how to walk with assistive devices at home to allow the client to continue to live independently at home. When home care nurses successfully implement individualized teaching plans, clients and families may attain improved quality of life, make fewer physician visits, incur a reduction in overall costs of health care, and regain health or gain more control over an illness.

Evidence-Based Practice Trends

Clients need to understand how to manage their diseases and related care at home. However, knowledge alone does not necessarily predict a change in health-related behaviors (Falvo, 2004; Sedlak and others, 2000). As a result, researchers have investigated factors that lead to improved health behaviors in a variety of populations. Analysis of current research indicates that clients perceive teaching provided by nurses to be important. For example, in one study, clients with lower educational levels perceived that client education provided by nurses about illnesses, medications, and treatment options was very important. This group also identified that being able to call a nurse with questions was very important (Oermann and others, 2001). If a client has a lack of education, nurses need to be available and accessible to provide, clarify, and reinforce meaningful and relevant client education.

Clients who are informed are more likely to manage their health problems better than those who are not informed (Oermann and others, 2001). However, many times, people who are members of vulnerable populations do not pursue or have access to necessary health care. Two vulnerable populations in the community include people of lower socioeconomic status and people living with chronic illnesses. There are different educational strategies that enhance the outcomes of client education in these populations. For example, in low-income women, both group counseling and one-on-one approaches effectively improved breast cancer screening (Danigelis and others, 2001). In another example, adult clients with cancer preferred interactive communication with nurses and physicians as well as clearly presented information that was provided in print or on a CD-ROM (Agre and others, 2002; Harper Chelf and others, 2002). Finally, intensive, interdisciplinary teaching has helped children with type 1 diabetes and their parents transition to insulin pump therapy (Litton and others, 2002; Plotnick and others, 2003). The results of these studies indicate that educational interventions provided by nurses to meet the needs of vulnerable populations are successful in helping these clients attain positive outcomes.

Regardless of the population being taught or the skill or information being presented, the results of research indicate that individualized, interdisciplinary teaching efforts that are theoretically based are the most effective in promoting behavior change (Cooper and others, 2001). Therefore home care nurses should lead interdisciplinary teams to produce teaching interventions that will facilitate self-directed learning and problem solving in their clients. Evidence-based nursing strategies that facilitate positive client outcomes in client education are summarized in Box 42-1.

Skill Performance Guidelines

1. Assess the client's and caregiver's physical, cognitive, emotional, cultural, environmental, and social resources in regard to successful learning and skill performance.
2. Present information in an understandable and orderly manner directed toward the client's and caregiver's learning style and abilities.
3. Individualize the teaching care plan based on the assessed physical, psychosocial, cultural, educational and cognitive abilities of the client and caregiver.
4. Assess if the client in the home setting can safely perform a skill. If the client is unable to execute the skill independently, identify a care partner who can help provide the skill safely in the home setting.
5. Assess and determine if home medical equipment and hygiene needs can be supported in the home environment to promote successful self-care management.
6. Include teaching interventions for other persons in the household who may positively or negatively influence the client's self-care management.

BOX 42-1 **Strategies and Examples That Facilitate Positive Client Outcomes in Client Education**

- Individualize approaches to client teaching. Clients with similar problems and demographic characteristics do not learn the same way.
- For example, some clients learn better with verbal instructions, whereas others prefer to have information written down. Determining clients' preferences for education will enhance learning outcomes.
- Assess clients' present beliefs about health or disease-related management when designing teaching interventions for clients.
- For example, a client who believes that smoking cessation is an important step in becoming healthier will be more open to learning strategies to stop smoking when compared with a client who has no desire to stop smoking.
- Time teaching interventions to coincide with a client's readiness to learn and willingness to make health-related changes.
- For example, a mother who has an infant with an ear infection is ready to learn how to take her infant's temperature and to learn interventions that may help prevent ear infections in the future.
- Use of therapeutic communication and empathetic understanding will lay the foundation for effective teaching.

- For example, adolescent girls who are treated with respect learn the steps involved with self-breast examination (SBE) and are more likely to perform SBE monthly.
- Acknowledge and accept the client's fears, frustrations, and responses to illness in an understanding way.
- For example, the nurse accepts the frustrations of a client who is having trouble taking his pulse and patiently helps the client until he is able to take his pulse by himself.
- Design interventions that will facilitate problem solving, critical thinking, and goal setting.
- For example, a client with diabetes is encouraged to set a goal of weight loss. The nurse helps the client to develop a self-management plan by having the client review diet plans and identify foods that are acceptable and unacceptable.
- Provide frequent positive reinforcement and feedback whenever possible.
- For example, the nurse has family members provide frequent reinforcement and feedback when a child with asthma is learning how to use an inhaler for the first time.

Data from Cooper H and others: Chronic disease patient education: lessons from meta-analyses, *Patient Educ Couns* 44(2):107, 2001; Falvo DR: *Effective patient education: a guide to increased compliance*, ed 3, Boston, 2004, Jones & Bartlett Publishers; Norris SL and others: Effectiveness of self-management training in type 2 diabetes: a systematic review of randomized controlled trials, *Diabetes Care* 24(3):561, 2001.

SKILL 42-1 Teaching Clients to Measure Body Temperature

To practice health maintenance for themselves and their family members, clients need to know how to measure body temperature. An elevation in body temperature can be an early warning sign of serious health problems. Clients susceptible to temperature alterations should know how to measure their temperatures correctly so that they can seek medical attention early when alterations occur. Parents must know how to measure their children's temperature because children can develop seriously high fevers very quickly. Because older adults have impaired temperature-control mechanisms, a family caregiver should know the techniques for temperature measurement. Nurses teach clients the skills of measuring body temperature and lowering temperature when a febrile episode occurs at home and medical care is not immediately accessible.

There are a variety of body temperature measurement tools available for use, including mercury, disposable single-use, electronic digital, and tympanic thermometers. Mercury thermometers pose a significant risk to the environment and are becoming less available. If a mercury thermometer breaks,

and it is not disposed of properly, the mercury can get into the air, posing a major health risk in the home. Therefore cities throughout the nation (e.g., Duluth, Minn., and San Francisco) are banning the sale of mercury thermometers (Environmental Protection Agency [EPA], 2004b). Nurses throughout the nation have initiated mercury thermometer exchanges in their communities to reduce environmental exposure to mercury (Sattler, 2002). Nurses in home care need to educate their clients about the environmental hazards associated with mercury and encourage their clients to purchase mercury-free thermometers.

The nurse assists a client in choosing the best thermometer to use based on the client's dexterity, vision, and financial resources. For example, a client with visual changes from glaucoma or retinopathy may be able to read a thermometer with a large digital display more easily. The need for an oral, rectal, or axillary temperature is determined based on the client's age and health status. (See Chapter 17 for guidelines on use of all types of thermometers.)

DELEGATION CONSIDERATIONS

The skill of teaching clients to measure body temperature cannot be delegated to assistive personnel.

EQUIPMENT

- ❑ Thermometer
- ❑ Disposable probe cover if thermometer requires it
- ❑ Water-soluble lubricant (for rectal measurements only)
- ❑ Paper or logbook and pencil or pen if frequent measurements are to be taken
- ❑ Disposable gloves (for rectal temperature taken by a caregiver)

STEP	RATIONALE

ASSESSMENT

1. Assess client's ability to manipulate and read thermometer. Clients should wear eyeglasses if necessary.

   Physical restrictions in handling or reading thermometer may require nurse to instruct family member or significant other instead of client. Visual acuity impairment may prevent client from being able to read thermometer.

2. Assess client's knowledge of normal temperature range, symptoms of fever and hypothermia, and client's risk for body temperature alterations.

   Identifies client's ability to initiate preventive health measures and recognize alterations in body temperature.

3. Assess client's knowledge of criteria to determine appropriate type of thermometer to be used in varying situations (see Chapter 17).

   Determines knowledge of age-related or medical conditions that determine selection of oral, rectal, or axillary temperature.

4. Assess client's previous knowledge and experience in measuring temperature. Have client perform return demonstration if client indicates ability to measure temperature.

   Allows nurse to assess client's knowledge and use of safety precautions, aseptic technique, and time period for insertion.

NURSING DIAGNOSES

- Risk for imbalanced body temperature
- Health-seeking behaviors (temperature measurement)
- Hyperthermia
- Hypothermia

- Risk for infection
- Deficient knowledge regarding temperature measurement
- Readiness for enhanced therapeutic regimen management
- Ineffective thermoregulation

Related factors are individualized based on client's condition of needs.

PLANNING

1. Expected outcomes following completion of procedure:
   - Client is able to correctly measure temperature.

     Indicates skills are effectively learned.

   - Client demonstrates proper cleaning and storage of equipment.

     Prevents transfer of microorganisms and maintains integrity of thermometer.

   - Client states factors that affect temperature, signs and symptoms of fever and hypothermia, and measures to take with abnormal temperatures.

     Cognitive learning is achieved.

   - Client selects appropriate thermometer storage location.

     Preserves integrity of thermometer when not in use.

2. Select setting in home where client is most likely to measure temperature.

   Practicing in same environment where skill is routinely performed facilitates comprehension and learning.

3. Discuss and demonstrate with client or family member proper way to position client before thermometer insertion; instruct family member to remain with client if age or physical status requires.

   Promotes client's understanding of comfort and safety principles, as well as technique to ensure accurate measurement.

STEP	RATIONALE

IMPLEMENTATION

1. Demonstrate steps of thermometer preparation, insertion, and reading. Provide rationale for steps to client or caregiver.

2. If rectal temperatures are to be taken, instruct client to use only rectal thermometer for rectal temperatures.

3. Have client perform each step with guidance from nurse. Do not rush client.

Demonstration is best technique for teaching psychomotor skills (Falvo, 2004). Adults learn best when they understand purpose of procedure.

Prevents transmission of microorganisms.

Nurse is able to correct errors in technique as they occur and discuss implications.

• *Critical Decision Point*
Discuss normal temperature range for adult or child.

4. Instruct client to take temperature 20 to 30 minutes after smoking or ingesting hot or cold liquids or foods.

5. Discuss common symptoms of fever: warm, dry, flushed skin; feeling warm; chills; piloerection; malaise; and restlessness.

6. Discuss common signs and symptoms of hypothermia: cool skin, uncontrolled shivering, loss of memory, and signs of poor judgment. Explain that persons with inadequate home heating, older adults, or those unaware of potential dangers of cold conditions are at risk.

Client must understand factors that can alter temperature readings.

Client must be able to recognize onset of fever in self or family member.

Client must be able to recognize onset of hypothermia in self or family member

• *Critical Decision Point*
Teach client to take temperature after chills/shivering subsides to obtain an accurate temperature.

7. Discuss importance of notifying physician when temperature elevations occur, and review common therapies for temperature reduction that are safe to perform at home, including use of antipyretics, exposing the skin to air, reducing room temperature, increasing air circulation, applying cool moist compresses to the skin (e.g., forehead), and drinking fluids (Hockenberry and others, 2003).

8. Instruct client on proper method for storing thermometer (when applicable), and select suitable storage location.

9. Provide set of written guidelines for client's reference to promote client confidence in ability to implement the skill independently, and offer guidance regarding when additional action (such as notifying physician) should be taken.

10. Give client a logbook or piece of paper to record temperature and the time temperature was taken if client must measure temperatures frequently. Instruct client to use written record to report temperatures to health care provider.

Clients must understand danger of high temperature elevations.

Thermometer must be stored appropriately so that it does not break or become inaccurate when not in use.

Some clients need instructions written in clear, concise statements or pictures to minimize anxiety and support appropriate actions for health maintenance.

Keeping organized record of temperatures will assist client in validating temperature fluctuations and reporting important information to health care provider.

EVALUATION

1. Have client independently demonstrate technique for temperature measurement, including ability to read thermometer three separate times.

2. Observe client cleaning and storing equipment.

Feedback through return demonstration of psychomotor skill is best means of evaluating mastery of skill.

Proper cleaning prevents bacterial growth, and proper storage preserves accuracy of thermometer.

STEP	RATIONALE
3. Ask client to identify normal temperature range and influence of smoking and hot and cold liquids or foods on oral readings; discuss safety implications for temperature measurement.	Measures cognitive learning and confirms understanding of information.
4. Have client describe common signs and symptoms of fever and hypothermia and methods for control.	Measures cognitive learning.
5. *Optional:* Observe client recording temperature values and times in logbook. Review client's logbook periodically to ensure that temperatures are being recorded correctly.	Health care providers make changes in client care based on information provided by the client. To ensure changes are made appropriately, accurate information should be recorded.

Recording and Reporting

- Record information taught and client's response in home care record.
- Record temperature in home care record and home documentation system (e.g., logbook).

Unexpected Outcomes	Related Interventions
1. Client is unable to measure temperature or clean thermometer correctly.	• Plan for client to perform return demonstration during next scheduled home care visit, or plan to teach family caregiver. • Ask client to describe difficulties experienced while performing temperature measurement. • Review and/or redesign learning component with demonstration of that part of the skill.
2. Client is unable to explain factors affecting temperature, common signs and symptoms of fever and hypothermia, or measures to lower fever.	• Use a different teaching strategy. • Repeat instruction • Include family caregiver in instruction.
3. Client reports that mercury glass thermometer has broken.	• Instruct client on the following steps to safely dispose of the thermometer (EPA, 2004a): · If possible, close the room off from the rest of the house, and increase ventilation in the affected room by opening windows or turning on a fan. · Do not touch mercury. · Use an eyedropper or a piece of heavy paper (e.g., playing card) to pick up mercury. · Place mercury, material used to pick up mercury, and broken glass in a plastic bag that can be sealed tightly. Triple bag the contaminated objects (place in a total of three sealed bags). · Place bags in a sealable plastic container. · Call local health department to determine where to dispose of mercury safely. · If possible, keep windows open and room well ventilated for 2 days. · Instruct client not to use a vacuum cleaner, a broom, or household cleaners when cleaning up mercury spill.

Teaching Considerations

- Instruct client or family to never force thermometer into rectum and to never use rectal thermometer after rectal surgery, when the client has a rectal disorder such as tumor or severe hemorrhoids, or when client cannot be positioned for proper thermometer placement.
- Use caution in recommending aspirin or any other over-the-counter drug or antipyretic medicine in clients whose conditions contraindicate their use (e.g., gastric ulcer, bleeding tendencies, risk of Reye's syndrome in children, allergic reactions, drug interactions, liver or kidney dysfunction). Encourage client to contact health care provider before using over-the-counter antipyretics.
- Instruct to never use sponging with isopropyl alcohol to lower fever because of neurotoxic effects that have been reported (Hockenberry and others, 2003).

Pediatric Considerations

- Stage of growth and development of child will determine site of measurement and type of equipment used (see Chapter 17).
- Younger children should never be left unattended during procedure.
- Teach the family to take a child's temperature whenever a child feels warm to the touch, even if the temperature was recently determined to be normal. Rapid assessment of a child's temperature can positively affect the child's outcomes to a medical condition (Hockenberry and others, 2003).

Gerontological Considerations

- Mean oral temperature of older adults ranges from 36° to 37° C (96.9° to 98.6° F); therefore temperature considered within normal range may reflect a fever in the older adult (Eliopoulos, 2001).
- Older adults are more sensitive to temperature changes and have a tendency to demonstrate symptoms of delirium or dementia with variations of body temperature.
- Altered internal temperature regulation or dehydration may be seen in frail, debilitated clients. Temperature measurement becomes very important to prevent severe states of hypothermia or hyperthermia.
- Teaching sessions should involve active client participation. Learning will be best accomplished when client is rested and alert. Sessions may be shorter in duration depending on factors such as fatigue.
- Consider common age-related sensory changes in the older adult, and direct teaching strategies to compensate for any alterations, such as a magnifying glass to read thermometer.

Home Care Considerations

- Assess temperature and ventilation of environment to determine existence of any condition that may influence client's temperature.

SKILL 42-2 Teaching Clients to Measure Blood Pressure

Clients with underlying physical ailments such as cardiac, kidney, or vascular disease may be susceptible to wide variations in their blood pressure. They need to know how to correctly measure their blood pressure so they can seek medical attention early when alterations outside their acceptable ranges occur. Infrequent blood pressure measurements do not provide reliable data for treatment decisions (Evans and others, 2001). Therefore clients learn to regularly measure blood pressure to monitor their health, to assess medication regimen effectiveness, or as part of a rehabilitation or an exercise program.

Nurses teach clients the skill of measuring blood pressure and the important issues surrounding unusual readings. Nurses also teach clients about other factors that can affect blood pressure readings such as cuff placement, movement of the tubing, and position of the client. Specific actions to be taken to reduce the chance of negative outcomes that are

possible with poorly controlled blood pressure are equally important to the teaching plan (see Chapter 17).

Two types of sphygmomanometers are available to measure blood pressure (see Chapter 17). The mercury manometers are less commonly available due to the potential environmental risk associated with mercury. Aneroid manometers are safe, lightweight, compact, and portable. In the home, many clients choose to use electronic blood pressure reading devices that are commercially available. These devices produce a blood pressure measurement without needing to use a stethoscope. A cuff around the arm, the wrist, or a fingertip is used; and a reading is displayed electronically for the client. Although electronic monitors are easier to use, they are not always accurate (Campbell and others, 2001). For example, Altunkan and others (2002) found that although clients perceived that two different wrist blood pressure monitoring devices were comfortable and easy to use, the cuffs did not reliably measure systolic blood pressure. One factor that affects the accuracy of blood pressure monitoring is cuff size. Blood pressure cuffs that are too small tend to overestimate blood pressure, while cuffs that are too large tend to underestimate blood pressure (Jones and others, 2003). Bur and others (2003) found that current recommendations for cuff size yielded a significant number of inaccurate blood pressure readings. They concluded that current recommendations regarding cuff size and upper arm circumference should be reevaluated. Not all electronic home blood pressure monitors come with interchangeable cuff sizes, further compounding the problem of monitoring blood pressure at home. Home care nurses should help their clients investigate issues surrounding cuff size and calibration and accuracy of electronic equipment before the client determines which type of blood pressure monitor to purchase (Jones and others, 2003).

DELEGATION CONSIDERATIONS

The skill of teaching clients to measure blood pressure cannot be delegated to assistive personnel.

EQUIPMENT

❑ Sphygmomanometer or electronic blood pressure reading device (Figure 42-1) with bladder and cuff: bladder should completely encircle arm without overlapping; cuff should be secure and fit snugly (Table 42-1)
❑ Stethoscope (two-headed teaching stethoscope is ideal) if using sphygmomanometer
❑ Pen or pencil and logbook or paper for recording

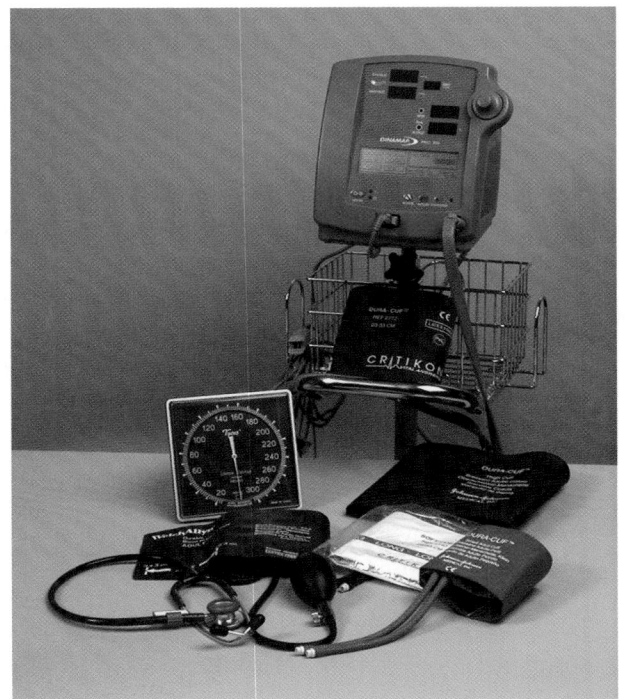

FIGURE **42-1** Home blood pressure monitoring device.

TABLE 42-1   GUIDE TO DETERMINING APPROPRIATE CUFF SIZE

CUFF SIZE	BLADDER WIDTH CM (IN)	BLADDER LENGTH CM (IN)	ARM CIRCUMFERENCE AT MIDPOINT CM (IN)
Newborn	3 cm (1 in)	6 cm (2½ in)	<6 cm (< 2½ in)
Infant	5 cm (2 in)	15 cm (6 in)	6-15 cm (2½-6 in)
Child	8 cm (3 in)	21 cm (8 in)	16-21 cm (6-8 in)
Small adult	10 cm (4 in)	24 cm (9½ in)	22-26 cm (9-10 in)
Adult	13 cm (5 in)	30 cm (12 in)	27-34 cm (11-13 in)
Large adult	16 cm (6 in)	38 cm (15 in)	35-44 cm (14-17 in)
Adult thigh	20 cm (8 in)	42 cm (16½ in)	45-52 cm (18-20½ in)

Data from Perloff D and others: Human blood pressure determination by sphygmomanometry [American Heart Association medical/scientific statement], *Circulation* 88(5):2460, 1993, http://www.americanheart.org/presenter.jhtml?identifier=3000861, American Heart Association, 2004, retrieved April 25, 2004.

STEP	RATIONALE

ASSESSMENT

1. Assess client's visual and auditory acuity as well as ability to manipulate and properly use blood pressure monitoring equipment.

2. Assess client's knowledge of normal blood pressure (BP) range and symptoms and common causes of hypotension and hypertension.

3. Assess client's knowledge of what BP measures, any specific medical issues that affect it, and why an awareness of variations is important to client's well-being.

4. Assess client's previous knowledge and experience in measuring BP. Have client perform return demonstration if client indicates ability to measure BP.

5. Assess home environment for a place conducive to measuring BP (e.g., quiet room with a comfortable place to sit).

Physical restrictions in handling, seeing, or hearing when using equipment may require nurse to instruct family member instead of client.

Identifies client's ability to know when to initiate preventive health measures and recognize alterations in BP.

Identifies client's understanding of potential cause-and-effect relationships between poorly controlled BP variations and health status.

Allows nurse to assess client's knowledge and skill performance.

Ensures more accurate measurement of BP.

NURSING DIAGNOSES

- Decreased cardiac output
- Deficient fluid volume
- Excess fluid volume

- Ineffective health maintenance
- Health-seeking behaviors (BP measurement)
- Deficient knowledge regarding blood pressure monitoring

Related factors are individualized based on client's condition or needs.

PLANNING

1. Expected outcomes following completion of procedure:
   - BP is accurately monitored by client.
   - BP is within range expected for client's age and condition.
   - Client explains purpose and implications of therapies and describes which alterations in BP require communication with health care provider to evaluate changes in treatment regimen.

2. Encourage client to perform measurements on routine schedule for a long-term monitoring plan.

3. Encourage client to avoid exercise, caffeine, and smoking for 30 minutes before assessment to avoid inaccurate reading.

4. Have client perform measurement in a comfortable position, with feet flat on floor, and in warm and quiet environment.

Learning has occurred.
Cardiovascular status is stable at level that is acceptable for client.
Measures cognitive learning.

Daily activities and many extrinsic and intrinsic factors affect BP fluctuations. A routine schedule allows for daily comparisons.
These factors can cause false elevations in BP.

Maintains client's comfort during measurement. Systolic and diastolic BP may increase with crossed-leg position.

- *Critical Decision Point*

  Eliminate extraneous noise such as television and conversation if client must use stethoscope to measure BP.

5. In teaching phase, explain procedure to client, and have client rest at least 5 minutes before measurement.

Reduces anxiety that can falsely elevate readings. BP readings taken at different times can be objectively compared when all are assessed with client at rest.

STEP	**RATIONALE**

6. Describe symptoms that indicate the need to perform BP measurement.

Promotes understanding of health status alterations that may need medical intervention.

IMPLEMENTATION

1. Discuss with client the best sites for assessing BP. For self-measurement, brachial artery is almost always used. Explain why client should avoid applying cuff to arm with:
   - Intravenous (IV) catheter with or without fluids infusing
   - Arteriovenous shunt
   - Breast or axillary surgery
   - Trauma, inflammation, or disease
   - Cast or bulky bandage

Most accessible sites are easiest to measure for accuracy of assessment. Appropriate site selection will promote accuracy in reading and minimize potential for trauma. Application of pressure from inflated bladder can temporarily impair blood flow and compromise circulation in extremity that already has impaired circulation.

2. Demonstrate steps for measuring BP (see Chapter 17):

Demonstration is best technique for teaching psychomotor skill (Falvo, 2004).

   a. Use of sphygmomanometer and stethoscope:
   (1) Teach palpation of artery, positioning of cuff, wrapping of cuff, placement of stethoscope, inflation and release of cuff, listening for Korotkoff sounds.

Learning is supported with appropriate information being received.

   (2) Describe sounds of measurement and relationship to observation of gauge during BP reading. Caution client about level and length of time appropriate for cuff inflation.

Ensures accurate reading. Prolonged inflation of cuff may damage circulation of limb.

   (3) Teach client to routinely clean diaphragm of stethoscope with rubbing alcohol or damp cloth.

Stethoscopes are frequently contaminated with microorganisms. Cleaning stethoscope routinely prevents transmission of microorganisms.

- **_Critical Decision Point_**
  If client must use stethoscope to take BP, use double-headed teaching stethoscope to verify accuracy of reading, or nurse should perform BP soon after client's attempt to verify accuracy.

   b. Use of electronic blood pressure monitor:
   (1) Teach correct placement of cuff, use of electronic equipment for proper cuff inflation, and procedure for changing batteries if used.

Using electronic equipment correctly helps ensure accurate BP readings.

3. Have client manipulate all equipment away from limb.

Proper equipment manipulation is required for accurate skill performance.

4. Have client attempt each step of skill on nurse or family member.

Nurse can correct any errors in technique as they occur.

5. Have client demonstrate techniques on self. Do not allow multiple repetitive attempts on any one limb.

Repeated attempts may affect measurement because of anxiety and repeated circulatory restriction.

6. Identify that skill performance teaching may need to be accomplished slowly, attempting each step of skill at different times until comfort is gained.

Psychomotor, cognitive, and affective learning may be impaired if teaching is attempted too quickly rather than in incremental steps.

7. Have client perform skill under observation, and record readings.

Verification of accuracy promotes confidence in client's abilities to successfully measure BP.

8. Provide client with printed instructions with written or pictorial guide, or provide client with a videotape demonstrating procedure if possible.

References for client will promote confidence for independent performance.

STEP	RATIONALE
9. Discuss desired BP range and when BP should be monitored.	Client must be able to identify desired and undesired BP values.

- **Critical Decision Point**
  Discuss importance of withholding antihypertensive medications when BP is low and notifying health care provider whenever BP is out of desired range and medications are not taken.

STEP	RATIONALE
10. Give client a logbook or piece of paper to record BP and the time BP was taken. In addition, client can record whether or not medications that affect BP were taken. Instruct client to use written record to report BP readings to health care provider.	Keeping organized record of BP readings and antihypertensive medications will assist client in reporting important information to health care provider.
11. Instruct client in proper care of BP equipment (e.g., storage, cleaning, and battery care).	Improper care and storage of equipment can affect accuracy of measurement.

EVALUATION

1. Observe client demonstrate technique for BP measurement on at least three different occasions, and verify client adds information to logbook correctly.	Feedback through return demonstration of psychomotor learning is best means to evaluate learning.
2. Ask client if blood pressure readings are within desired range and when to report abnormal readings to health care provider.	Determines client's ability to know when blood pressure obtained is within proper range and what to do when abnormal readings are obtained.
3. Ask client to describe reason for blood pressure monitoring and any related medications (e.g., antihypertensives) or treatment (e.g., diet and exercise).	Determines client's understanding of blood pressure monitoring and related therapies.
4. Have client demonstrate proper care of the BP equipment	Demonstrates learning.

Recording and Reporting

- Record teaching and client responses in home care record.
- Record BP in home care record and home documentation system (e.g., logbook).

Unexpected Outcomes	Related Interventions
1. Client or family member is unable to measure BP due to inability to manipulate equipment, accurately hear or palpate BP, or visualize numbers on equipment.	• Indicates need for alteration in teaching plan. • Review skill performance and recording of BP measurements client has performed between home care nursing visits. • Investigate other types of equipment that are easier to manipulate, see, or hear.
2. Client has difficulty in explaining purposes or implications of therapy.	• Review and reinforce information that client does not understand.

Unexpected Outcomes	**Related Interventions**
3. Blood pressure is inaudible or difficult to obtain with stethoscope.	• Have client wait 1 or 2 minutes and repeat BP reading. • Ensure that client is applying cuff appropriately and that the correct size cuff is being used. Determine correct placement of stethoscope, appropriate length of tubing, and correct use of equipment (e.g., cuff may have been deflated too quickly or too slowly; cuff may not have been pumped high enough for systolic readings). • If pressure is still inaudible or difficult to obtain, try alternative methods (e.g., use other arm, consider changing to electronic equipment for measurement).

Teaching Considerations

• Instruct client and/or family to report abnormal readings to physician.
• Educate client about risks for hypertension (see Chapter 17).
• Instruct client about specifics of treatment regimen, including potential side effects and interactions of any medication therapies.

Pediatric Considerations

• Understand that BP readings may be inaccurate if the infant or child is anxious and uncooperative or if the cuff size is inappropriate. Assistance from others in the form of providing diversionary tactics or taking the child's blood pressure while seated on the parent's lap may help calm the child (Hockenberry and others, 2003).
• Young children will be more apt to cooperate if allowed to manipulate and/or play with equipment before procedure. Another intervention that might enhance cooperation includes performing the procedure first on the parent or another person significant to child. This allows the child to observe that the procedure is safe.

Gerontological Considerations

• Musculoskeletal changes such as arthritis or other joint conditions may impair abilities to position limb comfortably and/or perform fine motor skills required for client to measure blood pressure (Lueckenotte, 2000).

• Older adults, especially those who are frail or who have lost upper arm mass, require a smaller BP cuff.
• Current national guidelines support that normal blood pressure limits should be the same regardless of age. Therefore, older adults should maintain a blood pressure less than 120/80 mm Hg. Clients with hypertension and diabetes or renal disease should have blood pressures less than 130/80 (National Institutes of Health [NIH], 2003).
• Home blood pressure monitoring is not a replacement for blood pressure monitoring by health care professionals in older adults, but it can help reduce the number of required office visits if the older adult client is able to accurately use the equipment and if the equipment is accurate (Broege and others, 2001).

Home Care Considerations

• Inaccurate home readings of BP can negatively affect client outcomes. Differences in blood pressure readings made at home and in an office or clinic setting tend to vary, with home readings often being much lower. To avoid discrepancies in blood pressure readings, clients should learn to be careful when using blood pressure equipment at home. Home equipment should also be calibrated to ensure that they are accurately measuring BP. Clients who have mastered the technique of BP monitoring at home with accurate equipment tend to experience improved outcomes (Campbell and others, 2001).

SKILL 42-3 Teaching Clients to Measure Pulse

Some clients benefit from knowing how to assess their own pulse. Persons taking medications that specifically affect heart function already have symptoms of heart disease and are susceptible to side effects of the medications. By being able to assess their own pulse rate and rhythm correctly, these clients can detect complications of their disease and any undesirable effects of their medications. Clients can thus seek prompt medical attention before serious problems occur.

Another group of clients who should learn how to assess their own pulse are those undergoing cardiovascular rehabil-

itation. For example, clients who have had myocardial infarction undergo exercise training to improve the strength of their heart muscle. Pulse rate and rhythm are the criteria used to determine how well these clients tolerate exercise.

There are many healthy persons who actively exercise and who can learn about their health from measuring their pulse. Exercise tolerance can vary depending on environmental conditions, intake of certain foods, and the overall physical condition of a person. By measuring pulse rate and rhythm, a person can learn how the body responds to strenuous exercise and when to cease further physical activity.

DELEGATION CONSIDERATIONS
The skill of teaching clients to measure pulse cannot be delegated to assistive personnel.

EQUIPMENT
❑ Wristwatch or clock with second hand
❑ Paper or logbook and pencil or pen

STEP	RATIONALE

ASSESSMENT

1. Identify client's understanding of purpose for assessing pulse and level of interest in performing skill.

Aids in identifying client's motivation to regularly assess pulse after learning skill. Also allows nurse to assess client's understanding of physical conditions and knowledge of medications prescribed.

2. Assess client's ability to feel arterial pulse by having client palpate own or nurse's artery. (Nurse palpates pulse of client or self simultaneously to see if client can successfully feel pulse wave.)

Physical impairment in sensation may necessitate nurse instructing family member or significant other instead of client.

3. Assess client's ability to visualize clock with second hand.

Client needs to have visual acuity to read clock with second hand.

4. Assess client's previous knowledge and experience in measuring pulse. Have client perform return demonstration if client indicates ability to measure pulse.

Reveals client's level of skill in assessing pulse.

NURSING DIAGNOSES
* Decreased cardiac output
* Deficient fluid volume
* Excess fluid volume

* Health-seeking behaviors (pulse measurement)
* Deficient knowledge regarding obtaining pulse
* Readiness for enhanced therapeutic regimen management

Related factors are individualized based on client's condition or needs.

PLANNING

1. Expected outcomes following completion of procedure:
   * Client is able to measure own pulse rate and rhythm correctly.
   * Client identifies normal range of pulse rate.
   * Client discusses importance of assessing pulse and best time for measurement.
   * Client discusses abnormalities and steps to take if pulse is not in desired range.
2. Select setting in home that client is most likely to use when assessing pulse.

Indicates skill was effectively learned.

Cognitive learning was achieved.
Ensures accurate monitoring of health status.

Client learns preventive health actions.

Practicing in same environment in which skill is routinely performed facilitates comprehension and learning.

STEP	RATIONALE

IMPLEMENTATION

1. Discuss with client the best sites for assessing pulse: radial and carotid.

Accessible sites are easiest to palpate for accuracy of assessment.

● *Critical Decision Point*

   If carotid site is chosen, caution client against vigorously massaging neck while attempting to locate pulse or attempting to locate both arteries at the same time. Stimulation of carotid sinus could lead to reflex slowing of heart rate from vagal stimulation. In addition, simultaneous occlusion of both carotid arteries decreases blood to brain, resulting in fainting.

2. Demonstrate steps for palpating pulse (see Chapter 17): position of artery on wrist or neck, how to locate artery, use of fingertips for palpation, compression of artery, palpation of pulse before counting, counting pulse, and calculating pulse rate.

   Demonstration is best technique for teaching psychomotor skills.

   a. Instruct use of gentle pressure; reinforce not to press hard over pulse site.

   Pressing too hard may occlude the artery.

   b. Instruct in use of watch or clock with a second hand to count pulse.

   Ensures correct timing of pulse.

   c. Instruct to count for a full 60 seconds, starting with second hand at 12:00 position.

   Consistent timing procedure will reduce confusion, forgetfulness about time period, or starting point used for pulse measurement. A full 60-second count increases accuracy of measure.

3. Have client perform each step with nurse's guidance (see illustration).

   Allows nurse ability to correct any errors in technique as they occur.

4. Discuss normal desired pulse range, purpose for monitoring pulse, and when pulse should be measured (e.g., before and after taking heart medications; before, during, and after exercise).

   Client must be able to determine when pulse or rhythm is not normal and when pulse should be taken.

● *Critical Decision Point*

   Discuss importance of notifying health care provider and withholding medication dose when pulse alterations occur. Client must understand preventive measures to take and prescriber's directions to be followed if alterations in pulse develop.

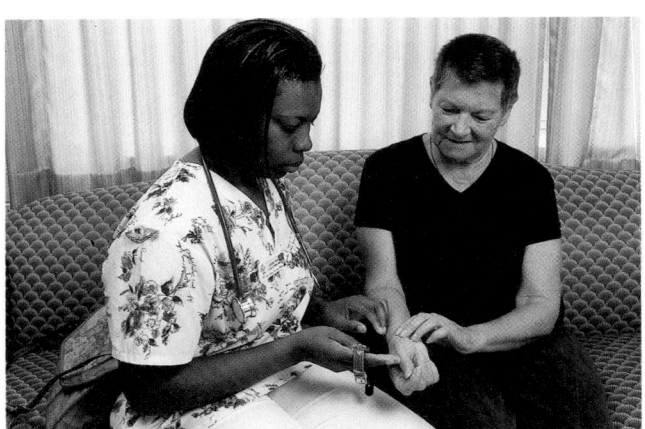

STEP 3 Nurse observing client checking pulse.

STEP	RATIONALE
5. Teach client to monitor pulse even though it remains in normal range.	Pulse staying within normal limits means medications are effective. Continual monitoring of pulse provides important information that supports effectiveness of medications or treatment.
6. Give client a logbook or piece of paper to record pulse rate and rhythm and the time pulse was taken. Have client document when medications that affect heart rate were taken. Instruct client to use written record to report pulse to health care provider.	Keeping organized record of pulse and heart medications will assist client in reporting important information to health care provider.

EVALUATION

1. Observe client independently demonstrate technique for pulse assessment and calculate pulse rate and rhythm three times.	Feedback through return demonstration of psychomotor skill is best means of evaluating learning of skill.
2. Have learner take radial pulse rate of nurse or other person at same time nurse is taking pulse of the individual.	Concomitant pulse taking will verify learner is able to accurately accomplish this skill.
3. Ask client to identify reasons for assessing pulse, normal pulse rate range, and steps to take when abnormalities are found.	Measures client's cognitive learning.
4. Pose situations involving changes in pulse rate, and ask client to describe when to withhold medication.	Confirms understanding of specific medical instructions received regarding withholding of certain prescribed medications with specific pulse rates.
5. Ask client to state time of day and activity level before taking pulse if purpose of measurement is for possible medication dosage adjustment.	Demonstrates understanding of relationships of time of day and activity levels with pulse rate variation.
6. Review client's logbook, and observe client as information about pulse is added.	Confirms client understands record keeping of pulse and medications that affect heart rate and rhythm.

Recording and Reporting

- Record information taught and client's response in home care record.
- Record pulse in home care record and home documentation system (e.g., log book).

Unexpected Outcomes	Related Interventions
1. Client is unable to palpate pulse or count rate correctly. May result from cognitive or sensory alteration, excess pressure, or the inability to locate artery or palpate it correctly. Clients with preexisting dysrhythmias often have difficulty learning to count pulse correctly.	• Reinforce information taught, and plan return demonstration to evaluate client's ability to perform skill. • Teach skill to a friend or family member.
2. Client is unable to discuss information related to pulse assessment.	• Anxiety, lack of interest, language barriers, or method of instruction may interfere with learning. • Review client's pulse assessment log to assess for significant issues or medication noncompliance.

Teaching Considerations

- Prescribers will recommend whether drug dose should be withheld in event of pulse alteration. Clients taking thyroid medications are often instructed to withhold medications when pulse is above 100 beats per minute; beta blockers (e.g., propranolol), calcium channel blockers (e.g., verapamil hydrochloride), or cardiac glycosides (e.g., digoxin) often are withheld if pulse is below 60 beats per minute. Specific drug dosage instructions are to be confirmed with prescriber, documented in home care record, and written clearly for the client.

Pediatric Considerations

- The radial pulse should be used in children over 2 years of age. Femoral or brachial pulse is best site for palpation of pulse for children under 2 (Hockenberry and others, 2003; White and others, 2004). The older the child, the easier it will be for the parent to assess heart rate (White and others, 2004).
- In infants, teach parents that pulse can be observed **(do not palpate)** and counted on anterior fontanel.

Gerontological Considerations

- Musculoskeletal changes such as arthritis or other joint conditions may impair a client's ability to palpate pulse for 60 seconds because of discomfort caused by positioning. Provide client with options for comfortable resting position of limbs when measuring pulse.
- Be aware of possible changes in visual acuity, and ensure environment and equipment used (clock or watch) support clear visualization.
- Older adult clients need to be taught how to exercise safely. Cardiac output is lower in older adults. Therefore the heart cannot adapt as well to sudden demands for increased oxygen (Ebersole and others, 2004). The following calculation can be used to determine a safe maximum heart rate during exercise in the older adult population: $(220 - \text{age}) \times 0.70$ (Eliopoulos, 2001). For example, if the client is 77 years old, using this formula would yield a safe maximum heart rate of 100 beats per minute.

SKILL 42-4   Using Home Oxygen Equipment

Home oxygen therapy is usually administered via nasal cannula or different types of masks (e.g., simple mask, reservoir mask, nonrebreather mask) (Petty, 2004). When a client has a permanent tracheostomy, however, a T tube or tracheostomy collar is used. Oxygen-conserving devices (OCD) are generally not covered by Medicare or insurance providers, but they reduce the amount of oxygen the client uses, resulting in an overall cost reduction to the client. The three types of OCDs are the reservoir nasal cannula, which stores oxygen in a chamber during the expiratory phase of respirations; demand oxygen delivery systems, which deliver a burst of oxygen only during inspiration; and the transtracheal oxygen catheter, which delivers oxygen through a catheter permanently inserted into the trachea, thus allowing the client to speak and bypassing anatomical dead space (Findeisen, 2001). Table 42-2 summarizes different oxygen devices and their uses.

In the home, three types of oxygen delivery systems are available: compressed oxygen, oxygen concentrators (Figure 42-2), and liquid oxygen (Figure 42-3, *A, B*). Some oxygen tanks are large and stationary, whereas smaller tanks may be classified as being either portable or ambulatory. Portable tanks are easily moved, weigh more than 10 pounds, are not designed to be carried, and deliver oxygen for about 5 hours at 2 L/min (Findeisen, 2001). Ambulatory tanks weigh less than 10 pounds, are designed to be carried,

---

TABLE 42-2	OXYGEN FLOW AND APPROPRIATE USES FOR OXYGEN DELIVERY DEVICES		
DEVICE	**FLOW (L/min)**	**FiO₂ RANGE (%)**	**USES**
Nasal cannula	¼-8	22-45	Clients receiving long-term oxygen therapy
Transtracheal catheter	¼-4	22-45	Clients who require high oxygen flow through a tracheostomy tube
Simple oxygen mask	6-12	35-50	Clients who require short-term oxygen therapy with moderate FiO₂ needs
Reservoir mask	6-10	35-60	Clients in acute respiratory distress with moderate FiO₂ needs
Nonrebreather mask	10-15	80-100	Clients in acute respiratory failure or in emergency situations

Data from Petty TL: *Guide to prescribing home oxygen: home oxygen options,* http://www.nlhep.org/resources/Prescrb-Hm-Oxygen/home-oxygen-options-4.html, National Lung Health Education Program, 2004, retrieved April 25, 2004.

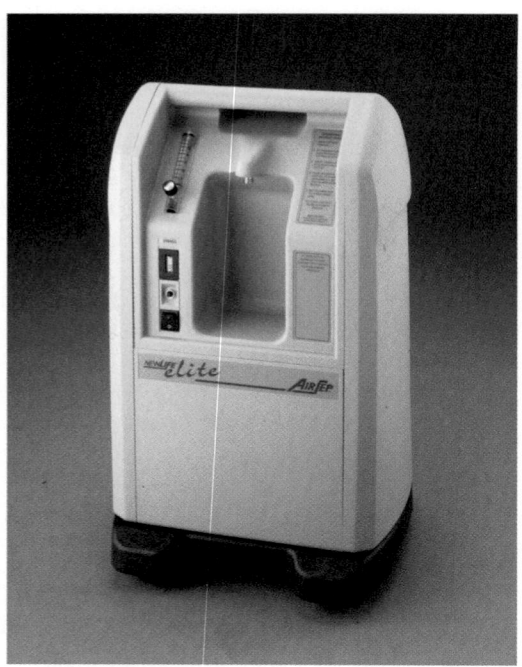

FIGURE **42-2** Oxygen concentrator. (Courtesy AirSep Corporation.)

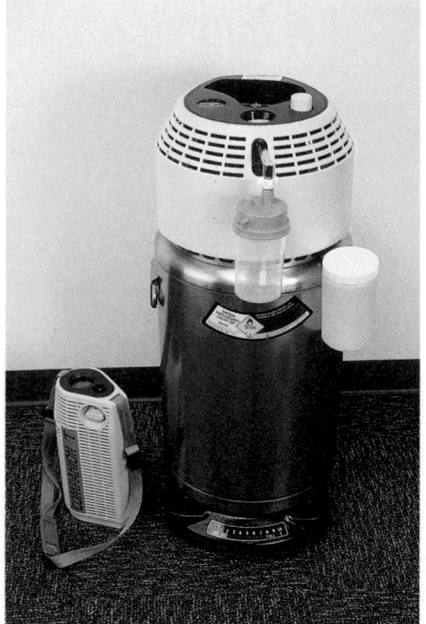

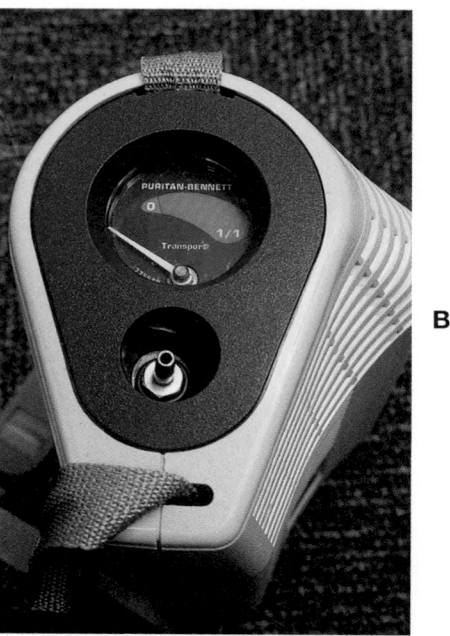

FIGURE **42-3 A,** Liquid oxygen containers. Smaller container is ambulatory unit, and larger container is stationary reservoir. **B,** Control panel.

and deliver oxygen for at least 4 hours at 2 L/min (Petty, 2004). Table 42-3 compares the different types of home oxygen delivery systems.

Compressed oxygen requires a regulator and flowmeter. The client receives delivery of several large oxygen tanks to the home. Large oxygen tanks last approximately 50 hours at 2 L/min. Liquid systems take up less space because oxygen is stored in a liquid state. Liquid oxygen is stored at or below −297° F and requires the use of a small ambulatory tank that is filled from a reservoir in the home. The oxygen concentrator method extracts oxygen from the room air and supplies oxygen to the client at prescribed flow rates. Table 42-4 shows how long a liquid oxygen system will last depending on the prescribed flow rate, and Table 42-5 shows how long compressed oxygen tanks will last. Oxygen concentrators deliver a lower percentage of oxygen to the flowmeter. Therefore, if a client is switched to a concentrator, the flow rate may need to be adjusted. The client who uses a concentrator must have a backup system, such as a portable oxygen tank, in case of power failure (Findeisen, 2001).

Home oxygen equipment is designated as durable medical equipment (DME) in the home care setting. Home oxygen therapy is often paid for by governmental or private insurance if there are written orders prescribed by the physician or advance practice nurse. A certificate of medical necessity (CMN) is required for clients who receive Medicare (Findeisen, 2001). Specific guidelines must be met before Medicare coverage can begin (Box 42-2).

Clients requiring home oxygen need extensive teaching to continue their oxygen therapy efficiently and safely. In preparation to initiate therapy, the home care nurse must coordinate efforts with the client, prescriber, caregivers, DME provider, and payer.

Common concerns of clients using oxygen at home include the fear of combustion, the concern of becoming oxygen dependent, and body image changes. Home care nurses provide client education and correct information when necessary (Findeisen, 2001).

TABLE 42-3   HOME OXYGEN SYSTEMS

PRIMARY USE	ADVANTAGES	DISADVANTAGES
COMPRESSED OXYGEN		
Intermittent therapy, such as for exercise or sleep only	100% oxygen stored in steel or aluminum cylinders; relatively inexpensive, no loss of gas during storage; relatively portable, delivery of up to 15 L/min; does not require electrical source; smaller tanks available	Bulky and heavy; frequent refilling necessary with continuous use; client must know how to read regulator and must understand when to call medical supplier for replacement cylinder; portable cylinders weigh 15 pounds and empty quickly when in use; may require weekly deliveries
LIQUID OXYGEN SYSTEMS		
System of choice for high-volume users and active clients	100% oxygen; more oxygen can occupy a smaller space; convenient ambulatory units refilled at home can be carried as a shoulder bag, backpack, or wheeled luggage cart; delivery of up to 6 L/min; client can be taught how to safely fill ambulatory units from larger reservoir; quiet and easy operation; does not require electricity for operation; requires relatively fewer deliveries of oxygen (as few as 8 times per year)	Evaporates, especially in warmer temperatures and when not in use; potential for connections to freeze together or form frost at connections if tight connection not maintained during filling; can be costly in set up and delivery fees
CONCENTRATORS		
Cost-effective for clients requiring low-flow continuous oxygen and clients with limited mobility inside or outside home	Inexpensive, fixed monthly costs; most units with delivery of up to 4 or 5 L/min; good choice for people who do not leave their homes frequently; no cylinders or tanks to refill	Oxygen concentration decreases as liter flow increases (usually 85% to 90%); power supply necessary; increased electrical costs (around $30 or more a month); is not an ambulatory unit, therefore requires second system for portability (usually gas cylinders); requires regular maintenance and a backup system

Data from Findeisen M: Long-term oxygen therapy in the home, *Home Healthc Nurse* 19(11):692, 2001; Petty TL: *Guide to prescribing home oxygen: home oxygen options,* http://www.nlhep.org/resources/Prescrb-Hm-Oxygen/home-oxygen-options-4.html, National Lung Health Education Program, 2004, retrieved April 25, 2004.

TABLE 42-4   LIQUID OXYGEN TIMETABLE

L/MIN	STATIONARY RESERVOIRS		PORTABLE UNITS	
	41 L	31 L	½ L	1 L
0.25	1400 hr	1060 hr	28 hr	44 hr
0.50	1125 hr	850 hr	18 hr	27 hr
1	560 hr	425 hr	9 hr	15½ hr
1.5	375 hr	283½ hr	6 hr	11½ hr
2	281 hr	213 hr	4½ hr	8½ hr
3	187½ hr	142 hr	3 hr	6 hr

TABLE 42-5 OXYGEN CYLINDER TIMETABLE*

L/MIN	LARGE (H-K) TANK		SMALL (E) TANK	
	2200 LB FULL	1000 LB ½ FULL	625 L FULL	284 L ½ FULL
1	115 hr	52 hr	10 hr	5 hr
2	56 hr	26 hr	5 hr	2 hr
3	37 hr	17 hr	3 hr	1 hr
4	28 hr	13 hr	3 hr	1 hr
5	22 hr	10 hr	2 hr	54 min
6	18 hr	8 hr	<2 hr	47 min

The following formulas can also be used to determine the length of time a tank will last:

FOR E CYLINDERS

Pressure on cylinder gauge (psi) − 500 psi (safety factor) × 0.3 (E cylinder factor) ÷ L/min = minutes

FOR H CYLINDERS

Pressure on cylinder gauge (psi) − 500 psi (safety factor) × 3.1 (H cylinder factor) ÷ L/min = minutes

EXAMPLE: If E cylinder reads 1500 psi and liter flow rate is 4 L/min
Time left: $1500 - 500 \times 0.3 \div 4 = 1000 \times 0.3 \div 4 = 300 \div 4 = 75$ minutes (1 hr 15 min)

NOTE: Do not allow oxygen cylinder pressure to fall below 500 psi, or the client may run out of oxygen.

*All times are approximate.

BOX 42-2 Medicare Qualifications for Home Oxygen Therapy

OXYGEN THERAPY AT REST

- $PaO_2 \leq 55$ mm Hg or $SaO_2 \leq 88\%$ at room air
- $PaO_2 = 56\text{-}59$ mm Hg or $SaO_2 \leq 89\%$ *and one of the following:*
  - Dependent edema suggesting congestive heart failure
  - Cor pulmonale or pulmonary hypertension as evidenced on ECG, echocardiogram, gated blood pool scan, or pulmonary artery pressure measurement
  - Erythrocythemia as evidenced by hematocrit >56%

NOCTURNAL OXYGEN THERAPY

- $PaO_2 \geq 56$ mm Hg or $SaO_2 \geq 89\%$ at room air while awake *and one of the following:*
  - $PaO_2 \leq 55$ mm Hg or $SaO_2 \leq 88\%$ during sleep
  - PaO_2 falls more than 10 mm Hg during sleep
  - SaO_2 falls more than 5% with signs and symptoms of hypoxemia during sleep

EXERCISE OXYGEN THERAPY

- $PaO_2 \geq 56$ mm Hg or $SaO_2 \geq 89\%$ at room air while at rest *and one of the following:*
  - $PaO_2 \leq 55$ mm Hg during exercise
  - $SaO_2 \leq 88\%$ during exercise

PaO₂, Arterial oxygen tension (partial pressure); *SaO₂,* oxygen saturation in blood; *ECG,* electrocardiogram.
Data from Findeisen M: Long-term oxygen therapy in the home, *Home Healthc Nurse* 19(11):692, 2001; Positive Air, Inc: *Medicare requirements for the home use of oxygen,* http://positiveair.com/medicare_home_use_of_oxygen.htm, 2004, retrieved Aug 8, 2004.

DELEGATION CONSIDERATIONS

The skill of teaching clients how to use home oxygen equipment cannot be delegated to assistive personnel.

EQUIPMENT

- ❑ Nasal cannula, oxygen mask (see Skill 22-1), OCD, or other prescribed delivery device
- ❑ Oxygen tubing
- ❑ Home oxygen delivery system (compressed oxygen, oxygen concentrator, or liquid oxygen) with all required equipment (varies with supplier and system used)

STEP	RATIONALE

ASSESSMENT

1. While client is still in the hospital, determine client's or family's ability to use oxygen equipment correctly (if appropriate and possible). In the home setting reassess for appropriate use of equipment.

   Physical or cognitive impairments may necessitate instructing family member or significant other how to operate home oxygen equipment. Enables nurse to determine specific components of skill that client or family can easily complete.

2. Assess home environment for adequate electrical service if oxygen concentrator is used.

   Oxygen concentrators require electricity to work (Findeisen, 2001). Continuous oxygen therapy must not be interrupted.

3. Assess client's and/or family's knowledge of purpose of oxygen and ability to observe for signs and symptoms of hypoxia: apprehension, anxiety, decreased ability to concentrate, decreased levels of consciousness, increased fatigue, dizziness, behavioral changes, increased pulse, increased respiratory rate, pallor, and cyanosis.

   Hypoxia can occur at home when client uses oxygen. Hypoxia may be caused by poor tubing connections or use of long oxygen tubing. It can also be caused by worsening of client's physical problem with a change in respiratory status.

STEP	**RATIONALE**
4. Determine appropriate resources in community for equipment and assistance, including maintenance and repair services, and medical equipment supplier.	Ensures readily available assistance for clients with home oxygen systems.
5. Determine appropriate backup systems, if compressor is used, in event of power failure (e.g., notify local emergency medical service [EMS]). Have a spare oxygen tank available for emergency use.	Many municipalities require that clients who have home oxygen equipment notify EMS before bringing the equipment home. When there is a power outage, EMS will call the home, and in some cases the home is on priority list for having power restored.

NURSING DIAGNOSES

- Anxiety
- Ineffective breathing pattern

- Ineffective health maintenance
- Deficient knowledge regarding home oxygen therapy

Related factors are individualized based on client's condition or needs.

PLANNING

1. Expected outcomes following completion of procedure:	
• Client receives oxygen at the prescribed rate.	Oxygen system set up correctly.
• Client and family will verbalize purpose and correct use of home oxygen.	Provides measurable criteria to determine level of understanding.
• Client and family will demonstrate how to maintain oxygen system.	Provides return demonstration of skills needed to use home oxygen system.
• Client and family will state indications for calling DME provider to replenish oxygen supply and re-order oxygen delivery supplies.	Client cannot run out of oxygen at home.
• Client and family will be able to verbalize safety guidelines for oxygen use (e.g., no smoking signs will be posted outside of home).	Provides measure of understanding of oxygen use.
• Client and family will be able to verbalize emergency plan of care.	Ensures safe, continuous delivery of home oxygen.
2. Select setting in home where client is most likely to use oxygen equipment.	Practicing in same environment where skill is routinely performed facilitates comprehension and learning.

IMPLEMENTATION

1. Perform hand hygiene.	Reduces transmission of microorganisms.
2. Place oxygen delivery system in a clutter-free environment that is well ventilated, away from walls, drapes, curtains, bedding, combustible materials, and at least 8 feet from heat sources.	Keeps system balanced and prevents injury.

• *Critical Decision Point*
Do not place oxygen delivery system in a closet.

3. Demonstrate steps for preparation and completion of oxygen therapy.	Demonstration is reliable technique for teaching psychomotor skill (Falvo, 2004) and enables client to ask questions.
a. *Compressed oxygen system:*	
(1) Turn cylinder valve counterclockwise two to three turns with wrench.	Turns on oxygen.
(2) Check cylinders by reading amount on pressure gauge.	Verifies adequate oxygen supply for client use.
(3) Store wrench with oxygen tank or in other safe place.	Storing wrench used to turn oxygen on in a safe place ensures it is available whenever needed.

STEP	RATIONALE

b. *Oxygen concentrator system:*

    (1) Plug concentrator into appropriate outlet.   Provides power safely to concentrator.

    (2) Turn on power switch.   Starts concentrator motor.

    (3) Alarm will sound for a few seconds.   Alarm turns off when desired pressure inside concentrator is reached.

c. *Liquid oxygen system:*

    (1) Check liquid system by depressing button at lower right corner and reading the dial on the stationary oxygen reservoir or the ambulatory tank (see Figure 42-3, *B*).   Verifies adequate oxygen supply for client use.

    (2) Collaborate with DME provider to provide instruction on refilling ambulatory tank.   Ambulatory tanks of liquid oxygen must be filled when empty.

• *Critical Decision Point*

Only fill ambulatory tanks when they are empty. Liquid oxygen is stored at or below −297° F inside reservoir, and the temperature inside the ambulatory tank is warmer. If cold oxygen from the reservoir mixes with warmer oxygen left in the ambulatory tank, the ambulatory tank may malfunction.

    (3) To refill liquid oxygen tank:

        (a) Wipe both filling connectors with a clean, dry, lint-free cloth.   Removes dust and moisture from system.

        (b) Turn off flow selector of ambulatory unit.

        (c) Attach ambulatory unit to stationary reservoir by inserting female adapter from ambulatory tank into male adapter of stationary reservoir (see illustration).   Secures connection between oxygen reservoir and ambulatory tank.

        (d) Open fill valve on ambulatory tank (e.g., lever, button, key), and apply firm pressure to top of stationary reservoir (see illustration). Stay with unit while it is filling. A loud hissing noise will be heard. Tank should be filled in about 2 minutes.   Prevents leakage of oxygen during filling process. If oxygen leaks during filling process, connection between ambulatory tank and reservoir could ice up and stick together.

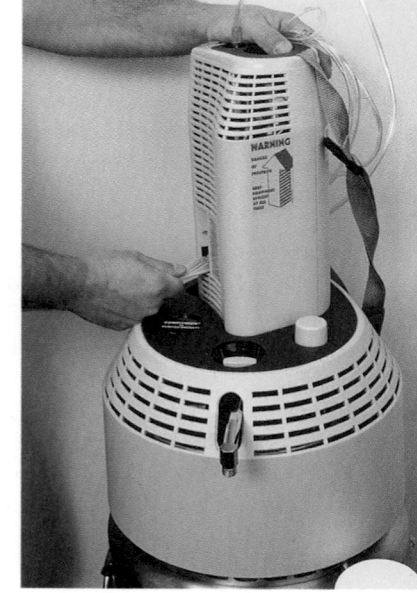

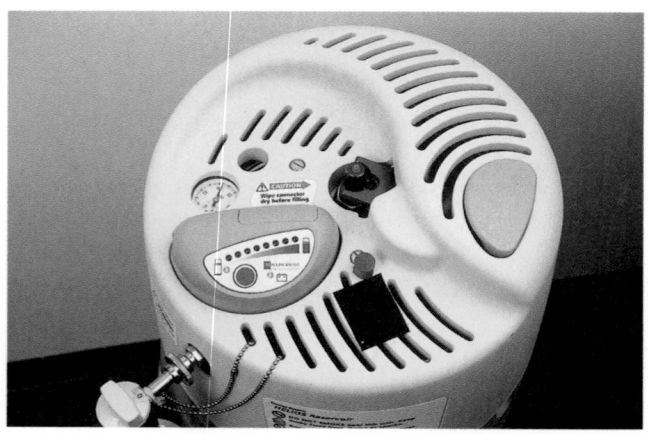

STEP **3c(3c)** Top view of stationary reservoir.

STEP **3c(3d)** Fill valve on ambulatory tank is opened while applying firm pressure to top of ambulatory tank.

STEP	RATIONALE

   (e) Disengage ambulatory unit from stationary reservoir when hissing noise changes and vapor cloud begins to form from stationary unit.

Overfilling may cause ambulatory unit to malfunction due to high pressure in tank.

- ### Critical Decision Point
  If ambulatory unit does not separate easily, valves from reservoir and ambulatory unit may be frozen together. Wait until valves warm to disengage (about 5 to 10 minutes). Do not touch any frosted areas because contact with skin may cause skin damage from frostbite.

   (f) Wipe both filling connectors with clean, dry, lint-free cloth.

Ice may form during filling process. Removes moisture from oxygen system.

4. Connect oxygen delivery device (e.g., nasal cannula) to oxygen delivery system (see Chapter 22) (see illustration).

Connects oxygen source to delivery method.

5. Adjust oxygen flow rate (L/min).

Ensures appropriate oxygen delivery.

6. Place oxygen delivery device (e.g., nasal cannula) on client (see Chapter 22).

Delivers oxygen to client.

7. Perform hand hygiene.

Reduces transmission of microorganisms.

8. Instruct client not to change oxygen flow rate.

Provides prescribed amount of oxygen.

9. Have client or family member perform each step with guidance from nurse. Provide written material for reinforcement and review.

Allows nurse to correct any errors in technique and discuss their implications.

10. Instruct client or family to notify physician if signs or symptoms of hypoxia or respiratory tract infection (e.g., fever, increased sputum, change in color of sputum, foul sputum odor) occur.

Respiratory tract infections increase oxygen demand and may affect oxygen transfer from lungs to blood. Can create severe exacerbation of client's pulmonary disease.

11. Discuss emergency plans for power loss, natural disaster, and acute respiratory distress. Have family, caregiver, or client call 911 and notify physician and home care agency.

Ensures appropriate response and can prevent worsening of client's condition.

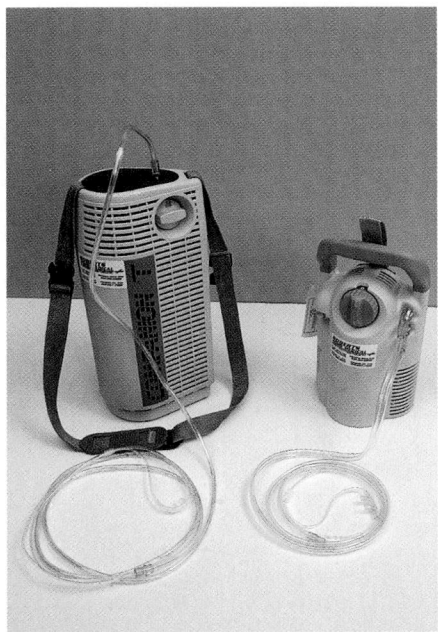

STEP 4 Oxygen delivery device and tubing attached to ambulatory oxygen tanks.

STEP	RATIONALE
12. Instruct client in safe home oxygen practices, including not allowing smoking in the house, keeping oxygen tanks away from open flames, and storing oxygen tanks upright.	Ensures safe use of oxygen in the home and prevents injury to client and family.
13. Record teaching plan, information given to client, and validation of learning.	Provides written documentation of teaching plan for client and family. Documents client learning.

EVALUATION

1. Monitor rate at which oxygen is delivered.	Determines if client is regulating oxygen at prescribed rate.
2. Ask client about ease or problems associated with home oxygen.	Determines ability of client or family to deal with stressors associated with home oxygen use. Also indicates client's risk for inappropriate oxygen use.
3. Ask client and family to state safety guidelines, emergency precautions, and emergency plan.	Determines client's knowledge of what to do if power fails, there is a failure in equipment, or client's status worsens.

Recording and Reporting

- Record teaching plan and information provided to client in home care record.
- Record validation of client or family learning.
- Communicate client's or family's learning progress to other health care providers involved.
- Record oxygen delivery system, related supplies, and prescribed oxygen flow rate.

Unexpected Outcomes	Related Interventions
1. Client has signs and symptoms associated with hypoxia (see Assessment, step 3).	• Determine if oxygen delivery device and oxygen source are delivering oxygen properly. • Determine if prescribed oxygen flow rate is set properly. • Assess client for change in respiratory status, such as airway plugging, respiratory tract infection, or bronchospasm. • Instruct client and family when to notify physician of signs of hypoxia.
2. Client uses unsafe practices with oxygen therapy, uses oxygen around fire or cigarette smoking, or sets incorrect flow rate.	• Reinforce client education, and perform follow-up reassessment (Box 42-3). • Include family caregiver in instruction, and set up problem-solving exercises with client.

BOX 42-3   Safe Home Oxygen Therapy Principles

FIRE SAFETY

- Although oxygen is not flammable, it will support combustion, therefore:
  - Use and store oxygen in a well-ventilated area.
  - Do not use petroleum-based ointments (e.g., Vaseline) around the nose—use of these ointments could cause burns.
  - Keep all oxygen equipment at least 8 feet from open flames (e.g., matches, fireplaces, stoves, space heaters, candles).
  - Do not allow smoking in the house.
  - Avoid using electrical appliances that produce sparks (e.g., electric razors).
  - Install smoke detectors and have a fire extinguisher available in the home.
  - Help client and family plan a fire evacuation route.

OXYGEN STORAGE AND HANDLING

- Store oxygen tanks upright in carts or stands to prevent tipping or falling, or place tanks flat on the floor when not in use.

- Do not store oxygen tanks in the trunk of a car.
- When transporting oxygen in a vehicle, ensure tanks are secured properly in the passenger area with the windows opened 2 to 3 inches to allow adequate ventilation.

CONCENTRATOR SAFETY

- Plug concentrators into properly grounded outlets.
- Do not use extension cords, power strips, or multioutlet adapters with concentrators.
- Ensure power supply or circuit meets or exceeds the amperage requirements of the concentrator.

LIQUID OXYGEN SAFETY

- Avoid direct contact with liquid oxygen because it can cause frostbite.
- Do not touch connectors that are frosted or icy.
- Keep ambulatory tanks upright; do not lay them down or place on their side.

Data from Findeisen M: Long-term oxygen therapy in the home, *Home Healthc Nurse* 19(11):692, 2001; Robb BW and others: Home oxygen therapy: adjunct or risk factor? *J Burn Care Rehabil* 24(6):403, 2003.

Teaching Considerations

- Potential for oxygen desaturation and decreased oxygen delivery to brain impairs client's ability to remember previous learning. Provide frequent teaching sessions and written or pictorial instructions to reinforce previous learning of teaching plan.
- Instruct client to observe level of oxygen in canister tank and to use portable or ambulatory tank when client leaves home.
- Instruct client and caregiver in appropriate cleaning, disinfecting, and maintenance of all oxygen delivery systems and supplies. Verify instructions with manufacturer's guidelines and DME provider's instructions.
- Instruct client and caregiver to check mask and tubing by placing hands or face over mask or cannula to feel air flow and to check to be sure mask is not too tight; it can leave marks on skin. Apply cotton or gauze sponge at pressure points.
- Instruct client to keep a bell handy for notifying primary caregiver when help is needed.

Pediatric Considerations

- Equipment must be kept out of reach of any children in home. Manipulation of dials or flow meters could have disastrous effects on oxygen delivery process.
- Instruct family of risk of fire and explosion when using oxygen equipment in the home. Caution against having oxygen near an open flame or when a family member is smoking.
- Home oxygen therapy in children may create a lot of stress in the family, especially when the child is a premature infant, because of the complex demands placed on the parents. Home visits by a nurse and other health care professionals and referral to support groups may help parents better cope with the demands of caring for a child requiring oxygen at home (McLean and others, 2000).

Gerontological Considerations

- Older adults have less efficient respiratory systems and less surface area for gas exchange, so their response to decreased oxygen and infection may cause cerebral anoxia, and they may experience confusion. They may be unable to recognize respiratory problems or problems with delivery system; therefore they must have frequent contact with a designated caregiver.
- Oxygen administration in older adults can have serious and even fatal consequences. Home care nurses need to ensure that the client is receiving oxygen at the prescribed rate and evaluate and recommend oxygen delivery systems that are the most effective for each client (Eliopoulos, 2001).

Home Care Considerations

- Provide two complete sets of oxygen delivery devices (e.g., nasal cannula, flowmeter [if used]) and tubing so the client has an extra set whenever equipment is being cleaned or in case equipment malfunctions.
- Home oxygen therapy is associated with a high risk of burns if not used correctly (Robb and others, 2003). Instruct client and family in the principles of safe oxygen use (see Box 42-3).
- Some clients are unable to fill ambulatory systems. In this case the nurse helps clients identify persons who can assist them.

SKILL 42-5 Teaching Home Tracheostomy Care and Suctioning

The indications for performing tracheostomy care and suctioning in the home are similar to tracheostomy care and suctioning in the hospital except for one key variable: the use of *medical asepsis or clean technique*. In the hospital, principles of surgical asepsis are used because the client is more susceptible to infection and because more virulent or pathogenic microorganisms are usually present than in the home setting. In the home setting the majority of clients use clean technique.

However, not all home care clients should use clean technique. The nurse must use judgment in choosing clients who are candidates for using clean or aseptic technique. For example, the immunocompromised client, who is at risk for severe infections, may need to continue to receive suctioning using principles of surgical asepsis. Clients who are infected (not colonized) should be suctioned using sterile technique until the infection is resolved. Caregivers who are infected with viral, bacterial, or fungal microorganisms should suction using principles of surgical asepsis. Clients living in nonhygienic (nonclean) conditions should be suctioned using sterile technique whenever possible, in hopes of preventing infection. All caregivers should use standard precautions when suctioning.

Caring for a tracheostomy (also called a trach) at home begins in the hospital with teaching and return demonstration. The client usually learns better when instruction on less invasive techniques such as tracheal stoma care precedes more invasive techniques such as inner cannula care and suctioning. The nurse continually develops, implements, and evaluates the teaching plan based on client performance. Some clients and their families learn quickly, whereas others do not. Therefore teaching should begin as soon as it is feasible. It is imperative that clients and their families have the ability to suction several times before discharge to develop confidence with skill performance; otherwise, arrangements to provide 24-hour care are necessary before discharge.

DELEGATION CONSIDERATIONS
The skill of teaching home tracheostomy (or trach) care and suctioning should not be delegated to assistive personnel.

EQUIPMENT
❏ Suction machine with connecting tube (Figure 42-4)
❏ Clean or sterile gloves
❏ 3 small basins
❏ Hydrogen peroxide, water (sterile water or boiled water preferred over tap water)
❏ Normal saline
❏ Clean 4 × 4 gauze pads (nonshredding)
❏ Appropriate size of sterile or clean and disinfected suction catheter (diameter should be no greater than half the diameter of the trach tube; e.g., if the trach tube is 8 mm, then the suction catheter should be no larger than a size 16 Fr)
❏ Tracheostomy care kit or clean 4 × 4 gauze pads (nonshredding)
❏ Small nylon bottle brush or pipe cleaners or disposable inner cannula
❏ Cotton-tipped applicators
❏ Tracheostomy ties (twill ⅜-inch preferably)
❏ Mirror

❏ Wet washcloth or paper towel (optional)
❏ Dry cloth, towel, or paper towel (optional)
❏ Protective eyewear (optional)
❏ Trash bag (plastic, nonleaking preferred)
❏ Disposable apron (optional)
❏ Bag-valve-mask (BVM) with oxygen supply (optional)

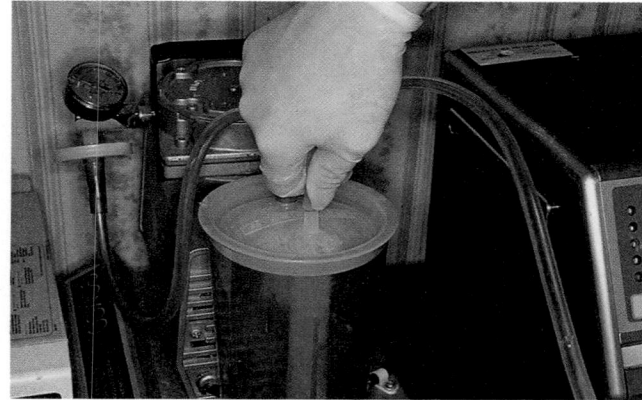

FIGURE **42-4** Suction machine.

STEP	RATIONALE

ASSESSMENT

1. Assess client's ability to properly perform tracheostomy care and suctioning, including level of consciousness, ability to attend and problem solve, and fine motor function.

Physical and cognitive impairment may necessitate instructing family member or significant other to perform tracheostomy care and suctioning. An emergency situation may also require family member or significant other to suction.

2. Assess client's and family member's knowledge of need to perform:
   a. Tracheostomy care, including presence of excess peristomal secretions, excess intratracheal secretions, soiled or damp tracheostomy dressing/ties, and diminished airway through tracheostomy tube.

   Allows client to accurately evaluate need to provide tracheostomy care. Signs and symptoms are related to presence of secretions at stoma site or within tracheostomy tube.

   b. Suctioning, including the presence of gurgling, tactile fremitus, wheezes or crackles on inspiration or expiration, restlessness, ineffective coughing, absent or diminished breath sounds, tachypnea, cyanosis, acutely decreased level of consciousness, hypertension or hypotension, tachycardia or bradycardia, acutely shallow respirations, or acute dyspnea.

   Allows client to accurately evaluate need to perform trach tube suctioning. Physical signs and symptoms result from lower airway obstruction and tissue hypoxia.

3. Observe client or family member performing complete trach tube care and suctioning.

Allows nurse to determine which specific components of skill client or family member can easily complete and which are more difficult and require instruction or reinforcement.

NURSING DIAGNOSES

- Ineffective airway clearance
- Ineffective breathing pattern
- Risk for caregiver role strain

- Risk for infection
- Deficient knowledge regarding tracheostomy care
- Impaired oral mucous membrane

Related factors are individualized based on client's condition or needs.

PLANNING

1. Expected outcomes following completion of procedure:
   - Client or family member identifies signs and symptoms indicating need for trach care and suctioning.
   - Client or family member states factors that normally influence tracheostomy airway functioning.
   - Client or family member correctly demonstrates complete trach tube care and suctioning in controlled setting.
   - Client or family member identifies signs of stoma inflammation or respiratory tract infection and when to notify physician.
   - Lower and upper airways are cleared of secretions, as evidenced by absent or diminished crackles, wheezes, tactile fremitus, and gurgles in large airways; return of breath sounds that were absent or diminished; normalization of vital signs; increased depth of respirations; absence of cyanosis; improved color; and decreased dyspnea.
   - Stoma site is clean and free of infection and transesophageal fistula; inner cannula is free of secretions.

2. Select setting in home that client or family member is most likely to use when completing trach tube care.

Client or family member is able to institute preventative means to maintain airway.
Tracheostomy can impair normal airway clearance, humidification, and gas exchange.
Provides documentation of ability to perform procedure.

Measures cognitive learning.

Suctioning is successful.

Tracheostomy care is successful.

Practicing skill in same setting where skill will be routinely performed facilitates comprehension and learning.

STEP	RATIONALE
3. Discuss and demonstrate with client or family member proper position for procedure (high-Fowler's position in front of a mirror).	Promotes understanding of comfort and safety principles and facilitates visibility.

IMPLEMENTATION

1. **Suctioning**

a. Verify health care provider's orders for suctioning.	Invasive procedure requires an order.
b. Perform hand hygiene.	Reduces transmission of microorganisms.
c. Demonstrate step-by-step preparation and completion of tracheostomy tube suctioning.	Demonstration is reliable technique for teaching psychomotor skill and enables client or family member to ask questions throughout procedure (Falvo, 2004).
d. Prepare suction equipment according to manufacturer's directions.	Preparation of equipment ensures orderly procedure.
(1) Place suction machine on level surface.	Maintains stability and integrity of suction machine.
(2) Plug into grounded outlet.	Ensures safe electrical power source for machine.
(3) Set continuous suction pressure between 80 and 150 mm Hg.	High levels of negative pressure can cause mucosal damage (Day and others, 2001).
e. Place client in high-Fowler's position.	Promotes lung expansion and allows client to view procedure.
f. Fill basin with ½ cup water or normal saline.	Supplies are used later in skill and are prepared in advance to allow for smooth performance of skill.
g. Apply gloves. *Optional:* Apply other protective equipment (e.g., eyewear, apron) if necessary.	Reduces transmission of microorganisms.

- *Critical Decision Point*

  Installation of normal saline before suctioning, once a common practice, is no longer recommended because it can cause a fall in PaO_2, an increased risk of infections, and tachycardia (Akgul and Akyolcu, 2002; Day and others, 2001).

h. Connect suction catheter to suction apparatus, and check that equipment is functioning by suctioning small amount of fluid from basin.	Ensures proper equipment function and suction levels before catheter insertion (Carroll, 2003).

- *Critical Decision Point*

  To minimize trauma to the airway, use a suction catheter with multiple side holes, and ensure the suction catheter does not exceed one half of the internal diameter of the tracheal tube (Day and others, 2001).

i. Remove oxygen delivery device if client uses one.	Provides access to trach tube for suctioning.

- *Critical Decision Point*

  If client has experienced hypoxia during previous suctioning, provide hyperoxygenation with bag-valve-mask before suctioning (Day and others, 2001; Oh and Seo, 2003).

j. Using dominant thumb and forefinger, gently but quickly insert catheter without applying suction to end of trach tube or until resistance is met (catheter touches tracheal carina) or client coughs. Then pull catheter back 1 cm.	Prevents trauma to tracheal tissues.

STEP	RATIONALE

k. Apply intermittent suction by placing and releasing thumb over catheter vent, and slowly withdraw catheter while rotating it between dominant thumb and forefinger (see illustration). Total suctioning time should be no more than 10 to 15 seconds (Oh and Seo, 2003).

Intermittent suction and rotation of catheter prevent injury to tracheal mucosal lining and hypoxia (Joanna Briggs Institute, 2000).

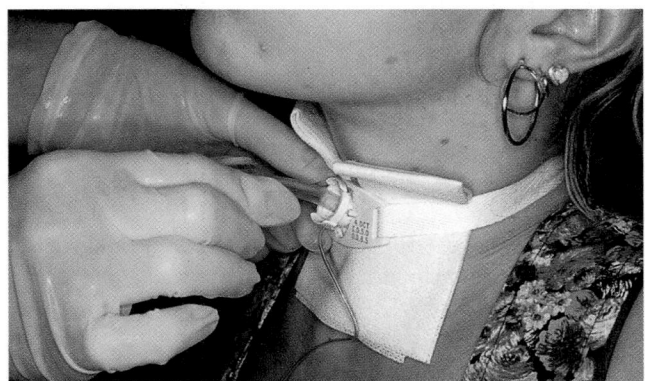

STEP **1k** Applying suction to catheter in tracheostomy tube.

l. Reapply oxygen delivery device to client's trach. Using continuous suction, rinse catheter with basin fluid until clean.

Removes secretions from catheter. Promotes patent catheter.

m. Allow client to rest for at least 1 full minute, and encourage client to take two to three deep breaths. Provide hyperoxygenation if necessary using a BVM (Taylor-Piliae, 2002).

Reduces oxygen loss and prevents hypoxia. Rest and hyperoxygenation prevent adverse effects of suctioning, including hypoxemia, hypertension, cardiac arrhythmias, and increased intracranial pressure (Joanna Briggs Institute, 2000).

n. Repeat steps i through m once or twice more if needed to clear secretions.

Repeated suctioning clears airway of excessive secretions and improves oxygenation.

o. Suction nasal and oral pharynx if needed (see Chapter 24).

Removes secretions from upper airway.

- **Critical Decision Point**
  Do not reinsert catheter into trachea after oral or nasal suction.

p. Rinse catheter by using continuous suction with basin fluid.

Removes secretions from catheter, reducing transmission of microorganisms and maintaining patency of catheter.

q. At conclusion of procedure have client take two to three deep breaths.

Reduces oxygen loss and prevents hypoxia.

r. Disconnect suction catheter; coil and discard catheter in appropriate receptacle. If catheter is to be cleaned and disinfected, set aside. Remove soiled gloves, and perform hand hygiene.

Prevents transmission of microorganisms.

2. Trach Care

a. Place impervious trash bag near work site, and create a clean field for equipment; place three basins on the field.

Ensures maintenance of standard precautions.

b. Perform hand hygiene. Apply clean gloves.

STEP	RATIONALE
c. Pour hydrogen peroxide in one container and water or normal saline in second container. Mix a solution of one-half hydrogen peroxide and one-half normal saline in third container. (*Optional:* Pour water or normal saline in third container.) Place 4 × 4 gauze pads and cotton-tipped applicators in third container. (*Optional:* May use washcloth or paper towels if other supplies are not available. Do not use tissues.)	Prepares work area and supplies for cleansing of trach tube.
d. Remove oxygen delivery device (e.g., trach mask) and old tracheostomy dressing. Discard dressing using standard precautions.	Reduces transmission of microorganisms.
e. Remove and discard contaminated gloves.	Reduces transmission of microorganisms.
f. Apply clean gloves.	
g. *For nondisposable inner cannula:*	
(1) While touching only the outer part of the tube, unlock and remove inner cannula; place in basin with hydrogen peroxide to soak.	Loosens secretions and encrustations adhered to inner cannula.
(2) Place oxygen delivery device near outer cannula of trach tube.	Maintains oxygen supply to client.
(3) Using nylon brush or pipe cleaners, gently scrub inner cannula.	Removes crusted secretions that adhere to tube.
(4) Holding inner cannula over basin, quickly and thoroughly rinse with normal saline or water for at least 15 seconds; shake off excess solution.	Removes secretions and hydrogen peroxide from inner cannula. Remaining solutions could cause airway or stoma irritation.
(5) Examine patency of cannula; if not clean, repeat cleansing process. Replace inner cannula in position and lock.	Ensures patent airway.
h. For disposable inner cannula:	
(1) Remove new cannula from manufacturer's packaging.	Prepares inner cannula for use.
(2) While touching only the outer aspect of the soiled inner cannula tube on the client, follow manufacturer's directions to remove the inner cannula, and dispose of cannula in trash bag.	Removes old inner cannula. Proper disposal of contaminated products prevents transmission of microorganisms.
(3) Following manufacturer's directions, quickly insert new inner cannula. Only touch outer aspect of new inner cannula.	Maintains sterility of inner aspect of new inner cannula.
i. Using presoaked 4 × 4 gauze sponges and damp applicators, wash skin gently around stoma, under trach ties and flanges, extending 5 to 10 cm (2 to 4 inches) in all directions from stoma (see illustration).	Removes secretions that predispose client to localized infection.

• **Critical Decision Point**

If hydrogen peroxide is used to clean stoma, rinse with cotton-tipped applicators and 4 × 4 gauze sponges soaked in water or saline.

j. Dry exposed outer cannula and skin with dry 4 × 4 gauze or cloth or paper towel.	Prevents moist environment for organism growth.
k. Change ties (see Chapter 24).	

STEP	RATIONALE

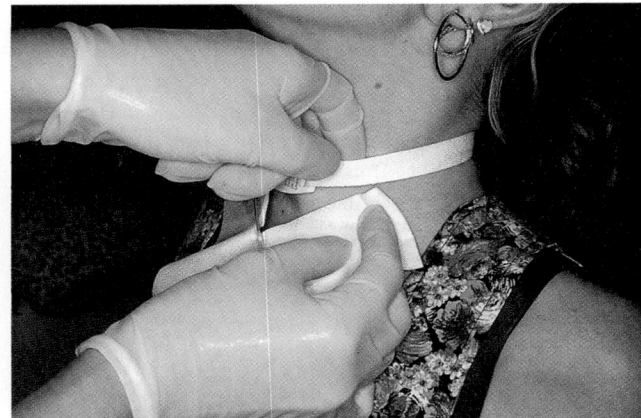

STEP **2i** Cleansing area around tracheal stoma.

STEP **2l** Applying clean tracheostomy dressing.

- ### *Critical Decision Point*
  Client is at risk for trach tube coming out as ties are changed. Two trach tubes, one the same size as the client's and one a size smaller, should be kept at the client's bedside so a new trach can be inserted if the tube comes out (Woodrow, 2002).

   l. Apply fresh trach dressing if ordered (see illustration).

Protects skin around stoma from pressure breakdown and collects secretions.

   m. Clean reusable supplies in warm soapy water. Rinse thoroughly, and dry between two layers of clean paper towels. Store supplies in loosely closed clear plastic bag.

Prevents transmission of microorganisms. Air must circulate, or humidity in bag can promote microorganism growth.

   n. Remove and discard gloves. Perform hand hygiene.

Reduces transmission of microorganisms.

   o. Reusable supplies should be disinfected at least weekly. To disinfect supplies use one of the methods described below:

Removes organisms and reduces risk for infection.

   (1) *Method 1:* Boil reusable (boilable) supplies for 15 minutes. Allow to cool and dry.

   (2) *Method 2:* Soak reusable supplies in equal parts of vinegar and water for 30 minutes. Remove, rinse thoroughly, and dry.

   (3) *Method 3:* Soak reusable supplies in prepared solutions of quaternary ammonium chloride compounds according to manufacturer's instructions. Rinse and dry.

3. Have client or family member perform each step with guidance from nurse.

Adult learners learn psychomotor skills best by active participation, and nurse can correct any errors in technique as they occur and discuss their implications (Falvo, 2004).

STEP	RATIONALE

4. Discuss signs and symptoms of:
   a. Stomal infection (redness, tenderness, drainage).
   b. Respiratory tract infection (fever, increased sputum, change in color of sputum, foul sputum odor, increased cough, chills, night sweats).
   c. Transesophageal fistula (air leaking through stoma, nose, or mouth with cuff properly inflated; more air needed to inflate cuff; aspiration of food or liquid during suctioning; excessive belching; coughing when swallowing) (Schreiber, 2001).

Client and caregiver must be able to recognize onset of complications associated with long-term tracheostomy use early so that medical treatment can begin, reducing risk of more serious negative outcomes. Emphasize importance of notifying physician when signs and symptoms of complications occur.

EVALUATION

1. Ask client to state all signs of stomal or respiratory tract complications.

   Prompt identification of symptoms results in early treatment and decreases risk of complications that may lead to hospital readmission.

2. Observe client or family member demonstrating technique for trach tube care and suctioning.

   Feedback through independent demonstration of psychomotor skill is reliable method to evaluate learning.

Recording and Reporting

- Record client instruction and accuracy of care delivered by client or family member.
- Develop a system of home care recording to be used by client or caregiver to provide information that compliance is achieved or maintained.

Unexpected Outcomes	Related Interventions
1. Stoma site is reddened or hard, with or without drainage.	• Evaluate cleaning regimen for continued use of clean technique. • Increase tracheostomy care frequency.
2. Copious colored secretions are present around stoma or when client is suctioned.	• Use sterile technique for suctioning and tracheostomy care. • Evaluate for adequate humidity (use room humidifier or tracheostomy collar humidity, if needed) (see Chapter 22). • Notify health care provider.
3. Bloody secretions are suctioned.	• Evaluate suctioning technique, suctioning frequency, and size of catheter used. • Assess for signs of infection. • Notify health care provider.
4. No secretions are suctioned.	• Evaluate fluid status, need for increased humidity. • Determine if appropriate size of suction catheter is used. • Reassess suction frequency.
5. Trach tube comes out.	• Replace trach tube to maintain an airway. • Activate emergency medical service system if needed.
6. Skin breakdown is present at stoma site.	• Assess site for pressure areas or site infection. • Remove pressure source.

Teaching Considerations

- Client may need mirror to visualize stomal area.
- Loss of upper airway functions with tracheostomy can predispose client to greater secretions.
- Ideally, home care nurse should participate in discharge teaching in hospital.

Pediatric Considerations

- Many physicians order child to receive 10% to 15% higher oxygen before tracheostomy tube changes.
- Parents should be encouraged to begin assisting with trach care as soon as child is stable in the hospital. The more time they have to practice these skills, the more comfortable they become in caring for the child at home.
- An additional adult should travel in the car with the child to assist if problems arise during drive home.
- The airways of infants and young children have smaller diameters. Awareness of level of parent's anxiety surrounding performance of this skill will require frequent support and assistance by the home care nurse until independence and comfort level are achieved.
- Suction pressure for preterm infants should range from 40 to 60 mm Hg, whereas suction pressure for infants and children should range from 60 to 100 mm Hg (Hockenberry and others, 2003).
- To prevent hypoxia, the child should be hyperoxygenated before and after suctioning with a BVM, and suctioning should not last more than 5 seconds. Allow the child to rest for at least 60 seconds between suctioning passes, and do not suction more than 3 times (Hockenberry and others, 2003).
- Families and significant others should be taught infant or child cardiopulmonary resuscitation, including use of bag-valve-mask or mouth-to-trach technique. They should also notify the local EMS of the child's condition and the presence of a trach, and provide EMS with a list of equipment in the home (Hockenberry and others, 2003).
- Importance of humidity should be stressed to keep secretions thin and decrease the likelihood of mucous plugging.
- Children with tracheostomies should be encouraged to socialize and play with other children who are close to their own age (Hockenberry and others, 2003).

Gerontological Considerations

- Manual dexterity may be limited due to arthritic changes of upper extremities.
- Skin integrity may be compromised and at risk for breakdown from secretions and/or tape.
- Older adults have lost some properties of elastic recoil and may have greater difficulty in clearing airway secretions through cough. As a result, they require more suctioning and airway care and have increased risk of infection (Ebersole and others, 2004).
- Diminished visual acuity may impair ability to detect early signs of infection and stomal changes.

- Anxiety accompanies decreased ability to breathe and may cause the older adult to become too nervous to perform suctioning independently.

Home Care Considerations

- Caregiver role strain is commonly found in caregivers of clients with tracheostomies. Rossi Ferrario and others (2001) found that younger caregivers, those caring for clients receiving ventilation at night, caregivers of clients who have had a tracheostomy for less than a year, and female caregivers tended to perceive high levels of strain that persisted over time. Home care nurses must assess the needs of the caregiver and provide interventions to relieve perceived caregiver role strain.
- Procedure must be performed at least daily in home setting. When tracheal secretions are copious, client or family member must perform procedure more frequently (such as every 4 hours).
- Clients should have two trach tubes available by their beds at all times in the home setting. One tube should be the same size as the tube the client currently has, and the other should be one size smaller. Ensure that appropriate-size tubes are available, especially if trach tube size is changed for any reason (Woodrow, 2002).
- Clients may benefit from proper room humidification. Be sure humidifier is clean and in optimal operating condition.
- Water in humidifier may grow *Pseudomonas,* and container must be cleaned daily.
- Trach tubes should be changed every 3 to 4 weeks in adults and every 1 to 2 weeks in children (Hockenberry and others, 2003; Schreiber, 2001). Two people are required to change the trach. Box 42-4 provides guidelines for changing a trach tube at home.

BOX 42-4 Procedural Guideline
Changing tracheostomy at home

EQUIPMENT

Clean gloves, suction catheter, suction machine, bag-valve-mask, face mask, new sterile tracheostomy tube

1. Client should be allowed nothing by mouth (NPO) or have tube feedings held for at least 1 hour before procedure.
2. Explain procedure to client before trach is changed to alleviate anxiety.
3. Perform hand hygiene, and put on clean gloves.
4. Suction trach, and have bag-valve-mask and face mask available.
5. Loosen trach ties, and deflate trach cuff (if trach has one).
6. One person pulls the old trach out with gentle, steady pressure in the same direction as an inner cannula would be removed.
7. Other person verifies patency and integrity of new cuff, puts on sterile gloves if available, and pushes new trach into tracheostomy site using gentle force, while pushing back and then down.
8. Attach new trach ties, inflate cuff, and place dressing around stoma if necessary.

Data from Schreiber D: Trach care at home: a how-to guide, *RN* 64(7):43, 2001.

SKILL 42-6 Teaching Clients Self-Medication Administration

Researchers estimate that over half of clients who are prescribed drug regimens at home fail to take medications correctly (Haynes and others, 2002). Consequently, a large portion of admissions to hospitals and nursing homes, medical malpractice suits, therapeutic failures, and medical emergencies result from inaccurate medication use (Schommer and others, 2002). Difficulty in taking prescribed medications regularly exists for several reasons: clients stop taking medications once symptoms subside, regimens involving multiple drugs at a variety of times are confusing, the consequences of not taking medications are poorly understood, prescriptions are costly, and many clients fear addiction. A large portion of

clients who do not comply are older adults, who frequently suffer psychomotor, cognitive, sensory, and mobility problems and who have poor social support, interfering with the ability to prepare and take medications correctly (Maddigan and others, 2003; McGraw and Drennan, 2001). Medication education has been associated with enhanced client outcomes (Chang and others, 2002; Johansson and others, 2002; Saounatsou and others, 2001). Educating clients about their medications could save 120,000 lives and $45.6 billion per year in the United States alone (Schommer and others, 2002).

The following skill is actually an outline to help prepare clients for following drug regimens in the home.

DELEGATION CONSIDERATIONS
The skill of teaching clients self-medication administration cannot be delegated to assistive personnel. However, assistive personnel, such as home care aides, are often in a situation to be able to see how clients are self-administering medications. Assistive personnel should be instructed to communicate problems clients are having with medication administration to the nurse.

EQUIPMENT
- ❑ Medication
- ❑ Liquid to take with medication
- ❑ Medication administration record, computer printout, or other up-to-date list of current medications from prescriber
- ❑ Container for daily or weekly preparation
- ❑ Measuring devices as needed (e.g., medicine cup, teaspoon)
- ❑ Teaching tools (e.g., charts, written instructions, color codes)

STEP	RATIONALE

■ ASSESSMENT

1. Assess client's cognitive, sensory, and motor function; level of consciousness, sight, hearing, touch, literacy, swallowing ability, mobility, activity tolerance, social support, and willingness to cooperate.

   Cognitive, sensory, and motor deficits may influence client's ability to take or prepare prescribed medication correctly and to participate in instruction (Maddigan and others, 2003).

2. Assess resources client has to obtain medications when needed: finances, social support, transportation.

   Lack of resources is a major factor that will negatively affect compliance with self-medication regimen (McGraw and Drennan, 2001).

3. Assess client's learning readiness and ability to attend; consider presence of pain, fatigue, client interest in instruction.

   Presence of significant illness, frailty, or confusion will affect teaching plan. Reliance on caregiver for learning and implementation (if available) may be necessary on a short- or long-term basis.

4. Assess client's knowledge regarding medication therapy: names of drugs, how to administer, purpose or action, daily doses and times to be taken, side effects to expect, and what to do if problems occur.

   Reveals client's level of understanding and need for instruction.

5. Assess family member's knowledge of medication therapy: why client takes medication, daily doses, side effects, and what to do if problems arise.

   Family member or support person is important resource to help client comply with or adhere to medication therapy.

6. Assess client's belief in need for drug therapy. Consider cultural values, religious beliefs, personal experiences with medications, and significant others' values about drugs.

   Many factors influence client's willingness to follow drug regimen.

STEP	RATIONALE
7. Check client's prescribed and over-the-counter (OTC) medications, including use of herbal supplements: Has more than one physician prescribed medications? Are medications obviously inappropriate? Are labels clearly marked? Are time schedules confusing? Do different drugs look alike? Does client store medications together or out of original containers? Are expiration dates on bottles still current?	Assists nurse in determining sources of confusion affecting client's compliance. Noncompliance with medication therapy (especially in older adults) may be aggravated by multiple chronic conditions, which are often treated with multiple medications sometimes prescribed by more than one physician (Lueckenotte, 2000). Compliance is more difficult when medication regimens are complex (Haynes and others, 2002).
8. Assess client's understanding of effects and interactions between prescribed medications and with ingestion of certain foods, over-the-counter drugs, and herbal supplements.	Medication interactions, including those with over-the-counter drugs, herbals, and certain foods, can seriously affect effectiveness and/or create negative side effects.

NURSING DIAGNOSES

- Anxiety
- Ineffective health maintenance
- Health-seeking behaviors (self medication)
- Deficient knowledge regarding medication administration

- Readiness for enhanced knowledge
- Ineffective individual or family therapeutic regimen management

Related factors are individualized based on client's condition or needs.

PLANNING

1. Expected outcomes following completion of procedure:	
• Client is able to state purpose of each medication and why it is beneficial.	Demonstrates cognitive learning.
• Client identifies common adverse effects and relief measures.	Enhances compliance with medication therapy (Savini and others, 2003).
• Client is able to state when to notify physician about medication problems.	Empowers client to participate in care.
• Client reads each label and explains when each drug should be taken.	Prevents medication administration errors.
• Client demonstrates self-administration of medication by prescribed route (see illustrations).	Demonstrates skill achieved.

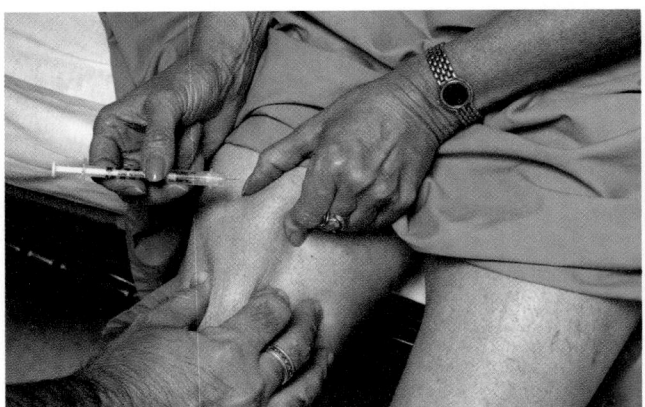 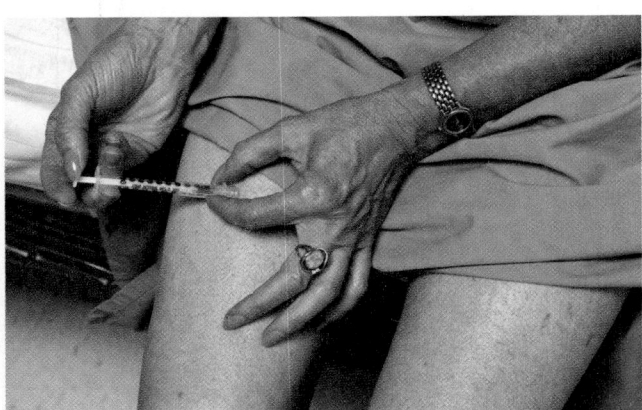

A   **B**

STEP **1 A, B,** Client demonstrating self-injection technique.

STEP	RATIONALE

2. Prepare environment for teaching session:
   a. Select room that is well lit.
   b. Provide comfortable seating.
   c. Be sure client is close and can see nurse clearly.
   d. Control sources of noise and distractions.

Room environment should be designed to minimize existing sensory alterations. Comfortable environment free of distractions promotes client's attention.

3. Prepare teaching materials:
   a. Materials should be printed in large bold letters (size 14 point or larger).
   b. Illustrations of safety guidelines should be provided.
   c. Written schedules or individualized instruction sheets are helpful.

Teaching materials should be designed to meet client's learning needs and client's capacity to learn.

4. Clients should wear glasses or hearing aids if needed during teaching session.

Use of glasses or hearing aids increases client's sensory perception and increases likelihood of attending to teaching session and understanding content.

5. Consult with prescriber to review medications client is receiving and to simplify regimen if possible.

Review of medications can help minimize risk of drug interactions from multiple medications and ensures accuracy of medication regimen. Simplification of regimen can improve compliance, particularly related to daily frequency of prescribed doses (Savini and others, 2003).

6. Arrange teaching time so that family members may participate (see illustration).

Family can serve as positive resource to client and often reinforce information provided.

IMPLEMENTATION

1. Present information clearly and concisely:
   a. Face learner; be sure nurse's face is illuminated.

Improves client's ability to attend and understand.

Allows nurse to see client's nonverbal responses to education. Client with hearing loss or visual problem will be able to see nurse's expressions, read written information, and hear voice more clearly.

   b. Use short sentences, and speak in slow, low-pitched voice.

Enhances understanding of information.

   c. Provide descriptions in understandable terms.

Prevents confusion of terminology. Clients learn more quickly when information is provided at the level of the learner.

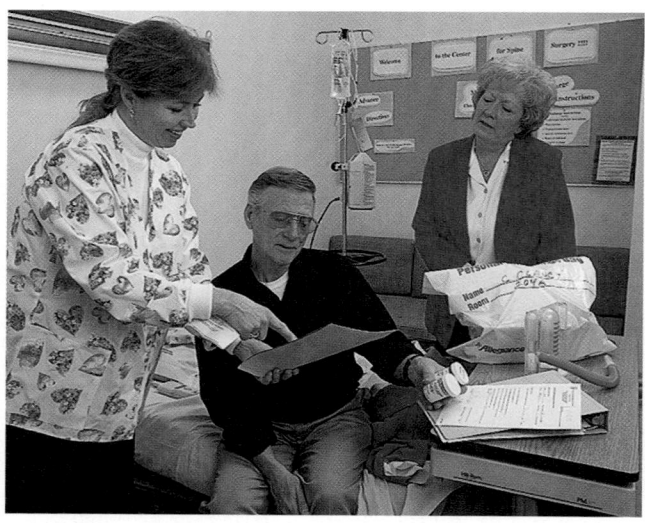

STEP 6 Family participating in self-medication teaching program.

STEP	RATIONALE

2. Provide frequent pauses so that client can ask questions and express understanding of content.

3. Instruct client on the following content: purpose of drugs and their positive effects, how drug works and why it helps, dosage schedules and rationale, common side effects, what to do to relieve side effects, what to do if dose is missed, when to call with problems, who to call with problems, drug safety guidelines, and implications when medications are not taken.

Increases client's participation in learning process. Ongoing feedback ensures nurse that client is acquiring information. Provides client with sufficient information to understand and take medications safely at home.

4. Instruct client on appropriate route of medication delivery, including oral, subcutaneous, intramuscular, topical, etc.

Client needs to be proficient in all routes of medication administration. Adverse effects may occur if medications are administered incorrectly.

5. Provide frequent, short teaching sessions. Learning about multiple medication regimens will probably require several teaching sessions. Leave instruction aids in the home for client to review if possible.

Client needs to learn extensive amount of information. Improves client's attention and retention of information discussed. Reference to charts, written information, and other teaching tools as a resource will assist client in learning.

- **Critical Decision Point**
Review previously taught information, and ask client to recall and relay information before proceeding to new teaching area.

6. Provide teaching about prescribed medications, over-the-counter medications, and herbal supplements that are used on a prn basis.

Consideration of knowledge and accessibility of prn medications must be given, because prn drugs are not included in routine, prepared medication delivery systems (i.e., daily or weekly pillbox systems).

7. Provide client with special charts, diagrams, learning aids, written information, and Internet/intranet resources (see illustration).

Clear written information, charts, and other resources, such as the Internet/intranet enhance client learning and allow for reinforcement of information (Institute of Safe Medical Practice [ISMP], 2003; Sorrentino and others, 2002).

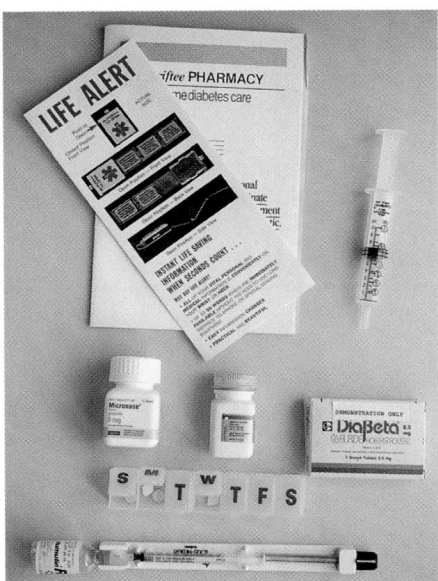

STEP 7 Examples of aids for client self-medication administration.

STEP	RATIONALE
8. Offer assistance as client practices preparing medication (e.g., "Let's prepare the medications you will take with your meals; or prepare the medicines you take first in the morning").	Nurse can observe client's ability to read labels correctly and prepare all medications for prescribed times.
9. Have pharmacy provide clear, large-print labels for medication bottles and medication teaching handouts if appropriate.	Improves client's ability to read and follow directions.
10. Have pharmacy provide containers that client can open independently if manual dexterity is limited.	Most pharmacies dispense pills in "childproof" containers, which the client with limited mobility of fingers/hands may find difficult to manipulate or open.

- **Critical Decision Point**

  If there are pets or small children in home or children who frequently visit home, help client establish a "safe place" for medication, to reduce risk of accidental ingestion by pets or children.

11. Facilitate arrangements for pharmacy to receive written prescriptions in a timely fashion if required for dispensing. Arrange for pharmacy to deliver medications to home if client is unable to reach pharmacy on own.	Availability of drugs influences compliance.

EVALUATION

1. Ask client and family member to explain information about each drug: purpose; actions; routes; timing of medications and maximum frequency of use of either prescribed or over-the-counter drug; side effects and interactions; and foods, herbals, or over-the-counter drugs to avoid.	Feedback measures client's cognitive learning and helps to ensure compliance with medication therapy.
2. Identify client's problem-solving initiatives if unsure of action to be taken (e.g., call health care provider, refer to printed information for resources).	Developing techniques to gain information and solve problems will assist in client compliance and reduce potential problems from medication regimen (Litton and others, 2002).
3. Have client or family member prepare doses for all prescribed medications.	Indicates understanding of medication dosages and schedules.
4. Ask client to verbalize any remaining questions regarding medication management.	Offers opportunity for clarification and minimizes any remaining confusion or misunderstanding.

Recording and Reporting

- Document instruction provided and learning outcomes achieved by client in home care record.
- Develop system of recording to be used by client or family member to provide information that compliance is achieved or maintained.
- Develop a client recording mechanism of dosage schedules and self-monitoring of regimen.

Unexpected Outcomes	Related Interventions
1. Client makes errors in preparing medications or is unable to recall and/or explain information discussed in teaching sessions.	• Provide additional instruction and/or teaching materials for consultation when information is forgotten or unclear. • Ensure written instructions are at reader's level of understanding. Some commercially prepared booklets may contain instructions that are too complex or contain medical jargon that is difficult to understand. • Consider use of pictures, color coding, diagrams, and tape-recorded instructions for the reading or sight impaired. • Periodically observe client demonstrate medication administration.
2. Self-medication plan is not possible due to client's self-care deficits. This is very commonly when changes in mentation exist.	• Develop alternative plan, which may rely on others, to provide safe administration of home medication regimen.
3. Client refuses to take medications as prescribed.	• Explore and identify reasons for noncompliance, which may include the following: cost, side effects, complexity of regimen, problems with swallowing, and cultural preferences. • See Box 42-5.

BOX 42-5   Evidence-Based Nursing Interventions to Enhance Compliance With Medication Therapy

- Be available for the client, and make frequent contacts, especially when a new therapy is initiated or changes are made (Litton and others, 2002).
- Collaborate with other disciplines when providing information (Norris and others, 2001).
- Involve the client in decisions made regarding treatment decisions (Savini and others, 2003).
- Carefully assess and provide information the client perceives as being important (Johansson and others, 2002).
- Instruct clients about complications that may happen if medications are not taken correctly or if they are not taken at all (Saounatsou and others, 2001).

- Provide interdisciplinary medication education in settings that are convenient for the client and enhance learning (Schommer and others, 2002).
- Identify clients who are at risk for noncompliance, and intervene early and frequently (Hudson and others, 2004).
- Strengthen nurse-client relationships by developing trust, partnership, and mutual respect (Rycroft-Malone and others, 2000).

Teaching Considerations

- See Chapter 41 for guidelines for medication safety.
- If it is difficult to plan a separate teaching session, instruct client while administering medications.
- Repetition, reinforcement, and positive feedback must be elements of teaching plan (Falvo, 2004).
- Assessment of an appropriate amount of information taught at each session is critical so as not to overwhelm client with task at hand (Falvo, 2004).
- Examples of learning aids include homemade calendars for each week that contain plastic bags containing medications to take at specific times, egg cartons divided into color-coded sections with medications for the day, clock faces for clients who cannot read or see clearly, color coding for drug types (e.g., blue for sedative, red for pain pill), and pillboxes that identify days of the week and times of day.

Pediatric Considerations

- All medications must be kept safely out of reach of children.
- Caregivers should not compare medications to treats, even artificially sweetened varieties, because this could add to risk of child overdosing by mistaking medicine for candy.
- All medications in homes with small children must be placed in safe, secure, out-of-reach location.
- Successful medication teaching should involve the child's parents or other caregivers and the child and siblings

whenever possible. Nurses who provide effective medication teaching to children take the child's developmental and cognitive abilities into consideration when planning teaching sessions (Hockenberry and others, 2003).

- Parents should supervise initial attempts as older children begin taking responsibility for their own treatment.

Gerontological Considerations

- Older adults commonly have reduced visual and hearing acuity and difficulty understanding language because high-frequency tones are less perceptible.
- Problems with dexterity may make it difficult for the older adult to open containers and handle, prepare, and administer medications.
- Capacity for learning new information remains as people age (in the absence of dementia); however, additional time is needed to accomplish learning. Allow adequate time and number of teaching sessions to support successful learning. Effective teaching strategies for older adults may include memory aids, information written in large letters (14 point is recommended), involvement of family member or caregiver, follow-up teaching sessions either over the telephone or in person, and computer-assisted teaching guides (Ebersole and others, 2004).

- Cognition problems coupled with complexity of medication regimens have a negative effect on safe self-medication in older adults. Efforts should be made to decrease the complexity of medication regimens in clients with cognitive deficits whenever possible to promote safe self-medication practices (Maddigan and others, 2003).
- Older adults often have to take medications in multiple routes (e.g., oral, inhaled, injections). Problems with physical dexterity, eyesight, cognitive skills, and memory can negatively affect adherence to medication schedules. Establishing a therapeutic nurse-client relationship in helping clients overcome these barriers to adherence is essential (McGraw and Drennan, 2001).

Home Care Considerations

- Discuss proper storage of medications (see Chapter 41).
- If client or family member cannot reliably fill weekly pillbox, nurse should make arrangements with pharmacy to deliver medications weekly.

SKILL 42-7 Enteral Nutrition in the Home

Enteral nutrition therapy in the home setting can be accomplished if several criteria are used to determine client eligibility. These criteria include the client's ability to tolerate 70% of feeding intake without complications, the client's medical stability, the client's capability of self-administering feedings and/or having a responsible and capable caregiver, and the client or caregiver having sufficient time in a controlled environment to learn the skill. The majority of clients requiring home enteral nutrition are older adults, people with disorders of the central nervous system, and people with dysphagia (Russell, 2002; Silver and others, 2004). Clients benefit from being able to see tube feeding equipment and devices when learning how to administer home enteral nutrition. Hands-on experience and client involvement with decision making about home enteral nutrition is recommended (Liley and Manthorpe, 2003).

This procedure in the home setting follows the guidelines and skills described in Chapter 30. This skill focuses on the teaching of the client or caregiver in the home. The nurse may be responsible in this setting for reinsertion of nasogastric and gastrostomy feeding tubes, and the physician may be responsible for reinsertion of jejunostomy tubes. See Skills 30-1 to 30-5 for insertion and replacement procedures.

DELEGATION CONSIDERATIONS

For this skill, feeding tube insertion or medication administration cannot be delegated to assistive personnel. However, administration of enteral tube feeding via syringe is a procedure that may be delegated to assistive personnel (verify agency policy). The nurse should verify feeding tube placement and assess for residual volume before feeding. The nurse should also instruct assistive personnel to report difficulty with feeding, coughing, gagging, respiratory distress, discomfort, or vomiting.

EQUIPMENT

See Skill 30-1 for equipment for insertion, Skills 30-1 and 30-2 for placement, and Skills 30-4 and 30-5 for administration and equipment.

❑ Documentation records (daily weights, intake and output [I&O], temperature, feeding residuals)

STEP	**RATIONALE**

ASSESSMENT

1. Assess client's health status, including presence of discomfort and fatigue and ability to successfully manage enteral feedings in the home.

2. Assess client's or caregiver's physical, emotional, financial, and community resources.

3. Assess environmental conditions of home (sanitation, storage of equipment, work area, supplies, and power source).

4. Assess client's and caregiver's understanding of purpose of enteral feedings and positive expected outcomes.

5. Assess client's and caregiver's understanding of storage and management of equipment and supplies and where and how to obtain supplies.

6. Assess client's and caregiver's ability to manipulate feeding equipment.

Increases successful home management with fewer complications.

Increases ability for self-care and home management.

Ensures safe environment and decreases risks of infection and complications.

Understanding rationale of treatment is critical to enhancing participation and cooperation in care.

Ensures safe home management and decreases risk of complications.

May require caregiver to administer all enteral feedings. Allows nurse to identify areas for teaching and support.

NURSING DIAGNOSES

- Anxiety
- Risk for aspiration
- Diarrhea
- Ineffective health maintenance
- Deficient knowledge regarding administration of enteral feedings

- Imbalanced nutrition: less than body requirements
- Feeding self-care deficit
- Readiness for enhanced therapeutic regimen management

Related factors are individualized based on client's condition or needs.

PLANNING

1. Expected outcomes following completion of procedure:
   - Client and caregiver will verbalize the purpose of enteral feedings and enhanced nutritional health.
   - Client and caregiver will demonstrate proper use of equipment and handling of formulas.
   - Client and caregiver will demonstrate accurate administration of enteral feedings and medications.
   - Client and caregiver will verbalize understanding of signs and symptoms and management of complications of feeding.

Provides measurable criteria to determine level of cognitive understanding.

Provides demonstration of skills needed to manage home enteral nutrition.

Provides demonstration of skills needed to administer home enteral nutrition.

Confirms client and caregiver can administer feeding safely.

IMPLEMENTATION

1. Perform hand hygiene.
2. Discuss with client and caregiver purpose of enteral feeding and enhanced nutritional health.
3. Assist client or caregiver in determining a feeding schedule that will maintain nutritional requirements and that will fit within the client's or family's schedule.

Reduces transmission of microorganisms.

Reinforces importance of regular feedings.

Promotes compliance with enteral nutrition therapy.

- ### *Critical Decision Point*
  Explain that feeding schedules may be changed to fit daily routines. However, changes the client or caregiver makes in feedings must be communicated to home care nurse or health care provider (Liley and Manthorpe, 2003).

STEP	RATIONALE
4. Demonstrate how to identify placement of feeding tube: aspiration of gastric fluid, checking pH of gastric fluid, and acceptable pH range (see Skill 30-2).	Nasally placed tubes can be inadvertently placed in respiratory system and can migrate to esophagus or into respiratory tract. Nurse may need to check pH periodically. Aspirated secretions with low pH are strong indicator of gastric placement. However, high pH cannot differentiate between aspirated secretions obtained from respiratory and intestinal tube placements (Metheny and Titler, 2001).

- *Critical Decision Point*
  Instruct that nothing (e.g., feedings, flushes, or medications) should be administered if there is any doubt as to placement of enteral feeding tube.

STEP	RATIONALE
5. Observe client and family in determining placement of nasally placed tube.	Identifies if there are areas for further teaching.
6. Observe client or caregiver aspirate gastric contents. Instruct to return gastric contents after aspiration.	Aspirates of ≥200 ml indicate need to initiate interventions such as changing from intermittent to continuous feedings, evaluating possibility of decreasing opioid analgesics and narcotics, and starting a medication that enhances gastric motility (e.g., metoclopramide) to reduce aspiration risk (Metheny and others, 2004).

- *Critical Decision Point*
  If gastric aspirates are ≥200 ml, instruct client or caregiver to return gastric contents and delay tube feeding for 1 hour. If aspirates remain ≥200 ml after an hour, instruct client or caregiver to contact home care nurse or health care provider.

STEP	RATIONALE
7. Discuss use of medical asepsis in setting up and changing administration sets, mixing formulas (do not add formula to hanging bag), refrigeration of unused formula, limiting amount of formula "hung" at one time to amount that can be infused in a 4- to 6-hour period (less time in warmer weather), and maintenance and care of bag.	Medical aseptic technique minimizes risk of microorganism contamination. Refrigeration and limiting "hang" time reduces microorganism proliferation. Changing administration sets every 24 hours reduces microorganism growth.

- *Critical Decision Point*
  Bott and others (2001) found that closed enteral feeding systems did not become contaminated despite manipulation errors that occurred during set up and reuse of the system 2 to 3 times in a 24-hour period. Open systems were associated with a significant risk of contamination. Therefore the client should use closed systems whenever possible to reduce the risk of exposure to microorganisms.

STEP	RATIONALE
8. Instruct client or caregiver that the client should sit up in a chair or have the head of the bed elevated at least 30 to 45 degrees while receiving feedings or medications or when tube is flushed. If this is not possible, the client may be placed in reverse Trendelenburg's position.	Decreases risk of aspiration (Metheny and others, 2004). Aspiration is indicated by increased coughing, difficulty in breathing, or vomiting.

STEP	RATIONALE
9. Observe client or caregiver mixing, administering, and storing formulas, changing administration sets, and cleaning bags. Discuss flushing of tube after administration of feedings or medications (see illustration).	Identifies competence and need for further teaching. Regular flushing of tube prevents clogging.
10. Observe client or caregiver administering medications and flushing tube (see Chapter 20).	Ensures medications are given correctly.

- *Critical Decision Point*
  Verify that medications to be administered do not include any sublingual, enteric-coated, or sustained-release medications.

STEP	RATIONALE
11. Discuss and observe use of infusion pump if client is receiving continuous feeding (see illustration and Chapter 30).	Use of tube feeding infusion pumps is complex and requires reinforcement.
12. Discuss measures to stabilize feeding tube in clients with abdominal tubes and to protect skin integrity.	Prevents tube from dislodging and prevents skin breakdown.
13. Discuss whom to contact for equipment and supplies or in case of equipment failure.	Ensures family can respond in an emergency.
14. Discuss emergency plan and actions to take for signs and symptoms of aspiration such as elevating the head of the bed and calling health care provider.	Ensures understanding of management of equipment, supplies, emergency plan, and collaboration.
15. Discuss whom to contact and when for signs of diarrhea, constipation, or weight loss.	Provides support to client and family.
16. Perform hand hygiene.	Reduces transmission of microorganisms.

EVALUATION

1. Ask client and caregiver to state purpose of home enteral nutrition therapy.	Demonstrates cognitive learning.
2. Observe client and caregiver performing medical asepsis techniques, checking tube placement, aspirating residuals, administering medications and solutions, and using equipment.	Demonstrates psychomotor learning.
3. Ask client and caregiver to state measures needed to be used to prevent complications (e.g., verification of tube position before each feeding, elevation of client during feeding, stabilization and flushing of tubing).	Ensures safe home management and identification of areas for teaching.

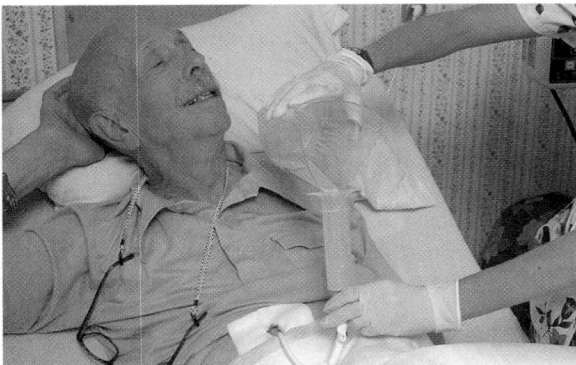

STEP **9** Administer enteral feeding to client.

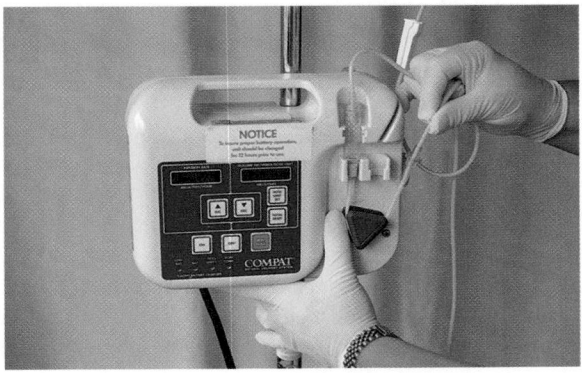

STEP **11** Family member threading feeding tubing through electric infusion pump.

STEP	RATIONALE
4. Ask client and caregiver how to care for open formula cans.	Ensures safe home management and identification of areas of teaching.
5. Ask client and caregiver about management of complications (e.g., signs of intolerance: nausea, abdominal distention, diarrhea, skin problems, and fluid deficit).	Ensures safe home management and identification of areas of teaching.

Recording and Reporting

- Record in home care record instructions given to client and caregivers and their response to them.
- Record specifics of enteral feeding plan, including type and size of tube in home, formula, and amounts to be administered in specific time frames.
- Client and caregivers need to document I&O, daily weights, amount of gastric fluid aspirated before each feeding (or every 4 hours if receiving continuous feeding), date and time of feedings, amount and type of formula, any additives, and date and time administration sets are changed.

Unexpected Outcomes	Related Interventions
1. Displacement of feeding tube occurs.	• Feeding tube must be repositioned and position verified before initiating any enteral feeding. • Instruct family to notify home care nurse whenever this happens.
2. Signs and symptoms of aspiration are present.	• Stop feeding. • Verify tube position. • Notify physician.
3. Client develops diarrhea.	• Notify physician. • May need to change strength or type of enteral feeding. • May need to administer antidiarrheal agents.
4. Skin surrounding stoma or tube insertion site (nares) breaks down, or drainage around insertion site develops.	• Reposition feeding tube at nares to avoid pressure. • Cleanse stoma area more frequently. • Apply antibiotic ointment around stoma as ordered. • Contact health care provider.

Teaching Considerations

- Teaching of enteral therapy skills begins in the hospital (Russell, 2002).
- Carrying out performance of skills without nurse in attendance is anxiety provoking. Always leave a phone number and instructions about how to reach home care nurse if needed.

Pediatric Considerations

- Parents should be encouraged to assist with feedings during a child's hospitalization. This includes tube placement for gavage feedings.
- A child's potential risk for aspiration and fluid and electrolyte imbalance is great and must be carefully monitored.
- Children who receive long-term home enteral feedings may experience developmental and growth delays.

Therefore these children require close follow-up and frequent nutritional monitoring (Puntis, 2001).

- Children who cannot sit up during or after a tube feeding should be positioned on their right side during the tube feeding and for at least 1 hour after the feeding (Hockenberry and others, 2003).
- Children with special health needs are living longer and are becoming adults. Many services for these children decrease dramatically when the child reaches 22 years of age. Nurses must carefully collaborate with interdisciplinary teams to ensure these individuals become as independent as possible (Dell'Olio and others, 2000).

Gerontological Considerations

- Assess for changes and limitations in sensory function, mobility, or dexterity that indicate a need to teach a significant other how to administer feedings.
- Home enteral therapy in older adults requires frequent monitoring, assessment, and intervention from interdisciplinary teams that include nurses and dietitians (Silver and others, 2004).

Home Care Considerations

- The provision of home enteral therapy raises many ethical questions. Families need to be informed of their choices, and their decisions should be supported if it is determined that the risks or burdens of enteral therapy outweigh the benefits or go against the client's wishes (Russell, 2002).

FOCUS *on* CLINICAL PRACTICE

You are scheduled to visit Mr. Anderson, a 75-year-old retired banker who is widowed. Mr. Anderson was recently hospitalized for atrial fibrillation, an abnormal heart rhythm, and was sent home on digoxin, a cardiac glycoside, to control his arrhythmia. Mr. Anderson has impaired visual acuity and is hard of hearing. However, he is very active and is very interested in learning about his new medical condition and medication. This is your first home visit.

1. What information would you like to have about Mr. Anderson before you go to his home to assist with safe medication administration?
2. You ask Mr. Anderson to show you the medications he is currently taking. The medications in his home do not match the list of medications you received from his physician. What should you do next?

3. You teach Mr. Anderson how to take his pulse before he takes his digoxin. How long should he take his pulse? Explain your choice.
   A. For 15 seconds and then multiply by 4
   B. For 30 seconds and then multiply by 2
   C. For a full minute
   D. For 2 minutes
4. If Mr. Anderson tells the nurse he cannot feel his pulse after repeated attempts, what should the nurse do?
5. Describe three teaching strategies that would enhance Mr. Anderson's learning.

NCLEX REVIEW QUESTIONS

1. A 7-year-old child who is receiving chemotherapy for acute lymphocytic leukemia is about to be discharged from the hospital. Which of the statements made by the child's mother indicates the need for follow-up by the nurse?
   1. "I should call the physician if my child starts to have chills."
   2. "I will have to learn how to take rectal temperatures with a glass thermometer."
   3. "I went to the drug store and bought a digital thermometer."
   4. "I should wait at least 20 minutes after my child has a cold drink to take his temperature."

2. Betty has purchased a new electronic blood pressure monitoring device. Which of the following nursing actions will verify the accuracy of the blood pressure monitor?
   1. Nothing needs to be done. Electronic blood pressure monitors are extremely accurate.
   2. Have Betty take her daughter's blood pressure with the new monitor.
   3. Take Betty's blood pressure with a manual aneroid sphygmomanometer right after Betty takes her blood pressure with her monitor.
   4. Ask Betty to describe when she should take her blood pressure, and have her locate an appropriate place in her home to store her monitor.

Continued

NCLEX REVIEW QUESTIONS

3. A group of clients are enrolled in an exercise class. Which pulse site would be the best for monitoring exercise tolerance?
   1. Femoral
   2. Brachial
   3. Antecubital
   4. Radial

4. Which of the following should the nurse teach a client who is being discharged from the hospital with home oxygen therapy?
   1. The client should not allow people in the home to smoke.
   2. The client should be able to attend his son's Boy Scout camp fire.
   3. The client should shave with an electric razor.
   4. The client should transport full oxygen tanks in the trunk of his car.

5. A client is using a concentrator oxygen delivery system at home. Which of the following statements when made by the client indicates understanding of client education?
   1. "If my concentrator does not reach the outlet in my house, I will use an extension cord."
   2. "I think I will move my concentrator into the closet because it is the first thing everyone who comes into my house sees."
   3. "I need to make sure my breaker box will meet the electrical requirements of the concentrator."
   4. "I don't need to worry about having a backup system because my concentrator will always work."

6. What step should the client do first when filling an ambulatory liquid tank from the stationary reservoir?
   1. Wipe the connectors of both tanks with a lint-free cloth
   2. Firmly attach the ambulatory tank to the reservoir
   3. Open fill valve on ambulatory tank
   4. Press down firmly on the top of the ambulatory tank

7. Which of the following nursing interventions will help prevent hypoxia during suctioning at home?
   1. Instilling normal saline before suctioning
   2. Setting the suction pressure on the suction machine to 180 mm Hg
   3. Applying suction for 20 seconds to the suction catheter
   4. Providing several breaths of 100% oxygen with a bag-valve-mask

8. When the nurse teaches a client's significant other how to suction, it is important for the nurse to stress that the significant other should:
   1. Place the client in a prone position
   2. Grasp the suction catheter with the nondominant hand
   3. Apply intermittent suction for no more than 15 seconds
   4. Repeat suctioning passes at least 4 times to ensure the airway is clear

9. When providing trach care at home, the nurse teaches the client to do all the following except:
   1. Wash hands before and after the procedure
   2. Boil reusable supplies for 15 minutes once a week
   3. Change trach ties whenever they get moist
   4. Save disposable inner cannulas for future use

10. Mr. Lyons is 83 years old and is caring for himself at home. Which of the following interventions will enhance compliance with his medication regimen?
    1. Teach him everything he needs to know in 1 day.
    2. Include him in making decisions about when he should take his medications.
    3. Provide handwritten instructions that are written in blue ink.
    4. Provide medication information when his daughter and small grandchildren are visiting him.

11. Which of the following statements when made by a mother of an 11-year-old boy diagnosed with diabetes would require that the nurse provide additional information?
    1. "I am not sure why my son has to take his insulin."
    2. "An important side effect of insulin I will need to watch for is low blood sugar."
    3. "My health insurance will pay for my son's insulin as well as his syringes."
    4. "I understand when my son needs to have his insulin."

12. Which of the following statements is true about the older adult and medication compliance?
    1. Compliance is dependent solely on the client's cognitive status.
    2. Problems with mobility, dexterity, and vision will not affect the client's compliance with medication therapy.
    3. Older adults with declining cognitive status should have simple medication regimens.
    4. The capacity for learning decreases with age. Therefore older adults tend to have many problems with medication administration.

NCLEX REVIEW QUESTIONS

13. A 60-year-old woman who is receiving home enteral nutrition begins to have difficulty breathing and is coughing. What should the nurse do first?
    1. Call the physician
    2. Put the head of the bed down
    3. Verify tube placement
    4. Stop the feeding

14. Which of the following statements when made by the wife of a man who is receiving home enteral therapy indicates that the wife is experiencing caregiver role strain?
    1. "I went out with my friends last night and played cards while my daughter stayed with my husband."
    2. "I think my husband wants to have the tube feedings stopped."

3. "I just don't think I can take care of my husband much longer."
4. "I am not sure how to program the feeding pump."

16. When teaching a client's caregiver administration of bolus tube feedings at home, the nurse teaches the caregiver to complete which of the following first?
    1. Verify feeding tube placement before administering the feeding.
    2. Crush all pills well, and dissolve them in warm tap water.
    3. Aspirate gastric contents.
    4. Perform hand hygiene.

References

American Diabetes Association: Standards of medical care in diabetes, *Diabetes Care* 27(suppl 1):S15, 2004.

American Hospital Association: *Patient care partnership: understanding expectations, rights, and responsibilities,* Chicago, 2003, The Association.

Carroll P: Improve your suctioning technique, *RN* 66(5):30ac2, 2003.

Dell'Olio J and others: Noah grows up: transitioning problems from special feeding routes to oral intake, *Nutr Rev* 58(4):118, 2000.

Dreger V, Trembeck T: Optimize patient health by treating literacy and language barriers, *AORN J* 75(2):280, 2002.

Ebersole P and others: *Toward healthy aging: human needs and nursing response,* ed 6, St. Louis, 2004, Mosby.

Eliopoulos C: *Gerontological nursing,* ed 5, Philadelphia, 2001, Lippincott.

Environmental Protection Agency: *Great Lakes toxics reduction: binational toxics strategy—frequently asked questions about mercury thermometers,* http://www.epa.gov/grtlakes/bnsdocs/hg/thermfaq. html#What%20should%20you%20do%20with%20a%20 broken%20mercury%20thermometer?, 2004a, retrieved April 24, 2004.

Environmental Protection Agency: *Great Lakes toxics reduction: binational toxics strategy—mercury thermometers,* http://www.epa.gov/ glnpo/bnsdocs/hg/thermometers.html, 2004b, retrieved April 24, 2004.

Falvo DR: *Effective patient education: a guide to increased compliance,* ed 3, Boston, 2004, Jones & Bartlett Publishers.

Findeisen M: Long-term oxygen therapy in the home, *Home Healthc Nurse* 19(11): 692, 2001.

Haynes R and others: Helping patients follow prescribed treatment: clinical applications, *JAMA* 288(22):2880, 2002.

Hockenberry MJ and others: *Wong's nursing care of infants and children,* ed 7, St. Louis, 2003, Mosby.

Institute of Safe Medical Practice: Helping to remove the barriers to patient education, *ISMP Medication Safety Alert* 8(20):1, 2003.

Joanna Briggs Institute for Evidence Based Nursing and Midwifery: Tracheal suctioning of adults with an artificial airway, *Best Practice* 4(4):1, 2000.

Jones DW and others: Measuring blood pressure accurately: new and persistent challenges, *JAMA* 289(8):1027, 2003.

Lueckenotte AG: *Gerontologic nursing,* ed 2, St. Louis, 2000, Mosby.

McGraw C, Drennan V: Self-administration of medicine and older people, *Nurs Stand* 15(18):33, 2001.

Metheny NA, Titler MG: Assessing placement of feeding tubes, *Am J Nurs* 101(5):36, 2001.

Metheny NA and others: Effect of gastrointestinal motility and feeding tube site on aspiration risk in critically ill patients: a review, *Heart Lung* 33(3):131, 2004.

National Institutes of Health: *The seventh report of the Joint National Committee on Prevention, Detection, Evaluation, and Treatment of High Blood Pressure,* http://www.nhlbi.nih.gov/ guidelines/hypertension/express.pdf, 2003, retrieved July 31, 2004.

Osborne H.: *In other words...can they understand? Testing patient education materials with intended readers,* http://www.healthliteracy. com/oncallnov2001.html, 2001, retrieved July 31, 2004.

Perloff D and others: Human blood pressure determination by sphygmomanometry [American Heart Association medical/scientific statement], *Circulation* 88(5):2460, 1993, http://www. americanheart.org/presenter.jhtml?identifier=3000861, American Heart Association, 2004, retrieved April 25, 2004.

Petty TL: *Guide to prescribing home oxygen: home oxygen options,* http://www.nlhep.org/resources/Prescrb-Hm-Oxygen/ home-oxygen-options-4.html, National Lung Health Education Program, 2004, retrieved April 25, 2004.

Positive Air, Inc: *Medicare requirements for the home use of oxygen,* http://www.positiveair.com/medicare_home_use_of_oxygen. htm, 2004, retrieved Aug 8, 2004.

Puntis JWL: Nutritional support at home and in the community, *Arch Dis Child* 84(4):295, 2001.

Redman B: *The practice of patient education*, ed 9, St. Louis, 2001, Mosby.

Russell CA: The needs of patients requiring home enteral tube feeding, *Prof Nurse* 17(8):500, 2002.

Sattler B: *Children's' health and the environment: environmental health in the health care setting*, http://nursingworld.org/mods/mod370/cehc03.htm, 2002, retrieved April 24, 2004.

Schreiber D: Trach care at home: a how-to guide, *RN* 64(7):43, 2001.

Sorrentino C and others: Using the intranet to deliver patient-education materials, *Clin J Oncol Nurs* 6(6):354, 2002.

Woodrow P: Managing patients with a tracheostomy in acute care, *Nurs Stand* 16(44):39, 2002.

Research References

Agre P and others: Creating a CD-ROM program for cancer-related patient education, *Oncol Nurs Forum* 29(3):573, 2002.

Akgul S, Akyolcu N: Effects of normal saline on endotracheal suctioning, *J Clin Nurs* 11(6):826, 2002.

Altunkan S and others: Wrist blood pressure-measuring devices: a comparative study of accuracy with a standard auscultatory method using a mercury manometer, *Blood Press Monit* 7(5):281, 2002.

Bott L and others: Contamination of gastrostomy feeding systems in children in a home-based enteral nutrition program, *J Pediatr Gastroenterol Nutr* 33(3):266, 2001.

Broege PA and others: Management of hypertension in the elderly using home blood pressures, *Blood Press Monit* 6(3):139, 2001.

Bur A and others: Factors influencing the accuracy of oscillometric blood pressure measurement in critically ill patients, *Crit Care Med* 31(3):793, 2003.

Campbell NRC and others: Self-measurement of blood pressure: accuracy, patient preparation for readings, technique, and equipment, *Blood Press Monit* 6(3):133, 2001.

Chang MC and others: Overcoming patient-related barriers to cancer pain management for home care patients, *Cancer Nurs* 25(6):470, 2002.

Cooper H and others: Chronic disease patient education: lessons from meta-analyses, *Patient Educ Couns* 44(2):107, 2001.

Danigelis NL and others: Two community outreach strategies to increase breast cancer screening among low-income women, *J Cancer Educ* 16(1):55, 2001.

Day T and others: An evaluation of a teaching intervention to improve the practice of endotracheal suctioning in intensive care units, *J Clin Nurs* 10(5):682, 2001.

Evans D and others: Vital signs in hospital patients: a systematic review, *Int J Nurs Stud* 38(6):643, 2001.

Harper Chelf J and others: Learning and support preferences of adult patients with cancer at a comprehensive cancer center, *Oncol Nurs Forum* 29(5):863, 2002.

Hudson TJ and others: A pilot study of barriers to medication adherence in schizophrenia. *J Clin Psychiatry* 65(2):211, 2004.

Johansson K and others: Patients' learning needs after hip arthroplasty, *J Clin Nurs* 11:634, 2002.

Liley AJ and Manthorpe J: The effect of home enteral tube feeding in everyday life: a qualitative study, *Health Soc Care Community* 11(5):415, 2003.

Litton J and others: Insulin pump therapy in toddlers and preschool children with type 1 diabetes mellitus, *J Pediatr* 141(4):490, 2002.

Maddigan SL and others: Predictors of older adults' capacity for medication management in a self-medication program: a retrospective chart review, *J Aging Health* 15(2):332, 2003.

McLean A and others: Quality of life of mothers and families caring for preterm infants requiring home oxygen therapy: a brief report, *J Paediatr Child Health* 36(5):440, 2000.

Norris SL and others: Effectiveness of self-management training in type 2 diabetes: a systematic review of randomized controlled trials, *Diabetes Care* 24(3):561, 2001.

Oermann MH and others: Teaching by the nurse: how important is it to patients? *Appl Nurs Res* 14(1):11, 2001.

Oh H, Seo W: A meta-analysis of the effects of various interventions in preventing endotracheal suction-induced hypoxemia, *J Clin Nurs* 12(6):912, 2003.

Plotnick LP and others: Safety and effectiveness of insulin pump therapy in children and adolescents with type 1 diabetes, *Diabetes Care* 26(4):1142, 2003.

Robb BW and others: Home oxygen therapy: adjunct or risk factor? *J Burn Care Rehabil* 24(6):403, 2003.

Rossi Ferrario S and others: Caregiver strain associated with tracheostomy in chronic respiratory failure, *Chest* 119(5):1498, 2001.

Rycroft-Malone J and others: Nursing and medication education, *Nurs Stand* 14(50):35, 2000.

Saounatsou M and others: The influence of the hypertensive patient's education in compliance with their medication, *Public Health Nurs* 18(6):436, 2001.

Savini CJ and others: Survey of patient and clinician attitudes on adherence in a rural HIV clinic, *J Assoc Nurses AIDS Care* 14(3):72, 2003.

Schommer JC and others: Interdisciplinary medication education in a church environment, *Am J Health Syst Pharm* 59(5):423, 2002.

Sedlak CA and others: Osteoporosis education programs: changing knowledge and behaviors, *Public Health Nurs* 17(5):398, 2000.

Silver HJ and others: Older adults receiving home enteral nutrition: enteral regimen, provider involvement, and health care outcomes, *JPEN J Parenter Enteral Nutr* 28(2):92, 2004.

Taylor-Piliae R: Review: several techniques optimize oxygenation during suctioning patients, *Evid Based Nurs* 5(2):51, 2002.

White J and others: Parents measuring pulses: an observational study, *Arch Dis Child* 89(3):274, 2004.

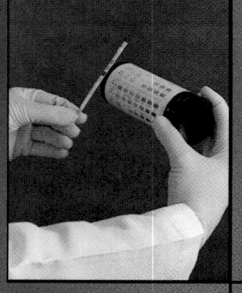

43

Specimen Collection

MEDIA RESOURCES

Evolve Site *evolve*

http://evolve.elsevier.com/Perry/skills
- Weblinks
- Video clips
- Mosby's Nursing Skills Video Exercises

Mosby's Nursing Skills Videos/CD-ROM

- *Specimen Collection Video:* Midstream urine specimen collection; fecal occult blood testing Hemoccult test; Gastroccult and gastric pH testing from an NG tube; sputum specimen collection; wound culture specimen; blood glucose testing; labeling, storage, and transfer of specimens to the laboratory; evaluating results of bedside tests

OBJECTIVES

Mastery of content in this chapter will enable the nurse to:

- Explain the rationale for the collection of each specimen.
- Identify special conditions necessary for satisfactory collection of each specimen.
- Describe the instructions to encourage client cooperation for successful collection of the specimen.
- Recognize the impact of sociocultural issues that may affect client's cooperation with collection of specimen.
- Identify measures to minimize anxiety and promote safety for selected techniques.
- Discuss nursing responsibilities for processing a specimen after collection.
- Chart appropriate information in the client's record after collection of the specimen.
- Discuss the precautions to prevent injury to the client during specimen collection.
- Properly collect clean-voided, timed, and catheterized urine specimens.
- Correctly measure glucose, ketones, protein, and blood in urine.
- Correctly measure for the presence of occult blood in a stool specimen.
- Correctly perform the analysis for the presence of occult blood in gastric secretions.
- Properly collect specimens for culture from the nose and throat, urethra and vagina, sputum, and wound.
- Properly perform venipuncture.
- Properly collect specimens for blood cultures.
- Correctly measure for blood glucose from a blood specimen collected by skin puncture.
- Use measures recommended for preventing transmission of pathogens.

KEY TERMS

Acetest
Aerobic
Anaerobic
Aseptic technique
Aspirate
Autolet
Blood culture
Clean-voided specimen
Clinitest
Culture
Double-voided specimen
Dysuria
Ecchymosis
Expectorate
Frequency
Glucose monitoring
Guaiac test
Hematoma
Hematuria

Hemolysis
Hemostasis
Ketones
Meatus
Melena
Midstream
Occult blood
pH
Platelet
Reagent
Renal
Sensitivity
Timed urine collection
Tourniquet
Urgency
Vacutainer tube
Venipuncture
Void

Proficiency in assisting with diagnostic testing and specimen analysis is important for the nurse. Skill and judgment in obtaining specimens affect client comfort and ensure accuracy and quality of diagnostic procedures. Accountability is increasing, and there is more attention to monitoring client outcomes. In addition, current health care economics insist that laboratory tests be performed accurately and in a timely manner.

Nurses often are responsible for collection of specimens. Depending on the type of specimen needed and skill required, the nurse might be able to delegate this task to assistive personnel. Laboratory examination of urine, stool, sputum, blood, and wound drainage specimens provides important information about body functioning and contributes to the assessment of the client's health status. Laboratory test results can aid in the diagnosis of health care problems, provide information about the stage and activity of a disease process, and measure a client's response to therapy.

Normal values for laboratory tests can be found in reference books, but the nurse should know that each laboratory establishes its own values for each test. These values are usually readily available on the laboratory slips of the agency. Any major deviations should be discussed with the provider immediately.

Clients often experience embarrassment or discomfort when giving a sample of body excretions or secretions. Excretion is the process by which the body eliminates or sheds substances by organs or tissues, whereas secretion is the release of chemical substances manufactured by cells of glandular organs. Gloves should be worn and hand hygiene performed as standard precautions. Excretions should be handled discreetly; therefore it is important to provide the client with as much comfort and privacy as possible. Anxiety is also provoked by the invasive nature of some collection procedures or by fear of unknown test results. Clients who are given a clear explanation about the purpose of the specimen and how it is to be obtained may be more cooperative in its collection. With proper instruction many clients are able to obtain their own specimens of urine, stool, and sputum, thus avoiding embarrassment.

Laboratory tests are often expensive. The nurse can prevent unnecessary costs by using the correct procedure for obtaining and processing specimens. When there are questions about laboratory tests, the nurse should consult the institution's procedure manual or call the laboratory.

The assurance of confidentiality is an important issue associated with testing. Disclosure of confidential information can result in discrimination in a variety of circumstances. Agencies must have clearly written and enforced policies regarding disclosure of test results and maintenance of confidentiality throughout the health care system (HIPAA Guidelines, 2003).

Evidence-Based Practice Trends

Positive patient identification is a term that means that the client is positively identified before the procedure. Before obtaining a laboratory specimen, usually via at least two identifiers, such as the identification number on the admission arm band and asking the client's name should be used. It is important to be aware of agency policies that govern obtaining laboratory specimens. Correct identification of clients for laboratory tests, as well as the delivery of care, are incorporated into the National Patient Safety Goals of the Joint Commission on Accreditation of Healthcare Organizations (see Chapter 19).

Advances in laboratory testing have resulted in bedside measures for some testing, such as arterial blood gases, urine testing via reagent test strip, and serum glucose testing. Point-of-care testing provides for timely results that the health care team can use to determine the client's response to therapy and to trend client progress (Malarkey and Morrow, 2000; Marx 2002). In addition, newer needleless and needle safety devices enable health care providers to collect blood specimens more safely with a lowered risk for needle-stick injuries (see Chapter 21).

Testing for fecal occult blood enables clients to obtain specimens in the privacy of their own homes and to send the testing cards to their physician. It remains possible to test for this at the bedside as well. The importance of collecting specimens in the home has increased the number of people who are adherent to this baseline screening, which is an initial test for colon health (Marx, 2002).

Cultural Considerations

Assess cultural beliefs associated with specimen collection. For example, Southeast Asians consider the blood as a vital life force that should not be wasted, and they may become anxious about a needle penetrating the skin, allowing blood and body fluids to seep out. The insertion of a foreign object into the mouth to collect specimens may be threatening to the Southeast Asian client who believes that diseases can be introduced through the mouth and the head as the seat of one's life force.

Consider both cultural and language barriers when delegating specimen collection to the client and family members. For example, Muslims and Hindus designate which hand is to be used for clean and dirty tasks. Collecting their own stool and urine specimens may be difficult because only the left hand can be used for "dirty" activities. Provide for hygienic needs of clients post procedure, including hand hygiene and cleansing of the anus and urinary meatus (Lawrence and Rozmus, 2001). Language barriers may make it difficult to explain the purpose of tests and collection techniques. Be sure to provide repeated return demonstrations to ensure the client or family member understands how to perform a procedure. Use of an interpreter can be helpful.

Whenever possible, use gender-congruent caregivers when collecting specimens (vaginal, rectal, urinary) from clients whose cultural values uphold distinct separation of gender roles and modesty. Provide privacy when giving instructions and during specimen collection.

Skill Performance Guidelines

1. Consider the client's need and ability to participate in specimen collection procedures.
2. Recognize that specimen collection may cause anxiety, embarrassment, or discomfort.
3. Provide support for clients who are fearful of the results of a specimen examination.
4. Consider age-related factors that may affect client's compliance with specimen collection.
5. Recognize that children require simple explanations of procedures and may benefit from support of parents/family members.
6. Consider sociocultural variations that may affect client's compliance with specimen collection.
7. Obtain specimens in accordance with specific prerequisite conditions (e.g., fasting, nothing by mouth [NPO]) as required.
8. Follow standard precautions (see Chapter 8) when collecting specimens of blood or other body fluids.
9. Collect specimens in appropriate containers, at the correct time, in the appropriate amount.
10. Properly label all specimens with the client's identification; complete laboratory requisition as necessary.
11. Deliver specimens to the laboratory within the recommended time, or ensure that they are stored properly for later transport.
12. Be aware of special conditions (e.g., iced specimens, special containers with preservatives) required for transport of specimens.

13. Know institutional policy regarding infection control practices for transportation of all specimen containers of body substances.
14. Be aware that some deviations from normal values occur as a result of medications or dietary intake.
15. Follow precautions for collecting specimens from clients who are in protective isolation.

SKILL 43-1 Collecting a Midstream (Clean-Voided) Urine Specimen

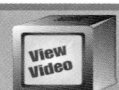

A common test performed on urine is a culture and sensitivity measurement. In the laboratory a few drops of urine are placed on a special medium to determine whether or not bacteria are present. Readings are made at 24- and 48-hour intervals, and the final reading is made after 72 hours. If bacteria are present, sensitivity testing reveals which antibiotics will be effective against the microorganisms.

With clients who are able to void voluntarily, the nurse collects a midstream urine specimen for culture and sensi-

tivity testing. The nurse may need to assist some clients who are unable to collect specimens independently. A client begins the urinary stream and then during the middle portion of voiding collects a specimen. The initial stream flushes the urethral orifice and meatus of any resident bacteria. It is easiest for a client to obtain a clean-voided specimen while using toilet facilities rather than a bedpan or urinal.

DELEGATION CONSIDERATIONS

The skill of collecting a midstream (clean-voided) urine specimen may be delegated to assistive personnel. Before delegating this skill the nurse must:
- Instruct assistive personnel if client has mobility restrictions that will affect collection technique.
- Instruct assistive personnel to report when blood, mucus, or foul odors are present in the specimen

EQUIPMENT

❑ Commercial kit (Figure 43-1) for clean-voided urine containing:
❑ Sterile cotton balls and/or 2 × 2 inch gauze pads, cleansing towelette, or two gauze pads
❑ Antiseptic solution (usually chlorhexidine or povidone-iodine solution)
❑ Sterile water or saline
❑ Sterile specimen container
❑ Sterile gloves
❑ Soap, water, washcloth, and towel
❑ Bedpan (for nonambulatory client), specimen hat (Figure 43-2) (if all urine needs to be measured), potty-chair (for young child)
❑ Completed specimen identification label
❑ Completed laboratory requisition form

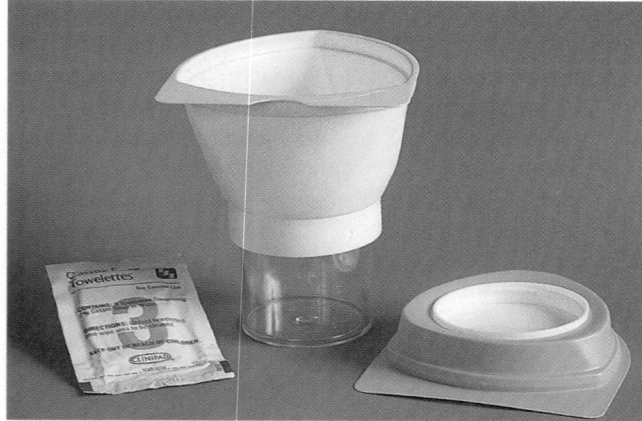

FIGURE **43-1** Clean-voided specimen collection kit.

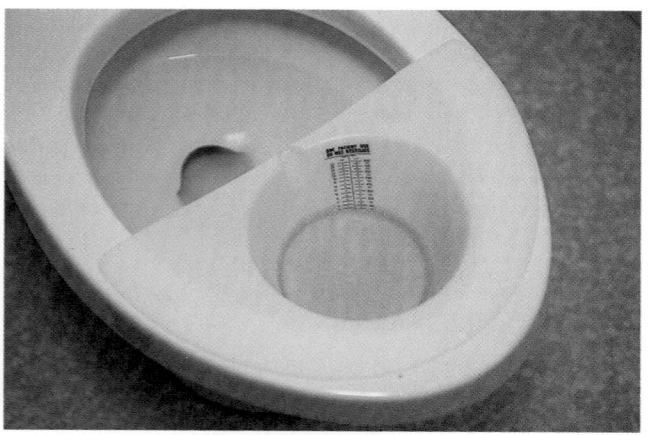

FIGURE **43-2** Specimen hat.

STEP	RATIONALE

◼ ASSESSMENT

1. Assess client's level of understanding of purpose of test and method of collection.

   Information allows nurse to clarify misunderstanding; promotes client compliance.

2. Assess client's mobility and balance in being able to use toilet facilities independently.

   Determines level of assistance required by client.

3. Refer to medical record for indications of urinary infection.

   Allows nurse to anticipate need to test client's urine for bacteria.

   a. Assess risks for urinary tract infection (e.g., poor perineal hygiene, improperly handled diagnostic instruments, previous urinary catheterization).

   Helps nurse explain purpose of specimen procedure for client.

   b. Observe for signs and symptoms of urinary tract infections: frequency, urgency, dysuria, hematuria, flank pain, fever, and cloudy, malodorous urine.

   Indicates bacteria in urine (Meredith and Horan, 2000).

   c. Refer to agency procedures for specimen collection methods.

   Agency policies may vary regarding collection or handling of specimens.

◼ NURSING DIAGNOSES

- Anxiety
- Risk for infection

- Deficient knowledge regarding specimen collection
- Acute pain

Related factors are individualized based on client's condition or needs.

◼ PLANNING

1. Expected outcomes following completion of procedure:
   - Client produces midstream urine specimen that is not contaminated with feces or toilet tissue.

   Proper collection technique prevents substances from changing normal characteristics of urine.

   - Urine has normal characteristics and does not reveal bacterial growth.

   Specimen collected correctly provides evidence of absence of infection.

   - Client will discuss purpose and benefits of midstream urine collection.

   Discussion can be used to evaluate client's learning.

2. Offer client fluids to drink (if permitted) before attempting to collect specimen.

   Enhances client's ability to void.

3. Explain procedure to client and/or family member.

   a. Reason midstream specimen is needed.

   Promotes cooperation and participation.

   b. How client/family member can assist.

   c. How to obtain specimen free of feces and tissue.

   Feces and tissue alter chemical composition of specimen.

   d. Use visual aids (if available) to explain procedure to client.

   Because this method of urine collection is somewhat complicated, clients benefit from illustrations emphasizing midstream collection technique.

◼ IMPLEMENTATION

1. Identify client. Perform hand hygiene.

   Proper hand hygiene reduces transfer of microorganisms.

2. Provide privacy for client who will give specimen in bed by closing curtain around bed or closing room door. Allow mobile clients to collect specimen in bathroom.

   Privacy allows client to relax and produce a specimen more easily.

3. Give client cleansing towelette or towel, washcloth, and soap to cleanse perineum, or assist client with cleansing perineum (if able).

   Clients prefer to wash their own perineal areas when possible. Cleansing prevents contamination of specimen after urine passes from urethra.

STEP	RATIONALE

4. Assist bedridden client onto bedpan (see illustration). Raise head of bed.

Provides easy access to perineal areas to collect specimen. Semi-sitting position eases voiding.

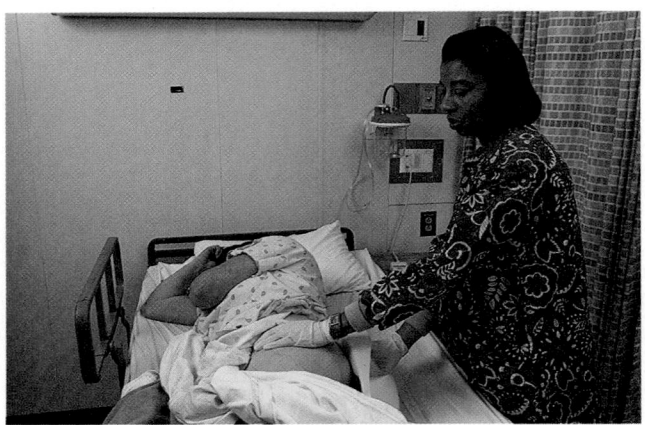

STEP **4** Nurse assisting client on a bedpan.

5. Using surgical asepsis, open sterile kit or prepare sterile tray.

Maintains sterility of equipment.

6. Apply sterile gloves.

Prevents introduction of microorganisms on nurse's hands into specimen.

7. Pour antiseptic solution over cotton balls (unless kit contains prepared gauze pads in antiseptic solution).

Cotton ball or gauze is used to cleanse perineum.

8. Open specimen container, and place cap with sterile inside surface up, and do not touch inside of container.

Contaminated specimen is most frequent reason for inaccurate reporting on urine cultures and sensitivities.

9. Perform urine collection by assisting or allowing client to independently cleanse perineum and collect specimen. The amount of assistance needed varies with each client. The nurse will assess client's ability to perform procedure and assist as needed.

Maintains client's dignity and comfort.

  a. Male client

    (1) Either nurse or client will hold client's penis with one hand. Using circular motion and antiseptic swab, cleanse meatus, moving from center to outside (see illustration).

Reduces number of microorganisms at urethral meatus and moves from areas of least to most contamination.

    (2) If agency procedure indicates, rinse area with sterile water and dry with cotton balls or gauze pad.

Prevents contamination of specimen with antiseptic solution.

    (3) After client has initiated urine stream into toilet or bedpan, pass urine specimen container into stream and collect 30 to 60 ml of urine (see illustration).

Initial urine flushes out microorganisms that normally accumulate at urinary meatus and prevents collection in specimen.

  b. Female client

● **Critical Decision Point**

If client is menstruating, record this information on laboratory slip.

    (1) Either nurse or client will spread client's labia minora with thumb and forefinger of nondominant hand.

Provides access to urethral meatus.

STEP	RATIONALE

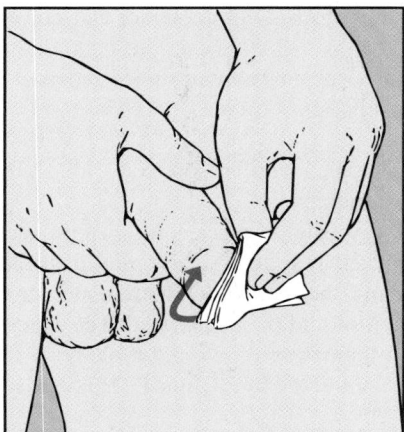

STEP **9a(1)** Cleansing urinary meatus. (Modified from Grimes D: *Infectious diseases,* Mosby's clinical nursing series, St. Louis, 1991, Mosby.)

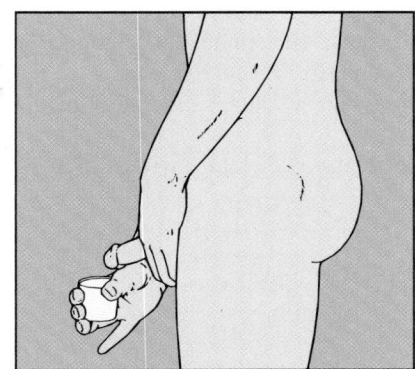

STEP **9a(3)** Collecting midstream urine specimen.

(2) Use dominant hand to cleanse urethral area with swab (cotton ball or gauze), moving from front (above urethral orifice) to back (toward anus). Using a fresh swab each time, repeat front-to-back motion three times (begin with center, then do left side, then do right side) (see illustration).	Prevents contamination of urinary meatus with fecal material.
(3) If agency procedure indicates, rinse area with sterile water and dry with cotton ball.	Prevents contamination of specimen with antiseptic solution.
(4) While continuing to hold labia apart, client should initiate urine stream into toilet or bedpan; after stream is achieved, pass specimen container into stream and collect 30 to 60 ml of urine (see illustration).	Initial stream flushes out resident microorganisms that accumulate at urethral meatus.
10. Remove specimen container before flow of urine stops and before releasing labia or penis. Client finishes voiding into bedpan or toilet.	Prevents contamination of specimen with skin flora.

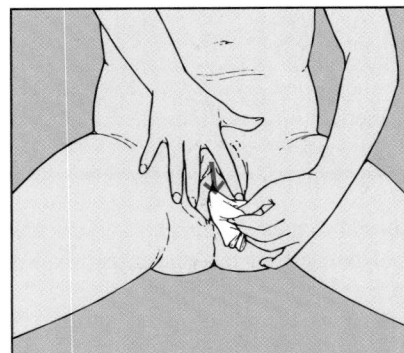

STEP **9b(2)** Cleansing urinary meatus with front-to-back motion. (Modified from Grimes D: *Infectious diseases,* Mosby's clinical nursing series, St. Louis, 1991, Mosby.)

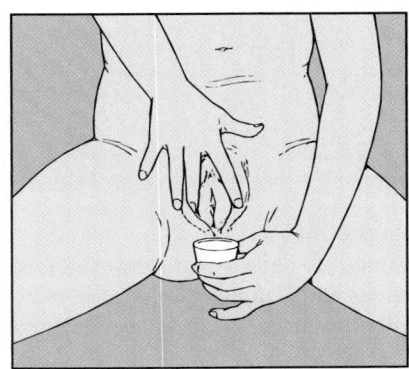

STEP **9b(4)** Collection of midstream urine specimen. (Modified from Grimes D: *Infectious diseases,* Mosby's clinical nursing series, St. Louis, 1991, Mosby.)

STEP	RATIONALE
11. Replace cap securely on specimen container (touch only outside).	Retains sterility of inside of container and prevents spillage of urine.
12. Cleanse urine from exterior surface of container.	Prevents transfer of microorganisms to others.
13. Empty bedpan (if applicable), remove and discard gloves, and perform hand hygiene.	Reduces transmission of microorganisms.
14. Label specimen and attach laboratory requisition.	Prevents inaccurate identification that could lead to errors in diagnosis or therapy.
15. Take specimen to laboratory within 15 to 20 minutes.	Urine specimens should arrive promptly in the laboratory and be analyzed as soon after arrival as possible. If a delay of more than 2 hours after collection cannot be avoided, the specimen should be refrigerated. The specimen should be at room temperature before the analysis is performed (National Committee for Clinical Laboratory Standards [NCCLS], 2001).

EVALUATION

1. Observe specimen for contaminants such as toilet paper or feces.	Contaminants prevent specimen from being used.
2. Assess client's urine culture and sensitivity report for bacterial growth.	Routine cultures identify organism(s), and sensitivity study identifies antimicrobial medications that may be effective against pathogen (Malarkey and McMorrow, 2000).
3. Ask client to describe midstream urine collection procedure.	Validates client's understanding.

Recording and Reporting

- Record appearance and odor of urine and evidence of dysuria in nurses' notes.
- Notify physician of any significant abnormalities.

Unexpected Outcomes	Related Interventions
1. Urine specimen is contaminated with feces or toilet paper.	• Repeat client instruction and specimen collection. If unable to obtain specimen through clean voiding, client may require catheterization (see Skill 43-3).
2. Urine specimen is accidentally discarded.	• Repeat specimen collection.
3. Client is unable to urinate on demand.	• Offer fluids if permitted. Allow more time for urine to accumulate in bladder. Try obtaining specimen after 30 minutes.
4. Urine culture reveals bacterial growth (determined by colony count of more than 10,000 organisms per milliliter).	• Report findings to physician. • Administer medications as ordered. • Monitor client for fever and dysuria.

Teaching Considerations

- Use visual aids to describe collection of specimen.
- Discuss signs and symptoms of urinary tract infection.
- Explain significance of cleansing genital area before collecting specimen.
- Explain to female client importance of cleansing labia from front to back.
- Discuss client's role in collecting specimen.

- Nurses should request feedback to assess client's understanding of purpose of test and directions for collecting specimen.

Pediatric Considerations

- It is not possible to obtain midstream urine collection on non–toilet-trained child; consequently, urine for culture should be obtained by use of sterile plastic urine-collecting

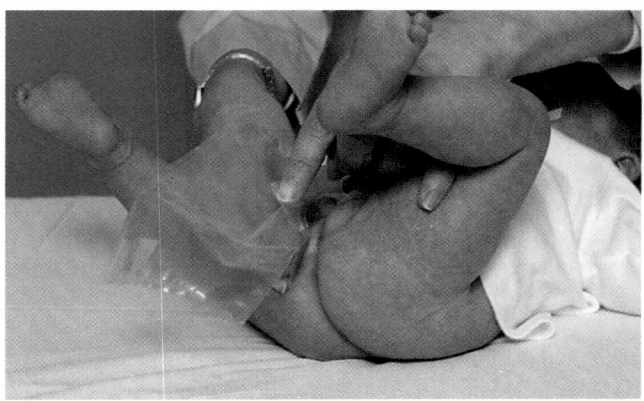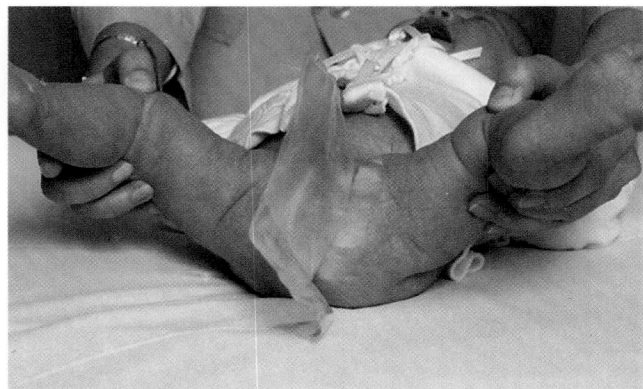

FIGURE **43-3** Application of urine collection bag. (From Hockenberry MJ and others: *Wong's nursing care of infants and children*, ed 7, St. Louis, 2003, Mosby.)

bag that adheres to perineum (Figure 43-3). Cleansing procedures have not been found to be of great benefit before the urine collection (Behrman and others, 2004).

- Instructions and/or explanations regarding cleansing and collecting the specimen should be given to children in an age-appropriate manner. This will encourage cooperation and decrease anxiety during the collection process.
- It may be easier to collect a midstream urine specimen in a young female child by having them sit facing the back of the toilet. In this position the labia are naturally separated, decreasing the chance of contamination (Hockenberry and others, 2003).
- Procedures involving genitals in preschool children cause anxiety (Hockenberry and others, 2003).

Gerontological Considerations

- Special assistance should be given to older adults. A clear and concise explanation should be given about procedure and reason for sample to be obtained. All equipment should be available at bedside to allow proceeding with obtaining specimen when client needs assistance.

Home Care Considerations

- Ideally, specimen for culture should not be collected at home because time delay before applying it to culture medium in laboratory setting would greatly enhance bacterial growth. If urine specimen is collected, it should be kept on ice until it reaches laboratory and is placed on medium.

SKILL 43-2 Collecting a Timed Urine Specimen

Some tests of renal function and urine composition require urine to be collected over 2 to 72 hours. The 24-hour timed collection is most common. The tests allow for the measurement of elements such as amino acids, creatinine, hormones, glucose, and adrenocorticosteroids, whose levels change over time. A timed urine collection can also provide a means to measure the concentration or dilution of urine.

Timed urine collections begin after a client urinates. The nurse discards the first specimen and then collects every successive specimen until the time period has ended. Each specimen is transferred immediately to a large collection bottle kept in the client's bathroom. Any missed specimens make test results inaccurate. The client should always provide the last specimen as close as possible to the end of the collection period.

DELEGATION CONSIDERATIONS

The skill of collecting a timed urine specimen may be delegated to assistive personnel. The nurse must:

- Instruct assistive personnel as to when timed collection is to begin and the proper way to store the specimen during the collection period
- Remind assistive personnel to place signs in client's toileting area that a timed urine collection is taking place and not to discard any urine
- Instruct assistive personnel to report when blood, mucus, or foul odors are present in the specimen

EQUIPMENT

- ❑ Large collection bottle with cap that may contain a chemical for urine preservation (consultation with laboratory is usually necessary to obtain bottle and determine appropriate chemical additive [e.g., toluene, acetic acid])
- ❑ Bedpan, urinal, specimen hat, bedside commode, or pediatric potty-chair if client does not have indwelling catheter
- ❑ Graduated measuring cup if intake and output are to be measured
- ❑ Basin large enough to hold collection bottle surrounded by ice if immediate refrigeration is required
- ❑ Completed specimen identification label
- ❑ Completed laboratory requisition with client's name, date, and time of collection
- ❑ Instructional signs that remind client and staff to save urine for timed specimen collection
- ❑ Clean disposable gloves

STEP	RATIONALE

▌ ASSESSMENT

1. Determine purpose of timed urine specimen collection for client and period collection is to include.

Most collection periods are for 24 hours because this provides average excretion rate for substances such as hormones or proteins excreted in small variable amounts in urine. If these substances are to be accurately measured and yield quantities of diagnostic value, urine may need to be collected over an extended period. Challenge dose of a chemical such as insulin may be given, and then timed urine specimen collection may be begun to detect renal disorders.

2. Determine if fluid or dietary requirements or medications need to be administered in conjunction with test.

Certain substances affect excretion and levels of urinary constituents. Glucose solution may be given for glucose tolerance test. Specific amounts of fluid may be required when collecting concentration/dilution tests.

3. Determine that client is taking correct diet.

Client's compliance is necessary for accurate test.

4. Assess client's ability to collect specimens independently.

Because timed specimens are difficult to collect, specimen collection must be a priority in client's care.

5. Assess client's or family members' understanding of purpose of test and need to collect urine over extended period.

Compliance is facilitated by degree of understanding.

6. Refer to agency policy for specimen collection procedure.

Agency policies may vary regarding collection or handling of specimens.

▌ NURSING DIAGNOSIS

- Deficient knowledge regarding urine collection procedure

Related factors are individualized based on client's condition or needs.

▌ PLANNING

1. Expected outcomes following completion of procedure:
   - All of client's urine voided during the time period is saved.
   - Urine specimen is not contaminated with feces or toilet tissue.

Necessary for satisfactory completion of test.

Proper testing procedure prevents results of urine test from being adversely affected by these substances.

STEP	RATIONALE
• Urine has expected constituents.	Test measured without contamination or break in protocol.
• Client explains purpose of and procedure for urine collection.	Validates learning and increases compliance.
2. Have client drink two to four glasses of water about 30 minutes before timed collection is to begin (if not contraindicated).	Enables client to void old urine (collected in bladder) at time test begins.
3. Explain procedure to client and/or family member. Discuss reason for specimen collection and how client can assist. Explain that urine must be free of feces and tissue.	A client who understands procedure is more likely to cooperate and may be able to obtain specimen independently. It also prevents accidental disposal and chemical changes resulting from feces and tissue.

IMPLEMENTATION

STEP	RATIONALE
1. Provide privacy for and assist the client in collecting specimen.	Clients prefer collecting specimens themselves. Timed specimens are not sterile.
2. Wear gloves when handling urine.	Prevents transmission of microorganisms.
3. Discard this first specimen as test begins. Indicate time that test began on laboratory requisition.	Collection period begins with empty bladder.
4. Certain urine tests are done to measure metabolites that are unstable in urine and require special conditions be adhered to and/or that preservatives be added to the specimen container (i.e., a 24-hour urine test for catecholamines requires that hydrochloric acid be added to container by laboratory and specimen be kept refrigerated or on ice during collection) (NCCLS, 2001). Check agency policy for specific guidelines and collection protocols.	Maintains integrity of urine specimen.
5. When applicable, have client drink required amount of liquid or take ordered medication.	Required for specific types of tests to measure elimination of urine constituents.
6. Place signs on client's door and toileting area indicating that timed urine specimen collection is in progress. If client leaves unit for test or procedure, be sure that personnel in that area collect and save all urine.	Prevents health care team members from accidentally discarding urine specimens.
7. Measure volume of each voiding if output is to be recorded.	Measures client's fluid balance.
8. Place all voided urine in labeled specimen bottle with appropriate additive.	Additives preserve urine specimen and prevent deterioration.
9. Unless instructed otherwise, keep specimen bottle in specimen refrigerator or in container of ice in client's bathroom.	Cold temperature prevents decomposition of urine.
10. Perform hand hygiene, and discard gloves after collection of each voiding.	Reduces transmission of microorganisms.
11. Encourage client to drink two glasses of water 1 hour before timed urine collection ends. If client's condition warrants fluid restrictions, be cautious in encouraging fluids.	Facilitates client's ability to void at end of collection period.
12. Encourage client to empty bladder during last 15 minutes of urine collection period.	Ensures urine collected for precise amount of time.
13. At end of period, send labeled specimen to laboratory with appropriate requisition.	Ensures laboratory results credited to correct client.
14. Remove signs, and remind client that specimen collection period is completed.	Allows client to resume usual voiding habits.

STEP	RATIONALE

▌ EVALUATION

1. Intermittently during collection period, observe client's compliance with saving of all urine.

2. Inspect urine for contamination from feces or toilet tissue.

3. Compare results of client's timed measurement with normal expected laboratory values.

Clients often benefit from being reminded to save urine.

Ensures specimen is not contaminated.

Reveals deviations from normal and may indicate need for further testing.

Recording and Reporting

- Record starting time of urine collection in client's chart.
- Report to oncoming shift that 24-hour urine collection is in progress.
- At completion of test, record time urine collection is finished; appearance, amount, and odor of urine; and disposition of specimen to laboratory.
- Discuss abnormal test results with physician.

Unexpected Outcomes	Related Interventions
1. A portion of urine specimen is accidentally discarded.	• Reinforce importance of saving the total specimen. • Notify laboratory to determine if collection must be restarted.
2. Urine specimen is contaminated by feces or toilet tissue.	• Notify laboratory to determine if collection must be restarted. • Assist client with specimen collection as needed.
3. Laboratory results reveal abnormal values for urine constituents.	• Notify physician of findings. • Continue to monitor client.

Teaching Considerations

- Explain fluid or dietary recommendations or restrictions to client and family.
- Explain how specimen is obtained and duration of collection.
- Instruct client in how specimen is stored.

Pediatric Considerations

- For infants and young children who are not yet potty trained, special plastic urine-collection bags with self-adhesive are designed to attach to perineal area.
- Toilet-trained young child may not be able to void on request and may be more successful if bedpan or potty-chair is placed on toilet. Use terms familiar to child such as "tinkle" or "wee wee." Enlist parent's support (Hockenberry and others, 2003).

- Toilet-trained older child is cooperative and appreciates explanation of why specimen is needed. Provide privacy and receptacle to conceal specimen, such as a paper bag (Hockenberry and others, 2003).

Gerontological Considerations

- A reminder should be placed in bathroom on mirror for ambulatory client.
- Verbal reminders will further enhance continuing sample collection.

Home Care Considerations

- Depending on type of specimen collected, instruct client regarding need to refrigerate specimen.

SKILL 43-3 Collecting a Sterile Urine Specimen From an Indwelling Catheter

It is often necessary to collect urine specimens from a client who has an indwelling catheter. Strict aseptic technique should be used to ensure sterility and to avoid introducing infection into the urinary tract.

A urine specimen for culture tests should not be collected from a urine drainage bag unless it is the first urine to drain into a new sterile bag. Bacteria grow rapidly in drainage bags and can give a false measurement of bacteria in the urine.

DELEGATION CONSIDERATIONS

The skill of collecting a sterile urine specimen from an indwelling catheter may be delegated to assistive personnel. The client must first be assessed to determine patency and functioning of the indwelling catheter system. The nurse should instruct assistive personnel:

- When the specimen should be obtained
- To report when blood, mucus, or foul odors are present in the specimen

EQUIPMENT

- ❑ 3-ml syringe with 1-inch needle (21 gauge) (for culture) or 20-ml syringe with 1-inch needle (21 gauge) (for routine urinalysis)
- ❑ Alcohol, chlorhexidine, or other disinfectant swab
- ❑ Clamp or rubber band
- ❑ Specimen container (nonsterile for routine urinalysis, sterile for culture)
- ❑ Completed specimen identification label
- ❑ Completed laboratory requisition (client's name, date, time of collection)
- ❑ Clean disposable gloves

STEP	RATIONALE

ASSESSMENT

1. Assess client's or family members' understanding of need to collect urine from indwelling catheter.
2. Assess for signs and symptoms of urinary tract infection: frequency, urgency, dysuria, and changes in urine color or odor, hematuria, and flank pain.
3. Assess indwelling catheter for built-in sampling port and type of material from which it is made.

Reveals knowledge of procedure and willingness to cooperate.

Indicates bacteria in urine (Meredith and Horan, 2000).

Provides appropriate place for removal of urine from catheter. Port prevents leakage of urine from catheter. It is safe to insert needle directly into self-sealing rubber catheter. Silastic, silicone, or plastic catheters are not self-sealing and thus should not be punctured with needle for aspiration of urine.

NURSING DIAGNOSES

- Risk for infection
- Acute pain
- Toileting self-care deficit

Related factors are individualized based on client's condition or needs.

PLANNING

1. Expected outcomes following completion of procedure:
   - Urine specimen is obtained from catheter without contamination.
   - Urinary catheter and drainage system remain intact.

   - Urine has normal characteristics and no bacterial growth.

Procedure is safely performed.

There is no indication (e.g., leaking of urine) that catheter or drainage system was punctured by needle during specimen collection.

Client is free of urinary abnormality. There are no signs of nosocomial infection.

STEP	RATIONALE
2. Explain why catheter will need to be clamped for 30 minutes before obtaining urine specimen and why it is not obtained from drainage bag.	Prevents development of anxiety over catheter clamping and promotes understanding of need for urine to collect within bladder.
3. Explain procedure to client and/or family member. Emphasize that although a syringe with a needle is used to remove urine from the catheter, the client will not experience any discomfort.	Prevents anxiety when nurse manipulates catheter and aspirates urine with syringe and needle. Promotes client cooperation.

IMPLEMENTATION

1. Perform hand hygiene.	Reduces transfer of microorganisms.
2. Clamp drainage tubing with clamp or rubber band for 30 minutes (see illustration).	Permits collection of fresh sterile urine in catheter tubing rather than draining into bag.
3. Return to room, and inform client that procedure to collect specimen from catheter will begin.	Allows client to anticipate manipulation of urinary catheter and cope more effectively with discomfort that may occur when catheter is moved.
4. Perform hand hygiene, and put on gloves.	Reduces transfer of microorganisms.
5. Position client so that catheter is easily accessible.	Allows for easy collection of specimen.
6. Cleanse entry port for needle with disinfectant swab. Wait until disinfectant is dry.	Prevents entry of microorganisms into catheter.
7. Insert needle at 45-degree angle just above where catheter is attached to drainage tube in self-sealing rubber catheter or at built-in sampling port in Silastic, silicone, or plastic catheter (see illustration).	Ensures entrance of needle into catheter lumen and prevents accidental puncture of lumen leading to balloon that holds catheter in place in bladder. Aspiration of water from lumen can result in catheter slipping out of bladder.
8. Draw urine into 3-ml syringe (for culture), or draw urine into 20-ml syringe (for routine urinalysis).	Allows collection of urine without contamination. Proper volume is needed to perform test.
9. Transfer urine from syringe into sterile urine container for culture or into nonsterile urine container for routine urinalysis.	Prevents contamination of urine during transfer procedure.
10. Place lid tightly on container.	Prevents contamination of specimen by air and loss by spillage.
11. Unclamp catheter, and allow urine to flow into drainage bag.	Allows urine to drain by gravity and prevents stasis of urine in bladder, which can cause much discomfort and potential damage to kidneys.

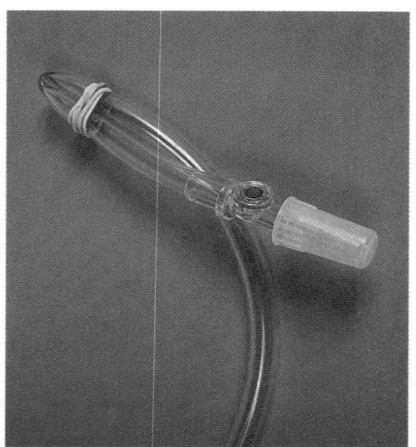

STEP **2** Clamped urinary drainage tubing.

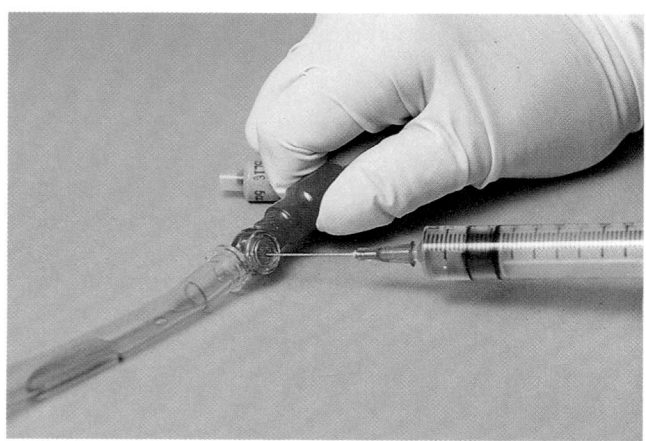

STEP **7** Insertion of needle through self-sealing port.

STEP	RATIONALE
12. Dispose of soiled supplies, remove and discard gloves, and perform hand hygiene.	Reduces transmission of microorganisms.
13. Securely attach properly completed identification label and laboratory requisition to specimen.	Incorrect identification of specimen could result in diagnostic or therapeutic errors.
14. Send specimen to laboratory immediately, or place in specimen refrigerator.	Transport specimen to laboratory immediately. If this is not possible, specimen may be refrigerated (NCCLS, 2001).

EVALUATION

1. Observe characteristics of urine and any signs of client discomfort.	Symptoms need to be further explored (Meredith and Horan, 2000).
2. Observe urinary drainage system to ensure that it is intact and patent.	System must remain closed to remain sterile.
3. Compare results of client's laboratory report with normal laboratory values, and report any abnormalities to physician.	Reveals deviations from normal and indicates need for further testing and intervention.

Recording and Reporting

- Record collection of specimen in nurses' notes or per agency policy; note time and date, appearance, odor and color of urine, and disposition to laboratory.
- Report any significant differences in urine.

Unexpected Outcomes	Related Interventions
1. Urine specimen is contaminated during procedure.	• Recollect specimen.
2. Lumen that leads to balloon that holds catheter in bladder is punctured.	• Notify physician and prepare for reinsertion of new catheter. • Collect specimen.
3. Urine has abnormal constituents.	• Continue to monitor client. • Notify physician of findings for further orders.
4. Client has pain during procedure.	• Continue to monitor client. • Notify physician. • Administer pain medication if ordered.

SKILL 43-4   Measuring Chemical Properties of Urine: Glucose, Ketones, Protein, Blood, and pH

Tests for chemical properties of urine, which are a part of the routine urinalysis done by the laboratory, can be performed quickly at the bedside or in the house. Normally, glucose and ketones are not present in the urine, and the appearance of either element generally indicates that glucose is not effectively reaching the body's cells. When this screening test for the presence of glucose in the urine is positive, other tests (e.g., glucose tolerance) are used to determine the diagnosis of diabetes mellitus.

Urine testing for glucose and acetone has been used for many years to monitor glucose control by diet, exercise, and medication. The test is acceptable to clients because it is easily performed and causes no pain; however, it is being replaced by testing capillary blood, which is obtained by skin puncture of the fingertip (see Skill 43-12). This change is being made because capillary blood monitoring directly reflects current serum glucose levels and is not affected by the renal threshold for glucose or fluid volume. Sampling of serum glucose may identify hypoglycemia, which cannot be detected by urine testing.

Assessing the chemical properties of urine can be done by immersing a special chemically prepared strip of paper into a clean urine specimen or by combining drops of urine with chemically prepared tablets. The change in color of the strip or tablet indicates the presence of any of these substances.

DELEGATION CONSIDERATIONS

Assistive personnel instructed in performing the skill may obtain this specimen, perform the test, and report the results of the test. In addition, the nurse should:

* Instruct assistive personnel to report any odor, blood, or mucus in specimen

EQUIPMENT

❏ Specimen hat, bedside commode, bedpan, urinal, or pediatric potty-chair
❏ Watch with second hand or digital counter
❏ Clean disposable gloves (if person other than client tests urine)
   Reagent Strip Testing (Figure 43-4)
❏ Reagent test strip
❏ Test strip color chart

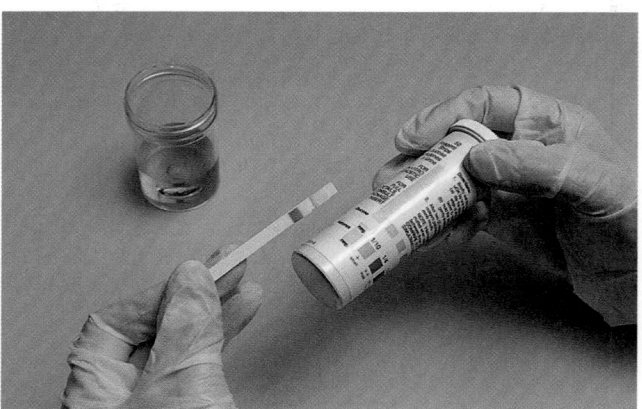

FIGURE **43-4** Testing urine using a reagent strip.

STEP	RATIONALE

ASSESSMENT

1. Determine rationale for physician request of this particular urine test.

2. Assess if client or family member performs urine testing at home or if there is need for client to learn skill.

3. Determine if physician has recommended specific type of reagent test for client to use.

4. Assess whether client, if diabetic, is familiar with double-voided specimen and uses technique regularly.

5. Assess type of medications client receives; check drug literature for effects on reagent strips.

6. Assess client for signs and symptoms of diabetes mellitus: polydipsia, polyuria, and polyphagia.

7. Assess client's ability to perform urine test.

Allows nurse to consider other significant assessments to make.

Client accustomed to testing own urine may prefer continuing to do so.

Variety of reagent strips permit fast, accurate monitoring of urine constituents.

A double-voided specimen is preferable for accuracy of glucose test (Pagana and Pagana, 2002). Clients often do not perceive importance of procedure.

Certain drug components create false-positive glucose readings.

Presence of these symptoms is often accompanied by glucosuria (Linton and others, 2000).

Determines level of instruction or assistance required from nurse. Diabetic clients may suffer from visual alterations or peripheral nerve damage that interfere with their ability to accurately perform test.

NURSING DIAGNOSES

* Acute or chronic confusion
* Deficient knowledge regarding urine testing procedure

* Noncompliance
* Readiness for enhanced knowledge

Related factors are individualized based on client's condition or needs.

STEP	RATIONALE

PLANNING

1. Expected outcomes following completion of procedure.
   - Client who requires daily or more frequent testing will be able to perform test independently.
   - Test results are negative for glucose, ketones, protein, and blood; pH is between 4.5 and 8.

   - Urine is not contaminated with feces or toilet tissue.

2. Offer client fluids to drink (if permitted) about 30 minutes before collecting urine.
3. Explain procedure to client and/or family member. Discuss reason for specimen collection, how client can assist, and fact that specimen must be free of feces and tissue.

Demonstrates learning and independence in own health maintenance.

Urine glucose is normally negligible and is reported as none. Ketones, protein, and blood are not normally found in urine (Malarkey and McMorrow, 2000).

Demonstrates client's ability to collect urine specimen correctly.

Enhances client's ability to void at requested times.

Client who understands procedure is more likely to cooperate and may be able to obtain specimen independently. Also prevents accidental disposal.

IMPLEMENTATION

1. Obtain double-voided specimen when testing urine for glucose:

   a. Ask client to collect random urine specimen and discard.

   b. Have client drink a glass of water.
   c. Have client collect another specimen 30 to 45 minutes later.

2. Apply disposable gloves.
3. Measure urine for glucose or ketones.
   a. Perform glucose/ketone reagent test strip test:
      (1) Immerse end of strip impregnated with chemical reagent into urine specimen.

      (2) Remove strip immediately from container, and tap it gently against container's side.
      (3) Hold strip in horizontal position.
      (4) Time for number of seconds specified on container, and compare color of strip with color chart (see Figure 43-4).

      (5) Dispose of reagent strip in trash.
   b. Use Multistix reagent test strip to assess for chemical properties of pH, protein, glucose, ketones, and/or blood simultaneously:
      (1) Immerse end of chemically impregnated test strip into urine.
      (2) Remove strip from container immediately, and tap it gently against side of container.

A fresh specimen should be used because stagnant urine that has been in bladder for several hours will not accurately reflect serum glucose level at testing (Pagana and Pagana, 1999).

Stagnant urine stored in bladder overnight or for long periods does not reveal amount of glucose and ketones excreted by kidney at time of testing.

Facilitates ability to void again within short time period.

Fresh specimen will provide accurate test measurements. If client is catheterized, single fresh specimen from catheter is adequate.

Reduces transmission of microorganisms.

Strip test provides reliable measure of glucose and ketones.

Immersion exposes reagent to urine constituents. Although Diastix, Clinistix, and Tes-Tape all measure quantity of glucose in urine, measurement scales are not interchangeable.

Excess urine can dilute reagents.

Prevents possible mixing of chemical reagents.

Accurate interpretation of results depends on precise timing: Ketostix, 15 seconds; Clinistix, 10 seconds; Diastix, 30 seconds; Tes-Tape, 60 seconds. Compare darkest part of tape with color chart. If results exceed 0.5%, wait another 60 seconds and compare with second color chart.

Maintains neat environment and reduces spread of infection.

Eliminates need for test described above. Presence of these elements may indicate renal or other systemic diseases.

Exposes reagent to urine.

Excess urine can dilute reagents.

STEP	RATIONALE
(3) Hold strip in horizontal position.	Prevents possible mixing of chemical reagents.
(4) Time for number of seconds specified on container, and compare color of strip with color chart (Table 43-1).	Accurate interpretation of results depends on precise timing.

TABLE 43-1 COLOR CHART FOR REAGENT STRIP

TEST	WHEN TO READ	RANGE OF RESULTS
pH	Anytime	5-9
Protein	Anytime	(1) to + 4
		(72,000 mg/100 ml)
Glucose	10 seconds (qualitative)	(−) to + 4
	30 seconds (quantitative)	(−) to + 4 (270)
Ketones	15 seconds	(−) to + 3 (large)
Blood	25 seconds	(−) to + 3 (large)

4. Remove and discard gloves; perform hand hygiene.	Reduces transmission of microorganisms.
5. When appropriate, discuss test results with client.	Client should participate in care to improve understanding and compliance.

EVALUATION

1. If client is to be responsible for self-testing, have client demonstrate proficiency.	Return demonstration is best evidence of proficiency.
2. Note presence of blood, protein, glucose, or ketones in urine.	None of these substances should be in urine; pH should be slightly acidic (average, 6; normal, 4.5 to 8).
3. Observe that sample is not contaminated with feces or toilet tissue.	May affect accuracy of measurement.

Recording and Reporting

- Record results immediately in nurses' notes or glucose testing flow sheet.
- If client is diabetic, nurse should determine if insulin should be given. If capillary glucose monitoring is impossible, urinary glucose level may be measured to determine dietary needs and insulin requirements (Malarkey and McMorrow, 2000).
- Have client in home setting record results of test on flow sheet. Encourage client to take samples at same time each day.
- Diabetic flow sheets often require charting of medications and amount of urine, as well as results of urine tests.

Unexpected Outcomes	Related Interventions
1. Client or family member is unable to perform urine test correctly.	• Reinforce need for regular monitoring.
	• Repeat teaching as needed; include return demonstration.
2. Test results are positive for glucose, ketones, protein, blood, and/or alterations in pH.	• Continue to monitor client.
	• Report findings to physician.
	• Follow new orders.

Teaching Considerations

- Instruct client about proper method for collecting random urine sample.
- Teach client to check expiration date on bottle of test strips.
- Teach clients to close bottles tightly after removing reagent strips to prevent them from absorbing moisture and altering future results.
- Explain rationale for double-voided specimen, and seek appropriate client feedback.
- Explain relationship of urinary findings of glucose with blood glucose when indicated.
- Discuss possible reasons for finding acetone, blood, and protein in urine.
- Discuss relationship of urinary pH to urinary tract infection and formation of renal calculi when appropriate.
- Have client return demonstrations on urine testing until client uses correct technique.
- Discuss client's plans for testing urine at home, if indicated.

Pediatric Considerations

- School-age children can learn to test urine accurately, but parents should continue to provide backup.
- Parents are usually very helpful in guiding young children through procedure.

Gerontological Considerations

- Older adults may have difficulty seeing color chart.
- Older adults with musculoskeletal alterations may not have fine motor coordination necessary to obtain samples for specimen collection.
- In older adults, urine testing is considered unreliable because of age-related renal function changes (Lueckenotte, 2000).

Home Care Considerations

- Most kits sold in drug stores contain all equipment necessary for testing urine except specimen container.
- Clients at home may prefer to use large clock with second hand for timing urine tests.
- Reagent strip method is most frequently used at home (Malarkey and McMorrow, 2000).

SKILL 43-5 Measuring Occult Blood in Stool

A common fecal laboratory test is the guaiac test for fecal occult blood. Fecal occult blood testing detects blood in the stool and is useful as a colorectal cancer screening test because cancers and adenomatous polyps bleed more than normal mucosa. The test measures microscopic amounts of blood in the feces. Normally a person loses small amounts of blood daily in the feces as a result of minor abrasions of the nasopharyngeal or oral mucosa. If greater than 50 ml of blood enters the feces from the upper gastrointestinal tract, the blood can be visualized as melena (darkening of feces). The guaiac test helps to reveal blood that is visually undetectable.

The test is a useful diagnostic tool for conditions such as colon cancer, upper gastrointestinal ulcers, and localized gastric parasitic infections or intestinal irritation. The amount of bleeding increases with the size of the polyp and stage of cancer. People with small polyps (less than 1 cm in diameter) bleed scarcely more than those without polyps.

The test is easy to perform. Clients are often instructed in how to collect fecal specimens for the test in the home. Only a small amount of stool is needed to perform the test successfully. The most common guaiac tests are the Hemoccult slides and the Hematest tablets.

DELEGATION CONSIDERATIONS

Assistive personnel may obtain and test stool for occult blood. The nurse should:

- Instruct assistive personnel to report immediately if blood is detected and not to discard stool from a positive test, so that the nurse may repeat the testing

EQUIPMENT

- ❏ Paper towel
- ❏ Disposable gloves
- ❏ Wooden applicator
  Hemoccult Test (Figure 43-5)
- ❏ Cardboard Hemoccult slide
- ❏ Hemoccult developing solution
  Hematest
- ❏ Hematest tablets (tablets must be protected from moisture, heat, and light)
- ❏ Guaiac paper (reagent tablet produces blue reaction on guaiac paper if fecal smear contains blood)
- ❏ Sink with running water

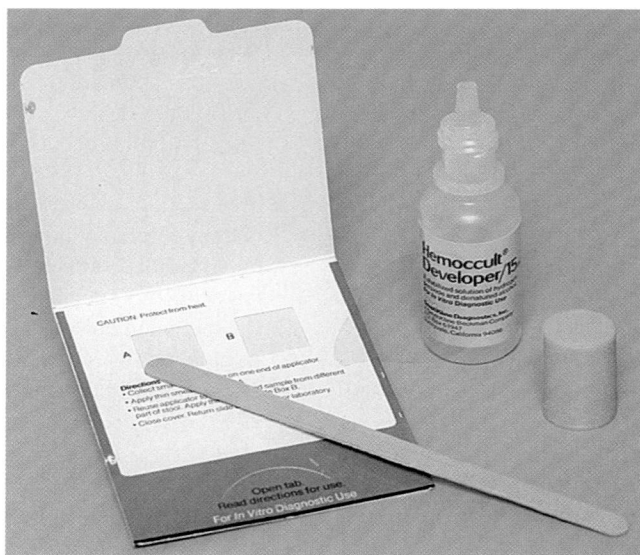

FIGURE **43-5** Hemoccult testing kit for measuring occult blood.

STEP	RATIONALE

ASSESSMENT

1. Assess client's or family members' understanding of need for stool test.

2. Assess client's ability to cooperate with procedure and collect specimen.

3. Assess client's medical history for bleeding, gastrointestinal disorder, or hemorrhoids.

4. Obtain client's medication history. Note drugs that can cause gastrointestinal mucosal bleeding.

5. Refer to physician's orders for medication or dietary modifications or restrictions before test.

Provides nurse with information on which to base necessary health teaching.

To avoid embarrassment, clients often prefer to collect own stool specimen. Some clients require assistance.

Nurse can institute routine screening. Hemorrhoids can cause bleeding that may be misinterpreted as upper gastrointestinal bleeding.

Anticoagulants increase risk of bleeding in gastrointestinal tract, even from minor trauma to mucosa. Long-term use of steroids, nonsteroidal antiinflammatory drugs (NSAIDs), and acetylsalicylic acid (aspirin) can irritate mucosa.

Specimens will be positive if contaminated by menstrual blood or hemorrhoidal blood or povidone-iodine. Diets rich in meats, green leafy vegetables, poultry, and fish may produce false-positive results. Drugs that affect results include alcohol, antiinflammatory agents, ascorbic acid (vitamin C), and nonsteroidal agents (Marx, 2002).

NURSING DIAGNOSES

- Anxiety
- Bowel incontinence
- Constipation

- Diarrhea
- Deficient knowledge regarding collection and testing of stool specimen

Related factors are individualized based on client's condition or needs.

PLANNING

1. Expected outcomes following completion of procedure:
   - Test for occult blood is negative.

Client has only small amount of blood in feces because of normal nasopharyngeal and oral mucosa abrasions.

STEP	RATIONALE

- Client will discuss purpose and benefits of testing stool for blood.

Validates learning.

2. Explain procedure to client and/or family member. Discuss reason for specimen collection and how client can assist. Explain that feces must be free of urine and tissue.

Client who understands procedure is more likely to cooperate and may be able to obtain specimen independently. Also prevents accidental disposal of specimen.

3. Arrange for any needed dietary or medication restrictions.

Ensures accuracy of test results.

■ IMPLEMENTATION

1. Perform hand hygiene, and apply clean disposable gloves.

Reduces transmission of microorganisms.

2. Obtain uncontaminated stool specimen

Specimen is obtained in clean, dry container and not contaminated with urine, water, or toilet tissue.

- *Critical Decision Point*
  Observe fecal specimen. If frank red blood is observed within stool itself, report these findings immediately.

3. Use tip of wooden applicator to obtain small portion of feces.

Small specimen is sufficient for measuring blood content.

4. Measure for occult blood.
   a. Perform Hemoccult slide test:
      (1) Open flap of slide, and apply thin smear of stool on paper in first box.

Guaiac paper inside box is sensitive to fecal blood content.

      (2) Obtain second fecal specimen from different portion of stool, and apply thinly to slide's second box (see illustration).

Occult blood from upper gastrointestinal tract is not always equally dispersed throughout stool.
Findings of occult blood are more conclusive for gastrointestinal bleeding when entire specimen is found to contain blood.

      (3) Close slide cover, and turn slide over to reverse side. Open cardboard flap, and apply 2 drops of Hemoccult developing solution on each box of guaiac paper (see illustration).

Developing solution penetrates underlying fecal specimen. Blood is indicated by change in color of guaiac paper.

      (4) Read results of test after 30 to 60 seconds. Note color changes.

Bluish discoloration indicates occult blood (guaiac positive). No change in color of guaiac paper indicates negative results.

      (5) Dispose of test slide in proper receptacle.

Reduces transfer of microorganisms.

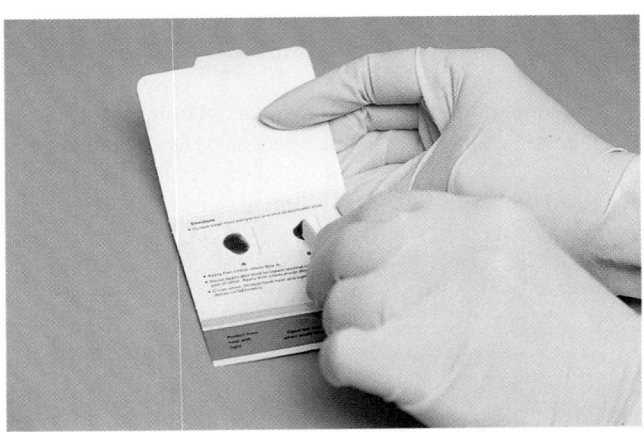

STEP **4a(2)** Application of stool specimen.

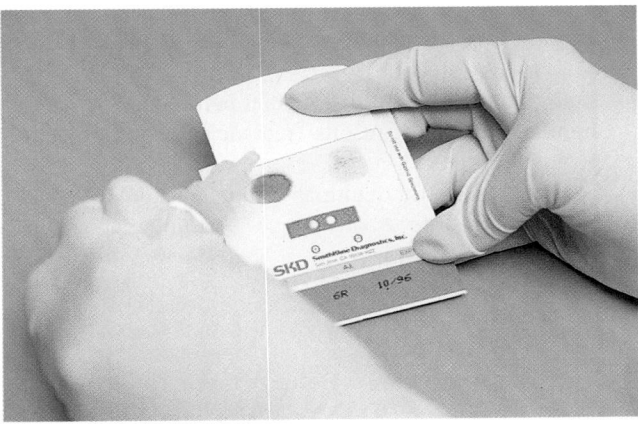

STEP **4a(3)** Application of solution.

STEP	RATIONALE
b. Perform test using Hematest tablets:	
(1) Place stool on guaiac paper and Hematest tablet on top of stool specimen.	Tablet contains solid form of developing solution.
(2) Apply 2 to 3 drops of tap water to tablet, allowing water to flow onto guaiac paper.	Tap water dissolves Hematest tablet and thus dispenses developing solution over specimen and guaiac paper.
(3) Observe color of guaiac paper within 2 minutes.	Bluish discoloration is guaiac positive. Do not read color after 2 minutes. False findings may occur.
(4) Dispose of tablet and paper in proper receptacle.	Reduces transmission of microorganisms.
(5) Wrap wooden applicator in paper towel, and dispose in proper receptacle.	Reduces transmission of microorganisms.
(6) Perform hand hygiene after removing and discarding gloves.	Reduces spread of infection.

EVALUATION

1. Ask client to explain collection procedure.	Documents level of learning.
2. Note color changes in guaiac paper.	Reveals blood in feces.

• *Critical Decision Point*
Single positive test result does not confirm bleeding or indicate colorectal cancer. For confirmed positive results, test must be repeated at least three times while client is on meat-free, high-residue diet. More in-depth diagnosis is needed with positive results.

3. Note character of stool specimen.	Certain abnormal constituents of stool may be visible.

Recording and Reporting

- Record results of test in nurses' notes.
- Record any unusual characteristics of stool in nurses' notes
- Report positive test results to physician.

Unexpected Outcomes	Related Interventions
1. Test for occult blood is positive.	• Continue to monitor client. • Notify physician.

Teaching Considerations

- Explain rationale regarding why client should obtain specimens from two different areas of stool specimen.
- If client has been on long-term steroid or anticoagulant drug therapy, explain how these drugs may result in occult blood in stools.
- If physician orders meat-free diet before test, explain its significance to test results (red meats can cause false-positive results).
- Discuss reason for multiple testing of stool for occult blood. Clients are usually requested to obtain specimen every day for 3 days.

Pediatric Considerations

- Children of school age and older are often very curious and may ask many questions about test. Questions should be answered honestly and at child's level of understanding. Allow child to watch, if desired, while test is performed.
- Encourage active participation in the school-age child (e.g., handling equipment, opening packages) (Hockenberry and others, 2003).
- Testing reagent is often poisonous so must be kept out of reach of the small child.

Gerontological Considerations

- If serial fecal specimens are required, older adult may need assistance from family member or friend.

Home Care Considerations

- Many clients are instructed to collect specimens at home and return them to clinic or physician's office.
- Clients who collect specimen at home are asked to prepare slide with feces, close cardboard slide, and return it to office or clinic.

- Alert client that presence of toilet bowl cleaner, disinfectant, or deodorizer will interfere with the results (Malarkey and McMorrow, 2000).

SKILL 43-6 Measuring Occult Blood in Gastric Secretions (Gastroccult)

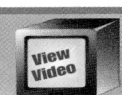

Analysis of gastric secretions or emesis can detect blood that is not always visible. Gastroccult testing could help to reveal bleeding in the esophagus or stomach. The test can verify the presence of blood when red or black coloration of the gastric contents is noted or when the gastric contents or emesis has the appearance of coffee grounds. The test measures microscopic amounts of blood in the gastric secretions. The guaiac test helps to reveal blood that is visually undetectable. The test is a useful diagnostic tool for conditions such as upper gastrointestinal ulcers or bleeding. The test is easy to perform. Clients are often instructed in how to test emesis in the home.

DELEGATION CONSIDERATIONS

This skill should not be delegated to assistive personnel if the specimen is collected from a nasogastric (NG) or nasoenteral tube. Assistive personnel can be delegated to perform the test on emesis. The nurse should:

- Instruct assistive personnel to report immediately if blood is detected in emesis.

EQUIPMENT

- ❑ Facial tissues
- ❑ Emesis basin
- ❑ Wooden applicator or 3-ml syringe
- ❑ 60-ml bulb or catheter tip syringe
- ❑ Gastroccult test cardboard slide
- ❑ Gastroccult developing solution

STEP	RATIONALE

ASSESSMENT

1. Assess client's or family members' understanding of need for test.
2. Assess client's medical history for bleeding or gastrointestinal disorders.
3. Obtain client's medication history. Note drugs that can cause gastrointestinal mucosal bleeding.

Provides nurse with information on which to base necessary health teaching.
Nurse can institute routine screening.

Anticoagulants increase risk of bleeding in gastrointestinal tract, even from minor trauma to mucosa. Long-term use of steroids, NSAIDs, and acetylsalicylic acid (aspirin) can irritate mucosa.

NURSING DIAGNOSES

- Anxiety
- Fear

- Deficient knowledge regarding occult blood testing.

Related factors are individualized based on client's condition or needs.

PLANNING

1. Expected outcomes following completion of procedure:
   - Test for occult blood is negative.
   - Client will discuss purpose and benefits of testing gastric contents for blood.

Client has only small amount of blood in gastric secretions. Validates learning.

STEP	RATIONALE

2. Explain procedure to client and/or family member. Discuss reason for specimen collection.

Client who understands procedure is more likely to be less anxious.

IMPLEMENTATION

1. Perform hand hygiene.

Reduces transmission of microorganisms.

2. Obtain specimen by aspirating 5 ml of fluid from nasogastric or nasoenteral tube using a bulb or catheter tip syringe or obtain 5 ml of emesis.

Aim is to test gastric contents.

• *Critical Decision Point*

Observe specimen. If frank red blood is observed or coffee-ground material is seen, report these findings immediately.

3. Use tip of wooden applicator to obtain small portion of secretions obtained from the enteral tubes or emesis collection.

Small specimen is sufficient for measuring blood content.

4. Measure for occult blood.
   a. Perform Gastroccult slide test:
      (1) Using applicator or syringe, apply 1 drop of gastric sample to Gastroccult blood test slide.

Sample must cover test paper for test reaction to occur.

      (2) Apply 2 drops of commercial developer solution over sample and 1 drop between positive and negative performance monitors. (see illustration)
      (3) Verify that performance monitor turns blue in 30 seconds, which indicates slide is working properly.
      (4) Dispose of test slide, wooden applicator, and syringe in proper receptacle.

Reduces spread of infection.

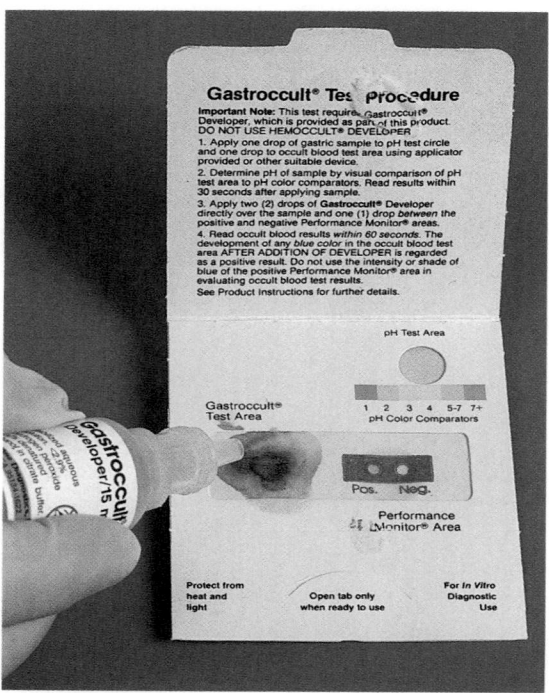

STEP **4a(2)** Apply developing solution to Gastroccult test area.

STEP	RATIONALE

EVALUATION

1. Ask client to explain reason for procedure.
2. Note color changes in guaiac paper.
3. Note character of gastric secretions.

Validates level of understanding.
Reveals blood in gastric secretions.
Blood may be visible or coffee-ground material denoting blood may be observed.

Recording and Reporting

- Record results of test in nurses' notes.
- Record any unusual characteristics of gastric contents in nurses' notes.
- Report positive test results to physician.

Unexpected Outcomes	Related Interventions
1. Test for occult blood is positive.	• Continue to monitor client. • Notify physician.

Teaching Considerations

- Explain rationale regarding why specimen is being obtained.
- If client has been on long-term steroid or anticoagulant drug therapy, explain how these drugs may result in occult blood.

Pediatric Considerations

- Children of school age and older are often very curious and may ask many questions about test. Questions should be answered honestly and at child's level of understanding. Allow child to watch, if desired, while test is performed.

- Encourage active participation in the school-age child (e.g., handling equipment, opening packages) (Hockenberry and others, 2003).

Gerontological Considerations

- Reassurance may be needed to reinforce that the specimen collection procedure is not uncomfortable if being obtained from an NG or nasoenteral tube.

Home Care Considerations

- Many clients are instructed to perform the Gastroccult test on emesis.

SKILL 43-7 Collecting Nose and Throat Specimens for Culture

Clients frequently have signs or symptoms of upper respiratory or sinus infections. A nose or throat culture specimen is a simple diagnostic tool for determining the nature of the client's problem. The laboratory personnel place the specimen on a culture medium to determine if pathogenic organisms will grow.

This specimen collection can cause discomfort to sensitive mucosal membranes. Likewise, collection of a throat culture may cause gagging. Clients should clearly understand how each specimen is to be collected to minimize anxiety or discomfort.

DELEGATION CONSIDERATIONS

This skill should not be delegated to assistive personnel.

EQUIPMENT

❑ Two sterile swabs in sterile culture tubes (flexible wire swab with cotton tip may be used for nose cultures)
❑ Nasal speculum (optional)

❑ Emesis basin or clean container (optional)
❑ Tongue blades
❑ Penlight
❑ Completed identification labels
❑ Completed laboratory requisition (date, time, name of test, source of culture)
❑ Facial tissues
❑ Clean disposable gloves

STEP	RATIONALE

ASSESSMENT

1. Assess client's understanding of purpose of procedure and ability to cooperate. Nurse may need assistance to obtain throat cultures from confused, combative, or unconscious clients.

Provides basis to determine need for health teaching and need for assistance.

2. Assess condition of and drainage from nasal mucosa and sinuses.

Reveals physical signs that may indicate infection or allergic irritation. Clear drainage usually indicates allergy. Yellow, green, or brown drainage usually indicates infection.

3. Determine if client has experienced postnasal drip, sinus headache or tenderness, nasal congestion, or sore throat.

Symptoms help reveal nature of problem.

4. Assess condition of posterior pharynx.

Local inflammation or lesions of pharynx may be revealed.

• *Critical Decision Point*

Pay particular attention to areas of inflammation or purulent drainage. Identification of inflamed or purulent areas allows nurse to swab those sites quickly.

5. Assess client for systemic signs of infection: fever, chills, and/or fatigue.

Infection originating within nasopharynx can become systemic, requiring antibiotic therapy.

6. Review physician's orders to determine if nose, throat, or both cultures are needed.

Prevents exposing client to unnecessary discomfort of repeated cultures.

NURSING DIAGNOSES

• Risk for infection
• Deficient knowledge regarding specimen collection
• Pain (acute or chronic)

Related factors are individualized based on client's condition or needs.

PLANNING

1. Expected outcomes following completion of procedure:
   • There is no bacterial growth in specimens.
   • Client does not experience bleeding of nasal mucosa.
   • Specimen is not contaminated.
   • Client will discuss purpose of nose and throat cultures.

Absence of infection.
Procedure is atraumatic.
Evidenced by results of laboratory analysis.
Validates learning.

2. Plan to do culture before mealtime or at least 1 hour after eating.

Because gagging may be induced by procedure, incidence of vomiting is decreased.

3. Explain procedure to client and/or family member. Discuss reason for specimen collection and how client can assist.

Understanding of procedure usually decreases anxiety and promotes cooperation.

4. Explain that client may have tickling sensation or gag during swabbing of throat. Nasal swab may create urge to sneeze. Both procedures require only a few seconds.

May help client to relax.

STEP	RATIONALE

IMPLEMENTATION

1. Ask client to sit erect in bed or chair facing nurse. Acutely ill client or young child may lie back against bed with head of bed raised to 45-degree angle.

Provides easy access to nasal or oral structures.

2. Have swab in tube ready for use. Nurse may wish to loosen top so that swab can be removed easily.

Nurse should be able to grasp swab easily without danger of contaminating it. Most commercially prepared tubes have tops that fit securely over end of swab, which allows nurse to touch outer tops without contaminating swab stick.

3. Collect throat culture:
   a. Perform hand hygiene, and put on gloves.
   b. Instruct client to tilt head backward. For clients in bed, place pillow behind shoulders.
   c. Ask client to open mouth and say "ah."

Reduces transmission of microorganisms.
Facilitates visualization of pharynx.

Permits exposure of pharynx, relaxes throat muscles, and minimizes gag reflex.

- ### *Critical Decision Point*
  If pharynx is not visualized, depress tongue with tongue blade and note inflamed areas of pharynx or tonsils. Depress anterior third of tongue only. (Illuminate with penlight as needed.) Area to be swabbed should be clearly visualized. Placement of tongue blade along back of tongue more likely initiates gag reflex. If client gags, remove tongue blade and allow client to relax before reinserting. Place pressure only on anterior third of tongue.

   d. Insert swab without touching lips, teeth, tongue, cheeks, or uvula.
   e. Gently but quickly swab tonsillar area side to side, making contact with inflamed or purulent sites (see illustration).
   f. Carefully withdraw swab without striking oral structures. Immediately place swab in culture tube. Place gauze around ampule, and crush ampule at bottom of tube. Push tip of swab into liquid medium (see illustration).

Poor technique will cause a false-positive result (Malarkey and McMorrow, 2000).
These areas contain most microorganisms.

Retains microorganisms within culture tube. Mixing swab tip with culture medium ensures life of bacteria for testing.

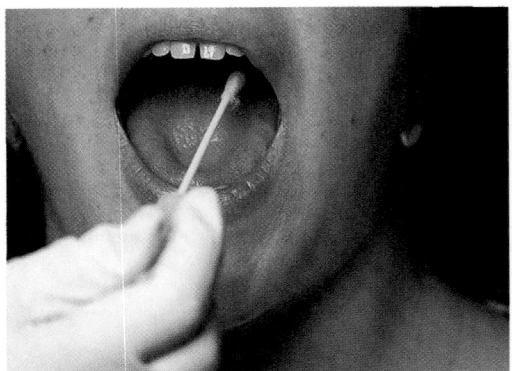

STEP 3e Obtaining tonsillar swab.

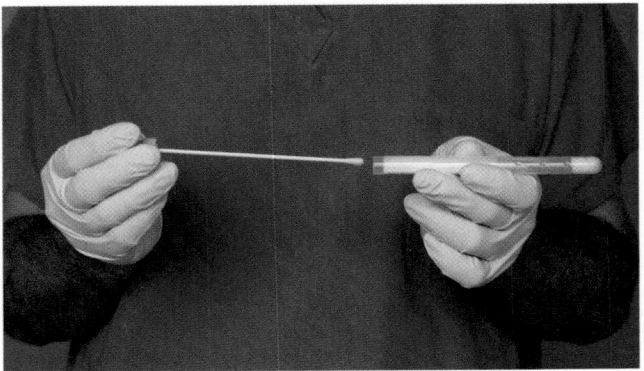

STEP 3f Activating culture tube.

STEP	RATIONALE
g. Place top on culture tube securely.	Prevents contamination from microorganisms.
h. Discard tongue depressor into trash; remove gloves and discard.	Reduces transmission of microorganisms.
4. Collect nose culture:	
a. Perform hand hygiene, and put on gloves.	Reduces transmission of microorganisms.
b. Encourage client to blow nose, and check nostrils for patency with penlight.	Clears nasal passages of mucus containing resident bacteria.

- **Critical Decision Point**

Ask client to alternatively occlude each nostril and exhale. Determines nostril with greater patency, from which specimen will be collected.

c. Ask client to tilt head back. Clients in bed should have pillow behind shoulders.	Facilitates visualization of nasal septum and sinuses (Malarkey and McMorrow, 2000).
d. Gently insert nasal speculum in one nostril (optional).	Allows retraction of mucosa for easier swab insertion.
e. Carefully pass swab through center of speculum (if used) into nostril until it reaches that portion of mucosa that is inflamed or containing exudate. Rotate swab quickly.	Swab should remain sterile until it reaches area to be cultured. Rotating swab covers all surfaces where exudate is present.
f. Remove swab without touching sides of speculum.	Prevents contamination of swab by resident bacteria.
g. Carefully remove nasal speculum (if used), and place in basin. Offer client facial tissue.	Minimizes period of time client will experience discomfort.
h. Insert swab into culture tube. Crush ampule at bottom of tube, and push tip of swab into liquid medium.	Retains microorganisms within culture tube. Mixing swab tip with culture medium ensures life of bacteria for testing.
i. Place top on tube securely.	Prevents contamination from microorganisms.
j. Remove gloves, discard, and perform hand hygiene.	Reduces transmission of microorganisms.
5. Collection of nasopharyngeal culture:	
a. Follow step 4, a through j, except use a special swab on a flexible wire that can be flexed downward to reach nasopharynx via nose.	Only this specially designed swab allows access to difficult-to-reach nasopharyngeal area.

- **Critical Decision Point**

This swab must advance into nasopharynx to ensure that culture has been obtained correctly.

6. Securely attach properly completed identification label and laboratory requisition to culture tube. Agency policy may dictate type of information to place on label. Note on laboratory requisition if client is taking antibiotic or if specific organism is suspected (e.g., *Bordetella pertussis*).	Incorrect identification of specimen could result in diagnostic or therapeutic errors.
7. Send specimen to laboratory immediately, or refrigerate.	Fresh specimen provides most accurate test results.

EVALUATION

1. Check laboratory record for results of culture test.	Results reveal type of organisms in nose or pharynx and antibiotics most likely to be effective.

Recording and Reporting

- Record specimen collection, date, time, and disposition in nurses' notes.
- Describe appearance of nasal and oral mucosal structures in nurses' notes.
- Report unusual test results to physician.

Unexpected Outcomes	Related Interventions
1. Nose and throat cultures reveal bacterial growth.	• Notify physician of findings. • Administer medications as ordered.
2. Client experiences minor nasal bleeding.	• Apply mild pressure and ice pack over bridge of nose. • Notify physician of client's condition.
3. Specimen is contaminated.	• Repeat specimen collection.

Teaching Considerations

- Clients should be instructed that procedure is painless but the gag reflex is commonly stimulated during procedure.
- Discuss client's role in collecting specimen.
- Explain how and why specimen is being obtained.
- Discuss relationship between culture results and medication.
- Discuss reason for time delay in receiving culture results.

Pediatric Considerations

- Allowing young children to visualize and examine speculum decreases their fear of it.
- Immobilization of child's head and arms is important when obtaining nose or throat culture and should be done in firm, gentle, kind manner. Ask another nurse to assist, if necessary.
- Ask parents to act as coach with their child.

- Showing tongue blade and penlight to child and demonstrating how to say "ah" helps to decrease anxiety.
- School-age child will be more cooperative if given opportunity to ask questions about procedure and results.
- Respiratory syncytial virus (RSV) is detected directly in respiratory secretions, usually obtained by nasopharyngeal aspiration (Hockenberry and others, 2003).
- Throat cultures should not be attempted if acute epiglottitis is suspected because trauma from swab might cause increase in edema and resulting occlusion of airway (Hockenberry and others, 2003).

Gerontological Considerations

- Older adults may need assistance in keeping mouth open to obtain specimen.
- In confused clients, assistive personnel may be necessary to hold client's hands while sample is being obtained.

SKILL 43-8   Obtaining Vaginal or Urethral Discharge Specimens

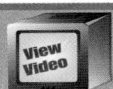

Normally there is minimal discharge from the vagina or urethra. Poor hygiene practices may cause an accumulation of discharge. However, if a client develops an increased amount of discharge or if there is a change in the character of discharge from the vagina or urethra, medical follow-up is necessary.

Drainage from the vagina or urethra is normally thin, nonpurulent, whitish or clear, and small in amount. A woman will have bloody discharge during menstruation. A newborn infant may have bloody discharge from the vagina for 2 to 4 weeks after birth because of the abrupt decrease in maternal hormones at birth.

The clients most commonly requiring cultures of vaginal or urethral discharge have signs and symptoms of sexually transmitted disease or urinary tract infection. Clients suspected of having a sexually transmitted disease may be embarrassed by their condition. The nurse must show respect and understanding toward the client. If the client undergoes a complete diagnostic workup, the many questions can be exhausting and may cause anxiety. When collecting vaginal or urethral specimens, the nurse should work quickly and calmly, maintaining the client's privacy at all times.

DELEGATION CONSIDERATIONS

The skill of obtaining vaginal and urethral discharge culture samples should not be delegated to assistive personnel.

EQUIPMENT

❑ Sterile swab in sterile culture tube (commercially available culture tubes have swab and tube with ampule containing special transport medium)

❑ Sheet, blanket, or paper drape
❑ Clean disposable gloves
❑ Penlight or gooseneck lamp
❑ Completed identification labels
❑ Completed laboratory requisition (date, time, name of test, type of culture)

STEP	RATIONALE

ASSESSMENT

1. Assess understanding of need for culture and ability to cooperate with procedure.

2. Perform hand hygiene and apply gloves. Assess condition of external genitalia. Observe urethra, meatus, and vaginal orifice for redness, swelling, tenderness, and discharge that is whitish, mucoid, and purulent.

3. Ask client if dysuria, localized pruritus of genitalia, or lower abdominal pain have been experienced.

4. If symptoms suggest sexually transmitted disease, record sexual history of client.

5. Refer to physician's order to determine if culture is to be vaginal or urethral.

Provides nurse with information on which to base necessary health teaching.
Assessment findings and specimen test results reveal nature of problem.

Symptoms of urinary tract or vaginal infection.

Determine sexual activity and if there has been sexual contact with a person known to have a sexually transmitted disease (Linton and others, 2000). If culture results are positive, tell client to receive treatment and to have sexual partners evaluated.
Client may require one or both types of cultures.

NURSING DIAGNOSES

• Anxiety
• Risk for infection

• Deficient knowledge regarding specimen collection
• Acute pain

Related factors are individualized based on client's condition or needs.

PLANNING

1. Expected outcomes following completion of procedure.
   • Specimen is not contaminated.

   • Vaginal or urethral cultures do not reveal growth of microorganisms.

2. Explain procedure to client and/or family member. Discuss reason for specimen collection and how client can assist. Instruct female client not to douche before culture is obtained.

3. Maintain nonjudgmental attitude while obtaining data.

Results on laboratory test can reveal whether skin cells or mucosal cells have contaminated specimen.
Evidence of absence of infection.

Client who understands procedure is less anxious and more likely to cooperate. Douching of vaginal canal would remove discharge containing pathogens.

Demonstrates respect for client.

IMPLEMENTATION

1. Perform hand hygiene.

2. Draw bedside curtains, or close room door. Place "Do Not Enter" sign on door (if available).

3. Assist client to proper position, raise gown, and drape body parts to be exposed:
   a. *Female:* Dorsal recumbent position with sheet draped over each leg and genitalia.
   b. *Male:* Sit on chair or bed or lie supine with sheet draped across lower trunk and genitalia.

Reduces transmission of microorganisms.
Provides privacy for client and demonstrates nurse's respect for client's well-being.
Provides easy access to perineal area. Draping minimizes exposure of body parts, minimizing anxiety.

STEP	RATIONALE
4. Apply clean disposable gloves.	Prevents contamination of nurse's hands from discharge.
5. Direct light source onto perineum (may not be needed for male client).	Allows better visualization of urethral or vaginal structures.
6. Open culture tube, and hold swab in dominant hand.	Provides for easier manipulation of swab during culture collection.
7. Instruct client to slowly deep breathe.	Helps client to relax. Tensing of muscles around pelvic floor may cause discomfort during swabbing.

8. Obtain necessary specimens:

   a. Female

(1) With nondominant hand, fully separate labia to expose vaginal orifice.	Exposes perineum and ensures specimen is of vaginal discharge.
(2) Touch tip of swab into discharge pool, being careful not to touch skin or mucosa along perineum or vaginal canal. If no discharge is visible, gently insert swabs 1 to 2.5 cm ($\frac{1}{2}$ to 1 inch) into vaginal orifice and rotate before removal.	Discharge contains the greatest concentration of microorganisms.
(3) To expose urethral meatus, use nondominant hand to pull gently on labia minora upward and back.	Allows better visualization of urethral orifice.
(4) Use clean swab, and gently apply to tip of meatus where discharge is visible. Avoid touching labia.	Discharge contains greatest concentration of microorganisms.

- **Critical Decision Point**

   If discharge near vagina appears different from discharge along perineum, collect separate specimens from each area because if there are two organisms present, they could be cross contaminated on a single swab.

   b. Male

(1) Hold client's penis near tip with nondominant hand; if male is uncircumcised, gently retract foreskin.	Provides clear exposure of urethral meatus.
(2) Use dominant hand to hold swab. Apply gently to area of discharge at urinary meatus.	Discharge contains greatest number of microorganisms.
(3) If no discharge is apparent, physician may order swab to be introduced into urinary meatus. Hold male genitalia gently.	Excess manipulation can cause erection.
(4) Return foreskin to natural position.	Tightening of foreskin around shaft of penis can cause localized discomfort and edema and potential necrosis.

STEP	RATIONALE
9. Return each swab to culture tube, and secure top.	Retains microorganisms within tube.
10. Remove and discard gloves.	Reduces spread of microorganisms.
11. If using commercial culture tube, wrap ampule with gauze to prevent injury to nurse's fingers while crushing. Immediately squeeze end of tube to crush ampule (see Skill 43-7, Implementation, step 3f). Push tip of swab into fluid medium.	Medium supports life of microorganisms until culture is obtained.
12. Label each culture tube with identification label, and affix completed requisition.	Incorrect specimen identification could lead to diagnostic or therapeutic error.
13. Send specimen immediately to laboratory, or refrigerate.	Bacteria multiply quickly; specimen should be analyzed quickly for accurate results.
14. Assist client to comfortable position, replace gown, and remove drape.	Reinforces client's sense of self-esteem.
15. Perform hand hygiene.	Reduces transmission of microorganisms.

STEP	RATIONALE

■ EVALUATION

1. Review laboratory results for evidence of pathogens.

   Results will reveal type of organisms present. Certain organisms are common to vaginal tract. Urethra should be free of microorganisms.

2. Continue to monitor whether discharge is present, and if so, observe color and amount.

   Characteristics of discharge can indicate specific type of infection.

3. Observe specimen for presence of feces.

   If feces are observed, obtain another specimen.

Recording and Reporting

- In nurses' notes record types of cultures obtained and date and time sent to laboratory.
- Describe character of discharge and appearance of vaginal orifice or urethral meatus.
- Report laboratory results to nurse in charge or physician.

Unexpected Outcomes	Related Interventions
1. Vaginal or urethral cultures reveal growth of pathogenic microorganisms.	• Notify physician of findings, and follow new orders. • Continue to monitor client.
2. Specimen is contaminated with epidermal cells.	• Repeat specimen collection.

Teaching Considerations

- Discuss symptoms of vaginal or urethral infection with client as appropriate.
- Explain relationship between genital discomfort and infection of vaginal or urinary tract.
- Explain time required to obtain results of culture.
- Discuss sexuality and safe sexual practices with client if appropriate.
- Clients with urethral or vaginal discharge may require instruction about perineal hygiene measures.
- If topical treatments (e.g., suppositories) are ordered, instruct client in proper administration of medication (see Chapter 20).

Pediatric Considerations

- Young child will probably desire parents' presence, whereas adolescent usually will not.
- In collection from infant or young child, another nurse can assist with specimen by gently holding child's legs apart in froglike position. Have parent present to encourage cooperation.
- Parents should understand that obtaining specimen would not affect virginity of child.
- Be sensitive to cultural variations and beliefs pertaining to genitalia (i.e., female circumcisions).
- In addition to collecting the specimen on adolescent clients, this may also open up the possibility of discussions related to sexuality in which they may have questions, but are not comfortable opening discussions on their own.

Gerontological Considerations

- When obtaining sample from older adult, assist client to comfortable position.
- Clear explanation regarding importance of obtaining sample is extremely helpful to alleviate or diminish anxiety and to gain cooperation.

SKILL 43-9 Collecting Sputum Specimens

Sputum is produced by cells lining the respiratory tract. Although production is minimal in the healthy state, disease states can increase the amount or change the character of sputum. Examination of sputum may aid in the diagnosis and treatment of several conditions ranging from simple bronchitis to lung cancer.

Suctioning may be indicated to collect sputum from the client who is unable to spontaneously produce a sample for laboratory analysis. Suctioning may provoke violent coughing, which can cause vomiting and aspiration of stomach contents, and induces constriction of pharyngeal, laryngeal, and bronchial muscles. In addition, suctioning may cause di-

rect stimulation of vagal nerve fibers in the airway and may cause cardiac arrhythmias and increases in intracranial pressure (Murray and Nadel, 2001).

Three major types of sputum specimens are sputum for cytology, culture and sensitivity, and acid-fast bacilli (AFB). Cytological or cellular examination of sputum may identify aberrant cells or cancer. Sputum collected for culture and sensitivity testing can be used to identify specific microorganisms and to determine antibiotics to which they are most sensitive. The AFB smear is used to support the diagnosis of tuberculosis (TB). A definitive diagnosis of TB requires a sputum culture and sensitivity.

DELEGATION CONSIDERATIONS

The skill of collecting expectorated sputum specimens may be delegated to assistive personnel. It is the nurse's responsibility to assess the client's respiratory status and sputum production. If a sterile suction method is needed to obtain the sputum specimen, this skill should not be delegated to assistive personnel. The nurse must instruct assistive personnel to:

* Notify the nurse when the client expectorates bloody sputum.

EQUIPMENT

Expectorated Specimen
❑ Sterile specimen container with cover
❑ Clean disposable gloves
❑ Facial tissues
❑ Emesis basin (optional)

❑ Toothbrush (optional)
❑ Completed identification labels
❑ Completed laboratory requisition (date, time, name of test, source of culture)
❑ Small plastic bag for delivery of specimen to laboratory (or a container as specified by agency)
Suctioned Specimen
❑ Suction device (wall or portable)
❑ Sterile suction catheter (size 14, 16, or 18 Fr—not large enough to cause trauma to nasal mucosa)
❑ Sterile gloves
❑ Sterile saline in container
❑ In-line specimen container or sputum trap
❑ Small plastic bag for delivery of specimen to laboratory (or a container as specified by agency)
❑ Oxygen therapy equipment if indicated
❑ Protective eyewear

STEP	RATIONALE

ASSESSMENT

1. Check physician's orders for type of sputum analysis and specifications (e.g., amount of sputum, number of specimens, time of collection, method to obtain). Specimens for AFB require three consecutive morning samples, and cultures can take up to 8 weeks.

2. Assess client's level of understanding of procedure and its purpose.

3. Assess client's ability to cough and expectorate specimens.

4. Assess when client last ate a meal (or had a tube feeding). Wait 1 to 2 hours after eating.

Specific test to be performed may dictate when or how frequently specimens are collected. Ideal time to collect sputum is early morning because bronchial secretions tend to accumulate during the night. Bacteria also accumulate as secretions pool.

Provides baseline for nurse to establish teaching plan.

Adequate cough is essential in production of mucus from tracheobronchial tree. Client may have nonproductive cough associated with abdominal or chest pain. Simple clearing of throat is unacceptable.

Client may gag, vomit, and aspirate stomach contents during procedure.

STEP	RATIONALE
5. Determine type of assistance needed by client to obtain specimen.	Positioning, postural drainage, deep breathing, and coughing exercises may improve ability to cough productively. Suctioning may be indicated if client is unable to cough and expectorate.
6. Assess client's respiratory status, including respiratory rate, depth, pattern, and color of mucous membranes.	Active coughing may alter respiratory status. Respiratory status can depend on amount of sputum in tracheobronchial tree.

NURSING DIAGNOSES

- Ineffective airway clearance
- Risk for aspiration
- Ineffective breathing pattern

- Risk for infection
- Deficient knowledge regarding specimen collection procedures

Related factors are individualized based on client's condition or needs.

PLANNING

1. Expected outcomes following completion of procedure:
   - Client's respirations are same rate and character as before procedure.
   - Client is relaxed, able to answer questions (if no artificial airway present).
   - Sputum is not contaminated by saliva or oropharyngeal flora.
   - Laboratory tests do not reveal abnormal cells or microorganisms.
   - Client will discuss purpose and benefit of sputum collection.
2. Explain steps of procedure and purpose. Specimen should not contain saliva. Secretions from oropharynx contain numerous bacteria that will contaminate sputum. Client who is to be suctioned should breathe normally to prevent hyperventilation.

Specimen collection did not alter respiratory status.

Suctioning tends to cause anxiety.

Sputum must originate from tracheobronchial tree for accurate results.

Absence of infection or abnormal cells.

Validates learning.

Promotes understanding and cooperation.

- *Critical Decision Point*
  When client is expectorating sputum, stress importance of deep coughing and need to avoid clearing of throat. If client is to be suctioned, stress importance of relaxing and breathing at normal rate.

3. For expectorated specimen, have client rinse mouth or brush teeth with water.

Reduces number of oral contaminants that can alter test results.

- *Critical Decision Point*
  Client should not use mouthwash or toothpaste because they may decrease viability of microorganisms and alter culture results.

IMPLEMENTATION

1. Perform hand hygiene.
2. Close curtains or room door.
3. Position client: semi-Fowler's position, sitting on side of bed or chair, standing for coughing and expectorating specimen; high or semi-Fowler's position for suctioning.

Reduces transmission of microorganisms.
Provides privacy.
Promotes full lung expansion and facilitates ability to cough.

STEP	RATIONALE

- *Critical Decision Point*
  If client has surgical incision or localized area of discomfort, have client place hands firmly over affected area or place pillow over area. Splinting of painful area minimizes muscular stretching and discomfort during coughing and thus makes cough more productive.

4. Collect specimen:
   a. Coughing and expectoration

(1) Apply clean disposable gloves.	Reduces risk of exposure to pathogens.
(2) Provide client with specimen container, and instruct client not to touch inside. Refer to agency policy, and provide type of specimen container indicated.	Prevents risk of contamination.
(3) Instruct client to take three to four slow deep breaths.	Helps to open airways, loosen secretions, and stimulate cough reflex.
(4) Instruct client to emphasize slow, full exhalation.	Moves secretions into large airways.
(5) After series of deep breaths, ask client to cough after full inhalation.	Full inhalation provides force to move secretions out of airways up to pharynx.
(6) Instruct client to expectorate sputum directly into specimen container.	Retains microorganisms in sterile container.
(7) Have client repeat coughing until an adequate amount of sputum has been collected.	Usually 2 to 10 ml ($\frac{1}{2}$ to 2 teaspoons) is required to ensure accurate analysis of specimen.

   b. Suctioning

(1) Prepare suction machine or device, and determine if it functions properly.	Adequate amount of suction is necessary to aspirate sputum.
(2) Connect suction tube to adapter on sputum trap.	Establishes suction that passes through sputum trap to aspirate specimen.
(3) Apply sterile gloves (required only for dominant hand).	Tracheobronchial tree is sterile body cavity. Allows nurse to manipulate suction catheter without contamination.
(4) With gloved hand, connect sterile suction catheter to rubber tubing on sputum trap.	Aspirated sputum will go directly to trap instead of to suction tubing.
(5) Other hand should have glove on for application of suction. Thumb should be on trap prepared to provide suction, and trap should be covered.	
(6) Gently insert tip of suction catheter through nasopharynx, endotracheal tube, or tracheostomy tube without applying suction (see Chapter 24).	Minimizes trauma to airway as catheter is inserted.
(7) Advance catheter into trachea.	Entrance of catheter into larynx and trachea triggers cough reflex.
(8) As client coughs, apply suction for 5 to 10 seconds, collecting 2 to 10 ml sputum.	Ensures collection of sputum from deep within tracheobronchial tree. Suctioning longer than 10 seconds can cause hypoxia and mucosal damage (Murray and Nadel, 2001).
(9) Remove catheter without applying suction, then turn off suction.	Suction can damage mucosa if applied during withdrawal.
(10) Detach catheter from specimen trap, and dispose of catheter in appropriate receptacle.	Decreases risk of spreading microorganisms.

STEP	RATIONALE
5. Secure top on specimen container tightly. For sputum trap, detach suction tubing and connect rubber tubing on sputum trap to plastic adapter (see illustration).	Contains microorganisms within container, preventing exposure to personnel handling specimen.

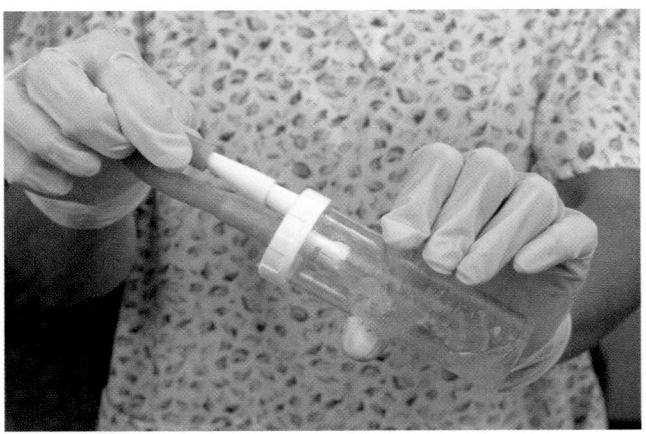

STEP **5** Securing top on sputum specimen container.

STEP	RATIONALE
6. If any sputum is present on outside of container, wash it off with disinfectant.	Prevents spread of infection to persons handling specimen.
7. Offer client tissues after expectorating. Dispose of tissues in emesis basin or trash container.	Maintains cleanliness and comfort.
8. Remove and dispose of gloves.	Reduces transmission of microorganisms.
9. Offer client mouth care, if desired.	Promotes comfort.
10. Perform hand hygiene.	Reduces spread of microorganisms.
11. Label specimen with identification label.	Incorrect identification could lead to diagnostic or therapeutic error.
12. Place specimen in small plastic bag (or container specified by agency), and attach requisition.	Plastic bag or container reduces risk of health care worker's exposure to sputum.
13. Send specimen immediately to laboratory, or refrigerate.	Bacteria multiply quickly. Specimen should be analyzed promptly for accurate results.

EVALUATION

1. Observe client's respiratory status throughout procedure, especially during suctioning.	Excessive coughing or prolonged suctioning can alter respiratory pattern and cause hypoxia.
2. Note anxiety or discomfort in client.	Procedure can be uncomfortable. If client becomes short of breath, anxiety will develop.
3. Observe character of sputum: color, consistency, odor, volume, viscosity, and/or presence of blood.	Characteristics may indicate disease entities.
4. Refer to laboratory reports for test results.	Indicates if abnormal cells or microorganisms in sputum.
5. Evaluate client's ability to describe/demonstrate sputum collection process.	Reinforces client's ability to collect future expectorated specimens.

Recording and Reporting

- Record method used to obtain specimen, date and time collected, type of test ordered, and laboratory receiving specimen in nurses' notes.
- Describe characteristics of sputum specimen.
- Describe client's tolerance of procedure.
- Report unusual sputum characteristics and client response to nurse in charge or physician.
- When laboratory reports are available, report abnormal findings. If AFB sputum culture is positive, initiate appropriate isolation techniques.
- Many agencies require nurse to note on specimen requisition if client is receiving antibiotics.

Unexpected Outcomes	Related Interventions
1. Client becomes hypoxic; increased respiratory rate and effort are necessary; client feels short of breath.	• Discontinue procedure until stable. • Provide oxygen therapy as needed (if ordered). • Notify physician of client's condition. • Continue to monitor client's vital signs and pulse oximetry.
2. Client remains anxious or complains of discomfort from suction catheter	• Discontinue procedure until stable. • Provide oxygen therapy as needed (if ordered). • Notify physician of client's change in condition. • Continue to monitor client's vital signs and pulse oximetry.
3. Specimen contains saliva.	• Repeat specimen collection after client takes several deep breaths and coughs.
4. Inadequate amount of sputum collected.	• Repeat specimen collection after client takes several deep breaths and coughs.
5. Specimen contains blood, pathogenic organisms, or abnormal cells.	• Stop suctioning further. • Report findings to physician.
6. Client complains of pain when coughing to produce sputum.	• Encourage client who is recovering from a surgical procedure to splint incision before coughing. • Obtain order for pain medication as needed (prn). • Inform physician of changes in client's condition.

Teaching Considerations

* Nurse may demonstrate effective coughing techniques versus clearing of throat.
* Nurse can demonstrate proper splinting technique for postoperative clients.
* Explain purpose of avoiding use of mouthwashes and toothpaste before sputum expectoration (to prevent decreasing viability of microorganisms).
* Explain purpose of obtaining specimen before breakfast (specimen will be most concentrated and free of food particles).
* If aerosol treatment is indicated, teach client purpose of procedure, explaining that it will stimulate coughing and sputum expectoration.
* Nurse can teach client to avoid contaminating outside of specimen cup to reduce risk of spread of infection.

Pediatric Considerations

* Children need very clear instructions or demonstration for deep breathing. Infants and young children will be unable to cooperate; aerosol treatment or suctioning may be indicated.
* Another nurse can assist nurse in restraining young child's head and arms during suctioning; parent may assist to give support.
* Young children often swallow secretions instead of expectorating. Use smaller catheter size for young children.
* It may be possible to elicit a cough by tickling the back of the throat with the suction catheter.

Home Care Considerations

* If client is to produce sputum specimen at home, instruct client and/or family member regarding proper technique and importance of having specimen sent to laboratory in timely manner.

SKILL 43-10 Obtaining Wound Drainage Specimens

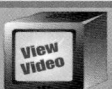

When caring for a client with a wound, the nurse assesses the wound's condition and observes for the development of infection. Localized inflammation, tenderness, and warmth at the wound site, in addition to purulent drainage, usually signify wound infection. Infection cannot be confirmed or treated accurately unless the causative organism is identified. A specimen of wound drainage is analyzed to determine the type and number of pathogenic microorganisms.

The nurse should never collect a wound culture sample from old drainage. Drainage devices should be emptied, and fresh drainage should be collected for the specimen. Resident colonies of bacteria on the skin grow in wound exudate and may not be the true causative organisms of infection. Separate techniques are used to collect specimens for measuring aerobic versus anaerobic microorganisms. Aerobic organisms grow in superficial wounds exposed to the air. Anaerobic organisms grow deep within body cavities, where oxygen is not normally present.

DELEGATION CONSIDERATIONS
Obtaining wound drainage specimens should not be delegated to assistive personnel.

EQUIPMENT
- ❏ Culture tube with swab and transport medium for aerobic culture
- ❏ Anaerobic culture tube with swab (tubes contain carbon dioxide or nitrogen gas)
- ❏ 5- to 10-ml syringe and 21-gauge needle
- ❏ Disposable gloves
- ❏ Sterile gloves
- ❏ Protective eyewear
- ❏ Antiseptic swab
- ❏ Sterile dressing materials (determined by type of dressing)
- ❏ Paper or plastic disposable bag
- ❏ Completed specimen identification label (according to institutional policy)
- ❏ Completed laboratory requisition (date, time, name of test)
- ❏ Small plastic bag for delivery of specimen to laboratory (or container specified by agency)

STEP	RATIONALE

▎ASSESSMENT

1. Assess client's understanding of need for wound culture and ability to cooperate with procedure.

2. Assess client for signs of fever, chills, or excessive thirst. Note in laboratory results if white blood cell count is elevated.

3. Ask client about extent and type of pain at wound site. If client requires analgesic before dressing changes, ideally medication is given 30 minutes before to reach peak effect.

4. Review physician's orders for aerobic or anaerobic culture.

5. Wear disposable gloves to remove any soiled dressings covering wound. Apply sterile gloves, and assess condition of wound carefully. Observe for swelling, opening of wound edges, inflammation, and drainage. Palpate gently along wound edges and note tenderness or drainage. While dressing is being changed, client may prefer not to see wound or soiled dressing.

6. Determine when dressing change is scheduled (see Chapter 38). This step may be performed as part of the actual procedure.

Nurse uses data to develop teaching plan. Wound is painful site. Collection of specimen may arouse anxiety or fear.

Signs and symptoms indicate systemic infection.

Pain at wound site often increases with infection.

Specimens are taken from different sites and placed in different containers, depending on type of culture.

Surface of open wound is considered sterile. Sterile gloves allow nurse to palpate area without wound contamination. Signs indicate wound infection. Gloves minimize exposure to microorganisms.

STEP	**RATIONALE**

NURSING DIAGNOSES

- Anxiety
- Risk for infection
- Risk for injury
- Deficient knowledge regarding wound drainage culture procedure

- Pain (acute or chronic)
- Impaired tissue integrity

Related factors are individualized based on client's condition or needs.

PLANNING

1. Expected outcomes following completion of procedure:
   - Wound culture does not reveal bacterial growth.
   - Culture swab is not contaminated by bacteria from skin.
   - Client will discuss purpose and procedure for specimen collection.
2. Determine if client may receive analgesic before dressing change or specimen collection. Administer as ordered.
3. Explain reason for wound culture and how it will be collected.
4. Explain that client may feel tickling sensation when wound is swabbed.

Wound remains free of pathogenic microorganisms.
Test results indicate type of cells present.

Validates learning.

Minimizes discomfort during procedure.

Promotes understanding and cooperation and eases anxiety.

Anticipation of expected sensations minimizes anxiety.

IMPLEMENTATION

1. Perform hand hygiene.
2. Close bedside curtains or door to room.
3. Apply disposable gloves, and remove old dressing. Observe drainage. Fold soiled sides of dressing together, and then dispose of dressing in bag.
4. Cleanse area around wound edges with antiseptic swab. Remove old exudate.
5. Discard swab, and dispose of soiled gloves in bag.
6. Open packages containing sterile culture tube and dressing supplies.
7. Apply sterile gloves.

8. Collect cultures:
   a. Aerobic culture
      (1) Take swab from culture tube, insert tip into wound in area of drainage, and rotate swab gently. Remove swab, and return to culture tube. (Wrap ampule with gauze to prevent injury to nurse's fingers.) Crush ampule of medium, and push swab into fluid.
   b. Anaerobic culture
      (1) Take swab from special anaerobic culture tube, swab deeply into draining body cavity, and rotate gently. Remove swab, and return to culture tube. OR Insert tip of syringe (without needle) into wound, and aspirate 5 to 10 ml of exudate. Attach 21-gauge needle, expel all air, and inject drainage into special culture tube.

Reduces transfer of microorganisms.
Provides privacy.
Protects hands from contact with drainage.

Removes skin flora, preventing possible contamination of specimen.
Reduces spread of infection.
Provides sterile field from which nurse can pick up and handle sterile supplies.
Allows nurse to maintain sterility of items while collecting specimen.

Swab should be coated with fresh secretions from within wound. Medium keeps bacteria alive until analysis is complete.

Specimen is taken from deep cavity where oxygen is not present. Carbon dioxide or nitrogen gas keeps organisms alive until analysis is complete. Air injected into tube would cause organisms to die.

STEP	RATIONALE

- *Critical Decision Point*
  Never collect exudate from skin unless it is separate culture and labeled as such.

STEP	RATIONALE
9. Place each culture tube on correct specimen label.	Ensures correct results for correct client.
10. Ask another nurse to attach labels and proper requisitions to each tube. Note on specimen requisition if client is receiving antibiotics. Send specimens to laboratory immediately.	Bacteria grow rapidly. Cultures should be prepared quickly for accurate results.
11. Clean wound as ordered, and apply new sterile dressing.	Protects wound from further contamination and aids in absorbing drainage and debriding wound.
12. Remove gloves by pulling inside out, and dispose of gloves in trash. Dispose of soiled supplies according to agency policy.	Reduces spread of infection.
13. Secure dressings with tape or ties.	Keeps dressing securely in place over wound.
14. Assist client to comfortable position.	Promotes client's ability to relax.
15. Perform hand hygiene after procedure.	Reduces transmission of microorganisms.

EVALUATION

1. Obtain laboratory report for results of cultures.	Report indicates if pathogenic organisms are identified.
2. Observe character of wound drainage.	Characteristics can reveal abnormal status.
3. Observe edges of wound for redness and bleeding.	Indicates trauma to healing tissue.
4. Ask client about purpose of wound culture.	Validates learning.

Recording and Reporting

- Record types of specimens obtained, source, and time and date sent to laboratory in nurses' notes.
- Describe appearance of wound and characteristics of drainage in nurses' notes.
- Report any evidence of infection to nurse in charge and physician.
- Record client's tolerance of toleration of procedure and response to analgesics.

Unexpected Outcomes	Related Interventions
1. Wound cultures reveal heavy bacterial growth.	• Monitor client for fever, chills, or excessive thirst, which may indicate systemic infection. • Inform physician of findings.
2. Wound culture is contaminated from superficial skin cells.	• Monitor client for fever and pain. • Inform physician of findings. • Repeat collection of specimen as ordered.
3. Client describes increased pain.	• Provide analgesia. • Repeat culture.

Teaching Considerations

- Notify client before possible discomfort during procedure.
- Instruct client to inform nurse if procedure causes pain.
- Teach client to assess status of wound for changes.
- Discuss signs and symptoms of infection.

Pediatric Considerations

- If procedure is to be performed on a child and is anticipated to be painful, some agencies prefer performing procedure in area other than child's room, thus maintaining feeling that child's room is safe place (Hockenberry and others, 2003).
- It may be helpful to have an additional nurse or other adult available to assist with a specimen collection in a young child or infant.

Home Care Considerations

- When applicable, discuss ways to prevent infection.
- Teach client antiseptic practices (e.g., handwashing, disposal of dressings, and clean technique for applying dressing).

Long-Term Care Considerations

- Carefully monitor wound drainage to prevent spread of infection to other residents (e.g., in a nursing home).

SKILL 43-11   Collecting Blood Specimens and Culture by Venipuncture (Syringe Method and Vacutainer Method)

Blood tests are one of the most commonly used diagnostic aids in the care and evaluation of clients. In any health care setting blood tests can yield valuable information about nutritional, hematological, metabolic, immune, and biochemical status. Tests allow physicians to screen clients carefully for early signs of physical alterations, plot the course of existing disease, and monitor responses to therapies.

The nurse is often responsible for collecting blood specimens; however, many institutions have specially trained phlebotomists who are responsible for drawing blood. Nurses must be familiar with their institution's policies and procedures and their state's Nurse Practice Act regarding guidelines for drawing blood samples.

The three primary methods of obtaining blood specimens are venipuncture, skin puncture, and arterial stick. Venipuncture, the most common method, involves inserting a hollow-bore needle into the lumen of a large vein to obtain a specimen. The nurse may use a needle and syringe or a special Vacutainer tube that allows the drawing of multiple blood samples. Because veins are major sources of blood for laboratory testing and routes for intravenous (IV) fluid or blood replacement, maintaining their integrity is essential. The nurse must be skilled in venipuncture to avoid unnecessary injury to veins.

Skin puncture, also called capillary puncture (Malarkey and McMorrow, 2000), is the least traumatic method of obtaining a blood specimen. A sterile lancet or needle is used to puncture a vascular area on a finger, toe, or heel. A drop of blood is placed on a test slide or collected within a thin glass capillary tube for laboratory analysis. Skin puncture is used to obtain blood glucose levels and blood samples in newborns.

Regardless of the method used to obtain a blood specimen, the nurse must anticipate the client's anxiety. The procedures can be painful, and often just the appearance of a needle is frightening, especially to children. The nurse's calm approach and skilled technique help to limit anxiety.

Blood cultures aid in detection of bacteria in the blood. It is important that at least two culture specimens be drawn from two different sites. Because bacteremia may be accompanied by fever and chills, blood cultures should be drawn when the client is experiencing these clinical signs (Pagana and Pagana, 1999). If only one culture produces bacteria, the assumption is that the bacteria are contaminants rather than the infectious agent. Bacteremia exists when both cultures grow the infectious agent.

Because culture specimens obtained through an IV catheter are frequently contaminated, tests using them should not be performed unless catheter sepsis is suspected. Cultures should be drawn before antibiotic therapy is started, because the antibiotic may interrupt the organism's growth in the laboratory. If the client is receiving antibiotics, the laboratory needs to be notified and told what specific antibiotics the client is receiving (Pagana and Pagana, 1999).

DELEGATION CONSIDERATIONS

The skill of collecting blood specimens by venipuncture is often delegated to specially trained assistive personnel. In some institutions, phlebotomists are the persons responsible for obtaining venipuncture samples. Agency policies differ regarding personnel who may draw blood specimens.

EQUIPMENT

- ❏ Alcohol or antiseptic swab
- ❏ Disposable gloves
- ❏ Small pillow or folded towel
- ❏ Sterile gauze pads (2 × 2 inch)
- ❏ Rubber tourniquet
- ❏ Adhesive bandage or adhesive tape
- ❏ Appropriate blood tubes
- ❏ Completed identification labels according to agency policy
- ❏ Completed laboratory requisition (date, time, type of test)
- ❏ Plastic bag for delivery of specimen to laboratory (or container as specified by agency)

Syringe Method
- ❏ Sterile needles: 20- to 21-gauge for adults; 23- to 25-gauge for children
- ❏ Sterile syringe of appropriate size

Vacutainer Method
- ❏ Vacutainer tube with needle holder
- ❏ Sterile double-ended needles: 20- to 21-gauge for adults; 23- to 25-gauge for children

Blood Cultures
- ❏ Antiseptic swabs (check agency policy for specific antiseptic solution)
- ❏ 70% alcohol (check agency policy)
- ❏ Sterile needles: 20- to 21-gauge for adults; 23- to 25-gauge for children
- ❏ Anaerobic and aerobic culture bottles

STEP	RATIONALE

ASSESSMENT

1. Determine understanding of purpose of procedure and method to be used.

Provides data for nurse to establish teaching plan and provide emotional support. Many clients may have past experiences that increase anxiety.

2. Determine if special conditions need to be met before specimen collection.

Some tests require meeting specific conditions to obtain accurate measurement of blood elements (e.g., fasting blood sugar, drug peak and trough level, and timed endocrine hormone levels).

3. Assess client for possible risks associated with venipuncture: anticoagulant therapy, low platelet count, bleeding disorders (history of hemophilia). Review medication history.

Client history may include abnormal clotting abilities caused by low platelet count, hemophilia, or medications that increase risk for bleeding and hematoma formation.

4. Determine client's ability to cooperate with procedure.

Some clients may need assistance of another caregiver. Procedure may appear threatening to client. Reassure child that blood entering tube or syringe will not hurt (Hockenberry and others, 2003).

5. Assess client for contraindicated sites for venipuncture: presence of IV fluids, hematoma at potential site, arm on side of mastectomy, or hemodialysis shunt.

Drawing specimens from such sites can result in false test results or may injure client. Samples taken from vein near IV infusion may be diluted or may contain concentrations of IV fluids. Postmastectomy client may have reduced lymphatic drainage in arm on operative side, increasing risk of infection from needle sticks. Arteriovenous shunt should never be used to obtain specimens because of risks of clotting and bleeding. Hematoma indicates existing injury to vessel's wall.

6. Review physician's orders for type of tests.

Multiple samples may be needed; physician's order is required.

STEP	RATIONALE

- ### *Critical Decision Point*
  Some specimens require special collection requirements before or following specimen collection, for example:
  - *Cryoglobulin levels: Use prewarmed test tubes.*
  - *Ammonia levels: Tube must be placed in ice for delivery to laboratory.*
  - *Lactic acid levels: Do not use tourniquet.*
  - *Vitamin levels: Avoid exposure of test tube to light.*

NURSING DIAGNOSES

- Anxiety
- Fear
- Risk for infection
- Risk for injury
- Deficient knowledge regarding blood specimen collection process

Related factors are individualized based on client's condition or needs.

PLANNING

1. Expected outcomes following completion of procedure:
   - Venipuncture site shows no evidence of continued bleeding or hematoma after specimen collection.
   - Client denies anxiety or discomfort.

   - Laboratory tests show normal findings.
   - Client will discuss purpose, procedure, and benefits of venipuncture.
2. Explain procedure to client: describe purpose of tests; explain how sensation of tourniquet, alcohol swab, and needle stick will feel.

Indicates hemostasis achieved.

Removal of painful stimulus lessens anxiety. Some clients are not anxious about procedure.
No abnormalities are found in blood elements.
Validates learning.

Anticipatory guidance helps to reduce anxiety.

IMPLEMENTATION

1. Perform hand hygiene.
2. Bring equipment to bedside.
3. Close bedside curtain or room door.
4. Raise or lower bed to comfortable working height.

5. Assist client to supine or semi-Fowler's position with arms extended to form straight line from shoulders to wrists. Place small pillow or towel under upper arm. If in clinic or physician's office, chair with special arm extension may be used.
6. Apply disposable gloves. If glove(s) become contaminated with blood, replace with clean pair after proper disposal of contaminated gloves.
7. Apply tourniquet 5 to 10 cm (2 to 4 inches) above venipuncture site selected (antecubital fossa site is most often used). Encircle extremity, and pull one end of tourniquet tightly over other, looping one end under other. Apply tourniquet so it can be removed by pulling end with single motion.

Reduces transfer of microorganisms.
Facilitates organized procedure.
Provides for privacy.
Reduces strain on nurse's back muscles and improves access to venipuncture site.
Helps to stabilize extremity because arms are most common sites of venipuncture. Supported position in bed reduces chance of injury to client if fainting occurs.

Reduces risk of exposure to blood-borne bacteria.

Tourniquet blocks venous return to heart from extremity, causing veins to dilate for easier visibility.

- ### *Critical Decision Point*
  Palpate distal pulse (e.g., brachial) below tourniquet. If pulse is not palpable, reapply tourniquet more loosely. If tourniquet is too tight, pressure will impede arterial blood flow.

STEP	**RATIONALE**

8. Keep tourniquet on client no longer than 1 minute.

Prolonged tourniquet application may cause stasis, localized acidemia, and hemoconcentration (Malarkey and McMorrow, 2000).

9. Ask clients to open and close fist several times, finally leaving fist clenched.

Facilitates distention of veins by forcing blood up from distal veins.

10. Instruct client to avoid vigorous opening and closing of fist.

May cause erroneous laboratory results of hemoconcentration.

11. Quickly inspect extremity for best venipuncture site, looking for straight, prominent vein without swelling or hematoma.

Straight and intact veins are easiest to puncture.

12. Palpate selected vein with fingers. Note if vein is firm and rebounds when palpated or if vein feels rigid and cordlike and rolls when palpated (see illustration).

Patent, healthy vein is elastic and rebounds on palpation. Thrombosed vein is rigid, rolls easily, and is difficult to puncture.

13. Select venipuncture site. In case of blood cultures, two different sites are selected. If tourniquet has been in place longer than 1 minute, remove and assess other extremity, or wait 60 seconds before reapplying. (If vein cannot be palpated or viewed easily, remove tourniquet and apply warm, wet compress over extremity for 10 minutes.)

Prevents discomfort to client and inaccurate test results (Malarkey and McMorrow, 2000). Heat causes local dilation.

14. Obtain blood sample:
  a. Syringe method
    (1) Have syringe with appropriate needle securely attached.

Needle must not dislodge from syringe during venipuncture.

    (2) Cleanse venipuncture site with antiseptic swabs, moving in circular motion from site for approximately 5 cm (2 inches) (see illustration). Allow to dry.

Antimicrobial agent cleans skin surface of resident bacteria so organisms do not enter puncture site. Allowing antiseptic to dry completes its antimicrobial task and reduces "sting" of venipuncture. Alcohol left on skin can cause hemolysis of sample.

      (a) If drawing sample for blood alcohol level or blood cultures, use only antiseptic swab rather than alcohol swab.

Ensures accurate test results.

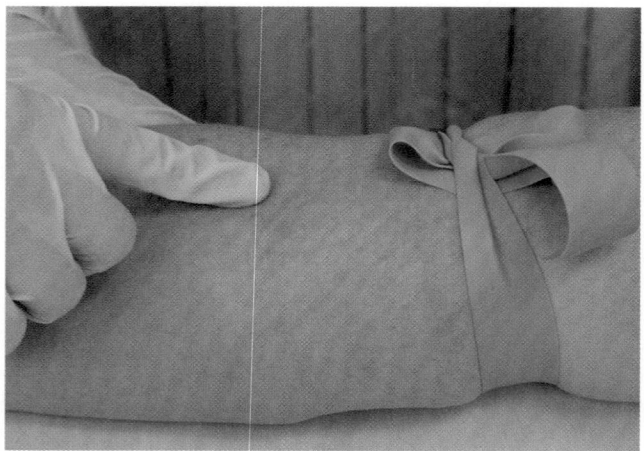

STEP **12** Palpation of vein.

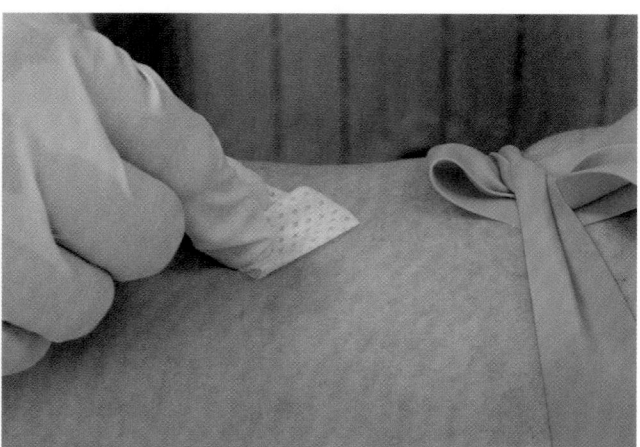

STEP **14a(2)** Cleansing site.

STEP	RATIONALE
(3) Remove needle cover, and inform client that "stick" lasting only a few seconds will be felt.	Client has better control over anxiety when prepared about what to expect.

• **Critical Decision Point**
Observe needle for defects, such as burrs, which can cause increased discomfort and damage to the client's vein.

STEP	RATIONALE
(4) Place thumb or forefinger of nondominant hand 2.5 cm (1 inch) below site, and gently pull skin taut. Stretch skin down until vein is stabilized.	Stabilizes vein and prevents rolling during needle insertion.
(5) Hold syringe and needle at 15- to 30-degree angle from client's arm with bevel up.	Reduces chance of penetrating both sides of vein during insertion. Keeping bevel up reduces vein trauma.
(6) Slowly insert needle into vein (see illustration).	Prevents puncture through vein to opposite side.
(a) With experience nurse will feel "pop" as needle enters vein. If plunger is pulled back too quickly, pressure may cause vein to collapse.	
(7) Hold syringe securely, and pull back gently on plunger (see illustration).	Syringe held securely prevents needle from advancing. Pulling on plunger creates vacuum needed to draw blood into syringe.
(8) Look for blood return.	If blood flow fails to appear, needle is not in vein.
(9) Obtain desired amount of blood, keeping needle stabilized.	Test results are more accurate when required amount of blood is obtained. Some tests cannot be performed without minimal blood requirement. Movement of needle increases discomfort.
(10) After specimen is obtained, release tourniquet.	Reduces bleeding at site when needle is withdrawn.

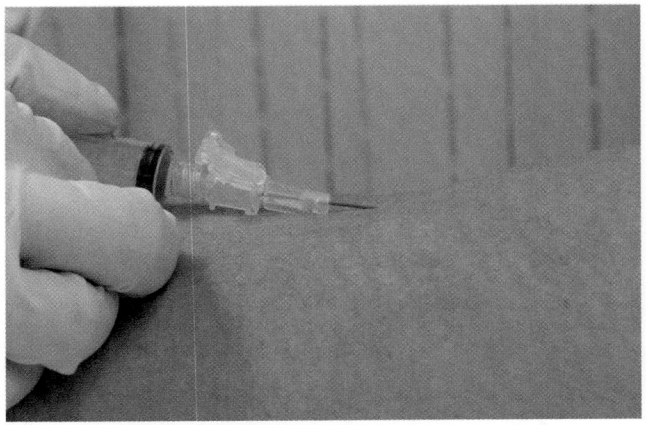

STEP **14a(6)** Inserting needle into vein.

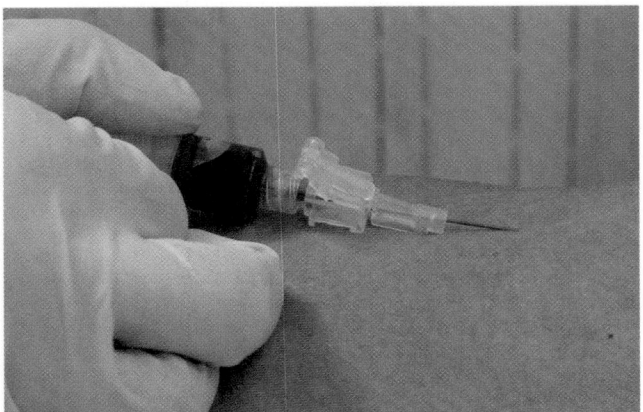

STEP **14a(7)** Pulling back on plunger.

STEP	RATIONALE
(11) Apply 2 × 2 inch gauze pad or alcohol swab over puncture site without applying pressure. Quickly but carefully withdraw needle from vein, and apply pressure following removal of needle (see illustration).	Pressure over needle can cause discomfort. Careful removal of needle minimizes discomfort and vein trauma.
(12) Activate needle safety cover and discard needle in proper receptacle.	Reduces risk of needle-stick injury.
b. Vacutainer method (vacuum tube system method)	
(1) Attach double-ended needle to Vacutainer tube (see illustration).	Long end of needle is used to puncture vein. Short end fits into blood tubes.
(2) Have proper blood specimen tube resting inside Vacutainer, but do not puncture rubber stopper.	Puncturing causes loss of tube's vacuum.
(3) Cleanse venipuncture site with antiseptic swab, moving in circular motion out from site for approximately 5 cm (2 inches). Allow to dry.	Cleans skin surface of resident bacteria so that organisms do not enter puncture site.
(4) Remove needle cover, and inform client that "stick" lasting only a few seconds will be felt.	Client has better control over anxiety when prepared about what to expect.
(5) Place thumb or forefinger of nondominant hand 2.5 cm (1 inch) below site, and pull skin taut. Stretch skin down until vein is stabilized.	Helps to stabilize vein and prevent rolling during needle insertion.
(6) Hold Vacutainer needle at 15- to 30-degree angle from arm with bevel up.	Reduces chance of penetrating both sides of vein during insertion. Keeping bevel up causes less trauma to vein.

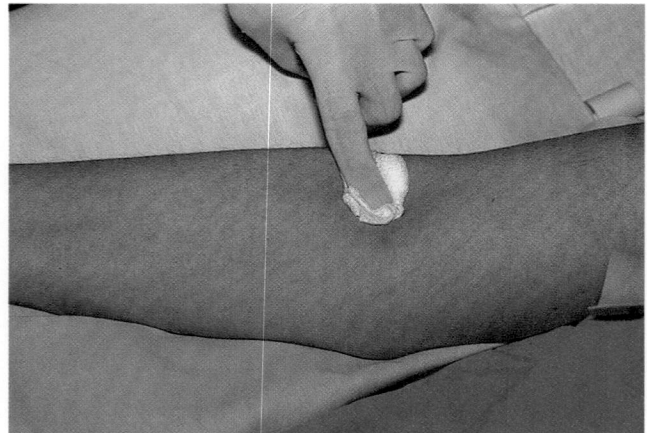

STEP **14a(11)** Application of gauze to puncture site.

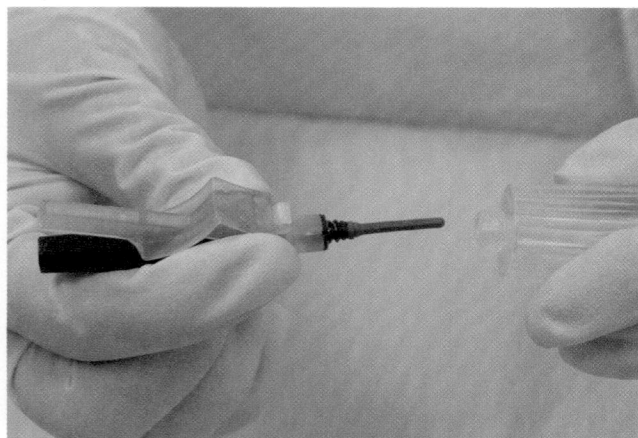

STEP **14b(1)** Attaching needle to Vacutainer tube.

STEP	RATIONALE
(7) Slowly insert needle into vein (see illustration).	Prevents puncture on opposite side.
(8) Grasp Vacutainer securely, and advance specimen tube into needle of holder (do not advance needle in vein).	Pushing needle through stopper breaks vacuum and causes flow of blood into tube. If needle in vein advances, vein may become punctured on other side.
(9) Note flow of blood into tube (should be fairly rapid) (see illustration).	Failure of blood to appear indicates that vacuum in tube is lost or needle is not in vein.
(10) After specimen tube is filled, grasp Vacutainer firmly and remove tube. Insert additional specimen tubes as needed.	Prevents needle from advancing or dislodging. Tube should fill completely because additives in certain tubes are measured in proportion to filled tube. Tubes with additives should be inverted as soon as possible.
(11) After last tube is filled and removed from Vacutainer, release tourniquet.	Reduces bleeding at site when needle is withdrawn.
(12) Apply 2 × 2 inch gauze pad over puncture site without applying pressure, and quickly but carefully withdraw needle from vein.	Pressure over needle can cause discomfort. Careful removal of needle minimizes discomfort and vein trauma.
15. Immediately apply pressure over venipuncture site with gauze or antiseptic pad for 2 to 3 minutes or until bleeding stops (see step 14a[11]). Apply pressure over site, and tape gauze dressing securely.	Direct pressure minimizes bleeding and prevents hematoma formation. Pressure dressing controls bleeding.
16. For blood obtained by syringe, transfer specimen to tubes:	
a. Using one-handed technique, insert needle through stopper of blood tube and allow vacuum to fill tube. Do not force blood into tube.	Prevents needle-stick injury.
b. Alternative method is to remove needle from syringe and stopper to each test tube. Gently inject required amount of blood into each tube. Reapply stopper.	Forcing blood into tube may cause hemolysis of red blood cells.

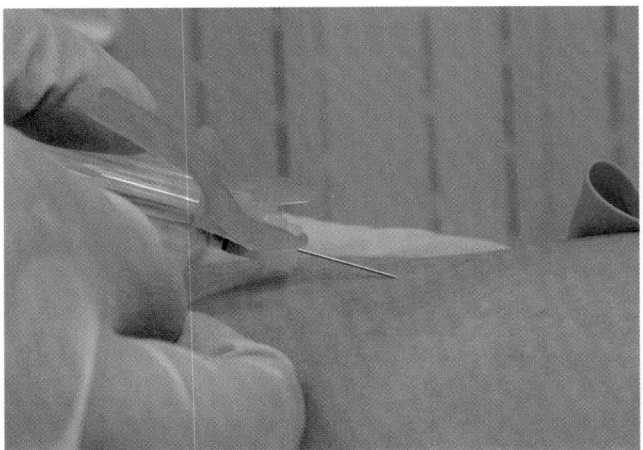

STEP **14b(7)** Inserting Vacutainer needle into vein.

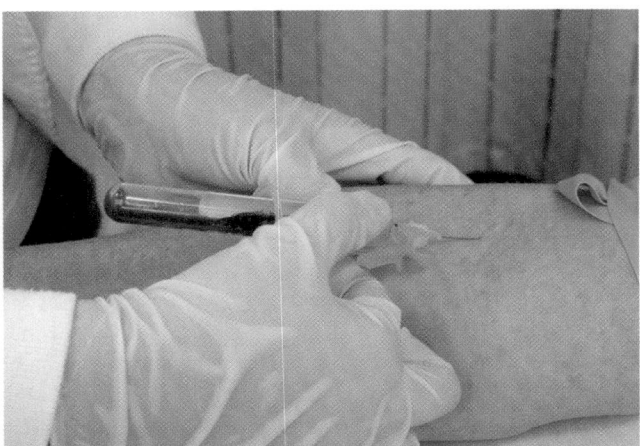

STEP **14b(9)** Blood flowing into tube.

STEP	RATIONALE
17. Take blood tubes containing additives; gently rotate back and forth 8 to 10 times.	Additives should be mixed with blood to prevent clotting. Shaking can cause hemolysis of red blood cells, producing inaccurate test results.
18. Inspect puncture site for bleeding, and apply adhesive tape with gauze.	Keeps puncture site clean and controls any final oozing.
19. Check tubes for any sign of external contamination with blood. Decontaminate with 70% alcohol if necessary.	Prevents cross contamination. Reduces risk of exposure to pathogens present in blood.
20. Assist client to comfortable position.	
21. Securely attach properly completed identification label to each tube, and affix proper requisition.	Incorrect identification of specimen could result in diagnostic or therapeutic errors.
22. Dispose of needles, syringe, and soiled equipment in proper container. Do not cap needles.	Prevents cross contamination through needle sticks and contact with blood.
23. Place specimens in bag to be sent to laboratory.	
24. Remove disposable gloves after specimen is obtained and any spillage is cleaned.	Reduces risk of exposure to blood-borne pathogens.
25. Perform hand hygiene after procedure.	Reduces transfer of microorganisms.
26. Send specimens immediately to laboratory.	Fresh specimen ensures accurate results.

BLOOD CULTURES

STEP	RATIONALE
1. Carefully prepare proposed sites with antiseptic swab (check agency policy). Allow antiseptic to dry.	Antimicrobial agent cleans skin surface so organisms do not enter puncture site or contaminate culture. Drying ensures complete antimicrobial action.
2. Clean bottle tops of vacuum tubes or culture bottles. Check agency policy regarding cleaning with 70% alcohol after cleaning with antiseptic solution and air-drying.	Ensures specimen is sterile.
3. Collect 10 to 15 ml of venous blood by venipuncture in 20-ml syringe from each venipuncture site.	Culture specimens must be obtained from two sites. If one site produces bacteria, but not the other, assumption is that bacteria in first culture may be a contaminant and not the infecting agent. When infecting agent grows in both cultures, bacteremia exists and is due to organism in culture (Pagana and Pagana, 2002).
4. Discard needle on syringe; replace with new sterile needle before injecting blood sample into culture bottle.	Maintains sterile technique and prevents contamination of specimen.
5. If both aerobic and anaerobic cultures are needed, inoculate anaerobic first (Pagana and Pagana, 2002).	Anaerobic organisms may take longer to grow (Pagana and Pagana, 1999).
6. Mix gently after inoculation.	Mixes medium and blood.
7. Immediately apply pressure over venipuncture site with gauze or antiseptic pad for 2 to 3 minutes or until bleeding stops. Apply pressure over site, and tape gauze dressing securely.	Direct pressure minimizes bleeding and prevents hematoma.
8. Label the specimen with the client's name, date, time, and tentative diagnosis. Indicate on laboratory slip any medications (e.g., antibiotics) taken. Place in appropriate bag for transfer.	Ensures correct processing and accurate reporting of results. Antibodies may affect results.
9. Transport the culture bottles immediately to the laboratory (or at least within 30 minutes) (Pagana and Pagana, 1999).	Cultures should be prepared quickly for accurate results.

EVALUATION

1. Reinspect venipuncture site.	Determines if bleeding has stopped or hematoma has formed.
2. Determine if client remains anxious or fearful.	Client may require more blood tests in future. Anxiety or concerns should be expressed and addressed.

STEP	RATIONALE
3. Check laboratory report for test results.	Reveals constituents of blood specimen.
4. Ask client to explain purposes of tests.	Validates learning.

Recording and Reporting

- Record date and time of venipuncture, samples obtained, and disposition of specimen.
- Describe venipuncture site.
- Report any "stat" test results to physician.
- Report any abnormal test results to physician.

Unexpected Outcomes	Related Interventions
1. Hematoma forms at venipuncture site.	• Apply pressure. • Continue to monitor client for pain and discomfort.
2. Bleeding at site continues.	• Apply pressure to site. • Instruct client to apply pressure. • Monitor client. • Notify physician.
3. Signs and symptoms of infection at venipuncture site occur.	• Notify physician. • Apply heat to site.
4. Client becomes dizzy or faints during venipuncture.	• Assist client into chair. • Lower client's head between knees. • Remain with client.
5. Laboratory tests reveal abnormal blood constituents.	• Notify physician.

Teaching Considerations

- Instruct client to apply pressure to venipuncture site briefly. Clients with bleeding disorders or those undergoing anticoagulant therapy should apply pressure for at least 5 minutes.
- Instruct client to notify nurse or physician if persistent or recurrent bleeding or expanding hematoma occurs at venipuncture site.

Pediatric Considerations

- Explain procedure to child as developmentally appropriate and provide atraumatic care (Hockenberry others, 2003).
- Because children often fear that loss of their blood is a threat to their lives, explain to them that their blood is continually being produced. Adhesive bandage gives them assurance that their blood will not leak out through puncture site (Hockenberry and others, 2003).
- At times it is advantageous to draw children's blood specimens in treatment room instead of in bed or room to maintain feeling that room is safe place.

- Restrain child only as necessary to prevent injury (Hockenberry and others, 2003).
- When performing venipuncture on children, nurse needs to explore a variety of sources for vein access: scalp, antecubital fossa, saphenous, and hand veins.
- Application of EMLA cream may be ordered to reduce pain in infants and young children (Hockenberry and others, 2003).
- Vacutainers are not recommended in children under 2 years of age due to possible vein collapse with their use.

Gerontological Considerations

- Older adults have fragile veins that are easily traumatized during venipuncture. Sometimes application of warm compresses may help in obtaining samples. Using small-bore catheter also may be beneficial.

Home Care Considerations

- In home care setting a blood pressure cuff, rather than a tourniquet, can be used for venipuncture.

SKILL 43-12 Measuring Blood Glucose Level After Skin Puncture (Capillary Puncture)

Obtaining capillary blood by skin puncture is an alternative when venipuncture cannot be performed or when reducing the frequency of needle sticks is desirable. The procedure is also less painful than venipuncture, and the ease of the skin puncture method to obtain blood samples makes it possible for clients to perform this procedure. Along with the development of reagent strips and home glucose monitors, the skin puncture method has revolutionized home management care of clients with diabetes. Although not all blood tests can be performed on capillary samples, it is a viable alternative to venipuncture in many situations.

Self-testing of blood glucose level can be performed by two methods. Both methods require obtaining a large drop of blood by skin puncture. A hand-held single-use lancet or one of many automatic lancet-holding devices available on the market today may be used. The blood is applied to a specially prepared chemical reagent strip.

The first method involves visually reading the reagent strip by comparing it to the color chart on the container. Examples of such strips include Chemstrip BG, Glucostix, and Trendstrips. If the color on the strip falls between two reference blocks on the chart, the results may need to be estimated. Thus accurate results of blood glucose measurement may not always be obtained.

The second type of blood glucose monitoring is done by the use of reflectance meters (Figure 43-6). A variety of meters are on the market, including the Glucometer II (Ames), Accu-Check III (Boehringer Mannheim), Glucoscan 3000 (LifeScan), and OneTouch (LifeScan). After a drop of blood from the skin puncture is dropped onto the reagent strip, the meter provides an accurate measurement of blood glucose level in less than 60 seconds.

The meters use a wet-wash or dry-wipe method of testing. To perform a wet wash, the user flushes the blood-coated reagent strip with water before inserting the strip into the glucose meter. The dry-wipe method is somewhat simpler, requiring the user to wipe off the blood-coated reagent strip with a dry cotton ball before making a reading. Some products do not require blood to be wiped before a reading is given. The various methods allow measurement of blood

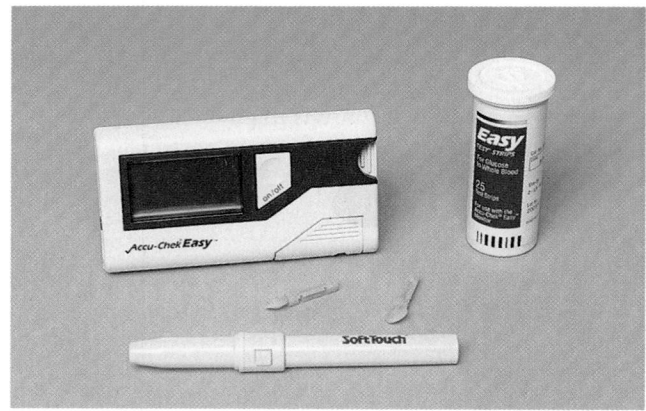

FIGURE **43-6** Accu-Check Easy glucose monitoring equipment.

glucose between 20 and 800 mg/100 ml, thus providing a sensitive measure of blood glucose level.

A variety of glucose meters are currently available. The size of the meters range from 2.1 × 3.3 inches to 6.5 × 2.4 inches. The larger meters are voice activated, which is a nice support for the older adult client with visual impairments. The meters weigh 1.1 to 5.3 ounces. The larger voice-activated meters are 10.94 ounces. Glucose readings will be measured from 0 to 600 mg/100 ml. The amount of time to complete the glucose testing with the current glucose meters varies from 5 seconds to 50 seconds. Some meters can be programmed to monitor the glucose levels for a continuous 72 hours. The meters have memory for the storage and reference of glucose levels (American Diabetes Association [ADA], 2003).

The skill describes the techniques used to measure blood glucose level with a meter using the dry-wipe method. Figure 43-6 depicts an Accu-Check Easy glucose monitor. When the nurse measures blood glucose, gloves are worn according to the Centers for Disease Control and Prevention's (CDC's) standard precautions (CDC, 1996) and Occupational Safety and Health Administration's (OSHA's) recommendations (OSHA, 1991).

DELEGATION CONSIDERATIONS

The skill of measuring blood glucose level after skin puncture (capillary puncture) may be delegated to assistive personnel who have been instructed in performing the skill. The nurse must first assess the client to determine that serum glucose monitoring is appropriate for delegation. When the client's condition changes frequently, this skill should not be delegated to assistive personnel.

EQUIPMENT

- ❑ Antiseptic swab
- ❑ Cotton ball
- ❑ Sterile lancet or blood-letting device
- ❑ Heel-warming device (optional)
- ❑ Paper towel
- ❑ Glucose testing meter
- ❑ Blood glucose reagent strips (brand determined by meter used)
- ❑ Disposable gloves

STEP	RATIONALE

ASSESSMENT

1. Assess understanding of procedure and purpose. Determine if clients with diabetes understand how to perform test and realize importance of glucose monitoring.

   Data set guidelines for nurse to develop teaching plan.

2. Determine if specific conditions need to be met before or after sample collection (e.g., with fasting, after meals, or after certain medications or before insulin doses).

   Dietary intake of carbohydrates and ingestion of concentrated glucose preparations alter blood glucose levels.

3. Determine if risks exist for performing skin puncture (e.g., low platelet count, anticoagulant therapy, bleeding disorders).

   Abnormal clotting mechanisms increase risk for local ecchymosis and bleeding.

4. Assess area of skin to be used as puncture site. Inspect fingers, toes, and heel. Avoid areas of bruising and open lesions.

   Sides of fingers, toes, and heels are commonly selected because they have fewer nerve endings and are highly vascular. The puncture site should not be edematous, inflamed, or recently punctured because these factors cause increased interstitial fluid and blood to mix and also increase the risk of infection (Malarkey and McMorrow, 2000).

5. Review physician's order for time of frequency of measurement.

   Physician determines test schedule on basis of client's physiological status and risk for glucose imbalance.

6. For diabetic client who performs test at home, assess ability to handle skin-puncturing device. If client chooses, he or she may wish to continue self-testing while in hospital.

   Client's physical health may change (e.g., vision disturbance, fatigue, pain, disease process), preventing client from performing test.

NURSING DIAGNOSES

- Anxiety
- Ineffective health maintenance
- Deficient knowledge regarding blood glucose monitoring

- Disturbed sensory perception (tactile)
- Ineffective therapeutic regimen management

Related factors are individualized based on client's condition or needs.

PLANNING

1. Expected outcomes following completion of procedure:
   - Puncture site shows no evidence of bleeding or tissue damage.

     Hemostasis achieved. Lancet or needle did not puncture skin too deeply.

   - Blood glucose level is normal.

     Normal fasting glucose is 70 to 110 mg/100 ml, indicating good metabolic control.

   - Client demonstrates procedure.

     Demonstrates psychomotor learning.

   - Client explains test results.

     Validates knowledge.

2. Explain procedure and purpose to client and/or family. Offer client and family opportunity to practice testing procedures. Provide resources/teaching aids for client.

   Promotes understanding and cooperation.

STEP	RATIONALE

IMPLEMENTATION

1. Perform hand hygiene before procedure.
2. Instruct adult to perform hand hygiene with soap and warm water, if able.

3. Position client comfortably in chair or in semi-Fowler's position in bed.

4. Remove reagent strip from container; then tightly seal cap.

5. Turn on glucose meter.
6. Insert strip into glucose meter (see manufacturer's directions), and make necessary adjustments.

7. Remove unused reagent strip from meter, and place on paper towel or clean, dry surface with test pad facing up.
8. Apply disposable gloves.
9. Choose puncture site. Puncture site should be vascular. In adult, select lateral side of finger; be sure to avoid central tip of finger, which has more dense nerve supply (Malarkey and McMorrow, 2000).

10. Hold finger to be punctured in dependent position while gently massaging finger toward puncture site (Malarkey and McMorrow, 2000).

11. Clean site with antiseptic swab, and *allow it to dry completely.*

12. Remove cover of lancet or blood-letting device. Some agencies use lancet devices with an automatic blade retraction system (Microtainer Brand Safety Flow Lancet [Becton Dickinson]). This reduces the possibility of self-sticks, preventing exposure to blood-borne pathogens.

13. Place blood-letting device firmly against side of finger and push release button, causing needle to pierce skin (see illustration). Hold lancet perpendicular to puncture site, and pierce finger or heel quickly in one continuous motion (do not force lancet).

Reduces transfer of microorganisms.

Promotes skin cleansing and vasodilation at selected puncture site. Hand washing establishes practice for client when test is performed at home.

Ensures easy accessibility to puncture site. Client will assume position when self-testing.

Protects strips from accidental discoloration due to exposure to air or light.

Activates meter.

Some machines must be calibrated; others require zeroing of timer. Each meter is adjusted differently.

Moisture on strip can change its color, altering reading of final test results.

Reduces risk of contamination by blood.

Ensures free flow of blood following puncture.

Increases blood flow to area before puncture.

Alcohol can cause blood to hemolyze.

Cover keeps tip of lancet/needle sterile.

Blood-letting devices are designed to pierce skin for specific depth, ensuring adequate blood flow. Perpendicular position ensures proper skin penetration.

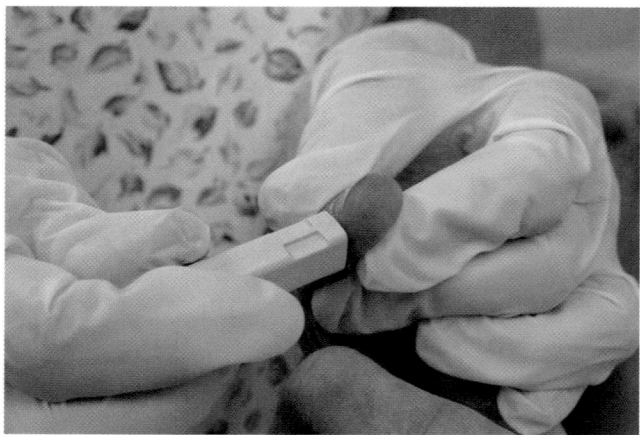

STEP **13** Piercing of fingertip.

STEP	RATIONALE

14. Wipe away first droplet of blood with cotton ball. (See manufacturer's directions for meter used.)

First drop of blood contains tissue fluids (Malarkey and McMorrow, 2000).

15. Lightly squeeze puncture site (without touching) until large droplet of blood has formed. Some agencies use capillary tubes or pipettes to collect the blood sample, reducing risk of direct contact with blood.

Ensures proper coverage of test pad on reagent strip. Excessive squeezing of tissues during blood sample collection may contribute to pain, bruising, scarring, and hematoma formation (Malarkey and McMorrow, 2000).

16. Hold reagent strip test pad close to drop of blood, and lightly transfer droplet to test pad (see illustration). Do not smear blood. Repuncturing may be necessary if large enough droplet does not form to ensure accurate test results.

Droplet must be absorbed by test pad to ensure proper chemical reaction. Smearing causes inaccurate test results.

- **Critical Decision Point**
  Diabetic clients frequently have peripheral vascular disease, making it difficult to produce a large droplet of blood after a finger stick. Be sure that finger is held in dependent position before stick is done to improve blood flow to area.

17. Immediately press timer on glucose meter, and place reagent strip on paper towel or on side of timer. (See manufacturer's directions for meter used.)

Blood must be exposed to test strip for prescribed time to ensure proper results. Strip should lie flat so that blood does not pool on only one part of pad.

- **Critical Decision Point**
  Some meters (such as OneTouch [LifeScan]) require blood sample to be applied to test strip, which is already in meter.

18. Apply pressure to skin puncture site.

Promotes hemostasis.

19. When timer displays 60 seconds (for Accu-Check III model), use moderate pressure to wipe blood from test pad with dry cotton ball. No blood should remain on test pad for some meters. (See manufacturer's directions for meter used.)

For meter to read glucose levels, some strips must be dry. Refer to product directions for timing used with each type of meter.

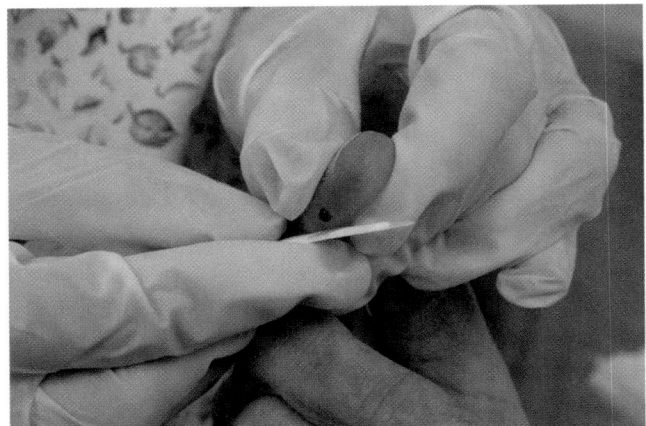

STEP **16** Transferring droplet to test pad.

STEP	RATIONALE

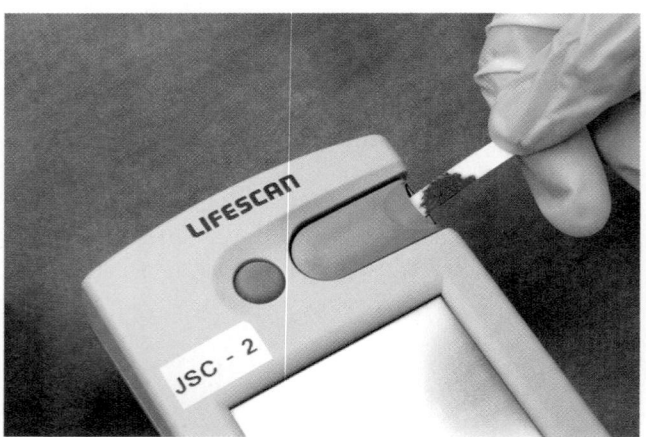

STEP **20** Placing reagent strip into meter.

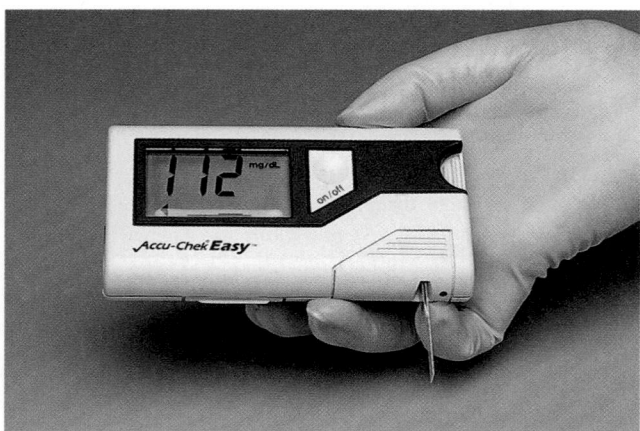

STEP **21** Reading meter.

20. While timer continues to count, place reagent strip into meter (see illustration). — Strip must be inserted correctly to obtain accurate reading.

21. Read meter, noting reading on display (see illustration). — Each meter has specified time for reading glucose level.

22. Turn meter off. Dispose of test strip, cotton balls, uncapped lancet or Autolet, and platform from lancet device (if indicated) in proper receptacle. — Meter is battery powered. Proper disposal reduces spread of microorganisms. Lancets and platforms need to be disposed of after each client use.

23. Remove disposable gloves, and dispose of them properly. Perform hand hygiene. — Reduces transmission of infection.

24. Share test results with client. — Promotes participation and compliance with therapy.

EVALUATION

1. Reinspect puncture site for bleeding or tissue injury. — Can be source of discomfort.

2. Compare glucose meter reading with normal blood glucose levels. — Determines if glucose level is normal.

3. Ask client to discuss procedure. — Validates level of learning.

4. Ask client to explain test and results. — Results of test may cause anxiety. Client may misunderstand specific step of procedure.

Recording and Reporting

- Record procedure and glucose level in nurses' notes or special flow sheet and action taken for abnormal range.
- Describe response, including appearance of puncture site, in nurses' notes.
- Describe explanations or teaching provided in nurses' notes.
- Record and report abnormal blood glucose levels.

Unexpected Outcomes	Related Interventions
1. Puncture site is bruised or continues to bleed.	• Apply pressure. • Notify physician.
2. Blood glucose level is above or below normal range.	• Continue to monitor client. • Check if there are medication orders for deviations in glucose level. • Administer insulin or carbohydrate source as ordered depending on glucose level. • Notify physician.
3. Glucose meter malfunctions.	• Review instructions for troubleshooting glucose meter. • Repeat test.
4. Client expresses misunderstanding of procedure and results.	• Repeat instructions to client. • Have client demonstrate procedure.

Teaching Considerations

- Provide information on where client with diabetes can obtain testing supplies if applicable.
- Provide client with information on where to obtain assistance if glucose meter has malfunctioned.
- Instruct client in what to do and whom to contact if glucose meter malfunctions.
- Stress importance of testing blood glucose level, particularly in diabetic clients.

Pediatric Considerations

- Young children should be allowed to choose puncture site.
- Heel and great toe are frequently used as puncture sites in infants.
- To avoid osteochondritis, puncture of heel in infant must be no deeper than 2.4 mm and should be made at outer aspect of heel (Hockenberry and others, 2003).
- Assess for localized complications in heels of premature infants who must have blood drawn repeatedly.
- Heel warming can be used to facilitate obtaining specimen from neonate.

- Infection is the most serious complication of heel-stick puncture in infants (Malarkey and McMorrow, 2000).
- Earlobe may be used to obtain blood in older pediatric clients (Pagana and Pagana, 2002).
- Allow young child with parent to demonstrate technique; incorporate a play activity for further understanding.

Gerontological Considerations

- Warming fingertips may facilitate obtaining specimen.
- Older adults may have vision or dexterity problems that may interfere with performing self-finger stick (Lueckenotte, 2000).

Home Care Considerations

- Glucose meters may be used routinely by clients in their homes.
- Suggest client attend diabetic support group if needed.

SKILL 43-13 Obtaining an Arterial Specimen for Blood Gas Measurement

Oxygenation and ventilation can be assessed by measuring arterial blood gases (ABGs). Measurement of ABGs provides valuable information in assessing and managing a client's respiratory and metabolic disturbances (Pagana and Pagana, 1999). The parameters measured include arterial blood pH, partial pressure of oxygen (PaO_2), partial pressure of carbon dioxide ($PaCO_2$), and arterial oxygen saturation (SaO_2). The ABG sample is easily obtained and can be quickly analyzed to provide the nurse with a clear picture of acid-base balance, oxygenation, and ventilation. Alterations from normal show the nurse how the client is adapting to the disease process.

Measuring ABGs aids the nurse in assessment. Nurses should check agency policy regarding who is allowed to obtain ABG samples. Many institutions allow only nurses in critical care areas to obtain ABG samples and require institutional certification of this skill. A decision to draw ABG samples frequently may be a direct result of the nurse's physical assessment (see Chapter 18).

DELEGATION CONSIDERATIONS
The skill of obtaining an arterial blood sample should not be delegated to assistive personnel. The nurse should:
- Instruct assistive personnel to report any bleeding from puncture site of the specimen obtained.

EQUIPMENT
- ❏ 3-ml heparinized syringe
- ❏ 23- or 25-gauge needle
- ❏ Syringe cap
- ❏ Alcohol swabs (2)
- ❏ 2 × 2 inch gauze pad
- ❏ Tape
- ❏ Heparin (1:1000 solution)
- ❏ Cup or plastic bag with crushed ice
- ❏ Label with client identification
- ❏ Laboratory requisition
- ❏ Disposable gloves
- ❏ Protective eyewear
- ❏ Commercial blood gas kits are available

STEP	RATIONALE
ASSESSMENT	
1. Determine need to obtain ABG sample and presence of physician's order. Signs and symptoms of alteration in respiratory status requiring sampling may include dyspnea, sudden change in respiratory rate or pattern, unequal breath sounds, unequal chest expansion, cyanosis, change in level of consciousness, self-extubation without need for immediate reintubation, and increased work of breathing.	Some situations and medical conditions place clients at risk for alteration in acid-base balance and ventilation status. Physician's order is required for ABG sample.

2. Assess for factors that influence ABG measurements:
  a. Client who has just awakened
  b. Immediately after suctioning
  c. Less than 20 to 30 minutes after oxygen therapy or ventilator setting change
  d. Client whose oxygen has not been in place continually for at least 20 to 30 minutes
	Allows nurse to eliminate factors that cause inaccurate results.

3. Perform physical assessment of thorax and lungs.	Physical signs and symptoms may indicate need for ABG sample.

STEP	**RATIONALE**

4. Review criteria for choosing site for ABG sample.

Prevents causing compromised circulation from puncture.

● *Critical Decision Point*

Factors that contraindicate use of arterial site include amputation, contractures, localized infection, dressing or cast, mastectomy, or arteriovenous shunts.

a. Assess collateral blood flow. Perform Allen's test:

Allen's test is performed to assess collateral circulation before performing arterial puncture on radial artery. Positive Allen's test ensures there is collateral circulation to hand in case thrombosis of radial artery occurs following puncture (Pagana and Pagana, 1998).

(1) Have client make tight fist and raise hand above heart.

Removes as much blood from hand as possible.

(2) Apply direct pressure to both radial and ulnar arteries (see illustration).

Obstructs arterial blood flow to hand.

(3) Have client lower hand and open hand (see illustration).

Fingers and hand should be pale and blanched, indicating lack of arterial blood flow.

(4) Release pressure over ulnar artery; observe color of fingers, thumbs, and hand (see illustration).

Flushing can be seen immediately if flow through ulnar artery is good. Allen's test is positive, verifying ulnar artery alone is capable of providing blood supply to entire hand. Therefore radial artery can be used for puncture. If there is no flushing in 15 seconds, Allen's test is negative, and this test should be repeated on other arm. When both arms give a negative result, another artery (femoral) needs to be chosen for puncture (Pagana and Pagana, 1998).

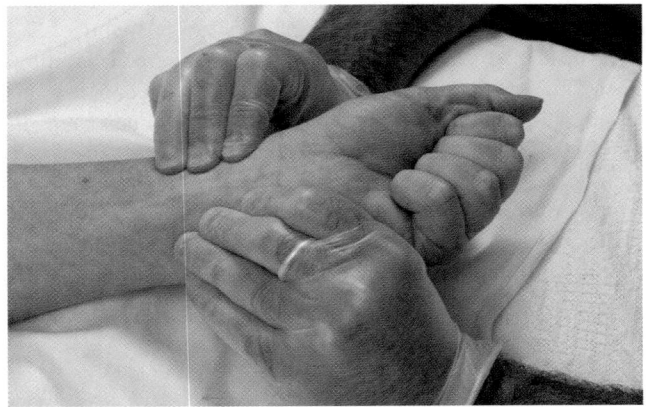

STEP **4a(2)** Applying pressure to radial and ulnar arteries.

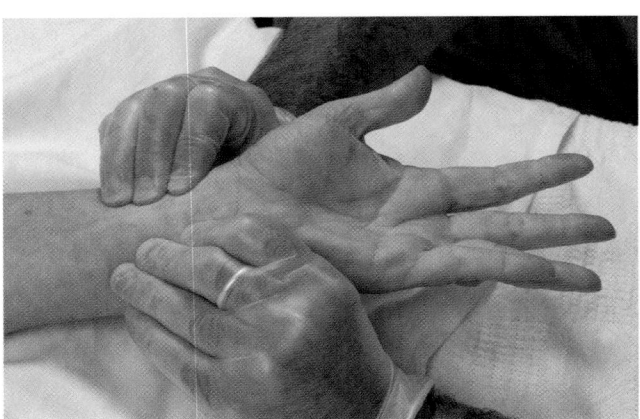

STEP **4a(3)** Client opening hand.

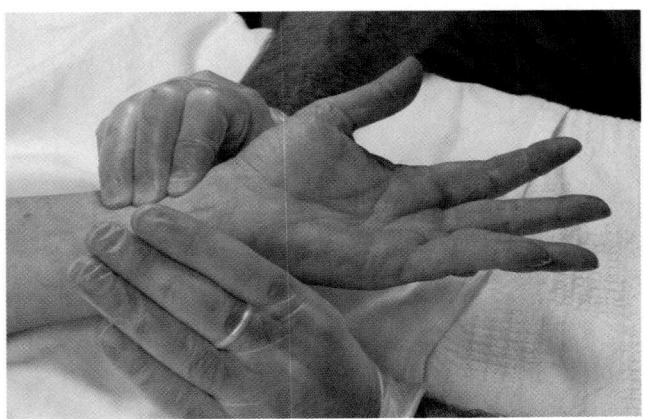

STEP **4a(4)** Releasing pressure over ulnar artery.

STEP	RATIONALE
b. Accessibility of vessel.	Palpating, stabilizing, and performing venipuncture of a superficial artery is easier. Superficial arteries are located at distal ends of extremities.
c. Tissue surrounding artery.	Muscle, tendon, and fat have decreased sensation to pain. Bony periosteum and nerves are highly sensitive to pain.
d. Arteries not directly adjacent to veins.	Helps reduce chance of venous puncture and possibility of inaccurate samples.
5. Assess best arterial sites for use in obtaining specimen.	Arterial blood may be obtained from areas where strong pulses are palpable (i.e., radial, brachial, or femoral artery) (Pagana and Pagana, 2002).

• *Critical Decision Point*
Previous puncture sites or preexisting conditions may eliminate potential sites. Artery should be easily accessible.

a. Radial artery	Safest, most accessible site for puncture; is superficial, is not adjacent to large veins, usually has adequate collateral circulation by ulnar artery, is relatively painless if periosteum is avoided, is used when Allen's test is positive.
b. Brachial artery	Has reasonable collateral blood flow, is less superficial, is more difficult to palpate and stabilize, carries increased risk of venous puncture, and results in increased discomfort for client if brachial nerve is punctured, is used when radial artery is inaccessible or Allen's test is negative.
c. Femoral artery	Should not be used by nurses without specialized training. Has no adequate collateral flow if obstructed below inguinal ligament, is difficult to stabilize, is deep, and directly adjacent to femoral vein. Is best artery to use in emergency (e.g., cardiac arrest or hypovolemic shock when pulses are difficult to palpate).
6. Determine baseline ABG values for client.	Provides basis for comparison and evaluation of therapies.
7. Determine client's knowledge about ABG procedure.	Obtaining blood specimen is painful. Client who is knowledgeable will be more cooperative.

NURSING DIAGNOSES

- Anxiety
- Ineffective airway clearance
- Ineffective breathing pattern
- Impaired gas exchange

- Risk for injury
- Deficient knowledge regarding arterial blood gases
- Ineffective peripheral tissue perfusion

Related factors are individualized based on client's condition or needs.

STEP	RATIONALE

PLANNING

1. Expected outcomes following completion of procedure:
   - Client's ABG values are within normal ranges.

   - Client's extremity distal to puncture remains warm, pink, and free of pain and has adequate capillary refill.
   - Client denies anxiety, and respiratory rate remains within baseline.
   - Client discusses ABG procedure.
2. Prepare heparinized syringe (if heparinized syringes are unavailable).
3. Aspirate 0.5 ml sodium heparin (1000 units/ml) into syringe from vial or ampule.
4. Withdraw plunger entire length of syringe and maintain asepsis.
5. Eject all heparin in barrel out of syringe.

6. Explain steps and purpose of procedure to client.

Determining normal values is essential for accurate interpretation.
Documents adequate arterial circulation to extremity.

Anxiety can increase respiratory rate, which can alter ABG results.
Documents learning.
Heparin mixes with specimen to prevent clotting.

Prevents blood sample from clotting before reaching laboratory. Excessive heparin can affect pH of arterial sample.
Coats barrel of syringe with heparin.

In hub of syringe 0.15 to 0.25 ml of sodium heparin remains; 0.05 ml of sodium heparin adequately anticoagulates 1 ml of blood; 0.15 ml adequately anticoagulates 3 ml without affecting pH level.
Reduces anxiety and promotes understanding and cooperation.

IMPLEMENTATION

1. Perform hand hygiene, and apply gloves.
2. Palpate selected radial site with fingertips.
3. Stabilize artery by hyperextending wrist slightly.

4. Clean area of maximal impulse with alcohol swab, wiping in circular motion.
5. Hold 2 × 2 inch gauze pad with same fingers used to palpate artery.
6. Keep fingertip on artery, just above chosen puncture site.
7. Hold needle bevel up and insert at 45-degree angle into artery, with bevel directed proximally. Prepare client for needle stick because radial sticks are painful.
8. Stop advancing needle when blood is noted returning into hub of needle or syringe.

Reduces transmission of infection.
Determines area of maximal impulse for puncture site.
Reduces mobility of artery and makes insertion of needle easier.
Reduces number of resident bacteria on skin's surface.

Keeps gauze pad accessible when covering of puncture site becomes necessary.
Maintaining location of artery improves likelihood of successful puncture.
Angle allows for better arterial flow into needle. Oblique hole in artery seals more easily. Prepared client will be less likely to withdraw arm.
Quick return of blood indicates that arterial flow is obtained. Prevents puncturing through both sides of artery.

STEP	RATIONALE
9. Allow arterial pulsations to pump 2 to 3 ml of blood into heparinized syringe slowly (see illustration).	Allowing pulsations to assist in filling syringe reduces presence of air bubbles in sample. Bubbles can alter ABG results.
10. When sampling is complete, hold 2 × 2 inch gauze pad over puncture site and withdraw needle.	Pad minimizes pulling of skin as needle is withdrawn.
11. Apply pressure over and just proximal to puncture site with pad (see illustration).	Insertion of needle into artery is just proximal to insertion site through skin. Gauze absorbs any blood that might ooze from site.
12. Maintain continuous pressure on and proximal to site for 3 to 5 minutes (approximately 15 minutes if client is undergoing anticoagulant therapy or has bleeding disorder) (Pagana and Pagana, 1998).	To avoid hematoma formation, hold pressure, apply pressure, or a pressure dressing to the arterial puncture site for 3 to 5 minutes (Pagana and Pagana, 2002).
13. Visually inspect site for signs of bleeding or hematoma formation.	Determines if continued need exists to exert pressure. Because an artery rather than a vein has been accessed, puncture site needs to be monitored for bleeding.
14. Palpate artery below or distal to puncture site.	Determines if pulse quality has changed, indicating alteration in arterial flow.
15. Remove gloves, and perform hand hygiene.	Reduces transmission of microorganisms.
16. Expel air bubbles from syringe.	Failure to expel air from the syringe will result in falsely elevated PaO_2 and falsely decreased $PaCO_2$ (Chernecky and Berger, 2001).

17. Prepare syringe for laboratory analysis according to agency policy. Common principles include:
  a. Place client identification label on syringe.
  b. Place syringe in cup of crushed ice.
 	
  c. Attach properly labeled requisition to blood gas sample.
  d. Indicate amount of any supplemental oxygen (e.g., 2 L O_2, 70% by mask, room air) on requisition.
  e. Indicate client's temperature.
	Permits proper identification of sample for laboratory.
	Failure to place the ABG sample in an ice bath may result in decreased pH, PaO_2, and oxygen saturation (Chernecky and Berger, 2001).
	Prevents mislabeled specimens in laboratory. Ensures correct results received for correct client.
	Documents FIO_2 (fraction of inspired oxygen) at the time specimen was collected (Linton and others, 2000).
	Elevated body temperature decreases the oxygen saturation result (Chernecky and Berger, 2001).

18. Send sample to laboratory immediately.	A prolonged time lapse between collection and testing may result in a decreased pH (Chernecky and Berger, 2001).

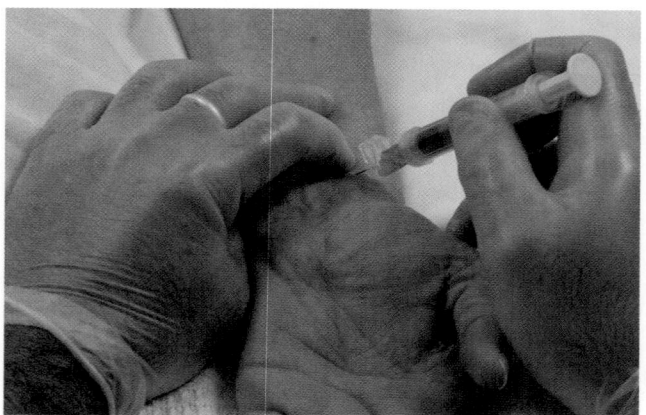

STEP **9** Blood flow into syringe.

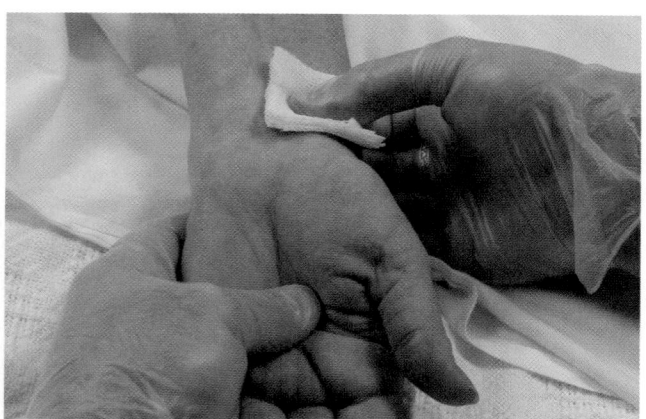

STEP **11** Apply firm pressure to arterial puncture site.

STEP	RATIONALE

▎ EVALUATION

STEP	RATIONALE
1. Inspect area distal to puncture site for complications.	Obstruction of artery can develop from hematoma or damage to vessel wall, reducing arterial flow (Pagana and Pagana, 2002).
2. Review results of sample as soon as possible.	Identifies any abnormality and expedites initiation of treatment.

Recording and Reporting

- Record puncture site and disposition of specimen to laboratory in nurses' notes.
- Report ABG results to physician as soon as available.
- Report client's FIO_2 and any ventilator settings (e.g., tidal volume [V_T], respiratory frequency [RF] mode of ventilation).
- Record results of test and condition of puncture site in nurses' notes.

Unexpected Outcomes	Related Interventions
1. Client has abnormal ABG values.	• Continue to monitor client. • Notify physician of findings, and obtain further orders.
2. Client has hematoma formation at puncture site.	• Apply warm compresses to enhance absorption of blood (Pagana and Pagana, 2002). • Continue to monitor client. • Notify physician.
3. Puncture site is bruised or continues to bleed.	• Apply pressure. • Notify physician.

Teaching Considerations

- Client is taught to report numbness, burning, and/or tingling in hand that had radial artery puncture.

Pediatric Considerations

- In neonatal and pediatric clients, capillary blood gas may also be used. Procedures are similar to those for obtaining heel sticks.
- When dealing with neonatal clients, especially premature infants, normal values for ABGs may differ from those of adults.

- Arterial blood samples from punctures are painful and cause crying and breath holding that affect the accuracy of blood gas values (decreases PO_2) (Hockenberry and others, 2003).

Gerontological Considerations

- Special attention in interpretation of ABGs must be devoted to clients with chronic pulmonary conditions. In these clients compensatory mechanisms may allow normal pH in face of markedly elevated PCO_2.

FOCUS on CLINICAL PRACTICE

Mrs. Kramer is a 72-year-old diabetic client with previous normal bowel function. She now presents with constipation, rectal bleeding, upper abdominal pain, and active vomiting. You have provided her with an emesis basin.

1. Which of the following tests would you expect to be ordered?
   A. Occult blood analysis of stool and emesis
   B. Mid-stream urine collection
   C. Sputum culture
   D. Blood specimens via venipuncture (CBC, chemical profile)
   E. Choices A and D
   F. All of the above
2. Immediate results will be available for which of the tests?
3. Describe the differences between testing materials for emesis and stool.
4. What supplies will the client need to continue home testing?

NCLEX REVIEW QUESTIONS

1. The middle portion of voiding is collected for a culture and sensitivity because:
   1. The urine has more bacteria
   2. The initial stream flushes the urethral orifice and meatus of any resident bacteria
   3. It gives the client more time to be prepared to collect the urine sample
   4. The initial stream flushes the cleansing agent away from the meatus
2. How much urine is needed for a culture and sensitivity specimen?
   1. 10 to 20 ml
   2. 20 to 40 ml
   3. 40 to 60 ml
3. When obtaining a timed urine collection the nurse:
   1. Discards the first urine specimen
   2. Includes the first specimen for the test
   3. Discards both the first and last specimen
   4. Discards the last specimen
4. A sterile urine specimen from an indwelling catheter is obtained from:
   1. The drainage bag at the end of the shift when the output is measured
   2. The sterile self-sealing specimen port on the catheter
   3. The connection between the catheter and the drainage bag
   4. The tip of the discontinued Foley catheter

5. Which of the following is not necessary to observe and document when obtaining urine from an indwelling catheter?
   1. Characteristic of urine (color and clarity)
   2. Patency of the urinary drainage system
   3. Patient discomfort
   4. Total output
6. Glucose present in the urine may be indicative of:
   1. Urinary tract infection
   2. Diabetes
   3. Kidney stones
   4. Urinary retention
7. A double voided specimen is used for testing urine for glucose. A double voided specimen:
   1. Is a procedure to check 2 urine samples
   2. Is a procedure to obtain fresh urine
   3. Is a procedure similar to mid-stream collection
   4. Is a procedure similar to residual urine collection
8. A stool for guaiac tests for:
   1. Bacteria
   2. Protein
   3. Blood
   4. Parasites
9. Which foods can alter the results of a stool for occult blood?
   1. Potatoes
   2. Tomatoes
   3. Bananas
   4. Apples

NCLEX REVIEW QUESTIONS

10. Gastroccult testing could help to reveal bleeding in the:
    1. Stomach, esophagus
    2. Liver
    3. Intestine
    4. Gallbladder
11. Gastric secretions can be obtained from:
    1. NG, nasoenteral tube
    2. Tracheal secretions
    3. Saliva
    4. Diarrhea
12. When obtaining a nasal or throat collection, it is preferred to have the client:
    1. Lying flat in bed
    2. Sitting upright or at a 45-degree angle
    3. Leaning his or her head forward
    4. Lying on his or her side
13. When obtaining a throat culture, the nurse should swab the:
    1. Uvula
    2. Tonsillar area
    3. Side of either cheek
    4. Base of the tongue
14. The ampule at the end of the culture tube should be:
    1. Moistened
    2. Crushed
    3. Left intact
    4. Discarded
15. When obtaining a urethral discharge culture, the genital area for both male and female clients should be observed for:
    1. Redness, swelling, and discharge
    2. Discharge
    3. Foul-smelling urine
    4. Redness and itching
16. Sterile sputum specimens are collected by:
    1. The client coughing (expectorating)
    2. Oral suctioning
    3. Tracheal suctioning
    4. Nasopharyngeal suctioning
17. How long is it necessary to wait after a meal before collecting a sputum specimen?
    1. $\frac{1}{2}$ to 1 hour
    2. 1 to 2 hours
    3. 2 to 3 hours
    4. 3 to 4 hours
18. When obtaining a wound culture sample the nurse should collect the sample from:
    1. Old drainage (exudate)
    2. Old dressing

3. New drainage (exudate)
4. New dressing
19. Aerobic organisms commonly grow in:
    1. Superficial wounds exposed to the air
    2. Deep wounds within body cavities
    3. Fresh wounds
    4. Poorly oxygenated wounds
20. Clients with the following medical history are at greater risk for complications from venipuncture:
    1. Bleeding disorder
    2. Anticoagulant therapy
    3. Low platelet count
    4. Polycythemia
21. Before performing a venipuncture, ask the client to open and close his or her fist several times. This helps to:
    1. Facilitate distention of veins
    2. Relieve anxiety
    3. Oxygenate the blood
    4. Reduces needle stick pain
22. Patent and healthy veins:
    1. Roll easily when palpated
    2. Feel strong and rigid when palpated
    3. Are elastic and rebound when palpated
    4. Are inelastic and rebound when palpated
23. When performing a venipuncture, the nurse should release the tourniquet:
    1. Immediately after the needle is inserted and there is a blood return
    2. After the blood sample is obtained
    3. Before the stick with the needle
    4. After the venipuncture site is selected
24. For blood obtained by syringe, the one-handed technique is used to transfer the blood specimen to the laboratory tube. This helps to:
    1. Prevent needle-stick injury
    2. Show the client your level of competency with the procedure
    3. Decrease contamination
    4. Reduce delivery time to the laboratory
25. Skin puncture sites for obtaining a glucose level are:
    1. Sides of the fingers, toes, heels
    2. Abdomen
    3. Arms
    4. Hands
26. After a capillary stick (finger stick) is performed:
    1. Wipe away the first droplet of blood with alcohol
    2. Immediately place the droplet of blood on the reagent strip
    3. Wipe away the first droplet of blood with a cotton ball
    4. Immediately discard the lancet

References

Adams CR: Lessons learned from urban Latinas with type 2 diabetes mellitus, *J Transcult Nurs* 14(3):255, 2003.

American Diabetes Association: Diabetes forecast. In *ADA resource guide 2003: blood glucose monitors and data management,*

Behrman RE and others: *Nelson textbook of pediatrics,* Philadelphia, ed 17, 2004, Elsevier.

Centers for Disease Control and Prevention: Standard Precautions, *AM J Infect Control,* Feb 24, 1996.

Chernecky C, Berger B: *Laboratory tests and diagnostic procedures,* ed 4, St. Louis, 2001, WB Saunders.

Grimes D: *Infectious diseases,* Mosby's clinical nursing series, St. Louis, 1991, Mosby.

HIPAA guidelines, *Federal Register,* 2003.

Hockenberry MJ and others: *Wong's nursing care of infants and children,* ed 7, St. Louis, 2003, Mosby.

Lawrence P, Rozmus C: Culturally sensitive care of the Muslim patient, *J Transcult Nurs* 12(3):228, 2001.

Linton A and others: *Introductory nursing care of adults,* ed 2, Philadelphia, 2000, WB Saunders.

Lueckenotte A: *Gerontologic nursing,* ed 2, St. Louis, 2000, Mosby.

Malarkey LM, McMorrow ME: *Nurse's manual of laboratory tests and diagnostic procedures,* ed 2, Philadelphia, 2000, WB Saunders.

Marx JA and others: *Rosen's emergency medicine: concepts and clinical practice,* ed 5, 2002, Mosby.

Meredith P, Horan N: *Adult primary care,* Philadelphia, 2000, WB Saunders.

Murray JF, Nadel JA: *Textbook of respiratory medicine,* ed 3, 2001, WB Saunders.

National Committee for Clinical Laboratory Standards: *Urinalysis and collection, transportation and preservation of urine specimens,* vol. 18, no. 7, ed 2, 2001.

Occupational Safety and Health Administration: Occupational exposure to bloodborne pathogens: final rule, 29 CFR 1919:1030, *Federal Register* 56:64003, 1991.

Pagana K, Pagana T: *Diagnostic testing and nursing implications: a case study approach,* ed 5, St. Louis, 1999, Mosby.

Pagana K, Pagana T: *Mosby's manual of diagnostic and laboratory tests,* St. Louis, 2002, Mosby.

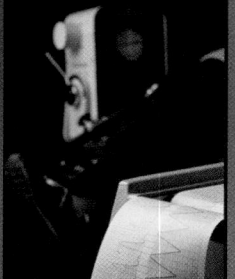

44

Diagnostic Procedures

MEDIA RESOURCES

Evolve Site *evolve*
http://evolve.elsevier.com/Perry/skills
• Weblinks

OBJECTIVES

Mastery of content in this chaper will enable the nurse to:

- Identify physiological indications for diagnostic procedures.
- Demonstrate organizational skills in planning procedures.
- Describe the procedural responsibilities of the nurse, physician, and assistive personnel.
- Perform appropriate physical and psychological assessments before, during, and after related procedures.
- Effectively assist the physician or other health professional with angiography, cardiac catheterization, intravenous pyelogram, bone marrow aspiration/biopsy, lumbar puncture, paracentesis, thoracentesis, bronchoscopy, endoscopy, and cardiogram.
- Demonstrate understanding of nursing responsibilities related to the use of IV sedation during any procedure.

KEY TERMS

Abdominal girth	Lavage
Aldrete score	Lumens
ASA classification	Manometer
Ascites	Medullary
Aspiration	Megakaryocyte
Biopsy	Minimal sedation
Bone marrow	Moderate sedation
Cannula	Modified Ramsay sedation
Cerebrospinal fluid (CSF)	scale
Coagulopathy	Percutaneous coronary
Cytological	intervention
Deep sedation	Peritoneal fluid
Epidural blood patch	Portal hypertension
Fiberoptic	Positive patient identification
Glomerular filtration	Precordial
rate (GFR)	Radiopaque
Herniation	Stopcock
Intestinal obstruction	Subarachnoid space
Intraabdominal pressure	Thrombocytopenia
Intracranial pressure (ICP)	Tracheobronchial tree
Intravenous conscious	Trocar
sedation (IV sedation)	

Diagnostic tests are performed at the client's bedside or in specially equipped rooms within a hospital or ambulatory care setting. Responsibilities of the nurse include assessing the client's knowledge of the procedure, preparing the client, providing a safe environment and emotional support throughout the procedure, and providing postprocedural assessment and care. The nurse supervises any nursing care delegated to assistive personnel. If testing was done on an ambulatory care basis, the nurse provides detailed printed home care instructions. In some instances, the nurse may provide teaching regarding postprocedure care needs that must be performed by the client or caregiver. Knowledge of each test and application of the nursing process ensures safe performance of the procedure.

Evidence-Based Practice Trends

Positive patient identification is a term that means that a client is positively identified, usually via at least two identifiers, before the delivery of care. Agencies vary in their policies that describe what information is required to positively identify a client. As a client safety initiative, use of positive client identification methods has been increasing over the last several years. It has resulted from an increasing national awareness of the volume of medical errors of types involving wrong client/wrong drug/wrong procedure. The term and concept have been incorporated into the National Patient Safety Goals of the Joint Commission on Accreditation of Healthcare Organizations. For the invasive procedures described in this chapter, positive client identification before the procedure is essential.

The process of obtaining informed consent for procedures has become much more consistent and thorough. Clients are usually "consented" multiple times by more than one person for different aspects of the same procedure. For example, a client awaiting surgery may give consent for the surgical procedure after speaking with the surgeon and give consent for sedation or anesthesia after speaking with the anesthesiologist. He or she may also give separate consent for blood administration during the procedure and a general consent for treatment to cover all other care. These changes have evolved as a result of evolving focuses of accrediting agencies on specific areas of practice, as well as improvements in practitioners' processes for reducing liability by fully informing the client (Fleming and Souba, 2004).

The recommended terminology for procedural sedation is becoming more specific. This has come about because the term *conscious sedation* may be misinterpreted. Procedural sedation is now classified as "minimal," "moderate," and "deep" sedation, with *moderate* corresponding to the older term of *conscious* sedation. (American Academy of Pediatrics, 2002; American Society of Anesthesiologists, 1999). In procedures using sedation, objective standards for preassessment, preparation, and monitoring have been implemented in many agencies. Sedation standards often take the form of scales with associated objective criteria that give guidance to physicians and nurses to help gauge client risk and status. These scales are published evidence-based criteria that, when followed, help reduce the risk of complications. For example, the American Society of Anesthesiologists (ASA) classification is used to help determine whether an anesthesiology consultation should be considered before a procedure in which a client will receive intravenous sedation. It may also be used to quantify a client's level of sedation (Hoffman and others, 2002).

The use of a vascular closure device is now common after procedures that involve an arteriotomy. The devices apply manual compression to prevent bleeding at an arterial site. Vascular closure devices are available in varieties that mechanically "plug" the arteriotomy or that percutaneously apply pressure over the site. Research findings vary on whether the risk of bleeding and thrombosis is decreased or increased compared with manual compression (Hoffer and Bloch, 2003).

Emerging technologies are sometimes substituted for a number of procedures included in this chapter. These include virtual endoscopic magnetic resonance colonography in place of colonoscopy, endoscopic ultrasound in place of gastrointestinal studies involving contrast, and studies that combine computed tomography with emission tomography to simultaneously evaluate both structure and function of organs (Hasegawa and others, 2002). In general, these emerging technologies are less invasive and thus pose less risk to the client. Diagnostic usefulness of these techniques often, but not always, equals the more traditional procedures. The nurse should expect traditional diagnostic procedures to continue to be heavily used. However, as the cost of the newer technologies decreases and the studies of usefulness become more common, expect to see gradual integration of less invasive testing into client care.

Knowledge about the causes of postpuncture headache after lumbar puncture (LP) has evolved. Evans and others (2000) demonstrated in a review article containing practice guidelines for lumbar puncture that client demographics, equipment used, and procedure technique, rather than postprocedure care interventions were correlated with the frequency of postpuncture headache. Details are included in the lumbar puncture section of this chapter.

Skill Performance Guidelines

Before the procedure:

1. Perform the essential client safety step of proper identification of the client and procedure (and site, where applicable). Check agency policy for required steps. This may include verbal verification and documentation of the above upon client arrival, again in the procedure room, and just before starting the procedure (Healthcare Organizations, Joint Commission Perspectives on Patient Safety, 2003, 2002).

2. Perform a medication history, being careful to identify any medications for which uninterrupted dosing is required (e.g., anticonvulsants, antibiotics, certain cardiac medications). If the procedure requires a status of nothing by mouth (NPO), discuss such medications with the physician to determine whether the client may take them. If insulin or oral hypoglycemic medications have been administered to clients before diagnostic testing, arrange to have either the client's meal or other nutritional support available on completion of the test.

3. Determine client factors that can affect the procedure or the client's responses.

Factor	Possible Effect(s)
Level of anxiety, educational level, previous experience, language barrier, sensory deficits	Impaired ability to understand and give informed consent. Impaired ability to understand and cooperate with instructions during the procedure. Impaired ability to understand postprocedure instructions.
Previous positive or negative experience with diagnostic testing	May influence the amount of teaching and support needed. Intravenous (IV) or oral sedation may be needed.
Physical limitations	Impaired ability to maintain needed position during the procedure.
Cultural factors	May affect the client's acceptance and response to the procedure. Some cultures may be more or less expressive about communicating discomfort.

4. Because of age-related changes in the older adult, plan diagnostic testing schedules to provide rest periods between multiple tests performed on the same date.

5. Verify that informed consent has been obtained. The physician performing the procedure is responsible for obtaining informed consent for the procedure from the client (see Chapter 35). In some agencies after the physician has the required discussion with and obtains verbal consent of the client, the nurse obtains the client's signature on the consent form. Check the agency's policy to find out whether a consent form is required and the expectations of the RN in this process. If there is no evidence of informed consent in the client medical record, hold any preprocedure medications that would alter the client's level of consciousness, and notify with the practitioner performing the procedure, as well as staff in any receiving area.

During the procedure:

1. Some of these procedures involve the use of radiation. Minimize the amount of radiation exposure to self by using protective shielding devices such as a lead apron and goggles, radioprotective gloves, and thyroid shield. Also, stay positioned as far away from the radiographic equipment as possible, while still being able to perform the required client care (National Council on Radiation Protection, 2000).

2. Provide reassurance to the client throughout the procedure. Most of these procedures cause moderate discomfort, and the client may tolerate the procedure better if a well-informed nurse remains in attendance at the client's bedside and explains each step.

3. Monitor physiological parameters as indicated by the procedure being performed.
4. Assist the physician with the procedure, repositioning client as needed, providing equipment and supplies, and obtaining and preparing specimens for testing.

After the procedure:
1. Monitor physiological parameters as indicated by the procedure being performed.

2. Provide the client and any caregivers with discharge instructions that include, at a minimum:
   - What complications to watch for
   - How to handle complications
   - Physical signs for which to call for help
3. Follow agency policy for disposal of waste materials from the procedure.

SKILL 44-1 Intravenous Moderate Sedation During a Diagnostic Procedure

IV moderate sedation (formerly referred to as conscious sedation) is a drug-induced depression of consciousness during which clients respond purposefully to verbal commands, either alone or accompanied by light tactile stimulation. No interventions are required to maintain a patent airway, and spontaneous ventilation is adequate. Cardiovascular function is usually maintained (American Society of Anesthesiologists, 1999). Moderate sedation improves the client's cooperation with the procedure and allows a rapid return to the preprocedure status, thus minimizing the risk of injury. In addition, it often raises the pain threshold and provides a welcome amnestic effect for the client concerning the actual procedural events.

A risk with moderate sedation is that the client's level of consciousness will be depressed past the point where he or she can maintain a patent airway, a state referred to as deep sedation. Because of this risk, the use of IV moderate sedation is closely controlled and normally restricted to physicians and nurses who have received special training or credentialing. Although a registered nurse may administer an IV sedative intended to produce moderate sedation, it is the responsibility of the physician to order the appropriate drugs and dosages.

Check agency policy for recommended and maximum doses of medications, as well as monitoring and documentation requirements when IV sedation is used.

The most common types of drugs used to achieve moderate sedation include benzodiazepines and opiates. Benzodiazepines reduce anxiety and promote muscle relaxation. Midazolam, in particular, also produces an amnestic effect. Opiates such as meperidine help control pain while achieving sedation.

Client risks during IV sedation include hypoventilation, airway compromise, hemodynamic instability, and/or altered levels of consciousness that may include an overly depressed level of consciousness or agitation and combativeness. Emergency equipment appropriate for the client's age and size (see Chapter 26) and staff prepared to perform emergency medical treatment must be immediately accessible in settings where IV sedation is administered. During and after the procedure, clients need continuous monitoring of heart rate and oxygen saturation by pulse oximetry (see Chapter 17) and continual checks for improving level of consciousness.

DELEGATION CONSIDERATIONS

The skill of assisting with IV sedation cannot be delegated to assistive personnel. In most agencies the client's level of sedation and level of consciousness must be directly assessed and monitored by a registered nurse or physician, and a registered nurse, respiratory therapist, or physician must assess the integrity of the client's airway. Roles in monitoring depend on scope-of-practice guidelines as determined by state regulations and by agency policy and practitioner credentialing. Check agency procedures regarding specific monitoring parameters and frequency required before, during, and after the procedure.

EQUIPMENT

- ❏ Emergency supplies: crash cart, defibrillator, and endotracheal equipment in various sizes
- ❏ Supplies for insertion of a peripheral intravenous catheter (see Chapter 27).
- ❏ Oxygen and airway supplies: bag and mask device, Oral/nasopharyngeal airways, suction equipment
- ❏ Sphygmomanometer or noninvasive blood pressure monitor
- ❏ Pulse oximeter
- ❏ Appropriate reversal drugs (e.g., flumazenil for reversal of benzodiazepines, naloxone for reversal of opiates)
- ❏ Pain medication for procedures anticipated to cause discomfort

STEP	RATIONALE

ASSESSMENT

1. Perform positive client identification according to agency policy.

Complies with National Patient Safety Goals issued by the Joint Commission on Accreditation of Healthcare Organizations (JCAHO).

2. Verify that a preprocedure history and physical examination was completed by the physician.

Accrediting agencies, such as the JCAHO, require a documented preprocedure history and physical before the administration of procedural IV sedation.

3. Verify that informed consent has been obtained.

Informed consent for procedure is required by federal regulations, many state laws, and accreditation agencies, such as the JCAHO.

4. Assess the client's past history of adverse reaction to IV sedation (e.g., hemodynamic instability, airway compromise, altered level of consciousness).

Clients who have had any of these reactions are at higher risk for procedural complications if IV sedation will be used.

5. Verify the client's ASA Physical Status Classification (Box 44-1).

The ASA recommends that clients receiving a classification of 3 or higher have an anesthesia consult before receiving IV sedation.

• *Critical Decision Point*

If the client is discovered to have an ASA classification of 3 to 6 or history of or evidence for difficult intubation, sleep apnea, or complications related to sedation/anesthesia, then consultation with an anesthesiologist may be required by the agency.

6. Assess the client's past history for a history of substance abuse.

A history of substance abuse may require dose adjustment of the sedative.

7. Verify that the client has not taken food or fluids, except for oral medications, for at least 4 hours. Verify specific agency requirements.

Because a risk of moderate sedation is client loss of airway protection, an empty stomach reduces the risk of aspiration.

8. Assess client's level of understanding of procedure, including any concerns.

Determines extent of instruction or level of support required.

9. Establish IV access.

Provides route for administration of IV sedation, as well as rapid IV access should emergency care be needed.

10. Assess baseline heart rate, respiratory rate, blood pressure, level of consciousness, pain level, and oxygen saturation.

Establishes a baseline to which the client's status during the procedure may be compared.

11. Assess and document the client's baseline status via the agency's designated scoring system. Many agencies use an "Aldrete score" (Table 44-1).

Establishes a baseline to which the client's status after the procedure may be compared.

BOX 44-1   Physical Status Classification

1 = Healthy client; no organic, physiologic or psychiatric disturbances.
2 = Presence of mild systemic disease without functional limitations.
3 = Presence of severe systemic disease with significant systemic effects and significant functional limitation.
4 = Presence of medical condition that is poorly controlled, associated with significant dysfunction and is a potential threat to life.
5 = Presence of critical medical condition associated with little chance of survival.
6 = Presence of brain death.

From American Society of Anesthesiologists: *Relative value guide*, 2004, The Society.

STEP	RATIONALE

TABLE 44-1 ALDRETE SCORING SYSTEM

		SCORE
Activity (Moving voluntarily on command)	4 extremities	2
	2 extremities	1
	0 extremities	0
Respiration	Able to deep breathe and cough freely	2
	Dyspnea, shallow or limited breathing	1
	Apneic	0
Circulation	BP $\pm$ 20 mm Hg of presedation level	2
	BP $\pm$ 20-50 mm Hg of presedation level	1
	BP $\pm$ 50 mm Hg of presedation level	0
Consciousness	Fully awake	2
	Arousable on having name called	1
	Not responding	0
Color	Normal	2
	Pale, dusky, blotchy, jaundiced or other change	1
	Cyanotic	0

From Aldrete JA: The postanesthesia recovery score revisited, *J Clin Anesth* 7:89, 1995.

NURSING DIAGNOSES
- Ineffective airway clearance
- Anxiety
- Risk for injury
- Deficient knowledge regarding purpose and steps of procedure
- Acute pain

Related factors are individualized based on client's condition or needs.

PLANNING

1. Expected outcome following completion of procedures involving IV moderate sedation:
   - Client's level of comfort is equivalent to a score of 4 or less on a pain scale of 0 to 10.

   Use of a standardized pain scale provides reliable detection of increasing pain and pain relief.

2. Explain to client that the IV sedation will cause relaxation, but that he or she will be awake during the procedure. If the client will not be able to verbalize due to the nature of the procedure, teach client agreed-upon nonverbal signals for things such as "yes," "no," and "pain."

   Encourages cooperation and minimizes risks and anxiety about the procedure.

3. Explain to client that close monitoring of vital signs and frequent checks to be sure the client is awake are normal during the procedure and do not mean that there are problems.

   Reduces client anxiety during the procedure.

4. Explain to client the major steps of the procedure.

   Reduces client anxiety during the procedure.

5. Position the client as needed for the procedure.

IMPLEMENTATION

1. Establish a peripheral intravenous infusion (see Chapter 27).

   Provides access for administration of sedation and any emergency changes (as needed).

STEP	RATIONALE

TABLE 44-2   MODIFIED RAMSAY SEDATION SCALE

Minimal sedation (anxiolysis)	1	Anxious and agitated or restless or both
	2	Cooperative, oriented, and tranquil
Moderate sedation/analgesia (conscious sedation)	3	Responds to commands spoken in a normal voice
Deep sedation/analgesia	4	Brisk response to a light forehead tap or loud auditory stimulus
	5	Sluggish response to a light forehead tap or loud auditory stimulus
	6	No response to a light forehead tap or loud auditory stimulus

Data from Ramsay MA and others: Controlled sedation with alphaxalone-alphadolone, *Br Med J* 2(920):656, 1974; American Society of Anesthesiologists: *Continuum of depth of sedation definition of general anesthesia and levels of sedation/analgesia,* Oct 31, 1999, http://www.asahq.org/publicationsAndServices/standards/20.htm, accessed Jan 18, 2004.

2. During the diagnostic procedure, monitor for heart rate and oxygen saturation continuously via pulse oximetry equipment. Monitor visually for level of consciousness and responsiveness.

- Monitor level of consciousness/responsiveness to verbal/physical stimulation. Level of sedation may be assessed using the Modified Ramsay Sedation Scale (Table 44-2), or other criteria adopted by the agency.

Vital signs are used for comparison to client's baseline status.

This is used to gauge the client's level of sedation. Use of a numeric rating scale ensures consistency in assessments and an accurate judgment of the client's changing status.

EVALUATION

1. Monitoring after use of IV sedation is tailored to the type of procedure performed and type of sedation that was used.

2. Continue close assessment and monitoring for airway patency, intact protective reflexes, and degree to which client meets discharge criteria on the Aldrete scale.

3. Assess heart rate, respiratory rate, blood pressure, oxygen saturation, pain score, and level of consciousness every 5 minutes for at least 30 minutes, then every 15 minutes for an hour, then every 30 minutes until client meets discharge criteria.

Provides data to verify client's expected return to baseline status.

Enables prompt detection of any suppression of airway and protective reflexes due to delayed action of medication.

Verifies client's tolerance of sedative.
Verifies client's level of comfort to determine need for pain medication.

Recording and Reporting

- Document the following items in the client's medical record:
  - Heart rate, respiratory rate, blood pressure, oxygen saturation, and sedation level at baseline, then every 5 minutes during the procedure, and every 15 minutes for at least 30 minutes after the procedure.
  - Dosage, route, time of drugs administered during and following the procedure, including the use of reversal agents. Include intravenous fluids and blood products, if administered.
  - Significant client reactions during the procedure.
  - Any other required monitoring specific to the procedure being performed.

Unexpected Outcomes	Related Interventions
1. Oversedation as demonstrated by: • Decreasing oxygen saturation • Tachycardia • Absence of patent airway • Sedation score of 4 or higher on the Modified Ramsay Sedation Scale	• Support client's breathing via positioning and manual bagging. • Be prepared to administer reversal agents. Naloxone is used for reversal of opioids, and flumazenil is used for reversal of benzodiazepines.

Teaching Considerations

- Explain that the client will receive sedation but will not be unconscious. The amount of sedation used is only enough to relax the client.
- Explain that it is unlikely that the client will remember the procedure, due to the amnestic effect of the sedative.

Pediatric Considerations

- Sedation is used in pediatric clients to attain their cooperation with procedures. For this reason, deep sedation is used more often than conscious sedation in children under age 6 or who have not progressed as expected through their developmental stages (American Academy of Pediatrics, 2002).
- Because deep sedation is used more often and because children are more likely than adults to slip from moderate to deep sedation, children are more likely than adults to sustain a serious complication resulting from anesthesia. Such complications are often linked to either the cardiovascular or respiratory system. For this reason the American Academy of Pediatrics recommends that personnel who are able to manage a child's airway must be present for the procedure (American Academy of Pediatrics, 2002).
- A preprocedure medical evaluation is required. One must consider anatomical and physiological variations, preprocedure assessments, and pharmacological techniques to safely administer sedation to the pediatric client (American Academy of Pediatrics, 2002).
- Before the procedure, verify that pediatric emergency equipment, appropriate for the age and weight of the child, is present and in working order (American Academy of Pediatrics, 2002).
- During the preprocedure assessment the physician and nurse participating in the client's care should answer the parent's questions in a relaxed and confident manner and tailor their communication with the child to the child's developmental stage.

Gerontological Considerations

- When providing IV sedation to the geriatric client, it is important to support the client's psychological well-being. Many geriatric clients rely on a daily routine to feel a sense of control in their lives, and the administration of IV sedation for minor procedures removes clients from their usual patterns of behavior.
- When the older adult client recovers from IV sedation, offer bedpan/urinal every 2 to 3 hours because of age-related changes in the urinary tract.
- Physical limitations of the client, including hearing and vision loss, may contribute to frustration and confusion, compounding the sense of loss of control.
- Be aware that NPO status in the older adult client may result in dehydration.

Home Care Considerations

- Driving is usually restricted for 24 hours after IV sedation has been used.
- The client should not participate in legally binding decisions until at least 24 hours after the procedure, if IV sedation was used.

SKILL 44-2 Contrast Media Studies: Angiogram, Cardiac Catheterization, and Intravenous Pyelogram

An angiogram (angiography, arteriography) permits radiographic visualization of the vasculature of the heart and arterial system after the intravascular injection of a radiopaque contrast medium. Arteriography is most frequently performed by a radiologist to aid in the diagnosis of occlusions, stenosis, emboli or thromboses, aneurysms, tumors, congenital malformations, or trauma of the arteries of the brain, heart, lung, kidneys, or lower extremities. A small incision or needle puncture is made in a peripheral artery (femoral, brachial, or carotid), and, under x-ray visualization, a small radiopaque catheter is threaded through the artery to the site. The iodinated contrast material is injected, and timed x-ray films are taken. Potential complications of angiography include hemorrhage or thrombosis at the catheter insertion site, infection, allergic reactions to the dye, embolism, and renal failure. In addition, the nurse must be alert for complications related to IV sedation.

Cardiac catheterization is a specialized form of angiography in which a catheter is inserted into either the left or right side of the heart to study pressures within the heart, cardiac volumes, valvular function, and patency of coronary arteries. Cardiac catheterizations are performed in specially equipped laboratories (Figure 44-1). A contrast medium is injected, and the structures and functions of the heart are assessed. In right-side heart catheterizations, usually the subclavian or femoral vein is used for vascular access.

Cardiac catheterizations may be contraindicated in clients who would refuse surgery if needed, who are allergic to io-

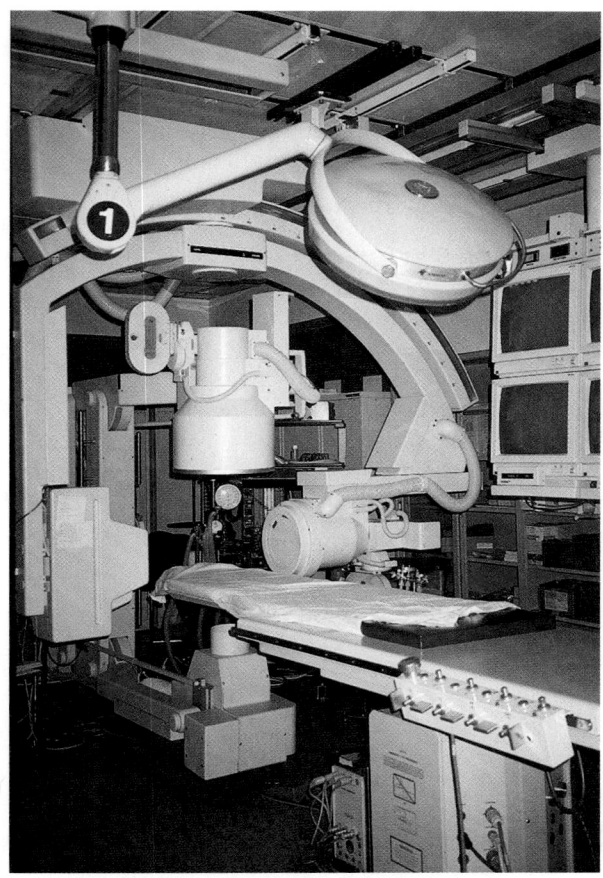

FIGURE 44-1 Cardiac catheterization laboratory. (From Hockenberry MJ and others: *Wong's nursing care of infants and children,* ed 7, St. Louis, 2003, Mosby.)

dine contrast media, who are uncooperative or cannot lie still during the entire procedure, or who are susceptible to dye-induced renal failure. Precautions to help prevent dye-induced renal failure include making sure the client is well-hydrated, premedicating with acetylcysteine (Mucomyst) before, during, and after the procedure, and using nonionic (instead of ionic) contrast media (Tepel and others, 2000).

Either ionic or nonionic contrast media may be used for these procedures. Ionic contrast media is considered less expensive but more risky than nonionic contrast media. Ionic contrast media usually contains iodine, which is highly osmotic. It poses a higher risk of allergic reactions, cardiac electrophysiological disruptions, hemodynamic alterations, and dye-induced renal impairment. Nonionic media has a much lower osmotic value. Because it costs approximately 10 times more than ionic media, it is often reserved for clients considered to be at moderate-to-high risk for renal impairment resulting from the procedure.

The procedures are usually elective but may be performed emergently in the event of sudden occlusion of an artery or in the case of an acute myocardial infarction. Cardiac catheterizations in infants have the highest risk for complications and death in infants weighing less than 5 kg (Cheatham, 2001; McMahon and others, 2003; Rhodes and others, 2000).

Intravenous pyelography (IVP) is a venographic examination of the flow of radiopaque contrast medium through the kidneys, ureters, and bladder to identify obstruction, hematuria, stones, bladder injury, or renal artery occlusion. Dye is injected into a peripheral vein, and serial radiographs are taken over the subsequent 30 minutes.

DELEGATION CONSIDERATIONS

The skill of assisting with angiography and intravenous pyelography may be delegated to assistive personnel if the client is stable and if no IV sedation is used. The nurse must instruct assistive personnel in:

- Obtaining vital signs and values to report to the nurse
- Signs and symptoms experienced by the client that must be reported
- Accompanying the client to the procedure room and assisting specially trained and licensed radiology personnel with the specific angiography procedure

The skill of assisting with cardiac catheterization may be delegated to specially trained assistive personnel with an RN continuously present. The RN presence is needed because of the required continuous assessment and monitoring for serious complications. Assistive personnel may help with client transport, positioning, and obtaining needed supplies.

EQUIPMENT

- ❑ Protective supplies: Mask, goggles, sterile gown and gloves
- ❑ Special packs containing various sizes and types of procedure catheters
- ❑ Intravenous equipment for establishing intravenous access
- ❑ Medications: diazepam, midazolam, or other sedative for IV sedation
- ❑ Emergency supplies: oxygen, emergency cart, defibrillator, cardiac monitor, pulse oximeter

STEP	**RATIONALE**

ASSESSMENT

1. Perform positive client identification according to agency policy.

2. Verify that informed consent has been obtained.

3. Determine if client is taking anticoagulants.

4. Assess client for conditions for which the procedure would be contraindicated:
   - Angiography contraindications: Anticoagulant therapy; bleeding disorders; thrombocytopenia; dehydration; uncontrolled hypertension; previous allergy to radiographic dye, iodine, or shellfish; renal insufficiency; and pregnancy (if iodinated contrast media is used, because media crosses the blood-placental barrier)
   - Cardiac catheterization contraindications: Pregnancy (due to radioactive iodine crossing the blood-placental barrier), severe cardiomyopathy, severe dysrhythmias, uncontrolled congestive heart failure
   - IVP contraindications: dehydration, known renal insufficiency (Chernecky and Berger, 2004)

5. Determine whether client has taken the drug metformin within the prior 48 hours. If so, notify the physician immediately.

6. Assess client for allergies, especially if allergic to iodine dye. If so, notify cardiologist or radiologist. Nonionic contrast media may be used, and steroids and/or diphenhydramine may be given before the procedure.

7. Obtain ordered laboratory tests (e.g., complete blood count [CBC], platelets, prothrombin time, electrolytes, blood urea nitrogen [BUN], creatinine levels) before the procedure.

8. For IVP, verify that client has completed the necessary bowel preparation of an orally administered evacuation preparation 24 hours before the test and evacuation enema 8 hours before test.

9. Remove all of client's jewelry and metal objects.

10. Obtain vital signs and peripheral pulses. For arterial procedures, mark client's peripheral pulses before the procedure. For cardiac catheterization, also auscultate heart and lungs and obtain weight.

11. Assess client's level of understanding of procedure, including any concerns.

Complies with National Patient Safety Goals issued by the Joint Commission on Accreditation of Healthcare Organizations (JCAHO).

Informed consent for procedure is required by federal regulations, many state laws, and accreditation agencies, such as the JCAHO.

Physician needs to be notified, and medication will need to be stopped before the procedure creates risk for bleeding.

Anticoagulants and bleeding disorders are contraindications for arterial procedures due to interference with the client's blood clotting abilities and risk of too much blood loss.

Dehydration and renal insufficiency are contraindications to the use of ionic radiographic contrast media because the client will have an impaired ability to excrete the contrast media via the kidneys.

Metformin taken within 48 hours before receiving iodinated contrast media can lead to lactic acidosis. Metformin is contained in the drugs Glucophage and Glucovance (Calabrese and others, 2002).

An iodine-based radiopaque contrast medium may be used during the procedure; however, a nonionic, hypoallergenic contrast medium is more frequently used. Clients with allergies to iodine, shellfish, or other contrast media may experience anaphylactic reactions.

Abnormal findings might contraindicate the procedure because hemorrhage and/or renal failure may be a complication. Report elevated BUN or creatinine levels because such clients are at risk for renal failure induced by contrast media (Malarkey and McMorrow, 2000).

An evacuated lower intestine and bowel improves visualization of urinary structure.

Eliminates objects that interfere with radiography visualization of the vessels.

Provides baseline data and locations for comparison with findings during and after procedure.

Determines extent of instruction or level of support required.

STEP	RATIONALE
12. Determine type of arteriogram to be performed— carotid, femoral, or brachial. If cardiac catheterization, determine whether right or left heart is being studied. For IVP, determine whether one or both kidneys will be studied.	Enables nurse to anticipate client teaching needs and post-procedure interventions.
13. For cardiac catheterization determine whether the site of catheter insertion needs to be shaved and prepped with antiseptic just before the procedure. Antiseptic should be allowed to dry.	Reduces risk of site-related infection. Drying promotes maximal antibacterial activity.
14. Assess that client has been NPO for 6 to 8 hours before the procedure. Exceptions may occur for clients at risk for contrast-media–induced renal impairment who are specifically instructed to drink increased fluids in the hours before the procedure.	Prevents possible aspiration because client is sedated. Excessive hydration causes dilution of the contrast medium, making structures more difficult to visualize. Good preprocedure hydration reduces the risk of renal impairment caused by contrast media (Tepel and others, 2000).
15. Review physician's orders for preprocedure medications (may be given on nursing unit or in radiology department) and medication for IV sedation:	Increased sedation may be necessary in anxious or confused clients.
a. Atropine	Decreases salivary secretions and increases heart rate when bradycardia is present.
b. Benadryl	Used prophylactically to block histamine and decrease allergic response.
c. Corlopram	Dopamine receptor agonist that promotes renal flow and augments natriuresis (Luther and others, 1997).
d. Preprocedural sedative	Decreases anxiety and promotes relaxation.
e. IV sedation during procedure	See Skill 44-1.

NURSING DIAGNOSES

- Anxiety
- Decreased cardiac output
- Fear
- Risk for infection

- Risk for injury
- Deficient knowledge regarding purpose and steps of procedure
- Acute pain

Related factors are individualized based on client's condition or needs.

PLANNING

1. Expected outcomes following completion of procedure:	
• Client has no significant changes in vital signs or peripheral pulses and no allergic response.	Procedure performed without complication.
• Client's level of comfort is equivalent to a score of 4 or less on a pain scale of 0 to 10. Normal discomfort, includes soreness at catheter insertion site and possible backache.	Client tolerates procedure. These are considered normal and expected. Use of a standardized pain scale provides reliable detection of increasing pain and pain relief.
• Client is able to tolerate increased fluid intake and void sufficient output (at least 30 ml/hour) to excrete the radiographic dye.	Renal function is adequate.
• Client recovers from IV sedation without respiratory complications or change in level of consciousness.	Level of sedation is appropriate.
2. Explain to client purpose of the procedure and what will happen during the procedure.	Helps to minimize client's anxiety.

STEP	**RATIONALE**
3. For cardiac catheterization, it is common to verify the availability of emergent cardiac surgery, due to the risk of complete coronary artery occlusion from dislodged plaque or inadvertent perforation of the vasculature (Chernecky and Berger, 2004). Check agency policy. This may not be a practice in freestanding cardiac catheterization facilities performing elective procedures on low-risk clients.	Prepares backup plan for serious procedure complications.

■ IMPLEMENTATION

NURSE'S RESPONSIBILITY

1. Perform hand hygiene, and apply clean gloves.

Reduces transmission of microorganisms.

2. For cardiac catheterization, provide IV access using large-bore cannula.

Provides access for delivery of intravenous fluids and/or drugs.

3. Monitor vital signs, obtain weight, and (for arterial procedures) palpate peripheral pulses.

Provides baseline data for comparison during and after procedure.

4. Assist client in assuming a comfortable supine position on x-ray table. Clients undergoing IVP may be placed supine or in a slight Trendelenburg's position. Immobilize the extremity to receive the injection.

For arterial procedures, position may need to be maintained for 1 to 3 hours.

5. Tell client that during the injection of the dye, he or she may experience some chest pain and a severe hot flash that is quite uncomfortable but lasts only a few seconds.

Dye causes a feeling of warmth, flushing, or a metallic taste shortly after injection.

6. Nurse administering IV sedation monitors level of sedation and level of consciousness (see Skill 44-1).

IV sedation should not cause loss of consciousness.

PHYSICIAN'S RESPONSIBILITY

1. Perform hand hygiene, and prepare area of catheter insertion (femoral, carotid, or brachial) with antiseptic.

Reduces transmission of microorganisms.

2. Apply mask and goggles, sterile gown, cap, and gloves. (All technologists and assistants do the same.) Drape client with sterile drapes.

Maintains surgical asepsis.

3. Anesthetize the skin overlying the arterial puncture site.

Provides local anesthetic to area of incision or puncture.

4. For arterial procedures:
   - Perform needle puncture of artery; insert guidewire through needle and angiographic (or cardiographic) catheter threaded over wire.

Permits access to artery and prevents coiling of catheter in artery.

   - Advance catheter to desired artery or cardiac chamber, and inject contrast medium.

Permits radiographic visualization of structures, aneurysms, occlusions, or anomalies.

5. During dye injection, specialized machinery takes rapid sequence of x-ray films.

Permits radiographic records of visualization of dye through artery and any abnormalities present.

6. For cardiac catheterization, also measure cardiac volumes and pressure.

Provides data related to cardiac output, central venous pressure (CVP), ventricular pressures, and pulmonary artery pressure. Pressure on puncture site promotes clotting and prevents bleeding.

- ***Critical Decision Point***
  Be prepared to end the cardiac catheterization procedure early in the event of severe unrelieved chest pain, neurological symptoms of a cerebrovascular accident, cardiac dysrhythmias, or hemodynamic changes (Chernecky and Berger, 2004).

STEP	RATIONALE

7. Withdraw catheter and apply pressure to puncture site for 5 to 15 minutes.

Five to fifteen minutes of manual pressure is often enough to stop active site bleeding. However, a certain amount of bed rest is needed to achieve reliable hemostasis. Check agency policy for postprocedure bed rest requirements. This is often up to 6 hours when no vascular closure device is used.

• *Critical Decision Point*
Before removing sheaths, check for physician's orders that give instructions on how to treat a vasovagal reaction. Manual pressure applied to the groin can sometimes stimulate the baroreceptors and cause a vasovagal reaction in which the client becomes bradycardic and hypotensive. Vasovagal reactions are usually brief and self-limiting, but quite dramatic. When applying pressure to the groin after sheath removal, be alert for a vasovagal reaction and be prepared to treat it by lowering the head of the bed to the flat position and giving a bolus of intravenous fluids.

8. Alternatively, a vascular closure device may be used.

Vascular closure devices include Angio-Seal, VasoSeal, Duett, and Perclose. Each has a unique method for providing closure of the arterial site. Angio-Seal uses a resorbable anchor in combination with a collagen plug and provides hemostasis in 2 to 4 hours. Duett uses a temporary balloon in combination with promotion of thrombus formation and provides hemostasis in 4 to 6 hours. VasoSeal uses a temporary J-wire in combination with a collagen plug and provides hemostasis in 5 to 13 hours. Perclose uses nonabsorbable sutures and provides hemostasis in 11 to 19 hours. In spite of the above times, time to ambulation may be anywhere from 2 hours (with the Duett device) to 6 to 8 hours (Silber, 2000).

9. If a percutaneous coronary intervention (PCI), such as a percutaneous transluminal coronary angioplasty (PTCA) or directional coronary atherectomy (DCA), was performed during the cardiac catheterization, a femoral sheath may be left in place and removed in several hours.

Postinterventional sheaths are left in place to provide emergency access to the vasculature in the event that the coronary artery occludes and to allow time for anticoagulants to wear off.

EVALUATION

1. Monitor vital signs, and assess for signs of cardiac complications. Auscultate heart and lungs if cardiac catheterization was done, and compare findings with preprocedure values.

Verifies client's physiological status and evaluates effect of procedure. Signs of cardiac complications include chest pain or pressure, new dysrhythmias, and/or shortness of breath.

2. Perform neurovascular checks by palpating peripheral pulses and affected extremity and by comparing right and left extremities for skin color, temperature, and sensation. Use a Doppler to locate pulses that are not palpable. To use a Doppler, apply a small amount of ultrasound transmission gel to the marked area where the pulse was located before the procedure started. Turn the volume to low, and gently press the tip of the Doppler over the gel, being careful to avoid displacing the entire cushion of gel. Slowly turn the volume up as you move the Doppler in an expanding circular motion. When the pulse is heard through the Doppler speaker, hold the Doppler steady to obtain a count of the pulse. When finished, turn off the Doppler and wipe the gel off the skin with a tissue.

Enables prompt detection of circulatory impairment caused by intravascular clotting or bleeding at the procedure site. Signs of reduced circulation include diminishing distal pulses and/or coolness, mottling, pallor, pain, numbness, and tingling in affected extremity. It is important to know if the peripheral pulses of the affected extremity were palpable before the procedure in order to know if the pulse has diminished when a Doppler is required after the procedure.

STEP	**RATIONALE**
3. Assess vascular access site for hemostasis and hematoma.	Verifies expected sealing of puncture.
4. For arterial procedures	
• Keep affected extremity immobilized for 2 to 8 hours after removal of sheath, according to agency protocol. Use orthopedic bedpan for female client as needed while on bed rest.	Allows time for the body's natural hemostatic mechanisms to form stable initial repair at the insertion site.
• Emphasize the need to lay flat for 6 to 12 hours (and possibly overnight if the sheath is left in the groin).	Helps disruption of hemostasis.
5. Encourage client to drink 1 to 2 L of fluid after procedure.	Facilitates elimination of contrast material and prevents renal damage (Chernecky and Berger, 2004).
6. Assess client for possible delayed reaction to iodine dye (if used)—dyspnea, hives, tachycardia, and rash (Pagana and Pagana, 2002).	Reaction may occur up to 6 hours after injection of dye.
7. Assess for level of sedation, level of consciousness, and oxygen saturation. Use the Aldrete scale (see Skill 44-1).	Determines client's response to IV sedation.
8. Assess postprocedure laboratory values—CBC, prothrombin time.	Detects changes in laboratory values that may indicate the onset of complications, such as bleeding.
9. Observe client for signs of discomfort.	May be early sign of complication.

• Critical Decision Point
Client's report of any feelings of pain, dyspnea, numbness or tingling, or other untoward symptoms may indicate cardiac complications or procedure site complications. Immediately report these to the physician.

Recording and Reporting

- Record client's status on return to nursing unit: vital signs, status of pulses for equality and symmetry, blood pressure (BP) especially for hypotension, temperature and color of catheterized extremity, condition of IV site, and level of client responsiveness.
- Record any drainage from puncture site, appearance of dressing, and condition of puncture site.
- Report to physician changes in vital signs, excessive bleeding or increasing hematoma at puncture site, decreased or absent peripheral pulses, persistent pain, altered neurological status, dysrhythmias, decreased oxygen saturation, or decreased responsiveness after sedation.
- Report to nurses on next shift all relevant physiological data and status of puncture site and dressing.

Unexpected Outcomes	**Related Interventions**
1. Client experiences marked changes in vital signs, evidenced by:	• Support airway.
• Tachycardia, bradycardia, hypertension, or hypotension	• Lower table or head of bed to flat or to the Trendelenburg's position.
2. Vasovagal response occurs (at time of femoral puncture or postprocedure with femoral pressure). Symptoms include feeling faint, dizzy, light-headed, and possible loss of consciousness for a few seconds. Pulse is bradycardic. Response is caused by stimulation of the vagus nerve via baroreceptors.	• Lower table or head of bed to flat position or to the Trendelenburg's position. • Be prepared to administer bolus of IV fluid.
3. Client experiences oversedation, evidenced by: • Prolonged reduced level of consciousness	• See Skill 44-1, p. 1473.

Unexpected Outcomes	Related Interventions
4. Hemorrhage is present at catheter insertion site, evidenced by: • Continuous bleeding	• Apply pressure to site. • Monitor catheter site every 30 minutes for 2 to 3 hours, then as needed. • Notify physician if interventions do not stop the bleeding of if client demonstrates symptoms of acute blood loss (hypotension, tachycardia).
5. Hematoma develops at catheter insertion site, evidenced by: • Unilaterally diminishing or absent distal pulses and/or coolness, mottling, pallor, pain, numbness, or tingling	• Continue to monitor. • Notify physician immediately. • Follow specific postprocedural orders related to findings. These may include reduction of mechanical pressure over the site.
6. Client has allergic reaction to contrast medium, evidenced by: • Symptoms of flushing, itching, and urticaria	• Continue monitoring. • Assess client for anaphylaxis. • Monitor vital signs. • Notify physician. • Follow specific postprocedural orders related to findings. • Administer antihistamine or epinephrine if ordered.
7. Client experiences cardiac dysrhythmias.	• Follow specific postprocedural orders. • Monitor vital signs. • Notify physician.
8. Early signs of infection/sepsis are present, evidenced by: • Confusion • Hypotension	• Continue to monitor temperature and vital signs. • Notify physician.
9. Renal toxicity from contrast medium occurs, evidenced by: • Urine output less than 30 ml/hour	• Place on strict intake and output monitoring. • Monitor closely for signs of fluid overload. • Review electrolyte, urea nitrogen, and creatinine levels.
10. Cerebrovascular accident occurs (left-sided heart catheterization), evidenced by sudden appearance of any of the following: • Numbness or weakness of the face, arm, or leg on one side of the body • Confusion, trouble speaking or understanding • Vision problems	• Notify physician immediately. • Provide symptomatic support. • Implement stroke protocol according to agency policy. This may include emergency notification of a stroke team, consideration of eligibility for thrombolytic therapy, and placement in an intensive care unit.
11. Myocardial infarction occurs (cardiac catheterization), evidenced by: • Dysrhythmias (tachycardia, bradycardia, premature ventricular contractions, ST-segment elevation or depression)	• Notify physician immediately. • Administer oxygen as ordered. • Initiate continuous cardiac monitoring. • Be prepared for administration of antithrombolytic, anticoagulant, and other cardiac medications. • Transfer to intensive cardiac care setting.
12. Pulmonary embolism occurs (right-sided heart catheterization), evidenced by: • Sudden onset of sharp chest pain, dyspnea, anxiety • Tachypnea and decreasing oxygen saturation	• Administer oxygen. • Initiate continuous cardiac monitoring. • Notify physician immediately. • Provide symptomatic support. • Be prepared for administration of anticoagulant. • Transfer to intensive care setting.

Continued

Unexpected Outcomes	Related Interventions
13. Client experiences retroperitoneal bleeding (when femoral access site is used), evidenced by: • Low back pain radiating to both sides of the body (hallmark sign)	• Prepare client for emergency surgery. • Monitor vital signs every 5 to 15 minutes. • Monitor distal pulses hourly.
14. Client experiences air embolus, evidenced by: • Sudden dyspnea • Hypoxia—oxygen saturation less than 90% or decreasing oxygen saturation	• Position client in left lateral position with head lower than feet to allow air embolus to stay in right ventricle. • Cap any open central lines. • Notify physician immediately. • Initiate continuous cardiac monitoring. • Provide symptomatic support. • Transfer client to intensive care setting.

Teaching Considerations

• Before the procedure, confirm that client has made arrangements for transportation home afterwards. In addition, the client needs to be prepared to stay overnight in a hospital if complications occur or if an intervention necessitates prolonged postprocedure vascular checks. Examples of procedures that typically involve an overnight stay include PTCA, atherectomy, and/or insertion of intracoronary stent(s).

• Instruct client when to start NPO status.

• Instruct client about coughing and breath holding when asked to do so during the cardiac catheterization procedure. Coughing can sometimes eliminate potentially life-threatening supraventricular dysrhythmias that may occur during the procedure.

• Explain to client that, during the arteriogram or cardiac catheterization procedure, lying in one position for 1 to 3 hours is expected. During the IVP procedure, lying still for 30 to 45 minutes is expected.

• Explain that the client might experience a feeling of falling when the table is rotated from side to side.

• Explain the necessity of bed rest and immobility following the arteriogram and cardiac catheterization procedures.

• Explain that after the procedure the client's vital signs will be taken and the puncture site will be inspected at frequent intervals.

• Teach women who are breast-feeding to substitute formula for breast milk for 24 hours after the procedure (Chernecky and Berger, 2004).

• Some institutions provide written discharge instructions.

Pediatric Considerations

• Infants and children are particularly susceptible to the diuretic effects of radiocontrast dyes, due to their small body size. In addition, those with congenital cardiac anomalies may have developed compensatory erythrocytosis and thus will experience complications from dehydration very quickly. Emphasize the importance of fluid intake with the child and parent(s) (Nagelhout and others, 2001).

• Blood loss from the procedure occurs from the cutdown site and bleeding into surrounding tissues. Fluid boluses IV may be required to maintain acceptable circulating plasma volume (Nagelhout and others, 2001).

• See Skill 44-1 on IV sedation.

Gerontological Considerations

• Physical exposure and room temperature may contribute to hypothermia in frail older adults, who may not be able to communicate that they are cold. Use heated blankets or forced air heat to maintain core temperature at comfortable, safe levels (Negishi and others, 2003).

• In the older adult, slight alterations in vital signs or behavior may be precursors to impending problems; therefore close monitoring is very important.

• Older adult clients may have reduced drug clearance from decreased glomerular filtration rate (GFR) and nephron activity or decreased hepatic function with resulting delayed excretion of consciousness-altering medications. Therefore the nurse must monitor the effects of medications given to the older adult client (Phipps, and others, 2003).

• The older adult with preexisting dehydration or renal insufficiency in combination with NPO status is at greater risk for dye-induced renal failure. Careful attention to intake and output is essential.

• Because of the normal aging process, an older adult is at risk for skin breakdown and joint stiffness. The client may require assistance with frequent position changes.

• Offer bedpan or urinal every 2 to 3 hours because of age-related changes in the urinary tract.

Home Care Considerations

• On discharge, client will be instructed to contact the physician (or affiliated emergency department) if the following occur after arteriogram or cardiac catheterization:
   · Bleeding from the catheterization puncture site; apply gentle pressure with a clean gauze or cloth
   · Formation of a knot or lump under the skin that increases in size

- Worsening of a bruise or its movement down the extremity rather than disappearing
- Pain at puncture site or in the extremity used for the catheterization
- Pale and cool-to-the-touch extremity where arterial puncture is made
- Appearance of redness, swelling, or warmth of the affected extremity

• Although bathing or showering may be allowed the day after the catheterization, the client should be cautioned to avoid slipping because the leg (if this extremity was used) may feel stiff.

• After arteriogram or cardiac catheterization, instruct client not to drive or climb stairs for 24 hours; to avoid sports, strenuous housework, and lifting for 3 days; and to avoid taking baths until wound is healed.

• After arteriogram or cardiac catheterization, client's urinary output needs to be monitored. Encourage fluid intake because dehydration may result from diuretic action of the dye.

• After arteriogram or cardiac catheterization, instruct client to keep follow-up appointments.

• On discharge after an IVP, client will be instructed to:
- Drink at least three 8-ounce glasses of water to help flush the contrast media through the kidneys
- Watch for signs of a delayed reaction to the contrast medium for 24 hours after the procedure and call his or her physician or go to the nearest emergency department should they occur

---

SKILL 44-3   Assisting With Aspirations: Bone Marrow Aspiration/Biopsy, Lumbar Puncture, Paracentesis, and Thoracentesis

Bone marrow aspiration is the removal of a small amount of the liquid organic material in the medullary canals of selected bones, in particular the sternum and the posterior superior iliac crests (Figure 44-2). In children the proximal tibia may be used (Pagana and Pagana, 2002). A biopsy is the removal of a core of marrow cells for laboratory analysis. Both aspiration and biopsy are used to diagnose and differentiate leukemias, certain malignancies, anemias, and thrombocytopenia. The marrow is examined in a laboratory to reveal the number, size, shape, and development of red blood cells (RBCs) and megakaryocytes (platelet precursors). Culture of bone marrow can help differentiate infectious diseases such as tuberculosis or histoplasmosis.

The sterile procedure is usually performed by a physician assisted by a nurse or assistive personnel at the client's bedside and takes approximately 20 minutes. The sternal site is the preferred site in adults when a bone marrow biopsy is planned, or the posterior superior iliac spine if the method used will be a needle biopsy. Other sites sometimes used are the anterior iliac crest and the vertebral spinous process.

Potential complications of bone marrow aspiration or biopsy are bleeding, especially if a coagulopathy is present, infection, and less commonly organ puncture. The nurse should know normal hematological laboratory values before assisting with the procedure.

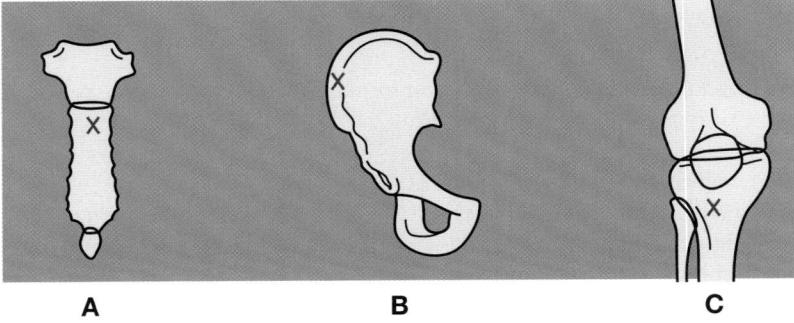

FIGURE 44-2 Anatomical sites (*X*) for bone marrow aspiration. **A,** Sternum between the second and third intercostal spaces. **B,** Iliac crest on the rim or upper posterior surface. **C,** Proximal tibia about 1 to 2 inches below the patella of the infant or small child.

DELEGATION CONSIDERATIONS

The skill of assisting with bone marrow aspiration may be delegated to assistive personnel if the client is stable (check agency policy). The nurse must instruct assistive personnel about:

- Proper positioning of client during the procedure
- Taking baseline, as well as postprocedure, vital signs and reporting these vital signs to the nurse
- Signs and symptoms experienced by the client and reporting these signs to the nurse

EQUIPMENT

- ❑ Antiseptic solution
- ❑ Bone marrow aspiration tray, if available from central supply, which may include: antiseptic solution (e.g., povidone-iodine); gauze sponges (4 × 4); sterile towels for draping; local anesthetic solution (e.g., lidocaine 1%); sterile syringes: two 3-ml, 23- to 25-gauge needles for anesthetic; two 10- and 50-ml syringes for marrow aspiration; two bone marrow needles with inner stylus (see Figure 44-3)
- ❑ Test tubes and/or glass slides, along with any staining solutions needed
- ❑ Sterile gloves of proper size for physician
- ❑ Protective equipment: masks, goggles, and gowns for physician and nurse (check institution's policy) (masks are used for immunocompromised clients, including those receiving chemotherapy or high-dose steroid therapy)
- ❑ Gauze (2 × 2), tape, and antiseptic ointment
- ❑ Pain medication, if ordered (given 30 minutes before procedure)

STEP	RATIONALE

ASSESSMENT

1. Perform positive client identification according to agency policy.

Complies with National Patient Safety Goals issued by the JCAHO.

2. Determine purpose of procedure.

Allows nurse to determine whether aspiration or biopsy will be performed and to anticipate laboratory requisitions.

3. Determine client's ability to assume position required for procedure and ability to remain still. Discuss with the physician the need for premedication for very anxious clients.

Movement during the procedure can cause complications. The required position depends on site used for bone marrow aspiration (e.g., for sternal or tibial biopsy use supine position; for iliac crest biopsy use prone or lateral recumbent position; for vertebral biopsy have client in a seated position).

4. Obtain vital signs.

Provides baseline for comparison with postprocedure vital signs.

5 Assess client's coagulation status: use of anticoagulants, platelet count, and prothrombin time.

Invasive bone marrow procedures are contraindicated in clients with coagulation disorders due to risk of bleeding (Chernecky and Berger, 2004).

6. Determine whether client is allergic to antiseptic or anesthetic solutions.

Decreases chance of allergic reactions.

7. Assess client's level of understanding of procedure, including any concerns.

Determines extent of instruction and level of support required.

NURSING DIAGNOSES

- Anxiety
- Fear
- Risk for infection
- Risk for injury

- Deficient knowledge regarding purpose and steps of procedure
- Acute pain

Related factors are individualized based on client's condition or needs.

PLANNING

1. Expected outcomes following completion of procedure:
   - Client can assume and maintain the required position.
   - Client has no bleeding at needle insertion site.
   - Amount of aspirate is sufficient to perform laboratory testing.
   - Client's level of comfort is equivalent to a score of 4 or less on a pain scale of 0 to 10.
2. Explain steps of skin preparation, anesthetic injection, needle insertion, position required.

Client tolerates procedure well.
Precautions during procedure prevent bleeding.

Use of a standardized pain scale provides reliable detection of increasing pain and pain relief.
Anticipation of expected sensations and procedural activities reduces anxiety.

STEP	RATIONALE

IMPLEMENTATION

NURSE'S RESPONSIBILITY

1. Perform hand hygiene.
2. Premedicate for pain, if ordered.
3. Set up sterile tray, or open supplies to make accessible for physician.
4. Assist client in maintaining correct position (see Assessment, step 2). Reassure client while explaining procedure. Emphasize to client to remain very still and avoid sudden movement throughout the procedure.
5. Explain to client that pain may occur when lidocaine is injected into the tissues. Pressure may also occur when the bone marrow is aspirated.

6. Assess client's condition during procedure, including respiratory status and vital signs if indicated.
7. Note characteristics of bone marrow aspirate (e.g., amount, color). Marrow may appear red or yellow.

Reduces transmission of microorganisms.
Reduces the discomfort of the procedure.
Maintains integrity of sterile field and promotes prompt completion of procedure.
Decreases chance of complications occurring during procedure. Explanations increase client comfort and relaxation.

Bone marrow aspiration is painful, but lasts for only a few moments. Preprocedure analgesia may be given to decrease the discomfort. A deep pressure feeling may be experienced as the bone marrow is withdrawn (Chernecky and Berger, 2004).
Identifies any changes that may indicate complication.

Characteristics are used for observation, reporting, and recording.

PHYSICIAN'S RESPONSIBILITY

1. Perform hand hygiene.
2. Select site to be used for bone marrow aspiration.

3. Apply sterile gloves, mask, and goggles. Disinfect skin with antiseptic solution and 4 × 4 gauze sponges.
4. Replace sterile gloves, and drape client with sterile towels.
5. Inject local anesthetic. Allow time for anesthesia to occur.

6. Insert bone marrow needle (Figure 44-3) with inner stylus into bone, then advance needle until it reaches area of spongy bone and remove stylus.
7. Attach 10-ml syringe to needle, and aspirate bone marrow. For biopsy, screw the core biopsy instrument into the bone and remove plug of tissue.

8. Remove needle or biopsy instrument, and apply pressure to puncture site. Apply antiseptic ointment and dressing.
9. Place the specimen on glass slides or in test tubes.

Reduces transmission of microorganisms.
Sites are chosen for direct access to area of spongy bone. These sites include anterior and posterior iliac spines, iliac crest, body of sternum, and tibia.
Removes surface bacteria from skin at area of puncture site.

Maintains surgical asepsis.
Provides optimal effect of local anesthesia at time of bone marrow aspiration.
Stylus is stiff and has long bevel to enable it to enter bone with ease. Spongy bone is location of bone marrow.

Amount aspirated is determined by purpose of procedure: small amount (approximately 0.5 to 2.0 ml) is obtained for laboratory test; larger amount, including cells, is obtained by biopsy.
Prevents bleeding from and bacterial growth at the puncture site.
Provides proper medium/container for laboratory analysis.

EVALUATION

1. Monitor vital signs. Check agency policy; may be as often as every 15 minutes for 2 hours.
2. Inspect dressing over puncture site for bleeding, swelling, tenderness, and erythema. Inspect area under client for bleeding. Use caution not to disrupt a healing clot at the site if a pressure dressing is present.
3. Assess pain score to determine if client's level of comfort is equivalent to a score of 4 or less on a pain scale of 0 to 10.

Verifies client's physiological status in response to potential blood loss.
Determines further blood loss from puncture site. Infection is a potential complication, especially if the client is leukopenic (Pagana and Pagana, 2002).

Use of a standardized pain scale provides reliable detection of increasing pain so that postprocedure analgesia may be given.

STEP	RATIONALE

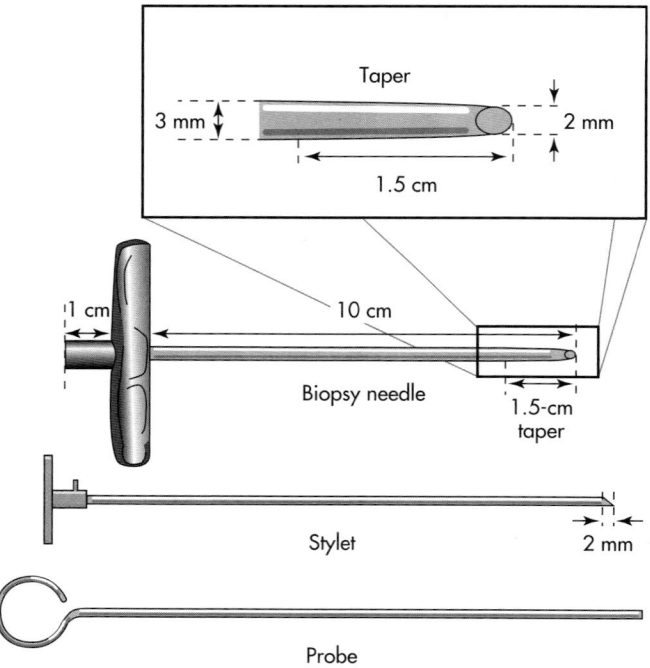

FIGURE **44-3** Bone marrow biopsy needle showing shape and size. (From Phipps W and others: *Medical-surgical nursing: health and illness perspectives,* ed 7, St. Louis, 2003, Mosby.)

Recording and Reporting

- Record in client's chart name of procedure, location of puncture site, amount and color of marrow aspirated, duration of procedure, client's tolerance to the procedure, vital signs and pain score before and after the procedure, any complications, laboratory tests ordered, specimen sent, type of dressing over puncture site, and whether drainage is present.
- Report to physician immediately any change in vital signs beyond client's normal limits and any excessive drainage from dressing over puncture site.
- Report results of procedure to nurses on the next shift.

Unexpected Outcomes	Related Interventions
1. Malpositioning occurs, evidenced by: • Client movement that disrupts the location or the sterile field	• Encourage client to remain still. • Seek additional help in immobilizing the client, if necessary.
2. Site complications occur, evidenced by: • Tenderness or erythema at bone marrow site	• Administer analgesic as ordered. • Continue to monitor site. • Notify physician, and obtain further orders.
3. Client experiences infection/sepsis, evidenced by: • Hypotension, tachycardia, and fever	• Notify physician, and obtain further orders.

Teaching Considerations

- After explaining this procedure, encourage client to verbalize concerns. Many clients are anxious about procedure.
- Teach client to contact physician if tenderness and/or redness appear at puncture site.
- Instruct client that some persons experience tenderness at the puncture site for several days after the study and that mild analgesia may be ordered by the physician.

Pediatric Considerations

- The site preferred in children is the iliac crest, and for infants the anterior tibia.
- This procedure can be frightening for child because it is done behind his or her field of vision.
- Conscious or unconscious sedation is commonly used. If unconscious sedation is used, an anesthesiologist will be needed for the procedure.

- Prepare child of preschool age before the procedure; make a game out of having child recall the next procedural step, which can serve as distraction mechanism (Haiat and others, 2003).

Gerontological Considerations

- Older adults with arthritis may need help to sustain the required position.
- Assess for pain; the older adult may not ask for pain relief.
- Be aware that older adults may have specific fears and anxiety related to postprocedure falling and fatigue.

Home Care Considerations

- If client is transferred to long-term care facility, ensure thorough communication between facilities regarding results of procedure and client condition.

Lumbar Puncture

A lumbar puncture, also called a spinal puncture or spinal tap, is a bedside procedure performed by a physician that involves the introduction of a spinal needle into the subarachnoid space of the spinal column. Lumbar punctures are done to measure cerebrospinal fluid (CSF) pressure in the subarachnoid space, to obtain CSF for visual and laboratory examination, to inject anesthetic, diagnostic, or therapeutic agents and to drain CSF volume in benign intracranial hypertension. Laboratory examination of CSF fluid helps diagnose spinal cord tumors, central nervous system infections, hemorrhage, autoimmune or demyelinating diseases, and degenerative brain disease.

The major contraindication for lumbar puncture is if there is evidence of greatly increased intracranial pressure (ICP) because the sudden release of pressure may cause her-

niation of the brain structures through the foramen magnum. This herniation compresses the brain stem, which contains the vital cardiac, respiratory, and vasomotor centers, and sudden death may result. In elective lumbar puncture, preprocedure computed tomography results are reviewed for evidence of brain shift to rule out increased intracranial pressure. However, when the need for diagnostic LP is urgent, such as in clients without brain shift who are comatose and suspected of acute meningitis, prior CT may be omitted (van Crevel 2002).

Other contraindications include spinal degenerative joint disease, spinal deformities, and coagulopathies. Finally, infection near the lumbar site not only risks introduction of infection into the CSF, but also affects the accuracy of the resulting CSF cytologic studies (Chernecky and Berger, 2004).

DELEGATION CONSIDERATIONS

The skill of assisting with a lumbar puncture may be delegated to assistive personnel if the client is stable. The nurse must instruct assistive personnel in:

- Proper positioning of client during the procedure
- Taking baseline and postprocedure vital signs and reporting these vital signs to the nurse
- Signs and symptoms experienced by the client to report to the nurse

EQUIPMENT

- ❏ Lumbar puncture tray, including: antiseptic solution; 10 gauze sponges (4 × 4); sterile towels; 3 spinal needles (various sizes) with inner obturators (5 to 12.5 cm long; infants need 5-cm needle); alcohol swabs; anesthetic agent (e.g., lidocaine 1%); syringes (3 to 5 ml); 2 rolled bath towels; needles (16 to 27 gauge; NOTE: incidence of postpuncture headache progressively decreases as needle gauge decreases [Evans and others, 2000])
- ❏ Protective equipment: masks and goggles (optional), sterile gloves (check physician's size)
- ❏ Glass or plastic manometer with three-way stopcock
- ❏ Four test tubes
- ❏ Antiseptic ointment
- ❏ Band-Aids or 2 × 2 gauze dressing
- ❏ Straight chair for physician

STEP	RATIONALE

ASSESSMENT

1. Perform positive client identification according to agency policy.

2. Verify that informed consent has been obtained.

3. Assess for client's ability to understand and follow directions.

4. Assess client's level of understanding of procedure, including any concerns.

5. Assess musculoskeletal flexibility of client to assume lateral decubitus (fetal) position, as well as his or her ability to remain in position.

6. Examine medical record for contraindications listed above.

7. Obtain vital signs and neurological status of lower extremities: movement, sensation, and muscle strength (see Chapter 18).

Complies with National Patient Safety Goals issued by the Joint Commission on Accreditation of Healthcare Organizations (JCAHO).

Informed consent for procedure is required by federal regulations, many state laws, and accreditation agencies, such as the JCAHO.

Procedure requires client to follow directions closely and assume proper position. Clients with neurological problems may have reduced level of consciousness.

Determines extent of instruction and level of support required

Lateral decubitus position is important to place spinal needle in proper position. Movement can cause injury from spinal needle.

Reduces risks of procedure complications.

Provides baseline data for comparison with postprocedural measurements.

NURSING DIAGNOSES

- Anxiety
- Fear
- Risk for infection
- Risk for injury

- Deficient knowledge regarding purpose and steps of procedure
- Acute pain
- Impaired mobility

Related factors are individualized based on client's condition or needs.

PLANNING

1. Expected outcomes following completion of procedure:
   - Client understood and cooperated with lateral positioning.
   - Only a small amount (1- to 2-cm circle) (½ to 1 inch) of clear or red drainage is present at puncture site.
   - Client does not experience postpuncture headache.

   - Test results of CSF are normal.

   - Client's level of comfort is equivalent to a score of 4 or less on a pain scale of 0 to 10.

Reduces risk of injury during the procedure due to client movement.

Small amount of CSF or bloody drainage is considered normal and expected.

Postpuncture headaches occur in about 32% of clients, but incidence can be reduced to 6% if certain preventive measures (described under Physician's Responsibility) are followed. These headaches usually appear within 48 hours and resolve within 1 week. Risk for postpuncture headache is highest in females, particularly ages 18 to 30 and is lowest in children and in adults over age 60. Risk is also elevated in those who have headaches before the procedure and in adults with low body weight (Chernecky and Berger, 2004; Evans and others, 2000).

Comparison of client's laboratory data with normal laboratory values shows no abnormal pressures, cells, organisms, or other constituents.

Use of a standardized pain scale provides reliable detection of increasing pain so that postprocedure analgesia may be given.

STEP	**RATIONALE**

2. Explain procedure to client.

3. Have client empty bladder and bowel before procedure begins.

Nurse tells client in understandable terms about potential discomfort associated with procedure and length of procedure. Avoids interruption of test and prevents discomfort.

IMPLEMENTATION

NURSE'S RESPONSIBILITY

1. Explain that client must lie in flexed position and remain still for entire procedure.

Client must remain still throughout procedure because movement may cause traumatic injury from the spinal needle within spinal column (Chernecky and Berger, 2004).

2. Position client in lateral recumbent (fetal) position with head and neck flexed (Figure 44-4). Bring both arms and knees toward center of body; client may grasp knees with hands. A pillow may be placed between the knees to help maintain position.

Gives spinal column full curvature. Spinal column should be flexed as much as possible to allow maximal space between vertebrae.

3. Caution client not to cough and to breathe slowly and deeply. Encourage client to relax.

4. Explain each step that may give discomfort.

Coughing or changes in breathing may result in injury and/or inaccurate readings.

Reassure client as needles are inserted. A stinging sensation results from administration of the anesthetic. Brief pain occurs when the spinal needle penetrates the dura and enters the subarachnoid space (Malarkey and McMorrow, 2000).

5. Apply gloves in preparation for assisting with filling test tubes with CSF.

Prevents transmission of microorganisms.

6. Properly label tubes with client information and name of test desired. Transport specimens to laboratory immediately.

The first specimen is discarded because it is likely to be contaminated with blood. The remaining test tubes are numbered in sequence of collection (e.g., mark the tubes "1," "2," "3," etc.). Tube 1 is used for chemical and immunological analysis because blood or tissue fluid will not alter these test results. Tube 2 is used for microbial analysis. Tube 3 is used for microscopic examination of cells (Malarkey and McMorrow, 2000). Analysis must be performed promptly on freshly obtained specimens (Chernecky and Berger, 2004).

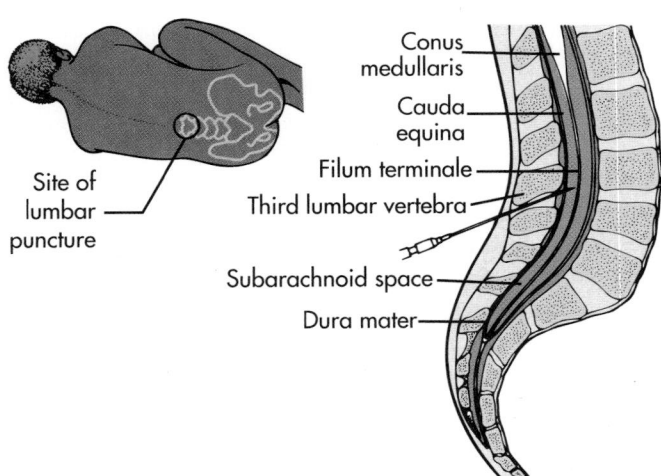

FIGURE 44-4 Client position for lumbar puncture. (Modified from Pagana K, Pagana T: *Mosby's diagnostic and laboratory test reference,* ed 5, St. Louis, 2000, Mosby.)

STEP	RATIONALE
7. Assist with placement of direct pressure and gauze dressing once needle is withdrawn from puncture site.	Pressure helps minimize CSF loss and bleeding.
8. Remove gloves; perform hand hygiene thoroughly after procedure.	Tubes might contain virulent organisms. Proper disposal of gloves reduces transmission of organisms.
9. Assist client in assuming comfortable position.	The duration of postprocedure bed rest has not been shown to be related to the incidence of headache (Evans and others, 2000).
10. Provide for client's comfort with medication if ordered, desirable, and not contraindicated.	Procedure is usually described as painful by client. Postprocedure headache may require that client be medicated.

- **Critical Decision Point**
  If client has a suspected CNS disorder, a sedative or analgesic may be contraindicated so as not to further cloud client's consciousness.

STEP	RATIONALE
11. During and after procedure, observe for:	
a. Changes in level of consciousness, pupil size and reaction, respiratory status, and vital signs.	Although an infrequent complication, increased intracranial pressure can occur (Malarkey and McMorrow, 2000). Changes in level of consciousness, pupil size and reaction, respiratory status, and vital signs indicate increasing intracranial pressure.
b. Numbness, tingling, or pain radiating down legs.	May result from spinal nerve irritation.
12. Client may return to regular diet.	The volume of fluid intake after LP has not been shown to be related to the incidence of headache (Evans and others, 2000).

PHYSICIAN'S RESPONSIBILITY

STEP	RATIONALE
1. Perform hand hygiene.	Reduces transmission of microorganisms.
2. Set up sterile field of equipment.	Provides sterile work area.
3. Apply sterile gloves (mask and goggles optional).	Reduces risk of procedure-related infection.
4. Prepare lumbosacral area with antiseptic solution and gauze sponges.	Prevents entry of microorganisms from skin to CSF in spinal canal.
5. Inject topical anesthetic agent.	Provides local anesthetic to skin surrounding puncture site.
6. Insert spinal needle containing an inner obturator into subarachnoid space (see Figure 44-4).	Care is taken to avoid trauma to spinal nerves. Factors that have been shown to reduce the incidence of postpuncture headache include using the smallest needle possible to achieve the procedure objective and inserting the bevel of the needle parallel (rather than perpendicular) to the dural fibers. In addition, using a cutting needle, such as a Quincke needle instead of a noncutting pencil-point needle may also reduce the incidence of postpuncture headache (Angle and others, 2003; Evans and others, 2000).
7. After entering subarachnoid space, obturator is removed.	Allows flow of CSF from subarachnoid space.
8. Attach manometer with stopcock, and read manometer for "opening pressure." Before the pressure reading is taken, ask client to relax and straighten the legs.	Manometer is calibrated in centimeters of water. Relaxing and straightening the legs reduces the intraabdominal pressure. This maneuver thus reduces risk of an increase in CSF pressure (Rosin and Rosenthal, 2001).
9. Turn stopcock to allow CSF to drip into test tubes to send for appropriate testing.	The volume of CSF fluid removed has not been shown to be related to the incidence of postpuncture headache (Evans, and others, 2000).

STEP	RATIONALE
10. Reinsert stylet, then remove spinal needle and place digital pressure on insertion site.	Decreases or stops CSF leakage from spinal canal. Replacing the stylet before withdrawing the needle has been shown to reduce the incidence of postpuncture headache. It is theorized that this prevents arachnoid strands from threading through the insertion site and allowing CSF leakage (Evans and others, 2000).
11. Place adhesive gauze or Band-Aid over insertion site.	Ensures sterility of insertion site.

EVALUATION

1. Assess needle insertion site for drainage.	Small amount of CSF (clear) or bloody (red) drainage is considered normal.
2. Assess level of consciousness, vital signs, pupils, and respiratory status; assess numbness, tingling, and ability to move the lower extremities.	Changes may indicate complications of brain herniation or irritation of spinal nerves.

Recording and Reporting

- Record in nurses' notes the procedure performed, including time, physician's name, client's tolerance (e.g., opening pressure, color of CSF, amount of drainage on dressing, and whether headache and leg tingling are present), and specimens sent to laboratory.
- Report pertinent findings to nurse in charge and to physician: changes in vital signs, nausea, vomiting, and changes in level of consciousness.

Unexpected Outcomes	Related Interventions
1. Postdural puncture headache (PDPH), evidenced by: • Headache • Blurred vision • Tinnitus (Drug Therapy Perspectives, 2001)	• Medicate for pain as ordered. • Notify physician, who may choose to inject a small amount of autologous blood into the epidural space. This is known as an "epidural blood patch" and is thought to relieve postpuncture headache through two mechanisms: adding volume to the CSF and interacting with CSF to cause closure of the puncture site through rapid clot formation (Drug Therapy Perspectives, 2001). • Intravenous caffeine sodium benzoate has been used with limited success in relieving PDPH (Yucel and others, 1999). NOTE: Increasing the fluid intake, a longstanding practice, has not been shown to prevent postpuncture headache.
2. Excessive drainage from insertion site, evidenced by: • More than 2 mm diameter of drainage on dressing	• Reinforce dressing. • Follow postprocedure orders related to this finding. • Continue to assess site and neurological status frequently. • Notify physician if accompanied by changing neurological status.
3. Hematoma at puncture site, evidenced by: • Lower extremity tingling	• Compare to baseline assessment. • Notify physician. • Continue frequent reassessments.
4. Excessive loss of CSF, evidenced by: • Large amount of CSF drainage from site • Reduced level of consciousness, dilated pupils, and increased blood pressure	• Maintain airway. • Notify physician immediately. • Prepare for transfer to intensive care setting.

Teaching Considerations

- Thoroughly explain procedure and postprocedure routine to client. Many clients have misconceptions regarding procedure. Emphasize that postprocedure headache for up to a week is common, but it is possible for a headache to linger for 4 weeks.
- Teach client the importance of drinking extra fluids after the procedure to replace CSF removed during the lumbar puncture.
- Teach client to inform physician of any unusual sensations in the legs, such as numbness and tingling.

Pediatric Considerations

- Apply topical anesthetic cream to the lumbar puncture site at least 1 hour before the procedure.

- Sedation is recommended, because of risk of injury due to movement of the client during the procedure. See Skill 44-1.

Gerontological Considerations

- Older adults may need assistance in assuming and maintaining the side-lying knee-to-chest position.

Home Care Considerations

- Provide written instructions to reinforce oral instructions.
- Client should seek medical attention immediately if he or she suddenly complains of severe headache or has change in level of consciousness.

Paracentesis

Abdominal paracentesis is a sterile, invasive procedure performed at the bedside or in a physician's office. In the aspiration paracentesis, peritoneal fluid is obtained via aspiration through a large-bore needle (or trocar and cannula) inserted percutaneously into the peritoneal cavity. The aspirated specimen then undergoes cytologic studies and analysis of the composition of bacteria, blood, glucose, and protein to help diagnose the cause(s) of abdominal effusion. Aspiration paracentesis may also be performed as a pallia-

tive measure to provide temporary relief of abdominal and respiratory discomfort caused by severe ascites. Lavage paracentesis, in which a lavage of solution is instilled then withdrawn, may be done to detect the presence of bleeding, as in cases of blunt abdominal trauma, or tumor cells, when cancer is suspected. Although not contraindicated, paracentesis should be performed with caution in clients with coagulopathies, with portal hypertension with abdominal collateral circulation, and in those who are pregnant.

DELEGATION CONSIDERATIONS

The skills of assisting with abdominal paracentesis may be delegated to assistive personnel if the client is stable. The nurse must instruct assistive personnel about:

- The proper way to position the client for a paracentesis
- Taking baseline and postprocedure vital signs and reporting these vital signs to the nurse
- Signs and symptoms experienced by the client that are to be immediately reported to the nurse

EQUIPMENT

- ❑ Antiseptic solution for hand hygiene
- ❑ Paracentesis tray, if available from central supply, which may include: antiseptic solution (e.g., povidone-iodine solution), sterile gauze sponges (4 × 4); local anesthetic solution for injection (e.g., lidocaine 1%); sterile syringes: two 3-ml, 23- to 25-gauge needles for anesthetic;

four 10- to 60-ml, 19- to 21-gauge needles; small, sterile knife blade; two sterile cannula needles, sizes 10 or 12, with inner trocar, or catheter

- ❑ 2 to 3 L IV fluids as ordered
- ❑ IV tubing, usually macrodrip size with three-way stopcock
- ❑ Sterile specimen containers and bag for containment
- ❑ Vacuum bottles as ordered
- ❑ Two packages of sterile gloves (check physician's preferred size)
- ❑ Masks and goggles for nurse, physician, and assistive personnel (check institution's policy)
- ❑ Sterile gauze sponges (2 × 2), tape, adhesive bandages, and antiseptic ointment
- ❑ Pain medication, if ordered (given 30 minutes before procedure)
- ❑ Laboratory requisitions and labels
- ❑ Measuring tape and marker

STEP	RATIONALE

ASSESSMENT

1. Perform positive client identification according to agency policy.

2. Verify that informed consent has been obtained.

3. Determine whether client has history of being uncooperative or has severe coagulopathy, thrombocytopenia, intestinal obstruction, abdominal wall infection, previous multiple abdominal surgeries, or portal hypertension with abdominal collateral circulation.
4. Perform hand hygiene.
5. Obtain vital signs, especially blood pressure. Check with physician regarding orders for hematocrit, prothrombin time, partial thromboplastin time, and platelet values before the procedure.

6. Palpate client's bladder for distention, or determine time of last voiding. Have client void before procedure.
7. Weigh client, assess abdomen (see Chapter 18), and measure abdominal girth in centimeters at largest point of abdomen. Use ink pen to mark where measuring tape lies.
8. Assess client's respiratory rate, diaphragmatic excursion, and chest wall motion.

9. Assess client's level of understanding of procedure, including any concerns.
10. Administer preprocedure medication if indicated.

Complies with National Patient Safety Goals issued by the Joint Commission on Accreditation of Healthcare Organizations (JCAHO).

Informed consent for procedure is required by federal regulations, many state laws, and accreditation agencies, such as the JCAHO.

These conditions will increase the risk of procedure-related complications.

Reduces transmission of microorganisms.

Baseline vital signs detect changes caused by complications from drainage of large fluid volumes. Obtaining laboratory values provides a baseline to compare values because of the risk of bleeding in the posttest period (Malarkey and McMorrow, 2000).

Chance of bladder trauma is decreased if bladder is not distended (Malarkey and McMorrow, 2000).

Abdominal girth is measured in same place to accurately note abdominal size before and after paracentesis.

Excess peritoneal fluid increases intraabdominal pressure, which in turn compromises respiration (Linton and others, 2003).

Determines extent of instruction and level of support required.

Clients who are anxious may benefit from preprocedure medications.

NURSING DIAGNOSES

- Anxiety
- Ineffective breathing pattern
- Risk for infection
- Risk for injury

- Deficient knowledge regarding purpose and steps of procedure
- Acute pain

Related factors are individualized based on client's condition or needs.

PLANNING

1. Expected outcomes following completion of procedure:
   - Client assumes positions without problems, has few changes in vital signs, and has no complications.
   - For peritoneal lavage and abdominal aspiration, aspirate is clear or slightly blood tinged.
   - For therapeutic treatment of ascites by paracentesis, fluid drainage results in decreased abdominal girth, skin tightness, and weight and improved respiratory status.
   - Client's level of comfort is equivalent to a score of 4 or less on a pain scale of 0 to 10.

2. Organize equipment on bedside table.

Client tolerates procedure well.

Slight amount of blood-tinged drainage may be caused by irritation to tissue by needle.

Clients usually experience transient relief of distention and dyspnea (Pagana and Pagana, 2002).

Use of a standardized pain scale provides reliable detection of increasing pain so that postprocedure analgesia may be given.

Ensures ease and success of procedure.

STEP	**RATIONALE**

3. Prepare client for procedure:

4. Explain purpose of and steps in the procedure. — Assists in minimizing anxiety and promoting relaxation and cooperation.

5. Have client void before procedure. — Full or distended bladder increases possibility of puncturing bladder (Chernecky and Berger, 2004).

• *Critical Decision Point*
If client is unable to void and bladder is distended, obtain an order for catheterization.

6. Client assumes position desired by physician, either semi-Fowler's in bed or sitting upright on side of bed or in chair with feet supported. Because of underlying physical condition (i.e., respiratory distress from increased fluid), client may be unable to assume required position for procedure and may require assistance of pillows or other positional devices (Figure 44-5). — These positions cause fluid to accumulate in the lower abdominal cavity and be drained more easily (see Figure 44-5).

IMPLEMENTATION

NURSE'S RESPONSIBILITY

1. Perform hand hygiene. — Reduces transmission of microorganisms.
2. Set up sterile tray, or open sterile supplies and make accessible for physician. — Ensures maintenance of sterility throughout procedure.
3. Prepare solution to be used for lavage; attach to IV tubing. — If fluid instillation is to be performed, as with blunt abdominal trauma, fluid is ready to attach to plastic tubing after cannula is in place in abdomen.
4. Ensure client's comfort, and assess for complications. — Assists client in tolerating procedure and identifies need to modify or discontinue procedure.

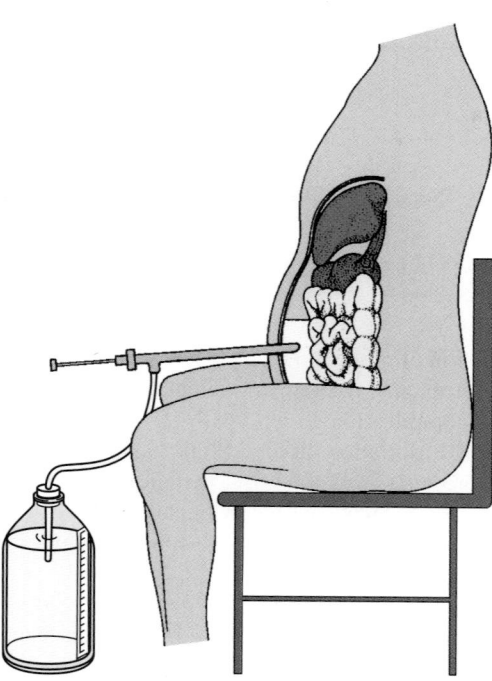

FIGURE **44-5** Paracentesis. (Pagana KD, Pagana TJ: *Mosby's manual of diagnostic and laboratory tests,* ed 6, St. Louis, 2003, Mosby.)

STEP	**RATIONALE**
5. Assess vital signs before, every 15 minutes during, and every 15 minutes for an hour after the procedure or according to agency policy.	Identifies hemodynamic changes and possible complications of procedure. Hypotension may occur if a large volume of fluid was removed.
6. Implement fluid instillation for lavage:	
a. Apply clean gloves (and mask and goggles, if required).	Reduces transmission of microorganisms.
b. After IV tubing is attached to cannula, administer physician-ordered amount of fluid at prescribed rate.	Promotes infusion of prescribed fluid into peritoneum.
c. Clamp IV tubing after fluid is instilled, and place drainage tubing below client's abdominal level.	Promotes gravitational drainage of fluid from peritoneal cavity.
d. Ascitic fluid is withdrawn by either gravity or vacuum drainage. Maximum amount of ascitic fluid usually allowed to drain is 1500 ml but may be as much as 5 L in cases of severe ascites.	Permits flow of fluid or solution from abdomen. Aspiration of more than 1500 ml of fluid may cause hypovolemic shock because of the sudden shift of fluid from the circulatory system to replace the aspirated fluid.
7. Collect any necessary laboratory specimens in sterile containers.	
8. Assess client's tolerance of procedure, including pain and mental status.	Enables nurse to evaluate client's tolerance of procedure and detects changes from preprocedure condition.
9. Assist client in assuming comfortable position in bed.	Maintains comfort.
10. Carefully dispose of equipment, remove gloves, and perform hand hygiene. Needles and other sharp objects should be placed in special containers. Dispose of peritoneal fluid not sent to laboratory according to hospital procedure.	Controls transmission of infection. Proper disposal of sharps prevents accidental injury to personnel.

PHYSICIAN'S RESPONSIBILITY

1. Perform hand hygiene. Prepare abdomen with antiseptic solution and 4 × 4 sponges.	Reduces transmission of microorganisms.
2. Wear mask (if required), apply sterile gloves and goggles, and drape client with sterile towels.	Maintains surgical asepsis.
3. Inject local anesthetic, and allow time for it to take effect.	Provides local anesthetic to area of puncture or incision.
4. If the purpose of the paracentesis is to drain ascitic fluid or to lavage, insert the large-bore needle or trocar through a small incision between the umbilicus and the symphysis pubis.	Facilitates placement of large-bore needle or trocar into abdominal cavity for instillation and drainage of fluid. Permits the removal of blood and/or fluid specimens.
5. Attach IV tubing to the cannula, and allow fluid to drain into a receptacle to a maximum of 1500 ml. The fluid may also be aspirated using a 60-ml syringe. For lavage, instill prescribed amount of sterile fluid and allow it to drain.	Fluid is drained slowly, to a maximum of 1500 ml to prevent hypovolemic shock.
6. If only specimens are needed and an incision is not made, insert 10-gauge needle attached to syringe, aspirate fluid, and place in specimen containers. Remove cannula, needle, or trocar.	Obtains sterile specimens for laboratory analysis.
7. Place manual pressure over insertion site until drainage ceases or apply pressure dressing.	Prevents excessive drainage from puncture site.
8. Place antiseptic ointment with 2 × 2 gauze sponge over insertion site.	Prevents growth of bacteria at puncture site.

STEP	RATIONALE

▌ EVALUATION

1. Take vital signs, including pain score, every 15 minutes for 1 hour and then every 30 minutes for 2 hours or according to agency policy; check for stability by comparing with preprocedure values.

   Helps detect hypotension due to fluid shifts.

2. Monitor urinary output for signs of bleeding for 24 hours.

   Verifies client's physiological status. Hematuria may indicate bladder trauma.

3. Check dressing over insertion site for bleeding or drainage.

   Provides for continued observation of puncture site. May indicate accumulation of blood or fluid in abdominal cavity. A major complication of this procedure is hemorrhage (Malarkey and McMorrow, 2000).

4. Measure abdominal girth and weight.

   Determines change after fluid drainage.

5. Inspect character of lavage or aspirate.

   For peritoneal lavage and abdominal aspiration, aspirate is clear or slightly blood tinged.

6. Observe and question if client is having acute abdominal pain.

   May indicate perforation of the bowel (Malarkey and McMorrow, 2000).

Recording and Reporting

- Record in client's medical record:
  - Time and type of procedure (aspiration or lavage)
  - Color, consistency, and amount of fluid withdrawn
  - Client's tolerance of procedure (pain level, vital signs)
  - Type of dressing over insertion site and whether drainage is present
  - Laboratory to which specimen was sent
  - Changes in abdominal girth, weight, and amount, color, and clarity of fluid
- Notify physician of significant deviations from client's baseline vital signs or if there is severe abdominal pain or excessive bloody drainage from insertion site.

Unexpected Outcomes	Related Interventions
1. Client experiences bowel perforation, evidenced by: • Acute abdominal pain	• Notify physician immediately. • Continue close reassessments of quantity and quality of drainage. • Anticipate need for emergency surgery.
2. There is fluid shift out of intravascular space and into peritoneum, evidenced by: • Hypovolemia	• Continue to monitor vital signs closely. • Position bed with knees elevated, if client is able to tolerate this position. • Notify physician. • Anticipate orders for hypertonic IV fluid administration such as salt-poor albumin or mannitol.
3. Change in color of drainage is observed.	• Continue to monitor closely. • Notify physician of findings.
4. Infection develops, evidenced by: • Increasing temperature to over 101.5° F (38.6° C)	• Monitor temperature and signs of chilling. • Assess site. • Notify physician of findings. • Anticipate orders for antibiotics.

Unexpected Outcomes	Related Interventions
5. Client has pathological condition, evidenced by: • Abnormal laboratory results on tests of the aspirated peritoneal fluid	• Notify physician of results.
6. Leakage of fluid occurs at aspiration site, evidenced by: • Continuously saturated dressings	• Reinforce dressing. Place collection bag over site, if needed. • Notify physician, who may place a small suture to stop the drainage.

Teaching Considerations

- Explain to client that procedure will be more safely performed if bladder is empty.
- Explain that although the local anesthetic will eliminate pain at the insertion site, a pressure type of discomfort may be experienced as the needle is inserted.
- Inform client with ascites that comfort will probably increase and breathing will be easier after paracentesis, but that the effect will be temporary and repeat procedures might be needed.
- Encourage client to check with physician regarding test results.

Gerontological Considerations

- If the older adult cannot tolerate sitting at the side of the bed, he or she is placed in high-Fowler's position.
- In older adults, skin is normally inelastic and thin; therefore special care should be used when removing adhesive bandages or tape at puncture site.

- Early signs of fluid shift such as confusion or restlessness may be hard to detect in the older adult, because they may be mistaken for baseline status. Be sure to obtain a thorough assessment of baseline mentation and abilities before this procedure for postprocedure comparison.

Home Care Considerations

- If paracentesis is done on an ambulatory care basis, inform client to notify physician of fever or any swelling, pain, or drainage at puncture site.
- In males, scrotal edema should be reported to the physician.

Long-Term Care Considerations

- If the client is received from a long-term care facility, obtain a thorough baseline report of mentation and cognitive abilities; use findings for comparison when assessing for signs of infection and fluid shift complications after the procedure.

Thoracentesis

Thoracentesis, an invasive procedure, is performed to analyze or remove pleural fluid or to instill medications intrapleurally. Specimens are examined for gross appearance and consistency and for protein, glucose, amylase, lactate dehydrogenase (LD), and cellular composition. Cytologic specimens are examined for malignancy, differentiated between transudative and exudative characteristics, and cultured for pathogens. Transudate in the pleural space may be caused by ascites, cirrhosis (hepatic), congestive heart failure, hypertension (pulmonary, systemic), nephritis, and nephrosis. Exudate in the pleural space may be caused by blocked lymphatic drainage, empyema, esophageal rupture, infarction (pulmonary), infection, neoplasm, pancreatitis, rheumatoid arthritis, systemic lupus erythematosus, thoracic duct disruption, accidental injury, and tuberculosis (Chernecky and Berger, 2004).

The procedure is performed by a physician and assisted by a nurse or assistive personnel using strict sterile technique. With the client positioned upright, a large-bore needle is passed through the chest wall into the pleural cavity. Excess pleural fluid resulting from injury, infection, or disease may be removed. The primary therapeutic purpose of thoracentesis is to relive pain and dyspnea caused by the resulting pleural pressure from the effusion.

Thoracentesis can generally be performed in less than 30 minutes at the client's bedside, in a procedure room, or in the physician's office. Thoracentesis poses a risk of causing pneumothorax or air embolism. Both complications require immediate emergency nursing and medical intervention.

DELEGATION CONSIDERATIONS

The skill of assisting with a thoracentesis may not be delegated to unaccompanied assistive personnel because this skill requires repeated performance of nursing assessments for client tolerance of the procedure and for life-threatening complications requiring emergency intervention. Assistive personnel may take baseline and postprocedure vital signs and assist with client positioning, as long as a nurse is continuously present during the procedure.

EQUIPMENT

❑ Antiseptic solution for hand hygiene
❑ Thoracentesis tray, if available from central supply, which may include: antiseptic solution; gauze sponges

(4 × 4); sterile towels; local anesthetic solution for injection (e.g., lidocaine 1%); sterile syringes: two 3-ml, 23- to 25-gauge needles for anesthetic; and two 50-ml, 14- to 17-gauge needles, 5 to 7 cm long (or 2 to 3 inches), for drainage of pleural fluid
❑ Collection receptacle(s) for fluid; three-way stopcock; two-way stopcock with extension tubing; test tubes
❑ Antiseptic (e.g., chlorhexidine or povidone-iodine)
❑ Protective equipment: sterile gloves of proper size for physician; masks and goggles for physician, nurse, and/or assistive personnel (check institution's policy)
❑ Gauze (4 × 4) pads, tape, and antiseptic ointment
❑ Cough suppressant or pain medication if ordered

STEP	RATIONALE

▌ASSESSMENT

1. Perform positive client identification according to agency policy.

Complies with National Patient Safety Goals issued by the Joint Commission on Accreditation of Healthcare Organizations (JCAHO).

2. Verify that informed consent has been obtained.

Informed consent for procedure is required by federal regulations, many state laws, and accreditation agencies, such as the JCAHO.

3. Assess client's knowledge of procedure, including any concerns.

Determines level of health teaching and support required.

4. Assess client's ability to assume position required for procedure (Figure 44-6).

Client must remain immobile during the procedure to prevent needle damage to the lung or pleura. Clients with musculoskeletal or respiratory alterations may be unable to sit on side of bed with arms draped over high bedside table.

5. Obtain vital signs and oxygen saturation.

Provides baseline data for comparison.

6. Be aware of client's underlying medical condition, which may indicate presence of potential bleeding problems.

May contraindicate procedure because of risk of bleeding.

7. Assess respiratory function: symmetry of chest on inspiration and expiration, respiratory difficulty, and type of cough and sputum produced.

Provides baseline status for comparison with respiratory status during and after procedure.

8. Determine whether client is allergic to antiseptic or anesthetic solutions.

Decreases chances of allergic reactions.

9. Assess need for preprocedure pain medication.

Procedure can be painful, and client must remain still throughout it because of potential complications.

▌NURSING DIAGNOSES

• Anxiety
• Ineffective breathing pattern
• Fear
• Impaired gas exchange
• Risk for infection

• Risk for injury
• Deficient knowledge regarding purpose and steps of procedure
• Acute pain

Related factors are individualized based on client's condition or needs.

STEP	RATIONALE

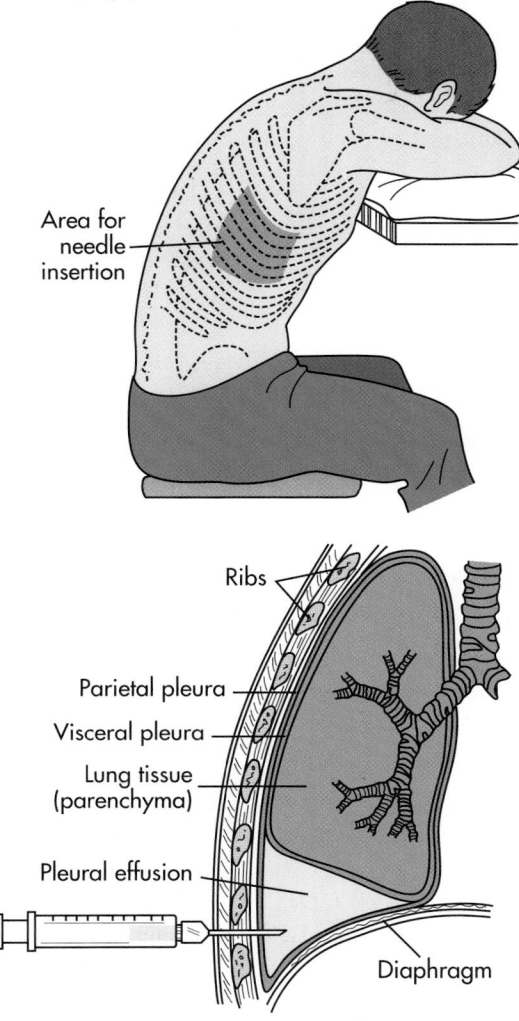

FIGURE **44-6** Thoracentesis.

PLANNING

1. Expected outcomes following completion of procedure:
   - Client describes purpose and steps of procedure as well as proper positioning.
   - Client tolerates procedure well.

   - Respiratory status is improved, evidenced by reduced labor of respirations, improved oxygen saturation, and improved comfort.
   - Client's level of comfort is equivalent to a score of 4 or less on a pain scale of 0 to 10.

2. Verify that chest x-ray results are available.

Demonstrates client understanding and improves likelihood of cooperation.

Client can assume position without problems and has little discomfort.

Optimal expansion of lungs improves gas exchange.

Use of a standardized pain scale provides reliable detection of increasing pain so that postprocedure analgesia may be given.

A decubitus chest x-ray examination is done before a thoracentesis to ensure the mobility and accessibility of the pleural fluid.

STEP	RATIONALE

3. Explain that, although a local anesthetic will be given at the insertion site, the client may feel a pressure-like pain when the pleura is entered for fluid removal (Malarkey and McMorrow, 2000).

Reinforces that sensation of pressure is related to entrance of catheter into pleura and not lack of adequate anesthesia. Client should not feel pain.

4. Have client void just before procedure.

Prevents interruption of procedure and promotes client's comfort.

5. Assess for presence of coughing.

Coughing during the procedure increases the risk of lung perforation. If client has a cough, preprocedure cough medicine may be ordered to be given.

6. Assist client in assuming the orthopneic position (an upright position with arms and shoulders raised and supported on a padded over-bed table) (see Figure 44-6). If unable to tolerate this position, assist client to side-lying position with the procedure-site side positioned upward.

Expands intercostal space for needle insertion.

IMPLEMENTATION

NURSE'S RESPONSIBILITY

1. Perform hand hygiene.

Reduces transmission of microorganisms.

2. Set up sterile tray, or open supplies to make them accessible for physician.

Prevents introduction of pathogens into the pleural space.

3. Assist client in maintaining correct position. If necessary, hold client's shoulders or sides, and provide reassurance.

Prevents sudden movement on part of client.

- *Critical Decision Point*
  Emphasize the importance of remaining immobile during the procedure to prevent trauma to the visceral pleura. Client must not cough, sneeze, or breathe deeply during procedure because it could cause trauma to visceral pleura.

4. Assess client's pulse for reflex bradycardia, diaphoresis, and feeling of faintness.

Evaluates tolerance to procedure.

5. Assess client's respiratory status during procedure: rate, effort to breathe, and color of mucous membranes and nail beds.

Evaluates tolerance to procedure and detects complications.

6. After thoracentesis, assist client in assuming comfortable position in bed.

If leakage into pleural space is suspected, client is positioned recumbent with punctured chest side up.

7. Label specimens, and send to the laboratory for any ordered testing.

A delay in processing may lead to erroneous laboratory findings, due to specimen deterioration (Chernecky and Berger, 2004).

PHYSICIAN'S RESPONSIBILITY

1. Perform hand hygiene.

Reduces transmission of microorganisms.

2. Disinfect skin with antiseptic solution and 4 × 4s.

Removes surface bacteria on skin.

3. Locate the upper border of the effusion by the loss of fremitus and the presence of flat percussion. The thoracentesis will be performed in the interspace below this level and 5 to 10 cm lateral to the spine (Chernecky and Berger, 2004).

Identifies correct needle insertion site. If needle is inserted too low, liver or spleen may be punctured, causing serious complications (Chernecky and Berger, 2004).

4. Apply mask, goggles, and sterile gloves, and drape client with sterile towels.

Maintains surgical asepsis.

5. Inject anesthetic, and allow time for it to take effect.

Provides local anesthesia at needle insertion site.

STEP	RATIONALE
6. Attach thoracentesis needle to three-way stopcock, which is turned off to needle lumen.	Ensures that no air enters pleural space when needle is introduced.
7. Slowly insert needle above the superior aspect of the lower rib of the intercostal space until the pleural space is reached, and then slowly aspirate fluid. Up to 1000 ml of pleural fluid can be removed at one time. At least 50 ml is required for diagnostic sampling.	Places needle in pleural space. Fluid is aspirated slowly to decrease risk of aspirating lung tissue into needle. Limitations on the amount of fluid removed are to prevent mediastinal shift and compromised venous return (Lewis and others, 2004).
8. Remove needle, and apply pressure and sterile dressing to puncture site.	Pressure assists in sealing puncture site. Dressing ensures sterility of site.
9. Order chest x-ray film and blood work (e.g., hematocrit and hemoglobin, serum electrolytes).	Chest x-ray film may show decreased fluid level in pleural space. Blood work is performed to check cell count and electrolytes in case replacement is needed.

EVALUATION

1. Note amount and color of pleural fluid. Apply small bandage over needle site. Turn client on unaffected side for 1 hour.	Characteristics are used for observation, reporting, and recording. Allows pleural puncture site to heal (Pagana and Pagana, 2002).
2. Monitor vital signs, oxygen saturation, and auscultate lung sounds every 5 minutes for $\frac{1}{2}$ hour, then every 30 minutes for 2 hours or as per agency policy. Compare with prethoracentesis data. Monitor for decreased lung sounds or shortness of breath (SOB) if large volume of fluid removed.	Monitors physiological status as compared with baseline. Assesses for reduction in labor of breathing as a result of the procedure.
3. Monitor client for complications from the thoracentesis listed in unexpected outcomes section.	Detects procedure complications.

- **Critical Decision Point**

  The complications of diaphragmatic, liver, or spleen perforation are less common than lung perforation. The risk of this occurring is greatest when the thoracentesis is performed below the tenth intercostal space. Symptoms of diaphragmatic perforation include ipsilateral shoulder pain during the procedure (Chernecky and Berger, 2004). Symptoms of liver or spleen perforation are more subtle and may not be noted for several days. Symptoms include decreasing hemoglobin and hematocrit values and possibly abdominal pain, hypotension, and tachycardia.

4. Follow up on postthoracentesis chest x-ray film as indicated.	Determines presence of pneumothorax.
5. Ask client to describe and demonstrate postprocedure limitations and positioning.	Evaluates learning.

Recording and Reporting

- Record in nurse's notes the name of procedure, name of person performing procedure, location of puncture site, amount and color of fluid drained, duration, tolerance (e.g., vital signs, pain, respiratory status, complications), laboratory tests ordered and sent, type of dressing over puncture site, and drainage.
- Report to physician immediately:
  - Decreased respiratory function
  - Changes in vital signs beyond normal limits
  - Changes in postprocedure hemoglobin, hematocrit, or serum electrolyte values
- Document completion of postprocedure chest x-ray examination; notify physician if any complications were detected.
- Report to nurses on next shift all data that have been recorded in nurses' notes and reported to physician.

Unexpected Outcomes	Related Interventions
1. Client does not assume position well, evidenced by: • Inability to comprehend instructions • Mechanical difficulty with positioning	• Reassess and assist client in proper position.
2. Needle displacement occurs, caused by: • Client movement or coughing during procedure	• Reassess and instruct client in importance of maintaining position and not moving. • Alert physician to the client's need to cough.
3. Pneumothorax occurs, evidenced by: • Sudden dyspnea and tachypnea • Anxiety • Asymmetrical chest excursion	• Administer oxygen. • Anticipate chest x-ray examination. • Anticipate possible chest tube insertion. • Monitor vital signs and respiratory status frequently.
4. Client experiences shock, evidenced by: • Hypotension • Tachycardia • Cool, clammy skin • Altered level of consciousness	• Place on oxygen and continuous cardiac monitoring. • Notify physician. • Obtain emergency equipment and supplies. • Anticipate transfer to intensive care setting. • Anticipate orders for administration of fluids and possibly vasopressors.
5. Subcutaneous emphysema is present, evidenced by: • Soft tissue edema around site • Palpation of crepitations over the affected area	• Cover site with Vaseline gauze. • Notify physician. • Monitor frequently to determine whether the amount is increasing.
6. Pyogenic infection develops, evidenced by: • Fever • Tachycardia • Chills	• Notify physician. • Anticipate orders for antibiotics. • Monitor for signs of progression to sepsis (hypotension, tachycardia, reduced level of consciousness, reduced urine output).

Teaching Considerations

• After explaining procedure, make certain client knows that movement or coughing can damage the lung or pleura. Cough suppressant may be administered before procedure if client has cough.

• Explain to client that chest x-ray film is often ordered after procedure to check for adequate lung expansion.

• Encourage client to report any dyspnea, chest pain, or cough after procedure.

• Inform the client that no food or fluid restrictions are necessary before or after the test.

• Encourage client to check with physician regarding test results.

Gerontological Considerations

• During all aspects of this procedure, be aware of ineffective breathing patterns in the older adult because of age-related changes such as reduced elastic lung recoil, declining chest expansion, reduced cough efficiency, and weaker thoracic and diaphragmatic muscles.

• Older adult clients may demonstrate restlessness as an early indication of hypoxia.

• Age-related changes of the musculoskeletal system may restrict movement during positioning and during procedure.

• After the procedure, be aware of need to change positions slowly in older adult clients to minimize safety risks and possible postural hypotension.

Home Care Considerations

• Teach client symptoms of complications related to liver and spleen perforation that may not be present for several days after procedure and to notify the physician. The client should report any new abdominal pain to the physician.

SKILL 44-4 Assisting With Bronchoscopy

Bronchoscopy is the examination of the tracheobronchial tree through a lighted tube containing mirrors. The tube, or bronchoscope, most commonly used is a flexible fiberoptic bronchoscope that allows both visualization and simultaneous administration of oxygen (Figure 44-7). The fiberoptic bronchoscope has lumens for visualization and for obtaining sputum, foreign bodies, and biopsy specimens. Laser ablation of endotracheal lesions may be performed through the bronchoscope.

Bronchoscopy may be an emergency or elective procedure and is performed for diagnostic or therapeutic reasons. The main purposes of this procedure are to aspirate excessive sputum or mucous plugs that cannot be sufficiently suctioned nasotracheally; to visualize the tracheobronchial tree for assessment of abnormalities of the mucosa, abscesses, aspiration pneumonia, strictures, and tumors; to obtain deep tissue biopsy and sputum specimens; and to remove foreign bodies (Chernecky and Berger, 2004). This procedure is contraindicated in clients who cannot tolerate interruption of high-flow oxygen unless intubated. Potential complications of bronchoscopy may include fever, infection, hypoxemia, bronchospasm and laryngospasm, pneumothorax, aspiration, dysrhythmias and hypotension, hemorrhage (after biopsy), and cardiac arrest. The nurse should be able to perform nasotracheal and orotracheal suctioning before assisting with the procedure.

This procedure is usually performed by a physician, usually a pulmonary specialist or surgeon, in about 30 to 45 minutes. The procedure may be performed at the bedside or in a specially equipped endoscopy room.

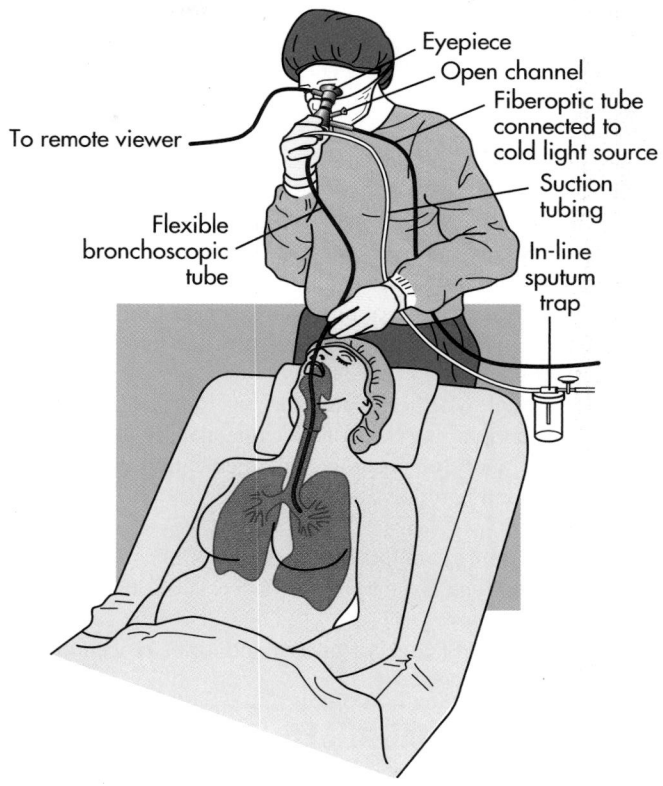

FIGURE **44-7** Flexible fiberoptic bronchoscopy.

DELEGATION CONSIDERATIONS

The skill of assisting with bronchoscopy may NOT be delegated to unaccompanied assistive personnel because this skill requires repeated performance of nursing assessments for client tolerance of the procedure and for life-threatening complications requiring emergency intervention. Assistive personnel may take baseline and postprocedure vital signs and assist with client positioning, as long as a nurse is continuously present during the procedure. In addition, this procedure often involves the use of IV moderate sedation, which requires the continuous presence of a nurse.

EQUIPMENT

❑ Bronchoscopy tray, if available from central supply, which may include: flexible fiberoptic bronchoscope (see Figure 44-7); gauze sponges (4 × 4); local anesthetic spray (lidocaine); sterile tracheal suction catheters (see Chapter 24); diazepam, midazolam, or other sedative for IV sedation; oxygen, resuscitative equipment, pulse oximeter, cardiac monitor; sterile gloves; sterile water-soluble lubricating jelly. Petroleum-based lubricants should not be used because of the hazard of aspiration and subsequent pneumonia.
❑ Mask and goggles for physician and nurse
❑ Emesis basin
❑ Oxygen equipment

STEP	**RATIONALE**

ASSESSMENT

1. Perform positive client identification according to agency policy.

2. Verify that informed consent has been obtained.

3. Obtain vital signs and oxygen saturation.

4. Assess respiratory status: type of cough, sputum produced, and lung sounds.

5. Determine purpose of procedure: for sputum aspiration, for assessment, for tissue biopsy, or for removal of foreign body.

6. Determine whether client is allergic to local anesthetic used for spraying throat (lidocaine usually used).

7. Assess need for preprocedure medication (usually atropine and narcotic or sedative).

8. Assess time client last ingested food. Client should have taken nothing by mouth for at least 8 hours before a bronchoscopy.

9. Assess client's level of understanding of procedure, including any concerns.

Complies with National Patient Safety Goals issued by the Joint Commission on Accreditation of Healthcare Organizations (JCAHO).

Informed consent for procedure is required by federal regulations, many state laws, and accreditation agencies, such as the JCAHO.

Baseline data provides for comparison with findings during and after procedure.

Provides for comparison with respiratory status during and after procedure.

Enables nurse to anticipate needs of client and physician.

Allergy could cause laryngeal edema or laryngospasm.

Atropine decreases secretions and inhibits vagally stimulated bradycardia; narcotics or sedatives relieve anxiety and decrease discomfort.

Reduces risk of aspiration.

Determines extent of instruction and level of support required.

NURSING DIAGNOSES

- Anxiety
- Risk for aspiration
- Ineffective breathing pattern
- Fear
- Impaired gas exchange

- Ineffective airway clearance
- Risk for infection
- Risk for injury
- Deficient knowledge regarding purpose and steps of procedure

Related factors are individualized based on client's condition or needs.

PLANNING

1. Expected outcomes following completion of procedure:
    - Client has no respiratory complications.
    - Client's level of comfort is equivalent to a score of 4 or less on a pain scale of 0 to 10.

    - Physician is able to observe, suction, and obtain specimens from tracheobronchial tree.
    - Client recovers from sedation without respiratory complications or change in level of consciousness.
    - Client explains procedure and position to be assumed.
2. Explain procedure to client.
3. Assist client in maintaining position desired by physician: side-lying, semi-Fowler's, or supine.
4. Remove and safely store client's dentures.

Client tolerates procedure well.

Minimal trauma caused by bronchoscope.

Use of a standardized pain scale provides reliable detection of increasing pain so that postprocedure analgesia may be given.

Indicates that purpose of procedure was achieved.

Sedation adequate.

Demonstrates client's understanding.

Reduces anxiety and increases cooperation.

Provides maximal visualization of lower airway and adequate lung expansion.

Minimizes chance of airway obstruction.

STEP	RATIONALE

IMPLEMENTATION

NURSE'S RESPONSIBILITY

1. Perform hand hygiene.
2. Instruct client not to swallow local anesthetic; provide emesis basin for expectoration of local anesthetic.
3. Assist client through procedure with explanations.

4. Assess client's respiratory status during procedure: observe degree of restlessness and respiratory rate; observe capillary refill, color of nail beds, and pulse oximetry.

5. Note the characteristics of suctioned material. A small amount of blood mixed with the aspirate is expected because of tissue trauma.
6. Using gloved hand, wipe client's mouth and nose to remove lubricant after bronchoscope is removed.
7. Do not allow client to eat or drink until the tracheobronchial anesthesia has worn off and gag reflex has returned, usually 2 hours. Use tongue depressor to touch pharynx to test for presence of gag reflex.

Reduces transmission of microorganisms.
Reduces unintended anesthesia of esophagus.

Although premedicated and drowsy, clients need to be reminded not to change position and to cooperate. Reinforce that client will be able to breathe during procedure.
Bronchoscope may cause feelings of suffocation and vasovagal response, as well as laryngospasm; in addition, because airway is partially occluded, client may become hypoxic during observations.
Information used to record and report and to make further client observations.

Promotes hygiene and comfort.

Prevents aspiration.

PHYSICIAN'S RESPONSIBILITY

1. Perform hand hygiene.
2. Spray nasopharynx and oropharynx with topical anesthetic. Lidocaine is commonly used. When a client is intubated or has a tracheostomy, anesthetic spray may not be needed.
3. Attach bronchoscope to machine for light source.

4. Apply goggles, mask, and sterile gloves; then introduce bronchoscope into mouth to pharynx, and pass through glottis (see Figure 44-7). For intubated clients, the flexible bronchoscope is introduced through the endotracheal tube. May use more anesthetic spray at glottis to prevent cough reflex. Pass tube into trachea and bronchi.
5. Mucus may be suctioned, and bronchial washing performed with cytologic specimens taken with a wire brush or curette. Biopsy specimens may also be taken.

Reduces transmission of microorganisms.
Provides swift anesthesia of oropharynx.

Another physician, surgery personnel, or nurse attaches machine cable to bronchoscope.
Bronchoscope must be passed through upper airway structures to promote visualization of lower airways. Trachea and bronchi are observed for lesions and obstructions. Adaptor accompanies bronchoscope and may be used for bag-valve-mask or ventilator use.

Cytologic specimens are obtained to diagnose carcinoma.

EVALUATION

1. Monitor vital signs.
2. Observe character and amount of sputum. Physician may order serial sputum collection for 24 hours for cytologic examination.
3. Observe respiratory status closely, particularly for facial or neck crepitus.

Verifies physiological response.
Assesses for complication of bronchial perforation, which would be indicated by severe hemoptysis. Slight blood-tinged sputum is normal after this procedure.
Detects an early sign of bronchial perforation (Chernecky and Berger, 2004).

STEP	RATIONALE
4. Instruct client not to try to swallow sputum until gag reflex returns. Provide emesis basis for expectoration of sputum. Assess for return of gag reflex. Gag reflex usually returns in approximately 2 hours.	Helps prevent aspiration pneumonia, which is a risk until gag reflex returns.
5. Ask client to describe postprocedure normal and abnormal symptoms.	Evaluates client's understanding.

Recording and Reporting

- Record in nurses' notes name of procedure (include biopsy if performed), duration of procedure, client's tolerance of procedure and complications, and collection and disposition of specimen.
- Report excessive bleeding or respiratory difficulty after procedure or changes in vital signs beyond client's normal limits to physician immediately.
- Report results of procedure to nurses on the next shift.

Unexpected Outcomes	Related Interventions
1. Vasovagal response caused by stimulation of the baroreceptors during bronchoscope insertion, evidenced by: • Feeling faint, dizzy, and light-headed • Diaphoresis with a slow, steady pulse • A few seconds of unconsciousness	• Lower head of table. • Support airway.
2. Laryngospasm and bronchospasm, evidenced by: • Sudden, severe shortness of breath	• Call physician immediately. • Prepare emergency resuscitation equipment. • Anticipate possible cricothyrotomy.
3. Hypoxemia, evidenced by: • Gradual shortness of breath • Decreasing level of consciousness	• Maintain airway and breathing. • Notify physician immediately. • Monitor oxygen saturation.
4. Hemorrhage, evidenced by: • Acute blood loss • Hypotension and tachycardia • Decreasing level of consciousness	• Notify physician immediately. • Follow specific postprocedural orders related to findings.
5. See section on intravenous sedation.	

Teaching Considerations

- Before the procedure, instruct client to perform good mouth care to decrease risk of introducing bacteria into lungs during procedure.
- Instruct client to arrange for transportation home after an ambulatory procedure because (at most agencies) client will not be permitted to drive for 24 hours after receiving sedation.
- Instruct client in how to perform controlled coughing techniques for obtaining serial sputum samples, if ordered (see Chapter 43).

Pediatric Considerations

- In children the procedure is most frequently performed to remove foreign bodies from larynx or trachea and is often performed under general anesthesia. Client is placed in the lateral position after the procedure to prevent aspiration.
- Children are at higher risk of hypoxemia than adults because their bronchus is smaller and the bronchoscope decreases the available breathing space (Pagana and Pagana, 2002).
- Follow-up care after the foreign body is removed includes chest physiotherapy as needed, monitoring for respiratory distress, and education of parents.

Gerontological Considerations

- Physical exposure and room temperature may contribute to hypothermia in frail older adults, who may not be able to communicate that they are cold. Use heated blankets or forced air heat to maintain core temperature at comfortable, safe levels (Negishi and others, 2003).
- Be aware that NPO status in the older adult client may result in dehydration.
- Postoperative restlessness could indicate hypoxemia, not pain.
- Older adult client may experience postprocedure pain related to positioning.

- Because of multiple medications the older adult client may be taking, be aware of alterations in administration schedules necessary as a result of the NPO status for the diagnostic test.

Home Care Considerations

- Ambulatory care clients should be instructed to notify the physician if the following symptoms develop: fever, chest pain or discomfort, dyspnea, wheezing, or hemoptysis.
- Written instructions regarding names and phone numbers of persons to contact reinforce oral instructions.
- Throat discomfort may be managed with throat lozenges.

SKILL 44-5 Assisting With Endoscopy

Endoscopy is any study that allows direct visualization of an internal organ or structure by means of a long, flexible fiberoptic scope with a light source attached (Figure 44-8). For visualization of the upper gastrointestinal (GI) tract, esophagoscopy, gastroscopy, gastroduodenojejunoscopy (GJD) or duodenoscopy is performed, or more frequently, esophagogastroduodenoscopy (EGD), which permits visualization of esophagus, stomach, and duodenum in one examination. Besides direct observation, endoscopy enables biopsy of suspicious tissue, polyp removal, and performance of many other procedures, such as direct visual guidance for fine-needle aspiration biopsies and dilation and stenting of strictures. For visualization of the hepatobiliary tree and pancreatic ducts, an endoscopic retrograde cholangiopancreatography (ERCP) is performed. For visual examination of the lower GI tract, a proctoscopy, sigmoidoscopy, or colonoscopy may be performed. Typically these clients receive IV moderate sedation.

EGD is contraindicated in clients with Zenker's diverticulum or a large aortic aneurysm. Colonoscopy is contraindicated after a recent myocardial infarction or pulmonary embolus, during pregnancy, and when the client's lower gastrointestinal tract contains retained barium from an upper endoscopic study or barium enema.

Risks of endoscopic procedures include intestinal perforation, hemorrhage, peritonitis, aspiration, respiratory depression, and myocardial infarction secondary to vasovagal response. Both upper and lower GI endoscopic examinations are performed in a specially equipped endoscopic unit.

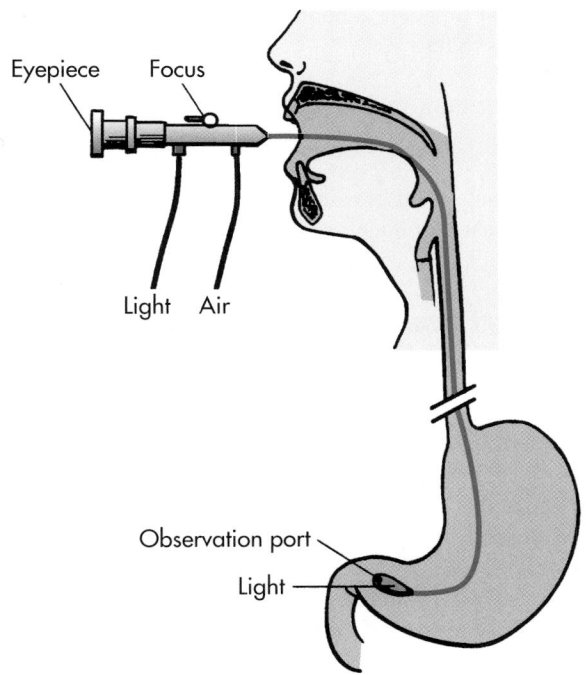

FIGURE 44-8 Stomach may be visualized by means of a fiberscope.

DELEGATION CONSIDERATIONS

The skill of assisting with endoscopy may NOT be delegated to unaccompanied assistive personnel because this skill requires repeated performance of nursing assessments for client tolerance of the procedure and for life-threatening complications requiring emergency intervention. Assistive personnel may take baseline and postprocedure vital signs and assist with client positioning, as long as a nurse is continuously present during the procedure. In addition, this procedure often involves the use of IV moderate sedation, which requires the continuous presence of a nurse.

EQUIPMENT

- ❑ Antiseptic solution for hand hygiene
- ❑ Endoscopy tray
- ❑ Fiberoptic endoscope (see Figure 44-8)
- ❑ Camera
- ❑ Solutions for biopsy specimens
- ❑ Local anesthetic spray
- ❑ Tracheal suction equipment (see Chapter 24)
- ❑ Blood pressure equipment
- ❑ Sterile water-soluble jelly
- ❑ Sterile gloves for physician
- ❑ Emesis basin
- ❑ Intravenous fluid and equipment for IV start (optional)
- ❑ Diazepam, midazolam, or other sedative for IV sedation (optional)
- ❑ Carbon dioxide source (for lower GI procedures)
- ❑ Oxygen, resuscitative equipment, and pulse oximeter
- ❑ Protective equipment: mask, gown, gloves, goggles

STEP	RATIONALE

ASSESSMENT

1. Perform positive client identification according to agency policy.

Complies with National Patient Safety Goals issued by the Joint Commission on Accreditation of Healthcare Organizations (JCAHO).

2. Verify that informed consent has been obtained.

Informed consent for procedure is required by federal regulations, many state laws, and accreditation agencies, such as the JCAHO.

3. Determine if GI bleeding is present. Observe character of emesis, stool, and nasogastric tube drainage.

Test is contraindicated in clients with severe upper GI bleeding because viewing lens may become covered with blood clots, preventing visualization (Pagana and Pagana, 2002).

- **Critical Decision Point**
  If client is actively bleeding, physician may order that the stomach be lavaged and aspirated clear of clots before procedure is attempted.

4. Determine purpose of procedure: biopsy, examination, or coagulation of bleeding sites.

Enables nurse to anticipate equipment needs.

5. Verify that client has been NPO for at least 8 hours for endoscopy of upper GI tract.

Introduction of endoscope can induce vomiting due to stimulation of the gag reflex. Empty stomach reduces risk of aspiration of stomach contents.

6. For lower GI studies (proctoscopy, sigmoidoscopy, or colonoscopy), verify that the client has followed a clear liquid diet for 2 days and has completed any ordered bowel cleansing regimen.

An empty intestinal tract is necessary to allow the endoscope insertion and good visualization of the interior walls.

7. Assess client's level of understanding of procedure, including any concerns.

Determines extent of instruction and level of support required.

NURSING DIAGNOSES

- Anxiety
- Risk for aspiration
- Ineffective breathing pattern
- Fear
- Impaired gas exchange

- Risk for infection
- Risk for injury
- Deficient knowledge regarding purpose and steps of procedure
- Acute pain

Related factors are individualized based on client's condition or needs.

STEP	RATIONALE

PLANNING

1. Expected outcomes following completion of procedure:
   - Client does not aspirate and has no postprocedure bleeding.

   Indicates absence of complications and tolerance of procedure.

   - Client's level of comfort is equivalent to a score of 4 or less on a pain scale of 0 to 10.

   Use of a standardized pain scale provides reliable detection of increasing pain so that postprocedure analgesia may be given.

   - Client is without respiratory complications or change in level of consciousness.

   Recovers from sedation.

   - Client describes purposes and steps of procedure.

   Documents client understanding.

2. Prepare client.
   a. Explain steps of procedure, including sensations to expect.

   Nurse can relieve anxiety and answer client's questions.

   b. Administer pain medication or preprocedure medication.

   Promotes relaxation and reduces anxiety.

IMPLEMENTATION

NURSE'S RESPONSIBILITY

1. Perform hand hygiene, and apply gloves, goggles, and mask.

   Reduces transmission of organisms.

2. Remove client's dentures or other dental appliances.

   Prevents dislodgement of dental structures during intubation phase.

3. For upper GI procedures, assist client in maintaining left lateral Sims' position. For lower GI procedures, assist client in maintaining left lateral decubitus position. Drape client for privacy and comfort.

   Position allows easy passage of upper or lower endoscope.

4. Ensure IV line is patent.

   Provides route for emergency medications.

5. Administer atropine, if ordered (upper GI studies).

   Atropine reduces the quantity of secretions, therefore reducing risk of aspiration for upper GI endoscopic procedures

6. Position tip of suction cannula for easy access in the client's mouth (upper GI studies).

   Drains oral secretions to reduce risk of aspiration.

7. Assist client through procedure:
   a. Anticipate needs, and promote comfort.

   Client is unable to speak after tube is passed into throat.

   b. Tell client what is happening as each portion of the procedure is carried out.

   Reassures client about procedure and how long it will last.

   c. Place tissue specimens in proper laboratory containers.

   Ensures proper labeling and preparation of specimens for microscopic examination.

   d. Assist client to comfortable position, then perform hand hygiene.

   Promotes rest and relaxation.

8. Provide slides and containers for specimens, and fix or seal as needed.

   Provides specimen preservation for accurate histopathological examination.

PHYSICIAN'S RESPONSIBILITY

1. Perform hand hygiene.

   Reduces transmission of microorganisms.

2. For upper endoscopic procedures, spray nasopharynx and oropharynx with local anesthetic.

   Topical anesthetic decreases the gag reflex caused by passage of the endoscope, thus improving safety and comfort.

3. Apply gown, mask, goggles, and gloves.

   Adheres to standard precautions.

STEP	RATIONALE
4. Attach distal end of endoscope to light source (see Figure 44-8).	Provides for direct visualization of upper GI tract.
5. Position client in left lateral (Sims') position (upper GI studies) or left lateral decubitus position (lower GI studies).	Provides for airway clearance if client gags and vomits gastric contents. Provides access to lower GI tract. Provides visualization of structures.
6. For upper GI studies, slowly pass endoscope into mouth, esophagus, stomach, or duodenum, and advance to desired depth while visualizing the walls. For lower GI studies, apply lubricant to the flexible fiberoptic endoscope, and insert it through the anus. Slowly advance the endoscope through the rectum and colon, while visualizing the walls.	
7. Insufflate air through endoscope into upper GI tract. For colonoscopies, carbon dioxide is used.	Distends GI structures for better visualization. Carbon dioxide insufflation produces less postprocedure abdominal cramping than air insufflation (Chernecky and Berger, 2004).
8. Examine, photograph, or perform biopsy of structures.	Provides data from which diagnosis is made.
9. Slowly remove the endoscope.	

EVALUATION

1. Monitor vital signs and oxygen saturation according to agency policy. May be as often as every 15 minutes for 2 hours.	Can identify change in vital signs that may indicate new bleeding in GI tract or oversedation.
2. Assess for level of sedation and level of consciousness.	Determines client's response to IV sedation.
3. Observe for pain.	Monitors for sudden abdominal pain, which can indicate rupture of abdominal organs.
4. Evaluate emesis or aspirate for frank or occult blood (see Chapter 43).	Monitors for gastrointestinal bleeding.
5. Assess for return of gag reflex, usually in 2 to 4 hours. Provide oral hygiene when gag reflex returns.	Determines when effects of anesthetic have disappeared. Gag reflex prevents aspiration.
6. Ask client to state postprocedure dietary and activity limitations.	Evaluates client understanding.

Recording and Reporting

- Record in nurses' notes the procedure, duration, client's tolerance, complications and interventions, and collection and disposition of specimen.
- Report onset of bleeding, abdominal pain, dyspnea, and vital sign changes to physician.
- Report to nurse in charge the duration of procedure, client's tolerance, and changes in vital signs or condition.

Unexpected Outcomes	Related Interventions
1. Vasovagal response caused by stimulation of the baroreceptors during endoscope insertion, evidenced by: • Feeling faint, dizzy, and light-headed • Diaphoresis with a slow, steady pulse • A few seconds of unconsciousness	• Lower head of table. • Support airway.
2. Damage to the intestinal wall, evidenced by: • Abdominal pain, fever, or bleeding	• Continue to monitor vital signs. • Notify physician of findings.

Unexpected Outcomes	Related Interventions
3. Aspiration pneumonia, evidenced by: • Dyspnea, tachypnea • Decreasing trend in oxygen saturation • Fever	• Support airway. • Follow specific postprocedural orders related to findings. • Notify physician.
4. Oversedation, evidenced by: • Decreasing level of consciousness	• See section on intravenous sedation.

Teaching Considerations

• Inform client of preprocedure medication and anticipated effects.
• Upper GI endoscopy:
  · Explain method for endoscope insertion. Prepare the client for a slight feeling of not being able to breathe. Assure client that this feeling is common, but that air is delivered through the endoscope and suffocation will not occur.
  · Teach the client simple hand signals for pain or discomfort, because he or she will not be able to speak after the endoscope is positioned in the esophagus.
  · Instruct client not to eat or drink after the procedure until the gag reflex returns, which is usually about 2 hours after the procedure.
• Lower GI procedures (colonoscopy, sigmoidoscopy, proctoscopy):
  · Explain that it is normal to experience increased flatus and abdominal cramping.
  · Small amounts of blood in the stool might be seen if a biopsy was taken.

Pediatric Considerations

• Child requires deep sedation or general anesthesia (American Academy of Pediatrics, 2002).
• Introduction of the endoscope in infants and small children who have a narrow and collapsible airway may result in respiratory distress.

Gerontological Considerations

• Removal of dentures may cause embarrassment to client.
• Older adult clients may have reduced drug clearance from decreased GFR and nephron activity or decreased hepatic function. Therefore the nurse must monitor the effects of medications given to the older adult client (Phipps, and others, 2003).
• Because of age-related changes in the older adult, the gastric mucosa is thinner, which increases the incidence of irritation and ulceration (Phipps and others, 2003).
• Assess skin integrity of client who has been lying still on examining table. Older adult clients are at greater risk for skin breakdown.
• Physical exposure and room temperature may contribute to hypothermia in frail older adults, who may not be able to communicate that they are cold. Use heated blankets or forced air heat to maintain core temperature at comfortable, safe levels (Negishi and others, 2003).
• Be aware that NPO status in the older adult client may result in dehydration.
• Because of multiple medications the older adult client may be taking, be aware of alterations in administration schedules necessary as a result of the NPO status for the diagnostic test.
• The older adult may experience dehydration, electrolyte imbalance, and exhaustion from test preparation. If the procedure is done on an ambulatory care basis, it may be helpful to have someone stay with the client.

Home Care Considerations

• Explain that client may be hoarse or have sore throat after procedure. Ice chips or anesthetic lozenges can be given after gag reflex returns.
• Instruct client to drink fluids to promote dye excretion.
• A warm tub bath may be soothing if rectal discomfort occurs after lower GI tract endoscopy.

SKILL 44-6 Assisting With Cardiogram

An electrocardiogram (ECG or EKG) is a graphic representation of the electrical impulses generated by the heart during the cardiac cycle of contraction and relaxation. The electrical impulses are conducted to the body's surface, where they are detected by electrodes placed on the limbs and torso. The electrodes carry these impulses to a continuously running graph that plots the ECG wave pattern. The appearance of the ECG pattern helps diagnose whether there are any abnormalities in the electrical conduction through the heart. The 12-lead ECG equipment is composed of 10 electrodes that are connected to the 10 lead wires of an ECG machine. One electrode is placed on each of the four extremities, and 6 electrodes are placed at specific sites on the chest. The 12 "leads" that are produced are 12 different graphical pictures, based on how the electricity flows between specific electrodes. They are the bipolar limb leads I, II, III; augmented limb leads aV_R, aV_L, aV_F; and precordial chest leads V_1 to V_6. Because the leads are specific to portions of the heart's anatomy, abnormalities in conduction can be correlated to help determine which part of the heart has sustained damage.

Single-lead tracings are used during emergencies and during pacemaker insertion. In a single-lead procedure, one electrode is substituted sequentially for the six chest electrodes. If a continuous ECG recording is needed over an extended period of time, a Holter monitor is used. A Holter monitor is a small, portable device that records electrical activity of the heart for up to 24 hours. The ECG is recorded on magnetic tape or in a digital record and monitors cardiac rhythm during activity, rest, and sleep.

DELEGATION CONSIDERATIONS

Because an ECG is noninvasive and poses no risk to the client, the skill of assisting with the electrocardiogram is routinely delegated to assistive personnel who are specifically skilled in obtaining the measurement.

- Instruct assistive personnel to summon the nurse immediately if the client states that he or she is having pain, or if the client appears anxious.

EQUIPMENT

- ❏ ECG machine
- ❏ ECG leads or electrodes (self-stick adhesive)
- ❏ Electrode gel (optional)
- ❏ Alcohol wipes
- ❏ Scissors

STEP	RATIONALE
ASSESSMENT	
1. Determine rationale for obtaining ECG.	ECG may be done to determine baseline cardiac function (e.g., preoperative, prediagnostic testing), to help evaluate response to cardiac medications, to help monitor recovery after a myocardial infarction, or when client experiences chest discomfort (Chernecky and Berger, 2004). If the ECG is being done for active chest pain, it should be performed right away.
2. Assess client's level of understanding of procedure, including any concerns.	Determines extent of instruction and level of support required.

NURSING DIAGNOSES

- Anxiety
- Fear
- Deficient knowledge regarding purpose and steps of procedure
- Acute pain

Related factors are individualized based on client's condition or needs.

STEP	RATIONALE

PLANNING

1. Expected outcomes following completion of procedure:
   - Client tolerates procedure without anxiety or discomfort.

   Appropriate preparation decreases anxiety.

   - Normal ECG waveform.

   A normal ECG waveform (Figure 44-9) consists of specific waves P, Q, R, S, T that are plotted on graph paper. Each small block on the graph paper measures 0.04 second. A "normal" ECG waveform demonstrates the following characteristics:

   PR interval = 0.12 to 0.20 second
   QRS width = less than 0.10 second
   QT interval = less than 0.38 second
   ST-segment is isoelectric (on the same horizontal level as the PR interval)

2. Close room door or bedside curtains.

   Provides privacy.

3. Prepare client for procedure:
   a. Remove or reposition client's clothing to expose only the client's chest and arms. Keep the abdomen and thighs covered.

   Facilitates correct placement of cardiac leads and minimizes client's embarrassment. Improper lead placement produces artifact, which may necessitate repeating the test (Chernecky and Berger, 2004).

   b. Place client in supine position.

   Exposes client for lead placement.

   c. Instruct client to lie still without talking (12-lead ECG only) and to not cross legs.

   Body movement produces artifact, which may necessitate repeating the test (Chernecky and Berger, 2004).

IMPLEMENTATION

1. Perform hand hygiene.

   Reduces transmission of microorganisms.

2. Cleanse and prepare skin; wipe sites with alcohol. It may be necessary to shave or clip hair from the chest if large amounts of hair are present. In clients who are very thin and emaciated, it may be difficult to secure electrodes because of bony structure and decreased amount of subcutaneous tissue.

   This skin preparation helps remove oils that would prevent adherence of the electrodes.

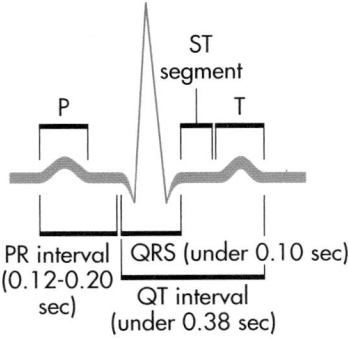

FIGURE **44-9** Normal ECG waveform. (From Pagana KD, Pagana TJ: *Mosby's manual of diagnostic and laboratory tests,* ed 2, St. Louis, 2002, Mosby.)

STEP	RATIONALE

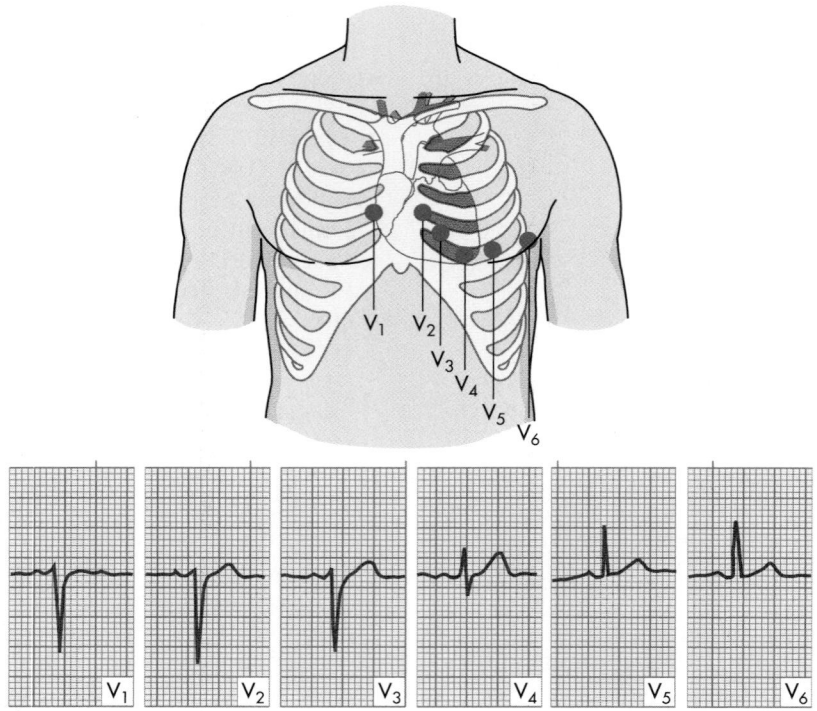

FIGURE **44-10** Anatomical placement of precordial leads. (From Phipps W, Sands J, Marek J: *Medical-surgical nursing: health and illness perspectives*, ed 7, St. Louis, 2003, Mosby.)

3. Apply self-sticking electrode, being careful to use pressure on the perimeter only, and attach leads. (If self-sticking leads are not available, apply electrode paste to skin before attaching leads.) For 12-lead ECG:

   a. Chest (precordial leads) (Figure 44-10): V_1—Fourth intercostal space (ICS) at right sternal border. V_2—Fourth ICS at left sternal border. V_3—Midway between V_2 and V_4. V_4—Fifth ICS at midclavicular line. V_5—Left anterior axillary line at the fifth intercostal space. V_6—Left midaxillary line over the fifth intercostal space.

   b. Extremities: one lead on each extremity. Place on upper arms and upper legs.

4. Obtain tracing.

   a. *Simultaneous 12-channel recording:* Enter client's name and medical record number into the ECG machine menu. Obtain test tracing. Reposition leads as needed. Activate machine to obtain a simultaneous tracing of all 12 leads. If client experiences chest pain during the procedure, document occurrence of chest pain on the resulting printout.

Position of leads promotes proper display of ECG on paper. Pressure on the center of the lead displaces the electroconductive gel and may result in a poor tracing.

Careful placement assures a reliable basis for comparison of this ECG to prior ECGs.

Upper portions of extremities produce less artifact because there is less chance of movement during the procedure.

Transfers electrocardiac conduction to ECG tracing paper for subsequent analysis by cardiologist. Chest pain experienced during the study may be correlated to an arrhythmia on the ECG (Pagana and Pagana, 2002).

STEP	RATIONALE

b. *Single-channel recording:* After the limb electrodes are placed, electroconductive gel is dispensed over the V_1 to V_6 locations (described above). The lead selector is turned to lead "1," the machine is turned on, and the recording is begun. If the tracing is clear, run sequential 6-second tracings for leads I, II, III, aV_R, aV_L, and aV_F by turning the lead selector to the corresponding settings. Then stop the machine, position the V electrode over the V_1 position and run a 6-second tracing. Repeat sequentially by moving the V electrode over V_2, V_3, V_4, V_5, and V_6 positions.

5. Inspect resulting printout for clarity. Repeat the procedure if tracings contain artifact. Disconnect leads, wipe excess electrode paste from chest, and perform hand hygiene.

   Promotes comfort and hygiene. Reduces transmission of microorganisms.

6. Deliver ECG tracing to appropriate laboratory, physician, or nurse.

   Provides for review of ECG by cardiologist.

EVALUATION

1. Although the procedure is painless, it is important to note and document if the client is experiencing any chest discomfort during the procedure.

   Helps correlate ECG changes to symptoms of chest pain.

Recording and Reporting

- Record in nurses' notes when ECG was obtained (date and time) and where tracing was sent, rationale for obtaining ECG (e.g., pain, discomfort, preoperatively, postoperatively), and baseline vital signs.
- Report any unexpected outcomes immediately.

Unexpected Outcomes	Related Interventions
1. Uninterpretable ECG, evidenced by: • Absence of tracing in one or more leads • The presence of artifact in the ECG tracings	• Inspect electrodes for secure placement. • Reposition any wires that are moving as a result of client breathing or movement, or vibrations in the environment. • Remind client who is moving that lying still is necessary to obtain a good tracing. Manually hold any extremities, if needed. • If artifact looks like 60-cycle interference (looks like a very thick–lined waveform), unplug battery-operated equipment in the room one item at a time to see if the interference disappears. NOTE: 60-cycle interference is rare. • Repeat the tracing.
2. Cardiac deterioration secondary to anxiety, evidenced by: • Chest pain or pressure	• Continue to monitor. • Reassess factors contributing to anxiety. • Follow specific postprocedural orders related to findings. • Notify physician.

Teaching Considerations

- After explaining procedure, assure client that flow of electric current is from client to machine. Client will not feel anything during procedure.
- If Holter monitoring is selected, instruct client to maintain an accurate diary of activities (detailed documentation of activities and occurrence of chest pain assist in diagnoses of condition).

- Inform client that the Holter monitoring interpretation will be available in a few days.

Gerontological Considerations

- Be aware that medications can affect results, including digitalis and antiarrhythmics.

FOCUS *on* CLINICAL PRACTICE

One of your clients this morning is Mr. Hall, a 67-year-old black man who is a retired executive. He will be having a cardiac catheterization procedure in the ambulatory care department of your hospital. The prescription for the procedure that was faxed from the physician's office lists "new-onset chest pain" as the clinical indication for the procedure.

1. What other information would you assess about this client?
2. What laboratory data would you review as part of your preparation of Mr. Hall for his procedure?
   A. CBC, levels of prealbumin and blood gases
   B. Complete blood count, prothrombin time, levels of BUN and creatinine, urine specific gravity
   C. Lipid panel, blood glucose level, and electrolyte levels
3. Describe the steps you would take to perform client verification safety procedures for Mr. Hall.
4. Cardiac catheterization often involves the use of intravenous moderate sedation. The physician has not requested the presence of an anesthesiologist during the procedure. You are responsible for assessing Mr. Hall's ASA classification before the procedure. What ASA classification would you consider appropriate for Mr. Hall?
   A. 1
   B. 2
   C. 3
   D. 4
   E. 5
   F. 6

5. When you review Mr. Hall's chart, you see that the consent form for the procedure is unsigned. When you inquire of him whether the physician explained the procedure and the risks, and ask if he has any questions, he replies, "My doctor told me that I needed this to find out why my chest pain is happening. But I don't know how risky it is." What would you do?
   A. Ask Mr. Hall to sign the consent form, and tell him to ask about the risks when the doctor arrives.
   B. Hold the consent form to be signed after the physician arrives to speak with Mr. Hall Proceed with preparation by administering the preprocedure valium to Mr. Hall.
   C. Hold the consent form to be signed after the physician arrives to discuss the information needed for informed consent. Hold the preprocedure valium until after informed consent has been obtained.
6. Mr. Hall's cardiac catheterization procedure is finished. You receive him back into his bed and learn that the right femoral site was used for catheter insertion. Which items should take priority in your postprocedure assessments of Mr. Hall?
   A. Heart rate and rhythm, respiratory effort, oxygen saturation, procedure site for bleeding control, pedal pulses
   B. Blood pressure, pain level, neurological checks, complete blood count, electrolytes
   C. Pupil checks, level of consciousness, breath sounds, bowel sounds

NCLEX REVIEW QUESTIONS

1. Intravenous moderate sedation has what *desired* effect on a client who will undergo a procedure?
   1. Induces a state of sleep
   2. Relaxes the client
   3. Improves oxygenation
   4. Eliminates client's ability to maintain/protect own airway

2. During a procedure, nursing assessments of a client who has received intravenous moderate sedation should include:
   1. Breath sounds
   2. Neurological checks
   3. Heart sounds
   4. Pulse oximetry values

3. Which statement concerning an angiogram procedure is *false?*
   1. Assisting with an angiogram may be delegated to unlicensed assistive personnel.
   2. The angiogram procedure always involves the use of intravenous moderate sedation.
   3. A client may ambulate as soon as an angiogram is completed.
   4. An angiogram is usually done by the client's attending physician.

4. Mrs. S. is recovering after a cardiac catheterization. Which set of postprocedure signs would you report *immediately* to the physician for a client who has had a cardiac catheterization?
   1. Heart rate increased from 92 to 106 beats per minute, low back pain radiating to the sides, other assessments unchanged
   2. Occasional premature ventricular contractions (PVCs), mild tenderness at catheter insertion site
   3. Urine output of 40 ml in the first hour postcatheterization, oxygen saturation decreased from 99% to 96%
   4. Blood drainage visible at edge of dressing, partial thromboplastin time (PTT) decreased from baseline

5. Mrs. S. experiences a postcatheterization vasovagal reaction because of the manual pressure placed over her right femoral procedure site. Your *immediate* interventions should include which of the following?
   1. Turn her on her left side, and elevate the head of the bed.
   2. Place her in a high-Fowler's position, and give her an emesis basin.
   3. Place the bed in a reverse Trendelenburg's position, and give her an emesis basin.
   4. Place the bed in Trendelenburg's position, and support her airway.

6. What is a contraindication for an intravenous pyelogram?
   1. Renal failure
   2. Peripheral vascular disease
   3. Diabetes mellitus
   4. Urinary tract infection

7. Client teaching before a bone marrow aspiration or biopsy should include which of the following?
   1. The procedure is painful, but only briefly.
   2. It is acceptable for the client to move during the procedure.
   3. General anesthesia is used for the procedure when it is done on an adult.
   4. Informed consent is not required because the procedure does not pose risk of client injury.

8. Diagnostic testing before performing a lumbar puncture usually includes which of the following?
   1. Cerebral ultrasound
   2. Cerebral angiogram
   3. Magnetic resonance imaging of the brain
   4. Computed tomography scan of the brain

9. Desired outcomes from a paracentesis include:
   1. Increased abdominal girth and decreased respiratory effort
   2. Increased abdominal girth and increased respiratory effort
   3. Decreased abdominal girth and decreased respiratory effort
   4. Decreased abdominal girth and increased respiratory effort

10. Which of the following statements are *true* about the thoracentesis procedure?
    1. Assisting with a thoracentesis may be delegated to unlicensed assistive personnel.
    2. The client is positioned lying face down on a bed or table for the procedure.
    3. The amount of fluid removed is usually no more than 1.5 L.
    4. A chest tube is inserted at the end of the procedure to collect samples for testing.

11. Expected outcomes of a bronchoscopy procedure include which of the following?
    1. Facial crepitus is no higher than level of the mouth.
    2. Sputum is clear or slightly blood tinged.
    3. Gag reflex returns within 45 minutes after the procedure.
    4. Client is able to drive self home after the procedure.

Continued

NCLEX REVIEW QUESTIONS

12. The cooperation of the adult client during the procedure is achieved by which of the following methods?
    1. Intravenous minimal sedation
    2. Intravenous moderate sedation
    3. Intravenous deep sedation
    4. No sedation is needed. The physician explains each step, and the client cooperates.
13. You are giving Mr. J., a 77-year-old man, instructions about how to prepare for his colonoscopy the following week. Your instructions should include:
    1. Soft foods only for 3 days before the day of the procedure. A cleansing enema in the morning before the test. No food or fluids for 4 hours before the procedure.
    2. Full liquid diet the day before the procedure. Drink a bowel cleansing preparation the night before the procedure. Take the prescribed antibiotic the morning of the procedure.
    3. No diet modifications needed in the days before the procedure. Fast from food and fluids, except for medications, the night before the procedure. Have a bowel movement the morning before the procedure.
    4. Clear liquids only for 2 days before the procedure. Complete the bowel preparation the night before the procedure. Fast from food and fluids for 8 hours before the procedure.
14. When Mr. J. arrives for his colonoscopy, he states that he forgot to skip breakfast and had eaten two bites of toast and half of a cup of coffee before he remembered the fasting instructions. What would you do?
    1. Reschedule the procedure, and send Mr. J. home, telling him that he will have to start his instructions all over again.

2. Ask a nurse with more experience whether she thinks it would be all right for Mr. J. to have his colonoscopy, because he took such a small amount of food.
3. Tell Mr. J. that the small amount of food and coffee he took should not keep him from having the procedure. Continue your preprocedure preparations, then tell the physician about the food and fluid intake when he or she arrives.
4. Proceed no further with preparation for the test. Inform Mr. J. that there is a chance that his procedure might have to be rescheduled. Then notify the physician, and await instruction about how to proceed.
15. The type of cardiogram that is most commonly used to help diagnose the cause of an acute episode of chest pain is:
    1. Holter monitor
    2. Single-channel recording
    3. 12-lead ECG
    4. Continuous bedside cardiac monitor
16. You are troubleshooting the reasons for artifact in a client's cardiogram waveform. Which of the following is *not* likely to be a cause of the artifact?
    1. Electrode wire draped over ventilator tubing
    2. Electrode gel dried out or too thinly smeared
    3. Client movement
    4. 60-cycle interference from other equipment plugged into outlets in the same room

References

American Society of Anesthesiologists: *Continuum of depth of sedation definition of general anesthesia and levels of sedation/analgesia,* Oct 31, 1999, http://www.asahq.org/ publications AndServices/standards/20.pdf, accessed Jan 18, 2004.

American Society of Anesthesiologists: *Relative value guide,* 2004, The Society.

Beare P, Myers J: *Adult health nursing,* ed 3, St. Louis, 1998, Mosby.

Chernecky CC, Berger BJ: *Laboratory tests and diagnostic procedures,* ed 4, Philadelphia, 2004, Elsevier.

Healthcare organizations, *Joint Commission Perspectives on Patient Safety,* 2(3), 2002.

Healthcare organizations, *Joint Commission Perspectives on Patient Safety,* 3(1), 2003.

Lewis S and others: *Medical-surgical nursing,* ed 6, St. Louis, 2004, Mosby.

Linton A and others: *Introduction to medical/surgical nursing,* ed 3, Philadelphia, 2003, WB Saunders.

Malarkey L, McMorrow M: *Nurse's manual of laboratory tests and diagnostic procedures,* ed 2, Philadelphia, 2000, WB Saunders.

Nagelhout JJ and others: *Handbook of nurse anesthesia,* ed 2, St. Louis, 2001, Elsevier.

National Council on Radiation Protection: The application of ALARA for occupational exposures NCRP Statement No. 8, issued June 8, 1999, *Health Phys* 78(5 Suppl):S76, 2000.

Pagana KD, Pagana TJ: *Mosby's manual of diagnostic and laboratory tests,* ed 6, St. Louis, 2003, Mosby.

Phipps WJ and others: *Medical surgical nursing: health and illness perspectives,* ed 7, St. Louis, 2003, Mosby.

Silber S: Vascular closure devices for immediate sheath removal after coronary interventions: luxury or necessity? In *Handbook of coronary stents,* ed 3, London, 2000, Dunitz Publishers Ltd.

Research References

Aldrete JA: The postanesthesia recovery score revisited, *J Clin Anesth* 7:89, 1995.

American Academy of Pediatrics: Policy guidelines for monitoring and management of pediatric patients during and after sedation for diagnostic and therapeutic procedures: addendum, *Pediatrics* 110(4):836, 2002.

Angle PJ and others: Dural tissue trauma and cerebrospinal fluid leak after epidural needle puncture: effect of needle design, angle, and bevel orientation, *Anesthesiology* 99(6):1376, 2003.

Calabrese A and others: Evaluation of prescribing practice: risk of lactic acidosis with metformin therapy, *Arch Intern Med* 162:4, 2002.

Cheatham JP: Intervention in the critically ill neonate and infant with hypoplastic left heart syndrome and intact atrial septum, *J Interv Cardiol* 14(3):357, 2001.

Drug therapeutic perspectives: prevention is key but an epidural blood patch is standard treatment in postdural puncture headache, *Anesthesiology* 95(2):334, 2001, accessed 1/06/2004.

Evans RW and others: (2000). Assessment: prevention of post-lumbar puncture headaches—report of the Therapeutics and Technology Assessment Subcommittee of the American Academy of Neurology, *Neurology* 55(7):909, 2000.

Fleming GH, Souba WW: Minimizing the risk of malpractice claims, *ACS Surgery: Principles & Practice*, MD Consult.

Haiat H and others: The world of the child: a world of play even in the hospital, *J Pediatr Nurs* 18(3):209, 2003.

Hasegawa BH and others: (2002). Dual-modality imaging of function and physiology, *Acad Radiol* 9:1305, 2002.

Hoffer EK, Bloch RD: Percutaneous arterial closure devices, *J Vasc Interv Radiol* 14(7):865, 2003.

Hoffman GM and others: Risk reduction in pediatric procedural sedation by application of an American Academy of Pediatrics/American Society of Anesthesiologists process model, *Pediatrics* 109(2):236, 2002.

Luther R and others: The selective DA_1 agonist corlopram® for the treatment of acute renal failure: evidence for augmentation of renal blood flow and natriuresis, *Am J Hypertens* 10(4):187A, 1997.

McMahon CJ and others: Cardiac catheterization in infants weighing less than 2500 grams, *Cardiol Young* 13(2):117, 2003.

Negishi C and others: Resistive-heating and forced-air warming are comparably effective, *Anesth Analg* 96(6):1683, 2003.

Ramsay MA and others: Controlled sedation with alphaxalone-alphadolone, *Br Med J* 2(920):656, 1974.

Rhodes JF and others: Impact of low body weight on frequency of pediatric cardiac catheterization complications, *Am J Cardiol* 86(11):1275, 2000.

Rosin D, Rosenthal RJ: Adverse hemodynamic effects of intraabdominal pressure: is it all in the head? *Int J Surg Investig* 2(5):335, 2001.

Tepel M and others: Prevention of radiographic-contrast-agent-induced reductions in renal function by acetylcysteine, *N Engl J Med* 343(3):180, 2000.

van Crevel H and others: Lumbar puncture and the risk of herniation: when should we first perform CT? *J Neurol* 249:129, 2002.

Yucel A and others: Intravenous administration of caffeine sodium benzoate for postdural puncture headache, *Reg Anesth Pain Med* 24(1):51, 1999.

Answer Key

Chapter 1

Focus on Clinical Practice Answers

1. Additional information that would be helpful as the nurse assumes care for this client includes:
   - Level of consciousness and confusion, findings from neurological assessment completed by ED nurse and physician
   - Client's medical history, including medications; information regarding any recent changes in medication or treatment plan
   - Blood sugar level, home insulin schedule and dosages, whether home insulin was administered before presenting to hospital, time and substance of last meal
   - Results of any testing completed in ED such as computed tomography (CT) scan of head
2. You are aware that Mr. Johnston is experiencing confusion and has a history of falls. Assign Mr. Johnston to a room near the nurses' station, and implement fall precautions.
3. Allow Mrs. Johnston to participate in the care of Mr. Johnston to the extent that she is comfortable. Allow Mrs. Johnston to assist while you get Mr. Johnston undressed and into bed. Provide Mrs. Johnston with a comfortable chair, and support her interactions with her husband.
4. Ask Mrs. Johnston to bring a copy of the advance directive to the hospital. Notify the physician that the client has an advance directive. Document in the medical record the presence of an advance directive and the request made for Mrs. Johnston to bring the document to the hospital. Because Mr. Johnston is confused, the nurse will not be able to ask him the substance of the advance directive.

Answers to NCLEX Review Questions

1. 4. Allergy band
2. 1. Team members of each discipline involved in the care of the client

3. 2. Identify any potential changes in clinical needs of the client that may prevent transfer/discharge or may require nursing intervention to provide for client safety during transport

Chapter 2

Focus on Clinical Practice Answers

1. Additional information may include the following:
   - History:
     - Client is originally from Mexico and has lived in the United States for the past 10 years. English is her second language, and she mainly communicates in Spanish. She lives with her daughter.
     - Her baseline level of functioning is as follows: before her fall, she was independent in her ADLs and walked without assistance.
     - Her general health is good, although she has a history of hypertension and osteoarthritis.
     - She takes over-the-counter (OTC) medications to manage her pain related to osteoarthritis.
     - Currently client is alert and oriented to person, place, and time but has difficulty communicating to members of the health care team because of her language barrier.
   - Current postoperative pain control regimen:
     - Mrs. Garcia has been taking intramuscular (IM) narcotic analgesics for pain since her surgery. Because of the language barrier, the nurses have not adequately evaluated the success of her pain control.
2. A, B, C, and D are all correct. Because Spanish is the client's primary language, it will be helpful to use an interpreter to care for the client. In addition, it is beneficial to involve the daughter in her mother's care. Because the client lives with her, the daughter may provide valuable information regarding the client's baseline status and usual health habits. Managing the client's pain both pharmacologically and nonpharmacologically is helpful to help the client return to her highest level of functioning.

3. A. Use interpreter or daughter when communicating with client.

4. A, B, and C are correct. Clear communication with client can be achieved with the aid of an interpreter. Setting limits with client's negative behaviors helps to inform the client about negative behaviors and reinforce acceptable behaviors. It is important the nurse remain calm and not react to the client's anger, because this will only exacerbate the situation. It is not therapeutic to tell a client you will refuse to care for her.

5. A, B, C, and D are all correct. Clear communication can be achieved with the aid of an interpreter. By conveying empathy and displaying a nonjudgmental attitude, the nurse can facilitate a positive experience with the client. Involving the daughter in the client's care assists the nurse to obtain baseline information about the client's ADLs status and any health habits the client prefers. Providing privacy is essential when taking care of personal needs.

Answers to NCLEX Review Questions

1. 4. Avoiding issues that are uncomfortable for clients
2. 1. "I think your doctor needs to know that you are still in pain."
3. 3. "Why do you feel depressed and worthless?"

Chapter 3
Focus on Clinical Practice Answers

1. Vital signs (VS) and ambulation can be recorded by assistive personnel on flow sheet. It is appropriate for the assistive personnel to document repetitive care aspects. As a nurse you must give the assistive personnel specific information as to when you want to be notified about VS data (e.g., temperature above 99° F orally, heart rate greater than 100 beats per minute, blood pressure less than 100/70 mm Hg or greater than 130/85 mm Hg). Wound assessment must be done and recorded by the nurse.

2. The nurse would include information pertaining to the dressing (e.g., dry and intact, no drainage or drainage that is dark in color about the size of a quarter). The nurse would also need to specify in her report to the assistive personnel that the assistive personnel was to notify the nurse if the dressing loosened, if there was any drainage, if the client complained on any new-onset incision pain, or "felt something give" under the dressing.

3. Elements to include: wound intactness, drainage, pain/discomfort, odor, information obtained from palpation of area, client comments, integrity of the dressing or drains.

4. The following are the nurse's actions in order of priority:
   a. Fully assess Mr. Klein.
      (i) History: Determine what he means by "feels funny." He could be weak and feel faint; he could feel increased incision pain; or because of his degenerative neuromuscular condition, he could feel unbalanced.
      (ii) Physical assessment: Obtain VS; auscultate chest, heart, and abdomen.
      (iii) Observe Mr. Klein walking if possible, and assess after his walk.

   b. Notify the supervisor/physician. Rationale: Notification of physician after your assessment of Mr. Klein provides some objective data for the physician to evaluate. Merely calling the supervisor/physician and reporting that the assistive personnel reported that Mr. Klein felt funny provides no objective information. Remember, it is the nurse's responsibility to assess the client and to report and document the findings.
   c. Perhaps you may want to increase the frequency of Mr. Klein's VS measurements until he is seen by his physician. Provide the assistive personnel with specific instructions about what information you want reported and when you want the information reported to you about these VS.

5. The following are the nurse's actions in order of priority:
   a. Fully assess Mr. Klein.
      (i) History:
         (a) If possible, gather data about what occurred before falling out of chair (e.g., did he become dizzy, did he attempt to get up and lost his balance?).
         (b) Ask questions to determine his level of consciousness and orientation. Did he hit his head, does it hurt, is he oriented to time, place, and person? Does he have pain anywhere? Does he have restricted movement?
      (ii) Physical assessment: Obtain VS; auscultate chest, heart, and abdomen.
      (iii) Observe Mr. Klein's incision.
   b. Notify the supervisor/physician. Rationale: Notification through the nursing office and physician is necessary when a client has an incident, such as a fall.
   c. Complete an incident report according to agency policy.
   d. Implement and document any postincident procedures.

Answers to NCLEX Review Questions

1. 2. Record information provided by another nurse
2. 3. 1600
3. 1. Data-Action-Response
4. 3. Identify trends in clinical care
5. 3. Provide continuity of care
6. 3. Identify high-risk trends

Chapter 4
Focus on Clinical Practice Answers

1. Mrs. Dean's risk includes history of parkinsonism with altered gait, fatigue that would accompany melanoma, and decreased hearing.
2. The diuretic Lasix, antihypertensive Catapres
3. The correct answer is C. The "Get Up and Go" test measures a person's balance and gait.
4. The elevation of all four side rails can be considered a restraint. Side rails should not be used to prevent an alert and functional client from getting out of bed. Explain to the daughter that side rails are designed to help the client move and reposition in bed.

5. Physical therapy can instruct Mrs. Dean in gait training and muscle strengthening exercises. These interventions have been show to help older adults reduce their incidence of falling.

Answers to NCLEX Review Questions

1. 4. A safe environment is important, but the client's risks must be matched with appropriate interventions. Restraints are always used as a last resort and are not considered a safe fall prevention strategy. A bed alarm can be useful in fall prevention but should be combined with appropriate behavioral therapies.
2. 2. Do not engage a client in securing a fire. Have the client evacuated as quickly and safely as possible.
3. 2. The correct answer is 2. The most appropriate method for evacuating Mr. Joseph due to his weight and mobility restriction would be by bed. Attempting to carry him or lift him onto one's back would increase the risk of injury to a nurse.
4. 4. A physician's restraint order must include time limitations, type of restraint, and the behavior that warrants use of the restraint. Although it is helpful for the physician to be involved in the selection of restraint alternatives, this is not part of a restraint order.

Chapter 5
Focus on Clinical Practice Answers

1. Focused assessment:
   a. Pulmonary system
      (i) Pulse oximetry
      (ii) Observe breathing pattern
      (iii) Observe for use of accessory muscles and nasal flaring
      (iv) Auscultate lungs for adventitious sounds
      (v) Auscultate lungs to determine if adventitious lung sounds clear with coughing
      (vi) Observe sputum for color, thickness, amount, and client ability to clear airway
   b. Cardiac system
      (i) Vital signs
      (ii) Heart rate and rhythm
   c. Neurological system
      (i) Level of consciousness (LOC)
      (ii) Orientation
      (iii) Ability to follow instructions
      Rationale: The clients are admitted with fever, cough, chills, and in some cases confusion, which are relatively vague symptoms suggestive of numerous diagnostic possibilities. Obtaining cardiopulmonary data through a focused assessment enables the nurse to identify pertinent data about the client's status before initiating treatment. In addition, a brief neurological examination obtains baseline LOC and orientation and assists in determining the client's ability to follow instructions. The baseline data help to determine the client's present cardiopulmonary and oxygenation status without increasing the client's level of fatigue. Remember, in clients without underlying cardiac disease, the body adapts to decreased oxygenation or increased oxygen demands by increasing heart rate and blood pressure. In addition, the nurse has a sense of the client's understanding of care and ability to participate in care through coughing and deep breathing, anticipated oxygen therapy, and implementation of isolation precautions, as needed.

2. Priority actions for health care personnel:
   a. Notify the hospital disaster incident commander.
   b. Institute appropriate isolation precautions; because a diagnosis of the cause for the client symptoms has not been made, the following precautions should be considered.
      (i) Standard precautions
      (ii) Airborne precautions

3. Action to be taken:
   a. Obtaining additional resources and supplies is not part of the role that the nurse performs while caring for clients in the event of an MCI. This function is the responsibility of the incident commander, who will delegate the function to the appropriate support personnel.
   b. In preparation for an MCI most hospitals will have developed mutual aid agreements. These agreements will allow the hospital to access needed resources and supplies. Furthermore, through these types of agreements clients can be diverted to hospitals where the needs do not exceed resources and supplies.

4. The rationale includes the following:
   a. At this point, staff education is important regarding precaution to avoid self-contamination; furthermore, staff should be comforted and counseled to reduce levels of anxiety.
   b. Health care needs already exceed supplies and resources. Sending anxious staff home will only further diminish the valuable health care resource these personnel provide.
   c. In the case of anthrax, staff are exposed only if the biological agent has been brought to the ED (e.g., on the clothing of the clients). In the unlikely event that the biological agent has been brought to the ED, it could be spread to other sites, thus further contaminating an already unknown geographical area of contamination.
   d. Postexposure prophylaxis would include one of the fluoroquinolones (e.g., ciprofloxacin, levofloxacin, ofloxacin), or in the event these drugs are unavailable, doxycycline is used.

5. Preparations that should be made for the transport and admission of these clients includes the following:
   a. The method of disease transmission must be considered. For patients diagnosed with anthrax, the disease is spread by contact with the aerosolized spores rather than by contact with infected individuals.
   b. Standard precautions are appropriate once a diagnosis of anthrax is made.
   c. When the client is transported to an in-patient unit, no restrictions are necessary regarding the transport.

d. Cleaning of equipment used should include disinfecting surfaces with a 1:9 bleach/water solution (10% solution). Undiluted bleach can result in inhalation and contact injury to personnel.

e. Management of linen is the same as with any other client.

Answers to NCLEX Review Questions

1. 1. Practice makes staff more familiar with disaster protocols in the event of a true disaster.
2. 4. An experienced nurse who must inform a mother that her three children ages 2, 3, and 4 years of age did not survive the plane crash
3. 2. A disaster victim who arrives at the ED with labored respirations, cool skin, a pulse of 120, and a blood pressure of 90/60
4. 2. Contact

Chapter 6
Focus on Clinical Practice Answers

1. The correct answer is C. Mr. Johnson is unable to understand or speak; therefore the best approach is to observe for nonverbal pain behaviors. It is very important to assess for these behaviors during activity because lying still usually does not aggravate the pain; however, the body is meant to move and when not moving is at higher risk for deconditioning and for hazards of immobility.
2. Remove the PCA from the maintenance IV line. With another nurse, measure and discard the remaining morphine from the cassette, syringe, or bag. Record amount discarded on agency form. Both nurses should sign form. Complete agency PCA form. Notify pharmacy per agency policy. Discard PCA tubing according to agency policy. Return infuser to appropriate department.
3. The correct answer is A. You have assessed his pain via nonverbal behaviors and with movement. If there were a loved one available, you could also seek a proxy rating. The 1 mg of morphine does not last longer than 4 hours. It is appropriate to administer 1 Percocet tablet and then reassess for pain within 1 hour. If your assessment reveals continued pain, you should give another tablet. Because of his age and because he has not had any Percocet, it is wiser to begin with a small dose and increase it as necessary.
4. The correct answer is B. You are right to be concerned. Because Mr. Johnson is unable to request pain medication, it would be appropriate to place him on an around-the-clock analgesic regimen and continue to reassess the pain on a regular basis. Just because a person cannot verbalize presence of pain, this does not mean he or she is not in pain. Acetaminophen is probably not a good drug in this situation because Mr. Johnson has had recent surgery and thus is experiencing some inflammation. Acetaminophen has no antiinflammatory properties. At a later date, acetaminophen might be appropriate.

5. The correct answer is B. Your assessment indicates reduced peristalsis, but no obstruction. The combination of morphine and immobility has most likely slowed peristalsis. A simple stool softener will not increase peristalsis. A stimulant laxative is necessary. Increasing his fluid intake would be beneficial, as well as moving him out of bed as much as possible.

Answers to NCLEX Review Questions

1. 3. Physical dependence
2. 3. Movement
3. 1. Drifts off to sleep while talking
4. 3. Not pushing button for the client
5. 4. Sepsis
6. 4. Povidone-iodine
7. 4. Severe itching
8. 1. Bring removed catheter to the first postoperative physician visit
9. 1. With analgesics
10. 2. Taking rest periods between strategies

Chapter 7
Focus on Clinical Practice Answers

1. The correct answer is B. Mr. Weiss's heart attack was sudden and without warning. The family has had no time to prepare for the sudden change in family relationships.
2. The correct answer is C. It is imperative that you as the nurse collect more information regarding Mrs. Weiss's response to this loss. It is premature to make a nursing diagnosis. You cannot assume Mrs. Weiss is in any one stage of grief. Your assessment should validate the actual stage of grief Mrs. Weiss is experiencing. Remember, Mrs. Weiss will likely move back and forth between different stages.
3. Your approach to assessment should encourage Mrs. Weiss to tell her story. As you talk, note when Mrs. Weiss exhibits a behavior or expresses what appears to be a concern. Then use communication techniques to confirm your observation (e.g., summarizing, paraphrasing, clarifying, sharing observations). Next, determine the quality and meaning of the relationship severed by the client's grief experience. This will require more detailed information about Mr. Weiss and his role as father and husband. Also, be sure to have Mrs. Weiss explain how this loss is affecting her now. As you identify behaviors that suggest the stage of grief Mrs. Weiss is experiencing, allow this information to guide the assessment.
4. The correct answer is A. An advance directive sets forth a client's choices for medical treatment when a situation occurs that medically prevents him or her from being able to make decisions. An advance directive is not a document that simply defines which family members have a legal right to decide about end-of-life care. However, an advance directive may identify a proxy family member who is given the right to make treatment decisions. Usually an advance directive outlines the client's

choices rather than listing options from which the family chooses. An advance directive is more comprehensive than a document giving consent for organ donation. However, an advance directive may include the deceased's wishes regarding organ donation.

5. You will need to explain to the daughter the concept of brain death. She and her mother and sister must understand that her father, once legally determined as brain dead, could be maintained on life support until organs are successfully retrieved. This ensures the viability of the organs. The daughter is not the one to approach for organ donation. Request should be made of Mrs. Weiss.

Answers to NCLEX Review Questions

1. 1. Maturational loss
2. 1. Reviewing laboratory values
3. 3. Buddhism
4. 1. Recognize that the dying client's symptoms are very real

Chapter 8
Focus on Clinical Practice Answers

1. Joe should wash his hands with soap and water and then put on gloves to continue his assessment, explaining the rationale for this to Mr. Nesbitt. He should put Mr. Nesbitt under contact precautions because the drainage from his sacral wound may contain pathogens. His gloves should be changed if they become soiled during the assessment to avoid spreading microorganisms to other parts of Mr. Nesbitt's body.
2. Joe's hands are probably not visibly soiled after checking Mr. Nesbitt's catheter and removing his gloves. He should use an alcohol-based antiseptic hand rub.
3. By putting on gloves and performing hand hygiene, Joe broke the chain of a mode of transmission.

Answers to NCLEX Review Questions

1. 3. After contact with the environment close to the client
2. 1. Consider that the client may feel lonely and provide opportunity for social interaction
3. 2. Droplet precautions

Chapter 9
Focus on Clinical Practice Answers

1. Insertion of the peripheral intravenous catheter requires wearing sterile gloves.
2. Because Mrs. Smith is blind, explain the activities you are performing in detail to her to attempt to alleviate any anxiety she may have and to provide as much information as possible. In addition, ask her if she has questions regarding the procedures you will be performing.
3. Discard the used catheter, reprepare the skin at a new site, and open a new catheter for insertion into the vein.
4. Ask Mrs. Smith if she has ever had a previous reaction to the following items within hours of exposure: adhesive tape, dental or face mask, golf club grip, ostomy bag, rubber band, balloon, bandage, elastic underwear, IV tubing, rubber gloves, condom. Use latex-free products when caring for Mrs. Smith.
5. Nothing. Only 1 inch from the border of the drape to the edge is considered contaminated.

Answers to NCLEX Review Questions

1. 1. Gloves, then mask, eyewear, and cap
2. 2. Holding or moving the object below the waist
3. 1. Grab only the inside of the glove with your bare hand

Chapter 10
Focus on Clinical Practice Answers

1. Additional information may include the following:
   a. Focused examination, for example
      (i) Vital signs: blood pressure, 148/72 mm Hg; pulse, 100 beats per minute; respirations, 24 breaths per minute, unlabored
      (ii) Level of orientation and alertness
      (iii) Medicated for pain with morphine sulfate 5 mg intravenously 2 hours before admission to unit
      (iv) Level of sedation, for example, numbness and tingling in lower extremities
      (v) Type of injury, for example, spinal fracture considered unstable until further testing:
   b. Past medical history
      (i) No chronic illnesses reported or conditions affecting positioning
2. A, B, and C are correct answers. Mr. Clark is in pain most likely related to his lacerations and fractures. Pain management is a priority at this time. In addition to pain management, explaining to Mr. Clark the purpose of the CT scan will help elicit his cooperation. Mr. Clark is most likely fearful of movement due to his pain and uncertainty of his condition. Describing the method of transfer along with showing him that there will be additional personnel to help transfer him to the stretcher will increase his trust and cooperation.

   D is incorrect. You may inform Mr. Clark that it is a physician's order, but the client has the right to refuse treatment. You are more likely to elicit Mr. Clark's cooperation by determining the underlying reasons for Mr. Clark's refusal to transfer.
3. Logrolling Mr. Clark will maintain proper alignment by moving all body parts at the same time, preventing tension or twisting of the spinal column.
4. A nurse must supervise and aid assistive personnel when moving a client who has suffered a spinal cord injury to keep the spinal column in straight alignment to prevent further injury.

Answers to NCLEX Review Questions

1. 4. Risk for injury
2. 3. "I will keep my knees bent and trunk erect so my muscles work together."

3. 1. Apply a transfer belt around Mrs. Jones's waist.
4. 3. "I'll go get the slide board; it is more comfortable for the client, and it will protect us from injury."
5. 2. Pain
6. 2. Logroll the client with the assistance of three nurses.

Chapter 11
Focus on Clinical Practice Answers

1. Mr. Timber reports a pain level of 8 on a scale of 0 to 10. A nursing priority is to provide pain management strategies and lower his level to an agreed-upon range. In addition, Mr. Timber may have concerns about his ability to safely ambulate without falling or injuring himself. Spending time with Mr. Timber explaining about and demonstrating the use of crutches will assist in minimizing his anxiety and concerns.

2. Mr. Timber has at least two major risk factors associated with orthostatic hypotension: his history of diabetes mellitus and his age. To minimize the complications, allow Mr. Timber to sit with the head of the bed elevated for several minutes before dangling him on the side of the bed. During dangling, instruct Mr. Timber to take several deep breaths and move his feet up and down and in a circular motion to promote venous return via intermittent contraction and relaxation of the skeletal leg muscles.

3. Assess the safety of the CPM machine by inspecting the electrical cord for fraying and damage. In addition, put the CPM machine through one full cycle before applying to client to ensure the machine is functioning properly. Assess the setup of the machine before placing on the client's bed: check the stability of the frame, the flexion/extension controls, padding to exposed metal parts or hard surfaces, and the on/off switch.

4. The appropriate crutch gait for Mr. Timber is the three-point alternating, or three-point gait that requires the client to bear all of his weight on one foot. Several teaching considerations are needed for Mr. Timber. It is important that these considerations are individualized to meet the learning needs of the client. Some examples of teaching considerations for Mr. Timber are:
   - Instruct client with axillary crutches about the dangers of pressure on the axillae that occurs when leaning on the crutches to support body weight.
   - Explain why client must use crutches measured for him or her.
   - Demonstrate how to routinely inspect crutch tips. Rubber tips should be securely attached to the crutches. When tips are worn, they should be replaced. Rubber crutch tips increase surface friction and help prevent slipping.

Answers to NCLEX Review Questions

1. 2. Orthostatic hypotension
2. 2. Perform range of motion to the left elbow only until resistance is met

3. 2. Active range of motion is encouraged if the client's health status allows because it promotes independence and assists in maintaining muscle tone as well as joint mobility.
4. 1. Always exhale when exerting effort during isometric exercises
5. 4. Risk for activity intolerance
6. 1. The CPM machine provides continuous passive motion.
7. 2. Determine if hard surfaces on CPM machine are well padded.
8. 4. Facilitate the return of venous blood to the heart to prevent venous stasis.
9. 3. Prepare the client for radiological studies such as a Doppler compression ultrasonogram.
10. 2. Pulmonary emboli
11. 3. Inspect environment for potential threats to client safety such as spills or clutter.
12. 2. The client can use a cane, but you stand on the right side.

Chapter 12
Focus on Clinical Practice Answers

1. The correct answer is D. Only the palms are used to move the cast to prevent indentations that fingertips may cause. Covering with plastic wrap will delay drying and may generate heat that will burn the underlying tissues. The cast should be open to air to promote drying.

2. The correct answer is D. Neurovascular assessment includes the 6 P's (pain, pallor, pulselessness, paresthesia, paralysis, pressure). The neurological findings of numbness and tingling may indicate pressure from swelling on the nerves in the compartment. Warm skin distal to the cast and capillary refill less than 3 seconds in the toes are normal findings.

3. The correct answer is B. To bivalve the cast, cut it in two lengthwise along each side. In addition, the wadding underneath is cut to relieve the pressure. Although a window may be cut in a cast to visualize a wound underneath, it does not relieve pressure.

4. The correct answer is A. Redness (erythema), swelling (edema), and purulent (infectious) drainage all indicate a possible pin site infection. Clear drainage and/or crusting are to be expected with skeletal pins.

5. The correct answers are B, D, and E. The pulley, spreader bar, or foot plate should not rest against the foot of the bed because this will interfere with the pull of the weights. Traction rope rests in grooves of the pulley and moves easily to allow up and down movement of the weights as needed. The rope must have knots that are secured and taped to prevent slippage. The client must have correct body alignment to ensure correct line of pull.

Answers to NCLEX Review Questions

1. 2. Every 1 to 2 hours
2. 1. Explaining the purpose of the traction to the client
3. 4. "Scratching can cause skin breaks and infection. I'll get you some medication for the itching."
4. 3. Teach the client how to use the trapeze bar
5. 1. Elevation and ice
6. 1. Fifteen minutes following application of the skin traction
7. 1. Inspect the underlying tissues for redness or drainage
8. 2. Pressure
9. 1. To decrease muscle spasms in the leg
10. 3. Report purulent pin site drainage to the doctor.
11. 4. Pain on passive motion of the affected foot
12. 3 and 4. Keep the brace clean, dry, and in good working order. Inspect the skin under the brace daily for reddened areas.

Chapter 13
Focus on Clinical Practice Answers

1. Complete assessment with emphasis on pressure ulcer risk, current mobility status, and skin integrity.
2. Determine client's level of pressure ulcer risk, and then determine whether pressure reduction or relief is needed. Mr. Kline is at high risk for pressure ulcers. He has decreased mobility and sensation.
   a. Mr. Kline needs pressure relief. The rationale is that he has no ability to independently change position. In addition, because of impaired sensation, he cannot perceive pressure on his skin and tissues.
3. Anxiety and nausea are common with air-suspension beds; the client's comfort can be improved with pharmacological agents to reduce anxiety and nausea. In addition, when lateral rotation is also used, a client's nausea increases. When clients are prescribed an antiemetic, such as Compazine, the nurse should be sure that this medication is given routinely as opposed to an "as needed" (prn) order. Explaining to the client that these sensations are temporary and will gradually improve is important. However, the client cannot really process this information unless he or she is comfortable. For these reasons pharmacological agents to control anxiety, nausea, and any pain are beneficial to clients on support surfaces.
4. She may not express pain and try to "not complain." It is important to talk to her about comfort measures and pain control. You may also need to reassure her that she will not become addicted to the pain medication. As her pain resolves, her need for pain medication will decrease.
5. When she receives the tube feeding, adaptations need to be made so that the head of the bed remains elevated. This can be achieved with intermittent use of foam wedges or a bed that is modified to maintain pressure relief when the head of the bed is elevated.
6. Talk to Ms. Long about her inner ear problem, and determine the presence of dizziness and if the dizziness increases with position change. If this symptom cannot be controlled, Ms. Long may not be a candidate for Rotokinetic therapy. In addition, determine Ms. Long's level of knowledge about her condition and the importance of change of position and improving pulmonary functioning.

Answers to NCLEX Review Questions

1. 3. Air-fluidized bed. Rationale: Clients tend to perspire on this bed. The surface of the bed quickly removes fluids from contact with the client's skin, so the evidence of perspiration may be minimized. The perspiration and/or diaphoresis can go undetected and the increase in insensible fluid loss may not be noticed until the client develops dehydration or electrolyte changes.
2. 2. Stop the rotation of the bed and assess the client further. Rationale: The client may experience orthostatic hypotension when the bed rotates. Stopping rotation while remaining with the client and conducting further BP assessments will indicate if the problem diminishes. The rotation can begin again, perhaps at a decreased angle and at a slower cycle.
3. 4. Consider changing to a pressure-relief device. Rationale: The air-filled mattress overlay is a pressure-reducing device used with meticulous skin care and repositioning. This client is not responding to pressure reduction and needs to move to a pressure-relief system because he is developing pressure ulcers on more than one position area (e.g., supine and left lateral positions).
4. 1. Client's ability to assist with transfer to the bed. Rationale: The ability of the client to assist with the transfer to the bed is never a consideration. The severely overweight client has problems with mobility and therefore needs a bed that will enable the caregiving staff to reposition and provide care while relieving pressure on the skin.

Chapter 14
Focus on Clinical Practice Answers

1. The correct answer is B. Mrs. Giles is self-sufficient and not totally dependent on the nurse for assistance. For this reason a sponge bath at the sink would be appropriate. A complete bath is not necessary. A tub bath and shower are probably safety risks because of her gait, rigidity, and slow movement.
2. Assist client with turning or repositioning. Offer short rest periods while changing the bath water, and offer a bath in the evening instead of the day.
3. The correct answer is C. Mrs. Giles's intentional hand tremors and rigidity of hands make it important to assess how difficult it is for her to manipulate a toothbrush. She might be able to manipulate a large-grip toothbrush more easily. She is a young older adult but is beginning to reach the age when changes in her oral cavity might develop.

4. Encourage Mrs. Giles to rinse her mouth thoroughly with an essential oil antiseptic mouthrinse a minimum of twice daily.

5. Have the sister inspect all surfaces of fingers, toes, feet, and nails at least weekly. Pay particular attention to areas of dryness, inflammation, or cracking. Also inspect areas between toes, heels, and soles of feet. Inspect socks for stains.

6. The correct answers are as follows:
   B. True, testing of the water temperature prevents accidental burns.
   D. True, never cut a diabetic client's nails. Use only a nail file.

Answers to NCLEX Review Questions

1. 3. To cleanse and remove the outer skin of dead skin cells
2. 4. Clients with neck injuries and vertigo
3. 2. Increased glucose levels in the saliva
4. 1. A buildup of gram-negative bacteria in the oral cavity
5. 4. Provide a thermal bath in bed
6. 3. Bag infested clothing until laundered

Chapter 15
Focus on Clinical Practice Answers

1. Ms. Malles has right-sided weakness following the cerebral vascular accident. This weakness may limit her degree of physical activity, possibly limiting her to bed rest. Immobility will prevent her from making significant changes in her position. These two factors of immobility and prolonged bed rest place her at risk for skin breakdown, because she will be unable to independently reposition herself. She will be at risk for pressure ulcer development because of unrelieved pressure as her skin is compressed between a bony prominence and the bed. Fecal incontinence will cause the skin to become moist and contribute to impaired skin integrity. Ms. Malles will be unable to communicate with the staff if she feels pain or discomfort; thus if she remains in one position for a prolonged period of time, she will be at risk for skin breakdown.

2. The correct answer is B. The Braden Scale for Predicting Pressure Sore Risk identifies the specific risk factors that place Ms. Malles at risk for skin breakdown. The client will be assessed for the presence of the risk factors, sensory perception, moisture, activity, mobility, nutrition, shear and friction. Once the factors are identified, specific interventions can be targeted that can reduce or eliminate the factors. The Braden scale will not provide an assessment of any existing skin breakdown, nor will it provide information on diabetes or nutritional management.

3. The correct answer is B. In evaluating the moisture subscale of the Braden scale the most appropriate subscale would be "2. Very moist: Skin is often, but not always, moist. Linen must be changed at least once a shift."

Ms. Malles has been noted to have loose stools at least once every 6 hours, and she is wearing an absorbent diaper. The presence of loose stools will keep her skin moist, not at all times but at least once per shift. This risk factor can cause maceration, softening her skin, making it susceptible to skin breakdown.

4. The correct answer is B. The use of the Braden scale will provide you with risk factors that place the client at risk for skin breakdown. You will need to do a skin and wound assessment as a second assessment to obtain wound length and depth.

Answers to NCLEX Review Questions

1. 2. Upon admission to the unit and as their condition changes
2. 2. Consult with the wound clinical nurse specialist about the most appropriate bed surface to reduce pressure.
3. 4. This pressure ulcer cannot be staged because you must be able to see the wound base to assess the depth of tissue destruction.
4. 2. Hydrocolloid dressings protect the wound base and provide a moist environment.

Chapter 16
Focus on Clinical Practice Answers

1. Presence and position of lenses; availability of eyeglasses; client ability to remove lenses; time since insertion of lenses and wear schedule; signs and symptoms of infection or injury such as pain, redness, discharge, swelling, excessive tearing, or changes in visual acuity.

2. The correct answer is C. It is important to locate the lenses of a contact lens wearer on admission to the health care system to prevent eye injury from overwear or displacement. Periodic examinations during hospitalizations (answer A) are not likely unless admission is for a vision related issue. The therapeutic relationship (answer B) could best be fostered in more direct ways. It is not necessary to distract the client to inspect the eye (answer D).

3. The correct answer is C. It is not uncommon for a lens to be displaced to the sclera. It may, however, be obscured by the eyelid or eyeball. An undetected displaced lens can cause serious injury. Expert examination may be necessary to rule out the presence of a lens. The nurse is responsible for documenting direct observations and nursing diagnoses and interventions, not suspicions (answer A). The client's past experience cannot address the current issue (answer B). Consultation (answer D) is premature until careful assessment has been conducted.

4. The correct answer is B. Sterile saline is an acceptable emergency substitute for lens storage solution. Saliva is not an acceptable substitute for a lens solution (answer A). Storage of the lenses in the same container (answer C) may cause problems if the lenses are different prescriptions and unnecessarily deprives the client of corrected vision in both eyes. Completing the client's forms (answer D) would be unnecessary if he is allowed to keep

one lens in place and emphasizes his dependence, which could affect his self-esteem.

Answers to NCLEX Review Questions

1. 2. Client will be unable to care for contact lenses immediately after surgery. Although anxiety may be present (answer 1), no signs or symptoms have been presented to justify this choice. Neither "alteration in nutrition" nor "sensory perceptual alterations" represents a NANDA nursing diagnosis.
2. 4. Answers 1, 2, and 3 represent accurate knowledge. Answer 4 requires educator clarification because some disposable contacts are intended to be cleaned and reused. Furthermore, there is increased risk of infection with any contact lens use.
3. 1. The artificial eye should be cleaned only as often as necessary to prevent discomfort. The other statements are correct and indicate adequate teaching.
4. 3. An artificial pupil will not react to stimuli. Movement (answer 2) is present if the eye muscles have been attached to the ocular implant beneath the artificial eye. Veins (answer 4) may be drawn on the prosthesis by the ocularist. The tissues of the eye socket will continue to produce secretions (answer 1).
5. 4. The chemical should be removed as soon as possible to minimize the risk of permanent damage to the eye. Although a basin may be positioned to catch a dislodged contact lens, taking time to remove the lens (answer 1) delays removing the chemical from the eye and increases the risk of permanent damage. Testing the pH of secretions may be performed after an initial period of irrigation to determine the need to continue (answer 3).
6. 2. Unless asked to do otherwise, address the client in a normal tone of voice. Raising voice volume (answer 1) distorts the voice and may make understanding more difficult. If the client appears not to understand, a different choice of words may help, but a rapid series of statements or questions (answer 3) deprives the client of the longer processing time needed to compensate for a hearing impairment. Speaking toward the better ear may facilitate understanding (answer 4).
7. 3. "Dressing" may involve washing the face, applying hair spray or cologne, or using a hair dryer, each of which may damage hearing aids. Daily adjustment to hearing aids is not usually necessary. Adjustment over time (answer 4) will usually help the client learn to hear in spite of background noises or conversations with several people at once. Desiccant (answer 1) dries the hearing aids and prolongs life. Increased earwax (answer 2) may be a sign of irritation.

Chapter 17
Focus on Clinical Practice Answers

1. All of the routine vital signs can be delegated. Temperature should be tympanic, because client is sleepy and will not be able to hold an oral thermometer. Blood pressure should be obtained on the left arm or lower extremity. Oximeter probe should be attached to fingers of the left hand to avoid any circulation compromise caused by the fracture.
2. Possible explanations for differences are technique, equipment, and client-related findings. Technique includes site of blood pressure measurement and whether the nursing assistant used the proper method. The nurse may want to observe the nursing assistant's technique in blood pressure measurement. Equipment differences include using a cuff that is too small. An example of a client-related finding is that the client may have abnormally low blood pressure and preoperatively was anxious and in pain, thus raising blood pressure. The intervention indicated is for the nurse to repeat the blood pressure.
3. The priority action is to reposition the oximeter sensor on the left hand and more carefully assess the tissue perfusion to the right arm and hand. The arm may be swelling under the cast, resulting in a poor waveform and inaccurate pulse rate and SpO_2 value.

Answers to NCLEX Review Questions

1. 4. Tympanic and rectal
2. 3. Obtain a temperature using a tympanic thermometer on the infant.
3. 4 Remove extra clothing and bed covers, and evaluate the client's complaints.
4. 4. Irregular rate
5. 1. Assess right radial pulse for symmetry.
6. 3. Carotid
7. 4. During routine vital sign measurement
8. 4. Sleeping
9. 2. It reflects the cardiac apex.
10. 3. Ask the nursing assistant for help in obtaining apical-radial pulse.
11. 4. Narcotic analgesics
12. 4. Decrease in chest expansion
13. 3. 72
14. 2. Produces false high systolic pressure
15. 3. Repeat the blood pressure measurement again at the end of the assessment after the client has been resting quietly.
16. 4. When the fourth Korotkoff sound has changed character
17. 2. Demonstrate the one-step blood pressure technique on the client's other arm.
18. 3. Retake the client's blood pressure observing the electronic device.
19. 1. Reposition the oximeter sensor.
20. 4. Least affected by decreased blood flow

Chapter 18
Focus on Clinical Practice Answers

1. Focused systems assessments would include cardiovascular and peripheral vascular, respiratory, abdominal and perineal, I&O.
    a. Key elements of each system:
        (i) Cardiovascular: blood pressure (BP); heart rate (HR); inspection, palpation, and auscultation of the heart
        (ii) Peripheral vascular: inspection and palpation of extremities; checking peripheral pulses, edema, skin color temperature, capillary refill of nailbeds
        (iii) Respiratory: checking rate and depth of respirations, chest excursion
        (iv) Abdominal: checking size and shape of abdomen, palpating bladder, assessing bowel sounds
2. A crackling noise upon inspiration indicates crackles. Crackles indicate fluid in the alveoli and small airways. Priority nursing diagnosis is ineffective airway clearance.
3. The correct answer is A. A heart rate between 60 and 100 beats per minute, regular rate and rhythm, is normal.
4. The correct answer is B. The nurse must listen for 5 minutes over each quadrant before deciding bowel sounds are absent. It is common for bowel sounds to be hypoactive postoperatively for 24 hours or more following abdominal surgery.
5. The correct answer is C. The nurse should be concerned and report finding to physician. Unilateral leg edema is one of the most reliable findings of deep vein thrombosis (DVT). Other symptoms include pain or tenderness, erythema, increased warmth, firmness of affected area. Testing for Homans' sign is contraindicated if any of these symptoms are present.
6. • Questions to ascertain risk for osteoporosis:
    · Family history?
    · Presence of osteoporosis risk factors? (See Skill 18-5, Assessment, step 1.)
    · Level of activity/exercise? Ability to perform self-care?
    · Alcohol/caffeine intake/smoking?
    · History of fractures/presence of pain/history of falls?
    · Calcium intake?
    · Onset of menopause? Use of estrogen replacement therapy (ERT)?
   • Physical examination techniques:
    · Musculoskeletal system checking for kyphosis, gait impairments.

Answers to NCLEX Review Questions

1. 1. Appearance and behavior
2. 3. Are blue/black or variegated in color
3. 1. Side to side
4. 1. Presence of fremitus
5. 3. Rhonchi
6. 3. Aortic and pulmonic valves
7. 1. Sinus bradycardia
8. 4. Observe the amount of time it takes for normal color to return to fingernail after pressure has been applied for a few seconds
9. 2. Prevent distortion of the bowel sound
10. 4. Notify the physician immediately
11. 3. Internal rotation
12. 3. VII—facial
13. 3. Compare symmetrical areas
14. 4. Lateral to the extensor tendon of the great toe
15. 3. Deficient fluid volume

Chapter 19
Focus on Clinical Practice Answers

1. The correct answer is D.
2. Altered gastrointestinal (GI) function (e.g., nausea/vomiting), reduced GI motility, surgical resection of portion of gastrointestinal tract, clients who are NPO and unable to swallow, clients with gastric suction. Oral medications are also contraindicated in clients before some tests or surgery. An unconscious or confused client may be unable or unwilling to swallow.
3. The correct answer is C.
4. Remember, the formula is:

$$\frac{\text{Dose ordered}}{\text{Dose on hand}} \times \text{Amount on hand} = \text{Amount to administer}$$

$$\frac{0.5 \text{ mg}}{0.25} \text{ mg} \times 1 \text{ tablet} = 2 \text{ tablets}$$

5. A. Six rights
   B. Three times
   C. As soon as it is given

Answers to NCLEX Review Questions

1. 3. Related to dose
2. 2. The point at which the lowest amount of drug is detected in the serum
3. 4. On the skin
4. 1. Right route. Because Mrs. Ramirez is nauseated, it is important to judge which route is best for the client. Giving an analgesic orally might be ineffective if the client is nauseated, as she very easily could vomit the medication.

Chapter 20
Focus on Clinical Practice Answers

1. Assessments before giving medications include:
   - Contraindication to the medications ordered
   - Risk for aspiration
   - Drug and food allergies
   - Medication history
   - Vital signs
   - Renal and liver function studies
   - Client's knowledge regarding health and medication use

2. The diltiazem is an extended-release formulation and therefore should not be crushed.

3. Interventions to proper use of metered-dose inhaler
   A. Use of a spacer device is helpful when weakened grasp or inability to coordinate actuation of the canister with inhalation occurs.
   B. The mouth should be rinsed after inhaling corticosteroids to prevent oral candidiasis.
   C. Teach the client that inhaled corticosteroids (such as the Flovent) are useful for maintenance therapy for asthma but not useful for acute bronchospasm. Bronchodilators, such as the Proventil, are indicated for treatment of acute bronchospasms.

4. Mrs. K.L. needs to be reminded that the wound area should be cleansed thoroughly before each application of the cream and that the old medication should be removed. The client should use the amount of cream specified by the instructions, followed by a dry dressing to cover the area. The nurse should watch as Mrs. K.L demonstrates wound care. If Mrs. K.L. is unable to perform the wound care, then a family member should be included in the demonstration and practice session.

Answers to NCLEX Review Questions

1. 4. Oral-dosing syringe
2. 3. The tablet should not be crushed, broken, or chewed.
3. 4. Flush tube with 30 to 60 ml of water after the last dose of medication.
4. 2. Attempt to irrigate it gently with tepid water.
5. 2. Use sterile gloves when applying medication.
6. 1. "I will apply the patch to a different area each time."
7. 4. Apply gentle pressure to the client's nasolacrimal duct for 30 to 60 seconds after giving the drops.
8. 2. The drops should be instilled into the conjunctival sac.
9. 3. Straighten the ear canal by pulling the auricle down and back.
10. 2. Run warm water over the medication bottle.
11. 2. Removal of cerumen
12. 3. Hold the tip of the syringe 1 cm ($\frac{1}{2}$ inch) above the opening to the ear canal.
13. 4. Increased congestion and swollen mucosa
14. 3. 20 to 30 minutes before feeding.
15. 2. Inhale slowly while pressing down to release the medication.
16. 3. Provide a spacer device for clients who have trouble pressing the canister.
17. 3. Pulse rate
18. 2. Clients should rinse their mouths with water after receiving inhaled steroids.
19. 2. After administration she should remain on her back for at least 10 minutes.
20. 3. Dorsal recumbent
21. 4. Encourage the client to lie on his or her left side for 15 to 20 minutes after insertion.
22. 1. Diarrhea

Chapter 21
Focus on Clinical Practice Answers

1. Before you give the medication, you would need the following information:
   - The drug classification, desired effect, and nursing implications associated with Neupogen therapy, such whether or not a filter needle is needed with medication preparation
   - The safe dose for the medication and compare it with the ordered dose
   - The amount of medication in ml to be administered
   - If Neupogen comes in a vial or an ampule
   - If any of Mrs. Stevens's current medications have potential drug-drug interactions with Neupogen
   - The anticipated adverse effects of Neupogen

2. You would need to know:
   - Mrs. Stevens's height and weight
   - If anything is affecting the blood flow to Sub-Q tissues
   - Nutritional and fluid status and skin turgor
   - White blood count to evaluate the desired effect

3. The correct answer is C. A small gauze pad or unopened alcohol swab should be wrapped around the neck of the ampule to prevent the glass from cutting your fingers. Opened alcohol swabs should not be used because alcohol may leak into the ampule.

4. The correct answer is D. You should always use the smallest syringe possible when preparing medication. Usually, a 25-gauge $\frac{1}{2}$- to $\frac{5}{8}$-inch needle will deposit medication into the Sub-Q tissue of a normal-sized client.

5. All of the answers are correct responses. Answer A: It is important to know if a medication needs to be diluted before you administer it IV push. Many medications, including morphine, have a rapid onset of action when administered IV push. Medications may also be irritating to the veins. Diluting the medication will enhance the client's tolerance to the medication and will diminish irritation at the site of injection. Answer B: Giving medications too quickly can lead to poor client outcomes. Pushing morphine too quickly could cause respiratory depression. Answer C: Some people are allergic to morphine. It is important to assess the client's medication allergies before administering any medication. Answer D: You need to assess the compatibility of IV medications

with IV fluids before administering the medication. If an IV medication is not compatible with the maintenance fluids that are hanging, you should stop the IV fluids, flush the site, give the medication, flush the site, and restart the maintenance fluids; or you should initiate a new IV site.

Answers to NCLEX Review Questions

1. 4. Evaluates the medication's concentration after the diluent and powder are mixed
2. 1. Prepares the medication in the vial first
3. 2. An induration of 18 mm
4. 3. Administer the injection over 30 seconds
5. 1. Pain, numbness, and tingling at the injection site 2 hours after the injection
6. 2. 22-gauge, $1\frac{1}{2}$ inch
7. 1. Infiltration
8. 4. The pump allows small amounts of fluid to be infused within a specified amount of time.
9. 3. Using the term *IV push* with medications that are to be given over more than 1 minute.
10. 1. Assess the condition of the IV insertion site
11. 4. Pinch the skin with the nondominant hand before inserting the needle.

Chapter 22
Focus on Clinical Practice Answers

1. Additional information may include the following:
   a. Pulmonary system
      (i) Pulse oximetry
      (ii) Observe breathing pattern
      (iii) Observe for use of accessory muscles and nasal flaring
      (iv) Auscultate lungs for adventitious sounds
      (v) Auscultate lungs to determine if adventitious lung sounds clear with coughing
      (vi) Observe sputum for color, thickness, amount, and client ability to clear airway
   b. Cardiac system
      (i) Vital signs
      (ii) Heart rate and rhythm
   c. Neurological system
      (i) Level of consciousness (LOC)
      (ii) Orientation
      (iii) Ability to follow instructions
   Rationale: Mr. Landon is very fatigued and short of breath, which makes taking a history difficult. Obtaining cardiopulmonary data through a focused assessment enables the nurse to identify pertinent data about the client's status before treatment. In addition, a brief neurological examination obtains baseline LOC and orientation and assists in determining the client's ability to follow instructions. These baseline data help to determine the client's present cardiopulmonary and oxygenation status without increasing client's level of fatigue. Remember, in clients without underlying cardiac disease, the body adapts to decreased oxygenation or increased oxygen demands by increasing heart rate and blood pressure. In addition, the nurse has a sense of the client's understanding of care and ability to participate in care through coughing and deep breathing, anticipated oxygen therapy, etc.

2. Administration of oxygen therapy
   a. FiO_2 level is between 24% and 28%.
   b. Hypercarbia is a risk for clients with COPD because the oxygen therapy may override the adapted respiratory drive. As a result, CO_2 is retained, and there is an increased risk for respiratory failure in this client.

3. Comfort measures to use with oxygen therapy
   a. The strap on the cannula may be too tight or placed incorrectly. Inspect the external ears where the cannula strap rested to observe for any skin irritation. Adjust the fit of the cannula, and place pressure-relieving devices (e.g., ear protectors or folded 4×4) under the cannula's elastic strap.
   b. The oxygen may dry out the nasal mucosa, and the cannulas themselves can irritate the client's nares. Inspect nares for skin irritation; apply a water-soluble lubricant to areas of nasal irritation. Evaluate the humidification level of the oxygen therapy; perhaps more humidification is needed.

4. The correct answer is D. Partial rebreather masks mix exhaled carbon dioxide with oxygen. Because Mr. Landon has underlying COPD and pneumonia, he is at risk for carbon dioxide retention, and this risk is further increased via the partial rebreather mask.

5. Worsening of client's oxygenation status
   A. Mr. Landon is confused at times, and his level of consciousness is decreased. The BiPAP requires a snug-fitting facemask. It is possible that the client will feel claustrophobic or be so confused that he will continually attempt to remove the mask. It is important that someone (e.g., assistive personnel, family) be with him to reinforce why the mask is in place and to help relieve anxiety. If BiPAP is effective in this client, his LOC and oxygenation levels should improve within 20 to 30 minutes of therapy.
   B. There is a risk of carbon dioxide retention. Monitoring of continuous pulse oximetry provides oxygen saturation trends. Serial ABGs (e.g., ABGs taken every hour) provide data to monitor carbon dioxide and pH levels.

6. The correct answer is B. As clients' oxygenation declines, they work harder; therefore the respiratory rate is increased. But the results of this work are ineffective, and the oxygen saturation falls, and they retain more carbon dioxide. As a result of the carbon dioxide retention, clients develop a CO_2 narcosis in which they become very sleepy.

   As clients improve, answer D would reflect part of the clinical picture.

Answers to NCLEX Review Questions

1. 3. Chest x-ray
2. 2. Reduce the risk of carbon dioxide retention
3. 1. Prevent drying of the nasal mucosa
4. 4. It uses positive pressure during inhalation and exhalation
5. 3. Clients with an underlying diagnosis of chronic obstructive pulmonary disease
6. 1. Begin manual ventilation and obtain vital signs and pulse oximetry as soon as possible
7. 3. Suction the client's airway.

Chapter 23
Focus on Clinical Practice Answers

1. Place bed in Trendelenburg's, and use three positions: left side-lying to drain right lower lobe bronchus, right side-lying to drain left lower lobe bronchus, and left side-lying with one-quarter turn back onto pillow to drain right middle lobe.
2. Chest examination revealed decreased breath sounds at bases posteriorly and over right lateral chest wall. There was decreased chest wall excursion, which was more pronounced on the right side. Client complained of increased cough and sputum production and dyspnea. Respiratory rate increased to 30 breaths per minute, and oxygen saturation decreased to 85% on room air.
3. Improvement of lobar collapse on chest x-ray film is a common clinical finding after the successful application of CPT (Stiller, 2000). In addition, oxygenation usually improves, and dyspnea, tachypnea, fever, and leukocytosis begin to resolve.
4. Documentation should include the following: (a) tolerated CPT to bilateral lower lobes and right middle lobe using Trendelenburg's position; (b) breath sounds increased at both bases and right middle lobe area after treatment with decreases in rhonchi and palpable fremitus; (c) coughed up 30 ml thick yellow secretions and drank two 8-oz glasses of water during therapy session; (d) instructed family in how to position client at home and how to do percussion and vibration; they performed an excellent return demonstration; and (e) repeat chest x-ray film showed reexpansion of right middle lobe and increased aeration of bilateral lower lobes.

Answers to NCLEX Review Questions

1. 1. Right side-lying Trendelenburg's
2. 1. Sitting up in a chair and leaning backward onto a pillow
3. 3. Cystic fibrosis

Chapter 24
Answers to NCLEX Review Questions

1. Additional information may include the following:
   - History, for example:
     - 60 pack-year (2 packs a day times 30 years) smoking history
     - Quit 1 year ago
   - Sputum is yellow, blood tinged, and increased volume
   - She reports difficulty in clearing her airway
   - Past medical history, for example:
     - No allergies
     - Occasional bronchitis treated as an outpatient with antibiotics
     - No history of asthma
     - No family history for cardiac disease, cancer, or diabetes mellitus
   - Focused physical examination, including:
     - Level of orientation
     - VS: blood pressure, 140/86 mm Hg; pulse, 110 beats per minute; respirations, 34 breaths per minute; temperature, 102.6° F (orally); oxygen saturation is 86%, baseline is 89%
     - Condition of skin: for example, pale, diaphoretic, warm to touch
     - Pulmonary status: for example, decreased breath sounds, crackles throughout lower lung fields; crackles do not clear with coughing; sputum thick, yellow
     - Cardiac status: within normal limits
     - Extremities: for example, pulses palpable, no edema
2. The correct answer is A. Rationale: Yankauer suctioning is the method of choice; this enables the client to clear oral secretions as needed, and it is a clean, nonsterile procedure.
3. The correct answer is B. The client's pulmonary secretions are deep within the lungs, and the suction catheter must enter the trachea. The Yankauer suction device is not designed to clear secretions within the lungs. Orotracheal suction runs the risk of introducing oral bacteria into the lungs, thus worsening the client's pulmonary infections.
4. The correct answers are A, B, and C. Hand hygiene has a direct benefit in reducing nosocomial infections and the transfer of microorganisms to health care professionals. Sterile suction technique reduces nosocomial infection in clients in acute care settings, those with new artificial airways or new tracheostomies, or those clients with acute illnesses/trauma. Clean suction technique can be used in clients who have permanent airways, usually a tracheostomy, and are free of any pulmonary infections. Frequently clean technique is used in the home environment.
5. The correct answers are A, C, and E. Answer A: It is important to notify the physician or the charge nurse because new care orders may be necessary for this client; these orders may include antibiotics, chest physiotherapy, or diagnostic tests such as bronchoscopy. Answer C: In some clients increasing fluids may assist in liquefying pulmonary secretions. Before increasing fluids be sure to determine that it is not contraindicated for this client. For example, clients with cardiac or renal diseases may not be able to tolerate an increase in fluids. Answer E: A sputum specimen for culture and sensitivity is needed because a change in thickness and/or sputum color frequently indicates an infectious process. The type of infection needs to be determined before administering an antibiotic.

Frequently clients will have a sputum specimen obtained and then be treated with a very broad-spectrum antibiotic. Following the results of the sputum specimen the antibiotics may be changed if necessary.

Answers to NCLEX Review Questions

1. 1. Hypoxia
2. 1. Oropharyngeal
3. 2. Oropharyngeal
4. 3. Oral cavity is dirtier that the tracheal area and is suctioned last.
5. 2. Decrease airway size and increase the work of breathing
6. 3. Presence of patent airway
7. 3. Suction the airway
8. 1. Liquefies and thins secretions

Chapter 25
Focus on Clinical Practice Answers

1. Vitals signs will document client's cardiopulmonary status and identify any early changes. Prompt detection and correction of air leaks related to the chest tube decrease the risks for chest tube complications and duration of chest tube placement. The hourly monitoring of chest tube drainage is to provide timely observations on the amount and type of drainage. During the first 3 hours 100 ml/hr is expected, and client coughing and position changes can result in a temporary increase in drainage.

2. Avoid dependent chest tube loops; change position of client and drainage tubes to prevent drained blood from pooling in the chest or tube.

3. This drainage is dark red, not bright red; it is not a large volume; and it is probably due to the rapid discharge of accumulated drainage from the chest. This discharge of fluid was probably stimulated by the client's activity from bed to chair. However, because this is a fresh postoperative client, you would take his vital signs to determine his tolerance to activity and to monitor cardiopulmonary status. You would also monitor chest tube drainage to be sure that the volume did not increase excessively, and you would implement measures to assist in maintaining chest tube patency (see answer 2).

4. This is an emergent situation. Your client could have a recurrence of a pneumothorax or hemothorax, or he could have another unrelated problem such as a myocardial infarction. Your actions are as follows: Notify physician of your findings, remain with client, and get assistance in getting Mr. Robert into bed. It would also be important to make sure that supplemental oxygen is available and on and to verify that there is an adequate IV line. If the client has had his oxygen and IV fluids discontinued, have someone bring the necessary equipment to the client's bedside.

Answers to NCLEX Review Questions

1. 2. Explaining that by controlling pain he will be able to be active and cough well

2. 3. Worsening pneumothorax
3. 1. Monitoring chest tube drainage and maintaining chest tube patency
4. 1. Pleural tubes placed in the 2-3 intercostal space
5. 3. Place an occlusive dressing over chest tube site and take vital signs

Chapter 26
Focus on Clinical Practice Answers

1. The correct answer is B. Rationale: Upon finding an unconscious client, you must call for help immediately to ensure that the required equipment for defibrillation is brought to the client as soon as possible. Adults suffering from cardiac arrest frequently required defibrillation. Statistics show that defibrillation within 1 minute can result in a successful rescue as high as 90%; however, statistics drop off rapidly to 50% after 5 minutes, 30% after 7 minutes, and 10% after 9 to 11 minutes (AHA, 2000). An AED would need to be applied quickly but only after assessing that the client is unconscious, breathless, and pulseless. Therefore the first action would be call for help; the second, open airway and provide artificial ventilations; the third, check a pulse; then the AED would be applied.

2. The correct answer is A. Rationale: In a hospital setting where protected methods of artificial ventilation are available, mouth-to-mouth without a barrier device is not recommended because of the risk of microbial contamination.

3. The correct answer is A. Rationale: Need to verify that after successful ventilation, the client still remains pulseless before initiation of chest compressions or AED.

4. The correct answer is B. Cardiopulmonary resuscitation is interrupted when changing CPR personnel, during defibrillation, or when transporting victim. During intubation, CPR may be interrupted for more than 5 seconds but interruption should not exceed 30 seconds. Nurse should remind rescue team of number of seconds elapsing during intubation.

5. The primary ABCD's will continue even after the code team has arrived. Assisting the code team with performance of the secondary ABCD's may include handing off the requested supplies from the crash cart for intubation or medications, setting up suction, inserting a peripheral or central IV, chest auscultation upon intubation, connection to monitor/defibrillator, relaying significant client information to the code team, administering or handing off medications. Delegation of other actions may include assisting the victim's roommate or visitors away from the code scene, assigning pastoral care or other nurses to communicate with family, delegating someone to remove excess furniture or equipment from the room, having someone bring client's chart to the bedside, assigning a fresh person to perform chest compressions, or assigning another nurse to record/document the events of the code.

Answers to NCLEX Review Questions

1. 4. It may stimulate vomiting or laryngospasm if inserted in the semiconscious patient.

2. 3. Call for help, get the AED, open the airway, provide two breaths if needed, check for a pulse, and if no pulse is present, attach the AED.
3. 3. Jaw thrust
4. 4. All of the above
5. 2. 3 minutes

Chapter 27
Focus on Clinical Practice Answers
1. The correct rate would be 60 gtt/min.
2. The following steps are necessary before initiating the IV:
   - The nurse should first check the physician's order to ensure that a written order for the initiation of the IV, solution, rate of administration, and any other instructions related to the IV is recorded.
   - Check the IV solution for integrity, including, but not limited to, discoloration, cloudiness, leakage, expiration date.
   - Obtain IV history from the client. Provide explanation of the procedure to the client. Allay any anxieties, and answer any questions the client may have.
   - Obtain all equipment necessary for the procedure.
   - Check laboratory data to evaluate any abnormalities, such as K^+, that should be considered before starting the IV solution.
3. The nurse should take the following measures before another attempt is made:
   - Place pressure on the unsuccessful venipuncture site, and allow time for bleeding to stop.
   - Explain to the client the need to perform another venipuncture.
   - Use another sterile cannula for the venipuncture.
   - Repeat the steps of assessing the vasculature and selecting a suitable site for the venipuncture.
   - Strategies that may assist in venous dilation if veins are difficult to see or palpate are as follows: application of warm, moist heat to the extremity for 5 to 10 minutes; placing the extremity in a dependent position to facilitate gravity fill; milking the extremity downward.
   - Obtain necessary equipment for venipuncture.
4. The following are teaching considerations for the nurse:
   - Instruct the client in the signs and symptoms of complications of IV cannulas, such as tenderness and pain at site, redness, swelling.
   - Instruct the client in the need to keep IV tubing unobstructed and free of kinks, to notify the nurse if tubing comes disconnected, and to place pressure on site if bleeding occurs at the site.
   - Instruct the client in how to ambulate with the IV using a rolling IV pole and keeping the IV solution container in a gravity-dependent position with the IV site.
   - Instruct the client in any complications associated with the infusing of the IV solution, such as free-flow, flow stoppage, blood noticed in tubing.

Answers to NCLEX Review Questions
1. 2. 21
2. 3. Phlebitis
3. 4. Superior vena cava
4. 1. A Huber needle
5. 2. Use aseptic technique in related procedures.
6. 1. 24-gauge catheter
7. 3. Use an electronic infusion device.
8. 1. Apply pressure to the IV site for 5 minutes.

Chapter 28
Focus on Clinical Practice Answers
1. Assessments that are necessary before initiating the transfusion:
   - Verify the patency of existing IV line and that an appropriate-gauge cannula is in place.
   - Verify that IV site is free of complications (e.g., phlebitis, infiltration).
   - Review client's transfusion history (e.g., types of products, allergic reactions, complications).
   - Obtain baseline vital signs.
   - Obtain baseline body temperature.
   - Document and obtain baseline laboratory values (e.g., hemoglobin, hematocrit).
   - Verify physician order.
   - Review client's condition and indication for blood product.
   - Determine client's level of comfort.
   - Determine client's knowledge of procedure.
2. The nurse should do the following:
   - Correctly verify product, and identify client with a person considered qualified by your agency (e.g., RN, LPN, client care technician).
   - Check client's first and last names by having client state name, if able. Also check client's identification number and date of birth on arm band and client record.
   - Verify that component received from blood bank is component ordered by physician.
   - Check that client's blood type and Rh type are compatible with donor blood type and Rh type. Be sure that transfusion is not discolored, clotted, or leaking and does not have bubbles present.
   - Check that unit number on unit of blood and on form from blood bank match.
   - Check expiration date and time on unit of blood.
   - Record verification process as directed by agency policy.
   - Check appearance of blood product for leaks, bubbles, clots, or purplish color.
3. The nurse's responsibilities:
   - Remain with client during the first 5 to 15 minutes of a transfusion. Initial flow rate during this time should be 2 ml/min, or 20 gtt/min.

- If signs of a transfusion reaction occur, stop the transfusion, start normal saline with new primed tubing directly to the VAD at KVO, and notify the physician immediately.
- Monitor client's vital signs 5 minutes after the blood product has begun infusing and per agency policy after that.
- Regulate rate of transfusion according to physician's orders.
  - Verify that PRBCs will infuse in less than 4 hours.
  - If infusion time is greater than 4 hours, contact the physician.

4. The nurse's actions:
   - Suspect a transfusion reaction.
     - Stop transfusion.
     - Normal saline should be connected at VAD hub to prevent any subsequent blood from infusing from tubing.
     - Disconnect blood tubing at VAD hub, and cap distal end with sterile connector to maintain sterile system.
     - Keep vein open (KVO) with slow infusion of normal saline at 10 to 12 gtt/min to ensure venous patency and maintain venous access for medication or to resume transfusion. It is important to regulate flow rate to minimize administration of excess IV fluid, especially in clients who are prone to fluid overload such as clients with cardiac and renal disorders, pediatric clients and older adults.
     - Notify physician.
     - Remain with client, and monitor vital signs.
     - Verify that there is a patent IV line in case emergency medications are needed.

Answers to NCLEX Review Questions

1. 3% Normal saline
2. 2. A.
3. 4. 72-year-old scheduled for total hip replacement
4. 2. Comparing the client's identification bracelet with the blood bag label number

Chapter 29
Focus on Clinical Practice Answers

1. Concerns related to her nutrition risk:
   a. Does this patient have dysphagia?
   b. Has a diet been ordered?
      (i) If not, why?
      (ii) If so, is the consistency appropriate?
   c. What is the client's weight and height?
      (i) Has her weight recently changed? If so, was it intentional?
   d. Has laboratory work been ordered?
      (i) Albumin
      (ii) Prealbumin
      (iii) Complete blood count
      Other information:
   b. What is the client's past medical history?
   c. Does she have any food or drug allergies?

2. Further testing:
   a. Cranial nerve examination results
   b. Assessment of ADLs
   c. Laboratory analysis: albumin, prealbumin, complete blood count, cholesterol
   d. Dysphagia screening
3. Aspiration precautions
4. Referrals:
   a. Speech therapist
   b. Registered dietitian
   c. Occupational therapist
   d. Physical therapist
   e. Social work

Answers to NCLEX Review Questions

1. 4. All of the above
2. 1. A federally funded program aimed at identifying older adults at nutrition risk
3. 1. She has glossitis and a possible B_{12} deficiency.
4. 2. Protein malnutrition because albumin has a long half-life and prealbumin a short half-life.
5. 2. Aspiration
6. 3. Is a measure of body weight in proportion to height

Chapter 30
Focus on Clinical Practice Answers:

1. Additional information may include the following:
   a. Report information:
      (i) Did she hit her face or head? She does not remember, but she has some minor bruises and scrapes.
      (ii) Are there any known fractures to her face or neck? None.
      (iii) Did she already have x-ray films of the head, face, and neck? Yes, all negative; and she sustained no spinal fractures either.
      (iv) What is her current level of consciousness? She is sedated.
      (v) Was there any other type of surgical procedure besides what was done to her legs and arm? No.
      (vi) Is she mechanically ventilated or breathing on her own? She is mechanically ventilated. The physician had planned to remove the breathing tube; however, Mrs. L had some cardiac abnormalities at the end of the surgery; she sustained some blunt chest trauma and blunt abdominal trauma. Consequently, the physician wants to have her monitored overnight in the intensive care unit and extubate her in the morning.
      (vii) What is her height and weight? 5'5″ and 110 pounds.
      (viii) Is there a family member who can provide history? Yes, her husband.

b. History:
  (i) No significant medical or surgical history.
  (ii) No known allergies.
2. Bowel sounds, distention, evidence of internal injury (e.g., bleeding).
3. Assess the nose for injury (it is possible that a fracture was missed). If there were concern of a possible break, or excessive soft tissue injury around the nares, the tube could be placed orally. Because the client is sedated and not able to cooperate with the procedure, obtain assistance for positioning. Do not force the tube if resistance is met. Notify the physician immediately if blood is aspirated from the tube. Check placement of the tube.
4. Irrigate the tube per hospital policy. Check placement of the tube before irrigation. Monitor the insertion site for breakdown.
5. Verify that there has been an x-ray film showing that the tube is in the stomach and not the respiratory tract. Check placement by aspirating fluid from the tube, observing its appearance, and testing the pH. Check to see if there is excessive residual volume in the stomach. Make sure the tube can be easily irrigated (no resistance to flushing the tube). Assess the client's height, weight, fluid, and electrolyte levels. Assess bowel sounds. Position the client with the head of the bed elevated at least 30 degrees.
6. Placement of a small-bore NG tube

Answers to NCLEX Review Questions

1. 1. Radiographic confirmation of nonrespiratory placement
2. 3. Intestine
3. 2. Stomach
4. 2. Stomach
5. 3. J-tube
6. 2. Sodium
7. C. Aspiration pneumonia
8. Perform hand hygiene

Chapter 31
Focus on Clinical Practice

1. Vital signs, electrolyte levels, weight, and fluid status (lung sounds, checking for edema)
2. Provides baseline for measuring tolerance to high concentration of glucose infusion
3. Amino acids, carbohydrates, and fats
4. The nurse's explanation is incorrect. A Valsalva maneuver involves holding the breath and also straining. The maneuver causes an increase in intrathoracic pressure, preventing an air embolus from entering the central circulation at the time of catheter insertion.
5. The correct answer is D, hyperglycemia.
6. You would caution Mr. Giles about his enthusiasm and explain that it is unlikely he has gained all of the weight from a restoration in nutritional status. It is likely that some of the weight gain is from fluid retention. Your assessment would include lung sounds, checking for edema in the extremities, and comparing heart rate with baseline.

Answers to NCLEX Review Questions

1. 3. Hyperosmolar
2. 1. Use of full sterile-barrier precautions during insertion
3. 4. Supine with pillow under shoulder
4. 2. Determine position of catheter tip
5. 4. 10.0%
6. 1. Increased temperature, chills, headache, nausea and vomiting, and chest pain

Chapter 32
Focus on Clinical Practice

1. Other assessment data:
   • Level of consciousness, level of understanding, mobility, and any physical limitations because of the arthritic joints.
   • Determine if the client has a distended bladder.
   • Ask when the client last voided.
   • Assess client's knowledge of condition.
2. Teaching would include the reason the client needs to void before the procedure and that the procedure includes catheterization. You might also explain the type of discomfort caused by catheterization.
3. The correct answer is D. The most common catheter size for a woman of her age would be a 16 Fr.
4. The procedure requires a straight catheter because the purpose is to assess how much urine is in the bladder after the client voids. An indwelling catheter is for long-term use. In this case, no order for an indwelling catheter was written if the residual exceeded a certain amount.
5. The correct answer is A. Sims'. The client has arthritic joints, and if the hips are involved, she may not be able to assume a dorsal recumbent position with the hips abducted.

Answers to NCLEX Review Questions

1. 4. Ensure the elastic adhesive is not tight.
2. 1. Replace foreskin over the glans penis.
3. 2. Secure catheter tubing to the thigh.
4. 3. Have the client void before obtaining the specimen.
5. 1. The catheter must be inserted 1 to 2 inches after urine flows.
6. 3. Possible urethral trauma
7. 4. Deflate the balloon
8. 4. Using a single sterile cotton ball for each wipe
9. 3. Before lubricating the catheter
10. 3. Inserting the catheter to the bifurcation of the catheter ports
11. 1. Balloon is inflated
12. 4. If strong resistance is noted, do not force the irrigation.

13. 2. Maintain fluid intake of at least 2000 ml
14. 1. Starts close to the drain site and cleans in a circular motion outward
15. 1. The client is losing fluid weight
16. 1. Use strict aseptic technique.

Chapter 33
Focus on Clinical Practice Answers

1. A fracture bedpan is best; it is easier to place in clients with restricted mobility. Mrs. Feld can assist with placement by using a side rail or a trapeze bar. A commode is contraindicated because Mrs. Feld is not able to bear weight and cannot transfer from bed to commode.

2. It is expected that the Fleet enema would stimulate a bowel movement, and the fecal material expelled may be hard or range from hard to soft stool. In addition, Mrs. Feld may have subsequent bowel movements throughout the day. You must instruct the assistive personnel about the expected outcome of the enema. In addition, you must instruct the assistive personnel to immediately report to you any complaints of abdominal pain or discomfort. You must also instruct the assistive personnel to report any rectal bleeding, blood in the stool, enlarged abdomen, or changes in vital signs.

3. These first three actions will occur rapidly.
   1. D. Perform an abdominal assessment. Her pain could be due to many factors ranging from benign gas to perforation. You need to collect data as baseline to monitor progression of pain and other abdominal signs and symptoms. In addition, you need data when you call her physician.
   2. E. Obtain vital signs, and instruct assistive personnel to obtain vital signs every 15 to 30 minutes thereafter. You need to obtain the first set of VS as a baseline and compare with the client's range of VS. The assistive personnel then monitors these VS at your direction for frequency. This obtains valuable information while you are contacting the physician.
   3. A. Notify the physician. You should now have abdominal assessment and your VS measurement data to report.

You do not:
   B. Instruct assistive personnel to palpate Mrs. Feld's abdomen. Assessment is a nursing responsibility. You may, however, instruct assistive personnel to notify you if it appears that Mrs. Feld's abdomen is getting bigger or her level of pain changes.
   C. Give postoperative pain medication as ordered. Although Mrs. Feld indeed has pain medication, that medication is to control postoperative hip pain. It will take away or diminish her abdominal pain. Until the cause of Mrs. Feld's abdominal pain is identified, the presence of pain and changes in quality and intensity are important clinical assessment findings that should not be masked by analgesia.

4. Mr. Dale's NG tube is probably obstructed or resting against the abdominal wall and cannot drain. As the gastric secretions accumulate, he becomes nauseated, and if these secretions are not removed, vomiting occurs. Irrigate the NG tube with 30 to 60 ml of normal saline, being careful to note the volume of irrigation on the intake and output record. Following irrigation, observe NG tube and suction equipment, and monitor output. Follow up with abdominal assessment, observe NG tube drainage, and determine if client's nausea is relieved. Instruct assistive personnel to report any nausea, vomiting, and changes in vital signs, stomach pain, and increased abdomen.

Answers to NCLEX Review Questions

1. 4. Absent bowel sounds
2. 1. Lifestyle changes, bulk-forming laxatives, saline or osmotic laxatives, stimulating laxatives
3. 2. Dietary fiber decreases intestinal transit time and increases bulk of fecal contents.
4. 3. 5 to 35 per minute
5. 4. Peritonitis and paralytic ileus
6. 3. Reflex bradycardia
7. 3. Determine pH of gastric contents

Chapter 34
Focus on Clinical Practice Answers

1. Additional information may include:
   - History:
     - No previous surgery or anesthesia experience
     - Nonsmoker
     - Takes a multiple vitamin, a birth control pill, and a calcium tablet daily
     - Wears soft contact lenses
   - Past medical history:
     - No known drug or food allergies
     - Had bacterial pneumonia at age 15
     - Family history of colon cancer (grandmother died at age 58)
   - Focused physical examination:
     - Alert and oriented
     - Vital signs: temperature, 98.2° F; pulse, 102 beats per minute; respirations, 26 breaths per minute; blood pressure, 120/80 mm Hg
     - Height 5′6″; weight 110 pounds
     - Skin: warm and moist
     - Pulmonary: lungs clear to auscultation bilaterally
     - Cardiac: 102 beats per minute and regular
     - Gastrointestinal: bowel sounds present all four quadrants
     - Extremities: pulses present bilaterally
   - Additional:
     - Potential stoma site marked by enterostomal therapist

2. The correct answer is A. A Kock internal reservoir is constructed in a way that uses the walls of the ileum as a

valve to contain the effluent until a catheter is inserted to allow drainage. The effluent will never be formed but may become a thickened liquid in time. A healthy stoma is normally reddish and moist.

3. The correct answers are A, C, and D. The ileum normally produces a mucous coating, and a healthy stoma should be red, indicating a good blood supply. Initially a catheter is placed into the stoma to allow for continuous drainage and healing. The stoma should protrude above the skin level but will shrink as edema lessens and will be smaller and flatter in time.

4. The correct answer is C. Although equipment used in the hospital on a newly created pouch is sterile, in the home clean equipment is satisfactory. Only water-soluble lubricant or water should be used for catheterization. Initially, intermittent catheterization of pouch should be done every 3 to 4 hours. As the reservoir heals, the capacity increases, and 3 to 4 times a day is usually satisfactory.

Answers to NCLEX Review Questions

1. 2. Gently insert catheter a little more
2. 4. Holds the gauze wick on stoma during a pouch change
3. 3. Urine drains continuously
4. 3. Using karaya barrier
5. 1. As normal a diet as possible
6. 4. Invite a person with an ostomy to speak with client
7. 2. 30 to 60 ml of warm tap water

Chapter 35
Focus on Clinical Practice Answers

1. Client is provided with the risks, benefits, and alternatives to having a procedure and agrees to proceed. The physician is responsible for obtaining consent from the client. The nurse may act as a witness to the consent.

2. Client would most likely receive antibiotic prophylaxis in the holding area outside of the operating room 30 minutes before incision to aid in prevention of surgical site infection.

3. Topics included should be instructions to remain NPO and to empty bladder before leaving the client care unit to go to the operating room, what to expect in the preoperative holding area/operating room and recovery room, pain control, dressings, drains, diet, and wound healing process with rationale for each. In addition, Mrs. Edmonds should learn postoperative exercises.

4. Given her history of smoking, she is at an increased risk for pulmonary complications. A history of obesity, taking birth control pills, and undergoing pelvic surgery place her at an increased risk of DVT.

5. Client should ask for pain medications 30 minutes before ambulating/performing exercises or be instructed to use PCA as well as to splint incision with small pillow to decrease incisional discomfort.

Answers to NCLEX Review Questions

1. 1. An explanation of the risks of having the procedure

2. 3. Physicians should discuss and document issues with the client and/or family to determine whether DNR orders are to be maintained or modified during surgical procedures.
3. 1. Within 30 minutes of incision
4. 3. Applying an intermittent pneumatic compression device
5. 2. Crohn's disease
6. 1. Positive Homans' sign
7. 2. Using a black pen, mark the dressing with a circle around the drainage.
8. 2. Provide the client with mouth care only by swabbing oral mucosa with a dampened swab.
9. 3. Cardiac-respiratory monitor

Chapter 36
Focus on Clinical Practice Answers

1. The correct answer is B. Rationale: The surgical hand scrub is now contaminated and needs to be started over.
2. The correct answer is C. Rationale: Artificial nails may not be worn because they may harbor gram-negative microorganisms and fungus, therefore increasing the risk of the client's developing a surgical wound infection.
3. The correct answer is A. Rationale: A short prescrub wash/rinse removes gross debris and superficial microorganisms and is an essential step before surgical antisepsis, with or without using a brush.
4. The correct answer is C. Rationale: Any break in sterile technique must be communicated and acted upon immediately to decrease the risk of the client's developing a surgical wound infection.

Answers to NCLEX Review Questions

1. 3. Conduct perioperative assessment, review medical record, verify consent forms
2. 1. The surgical hand scrub
3. 2. Inspect fingernails, cuticles, hands, and forearms for presence of abrasions, cuts, or open lesions
4. 1. Both hands should be covered with the cuffs of the gown
5. 4. Before scrub nurse dries hands with a towel, she drips water on the sterile gown she is about to put on but does not replace the gown

Chapter 37
Focus on Clinical Practice Answers

1. The correct answers are A, B, and E. Rationale:
   - Prednisone is a steroid. Steroids decrease the inflammatory response and slow collagen synthesis, impairing wound healing.
   - Diabetes mellitus impairs wound healing by decreasing tissue perfusion and hindering the release of oxygen at the tissue level.
   - Age impairs wound healing. Vascular changes, diminished pliability in collagen tissue, and scar tissue tightness contribute to impaired wound healing.

2. You explain to Mrs. Tobias that wound irrigation is a therapy that uses a stream of solution as a way to clean the open wound on her abdomen. The stream is delivered under an appropriate constant pressure. Irritation helps to remove debris, dead tissue and cells, and bacteria from the wound. This keeps the wound clean and allows healing to occur.

3. The correct answer is C. Rationale: This is the position of choice for abdominal wound irrigation. This position allows the flow of irrigation solution to go from the area being cleansed to an area that is distal and lower. The solution flows from a clean to a contaminated area. The collection basin helps to keep the client's bed dry.

4. The correct answers are A and B. Use sterile technique, and direct the flow of solution from healthy tissue to infected tissue.

5. The correct answer is D. Rationale: The bleeding that occurs during irrigation can be caused by irrigation pressures that are too high. The high pressures cause tissue trauma and bleeding. Decreasing the pressure will decrease the risk of this occurring. You should notify the physician if bleeding does occur during the irrigation.

Answers to NCLEX Review Questions

1. 4. I'll irrigate the wound starting at the bottom and move to the top.
2. 2. Red
3. 3. 35-ml syringe with 19-guage angiocatheter.
4. 2. Obtain the physician's order for removal.
5. 1. Snips suture at end proximal to knot.
6. 3. Administer an analgesic 30 minutes before staple removal.
7. 4. To remove drainage from the wound area to promote healing.
8. 2. Pin the drainage tubing to the client's gown.
9. 1. Continue to monitor the color and amount of drainage.

Chapter 38
Focus on Clinical Practice Answers

1. You explain to the client that wounds heal best in a moist environment. Hydrocolloid dressings like the dressing the physician ordered for your leg ulcer are used frequently to treat this type of ulcer because it is a clean, shallow wound. This type of dressing will help keep the wound bed moist to improve healing, absorb wound drainage into the dressing for removal, and remove dead tissue and debris from the wound.

2. The correct answer is C. Because hydrocolloid dressings remain moist and keep the wound bed moist, there is less pain and discomfort for the client when the dressing is removed. Wet-to-dry dressings when removed debride the wound and often cause client pain and discomfort because the dried dressing pulls on the newly granulated wound bed. Bleeding can also occur during removal.

3. The correct answer is B. Healing that occurs due to formulation of granulation tissue and epithelialization is called secondary intention. This type of healing is generally used in the treatment of venous ulcers.

4. The correct answer is A. The wound should be cleansed with the prescribed cleaner and then dried thoroughly. Drying the wound bed and surrounding skin will increase the adherence of the dressing and prevent breakdown of skin surrounding the wound. The dressing is removed using clean gloves not sterile gloves. Hydrocolloid dressings do not require soaking before insertion. You would need to soak gauze dressings that are used for wet-to-dry dressings. The hydrocolloid dressing should not be stretched to fit the wound. This puts tension on the wound bed and wound edges. Cut a dressing that is the appropriate size for the wound.

5. You would need to report options B, E, F, and G. A strong unpleasant odor can be an indication of a possible wound infection. Brisk bleeding in the wound bed should not occur. This is an indication that there is a problem with the wound healing. Thick, creamy yellow drainage is an indication of possible wound infection. Remember, with hydrocolloid dressings, you may see whitish-yellow gel in the wound. This occurs as the dressing absorbs exudate and is normal. Wound edges that are black and dry are an indication of necrotic tissue, indicating poor wound healing. With the hydrocolloid dressings, you would expect the wound to be pink and moist. This indicates healthy tissue and adequate wound healing.

6. The correct answer is D. Hydrocolloid dressings do not need to be moistened before removal. The purpose of this type of dressing is to keep the wound bed moist, so drying is not a problem. The other three statements are statements that indicate correct technique and client understanding of changing hydrocolloid dressings.

Answers to NCLEX Review Questions

1. 2. Remove unhealthy or dead tissue from the wound
2. 4. Pull off tape parallel to skin toward the dressing.
3. 3. Packing removed from wound has strong foul odor.
4. 3. Apply direct pressure.
5. 1. Tape is wrapped around the leg to secure the dressing.
6. 4. Elevate the area of bleeding.
7. 2. Small wound with no exudate
8. 3. Press out wrinkles by applying outward strokes.
9. 1. Instill 10 to 30 ml of saline into the foam, and remove dressing in 15 minutes.
10. 3. Shave hair around wound edges.
11. 4. Increased drainage and odor

Chapter 39
Focus on Clinical Practice Answers

1. Assessment should include the following areas:
   - Respiratory system
     - Ability to breathe deeply
     - Ability to cough
   - Skin for actual or potential alterations
     - Irritation
     - Abrasions

- Skin surfaces that rub against each other
- Allergic response to adhesive tape from dressing
  - Surgical dressing
    - Dressing intact
    - Presence of drainage
    - Coverage of incision
  - Comfort level
    - Compare levels before and after application
    - Measure client for appropriate binder size according to manufacturer's instructions

2. Explain to Mr. Dodson that the purpose of the binder is to:
   - Support the underlying muscles after surgery
   - Promote comfort by supporting the incision when turning, walking, or deep breathing
   - Decrease tension on the suture line to promote healing
   - Support the incision line to keep suture line intact

3. The correct answers are A, D, F, and G.

4. 08:30 Abdominal binder applied. Surgical dressing dry and intact. Client rates pain level as 2/10. Respirations deep and nonlabored. Respiratory rate 14. Client effectively demonstrated deep breathing and coughing.

5. Your first action should be to remove the abdominal binder. The assessment findings indicate that Mr. Dodson is experiencing increased discomfort and impaired breathing. This can occur if the binder is too tight or applied incorrectly. After removing the binder, reassess for improved breathing and decreased discomfort. The binder can be reapplied. Check to make sure that you use correct technique when reapplying the binder.

Answers to NCLEX Review Questions

1. 4. Promote venous return
2. 1. 4 hours
3. 2. Abraded chaffed skin on the lower leg
4. 3. Support the abdominal muscles
5. 4. Remove the binder, and reapply it.
6. 2. Supine

Chapter 40
Focus on Clinical Practice Answers

1. Additional information may include the following: level of client's discomfort, pressure of swelling of ankle, stiffness and difficulty walking, range of motion in right ankle. Also assess sensitivity of skin to light touch and pain.
   - History
     - Extremities: pulses 2+ bilaterally; right foot and ankle edematous and tender to touch; no abrasions noted

2. The correct answers are B, C, and D. Physician's order is required for all cold applications. Assessing current pain level provides a baseline for determining pain relief with therapy. Assessing the condition of the injured body part provides a baseline for determining the change in condition of injured tissues.

3. Instruct the client in the proper techniques for performing a cold application. Inform the client about what to expect during therapy. Describe part of the rationale for performing the treatment.

4. The correct answer is B. Vasodilation improves blood flow to the injured body part, decreasing venous congestion in injured tissues.

Answers to NCLEX Review Questions

1. 2. Moist heat penetrates deeper into tissue layers
2. 3. Peripheral vascular disease
3. 2. Skin is reddened and sensitive to touch.
4. 4. Monitor the condition of the skin every 5 minutes during the application.
5. 1. Affected area is slightly pale and cool to touch.
6. 2. Causing vasoconstriction, which decreases blood flow
7. 1. Decrease the time of the cold applications
8. 3. Increasing metabolic rate and heat production

Chapter 41
Focus on Clinical Practice Answers

1. Hypertension and use of antihypertensive medications may predispose client to postural hypotension. Visual alterations increase risk of client being unable to see obstacles or barriers in the home. Arthritis may minimize mobility or range of motion, increasing risk of slips or tripping.

2. The correct answer is B.

3. Despite older adults' risks, they learn how to negotiate their environments relatively well and are usually more aware of potential dangers. Thus older adults may often be more cautious than younger persons. Usually an older adult will be amenable to changes that bring a sense of security and safety. Encourage the daughter to discuss with her mother what might provide a greater sense of security for both of them. It is important to maintain the mother's autonomy in deciding what, if anything, to change. Offer a home safety assessment.

4. Rationales: Answer A: If stairs are of uniform size, installing a tread prevents client from having to continually adjust vision or stride. Answer B: This creates an unobstructed pathway for ambulation. Answer C: Because of her glaucoma, Mrs. Gleason may adjust appliance to wrong setting, creating potential risk of fire or burning. Colored knobs improves visibility. Answer D: Grab bar provides stability for maneuvering in bathroom, which will be helpful for a client with arthritis. Answer E: Mrs. Gleason will likely have difficulty seeing edges of stairs. Handrail provides stability while she places foot down a step.

5. Mrs. Gleason might have difficulty with opening medication containers and manipulating an eye dropper.

6. Have the daughter count the number of pills in the medicine containers each day or at end of week.

Answers for NCLEX Review Questions

1. 1, 2, and 3 are all characteristic behaviors of Alzheimer's disease. 4 is symptomatic of depression. NOTE: Over time Alzheimer's clients can develop depression.
2. 2. Short-term exercises are the most effective, as long as a client maintains the regular regimen.
3. 2. The MMSE is used to screen for cognitive changes. SPLATT is an acronym used to assess actual falls. A fall diary is used to record the events surrounding an actual fall.
4. 4. Soiled dressings should be double bagged in impervious plastic.

Chapter 42
Focus on Clinical Practice Answers

1. Additional information needed:
   - List of current medications
   - Cognitive status
   - Problems with sensation or mobility
   - Recent vital signs, especially heart rate and rhythm
2. When the client's medications at home do not match the medications the prescriber believes the client is taking, the nurse should contact the prescriber to ensure the nurse has accurate information about the client's prescribed medications. The nurse may need to employ the assistance of the client's pharmacist to ensure that the client receives only prescribed medications. Medications that the client should not be taking should be discarded or removed from the area where current medications are stored. The nurse needs to educate the client and provide a written list of which medications should be taken, including their dosages and times for administration.
3. The correct answer is C. The pulse of a client with an arrhythmia should be taken for a full minute in case the pulse is irregular.
4. Mr. Anderson may be pressing too hard over the artery or is unable to locate it. Coach him in his technique and reinstruct about artery location. If a cognitive deficit exists, teach a family member or friend how to check the pulse.
5. There are many teaching strategies a nurse can employ to facilitate successful medication education in older adults (see Box 42-5). Some strategies to enhance Mr. Anderson's learning include the following:
   - Provide typewritten information in large print.
   - Provide information to the client that he feels is important.
   - Repeat information that is important in the beginning and at the end of teaching sessions.
   - Develop a trusting relationship with Mr. Anderson.
   - Use a memory aid, such as a daily checklist, to help him remember to take his medications.

Answers to NCLEX Review Questions

1. 2. "I will have to learn how to take rectal temperatures with a glass thermometer."
2. 3. Take Betty's blood pressure with a manual aneroid sphygmomanometer right after Betty takes her blood pressure with her monitor.
3. 4. Radial
4. 1. The client should not allow people in the home to smoke.
5. 3. "I need to make sure my breaker box will meet the electrical requirements of the concentrator."
6. 1. Wipe the connectors of both tanks with a lint-free cloth.
7. 4. Providing several breaths of 100% oxygen with a bag-valve-mask.
8. 3. Apply intermittent suction for no more than 15 seconds.
9. 4. Save disposable inner cannulas for future use.
10. 2. Include him in making decisions about when he should take his medications.
11. 1. "I am not sure why my son has to take his insulin."
12. 3. Older adults with declining cognitive status should have simple medication regimens.
13. 4. Stop the feeding.
14. 3. "I just don't think I can take care of my husband much longer."
15. 4. Perform hand hygiene.

Chapter 43
Focus on Clinical Practice Answers

1. The correct answer is E: choices A and D are correct. Testing for occult blood of the client's stool and emesis would be important to assess for gastrointestinal bleeding. Blood samples will provide the physician with a blood count, which could detect evidence of active bleeding. Because the client is diabetic, it is important to monitor her glucose level.
2. The stool for guaiac and the emesis specimen for Gastroccult analysis will provide immediate test results.
3. Gastric emeses must be tested with Gastroccult reagent, and stool is tested with Hemoccult reagent. Mixing up these two reagents has the potential of leading to false negative or false positive results. This is because the pH of the specimens is different, gastric being more acidic.
4. The client could be requested to continue testing of stool and emesis for occult blood. She would need the following supplies:
   - Stool for occult blood testing kit (cardboard Hemoccult slide, wooden applicator, and Hemoccult developing solution)
   - Gastroccult kit (cardboard slide, wooden applicator, and developing solution)

Answers to NCLEX Review Questions

1. 2. The initial stream flushes the urethral orifice and meatus of any resident bacteria
2. 3. 40 to 60 ml
3. 1. Discards the first urine specimen
4. 2. The sterile self-sealing specimen port on the catheter
5. 4. Total output
6. 2. Diabetes
7. 2. Is a procedure to obtain fresh urine
8. 4. Parasites
9. 2. Tomatoes
10. 1. Stomach, esophagus
11. 1. NG, nasoenteral tube
12. 2. Sitting upright or at a 45-degree angle
13. 2. Tonsillar area
14. 2. Crushed
15. 1. Redness, swelling, and discharge
16. 3. Tracheal suctioning
17. 2. 1 to 2 hours
18. 3. New drainage (exudate)
19. Superficial wounds exposed to the air
20. 4. Polycythemia
21. 1. Facilitate distention of veins
22. 4. Are elastic and rebound when palpated
23. 2. After the blood sample is obtained
24. 1. Prevent needle stick injury
25. 1. Sides of the fingers, toes, heels
26. 1. Wipe away first droplet of blood with alcohol ball.

Chapter 44
Focus on Clinical Practice Answers

1. Additional information may include the following:
   - History
   - Mild congestive heart failure
   - Chronic atrial fibrillation
   - Hyperlipidemia
   - Past medical history
   - Chronic back pain secondary to spinal stenosis
   - Relevant recent diagnostic testing
   - Echocardiogram results that showed a 45% ejection fraction
   - Positive pharmacological stress test.
   - Home medications
   - Furosemide
   - Lisinopril
   - Warfarin
   - Tylenol
   - Lifestyle assessment
   - Lives in own home with spouse
   - Active mobility (walks in stores, volunteers at local school)
   - Focused physical examination
   - Alert and oriented.

   - Vital signs: blood pressure, 122/67 mm Hg; heart rate, 86 and irregular; respiratory rate, 20 breaths per minute; temperature, 36.8° C
   - Pulmonary: breath sounds with faint crackles over bases, but unlabored breathing with activity; pulse oximetry reading of 98%
   - Cardiac: heart rate irregular, mild bilateral pedal edema, pedal pulses palpable
   - Integumentary: skin warm and dry
   - GI: within normal limits
   - Genitourinary: states he urinates "a lot, especially after taking my furosemide and lisinopril"

2. The correct answer is B. Rationale: Cardiac catheterization poses a risk of blood loss, and a risk of complications that would require emergency coronary artery bypass graft surgery. H&H is needed to obtain a baseline hematologic status that will be compared with possible repeat testing. PT/INR is affected by warfarin, which Mr. H is taking for chronic atrial fibrillation. The physician should have instructed Mr. H. to stop his warfarin 1 to 2 nights before this procedure. A current PT/INR is needed to determine whether Mr. H. is at risk for uncontrolled bleeding. BUN and Cr are needed to evaluate Mr. H.'s renal function and along with urine specific gravity to help determine whether Mr. H. is dehydrated. Clients with baseline dehydration or impaired renal function are at risk for impaired excretion of the radiographic dye used during the cardiac catheterization procedure.

3. In the presence of another nurse, ask Mr. H. the following upon arrival and just before starting the procedure: name; identifying number, such as birth date; purpose of visit. Also compare the information given verbally by Mr. H. to his wrist identification band. Document both instances in Mr. H.'s medical record.

4. The correct answer is B. Mr. H. falls into an ASA classification of "2—presence of mild systemic disease without functional limitations." Although he has mild congestive heart failure and chronic atrial fibrillation, he lives independently and is able to be active in his community. After documenting the ASA score, no further action is needed.

5. The correct answer is C. Clients who have not yet given informed consent should not be asked to sign a consent form. In addition, they should not receive any medication that can reduce their level of consciousness, because it will impair their ability to give legal informed consent.

6. The correct answer is A. These assessments are in order of threat to life and tailored to the procedure that was done. Heart rate and rhythm can be affected because of catheter irritation or injury to the heart. Respiratory effort and oxygen saturation can be insufficient if the intravenous sedation suppressed Mr. H. past the level of "moderate" sedation. The procedure site can easily bleed if mechanically disrupted when Mr. H. is transferred

from the procedure table to a cart and them to his bed. A visual check is essential to make sure that the dressing, sandbag, or closure device is secure to prevent arterial bleeding. Frequent pedal pulse checks help promptly detect any intravascular clotting that might occur at the procedure site and cause reduced circulation to the legs.

Answers to NCLEX Review Questions

1. 2. Relaxes the client
2. 4. Pulse oximetry values
3. 1. Assisting with an angiogram may be delegated to unlicensed assistive personnel.
4. 1. Heart rate increased from 92 to 106 beats per minute, low back pain radiating to the sides, other assessments unchanged
5. 4. Place the bed in Trendelenburg's position, and support her airway.
6. 1. Renal failure
7. 1. The procedure is painful, but only briefly.
8. 4. Computed tomography scan of the brain
9. 3. Decreased abdominal girth and decreased respiratory effort
10. 3. The amount of fluid removed is usually no more than 1.5 liters.
11. 2. Sputum clear or slightly blood-tinged
12. 2. Intravenous moderate sedation
13. 4. Clear liquids only for 2 days before the procedure. Complete the bowel prep the night before the procedure. Fast from food and fluids for 8 hours before the procedure.
14. 4. Proceed no further with preparation for the test. Inform Mr. J. that there is a chance that his procedure might have to be rescheduled. Then notify the physician, and await instruction about how to proceed.
15. 3. 12-lead ECG
16. 2. Electrode gel dried out or too thinly smeared

Terminology/Combining Forms: Prefixes and Suffixes

Medical terminology is similar to a foreign language. Many medical terms are derived from Latin and Greek sources. They often consist of two or more simple words or word elements. A word root or *combining form* may be put together with a *prefix* and a *suffix*.

Root—the basis of a word
Example: *nephr*/o/tic (degenerative changes in the kidney)
Root: nephr- (kidney)

Linking vowel—a vowel that joins the combining form to the suffix or another combining form
Example: nephr/*o*/sis (disease of the kidneys)
Linking vowel: o

Prefix—the beginning of a word
Example: *hyper*/active (excessively active)
Prefix: hyper- (excessive)

Suffix—the ending of a word
Example: nephr/itis (inflammation of the kidney)
Suffix: -itis (inflammation)

Combining form—the union of a word root with a linking vowel
Example: *hepato*/megaly (enlargement of the liver)
Combining form: hepato- (liver)

The following table provides some of the most commonly used terminology for your reference.

Common Prefixes

PREFIX	DEFINITION
a-	without
ab-	away from
abd-	abdominal
acu-	sharp
ad-	toward
adip-	fat
ad lib-	freely, as wanted
aero-	air, gas
al-	toward
ambi-	both
an-	not
ana-	up

PREFIX	DEFINITION
ante-	before, in front of
anti-	against
arteri-	artery
arthro-	joint
auto-	self
bi-	two
brady-	slow
cata-	down
chole-	bile
cili-	eyelid
circum-	around
co-	with, together
cogni-	know
colo-	colon
con-	with, together
contra-	against
crani-	skull
cut-	skin
cyt-	cell
de-	from, lack of
demi-	half
dent-	tooth
derm-	skin
dia-	through, across
diplo-	double, twofold
dis-	to free or undo
dors-	back
dur-	hard
dy-	two
dys-	bad, painful, difficult, abnormal
ec-	out, out from
ecto-	outside
em-	in
embol-	to insert
encephalo-	brain
endo-	in, within
entero-	intestine
epi-	above, upon

PREFIX	DEFINITION
erythro-	red
eso-	within, inward
et-	and
eu-	good, normal
ex-	out, away from
exo-	outside
extra-	outside
faci-	face
fiss-	split, cleft
fore-	before, in front of
gastro-	stomach
glosso-	relating to the tongue
glyco-	sugar
haplo-	simple, single
heme-	iron-based
hemi-	one half
hepat-	liver
hetero-	different
histo-	tissue
homo-	same
hydro-	wet, water
hyper-	excessive, above normal
hypo-	under, below
im-	not
in-	in, not
infra-	under, below
inter-	between
intra-	in, within
isch-	deficiency
iso-	equal, alike
lapra-	loin or flank, sometimes abdomen
lapis-	stone
latero-	side
macro-	large
mal-	bad
meato-	opening
medi-	middle
melano-	black
mesa-	middle
meso-	middle
meta-	beyond, change
micro-	small
mono-	one
morpho-	form, structure
multi-	many, much
neo-	new
nephro-	kidney
oculo-	eye
onco-	tumor
oro-	mouth
osteo-	bone
pan-	all
para-	beside, beyond
per-	through, by
peri-	around

PREFIX	DEFINITION
phago-	eating
poly-	many, much
post-	after, behind
pre-	before, in front of
primi-	first
pro-	before, in front of
pseudo-	false
quadri-	four
re-	again, backward
retro-	backward, behind
rhabdo-	rod-shaped, striated
rhodo-	red
scler-	hardening
semi-	one half
sub-	under, below
super-	above, excessive
supra-	above, excessive
stetho-	chest
sym-	together
syn-	union, together, joined
tachy-	rapid
tetra-	four
therm-	heat
trans-	through, across
tri-	three
ultra-	beyond, excess
uni-	one
vas-	vessel or duct
xantho-	yellow
xero-	dry

Common Suffixes

SUFFIX	DEFINITION
-ac	pertaining to
-agra	excessive pain
-al	pertaining to
-algia	painful condition, pain
-apheresis	removal
-ar	pertaining to
-ary	pertaining to
-ase	enzyme
-bi	two, double
-blast	developing cell
-cele	hernia, swelling, sac
-centesis	puncture of a cavity
-clasis	break, fracture
-clysis	irrigation, washing
-coccus	berry shaped
-crit	to separate
-cyte	cell
-desis	fusion, binding, fixation
-drome	to run
-dynia	pain
-ectasis	expansion, dilation

SUFFIX	DEFINITION	SUFFIX	DEFINITION
-ectomy	excision, removal of a body part	-pathy	disease, suffering
-emesis	vomiting	-penia	deficiency, lack of, decrease
-emia	blood	-pexy	fixation
-er	one who	-phagia	eating, swallowing
-gen	forming, producing, origin	-phasia	speech
-genesis	forming, producing, origin	-philia	attraction for
-genic	origin, formation	-phobia	fear
-grade	to go	-physis	to grow
-gram	the record made, mark	-plasia	formation, growth
-graph	instrument for recording, machine	-plasm	growth, formation
-graphy	the process, process of recording	-plasty	mold, shape, repair
-ia	condition	-plegia	paralysis
-iasis	morbid condition	-poiesis	formation, production
-iatry	treatment, medicine	-ptosis	downward displacement, falling
-ic/-ical	pertaining to	-ptysis	spitting
-icle	small, minute	-rrhage	bursting forth, rupture
-ism	condition	-rrhaphy	suturing in place
-ist	one who specializes in, specialist	-rrhea	flow, discharge
-itis	inflammation	-rrhexis	rupture
-lith	stone, calculus	-scope	instrument to visually examine
-logist	specialist in the study of	-scopy	process of examining, visual examination
-logy	process of study	-sepsis	infection
-lysis	dissolution, setting free	-sis	state of, condition
-malacia	softening, soft	-spasm	involuntary spasm
-megaly	enlargement	-stalsis	constriction
-meter	instrument for measuring	-stasis	control, constant level, stop
-metry	act of measuring	-stenosis	narrowing, stricture
-odynia	pain	-stomy	creation of an opening
-oid	form, shape	-therapy	treatment
-ole	small, minute	-tic	pertaining to
-ology	study or science of	-tome	instrument for cutting
-oma	tumor	-tomy	process of cutting, incision
-opsy	to view	-toxic	poison
-or	one who	-tresia	opening
-orrhea	flow, discharge	-tripsy	surgical crushing
-osis	condition or state	-trophy	nourishment
-ous	pertaining to	-ula	small, minute
-para	to bear (offspring)	-ule	small, minute
-paresis	partial paralysis	-y	process

Glossary

abdominal girth The measurement of the abdomen's circumference, taken at the same place with each measurement.

abduction Movement of an extremity away from the midline of the body.

accommodation reflex Adjustment of the eyes for near vision, composed of pupillary constriction, convergence of the visual axes, and increased convexity of the lens.

accurate empathy Communication technique used by nurse to show understanding of client's feelings and experiences.

Acetest A test that measures the presence of ketone (acetone) bodies in the urine. A large quantity of acetone causes rapid change in the color of the Acetest tablet.

active listening An interpersonal process whereby a person hears a message, decodes the meaning, and conveys an understanding about the meaning to the sender.

active range-of-motion exercises Exercises of the joints performed by an individual without assistance.

active-assisted range-of-motion exercises Exercises of the joints performed by an individual with some assistance. A nurse, for example, helps support an extremity.

activity tolerance Kind and amount of exercise or work that a person is able to perform.

actual loss Any loss of a person or object that can no longer be felt, heard, known, or experienced.

acuity records Documentation that quantifies the level of care required by a client in a health care setting.

acute pain Severe pain with a rapid onset and of short duration.

addiction A compulsive physiological need for a habit-forming drug.

adduction Movement of an extremity toward the midline of the body.

adjuvant therapy The treatment of a disease with substances that enhance the action of drugs, especially drugs that promote the production of antibodies.

adrenergic drug A medication that mimics the effects of sympathetic nerve stimulation of the autonomic nervous system.

advance directives Document defining the client's end-of-life care decisions.

adverse drug reactions (ADRs) Nontherapeutic effects of medications.

aerobe A microorganism that lives and grows in the presence of free oxygen.

aerobic Pertaining to the presence of air or oxygen.

afebrile Without fever.

agglutinate A process by which cells that display antigens (red blood cells, bacteria) adhere to each other, or clump together.

air embolus A quantity of air that circulates in the bloodstream to eventually lodge in a blood vessel.

air fluidization The process of blowing warm air through a collection of microspheres to create a fluidlike environment; used in special mattresses designed to reduce pressure against a person's skin.

air leak Escaping air in closed chest drainage; may be client centered or within the chest tube system.

air-fluidized bed A special bed designed to distribute weight evenly over its support surface. Fluidization is created by forcing a gentle flow of temperature-controlled air upward through a mass of fine ceramic microspheres.

air-suspension bed A device that supports a client's weight on air-filled cushions, minimizing tissue damage from pressure and shear.

albumin An acute phase protein involved in nutrient transport and the maintenance of oncotic pressure. Used as a measure of visceral protein status. Has a half-life of 14 to 20 days.

aldosterone A steroid hormone produced by the adrenal cortex that causes the kidney tubules to excrete potassium and reabsorb sodium and water.

allergen A substance that can produce a hypersensitive reaction in the body but that is not necessarily intrinsically harmful.

all-hazards event Multiple manmade or natural events with destructive capacity to cause multiple casualties.

all-hazards preparedness The comprehensive preparedness necessary to manage casualties resulting from a disaster regardless of etiology.

allogenic Denoting a cell type that is from the same species but genetically distinct.

alopecia Partial or complete lack of hair.

Alzheimer's disease Presenile dementia, characterized by progressive confusion, memory failure, disorientation, restlessness, and speech disturbances. Cause is not fully understood.

amino acid An organic compound composed of one or more basic amino groups and one or more carboxyl groups. Amino acids are the building blocks that construct proteins and the end products of protein digestion.

amnesic syndrome Memory impairment in the absence of other cognitive impairments.

ampule Small sterile glass or plastic container that usually contains a single dose of solution to be administered parenterally.

anaerobic Pertaining to absence of air or oxygen.

analgesia A decreased or absent sensation of pain.

anaphylactic reaction Exaggerated hypersensitivity reaction to a previously encountered antigen. It is a severe and sometimes fatal systemic reaction characterized by itching, hyperemia, angioedema, and in severe cases vascular collapse, bronchospasm, and shock.

anaphylaxis An exaggerated hypersensitivity reaction to a previously encountered antigen. The reaction may be localized or generalized.

anastomosis A surgical joining of two ducts or blood vessels to allow flow from one to the other.

anemia A disorder characterized by a decrease in hemoglobin in the blood to levels below the normal range, decreased red cell production, or increased red cell destruction or blood loss.

anesthesia The absence of normal sensation, especially sensitivity to pain.

anesthetics Drugs or agents capable of producing a complete or partial loss of feeling.

anions Negatively charged ions.

anthropometry The science of measuring the human body as to height, weight, and size of component parts, including measurement of skinfolds.

antianginal A medication that dilates coronary arteries, improving blood flow to the myocardium to prevent angina.

antidysrhythmic A class of medications that possesses properties for controlling abnormal cardiac rhythms, (e.g., quinidine and propranolol [Inderal]).

antiemetic Of or pertaining to a substance or procedure that prevents or alleviates nausea and vomiting.

antipyretic Pertaining to a substance, such as a medication, that reduces fever.

apical pulse Measurement of the heartbeat as taken with the stethoscope placed over the apex of the heart.

apnea An absence of spontaneous respirations.

approximate To come together, as in the edges of a wound.

aqueous Watery or waterlike; referring to a medication prepared with water.

artificial airway Plastic or rubber device inserted into the upper or lower respiratory tract to facilitate ventilation or secretion removal.

ascites Effusion and accumulation of serous fluid in the abdominal cavity.

asepsis The absence of disease-producing (pathogenic) organisms.

aseptic technique The methods used during client care to prevent microbial contamination. They can be either clean (medical asepsis) techniques or sterile (surgical asepsis) techniques.

aspirant Fluid or particulate that is aspirated.

aspirate Withdrawal of fluid or air into the barrel of a syringe or suction device.

aspiration The entry of gastric contents into the tracheobronchial passages. This increases a client's risk for aspiratory pneumonia.

astigmatism Abnormal condition of the eye in which the light rays cannot be focused clearly in a point on the retina because the spherical curve of the cornea is not equal in all meridians. Vision is blurred, and use of the eyes causes discomfort.

astringent A topical substance that causes constriction of tissues upon application; commonly used for cleansing the skin.

atelectasis An abnormal condition characterized by the collapse of lung tissue, preventing the respiratory exchange of carbon dioxide and oxygen.

atmospheric pressure Pressure exerted by the atmosphere. (Atmospheric pressure at sea level is 760 mm Hg.)

atrophy Wasting or diminution of size or physiological activity of a part of the body caused by disease or other influences.

audiologist A health professional with at least a master's degree who studies sense of hearing defects and diagnoses hearing loss and works to provide rehabilitation of individuals with hearing loss.

auscultation The act of listening for sounds within the body to evaluate the condition of the heart, lungs, pleura, intestines, or other organs or to detect fetal heart sounds. Performed directly or most commonly through use of a stethoscope.

auscultatory gap The temporary disappearance of Korotkoff sounds when blood pressure is being auscultated. Occurs in hypertensive clients and may cause an underestimation of blood pressure.

autoclave An appliance used to sterilize medical instruments or other objects with steam under pressure.

Autolet A small instrument with a lancet used to obtain a capillary blood specimen.

autologous blood transfusion Transfusion of a client's own blood through either predeposit, blood salvaged intraoperatively by a cell saver, or blood shed postoperatively.

automated external defibrillator (AED) Device used by basic CPR providers to treat fast, irregular dysrhythmias with electrical shock to the heart using automated rhythm analysis and simplified functions.

autopsy Examination of the deceased's body performed after a person's death to confirm or determine the cause of death.

autotransfusion The collection, anticoagulation, filtration, and reinfusion of blood from an active bleeding site. Used in cases of trauma and major surgery.

axillary Pertaining to the pyramid-shaped space that forms the underside of the shoulder between the upper part of the arm and the side of the chest.

bacteremia Presence of bacteria in the blood.

bacteriostatic Tending to inhibit development or reproduction of bacteria

bag-valve-mask (BVM) or Ambu-bag Bag attached to a mask that provides artificial ventilations to the client when squeezed.

balance Position in which the person's center of gravity is correct so that the risk of falling is reduced.

bariatric bed A specialized surface equipped with hand controls to allow for self-positioning, providing a stable, adaptable surface for managing the morbidly obese client.

basal energy expenditure (BEE) The amount of energy required at rest for basic life processes such as breathing, maintaining body temperature, and cardiac function. Basal energy expenditure can be estimated or measured.

basal metabolism Energy needed to maintain the body's basic processes such as respiration, circulation, and temperature.

base of support Surface area on which an object rests.

bed rest Placement of the client in bed for a prescribed period for therapeutic reasons.

belt restraints Type of restraint used to secure a client on a stretcher.

binder Bandage made of a large piece of material to fit and support a specific body part.

bioavailability The extent to which a dose of a drug reaches its site of action to produce an effect.

biological agent Bacteria or virus that, when released into the environment, has the potential to cause widespread and continuing infection and mass casualties.

biological disaster The unexpected release of a biological agent capable of causing widespread illness or contamination into the environment.

biopsy The removal and microscopic examination of tissue, performed to establish precise diagnosis.

bioterrorism/bioterrorist attack The release of a biological agent into a specified environment with the intent of causing mass casualties.

blood culture A laboratory test on serum to determine presence of infection in the blood.

blood group Classification of blood based on the presence or absence of genetically determined antigens on the surface of the red cell.

blood plasma The liquid portion of the blood, free of its formed elements and particles.

blood transfusion Administration of whole blood or a blood component as cells to replace blood lost through trauma, surgery, or disease.

blood type Blood groups identified by genetically determined antigens on the surface of red blood cells.

body alignment Refers to the condition of joints, tendons, ligaments, and muscles in various body positions.

body mass index (BMI) A measurement of weight in comparison to height. Used to categorize an individual's degree of adiposity.

body mechanics Coordinated efforts of the musculoskeletal and nervous systems to maintain proper balance, posture, and body alignment.

bolus A large, round preparation of medicinal material for oral ingestion; a dose of a medication or a contrast material injected all at once intravenously.

bone marrow Specialized, soft tissue filling the spaces in cancellous bone of the epiphyses; responsible for red blood cell production.

borborygmus Audible abdominal sound produced by hyperactive intestinal peristalsis.

bradycardia An abnormality in heart rate in which the heart contracts steadily at a rate less than 60 contractions per minute.

bradypnea Breathing that is normal in rate but abnormally slow (less than 12 breaths per minute).

bronchophony An increase in intensity and clarity of vocal resonance that may result from an increase in lung tissue density, such as in the consolidation of pneumonia.

bronchospasm Abnormal contraction of the smooth muscles of the bronchi.

bronchus One of several large air passages in the lungs through which pass inspired air and exhaled gases.

bruit Abnormal sound or murmur created by turbulent blood flow heard while auscultating an organ, gland, or artery.

buccal Of or pertaining to the inside of the cheek; surface of a tooth or gum next to the cheek.

cadence Pace or rate of verbal communication.

calorie (Kcal) A calorie is the amount of heat required to raise the temperature of 1 g of water 1° C at atmospheric pressure.

cannula A flexible tube containing a stiff, pointed trocar; the tube may be inserted into the body, guided by the trocar. As the trocar is removed, a body fluid may pass through the cannula.

capillary closing pressure The amount of external pressure required to close off the blood flow to the capillaries.

carcinoma Malignant epithelial neoplasm that tends to invade surrounding tissue and spread to distant regions of the body.

cardiac Pertaining to the heart; pertaining to a person with heart disease.

cardiac arrest The cessation of circulating blood flow that eliminates oxygen transport or perfusion, usually precipitated by ventricular fibrillation or ventricular asystole.

cardiac output Volume of blood ejected by the ventricles of the heart in 1 minute; equal to stroke volume times heart rate.

cardiomegaly Enlargement of the heart; typical sign of heart failure.

cardiopulmonary arrest Sudden cessation of respirations, pulse, and circulation.

cardiopulmonary resuscitation (CPR) Basic emergency procedure for life support, consisting of artificial respiration and manual external cardiac massage.

caries Decay of a tooth; progressive decalcification of enamel and dentin of a tooth.

case management The assignment of a health care provider to assist a client by assessing need for health care and social service systems and to ensure that required services are obtained.

cast Rigid plaster or fiberglass application molded over skin tissues to hold musculoskeletal tissues to permit healing of injuries.

cast brace Combination of a brace within a cast at a joint.

cast saw Saw used to cut through plaster to remove cast.

cast shoe Shoe worn over the foot encased in plaster.

cast syndrome A series of client signs indicative of an untoward (claustrophobic) reaction to being in a cast.

casualty Any individual who is ill, injured, missing, or killed as a result of a mass casualty incident.

cathartic Drug that acts to promote bowel evacuation.

catheterization Introduction of a rubber or plastic tube through the urethra and into the bladder.

cations Positively charged ions.

cell cycle The sequence of events that occurs during the growth and division of tissue cells.

center of gravity Midpoint or center of body weight. In the adult it is the midpelvic cavity between the symphysis pubis and the umbilicus.

centigrade Temperature scale in which 0 degrees is the freezing point of water and 100 degrees is the boiling point of water at sea level; also called Celsius.

central venous catheter (CVC) A catheter that is threaded through the internal jugular, antecubital, or subclavian vein, usually with tip resting in the superior vena cava or right atrium.

central venous pressure (CVP) Pressure in the great veins (superior and inferior vena cava) as blood returns to the heart.

cephalic vein One of the four superficial veins of the upper limb.

cerebrospinal fluid (CSF) Substance contained within the four ventricles of the brain, the subarachnoid space, and the central canal of the spinal cord.

cerumen Earwax; a waxy secretion produced by apocrine sweat glands in the external ear canal.

cervical halter Support for the head, made of cotton material, used for traction.

change-of-shift report Means through which nurses report information about their assigned clients to the nurses working the next shift for the purpose of providing continuity of care for the client. May be given orally in person, by audiotape recording, or during "walking-planning" rounds at each client's bedside.

charting by exception (CBE) A charting methodology in which data are entered only when there is an exception from what is normal or expected. Reduces time spent documenting.

cheilosis Disorder of the lips and mouth characterized by scales and fissures.

chemical decontamination The process of removing or netralizing contaminating chemical agents.

chemotherapy Use of drugs to prevent cancer cells from multiplying, invading adjacent tissue, and metastasizing.

chest physiotherapy Physical maneuvers, including postural drainage, chest percussion, vibration, rib shaking, and cough, to improve airway mucus clearance in clients with retained tracheobronchial secretions.

chest tube Catheter inserted through the chest wall into the intrapleural space by the physician.

chronic pain Pain that persists beyond the period of healing, ceases to serve a protective function, degrades client function, and serves no adaptive purpose.

chronic venous insufficiency Abnormal circulatory condition characterized by decreased return of the venous blood from the legs to the trunk of the body.

circulating nurse An RN considered to be the charge nurse in the operating room during a surgical procedure.

circumduction The circular movement of a limb; the motion of the head of a bone within an articulating cavity such as the hip joint.

clarifying An attempt to put into words vague ideas or unclear thoughts of the client to enhance the nurse's understanding, or asking the client to explain what he or she means.

clean technique (medical asepsis) The purposeful prevention of the transmission of microorganisms by using procedures such as hand washing and disinfection of equipment to reduce the number of microorganisms.

cleansing enema An enema, usually soapsuds, administered repeatedly until the colon is free of all formed fecal material.

clean-voided specimen A technique used to collect a urine specimen as free from bacterial contamination as possible without catheterizing the client.

Clinitest A test that measures the amount of glucose and acetone in a urine specimen.

closed system suction catheter   A suction catheter that is attached to the mechanical ventilator circuit encased within a sterile sheath. The catheter system permits sterile airway suctioning without interrupting mechanical ventilation or requiring the nurse to apply sterile gloves.

coagulopathy   A pathological condition affecting the ability of the blood to coagulate.

colon   Portion of large intestine from the cecum to the rectum.

colon conduit   A surgical urinary diversion in which the ureters are implanted into a 4- to 6-cm piece of large intestine that has been removed from the rest of the bowel and will now serve as a passageway for the urine. The distal end of this piece of colon is sutured closed, and the other end of the colon is brought out onto the client's abdomen as a stoma.

colonization   The reproduction of microorganisms at a specific site without the signs/symptoms of a disease or tissue invasion.

colonized   The presence of bacteria on the surface or in the tissue of a wound without indications of infection such as purulent exudate, foul odor, or surrounding inflammation. All stage II, III, and IV pressure ulcers are colonized.

colostomy   Surgical formation of an opening of the colon onto the surface of the abdomen through which fecal matter is emptied.

comforting   Any nursing action taken to promote comfort of the client, such as a back rub, change in position.

compartment syndrome   Insufficient arterial perfusion to an extremity caused by trauma or stasis; leads to ischemia and tissue necrosis if not reversed.

compatibility   The quality or state of existing together in harmony. The formation of a stable chemical or biochemical system, specifically in medication, so that two or more drugs can be administered at same time without producing side effects.

compliance   Fulfillment by the client of the caregiver's prescribed course of treatment.

compound   A substance composed of two or more different elements, chemically combined, that cannot be separated by physical means.

compress   Soft pad of gauze or cloth used to apply heat, cold, or medications to the surface of a body part.

computer-based patient care record (CPCR)   A new comprehensive system that uses many components of data collection. This system permits the nurse to have an instrumental role in developing this method of documentation.

condition of participation   A requirement that all clients be notified of their rights when entering a health care facility. Part of the Key Principles of Patient's Rights documentation.

conduction   Mechanism of heat transfer involving flow of heat from one object to another with which it is in contact.

conjunctiva   Mucous membrane lining the inner surfaces of the eyelids and anterior part of the sclera.

conjunctivitis   A highly contagious eye infection. The crusty drainage that collects on eyelid margins can easily spread from one eye to the other.

constipation   Condition characterized by difficulty in passing stool or an infrequent passage of hard stool.

consultation   A process in which the help of a specialist is sought to identify ways to handle problems in client management or in the planning and implementation of health care programs.

contact lens   A small, transparent, curved glass or plastic lens shaped to fit over a person's cornea; the lens floats on a precorneal tear film.

contamination   The introduction of infectious material on normally clean or sterile sites.

continent ostomy or diversion   Results from a surgical procedure that leaves the client with an internal pouch where either stool or urine is temporarily stored and the effluent is removed by intubation through the external stoma. It is continent because the effluent does not drain spontaneously from the stoma; instead a catheter must be inserted through the stoma to drain the effluent from the internal pouch.

continuous subcutaneous infusion (CSQI or CSCI)   A method of medication administration in which medication is administered continuously into the subcutaneous tissue using a medication infusion pump.

continuum of care   Matching an individual's ongoing needs with the appropriate level and type of medical, psychological, health, or social care or services within an organization or across multiple organizations.

contractures   Abnormal condition of a joint, characterized by flexion and fixation and caused by atrophy and shortening of muscle fibers or by loss of normal elasticity of the skin.

core temperature   Temperature of deep body tissues and organs.

costovertebral angle (CVA) tenderness   Palpation over this region can elicit tenderness. Tenderness is common with kidney infection or trauma to the region.

cough   Forced exhalation following this normal series of events: (a) partial or full inhalation; (b) closure of the glottis; (c) active contraction of expiratory muscles; and (d) rapid glottic opening.

countertraction   Use of client's body weight or other weights, ropes, and pulleys to counter the pull of the traction weight.

crackles   Fine bubbling sound heard on auscultation of the lung.

crepitation   The sound and/or feeling produced when bone ends rub against each other. The client describes the sound and feeling.

critical pathway   A schedule of critical care medical and nursing procedures, including diagnostic tests, medications, and consultations designed to effect an efficient coordinated program of treatment.

crutch gait   Gait assumed by a person on crutches by alternately bearing weight on one or both legs and on the crutches.

crutch palsy   Temporary or permanent loss of sensation or movement resulting from pressure on axilla from crutch.

cryotherapy   Therapy in which the skin is exposed to cool or cold temperatures; used to treat localized inflammatory responses.

cuff   A plastic, air, or foam and air-filled balloonlike attachment on the distal end of the endotracheal tube or tracheostomy tube that prevents loss of air from the lung and inhalation of foreign bodies around the tube.

culture   Laboratory test involving the cultivation of microorganisms or cells in a special growth medium.

cutaneous stimulation   Stimulation of the skin.

cuticle   A thin edge of cornified epithelium at the base of a nail.

cyanosis   Bluish discoloration of the skin and mucous membranes caused by an excess of deoxygenated hemoglobin in the blood or a structural defect in the hemoglobin molecule.

cycloplegic   Pertaining to a drug that paralyzes ciliary muscles of the eye, causing pupillary dilation for ophthalmological examination or surgery.

cystectomy   The surgical removal of the bladder.

cytology   The study of cells, including their formation, origin, structure, function, biochemical activities, and pathology.

dangling   To sit on the side of a bed with legs dependent or feet on the floor.

DAR   An acronym for a method of documentation that includes data (subjective and objective), action (nursing interventions), and response of the client (evaluation of effectiveness).

dead space   A cavity remaining in a wound.

debride   To remove dead or damaged tissue from a wound; to remove dirt, foreign objects, damaged tissue, and cellular debris from a wound or burn to prevent infection and promote healing.

debridement   Removal of dead tissue in a wound.

decompression   Removal of pressure as from gas and fluid in the stomach and intestinal tract.

decontamination   The process of removing foreign material such as blood, body fluids, chemical, biological, or radioactive contaminents. It does not eliminate microorganisms but is a necessary step preceding disinfection or sterilization.

deep vein thrombosis   A thrombus in one of the deep veins of the body, most often the iliac or femoral vein. Symptoms include tenderness, pain, swelling, warmth, and discoloration of the skin. It is potentially life-threatening.

de-escalation   A communication strategy involving the reduction of anxious and/or agitated behaviors exhibited verbally or nonverbally by the client; using a calm yet firm approach diffuses the client's increasing anxiety and/or agitated state, thereby minimizing potentially violent outbursts.

defecation   Passage of feces from the digestive tract through the rectum.

dehiscence   The separation or opening of wound layers.

dementia   A term used to describe a group of symptoms related to a loss or impairment of mental powers. These symptoms appear in a person who is awake and are demonstrated by symptoms of mental confusion, memory loss, disorientation, intellectual impairment, or similar problems.

dental caries   Chalky white discoloration of teeth or presence of brown or black discoloration.

dentifrice   A pharmaceutical compound used with a toothbrush for cleaning and polishing teeth.

dermatitis   An inflammatory condition of the skin characterized by erythema and pain or pruritus.

dermatological   Pertaining to the skin.

detection and surveillance   Awareness of the environment, recognizing what might be unusual or different, and knowing what these differences mean in terms of terrorism preparedness.

devitalized   Tissues with reduced oxygen supply and blood flow.

dialysis   A procedure that removes fluid and solid wastes from the blood or lymph.

diaphoresis   Secretion of sweat typically associated with hyperthermia, physical exertion, and emotional stress.

diastolic pressure   The lower blood pressure measurement, which reflects the pressure consistently exerted within the arterial system during the period of ventricular relaxation.

diffusion   Movement of oxygen to the red blood cells at the alveolar level.

diluent   Agent that makes a solution or mixture thinner or more liquid by admixture.

disaster   A catastrophic and/or destructive event that disrupts normal functioning; it may include any anticipated or unexpected event whose effects lead to significant destruction and/or adverse consequences.

disaster triage   A model for sorting individuals by the seriousness of their condition and the likelihood of their survival.

discharge planning   The process by which the nurse plans for a client's eventual release from a health care agency; the process begins on a client's admission to the agency.

distraction   A pain-reduction technique that diverts an individual's attention away from the pain sensation.

documentation   Anything written or printed that is relied on as record or proof for authorized persons. It is a vital aspect of nursing practice and is a vital link between the provision and evaluation of health care.

dorsal   Pertaining to the back or posterior.

dorsiflexion   Flexion toward the back, as accomplished by a muscle (e.g., in the hand or foot).

dorsum   The back of the hand.

double-void   A procedure of discarding the first urine specimen and testing the second urine specimen that was obtained 30 to 45 minutes later; this procedure gives amore accurate amount of glucose being spilled into the urine at that particular time.

drawsheet A special sheet placed over the regular sheet on a bed and used to move a person in bed.

drop factor Refers to the calibration of IV tubing (IV infusion set) in drops per milliliter. For example, the drop factor of microdrip IV tubing is 60 gtt/ml.

drug tolerance (see Table 6-1) A decreased physiological response after repeated administration of a drug or a chemically related substance.

duration of action Length of time during which a drug is present in a concentration great enough to produce a therapeutic effect.

dysphagia Difficulty swallowing.

dyspnea Difficulty in breathing.

dysrhythmia An irregular, fast or slow heart rhythm.

dysuria Pain or burning on urination, may also be accompanied with difficulty in urination. Usually indicates an urinary tract infection.

ecchymosis Discoloration of an area of the skin or mucous membrane resulting from extravasation of blood into the subcutaneous tissues as a result of trauma to the underlying blood vessels or of fragility of the vessel walls.

eczema Superficial dermatitis of unknown cause.

edema Abnormal accumulation of fluid in interstitial spaces of tissues.

effleurage A type of massage stroke that glides without manipulating deep muscles, smoothes and extends muscles, increases nutrient absorption, and improves lymphatic and venous circulation.

effluent The drainage that is expected from an ostomy.

egophony A change in the voice sound as heard on auscultation of a client with pleural effusion. When client is asked to make e-e-e sounds, the sound is heard over the peripheral chest wall as a-a-a.

elastic bandage Bandage of elasticized fabric that provides support and allows movement.

electrolyte An element or compound that, when melted or dissolved in water or another solvent, dissociates into ions and is able to carry an electric current.

electronic infusion device (EID) Used to infuse IV fluid at a prescribed rate. There are two types: an infusion pump, which is designed to deliver a measured amount of fluid over a period of time, and an IV controller, which delivers fluid with the aid of gravity.

embolus (emboli) A foreign object, a quantity of air or gas, a bit of tissue or tumor, or a piece of thrombus that circulates in the bloodstream until it becomes lodged in a vessel.

emergency responders Those individuals whose job it is to respond to an emergency situation—typically police, fire, hazmat, and EMS personnel.

empathy Ability to recognize and to some extent share the emotions and state of mind of another and to understand the meaning and significance of that person's behavior.

end-of-life-care The human provision of physical, psychological, social, and spiritual support to a client and client's family at the end of life.

endotracheal intubation Placement of plastic tube into the trachea to provide artificial ventilations on a continuous basis.

endotracheal tube Artificial airway inserted through the mouth into the trachea.

enema Procedure involving introduction of a solution into the rectum for cleansing or therapeutic purposes.

enteral nutrition The administration of nutrition via the gastrointestinal tract (i.e., by mouth, tube feeding, or oral supplement).

enteral tube feeding The introduction of food or nutritive material directly into the digestive tract by nasogastric or gastric tube.

enteric coated Tablets coated with a substance that does not dissolve until reaching the intestine. Used when drug constituents are irritating to oral and gastric mucosa.

enterostomy Surgical procedure that produces an artificial anus or fistula in the intestine by incision through the abdominal wall.

enucleation Removal of the eyeball, performed in cases of malignancy, severe infection, extensive trauma, or to control pain in glaucoma.

epidemiology Study of the occurrence, distribution, and causes of disease.

epidural Administration of local anesthetic by way of a catheter into the epidural space of the spinal column. Designed to produce anesthesia of the pelvic, abdominal, or genital areas.

epidural blood patch Procedure whereby a physician injects a small amount of autologous blood into the epidural space.

episiotomy A surgical procedure in which an incision is made in a woman's perineum to enlarge her vaginal opening for delivery of an infant; procedure prevents tearing of perineum.

epithelialization The process by which epidermal cells migrate (move) over the wound's surface to close the top or "resurface" the wound.

erythema Redness or inflammation of the skin or mucous membranes, result of dilation and congestion of superficial capillaries.

eschar Scab or dry crust that results from excoriation of the skin.

evaporation Mechanism of heat loss whereby moisture from the body's surface changes to vapor and transfers heat to the surrounding air.

eversion Turning outward or inside out, such as turning the foot outward at the ankle.

evidence-based practice Recommended nursing interventions that have been shown to be effective when tested in clinical research.

evisceration The separation of wound layers with the protrusion of abdominal organs through the wound layers.

excoriation An injury to the surface of the skin or other part of the body caused by scratching or abrasion.

excretion   The process of eliminating, shedding, or getting rid of substances by body organs or tissues.

exercise   Performance of any physical activity for the purpose of conditioning the body, improving health, maintaining fitness, or as a therapeutic measure.

exit site   Point at which a catheter leaves a body site.

exophthalmos   Abnormal protrusion of one or both eyeballs caused by trauma, intracranial lesions, intraorbital disorders, or systemic disease, most commonly hyperthyroidism.

expectorant   An agent that facilitates removal of bronchopulmonary secretions.

expectorate   The act of coughing and spitting out mucus from the respiratory tract. Maneuver is useful in assisting a client with clearing the airways of pulmonary secretions.

extended wear contact lens   Type of contact lens to be worn continuously for up to a week or even a month depending on the model.

extension   Movement increasing the angle between two adjoining bones.

external fixation   Skeletal traction applied through the use of pins attached to a frame rather than weights.

external rotation   Rotation of a joint outward.

external urethral sphincter   Voluntary muscle that must relax in order for the client to void or completely empty the bladder.

extravasation   The inadvertent infiltration of intravenous fluids or medications into the subcutaneous tissues surrounding the infusion site.

extremity restraints   Restraints used to immobilize one or all extremities.

exudate   Any fluid that has been extruded from a tissue or its capillaries, more specifically because of injury or inflammation. It is characteristically high in protein and white blood cells.

Fahrenheit   Temperature scale in which 32 degrees is the freezing point of water and 212 degrees is the boiling point of water at sea level.

fascia   Fibrous connective tissue.

febrile   Pertaining to or characterized by fever or an elevation in body temperature.

fenestrated drape   A drape with a round or slitlike opening in the center.

fenestrated tracheostomy tube   A tracheostomy tube containing a hole (fenestration) on the posterior aspect of the outer cannula that allows airflow over the vocal cords and speech in spontaneously breathing clients.

fenestration   Surgical procedure in which an opening is created to gain access to the cavity within an organ or a bone.

fever   An abnormal elevation of body temperature.

fiberoptic   Pertaining to fiberoptics; referring to the transmission of an image along flexible bundles of coated glass or plastic fibers having special optical properties.

first responders   Those public service providers required to be the first on the scene of a disaster, typically EMS, fire, or police personnel.

flexion   Movement decreasing the angle between two adjoining bones; bending of a limb.

floor stock   A term applied to medications that are distributed by the pharmacy to the nursing unit in bulk. Generally, floor stock medications are ones that are commonly used and are often obtainable as over-the-counter preparations. Examples include Tylenol, Milk of Magnesia, antacids, and stool softeners.

flora   Microorganisms that reside on and within the body to compete with disease-producing microorganisms to provide a natural immunity against certain infections.

flossing   Mechanical cleansing of tooth surfaces with the use of stringlike waxed or unwaxed dental floss.

flotation device   A foam mattress with a gel-like pad located in its center, designed to protect bony prominences and distribute pressure more evenly against the skin's surface.

flotation pad   A device constructed of foam or a silicone or polyvinal chloride gel encased in a vinyl-covered square, protects bony prominences and distributes pressure more evenly against the skin's surface.

flow sheet   A recording form used to document the same type of repeated measurements, procedures, or observations over time. Data on flow sheets allow the user to see trends over time.

fluid volume deficit (FVD)   An alteration characterized by the loss of fluids and electrolytes in an isotonic fashion.

fluid volume excess (FVE)   An alteration characterized by the abnormal retention of fluids and electrolytes in an isotonic fashion.

focus charting   A charting methodology for structuring progress notes according to the focus of the note, for example, symptoms and nursing diagnosis. Each note includes data, action, and client response.

fontanel   A space covered by tough membranes between the bones of an infant's cranium.

footboard   Board placed perpendicular to the mattress, parallel to and touching the plantar surface of the client's feet and used to maintain dorsiflexion of the feet.

footdrop   A falling or dragging of the foot from paralysis of the flexors of the ankle.

foramen magnum   The large opening in the anterior and inferior part of the occipital bone, interconnecting the vertebral canal and cranial cavity.

four-poster cast   Cast placed over the shoulders; contains four vertical posts or poles on the anterior and posterior lateral sides of the head to immobilize the cervical vertebrae.

Fowler's position   Posture assumed by a client when the head of the bed is raised approximately 45 to 90 degrees, as though the client is sitting upright.

fracture pan   A bedpan designed for clients with body or leg casts or clients restricted from raising their hips. It has a shallow upper end that slips easily under a client.

frequency   Symptom of urinary disorder involving repetitive voidings over a fixed time period.

friction   Effect of rubbing, or the resistance that a moving body meets from the surface on which it moves; a force that occurs in a direction to oppose movement; in massage, technique in which deeper tissues are stroked or rubbed, usually through strong circular movements of the hand.

friction rub Dry grating sound heard during auscultation, caused by rubbing of tissue surfaces.

gag reflex A normal neural reflex elicited by touching the soft palate or posterior pharynx, the response being the elevation of the palate, retraction of the tongue, and contraction of the pharyngeal muscles. Tests for function of the vagus and glossopharyngeal nerves.

gait Manner or style of walking, including rhythm, cadence, and speed.

gait belt A leather or heavy canvas belt that encircles the client's waist, it may or may not have handles. The purpose of the belt is for the nurse to hold when ambulating the unsteady client, to reduce risk of fall.

gastrostomy feeding tube Long, hollow, flexible tube inserted into the stomach through a stab wound in the upper left abdominal quadrant.

gingivae The gums of the mouth.

gingivitis Inflammatory condition in which the gums are red, swollen, and bleeding.

glaucoma An abnormal condition of elevated pressure within the anterior chamber of an eye that occurs as a result of the obstruction of outflow of aqueous humor.

glomerular filtration rate (GFR) A kidney function test that determines the amount of ultrafiltrate formed by plasma flowing through the glomeruli or the kidney. It may be calculated from insulin and creatinine and blood urea nitrogen.

glucose monitoring A diagnostic test to determine the blood glucose level.

granulation The presence of red, granular, moist tissue that appears during the healing of open wounds; type of tissue containing new blood vessels that bleed readily.

granulation tissue Soft, pink, fleshy projection of tissue that forms during the healing process in a wound not healing by primary intention.

graphical user interface Program interfaces, such as touch pads, mouse, and icons, that make computer programs easier to use.

gravity The heaviness or weight of an object resulting from the effect of the attraction between any body of matter and any planetary body.

guaiac test Diagnostic test to detect blood in the stool.

guided imagery Technique in which client focuses on an image, becoming less aware of pain.

gurgle Abnormal coarse sound heard during auscultation of the lung; produced by air entering large mucus-containing airways.

halitosis Offensive breath resulting from poor oral hygiene, dental or oral infections, ingestion of certain foods, or systemic diseases.

hand rolls Cylindrical rolls of cloth or gauze placed against the palmar surface of a client's hand to maintain hand, thumb, and fingers in a functional position.

Harris splint Expandable splint that supports the thigh in skeletal traction.

hazard/hazard identification A condition or phenomenon that increases the probability of a loss that may result in injury or illness/recognition of conditions or agents creating risk.

healing ridge Induration of collagen deposits beneath the skin extending to about 1 cm on each side of the wound.

Health Insurance Portability and Accountability Act (HIPAA) A federal law designed to protect the privacy of client health information.

heatstroke Condition characterized by core body temperature of 47° C (113° F).

heave A lift or thrust felt during palpation of the heart.

hematemesis Vomiting of blood.

hematology The study of blood cells.

hematoma Collection of extravasated blood trapped in the tissues of the skin or in an organ; results from trauma or incomplete coagulation.

hematopoiesis The formation and development of blood cells in bone marrow.

hematuria Abnormal presence of blood in the urine.

hemiparesis Muscular weakness of one half of the body.

hemiplegia Paralysis of one side of the body.

hemoconcentration The concentration of red blood cells in one area.

hemodialysis A procedure in which impurities or wastes are removed from the blood; used in treating renal insufficiency and various toxic conditions.

hemodynamics The study of movements of the blood and of the forces concerned therein.

hemolysis The destruction of red blood cells.

hemopneumothorax An accumulation of both air and blood in the intrapleural space. This condition is characterized by the signs and symptoms listed with pneumothorax and hemothorax.

hemoptysis Coughing up of blood from the respiratory tract.

hemorrhoids A varicosity in the lower rectum or anus caused by congestion in the hemorrhoidal veins.

hemostasis Termination of bleeding by mechanical or chemical means or by the coagulation process of the body.

hemothorax An accumulation of blood in the intrapleural space caused by a pulmonary infarction, tissue damage that occurs as a result of lung cancer or other chest trauma, or a complication of anticoagulant therapy after chest surgery.

Hemovac drain A type of closed drain system.

heparin lock An intravenous needle connected to a small "well" that allows for the intermittent injection of medication without the need for repeated venipuncture.

herniation The abnormal protrusion of an organ or other body structure through a defect or natural opening in a covering, membrane, muscle, or bone.

high-Fowler's position Placement of a client in a semisitting position by raising the head of the bed more than 45 to 60 degrees

hirsutism Excessive body hair in a masculine distribution, caused by heredity, hormonal dysfunction, or medication.

Homans' sign In the presence of phlebitis or when phlebitis is suspected, dorsiflexion of the foot elicits pain in the calf.

homeostasis The state of equilibrium (balance between opposing pressures) in the internal environment of the body, naturally maintained by adaptive responses that promote healthy survival.

hospice A system of family-centered care designed to assist the terminally ill person to be comfortable and to maintain a satisfactory lifestyle through the phase of dying.

Hoyer lift (mechanical/hydraulic lift) Mechanical device that uses a canvas sling to easily lift dependent clients for transferring.

Huber needle Special needle with a deflected point designed to prevent damage to the silicone septum of implanted infusion ports.

humectant A substance that promotes retention of moisture.

hydrocolloid An adhesive, moldable wafer made of a carbohydrate-based material, usually with a waterproof backing. This dressing usually is impermeable to oxygen, water, and water vapor and has some absorptive properties.

hydrogel A water-based, nonadherent, polymer-based dressing that has some absorptive properties.

hygiene The science of health. Self-care measures people use to maintain their health are called personal hygiene.

hypercalcemia Greater than normal amounts of calcium in the blood.

hypercapnia Elevated arterial pCO_2 greater than 45 mm Hg, also called hypercarbia.

hyperemia Increased blood flow in part of the body, as in the inflammatory response, local relaxation of arterioles, or obstruction of the outflow of blood from an area.

hyperextension Movement of a body part beyond its normal resting extended position.

hyperkalemia Refers to solutions with potassium concentrations greater than 5.0 mEq/L.

hypermagnesemia Refers to solutions with magnesium concentrations greater than 2.5 mEq/L.

hypernatremia Refers to solutions with sodium concentrations greater than 147 mEq/L.

hyperopia A refractive error of the eye in which parallel rays of light focus behind the retina; causes difficulty seeing near objects.

hyperphosphatemia Refers to a higher than normal range of serum phosphorus. Normal range for serum phosphorus is 2.5 to 4.5 mg/100 ml (1.7 to 2.6 mEq/L).

hyperpigmentation Unusual darkening of the skin.

hypertension Condition characterized by an elevated blood pressure persistently exceeding 150/90 mm Hg.

hyperthermia Condition characterized by body temperature over 38° C (100.4° F).

hypertonic Having a greater concentration of solute than another solution, hence exerting more osmotic pressure: a total electrolyte content of 375 mEq/L or greater.

hypodermoclysis The injection of an isotonic or hypotonic solution into subcutaneous tissue to supply a continuous and large amount of fluid, electrolytes, and nutrients.

hypokalemia Refers to solutions with potassium concentrations less than 3.5 mEq/L.

hypomagnesemia Refers to solutions with magnesium concentrations less than 1.5 mEq/L.

hyponatremia Refers to solutions with sodium concentrations less than 137 mEq/L.

hypoosmolar State in which there is an abnormal gain in water or loss of sodium-rich fluids with replacement by water only. As a result, there is a low concentration of solutes in the body fluids.

hypophosphatemia Refers to a lower than normal range of serum phosphorus. Normal range of serum phosphorus is 2.5 to 4.5 mg/100 ml (1.7 to 2.6 mEq/L).

hypotension Condition characterized by a low blood pressure that is inadequate to perfuse and oxygenate body tissue.

hypothermia Condition characterized by body temperature below 36° C (96.8° F).

hypothermia therapy Techniques used to reduce elevated body temperature.

hypotonic Having a smaller concentration of solute than another solution, hence exerting less osmotic pressure.

hypovolemic shock State of physical collapse caused by massive blood loss, circulatory dysfunction, and inadequate tissue perfusion.

hypoxemia Abnormal deficiency of oxygen in arterial blood.

hypoxia Insufficient oxygen available to meet the metabolic needs of tissues and cells.

idiosyncratic reaction A response to a medication or therapy that is unique to an individual.

ileal conduit A method of urinary diversion through intestinal tissue. Ureters are implanted in a section of dissected ileum that is then sewed to an ostomy in the abdominal wall.

ileostomy Surgical formation of an opening of the ileum onto the surface of the abdomen, through which fecal matter is emptied.

immobility Pertaining to the inability of a body part or limb to be moved.

immunocompromised A state of defective or failed immune response that makes a person more likely to acquire an infection.

impaction Presence of large or hard fecal mass in the rectum or colon.

implanted infusion port A self-sealing silicone septum encased in a metal or plastic case with an attached silicone catheter threaded into a large vein. Used to administer chemotherapy and other irritating intravenous medications.

incentive spirometer Individual client device used to encourage full lung expansion. Reduces the risk of atelectasis in the immobilized or postoperative client.

incentive spirometry Method of deep breathing providing visual feedback to clients concerning their inspiratory volume.

incident report Confidential document that describes any client accident while the person is on the premises of a health care agency.

incompatibility Describes two medications of different chemical makeup that cannot be mixed together.

incontinence Inability to control urination or defecation.

incontinent diversion A urinary diversion that does not give the client the ability to control when urine exits the stoma, requiring the use of an external ostomy pouch.

incubation period Period between exposure to a pathogenic organism and the appearance of symptoms. The client is often contagious during this time and capable of spreading disease without realizing it.

induration Hardening of a tissue, particularly the skin.

infection The invasion and reproduction of microorganisms in a body tissue that can result in a local or systemic clinical response such as cellulitis or fever.

infiltration Presence of intravenous fluids within the subcutaneous space surrounding a venipuncture site.

informed consent Permission obtained from a client to perform a specific test or procedure.

infusate Volume of parenteral fluid infused into a client over an established period of time.

infusion Introduction of a fluid such as a drug, electrolyte, or nutrient directly into a vein by means of gravity flow.

infusion pump Device designed to deliver a measured amount of fluid over a period of time.

injection Act of forcing a liquid into the body by means of a syringe.

injection cap A rubber diaphragm covering a plastic cap. Permits needle insertion into a catheter or vial.

inspection A physical examination skill involving the examiner's looking at external and internal body parts for physical characteristics.

insulator A substance that conducts temperatures poorly used to protect skin and tissues from hot or cold therapies.

intake Measurement of the ingestion or infusion of liquids into the body, including all liquids and semiliquids, liquid medications, enteral tube feedings, intravenous therapy, blood components, and parenteral nutrition.

intake and output record Measuring and recording of all liquid intake and output over a 24-hour period of time.

integument Skin and its appendages: hair, nails, and sweat and sebaceous glands.

intercostal space (ICS) Space found between adjoining ribs.

internal rotation Rotation of a joint inward.

interviewing The process of conducting an organized, systematic conversation with a client. Designed to gather information regarding a client's level of health, response to care, or perception of symptoms or events.

intestinal obstruction Any obstruction that results in failure of the contents of the intestine to pass through the lumen of the bowel.

intraabdominal pressure Amount of tension within the abdominal cavity.

intracavitary Within a body cavity.

intracellular fluid Liquid within the cell membrane.

intraclavicular fossa Small pocket area or indentation just below the clavicle on both sides of the neck.

intracranial pressure Pressure exerted by cerebrospinal fluid within the subarachnoid space surrounding the brain and spinal cord.

intradermal (ID) injection Form of injection in which a solution is introduced into the dermal skin layer.

intramuscular (IM) injection Form of injection in which a solution is introduced into the body of a muscle.

intrapleural Pertaining to, or affecting, the potential space between the parietal and visceral pleurae.

intrapulmonic Pertaining to, or affecting, the spaces within the lungs.

intraspinal Referring to both the epidural and intrathecal routes of medication administration.

intrathecal Of or pertaining to a structure, process, or substance within a sheath, as within the spinal canal.

intravenous conscious sedation (IVCS) The intravenous administration of pharmacological agents to provide a minimally depressed level of consciousness to provide comfort during diagnostic or treatment procedures.

intravenous (IV) injection Form of injection in which a solution is introduced into a vein.

introitus An entrance or orifice into a cavity.

intubation Passage of a tube into a body aperture.

invasive Referring to procedures that involve puncture, incision, or insertion of a foreign object into the body.

invasive procedure A procedure in which the normal protective barrier of the skin or mucous membrane is broken or compromised (e.g., an intravenous puncture or a bladder catheterization).

inversion Turning something upside down.

irrigate To flush with a fluid, usually with a slow, steady pressure on a syringe plunger. Done to cleanse a wound or clear tubing.

irrigation Gentle washing of an area with a stream of solution.

ischemia A decreased supply of oxygenated blood to a body organ or part.

isolation Infection control and prevention methods such as barrier technique that are used to decrease the transmission of microorganisms.

isometric contraction Increased muscle tension without muscle shortening.

isometric exercise The tightening or tensing of muscles without moving body parts.

isotonic A solution with a total electrolyte content of approximately 310 mEq/L.

isotonic solution   Having the same concentration of solute as another solution, hence exerting the same amount of osmotic pressure as the solution.

IV plug   A small rubber or plastic cap that connects to the open end of a client's IV access catheter. Also referred to as injection cap because a needle can be inserted into the rubber cap for the administration or aspiration of fluids.

jacket restraints   Vestlike restraints that usually cross in the back of the client but may also cross in the front.

Jackson-Pratt drain   A closed drain system.

jejunostomy feeding tube   A hollow tube inserted into the jejunum through the abdominal wall for administration of liquefied foods.

joint   Any one of the connections between bones.

Joint Commission on Accreditation of Healthcare Organizations (JCAHO)   A private, nongovernmental agency that establishes guidelines for the operation of health care facilities. The guidelines are the basis of accreditation, generally required for Medicare reimbursement.

karaya   A natural gum product that softens with body heat and conforms to the contours around the stoma.

Kardex   Trade name for card filing system that allows quick reference to the particular need of the client for certain aspects of nursing care.

keloid   An overgrowth of scar tissue at the site of skin injury, such as a wound or surgical incision.

ketones   An organic chemical compound with two compounds attached to it.

kilogram   The metric conversion for a pound; weight (pounds) $\div$ 2.2 = kilograms.

kinesthetic   Related to the ability to perceive the existence or direction of weight or movement.

laryngospasm   Spasm of the muscles surrounding the larynx causing airway narrowing and stridorous breathing.

lateral flexion   A range of joint motion exercise during which the head is tilted as far as possible toward each shoulder, maintains neck mobility.

latex allergy reaction   Allergic response to products containing latex (e.g., gloves, medical devices). Can present as contact dermatitis, allergic rhinitis, or immediate life-threatening reactions leading to urticaria, bronchospasm, edema, etc.

lavage   The irrigation or washing out of an organ or cavity.

let-down reflex   A normal reflex in a lactating woman often elicited by tactile stimulation of the nipple, resulting in release of milk from the glands of the breast.

leukopenia   A decrease in circulating white blood cells.

leverage   Occurs when specific bones, such as the humerus, ulna, and radius, and the associated joints, such as the elbow joint, act together as a lever.

line of gravity   An imaginary line that goes from the center of gravity to the base of support.

lipid emulsion   A soybean oil.

lipodystrophy   Any abnormality in metabolism and deposition of fat.

logrolling   Maneuver used to turn a reclining client from one side to the other or completely over without flexing the spinal column.

loss   Absence of a significant other, object, or state of health to which the person must adapt through the grieving process.

lotion   Liquid preparation applied externally to protect the skin or treat a dermatological disorder.

lumen   The hollow channel within a tube.

lunula   A semilunar structure, such as the crescent-shaped pale area at the base of the nail of a finger or toe.

macerate   To soften, usually by soaking in water.

maceration   Skin that becomes abnormally soft and breaks down because of prolonged exposure to moisture.

maculopapular   Discolored elevated lesions on the skin.

malabsorption   Impaired absorption of nutrients from the GI tract.

malignant hyperthermia   An autosomal dominant trait characterized by often fatal hyperthermia with rigidity of the muscles occuring in affected people exposed to certain anesthetic agents.

malnutrition   Any disorder of nutrition.

manmade disaster   A catastrophic event whose principle direct cause is attributable to human action.

manometer   An instrument for measuring pressure or tension of liquids or gases.

manual defibrillator   Device used by trained personnel to treat fast, irregular dysrhythmias with electrical shock to the heart.

mass casualty disaster/event/incident (MCI)   Any event or situation that results in multiple casualties and/or deaths; an MCI exists when health care needs exceed health care resources.

mass casualty triage   *M*ove, *A*ssess, *S*ort, and *S*end (MASS) approach to triage initially sorts victims into groups, which are then evaluated for transportation to treatment.

massage   A form of cutaneous stimulation that involves the application of touch and movement to muscles, tendons, and ligaments.

mastication   Chewing, tearing, or grinding food with the teeth while it mixes with saliva.

maturational loss   A loss expressed as any change in a person's developmental process that is normally expected during a lifetime.

meatus   Any opening or tunnel through any part of the body (e.g., the point at which the urethra opens to the skin).

mediastinal shift   A condition in which the mediastinal contents move toward the unaffected side in the presence of a pneumothorax, hemothorax, or hemopneumothorax. The mediastinal shift causes compression of the organs and is a life-threatening situation.

medical asepsis   The techniques used to reduce and prevent the spread of microorganisms (clean technique).

medical disaster A catastrophic event that results in human casualties that overwhelm the available health care resources.

medicated enema Administration of a medication via an enema. Usually used preoperatively with clients scheduled for bowel surgery.

medication dependence Two types of medication dependence exist: psychological (or addiction) and physical. In psychological dependence the client desires the medication for some benefit other than the intended effect. The individual believes a desirable effect will result when taking the medication. Physical dependence involves a physiological adaptation to a medication that manifests itself by intense physical disturbance when the medication is withdrawn.

medication plateau Blood serum concentration reached and maintained after repeated, fixed doses.

medication polymorphism The exhibition of a variation in response to a medication by an individual client; may be caused by environmental or cultural factors.

medication tolerance Decreased physiological response after repeated administration of a medication or a chemically related substance.

medullary Of or pertaining to the medulla of the brain.

megakaryocyte Precursor of platelets found in blood marrow.

melanin Black or dark brown pigment that occurs naturally in the skin, hair, and iris.

melanocyte A body cell capable of producing melanin, the pigment of the skin.

melena Darkening of the feces by blood pigments.

metastasis Process by which tumor cells are spread to distant parts of the body.

metered-dose inhaler (MDI) A device designed to deliver a measured dose of an inhalation drug.

microorganisms Any microscopic entity capable of sustaining living processes, such as bacteria, virus, fungi, only some of which typically cause human disease.

microvasculature The portion of the circulatory system composed of the capillary network.

micturition Urination; act of passing or expelling urine voluntarily through the urethra.

midarm circumference (MAC) A measurement of the circumference of the upper arm used to estimate muscle mass.

midstream collection Procedure in which the client initiates a stream of urine, inserts a sterile collection cup into the stream, and then withdraws the cup before the stream of urine stops.

milliequivalent per liter (mEq/L) Number of grams of a specific electrolyte dissolved in 1 L of plasma.

Minerva jacket Cast encasing the head (with face and ears exposed), continuing over the thorax and back to the iliac crests.

minimal sedation Lightest level of sedation; includes local and topical anesthetics and peripheral nerve blocks.

mitten restraints Thumbless mitten devices used to restrain a client's hands.

mobility The amount and quality of physical activity.

moderate sedation A drug-induced depression of consciousness during which clients respond purposefully to verbal commands, either alone or accompanied by light tactile stimulation.

Modified Ramsey Sedation Scale A numeric rating scale used to evaluate clent's level of sedation.

moleskin Adhesive-backed tape used for some forms of skin traction.

morgue A unit of a hospital with facilities for the storage and autopsy of the dead.

mucociliary transport Process in which cilia lining the tracheobronchial tree sweep mucus upward toward the esophagus to keep airways clear of inhaled particulate.

mucopurulent Characteristic of a combination of mucus and pus.

mummy restraints Blanket or sheet folded in such a manner as to restrain a small child or infant.

mutual aid agreement Reciprocal agreement to provide help between two or more agencies.

mydriasis Dilation of the pupil of the eye caused by contraction of dilator muscles of the iris.

mydriatics Ophthalmic preparations that stimulate the sympathetic nerve fibers or block parasympathetic nerve fibers of the eye, temporarily paralyzing the iris sphincter muscle.

myelosuppression A decrease in the cellular components of the bone marrow.

myopia A refractive error of the eye in which parallel rays of light focus in front of the retina; causes difficulty seeing far objects clearly.

nares The pairs of anterior and posterior openings in the nose that allow for passage of air to the pharynx and lungs.

nasal Of or pertaining to the nose and nasal cavity.

nasal cannula A device for delivering oxygen by way of two small, short tubes that are inserted into the nares.

nasogastric (NG) feeding tube A small tube that is passed via the nares into the stomach.

nasointestinal (NI) feeding tube Tungsten-weighted tube inserted through the naris to allow natural peristaltic movement of the tube through the pyloric sphincter into the duodenum or jejunum.

National Dysphagia Diet Released in October 2002, the National Dysphagia Diet provides recommendations for uniformity of dysphagia diets for all health care facilities. Solid and liquid diets are separated into four levels.

natural/environmental disaster A catastrophic event that results from an ecological event that exceeds the capacity of the community.

nebulization Vaporization or dispersion of a liquid in a fine spray.

nebulizer Device used to distribute medication throughout nasal passages and tracheobronchial airway.

necrosis Localized tissue death.

necrotic   Related to death of a portion of tissue.

negative pressure   Pressure, measured in mm Hg, that is less than atmospheric pressure.

negative pressure ventilation   Therapy used for clients with primary neuromuscular illnesses that interfere with normal respiratory muscle function. The client is fitted with a poncho or shell that is connected to the ventilator. Air is removed from between the client's chest wall and the interior wall of the poncho or shell, causing the client to inhale.

negligence   Omission of care.

neovascular assessment   Series of eight observations required to measure neurological and circulatory status of a client's peripheral tissue.

neovascularization   The process by which the vascular network in a wound is generated. This can also be called angiogenesis.

neurological   Pertaining to the study and treatment of the nervous system.

neuropathy   An abnormal condition characterized by inflammation and degeneration of the peripheral nerves.

neurovascular assessment   Series of eight observations (assessments) required to measure neurological and circulatory status of a client's peripheral tissues.

neutropenia   An abnormal decrease in the number of neutrophils in the blood.

neutropenic   Having an abnormal decrease in the number of neutrophils, white blood cells, in the blood.

nitroglycerin   Medication that causes dilation of coronary arteries.

noncontinent (incontinent) ostomy/diversion   Results from a surgical procedure that leaves the client with an external stoma through which either stool or urine drains. It is noncontinent/incontinent because the effluent drains spontaneously from the stoma and the client must continuously wear an external ostomy pouch over the stoma.

noncoring Huber needle   A specially designed needle (straight or a 90-degree needle) intended for use with a vascular access device. This needle permits penetration into the chamber of the vascular access device without causing damage and thus permits repeated administration of medication directly into the client's bloodstream.

noninvasive ventilation (NIV)   Noninvasive ventilation (NIV) maintains positive airway pressure and improves alveolar ventilation without the need for an artificial airway. In addition, this mechanical ventilator alternative reduces and reverses atelectasis, improves oxygenation, reduces pulmonary edema, and improves cardiac function.

nonopioids   Analgesics that do not contain opioids.

nonpharmacological aids   Interventions used to prevent illness and promote health without the use of or in addition to the use of medications.

nosocomial (hospital-acquired) infection   An infection that developed during a stay or work in a health care facility and was not present or incubating at the time of admission.

noxious   Harmful, injurious, or detrimental to health.

NPO   Nothing to be taken or given by mouth.

nuclear event   The release of radiation by a device in an explosive manner as a result of a nuclear chain reaction.

nutritional risk   The potential to become malnourished because of factors that are primary (e.g., inadequate intake), or secondary (e.g., disease).

nutritional screening   The systematic process of identifying risk factors related to nutritional problems and malnutrition.

nutritional support nursing   The care of individuals with potential or known nutrition alterations. The goal is to assist individuals to restore and maintain optimal nutritional health

objective data   Data obtained by an observer (nurse) through direct physical examination, including observation, palpation, and auscultation, and by laboratory analyses and radiological and other studies.

obstipation   The absolute inability to pass stool.

obturator   Small dull-pointed introducer inserted in outer cannula that facilitates insertion of tracheostomy tube by gradually widening or dilating stoma to width of tracheostomy tube.

occlusive dressing   A dressing that prevents air from reaching a wound or lesion and retains moisture, heat, body fluids, and medication.

occult blood   Blood that appears from a nonspecific source, with obscure signs and symptoms. May be detected by means of a chemical test or microscopic examination.

ocular   Of or pertaining to the eye.

ocularist   Specialist in the fabrication and care of artificial eyes.

oil-retention enema   An enema containing a small volume of an oil-based solution; used to soften fecal mass.

ointment   A semisolid externally applied preparation, usually containing a drug.

olfaction   The sense of smell.

oncology   A branch of medicine regarding the study of tumors.

onset of medication action   Period of time after a drug is administered for it to produce a response.

opening pressure   The amount of tension measured in a manometer following insertion of a spinal needle into the subarachnoid space.

ophthalmic   Of or pertaining to the eye.

ophthalmologist   A medical doctor whose practice is limited to diseases, conditions, and trauma to the eyes. An ophthalmologist also prescribes corrective lenses for clients whose visual acuity is impaired.

opioids   Pertaining to natural and synthetic chemicals that have opiumlike effects although they are not derived from opium.

opposition   The relation between the thumb and the other digits of the hand for the purpose of grasping objects between the thumb and fingers. This maneuver is used during range-of-joint-motion exercises to maintain grasping ability of the client.

optometrist A person who practices optometry, tests the eyes for visual acuity, prescribes corrective lenses, and recommends eye exercises.

oral airway Minimally flexible curved piece of plastic extending from the exterior of the lips over the tongue to the pharynx.

Organ Procurement Agency (OPA) Community-based agency whose focus is to obtain donated organs for transplantation.

organ/tissue donation Families and significant others are offered the option of organ and/or tissue donation. This process includes, but is not limited to, the donation of heart, lung, kidneys, liver, corneal tissue, and bone.

orientation phase Period in the nurse-client relationship when the nurse and client first meet and set the tone for the rest of their relationship, assessing the client's situation and setting goals.

orifice Entrance or outlet of any cavity in the body.

orthopedics Branch of medicine devoted to the study and treatment of the skeletal system, its joints, muscles, and associated structures.

orthopnea An abnormal condition in which a person must sit or stand to breathe deeply or comfortably.

orthostatic hypotension A drop in blood pressure of 15 mm Hg or more when an individual rises from a sitting to a standing position.

osteoblastic Physiological activity that leads to the formation of specific bone tissue, osteoblasts.

osteoblasts Osteoblasts synthesize the collagen and glycoproteins to form the matrix for bone formation.

osteoclastic Physiological activity producing osteoclast bone cells that function in the development and periods of bone growth and repair, such as the breakdown and resorption of osseous tissue.

ostomy A surgical procedure where the elimination of stool or urine is re-routed from the usual exiting part of the client. Instead, the stool or urine exits the body through a surgically created opening called a stoma.

otic Of or pertaining to the ear.

otitis media Inflammation or infection of the middle ear, a common childhood affliction.

ototoxic Having a harmful effect on the eighth cranial nerve or the organs of hearing and balance.

outer cannula Main portion of tracheostomy tube through which client breathes that stays in place at all times. The pilot balloon and faceplate are connected to the outer cannula.

output Includes all liquids excreted, such as urine, vomitus, and diarrhea, and drainage from wounds, fistulas, and suction equipment.

overdose Oral or parenteral ingestion of an excessive quantity of a medication or drug.

over-the-counter medication (OTC) Drug available to a consumer without a prescription.

over-the-needle catheter (ONC) A type of angiocatheter. The needle used for peripheral IV access is encased in a catheter made of Teflon, plastic, or another flexible material. After the needle pierces the skin, the catheter is threaded into a vein and the needle is withdrawn. The catheter remains in the vein for the instillation of fluid.

oximetry Procedure used to measure amount of oxygenated hemoglobin.

oxygen mask A flexible mask that fits snugly and securely over the client's nose and mouth for delivery of oxygen.

oxygen saturation Amount of hemoglobin that is fully saturated with oxygen expressed as percent of total available hemoglobin.

oxygen therapy Administration of oxygen by any route to a client, to prevent or relieve hypoxia.

oxygen toxicity Administration of oxygen level greater than 50% for greater than 24 hours resulting in increased permeability of the alveolar wall, alveolar-capillary leakage, noncardiogenic pulmonary edema, decreased lung compliance, and respiratory failure

pain Subjective, unpleasant sensation caused by noxious stimulation of sensory nerve endings.

pain intensity The degree or extent of pain perceived by an individual.

pain rating scales Graphic or numeric representations that allow clients to quantify their pain experience.

pain threshold The amount of pain stimulus required to produce a physical or psychological response.

pain tolerance Point at which a person is not willing to accept pain of greater severity or duration.

palliative care The prevention, relief, reduction or soothing of symptoms of disease or disorders without effecting a cure.

pallor Unnatural paleness or absence of color in the skin.

palpation A technique used in physical examination in which the examiner feels the texture, size, consistency, and location of certain parts of the body with the hands.

palpebra Portion of the conjunctiva that lines the inner surface of the eyelids; it is thick, opaque, and highly vascular.

paralysis An abnormal condition characterized by loss of muscle function or the loss of sensation.

paralytic ileus A decrease in or absence of intestinal peristalsis that may occur after abdominal surgery, illness, or trauma.

paraphrasing Transforming the client's words into the nurse's words, keeping the meaning intact.

parenteral Not in or through the digestive system.

parenteral nutrition (PN) The administration of nutrition into the vascular system.

paresis Slight or partial paralysis related in some cases to local neuritis.

parietal pleura The pleural membrane that lines the thoracic cavity.

passive range-of-motion exercises Exercises of the joints performed for an individual by someone else.

patency Absence of obstruction such as clots within an intravenous needle or kinks within intravenous tubing; the state of being open and unblocked.

pathogen Microorganism capable of producing disease.

pathogenic microorganisms Those capable of producing an infection or disease.

patient care profile (PCP) A report that is automatically updated each shift within a computerized medical record.

Patient Self-Determination Act Legislation that requires all Medicare and Medicaid recipient hospitals to provide clients with information on advance directives and their right to accept or reject medical treatment.

patient-controlled analgesia Technique that allows clients to self-administer small, continuous doses of IV or subcutaneous opioids as they feel the need.

A Patient's Bill of Rights A list of patient's rights promulgated by the American Hospital Association; it offers some guidance and protection to clients by stating the responsibilities that a hospital and its staff have toward clients and families during hospitalization; it is not a legally binding document.

peak action Time it takes for a drug to reach its highest effective concentration.

peak airway pressure The highest amount of positive pressure needed to inflate the lung.

peak concentration The highest effective concentration of a drug in the serum.

Pearson attachment The support used under the leg in balanced-suspension skeletal traction.

pediculosis Infestation of the integument with blood-sucking lice.

PEH Acronym for "pseudoepitheliomatous hyperplasia"; maceration of skin surrounding the stoma.

pelvic belt Girdle-shaped cotton belt or support that fits around the hips, lumbosacral area, and abdomen for attaching ropes and weights in pelvic belt traction.

pelvic sling A hammocklike sling that fits under the client's lumbosacral area and hips and is then connected to ropes and weights; it suspends the pelvis off the bed as treatment for fractures of pelvic bones.

Penrose drain An open drain system.

perceived loss Any loss that is tangible and uniquely defined by the grieving client. It may be less obvious to others.

percussion A technique in physical examination used to assess the size, borders, and consistency of some of the internal organs and to discover the presence and to evaluate the amount of fluid in a cavity of the body.

percutaneous Performed through the skin, such as a biopsy or the aspiration of fluid from a space below the skin using a needle, catheter, and syringe.

percutaneous coronary intervention Procedures such as percutaneous transluminal coronary angioplasty (PTCA) or directional coronary atherectomy (DCA) performed during cardiac catheterization.

perfusion Effect of pulmonary circulation in moving blood to and from the blood-gas barrier so gas exchange can occur.

periodontal Referring to tissues surrounding the teeth, such as the gums and buccal mucosa.

periodontitis Receding gum lines, inflammation, gaps between teeth.

perioperative Related to the entire surgical experience.

peripherally inserted central catheter (PICC) A peripherally inserted catheter that extends to the superior vena cava or right atrium.

peristalsis The coordinated, rhythmical, serial contraction of smooth muscle that forces food through the digestive tract.

peristomal Referring to the area of skin surrounding a surgically created stoma.

peritoneal fluid Substance in the abdominal cavity for lubrication of peritoneal membrane and internal organs.

peritonitis Inflammation of peritoneum produced by bacteria or irritating substances introduced into the abdominal cavity by a penetrating wound or perforation of an organ in the gastrointestinal or reproductive tract.

PERRLA Acronym for "pupils equal, round, reactive to light, and accommodation"; the acronym is recorded in the physical examination if pupil assessment is normal.

petaling Finishing the raw or ragged edges of a plaster cast to prevent skin irritation or pressure.

pétrissage A massage technique in which the skin is gently lifted and squeezed.

pH Reflection of the hydrogen ion concentration of a liquid.

pharmacological agents Oral, parenteral, or topical substances used to alleviate symptoms and treat or control illness.

pharynx The throat.

phlebitis Inflammation of a vein.

phlebitis solution A hypertonic solution capable of causing inflammation of a vein.

phlebothrombosis Blood clot formation.

phlebotomy The incision of a vein for the letting of blood, as in collecting blood from a donor.

physical dependence A physiological state in which abrupt cessation of a drug results in a withdrawal syndrome.

physical restraint Any device, garment, material, or object that restricts a person's freedom of movement or access to one's body.

PIE An acronym for "problem, intervention, and evaluation," used as an organizing framework for narrative nurses' notes.

piggyback infusion Method for administering intravenous medications intermittently; a piggyback IV set is a supplementary set that connects with the primary IV tubing.

piloerection Erection of hair due to the action of the arrectores pilorum muscles, the smooth muscles attached to the hair follicles; commonly referred to as goose bumps.

plantar flexion Flexion of the foot and toes toward the sole.

plaque (dental) A thin film on teeth made up of mucin and colloidal material found in saliva and often secondarily invaded by bacteria.

plateau Blood serum concentration reached and maintained after repeated, fixed doses of a drug.

platelet Formed particle found in blood that relates directly to the ability of the blood to clot.

pleura Delicate serous membrane enclosing the lung.

pleural cavity Space between visceral and parietal pleurae; pressure within the cavity is negative when compared with atmospheric pressure.

pleural fluid Substance contained between visceral and parietal pleurae for lubrication of the membranes.

pneumonitis Inflammation of the lung; may be caused by a virus or may be a hypersensitivity reaction that occurs as a result of allergy to chemical or organic dusts.

pneumothorax An accumulation of air in the intrapleural space caused by a severe blow to the chest, extremely forceful cough, chest trauma, or open chest surgery.

podiatrist A health care professional trained to diagnose and treat diseases and disorders of the feet.

point of maximal impulse (PMI) Point at which the heartbeat can most easily be palpated through the chest wall, usually along the left-midclavicular line at the fourth or fifth intercostal space.

polypharmacy Concurrent prescription, administration, or use of multiple medications, some of which may not be indicated clinically.

POMR An acronym for "problem-oriented medical record," used as an organizing framework for a client's complete medical record.

portal hypertension An increased venous pressure in the portal circulation caused by compression or by occlusion at the portal or hepatic vascular system.

positive patient identification A term that means the client is positively identified, usually via at least two identifiers, before the delivery of care.

positive pressure Pressure, measured in mm Hg, that is greater than atmospheric pressure.

positive-pressure ventilation Mechanical ventilation that delivers compressed gas to the airways at greater than ambient pressure.

postanesthesia care unit (PACU) Postsurgical recovery area where clients are closely monitored and stabilized before discharge to a specific nursing unit or in the case of same day surgery, to home.

postcast care Nursing interventions performed for and with clients in casts or after cast removal.

postoperative Period of time after completion of a surgical procedure wherein the nurse monitors the client's recovery.

postmortem care Care provided to the body after death.

postural Position of body, usually refers to change of position from supine to sitting, sitting to standing.

postural drainage Gravitational clearance of airway secretions by assumption of one or more of 10 different body positions for 5 to 15 minutes each; each posture corresponds to specific segments of bronchi in the lung.

postural hypotension Condition in which a normotensive person becomes light-headed or dizzy and experiences low blood pressure when rising to an upright position.

posture Position of the body in relation to the surrounding space.

prealbumin A plasma protein with a half-life of only 2 days, used as a marker of nutritional status.

precordial Of or pertaining to the precordium, which forms the region over the heart and the lower part of the thorax.

preemptive analgesia A method of preventing pain while reducing opioid use.

premature ventricular contraction (PVC) A cardiac dysrhythmia characterized by a ventricular contraction preceding the expected contraction; it appears on an electrocardiogram as an early, wide QRS complex without a preceding P wave.

preoperative The period of time preceding induction of anesthesia and the beginning of a surgical procedure.

preoperative checklist Agency-specific list of guidelines for ensuring completion of nursing interventions. This list includes items to be assessed or verified, for example, verification that preoperative orders are written and completed, laboratory work is in the client's medical record, the client has voided, current vital signs are documented.

presbycusis Loss of hearing sensitivity and speech intelligibility, associated with aging.

presbyopia Farsightedness resulting from a loss of elasticity of the lens of the eye. The condition commonly develops with advancing age.

pressure dressing A temporary treatment for the control of excessive bleeding; pressure dressings require elastic bandages to maintain the pressure and may also require the application of sandbags adjacent to the dressing to augment pressure.

pressure ulcer A lesion that develops in the skin as a result of prolonged, unrelieved pressure.

primary dressing A dressing that comes in direct contact with the wound bed.

primary intention Primary union of the edges of a wound, progressing to complete scar formation with granulation.

prn Abbreviation for *pro re nata,* a Latin phrase meaning "as needed." The times of administration are determined by the needs of the client.

problem-oriented medical record (POMR) Method of recording data about the health status of a client that fosters a collaborative problem-solving approach by all members of the health care team.

procedural sedation An anesthetic procedure in which analgesia and anesthesia are accomplished without loss of consciousness.

pronation Movement of a body part so the front or ventral surface faces downward.

proprioceptive function Sensation that is achieved through stimuli originating from within the body regarding spatial position and muscular activity.

prosthesis An artificial replacement for a missing part of the body.

pruritus The symptom of itching.

Pseudomonas A genus of gram-negative bacteria that includes several free-living species of soil and water and some opportunistic pathogens, isolated from wounds and sputum; may produce blue and yellow pigments.

pseudoaddiction Exhibition of drug-seeking behaviors though the true driving factor is pain relief not physical addiction.

pulleys Mechanical round, grooved disks over which ropes can move freely for traction pull.

pulmonary edema Accumulation of extracellular fluid in a client's lung tissue and alveoli, commonly caused by left-sided heart failure, fluid overload.

pulse deficit Condition characterized by difference between apical pulse rate and peripheral pulse rate that results in a lack of peripheral perfusion.

pyrogen Any substance or agent that tends to cause a rise in body temperature, such as some bacterial toxins.

quality assurance In health care, any evaluation of services provided and of the results achieved as compared with accepted standards.

radial flexion A range-of-motion exercise during which there is a bending of the wrist medially toward the thumb; maintains wrist mobility.

radiopaque Not permitting the passage of x-rays or other radiant energy. Bones are relatively radiopaque and therefore show as white areas on an exposed x-ray film.

random voided specimen A urine specimen obtained at any point of a 24-hour period.

reactive hyperemia The return of blood to an area of tissue upon the release of externally applied pressure.

reagent Chemical used to indicate the presence of a particular substance.

reduction The alignment of fracture fragments through manipulation. Closed reduction is accomplished through manual manipulation and casting or traction.

reflecting A cognitive strategy that involves reappraisal of one's actions to evaluate outcomes. A communication strategy used to clarify what a client is feeling and to affirm that the client's feelings are acceptable.

refractive error Condition in which parallel rays of light are not brought to focus on the retina.

registered dietitian A health care professional who has successfully completed an examination and maintains continuing education requirements in nutritional care for individuals and groups.

registered nurse first assistant (RNFA) A nurse with advanced education who assists the surgeon with surgical procedures, performing a combination of nursing and medical functions.

reinfusion device An apparatus that is placed, usually intraoperatively during orthopedic or vascular procedures, into a space where significant blood loss is anticipated. This device collects the blood, filters it, and is then used to reinfuse that blood intravascularly.

relaxation A cognitive strategy that provides mental and physical pain relief or reduces pain.

reminiscing A form of therapy for older adults that provides a life review. Individual talks about remote memories, expression of related feelings, and recognition of positive experiences, as well as conflicts.

remission The partial or complete disappearance of the clinical and subjective characteristics of a chronic or malignant disease.

renal Pertaining to the kidney.

renal insufficiency Partial kidney failure characterized by less than normal urinary excretion and abnormal urinary laboratory results (e.g., creatinine, blood urea nitrogen level).

resident A client in a long-term or extended care facility.

residual urine The volume of urine in the bladder after a normal voiding.

residual volume The amount of fluid that pools in the stomach or intestine that is able to be aspirated from a gastric or intestinal tube at any given time.

resistive isometric exercise Contracting of muscles while pushing against a stationary object or resisting the movement of an object.

respiratory arrest Cessation of respirations.

respiratory distress Difficulty breathing that may be associated with abnormal blood oxygen or carbon dioxide levels and may require supportive measures to preserve life.

respite care Provision of short-term relief or time off for people providing home care to an ill, disabled, or frail older adult.

restating A communication strategy involving the reiteration of the client's verbal statements and/or questions using similar words; this affirms that the message was acknowledged by the nurse.

restating The process of verbally clarifying information provided by the client or family.

restraint Device used to immobilize a client or an extremity.

reverse Trendelenburg's position Position in which the lower extremities are low and the body and head are elevated on an inclined plane.

right atrial catheter An indwelling intravenous catheter inserted centrally or peripherally and threaded into the superior vena cava or right atrium.

rigidity Condition of hardness, stiffness, or inflexibility.

rigor mortis The rigid stiffening of skeletal and cardiac muscle shortly after death.

risk assessment tool for pressure ulcers Evaluation protocols for assessing the likelihood for the development of pressure ulcers; two such protocols are the Braden scale and the Norton scale, which assess the following five risk factors: physical condition, mental state, activity, mobility, and incontinence.

rooting reflex A normal response in newborns when the cheek is touched or stroked along the side of the mouth to turn the head toward the stimulated side and begin to suck.

rotation A basic range of joint motion allowed by various joints: the rotation of a bone around its central axis, such as shoulder rotation.

Rotokinetic bed A special bed equipped with an automatic turning device that completely immobilizes clients while rotating them from 90 to 270 degrees along a horizontal axis.

S$_1$ Symbol for the first heart sound in the cardiac cycle occurring with ventricular systole; it is associated with the closure of the mitral and tricuspid valves.

S$_2$ Symbol for the second heart sound in the cardiac cycle; it is associated with closure of the aortic and pulmonary valves just before ventricular diastole.

saline lock See heparin lock.

sclerosis Condition characterized by hardening of tissue resulting from any of several causes, including inflammation, the deposit of mineral salts, and infiltration of connective tissue cells.

scrubbed team members Includes the surgeon and scrub nurse or technician and assisting physicians who are scrubbed.

scrub nurse Provides the surgeon with instruments and supplies, which requires strict surgical asepsis. In addition, this nurse along with the circulating nurse disposes of soiled sponges and accounts for sponges, needles, and instruments on the surgical field.

sebaceous gland One of the small glands in the dermis that secretes an oily substance (sebum) on the skin's surface and in the hair.

seborrheic dermatitis A common and chronic, inflammatory skin disease characterized by dry or moist greasy scales and yellow crusts.

sebum Oily secretion of the sebaceous glands of the skin. When combined with sweat, sebum forms a moist, oily, acidic film that is antibacterial and antifungal and protects the skin against drying.

secondary dressing A dressing used to cover or hold primary dressings in place.

secondary intention Wound closure in which the edges are separated, granulation tissue develops to fill the gap, and, finally, epithelium grows in over the granulation, producing a larger scar than results with primary intention.

secretion A product produced by a gland of the body.

seizure A hyperexcitation of neurons in the brain leading to a sudden, violent, involuntary series of muscle contractions that may be paroxysmal and episodic, as in a seizure disorder, or transient and acute, as after a head injury.

seizure precautions Measures that protect the client from injury during a seizure.

self-catheterization The ability of individuals to insert a urinary catheter into their urinary meatus.

semi-Fowler's position Placement of client in an inclined position, with the upper half of the body raised by elevating the head of the bed approximately 30 to 45 degrees.

sensitivity Laboratory test used in conjunction with culture; it measures the response of microorganisms to antibiotics that have been placed on a culture plate.

sepsis Infection, contamination.

serology Branch of medicine dealing with serum and blood products.

shaking Physiotherapy technique in which a concurrent, compressive force is supplied to the chest wall.

sharps container A puncture-proof container that is used for the disposal of any used sharp items such as needles, disposable scissors, and scalpels.

shearing Pressure exerted against the surface and layers of the skin as tissues slide underneath the body as it moves against a surface.

shearing force An applied force or pressure exerted against the surface and layers of the skin as tissues slide in opposite but parallel planes.

sheet wadding Stretchable sheets of cotton padding used to cover skin before a cast is applied.

shelter-in-place To take refuge in a small interior room with no or few windows.

side effect An effect caused by a drug that is different from the therapeutic (desired) action; the effect may be harmless or injurious.

sigmoid colon The part of the large intestine that extends from the descending colon to the rectum.

sign Objective finding perceived by an examiner, such as a fever, rash, abnormal reflex, or abnormal breath sound.

silicone septum Silicone partition that covers the port chamber housed in the metal or plastic body of the implanted infusion port.

situational loss Loss due to any sudden, unpredictable external event.

sitz bath Special bath in which only the hips and buttocks are immersed in fluid.

skin barrier An artificial layer of skin, made of plastic or vinyl-like material, applied to skin before application of tape or ostomy drainage bags. Protects skin from chronic irritation.

sling Device used to support or limit movement, enhance circulation, and prevent edema of the arm, hand, or wrist.

slough Necrotic (dead) tissue in the process of separating from viable portions of the body.

SOAP Acronym for "subjective, objective, assessment, and plan," the four parts of the written account of a client's health problem in a problem-oriented record.

SOAPIE See SOAP—Alternative acronym includes intervention and evaluation.

solute A substance dissolved in a solution.

solute solution   Solutes are dissolved particles and are either electrolytes or nonelectrolytes. Solute solution refers to these particles when they are found in body fluids or plasma (i.e., solution).

solution   A mixture of one or more substances dissolved in another substance.

spasm   Involuntary muscle contraction.

speculum   A retractor used to separate the walls of a cavity (e.g., the vaginal cavity).

sphygmomanometer   Device used for noninvasive measurement of arterial blood pressure consisting of cuff, air bladder, inflation bulb, and gauge to indicate amount of air pressure being exerted.

spica cast   An orthopedic cast applied to immobilize part or all of the trunk of the body and part or all of one or more extremities.

splinting   Supporting the abdominal area to reduce pain caused by coughing or sneezing after surgery.

sponge   Gauze dressing used to absorb blood in a surgical wound.

spore   An inactive but viable state of microorganisms.

spreader bar   A metal bar with curved hoop areas for attaching hooks or pins for traction.

sputum   Lung mucus; normally thin, watery, and white or clear and watery.

standard precautions   Techniques used to reduce the risk of the transmission of blood-borne pathogens or microorganisms present in moist body substances regardless of the client's diagnosis or infection status.

standardized care plan   Documentation that uses the nursing process format in specifying the plan of care for client problems.

staples   Stainless steel wire used to close a surgical wound.

stent   A straw or tubelike device that is placed through the stoma into bowel to keep open the flow of effluent.

sterile   Free from all life forms, including spores.

sterile conscience   One's personal principles and morals that guide one to maintain strict asepsis and sterile techniques at all times.

sterile field   A specified area, such as within a tray or a sterile drape, that is considered free from microorganisms.

sterilization   Process by which microorganisms, including spores, are killed.

stockinette   Stretchable cotton materials of various sizes and widths used immediately over the skin to protect tissues from the irritation of felt or plaster.

stoma   Surgically created opening between a body cavity and the body's surface, such as a colostomy.

stomatitis   Any inflammatory condition of the mouth.

stopcock   A valve that controls the flow of fluid or air through a tube.

strike through   Source of contamination by which moisture permeates a sterile field or barrier.

stroke volume (SV)   The volume of blood ejected from the left ventricle with each ventricular contraction.

subarachnoid space   Situated or occurring between the arachnoid and the pia mater membranes, which cover the brain and spinal cord.

subcutaneous emphysema   The presence of free air or gas in the subcutaneous tissues.

subcutaneous (Sub-Q) injection   Form of injection in which a solution is introduced into subcutaneous tissues.

subcutaneous tunnel   A tunnel under the skin between the exit site of a catheter and the entrance into a body cavity (such as the epidural space) or vein.

subjective data   Data collected from a client.

sublingual   Route for administering a drug beneath the tongue.

suction   The act of sucking up a substance by reducing air pressure over its surface.

suction catheter   Thin plastic or rubber tubing used to remove secretions.

summarization   Reworking a lengthy interaction or discussion into a few brief sentences.

summarizing   A process in which an interviewer organizes and condenses information provided and verifies with the client that the information is correctly interpreted.

summation   Occurs when the combined effect of two drugs produces a result that equals the sum of the individual effects of each drug.

supination   Movement of a body part so the front or ventral surface faces upward.

suppository   A solid form of medication inserted into a body cavity (e.g., the rectum or vagina). The drug is absorbed after it dissolves in the cavity.

surgical asepsis   Practices or techniques designed to render and maintain objects and areas free from pathogenic microorganisms. Also referred to as sterile techniques.

surgical scrub   Process of removing as many microorganisms as possible from the hands and arms by mechanical washing and chemical antisepsis.

suspension   A liquid in which small particles of a solid are dispersed, but not dissolved, and in which the dispersal is maintained by stirring or shaking the mixture.

sympathomimetic   A pharmacological agent that mimics the effects of stimulation of organs and structures by the sympathetic nervous system.

synergistic reaction   An undesired reaction that occurs when one drug potentiates the effect of another.

systemic   Of or pertaining to the whole body rather than to a localized area.

systolic pressure   The higher blood pressure measurement; reflects pressure within the arterial system during the period of ventricular contraction (systole).

T tube   A T-shaped device that is attached to an endotracheal or tracheostomy tube for delivery of humidified air.

tachycardia   An abnormality in heart rate in which the myocardium contracts regularly, but at a rate over 100 beats per minute.

tachypnea   Condition characterized by respiratory rate greater than 20 breaths per minute.

tartar A hard, gritty deposit that collects on the teeth.

technological disaster A catastrophic event in which people, property, community infrastructure, and economic welfare are adversely affected by the disruption of technology (e.g., industrial accidents and unplanned release of nuclear waste).

TENS Transcutaneous electrical nerve stimulation. A mild electrical stimulation that interferes with the transmission of painful stimuli.

tepid Moderately warm to the touch.

termination phase The period in the nurse-client relationship when the nurse and client examine and evaluate their relationship and its goals and results; the time when they deal with the emotional content involved in saying good-bye.

tertiary intention Wound healing that occurs when surgical wounds are not closed immediately, but left open for 3 to5 days to allow edema or infection to diminish.

therapeutic Treatments or interventions implemented to prevent illness and/or promote health.

therapeutic effect The intended or desired physiological response of a medication.

therapeutic silence The use of silence that encourages verbal description and reflection; avoidance of premature verbal communication that may be due to the nurse's anxiety.

thermoregulation Ability to control temperature within acceptable range.

third party payer An insurance plan, HMO, or PPO that reimburses for health care services.

Thomas splint A long splint with a half or full ring at one end; covered with towels and lined with felt or other soft material, it is used to suspend the thigh in skeletal traction.

thrill A fine vibration felt by an examiner's hand on the body of a client over the site of an aneurysm or on the precordium.

thrombocytopenia A decrease in circulating platelets.

thrombophlebitis Inflammation of a vein, often accompanied by formation of a clot.

thrombosis An abnormal vascular condition in which thrombus develops within a blood vessel of the body.

thrombus Accumulation of platelets, fibrin, clotting factors, and the cellular elements of the blood attached to the interior wall of a vein or artery, sometimes occluding the lumen of the vessel.

tidal volume Amount, in milliliters, of air inhaled with each breath. Spontaneous tidal volume is 5 to 10 ml/kg body weight.

tidaling A normal gentle rocking of fluid in a chest tube water-seal system or in the diagnostic indicator of water-less units. Indicates that the system is functioning properly.

timed collection The collection of a substance such as urine or stool for a specific period of time.

tinnitus Ringing heard in one or both ears.

tissue ischemia Decreased blood supply to body tissues.

TLC 1. Abbreviation for total lung capacity. 2. Informal abbreviation for tender loving care.

tolerance A phenomenon by which the body becomes increasingly resistant to a drug or other substance through continued exposure to the substance.

tongue-thrust reflex An immature form of swallowing in which the tongue is projected forward instead of retracted during swallowing.

topical Of or pertaining to a drug or treatment applied to the surface of a body part.

topical agents Pertaining to a drug or treatment applied to the surface part of the body.

tourniquet An item used for the compression of blood vessels.

toxic effects Severe and progressive negative effects of drugs.

tracheobronchial tree Anatomical divisions of the respiratory tract, including the combination of trachea, bifurcations into the right and left mainstem bronchi, and subsequent bifurcations into smaller bronchi and bronchioles.

tracheostomy Opening through the neck into the trachea with an indwelling tube inserted; created surgically to produce an airway.

tracheostomy collar Curved oxygen delivery device with an adjustable neck strap that fits around the tracheostomy.

traction Force or pull applied to limbs, bones, or other tissues to pull the tissues apart, often for realignment.

traction boot A foam rubber boot shaped to fit a forearm or leg, used for a type of skin traction.

transdermal Refers to a form of medication that is applied to the skin's surface and is absorbed across the dermal or outer skin layer.

transfusion reaction Systemic response by the body to the administration of blood incompatible with that of the recipient.

transmission-based precautions Techniques used to prevent the transmission of microorganisms from clients documented or suspected to be infected with highly transmissible pathogens for which additional precautions are needed beyond standard precautions. The three types are airborne, droplet, and contact precautions.

transtracheal oxygen therapy (TTOT) A method of administering oxygen to a client by establishing a low-flow catheter route directly in the trachea.

Trendelenburg's position Position in which the head is low and the body and legs are elevated.

triage Establishing priorities of client care for urgent treatment based on the seriousness of injuries and likelihood for survival; used in an emergency situation to maximize effectiveness of available resources.

trocar A sharp, pointed rod that fits inside a tube; used to pierce the skin and the wall of a cavity or canal in the body to aspirate fluids, to instill a medication or solution, or to guide the placement of a soft catheter.

trough concentration The point at which the lowest amount of drug is detected in the serum.

tuberculosis A chronic granulomatous infection caused by an acid-fast bacillus, Mycobacterium tuberculosis, generally transmitted by the inhalation or ingestion of infected droplets and usually affecting the lungs.

turning sheet Bed sheet folded in half, placed under the client between shoulders and below the hips. Used by health care providers to lift, turn, and position the client.

tympanic Pertaining to a structure that resonates when struck; drumlike.

ulnar flexion A range-of-motion exercise during which there is a lateral bending of the wrist toward the fifth finger; maintains wrist mobility.

undermining Condition of a wound in which the loss of underlying tissues is greater than the loss of the skin.

unit-dose system System of drug distribution in which a portable cart containing a drawer for each client's medications is prepared by the pharmacy with a 24-hour supply of medications.

unscrubbed team members Includes the anesthesiologist or anesthetist and the circulating nurse, who wear surgical attire but are not gowned or gloved.

upper airway respiratory system All respiratory structures above the epiglottis, including nose, sinuses, mouth, and pharynx.

ureterostomy An ostomy site in which one or both ureters are surgically brought to the abdominal surface for the excretion of urine.

urethral meatus The opening to the canal for the discharge of urine.

urethral sphincter Voluntary muscle at the neck of the bladder that relaxes to allow micturition.

urgency The need to void immediately.

urinal Plastic or metal receptacle for urine.

urinary diversion A surgical procedure in which the ureters are removed from the urinary bladder and surgically anastomosed directly to the skin or to either a conduit or internal pouch made of bowel with the other end brought out onto the client's skin as a stoma so that the urine can exit the body.

urinary retention Inability to empty the bladder, resulting from a number of possible causes.

urinary tract infection Greater than normal level of pathogens in the urinary tract.

urine Fluid secreted by the kidneys, transported by the ureters, stored in the bladder, and voided through the urethra.

urine specific gravity Measurement of the degree of concentration of the urine.

urinometer Device used for determining specific gravity of urine.

urostomy The diversion of urine away from a diseased or defective bladder through a surgically created opening, or stoma, in the skin.

Vacutainer tube A glass tube with a rubber stopper; air has been removed to create a vacuum.

valgus An abnormal position in which a part of a limb is bent or twisted outward, away from the midline, such as the heel of the foot.

Valsalva maneuver Any forced expiratory effort against a closed airway, as when an individual holds the breath and tightens the muscles in a concerted, strenuous effort to move a heavy object or to change position in a bed.

variance Positive or negative changes in client progress toward expected outcomes on a critical pathway. Deviations from the critical path plan most often used in the case management model of delivering health care.

varices Tortuous, dilated veins.

varus An abnormal position in which a part of a limb is turned inward toward the midline, such as the heel and foot.

vascular access device (VAD) An indwelling catheter, cannula, or other instrumentation used to obtain venous or arterial access.

vasoconstriction Narrowing of the lumen of any blood vessel, especially the arterioles and the veins in the blood reservoirs of the skin and abdominal viscera.

vasodilation An increase in the diameter of a blood vessel caused by inhibition of its vasoconstrictor nerves or stimulation of dilator nerves.

vein lumen Central opening through which blood flows in a vein.

vellus Soft, fine hair covering all parts of the body except the palms, soles, and areas where other types of hair are normally found.

venipuncture Technique in which a vein is punctured transcutaneously by a sharp rigid stylet (such as a butterfly needle), a cannula (such as an angiocatheter that contains a flexible plastic catheter), or a needle attached to a syringe.

venous thrombosis A condition characterized by the presence of a clot in a vein in which the wall of the vessel is not inflamed.

ventilation Respiratory process by which gases are moved into and out of the lungs.

ventral Of or pertaining to an anterior position, toward the abdomen.

verbal order A physician or nurse practitioner's order for a medication or other therapy that is spoken to the RN to be entered into the client's medical records.

vertigo A sensation of faintness or an inability to maintain normal balance in a standing or seated position, sometimes associated with giddiness, mental confusion, nausea, and weakness.

vesicant A drug capable of causing tissue necrosis when extravasated.

vial Glass container with a metal-enclosed rubber seal.

vibration Physiotherapy technique performed by contracting all the muscles in the caregiver's upper extremities to cause vibration while applying pressure to the chest wall.

viscera The internal organs enclosed within a body cavity, primarily the abdominal organs.

visceral pleura A serous membrane lining both lungs.

visceral protein status The amount of protein that pertains to the internal organs (e.g., abdominal).

vital signs Physiological parameters that reflect key body processes; refers to temperature, blood pressure, heart rate, respiratory rate, and oxygen saturation.

void The process of emptying the bladder of urine; urinate; micturate.

walking heel Plastic or rubber heel placed in the sole of a leg cast to allow weight bearing.

wandering Meandering, aimless, or repetitive locomotion that exposes the individual to harm and is frequently incongruent with boundaries, limits, or obstacles.

weight Force exerted on a body by the gravity of the earth.

weight holder A metal, T-shaped bar that holds weights for traction.

weights Filled bags or metal disks of varying poundage used for traction.

whispered pectoriloquy The transmission of a whisper through the pulmonary structures so that it is heard as normal audible speech on auscultation.

windowing Cutting a small area of a cast to permit inspection of the tissues below.

working phase The period in the nurse-client relationship when the focus is on communication strategies, interventions for problem resolution, and enhancement of self-concept.

Wound Vacuum Assisted Closure A type of therapy that speeds wound healing by applying localized negative pressure to draw the edges of a wound together.

xerostomia Dryness of the mouth caused by the cessation of normal salivary secretions. It is a common symptom of a number of diseases such as diabetes, acute infections, and Sjögren's syndrome and is a common adverse reaction to drugs.

Yankauer suction A large filter-tipped rigid plastic suction catheter used mainly in the mouth or other large body cavity.

Z-track method Method for injecting irritating medications into muscle without tracking residual medication through sensitive tissues.

Index

The letter *b* indicates box, *f* indicates figure, and *t* indicates
table.

Index of Skills